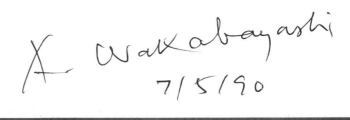

Surgery of the Chest

FIFTH EDITION

Volume II

David C. Sabiston, Jr., M.D.

James B. Duke Professor of Surgery
Chairman, Department of Surgery
Duke University Medical Center
Durham, North Carolina

Frank C. Spencer, M.D.

George David Stewart Professor and
Chairman, Department of Surgery
New York University School of Medicine
New York, New York

1990
W. B. SAUNDERS COMPANY
Harcourt Brace Jovanovich, Inc.
Philadelphia ■ London ■ Toronto ■ Montreal ■ Sydney ■ Tokyo

W. B. SAUNDERS COMPANY
Harcourt Brace Jovanovich, Inc.

The Curtis Center
Independence Square West
Philadelphia, PA 19106-3399

Library of Congress Cataloging-in-Publication Data

Surgery of the chest.

Includes bibliographies and index.

1. Chest—Surgery.   I. Gibbon, John Heysham.
II. Sabiston, David C., 1924–   III. Spencer, Frank
Cole.   [DNLM: 1. Thoracic Surgery.   WF 980 S961]

RD536.S86   1990   617.5'4   89–10150

ISBN 0–7216–2217–8

Editor: Edward H. Wickland, Jr.

Developmental Editor: David Kilmer

Designer: Maureen Sweeney

Cover Designer: Joanne Carroll

Production Manager: Carolyn Naylor

Manuscript Editors: Marjory I. Fraser, Wendy Andresen, and Mary Prescott

Illustration Coordinator: Peg Shaw

Indexer: Ann Cassar

Surgery of the Chest, 5/e

0–7216–2218–6 Volume I
0–7216–2219–4 Volume II
ISBN   0–7216–2217–8 Set

Last digit is the print number: 9   8   7   6   5   4   3   2   1

CONTRIBUTORS

Robert W. Anderson, M.D.
Professor of Surgery and Biomedical Engineering, Northwestern University, Chicago, Illinois. Senior Attending Surgeon and Chairman, Department of Surgery, Evanston Hospital, Evanston, Illinois.
Shock and Circulatory Collapse

W. Gerald Austen, M.D.
Edward D. Churchill Professor of Surgery, Harvard Medical School, Boston, Massachusetts. Surgeon-in-Chief, Massachusetts General Hospital, Boston, Massachusetts.
Acquired Aortic Valve Disease

John A. Bartlett, M.D.
Assistant Professor of Medicine, Duke University Medical Center, Durham, North Carolina.
Thoracic Disorders in the Immunocompromised Host

Thomas M. Bashore, M.D.
Associate Professor of Medicine and Director, Cardiac Catheterization Laboratory, Duke University Medical Center, Durham, North Carolina.
Cardiac Catheterization, Angiography, and Balloon Valvuloplasty; Coronary Arteriography

Harvey W. Bender, Jr., M.D.
Professor of Surgery, Vanderbilt University School of Medicine. Chairman, Department of Cardiac and Thoracic Surgery, Vanderbilt University Medical Center, Nashville, Tennessee.
Major Anomalies of Pulmonary and Thoracic Systemic Veins

William N. Bernhard, M.D.
Associate Professor of Anesthesiology, University of Maryland, Baltimore, Maryland. Director, Maryland Institute for Emergency Medical Service Systems, Baltimore, Maryland.
Mechanical Ventilation; Tracheal Intubation and Mechanical Ventilation

Arthur D. Boyd, M.D.
Professor of Surgery, New York University School of Medicine, New York, New York. Attending Surgeon, Tisch Hospital of the New York University Medical Center; Attending Surgeon, Bellevue Hospital Center; Attending Surgeon, Manhattan Veterans Administration Center, New York, New York.
Endoscopy: Bronchoscopy and Esophagoscopy; Mechanical Ventilation; Tracheal Intubation and Mechanical Ventilation

Henry Buchwald, M.D., Ph.D.
Professor of Surgery and Biomedical Engineering, University of Minnesota. Professor of Surgery and Biomedical Engineering, University of Minnesota Health Sciences Center, Minneapolis, Minnesota.
Partial Ileal Bypass for Control of Hyperlipidemia and Atherosclerosis

Robert M. Califf, M.D.
Associate Professor of Medicine and Director, Cardiac Care Unit, Duke University Medical Center, Durham, North Carolina.
Fibrinolytic Therapy in the Management of Acute Myocardial Infarction

Christian T. Campos, M.D.
Medical Fellow, Department of Surgery, University of Minnesota Health Sciences Center, Minneapolis, Minnesota.
Partial Ileal Bypass for Control of Hyperlipidemia and Atherosclerosis

Aldo R. Castaneda, M.D.
Professor of Surgery and Cardiovascular Surgery, Harvard Medical School, Boston, Massachusetts. Chief of the Departments of Surgery and Cardiovascular Surgery, The Children's Hospital, Boston, Massachusetts.
Anatomic Correction of Transposition of the Great Arteries at the Arterial Level

William A. Check, Ph.D.
President, Medical and Scientific Communications, Inc., Atlanta, Georgia.
Infection, Thrombosis, and Emboli Associated with Intracardiac Prostheses

Lawrence H. Cohn, M.D.
Professor of Surgery, Harvard Medical School, Boston, Massachusetts. Chief, Division of Cardiac Surgery, Brigham and Women's Hospital, Boston, Massachusetts.
Thoracic Aortic Aneurysms and Aortic Dissection

Joel D. Cooper, M.D., F.A.C.S., FRCS(C)
Professor of Surgery, Head of Thoracic Surgical Section, Washington University School of Medicine. Head, Thoracic Surgical Section, Barnes Hospital, St. Louis, Missouri.
Lung Transplantation

James L. Cox, M.D.
Professor of Surgery and Chief, Division of Cardiothoracic Surgery, Washington University School of Medicine, St. Louis, Missouri. Cardiothoracic Surgeon-in-Charge, Barnes Hospital, St. Louis, Missouri.
The Surgical Management of Cardiac Arrhythmias

Fred A. Crawford, Jr., M.D.
Professor of Surgery and Chairman, Department of Surgery; Chief, Division of Cardiothoracic Surgery, Medical University of South Carolina, Charleston, South Carolina. Medical University Hospital; Charleston Veterans Administration Hospital; Charleston Memorial Hospital; Roper Hospital, South Carolina.
Thoracic Incisions

Thomas A. D'Amico, M.D.
Research Fellow, Duke University Medical Center, Durham, North Carolina.
Kawasaki's Disease

Gordon K. Danielson, M.D.
Joe M. and Ruth Roberts Professor of Surgery, Mayo Medical School, Rochester, Minnesota; Chairman, Division of Thoracic and Cardiovascular Surgery, Mayo Clinic and Foundation, Rochester, Minnesota. St. Mary's Hospital and Rochester Methodist Hospital, Rochester, Minnesota.
Atrioventricular Canal; Ebstein's Anomaly

Charles J. Davidson, M.D.
Assistant Professor of Medicine, Duke University Medical Center, Durham, North Carolina. Associate Director, Cardiac Catheterization Laboratory, Duke University Medical Center, Durham, North Carolina.
Cardiac Catheterization, Angiography, and Balloon Valvuloplasty; Coronary Arteriography

R. Duane Davis, Jr., M.D.
Senior Assistant Resident, Department of Surgery, Duke University Medical Center, Durham, North Carolina.
The Mediastinum

Tom R. DeMeester, M.D., F.A.C.S.
Professor and Chairman, Department of Surgery, Creighton University School of Medicine, Omaha, Nebraska.
The Pleura

Roberto M. Di Donato, M.D.
Former Senior Resident, Department of Cardiovascular Surgery, The Boston Children's Hospital. Currently, Staff Surgeon, Dipartimento Medico-Chirurgico di Cardiologia Pediatrica, Ospedale Bambino Gesù, Rome, Italy.
Anatomic Correction of Transposition of the Great Arteries at the Arterial Level

John J. Downes, M.D.
Professor of Anesthesia and Pediatrics, The Children's Hospital of Philadelphia School of Medicine, Philadelphia, Pennsylvania. Anesthesiologist-in-Chief and Director, Department of Anesthesiology and Critical Care Medicine, The Children's Hospital of Philadelphia, Philadelphia, Pennsylvania.
Respiratory Support in Infants

Fredrick L. Dunn, M.D.
Assistant Professor of Medicine, Duke University Medical Center, Durham, North Carolina. Director, Lipid Clinic, Duke University Medical Center, Durham, North Carolina.
Dietary and Pharmacologic Management of Atherosclerosis

Paul A. Ebert, M.D.
Executive Director, American College of Surgeons, Chicago, Illinois.
The Pericardium

L. Henry Edmunds, Jr., M.D.
W. M. Measy Professor of Surgery and Chief, Cardiothoracic Surgery, University of Pennsylvania, Philadelphia, Pennsylvania. Hospital of the University of Pennsylvania and Children's Hospital of Philadelphia, Philadelphia, Pennsylvania.
Respiratory Support in Infants

F. Henry Ellis, Jr., M.D., Ph.D.
Clinical Professor of Surgery, Harvard Medical School. Senior Consultant, Department of Thoracic and Cardiovascular Surgery, Lahey Clinical Medical Center, Burlington, Massachusetts; Chief, Division of Thoracic and Cardiovascular Surgery, New England Deaconess Hospital, Boston, Massachusetts.
Disorders of the Esophagus in the Adult; The Nissen Fundoplication

T. Bruce Ferguson, Jr., M.D.
Assistant Professor of Cardiothoracic Surgery, Washington University School of Medicine. Attending Thoracic and Cardiovascular Surgeon, Barnes Hospital, and St. Louis Children's Hospital, St. Louis, Missouri.
Congenital Lesions of the Lung and Emphysema

Thomas B. Ferguson, M.D.
Professor of Cardiothoracic Surgery, Washington University School of Medicine. Attending Thoracic and Cardiovascular Surgeon, Barnes Hospital and St. Louis Children's Hospital, St. Louis, Missouri.
Congenital Lesions of the Lung and Emphysema

Robert M. Freedom, M.D., F.R.C.P.C., F.A.C.C.
Professor of Pediatrics and Pathology, University of Toronto Faculty of Medicine. Director,

Division of Cardiology, The Hospital for Sick Children, Toronto, Ontario, Canada.
The Mustard Procedure

Derek A. Fyfe, M.D., Ph.D.
Associate Professor of Pediatric Cardiology; Assistant Professor of Obstetrics and Gynecology, Medical University of South Carolina. Attending in Pediatrics, Division of Pediatric Cardiology, Medical University Hospital, Charleston, South Carolina.
Tricuspid Atresia

William A. Gay, Jr., M.D.
Professor and Chairman, Department of Surgery, School of Medicine, University of Utah, Salt Lake City, Utah. Chief of Surgery, University of Utah Hospital, Salt Lake City, Utah.
Cardiac Transplantation

J. William Gaynor, M.D.
Senior Resident in Surgery, Duke University Medical Center, Durham, North Carolina.
Patent Ductus Arteriosus, Coarctation of the Aorta, Aortopulmonary Window, and Anomalies of the Aortic Arch

Lawrence D. German, M.D.
Attending Cardiologist, St. Thomas Hospital, Nashville, Tennessee.
Cardiac Pacemakers and Cardiac Conduction System Abnormalities

Vincent L. Gott, M.D.
Professor of Surgery, Johns Hopkins University School of Medicine, Baltimore, Maryland. Staff Cardiac Surgeon, The Johns Hopkins Hospital, Baltimore, Maryland.
Heparinized Shunts for Thoracic Vascular Operations

William J. Greeley, M.D.
Assistant Professor of Anesthesiology and Pediatrics, Medical Director of Pediatric Intensive Care Unit, Duke University Medical Center, Durham, North Carolina.
Anesthesia and Supportive Care for Cardiothoracic Surgery

Lazar J. Greenfield, M.D.
Professor and Chairman, Department of Surgery, University of Michigan. Executive Director, University of Michigan Operating Rooms, University of Michigan Hospital, Ann Arbor, Michigan.
Benign Tumors of the Lung and Bronchial Adenomas

Hermes C. Grillo, M.D.
Professor of Surgery, Harvard Medical School. Chief of General Thoracic Surgery, Massachusetts General Hospital, Boston, Massachusetts.
Congenital Lesions, Neoplasms, and Injuries of the Trachea

John W. Hammon, Jr., M.D.
Professor of Surgery, Vanderbilt University School of Medicine. Director, Division of Cardiac and Thoracic Surgery, Nashville Veterans Administration Medical Center; Attending Surgeon, Vanderbilt University Medical Center, Nashville, Tennessee.
Major Anomalies of Pulmonary and Thoracic Systemic Veins

Alden H. Harken, M.D.
Professor and Chairman, Department of Surgery, University of Colorado, Denver, Colorado. Staff Surgeon, Veterans Administration Hospital, Denver, Colorado; Staff Surgeon, Cardiovascular Surgery, University of Colorado, Denver, Colorado; Staff Surgeon, Rose Medical Center, Denver, Colorado.
Left Ventricular Aneurysm

Charles R. Hatcher, Jr., M.D.
Professor of Surgery and Chief of Cardiothoracic Surgery, Emory University School of Medicine, Atlanta, Georgia. Vice President for Health Affairs and Director of the Robert W. Woodruff Health Sciences Center, Emory University, Atlanta, Georgia.
Infection, Thrombosis, and Emboli Associated with Intracardiac Prostheses

Robert J. Herfkens, M.D.
Clinical Associate Professor of Radiology, UCLA School of Medicine. Cedars-Sinai Medical Center, Los Angeles, California.
Role of Computed Tomographic Scans in Cardiovascular Diagnosis; Role of Magnetic Resonance Imaging in Cardiovascular Diagnosis

Lucius D. Hill, M.D.
Clinical Professor of Surgery, Department of Surgery, University of Washington. Staff Surgeon, Virginia Mason Hospital and Swedish Hospital Medical Center, Seattle, Washington.
The Hill Repair; Paraesophageal Hiatal Hernia

William L. Holman, M.D.
Assistant Professor of Surgery, University of Alabama at Birmingham, Division of Cardiothoracic Surgery. University of Alabama Hospital, Veterans Administration Medical Center, Birmingham, Alabama.
Aneurysms of the Sinuses of Valsalva

E. Carmack Holmes, M.D.
Professor of Surgery, UCLA School of Medicine, Los Angeles, California.
Immunology and Immunotherapy of Carcinoma of the Lung

R. Maurice Hood, M.D.
Clinical Professor of Surgery, New York University School of Medicine. Attending Surgeon at New York University Hospital; Bellevue

Hospital; and Manhattan Veterans Administration Hospital, New York, New York.
Trauma to the Chest

O. Wayne Isom, M.D.
Professor of Surgery, Cornell University Medical College. Chairman, Division of Cardiothoracic Surgery; Surgeon-in-Chief, The New York Hospital, New York, New York.
Aortic Grafts and Prostheses; Occlusive Disease of Branches of the Aorta

Marshall L. Jacobs, M.D.
Associate Professor of Surgery, George Washington University School of Medicine. Attending Cardiovascular Surgeon, Children's National Medical Center, Washington, D.C.
Acquired Aortic Valve Disease

Ellis L. Jones, M.D.
Professor of Surgery, Emory University School of Medicine, Atlanta, Georgia. Emory University Hospital; Henrietta Egleston Hospital for Children; Piedmont Hospital; Crawford W. Long Hospital of Emory University; Grady Memorial Hospital.
Infection, Thrombosis, and Emboli Associated with Intracardiac Prostheses

Robert H. Jones, M.D.
Mary and Deryl Hart Professor of Surgery, Associate Professor of Radiology, Duke University School of Medicine. Attending Surgeon, Duke University Medical Center, Durham, North Carolina.
Radionuclide Imaging in Cardiac Surgery

Allen B. Kaiser, M.D.
Associate Professor of Medicine, Vanderbilt University School of Medicine. Vice Chairman, Department of Medicine, Vanderbilt University Hospital, Nashville, Tennessee.
Use of Antibiotics in Cardiac and Thoracic Surgery

Robert B. Karp, M.D.
Professor of Surgery, Chief of Cardiac Surgery, University of Chicago, Chicago, Illinois.
Acquired Disease of the Tricuspid Valve

James K. Kirklin, M.D.
Professor of Surgery, University of Alabama at Birmingham School of Medicine, Birmingham, Alabama. University of Alabama at Birmingham Medical Center, Birmingham, Alabama.
Cardiopulmonary Bypass for Cardiac Surgery; Surgical Treatment of Ventricular Septal Defect

John W. Kirklin, M.D.
Faye Fletcher Kerner Professor of Surgery, University of Alabama at Birmingham School of Medicine, Birmingham, Alabama. Surgeon, Division of Cardiothoracic Surgery, University of

Alabama at Birmingham Medical Center, Birmingham, Alabama.
Cardiopulmonary Bypass for Cardiac Surgery; Surgical Treatment of Ventricular Septal Defect

Joseph A. Kisslo, M.D.
Professor of Medicine, Division of Cardiology; Director of Adult and Pediatric Echocardiography; Assistant Professor of Radiology, Duke University Medical Center, Durham, North Carolina.
Ultrasound Applications in Cardiac Surgery: Echocardiography

John M. Kratz, M.D.
Associate Professor of Surgery, Medical University of South Carolina, Charleston, South Carolina.
Thoracic Incisions

Edwin Lafontaine, M.D., F.R.C.S.(C)
Assistant Professor of Surgery, Department of Surgery, University of Montreal. Attending Surgeon, Department of Surgery, Hopital Hotel-Dieu, Montreal, Quebec, Canada.
The Pleura

Hillel Laks, M.D.
Professor and Chief, Cardiothoracic Surgery, UCLA Medical Center, Los Angeles, California.
Congenital Malformations of the Mitral Valve

John Leslie, M.D.
Assistant Professor of Anesthesiology, Duke University School of Medicine, Durham, North Carolina.
Anesthesia and Supportive Care for Cardiothoracic Surgery

Gary K. Lofland, M.D.
Associate Professor of Surgery and Associate Professor of Pediatrics, Medical Collage of Virginia, Virginia Commonwealth University. Director, Pediatric Cardiac Surgery, Medical College of Virginia, Richmond, Virginia.
Truncus Arteriosus

Floyd D. Loop, M.D.
Professor and Chairman, Department of Thoracic and Cardiovascular Surgery, The Cleveland Clinic Foundation, Cleveland, Ohio.
Repeat Coronary Artery Bypass Grafting for Myocardial Ischemia

Donald E. Low, M.D.
Thoracic Surgery Fellow, Royal Devon and Exeter Hospital, Exeter, Devon, England.
The Hill Repair; Paraesophageal Hiatal Hernia

James E. Lowe, M.D.
Associate Professor of Surgery and Pathology, Duke University Medical Center, Durham,

North Carolina. Director, Surgical Electrophysiology Service, Duke University Medical Center, Durham, North Carolina.
Bronchoplastic Techniques in the Surgical Management of Benign and Malignant Pulmonary Lesions; Cardiac Pacemakers and Cardiac Conduction System Abnormalities; Congenital Malformations of the Coronary Circulation; Prinzmetal's Variant Angina and Other Syndromes Associated with Coronary Artery Spasm

Philip D. Lumb, M.D., B.S.
Associate Professor of Anesthesiology and Associate Professor of Surgery, Duke University Medical Center, Durham, North Carolina. Vice-Chairman, Department of Anesthesiology, and Co-Director, Surgical Intensive Care Unit, Duke University Medical Center, Durham, North Carolina.
Perioperative Pulmonary Physiology

H. Kim Lyerly, M.D.
Chief Resident in Surgery, Duke University Medical Center, Durham, North Carolina. Duke University Hospital, Durham, North Carolina.
Thoracic Disorders in the Immunocompromised Host; Chronic Pulmonary Embolism; Pulmonary Arteriovenous Fistulas

George W. Maier, M.D.
Chief Resident in Surgery, Duke University Medical Center, Durham, North Carolina.
Cardiopulmonary Resuscitation

James R. Malm, M.D.
Professor of Surgery, Columbia University, College of Physicians and Surgeons, New York, New York. Chief of Thoracic and Cardiac Surgery, Columbia-Presbyterian Medical Center, New York, New York.
Pulmonary Atresia with Intact Ventricular Septum; Univentricular Heart

James B. D. Mark, M.D.
Johnson and Johnson Professor of Surgery and Head, Division of Thoracic Surgery, Stanford University School of Medicine. Chief of Thoracic Surgery and Chief of Staff, Stanford University Hospital, Stanford, California.
Surgical Management of Metastatic Neoplasms to the Lungs

Dwight C. McGoon, M.D.
Professor of Surgery, Mayo Medical School, Rochester, Minnesota (Retired).
Atrioventricular Canal

Eli Milgalter, M.D.
Visiting Assistant Professor, Cardiothoracic Surgery, UCLA Medical Center, Los Angeles, California.
Congenital Malformations of the Mitral Valve

Jon F. Moran, M.D.
Chairman and Associate Professor, Department of Thoracic and Cardiovascular Surgery, University of Kansas Medical Center, Kansas City, Kansas.
Surgical Treatment of Pulmonary Tuberculosis

Pamela B. Morris, M.D.
Assistant Professor of Medicine, Duke University Medical Center. Director, Duke University Preventive Approach to Cardiology, Duke University Medical Center, Durham, North Carolina.
Dietary and Pharmacologic Management of Atherosclerosis

Eldred D. Mundth, M.D.
Professor of Surgery, Hahnemann University, Philadelphia, Pennsylvania. Senior Attending Surgeon and Director, Division of Cardiac Surgery, The Bryn Mawr Hospital, Bryn Mawr, Pennsylvania.
Assisted Circulation

John D. Murphy, M.D.
Assistant Professor of Pediatrics, University of Pennsylvania School of Medicine. Director of Invasive Cardiovascular Laboratories, The Children's Hospital of Philadelphia, Philadelphia, Pennsylvania.
Hypoplastic Left Heart Syndrome

Hassan Najafi, M.D.
Professor of Surgery, Rush Medical College. Senior Attending Surgeon and Chairman, Department of Cardiovascular-Thoracic Surgery, Rush-Presbyterian-St. Luke's Medical Center, Chicago, Illinois.
The Pericardium

Kurt D. Newman, M.D.
Assistant Professor, Departments of Surgery and Child Health and Development, George Washington University. Attending Surgeon, Children's Hospital, National Medical Center, Washington, D.C.
Surgical Problems of the Esophagus in Infants and Children

William I. Norwood, M.D., Ph.D.
Professor of Surgery, University of Pennsylvania School of Medicine. Chief, Division of Cardiothoracic Surgery, Children's Hospital of Philadelphia, Philadelphia, Pennsylvania.
Hypoplastic Left Heart Syndrome

John B. O'Connell M.D.
Associate Professor of Medicine, Division of Cardiology, University of Utah School of Medicine. Medical Director, Utah Cardiac Transplant Program, Salt Lake City, Utah.
Cardiac Transplantation

C. Warren Olanow, M.D.
Professor of Neurology and Professor of Pharmacology and Experimental Therapeutics, University of South Florida, Tampa, Florida. Tampa General Hospital, Chief of Neurology, Tampa, Florida.
Surgical Management of Myasthenia Gravis

H. Newland Oldham, Jr., M.D.
Professor of Surgery, Duke University Medical Center, Durham, North Carolina.
The Mediastinum

Mark B. Orringer, M.D.
Professor and Head, Section of Thoracic Surgery, University of Michigan Medical Center, Ann Arbor, Michigan.
Short Esophagus and Peptic Stricture

A. D. Pacifico, M.D.
John W. Kirklin Professor of Surgery, Division of Cardiothoracic Surgery, University of Alabama at Birmingham School of Medicine, Birmingham, Alabama. Director, Division of Cardiothoracic Surgery, and Vice Chairman, Department of Surgery, University of Alabama at Birmingham Medical Center, Birmingham, Alabama.
Surgical Treatment of Ventricular Septal Defect; The Senning Procedure for Transposition of the Great Vessels

Peter C. Pairolero, M.D.
Professor of Surgery, Mayo Medical School. Staff Surgeon at St. Mary's Hospital and Rochester Methodist Hospital, Rochester, Minnesota.
Surgical Management of Neoplasms of the Chest Wall

Robert B. Peyton, M.D.
Raleigh, North Carolina
Aortic Grafts and Prostheses; Occlusive Disease of Branches of the Aorta

William S. Pierce, M.D.
Staff Surgeon at University Hospital, The Pennsylvania State University, The Milton S. Hershey Medical Center, Hershey, Pennsylvania.
The Artificial Heart

R. W. Postlethwait, M.D.
Professor of Surgery Emeritus, Duke University School of Medicine, Durham, North Carolina. Retired.
Hiatal Hernia, Reflux, and Dysphagia after Vagotomy

Francisco J. Puga, M.D.
Professor of Surgery, Mayo Medical School. Head of Cardiac Surgery Section, Mayo Clinic, Rochester, Minnesota.
Atrioventricular Canal

Judson Randolph, M.D.
Professor of Surgery and Child Health and Development, George Washington University. Surgeon-in-Chief, Children's Hospital, National Medical Center, Washington, D.C.
Surgical Problems of the Esophagus in Infants and Children

J. Scott Rankin, M.D.
Associate Professor of Surgery, Duke University Medical Center, Durham, North Carolina.
Cardiopulmonary Resuscitation; Physiology of Coronary Blood Flow, Myocardial Function, and Intraoperative Myocardial Protection; Utilization of the Internal Mammary Arteries for Coronary Artery Bypass

Russell C. Raphaely, M.D.
Professor of Anesthesiology and Pediatrics, The Children's Hospital of Philadelphia, School of Medicine, University of Pennsylvania. Associate Director, Department of Anesthesiology and Critical Care Medicine, The Children's Hospital of Philadelphia, Philadelphia, Pennsylvania.
Respiratory Support in Infants

Maruf A. Razzuk, M.D.
Clinical Associate Professor in Thoracic and Cardiovascular Surgery, University of Texas Southwestern Medical School, Dallas, Texas. Baylor University Medical Center; R.H.D. Memorial Hospital; Parkland Memorial Hospital, Dallas, Texas.
Thoracic Outlet Syndrome

Bruce A. Reitz, M.D.
Professor and Instructor in Surgery, Johns Hopkins University School of Medicine. Cardiac Surgeon-in-Charge, The Johns Hopkins Hospital, Baltimore, Maryland.
Heart and Lung Transplantation

J. G. Reves, M.D.
Professor of Anesthesiology and Director, Heart Center, Duke University School of Medicine. Duke University Hospital, Durham, North Carolina.
Anesthesia and Supportive Care for Cardiothoracic Surgery

William C. Roberts, M.D.
Clinical Professor of Pathology and Medicine (Cardiology), Georgetown University, Washington, D.C. Chief, Pathology Branch, National Heart, Lung, and Blood Institute, National Institutes of Health, Bethesda, Maryland.
Pathology of Coronary Atherosclerosis

Bradley M. Rodgers, M.D.
Professor of Surgery and Pediatrics, Chief, Division of Pediatric Surgery, University of Virginia Health Sciences Center, Charlottesville, Virginia.
Management of Infants and Children Undergoing Thoracic Surgery

David C. Sabiston, Jr., M.D.
James B. Duke Professor and Chairman, Department of Surgery, Duke University Medical Center, Durham, North Carolina.
Congenital Deformities of the Chest Wall; The Mediastinum; Carcinoma of the Lung; Bronchoplastic Techniques in the Surgical Management of Benign and Malignant Pulmonary Lesions; Pulmonary Embolism; Chronic Pulmonary Embolism; Pulmonary Arteriovenous Fistulas; Patent Ductus Arteriosus, Coarctation of the Aorta, Aortopulmonary Window, and Anomalies of the Aortic Arch; Tetralogy of Fallot; Physiology of Coronary Blood Flow, Myocardial Function, and Intraoperative Myocardial Protection; Congenital Malformations of the Coronary Circulation; Kawasaki's Disease; Tumors of the Heart

Robert M. Sade, M.D.
Professor of Surgery (Cardiothoracic) and Professor of Pediatrics, Medical University of South Carolina. Chief of Pediatric Cardiac Surgery, Medical University Hospital, Charleston, South Carolina.
Tricuspid Atresia

Edwin W. Salzman, A.B., M.A., M.D.
Professor of Surgery, Harvard Medical School. Surgeon, Beth Israel Hospital, Boston, Massachusetts.
Thromboembolic Complications of Cardiac and Vascular Prostheses

Stephen W. Schwarzmann, M.D.
Associate Professor of Medicine, Infectious Diseases, Emory University School of Medicine. Chief of Infectious Diseases, Emory University Hospital, Atlanta, Georgia.
Infection, Thrombosis, and Emboli Associated with Intracardiac Prostheses

David B. Skinner, M.D.
Professor of Surgery, Cornell University Medical College. President and Chief Executive Officer, The New York Hospital, New York, New York.
Esophageal Hiatal Hernia: I. The Condition: Clinical Manifestations and Diagnosis; The Belsey Mark IV Antireflux Repair

L. Richard Smith, Ph.D.
Assistant Professor, Division of Biometry and Medical Information, Duke University Medical Center, Durham, North Carolina.
Utilization of the Internal Mammary Arteries for Coronary Artery Bypass

Peter K. Smith, M.D.
Assistant Professor of Surgery and Biomedical Engineering, Duke University Medical Center, Durham, North Carolina.
Preoperative Assessment of Pulmonary Function: Quantitative Evaluation of Ventilation and Blood Gas Exchange; Postoperative Care in Cardiac Surgery; Computer Applications in Cardiothoracic Surgery; Ultrasound Applications in Cardiac Surgery: Echocardiography

Robert J. Sparaco, B.S., J.D., R.R.T.
Assistant Professor, Nassau Community College, Department of Allied Health Services, Garden City, New York. Educational Coordinator, Respiratory Care Department, Tisch Hospital of New York University Medical Center, New York, New York.
Tracheal Intubation and Mechanical Ventilation; Mechanical Ventilation

Frank C. Spencer, M.D.
George David Stewart Professor of Surgery and Chairman, Department of Surgery, New York University Medical Center, New York, New York.
Atrial Septal Defect, Anomalous Pulmonary Veins, and Atrioventricular Septal Defects (AV Canal); Acquired Disease of the Mitral Valve; Bypass Grafting for Coronary Artery Disease

Richard S. Stack, M.D.
Associate Professor of Medicine, Duke University Medical Center. Director, Interventional Cardiovascular Program, Duke University Medical Center, Durham, North Carolina.
Percutaneous Transluminal Coronary Angioplasty

Mack C. Stirling, M.D.
Assistant Professor of Surgery, Department of Surgery, Section of Thoracic Surgery, University of Michigan. Chief of Thoracic Surgery, Ann Arbor Veterans Hospital, Ann Arbor, Michigan.
Benign Tumors of the Lung and Bronchial Adenomas; Short Esophagus and Peptic Stricture

George A. Trusler, M.D.
Professor of Surgery, University of Toronto. Senior Staff Surgeon and Former Head, Cardiovascular Surgery, The Hospital for Sick Children, Toronto, Ontario, Canada.
The Mustard Procedure

Ross M. Ungerleider, M.D.
Assistant Professor of General and Thoracic Surgery; Chief, Pediatric Cardiac Surgery, Duke University Medical Center, Durham, North Carolina.
Tetralogy of Fallot; Congenital Aortic Stenosis

Harold C. Urschel, Jr., M.D., D.Sc. (Hon.), LL.D.(Hon.)
Professor of Thoracic and Cardiovascular Surgery, Baylor University Medical Center, Dallas, Texas; University of Texas Southwestern Medical School, Dallas, Texas. Senior Attending Surgeon, Baylor University Medical Center, Dallas, Texas; Attending Surgeon, St. Paul Hospital, Dallas, Texas; Consultant, Children's Medical Center, Dallas, Texas; Senior Attending, Presbyterian Hospital, Dallas, Texas.
Thoracic Outlet Syndrome

Peter Van Trigt, M.D.
Assistant Professor of Surgery, Duke University Medical School. Duke University Medical Center, Durham, North Carolina.
Lung Infections and Diffuse Interstitial Lung Disease; Diaphragm and Diaphragmatic Pacing; Tumors of the Heart

Marc S. Visner, M.D.
Associate Professor of Surgery, University of Massachusetts. Attending Surgeon, University of Massachusetts Medical Center, Worcester, Massachusetts.
Shock and Circulatory Collapse

J. Anthony Ware, M.D.
Assistant Professor of Medicine, Harvard Medical School. Associate Director, Morse Intensive Care Unit, Beth Israel Hospital, Boston, Massachusetts.
Thromboembolic Complications of Cardiac and Vascular Prostheses

Andrew S. Wechsler, M.D.
Stuart McGuire Professor of Surgery, Professor of Physiology, and Chairman, Department of Surgery, Medical College of Virginia. Chairman, Department of Surgery, Medical College of Virginia Hospitals; Consulting Surgeon, Hunter Holmes McGuire Veterans Administration Hospital; Attending Surgeon, Richard Memorial Hospital, Richmond, Virginia.
Surgical Management of Myasthenia Gravis

Walter G. Wolfe, M.D.
Professor of Surgery, Duke University Medical Center, Durham, North Carolina.
Preoperative Assessment of Pulmonary Function: Quantitative Evaluation of Ventilation and Blood Gas Exchange; Pulmonary Embolism

PREFACE

It is remarkable to review the many advances made in the field of cardiac and thoracic surgery since the fourth edition of this text was published in 1983. Extraordinary progress has been achieved, especially increased accuracy in diagnostic capabilities, improved myocardial protection, newer antibiotics, additional inotropic agents, and many improvements in specialized equipment. Moreover, the role of computers in cardiothoracic surgery has emerged to a new state of application. Other advances that deserve special emphasis include the role of invasive cardiology with balloon dilatation and percutaneous coronary angioplasty, the widespread and successful use of thrombolytic agents for acute myocardial infarction and pulmonary embolism, and the emerging significance of diet and medications in the prophylaxis of atherosclerosis.

In this edition, *Surgery of the Chest* has maintained its emphasis on the integration of the fundamental medical sciences, including pathology, physiology, biochemistry, pharmacology, immunology, and genetics, and their relationship to the diagnosis and management of cardiothoracic disorders. In fact, inclusion of these subjects is required in daily surgical practice by the discriminating student, resident, and cardiothoracic surgeon.

New chapters have been added, including "Computer Applications in Cardiac Surgery" by Peter K. Smith, "Thoracic Disorders in the Immunocompromised Host" by H. Kim Lyerly and John A. Bartlett, "Role of Magnetic Resonance Imaging in Cardiovascular Diagnosis" by Robert J. Herfkens, and "Dietary and Pharmacologic Management of Atherosclerosis" by Fredrick L. Dunn and Pamela B. Morris. A number of new authors have been added in this edition including Allen B. Kaiser on "Use of Antibiotics in Cardiac and Thoracic Surgery," J. G. Reves and associates on "Anesthesia and Supportive Care for Cardiothoracic Surgery," Bradley M. Rodgers for "Management of Infants and Children Undergoing Thoracic Surgery," and Peter C. Pairolero on "Surgical Management of Neoplasms of the Chest Wall." For the subject of "Special Diagnostic and Therapeutic Procedures in Cardiac Surgery," Thomas M. Bashore and Charles J. Davidson have contributed "Cardiac Catheterization, Angiocardiography, and Balloon Valvuloplasty"; Richard S. Stack has edited "Percutaneous Transluminal Coronary Angioplasty"; Robert M. Califf has prepared "Fibrinolytic Therapy in the Management of Acute Myocardial Infarction"; and Peter K. Smith and Joseph A. Kisslo have introduced a new and important field: "Ultrasound Applications in Cardiac Surgery: Echocardiography." Robert B. Peyton and O. Wayne Isom have contributed "Aortic Grafts and Prostheses" and "Occlusive Disease of Branches of the Aorta"; J. William Gaynor has edited "Patent Ductus Arteriosus, Coarctation of the Aorta, Aortopulmonary Window, and Anomalies of the Aortic Arch"; Lawrence H. Cohn has written the section on "Thoracic Aortic Aneurysms and Aortic Dissection"; and Ross M. Ungerleider has contributed "Congenital Aortic Stenosis" and "Tetralogy of Fallot." Eli Milgalter and Hillel Laks have prepared "Congenital Malformations of the Mitral Valve," and Roberto Di Donato and Aldo R. Castaneda have prepared "Anatomic Correction of Transposition of the Great Arteries at the Arterial Level." "Acquired Aortic Valve Disease" has been authored by Marshall L. Jacobs and W. Gerald Austen, and "Pathology of Coronary Atherosclerosis" by William C. Roberts. Robert B. Karp has contributed "Acquired Disease of the Tricuspid Valve," and William I. Norwood and John D. Murphy have authored the "Hypoplastic Left Heart Syndrome." Thomas A. D'Amico has written "Kawasaki's Disease," Peter Van Trigt has authored "Tumors of the Heart," and Bruce A. Reitz has contributed the section on "Heart and Lung Transplantation." William A. Gay, Jr., and John B. O'Connell prepared the chapter on "Cardiac Transplantation."

In the fifth edition the importance of illustrations has continued with a number of new additions. These new illustrations completely update the text with the most recent illustrations of procedures of proven value. Moreover, the bibliography has been completely updated with the most current listings. The *selected references* have accordingly been expanded and updated, permitting the reader to gain deeper insight into the meaning of the most outstanding publications in the field by reviewing a summary of their contents.

It is clear that the fifth edition is the result of much dedicated work by many authorities. The editors wish to express sincere thanks to each of the contributors for their tireless efforts. Special appreciation is due to Mr. Edward H. Wickland, Jr., of the W. B. Saunders Company who has been a prodigious co-worker in achieving the highest standards of excellence in contemporary publishing and whose distinct commitment and goals have been the creation of the very best text possible. Once again the reader will be impressed with the extraordinary talents of the W. B. Saunders Company because they continue their standard of perfection in every detail. Their unfailing attention to every aspect of this work is clearly apparent in this fifth edition and the editors are deeply appreciative.

DAVID C. SABISTON, JR.
FRANK C. SPENCER

ACKNOWLEDGMENTS

The fifth edition of *Surgery of the Chest* once again is comprised of contributions from a number of outstanding authorities in every field of cardiothoracic surgery. The editors owe special thanks to Ms. Carolyn Naylor and Ms. Marjory Fraser of the W. B. Saunders staff. As has been characteristic of their earlier participation, they have been completely cooperative in every request and have insisted on exacting detail in each endeavor. Together with their colleagues in the Production Department of W. B. Saunders, they have maintained the extraordinary quality of this text and have taken it to an even higher standard. In addition, Ms. Margaret Shaw has given special attention to the illustrations and has been certain that their quality and reproduction have been of the most outstanding character. Ms. Maureen Sweeney receives our thanks as the distinctive designer of this edition.

Most of all, the editors acknowledge their gratitude to Ms. Kathryn Slaughter. Through the years she has been a tireless worker who has reviewed every chapter in complete detail and has been of invaluable assistance in making this text outstanding from the point of view of accuracy, style, content, and expression. We have particularly appreciated her enthusiasm for every aspect of this work as well as her committed and enduring loyalty.

DAVID C. SABISTON, JR.
FRANK C. SPENCER

CONTENTS

Volume II

CHAPTER 29

DIAPHRAGM AND DIAPHRAGMATIC PACING

Peter Van Trigt

DIAPHRAGM

Historical Aspects

The first traumatic diaphragmatic hernia was reported in 1579 by Paré, who described the postmortem findings in two patients who died after a blunt injury and a gunshot wound, respectively (Sutton et al, 1967). In this report, Paré described an autopsy done on an artillery captain who died of a strangulated intestinal obstruction after incarceration of the intestine through a traumatic laceration of the diaphragm sustained 8 months earlier. In 1853, Bowditch published the first account of traumatic diaphragmatic hernia diagnosed antemortem in the United States. He established five criteria for the physical diagnosis of the lesion: (1) prominence and immobility of the left thorax, (2) displacement to the right of the area of cardiac dullness, (3) absent breath sounds over the left hemithorax, (4) bowel sounds audible in the chest, and (5) tympany to percussion over the left side of the chest (Bowditch, 1853). In 1886, Riolfi corrected a laceration of the diaphragm from a knife wound through which omentum had prolapsed (Grage et al, 1959). Naumann, in 1888, operated on a patient who had a traumatic diaphragmatic hernia and in whom the stomach had herniated into the left side of the chest (Grage et al, 1959). Before the 20th century, traumatic diaphragmatic hernia was a rarely reported condition.

Anatomy of the Diaphragm

The diaphragm consists of a central portion of a thin but strong aponeurosis and a peripheral muscular portion. The muscular components of the diaphragm are divided into those of sternal, costal, and lumbar origin. Embryologically, the middle leaflet of this central tendon develops from the transverse septum, which originates between the liver and the heart. It then grows caudad toward the dorsal mes-

entery of the foregut with which it ultimately fuses. The transverse septum fuses with the pleuroperitoneal membrane from the lateral chest wall, joining the muscular components of the diaphragm and separating the pericardial, peritoneal, and pleural cavities. Thus, in an adult, the diaphragm is composed of two portions: the peripheral muscular portion and a central tendinous portion shaped like an inverted capital V. This central tendinous portion is contiguous on its superior aspect with the pericardium (Fig. 29–1).

Three major openings in the diaphragm allow passage of structures from the chest to the abdomen: the aortic, esophageal, and vena cava openings. The aortic opening allows passage of the aorta, azygos vein, and thoracic duct. Through the esophageal hiatus pass the esophagus and vagus nerves, and the inferior vena cava passes alone through the caval opening.

Arterial supply to the diaphragm is predominantly from the abdominal aorta and is composed of the right and left phrenic arteries. The anterior branch of the phrenic artery supplies the central most tendinous portion, which is contiguous with the pericardium. Additional arterial supply to the posterior portion of the diaphragm rises from the superior phrenic arteries, which start from the lower portion of the thoracic aorta, and the pericardiophrenic and musculophrenic arteries, originating from the internal mammary artery. Venous drainage of the diaphragm is composed of the right and left inferior phrenic veins, which drain medially into the inferior vena cava. On the left side, a venous arcade that connects the phrenic vein with the left renal vein provides additional drainage.

The right and left phrenic nerves provide both motor and sensory supply to the diaphragm. The right phrenic nerve enters the diaphragm just lateral to the opening of the inferior vena cava in the diaphragm; the left phrenic nerve enters lateral to the left border of the heart (see Fig. 29–1). Once these nerves enter the diaphragmatic muscle, they divide into four trunks: sternal, anterolateral, pos-

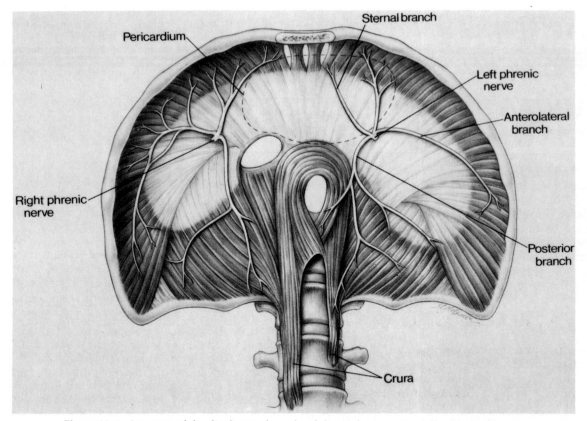

Figure 29–1. Anatomy of the diaphragm from the abdominal perspective, showing innervation.

terolateral, and crural. These trunks eventually course immediately below the peritoneal lining of the inferior surface of the diaphragm (see Fig. 29–1).

Congenital Diaphragmatic Hernia

There are three types of congenital diaphragmatic hernias: posterolateral (Bochdalek's) hernia, subcostosternal (Morgagni's) hernia, and esophageal hiatal hernia.

The posterolateral (Bochdalek's) diaphragmatic hernia is the result of a congenital diaphragmatic defect in the posterior costal part of the diaphragm in the region of the 10th and 11th ribs, which allows free communication between the thoracic and abdominal cavities. The defect is usually found on the left side (90%) but may occur on the right side, where the liver often prevents detection (Gravier, 1974). The male-female ratio is 2:1, and this particular congenital abnormality is usually isolated and not associated with other major congenital defects. Because of the negative intrathoracic pressure, herniation of abdominal contents occurs through left-sided defects with resultant collapse of the left lung, shifting of the mediastinum to the right, and compression of the contralateral right lung. This type of congenital diaphragmatic hernia is usually manifested by acute respiratory distress in newborns (Symbas et al, 1977).

Chest films establish the diagnosis, displaying intestinal gas patterns within the thorax and resultant shift of the relatively unstable and mobile neonatal mediastinum to the contralateral side. The clinical findings on examination include the presence of respiratory distress, absence of breath sounds on the left side, and presence of bowel sounds over the left side of the chest. Obstruction and strangulation of the bowel have been reported but are rare in the acute presentation of this entity, and the usual cause of morbidity and mortality is progressive hypoxemia as a result of increased pulmonary vascular resistance, decreased blood flow to the lungs, alveolar hypoxia, and further hypoxemia. Initial treatment consists of nasogastric decompression of the stomach and intestinal tract to reduce mediastinal shifting, replacement of fluids and electrolytes, correction of acid-base imbalance, positive-pressure respiratory support, and surgical correction of the diaphragmatic defect. For right-sided defects, repair is usually accomplished through a right-sided thoracotomy. For left-sided defects, an abdominal approach is preferred because of the malrotation and obstructing duodenal bands that can be present in this condition. Closure of the defect is accomplished by direct suture; chest tubes are placed in the involved hemithorax and are connected to underwater-seal drainage to assist expansion of the lung on the involved side.

Treatment of newborn infants who have congenital diaphragmatic hernia and who develop severe respiratory distress requiring operative repair within the first 24 hours of life represents one of the most challenging problems in pediatric surgery. Postoperative mortality varies between 30 and 50% (Harrison and De Lorimier, 1981; Shochat et al, 1979). Pathologic examination of the lungs of infants who have died with congenital diaphragmatic hernia reveals a decrease in size and weight, with the ipsilateral lung being the smaller and showing a distorted distribution of segmental airways. There is a reduction of total pulmonary volume due to a reduced total number of alveoli as a result of a deficiency in bronchial generation. These pathologic findings led to an earlier assumption that the high mortality after repair of a diaphragmatic hernia is due to pulmonary hypoplasia. However, despite a reduction in total pulmonary volume, the contralateral lung in infants with congenital diaphragmatic hernia is usually able to maintain ventilation, and in surviving infants, the small hypoplastic ipsilateral lung eventually expands and fills the thoracic cavity (Wohl et al, 1977). In those survivors, total pulmonary volume becomes normal but there is an abnormal distribution; the ipsilateral lung contributes only 40% (Hislop and Reid, 1976).

More recently, authors have emphasized the significance of an increase in pulmonary vascular resistance in these neonates with increased pulmonary artery pressure as the primary abnormality, which is responsible for the high postoperative morbidity and mortality (O'Callaghan et al, 1982). This hypothesis is supported by the clinical course of those neonates dying after repair of a diaphragmatic hernia. There is usually a great improvement in oxygenation in the immediate postoperative period, followed by deterioration 12 to 24 hours postoperatively, with progressive hypoxemia, acidosis, hypercarbia, and death despite all therapeutic manipulations to correct this progressive deterioration.

Cardiac catheterization studies have been done in children with a congenital diaphragmatic hernia and show pulmonary arterial hypertension with a right-to-left shunt across the ductus, raised right ventricular end-diastolic pressure, and raised right atrial pressure with shunting across the foramen ovale. Pulmonary arteriography shows a decreased total pulmonary flow with shunting across the ductus and almost no perfusion of the lung on the side of the diaphragmatic hernia. The pulmonary vasculature of infants who have died with congenital diaphragmatic hernia has been investigated, and a significant increase in smooth-muscle mass in the small pulmonary arteries has been documented (Naeye et al, 1976). Studies have established that this anatomically abnormal pulmonary vascular bed in infants with congenital diaphragmatic hernia (Levin, 1978) is capable of an exaggerated response to factors that are known to produce pulmonary vasoconstriction in newborns (hypoxemia, hypercarbia, acidosis, hypothermia, increase in transpulmonary pressure, and alveolar hypoxia) (Naeye et al, 1976). An exaggerated vasoconstrictive response of an abnormally hypertro-

phied pulmonary vascular bed leading to a rise of pulmonary vascular resistance appears to be the important mechanism leading to the often fatal hypoxemia in these neonates.

Pharmacologic interventions to break the vicious cycle of hypoxia, increased pulmonary vascular resistance leading to decreased pulmonary flow, and shunting across the ductus and foramen ovale leading to further hypoxia have been attempted with the use of vasodilators such as tolazoline (Levy et al, 1977; Sumner and Frank, 1981) and, more recently, prostaglandin E_1 (Cloutier et al, 1983; Ein et al, 1980). Earlier experience with tolazoline showed a significant incidence of complications associated with use of the drug, including hypotension, gastrointestinal bleeding, thrombocytopenia, seizures, and cardiac arrhythmias. Prostaglandin E_1 has been used clinically with significantly fewer complications, including fever, peripheral vasodilatation, and tremors.

In addition to pharmacologic interventions to alter pulmonary vascular resistance, extracorporeal membrane oxygenation (ECMO) has been used when more standard methods of support have failed to prevent progressive hypoxia and clinical deterioration (Hardesty et al, 1981; Redmond et al, 1987). ECMO is theoretically an ideal modality of support and therapy in this setting. It can immediately reduce or eliminate right-to-left shunting through the patent foramen ovale and ductus arteriosus and divert as much as 90% of the cardiac output from the right atrium into the extracorporeal circuit. Right atrial pressure and pulmonary blood flow are reduced, as is the volume of blood shunted across the atrium and through the ductus. Systemic hypoxemia and acidosis are reversed, and their vasoconstrictive effect on the pulmonary vasculature is eliminated. Transpulmonary pressures are reduced during ECMO, removing another potential pulmonary vasoconstricting factor. Reduction of pulmonary vascular resistance together with the improvement in systemic oxygenation and reduction in volume of ductal flow may lead to spontaneous closure of the ductus and resolution of the persistent fetal circulation that often occurs in the postoperative setting of these neonates. By using this type of extracorporeal support, neonates can be supported for several days, and pulmonary function and pulmonary vascular resistance can return to normal (Sawyer et al, 1986; Trento et al, 1986).

In 1769, Morgagni first described the findings of substernal herniation of abdominal contents into the thoracic cavity (Morgagni, 1769). Since that time, this entity has frequently been referred to as Morgagni's hernia; it has also been referred to as retrosternal hernia or Larrey's hernia. Larrey, Surgeon General for Napoleon, described the surgical approach to the pericardial cavity through an anterior diaphragmatic defect (Thomas, 1972). The more appropriate descriptive name, subcostosternal diaphragmatic hernia, is attributed to Harrington (1948). This type of hernia is uncommon and represents approximately 3% of all surgically treated diaphragmatic hernias. It is rarely symptomatic, unlike its posterior counterpart Bochdalek's hernia. With the increasing use of routine chest films and the need to exclude the possibility of a mediastinal neoplasm, most of these cases are brought to the attention of a thoracic surgeon. These hernias occur through a defect in the diaphragm just lateral to the xiphoid and are associated with a well-formed hernia sac. They rarely produce symptoms in childhood, and most patients with Morgagni's hernia become symptomatic later in life, usually after the age of 40. Increased intra-abdominal pressure caused by obesity, trauma, or pregnancy may precipitate internal herniation through this part of the diaphragm. Most frequently, the transverse colon, either alone or in combination with some omentum, is most commonly involved in a Morgagni's hernia (Fig. 29–2). Although most patients are not symptomatic and present only with an abnormal chest film, they may have symptoms of partial obstruction of the herniated viscus. Because the neck of the sac is usually small, the hernia may precipitate an acute or chronic colonic obstruction if it is left uncorrected, and this is an indication for surgical repair. An attempt to clearly define the hernia by preoperative diagnostic studies including contrast studies of the upper and lower intestine is indicated. An upper midline incision that extends into the

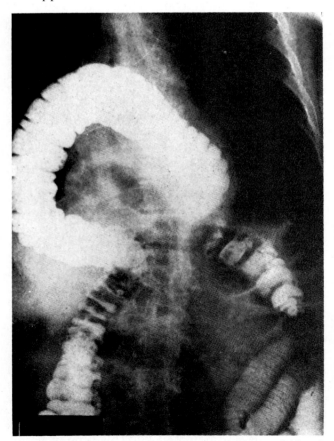

Figure 29–2. Subcostosternal (retrosternal, Morgagni's) hernia showing most of the transverse colon displaced retrosternally.

subxiphoid area allows the best approach for repair. However, if the presence of a hernia is uncertain and there is a possibility of an anterior mediastinal mass causing the abnormal findings on the chest film, a right anterior thoracotomy incision allows good exposure of the area. The subcostal sternal defect can usually be repaired by direct suture after the contents of the hernia sac have been reduced.

Esophageal hiatal hernia is a common finding in adults. A congenital defect in the esophageal hiatus leading to herniation of the stomach is less common. It is common, however, for neonates and infants to have gastroesophageal reflux, which in some is associated with esophageal hiatal hernia. In symptomatic infants, gastroesophageal reflux is associated with a high degree of morbidity (Lilly and Randolph, 1968). Vomiting, respiratory complications, anemia, and failure to thrive are the four main diagnostic features of neonatal gastroesophageal reflux. The diagnosis is easily confirmed by esophagography, together with fluoroscopy revealing free reflux of gastric contents into the esophagus, and by pH monitoring of the distal third of the esophagus. Esophagoscopy is not necessary for the diagnosis but is useful in evaluating the presence and severity of esophagitis. Conservative management consists of maintaining the infant in an upright prone position, usually at an angle of 60 degrees for 24 hours a day (Cahill et al, 1969; Lilly and Randolph, 1968). If medical management is unsuccessful, surgical repair is indicated. The type of repair is less important than the creation of a competent esophageal gastric sphincter and prevents the reflux of gastric contents into the esophagus.

Tumors of the Diaphragm

Although primary tumors of the diaphragm are rare, the diaphragm is frequently involved with malignant tumors extending from contiguous structures including the lungs, esophagus, stomach, liver, or retroperitoneum. Primary tumors of the diaphragm include cysts, inflammatory lesions, and benign or malignant neoplasms (Juvara and Priscu, 1966; Wiener and Chou, 1965).

In a review of 84 cases of primary tumor of the diaphragm (Olafsson et al, 1971), the male-female ratio was approximately equal (1:1.1). This also applied to involvement of either the right or left diaphragm, with the left side slightly predominating. The diagnosis is usually difficult to establish because of the rarity of these neoplasms and the nonspecific nature of the associated symptoms. The most common symptoms in order of frequency were epigastric or lower chest pain, cough, dyspnea, and gastrointestinal distress. Twenty per cent of the patients were asymptomatic, and in most the tumor was detected on the routine chest film. Routine chest films do not always provide a characteristic appearance, but computed tomography has been helpful in localizing the exact site of the tumor.

In Olafsson's series, most primary tumors were benign (60%), and the most frequently occurring benign tumors were cystic formations such as bronchial, mesothelial, or teratomal cysts. Most malignant tumors consisted of sarcomas, among which fibrosarcoma was the most common pathologic type. Trivedi (1958) reported three patients who had neurogenic diaphragmatic tumors and pulmonary osteoarthropathy and who were cured after resection. Radiographic manifestation of a diaphragmatic tumor consists of an enlarging mass on the diaphragmatic surface, usually remaining extrapleural (Anderson and Forrest, 1973).

Excision of the tumor is indicated whenever possible. Closure of the diaphragm by direct sutures is preferred, but when this is not possible, prosthetic material may serve as a replacement. In cases of inflammatory disease, such as hydatid disease or tuberculosis, treatment of the underlying condition is indicated.

Eventration and Unilateral Paralysis

Although previous authors disagree about the concept of the term, *eventration* is now generally recognized to be an abnormally high position of part or all of the diaphragm, usually associated with a sharp decrease in muscle fibers and a membranous appearance of the abnormal area. Eventrations of the diaphragm are divided etiologically into two groups: congenital or nonparalytic and acquired or paralytic (Thomas, 1968, 1970). Jean Louis Petit (1790) was the first person to recognize this entity during autopsy studies in 1774. Béclard (1829) first used the term *eventration*. In 1923, Morrison did the first successful repair of an eventrated diaphragm and used one of the techniques of plication now applied to remove the redundancy associated with the eventration. Bisgard (1947) did the first successful repair of congenital eventration of the diaphragm and provided the current definition of eventration as "an abnormally high or elevated position of one leaf of the *intact* diaphragm as a result of paralysis, aplasia, or atrophy of varying degrees of the muscle fibers." Bisgard emphasized that the unbroken continuity of the diaphragm differentiates this entity from diaphragmatic hernia, which is sometimes difficult to establish on a clinical basis. Bilateral congenital eventration has been reported (Avnet, 1962).

Traumatic Perforation

Traumatic diaphragmatic hernias are produced by either blunt thoracoabdominal trauma or penetrating wounds of the diaphragm. Traumatic diaphragmatic hernia due to blunt trauma is thought to be produced by a sudden increase in the pleuroperitoneal pressure gradient that occurs at areas of potential weakness along embryologic points of fusion (Childress and Grimes, 1961). Any patient with truncal penetrating trauma below the level of the nipples (fifth intercostal space) either anteriorly or posteriorly should be suspected of having diaphragmatic or intra-abdominal injuries. Automobile accidents are the most common cause of blunt traumatic diaphragmatic hernias, and in most series approximately 90% involve the left hemidiaphragm (Brooks, 1978; McElwee et al, 1984; Pomerantz et al, 1968). Traumatic rupture of the right hemidiaphragm is thought to be less common because of the presence of the liver in the right upper quadrant to cushion the force applied against the diaphragm (Estrera et al, 1985). Defects due to blunt trauma are large, usually between 10 and 15 cm, and are usually located in the posterior aspect of the left hemidiaphragm (De la Rocha et al, 1982; Rodriguez-Morales et al, 1986). Through these defects, abdominal viscera can easily herniate into the thorax, and the stomach, spleen, colon, small intestine, and liver are commonly located within the chest, in that order of frequency (Orringer et al, 1975) (Fig. 29–3). Respiratory insufficiency due to compressed lung and a shift of the mediastinum to the contralateral side are common in the early phase of the injury, whereas symptoms of chronic intestinal obstruction are more common when the hernia has been present for a considerable period (Iuchtman et al, 1977).

The diagnosis of diaphragmatic rupture can be elusive. Several centers have noted difficulty in diagnosing diaphragmatic injuries preoperatively because of the lack of specificity of chest film findings and clinical signs (Aronoff et al, 1982; Ebert et al, 1967; Miller et al, 1984). Although not pathognomonic, the chest film is still the best initial screening examination, and absence of complete visualization of the entire hemidiaphragm should raise an index of suspicion of injury (Carter et al, 1951; Ward et al, 1981). In patients sustaining blunt diaphragmatic hernias, the chest film in most series is diagnostic in approximately 50% and is abnormal (hydropneumothorax, pneumothorax) but not diagnostic of the specific disorder in the majority of the remaining patients (Strug et al, 1974). Small tears due to perforating trauma are often not evident on the chest film, and the diagnosis of traumatic diaphragmatic hernia resulting from penetrating injuries to the abdomen or chest is usually made at the time of operation (Wiencek et al, 1986). Those tears in the diaphragm are not as large as those resulting from blunt trauma, and herniation of the abdominal contents into the thorax does not always occur immediately after the injury (Ebert et al, 1967).

Barium contrast studies are contraindicated in patients who are suspected of having a diaphragmatic rupture with signs of obstruction, because the air and contrast introduced into the bowel can become trapped and transform a partial obstruction in the herniated loop into a complete obstruction (Adamthwaite et al, 1983).

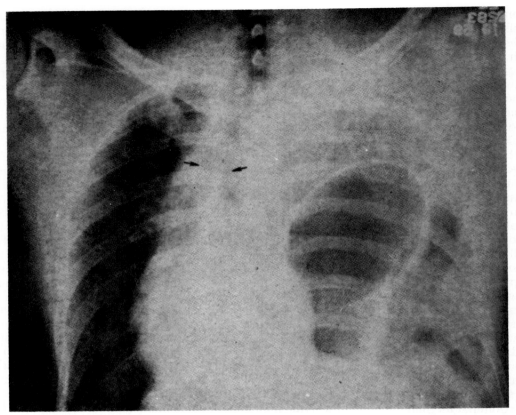

Figure 29–3. Blunt traumatic diaphragmatic hernia with stomach and bowel in left side of the chest. *Arrows* show lateral displacement of the tracheal shadow.

Almost all series reviewing traumatic diaphragmatic hernia report a few patients with overlooked diaphragmatic injuries and delayed diagnosis, which commonly lead to incarceration and strangulation of bowel (Brown and Richardson, 1985; Carter and Brewer, 1971). Some injuries can be overlooked even at operation, presumably because of diversion of attention to the frequently encountered associated injuries (Table 29–1). Complete thoracotomy or exploratory laparotomy for trauma should always include careful inspection and palpation of both hemidiaphragms to avoid the morbidity of later intestinal obstruction and strangulation, which appears to be common (85%) within 3 to 5 years of the injury (Hood, 1971; Pomerantz et al, 1968).

Several cases of traumatic *intrapericardial* diaphragmatic hernias have been reported (Larrieu et al, 1980; Morrison and Mullens, 1978; van Loenhout et al, 1986). The majority result from motor vehicle accidents. In these patients, chest films, computed tomographic scanning (Fagan et al, 1979), and echocardiography were helpful in establishing the diagnosis. Herniation of intra-abdominal organs into the pericardium results from a diaphragmatic tear in the transverse septum of the diaphragm. The most severe complication of intrapericardial diaphragmatic

TABLE 29–1. BLUNT DIAPHRAGMATIC RUPTURE—ASSOCIATED INJURIES*

Injury	No. of Injuries	Injury	No. of Injuries
Head	24	Femur fracture	5
Rib fracture	18	Pneumothorax	5
Pulmonary contusion	18	Humerus fracture	3
Spleen	18	Cervical spine fracture	2
Liver	18	Bladder rupture	2
Hemothorax	16	Myocardial contusion	2
Pelvic fracture	14	Lumbar spine fracture	1
Renal contusion	10	Pancreas	1
Hollow viscus	7	Shoulder dislocation	1
Pulmonary laceration	6	Clavicle fracture	1
Tibiofibular fracture	6	Aortic laceration	1

*From Beal, S. L., and McKennan, M.: Blunt diaphragmatic rupture. Arch. Surg., Vol. 123, p. 82. Copyright 1988, American Medical Association.

hernia is strangulation, which is more likely to develop in small tears than in larger hernias (Wetrich et al, 1969). By means of barium swallow and barium enema to delineate stomach and bowel, the diagnosis can be made (Figs. 29–4 and 29–5).

Mortality of patients sustaining traumatic diaphragmatic hernia varies between 15 and 40%; patients who sustain a blunt diaphragmatic hernia have the higher mortality because of the high incidence of associated injuries, which is almost 90% in most series (see Table 29–1).

Once the diagnosis of diaphragmatic hernia is made, repair should be made as soon as the patient is stabilized with regard to other significant injuries. Use of military antishock trousers with inflation of the abdominal compartment is contraindicated in a patient with suspected diaphragmatic hernia, because this will further aggravate the pulmonary compromise caused by the herniated bowel. Because there is a high incidence of associated intra-abdominal injuries with blunt left diaphragmatic ruptures, those patients whose injuries are diagnosed acutely after the injury should have transabdominal exploration so that associated injuries can be identified and corrected. If the diagnosis is delayed and there are no associated intra-abdominal injuries, repair is more easily accomplished by the transthoracic route. Right-sided herniations are often difficult to repair through an abdominal incision, because of the pres-

ence of the liver, and a right-sided thoracotomy may be required to correct the defect. Whatever approach is chosen, the surgeon must be prepared to do a combined thoracoabdominal operation through two different incisions (van Loenhout et al, 1986). Repair of the defect is accomplished by direct suture using a double layer of nonabsorbable suture and evacuation of the involved pleural cavity with a chest tube or with aspiration during the closure.

DIAPHRAGMATIC PACING

Historical Aspects

The fact that electricity could be used to stimulate movement of the diaphragm, the most important muscle of respiration, was first noted more than 200 years ago by Caldani, in 1786 (Schechter, 1970). In 1873 Hufeland proposed stimulating the phrenic nerve to treat asphyxia neonatorum. In 1818 Ure applied electricity from a voltaic battery to the phrenic nerve of a recently hung criminal. After observing "strong and laborious respirations," he proposed that if the spinal cord and blood vessels of the neck had not been damaged by the hangman's noose, resuscitation might have followed (Schechter, 1970). Duchenne (1872), an outstanding contributor to electrotherapy in the 19th century, clearly established phrenic nerve stimulation as the "best means of imitating natural respiration." Despite the early successes, electrophrenic stimulation did not become popular as a therapeutic technique, and when methods with negative- and positive-pressure ventilation became available, stimulation of the phrenic nerves to activate the diaphragm disappeared from clinical practice.

In the 1940s, Sarnoff and associates (1948) became interested in electrical stimulation of the phrenic nerves as a method of aiding respiration in victims of bulbar poliomyelitis. They showed in acute experiments the physiologic effects of electrical stimulation of the phrenic nerve and introduced the term *electrophrenic respiration*. Their experiments led to several important conclusions with regard to the technique, and these conclusions remain valid: (1) Artificial respiration by phrenic nerve stimulation can be done in humans. (2) A smooth, gradual diaphragmatic contraction occurs when an increased voltage is applied to the phrenic nerve. The diaphragm thus performs a motion closely resembling that which it does during natural inspiration. (3) Respiratory minute volumes in excess of the patient's spontaneous minute volumes can be readily obtained with the submaximal stimulation of one phrenic nerve. (4) The depth of inspiration is proportional to the peak voltage applied to the phrenic nerve in humans, such as in the experimental model. (5) Adequate oxygenation of the blood can be maintained by electrophrenic respiration in the absence of spontaneous respiration. (6) The patient completely relinquishes

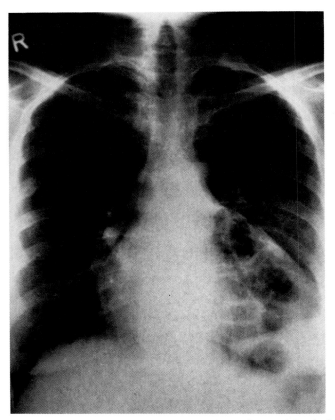

Figure 29–4. Chest film 1 year after blunt thoracoabdominal injury showing bowel gas patterns within the cardiac silhouette.

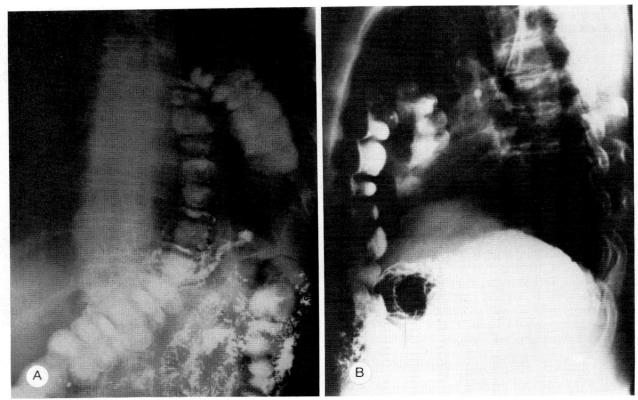

Figure 29–5. *A,* Contrast study showing barium-filled loops of colon intrapericardially (anteroposterior view). *B,* Lateral view locates the herniated colon to the anterior pericardial space.

spontaneous control of respiration when electrophrenic respiration is induced. The development of an effective vaccine against poliomyelitis and the lack of the availability of implantable electrical stimulators probably discouraged the investigation of long-term phrenic nerve stimulation.

Beginning in the late 1950s and continuing until the present, Glenn and associates were mainly responsible for the experimental development and clinical application of chronic diaphragmatic pacing by using radiofrequency signals to stimulate phrenic nerves through the intact skin (Farmer et al, 1978; Glenn et al, 1972). This group has acquired the greatest experience in using the technique and in doing so has defined the populations of patients in which chronic diaphragmatic pacing is efficacious. Moreover, their long-range interests and experience in this area have supplied information with regard to the safety of prolonged phrenic nerve stimulation and the mechanism of diaphragmatic fatigue by which effective pacing is usually limited to less than 24 consecutive hours (Kim et al, 1976).

Glenn, who is in the process of developing the technology of this field and applying those techniques to patients, has defined the relative indications and contraindications for successful electrophrenic stimulation. Diaphragmatic pacing is indicated for patients who have chronic ventilatory insufficiency and in whom function of the phrenic nerves, lungs, and diaphragm has proved to be adequate to sustain ventilation by electrical stimulation. This includes some patients with paralysis of the respiratory muscles (quadriplegia) and with a central alveolar hypoventilation also known as sleep apnea or "Ondine's curse." Diaphragmatic pacing is not indicated in cases of ventilatory insufficiency that result from respiratory paralysis due to lower motor neuron lesions involving the phrenic nerve, from muscular dystrophy affecting the diaphragm, or from extensive parenchymal pulmonary disease. By following these careful indications for the procedure, properly chosen patients clearly benefit and can be freed from cumbersome ventilatory support systems.

Apparatus

The diaphragmatic pacemaker commercially available is made by Avery Laboratory located in Farmingdale, New York, and consists of four components (Fig. 29–6). The receiver and electrode assembly are permanently implanted, and the transmitter and antenna remain external. The implanted radiofrequency receiver is inductively joined to the external transmitter and transforms the radiofrequency signals into an electrical impulse that is carried to the electrode placed behind the phrenic nerve (Fig. 29–7).

The transmitter-coded radiofrequency signals are generated by the external transmitter. Unlike cardiac

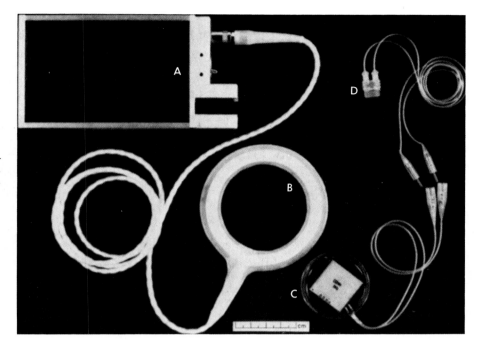

Figure 29–6. Components of the radiofrequency diaphragm pacemaker: *A,* transmitter; *B,* antenna; *C,* receiver; *D,* bipolar electrode.

pacemakers, which produce a single impulse, the output signal of the diaphragmatic pacer is a train of pulses lasting between 1.2 and 1.45 seconds (shorter intervals in infants). The duration of the pulse train corresponds to the length of inspiration, and the number of pulse trains per minute establishes the respiratory rate (Nochomovitz et al, 1988). The pulse interval is usually preset at 50 msec, which allows effective contraction of the diaphragm muscle without leading to rapid fatigue of diaphragmatic response (Bellemare and Bigland-Ritchie, 1987). Pulses have the same amplitude but differ in width with the result that each successive pulse transmitted in each train is wider than its predecessor. The width of each radiofrequency pulse, after demodulation by the receiver, determines the amplitude of the current delivered to the phrenic nerve, which determines the depth of inspiration. The gradual increase in energy delivered during the pulse train is required to provide a smooth excursion of the diaphragm by progressively recruiting more and more nerve fibers (Bear and Talonen, 1987).

The usual settings of the transmitter for an adult are a respiratory rate of 12 breaths per minute with an inspiration time of 1.3 seconds and a pulse interval of 50 msec. The amplitude of the final signal is selected by gradually increasing the stimulus until diaphragmatic excursion is noted to be maximal, such as that recorded during fluoroscopy.

Antenna

The antenna transfers the radiofrequency signal from the transmitter across the intact skin to the

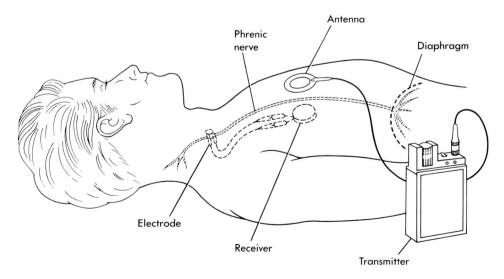

Figure 29–7. The relationship of the four components of the diaphragmatic pacer is shown, using a bipolar electrode. (From Avery Laboratories, Inc.: Diaphragm Pacer [product brochure 6011B–5/79]. Farmingdale, NY, Avery Laboratories, Inc., May 1979.)

subcutaneously implanted receiver. It is connected to a flexible wire lead that inserts into the transmitter. The antenna is placed directly over the implanted receiver and is secured in place with hypoallergenic tape. Because the intensity of the transmitted signal is determined by pulse width rather than by amplitude, the antenna can be displaced up to 2.5 cm from the center of the receiver without affecting operation.

Receiver

The implanted receiver (44-mm diameter, 15-mm thickness, 30.5-g weight) contains no batteries; an electronic integrated circuit obtains energy and stimulus information transcutaneously from the external transmitter by inductive electromagnetic coupling. The signal is demodulated into a unidirectional current, the amplitude of which varies directly with the width of the originally transmitted pulse. All components are hermetically sealed and encapsulated in an epoxy disk.

Electrode

The electrodes contain a ribbon of platinum embedded in a silicone rubber cuff (Fig. 29–8). The surface area is calculated to be 11.5 mm^2. The cuff of the electrode is designed to fit loosely around a 1.5-cm segment of phrenic nerve and to permit firm fixation to the adjacent tissues without injuring the nerve. The ribbon electrode is available as bipolar or monopolar, but monopolar is preferred in all cases

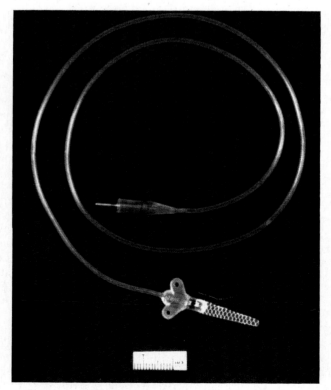

Figure 29–8. The newer platinum ribbon monopolar nerve electrode designed for phrenic nerve stimulation.

except when another electrical stimulation unit such as a cardiac pacemaker is in place. The advantage of the monopolar electrode is that it does not completely encircle the nerve and is therefore less likely to confine scar tissue that develops after implantation. The complete pacing system is shown in Figure 29–7.

Technique of Implantation

Although surgical techniques have been developed and used extensively for cervical implantation of the neuroelectrodes for diaphragmatic pacing, the thoracic approach is now preferred except occasionally in the patient with extensive thoracic deformity or pleural disease. This is because accessory nerve fibers often join the phrenic nerve as it courses through the thoracic inlet. The usual approach for implantation of the platinum ribbon electrode on the phrenic nerve in the chest is through the second intercostal space anteriorly. If bilateral implants are indicated, the two operations are done separately, at least 10 to 14 days apart to avoid the greater danger of infection from the longer operation required for simultaneous implantation (Glenn and Phelps, 1985).

After sterile preparation, a transverse incision is made in the second intercostal space from the sternal border to the anterior axillary line (Fig. 29–9). The incision is extended in a muscle-splitting manner through the pectoralis major, and the internal mammary artery and vein are exposed, fully ligated, and divided. The pleura is opened, and the mediastinum is exposed. A segment of phrenic nerve presenting on a relatively flat surface between the base of the heart and the apex of the chest is selected as the site of implantation. On the right side, this is usually just above the junction of the azygos vein and the superior vena cava where the phrenic nerve passes across the middle of the superior vena cava (Wetstein, 1987). On the left side, the preferred site is where the phrenic nerve passes between the aortic arch and the left pulmonary artery.

The phrenic nerve is isolated by making 1.5-cm parallel incisions on each side of the phrenic nerve through the pleura and underlying areolar tissue. Care is taken to keep 2 to 3 mm from the nerve to preserve the perineural blood supply. The electrode cuff is then inserted carefully beneath the nerve (monopolar) and secured to the surrounding structures (see Fig. 29–9). Preparation must ensure that the surface of the platinum electrode lies directly in contact with the perineurium of the phrenic nerve. The lead wires are then passed through a subcutaneous tunnel to join those from the receiver. The receiver is placed in a subcutaneous pocket, which is either over the upper chest in the midclavicular line for quadriplegics or over the lower chest in the midaxillary line for patients with central alveolar hypoventilation. In infants and children, the receiver is implanted subcutaneously over the lateral abdomen. The subcutaneous pocket should be made so

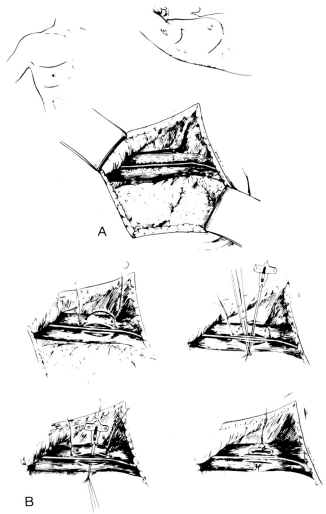

Figure 29–9. Transthoracic approach to the phrenic nerve. The mediastinum is exposed either through an incision in the second interspace anteriorly or through the third interspace in the axilla. The monopolar electrode is secured against the right phrenic nerve on the superior vena cava. If the nerve is isolated closer to the heart (within 5 cm), a bipolar electrode is required. (From Glenn, W. W. L., Hogan, J. F., and Phelps, M. L.: Ventilatory support of the quadriplegic patient with respiratory paralysis by diaphragm pacing. Surg. Clin. North Am., *60*:1055, 1980.)

that no part of the apparatus lies directly under the incision. The copper coil of the receiver faces outward toward the undersurface of the skin. If bilateral units are implanted, the receivers must be separated by at least 15 cm to avoid cross-interference. Before terminating the operation, the ability of the system to produce a diaphragmatic contraction should be shown by using a sterile antenna connected to an off-table transmitter, which lies directly over the implanted radio receiver. If a good response is obtained, the threshold to stimulation is noted; it should be in the range of 0.1 to 2 ma. A higher threshold may signal displacement of the electrode or interposition of tissue between the electrode and the phrenic nerve. A pacing schedule is not begun until 12 to 14 days postoperatively to allow time for

the wound to heal and for the resolution of perineural edema.

Preoperative Screening Tests

Proof of viability of the phrenic nerve is a prerequisite to implantation of a phrenic nerve electrode. To determine that viable phrenic neurons exist, the nerve in the neck is electrically stimulated percutaneously. The usual response, when most neurons are viable, is a brisk contraction of the diaphragm of at least several centimeters. The absence of contraction when stimulating in the anatomic location of the nerve almost always means nonviability of the nerve. If there is doubt that the probe locates the nerve correctly, direct exploration is planned, together with preparation to apply the nerve electrode if a viable nerve is found. Phrenic nerve conduction time is also measured preoperatively. The normal conduction time from the neck to the diaphragm is usually between 7 and 10 msec in adults; the interval is shorter in infants and children. Prolongation over 12 msec may indicate serious local or systemic disease.

Pacing Schedule

The electrical parameters for phrenic nerve stimulation currently used by Glenn and colleagues have evolved after many years of extensive laboratory and clinical trials. Glenn initially used electrical parameters that included a frequency of 25 Hz (40-msec pulse interval), inspiration duration of 1.35 seconds, and a pulse train repetition rate (respiratory rate) of 15 to 17 per minute.

The stimulus is pulse width modulated with the current amplitude, increasing from the initial contraction (threshold stimulation) to the maximal contraction of the diaphragm to obtain a smooth inspiratory diaphragmatic motion (Fig. 29–10). Clinical and experimental data acquired by Glenn show that when phrenic nerve stimulation is restricted to 12 hours daily, no harm is induced with respect to diaphragmatic fatigue. However, experiments in dogs with similar parameters have shown that if pacing is applied for several weeks or months without rest, diaphragmatic muscle function is reduced to less than 20% of normal and is accompanied by severe organic changes in the muscle that are irreversible (Ciesielski et al, 1983; Sato et al, 1970). The origination of fatigue after continuous electrophrenic stimulation in these studies was studied by measuring end-plate potentials after continued repetitive electrical stimulation. The cause of diaphragmatic fatigue was due to interference with transmission of impulses across the neuromuscular junction. Later, methods to reduce the electrical charge of the nerve and diaphragm were explored to reduce fatigue. Glenn and colleagues showed that pacing-induced fatigue of the diaphragm, such as that measured by

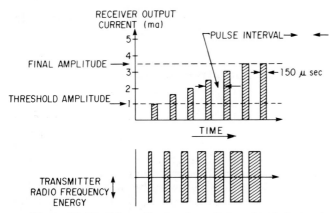

Figure 29–10. Schematic drawing of the electrical signals necessary to produce a single inspiration. The output of the transmitter is a train of biphasic pulses that vary progressively in width *(lower panel)*. The receiver modulates the signal and sends to the nerve-electrode a train of unidirectional impulses that vary in amplitude from 1 to 3.5 ma. The amplitude of the pulse is determined by the width of the corresponding biphasic signal. The first pulse is set at the threshold value and the final pulse at the current needed to produce a slightly submaximal contraction. A train of gradually increasing pulses is necessary to produce a smooth diaphragmatic contraction.

the tidal volume during stimulation of the phrenic nerves, was significantly less when (1) the current applied to the nerve was just under that required for maximal tidal volume, (2) the respiratory rate was 10 per minute instead of 20, and (3) the frequency of stimulation was 10 Hz compared with a higher frequency. The type of waveform and whether the electrode was monopolar or bipolar made no significant difference to the onset or duration of fatigue. Muscle fatigue becomes a greater issue when bilateral pacing is required for full-time ventilatory support in infants, when unilateral pacing is often inadequate to accomplish adequate ventilation because of the instability of the mediastinum and immaturity of the lungs and chest wall. As pacing is continued at a wide pulse interval (lower frequency) and the diaphragm muscle conditions to this lower stimulus frequency, there is fusion of the contractions. This results in muscle conditioning, which has been shown to be due to conversion of the fast-contracting fibers of the diaphragm (high glycolytic, white fibers) to slowly contracting fibers (low glycolytic, red fibers) (Salmons and Henriksson, 1981). When nocturnal ventilatory support alone is indicated in central alveolar hypoventilation or sleep apnea and only one hemidiaphragm is to be paced, the diaphragm must be paced more forcefully than for bilateral pacing. Because continuous pacing is not required and a period of several hours of rest is possible, this can be tolerated without inducing significant and irreversible muscle fatigue. The pulse interval is set at a relatively high frequency of approximately 50 msec (20 Hz) and a rate of 12 to 14 per minute. With the use of these parameters, pacing for 10 to 12 hours followed by a similar period of rest is well tolerated, and fatigue of the diaphragm is minimal (Oda et al,

1981). Consequently, the patient with central alveolar hypoventilation without respiratory muscle paralysis can, with these parameters, begin pacing for 8 to 10 hours nightly in the third week postoperatively.

Quadriplegic patients with respiratory muscle paralysis present a different problem in terms of initiating a pacing schedule. These patients do not present for pacing until several months after the injury that caused the paralysis. During this time, they have had full-time mechanical ventilatory support, and the diaphragm has become weak from disuse and is easily fatigued by electrical stimulation (Nochomovitz et al, 1984). In these patients, the technique for achieving full-time pacing can be complex and prolonged. After pacing parameters have been selected and the initial threshold and maximal determination of diaphragm motion have been obtained, pacing is begun usually at 2 to 3 minutes an hour while the patient is awake. The duration of pacing can be advanced each day by several minutes hourly, as long as the minute volume is not decreased by more than 25% from the beginning to end of the pacing period (Harpin et al, 1986). It may take 6 weeks to 8 months to accomplish full-time ventilatory support to condition the diaphragm according to such a pacing schedule. If ventilation cannot be maintained except by bilateral simultaneous pacing, an attempt must be made to convert the diaphragm muscle fibers to nonfatiguing fibers. This is done by gradually decreasing the frequency of stimulation to 10 Hz, the respiratory rate to 8 per minute, and the current amplitude to submaximal. A considerably longer period is required to condition the diaphragm muscle in children because of immaturity of respiratory components. In addition, a permanent tracheostomy is a necessity with full-time pacing to keep the airway clear and unobstructed. Diaphragmatic pacing can actually exacerbate upper airway obstruction because the usual coordinated pattern of simultaneous diaphragmatic and laryngeal muscle contraction during natural respiration is lost with artificial electrophrenic stimulation.

Selection of Patients for Diaphragmatic Pacing

Successful diaphragmatic pacing is possible only in the presence of a viable phrenic nerve that can stimulate a normal diaphragm to contract and allow expansion of parenchyma of the lung that is capable of satisfactory ventilation and oxygenation. Malfunction of any of these structures significantly reduces the effectiveness of diaphragmatic pacing. Thus, a thorough evaluation of the components of respiration must precede a recommendation to pace the diaphragm (Mier et al, 1987). Diaphragmatic pacing is contraindicated in cases of diaphragmatic paralysis that result from (1) destruction of the anterior horn cells at the level of the third, fourth, or fifth cervical vertebrae; (2) damage to the peripheral axons of the phrenic nerve; (3) impaired diaphragmatic function secondary to atrophy, eventration, myositis, or muscular dystrophy; or (4) severe damage to pulmonary parenchyma (Glenn, 1978). Direct electrical stimulation of diaphragmatic muscle without using phrenic innervation has not been successful because of ineffective diaphragmatic contraction and early fatigability (Mugica et al, 1987). Thus, paralysis or paresis of the diaphragm, commonly encountered after coronary bypass grafting operations, is not amenable to electrophrenic pacing of the involved diaphragm. The cause of the phrenic nerve dysfunction is based on cold or stretching injury or ischemia (Estenne et al, 1985; Markland et al, 1985), and because of peripheral nerve involvement, electrophrenic pacing would not be effective.

Central Alveolar Hypoventilation

Central alveolar hypoventilation occurs when the respiratory center fails to respond to hypercapnia by increasing minute ventilation. Alternatively, the carotid body chemoreceptors may also not respond to hypoxemia. Periodic apnea can occur especially during sleep. The clinical criteria for the diagnosis of central alveolar hypoventilation include the following: (1) clinical features of hypoventilation such as cyanosis, polycythemia, and cor pulmonale with right-sided heart failure; (2) hypoxemia and hypercapnia increasing during sleep; (3) hypoventilation during sleep, sometimes marked by periodic apnea; (4) almost normal results of ventilatory capacity tests; (5) reduced ventilatory response to induced hypoxemia and hypercapnia; and (6) absence of upper-airway obstruction during a sleep study or persistence of hypoventilation after relief of obstruction (Glenn, 1978). In the absence of an identifiable organic lesion of the respiratory centers, a cause of central alveolar hypoventilation may not be determined (Meisner et al, 1983). There frequently is a history of a previous attack of encephalitis or an undiagnosed febrile illness without an evident residual organic deficit. The presence of hypoventilation at birth or a history of apnea that suggests manifestations of the sudden infant death syndrome indicates the presence of a congenital defect in the respiratory center (Glenn, 1985).

Since 1966 Glenn and colleagues have used diaphragmatic pacing to treat 48 patients with defects in respiratory control secondary to the central alveolar hypoventilation syndrome. Since 1976 they have used the monopolar electrode in preference to the bipolar electrode for both unilateral and bilateral stimulation. Three cases were categorized as being congenital; 11 were idiopathic as the cause of the central alveolar hypoventilation syndrome; and the remainder were due to organic lesions of the brain stem or above, usually due to vascular accidents. The mean age of the patients with idiopathic central alveolar hypoventilation was 55 years, with a range between 44 and 67 years. These patients were paced with a mean of 95 months and with a range of 17 to 168 months. Four patients died in this group; the mortality was 36%. Of 33 patients with central alveolar hypoventilation treated with diaphragmatic pacing because of lesions of the brain stem or above, 19 ultimately died (a mortality of 58%) (Glenn and Phelps, 1985).

Quadriplegia

The fact that diaphragmatic pacing could provide total ventilatory support in humans was shown by Glenn in 1971 when he successfully transferred a ventilator-dependent quadriplegic patient to full-time electrophrenic respiration (Glenn et al, 1972). The patient was a 38-year-old man who sustained a spinal cord injury at the level of the first and second cervical segments. Five months after injury, he had a bipolar electrode placed around each phrenic nerve by using a cervical approach. Approximately 3 months after implantation, the patient was completely free of the mechanical respirator and was supported by radiofrequency electrophrenic respiration by alternating stimulation of the two phrenic nerves for 12 hours each. He was ultimately discharged from the hospital. Glenn reported a series of 20 quadriplegic patients (Glenn et al, 1980) in whom full-time ventilatory support was achieved by using diaphragmatic pacing in 8 patients and part-time support in an additional 8 patients. Similar results have been reported from other centers that specialize in the treatment of spinal cord injury (Oakes et al, 1980).

Use of the diaphragmatic pacing technique in quadriplegic patients requires special consideration of certain factors that have been well emphasized by Glenn and colleagues (1984).

1. The injury that produced quadriplegia must be localized to the first or second cervical segments of the spinal cord. If involvement of C3, C4, or C5 occurs, a portion of the anterior horn cells of the corresponding segments may be destroyed and the surviving neurons may become inadequate to achieve a satisfactory diaphragmatic function. Before permanent electrodes are implanted, nerve viability must be shown either by transcutaneous technique or by direct stimulation at the time of operation.

2. Some recovery of spontaneous ventilatory function may occur after spinal cord injury; therefore, the diaphragmatic pacing should be delayed until several months after injury to be certain that it is really indicated.

3. Disuse atrophy of the diaphragm that is the result of the cervical spinal cord injury requires slow and gradual conditioning before diaphragmatic pacing can be expected to provide adequate ventilation.

4. Fatigue of the diaphragm requires that pacing be periodically interrupted to permit recovery of the neuromuscular junction. Fatigue that is not recognized can result in permanent damage to the neuromuscular junction, which can preclude successful electrophrenic respiration later.

5. Diaphragmatic pacing is indicated only in patients who are good candidates for long-term rehabilitation after they have been supported by conventional positive-pressure ventilation following the first few months after injury.

Diaphragmatic Pacing in Infants

A series of phrenic nerve pacing in infants was reported by Ilbawi and associates (1985), who reviewed eight infants who ranged in age from 2.5 months to 8.5 months and who had central hypoventilation syndrome. Preoperative diagnosis was established by showing an inadequate ventilatory response to hypercapnia and hypoxia. Before placement of phrenic nerve electrodes, percutaneous measurements of phrenic nerve conduction time and diaphragmatic action potentials were done to evaluate the feasibility of diaphragmatic pacing. Bilateral anterolateral inframammary thoracotomy incisions were made, entering the chest through the third intercostal space. Unipolar electrodes were passed around each phrenic nerve and connected to the receiver in a subcutaneous pocket created in the flank.

Patients were followed postoperatively for 6 months to 8 years. In all patients, bilateral phrenic nerve stimulation allowed either a sharp decrease in or discontinuation of positive-pressure ventilation. Phrenic nerve conduction time and diaphragmatic action potential showed no evidence of nerve injury or muscle dysfunction after 8 years of pacing. This clinical experience confirms the previous work of Kim and associates (1976), who found that the histologic changes of phrenic nerves did not correlate with the duration of stimulation and that nerve injury was due to an inappropriate technique of electrode application (Fig. 29–11). The report by Ilbawi and colleagues (1985) suggested that diaphragmatic pacing in infants was safe, had no major side effects, and could be considered to be a viable long-term improvement to long-term positive-pressure ventilation. These conclusions were supported by other investigators (Cahill et al, 1983). The authors emphasized that tracheostomy is uniformly necessary in infants because pacing-related upper-airway obstruction is consistently observed as a result of failure to activate laryngeal and upper-airway muscles in synchrony with diaphragmatic contraction. This activation is necessary to counteract the negative pharyngeal pressure that is generated during inspiration. The authors also noted that it was uniformly necessary to use bilateral diaphragmatic pacing to sustain adequate ventilation in children. This was thought to be related to the mobile mediastinum in young children, which precluded successful unilateral diaphragmatic pacing (Brouillette et al, 1983).

Future Goals

The perfection of a totally implantable, battery-powered diaphragmatic pacemaker that can be programmed and interrogated from an exterior device similar to current cardiac pacemaker technology is a goal for the future (Glenn et al, 1986). An implanted energy source that could be developed from currently available technology would maintain an estimated battery life of 5 to 8 years for diaphragmatic pacing. Additionally, the development of a demand-type diaphragmatic pacemaker that would respond to ventilatory needs and act in synchrony with autonomic reflexes to maintain an open upper airway during respiration is the next goal in the evolution of artificial respiration by diaphragmatic pacing (Glenn, 1987). Perhaps the greatest contribution derived from the development of diaphragmatic pacing is the demonstration that peripheral nerves can be intermittently stimulated for extended periods by artificial pulses to achieve almost normal function of

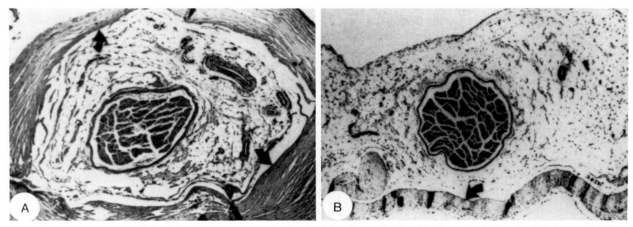

Figure 29–11. *A,* Section of the left phrenic nerve at the level of the electrode after bipolar stimulation for 126 days at 26 Hz. The epineural fibroadipose layer is surrounded completely by a thick fibrous capsule *(arrows)*, but the nerve fascicle is histologically unremarkable. *B,* Section of the right phrenic nerve at the electrode level after stimulation with a monopolar electrode for 154 days at 27 Hz. A band of fibrous tissue *(arrow)* has developed at the lower margin facing the electrode. The nerve fascicle is histologically unremarkable. (Hematoxylin and eosin stain, ×39.)

the neuromuscular unit without apparent damage. The development and application of diaphragmatic pacing represent a success story for neuroprosthetics and hopefully serve as the basis for the application of similar techniques to other neurologically impaired but otherwise functional units of the body.

Selected Bibliography

Anderson, L. S. and Forrest, J. V.: Tumors of the diaphragm. Am. J. Roentgenol. Radium Ther. Nucl. Med., *119*:259, 1973.

The authors present a radiographic analysis of diaphragmatic tumors in a classification of those tumors into the following groups: (1) primary benign neoplasms, (2) primary malignant neoplasms, (3) secondary malignant neoplasms, (4) cysts, (5) inflammatory lesions, and (6) endometriosis.

Beal, S. L., and McKennan, M.: Blunt diaphragmatic rupture. Arch. Surg., *123*:828, 1988.

A review of 37 patients sustaining traumatic diaphragmatic hernia from blunt injury during a 12-month period. Because of a high incidence of associated injuries (36 of 37 patients) and a high incidence of shock on initial presentation (54%), the overall mortality was 40%. The difficulty in diagnosis of traumatic diaphragmatic hernia was shown in that the rupture was not initially recognized in 69% of patients, and the initial chest film was often nondiagnostic. The authors recommend a high index of suspicion for the injury in patients sustaining blunt trauma and also prompt exploratory laparotomy with complete inspection of both hemidiaphragms and primary repair of the diaphragmatic tear.

Glenn, W. W. L., and Phelps, M. L.: Diaphragm pacing by electrical stimulation of the phrenic nerve. Neurosurgery, *17*:974, 1985.

In this review article, Glenn summarizes his personal experience with diaphragmatic pacing in 77 patients. The indications and contraindications for the procedure are outlined, and the authors discuss the preoperative screening tests, which should be carefully completed before initiating this type of therapy. The operative technique is discussed and illustrated. The authors recommend that bilateral units should be implanted at separate operations. A discussion of conduct of pacing as well as pacing schedules for diaphragmatic "conditioning" in quadriplegic patients is given. This is the most recent review of Glenn's experience in this area, which he has developed during the last 20 years, and it provides his views of application of this technology to patients with chronic ventilatory insufficiency.

Glenn, W. W. L., Hogan, J. F., Loke, J. S. O., et al: Ventilatory support by pacing of the conditioned diaphragm in quadriplegia. N. Engl. J. Med., *310*:1150, 1984.

This report updates the Yale group's experience with diaphragmatic pacing in quadriplegic patients. The group reports changes in the method of pacing used in the five most recent patients, techniques that minimized fatigue of the diaphragm and permitted uninterrupted simultaneous pacing of both hemidiaphragms to produce a more physiologic form of respiration. The patients included in the study had continuous electrical pacing of both hemidiaphragms simultaneously for 11 to 33 months. The strength and endurance of the diaphragm muscle increased with diaphragmatic pacing. Biopsy specimens taken from two patients who had uninterrupted stimulation for 6 and 16 weeks showed changes that suggested the development of fatigue-resistant muscle fibers. When comparing the results of continuing bilateral diaphragmatic pacing in the current group with a previous group of 17 patients with respiratory paralysis, continuous bilateral pacing using low-frequency stimulation was superior because of more efficient ventilation of both lungs, less electrical energy required to effect the same ventilation, and absence of myopathic changes in the diaphragm muscle. The authors conclude that for patients with respiratory paralysis and intact phrenic nerves, continuous simultaneous pacing of both hemidiaphragms with low-frequency stimulation at a slow respiratory rate is a satisfactory method of providing full-time ventilatory support.

Ilbawi, M. N., Idriss, S. S., Hunt, C. E., et al: Diaphragmatic pacing in infants: Techniques and results. Ann. Thorac. Surg., *40*:323, 1985.

This report reviews eight infants with central hypoventilation syndrome who were treated with phrenic nerve pacing for periods between 6 months and 8 years. The ages of the patients ranged from 2 1/2 to 8 1/2 months of age at the time of phrenic nerve diaphragmatic pacing. The preoperative diagnosis was established by showing an inadequate ventilatory response to hypercapnia and hypoxia. Preoperative screening tests were done on all patients and included measurement of phrenic nerve conduction time and diaphragmatic action potentials to assess the feasibility of diaphragmatic pacing. The electrodes were implanted through an anterior thoracotomy incision, with receiver implantation in the flank. There were no complications or deaths related to the procedure, and bilateral phrenic nerve stimulation allowed either sharp reduction in ventilatory requirement or discontinuation of positive-pressure ventilation. This report is encouraging in that it shows that prolonged phrenic nerve stimulation is safe in infants; in these selected patients, early initiation of diaphragmatic pacing can lead to an extended survival.

Miller, L., Bennett, E. V., Root, H. D., et al: Management of penetrating and blunt diaphragmatic injury. J. Trauma, *24*:403, 1984.

The authors review a 5-year experience with 102 patients with diaphragmatic injury, mostly penetrating trauma (93 of 102). Chest films were normal in 40% of the patients, and a peritoneal lavage was not useful in the diagnosis. Most of the injuries were diagnosed at exploration, because the authors followed a policy of exploratory laparotomy for all penetrating wounds of the abdomen and lower thorax. Although associated injuries occurred in 87% of the patients, only one death occurred.

Sawyer, S. F., Falterman, K. W., Goldsmith, J. P., and Arensman, R. M.: Improving survival in the treatment of congenital diaphragmatic hernia. Ann. Thorac. Surg., *41*:75, 1986.

This paper reviews 32 infants with congenital diaphragmatic hernia treated in the years 1979 to 1984. Twenty-four of the patients required immediate intubation and operative repair at less than 12 hours of age. The overall survival was 54% but was significantly influenced by the date of treatment, because the survival in the last 3 years of the series was 82% compared with 31% in the initial 3 years. The authors attribute the improved survival to more aggressive therapy to interrupt the vicious cycle of persistent fetal circulation that accompanies the disorder. The authors describe their indications and use of both pharmacologic agents (pulmonary vasodilators, inotropic agents, buffering agents to prevent and treat acidosis) and mechanical interventions including high-frequency jet ventilation and ECMO.

Thomas, T. V.: Congenital eventration of the diaphragm. Ann. Thorac. Surg., *10*:180, 1970.

This collective review outlines the etiology, symptoms and indications for operative intervention for diaphragmatic eventration. A classification separating congenital (nonparalytic) from acquired (paralytic) eventration is established. The author carefully differentiates between diaphragmatic eventration and congenital diaphragmatic hernia in terms of the pathologic features and also the differences in therapy.

Bibliography

Adamthwaite, D. N., Snijders, D. C., and Mirwis, J.: Traumatic pericardiophrenic hernia: A report of 3 cases. Br. J. Surg., 70:117, 1983.

Anderson, L. S., and Forrest, J. V.: Tumors of the diaphragm. Am. J. Roentgenol. Radium Ther. Nucl. Med., 119:259, 1973.

Aronoff, R. J., Reynolds, J., and Thal, E. R.: Evaluation of diaphragmatic injuries. Am. J. Surg., 144:671, 1982.

Avnet, N. L.: Roentgenologic features of congenital bilateral anterior diaphragmatic eventration. Am. J. Roentgenol., 88:743, 1962.

Beal, S. L., and McKennan, M.: Blunt diaphragm rupture: A morbid injury. Arch. Surg., 123:828, 1988.

Bear, G. A., and Talonen, P. P.: International symposium on implanted phrenic nerve stimulators for respiratory insufficiency. Ann. Clin. Res., 19:399, 1987.

Beclard, E.: Cited by J. Cruveilhier in Atlas d'Anatomie Pathologique. Paris: 1829. Vol. I, book 17, plate V, p.2.

Bellemare, E., and Bigland-Ritchie, B.: Central components of diaphragmatic fatigue assessed by phrenic nerve stimulation. J. Appl. Physiol., 62:1307, 1987.

Bisgard, J. D.: Congenital eventration of the diaphragm. J. Thorac. Surg., 16:484, 1947.

Bowditch, H. I.: Diaphragmatic hernia. Buffalo Med. J., 9:1, 65, 94, 1853.

Brooks, J. W.: Blunt traumatic rupture of the diaphragm. Ann. Thorac. Surg., 26:199, 1978.

Brouillette, R. T., Ilbawi, M. N., and Hunt, C. E.: Phrenic nerve pacing in infants and children: A review of experience and report on the usefulness of phrenic nerve stimulation studies. J. Pediatr., 102:32, 1983.

Brown, G. L., and Richardson, J. D.: Traumatic diaphragmatic hernia: Continuing challenge. Ann. Thorac. Surg., 39:170, 1985.

Cahill, J. L., Aberdeen, E., and Waterston, D. J.: Results of surgical treatment of esophageal hiatal hernia in infancy and childhood. Surgery, 66:597, 1969.

Cahill, J. L., Okamoto, G. A., Higgins, T., and Davis, A.: Experiences with phrenic nerve pacing in children. J. Pediatr. Surg., 18:851, 1983.

Caldani, L. M. A.: Institutiones Physiologicae. Venice, Pezzana, 1786. In Schechter, D. C.: Application of electrotherapy to noncardiac thoracic disorders. Bull. N.Y. Acad. Med., 46:932, 1970.

Carter, B. N., Giuseffi, J., and Felson, B.: Traumatic diaphragmatic hernia. Am. J. Roentgenol., 65:56, 1951.

Carter, R., and Brewer, L. A., III: Strangulating diaphragmatic hernia. Ann. Thorac. Surg., 12:281, 1971.

Childress, M. E., and Grimes, O. F.: Immediate and remote sequelae in traumatic diaphragmatic hernia. Surg. Gynecol. Obstet., 113:573, 1961.

Ciesielski, T. E., Fukuda, Y., Glenn, W. W. L., et al: Response of the diaphragm muscle to electrical stimulation of the phrenic nerve: A histochemical and ultrastructural study. J. Neurosurg., 58:92, 1983.

Cloutier, R., Fournier, L., and Levasseur, L.: Reversion to fetal circulation in congenital diaphragmatic hernia: A preventable postoperative complication. J. Pediatr. Surg., 18:551, 1983.

De la Rocha, A. G., Creel, R. J., Mulligan, G. W. N., et al: Diaphragmatic rupture due to blunt abdominal trauma. Surg. Gynecol. Obstet., 154:175, 1982.

Duchenne, G. B. A.: De l'electrisation localisée et de son application à la pathologie et à le therapeutique par courants induits et par courants galvaniques interrompus et continus, par le dr. Duchenne, 3rd ed. Paris, Bailliere, 1872.

Ebert, P. A., Gaertner, R. A., and Zuidema, G. D.: Traumatic diaphragmatic hernia. Surg. Gynecol. Obstet., 125:59, 1967.

Ein, S. H., Barker, G., Olley, P., et al: The pharmacologic treatment of newborn diaphragmatic hernia: A 2-year evaluation. J. Pediatr. Surg., 15:384, 1980.

Estenne, M., Yernault, J., De Smet, J., and De Troyer, A.: Phrenic and diaphragm function after coronary artery bypass grafting. Thorax, 40:293, 1985.

Estrera, A. S., Landay, M. J., and McClelland, R. N.: Blunt traumatic rupture of the right hemidiaphragm: Experience in 12 patients. Ann. Thorac. Surg., 39:525, 1985.

Fagan, C. J., Schreiber, M. H., Amparo, E. G., et al: Traumatic diaphragmatic hernia into pericardium: Verification of diagnosis by computed tomography. J. Comput. Assist. Tomogr., 3:405, 1979.

Farmer, W. C., Glenn, W. W. L., and Gee, J. B. L.: Alveolar hypoventilation syndrome: Studies of ventilatory control in patients selected for diaphragm pacing. Am. J. Med., 64:39, 1978.

Glenn, W. W. L.: Diaphragm pacing: Present status. Pace, 1:357, 1978.

Glenn, W. W. L.: Pacing the diaphragm in infants. Ann. Thorac. Surg., 40:319, 1985.

Glenn, W. W. L.: On diaphragm pacing. N. Engl. J. Med., 317:1477, 1987.

Glenn, W. W. L., Hogan, J. F., Loke, J. S. O., et al: Ventilatory support by pacing of the conditioned diaphragm in quadriplegia. N. Engl. J. Med., 310:1150, 1984.

Glenn, W. W. L., Hogan, J. F., and Phelps, M. L.: Ventilatory support of the quadriplegic patient with respiratory paralysis by diaphragm pacing. Surg. Clin. North Am., 60:1055, 1980.

Glenn, W. W. L., Holcomb, W. G., McLaughlin, A. J., et al: Total ventilatory support in a quadriplegic patient with radiofrequency electrophrenic respiration. N. Engl. J. Med., 286:513, 1972.

Glenn, W. W. L., and Phelps, M. L.: Diaphragm pacing by electrical stimulation of the phrenic nerve. Neurosurgery, 17:974, 1985.

Glenn, W. W. L., Phelps, M. L., Elefteriades, J. A., et al: Twenty years of experience in phrenic nerve stimulation to pace the diaphragm. PACE, 9:780, 1986.

Grage, T. B., MacLean, L. D., and Cambell, G. S.: Traumatic rupture of the diaphragm: A report of 26 cases. Surgery, 46:669, 1959.

Gravier, L.: Congenital diaphragmatic hernias. South. Med. J., 67:59, 1974.

Hardesty, R. L., Griffith, B. P., Debski, R. F., et al: Extracorporeal membrane oxygenation: Successful treatment of persistent fetal circulation following repair of congenital diaphragmatic hernia. J. Thorac. Cardiovasc. Surg., 81:556, 1981.

Harpin, R. P., Gignac, S. P., Epstein, S. W., et al: Diaphragm pacing and continuous positive airway pressure. Am. Rev. Respir. Dis., 134:1321, 1986.

Harrington, S. W.: Various types of diaphragmatic hernias treated surgically: Report of 430 cases. Surg. Gynecol. Obstet., 86:735, 1948.

Harrison, M. R., and De Lorimier, A. A.: Congenital diaphragmatic hernia. Surg. Clin. North Am. 61:1023, 1981.

Hislop, A., and Reid, L.: Persistent hypoplasia of the lung after repair of congenital diaphragmatic hernia. Thorax, 31:452, 1976.

Hood, R. M.: Traumatic diaphragmatic hernia. Ann. Thorac. Surg., 12:311, 1971.

Hufeland, C. W.: De usu vis electricae in asphyxia experimentis illustrato. Inaugural dissertation, Gottingae, 1873. In Schechter, D. C.: Application of electrotherapy to noncardiac thoracic disorders. Bull. N.Y. Acad. Med., 46:932, 1970.

Ilbawi, M. N., Idriss, F. S., Hunt, C. E., et al: Diaphragmatic pacing in infants: Techniques and results. Ann. Thorac. Surg., 40:323, 1985.

Iuchtman, M., Freire, E. C., and Jacob, E. R.: Acute diaphragmatic hernia caused by blunt trauma. Am. Surg., 43:460, 1977.

Juvara, I., and Priscu, A.: Primary congenital diaphragmatic tumors. Surgery, 60:255, 1966.

Kim, J. H., Manuelidis, E. E., Glenn, W. W. L., and Kaneyuki, T.: Diaphragm pacing: Histopathological changes in the phrenic nerve following long-term electrical stimulation. J. Thorac. Cardiovasc. Surg., 72:602, 1976.

Larrieu, A. J., Wiener, I., Alexander, R., et al: Pericardiodiaphragmatic hernia. Am. J. Surg., 139:436, 1980.

Levin, D. L.: Morphologic analysis of the pulmonary vascular bed in congenital left-sided diaphragmatic hernia. J. Pediatr., 92:805, 1978.

Levy, R. J., Rosenthal, A., Freed, M. D., et al: Persistent pulmonary hypertension in a newborn with congenital diaphragmatic hernia: Successful management with tolazoline. Pediatrics, 60:740, 1977.

Lilly, J. R., and Randolph, J. G.: Hiatal hernia and gastroesophageal reflux in infants and children. J. Thorac. Cardiovasc. Surg., 55:42, 1968.

Markland, O. N., Moorthy, S. S., Mahomet, Y., et al: Postoperative phrenic nerve palsy in patients with open-heart surgery. Ann. Thorac. Surg., 39:68, 1985.

McElwee, T. B., Myers, R. T., and Pennell, T. C.: Diaphragmatic rupture from blunt trauma. Am. Surg., 51:143, 1984.

Meisner, H., Schober, J. G., Struck, E., et al: Phrenic nerve pacing for the treatment of central hypoventilation syndrome—state of the art and case report. Thorac. Cardiovasc. Surg., 31:21, 1983.

Mier, A., Brophy, C., Moxxham, J., and Green, M.: Phrenic nerve stimulation in normal subjects and in patients with diaphragmatic weakness. Thorax, 42:885, 1987.

Miller, L., Bennett, E. V., Jr., Root, H. D., et al: Management of penetrating and blunt diaphragmatic injury. J. Trauma, 24:403, 1984.

Morgagni, G. B.: Seats and causes of diseases. Zellts 54, Monograph on Hernia of the Diaphragm, 1769.

Morrison, J. A., and Mullens, J. E.: Traumatic intrapericardial rupture of the diaphragm. J. Trauma, 18:744, 1978.

Morrison, J. M. W.: Elevation of one diaphragm, unilateral phrenic paralysis: A radiological study with special reference to differential diagnosis. Arch. Radiol. Electrother., 27:353, 1923.

Mugica, J., Dejean, D., Smits, K., et al: Direct diaphragm stimulation. PACE, 10:252, 1987.

Naeye, R. L., Shochat, S. J., Whitman, V., and Maisels, M. J.: Unsuspected pulmonary vascular abnormalities associated with diaphragmatic hernia. Pediatrics, 58:902, 1976.

Nochomovitz, M. L., Hopkins, M., Brodkey, J., et al: Conditioning of the diaphragm with phrenic nerve stimulation after prolonged disuse. Am. Rev. Respir. Dis., 130:684, 1984.

Nochomovitz, M. L., Peterson, D. K., and Stellato, T. A.: Electrical activation of the diaphragm. Clin. Chest Med., 9:349, 1988.

Oakes, D. D., Wilmot, C. B., Halverson, D., and Hamilton, R. D.: Neurogenic respiratory failure: A 5-year experience using implantable phrenic nerve stimulators. Ann. Thorac. Surg., 30:118, 1980.

O'Callaghan, J. D., Saunders, N. R., Chatrath, R. R., and Walker, D. R.: The management of neonatal posterolateral diaphragmatic hernia. Ann. Thorac. Surg., 33:174, 1982.

Oda, T., Glenn, W. W. L., Fukuda, Y., et al: Evolution of electrical parameters for diaphragm pacing: An experimental study. J. Surg. Res., 30:142, 1981.

Olafsson, G., Rausing, A., and Holen, O.: Primary tumors of the diaphragm. Chest, 59:568, 1971.

Orringer, M. B., Kirsh, M. M., and Sloan, H.: Congenital and traumatic diaphragmatic hernia exclusive of the hiatus. Curr. Probl. Surg., 12:33, 1975.

Petit, J. L.: Traite des Maladies Chirurgicales et des Opérations Qui Leur Conviennent: Ouvrage Posthume de J. L. Petit (Revised ed), Vol. II. Lesne, 1790, p. 233.

Pomerantz, M., Rodgers, B. M., and Sabiston, D. C., Jr.: Traumatic diaphragmatic hernia. Surgery, 64:529, 1968.

Redmond, C. R., Graves, E. D., Falterman, K. W., et al: Extracorporeal membrane oxygenation for respiratory and cardiac failure in infants and children. J. Thorac. Cardiovasc. Surg., 93:199, 1987.

Rodriguez-Morales, G., Rodriguez, A., and Shatney, C. H.: Acute rupture of the diaphragm in blunt trauma: Analysis of 60 patients. J. Trauma, 26:438, 1986.

Salmons, S., and Henriksson, J.: The adaptive response of skeletal muscle to increased use. Muscle Nerve, 4:94, 1981.

Sarnoff, S. J., Hardenbergh, E., and Whittenberger, J. L.: Electrophrenic respiration. Am. J. Physiol., 155:1, 1948.

Sarnoff, S. J., Hardenbergh, E., and Whittenberger, J. L.: Electrophrenic respiration. Science, 108:482, 1948.

Sato, G., Glenn, W. W. L., Holcombe, W. G., and Wuench, D.: Further experience with electrical stimulation of the phrenic nerve: Electrically induced fatigue. Surgery, 68:817, 1970.

Sawyer, S. F., Falterman, K. W., Goldsmith, J. P., and Arensman, R. M.: Improving survival in the treatment of congenital diaphragmatic hernia. Ann. Thorac. Surg., 41:75, 1986.

Schechter, D. C.: Application of electrotherapy to noncardiac thoracic disorders. Bull. N.Y. Acad. Med., 46:932, 1970.

Shochat, S. J., Naye, R. L., Ford, W. D. A., et al: Congenital diaphragmatic hernia: New concept in management. Ann. Surg., 190:332, 1979.

Strug, B., Noon, G. P., and Beall, A. C., Jr.: Traumatic diaphragmatic hernia. Ann. Thorac. Surg., 17:444, 1974.

Sumner, E., and Frank, J. D.: Tolazoline in the treatment of congenital diaphragmatic hernias. Arch. Dis. Child., 56:350, 1981.

Sutton, J. P., Carlisle, R. B., and Stephenson, S. E.: Traumatic diaphragmatic hernia. Ann. Thorac. Surg., 3:136, 1967.

Symbas, P. N., Hatcher, C. R., Jr., and Waldo, W.: Diaphragmatic eventration in infancy and childhood. Ann. Thorac. Surg., 24:113, 1977.

Thomas, T. V.: Congenital eventration of the diaphragm. Ann. Thorac. Surg., 10:180, 1970.

Thomas, T. V.: Nonparalytic eventration of the diaphragm. J. Thorac. Cardiovasc. Surg., 55:586, 1968.

Thomas, T. V.: Subcostosternal diaphragmatic hernia. J. Thorac. Cardiovasc. Surg., 63:278, 1972.

Trento, A., Griffith, B. P., and Hardesty, R. L.: Extracorporeal membrane oxygenation experience (ECMO) at the University of Pittsburgh. Ann. Thorac. Surg., 42:56, 1986.

Trivedi, S. A.: Neurolemmoma of the diaphragm causing severe hypertrophic pulmonary osteoarthropathy. Br. J. Tuberculosis, 52:214, 1958.

Ure, A.: Experiments made on the body of a criminal immediately after execution with physiological and philosophical observations. J. Sci. Arts, 12:1, 1818. In Schechter, D. C.: Application of electrotherapy to noncardiac thoracic disorders. Bull. N.Y. Acad. Med., 46:932, 1970.

van Loenhout, R. M. M., Schiphorst, T. J. M. J., Wittens, C. H. A., and Pinackaers, J. A.: Traumatic intrapericardial diaphragmatic hernia. J. Trauma, 26:271, 1986.

Ward, R. E., Flynn, T. C., and Clark, W. P.: Diaphragmatic disruption secondary to blunt abdominal trauma. J. Trauma, 21:35, 1981.

Wetrich, R. M., Sawyers, T. M., and Haug, C. A.: Diaphragmatic rupture with pericardial involvement. Ann. Thorac. Surg., 8:361, 1969.

Wetstein, L.: Technique for implantation of phrenic nerve electrodes. Ann. Thorac. Surg., 43:335, 1987.

Wiencek, R. G., Jr., Wilson, R. F., and Steiger, Z.: Acute injuries of the diaphragm. J. Thorac. Cardiovasc. Surg., 92:989, 1986.

Wiener, M. F., and Chou, W. H.: Primary tumors of the diaphragm. Arch. Surg., 90:143, 1965.

Wohl, M. E. B., Griscom, N. T., Strieder, D. J., et al: The lung following repair of a congenital diaphragmatic hernia. J. Pediatr., 90:405, 1977.

CHAPTER 30

SURGICAL MANAGEMENT OF MYASTHENIA GRAVIS

C. Warren Olanow
Andrew S. Wechsler

Myasthenia gravis is a disorder of neuromuscular transmission that is characterized by weakness and fatigue of voluntary muscles. It is now reasonably established to be due to an autoimmune attack directed against the postsynaptic nicotinic acetylcholine (ACh) receptors of voluntary muscles. Many detailed accounts of the clinical picture have been recorded before this century. The similarity of the clinical features of myasthenia gravis to those resulting from curare poisoning and the beneficial effect of prostigmine, shown by Mary Walker in 1934, focused attention on impaired neuromuscular transmission as the basis of the disorder.

Interactions between quanta of ACh released from the presynaptic terminal at the neuromuscular junction and acetylcholine receptors (AChR) on the postsynaptic membrane determine the likelihood of muscular contraction. The excessive number of potential interactions beyond that necessary to provide for maximal muscle contraction is referred to as the "safety factor" for neuromuscular transmission. Elmqvist and associates (1964) showed that patients with myasthenia gravis had reduced miniature end-plate potential amplitudes, reflecting fewer interactions between ACh and AChR and thus a reduced safety factor. Initially, this was thought to be due to inadequate release of ACh. More recent studies using specific neurotoxins (prepared from snake venom) have shown a reduction in the number of AChR in patients with myasthenia gravis, which has been suggested by histologic and electron microscopic studies. In 1960, Simpson proposed that myasthenia gravis was due to an autoimmune disorder. The recognition by Patrick and Lindstrom in 1973 of an experimental allergic myasthenia gravis after immunization of rabbits with purified AChR and the detection of specific AChR antibodies in 90% of patients with myasthenia gravis support this hypothesis.

A relationship between myasthenia gravis and the thymus gland has been appreciated since at least 1901. In 1912, Sauerbruch removed an enlarged thymus gland from a patient with myasthenia gravis who subsequently improved. In 1939, Blalock removed an enlarged thymus from a young woman with generalized myasthenia gravis. Encouraged by her response, in 1941, he made the important demonstration that removal of nontumorous thymus glands could lead to clinical improvement in patients with myasthenia gravis. His success stimulated subsequent investigators to examine the role of thymectomy in the treatment of myasthenia gravis. Although the role of the thymus gland in myasthenia gravis is incompletely defined, numerous reports suggest that thymectomy is an effective therapy. Studies in the authors' clinic have shown that the use of thymectomy as the sole method of treatment results in dramatic clinical improvement in many patients and suggests that a specific thymic factor contributes to the development of clinical weakness in myasthenia gravis.

CLINICAL FEATURES

Myasthenia gravis has a prevalence in the population of 1:75,000. There is a biphasic mode of distribution, with a tendency for populations of young women and elderly men to be affected. Women are involved twice as often as men, and in younger patients this ratio is increased to 4.5:1. The mean age of onset of symptoms is 26 years. Men tend to be affected at a later age and tend to have a higher incidence of thymoma. A genetic predisposition to develop myasthenia gravis is suggested by a high incidence of specific human leukocyte antigens (HLA).

Weakness and fatigue with activity are the hallmarks of myasthenia gravis (Fig. 30–1). Almost any muscle group in the body may be involved, and fluctuation daily in strength and even from hour to hour is common. Individual muscle groups may be selectively involved. Weakness tends to be more pronounced as the day progresses and after exercise. It may develop gradually or rapidly, and recovery

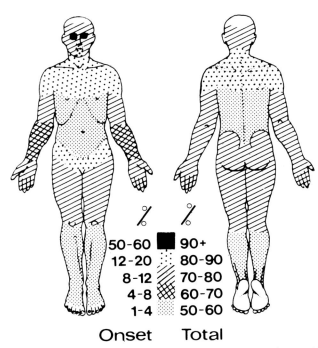

% / %

50-60 ■ 90+
12-20 ⠿ 80-90
8-12 ⧄ 70-80
4-8 ▨ 60-70
1-4 ░ 50-60

Onset   Total

Figure 30–1. Involvement of muscle groups in patients with myasthenia gravis at time of onset *(left column)* and during course of illness *(right column)*. (From Simpson, J. A.: *In* Walton, J. N. [ed]: Myasthenia gravis and myasthenic syndromes: Disorders of Voluntary Muscle, 4th ed. Edinburgh, Churchill Livingstone, 1978, pp. 585–624.)

may be total or incomplete. The ocular muscles are the most frequently affected muscle group and are the presenting feature in 50 to 60% of patients with myasthenia gravis and they are ultimately involved in 90% of patients. This is most often manifested by ptosis and diplopia and may be exaggerated by repetitive testing or sustained exercise. Ptosis may fluctuate during the course of the examination, and Cogan's sign (a downward fall of the levator palpebrae superioris after upward gaze) may be shown. Weakness of the orbicularis oculi is a frequent accompanying feature of ocular muscle involvement. Other cranial nerves may also be affected, which leads to potentially fatal complications such as dysphagia and respiratory distress. Impaired chewing, dysarthria, and nasal speech are particularly common in patients with late-onset myasthenia gravis. Facial weakness with a transverse smile and involuntary grimace may develop. The tongue may become atrophic with a characteristic triple furrow. Weakness of the flexor or extensor muscles of the neck may require that patients support their heads with their hands.

In the extremities, there is generally symmetric weakness, involving proximal muscles more than distal groups and the arms more than the legs. This pattern varies considerably, and in a specific patient, there may be asymmetric involvement, with any muscle group or even an isolated muscle being affected. The deep tendon reflexes tend to be preserved but may temporarily disappear with repetitive stimulation. The results of sensory examination are within normal limits, although patients may complain of nonspecific sensations. Autonomic system involvement with pupillary changes, bladder disturbances, and increased sweating have all been described but are uncommon.

The onset of symptoms may be insidious or sudden, spontaneous or precipitated by emotional stress, exercise, allergies, vaccinations, or pregnancy. Myasthenia gravis may also become manifest as prolonged weakness after the use of relaxant drugs and anesthesia during surgical therapy. Symptoms may be confined to the ocular muscles, but more than 80% of patients develop generalized weakness within 1 year of the onset of ocular disturbances. Grading systems to monitor clinical status are handicapped by difficulty in quantifying muscular strength and the variation that occurs in myasthenic patients, particularly after exposure to heat, exercise, stress, and drugs that interfere with neuromuscular transmission. The most widely used scale is the Osserman classification, which is given in Table 30–1. This is a clinical classification that is limited by its failure to consider dependency on medication or to reflect subtle clinical improvement, creating difficulty in monitoring response to treatment.

The incidence of spontaneous remission, without drug or other therapy, is not known but is thought to be uncommon and short-lasting and to occur in patients primarily with ocular involvement. The ultimate course cannot be predicted with certainty, and many variations, including spontaneous

TABLE 30–1. MODIFIED CLINICAL CLASSIFICATION OF PATIENTS WITH MYASTHENIA GRAVIS

Group I
　Ocular Myasthenia
　　Ocular muscles are involved, with ptosis and diplopia. Its form is very mild; no mortality is present.
Group II
　A. *Mild Generalized*
　　Onset is slow and frequently ocular, gradually spreading to skeletal and bulbar muscles.
　　Respiratory system is not involved. Response to drug therapy is good. Mortality is low.
　B. *Moderate Generalized*
　　Onset is gradual with frequent ocular presentations, progressing to more severe generalized involvement of the skeletal and bulbar muscles. Dysarthria, dysphagia, and difficult mastication are more prevalent than in mild generalized myasthenia gravis. Respiratory muscles are not involved. Response to drug therapy is less satisfactory; patients' activities are restricted, but mortality is low.
　C. *Severe Generalized*
　　1. *Acute fulminating.* Onset of severe bulbar and skeletal muscle weakness is rapid with early involvement of respiratory muscles. Progress is normally complete within 6 months. Percentage of thymomas is highest in this group. Response to drug therapy is less satisfactory, and patients' activities are restricted, but mortality is low.
　　2. *Late severe.* Severe myasthenia gravis develops at least 2 years after most of Group I or Group II symptoms. Progression of myasthenia gravis may be either gradual or sudden. The second highest percentage of thymomas occurs in this group. The response to drug therapy is poor, and the prognosis is poor.

remission in patients with long-standing disease or sudden deterioration in patients who have been asymptomatic for many years, have been recorded. A fixed myopathy late in the course of the disorder with permanent muscle weakness has been described. The authors have been concerned that this may be due to chronic anticholinesterase administration, but it has also been recorded in patients who have not received such medication.

A transient neonatal myasthenia gravis has been reported in infants of mothers with myasthenia gravis. Symptoms usually include diffuse weakness, impaired crying and sucking, poor swallowing, and, occasionally, feeble respiration. Symptoms are self-limited and generally resolve within 6 weeks. There are no clinical consequences as long as the initial symptoms are recognized and managed appropriately. Passive transfer of immunoglobulin across the placenta (presumably anti-AChR antibodies) is thought to be responsible. Interestingly, there is little correlation between the clinical status of the infant and that of the mother, despite comparable AChR antibody titers, supporting the hypothesis that host factors contribute to the development of clinical weakness.

A congenital myasthenia gravis that is more common in males has been described; it is often familial, but the mother is usually unaffected. The clinical configuration is usually not severe, and improvement occurs after 6 to 10 years of symptoms. Drugs and thymectomy are generally not effective. It has been postulated that a delay in the maturation of the neuromuscular apparatus results in a prolonged reduction of the safety factor for neuromuscular transmission. Another congenital myasthenic syndrome, due to a reduction of acetylcholinesterase in the subneural apparatus of the end-plate, has also been described. These patients do not have AChR antibodies and do not respond to anticholinesterase medications.

The myasthenic or Eaton-Lambert syndrome consists of weakness and fatigability of proximal muscles, particularly in the lower extremities. Ocular and bulbar involvement is mild or absent. Deep tendon reflexes tend to be depressed or absent, and there is a characteristic electrophysiologic abnormality on the electromyogram. This syndrome is usually seen in association with an underlying oat-cell carcinoma of the lung and may antedate recognition of the tumor. Less frequently, it occurs with other chronic disease states. The condition is due to the release of decreased quanta of ACh from nerve endings. Anticholinesterase drugs are less effective than they are in myasthenia gravis. Agents that facilitate the release of ACh from the presynaptic nerve terminal, such as guanidine, calcium, or 4-aminopyridine, may be helpful.

In general, the diagnosis of myasthenia gravis is not difficult to make if it is considered. Hysteria, thyroid disease, neuromyopathies, and other myasthenic conditions are occasionally mistaken for myasthenia gravis, but a Tensilon test, single-fiber electromyography, and determination of AChR antibody levels allow a definitive diagnosis to be made in most patients.

Associated Conditions

A number of conditions have been associated with myasthenia gravis. Many of these, such as rheumatoid arthritis, systemic lupus erythematosus, polymyositis, Sjögren's syndrome, and ulcerative colitis, are thought to be autoimmune. An association with vitamin B_{12} deficiency, thyroid disorders, diabetes mellitus, parathyroid disease, adrenal disorders, and vitiligo has been described as part of a polyglandular failure syndrome. These may be predetermined genetically, based on their linkage with histocompatibility antigens, particularly HLA-A1, HLA-B8, and HLA-Dw3. These may constitute genetic risk factors for autoimmune diseases by which a specific exposure triggers an abnormal immune response in a patient with a particular haplotype. This theory is supported by studies of monozygotic twins in which only one of the twins has been affected.

Thyroid dysfunction has been reported in 5% of patients with myasthenia gravis, and the overall incidence may be much higher. It may sometimes be difficult to distinguish features of thyroid disease from those of myasthenia gravis, because each can cause proximal muscle weakness and ocular disturbances. These conditions appear to be distinct, however, because it has been shown that increased quantities of thyroid hormone per se do not result in myasthenia gravis and that the relationship is more likely to be immunologic or genetic than hormonal. All forms of thyroid disease, including goiter, myxedema, Graves' disease, and Hashimoto's thyroiditis, have been associated with myasthenia gravis.

Thymic Abnormalities

Disorders of the thymus gland are found in 75 to 85% of patients with myasthenia gravis, and new staining techniques suggest that this incidence may be even higher. Ten to 15% of patients with myasthenia gravis have thymomas. In most cases, these are benign, well-defined, encapsulated lesions that may be cystic or calcified. They are generally composed of epithelial or lymphoid cells. However, two-thirds of thymomas have no association with myasthenia gravis and contain mainly spindle cells. Malignancy is usually defined by tumor infiltration into surrounding tissue such as pleura and pericardium rather than by changes in the histologic pattern. As many as 43% of thymomas were malignant in one series. However, in the authors' experience, malignancy is a rare occurrence, perhaps reflecting the tendency to do thymectomy earlier in the course of myasthenia gravis. Thymomas have not been described in children and are generally not seen before the age of 30 years. They are more common in male patients. A high-quality computed tomography (CT) scan of the mediastinum can detect almost all thymomas (Fig. 30–2). The authors have occasionally had a false-positive CT scan but have not failed to recognize a thymoma by CT scanning in the study in which all patients with myasthenia gravis have thymectomy, regardless of the interpretation of the CT scan.

Lymphoid hyperplasia of both the cortex and medulla is found in the thymus gland of most young patients with myasthenia gravis. The number of germinal centers may increase, but this is not unique to myasthenia gravis, and its significance is uncertain. Attempts to relate the numbers of germinal centers to the duration and severity of the disease and the response to treatment have been inconclusive. The T-cell composition of the thymus gland, in terms of both numbers and subsets, is generally normal. However, there is an increased number of B cells in the thymus glands of patients with myasthenia gravis.

Patients with late-onset myasthenia gravis (after the age of 55 years) most often have an atrophic involuted thymus gland. Occasionally, these can be recognized on CT scan by the existence of relatively low density (presumably fat) throughout the anterior mediastinum punctuated by dots of high density (presumably thymic tissue). There is evidence to suggest that an atrophic thymus gland may still be immunologically active, and thymic cells may be identified within the anterior mediastinal fat. This consideration is important with respect to the role of thymectomy in these patients. They have a relative

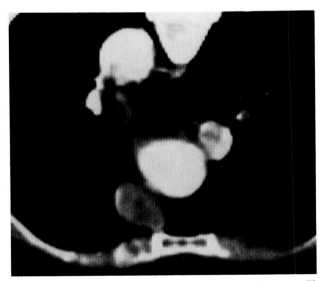

Figure 30–2. CT scan from a patient with a thymoma. The anterior mediastinal mass is easily visualized. With increasing experience, this test has become progressively more helpful in separating patients with thymomas from those with normal thymus glands and has even been able to identify islands of functioning thymus tissue within generally atrophic glands.

lymphopenia in the peripheral blood consisting primarily of a reduction in T lymphocytes and 3A1+ and OKT4 T-cell subsets. These changes are rapidly reversed after the removal of the "involuted" thymus gland.

DIAGNOSTIC STUDIES

Pharmacologic Agents

Anticholinesterase agents block the hydrolysis of ACh in the synaptic cleft, prolonging its action and increasing the likelihood of an interaction between ACh and the postsynaptic AChR. The result is an increase in the miniature end-plate potential and in the safety factor for neuromuscular transmission. These agents may reverse or improve the clinical and electrical abnormalities in myasthenia gravis. The most widely used anticholinesterase agent for diagnosis is edrophonium (Tensilon). This drug is short-acting and improves clinical or electrical abnormalities in 95% of patients with myasthenia gravis. Its use is widespread, and before more sophisticated laboratory evaluations, a positive response was central to the definition of myasthenia gravis. The response in individual patients differs from dramatic improvement, confirming the diagnosis, to subtle or no change. The ocular muscles are least sensitive to this drug and occasionally make it difficult to diagnose cases of myasthenia gravis confined to the ocular muscles. However, failure to respond to edrophonium does not exclude myasthenia gravis. It is recommended that the test be done at the end of the day or after exercise, when the patient's weakness is maximal.

Two to 10 mg of edrophonium are administered intravenously. The initial 2 mg may detect hypersensitivity so that the possibility of enhancing cholinergic weakness in patients receiving anticholinesterase medications may be avoided. Facilities to treat anaphylactic and respiratory complications should be available. A positive response generally develops within 30 to 60 seconds and lasts for approximately 1 to 5 minutes. It has been the authors' practice to do the edrophonium test in a triple-blind fashion with saline and nicotinic acid as control agents. Edrophonium generally causes a light-headed, hot sensation associated with lacrimation and flushing that patients may learn to recognize. Nicotinic acid reproduces some of these features without influencing neuromuscular transmission and thus serves as a suitable control substance.

Long-lasting anticholinesterase agents may be used when responses are too transient to record by standard bedside techniques. These agents have a longer latency and duration. Neostigmine may be used in a dosage of 1.5 mg administered intramuscularly. Improvement is seen within 10 to 30 minutes and lasts up to 4 hours. When the response is still

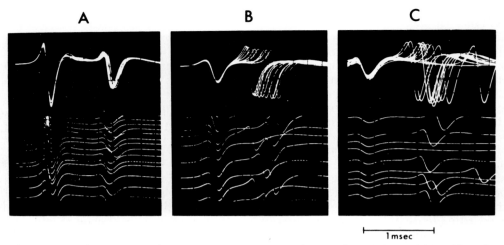

Figure 30–3. Electromyographic jitter recordings; traces are superimposed on top line. *A,* Normal jitter. Note the constant latency between the two muscle action potentials. *B,* Increased jitter but without impulse blocking in a patient with myasthenia gravis. *C,* Increased jitter with occasional blocking in a patient with severe myasthenia gravis. (From Stalberg, E., Trontel, J. V., and Schwartz, M. S.: Single muscle fiber recording of jitter phenomenon in patients with myasthenia gravis and in members of their families. Ann. N.Y. Acad. Sci., *274:*189, 1976.)

equivocal, a long-term trial of oral anticholinesterase agents over several weeks can be considered.

Patients with myasthenia gravis are highly sensitive to the neuromuscular blocking effect of curare and curare-like drugs. This heightened sensitivity has previously been used as a test to confirm the diagnosis. One-tenth of a curarizing dose may cause the patient to become significantly weak. An anesthetist must be present at this test because of the risk of respiratory decompensation and, consequently, this test is now rarely used.

An abnormal "dual response" after administration of decamethonium has been described, consisting of brief depolarization after a longer period of curare-like competitive block. Although interesting pharmacologically, this test is no longer used in practice.

Electrophysiologic Studies

The hallmark of myasthenia gravis is failure of neuromuscular transmission, which is characterized electrically by a reduction in the amplitude of the miniature end-plate potential. In 1895, Jolly recognized that faradic stimulation of a peripheral nerve resulted in muscle fatigue. He recognized that, in patients with myasthenia gravis, supramaximal repetitive stimulation of the nerve led to a gradual decrease of the evoked action potential without a change in antidromic conduction. The Jolly test consists of repetitive stimulation of a peripheral nerve. In normal patients, the safety margin is of such a magnitude that repeated stimulations can be tolerated to a rate of 40 to 50 per second. In patients with myasthenia gravis, abnormal diminution begins to occur at stimulation rates of 2 to 3 per second, particularly if these are done after tetanic contractions of muscle or the administration of regional curare.

This test has the advantage of being simple and inexpensive but, unfortunately, it is not particularly sensitive. Changes are not detected in more than 50% of patients with myasthenia gravis, particularly in the early stages.

The development of single-fiber electromyography has provided a more sensitive method of detecting impaired neuromuscular transmission. A single-fiber needle electrode is placed between two muscle fibers innervated by the same motor unit. The variation in the latency between the two action potentials is referred to as jitter (Fig. 30–3). The variation of neuromuscular transmission in myasthenia gravis leads to increased jitter or blocking of one of the action potentials in severe cases. Jitter measurements are abnormal in 95% of patients with myasthenia gravis if multiple muscle groups are studied. In patients with purely ocular symptoms, the frontalis or levator palpebrae superioris muscle should be examined. Jitter measurements must be analyzed in light of the clinical picture, because abnormalities can be seen in disorders other than myasthenia gravis. Because jitter is a function of the amplitude of the miniature end-plate potential, this test can be used to monitor the clinical course of patients with myasthenia gravis. Although it has the advantage of being sensitive in the early detection of myasthenia gravis, it requires expensive complex machinery and neurophysiologic expertise.

Stapedial reflex decay has been used as a diagnostic study in myasthenia gravis. Preliminary results indicate a high sensitivity in patients with ocular dysfunction, but results are less encouraging in patients with generalized weakness.

Serum Antibodies

A number of nonspecific antibodies have been described in patients with myasthenia gravis. These include antistriational, antinuclear, antithyroid, antigastric, antispermatogenic, and antineuronal antibodies.

The isolation of specific neurotoxins from the venom of elapid snakes such as cobras and kraits allowed the recognition of specific serum anti-AChR antibodies. Alpha-bungarotoxin, a specific neurotoxin from the banded krait, has been found to bind specifically and irreversibly to the active site of the AChR. This toxin can be used to measure the number of receptors, to purify receptors, and to assay for serum AChR antibody. The assay consists of the reaction between test serum and AChR antigen derived from human muscle that has been incubated with ^{125}I-labeled alpha-bungarotoxin. If serum AChR antibodies are present, they bind to the AChR and form a complex with the ^{125}I-labeled alpha-bungarotoxin, which is bound to an adjacent site on the receptor. Antihuman globulin then precipitates this complex, and the radioactivity in the precipitant allows for an estimation of the quantitative AChR antibody level. Serum AChR antibodies are present in 90% of patients with myasthenia gravis. These antibodies are highly specific for myasthenia gravis and have been found otherwise only after administration of penicillamine or inoculation with snake venom, but in no other disease state. Furthermore, AChR released from damaged muscle does not evoke the development of AChR antibodies. AChR antibody levels do not directly correlate with the clinical status of patients with myasthenia gravis, but patients with purely ocular disease tend to have the lowest antibody titers.

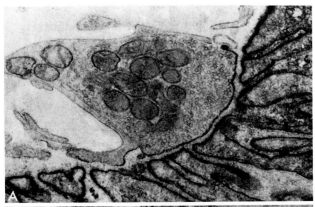
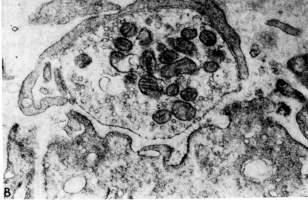

Figure 30–4. Neuromuscular junction with AChR stained by peroxidase-labeled alpha-bungarotoxin technique. *A*, Normal neuromuscular junction with normal quantity of AChR. *B*, Neuromuscular junction in a patient with moderately severe myasthenia gravis. Note the disorganization and destruction of the postsynaptic membrane, with reduction in staining for AChR. (Courtesy of A. G. Engel.)

PATHOGENESIS

Considerable evidence has accumulated since the original hypothesis by Simpson (1960) to support the concept that myasthenia gravis is an autoimmune disorder involving the postsynaptic nicotinic AChR. Histologically, the postsynaptic membrane is simplified and disorganized (Fig. 30–4). Alpha-bungarotoxin binding studies have shown quantitative reduction in the amount of AChR correlating with the reduction in the amplitude of the miniature end-plate action potential and the clinical severity of the condition. The detection of specific AChR antibodies in the serum of approximately 90% of patients with myasthenia gravis has focused attention on this antibody in the pathogenesis of myasthenia gravis. It has been postulated that these antibodies induce clinical weakness by reducing the number of functioning AChR, thus impairing neuromuscular transmission. Mechanisms proposed include (1) accelerated degradation of AChR on the postsynaptic membrane; (2) immunopharmacologic blockade in which the antibody hinders interactions between ACh and the AChR; (3) modulation or accelerated internalization with intracellular degradation of the

AChR-AChR antibody complex; and (4) reduced synthesis of AChR.

Passive transfer of serum, more specifically immunoglobulin (Ig) G from patients with myasthenia gravis to experimental animals, can induce a myasthenic syndrome characterized by clinical, electrical, and pharmacologic features similar to that of human myasthenia gravis. This syndrome may also be caused by specific monoclonal AChR antibodies. Passive transfer among animal species has been shown. Furthermore, IgG from patients with myasthenia gravis accelerates the degradation of AChR in myotube tissue culture. In human myasthenia gravis, plasmapheresis and steroids lead to clinical benefit in association with a reduction in the serum AChR antibody titer. The removal of thoracic duct lymph containing immunoglobulin also results in clinical improvement, and the readministration of this material results in rapid clinical deterioration. These observations support the hypothesis that AChR antibodies contribute to and may be the major mechanism responsible for receptor damage in myasthenia gravis.

Nevertheless, it is by no means clear that the AChR antibody is the sole factor responsible for clinical weakness. In studies at Duke University in which all patients were treated with thymectomy as the sole type of therapy and in which all drugs, including anticholinesterase agents, were avoided, dramatic clinical benefit was seen in most patients without a reduction in the AChR antibody titer. There was no direct correlation between the serum AChR antibody level and the clinical status of individual patients. The authors hypothesized that a thymic factor was essential to the development of clinical weakness in myasthenia gravis. This is supported by the development of transient neonatal myasthenia gravis in the infant of an asymptomatic thymectomized mother, with comparable levels and bioactivity of AChR antibody in each. Although steroids and plasmapheresis provide dramatic clinical improvement in many patients, the corresponding reduction in AChR antibody titer may be an independent phenomenon. It is presumptive to assume that this reduction is essential for clinical improvement, and clearly, more than AChR antibodies are removed by plasmapheresis. Furthermore, the reduction in the AChR antibody titer after plasmapheresis is often short-lived, whereas clinical benefit may persist for weeks or months.

Different AChR antibodies that react to different sites on the AChR have been identified, and it is possible that the current techniques fail to identify the specific subset that would better correlate with the clinical status of patients with myasthenia gravis. Furthermore, serum AChR antibody titers may not accurately reflect antibody activity at the neuromuscular junction. In the Duke drug-free group, no patient converted to a negative antibody titer after thymectomy, despite clinical improvement, and when antibody titers did fall, they did so gradually during a period of years rather than in direct correlation with the clinical status.

In an elegant series of experiments, Engel and associates (1977) showed deposits of IgG and C3 complement on segments of the postsynaptic membrane in the distribution of the AChR and on fragments of degenerating junctional folds in the synaptic space (Fig. 30–5). More severely affected myasthenic patients bind relatively smaller amounts of IgG and C3 complement, presumably because there are fewer residual AChR. The presence of C3 complement indicates activation of the complement reaction. Subsequent activation of the major or alternate pathway could then set the stage for a complement-mediated lysis of the membrane.

Sahashi and associates (1980), by using an immunoperoxidase method, showed the presence of the C9 terminal and lytic complement component at the postsynaptic junctional folds and in debris within the synaptic clefts in the same basic distribution as C3 complement. Once again, there was an inverse relationship between the structural integrity of the junctional folds and the abundance of C9. The areas of involvement were discrete and widely separated, supporting the concept of an autoimmune attack. C3

complement does not necessarily result in membrane damage and may be found over long portions of junctional membrane. Activation to C9, however, leads to irreversible damage to the membrane. Demonstration of C9 over only short portions of junctional folds and in abundance in the degenerated material of the synaptic cleft supports the role of the complement-mediated lysis as the mechanism of membrane damage in myasthenia gravis. This differs from other conditions such as Duchenne's muscular dystrophy in which degeneration of junctional folds occurs in the absence of IgG or C9 complement. It is possible that the AChR antibody marks the receptor for complement-mediated lysis, and some current evidence suggests that the thymus gland may activate the alternate complement pathway and may facilitate this reaction.

Although most attention has been focused on humoral immune mechanisms, cell-mediated immune mechanisms have not been excluded from having a role in the pathogenesis of myasthenia gravis. Studies in the authors' laboratories have shown a reduction in the number of peripheral blood T cells in patients with late-onset myasthenia gravis. This reduction consists primarily of T-cell subsets 3A1 and OKT4, and these changes normalize rapidly after thymectomy. Lymphocyte transformation has been described in several laboratories after exposure of peripheral blood and thymic lymphocytes to purified AChR antigen. This stimulation index has also been reported to be reduced after thymectomy. Alterations in mixed lymphocyte reactions and autologous lymphocyte reactions have been observed and are currently being studied. Although not a consistent finding, lymphorrhages, which are small groups of lymphocytes within muscle, are occasionally detected. All of these changes suggest that a cell-mediated mechanism has some role in the pathogenesis of myasthenia gravis, but its importance has not yet been defined. The possibility of multiple mechanisms and heterogeneous populations of patients must be considered.

Experimental Allergic Myasthenia Gravis

Using snake venom such as alpha-bungarotoxin, Patrick and Lindstrom (1973) were able to isolate AChR from homogenized muscle. Purified receptor was then injected into rabbits in an effort to provoke specific AChR antibodies. Several weeks after this immunization, the rabbits became weak and died. The weakness had clinical, electrical, and pharmacologic features resembling those seen in human myasthenia gravis, and this disorder is now known as experimental autoimmune myasthenia gravis. It is thought to be the result of AChR antibodies generated by immunization with AChR cross-reacting with the rabbits' own AChR, leading to impaired neuromuscular transmission. Histologic changes seen at the neuromuscular junction are similar to those seen

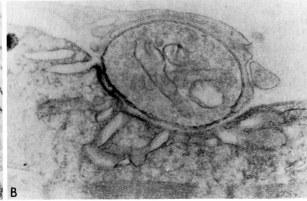

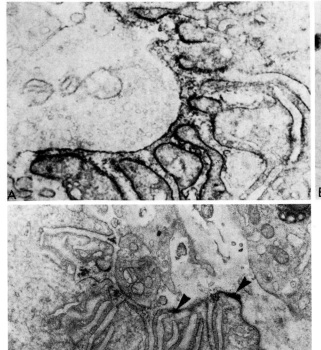

Figure 30–5. *A,* Ultrastructural localization of IgG in a patient with mild myasthenia gravis. Note the relative preservation of the postsynaptic region. *B,* Ultrastructural localization of C3 on postsynaptic membrane of a patient with myasthenia gravis. *C,* Ultrastructural localization of C9 at end-plates and on debris in synaptic folds in a patient with myasthenia gravis. *Arrows* indicate intense reaction for C9 over short segments of postsynaptic membrane. (*B,* from Engel, A. G., Lambert, E. H., and Howard, F. M., Jr.: Immune complexes [IgG and C3] at the motor end-plates in myasthenia gravis. Mayo Clin. Proc., *52:*267, 1977; *C,* from Sahashi, K., Engel, A. G., Lambert, E. H., and Howard, F. M., Jr.: Ultrastructural localization of the terminal and lytic 9th complement component [C9] at the motor end-plate in myasthenia gravis. J. Neuropathol. Exp. Neurol., *39:*160–172, 1980, Fig. 4-A, p. 166.)

in human patients, and passive transfer of serum or lymphocytes from these animals can induce the disease when injected into normal animals. An acute state occurs approximately 1 week after immunization and is characterized by severe muscle weakness and a cellular invasion of the neuromuscular junction with breakdown of the postsynaptic membrane and AChR. Approximately 3 weeks after immunization, a chronic stage develops in association with a rising AChR antibody titer. The postsynaptic membrane becomes decreased in area and simplified, with a consequent reduction in the total number of AChR. The chronic phase of experimental autoimmune myasthenia gravis is almost identical to that in the human disorder, but the experimental autoimmune condition differs from human myasthenia gravis in that the acute transient phase is not seen in human patients. This may reflect a differing nature of the immunizing event, with the human patient not being exposed to a massive bolus of antigen at one time, or differences in host response. It has also been suggested that the acute phase may be related to the adjuvant rather than the AChR.

Significantly, experimental autoimmune myasthenia gravis does not develop in animals that have been thymectomized before immunization. A thymic factor may be essential to the development of clinical weakness in this condition. Furthermore, C3 complement deficiency also attenuates the clinical and electrical features of experimental autoimmune myasthenia gravis and supports the hypothesis that

complement-mediated lysis may be the mechanism leading to membrane damage.

Role of the Thymus Gland

A relationship between the thymus gland and myasthenia gravis has been appreciated since the beginning of the 20th century. Seventy to 80% of patients with myasthenia gravis have pathologic changes in their thymus gland, and for 50 years thymectomy has been known to influence the clinical course of myasthenia gravis. It is therefore not surprising that thymic factors have been suggested to have a role in the pathogenesis of myasthenia gravis. The exact role that the thymus gland has, however, must still be defined. There are cells within the thymus gland (myoid cells) that have a striking similarity to embryonic muscle cells. These cells contain AChR on their surface and react with AChR antibodies. The thymic cells in culture can produce AChR antibody, and radiated thymic cells that have been thus rendered functionally inactive can augment the production of AChR antibody from peripheral lymphocytes. The thymus gland has a major part in lymphocyte maturation and is capable of influencing almost all humoral and cellular immune reactions. It has been proposed that an initiating event, possibly of a viral nature, induces a "thymitis." Because of the unique location of myoid cells in immediate proximity to maturing lymphocytes, an autoimmune reaction may develop directed against the AChR on myoid cells that later cross-reacts with AChR at the neuromuscular junction. The altered thymus gland might also generate a population of killer T cells, which destroy the neuromuscular junction, or a population of helper cells, which stimulate the production of AChR antibody by peripheral lymphocytes. More recently, it has been suggested that thymic factors may also have a role in activating the complement pathway leading to membrane lysis. The association of myasthenia gravis with other autoimmune disorders, particularly the polyglandular failure syndrome, suggests that the immunologic attack may be more widely directed than to the AChR alone in some patients. The relationship with HLA antigens in some patients with myasthenia gravis also suggests that there is a genetically predisposed population of patients whose immunologic tolerance may be altered in such a manner that a specific exposure results in altered immunologic responses.

The mechanism by which thymectomy leads to clinical benefit has not yet been elucidated. It has been shown that thymectomy influences cell-mediated immunity and peripheral T-cell counts in patients with late-onset myasthenia gravis, but the clinical relevance of this finding is not established. Thymectomy may serve to remove a source of (1) AChR antigen, (2) AChR antibody production, (3) sensitized killer T cells directed against the neuromuscular junction, (4) sensitized helper T cells that facilitate the production of AChR antibody by peripheral lymphocytes, and (5) a putative thymic factor that may activate the complement pathway leading to complement-mediated lysis at antibody-labeled receptor sites. It is also possible that thymectomy acts by multiple or unknown mechanisms.

Failure of thymectomy to induce clinical remission might be due to (1) incomplete thymectomy, (2) permanent irreparable damage to the neuromuscular junction, (3) a thymic influence exerted by extrathymic populations of lymphocytes within the spleen, lymph nodes, and so on that are unaffected by thymectomy, (4) the influence of long-lived peripheral T cells, and (5) heterogeneous disease mechanisms, by which the thymic influence differs in individual patients.

TREATMENT

Numerous methods of treatment have been used in the management of myasthenia gravis. Variations in the natural history and the lack of prospective control studies of the different treatment modalities prevent an absolute determination of the preferred form of treatment for a particular patient at the present time. Furthermore, it has been suggested that the natural history of myasthenia gravis as it is seen today follows a more benign course than that seen in previous decades. Improvement in supportive measures and surgical technique may contribute

to the improved statistics on patients, independent of the specific therapy chosen. The large number of variables to be controlled and physician bias favoring one form of therapy over another make it unlikely that a controlled study can be effected, and at least for the present, some judgment is required in instituting therapy.

The authors have favored total thymectomy done as early as possible after the development of generalized weakness. Drugs are avoided and used only when necessary rather than as a routine part of treatment. All patients are managed according to a prospective standardized treatment protocol to minimize variables and to avoid a physician bias. In the authors' practice, after a mean follow-up of 25.5 months, 87% of patients were free from generalized weakness, and 61% required no medication. The protocol does not compare thymectomy with other forms of treatment, but the excellent results and the possibility of avoiding additional medications lead the authors to prefer this form of treatment in patients with generalized myasthenia gravis. Before a more detailed discussion of thymectomy, the advantages and disadvantages of the major forms of treatment currently being used are considered. In each case, drugs that interfere with neuromuscular transmission (Table 30–2) should be avoided or used cautiously, because they may lead to a deterioration in the myasthenic status.

Medical Treatment

Anticholinesterase Agents. Anticholinesterase agents have been a standard form of medical treatment for myasthenia gravis since their introduction in the mid-1930s. They act by preventing the hydrolysis of ACh and increase the likelihood of interactions between ACh and the AChR. The safety margin for neuromuscular transmission is thus increased, providing temporary improvement in the clinical and electrical features of myasthenia gravis. These agents may result in considerable improvement with restoration of muscle strength. However,

TABLE 30–2. DRUGS THAT INTERFERE WITH NEUROMUSCULAR TRANSMISSION UNDER EXPERIMENTAL CONDITIONS

Antibiotics	*Psychotropics*
Amikacin	Amitriptyline
Paramycin	Amphetamines
Polymyxin A	Droperidol
Sisomicin	Haloperidol
Viomycin	Imipramine
	Paraldehyde
Antiarrhythmics	Trichloroethanol
Ajmaline	
	Others
Antirheumatics	Amantadine
Colchicine	Diphenhydramine
	Emetine
Anticonvulsants	Pindolol
Ethosuximide	Sotalol

this response is only symptomatic and these drugs in and of themselves do not lead to remission. Side effects of anticholinesterase drugs include abdominal colic, diarrhea, nausea, salivation, and lacrimation as a result of smooth muscle and glandular stimulation. These symptoms may be controlled by atropine. This is not recommended, however, because the symptoms may forewarn the patient and physician of developing "cholinergic crisis." Cholinergic crisis is the result of excessive stimulation of AChR with prolonged depolarization of receptors and consequent muscle weakness not directly related to myasthenia gravis. Cholinergic weakness can be differentiated from myasthenic weakness by administration of a test dose of Tensilon, because symptoms fail to respond or deteriorate after the administration of additional anticholinesterase medication. Treatment consists of discontinuation of anticholinesterase agents and appropriate support measures.

Neostigmine (Prostigmin) and pyridostigmine (Mestinon) are the most commonly used anticholinesterase agents. Neostigmine is available in 15-mg tablets, which are usually administered every 4 hours or more frequently when required. There is usually a 30-minute delay before maximal efficacy, and the optimal dosage is determined by trial and error. Parenteral administration of 0.5 mg is equivalent to 15 mg orally. Pyridostigmine is the more popular medication because it is thought to have a smoother effect and to be longer-acting, with a less abrupt loss of efficacy. Sixty milligrams of pyridostigmine is equivalent to 15 mg of neostigmine, and the time span of 180 mg is available for more prolonged use, such as at night.

Despite the popularity of these agents, the authors have preferred not to use them whenever possible. The symptomatic benefits that they provide may delay the introduction of early thymectomy, which is believed to be the preferred form of therapy. These agents increase bronchial and oropharyngeal secretions, which may lead to respiratory complications, particularly at the time of operation. Furthermore, after thymectomy, there appears to be an increased sensitivity to anticholinesterase medications, which may lead to cholinergic weakness, complicating the postoperative management. Thus anticholinesterase agents have been avoided in patients with thymectomy without an evident loss of clinical efficacy and with what appears to be a smoother operative and postoperative course.

Evidence in experimental animals indicates that chronic exposure to anticholinesterase agents independently leads to AChR damage and electron microscopic alterations identical to those seen in myasthenia gravis. Although there is no proof that a similar phenomenon occurs in human patients, there has been the concern that long-term use of these agents may lead to a fixed myopathic state unrelated to the myasthenia.

Corticosteroids. There have been many studies showing the beneficial effect of corticosteroids in patients with myasthenia gravis. The clinical response may be dramatic with total remission of symptoms, but it is important to appreciate that the introduction of steroids may be associated with a transient clinical deterioration (usually between the fourth and eighth days), and it is recommended that they be initiated in the hospital setting, where provisions for respiratory assistance are available. Prednisone has been most widely used, beginning with a dosage of 60 to 80 mg/day. Once an adequate response is obtained, patients are changed to an alternate-day dosage schedule, and the medication is gradually tapered as clinically appropriate. When an alternate-day dosage of 60 mg of prednisone has been reached, it is recommended that reductions in dosage should not exceed 5 mg every other day, no more frequently than once every other month, to minimize the risk of inducing myasthenic crisis.

Although many use steroids as a primary mode of therapy, particularly for patients with late-onset myasthenia gravis, the authors have preferred to use them only in patients who cannot or will not have a thymectomy or in patients who have had a clinically unsatisfactory response to thymectomy. Corticosteroids have also been used in a low-dose alternate-day schedule for patients with ocular myasthenia gravis or with residual ocular dysfunction after thymectomy. Corticosteroids have been used to prepare patients for thymectomy, but the same can now be accomplished with plasmapheresis without the risk of clinical deterioration and the difficulty in withdrawing steroid medication.

The mechanism of action of corticosteroids is not understood. Most attention has focused on immunosuppression. Several groups have reported a reduction in the AChR antibody titer that correlates with clinical improvement in patients with myasthenia gravis, raising the possibility that suppression of immunoglobulin is responsible for clinical benefit. However, studies of thymectomy as the sole treatment modality have failed to confirm a direct correlation between the clinical status of patients with myasthenia gravis and the AChR antibody titer. Although these studies suggest that an essential thymic factor contributes to the development of clinical weakness, the possibility exists that steroids and thymectomy act by different mechanisms. Steroids may have a thymolytic effect, although it is noteworthy that they may be effective in patients who have already had thymectomy. A direct effect on neuromuscular transmission has also been suggested by the transient deterioration during the off day reported by patients on an alternate-day steroid schedule.

Once steroids have been initiated, they may be difficult to discontinue. Although the dosage may be substantially reduced, in many patients steroids have to be maintained indefinitely. Aside from the risk of clinical deterioration related to dosage change, there are many side effects associated with sustained administration of steroids. These side effects include cataracts, psychosis, gastrointestinal bleeding, carbohydrate intolerance, hypertension, obesity, osteoporosis, growth failure in the juvenile population, and decreased resistance to infection. In one large series, as many as 50% of patients developed cushingoid features. Although the benefit of the steroids is not questioned, prospective control studies showing that they are superior to other forms of therapy such as thymectomy do not exist, and the authors have preferred to use these drugs only when necessary rather than on a routine basis in an effort to avoid these potential complications.

Plasmapheresis. Plasmapheresis is a technique that permits the selective removal of plasma or plasma components by a centrifugal method. The remaining red blood cells are then suspended in a solution such as lactated Ringer's solution and reintroduced to the patient. The procedure, which is easy to accomplish, produces a rapid transient clinical improvement in patients with myasthenia gravis and has proved to be a valuable method. The authors have used plasmapheresis primarily to optimize the medical status of patients before thymectomy. One to 3 liters of plasma is removed per run on an alternate-day basis until the maximal clinical benefit has been obtained (usually four to six runs). This clinical improvement facilitates the perioperative period while avoiding the need for additional medications. Except for occasional hypotension during the first or second run, plasmapheresis is generally well tolerated. Hypocalcemia and hypoalbuminemia may result from repeated runs and need to be identified and treated appropriately. Surgical intervention is not recommended within 48 hours of the last run of plasmapheresis to minimize the risk of bleeding and infection due to removal of clotting factors or immunoglobulins.

Plasmapheresis has been used in some centers as a primary therapeutic modality. Because plasmapheresis produces only temporary clinical benefit, immunosuppressive drugs must be used as well to obtain a stable clinical improvement, and it has not been established that plasmapheresis increases the likelihood of clinical remission compared with the use of immunosuppressive drugs alone. The authors have used this form of treatment only in patients whose symptoms are refractory to thymectomy or who have had acute deterioration after thymectomy.

The mechanism of action of plasmapheresis is presumably related to the removal of a specific plasma factor. The serum AChR antibody has been implicated because levels are dramatically reduced at the time of plasmapheresis in conjunction with clinical improvement. Clinical benefit, however, may persist for substantially longer periods than the AChR antibody remains depressed, and some patients respond to plasmapheresis who have no detectable serum anti-AChR antibodies. It must be emphasized that more than serum immunoglobulins are removed at the time of plasmapheresis, and the removal of additional factors may contribute to the improvement after plasmapheresis.

Immunosuppressive Agents. The evidence supporting an immunologic basis for myasthenia gravis and the response to plasmapheresis and thoracic duct drainage have fostered an interest in immunosuppressive drugs. Generally, these drugs have been used in patients who are refractory to more conventional therapies such as thymectomy or steroids. Azathioprine has been most widely used in a dose of 1.5 to 3 mg/kg. There is a latency period of 6 to 12 weeks before the onset of benefit, and maximal effect may not be obtained for 1 year or longer. European physicians have a wide experience with this drug and report favorable responses in the majority of their patients, although serious complications such as marrow suppression, gastrointestinal bleeding, decreased resistance to infection, and death have all been reported. The possibility of delayed side effects such as the development of malignancies must also be considered. Generally, the medication is well tolerated, although severe nausea, vomiting, and diarrhea have restricted its use in some patients. More potent cytotoxic drugs, such as cyclophosphamide, have not been widely studied, but there are occasional reports of benefit.

Immunosuppressant drugs may be more effective when combined with plasmapheresis, such as those described earlier. Antilymphocyte serum, antithymocyte serum, and splenic radiation have all been tried and have been reported to have some effectiveness in refractory cases of myasthenia gravis. Clearer delineation of the humoral or cellular immune mechanism directed against the AChR may allow more specific immunosuppression. Trials of monoclonal antibodies directed against the putative etiologic agents may be seen in the future.

Surgical Treatment

Thymectomy

Evidence suggesting the central role of the thymus gland in myasthenia gravis combined with the deficiencies of medical management has resulted in the increasing application of thymectomy in the management of myasthenia gravis. At Duke University Medical Center, thymectomy is used as the primary mode of therapy for myasthenia gravis. Patients with myasthenia gravis are considered for thymectomy as soon as possible after the development of generalized weakness. Plasmapheresis is used to optimize medical status before thymectomy if patients show significant weakness. Patients referred on anticholinesterase agents have these agents slowly withdrawn during plasmapheresis. It is rare to identify patients who cannot be withdrawn from anticholinesterase agents with plasmapheresis, and as a result, patients come to the operating suite without these supportive pharmacologic agents and consequently have a less complex perioperative course.

Patients receiving corticosteroids are maintained

on them throughout the perioperative period to prevent adrenal insufficiency; after this period attempts are made to gradually lower the dosage as tolerated.

Thymectomy should be done in an institution with an experienced treatment team. There must be a close working relationship between the neurologist, the anesthesiologist, the surgeon, and the intensive care unit personnel. When thymectomy is done under these conditions, the operative mortality should be below 1% and should occur only in high-risk patients with profound clinical weakness. Preoperative sedation may be given, but doses should be less than in patients without myasthenia gravis. Atropine is avoided. Most anesthesiologists use short-acting barbiturates for induction of anesthesia and maintain anesthesia with an inhalation agent. Succinyl chloride and curare are rarely necessary and are best avoided. Patients who have experienced significant respiratory difficulty or profound weakness before operation are generally managed with nasotracheal intubation, because it is more comfortable if ventilator support is required. When early extubation is anticipated, orotracheal intubation is used, which has the advantages of speed and avoidance of nasal mucosal trauma.

Surgical Anatomy of the Thymus Gland. Knowledge of the surgical anatomy of the thymus gland begins with an understanding of its embryonic differentiation. Human thymic primordium arises primarily from the third branchial pouch in close association with the inferior parathyroid gland, which affixes to the posterior side of the thyroid gland, whereas the thymus descends into the thorax. A portion of the thymic primordium may also develop from the fourth branchial pouch in association with the superior parathyroid gland. In the branchial complex stage, the pharyngobranchial duct closes and the communication between the pharynx and the thymus is loosened. Ultimately, the lobes of the thymus separate from the parathyroid glands and descend into the thorax. Controversy remains regarding ectopic portions of the thymus gland found in the neck, cephalad to the main body of the thymus gland. This thymic tissue may derive from the fourth branchial pouch along with parathyroid tissue. An alternative postulate suggests that this thymic tissue originates from the third branchial pouch but breaks off during its descent into the thorax. This complex migratory pattern of the thymus gland is thought to be responsible for the finding of ectopic thymic tissue in locations such as the left main bronchus, the parenchyma of the lung, the posterior mediastinum, and the hilum of the lung. This is shown in Figure 30–6A, which shows the branchial complex stage in which thymus is identified in close approximation to the cervical sinus and originating from the third branchial cleft before its descent into the thorax and before the formation of the gland from ectodermal cells surrounding the cervical sinus. In the definitive form stage (Fig. 30–6B), a separation of thymic tissue has occurred after migration of the thymic tissue from the third branchial cleft inferiorly, and residual thymus is identified superiorly in proximity to the superior parathyroid gland.

After the thymus gland has migrated into the inferior mediastinum, it relates to the major mediastinal structures (Fig. 30–7). It overlies the pericardium and great vessels at the base of the heart and is in

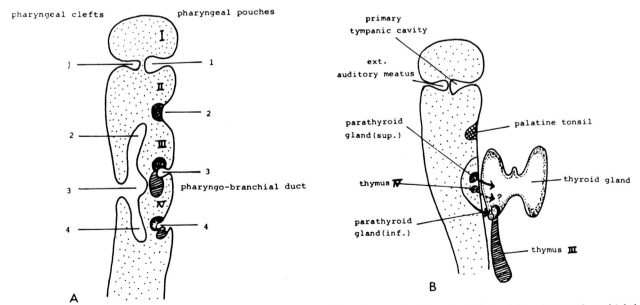

Figure 30–6. *A,* Primordial stage showing early development of the thymus gland in the vicinity of the pharyngobranchial duct and from the third branchial pouch. *B,* Definitive form showing later embryonic development of the thymus gland. By this stage, the close association of the thymus gland to the thyroid gland superiorly is shown as well as the overlapping anatomic areas for location of the parathyroid gland. Some minor controversy still exists regarding some contribution to thymic development from the fourth branchial pouch. (From Langman, J.: Medical Embryology, 2nd ed. Baltimore, Williams & Wilkins Co., copyright © 1969.)

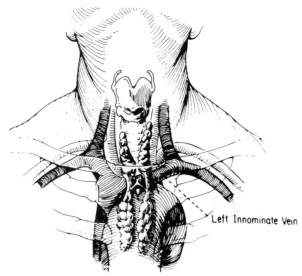

Figure 30–7. Location of the "normal" thymus gland in relation to other major intrathoracic structures. Of particular importance is the relationship of the thymus gland to the innominate vein. The draining veins from the thymus to the innominate vein are occasionally inconstant and may be a source of bleeding if not identified and carefully ligated. Occasionally, the thymus gland runs behind the innominate vein in proximity to the innominate artery. Various amounts of thymic fusion make the innominate vein more or less visible in the course of the dissection. (From Kark, A. E., and Kirschner, P. A.: Total thymectomy by the transcervical approach. Br. J. Surg., *58:*321, 1971.)

proximity to the left innominate vein. The thymus gland has an H-shaped configuration, with variable fusion of the right and left lobes at about the midportion of the gland. The superior poles of the gland are thinner than the inferior poles. The upper portion of the gland attenuates into the thyrothymic ligament, which connects the thymus gland to the thyroid gland. There are many variations in the regional anatomy of the thymus gland. It may lie posterior or anterior to the left innominate vein, and the superior pole of the gland may extend along the pretracheal fascia into the root of the neck. At the lateral extent of the gland, there is a fine capsule that separates it from the pleura and the parapleural mediastinal fat that lies proximal to the phrenic nerve. The arterial supply to the thymus gland comes from the internal mammary arteries via their pericardiophrenic branches. Venous drainage is through one or two large veins that drain into the anterior aspect of the left innominate vein. When the thymus gland lies posterior to the left innominate vein, drainage may be into the posterior portion of that vein. The thymus gland is largest relative to body size within the first or second year of life, when it may attain as much as 50% of its ultimate weight. The mass of the gland is usually greatest at the time of puberty and weighs 25 to 50 g. After puberty, there is gradual replacement of the densely packed lymphocyte architecture of the gland by adipose tissue, and in late life, thymic remnants may be detected only microscopically. Normally, there is a distinct thymic capsule that allows

its separation from surrounding mediastinal and cervical structures.

Some representative anatomic thymus configurations are shown in Figure 30–8. The degree of fusion and the extent of upper pole development vary to a great extent.

Surgical Technique. Various surgical techniques are available for the performance of thymectomy. The particular choice of technique varies as dictated by the personal preference of the surgeon and his beliefs concerning the pathogenesis of myasthenia and the role of thymectomy in the treatment of myasthenia gravis. Thymic tissue has been documented to be a normal component of perithymic fat, and if a diligent search for this tissue is made, it can be found approximately 75% of the time. Thymic tissue is frequently located in multiple sites within the anterior mediastinum, and thus the median sternotomy approach for thymectomy is preferred because it allows the most complete approach for total removal of thymic tissue. Surgical approaches for thymectomy include the following:

1. Transcervical thymectomy
2. Median sternotomy
3. Partial median sternotomy

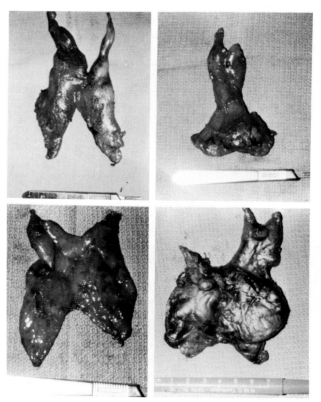

Figure 30–8. Operative specimens showing the broad range of anatomic variation in the normal thymus gland. The figure at the upper left represents the generally described "H" configuration. Other figures show greater fusion between the right and left portions of the gland, disproportionate development of the lower poles compared with the upper poles of the gland, and disproportionate development of one upper pole compared with the other pole. The number of upper poles varies, and careful anatomic dissection is required for complete removal of the gland.

4. Median sternotomy plus cervical incision

5. Upper median sternotomy combined with trans-sternal sternotomy

The technique of cervical thymectomy was initially described by Crotti in 1938, was reintroduced by Crile, and was extended by Kark and Kirschner. The technique is preferred by some surgeons because of the cosmetic incision, low morbidity, and minimal stay in the hospital. It has been advocated to be particularly useful in patients with significant respiratory distress and in whom no tracheostomy has been done. When cervical thymectomy is done, the patient is prepared and draped for a median sternotomy in the event of the occurrence of an intrathoracic complication requiring exploration or an unanticipated problem in removing the gland. The procedure is initiated by making a curvilinear incision approximately 2 cm above the supersternal notch and then extending this incision to the level of the strap muscles. After retraction of the strap muscles, the cervical fascia covering the thymus gland is entered, and the manubrium can be raised anteriorly. Special retractors have been devised that allow anterior traction to be placed on the sternum to facilitate the dissection. The thymus is mobilized from the innominate vein, and its venous attachment is divided between silver clips (Fig. 30–9). By traction on the upper pole of the gland, it is possible to continue mobilization, and the arterial supply to the gland is then divided by using electrocautery. Resection is generally limited to that portion of the gland enclosed within the thymic capsule. If the wound is dry,

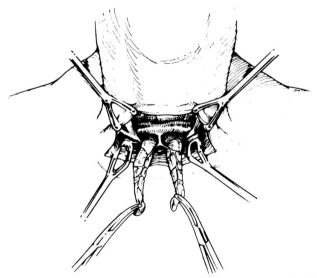

Figure 30–9. Transcervical thymectomy. The patient's head is at the upper portion of the picture and the figure shows the surgeon's view after retraction of the upper poles of the thymus gland to expose the venous drainage into the innominate vein. The use of specially constructed sternal retractors facilitates this procedure that generally results in removal of a good operative specimen, which is defined by the capsule of the gland. Thymic tissue in the mediastinum is more difficult to visualize and remove by using this technique. (From Kark, A. E., and Kirschner, P. A.: Total thymectomy by the transcervical approach. Br. J. Surg., *58*:321, 1971.)

drainage is generally not necessary. Inadvertent pleural entry can be treated by hyperinflation of the lungs as the deep tissue planes are closed. If the wound is not entirely free from bleeding at termination of the procedure, a small drainage catheter can be introduced into the superior mediastinum for several hours to a day to collect any residual blood. Advocates of this procedure generally cite remission rates for their patients comparable with those using the trans-sternal approach, although patients are usually preselected and the studies are neither standardized nor controlled. Further residual mediastinal thymic tissue has been found in up to 60% of patients after transcervical sternotomy. Recurrent myasthenia associated with significant amounts of residual thymic tissue and even thymomas have been reported after transcervical thymectomy. Although it is an aesthetically pleasing and technically feasible procedure, transcervical thymectomy achieves a less complete thymectomy than trans-sternal thymectomy. Although the importance of total thymectomy is unknown, there is concern that incomplete removal of the thymus may be associated with a higher recurrence rate of myasthenia gravis.

The initial concern with median sternotomy for thymectomy is related to impaired pulmonary mechanics after a major chest incision. Splinting of the chest, damage to the phrenic nerves, mediastinal infection, a higher pain medication requirement, a cosmetically less appealing incision, and postoperative pulmonary complications such as atelectasis and pneumonia have all been cited as disadvantages to the trans-sternal approach. Several factors have changed this situation. Patients are referred for thymectomy earlier in the course of their disease and tend to be less ill. Medical status can usually be improved by plasmapheresis before thymectomy so that even patients having respiratory difficulty come to thymectomy with good ventilatory potential. The better clinical state of patients before thymectomy has allowed early mobilization and has reduced the incidence of pulmonary complications after the procedure. For patients requiring tracheostomy, an incision can be used that is anatomically separated from the tracheostomy stoma and that minimizes the risk of contamination and mediastinal sepsis.

A composite drawing constructed from the work of Jaretzki and associates (1977), who did a careful anatomic and histologic examination of the mediastinal and cervical regions at the time of thymectomy, is shown in Figure 30–10. The normal location of the thymus gland is shown along with the variety of other locations for thymic tissue that were noted. The wide range of locations of thymic tissue in the mediastinum emphasizes the need for good exposure of both the mediastinal contents and the cervical extent of the thymus gland if thymectomy is to be attempted. This exposure can be obtained with a median sternotomy. In men, a short vertical skin incision can be made and can be mobilized adequately cephalad and caudad to allow median ster-

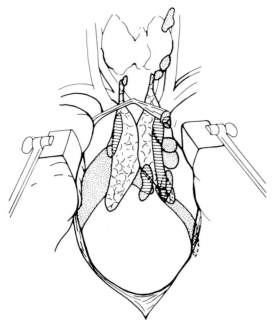

Figure 30–10. "Classic" location of the thymus gland. Based on the work of Jaretzki and associates (1977) the location of other thymic tissue is shown in the stippled or lined areas. Of particular importance is the location of thymic tissue deep in the lateral mediastinum and also superiorly in relation to the thyroid gland and frequently not in continuity with the remainder of the thymus gland.

notomy, sternal separation, and adequate cervical exposure by retraction of the skin. In women, a median sternotomy with excellent exposure of the superior extent of the thymus gland and the lower cervical region can be obtained by using supramammary or inframammary incisions that leave a cosmetically excellent scar. In these approaches, a curvilinear incision is made just over the breast and is extended inferiorly in the midline (supramammary incision) or beneath the breasts (inframammary incision).

By using skin hooks and electrocautery, it is possible to establish a bloodless plane of dissection that allows elevation of the anterior chest wall to well above the suprasternal notch superiorly and to the xiphoid inferiorly. The sternotomy is then done by using a saw and by taking care to remain in the midline of the sternum. This approach affords an excellent visualization of the thymus gland and its vascular attachments and is a cosmetically acceptable incision (Fig. 30–11). It also allows extensive removal of perithymic tissue and mediastinal fat.

The pleural reflections onto the thymus gland are pushed gently to the sides by blunt dissection. A plane is then established between the inferior aspect of the thymus gland and the anterior aspect of the pericardium. Starting in the midline and working toward the pleural spaces, each lobe of the inferior thymus gland is freed from its superficial pericardial attachments. As the gland gradually assumes form, gentle traction separates it from the

pleura. Efforts are made not to enter the pleural space, but if this occurs it is not a significant complication. As the dissection proceeds cephalad, the thymus gland is retracted superiorly to identify the thymic vein or veins on the posterior surface of the gland as they enter the left innominate vein. These veins are divided between silver clips, and the gland is separated from the innominate vein. Each of the superior poles of the thymus gland is then dissected from the surrounding fascial tissue until it is identified as an attenuated fibrous cord. Both fibrous cords are transected and the thymus is removed. This technique is shown in Figure 30–12.

Placement of a warm cotton pad in the anterior mediastinum for a few moments generally results in excellent hemostasis, after which a No. 28 chest tube is positioned in the mediastinum and the sternum is reapproximated. If the pleural space has been entered, the tip of the chest tube may be advanced into that pleural space, but a separate pleural drainage catheter is almost never necessary. Postoperative bleeding is usually minimal, and the tube can be removed several hours after the operation. The sternotomy wound is closed in layers, with a subcuticular skin closure.

Modification of Thymectomy for Thymoma. When the thymus gland appears to be unusually firm or is adherent to any of the surrounding structures, the surgeon should be highly suspicious that a thymoma is present. This may not have been appreciated in the preoperative assessment, even if CT scanning of the mediastinum was done. If a thymoma is present, infiltration into surrounding structures must be searched for carefully, because this is the major criterion for malignancy. Because there may be recurrences even after removal of a

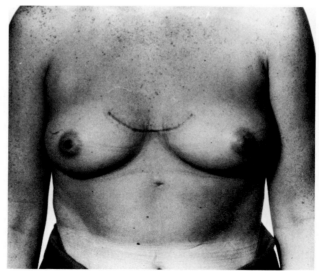

Figure 30–11. Cosmetic incision for median sternotomy in young women. The incision can be placed just on the superior surface of the breast as shown here, or it can be placed entirely in the inframammary region. In either case, the incision leaves an acceptable scar, and the resultant dissection allows excellent visualization of both the intrathoracic and cervical thymus gland.

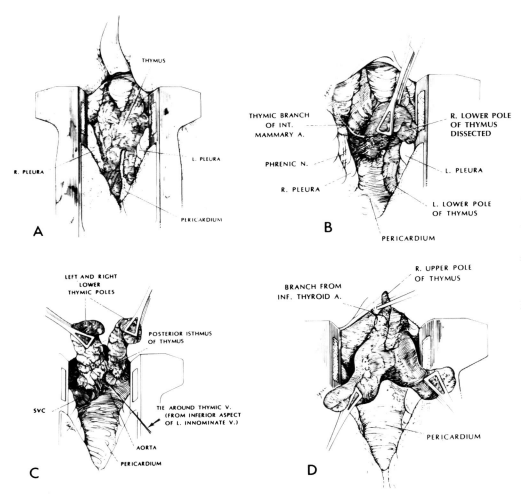

Figure 30–12. Procedure for removal of the thymus gland by using a median sternotomy. *A* to *D,* The important steps for safe and complete removal of the thymus gland. (From Wilkins, E. W.: Thymectomy. *In* Cohn, L. H. [ed]: Modern Techniques in Surgery. Cardiac/Thoracic Surgery. Mt. Kisco, NY, Futura Publishing Co., 1979.)

benign thymoma, a complete and careful dissection of the tumor mass is required. Care should be taken to avoid injury to the phrenic nerve; however, if it is incorporated within the tumor mass and complete resection is otherwise impossible, it may be sacrificed. Extensive involvement of the left innominate vein or of the internal surface of the pericardium is an ominous prognostic sign, and complete resection may not be possible. If a malignancy is suspected, however, an aggressive attempt at removal of the tumor is warranted, and removal of a portion of the pericardium, the left innominate vein, one of the phrenic nerves, and the pleural reflections should be done. Total surgical extirpation offers the best chance for long-term cure in cases of malignant thymoma. If removal of the tumor is impossible, radiation therapy is generally used, and the field can be better defined by marking the peripheral extent of tumor involvement with surgical clips. Frozen-tissue biopsies are of little help in diagnosing malignant thymomas because the determination of malignancy is primarily from the biologic behavior of the tumor.

Biopsy may, however, disclose the presence of cell types other than thymomas.

Postoperative Care. After thymectomy, the patient is returned to the intensive care unit to be observed by the physician and nursing team. The effects of the anesthetic agents are allowed to dissipate while the patient is supported with a ventilator, usually using intermittent mandatory ventilation at low-rate settings. The decision of when to extubate the patient is based mainly on the preoperative condition. In patients with disease of relatively short duration and mild symptoms, extubation is considered several hours after operation. Patients with more severe myasthenia gravis may require intubation for longer periods. Extubation is done when the patient is alert and shows a satisfactory vital capacity. The patient should be able to generate inspiratory negative pressure greater than 20 cm H_2O. After extubation, frequent measurements of vital capacity should be obtained by using a bedside digital spirometer. Patients must be watched carefully, because deterioration of ventilatory status may occur several days postoperatively. Preoperative preparation reduces the likelihood of prolonged intubation or subsequent ventilatory deterioration. The patient may be ambulated the morning after operation and, in most cases, is prepared for discharge within a few days.

Results of Thymectomy. Improvement after thymectomy has been reported in 57 to 86% of patients and permanent remission in 20 to 36%. This clinical improvement may be delayed from 3 to 5 years from the time of operation. Analysis of these data is hampered by differences in patients selected for operation, timing of thymectomy, choice of route, underlying pathologic conditions, and perioperative care. Furthermore, it is known that even without treatment, spontaneous remission may occasionally occur. There are no prospective controlled studies that allow comparison of the results of thymectomy versus medical therapy versus the natural history of myasthenia gravis in a particular population. Nonetheless, in reviewing most published articles, it has not been possible to find any reported series in which patients treated medically fared better than those treated surgically. A retrospective, controlled, matched, computerized study (Fig. 30–13) favored thymectomy over medical therapy with respect to remission and survival (Buckingham et al, 1976). It is difficult to determine which patients with delayed improvement after thymectomy might have experienced spontaneous remission without therapy. Although the data are confusing, it is the impression of most groups that the greatest chance for permanent remission is seen after thymectomy. In general, patients with nonthymomatous myasthenia gravis have better remission rates and long-term survival rates than those with thymomatous myasthenia gravis (Papatestas et al, 1971).

Only 10% of patients with a noninvasive thymoma are reported to have remission. When the tumor is invasive, remission is less likely, and more than 50% of patients die within 5 years. Most of these deaths occur in the first year after operation and are related to myasthenic complications. Because the primary feature of malignancy in thymoma is local invasion, the argument for early thymectomy has been advanced in an attempt to do thymectomy before the infiltration of surrounding tissues. This approach may result in a lesser percentage of malig-

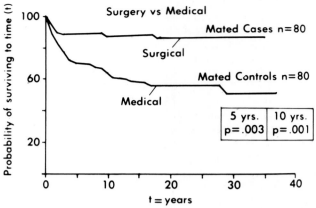

Figure 30–13. A matched, computerized, retrospective analysis of medical versus surgical management in myasthenia gravis. This work done at the Mayo Clinic provides the longest comparative follow-up for patients treated both medically and surgically in which the patients were matched for severity of disease as well as for their personal characteristics. The improved survival in the surgical group of patients was statistically significant at both 5 and 10 years, and this difference was maintained with additional passage of time. (From Buckingham, J. M., Howard, F. M., Bernatz, P. E., et al: The value of thymectomy in myasthenia gravis: A computer-assisted matched study. Ann. Surg., *184*:453, 1976.)

nant thymomas. The present ability to do thymectomy safely and to potentially avoid long-term drug side effects leads many experts to consider thymectomy as the treatment of choice for myasthenia gravis.

Eight years ago, a prospective management plan for patients with myasthenia gravis was established at Duke University Medical Center. All patients with evidence of generalized myasthenia gravis, regardless of severity, had thymectomy. Preoperative plasmapheresis was used to optimize medical status if necessary. Efforts were made to use thymectomy as the sole treatment modality and to use medications only if necessary rather than by routine. The results have been most gratifying and are indicated in Table 30–3. Thymectomy was not withheld because of age, and good results were obtained in all age groups with all types of thymic pathology. Residual myasthenic symptoms have been confined mainly to the ocular muscles. Forty-six of 47 patients were improved after thymectomy compared with their prethymectomy, preplasmapheresis state (mean follow-

TABLE 30–3. CLINICAL STATUS OF PATIENTS HAVING THYMECTOMY FOR TREATMENT OF MYASTHENIA GRAVIS IN THE DUKE MEDICAL CENTER SERIES

Before Thymectomy			No. of Patients After Thymectomy					
Clinical State	No. of Patients	No. Receiving Medication	Normal	I	IIA	IIB	IIC	Died
IIA	28	21	24	4				
IIB	9	8	4	2	3			
IIC	10	10	2	3	3	1		1
Number of patients receiving antimyasthenia drugs after thymectomy according to post-thymectomy clinical state.			1	1	3	1		

up 25.5 months). Thirty patients were functionally intact and free of generalized weakness at normal levels of activity. Nine patients had only residual ocular dysfunction. Thus 83% of patients were free of significant generalized weakness. The majority of these patients require no medication. Before thymectomy, AChR antibody titers generally correlated with the severity of the myasthenia. Postoperatively, there was no direct relationship between AChR antibody titer and clinical status, because AChR antibody levels did not change significantly, but there was dramatic clinical improvement in the patients.

Because the early results were encouraging, the series was continued and a second group of patients was analyzed (Olanow et al, 1987) in which 55 patients were treated for myasthenia gravis by using thymectomy as the primary therapy. None of these 55 patients were receiving long-term medical management for myasthenia gravis at the time of entry into the study and all patients were prepared for operation in an individualized manner by using plasmapheresis as the interim treatment modality when indicated. None of the patients had isolated ocular myasthenia and excluded from the study were patients with long-standing myasthenia thought to have a fixed neurologic deficit. Clinical status was assessed by using the modified Osserman grading system that was described earlier, and all patients were followed for at least 1 year. The mean follow-up for the group was 39.3 months.

Sixty-four per cent of the patients (35 of 55) were asymptomatic and had no functional neurologic deficit. Sixteen per cent (9 patients) had residual ocular dysfunction, but no generalized weakness. Thus 80% of the patients (44 of 55) were free of generalized weakness an average of 39.3 months after thymectomy. Ten patients continued to have mild generalized weakness, but none had residual bulbar dysfunction. Ninety-two per cent of the patients (50 of 55) were improved by at least one stage compared with their prethymectomy, preplasma exchange baseline status. Seventy-one per cent of patients (39 of 55) improved by two or more stages. Four patients did not improve, and there was one death related to management of an acute exacerbation with high-dose steroids, later development of a cushingoid state, and later pulmonary embolism. Thymic pathology included thymic hyperplasia, atrial thymic involution, thymoma, and thymic cysts. Improvement in patients was the rule regardless of the underlying thymic pathology. After thymectomy, drug therapy was avoided whenever possible. Fifty-five per cent of the patients (30 of 55) were not taking medication. Twenty-two per cent of the patients (12 of 55) required chronic prednisone therapy for generalized myasthenic symptoms and an additional 24% of patients (13 of 55) received low-dose, every other day, prednisone for management of ocular symptoms.

By using thymectomy as primary treatment for generalized myasthenia gravis, 92% of patients en-rolled in the series were improved and 80% were free of generalized weakness at the time of latest medical follow-up (mean of 39.3 months). Fifty-five per cent of patients received no medical therapy and 38% never received medical therapy in the course of their treatment. Particularly important for surgeons is the awareness that early use of thymectomy and avoidance of medical management avoided perioperative problems associated with the use of corticosteroid therapy. Specifically, slow wound healing, difficult postoperative management, and occasional postoperative deterioration seen in patients on steroid therapy were all avoided.

Previous series relating thymectomy to symptoms of myasthenia gravis have focused on the occurrence of pathology in the thymus gland and have considered involution to be an absence of pathology, but a normal consequence of aging. In evaluating patients with late onset myasthenia gravis, regardless of the mode of therapy, at the authors' institution, 10 of 11 patients had atrophic involuted thymus glands. Contrary to initial reports, there is accumulating evidence of immunologic competence even with atrophic involuted thymus glands. Thymic epithelial cells interspersed within anterior mediastinal fat stain for alpha$_1$-thymosin, which is an immunopotentiating peptide. Moreover, studies at Duke University have shown reduced numbers of peripheral blood T-cell subsets 3A1 and OKT4 compared with age-matched controls and patients with hyperplastic thymus glands. After thymectomy, these changes are corrected (Haynes et al, 1983).

Commitment to median sternotomy is still a consequence of the authors' belief that thymectomy may exert its beneficial effect by removal of a thymic factor leading to acceleration of the complement cascade that results in a complement-mediated lysis of the AChR previously marked by ACh antibodies (Olanow et al, 1981).

There has not been a prospective randomized study that compares the effects of thymectomy with the effects of other forms of management for myasthenia gravis. The Duke Medical Center study is unique in its use of thymectomy as the primary mode of therapy for all patients once they enter the program. It is difficult to compare these results with other thymectomy series, because in some institutions thymectomy is used only when medical management for treatment of myasthenia gravis has failed or when patients are suspected of having a thymoma. Because of the strict treatment protocol in the Duke series, no physician bias with regard to which patient should have thymectomy entered into the treatment decision. Rather than pursuing medical management, every effort was made to avoid the use of antimyasthenic medications. Optimization of the clinical state was by plasmapheresis without immunosuppression rather than with drug therapy when necessary. All thymectomies were done in a standardized manner, were radical in nature, and were done by the same surgeon. This approach showed that in most patients, thymectomy alone could result in dramatic and sustained clinical improvement without the need for additional medications. Moreover, reduction in the AChR antibody titer was not essential for clinical improvement. These observations support the hypothesis that a factor elaborated by or in the thymus gland has a role in AChR destruction. Further studies to identify, isolate, and characterize a putative thymic factor are necessary, because the identification of such a "thymic factor" could allow the development of special techniques to provide its removal or neutralization.

Because data continue to emerge relating the effects of thymectomy to the course of myasthenia gravis, it appears to be particularly important that a thymectomy that is as complete as possible be done. Assessment of long-term data should not be confused by uncertainty regarding the presence of residual thymic tissue.

Algorithms for Management of Patients with Myasthenia Gravis

Because of success with the ongoing treatment plans discussed in this chapter, a summary for the diagnosis and management of patients with myasthenia gravis is provided here.

As outlined in Figure 30–14, when a patient with myasthenic symptoms is examined, the first portion of the evaluation is a diagnostic phase, starting with a careful history and physical examination. One of the primary goals at this time is to determine whether the patient has myasthenia gravis or weakness associated with another clinical condition. The diagnosis of true myasthenia gravis is made by a combination of history, physical examination, and appropriate laboratory tests. The response to Tensilon, the Jolly and jitter tests, and determination of the level

of the AChR antibodies usually identify the disease correctly in more than 95% of cases. The patient is then placed in a subgroup according to functional classification, and careful distinction is made with regard to whether the patient has ocular or generalized myasthenia gravis. Many patients who seek the attention of a physician because of ocular symptoms have generalized myasthenia gravis but are unaware of it. Because the method of treatment for each type differs at this time, it is important to make this differentiation. Various laboratory tests are designed to determine whether there are associated conditions in addition to the clinical myasthenia gravis, and when present, these conditions are specifically treated. Radiographic studies are used to detect the presence of a thymoma.

Once the diagnosis of generalized myasthenia has been made, the therapeutic phase is entered, which is shown in Figure 30–15. In patients, who are thought to have isolated ocular myasthenia, a conservative treatment program is initiated, generally by using low-dose corticosteroids on an alternate-day schedule. These patients are followed carefully, because the majority develop generalized weakness and are then treated similarly to patients who initially present with generalized myasthenia gravis. In the authors' clinic, the primary treatment mode is thymectomy. For patients who are weak or who become weak when pharmacologic treatment is withdrawn, plasmapheresis is used to prepare the patient for thymectomy. If the patient's general condition is good, if weakness is not severe, and if there are no other contraindications, thymectomy is then done as the primary treatment. For those few patients with specific contraindications or reluctance to accept operation, medical therapy is used.

By using this overall treatment plan, the systemic complications of pharmacologic management of myasthenia gravis can be avoided or minimized.

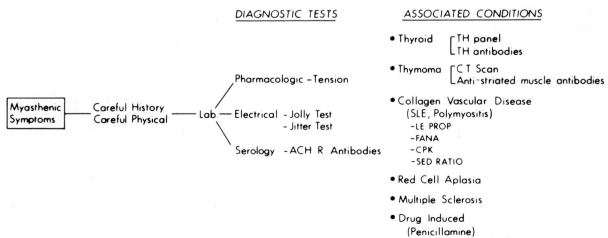

Figure 30–14. An algorithm for evaluating patients with myasthenia gravis. Identification of associated conditions is important for optimal management of patients with myasthenia gravis.

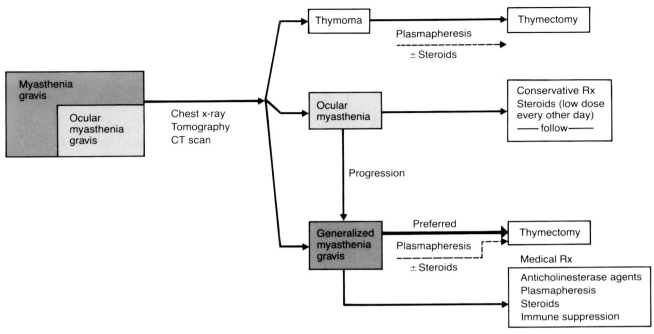

Figure 30–15. Therapeutic phase in the treatment of myasthenia gravis. The decision that isolated ocular myasthenia gravis exists is made only if careful single-fiber testing of peripheral muscles is entirely normal.

Thymectomy as the primary therapy for myasthenia gravis yields remission in most patients and allows reduced pharmacologic requirements in patients with residual symptoms after thymectomy.

Selected Bibliography

Blalock, A., Mason, M. F., Morgan, H. J., and Riven, S. S.: Myasthenia gravis and tumors of the thymic region. Ann. Surg., 110:544, 1939.

Blalock reports the first successful removal of a thymic tumor for the treatment of myasthenia gravis. He uses this case as the impetus for reviewing the literature and provides an excellent summary of the rationale for surgical extirpation of the thymus gland in the treatment of myasthenia gravis. The comments from the audience at the end of the manuscript are well worth reading.

Drachman, D. B.: Myasthenia gravis. N. Engl. J. Med., 298:136, 186, 1978.

This is a broad review of myasthenia gravis in which the disease process is discussed from the basic concepts of neuromuscular transmission to specific therapy. It serves as a good source of reference for the reader interested in pursuing certain areas of the subject in greater depth. It differs slightly from the views presented in this chapter in that treatment depends more on medical therapy and indications for thymectomy are more conservative.

Jaretzki, A., Bethea, M., Wolff, M., et al: A rational approach to total thymectomy in the treatment of myasthenia gravis. Ann. Thorac. Surg., 24:120, 1977.

This article is important for physicians interested in the surgical technique of thymectomy. The authors explore the completeness of thymectomy done by transcervical, median sternotomy, and combined transcervical and median sternotomy routes in a group of their own patients. There are extremely well done anatomic

drawings that show some of the atypical thymus gland locations encountered in the course of their clinical experience. There is also an excellent discussion that includes comments by proponents of other techniques of thymectomy and the reasons behind their arguments.

Lindstrom, J. M., Lennon, V. A., Seybold, M. E., et al: Experimental autoimmune myasthenia gravis and myasthenia gravis: Biochemical and immuno-chemical aspects. Ann. N.Y. Acad. Sci., 274:254, 1976.

This is a well-presented and comprehensive review of experimental work dealing with immune mechanisms in myasthenia gravis. It provides an excellent background for the understanding of current therapies designed to interfere with humoral and cell-mediated immunity.

Olanow, C. W., Wechsler, A. S., and Roses, A. D.: A prospective study of thymectomy and serum acetylcholine receptor antibodies in myasthenia gravis. Ann. Surg., 196:113, 1982.

This study, done at Duke University Medical Center, is unique in that every patient admitted with the diagnosis of myasthenia gravis was treated in accordance with a strict clinical protocol. For most patients, thymectomy was used as the primary and frequently the only method of therapy. High remission rates were reported with minimal reliance on drug therapy.

Bibliography

Abdou, N. I., Lisak, R. P., Sweiman, B., et al: The thymus in myasthenia gravis: Evidence for altered cell populations. N. Engl. J. Med., 291:1271, 1974.

Abramsky, O., Aharonov, A., Teitelbaum, D., et al: Myasthenia gravis and acetylcholine receptor: Effect of steroids in clinical course and cellular immune response to acetylcholine receptor. Arch. Neurol., 32:684, 1975.

Appel, S. H., Almon, R. R., and Levy, N.: Acetylcholine receptor antibodies in myasthenia gravis. N. Engl. J. Med., 293:760, 1975.

Argov, Z., and Mastaglia, F. L.: Disorders of neuro-muscular transmission caused by drugs. N. Engl. J. Med., *301*:409, 1979.

Castleman, B.: The pathology of the thymus gland in myasthenia gravis. Ann. N.Y. Acad. Sci., *135*:496, 1966.

Chang, C. C., Chen, T. F., and Chuang, S. -T.: Influence of chronic neostigmine treatment on the number of acetylcholine receptors and the release of acetylcholine from the rat diaphragm. J. Physiol., *230*:613, 1973.

Dau, P. C., Lindstrom, J. M., Cassel, C. K., et al: Plasmapheresis and immunosuppressive drug therapy in myasthenia gravis. N. Engl. J. Med., *297*:1134, 1977.

Drachman, D. B.: Myasthenia gravis. N. Engl. J. Med., *298*:136, 186, 1978.

Drachman, D. B., Kao, I., Pestronk, A., et al: Myasthenia gravis as a receptor disorder. Ann. N.Y. Acad. Sci., *274*:226, 1976.

Early thymectomy for myasthenia gravis (Editorial.) Br. Med. J., *3*:262, 1975.

Emeryk, B., and Strugalska, M. H.: Evaluation of results of thymectomy in myasthenia gravis. J. Neurol., *211*:155, 1976.

Frambrough, D. M., Drachman, D. B., and Satyamurti, S.: Neuromuscular junction in myasthenia gravis: Decreased acetylcholine receptors. Science, *182*:293, 1973.

Genkins, G., Papatestas, A. E., Horowitz, S. H., et al: Studies in myasthenia gravis. Early thymectomy: Electrophysiologic and pathologic correlations. Am. J. Med., *58*:517, 1975.

Goldman, A. J., Hermann, C., Jr., Keesey, J. C., et al: Myasthenia gravis and invasive thymoma: A 20-year experience. Neurology, *25*:1021, 1975.

Haynes, B. F., Harden, E. A., Olanow, C. W., et al: Effective thymectomy on peripheral lymphocytes subsets in myasthenia gravis: Selective effect on T-cells in patients with thymic atrophy. J. Immunol., *131*:773, 1983.

Jaretzki, A., Bethea, M., Wolff, M., et al: A rational approach to total thymectomy in the treatment of myasthenia gravis. Ann. Thorac. Surg., *24*:120, 1977.

Koelle, G. B.: Anticholinesterase agents. *In* Goodman, L. S., and Gilman, A. (eds): The Pharmacological Basis of Therapeutics, 5th ed. New York, Macmillan Company, 1975, pp. 445–466.

Langman, J.: Medical Embryology. Baltimore, Williams & Wilkins Co., 1969.

Legg, M. A., and Brady, W. J.: Pathology and clinical behavior of thymomas: A survey of 51 cases. Cancer, *18*:1131, 1965.

Lindstrom, J. M., Lennon, V. A., Seybold, M. E., et al: Experimental autoimmune myasthenia gravis and myasthenia gravis: Biochemical and immuno-chemical aspects. Ann. N.Y. Acad. Sci., *274*:254, 1976.

Matell, G., Bergstrom, K., Franksson, C., et al: Effects of some immuno-suppressive procedures on myasthenia gravis. Ann. N.Y. Acad. Sci., *274*:659, 1976.

Mittag, T., Kornfeld, P., Tormay, A., et al: Detection of antiacetylcholine receptor factors in serum and thymus from patients with myasthenia gravis. N. Engl. J. Med., *294*:691, 1976.

Mulder, D. G., Hermann, C., and Buckberg, G. D.: Effect of thymectomy in patients with myasthenia gravis: A sixteen year experience. Am. J. Surg., *128*:202, 1974.

Namba, T., Brown, S. B., and Grob, D.: Neonatal myasthenia gravis: Report of two cases and review of the literature. Pediatrics, *45*:488, 1970.

Olanow, C. W., Wechsler, A. S., and Roses, A. D.: A prospective study of thymectomy and serum acetylcholine receptor antibodies in myasthenia gravis. Ann. Surg., *196*:113, 1982.

Olanow, C. W., Wechsler, A. S., Sirotkin-Roses, M., et al: Thymectomy as primary therapy in myasthenia gravis. Ann. N.Y. Acad. Sci., *505*:595, 1987.

Papatestas, A. E., Alpert, L. I., Osserman, K. E., et al: Studies in myasthenia gravis. Effects of thymectomy: Results on 185 patients with nonthymomatous and thymomatous myasthenia gravis, 1941–1969. Am. J. Med., *50*:465, 1971.

Papatestas, A. E., Genkins, G., Horowitz, S. H., et al: Thymectomy in myasthenia gravis: Pathologic, clinical, and electrophysiologic correlations. Ann. N.Y. Acad. Sci., *274*:555, 1976.

Pinching, A. J., Peters, D. K., and Newsom, D. J.: Remission of myasthenia gravis following plasma-exchange. Lancet, *2*:1373, 1976.

Roses, A. D., Olanow, C. W., McAdams, M. W., and Lane, R. J. M.: There is no direct correlation between serum antiacetylcholine receptor and antibody levels and the clinical status of individual patients with myasthenia gravis. Neurology, *31*:220, 1981.

Rowland, L. P.: Controversies about the treatment of myasthenia gravis. J. Neurol. Neurosurg. Psych., *43*:644, 1980.

Stalberg, E., Trontel, J. V., and Schwartz, M. S.: Single muscle fiber recording of jitter phenomenon in patients with myasthenia gravis and in members of their families. Ann. N.Y. Acad. Sci., *274*:189, 1976.

van der Geld, H. W. R., and Strauss, A. J. L.: Myasthenia gravis: Immunological relationship between striated muscle and thymus. Lancet, *1*:57, 1966.

Wechsler, A. S., and Olanow, C. W.: Myasthenia gravis. Surg. Clin. North Am., *60*:946, 1980.

CHAPTER 31

SPECIAL DIAGNOSTIC AND THERAPEUTIC PROCEDURES IN CARDIAC SURGERY

I CARDIAC CATHETERIZATION, ANGIOGRAPHY, AND BALLOON VALVULOPLASTY

Thomas M. Bashore
Charles J. Davidson

HISTORICAL ASPECTS

Modern cardiac catheterization and angiography, like many advances in science, owes its origin and maturation to the merging of technologic advances on several fronts. The roots of cardiac catheterization lie in the development of x-ray equipment, contrast media, appropriate catheters, and a safe method of cannulating the vascular system.

Roentgen's discovery of the x-ray in 1895 quickly led to a surge of articles describing its use. The first angiogram (of a hand) was reported by Haschek and Lindenthol (1896), and in the same year Williams (1896) noted the pulsatile action of the heart on a newly developed fluoroscopic screen. X-ray motion pictures required the development of the motion picture concept and improved x-ray techniques. This advancement was highlighted by the development of a 16-mm cine camera in 1937 (Stewart et al, 1937) and a modern roll-film changer in 1953 (Rigler and Watson, 1953). Developmental changes continue today, and in the future there will likely be routine use of computerized storage of x-ray information in a digital format and the gradual shift from a cine-film-based medium to a computer-based system.

Paralleling the development of appropriate x-ray techniques was the discovery that the vascular system could be safely invaded using catheter systems. In the year 1929, the first human catheterization was done by Forssmann in a classic story of medical intrigue that was reviewed by Warren (1980). When Forssmann described his plan to pass a urethral catheter from his arm to his right atrium, his super-

visors intervened and refused to give him permission to do so. By enlisting the assistance of nurse Ditzen, he manipulated her into believing that he would use her for the first attempt at catheterization. She allowed him access to the venesection instruments in the surgical suite. After securing her, under the pretext that the local anesthesia might cause her to collapse, he inserted the urethral catheter into his own arm, then he walked to the basement, where an x-ray film was taken to show the catheter in his heart.

Others gradually realized the merit in Forssmann's adventure. Klein (1930) reported 11 patients in whom cardiac output was measured. Activity increased in the 1940s stimulated by the work of Cournand and Richards at Bellevue Hospital in New York. In 1956, Forssmann, Cournand, and Richards received the Nobel Prize in Medicine for their pioneering efforts.

Many other investigators contributed to the early development of cardiac catheterization. Brannon and associates (1948) described the findings in a patient with an atrial septal defect. In the laboratory of Dexter and colleagues (Hellems, 1949), the pulmonary capillary wedge was identified, and Zimmerman (1950) described the first left-sided heart catheterization in humans.

Left-sided heart catheterization continued to pose a formidable challenge, and numerous approaches were tried. These attempts included left atrial puncture during bronchoscopy (Facquet et al, 1952), a posterior transthoracic approach (Bjork et al, 1953), a suprasternal method (Radner, 1954), a left subcostal technique (Brock et al, 1956), and puncture

995

of the interatrial septum (Cope, 1959). The breakthrough in this area occurred when Seldinger described a method of percutaneous needle puncture with catheter exchange over a guidewire (Seldinger, 1953)—a modification of which is in general use today. Thus, retrograde left-sided heart catheterization became the standard.

Visualization of the coronary arteries posed problems and required innovative approaches. In humans, Radner (1945) is generally credited with first visualizing the coronary arteries with contrast media, and in 1962, Sones and colleagues described a practical method of selectively cannulating those arteries. The initial data of the Sones method that used a cutdown for isolation of the brachial artery were reported in 1962. By using the percutaneous femoral approach, Ricketts and Abrams (1962) suggested that a preformed catheter might be used. These were subsequently modified by Judkins (1967) and by Amplatz (1967). Other modifications, such as that by Schoonmaker and King (1974), are also used today.

The next advance in catheter design came in 1970 when balloon-tip catheters that could be inserted without fluoroscopy were introduced (Swan and Ganz, 1970). In the 1980s there has been a resurgence in catheter design and innovation with the advent of interventional cardiac catheter techniques. Newer catheter design allows the routine acquisition of myocardial biopsies (Mason, 1978), the performance of coronary angioplasty (Gruntzig et al, 1979), or percutaneous valvuloplasty (Cribier et al, 1986). Investigators currently are also exploring the use of laser technology to ''vaporize'' coronary artery plaques (Sanborn et al, 1987), ''Roto-Rooter'' atherectomy devices to drill open obstructed vessels (Perez, 1988), and intraluminal stents to maintain patency of vessels after these procedures (Sigwart et al, 1987).

The final step in the maturation of modern cardiac catheterization procedures was accomplished with the development of a safe x-ray contrast agent. Forssmann (1931) showed that a bolus of sodium iodomethamate (Uroselectan B) could be injected in the right atrium with only dizziness resulting. Other attempts to obtain x-ray contrast included notable methods such as using buckshot, air, bismuth and oil, potassium iodide, and so on (Miller, 1984). In the 1950s, the development of a safe, tri-iodinated benzoic acid contrast medium allowed a substantial reduction in contrast reactions with improved absorbance of the x-ray photons. Newer nonionic and low ionic contrast media that have been shown to be even safer (Bettman et al, 1984) than the diatrizoate compounds that have become the standard contrast agent have been introduced in the 1980s.

INDICATIONS FOR DIAGNOSTIC CARDIAC CATHETERIZATION

Diagnostic cardiac catheterization is indicated in almost all adult patients who have cardiac operative therapy (with few exceptions). The operating room is not the proper setting for diagnosing the severity of valvular or coronary lesions, because visual inspection or palpation cannot be expected to define disease severity adequately and reliably.

As with any diagnostic procedure, the decision to recommend cardiac catheterization is based on an appropriate risk-benefit ratio. Generally, diagnostic cardiac catheterization is recommended whenever it is clinically important to define the presence or severity of a suspected cardiac lesion. Because the mortality from cardiac catheterization is approximately 0.1% in most laboratories, there are few patients who cannot be studied safely in an active laboratory.

The indications for cardiac catheterization are changing and are likely to continue to evolve. The trend during the last 10 years in the United States has been in two broad directions. At the one extreme, many seriously ill and hemodynamically unstable patients are being studied during acute myocardial ischemia. At the other end of the spectrum, more and more studies are being done in an outpatient setting. The result has been the expansion of traditional indications for cardiac catheterization to include both the critically ill patients and the ambulatory patients.

Cardiac catheterization should be considered to be a diagnostic test to be used in combination with other complementary diagnostic tests in cardiology. For example, although coronary angiography is still the basis for defining the presence and severity of coronary disease (despite the substantial inaccuracy and variation of visual estimates of the severity of disease) (Marcus et al, 1988), the role of pharmacologic or exercise stress in defining the functional significance of anatomic lesions should not be overlooked when making clinical decisions. Cardiac catheterization in valvular or congenital heart disease is, likewise, best done with full knowledge of the echocardiographic and any other functional information. In this manner, catheterization can be directed, simplified, and shortened by not obtaining redundant anatomic information.

Identification and description of *coronary artery disease* are the most common indications for cardiac catheterization in adults. The information is crucial to the care of patients with various chest-pain syndromes. In addition, the presence of dynamic (e.g., spasm, thrombosis) coronary vascular lesions can be identified, as well as quantification of the consequence of coronary heart disease (e.g., the presence of ischemic valvular regurgitation or left ventricular aneurysm formation). In this era of active catheter intervention in coronary disease, many patients are being studied during myocardial infarction and others are being assessed in the early period after acute myocardial injury. The aggressiveness of individual centers in approaching these patients depends on local facilities and treatment philosophies as well as the availability of appropriate therapy and surgical support.

In patients with *myocardial disease*, cardiac catheterization provides useful information. In addition to identifying the etiologic role of coronary disease in patients with cardiomyopathy, cardiac catheterization permits detection of the presence of an active myocarditis by endomyocardial biopsy, quantification of the severity of both diastolic and systolic dysfunction, differentiation of myocardial restriction from pericardial constriction, assessment of the extent of valvular regurgitation, and observation of the response to acute pharmacologic intervention.

In patients with *valvular heart disease*, cardiac catheterization provides both confirmatory and complementary data to echocardiography and Doppler studies. The authors believe that only rarely should patients with valvular heart disease have cardiac surgical procedures without cardiac catheterization data available, despite controversy suggesting otherwise (St. John Sutton, 1981). There is agreement with Roberts' (1982) and Rahimtoola's (1982) editorial responses that the risk-benefit ratio of preoperative cardiac catheterization in these patients is weighted heavily in favor of cardiac catheterization. Catheterization may be unnecessary in some clinical situations, such as in patients with an atrial myxoma or young patients with endocarditis, acute mitral regurgitation, or acute aortic insufficiency. Nevertheless, additional confirmation of the severity of the valvular lesion, identification of associated coronary disease, quantification of the hemodynamic consequences of the valvular lesions, and occasionally the acute hemodynamic response to pharmacologic therapy all provide useful preoperative information that allows a safer and more directed surgical approach.

Finally, the role of cardiac catheterization in certain *congenital disease* states is less well defined, with the steady improvement in the accuracy and reliability of echo-Doppler techniques and the maturation of color-flow Doppler. Because gross cardiac anatomy can generally be well defined by echocardiographic methods, catheterization need only be done if certain hemodynamic information (e.g., shunt size or pulmonary vascular resistance) is important to the surgical procedure or if catheter interventional methods are contemplated. In children, it is particularly important that catheterization information be obtained in combination with the noninvasive data to avoid redundancy of data acquisition.

COMPLICATIONS ASSOCIATED WITH CARDIAC CATHETERIZATION

The overall risks of cardiac catheterization are difficult to define because of wide discrepancies in the methods used to collect this information and because of the recent advances in the procedure itself (such as the introduction of nonionic radiographic contrast or the use of the percutaneous brachial artery approach compared with brachial artery cutdown). For the purpose of this discussion, two large multi-

center trials, the American Heart Association's Cooperative Study on cardiac catheterization (Braunwald and Swan, 1968) and the Society of Cardiac Angiography's Registry (Kennedy, 1982) are considered representative. The former study was a prospective evaluation of 16 laboratories during a 2-year period that included 12,367 patients (only 3,312 had coronary angiography) and was published in 1968. The latter study was a registry report from 66 laboratories over a 14-month period that included 53,581 patients (41,204 had coronary angiography) and was published in 1982. Two studies evaluating the risk of coronary angiography are also available—a survey by Adams (1973) of 46,904 patients and the report from the Collaborative Study of Coronary Artery Surgery that included 7,553 prospectively studied patients reported in 1979 (Davis et al, 1979). The major complications reported in each of these studies are shown in Table 31–1.

Death from cardiac catheterization ranges from 0.14 to 0.75% depending on the population of patients and the era. The Registry report analyzed the characteristics of patients at highest risk for death, and these data are summarized in Table 31–2. The highest-risk patients in the adult population are those with significant disease in the left main coronary artery and poor left ventricular function. In addition, the extremes of age and the presence of associated valvular disease increase the observed risk of mortality during cardiac catheterization.

The risk of myocardial infarction varies from 0.07 to 0.06%, cerebrovascular accidents from 0.03 to 0.2%, and significant bradyarrhythmias or tachyarrhythmias from 0.56 to 1.3%. Reports of local arterial problems have varied widely, and most series suggest a slightly higher incidence of complications when the brachial approach is used. Women appear more likely to incur vascular complications than men (Bourassa and Noble, 1976). Local complications include thrombosis, subcutaneous hematoma formation (occasionally extensive), recurrent bleeding, pseudoaneurysm formation, and, rarely, cellulitis or phlebitis. Systemic reactions vary from mild vasovagal responses to severe vagal discharges that lead to cardiac arrest. Hypotension may also occur as a result

TABLE 31–1. COMPLICATIONS OF CARDIAC CATHETERIZATION

	Overall Complications		Coronary Angiography	
	Cooperative Study	*SCA* Registry*	*Adams Survey*	*CASS† Study*
Year reported	1968	1982	1973	1979
No. patients	12,367	53,581	46,904	7,553
Death	0.75%	0.14%	0.45%	0.2%
Myocardial infarction	NA	0.07%	0.61%	0.25%
Stroke	0.2%	0.07%	0.23%	0.03%
Vascular	0.3%	0.56%	NA	0.7%
Arrhythmias	1.3%	0.56%	0.77%	0.63%

*SCA = Society of Cardiac Angiography.
†CASS = Collaborative Study of Coronary Artery Surgery.

TABLE 31–2. HIGH-RISK PROFILE FOR MORTALITY FROM CARDIAC CATHETERIZATION

Parameter	%
Overall mortality	0.14
Age	
< 1 year	1.75
> 60 years	0.25
Coronary Disease	
One-vessel disease	0.03
Three-vessel disease	0.16
Left main disease	0.86
Heart failure	
NYHA* FC† I or II	0.02
NYHA FC III	0.12
NYHA FC IV	0.67
Valvular disease	
All valvular disease patients	0.28
Mitral disease	0.34
Aortic disease	0.19

*NYHA = New York Heart Association.
†FC = Functional class.

of various mechanisms that include the vasodepressor vagal response, vasodilation occurring after ionic contrast ventriculography, diuresis during the catheterization procedure, cardiac tamponade due to myocardial or coronary laceration, myocardial infarction, or an acute anaphylactoid reaction to the contrast media. Less common complications include the precipitation of pulmonary edema, the showering of cholesterol emboli (trash foot), and injury (dissection) of the coronary or pulmonary arteries.

After the procedure, diuresis from the radiographic contrast load and subsequent hypotension are common. Liberal use of fluids usually restores the blood pressure. Reactions to protamine sulfate can also occur if it is used to reverse the effects of heparin, and pulmonary emboli have been reported as a late sequela.

Controversy exists concerning the optimal vascular access approach (femoral or brachial), and whether heparin should be used routinely. It is also unclear if there is a minimal number of catheterization procedures that each physician must do to maintain proficiency (Fisher, 1983). The safety and efficacy of free-standing cardiac catheterization laboratories are also under close scrutiny (Kahn, 1985).

A final unresolved controversy exists regarding the use of nonionic versus ionic contrast media. By using ionic contrast media, several reviews have suggested an overall contrast-related toxicity in 1.4 to 2.26% of cases (Fareed et al, 1984; Shehadi, 1982). Ionic contrast produces various adverse hemodynamic and electrophysiologic effects during coronary angiography. Most of these adverse events are clearly related to the osmolality, sodium content, and calcium binding of the ionic contrast solutions. In addition, the observed myocardial depression, peripheral vasodilation, and increased coronary flow are due to these same characteristics (Fischer and Thom-

son, 1978). Nonionic contrast agents clearly reduce acute adverse hemodynamic and electrophysiologic reactions (Bashore et al, 1988; Higgins et al, 1980), experimentally may reduce nephrotoxicity (Humes et al, 1988), appear to release less histamine from mast cells, and potentially reduce allergic reactions (Salem et al, 1986). Clinical studies completed at Duke University Medical Center suggest no advantage of nonionic over ionic agents in the prevention of nephrotoxicity (Davidson et al, 1988; Schwab et al, 1989). The question of some inherent thrombogenicity of nonionic agents has also been raised (Grollman et al, 1988). A substantial difference in costs between ionic and nonionic media exists (up to a 15- to 20-fold difference), which makes the routine use of nonionic contrast controversial. Nonionic contrast is especially useful in patients at high risk for adverse events, and ongoing studies are attempting to identify these subsets.

BASIC CATHETER TECHNIQUES

Most cardiac catheterization procedures in the United States are now done by the femoral approach, with a minority done by the brachial artery. The relevant basic concepts are described (for further details, see Chapter 54).

The brachial (Sones) approach can be done either by cutdown or by percutaneous insertion of the catheter system in the brachial artery (Pepine et al, 1984). Systemic heparin is generally used in most laboratories. A catheter is then passed either directly into the artery or through a sheath placed in the vessel, and the catheter is advanced to the aortic root and eventually to the coronary arteries and left ventricle. Different catheters can be used to cannulate each coronary ostium as well as to obtain pressure data from the left ventricle by retrograde insertion across the aortic valve. Left ventriculography is done by power injection of the left ventricle with radiographic contrast; coronary angiography is usually done by hand injection of contrast. The Sones technique allows good catheter control but requires greater operator skill, and when an antecubital dissection is required to expose the artery, a vascular repair is required at the end of the procedure. The preformed catheters traditionally used for the femoral approach have been used with the brachial approach with good results.

The Judkins approach is less traumatic, allows the operator to be farther removed from the x-ray source (reducing operator exposure), and is done through a percutaneous needle puncture of the femoral artery. After insertion of a guidewire through the entry needle, either a sheath then a catheter or the catheter alone can be placed in the femoral vessel. The catheter is then advanced to the heart. Left-sided heart catheterization usually uses three preformed catheters—one for each coronary artery and a pigtail catheter with side holes for left ventriculography. Further advantages of the Judkins approach include the fact that there is no need for surgical repair of the vessel and the catheters generally seek the coronary ostia with minimal manipulation, requiring less skill on the part of the catheterizing physician who performs the catheterization. A single catheter system from the femoral artery is also used in some institutions (Schoonmaker and King, 1974).

Because some patients have severe iliac or aortic vascular disease that prohibits the femoral approach, cardiologists should have experience with both techniques. The more familiar the physician is with one procedure or the other appears to be a greater determinant of the risks of the brachial versus femoral approach than does the access site alone (Kennedy, 1982).

Trans-septal left-sided heart catheterization (O'Keefe et al, 1985) has become an infrequent procedure in many cardiac catheterization laboratories. However, with the growing popularity of some prosthetic valves in the aortic position (i.e., the disk and the St. Jude valves) that cannot be crossed retrograde at catheterization, and with the emerging technologic advances that allow balloon mitral valvuloplasty to be done, the trans-septal technique may be undergoing a revival. The trans-septal procedure can be done only through the right femoral vein. The trans-septal catheter is a short, curved catheter with a tapered tip and side holes. It is placed in the right atrium over a 70-cm curved Brockenbrough needle that is inserted through the catheter until it is just inside the catheter tip. Techniques vary, but in general the catheter-needle combination is manipulated into the fossa ovalis while usually continuously recording atrial pressure. Mere advancement of the catheter system against the fossa ovalis often results in entry of the catheter-needle apparatus into the left atrium. If this does not occur, a portion of the tip of the needle is abruptly advanced from the catheter into the left atrium. With the catheter in the left atrium, further manipulations are then used to advance the catheter into the left ventricle, and left ventricular pressures and angiograms are obtained. The major risk of trans-septal catheterization lies in inadvertent puncture of right atrial structures, such as the atrial free wall or coronary sinus, or entry into the aortic root.

Right ventricular endomyocardial biopsy is readily done with little risk (Mason, 1978). Either an internal jugular or femoral vein approach is available. The bioptome is directed without a sheath while monitoring the intracardiac electrogram or is guided with an appropriate guiding sheath to sample the interventricular septum. Approximately 1 mg of tissue is obtained with each biopsy. Multiple biopsy samples can be obtained at one setting.

Finally, catheterization of the coronary sinus can be readily achieved from brachial, subclavian, or femoral access sites. Coronary sinus flow and metabolism studies as well as oxygen content can be assessed (Baim et al, 1982) and may be useful after interventions. The coronary sinus may also provide a ''back door'' to the coronary circulation through which supportive therapy may be delivered to the ischemic myocardium.

BASIC FUNCTION OF THE X-RAY SYSTEM

High-quality cine film is essential for the appropriate diagnosis of angiographic catheterization results. Details of the manner in which this is achieved are available from other sources (Curry et al, 1984). A basic understanding is useful for every physician who is interested in examining the results of cardiac catheterization. A brief overview of this area is provided.

The major components of the cardiac catheterization x-ray system are shown schematically in Figure 31–1. This schematic ignores the complex interrelated electronics, switching devices, collimators, and so on required to produce eventual x-ray image. It concentrates on the practical aspects of how electrons are converted to x-rays and how these x-rays eventually produce a visual outline of the cardiac structures.

The story begins in the generator. Two types of

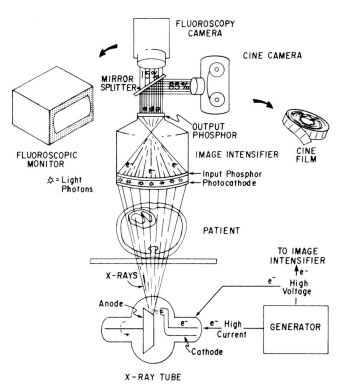

Figure 31–1. The cinefluoroscopy system. The current from the generator powers the image intensifier and x-ray tube. Electrons (e⁻) flow through the x-ray tube cathode, then ''jump'' to bombard the anode, where they are converted to x-rays. X-rays pass through the patient to the face of the image intensifier. From here they are converted to light, then electrons, then back to light at the output phosphor. The x-ray enhanced image is then picked up by the fluoroscopy camera or reflected to the cine camera.

current are produced by the generator—one high in voltage (the "strength" of the current) and one high in amperage (the number of electrons). The need for these two types of current becomes evident when one examines the mechanisms of the x-ray tube, a vacuum tube within which reside a cathode and an anode. The cathode is a coil through which the high-amperage current is passed. When high voltage (25,000 volts) is then applied across the x-ray tube, electrons in the cathode are encouraged to "jump" over to the anode.

These electrodes interact with tungsten material embedded in the anode, producing x-rays. By slanting the anode's surface, the resultant x-ray beam can be directed out of the x-ray tube and subsequently through the patient to the image intensifier. The system is inefficient, and only one x-ray is produced for each 100 electrons.

As the x-rays pass from the x-ray tube toward the image intensifier, they diverge. The patient absorbs some of the x-rays, some reach the image intensifier, and the remainder are scattered. Extensive measures to ensure protection from this scatter radiation are warranted and should be rigorously practiced in all laboratories. The various tissues absorb x-rays in a differential manner, and this variable penetration eventually results in certain body structures being outlined on the final image. Radiographic contrast containing iodine is used in all angiography specifically because the iodine atom absorbs x-ray photons so well.

The x-rays that reach the face of the image intensifier produce a faint image. The image intensifier strengthens this image by two methods—by a minification or shrinking of the size of the image and by electronic enhancement of the image by accelerating electrons through the intensifier (using the high voltage from the generator). The face of the image intensifier is covered by an input photocathode that first converts the x-ray photon energy to light, which then travels a minuscule distance before it meets a fluorescent screen (input phosphor). When light strikes the input phosphor, an electron is produced. The high-voltage field accelerates these electrons toward the output phosphor, where they are converted back to light. The result is a visible x-ray image.

The light next passes through a mirror splitter placed in the output path from the image intensifier. Differential silvering of the mirror allows a certain amount of light to pass through to the fluoroscopic video camera (usually about 15%), while the remainder of the image is reflected to the 35-mm cine camera. When cine film is to be recorded, the operator activates the cine camera by a foot switch, and film exposure begins (usually at speeds of 30 to 60 frames per second). The cine film is developed in a manner similar to the 35-mm film development process.

The final step in viewing the film is the cine projector, which is ostensibly one of the weaker links in the system. Because the eye is able to detect flicker at framing rates less than 50 frames per second, and because most cardiac catheterization laboratories expose film at 30 to 45 frames per second, flicker would be routinely seen in reviewing cine film. To avoid flicker during cine review, the cine projector projects each frame twice, thus misleading the eye and brain into perceiving that the true filming rate doubles. The result is a flicker-free image.

In the future, many changes will likely occur in this entire system. Some of those changes are imminent, but others are under active development at many sites around the world. There likely will be a gradual trend away from x-ray systems that produce only cine film to those that produce computerized digital images or enhanced video data. The advantages are numerous, but include flicker-free images even at very low frame rates, the ability to use less x-ray exposure, the ability to have immediate access to the image data without waiting for film processing, the ability to improve the images even after the catheterization study is completed, and the opportunity to apply quantitative computer algorithms to the image data. Thus, one can obtain quantitative and qualitative information in addition to the visual observations. This revolution requires a storage medium different from cine film, however, and that transition is still one of the major obstacles to the widespread application of routine digital angiographic systems.

HEMODYNAMIC MEASUREMENTS

Pressure Measurement

Methods

One of the major goals of cardiac catheterization is to record the pressure waveforms and their magnitude from various vascular structures. Although this may superficially appear readily obtainable, there are some important inherent errors in the measurement of these data that should be recognized to avoid overdependence on small variations in the values obtained.

It should be emphasized that any pressure data obtained from inside vascular organs reflects the sum of the pressures not only in the chamber being analyzed, but also in the contiguous structures that have influence on that chamber. For example, because the heart is located in the pericardium and both structures are surrounded by the lungs, changes in either pulmonary or pericardial pressure would be expected to alter intracardiac pressure measurements. Likewise, ventricular interaction results in the pressure of one ventricle affecting the pressure in the other. Physiologic variations such as simple respiration also affect all of the pressure data. The "hard" numbers reported from cardiac catheterization thus reflect only the average data at an arbitrary point in time. This does not imply that the data are incorrect, but rather that they represent only an average value considering the expected physiologic variation seen normally. Some pathologic states and conditions obviously affect these values to an even greater degree.

Sources of error in the measurement of pressures include the routine use of fluid-filled catheters, poor zeroing practices (in which the transducer diaphragm is not placed at midchest); air, kinking, or other obstructions in the tubing between the catheter and the diaphragm (resulting in damping of the pressure); and, perhaps most common, catheter whip artifact as the fluid-filled catheter tip is flexed inside the heart or great vessels. In addition, end-hole catheter pressure data may not be the same as side-hole pressure data, particularly in areas of streaming or high velocity. In small vessels or valvular orifices, the catheters themselves also become obstructive and the resultant pressures are altered.

Although micromanometer-tip catheters greatly reduce many of these errors, their use has been too impractical in most clinical situations. Therefore, the interpretation of pressure data from fluid-filled systems must be made with the appreciation of the inherent pitfalls in the actual data derived. When data do not agree with the clinical situation, it is wise to re-examine the pressure data to ensure that none of the artifacts mentioned are present.

Normal Pressure Waveforms

Appreciation of the normal waveforms is important if the effects of pathologic states are to be understood. Subtle alterations in pressure waveforms occasionally become important in the detection and quantitation of myocardial, valvular, and pericardial disease states.

The average and range for normal right-sided and left-sided heart pressures are outlined in Table 31–3. Whenever fluid is compressed within a chamber, the pressure rises; conversely, whenever there is either fluid loss from a chamber or the chamber goes into diastole, the pressure falls. This simple construction can explain all of various waveforms noted. Normal waveforms are outlined in Figure 31–2.

The *right atrial pressure waveform* consists of two major positive deflections that are called a and v waves. The a wave is due to atrial systolic contraction and follows electrical activation (represented by the P wave of the electrocardiogram). When atrial contraction occurs, the tricuspid valve is open. The height of the a wave thus reflects not only the vigor of the atrial contraction but also the resistance presented by the diastolic right ventricle. An increase in the height of the a wave occurs when there is poor compliance of the right ventricle. Ventricular systole begins immediately after atrial contraction. The pressure rise in the right ventricle closes the tricuspid valve, resulting in a protrusion of the valve into the

TABLE 31–3. NORMAL PRESSURES IN THE HEART AND VASCULATURE

	Range (mm Hg)	Average (mm Hg)
Cardiac Chambers		
Right atrium		
a wave	3–7	6
v wave	2–7	5
Mean	1–5	3
Right ventricle		
Peak systolic	17–30	26
End-diastolic	1–7	5
Pulmonary artery		
Peak systolic	17–30	25
End-diastolic	5–13	9
Mean	9–19	15
Pulmonary capillary wedge		
Mean	5–13	9
Left atrium		
a wave	4–16	10
v wave	3–12	8
Mean	6–21	13
Vasculature		
Aorta		
Peak systolic	85–140	125
End-diastolic	60–90	70
Mean	70–105	80
Right brachial		
Peak systolic	90–140	130
End-diastolic	60–90	70
Mean	70–105	85
Left brachial		
Peak systolic	85–140	125
End-diastolic	60–90	70
Mean	70–105	83
Femoral artery		
Peak systolic	95–150	135
End-diastolic	60–90	70
Mean	75–115	90

right atrium, reducing right atrial volume slightly and resulting in the c wave. As right ventricular contraction continues, the tricuspid annulus is pulled into the body of the right ventricle and the atrium concurrently goes into diastole. This combination results in a decline in right atrial pressure, the x descent. Atrial filling occurs during late ventricular systole and results in a gradual rise in atrial pressure and peaks at the v wave. The tricuspid valve then opens and atrial pressure falls (the y descent). The atrium and ventricle are then once again functioning as a common chamber, and atrial and ventricular diastolic pressures eventually equalize during the remainder of diastole. The height of the atrial v wave reflects both atrial compliance and the amount of blood returning to the atrium from the periphery.

The *left atrial pressure waveform* is similar to the right atrial waveform except that the v wave is usually higher than the a wave. This occurs because

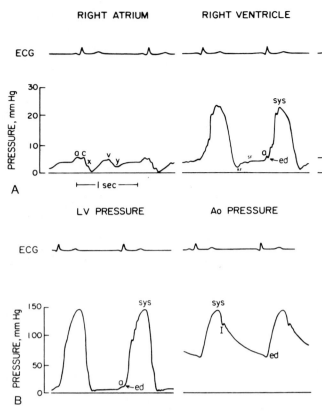

Figure 31–2. *A,* Normal right-sided heart pressures. Normal pressures and pressure waveforms are shown. *B,* Normal left-sided heart pressures. Normal pressures and pressure waveforms. (From Grossman, W., and Barry, W. H.: Cardiac catheterization. *In* Braunwald, E. [ed]: Heart Disease, 3rd ed. Philadelphia, W. B. Saunders Company, 1988.)

the left atrium is in a relatively confined space and is restricted posteriorly by the four pulmonary veins. However, the right atrium is readily decompressed by the inferior and superior venae cavae. Indeed, when left atrial compliance is poor and atrial flow high, a large left atrial v wave can be noted that must not be confused with the pathologic v wave due to mitral valve regurgitation (Fuchs et al, 1982).

The *pulmonary artery wedge pressure* has a waveform similar to that of the left atrial pressure, but it is usually dampened, and there is a delay in transmission of this waveform through the pulmonary capillary vessels. In particular disease states, and occasionally after procedures such as mitral valve replacement, it has been noted that the pulmonary artery wedge pressure may not accurately reflect left atrial pressure (Schoenfeld et al, 1985).

The diastolic phases of the *right and left ventricular pressures* differ primarily only in the magnitude of the waveforms. The ventricular diastolic pressure is characterized by a rapid initial decline followed by a brief rapid-filling phase then a longer slow-filling phase. At the most negative point in the ventricular early diastolic pressure tracing, almost half of the ventricle is filled. After the rapid-filling wave, approximately 25% of the blood enters the ventricle during the slow-filling period. A final 15 to 25% enters during atrial systolic contraction (Rankin et al, 1988). The rise in pressure during atrial systole is referred to as the ventricular a wave, and the pressure crossing at the end of the a wave and the rise

in the ventricular pressure is called the c point. This point is generally chosen as the ventricular end-diastolic pressure. When the c point is not well seen, the peak of the R wave from the simultaneous electrocardiogram is used to define the end-diastolic pressure.

The *pulmonary artery pressure waveform* reflects the systolic right ventricular pressure. When right ventricular pressure declines, the pulmonary pressure falls until the pulmonary valve closes. A notch or incisura is then evident. The low compliance in the pulmonary circuit often results in this incisura being delayed (referred to as *hangout*). A small dicrotic wave is usually seen and is followed by a slow fall in the pulmonary diastolic pressure until the initiation of ventricular systole again. A small systolic pressure gradient normally exists between the right ventricle and pulmonary artery. Right atrial contraction occasionally produces a small pressure deformation just before the minimal pulmonary artery pressure. This is reflected as an a wave in the pulmonary artery pressure tracing.

Arterial resistance is determined by the smaller arteries (<1,000 μ), the arterioles (20 to 200 μ), and the capillaries. An abrupt change in resistance occurs over a short path between the peripheral arteries and veins. The systolic *aortic pulse* is a composite of waves that results from forward flow (the percussion wave), a reflected wave from upper-extremity resistance (the tidal wave), and a reflected wave from lower body resistance after aortic valve closure (the dicrotic wave)

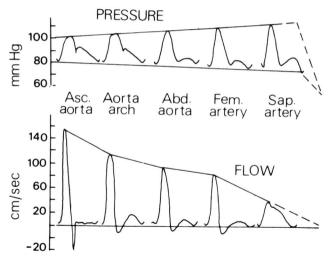

Figure 31–3. Arterial waveforms. The pulse pressure rises from the central aorta to the lower extremity as a result of the additive effects of reflected waves from the peripheral area of resistance. Note that the pulse pressure rises despite a decline in forward flow. The *broken line* represents decline in both flow and pressure within the arterioles. (From O'Rourke, M. F.: Wave reflections. *In* O'Rourke, M. F. [ed]: Arterial Function in Health and Disease. New York, Churchill Livingstone, 1982.)

(O'Rourke, 1982). As blood moves from the central aorta toward the periphery, the height of the pulse pressure increases because there is less elastic tissue in the descending aorta and because the wavefront approaches the areas of the resistance vessels at the periphery. The reflected wave thus summates with the forward wavefront, and the height of the pressure wave increases toward the periphery (McDonald and Taylor, 1959). Therefore, central aortic pressure may not be equal to the peripheral pressure. In addition, the relatively direct injection of blood into

the right subclavian artery often makes the systolic pressure in the right brachial artery slightly higher than in the left brachial artery. A representation of pressure recordings from the ascending aorta through to the femoral artery is shown in Figure 31–3.

Mean arterial pressure is calculated traditionally as the pressure at one-third of the value between diastole and systolic pressure (because the pressure wave has approximately a triangular shape). Although these mean pressure calculations are reasonably accurate in the peripheral circulation, the actual mean pressure may be closer to midway between systolic and diastolic pressure in the central aorta. In gross terms, the difference between systolic and diastolic pressure, or pulse pressure, reflects both stroke volume and arterial cushioning (compliance), whereas the mean pressure more closely represents conduit function (peripheral resistance). With aging, both the pulse pressure and the mean arterial pressure rise normally (Fig. 31–4).

Vascular Resistance Measurement

Clinically, the use of Ohm's law to represent steady-state vascular resistance has become acceptable. This law assumes that flow occurs only in systole, however. Fortunately this is not true, because systolic pressure would rise very high and diastolic pressure would fall to the level of the right atrium. Normal values are shown in Table 31–4 and the major assumptions are shown in Figure 31–5.

To determine the resistance across any particular vascular bed, the mean pressures just proximal and distal to the bed must be known. Pulmonary vascular resistance thus uses the mean pulmonary pressure, the mean pulmonary capillary wedge pressure, and the cardiac output. Systemic vascular resistance can

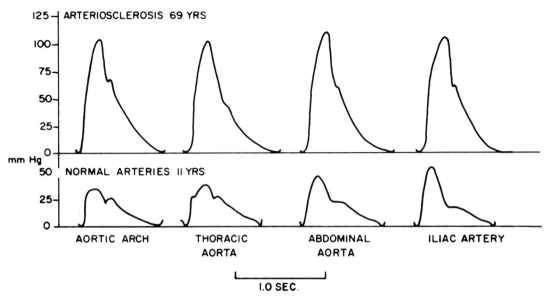

Figure 31–4. The effect of aging on the arterial pressure. The normal discrepancy between central aortic and peripheral pressure lessens with age. (From O'Rourke, M. F.: Wave reflections. *In* O'Rourke, M. F. [ed]: Arterial Function in Health and Disease. New York, Churchill Livingstone, 1982.)

TABLE 31–4. VASCULAR RESISTANCE UNITS—
NORMAL VALUES

Measurement	Absolute Units dyn · sec · cm^{-5}	Wood Units mmHg · min · liters^{-1}
Total pulmonary resistance	205 ± 51	2.5 ± 1.0
Pulmonary vascular resistance	67 ± 30	1 ± 0.5
Systemic vascular resistance	1170 ± 270	15 ± 3.5

be defined with the mean systemic pressure and the mean right atrial pressure; if the right atrial pressure is unknown, it can be dropped and the result is called total peripheral resistance. Resistance in the pulmonary circuit can not only be affected by pressure and flow, but also may vary with the "critical closing pressure" of the pulmonary vasculature (McGregor and Sniderman, 1985). The zones of the lung from which the pulmonary capillary wedge pressure is measured may also show a small variation.

To describe the arterial system accurately one must consider arterial compliance and the blood viscosity in a frequency-dependent model. Impedance calculations relate pressure to flow on a beat-to-beat basis. The relationship between pressure and flow cannot be readily obtained clinically, nor is this relationship readily apparent by inspecting either the pressure curve or the flow contour. Impedance measurements, therefore, have not been widely adopted because of the difficulty in obtaining simultaneous pressure and flow.

Cardiac Output Measurements

There is no accurate way to measure cardiac output in vivo. This is best done by using estimates of cardiac output based on various assumptions. Generally, the two major methods used for the measurement of cardiac output are the Fick method and thermodilution method. Cardiac output is often normalized for the patient's size based on the body surface area and is expressed as cardiac index. This assumption, like many "facts" in medicine, is open to question, but its use has generally been accepted clinically.

Indicator-Dilution Measures of the Cardiac Output

The indicator-dilution method has been used to measure cardiac output since introduction by Stewart (1897) with modifications by Hamilton and associates (1932). The basic equation commonly referred to as the Stewart-Hamilton equation is shown below:

$$\text{Cardiac output (l/min)} = \frac{\text{amount of indicator injected (mg)} \times 60 \text{ sec/min}}{\text{mean indicator concentration (mg/ml)} \times \text{curve duration}}$$

The assumption is made that the injection of a certain amount of an indicator into the circulation appears and then disappears from any downstream point in a manner commensurate with the cardiac output. For example, if the indicator rapidly appears at a particular point downstream and washes out quickly, the assumption is that the cardiac output is high. Although variation may occur, the site of injection is usually a systemic vein on the right side of the heart, and site of sampling is generally a systemic artery. The normal curve itself has an initial rapid upstroke followed by a slower downstroke and eventually the appearance of recirculation of the tracer. In reality, this recirculation creates some uncertainty at the end of the curve, and assumptions are made to correct for this distortion. Because the indicator concentration declines exponentially in the absence of recirculation, the initial data points from the descending limb are used to extrapolate the area under the ascending and descending limbs. The results, therefore, assume the ascending and descending limbs form a triangular shape. The base of this triangle then represents the total curve duration, and the mean area of the triangle can be assumed to be a function of the mean indicator concentration. Both of these can be used to determine the cardiac output by using the Stewart-Hamilton equation. A representative curve is shown in Figure 31–6.

There are several sources of error in this particular approach. When indocyanine green dye is used,

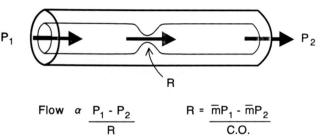

$$\text{Flow} \; \alpha \; \frac{P_1 - P_2}{R} \qquad R = \frac{\overline{m}P_1 - \overline{m}P_2}{C.O.}$$

Figure 31–5. The calculation of peripheral resistance. Flow is proportional to the difference in pressures from one end of the "pipe" to the other and inversely related to the resistance (R). Resistance measurements require knowledge of mean (static) pressures and flow (cardiac output [C.O.]).

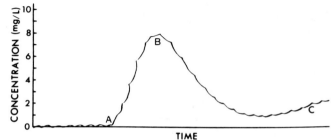

Figure 31–6. Representative normal indicator-dilation curve. The dye is injected on the right side and sampled on the left side of the circulation. The indocyanine green is first detected at *A* and initially peaks at *B*. After washout, recirculation of the dye occurs at *C*. (From Grossman, W.: Blood flow measurement: The cardiac output. *In* Grossman, W. [ed]: Cardiac Catheterization and Angiography, 3rd ed. Philadelphia, Lea & Febiger, 1986.)

fresh preparations are necessary because the dye is unstable over time and can be affected by light. The exact amount of dye is also critical to the performance of the study, and this must be accurately measured, generally in a tuberculin syringe, and injected as a single bolus over a brief period. The indicator, when injected, must also mix well before reaching the sampling site, and the dilution curve must have an exponential downpoint that occurs over a sufficient period so that extrapolation can occur. This latter problem is particularly significant if, for example, there is severe valvular regurgitation or a low-output state in which the washout decline of the indicator is so prolonged that recirculation begins well before there has been an adequate decline in the curve. Thus, the green dye method is inaccurate in patients with regurgitation lesions or low output. Intracardiac shunts may also greatly affect the shape of this curve.

Thermodilution Techniques

The rather tedious and time-consuming nature of doing indicator-dilution techniques has been replaced in most catheterization laboratories by the use of thermodilution techniques. The popularity of the Swan-Ganz catheter and its use have greatly expanded the ability to obtain thermodilution cardiac outputs in many clinical settings.

The thermodilution procedure requires the injection of a bolus of cooled liquid (saline or dextrose) into the proximal part of the catheter. The resultant change in temperature due to the iced liquid is then measured by a thermistor mounted in the distal end of the catheter. The change in temperature can be plotted in a manner similar to the dye-dilution method described. The cardiac output is then calculated by a rather complex equation that takes into consideration the temperature of the injectant and the temperature of the blood, together with the volume and the specific gravity. In addition, certain calibration factors are used. The basic concept is that the cardiac output is inversely related to the area under a thermodilution curve plotted as temperature versus time.

The thermodilution method has several advantages. Not only does it not require withdrawal of blood or arterial puncture, it is less affected by recirculation. Perhaps its greatest advantage is that the application of computers allows rapid display of results that can be used clinically. Computers use the washout rate of the downslope of the curve to obtain a decay constant. This method allows reconstruction of the complete triangular-shaped curve and the area under the curve. With knowledge of the injectant volume, temperature, and specific gravity, as well as the blood temperature and its specific gravity plus the area under the curve, the cardiac output can be calculated.

Thermodilution cardiac outputs are susceptible to similar problems of indicator-dilution methods using green dye. Because the data represent right-sided heart output, tricuspid regurgitation can be a particular problem. Thermodilution tends to overestimate the cardiac output in low cardiac output states because of the loss of the cold temperature to the surrounding cardiac structures and the later reduction in the total area under the curve. Other problems include fluctuations in blood temperature during respiratory or cardiac cycles and the warming of the temperature of the injectant before its injection into the catheter.

From a practical viewpoint, thermodilution cardiac outputs have become standard. Their range can be relatively broad, however, and small changes should not be overinterpreted. It is estimated that, overall, cardiac output data can only be defined to $\pm 15\%$ (Grondelle et al, 1983).

Fick Cardiac Output Principle

The Fick principle, first espoused by Adolph Fick (1870), assumes that the rate at which oxygen is consumed is a function of the rate of blood flow times the rate of oxygen pickup by the red blood cells. The basic assumptions are shown schematically in Figure 31–7. In simple terms, it is assumed that the same number of red blood cells that enter the lung leave the lung. If one knows how many oxygen molecules were attached to the red blood cells entering the lung, how many oxygen molecules were attached to the red blood cells leaving the lung, and how much oxygen was consumed during travel through the lung, then one can determine the rate of flow of these red blood cells as they passed through the lung. This can be expressed in the following terms:

Cardiac output (l/min) =

$$\frac{O_2 \text{ consumption (ml/min)}}{\text{A-VO}_2 \text{ difference (vol \%)} \times 10}$$

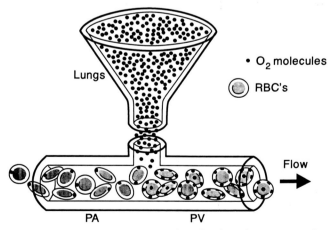

Figure 31–7. The Fick principle. The funnel represents the lungs. As the red blood cells (RBCs) pass through the lungs, oxygen (•) is picked up. The cardiac output is determined by knowing the hemoglobin and oxygen saturation in the pulmonary artery (PA), the oxygen consumption per minute and the oxygen saturation in the pulmonary veins (PV), the rate of flow = oxygen consumption/A-VO$_2$ difference.

Measurements must be done in steady state. Automated methods can accurately determine the oxygen content within the blood samples; the more difficult measurement is that of oxygen consumption. Van Slyke's method has traditionally been used; expiratory gas samples are collected in a large bag over a particular period of time. By measuring the oxygen consumption within the bag and by knowing the amount of room air oxygen, the amount of oxygen consumed per volume over time can be determined. Newer devices now allow for the measurement of oxygen consumption by using a polargraphic method in which expired oxygen can be quantitated by noting the change in electrical current between a gold cathode and silver anode embedded in a potassium chloride gel. These devices can be connected to the patient by use of a plastic hood or by a mouthpiece and tubing.

The Fick method suffers primarily from the vagaries of obtaining accurate oxygen consumption measurements and the inability to obtain a steady state under certain conditions. It requires considerable time and effort on the part of the catheterization laboratory to obtain the appropriate data. Some laboratories use an "assumed" Fick method in which oxygen consumption is assumed on the basis of the patient's age, sex, and body surface area. The advantage of the Fick method is that it is most accurate in patients in whom there is low cardiac output and thus provides better data in these situations. It is also independent of the factors that affect curve shape, as discussed earlier, by using thermodilution or indicator-dilution methods.

Shunt Determinations

Oximetric Method

Various techniques are now available to assist with the determination of intracardiac shunts. In most cases, intracardiac shunting is suspected before catheterization is done. Because fewer routine right-sided heart catheterizations are being done, the opportunity to detect small left-to-right shunts at catheterization has declined. The increased use of echocardiography, however, has clearly allowed the cardiac catheterization procedure to be more focused, which compensates for this loss. Shunts can be measured both noninvasively and invasively by various methods. In the invasive laboratory, shunts are most commonly measured by noting the presence of saturated blood in chambers supplied by the venous system (the oximetric method). A left-to-right shunt can be located and detected if a significant "step-up" in blood oxygen saturation or contents is observed in one of the right-sided heart chambers (Antman et al, 1980; Dexter et al, 1947). In addition, the continuous registration of oxygen saturation is now possible by using a fiberoptic catheter.

Before oxygen can be used as an accurate measure of abnormal shunting, however, a review of the normal chamber saturations is important. The inferior vena cava oxygen content is essentially always higher than the superior vena cava oxygen content because the kidneys use substantially less oxygen relative to cardiac output than other organs. Renal vein oxygen saturation is therefore high. As blood returns to the right atrium from the inferior vena cava, it is directed toward the interatrial septum by the eustachian valve, which creates turbulence and nonuniform mixing. In addition, very unsaturated blood flows in small amounts from the coronary sinus. Thus, the right atrium receives three different sources of blood with different saturations and has various flow patterns within it. For this reason, a great deal of physiologic variability in oxygen saturation is seen in the right atrium, and it is important to appreciate that random right atrial blood samples may vary considerably. More and more mixing occurs as blood enters the right ventricle and then the pulmonary artery. Therefore, mixed venous saturation is best measured in the pulmonary artery. As expected from the physiologic variability noted, the maximal allowable step-up in oxygen content also varies considerably from one chamber to another in the right side of the heart. This variability makes it more difficult to detect a small shunt at the atrial level than at the ventricular or pulmonary artery level. In fact, assuming a systemic cardiac index of 3 l/min/m², oximetry cannot accurately detect a shunt of less than 1.5:1 at the atrial level, whereas the smallest detectable shunt at the ventricular or great vessel level is 1.3:1.

To detect a shunt, one must obtain the oxygen saturation of blood just before it enters the chamber receiving the shunt and note the amount of oxygen step-up that occurs. This creates the most difficulty when assessing left-to-right flow into the right atrium, because the vessels supplying the right atrium (the superior vena cava [SVC] and inferior vena cava [IVC]) each contain differing amounts of

TABLE 31–5. MINIMUM VARIATION IN OXYGEN CONTENT AND SATURATION AMONG RIGHT-SIDED HEART STRUCTURES TO DETECT A SHUNT

Shunt	Step-up Sites	Minimal Change in Oxygen Content (Vol %)	Minimal Change in Oxygen Saturation Changes (%)
Patent ductus arteriosus	Right ventricle to pulmonary artery	0.5	5
Ventricular septal defect	Right atrium to right ventricle	0.9	7
Atrial septal defect	Mixed venous to right atrium	1.9	11

oxygen saturation. For this reason, several formulas have been devised to determine the mixed venous saturation at the levels of the SVC and IVC. The most common formula used (Flamm and colleagues 1969) is as follows:

$$\text{Mixed venous oxygen content} = \frac{3 \, (\text{SVC O}_2 \text{ content}) + 1 \, (\text{IVC O}_2 \text{ content})}{4}$$

Right atrial content should be the average of the high, low, and mid right atrial oxygen content; right ventricular oxygen content should be the average of the inflow and outflow right ventricular content. When these data are obtained, the presence or absence of a shunt can be defined and is shown in Table 31–5.

To determine the size of a left-to-right shunt, both pulmonary blood flow and the systemic blood flow determinations are required. The methods used are similar to the method described for Fick cardiac outputs. To understand how this occurs, the *effective pulmonary blood flow* (EPBF) must be considered. The effective pulmonary blood flow is defined as the fraction of mixed venous return received by the lungs without contamination by shunt flow. In the absence of a shunt, the effective pulmonary blood flow, the systemic blood flow, and the pulmonary blood flow are all equal. In the presence of a left-to-right shunt, however, pulmonary blood flow is equal to the effective pulmonary blood flow plus the left-to-right shunt. The effective pulmonary blood flow is defined from the Fick equation as the oxygen consumption divided by the pulmonary venous oxygen content minus the mixed venous oxygen content.

$$\text{EPBF} = \frac{\text{O}_2 \text{ consumption (ml/min)}}{\text{PV}_{\text{O}_2} - \text{MV}_{\text{O}_2} \text{ (vol \%)} \times 10}$$

By using this logic, pulmonary blood flow (PBF) is equal to oxygen consumption divided by the saturation difference across the pulmonary bed (pulmonary venous minus pulmonary arterial) and systemic blood flow (SBF) is defined by the oxygen consumption divided by the systemic arterial oxygen minus mixed venous oxygen. These equations are shown below:

$$\text{SBF} = \frac{\text{O}_2 \text{ consumption}}{\text{SA}_{\text{O}_2} - \text{MV}_{\text{O}_2} \text{ (vol \%)} \times 10}$$

$$\text{PBF} = \frac{\text{O}_2 \text{ consumption}}{(\text{PV}_{\text{O}_2} - \text{PA}_{\text{O}_2} \text{ (vol \%)}) \times 10}$$

The magnitude of a left-to-right shunt is thus defined as the pulmonary blood flow minus the effective pulmonary blood flow, and the blood samples used for an atrial septal defect are shown in Figure 31–8. Note that saturations are measured from the chamber

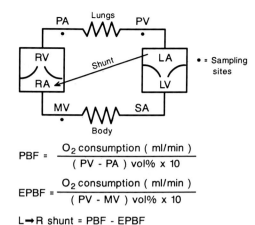

$$\text{PBF} = \frac{\text{O}_2 \text{ consumption (ml/min)}}{(\text{ PV} - \text{PA }) \text{ vol\%} \times 10}$$

$$\text{EPBF} = \frac{\text{O}_2 \text{ consumption (ml/min)}}{(\text{ PV} - \text{MV }) \text{ vol\%} \times 10}$$

L→R shunt = PBF - EPBF

Figure 31–8. Use of oxygen saturations to calculate a left-to-right shunt at the atrial level assuming an atrial septal defect with left-to-right shunt, the sampling sites required are those just before the origin of the shunt, the pulmonary vein (PV), and those before and after the destination, the mixed venous (MV) and pulmonary artery (PA). The left-to-right shunt plus the effective pulmonary blood flow (EPBF) combine to determine the pulmonary blood flow (PBF).

just before the shunt origin and on either side of the shunt destination.

This calculation is similarly applicable for right-to-left shunts. In a right-to-left shunt, the shunt flow is added to the pulmonary blood flow to obtain total systemic blood flow. As in the previous example, a right-to-left shunt at the atrial level requires oxygen saturation from the chamber just before the shunt (the mixed venous) and from the chamber just before and after the shunt (the pulmonary venous and left ventricular or systemic system), respectively. The method of calculating a right-to-left shunt at the atrial level is thus shown in Figure 31–9. By using the same logic, shunts at any level (ventricular, great vessel) can be determined. These same equations can be used to determine bidirectional shunts.

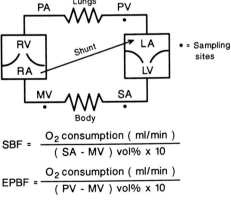

$$\text{SBF} = \frac{\text{O}_2 \text{ consumption (ml/min)}}{(\text{ SA} - \text{MV }) \text{ vol\%} \times 10}$$

$$\text{EPBF} = \frac{\text{O}_2 \text{ consumption (ml/min)}}{(\text{ PV} - \text{MV }) \text{ vol\%} \times 10}$$

R→L shunt = SBF - EPBF

Figure 31–9. Use of oxygen saturation to calculate a right-to-left shunt. As in Figure 31–8, the saturations required are those just before the shunt origin, mixed venous (MV), and those before and after the shunt destination (PV and SA). The systemic blood flow (SBF) is equal to the shunt plus the effective pulmonary blood flow (EPBF).

Indicator-Dilution Method

Shunt detection by indicator-dilution methods are more sensitive than those detected by oximetric methods but suffer from various limitations. There is a growing trend away from the use of indicator-dilution methods in the catheterization laboratories, thus lack of familiarity also presents some disadvantage. An indicator such as indocyanine green dye is injected into one chamber while sampling with a densitometer from another chamber. The density of dye over time is then displayed. Indicator-dilution methods are used more for qualitative than quantitative detection of shunt presence, but both the diagnosis and quantitation can be obtained by using these procedures.

To detect a left-to-right shunt, a bolus can be injected into the venous system and sampled in the arterial system. The first wavefront of dye is then observed, with a second wavefront normally appearing only after the sample has circulated throughout the body. If there is a left-to-right intracardiac shunt, the first wavefront of indicator to the brachial artery will rapidly be followed by a second wavefront because of the recirculation of dye through the shunt. This is referred to as *early recirculation*. If a right-to-left shunt is present, some dye will cross the shunt and appear in advance of the major bolus. The location of a shunt can be precisely located by various sites of injection and sampling. Examples of left-to-right and right-to-left shunt tracings are shown in Figure 31–10.

Calculation of Stenotic Valve Orifice Areas

Determination of Significant Valvular Stenosis

A normal cardiac valve offers little obstruction to forward flow. Abnormal leaflet structure or leaflet injury can result in turbulence of blood flow across the leaflet, which repeatedly injures the leaflet surface. Thus, leaflet injury initiates further injury and provides the substrate for calcium deposition, fibroblastic ingrowth, and scar formation. These processes stiffen the leaflet and narrow the effective orifice.

By using a fundamental hydraulic formula, Gorlin and Gorlin (1951) developed a method of determining the valvular orifice area. This method required knowledge only of the flow across the valve and the pressure gradient that occurs as a result of the stenosis. The basic formula was based on Torricelli's law:

$$\text{Effective orifice area} = \frac{\text{flow}}{\text{constant} \times 44.3 \times \sqrt{\text{mean gradient}}}$$

Gorlin observed that different constants corrected the resulting data for that observed at autopsy.

In the equation, flow is expressed in the number of seconds in a minute that flow occurs. For atrioventricular valves, only diastolic flow is used; for semilunar valves, only systolic flow is used. For mitral stenosis, the diastolic filling period is defined from mitral valve opening to mitral valve closure. For aortic stenosis, the systolic ejection period is defined from aortic opening to closure. To convert cardiac output measurements to flow during these intervals, the cardiac output is divided by heart rate times either the diastolic filling period or the systolic ejection period, respectively. The final equation is therefore defined as follows:

$$\text{Valve area} = \frac{\text{CO}/(\text{DFP or SEP}) \, (\text{HR})}{44.3 \times \text{constant} \times \sqrt{\text{mean gradient}}}$$

where CO = cardiac output, DFP = diastolic filling period, SEP = systolic ejection period, HR = heart rate, and 44.3 is a gravitation correction coefficient that also corrects for energy loss as pressure is converted to kinetic or velocity energy.

Gorlin validated the constant to be used for the mitral valve in 11 patients, and the maximal diameter observed varied by only 0.2 cm² when the constant 0.85 was used. For the aortic valve, a constant of 1.0 was used. Because there is no general clinical agreement with regard to what constitutes a significant effective orifice area in tricuspid or pulmonic valvular stenosis, the valve areas for these valves are usually not calculated.

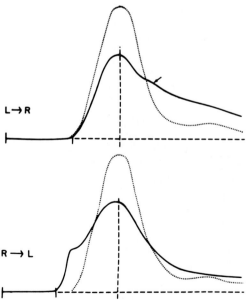

Figure 31–10. Examples of the identification of left-to-right or right-to-left shunts by using indicator-dilution methods. The *broken line* represents a normal forward curve after injection of indocyanine green in the right side of the heart and sampling in the brachial artery. If a left-to-right shunt is present *(upper panel)*, the onset of the curve is normal and recirculation of the dye appears prematurely *(arrow)*. If a right-to-left shunt is present, the dye that bypassed the lung will appear prematurely in the brachial artery *(lower panel)*.

The normal mitral valve (MV) orifice area in adults is generally considered to be 4 to 5 cm². Symptoms in mitral stenosis are a direct reflection of left atrial pressure and pulmonary venous hypertension. By rearranging the previous formula:

$$MV \text{ gradient} \propto \frac{\text{cardiac output}}{\text{diastolic filling period}}$$

Thus, the mitral valve gradient would be expected to rise with any high flow state or with any condition that shortens the diastolic filling period (e.g., during tachycardia). Because tachycardia tends to shorten diastolic filling time greater than systolic ejection time, tachycardia is particularly poorly tolerated in patients with mitral stenosis.

The relationship between the mitral gradient, the cardiac output, and the calculated mitral valve effective orifice area is complicated and important to understand if the surgeon is to interpret the results of procedures on the mitral valve. This relationship is shown in Figure 31–11. Note that when the orifice area declines to 1.5 to 1 cm², it becomes progressively more difficult to increase flow without causing high mitral valve gradients. This is generally considered the threshold for doing mitral valve procedures. Conversely, small changes in the mitral valve area in severely stenotic valves result in large declines in the resultant gradient.

The normal aortic valve area is considered to be 2.6 to 3.5 cm² in adults. As with the mitral valve, the aortic valve gradient is proportional to cardiac output and is inversely proportional to the systolic ejection period.

$$\text{Aortic gradient} \propto \frac{\text{cardiac output}}{\text{systolic ejection period}}$$

Because the systolic ejection period declines less than the diastolic filling period with tachycardia, patients with aortic stenosis are more susceptible to cardiac output demands (e.g., exercise) than they are to tachycardia alone. The relationship between gradient, flow, and the aortic valve area is shown in Figure 31–12. As with mitral stenosis, the aortic gradient depends on both the aortic valve effective orifice area and the cardiac output. At an aortic valve area of 0.8 cm² or less, the aortic gradient rises disportionately to the increase in cardiac output observed, and this level is usually considered the threshold for intervention.

Errors in Using Valvular Effective Orifice Area Measurements

Many potential errors are associated with the use of catheterization-derived valvular orifice area estimates (Carabello, 1987; Gorlin, 1987). These errors relate to both the difficulty in measuring the variables in Gorlin's equation and to a fundamental concern

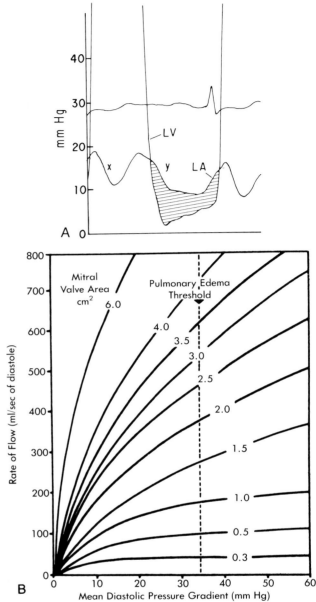

Figure 31–11. The mitral gradient and the relationship of gradient to flow and valve area. *A*, The gradient between the LA and LV in diastole in mitral stenosis. *B*, The dependence of the mitral gradient on both flow and the mitral valve area. (*A*, Adapted from Wallace, A. G.: Pathophysiology of cardiovascular disease. *In* Smith, L. H., and Thier, O. S. [eds]: Pathophysiology: The Biological Principles of Disease: The International Textbook of Medicine. Philadelphia, W. B. Saunders Company, 1981. *B*, From Schlant, R. C.: Altered cardiovascular function of rheumatic heart disease and other acquired valvular disease. *In* Hurst, J. W. [ed]: The Heart, 3rd ed. New York, McGraw-Hill, 1974.)

about the validity of this approach to estimate the orifice size. This concern also applies to prosthetic valve area estimations (Cannon et al, 1988).

The valvular orifice size estimate depends on accurate determination of cardiac output. This may be difficult at low-output states. If valvular regurgitation is present, the angiographically determined cardiac output must be used because the formula

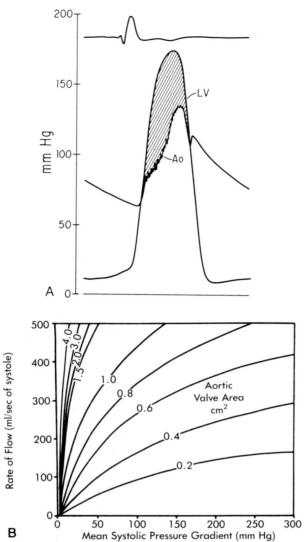

Figure 31–12. The aortic gradient and the relationship of gradient, flow, and valve area. *A,* Represents the relationship between the gradient, flow, and effective orifice area. *B,* The gradient between the aorta and LV. (*A,* Adapted from Wallace, A. G.: Pathophysiology of cardiovascular disease. *In* Smith, L. H., and Thier, O. S. [eds]: Pathophysiology: The Biological Principles of Disease: The International Textbook of Medicine. Philadelphia, W. B. Saunders Company, 1981. *B,* From Schlant, R. C.: Altered cardiovascular function of rheumatic heart disease and other acquired valvular disease. *In* Hurst, J. W., [ed]: The Heart, 3rd ed. New York, McGraw-Hill, 1974.)

depends on determining flow occurring across the valve of interest. If both aortic regurgitation and mitral regurgitation are present, neither the mitral nor the aortic valve area can be accurately assessed because flow across only a single valve cannot be determined.

Problems in the calculation of the effective orifice area of the mitral valve also include the use of pulmonary capillary wedge pressure as a substitution for left atrial pressure, calibration errors, and difficulty in defining the beginning and the end of the diastolic filling period. Estimation of the effective orifice area of the aortic valve is subject to the same

cardiac output errors as estimation of the mitral valve area. In aortic insufficiency, the total flow across the aortic valve can be estimated by using angiographic rather than Fick or thermodilution cardiac output. If associated mitral and aortic regurgitation is present, the aortic valve area cannot be determined. Additionally, because most catheterization laboratories use peripheral arterial pressure rather than central aortic pressure to define the aortic gradient, the delay between the onset of the peripheral waveform and the left ventricular pressure rise requires realignment for the data to be accurate (see Fig. 31–3). As discussed earlier, there may be a substantial difference in the height of the systolic pressure contour when the central aortic and peripheral arterial pressures are compared. If a discrepancy exists, the central aortic pressure can be determined by inserting a second catheter (preferred) or by use of a "pull-back" gradient. The catheter itself may also reduce the true valvular orifice area sufficiently to increase the gradient artifactually. Indeed, a rise in peripheral pressure has been observed with the removal of the catheter from the orifice of patients with aortic valve areas less than 0.5 cm² (Carabello et al, 1979).

The dependence of Gorlin's formula on cardiac output has been examined in patients with aortic stenosis, and the results have been particularly disturbing. By using inotropic agents such as dopamine (Casale et al, 1988) or isoproterenol (McCristin et al, 1988) to increase cardiac output, substantial changes in the calculated aortic valve areas can be shown. These results may be related to increased lifting of the heavily burdened calcific valve or to other inherent errors in the correction factor used in the in-vivo state. The dependence of the calculations of valve area on forward flow has been confirmed by Cannon and associates (1985); the "constant" used in the formula was found to be a linear function of the square root of the mean gradients and was not a constant at all.

Alternative Measures of the Effective Orifice Area of Stenotic Valves

Despite the dependence of valve gradients on flow, some institutions still rely solely on gradients to determine operability in most patients. For example, an aortic peak-to-peak gradient of more than 50 mm Hg or more or a mean mitral gradient of 15 mm Hg has been assumed to imply serious valvular stenosis and the need for operation. Similarly, a minimal mean gradient of 5 mm Hg across the tricuspid and 50 mm Hg gradient across the pulmonic valve is considered significant.

Because of the concerns in use of Gorlin's formula, other attempts to define the effective orifice area have been proposed. Hakki (1981) suggested a simplified formula that clinically appeared to be effective:

$$\text{Valve area} = \frac{\text{cardiac output (l/min)}}{\text{mean pressure gradient (mm Hg)}}$$

At normal heart rates, the effect of the systolic ejection period or the diastolic period was noted to be a relative constant; thus, this function was eliminated from the equation. The validity of this approach at higher heart rates was assessed by Angel and colleagues (1985); an empiric constant was added, depending on whether the heart rate was less than 75 beats per minute for mitral stenosis and more than 90 beats per minute for aortic stenosis. Rather than assume a given constant, Cannon and associates (1985) proposed the following:

$$\text{Valve area} = \frac{\text{flow (ml/sec)}}{K' \times \geq \text{mean gradient} + C}$$

where the valve orifice area is assumed to be inversely proportional to the actual mean gradient and K' and C are constants that vary depending on which valve is being studied. The acceptance of these alternative methods of estimating the orifice area of stenotic valves awaits the test of time.

ANGIOGRAPHIC DATA ANALYSIS

Angiographic Left Ventricular Volume Determination

The measurement of the volume of blood in the cardiac chambers and the relationship with both disease states and overall cardiac function have obvious clinical relevance. The major problems in determining cardiac volume lie with the difficulty of appropriately modeling the ventricles to a mathematically usable configuration. This is particularly true for cardiac chambers other than the left ventricle.

Several popular methods are used to measure left ventricular volumes, but most laboratories use an area-length determination (Dodge and Sheehan, 1983). Adequate opacification of the left ventricle without arrhythmia is required. The area-length method assumes that the left ventricle is shaped like a football (prolated ellipsoid). With knowledge of the corrected area of the silhouette and length, the volumes can be derived by using the following formula:

$$V = \frac{4}{3}\pi \times \frac{D(1)}{2} \times \frac{D(2)}{2} \times \frac{L}{2}$$

where D(1) = minor diameter in one view (anteroposterior [AP] or right anterior oblique [RAO]) and D(2) = minor diameter in the orthogonal view (lateral or left anterior oblique [LAO]), and L = long axis length. For biplane ventriculography, D(1) and D(2) are directly determined; for single-plane ventriculography, D(1) is assumed to be equal to D(2). The minor axes are calculated with knowledge of the planimetered area (A) of the left ventricular contour and L and by using the following formula:

$$D = \frac{4A}{\pi L}$$

where A = area of the projected image obtained by planimetry.

Because x-rays are divergent as they emerge from the x-ray tube and travel to the image intensifier, a correction factor must be determined to calculate actual area and length. This is generally obtained by measuring a known quantity (e.g., ball, bar, catheter markers, grid) at the level of the midventricle or by using various other geometric methods.

When these corrections are made, however, there still remains an offset between actual and calculated ventricular volumes. In the authors' laboratories, each x-ray suite has this offset determined by linear regression analysis of 20 human heart casts of known volume. This regression is slightly different for each x-ray room. In laboratories that are not equipped for this technique, the regression equation obtained by Kennedy and associates (1970) has generally proved to be satisfactory.

Angiographic volumes suffer greatly from many limitations, including the basic assumption that the shape of the left ventricular chamber is that of a prolated ellipsoid. Segmental wall motion abnormalities present particular problems. Errors in defining the silhouette of the left ventricle, errors in defining the appropriate correction factors, and the effects of arrhythmias all contribute to make the variation of these data as great as ±15 to 20%. Alternative methods, such as use of Simpson's rule, have not proved to be more accurate. Representative normal values are shown in Table 31–6 (Graham et al, 1971; Sandler and Dodge, 1968; Wynne et al, 1978).

Ejection Fraction Determination

From a practical clinical standpoint, the major advantage that has been derived from the ability to measure left ventricular volume has been the derivation of the most commonly used ejection phase index, the ejection fraction. Despite being dependent on both afterload and preload as well as inotropy, the ejection fraction remains the single most usable systolic performance characteristic derived at cardiac

TABLE 31–6. NORMAL LEFT VENTRICULAR VOLUMES AND EJECTION FRACTION DETERMINATIONS IN ADULTS AND CHILDREN

Patients	End-Diastolic Volume (ml/m²)	End-Systolic Volume (ml/m²)	Ejection Fraction (%)
Adults	72 ± 15	20 ± 8	0.72 ± 0.08
Children			
<2 years	42 ± 10	NA	0.68 ± 0.05
>2 years	73 ± 11	NA	0.63 ± 0.05

catheterization. The ejection fraction (EF) is simply the ratio of stroke volume (SV) to end-diastolic volume (EDV):

$$EF = \frac{EDV - ESV}{EDV} = \frac{SV}{EDV}$$

Because volumetric correction factors cancel each other in this ratio, errors in determining the correction factor for ventricular volumes become irrelevant in the ejection fraction determination. In most laboratories, a normal ejection fraction is defined as ≥55%. Minor variability is noted between biplane and single-plane methods and between groups who use a right anterior oblique (RAO) and left anterior oblique (LAO) view compared with those who use an AP and lateral view. Each individual laboratory group should establish its own normal values by using its own methods.

Assessment of Valvular Regurgitation

Regurgitant Fraction

The regurgitant fraction can be estimated by combining knowledge of forward cardiac output with angiographic output. If there is a single regurgitant valve, the difference between the angiographic stroke volume and the forward stroke volume can be defined as the regurgitant stroke volume by the following formula and regurgitant fraction (RF) determined:

$$RF = \frac{\text{angiographic SV} - \text{forward SV}}{\text{angiographic SV}} = \frac{\text{regurgitant SV}}{\text{angiographic SV}}$$

This formula incorporates many assumptions: that both the angiographic and forward cardiac output are correct, that heart rates are similar, that no changes have occurred in the hemodynamic state between the time the two measurements were made, and that only one valve is regurgitant. Because of these vagaries, the ratio provides only a gross estimate of the degree of valvular regurgitation.

Visual Assessment of Valvular Regurgitation

Valvular regurgitation is commonly assessed angiographically by visual estimation. When contrast is injected into the chamber distal to the regurgitant lesion, the amount of regurgitation into the proximal chamber can be assessed. The resultant opacity of the proximal chamber depends on the size and contractile properties of the proximal chamber. For example, a large, dilated proximal chamber appears less opacified by regurgitant contrast than a small chamber, despite a similar regurgitant volume. The basic classification of the degree of regurgitation

present was originally outlined by Sellers and associates (1964) and is essentially unchanged:

+	Minimal regurgitant jet seen. Clears rapidly from proximal chamber with each systole.
+ +	Moderate opacification of proximal chamber, clearing with subsequent systoles.
+ + +	Intense opacification of proximal chamber equal to that of the distal chamber.
+ + + +	Intense opacification of proximal chamber more dense than distal. Opacification often persists over entire series of images obtained.

In chronic mitral or tricuspid regurgitation, the atria are often greatly enlarged. In tricuspid regurgitation, contrast may be observed pulsating into the inferior vena cava during ventricular systole.

Regional Wall Motion Analysis

Adequate definitions of regional contractility have assumed greater importance with the advent of interventional procedures (coronary artery bypass or angioplasty) in patients with coronary artery disease. Both visual (qualitative) and quantitative methods have been applied.

Visual Interpretation of Segmental Wall Motion

Of five basic forms of segmental asynergy originally proposed by Herman and associates (1967), the following definitions have emerged in common use (Fig. 31–13):

Normal No abnormality seen
Hypokinesia A mild-to-moderate reduction in contraction with preservation of some degree of wall motion

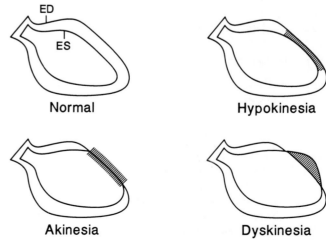

Figure 31–13. Regional definitions of wall motion. The end-diastolic (ED) and end-systolic (ES) contours are drawn, and the severity of regional wall motion is defined as shown.

Akinesia   Total absence of wall motion
Dyskinesia Paradoxical systolic expansion of the ventricular wall

In most laboratories, regional wall motion is assessed in three areas in the RAO or AP views (anterior, apical, inferior) and three areas of the lateral or LAO view (septal, apical, posterolateral). These regions are arbitrary, and several alternative divisions of the left ventricular silhouette are also used today.

Aneurysmal dilatation is difficult to define angiographically, but some guidelines are helpful (Cabin and Roberts, 1980). An aneurysm is probably present if there is a diastolic bulge in the left ventricular contour, discrete separation between the involved segment and the adjacent myocardium, and loss of trabeculation within the aneurysmal sac. The coronary artery supplying the aneurysmal area is usually poorly visualized or nonvisualized on selective injection. A false aneurysm or pseudoaneurysm may be present if a discrete area (neck) is seen between the aneurysmal sac and the remainder of the left ventricle in both systole and diastole. Pseudoaneurysms represent myocardial rupture with the formation of a localized pocket in the pericardium. The narrow neck represents the area of myocardial rupture between the normal left ventricular cavity and the pseudoaneurysm. Thrombus formation is a frequent observation in aneurysms.

Visual estimates of the severity of wall motion abnormalities are highly subjective. The precise delineations of various segments, the variability in wall motion even during one systole (tardokinesia is defined as normal but delayed contractility), the influence of chamber size, cardiac rotation, and systolic motion of the aortic and mitral valves all complicate visual analysis. In addition, the thin left ventricular apex results in wall stress at the apex, and because the majority of the stroke volume ejected is due to short-axis rather than long-axis shortening, the apex is particularly difficult to assess. Asynchrony in relaxation is also occasionally present (segmental early relaxation) (Gaasch et al, 1985).

Quantitative Segmental Wall Motion Analysis

To circumvent some of the difficulties with the visual interpretation of regional contraction abnormalities, various quantitative methods have been proposed. Each method requires certain inherent assumptions, and each has been variably accepted. In all of these methods, the end-systolic silhouette is superimposed on the end-diastolic silhouette, and segmental areas are then defined.

In the hemiaxial method, the realignment of the end-systolic and diastolic silhouettes is achieved by several methods, including aligning the aortic valve plane and the long axis of each and then constructing perpendicular chords to the long axis. Individual

chordal shortening can then be described. The radial method assumes that the ventricle contracts toward some predefined point. Chord lengths toward this point are then drawn and chordal shortening described. A variation of these methods uses the reduction of the areas enclosed by these hemiaxial or radial lines.

Sheehan and colleagues (1986) validated a centerline approach in which there was no realignment of the end-systolic or end-diastolic contours. The distance between the outer edges of these silhouettes is simply divided into half (the centerline) and 100 chords drawn perpendicularly to this centerline. After normalizing the data for the end-diastolic contour length, a plot of each chord motion is then displayed. Comparing patient data to a group of normal control ventriculograms, the motion of each chord can be defined in terms of standard deviation from the norm. Often selected chords (e.g., the 50% worst chords in an infarct area) are meaned and a single mean standard deviation number is reported. At Duke University Medical Center, a modification of this program is used clinically, and with more extensive analysis of the data it is also used for serial research studies (Fig. 31–14).

REPRESENTATIVE CLINICAL DATA

The following paragraphs briefly describe representative cardiac catheterization data for different disease states and are intended only to discuss pertinent hemodynamic observations.

Valvular Disease

Valvular Aortic Stenosis

Obstruction of the left ventricular outflow tract may occur at the level of the valve, above the valve (supravalvular stenosis), or below the valve (subvalvular stenosis). These stenoses can be observed angiographically and pressure gradients can be obtained. Valvular aortic stenosis is more common in men and rarely occurs as an isolated lesion in rheumatic disease. It is usually congenital or degenerative. Various degrees of commissural fusion, cusp malformation, and calcium deposition are seen in adult patients with aortic stenosis. Acquired aortic stenosis may be seen in rheumatic heart disease, in rheumatoid arthritis, in ochronosis, and with amyloid infiltration. Most adults with aortic stenosis have either a bicuspid aortic valve or tricuspid valves with "degenerative" calcific depositions that literally weigh the leaflets down. With obstruction to outflow, left ventricular pressures rise and left ventricular wall thickness increases to reduce wall stress:

$$\text{Wall stress} = \frac{\text{pressure} \times \text{radius}}{\text{wall thickness}}$$

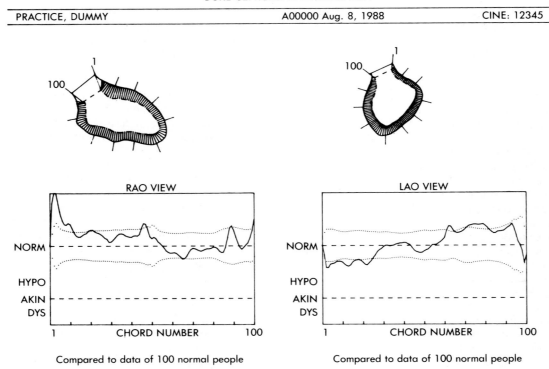

Figure 31–14. Duke centerline wall-motion program. This method of displaying regional wall motion by quantitative methods is a modification of that originally reported by Sheehan and associates (1986). The upper figures outline the end-diastolic (ED) and end-systolic (ES) silhouettes in the RAO *(left)* and LAO *(right)* views. The hatched area represents each of 100 chords drawn perpendicular to a centerline between the ED and ES contours. In the *bottom panels*, the normal (NORM) area is defined for each chord (within 1 standard deviation). Similarly, the areas of hypokinesia (HYPO), akinesia (AKIN), and dyskinesia (DYS) are plotted. Each chord motion relative to that observed in 100 normal patients is then shown.

Hypertrophy may become severe and is usually concentric. The resultant hypertrophy lowers wall stress and maintains the ejection fraction, but diastolic stiffness occurs, and symptoms of congestive failure and angina can result from the hypertrophic response despite preserved systolic performance. Atrial contraction becomes particularly important in an effort to fill these stiff ventricles, and the left ventricular a wave may be prominent. Cardiac output at rest is usually normal, although it may fail to increase appropriately during exercise. The ejection fraction, which may remain normal for many years, may decline as the "afterload mismatch" presented by the stenotic valve and high wall stress becomes dominant (Ross, 1976; Selzer, 1987). Because the ejection fraction and wall stress are inversely related (Gunther and Grossman, 1979), the reduction in ejection fraction noted in some patients with severe aortic stenosis may be a function of only high wall stress and not represent true myocardial failure. As a consequence, dramatic increases in ejection fraction may be observed after relief of the outflow obstruction when aortic valve replacement is performed.

The hypertrophy accompanying aortic stenosis is responsible for the congestive symptoms due to abnormal chamber stiffness, and although coronary flow per milligram of tissue is normal, the increased mass may alter transmural coronary flow, reduce coronary flow reserve (Marcus et al, 1982), and result in angina. Coronary arterial lesions of marginal significance under normal conditions may become flow limiting in the presence of such high coronary flow; this latter phenomenon makes it difficult at times to opacify coronary arteries adequately during angiography in patients with aortic stenosis. In general, an effective orifice area of ≤0.8 cm² and a peak systolic gradient of >50 mm Hg in the presence of a normal cardiac output are considered thresholds for performing surgical or other interventions in symptomatic patients.

Aortic Regurgitation

Although most adult patients with aortic stenosis have either bicuspid aortic valves or a degenerative calcific process, the causes of aortic regurgitation are more varied. Aortic regurgitation may result from a dilated aortic root (e.g., in Marfan's syndrome, Ehlers-Danlos syndrome, annuloaortic ectasia, cystic medial necrosis, hypertension, pseudoxanthoma elasticum), from primary aortic cusp involvement (e.g., endocarditis, rheumatic disease, alkylosing spondylitis, rheumatoid arthritis, sinus of Valsalva's aneurysm), from aortitis (e.g., syphilis, giant-cell arteritis) or from loss of commissural support (e.g., trauma, ventricular septal defect, aortic dissection).

Whatever the cause, the associated hemodynamics are directly related to the acuteness of the process. In *acute aortic regurgitation*, the left ventricle has had inadequate time to adapt to the sudden insult from the regurgitant volume. Diastolic left ventricular pressure increases dramatically (Morganroth et al, 1977) and may prematurely close the mitral valve in mid or late diastole. This "preclosure" can be readily observed by using echocardiography. Because stroke volume declines, the systemic pulse pressure may be narrow. To compensate for this, heart rates are often high. Because there may be little gradient between the aortic diastolic and left ventricular diastolic pressures, an aortic regurgitant murmur may not be audible. The patient is usually acutely ill. Representative hemodynamics are shown in Figure 31–15.

Compared with acute aortic regurgitation, the hemodynamics of *chronic aortic regurgitation* differ greatly. In chronic aortic regurgitation, the left ventricle hypertrophies and dilates over time. This gradual wall thickening in response to the dilated left ventricle maintains normal wall stresses in accordance with Laplace's equation (Grossman et al, 1975). The left ventricular chamber may greatly enlarge, and the ejection fraction may remain in the normal range for a long time. Although a decline in exercise ejection fraction has been used by some as a harbinger of impending myocardial failure (Kawanishi et al, 1986), the meaning of the exercise ejection fraction is complicated because of the shortened diastole (and less aortic regurgitation per beat) that occurs during stress testing.

The pulse pressure is usually wide and the left ventricular end-diastolic pressure is almost normal. When myocardial failure ensues, the resting ejection fraction falls and the end-systolic volume rises. Systolic wall tension increases late in the course, and afterload mismatch occurs as a result of inadequate hypertrophy (Ricci, 1982). Forward stroke volume ultimately declines. End-diastolic wall stress may then rise, and this can be estimated approximately by the echo end-diastolic radius/wall thickness ratio (Gaasch et al, 1978). With a fall in stroke volume and rise in end-diastolic volume, the end-systolic volume appears to be a sensitive indicator of both operative mortality and postoperative improvement after aortic valve replacement (Borow et al, 1980).

Mitral Stenosis

Mitral stenosis predominantly occurs secondary to rheumatic fever, although congenital forms (e.g., parachute mitral valve) and other acquired forms (e.g., carcinoid, lupus, rheumatoid arthritis, amyloid,

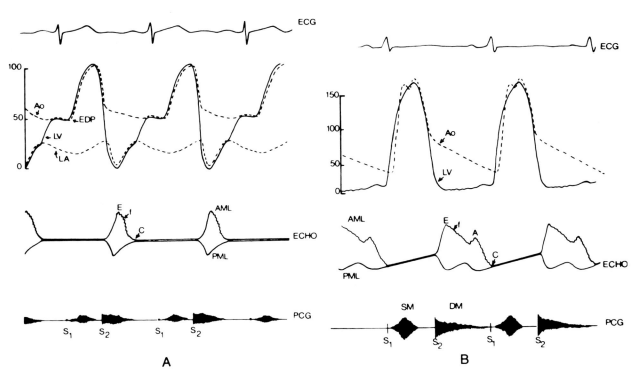

Figure 31–15. The hemodynamics of acute and chronic aortic regurgitation. *A,* Acute aortic regurgitation (AR) results in a sharp rise in the left ventricular end-diastolic pressure (LVEDP), a normal aortic (AO) pulse pressure, raised left atrial (LA) pressures, premature closure of the mitral valve (C point) on echo, and a relatively short and often soft diastolic murmur on phonocardiogram (PCG). *B,* Chronic AR is shown. In this situation, the LVEDP may be normal, the aortic pulse pressure is wide with a reduced aortic diastolic pressure, the mitral valve closes normally with the onset of LV systole, and the AR murmur is obvious. (Reproduced with permission from Morganroth, J., Perloff, J. K., Zeldis, S. M., and Dunkman, W. B.: Acute severe aortic regurgitation. Ann. Intern. Med., *87*:225, 1977.)

mitral annular calcification, tumor) are less commonly encountered.

When the normal mitral orifice (4 to 6 cm²) is reduced, a gradient occurs between the left atrium and left ventricle in diastole. Severe mitral stenosis is thought to be present when valve area is less than 1.5 to 1 cm². Atrial contraction helps to fill the left ventricle and can represent up to 30% of the gradient across the valve (Stott et al, 1970). With left ventricular filling reduced, the left ventricular end-diastolic volumes are often low or normal, and left ventricular mass is consequently normal or slightly reduced. A mild degree of global ventricular dysfunction may then result. In addition, scarring of the submitral apparatus and papillary muscle may result in regional wall-motion abnormalities (Colle et al, 1983). With exercise, symptoms in mitral stenosis are primarily related to the rise in the mitral gradient and not to exercise-induced left ventricular dysfunction (Johnston and Kostuk, 1986). The left atrial (pulmonary capillary wedge) pressure shows a prominent a wave and a blunted y descent as left ventricular filling from the left atrium is restricted (see Fig. 31–11).

Pulmonary hypertension eventually occurs not only as a result of the elevated left atrial pressure, but also as a result of arteriolar constriction and obliterative changes in the pulmonary vascular bed. There may be a reversible component to pulmonary hypertension (Halperin et al, 1985), and pressures usually fall rapidly after relief of the mitral valvular obstruction (Foltz et al, 1984). Pulmonary compliance is often reduced, blood flow is redistributed from the base to apex, and abnormal pulmonary function tests are observed. There is a poor correlation between the results of commissurotomy and symptoms, and restenosis may not always be present when symptoms recur after operation (Higgs et al, 1970).

Mitral Regurgitation

Normal function of the mitral valve apparatus involves the proper alignment and coaptation of the mitral leaflets, but it also requires appropriate function of the mitral annulus, the chordae tendineae, and the papillary muscles. Mitral regurgitation results whenever any component of this apparatus is abnormal.

The consequences of mitral regurgitation are due to both the magnitude and the acuteness of the process. When *acute mitral regurgitation* occurs, the left atrium is unable to accept the increased volume without a resultant greatly elevated left atrial pressure. A large v wave can then be seen in the pulmonary capillary wedge tracing and is even reflected into the pulmonary arterial pressure (Fig. 31–16). In *chronic mitral regurgitation*, the left atrium has usually enlarged over time and is able to absorb the effect of the regurgitant volume without greatly raising the pulmonary pressures.

Pathophysiologically, acute mitral regurgitation reduces the systolic workload on the left ventricle

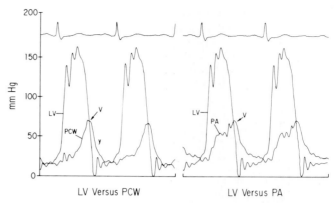

Figure 31–16. Mitral regurgitation and poor left atrial compliance. The left ventricular (LV) versus the pulmonary capillary wedge (PCW) pressure is shown on the left. The large regurgitant v wave is evident. This marked v wave is transmitted to the pulmonary arterial (PA) tracing and is seen to be superimposed in the *right panel.*

and allows it to empty more completely, increasing the measured ejection fraction. Over time the left ventricular end-diastolic volume gradually increases, and myocardial failure eventually ensues.

The "afterload sink" provided by the left atrium may maintain ejection fraction in the relatively normal range for a long time, however, which creates a dilemma in the timing of the operation in this situation. As with aortic regurgitation, the end-systolic volume or stress-volume ratio may provide the most useful information regarding operative outcome (Borow et al, 1980; Carabello et al, 1981). Patients who have chronic mitral regurgitation and who have even mild symptoms (Class II) should probably be operated on if exercise hemodynamics suggest inadequate compensation with stress or if resting left ventricular end-systolic volumes are increased. When the resting ejection fraction begins to decline, the surgeon must assume that myocardial dysfunction is well under way.

Right-Sided Heart Valvular Lesions

TRICUSPID STENOSIS

Tricuspid stenosis is generally the result of rheumatic heart disease or congenital atresia, although other causes (e.g., tumor, vegetations, carcinoid) may be etiologic. As the right atrial outflow obstruction increases, right atrial pressures rise, the y descent becomes blunted, and the a wave increases dramatically. A mean gradient in diastole of 5 mm Hg is considered significant. Most patients with tricuspid stenosis have associated valvular disease (usually mitral stenosis). Tricuspid regurgitation frequently accompanies tricuspid stenosis. Surgical approaches such as commissurotomy are infrequently effective, and valve replacement (often with a porcine heterograft) is required (Cobanoglu and Starr, 1986).

TRICUSPID REGURGITATION

The tricuspid valve apparatus differs in many ways from the mitral valve apparatus. In addition to three large leaflets, there are numerous chordae that attach to a variety of small papillary muscles and to the right ventricular endocardium directly. Papillary muscle dysfunction therefore is rarely a cause of tricuspid regurgitation compared with mitral regurgitation. Tricuspid annular dilatation may prevent adequate valvular coaptation (Come and Riley, 1985) and is the most common cause of tricuspid regurgitation—usually as a result of right ventricular failure from any of a number of causes. Various other diseases, both rheumatic and nonrheumatic, can affect the tricuspid leaflet primarily.

Right atrial pressure and the right ventricular end-diastolic pressure are usually increased in tricuspid regurgitation. As the condition worsens, the right atrial v wave occurs earlier and will gradually obliterate the x descent (c-v wave) as the regurgitation fills the atrium during ventricular systole. In severe tricuspid regurgitation there is "ventricularization" of the right atrium. Right atrial pressures may then lose the characteristic changes with respiration; in fact, an actual rise may occur during inspiration (Cha and Gooch, 1983).

When the right ventricular systolic pressure is greater than 40 to 45 mm Hg, one may assume that tricuspid regurgitation is functional. Right ventriculography is useful, although the right ventricular catheter may tend to hold the valve open during injection. Contrast injected into the right ventricle is seen jetting into the right atrium, and with proper positioning, the contrast may also be seen pulsating into the inferior vena cava or hepatic veins during ventricular systole. Various catheters and techniques (e.g., low injection rates) have been used to minimize catheter-induced tricuspid regurgitation during right-sided ventriculography (Ubago et al, 1981).

Tricuspid valvular prolapse may occasionally be seen on angiography by the posterior billowing of the tricuspid leaflets. In Ebstein's anomaly, the tricuspid valve ring is displaced into the right ventricle and there is atrialization of a portion of the right ventricle. Using simultaneous pressure recording and intracardiac electrocardiography, it can be shown that a catheter can be placed into a hemodynamically evident right atrium, yet record the right ventricular electrocardiographic changes in Ebstein's anomaly.

PULMONIC VALVE DISEASE

Most pulmonic stenosis occurs as a result of a congenitally abnormal pulmonic valve. Rarely acquired forms, such as rheumatic, carcinoid tumors, or contiguous structures, may obstruct the pulmonic outflow at the valvular level.

Pulmonic regurgitation is usually a result of dilatation of the pulmonic annulus. Dilatation can result from pulmonary hypertension or can be secondary to idiopathic pulmonary dilatation. Less frequently, collagen vascular diseases (e.g., Marfan's syndrome) or endocarditis rarely may occur. Surgical trauma to the valve may occur during repair of right-sided heart lesions. Other valvular lesions have been reported with congenitally malformed pulmonic leaflets—often in association with tetralogy of Fallot or ventricular septal defect. The use of pulmonary artery catheters has also been reported to cause pulmonic regurgitation (O'Toole et al, 1979).

Pulmonic stenosis is diagnosed by the simultaneous measurement of pulmonary artery and right ventricular pressures. A 50-mm Hg gradient is usually considered significant, and repair is recommended. The right ventricle is often greatly hypertrophied, and subpulmonic infundibular hypertrophy may be especially prominent. After sudden relief of pulmonary outflow obstruction (e.g., with valvuloplasty), the right ventricle may eject rigorously and fail to fill adequately on subsequent beats—the "suicide right ventricular phenomenon."

Pulmonic regurgitation is difficult to define by using commonly employed catheter techniques. When pulmonary systolic pressure is greater than 70 mm Hg, the pulmonary artery is often dilated and a Graham Steell's murmur of pulmonic regurgitation results. Intracardiac phonocardiography documents the presence of pulmonic regurgitation, although echo-Doppler methods are clearly superior to cardiac catheterization. Pulmonary angiography reveals pulmonic regurgitation, but catheter-induced valvular regurgitation makes the degree of regurgitation difficult to assess. Surgical intervention is rarely required as the right ventricle is designed for volume work and rarely fails as a result of pulmonic regurgitation alone (Emery et al, 1979).

Prosthetic Valve Assessment

All prosthetic valves are inherently obstructive to outflow or inflow, and some gradient can generally be detected across them. The effective orifice area and resultant pressure gradients across prosthetic valves can be approximated by in-vitro studies using a pulse duplicator (Gabby and Kresh, 1985). When mean effective orifice areas are evaluated for small prostheses at a common output (5 l/min), values from 1.2 to 1.9 cm^2 are common. Medium-sized prostheses have effective orifice areas in the range of 1.7 to 2.8 cm^2 and large prostheses from 1.9 to 3.4 cm^2. These prostheses carry mean gradients of 10 to 30 mm Hg for small, 5 to 19 mm Hg for medium, and 3 to 8 mm Hg for large valves, respectively.

The translation of in-vitro data to the clinical setting is difficult at best, but it is apparent that the prosthetic valve type and size are major factors in determining the potential degree of inherent stenosis. The determined effective orifice area is output dependent and Gorlin's formula may introduce bias in interpreting results (Cannon et al, 1988).

At catheterization, the ball valves and tissue

valves can usually be crossed in a retrograde manner without hemodynamic embarrassment. This is not true of disk valves (or the St. Jude valve) because the disks are held open by the crossing catheter. Gradient measurement with an aortic prosthesis in place must be accomplished by left ventricular pressure recording using a catheter placed trans-septally into the left ventricle. Ventriculography is accomplished using this same catheter.

Aortic prostheses are more inherently obstructive than mitral prostheses because of the smaller ring diameters. Resting hemodynamics may also fail to reflect the gradient potential observed during exercise. In patients with mitral valve replacement, the removal of the papillary muscles may also contribute to left ventricular dysfunction (Kazama et al, 1986), and newer attempts to preserve the native valve by valve repair are promising (Carpentier et al, 1980).

It is important to emphasize that the inherent stenotic nature of most prosthetic valves makes the use of valve replacement for stenotic lesions limited to severe valvular stenosis. Valvular replacement for mild to moderate stenosis may result in no effective hemodynamic change.

The fluoroscopic image for each prosthetic valve is unique to the device implanted and has been reviewed (Mehlman, 1988). Motion of the prosthetic valve ring in and out of the direction of flow should be considered normal whereas motion perpendicular to the direction of flow may imply valvular dysfunction. The acceptable tilt for most prosthetic aortic valves is less than 12 to 15 degrees (White et al, 1973).

A few comments regarding each prosthesis may be useful. Further details may be found in other sources (Morse et al, 1985). The evaluation of caged-ball valves should include poppet motion and configuration, the clearance between the ball and the struts or the ring, and the evenness of the stroke. The sewing ring on Starr-Edwards' valves may normally tilt from 2 to 6 degrees in the aortic position and from 5 to 21 degrees in the mitral position (White et al, 1973).

The hinged or tilting monocuspid valves, exemplified by the Björk-Shiley's prosthesis, should be observed to close completely against the sewing ring to ensure that no thrombosis is present. The base should tilt less than 6 degrees in the aortic and less than 10 degrees in the mitral position, and the opening angle should be 60 degrees (Heystraten and Paalman, 1981). Either low forward flow or thrombosis can affect the maximal opening angle.

Caged-disk prostheses, such as the Beall valve, are now used less commonly. The disk should be parallel to the suture ring at end-diastole and end-systole, although some cocking movement is seen normally. Disk sticking or cocking at end-diastole or end-systole is distinctly abnormal. Over time, disk shrinkage can occur and is noted by defining the disk-to-suture ring ratio. An abnormal ratio is less than 0.85 (Carlson et al, 1981).

Bileaflet prostheses, such as the St. Jude valve, are difficult to evaluate because the base ring is not radiopaque. When closed, the leaflets, which are radiopaque when viewed on end, meet the base at a 30 to 35-degree angle and open to an 85-degree angle. Valve orientation varies, and angulated views are usually required to observe the leaflets. In the aortic position, the LAO view with some angulation is often the best position for observing the thin lines of the leaflets in profile. The Duromedic bileaflet valve has an opaque base ring and is more readily assessed with fluoroscopy.

The fluoroscopic evaluation of heterografts is often difficult, although tilting of the base can be observed. Calcification may occasionally be seen and is indicative of degenerative changes within the leaflets. The large struts of the Carpentier-Edwards porcine or Ionescu-Shiley bovine pericardial valves are readily seen; however, only the metal supporting ring is opaque in the Hancock porcine valve.

Cardiomyopathies

Primary cardiac muscle disorders are now generally classified based on anatomic, hemodynamic, and functional features. Dilated (formerly congestive) cardiomyopathies are characterized by a dilated left ventricle (or right ventricle) chamber with large end-diastolic and large end-systolic volumes. Hypertrophy that should be present to reduce wall stress is not always achieved, and wall thickness is usually inappropriately in the normal range. Contractile performance is poor. Hypertrophic cardiomyopathies have inappropriately increased left ventricular hypertrophy with normal left ventricular diastolic volume and either normal or hypercontractile systolic function. Hypertrophy is usually asymmetric, with septal thickness greater than 1.3 times free-wall thickness, but apical and other regional hypertrophy may also occur. Restrictive cardiomyopathies have normal or almost normal systolic function, usually normal or mildly increased left ventricular end-diastolic volumes, and often greatly raised left ventricular end-diastolic pressures. Restrictive cardiomyopathies are primarily due to infiltrative processes. Restrictive myocardial disease almost always affects the left ventricle more than the right ventricle, and this distribution aids in differentiating restrictive hemodynamics from constrictive pericarditis.

The cause cannot be defined in most cases of *dilated cardiomyopathy*, and the condition likely reflects the final result of myocardial injury from a host of potential causes. Possible causes include infective myocarditis (usually viral), collagen vascular diseases, toxic agents (such as alcohol, cancer chemotherapeutic agents), chronic volume overload (atrioventricular shunts, sickle cell anemia), radiation, transplant rejection, genetic associations (such as Friedreich's ataxia). It has been described in the postpartum period and can be associated with obesity or other endocrine disorders (Johnson and Palacios, 1982).

At catheterization, in addition to defining the severity of the systolic and diastolic dysfunction and excluding coronary artery disease as causative, myocardial biopsies now can be done routinely. Myocardial biopsies can identify cardiac transplant rejection, myocarditis, sarcoidosis, amyloidosis, chemotherapy toxicity (due to high dose cyclophosphamide [Cytoxan] or doxorubicin [Adriamycin]), hemochromatosis, carcinoid, endocardial fibroelastosis, glycogen storage disease, or tumor (Laser et al, 1985).

Left ventriculography shows diffuse hypocontractility, although regional differences in the degree of wall motion abnormality occur frequently. Left ventricular thrombi can occasionally be identified.

In the normal left ventricle, the short-axis dimension at end-diastole is about one half the long axis, and approximately 85% of the stroke volume ejected is due to short-axis shortening. In dilated cardiomyopathy, the short-axis and long-axis diameters have almost equal dimensions (Krevlen et al, 1980). Teleologically, the thin left ventricular apex has greater wall stress (based on Laplace's equation), and as left ventricular systolic function declines, the left ventricle would therefore be expected to dilate more in the short-axis than in the long-axis dimension—thus becoming more spherical as failure occurs. A spherical left ventricular shape is common in dilated cardiomyopathies. The dilated left ventricular chamber is also associated with a dilated mitral annulus and malalignment of the mitral apparatus; therefore, mitral regurgitation of various amounts is usually present.

Hypertrophic cardiomyopathy is generally regarded as a genetic disorder (Clark et al, 1973). Because outflow obstruction of various degrees may be present, the terms *idiopathic hypertrophic subaortic stenosis (IHSS)* and *hypertrophic obstructive cardiomyopathy* are often used to describe this condition. Hypertrophy may not be confined to the septum, however, and an apical form is now frequently encountered. The unique dynamic nature of the left ventricular outflow obstruction observed has attracted the attention of most diagnosticians, but it is important to appreciate that although outflow tract obstruction may be hemodynamically interesting, the major symptoms experienced by the patient are due to the high ventricular filling pressures. Diastolic dysfunction results in symptoms of angina due to coronary underperfusion and to pulmonary congestion. The amount of outflow tract gradient has not been shown to correlate with either symptoms or survival.

The classic findings in hypertrophic cardiomyopathy include a raised left ventricular end-diastolic pressure caused by both increased ventricular stiffness and reduced active relaxation (Hanrath et al, 1980). Mitral regurgitation is relatively common, and the combination of mitral regurgitation and raised left ventricular end-diastolic pressure increases pulmonary pressures. Right ventricular outflow tract

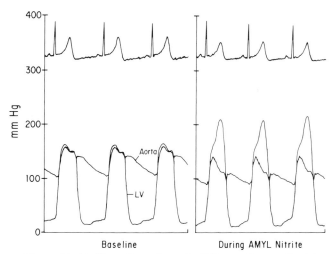

Figure 31–17. The effect of amyl nitrite on the gradient in hypertrophic cardiomyopathy. At baseline, little gradient is present although slight notching in the aortic contour is present. With amyl nitrite, the aortic pressure falls, the left ventricular (LV) pressure rises, and the gradient is increased.

obstruction can occasionally be noted. The subaortic jet may also cause aortic insufficiency over time.

The most interesting feature of hypertrophic cardiomyopathy is the dynamic nature of the left ventricular outflow gradient. Any maneuver that decreases left ventricular afterload, reduces left ventricular volume or that increases inotropy causes an increased gradient. The converse of this is also true. At catheterization, the dynamic nature of the systolic gradient is usually initiated by the Valsalva's maneuver, amyl nitrite, or isoproterenol (Fig. 31–17). Careful analysis of the gradient shows a subaortic chamber with no left ventricular to aortic gradient (Fig. 31–18). The pulse pressure in the beat following a single premature ventricular contraction would be

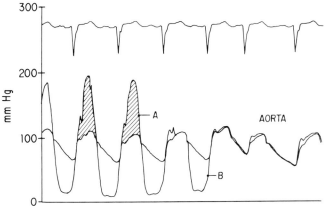

Figure 31–18. Left ventricular (LV) pressure during pullback from LV to the aorta in hypertrophic cardiomyopathy. By using a double-micromanometer catheter, the aortic tracing remains unchanged as the LV tracing shows a subaortic gradient *(A),* then no subaortic gradient *(B).* Despite the loss of an outflow tract gradient, the distal pressure still reflects LV pressure, confirming no valvular gradient.

expected to increase in normal patients, whereas it may decrease in patients with hypertrophic cardiomyopathy (an observation usually referred to as Brockenbrough's sign) (Brockenbrough et al, 1961) (Fig. 31–19).

The rapid emptying of the left ventricle results in a prominent percussion wave in the aortic tracing, and the early cessation of forward flow results in an initial decline, then a second, rounded tidal wave (the spike and dome configuration). The rapid ejection of blood from the ventricle through the narrowed outflow tract causes the anterior mitral leaflet to be drawn toward the septum during systole (systolic anterior motion). The role of the mitral valve in the creation of the outflow gradient is still controversial, however (Murgo et al, 1980; Wigle et al, 1985).

An angiogram indicates obvious left ventricular hypertrophy, and regional accentuation in the degree of hypertrophy (septal, midventricular, or apical) can usually be identified. An "empty ventricle" is sometimes present, with almost complete emptying of the left ventricle in systole. Systolic anterior motion of the mitral valve can be observed in the cranial LAO view in many patients. Mitral regurgitation of various amounts is seen, and aortic regurgitation is also present occasionally (presumably because of the jet from the subaortic stenosis injuring the aortic valve). Coronary angiography may demonstrate septal perforator compression (Pichard et al, 1979). Ventricular dilatation may develop if myocardial infarction occurs. Myocardial infarction has been reported in these patients despite normal epicardial coronary vessels (Maron et al, 1979).

Outflow tract obstruction under basal conditions is not required for the diagnosis of hypertrophic cardiomyopathy. Indeed, Maron and associates (1987) estimate that approximately only 25% of all patients have a gradient without provocation.

Restrictive cardiomyopathy due to infiltrative processes is uncommon. Differentiation from constrictive pericarditis may be difficult, but some guidelines are useful. In most patients, diastolic pressures in the left ventricle are higher than in the right ventricle when the pressures are simultaneously tracked (Tyberg et al, 1981). The abnormal left ventricular end-diastolic pressure results in raised pulmonary pressure to levels often more than 50 mm Hg (an uncommon finding in constriction) (Grossman, 1986). While early diastolic filling is excessively rapid in constrictive pericarditis, early filling may be blunted as a result of abnormal active relaxation in restrictive cardiomyopathy. Systolic performance (ejection fraction) may be normal or only slightly reduced in restrictive disease. Echocardiography and computed tomography may help to exclude pericardial disease.

Right ventricular pressure tracings during acute right ventricular infarction at times show the dip and plateau pattern similar to constrictive pericarditis (Lorell et al, 1979), which in effect mimics a form of right ventricular restriction. This pattern may be due to dilatation of the right ventricle to the extent that the pericardium becomes physiologically restrictive (Goldstein et al, 1982). Acute dilatation of any of the cardiac chambers, which may occur in tricuspid or mitral regurgitation (Bartle and Hermann, 1967), can also produce this dip and plateau pattern.

Pericardial Disease

One can conceptually visualize the pericardium as a balloon or sac. The heart can be then viewed as an organ pushed into the side of this sac. The visceral pericardium represents the portion of the sac that covers the heart and the parietal pericardium represents the remainder of the sac. The normal pericardium contains less than 50 ml of fluid produced by serosal cells that line the pericardium (Roberts and Spray, 1976). Lymphatics drain along the epicardial surface and eventually to the mediastinum and right-sided heart cavities (Miller et al, 1971).

The functions of the pericardium have been described as mechanical, membranous, and ligamentous (Spodick, 1983). Diseases of the pericardium cause restriction of diastolic filling of the heart. Cardiac tamponade causes compression of the ventricles and prevents filling both early and late in diastole. Constrictive pericarditis is characterized by rapid early filling of the left ventricle with sudden cessation in filling at mid and late diastole. Mixed disorders (effusive constriction) also exist.

Pericardial disorders are relatively common in the postoperative period after cardiac surgery. Pericardial tamponade and the postpericardiotomy syndrome are the most common complications that occur after open heart procedures (Engle et al, 1978). Other etiologies that result in pericarditis are numerous and include infections that mimic a form of right ventricular restriction. Intrapericardial pressure that occurs with fluid accumulation is a function of the compli-

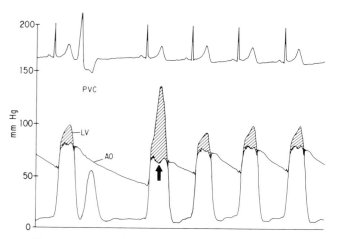

Figure 31–19. Brockenbrough's phenomenon in hypertrophic cardiomyopathy. After premature ventricular contraction (PVC), the left ventricular (LV) pressure gradient rises dramatically, but the aortic (AO) pulse pressure actually is less than the baseline pulse pressure. In addition, the "spike and dome" contour in the aortic pulse *(arrow)* becomes evident on the post-PVC beat.

ance of the pericardium, the size of the heart within the pericardium, the volume of the fluid, and the rapidity with which the fluid accumulates. When approximately 150 ml of fluid accumulates in a normal pericardium, the intrapericardial pressure rises sharply and pericardial tamponade may occur. The rise in intrapericardial pressure prevents right ventricular filling and results in the loss of the y descent in the right atrial tracing. Inspiratory changes are usually normal, with a normal fall in right atrial pressure during inspiration (i.e., no Kussmaul's sign is present). The inspiratory increase in right atrial and right ventricular filling, together with normal pooling of blood in the lungs, reduces left ventricular filling with inspiration. Left ventricular stroke volume thus declines during inspiration by more than 10 mm Hg (pulsus paradoxus). The high intrapericardial pressures result in end-diastolic right atrial, right ventricular, left ventricular, and pulmonary capillary wedge pressures all equalizing. The exception is when there is pre-existing left ventricular diastolic dysfunction (Reddy, 1978). The failure to transport blood from the right side of the heart to the left side of the heart results in normal or only modestly raised pulmonary artery pressures. Pulse pressure in the pulmonary artery and aorta may consequently be narrow.

Angiography is rarely necessary in cardiac tamponade. Right atrial angiography in the AP view may reveal a right atrial silhouette outside the right atrial angiographic border, confirming pericardial thickening or fluid. Echocardiography is clearly the most sensitive and useful diagnostic test to confirm pericardial fluid. Pericardiocentesis is easily done and is useful from both a diagnostic and therapeutic standpoint.

Pericardial constriction occurs when the two pericardial layers (parietal and visceral) fuse as a result of scar formation. The potential etiologies of constrictive pericarditis are extensive. Idiopathic causes, viruses, uremia, neoplasm, radiation, rheumatic disorders, and cardiac surgical intervention have replaced tuberculosis as the leading causes of constriction (Lorell and Braunwald, 1988). Fibrin and thrombus accumulation in the pericardium may result in a picture of constrictive pericarditis rapidly after heart operations (Cohen and Greenberg, 1979).

When the pericardium scars and fuses together, it acts physiologically like a cement vault. The heart within this vault can fill rapidly only in early diastole. As the heart fills, it expands against the walls of the vault and filling ceases. The high atrial pressures before atrioventricular valve opening result in a large early diastolic gradient and rapid early flow into the ventricles (the rapid y descent). The sudden cessation of inflow and the abrupt rise in ventricular diastolic pressure create a dip and plateau pattern in ventricular diastole. In severe constriction, inspiratory changes do not occur, and the right atrial pressure may even rise (Kussmaul's sign). Representative patient's hemodynamics are shown in Figures 31–20 and 31–21. This failure to fill the right side of the heart with inspiration differs from that observed in tamponade, and thus pulsus paradoxus is unusual in constrictive pericarditis. Pulmonary pressures are usually normal or only minimally increased, and the right ventricular diastolic pressure is usually greater than one-third of the right ventricular systolic. The hemodynamics can be confused with those in restrictive cardiomyopathy or those in severe atrioventricular valvular regurgitation as noted earlier.

Mixed effusive-constrictive physiology is also occasionally noted and becomes evident when constrictive hemodynamics persist after pericardiocentesis (Mann et al, 1978). In addition, it has been suggested that an occult pericardial constriction exists that can be identified by rapid volume loading in certain patients with normal baseline hemodynamics (Bush et al, 1977).

Angiography is rarely useful in pericardial constriction. Coronary angiography may reveal pericardial scarring that can compress or impede coronary flow (Navetta et al, 1988). Pericardial thickening can be seen by right atrial injection and by observation of the right atrial lateral wall thickness. When this is done, a slow, jerky pattern of forward flow of radiographic contrast is often observed due to the limited portion of the cardiac cycle when ventricular filling

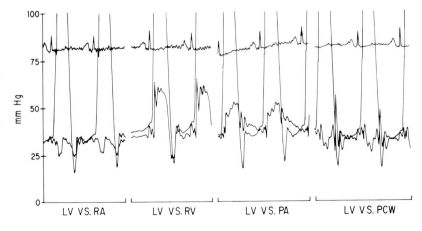

Figure 31–20. Equalization of diastolic pressures in constrictive pericarditis. When the left ventricle (LV) is tracked versus the right atrium (RA), right ventricle (RV), pulmonary artery (PA), and the pulmonary capillary wedge (PCW) pressure, diastolic pressures are similar. Note that the RV diastolic is half the RV systolic in the second panel. All diastolic pressures are greatly elevated in this example.

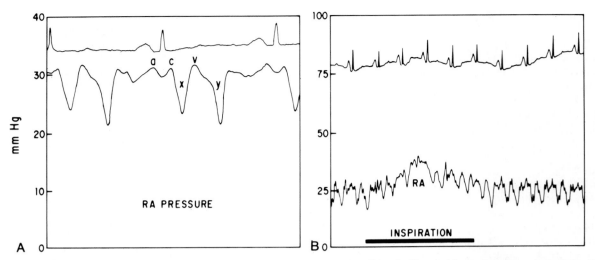

Figure 31–21. Representative right atrial (RA) tracings in constrictive pericarditis. *A,* The rapid x and y descents and the "square root" sign in diastole are evident in the left panel. *B,* Note the different scale. Inspiration results in a rise in the RA pressure. The rise or lack of fall in the RA pressure with inspiration is referred to as Kussmaul's sign.

can occur. Pericardial calcium may also be noted by fluoroscopy and usually spares the left ventricular apex (as opposed to left ventricular aneurysmal calcification).

Congenital Heart Disease

An outline of representative data in patients with congenital heart disease is beyond the scope of this discussion. Several brief comments are pertinent, however.

Techniques for catheterization of infants and children vary widely depending on the age of the child. The catheterization should be guided by the results of careful echo-Doppler examinations to prevent accumulation of redundant information. If the infant is less than 1 week old, an umbilical artery is generally catheterized for pressure monitoring. Venous access is usually easiest to achieve using the femoral vein, although the umbilical vein may be an option in neonates. The atrial septum may be readily crossed and left-sided heart catheterization is done through the patent foramen ovale. In children over 1 year of age, the femoral approach is routinely used in most laboratories. Various sedatives are used at the time of the procedure, depending on the child's age and whether cyanosis is present.

Cardiac catheterization in neonates carries a higher risk than in older children or in adults (Stanger et al, 1974). Urgent catheterization is generally done in cyanotic neonates, as interventional procedures (e.g., atrial septostomy) or the use of prostaglandin E_1 infusions to maintain the patient with a patent ductus arteriosus can be life-saving. A discussion regarding newer interventional procedures is included in the section on valvuloplasty and other invasive therapeutic procedures.

PERCUTANEOUS BALLOON VALVULOPLASTY AND OTHER INTERVENTIONAL TECHNIQUES

Rashkind and Miller (1968) initiated the use of balloon catheter techniques, reporting 31 children who had transposition of the great vessels and in whom catheter balloon atrioseptostomy was done. Since then, the field of catheter intervention has grown considerably, and its application has been broadened to include aortic coarctation (Lock et al, 1983; Morrow et al, 1988), obstructed intracardiac baffles (Lock et al, 1984), and stenosed pulmonary veins (Driscoll et al, 1982) and arteries (Lock et al, 1983). Catheter methods have also been used to insert devices to close atrial septal defects (King et al, 1976) and to close patent ductus arteriosus (Portsmann et al, 1967; Rashkind and Tait, 1985), arteriovenous fistulas (Terry et al, 1983) or even ventricular septal defects (Lock et al, 1988). Although a great deal must still be learned, balloon valvuloplasty procedures have steadily grown to be a significant case load for many busy pediatric cardiac catheterization laboratories (Lock et al, 1986).

Only recently have these procedures been applied in adult cardiac catheterization laboratories. The results are being investigated by national registry studies in both the United States and Europe. The initial results for pulmonic valvuloplasty have been so encouraging that the Food and Drug Administration has concluded that percutaneous valvuloplasty for pulmonic valve stenosis is an appropriate clinical option. It should be emphasized that percutaneous valvuloplasty is still experimental for all other valvular interventions and that research in the field has only just begun.

Sembh and associates (1979) generally are acknowledged to be the first surgeons to have successfully done balloon dilation of the pulmonic valve in a patient with pulmonary stenosis and severe tricuspid regurgitation. The procedure was accomplished by pulling an inflated balloon catheter back through the affected pulmonic valve. Kan and associates (1982) and Pepine and colleagues (1982) reported the procedure in isolated pulmonic stenosis. The number of reports has grown substantially since that time, and the technique has become widely used.

In 1984, the first attempts at percutaneous balloon valvuloplasty as therapy for mitral stenosis and aortic stenosis were reported. By using a single specially designed balloon catheter, Inoue and associates (1984) described successful dilatation of mitral stenosis in six patients with a trans-septal approach. In 1984 Lababidi and colleagues (1984) performed percutaneous aortic valvuloplasty in 23 children and young adults. These successes were followed by numerous other reports in young patients, most notably from Lock and associates (1985) and Al Zaibag and colleagues (1986) in rheumatic mitral stenosis and Rupprath and Neuhaus (1985) in aortic stenosis.

McKay and associates (1986) and Palacios and colleagues (1986) were the first physicians to report the successful application of percutaneous balloon valvuloplasty in adult patients with calcific mitral stenosis. In 1986 Cribier and co-workers described three elderly patients who had calcific aortic stenosis and in whom the procedure was successfully done.

Early follow-up results in patients with pulmonic or mitral stenosis are encouraging, but early restenosis appears evident in calcific aortic stenosis. The precise role these procedures will have in the future has yet to be clearly defined, although some guidelines are available.

The high rate of restenosis in elderly patients after aortic valvuloplasty is particularly frustrating, because this population also experiences the highest morbidity and mortality from open-heart procedures (Edmunds et al, 1988). Because all current prosthetic valves are responsible for significant morbidity over time, and many are inherently obstructive to cardiac inflow or outflow, the decision regarding surgical valve replacement is particularly difficult in very young and very old patients. Alternative approaches will certainly be eagerly sought until there are substantial improvements in the development and application of prosthetic valves.

Techniques and Immediate Results

PULMONIC BALLOON VALVULOPLASTY (Fig. 31–22)

Pulmonic valvuloplasty is usually done by using the percutaneous right femoral venous approach. The pulmonary artery catheter is replaced by a guidewire, and the balloon catheter is positioned over this wire. Balloon sizes have evolved over time, and most physicians now prefer oversized balloons based on both animal (Ring et al, 1984) and clinical (Radtke et al, 1987) data suggesting that maximal dilatation up

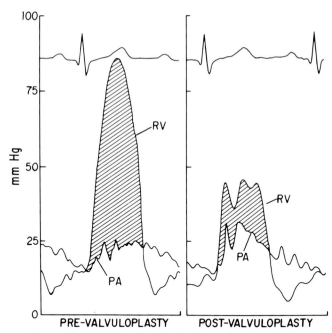

Figure 31–22. Pulmonic valvuloplasty. The sharply elevated right ventricular (RV) pressure and distorted low pulmonary artery (PA) pressure change dramatically and acutely after balloon pulmonic valvuloplasty.

to 30% larger than the pulmonic annulus can improve results. Balloons that inflate to 1.2 to 1.4 times the pulmonary annulus size, as assessed by echocardiography or angiography, are used. Either a double-balloon technique (Ali Khan et al, 1986) or a specially designed trefoil balloon catheter (Meier et al, 1986) is frequently required. If iliac vein obstruction is present, an axillary approach can be used (Sideris et al, 1988).

The immediate results from pulmonic valvuloplasty have been impressive. "Typical" results that have been reported are summarized in Table 31–7 (Ali Kahn et al, 1986; Cooke et al, 1987; Griffith et al, 1982; Kan et al, 1982, 1984; Marantz et al, 1988; Meier et al, 1986; Pepine et al, 1982; Radtke et al, 1987; Rao

TABLE 31–7. "TYPICAL" IMMEDIATE HEMODYNAMIC RESULTS AFTER PERCUTANEOUS VALVULOPLASTY PROCEDURES

Procedure and Measure	Before	After
Pulmonic valvuloplasty		
Peak right ventricular pressure (mm Hg)	100	50
Peak gradient (mm Hg)	80	30
Cardiac index (l/min/m²)	3	3
Mitral valvuloplasty		
Mean mitral gradient (mm Hg)	17	7
Mitral valve area (cm²)	1	2.2
Cardiac index (l/min/m²)	2.5	3
Aortic valvuloplasty		
Mean aortic gradient (mm Hg)	75	35
Aortic valve area (cm²)	0.6	0.9
Cardiac index (l/min/m²)	2	2.2

et al, 1988; Rocchini et al, 1984; Sembh et al, 1979). Immediate hemodynamic data would be expected to underestimate the final pulmonic gradient if transient right ventricular dysfunction occurred, but would overestimate the final gradient if subpulmonic obstruction transiently increased. Either of these situations may effect acute changes. Significant subpulmonic obstruction can occur immediately after the procedure, but fortunately this usually responds to beta-blocker therapy (Rao et al, 1988). This infundibular obstruction has been observed to regress over time after either pulmonary valvotomy (Engle, 1958; Griffith, 1982) or balloon valvuloplasty (Rao et al, 1988; Sullivan, 1986). If dysplasia of the pulmonic valve is present, balloon dilatation appears to be less effective, although larger balloon sizes may be satisfactory (Marantz et al, 1988; Rao et al, 1988). The true incidence of pulmonic regurgitation after pulmonic valvuloplasty ranges from 0 to 74%, depending on the methods used for assessment. Echo or Doppler studies suggest that pulmonic insufficiency of at least a mild degree is a frequent consequence of the procedure.

MITRAL VALVULOPLASTY (Fig. 31–23)

Mitral valvuloplasty can be accomplished by using several approaches. All require trans-septal catheterization. The original description by Inoue and associates (1984) used a specially designed balloon catheter that changes its shape in three stages facilitating insertion, placement, and finally balloon inflation. Inserted percutaneously in the right femoral vein, it has the major advantage of allowing large balloon sizes (from 25 to 29 mm in diameter) to be positioned in the mitral orifice by using a single-balloon technique. These sizes correspond to areas of 4.9 to 6.6 cm². A more widespread technique has been made popular by Al Zaibag and associates (1986), Lock and colleagues (1985), and Palacios and co-workers (1986): The interatrial septum is initially dilated with an 8-mm balloon to allow the passage of either one or two balloon dilatation catheters. The double-balloon catheter technique has rapidly become the more popular, based on reports of significantly lower residual valvular gradients following side-by-side balloon inflation (McKay et al, 1987).

A third approach has been championed by Babic and associates (1986, 1988) and involves positioning the balloons retrograde rather than antegrade across the mitral valve. This is accomplished by placing a trans-septal sheath through the mitral and aortic valves. A guidewire (or guidewires) inserted through this sheath is then snared by a retrieval catheter from the femoral artery (or arteries) and exteriorized. The trans-septal sheath is then withdrawn into the left atrium, and the balloon catheters are inserted from the femoral arteries retrograde over the guidewires. Although technically more complex, this method creates fewer atrial septal defects after the procedure and may be useful when larger balloons cannot be passed across a hypertrophied interatrial septum. Hemodynamic results appear similar to antegrade techniques (Babic et al, 1988).

Representative typical results of mitral valvuloplasty procedures are shown in Table 31–7 (Babic et al, 1988; Chen et al, 1988; DeUbago et al, 1987; McKay, 1988; McKay et al, 1987; Palacios et al, 1987). From the available data it appears evident that patients who are candidates for surgical commissurotomy are best suited for balloon mitral valvuloplasty. Calculated mitral valve areas are similar to those generally reported after surgical commissurotomy in similar patients (Bonchek, 1983; Mullin et al,

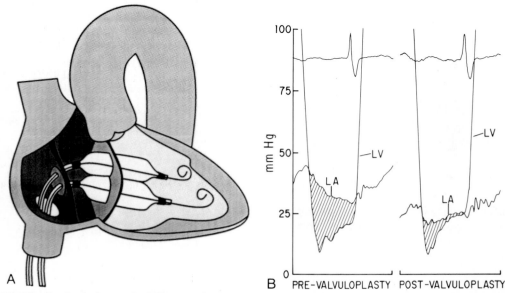

Figure 31–23. Mitral valvuloplasty. *A*, Schematically, the double-balloon technique is shown with the balloons traversing the interatrial septum and placed in position over guidewires in the left ventricle. *B*, A representative hemodynamic result is shown.

1972). Echocardiographic features may be useful in predicting the better candidates, because rigid calcific valves, chordae fusion, chronic atrial fibrillation, and significant mitral regurgitation all contribute to poorer initial results (Abascal et al, 1987; Reid et al, 1987).

Aortic Valvuloplasty (Fig. 31–24)

Unlike corresponding surgical procedures for mitral or pulmonic valve stenosis, efforts at aortic commissurotomy (Bailey et al, 1956; Hsieh et al, 1986) or mechanical debridement (Harken et al, 1958) have generally failed in aortic stenosis, primarily because of the creation of significant aortic regurgitation and a high rate of early restenosis. A new surgical alternative may be ultrasonic debridement, although only preliminary data are currently available (King et al, 1986; Worley et al, 1988).

Percutaneous aortic balloon valvuloplasty can be accomplished even in critically ill patients with acceptable morbidity and mortality (Davidson et al, 1988; Desnoyers et al, 1988; Schneider et al, 1987). The procedure is usually done through either a femoral or brachial artery approach and the aortic valve is crossed in retrograde fashion. Alternatively, a trans-septal method can be used and antegrade balloon dilatation is done when severe peripheral arterial disease prohibits the retrograde method (Block and Palacios, 1987). Aortic balloons are available in various shapes and sizes. In general, the maximal usable balloon size ranges from 18 to 23 mm in diameter for single-balloon procedures. Double balloons of various sizes are also used, and a trefoil balloon is available. Typical results from various sources are shown in Table 31–7 (Beekman et al, 1988; Choy et al, 1987; Cribier et al, 1986, 1987; Davidson et al, 1987, 1988; Dorros et al, 1987; Isner

et al, 1987; Lababidi et al, 1984; McKay et al, 1986; Safian et al, 1988; Schneider et al, 1987).

The obstruction of the left ventricular outflow by the balloon catheters can result in transient depression of left ventricular function, often shown by initial low cardiac outputs, decreased dP/dt, and evidence of diastolic dysfunction. Coronary sinus metabolism studies suggest that myocardial ischemia transiently occurs (Paulus, 1987). In addition, stimulation of left ventricular baroreceptors may initiate reflex peripheral vasodilation and lower systemic blood pressure. Sympathetic nervous system activity rapidly compensates, however, and the increased inotropic response that occurs, plus the reduction in the afterload mismatch, results in an improved ejection fraction in most patients. Overall, cardiac output changes minimally, but aortic gradients are generally reduced by 50 to 60% and the aortic valve area increases by about half. Compared with pulmonic and mitral valvuloplasty, aortic valvuloplasty frequently results in a final valvular effective orifice area still in the range of significant stenosis (<1 cm^2). Aortic regurgitation is usually not increased after the procedure.

Mechanisms, Complications, and Implications for Long-Term Efficacy

No long-term data are available by which to evaluate any of these procedures, although there are studies regarding the mechanisms involved. These studies, when combined with early follow-up data, provide insight into what might be expected on a long-term basis.

Pulmonic stenosis appears to respond to balloon dilatation by commissural splitting and by tearing or avulsion of the valve leaflets (Walls et al, 1984). The advantage of larger balloon sizes to overdilate the

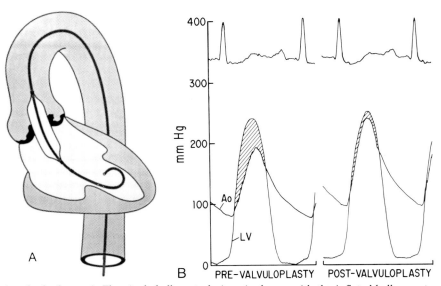

Figure 31–24. Aortic valvuloplasty. *A*, The single-balloon technique is shown with the inflated balloon retrograde across the aortic valve. *B*, A representative hemodynamic result is shown.

pulmonic valve is now clear. The potential disadvantage is that a significant amount of pulmonic insufficiency will likely occur in most patients. Because the right ventricle is basically structured to manage a volume load rather than a pressure load, the long-term result of this iatrogenic pulmonic insufficiency may not be of major consequence. The risks associated with the procedure are exceedingly small, and short-term (1 to 3 years) follow-up has indicated little restenosis or adverse effect from pulmonic regurgitation (Rao et al, 1988). Dysplastic pulmonary valves continue to present a challenge (DiSessa et al, 1987), although some excellent early results have been achieved in selected cases (Marantz et al, 1988).

Balloon valvuloplasty for mitral stenosis is associated with considerably more risk than valvuloplasty for pulmonic stenosis. In-hospital mortality has been reported in up to 4% (Palacios et al, 1986), and cerebrovascular accidents from dislodged thrombus or calcium probably occur with at least the same frequency (4 to 8%) that has been reported after closed commissurotomy (Mullin et al, 1972). To reduce the risk of this complication, most groups now place potential patients on warfarin therapy for 4 to 6 weeks before the procedure, even if they have a normal sinus rhythm. The trans-septal approach may result in a significant residual atrial septal defect, a form of iatrogenic Lutenbacher's syndrome. In addition, perforated or torn mitral cusps may produce severe mitral regurgitation, although this appears uncommon. Other reported complications include cardiac perforation and tamponade, conduction abnormalities and arrhythmias, blood loss, and the development of a vascular arteriovenous fistula.

The mechanism responsible for the improvement in the mitral gradient and the effective orifice area appears to be due primarily to commissural splitting, and fracture of leaflet calcium is less important (Block et al, 1987). In this regard, the selection of patients becomes important in interpreting long-term results. It is apparent that appropriate candidates for excellent long-term effects from percutaneous mitral valvuloplasty will be similar to those in whom surgical commissurotomy would have been effective. Shorter-term palliative procedures can be done in the elderly and in those with severe calcific rheumatic mitral stenosis, but the results are clearly inferior to those in the younger age group. Ongoing studies should provide guidance with regard to which patients benefit in the long run. Early follow-up studies (at 6 months) suggest that restenosis is uncommon when an adequate valvuloplasty has been achieved.

Aortic valvuloplasty appears to be initially effective either by separation of the aortic cusps along commissural lines or, more commonly in the elderly, by fracture of the valvular calcium (Isner et al, 1988; Kalan et al, 1988; McKay et al, 1986; Safian et al, 1987). At times, especially in younger patients, valvular mobility remains visibly impaired, however (Robicsek and Harbold, 1987). The early hemodynamic improvement usually results in improved symptomatic status for most patients, but early mortality remains high in the elderly and restenosis appears to be common, even as early as 6 months. This has rapidly led to the conclusion that aortic valvuloplasty should be reserved for those patients at highest risk for definitive surgical procedures (McKay, 1988; Rahimtoola, 1987), for those in whom a palliative procedure might be worthwhile (e.g., a "bridge" to definitive valve replacement in critically ill patients), for patients needing noncardiac surgical procedures urgently, or for those with severe left ventricular dysfunction or advanced age in whom a short-term improvement in the quality of life-style is a relevant therapeutic goal. Long-term clinical improvement is not likely to be sustained in adults (Litvack et al, 1988). In children, it is possible that the intrinsic difference in the etiology of the aortic stenosis will result in better long-term results than with the elderly (Sholler et al, 1988), although this remains unproven.

The complications of aortic valvuloplasty are significant but must be taken in light of the high-risk profile of the elderly patient population in whom it is normally being applied. Emboli are uncommon but have been reported in most large series, and they may be more common in patients with a bicuspid aortic valve and severe calcification (Davidson et al, 1988). In most series there is little change in the degree of aortic insufficiency observed compared with surgical valvotomy, perhaps because a less extensive valvotomy procedure is done by using percutaneous methods. Death occurs in 1 to 4% of patients either because of failure of the procedure to relieve the obstruction or because of acute aortic regurgitation, annular rupture, myocardial ischemia or infarction, cerebrovascular accident, ventricular arrhythmias, tamponade, or peripheral vascular injury (e.g., rupture of a pseudoaneurysm of the femoral artery). Many patients have severe coronary artery disease, and associated myocardial ischemia likely occurs with some frequency during and immediately after the procedure.

In the authors' initial experience with 125 patients, aortic valvuloplasty complications have occurred in 13%, including two deaths, five patients who suffered a cerebrovascular accident, two patients incurring a ventricular perforation that did not require surgical repair, and seven cases of procedure-related peripheral vascular trauma requiring surgical intervention.

At 6 months, a high percentage of patients have evidence of restenosis, but many patients do not have significant symptoms. Improvement in diastolic dysfunction is common in this latter group—possibly because of regression of left ventricular hypertrophy or improved coronary perfusion. The current national registries in the United States and France should help clarify the role of this procedure considerably. As long-term data become available, the value of these procedures in children will also become known.

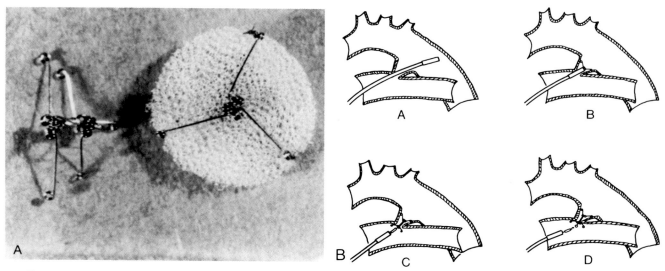

Figure 31–25. Closure of patent ductus arteriosus (PDA). *A,* Two double-disk, hookless PDA occlusion prostheses. The bare skeleton and the foam-covered prosthesis are shown. *B,* A diagram of its placement using catheter techniques. (From Rashkind, W. J., and Tait, M. S.: Interventional cardiac catheterization in congenital heart disease. *In* Schroeder, J. S. [ed]: Invasive cardiology. Cardiovasc. Clin., *15*:303, 1985.)

Other Investigational Interventional Techniques

COMBINATION PROCEDURES

It is now clear that certain situations may dictate the appropriateness of attempting more than one percutaneous balloon procedure in the same patient. This question most frequently arises when coronary artery disease is found concurrently in a patient with

severe calcific aortic stenosis. McKay and associates (1987) reported nine patients and Hamad and colleagues (1987) four patients in whom combined aortic valvuloplasty and coronary angioplasty were done successfully. The sequence in which the procedures can be done has obvious relevance. Recommendations can be made for proceeding with coronary angioplasty initially to prevent myocardial ischemia or for waiting until after the aortic valvuloplasty to prevent hypotension in patients with severe aortic stenosis—a recognizable, highly lethal situation. From these brief reports, there appears to be no real

Transcatheter Closure of Muscular VSDs

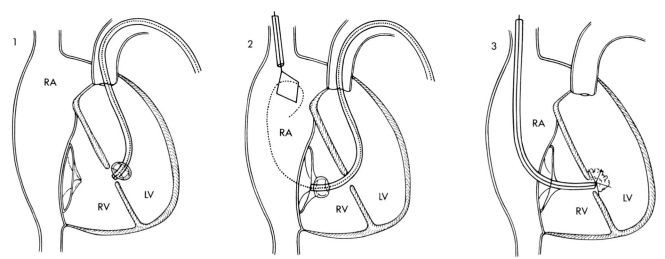

Figure 31–26. Transcatheter closure of ventricular septal defect (VSD). *1,* A balloon-tip catheter is shown transversing the VSD from the left ventricle. *2,* A wire is introduced through the balloon-tip catheter and is snared by a catheter in the right atrium (RA). The RA wire is then pulled through to the LV, and the guiding catheter with the umbrella prosthesis is inserted into the left ventricle (LV). *3,* The hooked umbrella is then allowed to open and is pulled back against the septum. (From Lock, J. E., Block, P. C., McKay, R. G., et al: Transcatheter closure of ventricular septal defects. Circulation, *78*:361, 1988. By permission of the American Heart Association, Inc.)

advantage with regard to which procedure is best done initially, although McKay and associates chose to do coronary angioplasty first in eight of their nine patients.

Combined procedures have also been reported in patients with both aortic and mitral stenosis (Berman et al, 1988) and in patients with combined tricuspid and pulmonic stenosis (Chen et al, 1988).

OTHER APPLICATIONS OF BALLOON CATHETER TECHNIQUES

Less common clinical situations have also been successfully approached by using balloon dilatation methods. Both aortitis (Khalilullah et al, 1987) and postoperative recurrent aortic coarctation (Saul et al, 1987) have been subjected to balloon dilatation techniques. Stenotic porcine prostheses are a particular problem, and although it would seem foolhardy to attempt dilatation of this bioprosthesis on the left side of the heart, several investigators have reported success on the right side of the heart. These reports have described reduction of bioprosthetic stenoses in modified Fontan's conduits (Pelikan et al, 1988), in Rastelli's conduits (Lloyd et al, 1987; Waldman et al, 1987) and in the tricuspid valve position (Feit et al, 1986). In addition, stenoses in peripheral pulmonary arteries of both children (Lock et al, 1983) and adults (Hoekenga et al, 1987), as well as in the superior vena cava (Ali et al, 1987), have been dilated by using balloon techniques.

OTHER EXPERIMENTAL TECHNIQUES UNDER INVESTIGATION

The use of a double-umbrella technique to close the patent ductus arteriosus has been shown to be effective (Rashkind, 1983) (Fig. 31–25). A similar approach has been applied in patients with atrial septal defect (King et al, 1976) and ventricular septal defect (Lock et al, 1988) with varied success (Fig. 31–26).

Finally, transcatheter closure of bronchial collaterals (redundant systemic pulmonary collaterals) can be accomplished in patients with tetralogy of Fallot and pulmonary atresia or similar lesions at the time of complete repair by using detachable balloons or preformed steel coils (Lock et al, 1986).

Selected Bibliography

Carabello, B. A.: Advances in the hemodynamic assessment of stenotic cardiac valves. J. Am. Coll. Cardiol., 10:912, 1987.

This review summarizes the concepts related to Gorlin's formula. It provides a review of the use of this formula and suggests where it might be changed. This article is followed by a response by Gorlin that is positive regarding the practical use of this formula for the determination of valve area.

Marcus, M. L., Skorton, D. J., Johnson, R. R., et al: Visual estimates of per cent diameter coronary stenosis: "A battered gold standard." J. Am. Coll. Cardiol., 11:882, 1988.

This review focuses on the difficulties in using the per cent stenosis in assessing the severity of coronary disease. It is brief and summarizes the vagaries in the use of visual data regarding coronary stenoses. The editorial is followed by a response by Gould commenting on functional tests that are currently available for the assessment of coronary stenoses.

McKay, R. G.: Balloon valvuloplasty for treating pulmonic, mitral and aortic valve stenosis. Am. J. Cardiol., 61:102G, 1988.

This is a brief review of advances in balloon valvuloplasty for pulmonic, mitral, and aortic valve stenosis. Although the data concentrate on the information from one institution, an overview of this evolving area is provided.

Mehlman, D. J.: A pictorial and radiographic guide for identification of prosthetic heart valves. Prog. Cardiovasc. Dis., 30:441, 1988.

This review summarizes the radiographic appearance of prosthetic heart valves and provides a useful review of this area. This reference guide is excellent for the identification of the prosthetic heart valve devices.

Perry, S. B., Keane, J. F., and Lock, J. E.: Interventional catheterization in pediatric congenital and acquired heart disease. Am. J. Cardiol., 61:1090, 1988.

This review presents the present status of catheter-directed therapy in pediatric congenital and acquired disease. Although it again focuses on a single institution's experience, it is well referenced and provides a concise summary of this area.

Sheehan, F. H., Bolson, E. L., Dodge, H. T., et al: Advantages and applications of the centerline method for characterizing regional ventricular function. Circulation, 74:293, 1986.

The use of the centerline method for determining regional ventricular function is described. This particular method has become popular because it allows the regional function to be analyzed statistically in a readily achievable manner.

Wigle, E. D., Sasson, Z., Henderson, M. A., et al: Hypertrophic cardiomyopathy. The importance of the site and the extent of hypertrophy: A review. Prog. Cardiovasc. Dis., 28:1, 1985.

This is a clinically relevant and complete review of hypertrophic cardiomyopathy. It discusses in depth many of the controversies regarding this disease process.

Bibliography

Abascal, V. M., Wilkins, G. T., Choung, C. Y., et al: Echocardiographic evaluation 6 months after percutaneous mitral valvotomy (Abstract). Circulation, 76:IV–92, 1987.

Adams, D. F., Fraser, D. B., and Abrams, H. L.: The complications of coronary arteriography. Circulation, 48:609, 1973.

Alday, L. E., and Juaneda, E.: Percutaneous balloon dilatation in congenital mitral stenosis. Br. Heart. J., 57:479, 1987.

Ali, M. K., Ewer, M. S., Balakrishnan, P. B., et al: Balloon angioplasty for superior vena cava obstruction. Ann. Intern. Med., 107:856, 1987.

Ali Khan, M. A., Yousef, S. A., and Mullins, C. E.: Percutaneous transluminal balloon pulmonary valvuloplasty for relief of pulmonary valve stenosis with special reference to double-balloon technique. Am. Heart J., 112:158, 1986.

Al Zaibag, M., Kabsab, S. A., Ribeiro, P. A., and Fagih, M. R.:

Percutaneous double balloon mitral valvotomy for the rheumatic mitral valve stenosis. Lancet, 1:757, 1986.

Amplatz, K., Formanek, G., Stanger, P., and Wilson, W.: Mechanics of selective coronary artery catheterization via femoral approach. Radiology, 89:1040, 1967.

Angel, J., Soler-Soler, J., Anivarro, I., and Domingo, E.: Hemodynamic evaluation of stenotic cardiac valves. II: Modification of the simplified formula for mitral and aortic valve calculation. Cathet. Cardiovasc. Diagn., 11:127, 1985.

Antman, E. M., Marsh, J. D., Green, L. H., and Grossman, W.: Blood oxygen measurements in the assessment of intracardiac left to right shunts: A critical appraisal of methodology. Am. J. Cardiol., 46:265, 1980.

Babic, V. V., Dorros, G., Pejcic, P., et al: Percutaneous mitral valvuloplasty: Retrograde transarterial double balloon technique utilizing the trans-septal approach. Cathet. Cardiovasc. Diagn., 14:229, 1988.

Babic, V. V., Pejcic, P., Djurisic, Z., et al: Percutaneous transarterial balloon valvuloplasty for mitral valve stenosis. Am. J. Cardiol., 57:1101, 1986.

Bailey, C. P., Bulton, H. E., Nichols, H. T., et al: The surgical treatment of aortic stenosis. J. Thorac. Surg., 31:375, 1956.

Baim, D. S., Rothman, M. T., and Harrison, D. C.: Simultaneous measurement of coronary venous flow and oxygen saturation during transient alterations in myocardial oxygen supply and demand. Am. J. Cardiol., 49:743, 1982.

Bartle, S. H., and Hermann, H. J.: Acute mitral regurgitation in man: Hemodynamic evidence and observations indicating an early role for the pericardium. Circulation, 36:839, 1967.

Bashore, T. M., Davidson, C. J., Mark, D. B., et al: Iopamidol use in the cardiac catheterization laboratory: A retrospective analysis of 3,313 patients. Cardiology, 5(Suppl.):6, 1988.

Beekman, R. H., Rocchini, A. P., Crowley, D. C., et al: Comparison of single and double balloon valvuloplasty in children with aortic stenosis. J. Am. Coll. Cardiol., 12:480, 1988.

Berman, A. D., Weinstein, J. S., Safian, R. D., et al: Combined aortic and mitral balloon valvuloplasty in patients with critical aortic and mitral valve stenosis: Results in six cases. J. Am. Coll. Cardiol., 11:1213, 1988.

Bettman, M. A., Bourdillon, P. D., Barry, W. H., et al: Contrast agents for cardiac angiography: Effects of a nonionic agent vs. a standard ionic agent. Radiology, 153:583, 1984.

Bjork, V. O., Balstrom, G., and Uggla, L. G.: Left auricular pressure measurements in man. Ann. Surg., 138:718, 1953.

Block, P. C., and Palacios, I. F.: Comparison of hemodynamic results of anteriograde versus retrograde percutaneous balloon aortic valvuloplasty. Am. J. Cardiol., 60:659, 1987.

Block, P. C., Palacios, I. F., Jacobs, M. L., and Fallon, J. T.: Mechanisms of percutaneous mitral valvotomy. Am. J. Cardiol., 59:178, 1987.

Bonchek, L. I.: Current status of mitral commissurotomy: Indications, techniques, and results. Am. J. Cardiol., 52:411, 1983.

Borow, K., Green, L. H., Mann, T., et al: End-systolic volume as a predictor of postoperative left ventricular performance in volume overload from valvular regurgitation. Am. J. Med., 68:655, 1980.

Bourassa, M. G., and Noble, J.: Complication rate of coronary arteriography. A review of 5250 cases studied by percutaneous femoral technique. Circulation, 53:106, 1976.

Brannon, E. S., Weens, H. S., and Warren, J. V.: Atrial septal defect: Study of hemodynamics by the technique of right heart catheterization. Am. J. Med. Sci., 210:480, 1948.

Braunwald, E., and Swan, H. J. C.: Cooperative study on cardiac catheterization. Circulation, 37(Suppl. III):1, 1968.

Brock, R., Milstein, B. B., and Ross, D. N.: Percutaneous left ventricular puncture in the assessment of aortic stenosis. Thorax, 11:163, 1956.

Brockenbrough, E. C., Braunwald, E., and Morrow, A. G.: A hemodynamic technique for the detection of hypertrophic subaortic stenosis. Circulation, 23:189, 1961.

Bush, C. A., Stang, J. M., Wooley, C. F., and Kilman, J. W.: Occult constrictive pericardial disease: Diagnosis by rapid volume expansion and correction by pericardiectomy. Circulation, 56:924, 1977.

Cabin, H. S., and Roberts, W. C.: Left ventricular aneurysm, intraaneurysmal thrombus and systemic embolus in coronary heart disease. Chest, 77:586, 1980.

Cannon, S. R., Richards, K. L., and Crawford, M.: Hydraulic estimation of stenotic orifice area: A correction of the Gorlin formula. Circulation, 71:1170, 1985.

Cannon, S. R., Richards, K. L., Crawford, M. H., et al: Inadequacy of the Gorlin formula for predicting prosthetic valve area. Am. J. Cardiol., 62:113, 1988.

Carabello, B. A.: Advances in the hemodynamic assessment of stenotic cardiac valves. J. Am. Coll. Cardiol., 10:912, 1987.

Carabello, B. A., Barry, W. H., and Grossman, W.: Changes in arterial pressure during left heart pullback in patients with aortic stenosis: A sign of severe aortic stenosis. Am. J. Cardiol., 44:424, 1979.

Carabello, B. A., Nolan, S. P., and McGuire, L. B.: Assessment of preoperative left ventricular function in patients with mitral regurgitation: Value of the end-systolic stress-end systolic volume ratio. Circulation, 64:1212, 1981.

Carlson, E. B., Mintz, G. S., and Bemis, C. E.: Hemodynamic significance of normal and abnormal fluoroscopic patterns of disc motion in the Beall mitral valve prosthesis. Radiology, 141:335, 1981.

Carpentier, A., Cherard, S., and Fahiani, J. N.: Reconstructive surgery of the mitral valve: Ten year appraisal. J. Thorac. Cardiovasc. Surg., 79:338, 1980.

Casale, P. N., Palacios, I. F., Abascal, V. M., et al: Gorlin valve area varies with cardiac output in aortic stenosis (Abstract). J. Am. Coll. Cardiol., (Suppl. II):63A, 1988.

Cha, S. D., and Gooch, A. S.: Diagnosis of tricuspid regurgitation: Current status. Arch. Intern. Med., 143:1763, 1983.

Chen, C., Lo, Z., Huang, Z., et al: Percutaneous transseptal balloon mitral valvuloplasty: The Chinese experience in 30 patients. Am. Heart J., 115:937, 1988.

Chen, C. R., Xiang, Z., Huang, Z. D., and Cheng, T. O.: Concurrent percutaneous balloon valvuloplasty for combined tricuspid and pulmonic stenoses. Cathet. Cardiovasc. Diagn., 15:55, 1988.

Choy, M., Beekman, R. H., and Rocchini, A. P.: Percutaneous balloon valvuloplasty for valvar aortic stenosis in infants and children. Am. J. Cardiol., 59:1010, 1987.

Clark, C. E., Henry, W. L., and Epstein, S. E.: Familial prevalence and genetic transmission of idiopathic and genetic transmission of idiopathic hypertrophic subaortic stenosis. N. Engl. J. Med., 289:709, 1973.

Cobanoglu, A., and Starr, A.: Tricuspid valve surgery: Indications, methods, and results. In Frankl, W. S., and Brest, A. N. (eds): Cardiovascular Clinics Valvular Heart Disease: Comprehensive Evaluation and Management. Philadelphia, F. A. Davis, 1986, pp. 375–388.

Cohen, M. Y., and Greenberg, M. A.: Constrictive pericarditis: Early and late complication of cardiac surgery. Am. J. Cardiol., 43:657, 1979.

Colle, J. P., Rahal, S., Ohayon, J., et al: Global left ventricular function and regional wall motion in pure mitral stenosis. Clin. Cardiol., 67:148, 1983.

Come, P. C., and Riley, M. F.: Tricuspid anular dilatation and failure of tricuspid leaflet coaptation in patients with tricuspid regurgitation. Am. J. Cardiol., 55:599, 1985.

Cooke, J. P., Seward, J. B., and Holmes, D. R.: Transluminal balloon valvotomy for pulmonic stenosis in an adult. Mayo Clin. Proc., 62:306, 1987.

Cope, C.: Technique for transseptal catheterization of the left atrium: Preliminary report. J. Thorac. Surg., 37:482, 1959.

Cournand, A.: Cardiac catheterization: Development of the technique, its contribution to experimental medicine, and its initial application in man. Acta Med. Scand. 579(Suppl.):7, 1978.

Cribier, A., Saoudi, N., Berland, J., et al: Percutaneous transluminal valvuloplasty of acquired aortic stenosis in elderly patients: An alternative to valve replacement? Lancet, 1:63, 1986.

Cribier, A., Savin, T., Berland, J., et al: Percutaneous transluminal balloon valvuloplasty of adult aortic stenosis: Report of 92 cases. J. Am. Coll. Cardiol., 9:381, 1987.

Curry, T. S., Dowdey, J. E., and Murry, R. C.: Christensen's Introduction to the Physics of Diagnostic Radiology. Philadelphia, Lea & Febiger, 1984.

Davidson, C. J., Skelton, T. N., Kisslo, K., et al: Percutaneous balloon valvuloplasty of calcific aortic stenosis. North Carolina Med. J., 48:249, 1987.

Davidson, C. J., Skelton, T. N., Kisslo, K., et al: A comprehensive evaluation of the risk of systemic embolization associated with percutaneous balloon valvuloplasty in adults. Ann. Intern Med., 108:557, 1988.

Davidson, C. J., Skelton, T. N., Morris, K. M., et al: Prospective evaluation of the nephrotoxicity of nonionic contrast following cardiac catheterization. Ann. Intern. Med., 110:119, 1989.

Davis, K., Kennedy, J. W., Kemp, H. G., et al: Complications of coronary arteriography from the collaborative study of coronary artery surgery (CASS). Circulation, 59:1105, 1979.

Desnoyers, M. R., Salem, D. N., Rosenfield, K., et al: Treatment of cardiogenic shock by emergency aortic balloon valvuloplasty. Ann. Intern. Med., 108:833, 1988.

DeUbago, J. L. M., DePrada, J. A. V., Bardaji, J. L., et al: Percutaneous balloon valvotomy for calcific rheumatic mitral stenosis. Am. J. Cardiol., 59:1007, 1987.

Dexter, L., Haynes, F. W., Burwell, C. S., et al: Studies of congenital heart disease. II: The pressure and content of blood in the right auricle, right ventricle and pulmonary artery in control patients, with observations on the oxygen saturation and source of pulmonary capillary blood. J. Clin. Invest., 26:554, 1947.

DiSessa, T. G., Alpert, B. S., Chase, N. A., et al: Balloon valvuloplasty in children with dysplastic pulmonary valves. Am. J. Cardiol., 60:405, 1987.

Dodge, H. T., Hay, R. E., and Sandler, H.: An angiographic method for determining left ventricular stroke volume in man. Circ. Res., 60:739, 1962.

Dodge, H. D., and Sheehan, F. H.: Quantitative contrast angiography for assessment of ventricular performance in heart disease. J. Am. Coll. Cardiol., 1:73, 1983.

Dorros, G., Lewin, R. F., King, J. F., and Janke, L. M.: Percutaneous transluminal valvuloplasty in calcific aortic stenosis: The double balloon technique. Cathet. Cardiovasc. Diagn., 13:151, 1987.

Driscoll, D. J., Hesslein, P. S., and Mullins, C. E.: Congenital stenosis of individual pulmonary veins: Clinical spectrum and unsuccessful treatment by transvenous balloon dilation. Am. J. Cardiol., 49:1767, 1982.

Edmunds, L. H., Stephenson, L. W., Edie, R. N., and Ratcliffe, M. B.: Open-heart surgery in octogenarians. N. Engl. J. Med., 319:131, 1988.

Emery, R. W., Landes, R. G., Moller, J. H., and Nicoloff, D. M.: Pulmonary valve replacement with a porcine aortic heterograft. Ann. Thorac. Surg., 27:148, 1979.

Engle, M. A., Holswade, G. R., Goldberg, H. P., et al: Regression after pulmonary valvotomy of infundibular stenosis accompanying severe valvular pulmonic stenosis. Circulation, 17:862, 1958.

Engle, M. A., Gay, W. A., Kaminsky, M. E., et al: The postpericardiotomy syndrome then and now. Curr. Probl. Cardiol., 3:1, 1978.

Facquet, J. M., Lemoine, J. M., Alhomme, P., and Fefebvre, J.: La measure de la pression auriculaire gauche par voie transbronchique. Arch. Mal. Coeur, 45:741, 1952.

Fareed, J., Moncada, R., Messmore, H. L., et al: Molecular markers of contrast-media induced adverse reactors. Semin. Thromb. Hemost., 10:306, 1984.

Feit, F., Stecy, P. J., and Nachamie, M. S.: Percutaneous balloon valvuloplasty for stenosis of a porcine bioprosthesis in the tricuspid valve position. Am. J. Cardiol., 58:363, 1986.

Fick, A.: Über die Messurg des Blutquantums in den Herzventrikeln. Sitz der Physik-Med ges Wurtzberg. 1870, p. 16.

Fischer, H. W., and Thomson, K. R.: Contrast media in coronary arteriography: A review. Invest. Radiol., 13:450, 1978.

Fisher, M. L.: Coronary angiography: Safety in numbers? Am. J. Cardiol., 52:898, 1983.

Flamm, M. D., Cohn, K. E., and Hancock, E. W.: Measurement of systemic cardiac output at rest and exercise in patients with atrial septal defect. Am. J. Cardiol., 23:258, 1969.

Foltz, B. D., Hessel, E. A., and Ivey, T. D.: The early course of pulmonary artery hypertension in patients undergoing mitral valve replacement with cardioplegic arrest. J. Thorac. Cardiovasc. Surg., 88:238, 1984.

Forssmann, W.: Experiments on myself: Memoirs of a surgeon in Germany. New York, Saint Martin's Press, 1974, pp. 84–85.

Forssmann, W.: Ueber kontrastdavstellung der hohler der lebenden vechten herzens und der lungenschlagader. Munch. Med. Wochenschr., 78:489, 1931.

Fuchs, R. M., Heuser, R. R., Yin, F. C. P., and Brinker, J. A.: Limitations of pulmonary wedge V waves in diagnosing mitral regurgitation. Am. J. Cardiol., 49:849, 1982.

Gaasch, W. H., Andvias, C. W., and Levine, H. J.: Chronic aortic regurgitation: The effect of aortic valve replacement on left ventricular volume mass and function. Circulation, 58:825, 1978.

Gaasch, W. H., Blaustein, A. S., and Bing, O. H. L.: Asynchronous (segmental early) relaxation of the left ventricle. J. Am. Coll. Cardiol., 5:891, 1985.

Gabby, S., and Kresh, J. Y.: Bioengineering of mechanical and biologic heart valve substitutes. In Morse, D., Steiner, R. M., and Fernandez, J. (eds): Guide to Prosthetic Cardiac Valves. New York, Springer-Verlag, 1985, pp. 239–256.

Goldstein, J. A., Vlahakes, G. J., Verrier, E. D., et al: The role of right ventricular systolic dysfunction and elevated intrapericardial pressure in the genesis of low output in experimental right ventricular infarction. Circulation, 65:513, 1982.

Gorlin, R.: Calculations of cardiac valve stenosis: Restoring an old concept for advanced applications. J. Am. Coll. Cardiol., 10:920, 1987.

Gorlin, R., and Gorlin, G.: Hydraulic formula for calculation of area of stenotic mitral valve, other cardiac valves and central circulatory shunts. Am. Heart J., 41:1, 1951.

Graham, T. P., Jr., Jarmakani, J. M., Canent, R. V., Jr., and Morrow, M. N.: Left heart volume estimation in infancy and childhood: Reevaluation of methodology and normal values. Circulation, 43:895, 1971.

Griffith, B. P., Hardesty, R. L., Siewers, R. D., et al: Pulmonary valvotomy alone for pulmonic stenosis: Results in children with and without muscular infundibular hypertrophy. J. Thorac. Cardiovasc. Surg., 83:577, 1982.

Grollman, J. H., Liu, C. K., Astone, R. A., and Lurie, M. D.: Thromboembolic complications in coronary angiography associated with the use of nonionic contrast medium. Cathet. Cardiovasc. Diagn., 14:159, 1988.

Grondelle, A. van, Ditchey, R. V., Groves, B. M., et al: Thermodilution method overestimates low cardiac low output in humans. Am. J. Physiol., 245:H690, 1983.

Grossman, W.: Profiles in constrictive pericarditis, restrictive cardiomyopathy, and cardiac tamponade, Chapter 27. In Grossman, W. (ed): Cardiac Catheterization and Angiography. Philadelphia, Lea & Febiger, 1986, p. 431.

Grossman, W., and Barry, W. H.: Cardiac catheterization. In Braunwald, E. (ed): Heart Disease. Philadelphia, W. B. Saunders Company, 1988, p. 250.

Grossman, W., Jones, W. D., and McLaurin, L. P.: Wall stress and patterns of hypertrophy in the human left ventricle. J. Clin. Invest., 56:56, 1975.

Gruntzig, A. R., Senning, A., and Siegenthaler, W. F.: Nonoperative dilation of coronary artery stenosis. Percutaneous transluminal coronary angioplasty. N. Engl. J. Med., 301:61, 1979.

Gunther, S., and Grossman, W.: Determinants of ventricular function in pressure-overload in man. Circulation, 59:679, 1979.

Hakki, A. H.: A simplified valve formula for the calculation of stenotic cardiac valve areas. Circulation, 63:1050, 1981.

Halperin, J. L., Brooks, K. M., Rothlauf, E. B., et al: Effect of nitroglycerin on the pulmonary venous gradient in patients after mitral valve replacement. J. Am. Coll. Cardiol., 5:34, 1985.

Hamad, N., Pichard, A., and Lindsay, J., Jr.: Combined coronary angioplasty and aortic valvuloplasty. Am. J. Cardiol., 60:1184, 1987.

Hamilton, W. F., Moore, J. W., Kinsman, J. M., and Spurling, R. G.: Studies on the circulation. IV: Further analysis of the injection method and of changes in hemodynamics under physiologic and pathologic conditions. Am. J. Physiol., 99:534, 1932.

Hanrath, P., Mathey, D. G., Siegert, R., and Bleifeld, W.: Left ventricular relaxation and filling pattern in different forms of left ventricular hypertrophy. Am. J. Cardiol., 45:15, 1980.

Harken, D. E., Black, H., Taylor, W. J., et al: The surgical correction of calcific aortic stenosis in adults: Results in the first 100 consecutive transaortic valvuloplasties. J. Thorac. Surg., 36:759, 1958.

Haschek, E., and Lindenthol, O.: Ein Beitrag Zur Proktischen Verwerthung Der Photographie Noch Rontgen. Wien. Klin. Wochenschr., 9:63, 1896.

Hellems, H. K., Haynes, F. W., and Dexter, L.: Pulmonary "capillary" pressure in man. J. Appl. Physiol., 2:24, 1949.

Herman, M. V., Heinle, R. A., and Klein, M. D.: Localized disorders in myocardial contraction asynergy and its role in congestive heart failure. N. Engl. J. Med., 277:222, 1967.

Heystraten, F. M. J., and Paalman, H.: Cineradiographic evaluation of the Bjork-Shiley mitral and aortic valves. Ann. Radiol., 24:346, 1981.

Higgins, C. B., Sovak, M., Schmidt, W. S., et al: Direct myocardial effects of intracoronary administration of new contrast agents with low osmolality. Invest. Radiol., 15:39, 1980.

Higgs, L. M., Glancy, D. L., O'Brien, K. P., et al: Mitral restenosis: An uncommon cause of recurrent symptoms following mitral commissurotomy. Am. J. Cardiol., 26:34, 1970.

Hoekenga, D. E., Stevens, G. F., and Ball, W. S.: Percutaneous angioplasty for peripheral pulmonary stenosis in an adult. Am. J. Cardiol., 59:188, 1987.

Hsieh, K. -S., Keane, J. F., Nadas, A. S., et al: Long term followup of valvotomy before 1968 for congenital aortic stenosis. Am. J. Cardiol., 58:338, 1986.

Humes, H. D., Cielinski, D. A., and Messana, J. M.: Effects of radiocontrast agents on renal tubule cell function: Implications regarding the pathogenesis of contrast-induced nephrotoxicity effects of contrast agents on renal function. Cardiology 5(Suppl.):14, 1988.

Inoue, K., Owaki, T., Nakamura, T., et al: Clinical application of transvenous mitral commissurotomy by a new balloon catheter. J. Thorac. Cardiovasc. Surg., 87:394, 1984.

Isner, J. M., Salem, D. N., Desnoyers, M. R., et al: Treatment of calcific aortic stenosis by balloon valvuloplasty. Am. J. Cardiol., 59:313, 1987.

Isner, J. M., Samuels, D. A., Slovenkai, G. A., et al: Mechanisms of aortic balloon valvuloplasty: Fracture of valvular calcific deposits. Ann. Intern. Med., 108:377, 1988.

Johnson, R. A., and Palacios, I.: Dilated cardiomyopathy of the adult. Part I. N. Engl. J. Med., 307:1051, 1982; Part II. N. Engl. J. Med., 307:1119, 1982.

Johnston, D. K., and Kostuk, W. J.: Left and right ventricular function during symptom-limited exercise in patients with isolated mitral stenosis. Chest, 89:186, 1986.

Jones, F. M., Jr., and Shirey, E. K.: Cine coronary arteriography. Mod. Concepts Cardiovasc. Dis., 31:735, 1962.

Judkins, M. P.: Selective coronary arteriography. I: A percutaneous transfemoral technic. Radiology, 89:815, 1967.

Kahn, K. L., with the Health and Public Policy Committee, American College of Physicians: The safety and efficacy of ambulatory cardiac catheterization in the hospital and free standing setting. Ann. Intern. Med., 103:294, 1985.

Kalan, J. M., Mann, J. M., Leon, M. B., et al: Morphologic findings in stenotic aortic valves that have had "successful" percutaneous balloon valvuloplasty. Am. J. Cardiol., 62:152, 1988.

Kan, J., White, R. I., Mitchell, S. E., and Gardner, T. J.: Percutaneous balloon valvuloplasty: A new method for treating congenital pulmonary valve stenosis. N. Engl. J. Med., 2307:540, 1982.

Kan, J. S., White, R. I., Jr., Mitchell, S. E., et al: Percutaneous transluminal balloon valvuloplasty for pulmonary valve stenosis. Circulation, 69:554, 1984.

Kawanishi, D. T., McKay, C. R., Chandraratna, A. N., et al: Cardiovascular response to dynamic exercise in patients with chronic symptomatic mild-to-moderate and severe aortic regurgitation. Circulation, 73:62, 1986.

Kazama, S., Nishiguchi, K., Sonoda, K., et al: Postoperative left ventricular function in patients with mitral stenosis. The effect of commissurotomy and valve replacement on left ventricular systolic function. Jpn. Heart J., 27:35, 1986.

Kennedy, J. W.: Complication associated with cardiac catheterization and angiography. Cathet. Cardiovasc. Diagn., 8:13, 1982.

Kennedy, J. W., Trenholme, S. E., and Kasser, I. S.: Left ventricular volume and mass from single-plane cineangiogram: A comparison of anteroposterior and right anterior oblique methods. Am. Heart J., 80:343, 1970.

Khalilullah, M., Tyagi, S., Lochan, R., et al: Percutaneous transluminal balloon angioplasty of the aorta in patients with aortitis. Circulation, 76:597, 1987.

King, R. M., Pluth, J. R., Giuliani, E. R., and Piehler, J. M.: Mechanical decalcification of the aortic valve. Ann. Thorac. Surg., 42:269, 1986.

King, T. D., Thompson, S. L., Steiner, C., and Mills, N. L.: Secundum atrial septal defect: Nonoperative closure during cardiac catheterization. J.A.M.A., 235:2506, 1976.

Klein, O.: Zur Bestimmung des zerkulatorischen minutens volumen nach dem fickschen prinzip. Munch. Med. Wochenschr., 77:1311, 1930.

Krevlen, T. H., Gorlin, R., and Herman, M. V.: Ventriculographic patterns and hemodynamics in primary myocardial disease. Circulation, 61:931, 1980.

Kyeselis, D. A., Rocchini, A. P., Beekman, R., et al: Balloon angioplasty for congenital and rheumatic mitral stenosis. Am. J. Cardiol., 57:348, 1986.

Lababidi, Z., Wu, J. R., and Walls, J. T.: Percutaneous balloon aortic valvuloplasty: Results in 23 patients. Am. J. Cardiol., 53:194, 1984.

Laser, J. A., Fowles, R. E., and Mason, J. W.: Endomyocardial biopsy. In Schroeder, J. S. (ed): Invasive Cardiology (Cardiovascular Clinics, Vol. 14.) Philadelphia, F. A. Davis, 1985, pp. 141–163.

Litvack, F., Jakubowski, A. T., Buchbinder, N. A., and Eigler, N.: Lack of sustained clinical improvement in an elderly population after percutaneous aortic valvuloplasty. Am. J. Cardiol., 62:270, 1988.

Lloyd, T. R., Marvin, W. J., Mahoney, L. T., and Laver, R. M.: Balloon dilation valvuloplasty of bioprosthetic valves in extracardiac conduit. Am. Heart J., 114:268, 1987.

Lock, J. E., Bass, J. L., Amplatz, K., et al: Balloon dilation angioplasty of aortic coarctations in infarcts and children. Circulation, 68:109, 1983.

Lock, J. E., Bass, J. C., Castanega-Zuniga, W., et al: Dilation angioplasty of congenital or operative narrowings of venous channels. Circulation, 70:457, 1984.

Lock, J. E., Block, P. C., McKay, R. G., et al: Transcatheter closure of ventricular septal defects. Circulation, 78:361, 1988.

Lock, J. E., Castaneda-Zuniga, W. R., Fuhrman, B. P., and Bass, J. L.: Balloon dilation angioplasty of hypoplastic and stenotic pulmonary arteries. Circulation, 67:962, 1983.

Lock, J. E., Keane, J. F., and Fellows, K. E.: The use of catheter intervention procedures for cardiac disease. J. Am. Coll. Cardiol., 7:1420, 1986.

Lock, J. E., Khalilullah, M., Shrnasta, S., et al: Percutaneous catheter commissurotomy in rheumatic mitral stenosis. N. Engl. J. Med., 313:1515, 1985.

Lorell, B. H., and Braunwald, E.: Pericardial disease, Chapter 44. In Braunwald, E. (ed): Heart Disease. Philadelphia, W. B. Saunders Company, 1988, pp. 1484–1534.

Lorell, B. H., Leinbach, R. C., Pohost, G. M., et al: Right ventricular infarction. Am. J. Cardiol., 43:465, 1979.

Mann, T., Brodie, B. R., Grossman, W., and McLaurin, L.: Effusive-constrictive hemodynamic pattern due to neoplastic involvement of the pericardium. Am. J. Cardiol., 41:781, 1978.

Marantz, P. M., Huhta, J. C., Mullins, C. E., et al: Results of balloon valvuloplasty in typical and dysplastic pulmonary valve stenosis: Doppler echocardiographic followup. J. Am. Coll. Cardiol., 12:476, 1988.

Marcus, M. L., Dot, D. B., Hiratzka, L. F., et al: Decreased coronary reserve: A mechanism for angina pectoris in patients with aortic stenosis and normal coronary arteries. N. Engl. J. Med., 307:1362, 1982.

Marcus, M. L., Skorton, D. J., Johnson, M. R., et al: Visual estimates of per cent diameter coronary stenosis: "A battered gold standard." J. Am. Coll. Cardiol., 11:882, 1988.

Maron, B. J., Bonow, R. O., Cannon, R. O., III, et al: Hypertrophic cardiomyopathy. Part I. N. Engl. J. Med., *317*:780, 1987; Part II. N. Engl. J. Med., *317*:844, 1987.

Maron, B. J., Epstein, S. E., and Roberts, W. C.: Hypertrophic cardiomyopathy and transmural myocardial infarction without significant atherosclerosis of the extramural coronary arteries. Am. J. Cardiol., *43*:1089, 1979.

Mason, J. W.: Techniques for right and left ventricular endomyocardial biopsy. Am. J. Cardiol., *41*:8874, 1978.

McCristin, J. W., Herman, R. L., Spaccavento, L. J., and Tomlinson, G. C.: Isoproterenol infusion increases Gorlin formula aortic valve area in isolated aortic stenosis (Abstract). J. Am. Coll. Cardiol., (Suppl. II):63A, 1988.

McDonald, D. A., and Taylor, M. G.: The hydrodynamics of the arterial circulation. Prog. Biophys. Biophys. Chem., *9*:107, 1959.

McGregor, M., and Sniderman, A.: On pulmonary vascular resistance: The need for a more precise definition. Am. J. Cardiol., *55*:217, 1985.

McKay, C. R., Kawanishi, D. T., and Rahimtoola, S. H.: Catheter balloon valvuloplasty of the mitral valve in adults using a double balloon technique. J.A.M.A., *257*:1753, 1987.

McKay, R. G.: Balloon valvuloplasty for treating pulmonic, mitral and aortic valve stenosis. Am. J. Cardiol., *61*:102G, 1988.

McKay, R. G., Lock, J. E., Keane, J. F., et al: Percutaneous mitral valvuloplasty in an adult patient with calcific rheumatic stenosis. J. Am. Coll. Cardiol., *7*:1410, 1986.

McKay, R. G., Lock, J. E., Safian, R. D., et al: Balloon dilation of mitral stenosis in adults: Post-mortem and percutaneous mitral valve studies. J. Am. Coll. Cardiol., *9*:723, 1987.

McKay, R. G., Safian, R. D., Berman, A. D., et al: Combined percutaneous aortic valvuloplasty and transluminal coronary angioplasty in adult patients with calcific aortic stenosis and coronary artery disease. Circulation, *76*:1298, 1987.

McKay, R. G., Safian, R. D., Lock, J. E., et al: Balloon dilatation of calcific aortic stenosis in elderly patients: Post-mortem, intraoperative and percutaneous valvuloplasty studies. Circulation, *74*:119, 1986.

Mehlman, D. J.: A pictorial and radiographic guide for identification of prosthetic heart valves. Prog. Cardiovasc. Dis., *30*:441, 1988.

Meier, B., Friedli, B., Oberhaeush, I., et al: Trefoil balloon for percutaneous valvuloplasty. Cathet. Cardiovasc. Diagn., *12*:277, 1986.

Miller, A. J., Pick, R., and Johnson, P. J.: The production of acute pericardial effusion: The effects of various degrees of interference with venous blood and lymph drainage from the heart muscle in the dog. Am. J. Cardiol., *28*:463, 1971.

Miller, S. W.: History of angiocardiography. *In* Miller, S. W. (ed): Cardiac Angiography. Boston, Little, Brown and Company, 1984, pp. 3–20.

Morganroth, J., Perloff, J. K., Zeldis, S. M., and Dunkman, W. B.: Acute severe aortic regurgitation. Ann. Intern. Med., *87*:225, 1977.

Morrow, W. R., Vick, G. W., Nihill, M. R., et al: Balloon dilation of unoperated coarctation of the aorta: Short- and intermediate-term results. J. Am. Coll. Cardiol., *11*:133, 1988.

Morse, D., Steiner, R. M., and Fernandez, J. (eds): A guide to prosthetic valves. New York, Springer-Verlag, 1985.

Mullin, E. M., Jr., Glaucy, D. L., Higgs, L. M., et al: Current results of operation for mitral stenosis: Clinical and hemodynamic assessment in 124 consecutive patients treated by closed commissurotomy or valve replacement. Circulation, *46*:298, 1972.

Murgo, J. P., Alter, B. R., Dorethy, J. F., et al: Dynamics of left ventricular ejection in obstructive and nonobstructive hypertrophic cardiomyopathy. J. Clin. Invest., *66*:1369, 1980.

Murgo, J. P., Westerhof, N., Giolma, J. P., and Altobelli, S. A.: Aortic input impedance in normal man: Relationship to pressure waveforms. Circulation, *62*:105, 1980.

Navetta, F. I., Barber, M. J., Gurbel, P. A., et al: Myocardial ischemia in constrictive pericarditis. Am. Heart J., *116*:1107, 1988.

O'Keefe, J. H., Jr., Vliestra, R. E., Hanley, P. C., and Seward, J. C.: Revival of the transseptal approach for catheterization of the left atrium and ventricle. Mayo Clin. Proc., *60*:790, 1985.

O'Rourke, M. F.: Pressure and flow waves in systemic arteries and anatomic design of the arterial system. J. Appl. Physiol., *23*:139, 1967.

O'Rourke, M. F.: Wave reflections. *In* O'Rourke, M. F. (ed): Arterial Function in Health and Disease. New York, Churchill Livingstone, 1982, pp. 134, 138.

O'Toole, J. D., Wurtzbacher, J. J., Wearner, N. E., and Jain, A. C.: Pulmonary valve injury and insufficiency during pulmonary-artery catheterization. N. Engl. J. Med., *301*:1167, 1979.

Palacios, I. F., Block, P. C., Brandi, S. C., et al: Percutaneous balloon volvatomy for mitral stenosis (Abstract). Circulation, *74*(Suppl. II):II–208, 1986.

Palacios, I., Block, P. C., Brandi, S., et al: Percutaneous balloon valvotomy for patients with severe mitral stenosis. Circulation, *75*:778, 1987.

Palacios, I., Lock, J. E., Keane, J. F., and Block, P. C.: Percutaneous transvenous balloon valvotomy in a patient with severe calcific mitral stenosis. J. Am. Coll. Cardiol., *7*:1416, 1986.

Paulus, W. J., Heyndrickx, G. R., Wyns, W., and Rousseau, M. F.: Occlusive balloon inflations during aortic valvuloplasty depress left ventricular function through global myocardial ischemia. Circulation, *76*:IV-546, 1987.

Pelikan, P., French, W. J., Ruiz, C., et al: Percutaneous double-balloon angioplasty of a stenotic modified Fontan aortic homograft conduit. Cathet. Cardiovasc. Diagn., *15*:47, 1988.

Pepine, C. J., Gessner, J. H., and Feldman, R. L.: Percutaneous balloon valvuloplasty for pulmonic valve stenosis in the adult. Am. J. Cardiol., *30*:1442, 1982.

Pepine, C. J., Gunten, C. V., Hill, J. A., et al: Percutaneous brachial catheterization using a modified sheath and new catheter system. Cathet. Cardiovasc. Diagn., *10*:637, 1984.

Perez, J. A., Hinohara, T., Quigley, P. J., et al: In-vitro and in-vivo experimental results using a new wire guided concentric atherectomy device (abstract). J. Am. Coll. Cardiol., *11*(Suppl. II):109A, 1988.

Pichard, A. D., Meller, J., Teichholz, L. E., et al: Septal perforator compression (narrowing) in idiopathic hypertrophic subaortic stenosis. Am. J. Cardiol., *39*:310, 1979.

Portsmann, W., Wierny, L., and Warnke, H.: Closure of persistent ductus arteriosus without thoracotomy. Thoraxchirurgie, *15*:199, 1967.

Radner, S.: Attempt at roentgenologic visualization of coronary blood vessels in man. Acta Radiol., *26*:497, 1945.

Radner, S.: Suprasternal puncture of the left atrium for flow studies. Acta Med. Scand., *148*:57, 1954.

Radtke, W., Keane, J. F., Fellows, K. E., et al: Percutaneous balloon valvotomy of congenital pulmonary stenosis using oversized balloons. J. Am. Coll. Cardiol., *8*:909, 1987.

Rahimtoola, S. H.: The need for cardiac catheterization and angiography in valvular heart disease is not disproven. Ann. Intern. Med., *97*:433, 1982.

Rahimtoola, S. H.: Catheter balloon valvuloplasty of aortic and mitral stenosis in adults: 1987. Circulation, *75*:895, 1987.

Rankin, J. S., Gaynor, J. W., Fenely, M. P., et al: Diastolic myocardial mechanics and the regulation of cardiac performance. *In* Grossman, W., and Larrell, B. H. (eds): Diastolic Relaxation of the Heart. Boston, Martinus Nijhoff, 1988, pp. 111–124.

Rao, P. S., Fawzy, M. E., Solymar, L., and Mardini, M. K.: Long-term results of balloon pulmonary valvuloplasty for valvar pulmonic stenosis. Am. Heart J., *115*:1291, 1988.

Rashkind, W. J.: Transcatheter treatment of congenital heart disease. Circulation, *67*:711, 1983.

Rashkind, W. J., and Miller, W. W.: Creation of an atrial septal defect without thoracotomy. J.A.M.A., *196*:173, 1966.

Rashkind, W. J., and Miller, W. W.: Transposition of the great arteries: Results of palliation by balloon atrioseptostomy in thirty-one infants. Circulation, *38*:453, 1968.

Rashkind, W. J., and Tait, M. S.: Interventional cardiac catheterization in congenital heart disease. *In* Schroeder, J. S. (ed): Invasive cardiology. Cardiovasc. Clin., *15*:303, 1985.

Reddy, P. S., Curtiss, E. L., O'Toole, J. D., and Shaver, J. A.: Cardiac tamponade: Hemodynamic observations in man. Circulation, *58*:265, 1978.

Reid, C. L., McKay, C. R., Chandraratna, P. A. N., et al:

Mechanisms of increase in mitral valve area and influence of anatomic features in double-balloon, catheter balloon valvuloplasty in adults with rheumatic mitral stenosis: A Doppler and two-dimensional echocardiographic study. Circulation, 76:628, 1987.

Ricci, D. R.: Afterload mismatch and preload reserve in chronic aortic regurgitation. Circulation, 66:826, 1982.

Ricketts, H. J., and Abrams, H. L.: Percutaneous selective coronary cine arteriography. J.A.M.A., 181:140, 1962.

Rigler, L. G., and Watson, J. C.: A combination film changer for rapid or conventional radiography. Radiology, 61:77, 1953.

Ring, J. C., Kulik, T. J., Burke, B. A., and Lock, J. E.: Morphologic changes induced by dilation of the pulmonary valve anulus with overlarge balloons in normal newborn lambs. Am. J. Cardiol., 55:210, 1984.

Roberts, W. C.: Reasons for cardiac catheterization before cardiac valve replacement. N. Engl. J. Med., 306:1291, 1982.

Roberts, W. C., and Spray, T. L.: Pericardial heart disease: A study of its causes, consequences and morphologic features. In Spodick, D. H. (ed): Pericardial Diseases, Vol. 7. Philadelphia, F. A. Davis, 1976, pp. 11–65.

Robicsek, F., and Harbold, N. B., Jr.: Limited value of balloon dilatation in calcified aortic stenosis in adults: Direct observations during open heart surgery. Am. J. Cardiol., 60:857, 1987.

Rocchini, A. P., Kveselis, D. A., Crowley, D., et al: Percutaneous balloon valvuloplasty for treatment of congenital pulmonary valvular stenosis in children. J. Am. Coll. Cardiol., 3:1005, 1984.

Ross, J., Jr.: Afterload mismatch and preload reserve: A conceptual framework for the analysis of ventricular function. Prog. Cardiovasc. Dis., 18:255, 1976.

Rupprath, G., and Neuhaus, K. L.: Percutaneous balloon valvulopasty for aortic valve stenosis in infancy. Am. J. Cardiol., 55:1655, 1985.

Safian, R. D., Berman, A. D., Diver, D. J., et al: Balloon aortic valvuloplasty in 170 consecutive patients. N. Engl. J. Med., 319:125, 1988.

Safian, R. D., Mandell, V. S., Thurer, R. E., et al: Post-mortem and intraoperative balloon valvuloplasty of calcific aortic stenosis in elderly patients: Mechanisms of successful dilation. J. Am. Coll. Cardiol., 9:655, 1987.

St. John Sutton, M. G., St. John Sutton, M., Oldershaw, P., et al: Valve replacement without preoperative cardiac catheterization. N. Engl. J. Med., 305:1233, 1981.

Salem, D. N., Findlay, S. R., Isner, J. M., et al: Comparison of histamine release effects of ionic and nonionic radiographic contrast media. Am. J. Med., 80:382, 1986.

Sanborn, T. A., Haudenschild, C. C., Garber, G. R., et al: Angiographic and histologic consequences of laser thermal angioplasty: Comparison to balloon angioplasty. Circulation, 75:1281, 1987.

Sandler, H., and Dodge, H. T.: The use of single plane angiocardiograms for the calculation of left ventricular volume in man. Am. Heart J., 75:325, 1968.

Saul, J. P., Keane, J. F., Fellows, K. E., and Lock, J. E.: Balloon dilation angioplasty of postoperative aortic obstructions. Am. J. Cardiol., 59:943, 1987.

Schneider, J. F., Wilson, M., and Gallant, T. E.: Percutaneous balloon aortic valvuloplasty for aortic stenosis in elderly patients at high risk for surgery. Ann. Intern. Med., 106:696, 1987.

Schoenfeld, M. H., Palachios, I. F., Hutter, A. M., et al: Underestimations of prosthetic mitral valve areas: Role of transseptal catheterization in avoiding unnecessary repeat mitral valve surgery. J. Am. Coll. Cardiol., 5:1387, 1985.

Schoonmaker, F. W., and King, S. B., III: Coronary arteriography by the single catheter percutaneous femoral technique. Circulation, 50:737, 1974.

Schwab, S., Davidson, C. J., Skelton, T. N., et al: A randomized study of the nephrotoxicity of ionic versus nonionic contrast following cardiac catheterization. N. Engl. J. Med., 320:149, 1989.

Seldinger, S.: Catheter replacement of the needle in percutaneous arteriography, a new technique. Acta Radiol., 39:368, 1953.

Sellers, R. D., Levy, M. J., Amplatz, K., et al: Left retrograde cardioangiography in acquired cardiac disease: Technique, indications and interpretations in 700 cases. Am. J. Cardiol., 14:437, 1964.

Selzer, A.: Changing aspects of the natural history of valvular aortic stenosis. N. Engl. J. Med., 317:91, 1987.

Sembh, B. K. H., Tjonneland, S., Stake, G., and Aabyholm, G.: Balloon valvotomy of congenital pulmonary valve stenosis with tricuspid insufficiency. Cardiovasc. Radiol., 2:239, 1979.

Sheehan, F. H., Bolson, E. L., Dodge, H. T., et al: Advantages and applications of the centerline method for characterizing regional ventricular function. Circulation, 74:293, 1986.

Shehadi, W. H.: Contrast media adverse reactions: Occurrence, recurrence and distribution patterns. Radiology, 143:11, 1982.

Sholler, G. F., Keane, J. F., Perry, S. B., et al: Balloon dilatation of congenital aortic valve stenosis: Results and influence of technical and morphological features in outcome. Circulation, 78:351, 1988.

Sideris, E. B., Baay, J. E., Bradshaw, R. L., and Jones, J. E.: Axillary vein approach for pulmonic valvuloplasty in infants with iliac vein obstruction. Cathet. Cardiovasc. Diagn., 15:61, 1988.

Sigwart, U., Piel, J., Mirkovitch, J., et al: Intravascular stents to prevent occlusion and restenosis after transluminal angioplasty. N. Engl. J. Med., 316:701, 1987.

Sones, F. M., and Shirey, E. K.: Cine coronary arteriography. Mod. Concepts Cardiovasc. Dis., 31:735, 1962.

Spodick, D. H.: The normal and diseased pericardium: Current concepts of pericardial physiology, diagnosis and treatment. J. Am. Coll. Cardiol., 1:240, 1983.

Stanger, P., Heymann, M. A., Tarnoff, H., et al: Complications of cardiac catheterization of neonates, infants and children. Circulation, 50:595, 1974.

Stewart, G. N.: Researches on the circulation time and on the influences which affect it. IV: The output of the heart. J. Physiol., 22:159, 1897.

Stewart, W. H., Hoffman, W. J., and Ghiselin, F. H.: Cineflurography. Am. J. Roentgenol., 38:465, 1937.

Stott, D. K., Marpole, D. G. F., Bristow, J. D., et al: The role of left atrial transport in aortic and mitral stenosis. Circulation, 41:1031, 1970.

Sullivan, I. D., Robinson, P. J., and MacArtney, F. J.: Percutaneous balloon valvuloplasty for pulmonary valve stenosis in infants and children. Br. Heart J., 54:285, 1986.

Swan, H. J. C., Ganz, W., Forrester, J. S., et al: Catheterization of the heart in man with use of a flow-directed balloon-tipped catheter. N. Engl. J. Med., 283:447, 1970.

Terry, P. B., White, R. I., Jr., Barth, K. H., et al: Pulmonary arteriovenous malformations: Physiologic observations and results of therapeutic balloon embolization. N. Engl. J. Med., 308:1197, 1983.

Tyberg, T. I., Goodyer, A. V. N., Hurst, V. W., et al: Left ventricular filling in differentiating restrictive amyloid cardiomyopathy and constrictive pericarditis. Am. J. Cardiol., 47:791, 1981.

Ubago, J. L., Figueroa, A., Colman, T., et al: Right ventriculography as a valid method for the diagnosis of tricuspid regurgitation. Cathet. Cardiovasc. Diagn., 7:433, 1981.

Waldman, J. D., Schoen, F. J., Kirkpatrick, S. E., et al: Balloon dilatation of porcine bioprostheses in the pulmonary position. Circulation, 76:109, 1987.

Wallace, A. G.: Pathophysiology of cardiovascular disease. In Smith, L. H., and Thier, O. S. (eds): Pathophysiology: The Biological Principles of Disease: The International Textbook of Medicine. Philadelphia, W. B. Saunders Company, 1981, pp. 1192, 1200.

Walls, J. T., Lababidi, Z., Curtis, J. J., and Silver, D.: Assessment of percutaneous balloon pulmonary and aortic valvuloplasty. J. Thorac. Cardiovasc. Surg., 88:352, 1984.

Warren, J. V.: Fifty years of invasive cardiology: Werner Forssmann (1904–1979). Am. J. Med., 69:10, 1980.

White, A. F., Dinsmore, R. E., and Buckley, M. J.: Cineradiographic evaluation of prosthetic cardiac valves. Circulation, 48:882, 1973.

Wigle, E. D., Sasson, Z., Henderson, M. A., et al: Hypertrophic cardiomyopathy. The importance of the site and the extent of hypertrophy: A review. Prog. Cardiovasc. Dis., 28:1, 1985.

Williams, F. H.: A method for more fully determining the outline of the heart by means of the fluoroscope together with other uses of this instrument. Boston Med. Surg. J., 135:335, 1896.

Worley, S. J., King, R. M., Edwards, W. D., and Holmes, D. R.: Electrohydraulic shock wave decalcification of stenotic aortic

valves: Post-mortem and intraoperative studies. J. Am. Coll. Cardiol., 12:458, 1988.

Wynne, J., Green, L. H., Grossman, W., et al: Estimation of left ventricular volumes in man from biplane cineangiograms filmed in oblique projections. Am. J. Cardiol., 41:726, 1978.

Zimmerman, H. A., Scott, R. W., and Becker, N. O.: Catheterization of the left side of the heart in man. Circulation, 1:357, 1950.

II PERCUTANEOUS TRANSLUMINAL CORONARY ANGIOPLASTY

Richard S. Stack

HISTORICAL ASPECTS

In 1963, Dotter inadvertently advanced a diagnostic catheter across a total iliac obstruction and initiated a new era in the treatment of atherosclerotic cardiovascular disease (Dotter, 1980). After this historic event, he observed

Perhaps it is wishful thinking, but in any event I am convinced that the relief of atheromatous obstruction in small arteries can best be accomplished by catheter technics.

A flexible guide introduced percutaneously into an artery proximal to an area of atheromatous narrowing can be manipulated so as to traverse the obstruction. A mechanical attack upon the lesion would then become feasible, perhaps by gradual direct dilatation.

DOTTER, 1963.

The first intentional angioplasty procedure was done by Dotter on January 16, 1964, in an elderly woman who had gangrene and refused an amputa-

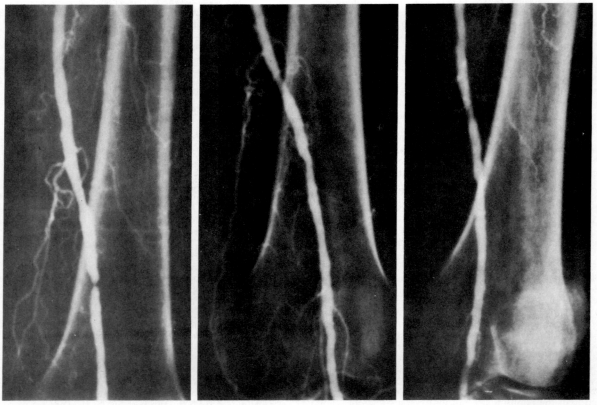

Figure 31–27. Femoral arteriogram of the first patient to receive percutaneous angioplasty. This 83-year-old woman had refused amputation for advanced gangrene due to a proximal popliteal stenosis and severe distal runoff disease. *Left panel,* Before dilatation; *middle panel,* immediately after dilatation; *right panel,* 2½ years after dilatation. The gangrene healed without operative therapy, and the patient became ambulatory. (From Dotter, C. T.: Transluminal angioplasty: A long view. Radiology, 135:561, 1980, with permission.)

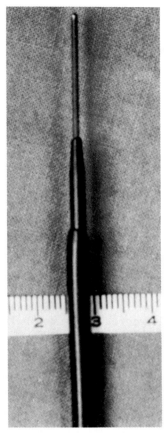

Figure 31–28. Dotter coaxial dilatation catheter and guidewire. (From Athanasoulis, C. A., Pfister, R. C., Greene, R. E., and Roberson, G. H.: Interventional Radiology. Philadelphia, W. B. Saunders Company, 1982.)

tion. An obstruction of the proximal popliteal artery was quickly passed with a guidewire and later dilated by means of several radiolucent, coaxial, polyethylene catheters (Fig. 31–27). The gangrene healed without operation, and the patient became fully ambulatory.

Later in 1964, Dotter and Judkins reported their clinical experience in the first 11 patients treated with percutaneous angioplasty. They advanced a 0.05-inch spring guidewire through an atherosclerotic obstruction followed by a tapered Teflon 0.1-inch dilating catheter over the wire. In appropriately sized vessels, this was followed by a 0.2-inch Teflon dilating catheter (Fig. 31–28). In the same year, Staple described a system of tapered catheters of increasing size passed sequentially over the guidewire to allow serial dilatations. A serial dilatation system was also introduced by van Andel (1976) by using gradually tapering catheters compared with the shorter bevelled designs used by Staple (Fig. 31–29). Each of these methods met with reasonable clinical success and became particularly popular in Europe (Waltman et al, 1982).

Initial experience with balloon-tip catheters with peripheral arterial dilatation was less satisfactory. Early balloon catheters used soft, compliant latex

balloons that were unable to generate sufficient radial force against the lesion (Waltman et al, 1982). Porstmann (1973) introduced a "corset" type of balloon catheter, which consisted of a latex balloon catheter within a Teflon outer catheter. The outer catheter had longitudinal openings located at the site of the inner balloon. This catheter served to stent the latex balloon and allowed adequate force to be applied to the lesion (Fig. 31–30). A problem with this design, however, was the potential for trapping endothelium between the Teflon struts during deflation.

Gruentzig (1974) introduced an ingenious new double-lumen catheter with a balloon constructed of noncompliant polyvinyl chloride (Fig. 31–31). The use of this balloon catheter system soon became popular in Europe after the successful experience of Gruentzig and Hopff in treating atherosclerotic lesions of the iliac and femoral arteries (Gruentzig et al, 1977).

Gruentzig first described the use of percutaneous balloon angioplasty in human coronary arteries in 1977 (Gruentzig, 1978). In 1979, he reported a series of 50 patients and initiated the modern era of percutaneous transluminal coronary angioplasty (PTCA) in the United States (Gruentzig et al, 1979).

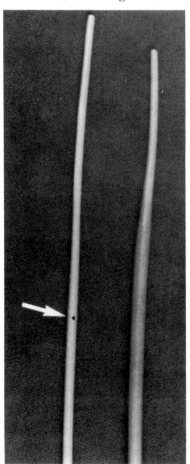

Figure 31–29. Staple–van Andel dilatation catheters. (From Athanasoulis, C. A., Pfister, R. C., Greene, R. E., and Roberson, G. H.: Interventional Radiology. Philadelphia, W. B. Saunders Company, 1982.)

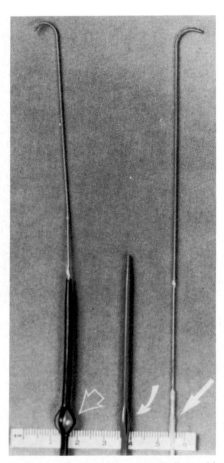

Figure 31–30. Porstmann corset-type balloon dilatation system. (From Athanasoulis, C. A., Pfister, R. C., Greene, R. E., and Roberson, G. H.: Interventional Radiology. Philadelphia, W. B. Saunders Company, 1982.)

A major improvement in balloon catheter system design was Simpson and colleagues' development of a maneuverable inner guidewire system in 1982. Since that time there has been a great expansion of technology and a rapid evolution of coronary angioplasty equipment and methods. Modern low-profile systems now allow the cardiologist to successfully maneuver the multiple turns and branches of the coronary arterial system with relative ease. An example of a modern low-profile catheter system is shown in Fig. 31–32.

PROCEDURE

Method of Dilatation

Procedural methods continue to evolve with further improvements in equipment and technique. The following is a summary of the routine procedures currently used in the author's laboratory.

Informed consent is obtained, and the patient is allowed nothing by mouth after midnight. A cardiothoracic surgeon is available at all times in the event of a failed angioplasty.

The patient is brought to the interventional cardiac catheterization laboratory and is prepared and draped in a sterile manner. Large-screen, high-resolution imaging systems, high-resolution stop-frame recorders, and digital subtraction angiography are examples of specialized equipment that are very helpful in making immediate decisions during interventional procedures without waiting for the development of cine films (Fig. 31–33). A dedicated intraaortic balloon pump console is also in the laboratory and is a useful feature in laboratories where emergency angioplasty procedures are done.

A No. 6 French introducer sheath is placed in the right femoral vein for placement of a No. 5 French balloon-directed pacing catheter in the event of bradyarrhythmias during balloon dilatation. A No. 8 (or 9) French angioplasty introducer sheath is placed in the right femoral artery, and a No. 8 (or 9) French thin-walled guiding catheter is advanced to the level of the coronary ostium over a 0.035-inch flexible wire guide. A balloon catheter with a movable guidewire is introduced through a Y connector into the guiding catheter and advanced to the coronary ostium. The

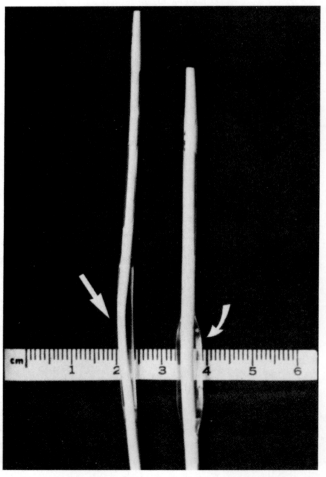

Figure 31–31. Gruentzig's polyvinyl chloride balloon dilatation catheter. (From Athanasoulis, C. A., Pfister, R. C., Greene, R. E., and Roberson, G. H.: Interventional Radiology. Philadelphia, W. B. Saunders Company, 1982.)

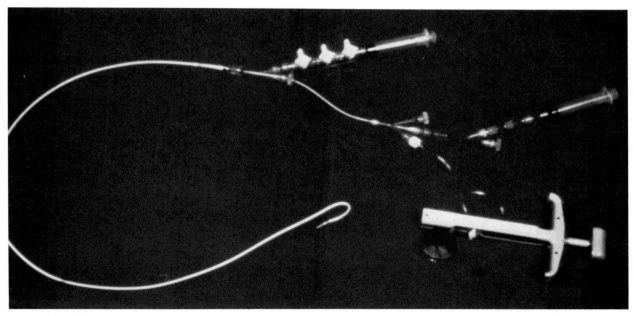

Figure 31–32. Modern steerable guidewire coronary angioplasty equipment. (Courtesy of Advanced Cardiovascular Systems.)

movable guidewire is then directed through the coronary tree and across the site of the atherosclerotic obstruction by a torque control device placed near the proximal end of the wire. After the lesion is successfully traversed with the wire under fluoroscopic control, the balloon is moved to the site of the lesion and placed directly across the obstruction with the aid of gold markers that are located at either end of the balloon (Fig. 31–34). At this point, some cardiologists record a pressure gradient from the distal tip of the balloon catheter and the proximal guiding catheter. One or more dilatations of the balloon are then done at pressures ranging from 5 to 9 atmospheres (atm) for 60 to 180 seconds. After adequate dilatation, the balloon is removed while the guidewire is retained across the lesion, and results of the dilatation are assessed arteriographically by using high-resolution fluoroscopy. The guidewire is

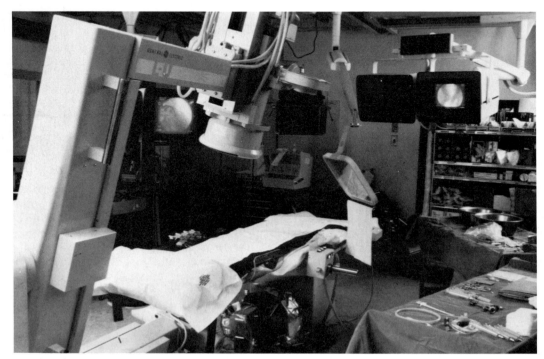

Figure 31–33. One of two dedicated procedure rooms in the interventional cardiac catheterization laboratory at Duke University Medical Center.

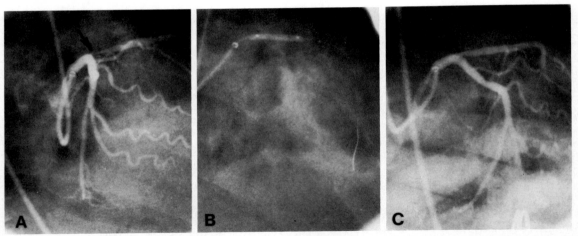

Figure 31–34. Coronary arteriogram in the right anterior oblique position. *A,* Proximal stenosis of the left anterior descending coronary artery. *B,* The balloon catheter is placed across the lesion. *C,* The post-PTCA result shows only a minor irregularity at the site of the previous stenosis.

then removed, and repeated arteriograms are done after 5 to 10 minutes to ensure that the targeted lesion is still widely patent.

The balloon may then be moved again across the lesion and a postdilatation pressure gradient may be recorded. Although many cardiologists rely on the use of pressure gradients across the obstruction to assess the results of the dilatation, there are several major limitations to the accuracy of these measurements (Feldman et al, 1985). These limitations include (1) the presence of the balloon catheter across the lesion, which contributes to the pressure gradient; (2) collateral flow distal to the obstruction; (3) the combination of long length and small catheter radius, which results in damping of the distal pressure tracing; (4) guidewire obstruction (if retained within the balloon catheter); and (5) the presence of viscous contrast material within the lumen, which causes further damping of the tracing. Each of these factors contributes to a very low natural frequency and severe damping of the dilatation catheter system. The signal often is so severely damped that even the mean pressure determination becomes inaccurate.

After withdrawal of the balloon catheter and guidewire from the lesion and clear arteriographic demonstration of successful dilatation, the guide catheter is removed from the sheath. The patient is returned to the regular cardiology ward for observation. Patients who are suffering from acute myocardial infarction and are treated with PTCA or other emergency angioplasty procedures or patients with significant dissection after the angioplasty procedure are admitted to the coronary care unit for observation.

Methods for Managing Failed PTCA

After initial dilatation, residual stenosis or abrupt vessel closure may occur as a result of plaque dissection, thrombosis, spasm, or any combination of these. In rare cases, a heavily calcified plaque may fail to dilate with 8 or 9 atm of pressure, the maximal pressure that can be applied routinely to standard balloons. In these cases, recently developed high-pressure balloons may be used to achieve inflation pressures up to 15 atm. In the more common case of reocclusion after initial dilatation, a repeated dilatation with the same size balloon for a longer duration (up to 5 minutes) is attempted. Intracoronary nitroglycerin and sublingual nifedipine are used to treat any potential component of coronary spasm. If these maneuvers are ineffective, repeated dilatations are done with a larger balloon if the native vessel size will permit. Prolonged dilatations (10 to 15 minutes) are sometimes successful in "tacking down" a dissection flap after failed PTCA and may be attempted by using recently developed flow-through catheters that allow continuous perfusion of the distal myocardium during balloon dilatation (Quigley, 1988). If all these maneuvers fail, emergency coronary artery bypass grafting (CABG) is indicated.

The safety of emergency CABG in this circumstance can be greatly increased by maintaining blood flow to the distal myocardium by a reperfusion catheter (Ferguson et al, 1986; Hinohara et al, 1988). The reperfusion catheter is a No. 4.5 French tapered polyethylene conduit with multiple side holes arranged in a spiral pattern over the distal 10 cm of the catheter. In the case of a failed angioplasty, the original guidewire is maintained across the stenosis and the original balloon catheter is moved over the guide to a point beyond the obstruction. A 300-cm coronary exchange wire is substituted for the original wire and is then moved through the original balloon catheter. The balloon catheter is removed while the exchange wire is maintained across the lesion. The reperfusion catheter is then moved through the obstruction, and the exchange wire is removed. Blood enters proximal side holes from the aorta and proximal coronary artery, passes through the central lumen of the reperfusion catheter, and out through the distal side holes to reperfuse the myocardium beyond the coronary obstruction (Figs. 31–35 and 31–36). Despite the availability of the reperfusion catheter, CABG should be done immediately to avoid potential interruption of flow through the reperfusion catheter due to thrombosis.

In a study by Ferguson and associates (1986), nine patients with failed angioplasty and impending infarction were reperfused by using the reperfusion catheter. All patients had emergency CABG. The reperfusion catheter was removed after aortic cross-clamping and delivery of cardioplegic solution. The presence of the catheter thus reduced the ischemic period to the interval from the onset of coronary occlusion after failed angioplasty until the reperfusion catheter could be placed across the lesion. In all patients, the catheter temporarily re-established coronary blood flow to the region of ischemic myocardium, resulting in resolution of symptoms. The catheter allowed antegrade delivery of cardioplegic solution infused into the aortic root to this area of myocardium, which in turn made it possible to do the subsequent CABG as a controlled optimal revascularization procedure.

In the author's institution, a dedicated emergency beeper is carried by the back-up surgeon and emergency coverage is provided on a rotational basis for all elective and emergency coronary angioplasty procedures. However, an operating room is not held in reserve for potentially failed angioplasty procedures. The anesthesiology team has an important role in coordinating the time of initiation of routine cardiothoracic procedures so that at any particular time a properly equipped cardiac operating suite is available in the event of a failed angioplasty.

The largest study of CABG conducted before the development of the reperfusion catheter was the National Institutes of Health (NIH) Registry report (Cowley et al, 1984). In this study, emergency CABG was done in 202 of the 3,079 patients (6.6% enrolled in the NIH PTCA Registry). The most frequent indication for emergency operation was coronary dissection in 46%, coronary occlusion in 20%, prolonged angina in 14%, and coronary spasm in 11%. Emergency CABG was most often necessary in patients in whom lesions could not be reached or traversed, but more than 25% of patients who required emergency operation had initially successful dilatation followed by abrupt reclosure of the vessel. The mortality in this study with emergency CABG was 6.4%, and nonfatal myocardial infarction occurred in 41% of patients, with Q waves developing in approximately 60% of those with infarction. However, in 52% of patients managed with emergency CABG and severe ischemic events with PTCA, there was no mortality or evidence of myocardial infarction and the patients had an uncomplicated postoperative course. No baseline clinical predictors of emergency CABG could be identified in this study.

SELECTION OF PATIENTS

Selection criteria of patients have continued to evolve with improvements in angioplasty equipment and technique. When PTCA was first introduced, selection of patients was limited to those with the following characteristics: (1) discrete, concentric lesions; (2) single-vessel involvement; (3) absence of calcification; (4) proximal location distant from major side branches; and (5) good left ventricular function (Levy et al, 1982). Today, modern steerable guidewire systems and low-profile balloons allow rapid and effective crossing of complicated lesions in multiple vessels and in more distal locations.

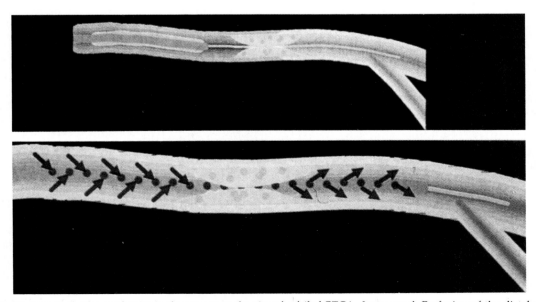

Figure 31–35. *Top panel,* The guidewire is shown across the site of a failed PTCA. *Lower panel,* Perfusion of the distal myocardium with the reperfusion catheter.

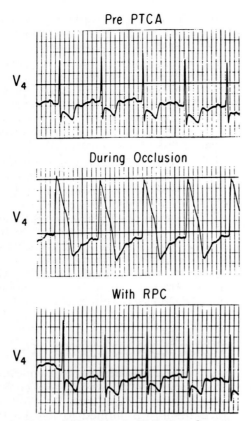

Figure 31–36. *A,* The chronic ST-T wave changes are shown before PTCA in a patient who was scheduled for elective angioplasty. *B,* Major ST segment elevation immediately after failed PTCA. *C,* Return to the baseline after insertion of a reperfusion catheter.

Although there has been a continued trend to broaden the criteria for selection of patients, each arteriogram must be carefully evaluated for the location, number, and configuration of the anatomic lesions. This information must be combined with physiologic exercise data and a patient's symptoms.

The following are selection criteria currently used in the author's laboratory: (1) patients with significant symptoms of angina pectoris or positive exercise tests in the presence of a significant (more than 75% luminal diameter narrowing) lesion on the coronary arteriogram; (2) patients with one-, two-, or three-vessel disease without significant left main stenosis; and (3) patients with acute myocardial infarction, who may be considered for mechanical balloon dilatation with or without previous thrombolytic therapy.

Patients with a large number of lesions or lesions that are very angular or exceedingly long may not be good candidates for PTCA. PTCA may be attempted for chronic total coronary occlusions, particularly if they are short and noncalcified, or for major bifurcation lesions, but protection of the opposite branch with a separate wire or balloon catheter is often required. Bifurcation lesions just distal to the left main artery involving the origin of the circumflex and left anterior descending arteries are not generally approached by PTCA.

In patients with multivessel disease, either multivessel angioplasty or CABG may be recommended. Presently, there are few data to help the clinician to determine the treatment of choice. Although angioplasty can be done less expensively and less traumatically, the long-term results are less satisfactory than with CABG. Until the results of current studies comparing CABG and PTCA are known, precise recommendations for either therapy in patients with multivessel disease must be individualized based on the experience of the institution and the individual physicians.

RESULTS

Histopathology

Preliminary theories attributed the mechanism of successful angioplasty to compression and local redistribution of atheromatous material with release of fluid constituents (Dotter, 1978; Dotter and Judkins, 1964; Lev and Gruentzig, 1978). Later studies involving animal models, atherosclerotic human cadaver coronary and peripheral arteries, and human postangioplasty autopsy studies were unable to document significant compression of atherosclerotic lesions (Baugham et al, 1981; Block et al, 1980b, 1981; Faxon et al, 1982; Waller et al, 1983). These studies suggest that as the balloon inflates, the plaque splits at its thinnest and weakest point. This break may extend through the internal elastic membrane so that further balloon dilatation stretches the more elastic media and adventitial tissue. The arterial lumen may continue to enlarge as the expanding balloon widens the disruption in the atheromatous plaque and further stretches the media and adventitia (Fig. 31–37).

Although the immediate postangioplasty healing process is not well understood, it may involve some dissolution of atheromatous material, fibrous retraction of the split plaque, and re-endothelialization. Further improvement in lumen diameter may also occur and may be due to plaque regression or progressive dilatation of the lumen under physiologic pressure (Zarins et al, 1982). A Duke study reported necropsy findings in four patients who died between 14 hours and 11 months after PTCA (Colavita et al, 1985). Three of the patients who died at 6 weeks or less from the time of the angioplasty had plaque disruption, intimal hemorrhage, and endothelial desquamation. One of these patients also had occlusion of a diagonal branch of the left anterior descending coronary artery due to plaque embolus, and another patient had a medial dissection. The third patient died 11 months after successful PTCA (25% residual stenosis by arteriography) and had a 50% residual cross-sectional area of stenosis at autopsy. No morphologic changes that could be attributed to PTCA were observed at the time of autopsy. The absence

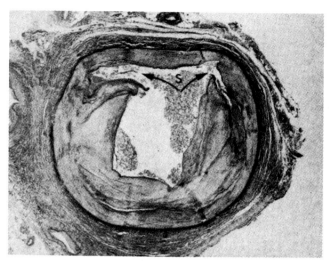

Figure 31–37. Postmortem cross-section of human atherosclerotic artery after PTCA showing splitting of the plaque. (From Block, P. C.: Mechanism of transluminal angioplasty. Am. J. Cardiol., 53:69C, 1984.)

of distinctive morphologic findings in patients who die several months after angioplasty has been described by Waller (Waller et al, 1984).

Procedural Results

Gruentzig (1978) reported an initial success rate (based on arteriographic or clinical evidence of improvement) in 80% of a group of highly selected patients. The original NIH PTCA Registry enrolled 3,248 patients from 105 clinical sites between 1979 and 1981. Arteriographic success was defined as a decrease of at least 20% in the luminal diameter narrowing. By using these criteria, the arteriographic success rate among all patients was 59% (Kent et al, 1982).

In August of 1985, the NIH reopened the PTCA Registry at its previous sites to document changes in angioplasty strategy and outcome. The new registry entered 1,802 consecutive patients who had not had a myocardial infarction in the 10 days before angioplasty (Detre et al, 1988). The selection of patients, technical outcome, and short-term major complications were compared with the 1979 to 1981 registry cohort. In addition, patients studied between 1977 and 1979 were retrospectively added to the original registry.

The new NIH Registry patients were older, and there was a significantly higher proportion of multivessel disease (53 versus 25%; p < 0.001), poor left ventricular function (19 versus 8%; p < 0.001), previous myocardial infarction (37 versus 21%; p < 0.001), and previous CABG (13 versus 9%; p < 0.01). The new registry cohort also had more complex coronary lesions. Attempts at angioplasty in these patients also involved more multivessel procedures.

Despite these differences, the in-hospital outcome in the new registry was better. Angiographic

success rates according to lesion increased from 67 to 88% (p < 0.001), and overall success rates (measured as a reduction of at least 20% in all lesions attempted without mortality, myocardial infarction, or CABG) increased from 61 to 78% (p < 0.001). In-hospital mortality for the new cohort was 1%, and the nonfatal myocardial infarction rate was 4.3%. These rates were similar to those of the old registry.

Changes in baseline characteristics between the old and new registry are shown in Table 31–8. Differences in PTCA strategy regarding the types of lesions attempted are shown in Table 31–9. A comparison of the angiographic and clinical success rates between the two registries is shown in Table 31–10. In the original registry, 22% of all lesions could not be crossed with available equipment and techniques. In the new registry, 92% of all lesions were successfully traversed. In the older registry, 68% of patients had one or more lesions reduced by at least 20%, whereas in the new registry, 91% of patients had successful dilatation of at least one lesion. The overall clinical success rate was 61% in the old registry and 78% in the new registry.

Untoward events in patients in the old and new registries are shown in Table 31–11. The incidence of death for patients with single-vessel disease was reduced from 1.3% to 0.2%. The incidence of emergency CABG was reduced from 6.1 to 2.9% in the same group. However, the incidence of death, nonfatal myocardial infarction, and emergency CABG for all patients combined was not different between the two registries (Table 31–12).

TABLE 31–8. BASELINE CHARACTERISTICS OF OLD- AND NEW-REGISTRY PATIENTS*

Characteristics	Old (n = 1155)	New (n = 1802)	p Value
	Registry		
Mean age (yr)	53.5	57.7	<0.001
Mean duration of chest pain (mo)	17	28	<0.001
	Number (%)		
Age ≥65	141 (12)	486 (27)	<0.001
Women	292 (25)	476 (26)	—
Unstable angina	431 (37)	890 (49)	<0.001
Vessel disease			<0.001
Single	863 (75)	839 (47)	
Double	203 (18)	568 (32)	
Triple	89 (8)	395 (22)	
Previous infarction	245 (21)	662 (37)	<0.001
Previous CABG	108 (9)	226 (13)	<0.01
Ejection fraction <50%†	76 (8)	270 (19)	<0.001
History of CHF‡	37 (3)	100 (6)	<0.01
History of diabetes†	101 (9)	244.(14)	<0.001
History of hypertension†	350 (35)	832 (47)	<0.001
Currently smoking†	398 (37)	519 (30)	<0.001

*Reprinted, by permission, from the New England Journal of Medicine, *318*:265, 1988.
†Data on these characteristics were missing for some patients. The percentages given are those of patients with known data.
‡CHF = congestive heart failure.

TABLE 31–9. PTCA STRATEGY IN OLD- AND NEW-REGISTRY PATIENTS, ACCORDING TO THE NUMBER OF DISEASED VESSELS*

Strategy	Single-Vessel (%) Old (n = 863)	New (n = 839)	Double-Vessel (%) Old (n = 203)	New (n = 568)	Triple-Vessel (%) Old (n = 89)	New (n = 395)	Total (%) Old (n = 1155)	New (n = 1802)
Two or more lesions attempted†	5.0	21.6	17.7	53.2	21.3	59.2	8.5	39.8
Arteries attempted†								
Right coronary only	22.8	26.7	31.0	20.2	29.2	15.4	24.8	22.2
Left anterior descending only	72.4	60.2	36.5	21.5	19.1	15.7	62.0	38.2
Left circumflex only	3.5	10.0	11.3	16.2	10.1	14.2	5.4	12.9
Right coronary + left anterior descending	0.1	1.4	6.9	16.0	6.7	7.1	1.8	7.3
Right coronary + left circumflex	—	0.1	1.0	7.7	1.1	6.8	0.3	4.0
Left anterior descending + left circumflex	0.1	0.2	3.0	13.0	3.4	12.9	0.9	7.0
Right coronary, left anterior descending, + left circumflex	—	0.1	0.5	0.5	1.1	11.6	0.2	2.8
Left main only	—	—	3.9	1.1	7.9	1.0	1.3	0.6
Left main and other‡	—	—	0.5	0.2	2.2	0.8	0.3	0.2
Bypass graft only	0.9	1.0	4.4	2.3	16.9	7.8	2.8	2.9
Bypass graft and other‡	0.1	—	1.0	1.4	3.4	7.1	0.5	2.0
Bypass graft attempted	1.0	1.0	5.4	3.7	20.2	14.9	3.3	4.9

*Reprinted, by permission, from The New England Journal of Medicine, 318:265, 1988.
†P < 0.001 for patients with single-vessel, double-vessel, and triple-vessel disease compared according to registry within each subgroup.
‡There is an overlap between these two categories of one case in the old registry and four cases in the new registry.

Restenosis

Long-term success of an angioplasty procedure may be limited by the development of restenosis at the original angioplasty site. The incidence of restenosis appears to be approximately 30%, although a wide range has been reported (13 to 47%) (Dangoisse et al, 1982; Jutzy et al, 1982; Meier et al, 1984; Williams et al, 1984). In the original NIH Registry study, follow-up angiography was done in 557 patients after successful PTCA in 27 selected clinical centers enrolled in the study (Holmes et al, 1984). The total recatheterization follow-up rate was 84% in these centers. The median time to repeat angiography was 188 days. Restenosis was defined as a 30% or greater increase in stenosis compared with the immediate post-PTCA result or loss of 50% or more of the gain achieved by the original PTCA. Restenosis by one or both of these definitions was documented in 33.6% of the patients studied. The incidence of restenosis in patients having follow-up angiography was highest within the first 6 months after PTCA. Among the patients with restenosis, 24% did not have symptoms of angina pectoris.

TABLE 31–10. ANGIOGRAPHIC AND CLINICAL SUCCESS IN OLD- AND NEW-REGISTRY PATIENTS, ACCORDING TO THE NUMBER OF DISEASED VESSELS*†

Outcome	Single-Vessel (%) Old	New	Double-Vessel (%) Old	New	Triple-Vessel (%) Old	New	Total (%) Old	New
Outcome by lesion†	(n = 910)	(n = 1060)	(n = 244)	(n = 985)	(n = 109)	(n = 847)	(n = 1263)	(n = 2892)
Unable to pass	21.5	6.8	23.4	9.6	20.2	7.2	21.8	7.9
Unable to dilate	6.3	4.2	10.7	4.0	10.1	4.8	7.4	4.3
Not successful, unknown reason	3.6	0.1	5.3	—	3.7	—	4.0	—
Dilated ≥20%	68.6	89.0	60.7	86.4	66.1	88.0	66.8	87.8
Outcome by patient	(n = 863)	(n = 839)	(n = 203)	(n = 568)	(n = 89)	(n = 395)	(n = 1155)	(n = 1,802)
One or more lesions reduced ≥20%†	68.7	90.7	62.1	90.5	68.5	90.9	67.5	90.7
All lesions reduced ≥20%‡	67.3	86.8	55.2	78.9	60.7	77.5	64.7	82.2
Clinical success§								
All lesions reduced ≥20% and no death, infarction, or CABG	63.6	84.3	51.2	74.6	58.4	70.9	61.0	78.3

*Reprinted, by permission, from The New England Journal of Medicine, 318:265, 1988.
†p < 0.001 for patients in all three groups compared according to registry within each subgroup.
‡p < 0.001 for patients with single- and double-vessel disease, and p < 0.01 for patients with triple-vessel disease.
§p < 0.001 for patients with single- and double-vessel disease, and p < 0.05 for patients with triple-vessel disease.

TABLE 31–11. UNTOWARD EVENTS AND ELECTIVE BYPASS GRAFTING IN OLD- AND NEW-REGISTRY PATIENTS, ACCORDING TO THE NUMBER OF DISEASED VESSELS*

Event or CABG	Single-Vessel (%)		Double-Vessel (%)		Triple-Vessel (%)		Total (%)	
	Old (n = 863)	New (n = 839)	Old (n = 203)	New (n = 568)	Old (n = 89)	New (n = 395)	Old (n = 1,155)	New (n = 1,802)
Death	1.3†	0.2†	0.5	0.9	2.2	2.8	1.2	1.0
Nonfatal infarction	5.0	3.5	3.9	5.1	6.7	5.1	4.9	4.3
CABG								
Emergency	6.1‡	2.9‡	5.4	3.7	3.4	4.3	5.8	3.4
Elective	19.5§	1.7§	27.6§	2.3§	16.9§	3.3§	20.7	2.2

*Reprinted, by permission, from The New England Journal of Medicine, 318:265, 1988.
†p < 0.05; ‡p < 0.01; §p < 0.001.

Repeated PTCA was done in 203 registry patients who were initially judged to have a successful acute PTCA but who later developed restenosis (Williams et al, 1984). Repeated PTCA was usually done within 6 months of the first procedure, and the success rate was 85.2%. As a direct result of PTCA, 1.5% of patients suffered acute myocardial infarction and 2% required emergency CABG. No mortality resulted from the attempted second procedure. One to 3 years of follow-up information was available in 94% of patients. Most patients (75.9%) did not have a subsequent PTCA, CABG, or interim myocardial infarction. The late mortality was 0.8%. Thus, with a high success rate and a low complication rate, repeat angioplasty appears to be a reasonable form of therapy for patients who have developed restenosis after an initially successful angioplasty procedure.

PTCA IN ACUTE MYOCARDIAL INFARCTION

Coronary reperfusion within 6 hours of the onset of acute myocardial infarction partially salvages jeopardized myocardium and significantly improves both short- and long-term survival (GISSI, 1986; Stack et al, 1985; Ritchie et al, 1985; Stadius et al, 1986). Thrombolytic therapy has become a standard therapeutic intervention in patients without contraindication to these medications. Despite the proven efficacy

of these agents, all available thrombolytic agents share two major limitations. First, even the best available agents fail to recanalize the coronary artery in 20 to 30% of patients (Stack et al, 1983; Topol et al, 1987). Second, even in patients who are reperfused there is a significant residual stenosis that often leads to reocclusion or symptomatic ischemia (Fung et al, 1986; Harrison, 1984). Unfortunately, noninvasive methods for identifying patients who have failed to reperfuse with thrombolytic therapy, such as chest pain, ST segment changes, or reperfusion arrhythmias, have been shown to be unreliable in several large trials (Califf et al, 1989; Kircher et al, 1987).

Because of the limitations of therapeutic efficacy of thrombolytic therapy and the inability to identify patients who fail to reperfuse, emergency cardiac catheterization with PTCA has been proposed as a more definitive treatment modality. Patients with total occlusion can be identified and reperfusion can be established directly with PTCA. Patients who have significant residual stenosis after reperfusion can have PTCA and achieve wider patency, reducing the likelihood for later reocclusion or other ischemic events. Although several trials have shown excellent results by using this approach, it is clear that angioplasty in the setting of an unstable plaque often results in a lower acute success rate and a higher in-hospital reocclusion rate compared with angioplasty

TABLE 31–12. WORST OUTCOMES OF PTCA IN OLD- AND NEW-REGISTRY PATIENTS, ACCORDING TO THE NUMBER OF DISEASED VESSELS*

Outcome	Single-Vessel (%)		Double-Vessel (%)		Triple-Vessel (%)		Total (%)	
	Old (n = 863)	New (n = 839)	Old (n = 203)	New (n = 568)	Old (n = 89)	New (n = 395)	Old (n = 1,155)	New (n = 1,802)
Death	1.3	0.2	0.5	0.9	2.2	2.8	1.2	1.0
Myocardial infarction	5.0	3.5	3.9	5.1	6.7	5.1	4.9	4.3
CABG								
Emergency	2.3	1.8	3.9	1.8	3.4	1.8	2.7	1.8
Elective	18.7	1.3	26.1	2.1	12.4	2.8	19.5	1.9
Lesions successfully dilated								
None	8.2	5.8	8.9	5.5	10.1	5.6	8.5	5.7
Some	0.9	3.1	5.4	10.0	6.7	11.1	2.2	7.0
All	63.6	84.3	51.2	74.6	58.4	70.9	61.0	78.3

*Reprinted, by permission, from The New England Journal of Medicine, 318:265, 1988.

in the elective setting. This is particularly true if angioplasty is applied in all cases regardless of the coronary anatomy.

On the basis of these data, the author and associates now use a treatment strategy designed to maximize both the efficacy of coronary reperfusion and the safety and long-term outcome of the procedure. Thrombolytic therapy is administered immediately at local community hospitals within a 150-mile radius of the interventional center, and the patient is transferred by helicopter or specialized cardiac ground transport units. Emergency cardiac catheterization is done by using small-bore (No. 6 French) arterial catheters. Infarct vessel patency status is documented arteriographically. In patients who are successfully recanalized with brisk antegrade flow, definitive angioplasty or operation is deferred until the plaque has stabilized later during the hospitalization. However, patients who have failed to reperfuse, patients with poor antegrade flow, and patients in cardiogenic shock immediately have emergency PTCA.

CONCLUSIONS

PTCA has become well established as an effective method for the management of selected patients with coronary artery disease. However, PTCA has at least three major limitations: (1) Many patients are not candidates for PTCA (e.g., patients with diffuse disease or chronic total occlusions). (2) The acute failure rate (>50% residual stenosis after PTCA) remains at 5 to 7%. (3) In approximately one-third of initially successful angioplasties, patients develop restenosis within 6 months.

In an effort to overcome these limitations, investigators have developed new devices to actually remove the plaque by using either laser or mechanical ablation by flexible catheters. Another new approach has been to place short conduits or stents made of stainless steel into dilated segments of arteries to prevent acute occlusion as well as chronic restenosis. Although initial studies with each of these new technologies are encouraging, they must each be tested in a prospective randomized manner against the current state-of-the-art methods of medical, interventional, and surgical therapy. In the future, it is likely that a number of excellent therapeutic options, both surgical and nonsurgical, will exist and can be tailored to the individual needs of the patient based on specific clinical and anatomic indications.

Selected Bibliography

Detre, K., Holubkov, R., Kelsey, S., et al: Percutaneous transluminal coronary angioplasty in 1985–1986 and 1977–1981. N. Engl. J. Med., *318*:265, 1988.

This important study compares the results of the original NIH PTCA Registry from 1977 through 1981 with the most recent NIH Registry from 1985 through 1986. The new registry entered 1,802 consecutive patients. The angiographic success rates according to lesion increased from 67 to 88% (p < 0.001), and the overall success rate (measured as a reduction of at least 20% in all lesions attempted, without death, myocardial infarction, or coronary bypass grafting) increased from 61 to 78% (p < 0.001) in the new registry.

Dotter, C. T.: Transluminal angioplasty: A long view. Radiology, *135*:561, 1980.

In this review article, Dotter gives a historical account of the development of percutaneous transluminal angioplasty. This is a very interesting perspective from the original developer of percutaneous dilatation techniques.

Dotter, C. T., and Judkins, M. P.: Transluminal treatment of arteriosclerotic obstruction. Circulation, *30*:654, 1964.

This is the original study describing the technique and preliminary report of the first group of patients treated with transluminal catheter dilatation for atherosclerotic arteries. Dotter describes the methods for dilating plaques with a guidewire and tapered Teflon catheters of increasing diameter. The outcomes of the first 11 patients treated in this manner are described in detail.

Ferguson, T. B., Hinohara, T., Simpson, J., et al: Catheter reperfusion to allow optimal coronary bypass grafting following failed transluminal coronary angioplasty. Ann. Thorac. Surg., *42*:399, 1986.

This study presents the results of a series of nine patients treated with the reperfusion catheter for failed PTCA. The article was written from the perspective of a cardiac surgeon and includes methods of use of the reperfusion catheter during the operative procedure, including the antegrade delivery of cardioplegic solution.

Gruentzig, A.: Transluminal dilatation of coronary-artery stenosis. Lancet, *1*:263, 1978.

In this study, the first five patients to have percutaneous transluminal coronary angioplasty are described. The original technique for coronary dilatation with a polyvinyl chloride balloon dilatation catheter is described. Seven dilatations were done in five patients in 1977, with a primary success achieved in six of the seven procedures.

Kent, K. M., Bentivoglio, L. G., Block, P. C., et al: Percutaneous transluminal coronary angioplasty: Report from the registry of the National Heart, Lung, and Blood Institute. Am. J. Cardiol., *49*:2011, 1982.

In this Registry, data were collected from 34 centers in the United States and Europe, where the initial series of angioplasty was done on 631 patients between 1977 and 1981. Coronary angioplasty was successful (more than 20% decrease of coronary stenosis) in 59% of the stenosed arteries. Emergency coronary bypass operation was required in 40 patients (6%). Myocardial infarction occurred in 29 patients (4%). In-hospital death occurred in six patients (1%), three with single-vessel disease and three with multivessel disease.

Kent, K. M., Mullin, S. M., and Passamani, E. R. (Guest eds.): Proceedings of the National Heart, Lung, and Blood Institute Workshop on the Outcome of Percutaneous Transluminal Coronary Angioplasty. Am. J. Cardiol., *53*:1–146C, 1984.

In this classic journal supplement, 35 articles are compiled from the proceedings of the National Heart, Lung, and Blood Institute Workshop on the outcome of PTCA. Articles in this volume include a report from the NIH Registry, experimental studies, technological considerations, surgical considerations, acute and chronic outcome of PTCA, and future directions of study.

Stack, R. S., Carlson, E. B., Hinohara, H., and Phillips, H. R.: Interventional cardiac catheterization. Invest. Radiol., *20*:333, 1985.

This review article describes historical developments in the field of PTCA, methods of procedure performance, complications, pathology, restenosis, use of PTCA in acute myocardial infarction, and new investigational interventional techniques.

Bibliography

Baughman, K. L., Pasternak, R. C., Fallon, J. T., and Block, P. C.: Transluminal coronary angioplasty of postmortem human hearts. Am. J. Cardiol., 48:1044, 1981.

Block, P. C., Baughman, K. L., Pasternak, R. C., and Fallon, J. T.: Transluminal angioplasty: Correlation of morphologic and angiographic findings in an experimental model. Circulation, 61:778, 1980a.

Block, P. C., Fallon, J. T., and Elmer, D.: Angioplasty: Lessons from the laboratory. Am. J. Radiol., 135:907, 1980b.

Block, P. C., Myler, R. K., Stertzer, S., and Fallon, J. T.: Morphology after transluminal angioplasty in human beings. N. Engl. J. Med., 305:382, 1981.

Colavita, P. G., Ideker, R. E., Reimer, K. A., et al: The spectrum of pathology associated with percutaneous angioplasty. J. Am. Coll. Cardiol., 5:525, 1985.

Cowley, M. J., Dorros, G., Kelsey, S. F., et al: Emergency coronary bypass surgery after coronary angioplasty: The National Heart, Lung, and Blood Institute's Percutaneous Transluminal Coronary Angioplasty Registry experience. Am. J. Cardiol., 53:22C, 1984.

Dangoisse, V., Guiteras, V. P., David, P. R., et al: Recurrence of stenosis after successful percutaneous transluminal coronary angioplasty (PTCA). Circulation, 66:331, 1982.

Detre, K., Holubkov, R., Kelsey, S., et al: Percutaneous transluminal coronary angioplasty in 1985–1986 and 1977–1981. N. Engl. J. Med., 318:265, 1988.

Dotter, C. T.: Cardiac catheterization and angiographic techniques of the future. Cesk. Radiol. 19:217, 1965; presented at the 1963 Czechoslovak Radiological Congress, Karlovy Vary, June 10, 1953.

Dotter, C. T.: Transluminal angioplasty-pathologic basis. In Zeitler, E., Gruentzig, A., Schoop, W. (eds): Percutaneous Vascular Recanalization. Berlin, Springer-Verlag, 3, 1978.

Dotter, C. T.: Transluminal angioplasty: A long view. Radiology, 135:561, 1980.

Dotter, C. T., and Judkins, M. P.: Transluminal treatment of arteriosclerotic obstruction. Circulation, 30:654, 1964.

Faxon, D. P., Weber, V. J., Haudenschild, C., et al: Acute effects of transluminal angioplasty in three experimental models of atherosclerosis. Arteriosclerosis, 2:125, 1982.

Feldman, R. C., and Anderson, D. J.: Gradients at PTCA: Physiological or artifactual? (Abstract). J. Am. Coll. Cardiol., 54:7C, 1985.

Ferguson, T. B., Hinohara, T., Simpson, J., et al: Catheter reperfusion to allow optimal coronary bypass grafting following failed transluminal coronary angioplasty. Ann. Thorac. Surg., 42:399, 1986.

Gruentzig, A., and Hopff, H.: Perjutane Rekanalisation chronischer arterieller Verschlusse mit einem neuen Dilatationstechnik. Baden-Baden, Witzstrock, 1977.

Gruentzig, A. R., Myler, R. K., Hanna, E. S., et al: Transluminal angioplasty of coronary artery stenosis (Abstract). Circulation, 56:III-84, 1977.

Gruentzig, A.: Transluminal dilatation of coronary-artery stenosis. Lancet, 1:263, 1978.

Gruentzig, A. R., Senning, A., and Siegenthaler, W. E.: Nonop-erative dilatation of coronary-artery stenosis. N. Engl. J. Med., 301:61, 1979.

Hinohara, T., Simpson, J. B., Phillips, H. R., and Stack, R. S.: Transluminal intracoronary reperfusion catheter: A device to maintain coronary perfusion between failed PTCA and emergency CABG. J. Am. Coll. Cardiol., 11:977, 1988.

Holmes, D. R., Vlietstra, R. E., Smith, H. C., et al: Restenosis after percutaneous transluminal coronary angioplasty (PTCA): A report from the PTCA Registry of the National Heart, Lung and Blood Institute. Am. J. Cardiol., 53:77C, 1984.

Jutzy, K. R., Berte, L. E., Alderman, E. L., et al: Coronary restenosis rates in a consecutive patient series one year post successful angioplasty. Circulation, 66:331, 1982.

Kent, K. M., Bentivoglio, L. G., Block, P. C., et al: Percutaneous transluminal coronary angioplasty: Report from the registry of the National Heart, Lung, and Blood Institute. Am. J. Cardiol., 49:2011, 1982.

Kober, G., Scherer, D., Koch, M., et al: Transluminal coronary angioplasty: Early and long-term results in 250 procedures. Herz, 6:309, 1982.

Lev, H. J., and Gruentzig, A.: Histopathologic aspects of transluminal recanalization. In Zeitler, E., Gruentzig, A., and Schoop, A. (eds): Percutaneous Vascular Recanalization. Berlin, Springer-Verlag, 39, 1978.

Levy, R. I., Mock, M. N., Willman, V. L. and Frommer, P. L.: Percutaneous transluminal coronary angioplasty. Am. J. Cardiol., 49:1216, 1982.

Meier, B., King, S. B., Gruentzig, A. R., et al: Repeat coronary angioplasty. J. Am. Coll. Cardiol., 4:463, 1984.

Porstmann, W.: Ein Neuer Korsett-Balloon Katheter zur transluminalen Rekanalisation nach Dotter unter besonderer Berucksichtigung von Obliterationen an den Bechenarterien. Radiol. Diagn. (Berl.), 14:239, 1973.

Quigley, P. J., Hinohara, T., Phillips, H. R., et al: Myocardial protection during coronary angioplasty in humans using an autoperfusion balloon catheter. Circulation (in press).

Scholl, J. M., David, P. R., Chaitman, B. R., et al: Recurrence of stenosis following percutaneous transluminal coronary angioplasty. Circulation, 64:193, 1981.

Simpson, J. B., Baim, D. S., Robert, E. W., and Harrison, D. C.: A new catheter system for coronary angioplasty. Am. J. Cardiol., 49:1216, 1982.

Staple, T. W.: Modified catheter for percutaneous transluminal treatment of arteriosclerotic obstructions. Radiology, 91:1041, 1968.

van Andel, G. J.: Percutaneous transluminal angioplasty: The Dotter procedure. Amsterdam, Excerpta Medica, 1976.

Waller, B. F., Gorfinkel, H. J., Rogers, R. J., et al: Early and late morphologic changes in major epicardial coronary arteries after percutaneous transluminal coronary angioplasty. Am. J. Cardiol., 53:42C, 1984.

Waller, B. F., McManus, B. M., Gorfinkel, H. J., et al: Status of the major epicardial coronary arteries 80 to 150 days after percutaneous transluminal coronary angioplasty. Am. J. Cardiol., 51:81, 1983.

Waltman, A. C., Greenfield, A. J., and Athanasoulis, C. A.: Transluminal angioplasty: General rules and basic considerations. In Athanasoulis, C. A., Greene, R. E., Pfister, R. C., and Roberson, G. H. (eds): Interventional Radiology. Philadelphia, W. B. Saunders, 1982, pp. 253–272.

Williams, D. O., Gruentzig, A. R., Kent, K. M., et al: Efficacy of repeat percutaneous transluminal coronary angioplasty for coronary restenosis. Am. J. Cardiol., 53:32C, 1984.

Zarins, C. K., Lu, C. T., Gewertz, B. L., et al: Arterial disruption and remodeling following balloon dilatation. Surgery, 92:1086, 1982.

III FIBRINOLYTIC THERAPY IN THE MANAGEMENT OF ACUTE MYOCARDIAL INFARCTION

Robert M. Califf

The evolution of an understanding of the fibrinolytic system, coinciding with safe techniques to evaluate the human coronary circulation during unstable ischemic heart disease syndromes, has led to a dramatic change in the therapy of unstable angina and acute myocardial infarction. Both mechanical and pharmacologic techniques to correct the underlying abnormality in coronary blood flow now form the basis for interventional therapy. Methods of restoring coronary blood flow after acute occlusion will continue for the foreseeable future to include the use of agents that lyse thrombi. Improved ability to exploit nature and more efficient and elaborate methods of production of human genetic products through technology involving recombinant genetic techniques will lead to increased flexibility in altering the structure of these molecules. Thus, a working understanding of the fibrinolytic system and the consequences of therapeutic manipulation of this system is essential to the cardiovascular practitioner.

HISTORICAL ASPECTS

The initial description of acute myocardial infarction by Herrick in 1912 described the clinical syndrome representing coronary thrombosis. Subsequent clinicians and researchers persisted in the description of the problem as involving a thrombosed coronary artery, until a series of pathologic studies failed to show thrombi in the coronary arteries of patients who died of acute myocardial infarction. These studies led many prominent cardiologists to doubt the primacy of thrombosis in the pathogenesis of the condition. This issue remained unsettled until the pioneering work of DeWood and colleagues, who reported in 1980 that when acute angiography was done in patients early in acute myocardial infarction, coronary occlusion was found in more than 80%. Moreover, when these patients were referred for coronary artery bypass grafting, thrombus could be removed surgically from the vessel.

In parallel with the development of understanding of the pathophysiology of myocardial infarction, knowledge concerning the fibrinolytic system was evolving. The instability of human blood clots has been recognized since 1838 when Denis described the dissolution of fibrin in human clots. Nolf and Yudin, from the Soviet Union, began the use of cadaveric blood for transfusion after they noted that clot dissolution occurred several hours after death. Tillett and Garner, at Johns Hopkins, initially described streptokinase in 1933. They showed that an isolate from beta-hemolytic streptococci could lyse plasma clots in humans. The possible role of this agent in pharmacologic treatment of thrombotic problems was not generally appreciated until experiments by Tillett and Sherry were reported in 1949 to 1952, showing that streptokinase could successfully lyse clots. Most of these applications were in diseases of the thorax caused by loculation of fluid by blood clots, and these experiments were reported in the surgical literature. In 1949, Johnson and Tillett reported the first model of in-vivo fibrinolysis in rabbits.

Nydick and colleagues (1948) reported a reduction in infarct size in the animal model with early treatment with streptokinase. The first clinical trial of thrombolytic therapy in acute myocardial infarction was reported by Fletcher (1958). These initial studies did not evoke tremendous enthusiasm from the clinical community, although a number of large studies of intravenous thrombolytic therapy were initiated in Europe in the 1960s and 1970s. The first large-scale trials of thrombolytic therapy in the United States were initiated by the National Institutes of Health to evaluate this treatment in pulmonary embolism, rather than acute myocardial infarction, mainly because of skepticism concerning the role of thrombus in the pathogenesis of myocardial infarction.

Despite the identification of tissue plasminogen activator (TPA) in the 1940s, the lack of a suitable method to produce sufficient quantities delayed its evaluation for clinical purposes. In 1979, in Collen's laboratory, a melanoma cell culture was used to isolate sufficient quantities to investigate the structure and biologic properties of TPA. The first patient was treated with TPA in 1981, and the resolution of renal vein thrombosis was shown in two patients after renal transplantation. Through a combination of industry and academic efforts, the TPA gene was cloned and expressed in a mammalian hamster ovary cell line. Large quantities of TPA were thus produced for laboratory and human investigation, beginning in February of 1984.

PATHOPHYSIOLOGY OF UNSTABLE ISCHEMIC HEART DISEASE SYNDROMES

Demonstration of complete coronary artery occlusion in humans at the time of acute myocardial infarction and pathologic documentation of abnormal plaque architecture in unstable angina, sudden death, and acute infarction have formed the basis for understanding the factors that produce unstable myocardial ischemia. Atherosclerotic plaques evolve from small yellow fatty streaks to complex lesions including smooth-muscle cell proliferation, connective tissue proliferation, and collagen and elastin in addition to pools of cholesterol. When detailed pathoanatomic studies have been done, plaques have varied considerably in architecture. Some plaques are predominantly composed of collagen (fibrous plaques) and others contain a large lipid pool, which is semifluid at body temperature. These lipid pools are covered by fibrous tissue, which is in turn covered by intact endothelium. Intracellular and extracellular lipid is also found throughout the plaque.

Although the precise mechanism remains to be defined, as "soft" atherosclerotic plaques evolve, sudden disruptions in the endothelium occur and are manifested pathologically as fissures on the surface of the plaques or more extensive disruption of the undersurface of the plaques, called "plaque rupture." Preliminary evidence has indicated that in some cases the fibrous plaque is eroded by macrophage digestion, whereas in other cases a sudden mechanical disruption occurs at stress points where the lipid pool and fibrous portion of the plaque adjoin. Exposure of the contents of the plaque to the bloodstream leads to a biochemical sequence that activates the clotting system. In most cases, the fissure is sealed off and significant compromise of the lumen of the vessel does not occur, but an intraluminal thrombus may occur, totally obstructing the artery. The occurrence of hemorrhage into the contents of the plaque along planes defined by the geography of the plaque may lead to significant alteration of the degree of lumen compromise without total occlusion (Fig. 31–38). Thus, the process of progressive atherosclerosis is now thought to involve a series of "plaque events" rather than a smooth progressive occlusion of the vessel. Finally, when the clotting system is activated and a thrombus projects into the lumen, the distal vessel may be subject to microemboli of platelets and fibrin.

The process of platelet activation is mediated by a series of events that are probably initiated through the exposure of platelet receptors to collagen and thrombin (Fig. 31–39). These receptors then activate biochemical pathways that lead to the secretion of vasoactive substances by the platelets. The initial phase in which platelets become attracted to form a layer on the disrupted endothelial surface is called platelet adhesion. Components that have been identified to be essential for normal platelet adhesion include von Willebrand's factor, the glycoprotein Ib receptor, and the glycoprotein IIb/IIIa receptor. When platelets adhere to the endothelial surface, a series of events occur, leading to platelet aggregation. The platelets secrete two types of granules: one containing adenine nucleotides, calcium, and serotonin and

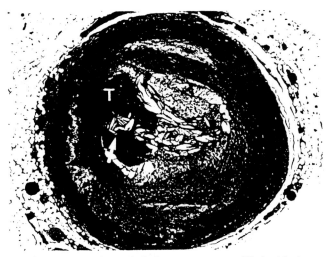

Figure 31–38. An occluded coronary artery filled with thrombus (T) is depicted. A fissure is present within an intimal pool of lipid, and the thrombus within the lumen contains cholesterol *(arrow)* that has extruded from the plaque. (From Davies, M. J.: Atherogenesis and thrombosis. *In* Califf, R. M., Mark, D. B., and Wagner, G. S. [eds]: Acute Coronary Care in the Thrombolytic Era. Chicago, Year Book Medical Publishers, 1988, p. 8. Reprinted with permission.)

the other containing adhesive and coagulation proteins and growth factors. Attention has focused on these growth factors (platelet-derived growth factor and beta growth factor) because of their ability to stimulate smooth-muscle cell proliferation and fibroblast migration. Large amounts of thromboxane A_2 are also produced and lead to vasospasm and further platelet aggregation.

As platelets are activated, a simultaneous activation of the blood coagulation system occurs (Fig. 31–40). A series of reactions involving coagula-

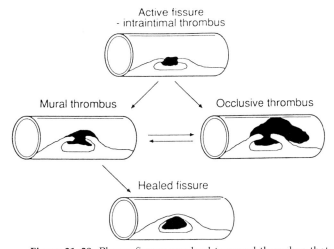

Figure 31–39. Plaque fissure can lead to mural thrombus that resolves or to an occlusive thrombus leading to myocardial infarction. (From Davies, M. J.: Atherogenesis and thrombosis. *In* Califf, R. M., Mark, D. B., and Wagner, G. S. [eds]: Acute Coronary Care in the Thrombolytic Era. Chicago, Year Book Medical Publishers, 1988, p. 9. Reprinted with permission.)

PLATELET ADHESION

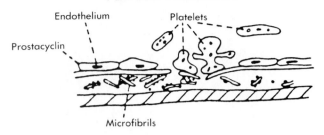

PLATELET AGGREGATION

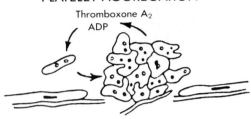

Figure 31–40. An overview of the process of primary hemostasis. The initial event is platelet adhesion to the vessel wall, which occurs when the subendothelium is exposed as a result of disruption or injury of endothelial cells. After adhesion, platelets become activated. Under the influence of mediators such as ADP and thromboxane A_2, circulating platelets are stimulated to the initial monolayer of platelets to form a platelet aggregate. (From Handen, R. I., and Loscalzo, J.: Hemostasis, thrombosis, fibrinolysis, and cardiovascular disease. *In* Braunwald, E.: Heart Disease, 3rd ed. Philadelphia, W. B. Saunders Company, 1988, p. 1758.)

tion proteins on the surface of the denuded endothelium leads to the production of thrombin. This process is regulated by antithrombin III, which inactivates many components in the coagulation cascade, and proteins C and S, which predominantly exert their action by inactivating Factors Va and VIIIa. The production of thrombin not only leads to the conversion of fibrinogen to fibrin, thus forming clot, but thrombin is also a potent stimulator of platelet activation.

This complex series of events can rapidly convert a "stable" atherosclerotic plaque to a primary initiator of acute ischemic heart disease syndromes (Fig. 31–41). The platelet and fibrin mass leads to a progressive narrowing of the arterial lumen. Vasoactive substances are produced, leading to further periodic fluctuations in vascular tone with accompanying unpredictable anginal episodes due to reduced blood supply to the distal myocardium. If the clotting process is not controlled, total occlusion of the vessel ensues, with necrosis downstream within 30 to 45 minutes of occlusion. If the process is controlled before total occlusion, a more high-grade stenosis results, with a more limited life-style for the patient.

FIBRINOLYTIC SYSTEM

The process of clot formation is actively opposed in nature by a system that acts to restore and main-

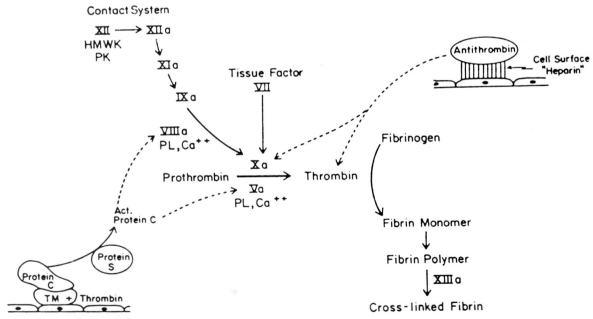

Figure 31–41. An overview of the coagulation cascade showing the two major pathways of activation. The intrinsic pathway involves Factors XII, XI, IX, and VIII, with the extrinsic or tissue factor system, which involves tissue factor and Factor VII. In both pathways, the conversion of inactive Factor X to its active form, XA, results in the formation of thrombin from prothrombin. Thrombin then converts fibrinogen to fibrin monomers, which are polymerized into cross-links by Factor XIIIA. This illustration also displays the two major anticoagulant systems. The binding of antithrombin to thrombin and Factor XA is accelerated by heparin on endothelial cells. Protein C is activated by thrombin after it is bound to the endothelial cell protein thrombomoduline. Activated protein C and protein S inactivate the two coagulation cofactors VIIIA and VA. (From Handen, R. I.: Bleeding and thrombosis. *In* Braunwald, E., Isselbacher, K. J., and Petersdorf, R. G.: Harrison's Principles of Internal Medicine, 11th ed. New York, McGraw-Hill Book Company, 1987, p. 270.)

tain vascular patency after thrombus formation. The process of clot formation and dissolution is ubiquitous, and the implications for normal biologic processes are now being realized. Just as the conversion of prothrombin to thrombin is the central process in clot formation, the conversion of plasminogen to plasmin is the focal event in clot dissolution (Fig. 31–42). Plasmin acts to degrade both fibrinogen and fibrin to components referred to as fibrin(ogen) degradation products. The action of plasmin to lyse clot is opposed by antiplasmins in the systemic circulation and is activated by a number of activators, just as thrombin is opposed by antithrombins and activated by the coagulation factors. The predominant antiplasmin in nature is alpha$_2$-antiplasmin, although a number of other antiplasmins have been described.

Plasminogen activators may be divided into three major classifications: exogenous, intrinsic, and extrinsic (Fig. 31–43). The exogenous activators are products from other organisms that can be administered from other biologic systems. The major exogenous activator is streptokinase, a streptococcal protein that forms a complex with plasminogen, leading to a shift in the configuration of the plasminogen, thus exposing the active site of the enzyme. The activated enzyme then converts circulating plasminogen to plasmin. The intrinsic pathway includes multiple molecules involved in coagulation and inflammation. The role of this system in nature or pathophysiology is poorly understood. The most clearly understood system is the extrinsic system, which is composed of a series of activators found in the human circulation. TPA is a glycoprotein produced by the vascular endothelium as well as other tissues. The molecular structure and function of this molecule have been defined in a series of eloquent experiments. The molecule contains a serine protease

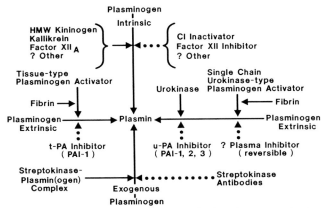

Figure 31–43. Major pathways of plasminogen activation. Plasma is formed indirectly from the exogenous administration of streptokinase but directly by activation of the intrinsic pathway. Direct plasmin generation also occurs through the action of the extrinsic plasminogen activators TPA and UPA. Note the distinction between the pathways of plasminogen activation and what are called "intrinsic" and "extrinsic" pathways of coagulation. (From Stump, D. C., and Collen, D.: Fibrinolytic system: Implications for thrombolytic therapy. *In* Califf, R. M., Mark, D. B., and Wagner, G. S. [eds]: Acute Coronary Care in the Thrombolytic Era. Chicago, Year Book Medical Publishers, 1988, p. 62.)

active site and two kringles with a configuration similar to the plasminogen molecule, a "finger" domain resembling the adhesive protein fibronectin, and a portion closely resembling epidermal growth factor. The close affinity of TPA for fibrin is probably conferred by the second kringle and the finger domain. TPA is produced in higher quantity by the vascular endothelium when stimulated by stress, including intravascular thrombus formation. In addition, regular exercise, lower body weight, and absence of cigarette smoking have been associated with a more responsive production of TPA by the endothelium. The other known extrinsic native human plasminogen activator is urokinase plasminogen activator (UPA). The role of UPA is less well understood, although it is present in the urinary tract in high concentrations and in the circulation in very low concentrations. In its proenzyme or single-chain form (SCUPA) the molecule has an affinity for fibrin, just as TPA. Each of these activators also has a specific rapid-acting inhibitor that has been isolated. Preliminary information suggests that imbalances between these activators and their inhibitors may be responsible for thrombotic tendencies in many disease states.

The conversion of plasminogen to plasmin and thus the degradation of fibrin and fibrinogen may occur in one of two compartments: on the surface of a clot (fibrin-specific activation) or in the systemic circulation (nonspecific activation) (Fig. 31–44). Fibrin-specific activation appears to be relatively more efficient, because large quantities of degradation products are not produced and coagulation factors distant from the site of the thrombus remain relatively intact. TPA is the prototypical fibrin-specific

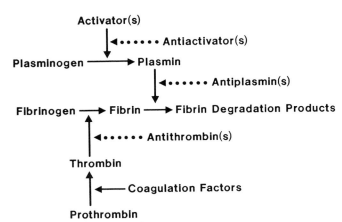

Figure 31–42. Major pathways of fibrin formation and dissolution. Fibrin is formed, and thrombin is generated by coagulation activation. Fibrin is dissolved when plasma is generated by fibrinolytic activation. (From Stump, D. C., and Collen, D.: Fibrinolytic system: Implications for thrombolytic therapy. *In* Califf, R. M., Mark, D. B., and Wagner, G. S. [eds]: Acute Coronary Care in the Thrombolytic Era. Chicago, Year Book Medical Publishers, 1988, p. 59.)

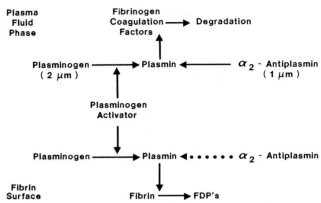

Figure 31–44. Schematic representation of the fibrin specificity of plasminogen activation. The fact that the activation of plasminogen is targeted to the fibrin surface leads to plasmin and is relatively protected from inhibition by alpha$_2$-antiplasmin. This targeting also avoids the generation of freely circulating plasmin that nonspecifically degrades normal plasma coagulation factors. (From Stump, D. C., and Collen, D.: Fibrinolytic system: Implications for thrombolytic therapy. *In* Califf, R. M., Mark, D. B., and Wagner, G. S. [eds]: Acute Coronary Care in the Thrombolytic Era. Chicago, Year Book Medical Publishers, 1988, p. 66.)

agent, and has affinity for plasminogen increased 400-fold when it is bound directly to fibrin; SCUPA is also relatively fibrin specific, although the mechanism for this effect is less well understood. However, streptokinase and urokinase have no special affinity for plasminogen in the presence of fibrin. In order for these agents to produce clot lysis, a sufficient amount is required to convert plasminogen to plasmin throughout the circulation, thus leading to destruction of not only the obstruction, but also depletion of fibrinogen, Factor V, and Factor VIII.

PATHOPHYSIOLOGY OF MYOCARDIAL NECROSIS

The basic concepts of the impact of coronary occlusion on myocardial necrosis and the pathophysiologic basis for salvage of myocardium have been elucidated by a number of investigators during the last 2 decades after the pioneering work of Reimer and Jennings (1979). In seminal experiments in the canine model, they showed that irreversible necrosis of the myocardium begins within 30 to 45 minutes of occlusion of an epicardial vessel and that this necrosis advances rapidly from the endocardium toward the epicardium (Fig. 31–45). This process has been called the *wavefront phenomenon of ischemic myocardial necrosis.* The same investigators showed that release of coronary artery occlusion at various points in time until about 3 hours after occlusion resulted in salvage of myocardium that would have become necrotic with continued occlusion. This myocardial salvage tended to occur from the epicardium toward the endocardium so that an epicardial rim of tissue is spared.

Another important contribution of these investigators was the demonstration that collateral circulation is an important determinant of the amount of myocardium that can be salvaged and the time frame in which salvage can be achieved (Fig. 31–46). The tremendous variation among species with regard to the time frame of myocardial necrosis and salvage is best explained by differences in collateral supply to the area at risk. Subsequent human studies have corroborated the importance of collateral supply as a mediator of myocardial salvage with reperfusion therapy.

Studies have focused on the process of necrosis

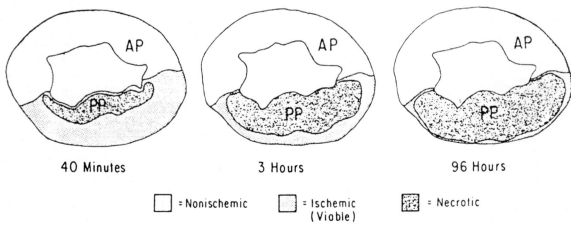

Figure 31–45. Progression of cell death versus time after left circumflex coronary artery occlusion. Necrosis occurs first in the subendocardial myocardium; with longer occlusions, the cell death moves from the subendocardial zone across the wall. This wavefront of ischemic cell death progressively involves more of the transmural thickness of the ischemic zone. (AP = anterior papillary muscle; PP = posterior papillary muscle.) (From Reimer, K. A.: The relationship between coronary blood flow in reversible and irreversible ischemic injury. *In* Califf, R. M., and Wagner, G. S. [eds]: Acute Coronary Care: Principles and Practice. Dordrecht, Martinus Nijhoff Publishers, 1985, p. 10.)

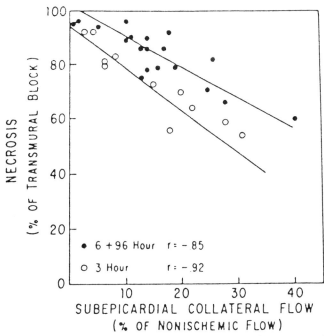

Figure 31–46. Relationship between transmural necrosis and subepicardial blood flow. Regression lines for permanent infarcts (96 hours) and infarcts reperfused at 6 hours were not significantly different and were combined. Infarcts reperfused at 3 hours were indicated by the *open circles*. In both groups the transmural extent of necrosis was inversely related to subepicardial flow measured at 20 minutes after left circumflex coronary occlusion. However, the 3-hour regression line shifted downward, indicating that reperfusion at 3 hours limited infarct size. (From Reimer, K. A.: The relationship between coronary blood flow in reversible and irreversible ischemic injury. *In* Califf, R. M., and Wagner, G. S. [eds]: Acute Coronary Care: Principles and Practice. Dordrecht, Martinus Nijhoff Publishers, 1985, p. 13.)

in the hope that manipulation of the biochemical substrate could lead to prolongation of the time frame for myocardial salvage. Many studies in laboratory models of acute occlusion and reocclusion of the coronary arteries have suggested that reperfusion of the acutely ischemic myocardium results in cellular damage that detracts from the beneficial overall effect of reperfusion. These deleterious effects appear to be mediated through a series of events resulting in myocardial and endothelial cell swelling and rapid accumulation of destructive metabolites and other byproducts of ischemia in the cell. A large overload of calcium occurs shortly after reperfusion, as well as explosive cell swelling, which may be caused by an inability of the cells to regulate cell volume. Hemorrhage into the area of infarction caused by loss of endothelial cell integrity also adds to mechanical decompensation. The oxygen free radical system as a potential mediator of increased cell death with reperfusion has received much attention. This system, which usually functions to rid tissues of superoxide anions through a reaction catalyzed by superoxide dismutase, becomes overwhelmed during reperfusion. Consequently, superoxide anions accu-

mulate within the cell, leading to rapid tissue destruction, especially to loss of structural integrity of the cell membrane. Whether this process of reperfusion injury actually increases infarct size or simply hastens the demise of cells initially destined to die remains unsettled. Another possible mechanism of increased damage due to reperfusion is the obstruction of distal arteriolar beds due to endothelial cell swelling or due to platelet and leukocyte accumulation and obstruction of distal vessels. Multiple pharmacologic manipulations of these systems are currently under investigation in animal and human studies.

Finally, demonstration of prolonged survival in patients treated beyond 6 hours from the onset of symptoms has focused attention on the process of healing of the myocardium. Human and animal studies have shown that during the recovery phase after acute infarction many ventricles go through a process of progressive dilatation that has been called *infarct expansion*. This phenomenon in its most extreme form leads to left ventricular aneurysm formation. In a less extreme form, infarct expansion leads to a larger end-diastolic volume, which has been associated with a high risk of death in the postinfarction period. Early reperfusion has prevented this process, presumably through greater epicardial sparing of tissue, thus preventing infarct expansion. However, in some animal models, even when reperfusion occurs after the point at which significant myocardial salvage can be expected, infarct expansion has been prevented. The pathophysiologic basis for this observation is not yet delineated.

FIBRINOLYTIC AGENTS

Streptokinase is currently the thrombolytic agent most commonly used on a worldwide basis. As described earlier, streptokinase is a streptococcal enzyme with nonfibrin specific lytic properties. The agent, which is administered in a dose of 1.5 million units for 45 to 60 minutes, has been associated with a 30 to 70% reperfusion rate in available studies. Because of its lack of fibrin specificity, it must be given in sufficient doses to create a systemic lytic state with its prolonged phase of fibrinogen and clotting factor depletion. In addition, because it is a bacterial enzyme, its use is associated with various systemic effects that are not observed with other thrombolytic agents. Hypotension with an average fall of systolic blood pressure of 30 mm Hg is observed in the average patient. This problem can be treated with volume in most patients, although pressor agents are required in some patients. Other acute problems range from a rash with fever and chills, to bronchospasm, to frank anaphylaxis. In addition, a late serum sickness-like reaction has been observed. An acylated plasminogen-streptokinase activator complex (APSAC) has been developed. It can be given as a bolus for 5 minutes without hypotension, although the other reactions may occur as the plasminogen deacylates in the circulation.

Urokinase has been available for many years. Because of its relative expense and lack of availability, however, it has not yet been approved for routine intravenous use in acute myocardial infarction. Current studies indicate that a dose of 3 million units for 90 minutes will achieve a reperfusion rate of 50 to 70% within 90 minutes of administration. The drug is not associated with hypotension or allergic phenomena because it is a human enzyme. However, it does create a systemic lytic state because it is a nonspecific fibrinolytic agent, like streptokinase.

TPA has now been produced on a large scale through recombinant genetic technology. The enzyme is fibrin specific at low doses, but as the dose is increased, a significant amount of systemic fibrinogenolysis occurs. The drug is usually administered in a dose of 60 mg in the first hour, with 10 mg as a bolus to produce rapid clot lysis. Efficacy rates are 60 to 75%. After the first hour, 20 mg/hr is given for 2 hours in an effort to continue clot lysis on the surface of the plaque and to prevent rethrombosis. Considerable controversy continues, however, concerning the weight-adjusted dose of TPA. Although the alpha half-life is short (5 to 10 minutes), the beta half-life is 55 minutes, and ongoing fibrinolysis has been shown several hours after the infusion has been discontinued.

A comparison of the clinical and hematologic effects of the drugs is shown in Table 31–13. Superior clot lysis rates have been shown with TPA compared with streptokinase in the only two double-blind trials to compare the agents. No significant difference was shown between TPA and urokinase in a similar trial. Because TPA has a shorter duration of biologic activity, a maintenance infusion is required to prevent reocclusion, although reocclusion is still a significant problem with all the agents. Although fibrin specificity was thought to confer a benefit with regard to a reduction in bleeding complication rates, randomized trials have failed to detect major differences among the different drugs. This finding probably is derived from the fact that the more potent fibrinolytic effects of fibrin-specific agents lead to greater lysis of vascular hemostatic plugs, whereas the systemic lytic

effect and clotting factor depletion are responsible for bleeding on non-fibrin-specific agents.

SELECTION OF PATIENTS

The early identification and treatment of candidates for fibrinolytic therapy have become major public health issues. Protocols are needed to rapidly assess and treat patients within 30 minutes of identification, because time is so important in determining the extent of myocardial salvage. Although a physician's supervision is required for use of these agents, pilot studies are being done to evaluate paramedic administration. Fibrinolytic therapy is currently reserved for patients with classic signs or symptoms of acute myocardial infarction and classic ST segment elevation on the electrocardiogram. In general, at least 30 minutes of symptoms without resolution with sublingual nitroglycerin is required. Patients with suspected acute myocardial infarction without these electrocardiographic criteria are subjected to coronary angiography to document the presence of coronary occlusion before treatment. Absolute contraindications to thrombolytic therapy include the following situations: known active bleeding sites or disorders, operation within 2 weeks, prolonged (>5 to 10 minutes) cardiopulmonary resuscitation, previous stroke, recent trauma (within 2 months), and persistent diastolic blood pressure more than 110 mm Hg or systolic more than 180 mm Hg. Based on the animal models of reperfusion and available human studies, a time limit of 6 hours from the onset of symptoms had classically been set for treatment. The recently released International Study of Infarct Survival (ISIS) II Trial (1987) has documented a benefit with regard to survival in patients treated with streptokinase within 24 hours after the onset of symptoms, causing a broadening of that time frame, although the mechanism for this late benefit is speculative.

The physical examination of patients before study should focus on excluding other diagnoses that could lead to a catastrophic outcome if confused with acute myocardial infarction. In particular, the cardiovascular examination should carefully assess the probability of aortic dissection or acute pericarditis. The alternative causes of electrocardiographic ST segment elevation should also be excluded if possible (early repolarization normal variant, coronary vasospasm, left ventricular aneurysm, pericarditis, and left ventricular hypertrophy). During infusion of a thrombolytic agent, the patient should have constant nursing supervision, with frequent vital sign determination, observation of neurologic status, and clinical and laboratory evaluation of bleeding status.

IMPACT OF THERAPY ON IMPORTANT CLINICAL OUTCOMES

The beneficial effect of fibrinolytic therapy on mortality has now been shown in multiple random-

TABLE 31–13. SUMMARY OF AGENTS

	Streptokinase (%)	TPA (%)
Speed of lysis	—	+ +
Coronary patency (90 minutes)	40–60	65–75
Coronary patency (24 hours)	80	80
Left ventricular function	+	+
Bleeding risk	+	+
Mortality	+	+ +

ized clinical trials. Although many smaller trials have shown a trend toward reduced mortality, the Italian GISSI Trial (1986) resolved the issue definitively by randomizing 11,806 patients to receive either 1.5 million units of streptokinase or conservative treatment. Mortality was reduced by 47% in patients treated within the first hour of the onset of symptoms and by 25% in the overall group of patients treated within 12 hours of the onset of symptoms. The longer treatment was delayed after the onset of symptoms, the less improvement there was in survival compared with conventional treatment. These findings have been replicated with streptokinase in the ISIS II Trial, with extension of the documentation of benefit to 24 hours from the onset of symptoms, although the magnitude of the benefit was less in patients treated later compared with earlier treatment. In addition, this trial clearly documented the benefit in elderly patients and patients with inferior myocardial infarction. Despite the wide time allowance for benefit, in both trials substantially more benefit was observed for patients treated promptly. A large, multicenter trial with APSAC has shown a similar reduction in mortality. No documentation of reduced mortality exists with regard to urokinase, because no large randomized trials have been done. Pooled data in TPA trials indicate a mortality reduction similar to that observed with streptokinase. Both the GISSI and ISIS groups are comparing streptokinase and TPA directly in large, randomized trials that have not yet been completed.

An important aspect of fibrinolytic therapy is that it can be initiated safely in the community hospital by a physician who has not had specialty training in cardiology. Thus, the treatment applies to most patients who are identified at an early stage of infarction without a major contraindication. Available information suggests that approximately 30 to 50% of patients with an eventual diagnosis of acute myocardial infarction reach medical care within 6 hours and do not have a contraindication to this form of treatment, and an additional 15 to 20% of patients come to medical attention within 24 hours. A major public health effort is being devoted to education about the signs and symptoms of myocardial infarction in an attempt to increase the proportion of patients who might benefit from treatment. Clinical trials are currently being done to evaluate the use of this form of treatment by paramedical personnel in the field.

A similar large body of data confirms the benefit of all of these agents with regard to the reduction of infarct size. Although an entirely satisfactory method of measuring infarct size in patients has not yet been developed, multiple data sources including enzyme release, left ventricular ejection fraction, and left ventricular volume determinations emphasize the same result. This outcome translates clinically into a lower incidence of heart failure and related complications and may be responsible for the apparent reduction in sudden death in these patients after they have been discharged from the hospital.

All available information indicates an increase in reinfarction rates in patients treated with thrombolytic therapy compared with conservative treatment. The reason for this observation relates most probably to the unstable atherosclerotic plaque that remains after fibrinolytic therapy has successfully achieved reperfusion through initial clot lysis. Multiple adjunctive therapies have been used in an attempt to prevent reocclusion and its often catastrophic outcome. Information from the ISIS group documents that aspirin has a dramatic effect on survival and essentially doubles the therapeutic benefit gained from streptokinase alone. The role of heparin is being investigated, although in the absence of definitive information intravenous heparin therapy has become standard treatment in the first several days after thrombolytic therapy is initiated. Intravenous nitroglycerin has also potentiated the effects of streptokinase on left ventricular function. Future efforts will concentrate on the role of other pharmacologic regimens that alter the coagulation system or platelet function.

Hemorrhagic complications are still the major drawback of this form of therapy. These complications can be divided into three different types: internal, access site, and intracranial. Careful attention to exclusion criteria can significantly reduce the risk of internal bleeding by not administering thrombolytic therapy to patients with active bleeding sources, particularly from the gastrointestinal tract. Nevertheless, a finite rate of such bleeding occurs from previously occult sources or new sources such as stress ulcers. Vascular intervention of patients immediately before and after thrombolytic therapy should be limited to procedures that are necessary to confer benefit, because a significant risk of bleeding occurs with any vascular puncture, particularly in an artery. Depending on the level of vascular invasion, the transfusion requirement after thrombolytic therapy has ranged from 2 to 35% of patients treated.

Intracranial bleeding that cannot be readily reversed is the major complication of this therapy. This event occurs in 0.2 to 0.6% of patients treated with current doses of fibrinolytic therapy despite the exclusion of patients with obvious central nervous system pathology. High-risk patients appear to be elderly or patients with a long history of poorly controlled hypertension or acute, severe hypertension with the acute infarction episode. When bleeding occurs, emergency measures for an accurate diagnosis must be taken (cranial tomography or magnetic resonance imaging) and all forms of anticoagulation and antiplatelet therapy must be discontinued. Early consideration of surgical hematoma evacuation may prevent a catastrophic outcome.

General measures to reduce bleeding, when it occurs, include discontinuation of anticoagulant and antiplatelet therapy, intravascular volume repletion, and compression of the involved site. Clotting factors may be replaced with fresh frozen plasma and cryoprecipitate. Early surgical intervention should be contemplated to repair sites of loss of vascular integrity if standard measures are unsuccessful. Epsilon-aminocaproic acid may be used in life-threatening bleeding, although the risk of rethrombosis of the coronary artery must be considered carefully.

ROLE OF INVASIVE PROCEDURES

Definition of the appropriate use of coronary angiography and coronary angioplasty in patients who have had thrombolytic therapy has been a topic of great research interest. Routine immediate angiography in acute myocardial infarction has now been shown to be safe and feasible. Between 30 and 50% of patients fail to achieve reperfusion after treatment with fibrinolytic agents. Unfortunately, accurate but noninvasive methods to detect failure to reperfuse have not been developed. Thus, early coronary angiography has been advocated as a method to recognize these patients so that angioplasty can be used to open the occluded artery. In addition, angiography identifies patients who have left main or severe three-vessel coronary disease and who might benefit from early surgical intervention. The routine use of angiography is expensive, however, and involves the transfer of many patients in the early phases of infarction from the community hospital to the interventional center. Several trials are being done to evaluate whether coronary angiography should be performed immediately, routinely after a delay to allow stabilization of the plaque, or only in the case of recurrent ischemia or hemodynamic distress after attempted thrombolysis.

Percutaneous transluminal angioplasty may be used either to replace thrombolytic therapy or as an adjunctive measure after thrombolysis. In patients with a contraindication to fibrinolytic agents, direct angioplasty may be used to achieve vessel patency. In patients who come directly to interventional centers with availability for rapid access to the catheterization laboratory, some researchers have suggested that direct angioplasty achieves superior recanalization rates with less bleeding. No direct comparative trials have yet been completed to resolve this issue.

Three multicenter randomized trials comparing immediate angioplasty with deferred angioplasty in the setting of therapy with TPA have now been completed. All three trials found no significant benefit of immediate angioplasty. An issue that has not yet been resolved is whether angioplasty only of vessels that have not been reperfused by the thrombolytic agent would result in a better overall result. Of course, such a strategy would require immediate angiography in all patients so that patients who had not responded to thrombolytic therapy could be identified. The current practice at this medical center involves precisely this strategy in an ongoing clinical trial to assess its efficacy relative to a conservative policy of deferred catheterization.

SURGICAL ISSUES

The current aggressive strategy of management of acute myocardial infarction almost certainly leads to earlier and more frequent identification of patients with high-risk anatomy and impaired left ventricular function. These findings promote earlier surgical intervention because of the convincing data from randomized trials that long-term survival is improved with surgical intervention in patients with multivessel disease and impaired left ventricular function. The multicenter TAMI group (1988) reported an experience with 24 patients having coronary bypass grafting while the TPA infusion was continued. The majority of these patients had a failed angioplasty with a reperfusion catheter inserted across the infarct lesion to maintain perfusion of the distal myocardial bed. Other patients had early operation for very high-risk anatomy (left main or combined proximal left anterior descending and circumflex obstruction) with hemodynamic deterioration. Although bleeding complications were more severe than encountered with elective operation, only three patients required reoperation and no lethal bleeding complications occurred. Only three in-hospital deaths occurred in the series, all from the eight patients in frank cardiogenic shock at the time of operation. The most dramatic improvement in global and regional left ventricular function observed in the trial occurred in these patients. In a review of the Duke experience, Ferguson and colleagues (1988) found that the complications, mortality, and length of stay were similar in patients who were referred for emergency operation during the acute phase of infarction compared with patients referred because of failure of elective angioplasty. The major difference was in the need for blood product replacement: The patients with acute infarction required 12.5 units of packed red blood cells, 8.7 units of frozen plasma, 0.9 platelet packs, and 1.2 units of cryoprecipitate. Equivalent figures for the patients with failed elective angioplasty were 8.8, 5.4, 0.48, and 0.48, respectively. Significantly, the internal mammary artery was used in half of the patients in each group, showing that even in emergency cases, this technique can be used.

An additional 72 patients in the TAMI I trial (1988) had coronary artery operations before being discharged from the hospital, but not in the acute phase of the infarction. The overall in-hospital mortality in all 94 operated patients was 6%, despite a risk profile significantly more adverse compared with patients treated without operation. In follow-up to 1 year, only one additional patient died, 86% were in functional Class I or II, and 76% rated their health as either excellent or good. This information confirms that coronary surgical procedures can be done safely in patients during the acute phase of infarction or during the subsequent hospitalization. Although the exact criteria must still be defined, these results have led the author to recommend operation early during hospitalization for patients identified as having multivessel coronary disease and impaired left ventricular function and for patients with ongoing ischemia and anatomy not suitable for angioplasty. Careful attention to repletion of clotting factors and meticulous operative technique lead to good results and a shorter stay in the hospital compared with a more deferred approach to operation.

An issue of growing importance is the proper management of patients with acute infarction after coronary artery bypass grafting. Thrombolytic therapy is contraindicated for the first several weeks because of the high risk of pericardial hemorrhage and subsequent tamponade. Beyond that point, however, thrombolytic therapy and acute angioplasty are still viable alternatives. Data from the randomized trials indicate that the risk of subsequent nonfatal infarction is not reduced by surgical therapy in patients with chronic angina. Particularly after the first 5 years, graft occlusion becomes a more substantial problem. For many reasons, clinical decision making in these patients is more complex than in patients without previous bypass grafting. The frequent occurrence of conduction disturbances makes the initial diagnosis more difficult than usual. The acute thrombus may be located in a bypass graft rather than in a native vessel. These two possibilities cannot be distinguished except by coronary angiography. The presence of a median sternotomy makes acute surgical intervention for failed angioplasty more difficult, especially after fibrinolytic therapy. A major practical problem is the frequent occurrence of extensive thrombus throughout the length of the graft. Inadequate data are available to delineate the proper course of action when a patient with previous grafting is identified in the early stages of acute infarction. The author's current practice is to initiate thrombolytic therapy in the emergency room and then to move quickly to coronary angiography to define the nature of the problem more clearly. Immediate angioplasty in these patients should be approached cautiously, although preliminary results in selected patients have been encouraging.

SUMMARY

Fibrinolytic therapy for acute ischemic syndromes has become a standard method of treatment. Despite its widespread use, many questions remain about the best agent(s), the most appropriate selection of patients, and the most beneficial combination of adjunctive therapies (Table 31–13). In addition, modifications of currently existing agents through recombinant genetic engineering offer the promise of more effective therapy with less risk. Improvement in acute survival rates and earlier identification of patients at high risk for recurrent ischemic events will almost certainly increase the frequency of cardiac surgical procedures in this setting.

Annotated Bibliography

Becker, L. C., and Ambrosio, G.: Myocardial consequences of reperfusion. Prog. Cardiovasc. Dis., 30:23, 1987.

This article reviews in detail the current concepts concerning reperfusion injury. In particular, the concepts of free radical scavengers and the influence of white blood cell accumulation on the final myocardial infarct size are emphasized. The article reviews both the clinical and basic science aspects of this topic.

Collen, D.: Human tissue-type plasminogen activator: From the laboratory to the bedside. Circulation, 72:18, 1985.

This editorial reviews the development of tissue plasminogen activator beginning with its initial isolation and early use in human studies. The use of recombinant DNA technology in the development of this pharmacologic agent is discussed.

Gruppo Italiano Per Lo Studio Della Streptochinasi Nell'Infarcto Miocardio (GISSI): Effectiveness of intravenous thrombolytic treatment in acute myocardial infarction. Lancet, 1:397, 1986.

This article reviews the initial findings of a randomized clinical trial comparing intravenous streptokinase with conservative treatment in more than 11,000 patients. A sharp reduction (47%) in mortality was observed in patients treated within the first hour of the onset of symptoms, and significant reductions in mortality were also observed in patients treated up to 6 hours after the onset of symptoms. This trial firmly establishes that thrombolytic therapy reduces mortality in acute myocardial infarction and addresses several important issues regarding specific subsets of patients.

Kereiakes, D. J., Topol, E. J., George, B. S., et al: Emergency coronary artery bypass surgery preserves global and regional left ventricular function after intravenous tissue plasminogen activator therapy for acute myocardial infarction. J. Am. Coll. Cardiol., 11:899, 1988.

This paper describes an experience with emergency surgical treatment of 27 patients during infusion of TPA for acute myocardial infarction. Although the bleeding complications were greater, the in-hospital and long-term mortality were low. Left ventricular function dramatically improved.

Laffel, G. L., and Braunwald, E.: Thrombolytic therapy: A new strategy for the treatment of acute myocardial infarction. N. Engl. J. Med., 311:710, 1984.

These review articles describe the approach to the selection and treatment of patients with thrombolytic therapy. A general discussion of important issues regarding salvage of myocardial function and the potential effects of thrombolytic therapy on mortality is included. Important unresolved issues in thrombolytic therapy administration are also identified.

Reimer, K. A., Lowe, J. E., Rasmussen, M. M., and Jennings, R. B.: The wavefront phenomenon of ischemic cell death. I: Myocardial infarct size vs. duration of coronary occlusion in dogs. Circulation, 56:786, 1977.

This important article describes the potential benefits of reperfusion on the salvage of myocardium. The authors used a canine model in which epicardial vessels were occluded and the occlusion was released at various times. A wavefront of myocardial cell death was described proceeding from the endocardium to the epicardium.

Stadius, M. L., Davis, K., Maynard, C., et al: Risk stratification for 1 year survival based on characteristics identified in the early hours of acute myocardial infarction. Circulation, 74:703, 1986.

This important paper describes the relationship between baseline characteristics and 1-year survival in a group of patients treated with intracoronary streptokinase. The importance of this manuscript is that it identified an important effect of coronary patency on mortality reduction that was independent of salvage of left ventricular function. The 1-year follow-up of these patients showed a dramatic improvement in survival in patients with a patent coronary artery at the time of initial therapy compared with patients without a patent coronary artery. This study has raised the issue of the effect of coronary patency during the phase of infarct healing compared with the initial salvage of myocardium.

TIMI Study Group: The thrombolysis in myocardial infarction (TIMI) trial. N. Engl. J. Med., 312:932, 1985.

This initial study directly compares the effects of TPA and streptokinase on coronary patency early in the phase of thrombolysis. A dramatic difference was found in favor of TPA in this trial. These results led the TIMI Study Group to abandon the use of streptokinase. Subsequent studies with streptokinase showing dramatic reductions in mortality, such as the GISSI Trial, have raised the issue of whether early coronary patency may not be the most important end point in trials of thrombolytic therapy.

Yusuf, S., Collins, R., Peto, R., et al: Intravenous and intracoronary fibrinolytic therapy in acute myocardial infarction: Overview of results on mortality, reinfarction and side-effects from 33 randomized controlled trials. Eur. Heart J., 6:556, 1985.

This review article combines 33 randomized controlled trials of intravenous intracoronary fibrinolytic therapy in a meta-analysis. The finding of this study was that mortality was reduced by 22% ± 5% and that the effects on mortality appeared to be present even in patients treated 12 hours after the onset of symptoms. This important analysis in combination with the GISSI Study firmly established the role of thrombolytic therapy as primary treatment for acute myocardial infarction.

Bibliography

AIMS Trial Study Group: Effect of intravenous APSAC on mortality after acute myocardial infarction: Preliminary report of a placebo-controlled clinical trial. Lancet, 1:545, 1988.

Ambrose, J. A., and Hjemdahl-Monsen, C. E.: Arteriographic anatomy and mechanisms of myocardial ischemia in unstable angina. J. Am. Coll. Cardiol., 9:1397, 1987.

Becker, L. C., and Ambrosio, G.: Myocardial consequences of reperfusion. Prog. Cardiovasc. Dis., 30:23, 1987.

Braunwald, E.: The aggressive treatment of acute myocardial infarction. Circulation, 71:1087, 1985.

Braunwald, E., and Kloner, R. A.: The stunned myocardium: Prolonged, postischemic ventricular dysfunction. Circulation, 66:1146, 1982.

Califf, R. M., Topol, E. J., George, B. S., et al: Characteristics and outcome of patients in whom reperfusion with intravenous tissue-type plasminogen activator fails: Results of the thrombolysis and angioplasty in myocardial infarction (TAMI) I trial. Circulation, 77:1090, 1988.

Chazov, E. I., Mateeva, L. S., Mazaev, A. V., et al: Intracoronary administration of fibrinolysin in acute myocardial infarction. Ter. Arkh., 48:8, 1976.

Chesebro, J. H., Knatterud, G., Roberts, R., et al: Thrombolysis in Myocardial Infarction (TIMI) Trial, Phase I: A comparison between intravenous tissue plasminogen activator and intravenous streptokinase. Circulation, 76:141, 1987.

Collen, D.: Human tissue-type plasminogen activator: From the laboratory to the bedside. Circulation, 72:18, 1985.

Ferguson, T. B., Muhlbaier, L. H., Salai, D. L., and Wechsler, A. S.: Coronary bypass grafting after failed elective and failed emergent percutaneous angioplasty. Relative risks of emergent surgical intervention. J. Thor. Cardiovas. Surg., 95:761, 1988.

Flameng, W., Sargeant, P., Vanhaecke, J., and Suy, R.: Emergency coronary bypass grafting for evolving myocardial infarction. J. Thorac. Cardiovasc. Surg. 94:124, 1987.

Gold, H. K., Leinbach, R. C., Garabedian, H. D., et al: Acute coronary reocclusion after thrombolysis with recombinant human tissue-type plasminogen activator: Prevention by a maintenance infusion. Circulation, 73:347, 1986.

Gruppo Italiano Per Lo Studio Della Streptochinasi Nell'Infarcto Miocardio (GISSI): Effectiveness of intravenous thrombolytic treatment in acute myocardial infarction. Lancet, 1:397, 1986.

Guerci, A. D., Gerstenblith, G., Brinker, J. A., et al: A randomized trial of intravenous tissue plasminogen activator for acute myocardial infarction with subsequent randomization to elective coronary angioplasty. N. Engl. J. Med., 317:1613, 1987.

Harrison, D. B., Ferguson, D. W., Collins, S. M., et al: Rethrombosis after reperfusion with streptokinase: Importance of geometry of residual lesions. Circulation, 69:991, 1984.

Herrick, J. B.: Clinical features of sudden obstruction of the coronary arteries. J.A.M.A., 59:2015, 1912.

Hochberg, M. S., Parsonnet, V., Gielchinsky, I., et al: Timing of coronary revascularization after acute myocardial infarction. J. Thorac. Cardiovasc. Surg., 88:914, 1984.

International Studies of Infarct Survival (ISIS) Pilot Study Investigators: Randomized factorial trial of high-dose intravenous streptokinase, of oral aspirin and of intravenous heparin in acute myocardial infarction. Eur. Heart. J., 8:634, 1987.

ISIS Steering Committee: Intravenous streptokinase given within 0–4 hours of onset of myocardial infarction reduced mortality in ISIS-2. Lancet, 1:502, 1987.

Kennedy, J. W., Ritchie, J. L., Davis, K. B., et al: The western Washington randomized trial of intracoronary streptokinase in acute myocardial infarction. N. Engl. J. Med., 312:1073, 1985.

Laffel, G. L., and Braunwald, E.: Thrombolytic therapy: A new strategy for the treatment of acute myocardial infarction. N. Engl. J. Med., 311:710, 1984.

National Heart Foundation of Australia Coronary Thrombolysis Group: Coronary thrombolysis and myocardial salvage by tissue plasminogen activator given up to 4 hours after onset of myocardial infarction. Lancet, 1:203, 1988.

O'Neill, W., Timmis, G., Bourdillon, P., et al: A prospective randomized clinical trial of intracoronary streptokinase versus coronary angioplasty therapy of acute myocardial infarction. N. Engl. J. Med., 314:812, 1986.

O'Neill, W. W., Topol, E. J., and Pitt, B.: Reperfusion therapy of acute myocardial infarction. Prog. Cardiovasc. Dis., 30:235, 1988.

Petrovich, J. A., Schneider, J. A., Taylor, G. J., et al: Early and late results of operation after thrombolytic therapy for acute myocardial infarction. J. Thorac. Cardiovasc. Surg., 92:853, 1986.

Rao, A. K., Pratt, C., Berke, A., et al: Thrombolysis in Myocardial Infarction (TIMI) trial. I: Hemorrhagic manifestations and changes in plasma fibrinogen and the fibrinolytic system in patients treated with recombinant tissue plasminogen activator and streptokinase. J. Am. Coll. Cardiol., 11:1, 1988.

Reimer, K. A., and Jennings, R. B.: The "wavefront phenomenon" of myocardial ischemic cell death. II: Transmural progression of necrosis within the framework of ischemic bed size (myocardium at risk) and collateral flow. Lab. Invest., 40:633, 1979.

Rentrop, K. P.: Thrombolytic therapy in patients with acute myocardial infarction. Circulation, 71:627, 1985.

Ritchie, J. L., Cerqueira, M., Maynard, C., et al: Ventricular function and infarct size: The western Washington intravenous streptokinase in myocardial infarction trial. J. Am. Coll. Cardiol., 11:689, 1988.

Ryan, T. J.: Angioplasty in acute myocardial infarction: Is the balloon leaking? N. Engl. J. Med., 317:624, 1987.

Schaer, D. H., Ross, A. M., and Wasserman, A. G.: Reinfarction, recurrent angina, and reocclusion after thrombolytic therapy. Circulation, 76:II-57, 1987.

Serruys, P. W., Simoons, M. L., Suryapranata, H., et al: Preservation of global and regional left ventricular function after early thrombolysis in acute myocardial infarction. J. Am. Coll. Cardiol., 7:729, 1986.

Sheehan, F. H., Braunwald, E., Canner, P., et al: The effect of intravenous thrombolytic therapy on left ventricular function: A report on tissue-type plasminogen activator and streptokinase from the thrombolysis in myocardial infarction (TIMI Phase I) Trial. Circulation, 75:817, 1987.

Sheehan, F. H., Mathey, D. G., Schofer, J., et al: Factors that determine recovery of left ventricular function after thrombolysis in patients with acute myocardial infarction. Circulation, 71:1121, 1985.

Sherry, S.: The development of thrombolytic therapy. J. Am. Coll. Cardiol., 10:933, 1987.

Simoons, M. L., Arnold, A. E. R., Betriu, A., et al: Thrombolysis with rt-PA in acute myocardial infarction: No beneficial effects of immediate PTCA. Lancet, 1:197, 1988.

Simoons, M. L., Brand, M. V. D., de Zwaan, C., et al: Improved survival after early thrombolysis in acute myocardial infarction. Lancet, 2:578, 1985.

Smith, B., and Kennedy, J. W.: Thrombolysis in the treatment of acute transmural myocardial infarction. Ann. Intern. Med., 106:414, 1987.

Sobel, B. E., Fields, L. E., Robison, A. K., et al: Coronary thrombolysis with facilitated absorption of intramuscularly injected tissue-type plasminogen activator. Proc. Natl. Acad. Sci. U.S.A., 82:4258, 1985.

Stack, R. S., Califf, R. M., Hinohara, T., et al: Survival and cardiac event rates in the first year following emergency angioplasty for acute myocardial infarction. J. Am. Coll. Cardiol., 6:1141, 1988.

Stack, R. S., O'Connor, C. M., Mark, D. B., et al: Coronary perfusion during acute myocardial infarction with a combined therapy of coronary angioplasty and high-dose intravenous streptokinase. Circulation, 77:151, 1988.

Stack, R. S., Phillips, H. R., Grierson, D. S., et al: Functional improvement of jeopardized myocardium following intracoronary streptokinase infusion in acute myocardial infarction. J. Clin. Invest., 72:84, 1983.

Stadius, M. L., Davis, K., Maynard, C., et al: Risk stratification for 1 year survival based on characteristics identified in the early hours of acute myocardial infarction. Circulation, 74:703, 1986.

The ISAM Study Group: A prospective trial of intravenous streptokinase in acute myocardial infarction (ISAM). N. Engl. J. Med., 314:1465, 1986.

The TIMI Study Group: The thrombolysis in myocardial infarction (TIMI) trial. N. Engl. J. Med., 312:932, 1985.

Topol, E. J., Bell, W. R., and Weisfeldt, M. L.: Coronary thrombolysis with recombinant tissue-type plasminogen activator: Hematologic and pharmacologic study. Ann. Intern. Med. 103:837, 1985.

Topol, E. J., Califf, R. M., George, B. S., et al: A randomized trial of immediate versus delayed elective angioplasty after intravenous tissue plasminogen activator in acute myocardial infarction. N. Engl. J. Med., 317:581, 1987.

Topol, E. J., Califf, R. M., George, B. S., et al: Coronary arterial thrombolysis with combined infusion of recombinant tissue-type plasminogen activator and urokinase in patients with acute myocardial infarction. Circulation, 77:1100, 1988.

Topol, E. J., Califf, R. M., Kereiakes, D. J., and George, B. S.: Thrombolysis and angioplasty in myocardial infarction (TAMI) trial. J. Am. Coll. Cardiol., 10:65B, 1987.

Verstraete, M., Bory, M., Collen, D., et al: Randomized trial of intravenous recombinant tissue-type plasminogen activator versus intravenous streptokinase in acute myocardial infarction. Lancet, 1:842, 1985.

Werns, S. W., Shea, M. J., and Lucchesi, B. R.: Free radicals and myocardial injury: Pharmacologic implications. Circulation, 74:1, 1986.

Yusuf, S., Collins, R., Peto, R., et al: Intravenous and intracoronary fibrinolytic therapy in acute myocardial infarction: Overview of results on mortality, reinfarction and side-effects from 33 randomized controlled trials. Eur. Heart. J., 6:556, 1985.

IV ROLE OF COMPUTED TOMOGRAPHIC SCANS IN CARDIOVASCULAR DIAGNOSIS

Robert J. Herfkens

Computed tomographic (CT) scanning for diseases of the body has developed rapidly during the last 15 years. The intrinsic advantages of CT scanning for the evaluation of central nervous system diseases were quickly realized. The extension of CT scanning into the body has depended on the development of imaging technologies that allow the acquisition of scans in short periods relative to most physiologic processes. Original CT scans had imaging times lasting minutes. Routine scans can now be obtained in as short a time as 1 to 4 seconds and, most recently, with the development of newer imaging techniques, in as short a time as 50 to 100 msec. The original long scan times led a number of investigators to suggest that CT scanning of the heart would never be possible. These more rapid scanning times and the improved contrast resolution of current CT scanners have proved that this prediction is inappropriate.

CT scanning has the specific advantage of providing high-contrast images in a tomographic manner. The tomographic ability of CT scanning eliminates the overlying structures and provides a detailed image of a cross-section of the body. CT scanning is sensitive to changes in density within the tissues themselves. The intrinsic contrast in the human body is mainly related to the electron density of the specific tissues. Basic soft-tissue contrast allows differentiation between fat, water-containing tissues, and calcium-containing tissues. With the addition of intravenous contrast material (iodinated), vascular structures can now be routinely visualized. This advance has expanded CT scanning to include a number of applications that are related specifically to cardiac and vascular lesions. Contrast imaging allows not only the sensitive detection of minor degrees of calcification but also facilitates delineation of vascular structures such as subtle coronary artery bypass grafts or, more generally, the distinction of endocardium and epicardium. The typical spatial resolution of CT scanners is excellent, now routinely allowing pixel elements as small as 0.3 mm throughout the chest in slices as thin as 3 to 5 mm. CT scanning techniques are generally limited to transaxial images of the thorax; however, when images are obtained in a series, computerized techniques have now allowed the reconstruction of images in almost any imaging plane.

ANATOMY

The spatial and density resolution provided by CT scanners allows delineation of cardiac and vascular structures. With the use of intravenous contrast material, the differentiation of vascular structures from soft-tissue abnormalities, or the relative changes in vascularity such as those in tumors versus cysts, permit characterization of a number of pathologic processes. Although the scan times currently available are relatively long in terms of cardiac motion, a general average of the cardiac cycle appears, showing images of the ventricles that mainly represent the diastolic phase of the cardiac cycle. These images sensitively differentiate epicardium and endocardium as well as such pathologic processes in the mediastinum as the presence of lymph nodes and vascular tumors. Additionally, nonvascular structural abnormalities such as thrombi within the ventricles, atria, or pulmonary arteries can be differentiated from the enhancing blood after intravenous administration of contrast materials. These basic principles have allowed CT scanning to provide a relatively noninvasive modality for the evaluation of many cardiovascular pathologies.

The basic technique for evaluation of cardiovascular processes involves the use of a CT scanner capable of relatively fast imaging techniques so that images can be obtained during a single inspiration. The intrinsic process of CT scanning involves rotating an x-ray tube about the patient, providing multiple projections into a detector system that can then be reconstructed by a computer into a two-dimensional slice of the patient. Basic analysis of cardiovascular structures requires administration of intravenous contrast material for differentiation of vascular from nonvascular structures (Fig. 31–47). A series of slices are obtained at separate inspirations throughout the structures of interest. To maximize the use of intravenous contrast material, current scanners are capable of rapidly repeating scans in a dynamic sequence, thus allowing the use of a bolus injection of contrast or a rapid drip infusion to contrast intravascular structures maximally from normal soft-tissue structures. This ability to maximize the information from a CT scan by using the highest concentrations of intravenous contrast material allows the differentiation of very subtle features such as coronary artery bypass grafts.

The contrast resolution provided by CT scanners also supplies physiologic information about the relative uptake of iodinated contrast in specific structures. Contrast enhancement has specifically been

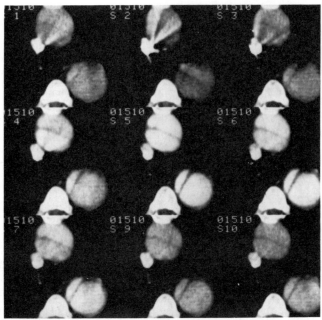

Figure 31–47. A series of nine transaxial images through the ascending aorta after the bolus injection of iodinated contrast material in a peripheral vein. On the early images, contrast can be seen entering into the superior vena cava. Note that there is little contrast in the ascending and descending aorta. By the fifth image, there is dense opacification of both the ascending and descending aorta. At this time, an intimal flap can clearly be seen in the ascending and descending aorta, allowing the accurate diagnosis of a Type A aortic dissection. The dense opacification seen on the fifth image is the level necessary for the accurate diagnosis of vascular pathology such as aortic dissections.

used to measure myocardial infarctions because of their lack of contrast uptake initially and ultimate delayed enhancement in the periphery of the infarct associated with capillary leaks in the periphery or border zone of the infarct itself.

CLINICAL APPLICATIONS

Ischemic Heart Disease

The basic technique for evaluation of acute myocardial infarction involves administration of rapid boluses of contrast materials and rapid scanning of the myocardium. An area of acute myocardial infarction appears initially as an area of hypoperfusion or decrease in signal intensity on a magnetic resonance image. Later images obtained over time show a general increase in signal intensity as contrast is washed out of the normal vascular structures and is trapped in the border zone or peri-infarct zone (Fig. 31–48). It has been proposed that measurements of myocardial size by CT scanning represent a strong prognostic indicator after acute myocardial infarction.

The sensitive detection of contrast differences between high intensity within the ventricular cavity, intermediate signal within the myocardium, and

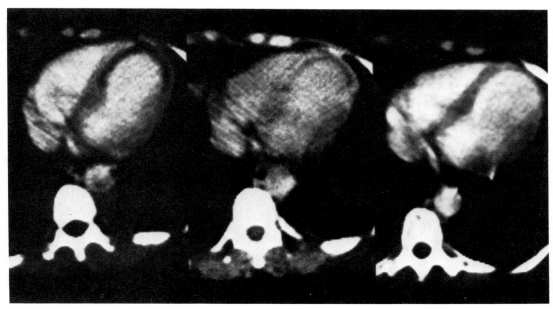

Figure 31–48. Three images obtained in a patient after left anterior descending coronary artery occlusion. The first image was obtained immediately after a bolus of contrast material. A deficit or decrease in signal, which can be seen in the endocardial portion of the distal septum and anterior wall, represents the nonperfused portion of this infarction. The second image was obtained 30 minutes after the first. There is some general clearance of contrast from the intervascular spaces, as well as an increase in signal intensity in the region of the peripheral zone of the infarct. This represents the associated capillary leak that is seen in acute myocardial infarction. The third image is an image obtained 6 weeks after the initial study. This third image shows no persistent myocardial deficit; however, there is an interval of marked thinning of the distal septum and anterior wall. The result in volume loss of myocardium can be clearly visualized when comparing this image with the first image.

greatly reduced signal in nonvascular structures such as thrombi allows differentiation of thrombus from normal ventricular wall. Unlike echocardiography, CT scanning does not depend on appropriate acoustic windows, nor is it directly interfered with by overlying calcific structures such as ribs or, in the presence of mitral valve disease, calcification within the mitral annulus. CT scanning is an effective method for evaluating thrombi in cardiac structures (Fig. 31–49).

Chronic myocardial infarction is characterized by a reduction in wall thickness and eventual fibrosis of the residual remaining tissue. After intravenous administration of contrast material, endocardial and epicardial borders can be identified, allowing demonstration of wall thinning associated with chronic myocardial infarction. Myocardial thinning may be visualized as early as 10 days after acute myocardial infarction. CT scanning clearly documents this wall thinning and can be used to measure and characterize the evolution of changes associated with acute myocardial infarction. The eventual development of an aneurysm or calcification with an aneurysm is shown well by the contrast resolution of CT scanning.

The development of newer imaging devices such as cine CT (Imatron) scanners potentially allows evaluation of functional abnormalities by obtaining scans in as little as 50 msec. This short scanning time then permits anatomic assessment of the myocardium as well as functional evaluation of motion-related defects.

Coronary Artery Bypass Grafts

Evaluation of patients with recurrent chest pain after coronary artery bypass grafting remains a vexing problem for clinicians. CT scanning provides a superior method for determining patency of coronary artery bypass grafts. Rapid, dynamic scanning after injection of a bolus of contrast material at the level just above the origin of the coronary arteries and below the origin of coronary artery bypass graft provides a sensitive method for assessing graft patency (Fig. 31–50).

This technique appears to be adequately sensitive for quantifying patency, although the ultimate determination of coronary graft flow is still elusive. The eventual evaluation of coronary artery flow may depend on the development of more rapid CT scanners such as cine CT scanning for correct evaluation of patent but stenotic grafts.

Congenital Heart Disease

Echocardiography is still a reliable method for evaluating congenital heart disease. In older age groups, however, the lack of an appropriate acoustic window may make appraisal of the grade vessels difficult. CT scanning does not depend on an acoustic window and provides a superior method for studying vascular structures such as operative shunts.

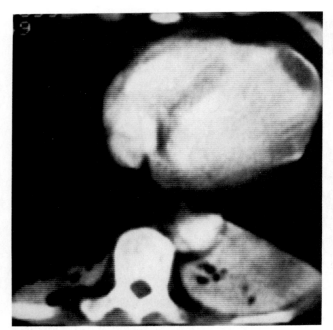

Figure 31–49. A transaxial slice through the midventricular level in a patient suspected of having a ventricular aneurysm. The endocardial and epicardial borders can be identified. There is a low-intensity area (unenhancing) in the left ventricular apex. This typical appearance after contrast material is diagnostic of thrombus within the apex of the left ventricle. The myocardium, seen to be thinned to approximately 2 mm, has marked increased density consistent with calcification in an apical aneurysm of the left ventricle.

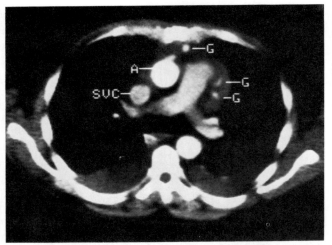

Figure 31–50. This transaxial image through the ascending and descending aorta was obtained after injection of a bolus of a small amount of intravenous contrast material. In the mediastinal fat adjacent to the aorta and pulmonary artery are three areas of contrast enhancement. In this particular patient, who had undergone coronary artery bypass graft, these areas represent enhancement in patent coronary artery bypass grafts.

The high-contrast tomographic capabilities of CT scanning provide an accurate method for measuring and determining patency of shunts. Atrial septal defects and ventricular septal defects can easily be measured by using the heightened contrast and spatial resolution of CT scanning. These methods do, however, require intravenous administration of contrast material to differentiate cardiac borders.

Pericardial Disease

The normal pericardium can be clearly identified on CT scanning and usually represents a 1 to 3-mm curvilinear density of intermediate signal separated by relatively low-intensity epicardial and pericardial fat. Although the pericardium may not be observed through its entire course, unless fat clearly separates it from the visceral pericardium of the heart, in pathologic conditions it is generally thick and well visualized. Echocardiography excels at documenting pericardial effusions but has significant limitations in assessing some patients with pulmonary disease and thoracic abnormalities. CT scanning is a superior method for sensitively quantifying pericardial thickness over the entire cardiac volume. It is superior for detecting subtle pericardial calcifications, which generally indicate significant pericardial disease. Some

reviews have suggested that CT scanning is an accurate method for differentiating constrictive pericarditis from restrictive cardiomyopathies (Fig. 31–51). The presence of pericardial abnormalities such as subtle thickening or calcification strongly suggests that pericardial constriction is the source of this hemodynamic abnormality. The absence of significant pericardial abnormality strongly suggests restrictive myocardial disease as the cause.

Congenital anomalies of the pericardium are rare. CT scanning has definite advantages for study-

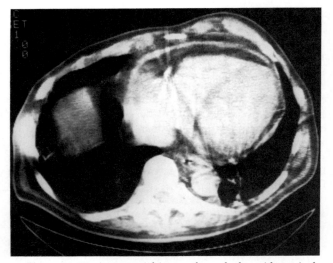

Figure 31–51. A transaxial image through the midventricular level shows a thick pericardium with an irregular nodular appearance that is separated from the normal ventricular structures by a water in density consistent with a pericardial effusion of moderate size. The transaxial format and excellent contrast resolution facilitate the evaluation of pericardial disease.

ing these entities and provides delineation of the normal ventricular and atrial structures and their relationship to the normal pericardium and potential cystic or diverticular structures.

Neoplastic or metastatic involvement of the pericardium is easily evaluated with contrast-enhanced CT scanning. The clear delineation of the normal pericardium is contrasted significantly by neoplastic involvement of the pericardium in which nodular changes or thickening of the pericardium can easily be evaluated. CT scanning not only permits evaluation of the intrinsic abnormalities of the pericardium but also serves as an accurate method for visualizing noncardiac structures such as pulmonary abnormalities or associated pleural changes, which may be helpful in estimating neoplastic involvement. Overall, CT scanning is excellent for documenting pericardial disease, both benign and malignant.

Myocardial Masses

Pericardial, myocardial, or thoracic masses associated with cardiovascular structures are evaluated well by CT scanning. The high-contrast resolution and tomographic format facilitate the staging of pericardial and myocardial masses. Thrombi can be differentiated from masses with the use of contrast-enhanced CT scanning. Cystic abnormalities or thrombi generally show little resemblance to a pericardiac or cardiac mass (Fig. 31–52). The relatively low density of fat, again, provides an additional method for characterizing fat-containing masses.

Vascular Diseases

Aneurysms of the aorta and dissections are rather difficult diagnostic problems for referring physicians. The tomographic format and high-contrast resolution of CT scanning provide an accurate method for noninvasive study of patients who are suspected of having aortic dissections. The use of a bolus of contrast material and serial transaxial scans through the ascending and descending aorta easily differentiates Type A from Type B dissections. This technique relies on administration of contrast material and, when appropriately done, is very sensitive for detection of abnormalities of the ascending and descending aorta. The contrast resolution allows delineation of clot within the lumen of either a dissecting hematoma or arteriosclerotic aneurysm within the aorta. The sensitive delineation of calcification either in the displaced intima of aortic dissection or in the wall of the aorta facilitates the differential diagnosis of aortic aneurysms.

Aneurysms can be identified as focal dilatations of the aorta. The presence of a small amount of calcification displaced in an intimal flap can easily identify a dissection. A cross-sectional format aids in assessing aortic pathology. This method also pro-

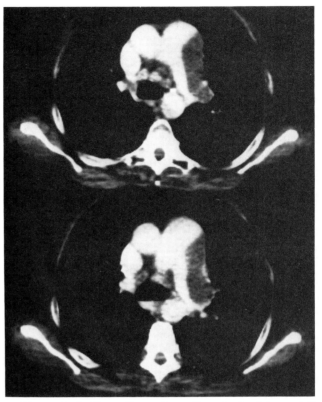

Figure 31–52. Two adjacent 1-cm slices obtained transaxially through the main pulmonary arteries in a patient with a questionable mediastinal mass. In this particular individual the widening of the mediastinum is clearly secondary to the enlargement of the main pulmonary artery. Within the pulmonary artery, in this contrast-enhanced scan, is a filling defect of low signal intensity. This unenhancing filling defect represents a chronic thrombus within the main pulmonary artery seen at two separate levels.

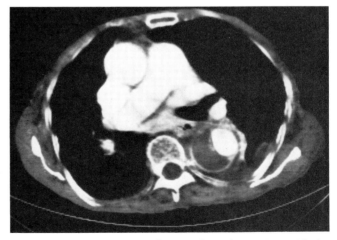

Figure 31–53. A transaxial image through a patient with the acute onset of chest pain shows a relatively normal ascending aorta and a descending aorta with a small displaced lumen. The medial two-thirds of the aortic lumen is filled with thrombus. Just medial to the aortic lumen within the thrombus can be seen some calcification representing a displaced intimal flap. CT has the advantage of showing extrathoracic pathology as well. In this case, a small mediastinal hematoma can be seen medially and a small pericardial effusion can be identified posteriorly.

vides a relatively noninvasive postoperative follow-up of these patients. The transaxial plane can easily be reproduced (Fig. 31–53).

CT scanning has a number of limitations for the evaluation of aortic pathology. The need to administer intravenous contrast material may make aortography difficult later on in the presence of significant renal disease. The inability of CT scanning to detect significant aortic insufficiency may be an additional limitation of this technique; however, its relatively noninvasive nature may provide an ideal method for studying relatively stable patients who are suspected of having aortic disease. Overall, CT scanning is a valuable method for appraising vascular abnormalities.

SUMMARY

CT scanning is an accurate method for evaluating cardiac diseases. The ability of CT scanning to visualize wall thickness, wall thinning, and associated changes in ischemic heart disease provides a means of characterizing ventricular abnormalities. The additional contrast sensitivity combined with rapid bolus infusions permits determination of coronary artery bypass graft patency and identification of aortic dissections. The eventual inclusion of rapid dynamic CT scanning, by using cine CT scans, for example, may provide the additional functional information necessary for complete evaluation of pathologic processes without requiring cardiac catheterization.

Selected Bibliography

Bank, E. R., and Hernandez, R. J.: CT and MR of congenital heart disease. Radiol. Clin. North Am., 26:241, 1988.

CT scanning and magnetic resonance imaging join echocardiography in the noninvasive evaluation of children with congenital heart disease. This article discusses the uses of these modalities in the assessment of the cardiovascular system in children.

Bateman, T. M., Gray, R. J., Whiting, J. S., et al: Prospective evaluation of ultrafast cardiac computed tomography for determination of coronary bypass graft patency. Circulation, 75:1018, 1987.

Twenty-five consecutive patients with 68 independent (single distal anastomosis) saphenous vein aortocoronary and 12 internal mammary bypass grafts (27 to left anterior descending, 10 to diagonal, 23 to left circumflex, 20 to right coronary artery) entered a reader-blinded, prospective, standardized study to establish the accuracy of ultrafast (cine) CT scanning for determining graft patency compared with invasive angiography. All patients had imaging after injection of 35 to 45 ml of meglumine diatrizoate (Renografin-76; 7 to 9 ml/sec for 5 sec) into a vein in the arm.

Electrocardiographically triggered images were acquired over 8 to 16 tomographic levels at 1-cm intervals from aortic arch to mid left ventricle. Criteria for graft patency were contrast opacification on at least two noncontiguous levels and contrast density-time curves that were morphologically similar to that of the aorta. Ultrafast CT scanning correctly determined that 46 to 48 bypass grafts were patent and 31 of 32 were occluded (sensitivity, speci-

ficity, and accuracy 96, 97, and 96%); there were no interpretation errors in 23 (92%) of the 25 patients. Accuracy was independent of the vessel bypassed and was not different for saphenous veins (96%) compared with internal mammary bypasses (100%). This study establishes a 20-minute outpatient intravenous injection technique that is highly accurate for determining the patency of coronary artery bypass grafts.

Conces, D. J., Jr., Tarver, R. D., and Augustyn, G. T.: Nonangiographic imaging of the pulmonary arteries: CT and MR. CRC Crit. Rev. Diagn. Imaging, 27:237, 1987.

CT scanning has provided an imaging modality by which the central pulmonary arteries can be studied noninvasively. CT scanning provides cross-sectional images that accurately show the pulmonary arteries and adjacent structures. Magnetic resonance imaging, with its ability to image vessels without contrast media, provides a potential noninvasive method of examining the pulmonary arteries. These modalities are well suited to evaluate pathology involving the central pulmonary arteries. Normal CT scanning and magnetic resonance anatomy is illustrated and discussed. The clinical presentation and appearance of pathologic processes involving the pulmonary arteries are described.

Godwin, J. D., Herfkens, R. J., Skioldebrand, C. G., et al: Evaluation of dissection in aneurysms of a thoracic aorta by conventional and dynamic CT scanning. Radiology, 136:125, 1980.

The authors evaluated the use of CT scanning methods for the prospective diagnosis of aneurysm of the aorta. They define excellent sensitivity and specificity when adequate contrast material is given. The basic technique for examining the aorta with CT scanning and its potential pitfalls are described.

Lipton, M. J.: Quantitation of left ventricular anatomy and function by ultrafast CT. Cardiovasc. Intervent. Radiol., 10:348, 1987.

Ultrafast CT scanning provides cross-sectional millisecond tomography, similar in many ways to cineangiography. The technique, which combines digital imaging and high resolution without the need for cardiac catheterization, is rapidly being validated. Fifty-millisecond scans at rates of 34 per second allow quantitation of left ventricular function by using typical calculations including global and regional ejection fraction, but ultrafast CT scanning also has the potential for providing unique data concerning regional wall thickening, mass, and even regional myocardial perfusion. Furthermore, interventional studies with exercise and pharmacologic agents have commenced and are being evaluated.

Moncada, R., Baker, M., Slinia, M., et al: Diagnostic role of computed tomography in pericardial heart disease: Congenital defect, thickening, neoplasm and effusions. Am. Heart J., 103:263, 1982.

The authors evaluate the use of CT scanning for investigation of pericardial abnormalities. They examined a group of normal persons and compared them with patients having a pathologically proven spectrum of pericardial diseases.

Parmley, L. F., Salley, R. K., Williams, J. P., and Head, G. B., III: The clinical spectrum of cardiac fibroma with diagnostic and surgical considerations: Noninvasive imaging enhances management. Ann. Thorac. Surg., 45:455, 1988.

A cardiac fibroma was successfully resected from the interventricular septum of a 25-year-old woman. The clinical data were correlated with a review of the data on 144 other patients, thus providing a clinical profile and management strategy for this type of tumor. Initial manifestations of a fibroma were determined to be congestive heart failure (21%), tachyarrhythmias (13%), and chest pain (3.5%). Most patients were asymptomatic (36%) but had abnormal physical findings or an abnormal chest film. Finding the tumor at autopsy incidentally or on sudden death (23%)

indicated the lethal potential. A few (3.5%) of the reports on patients with cardiac fibroma had no clinical data. Noninvasive imaging by echocardiography, CT scanning, and magnetic resonance imaging improved the diagnosis. Surgical treatment was successful in 53 of the 84 patients for whom it was attempted.

Takasugi, J. E., Godwin, J. D., and Chen, J. T.: CT in congenitally corrected transposition of the great vessels. Comput. Radiol., 11:215, 1987.

Congenitally corrected transposition of the great vessels (CTGV) may be detected de novo in adulthood, and the plain radiographic findings may be ambiguous or may be mimicked by a mediastinal mass. CT scanning readily shows the malposition of the aorta and pulmonary artery and may also show associated congenital heart lesions. The cases discussed show the CT findings in CTGV and the distinction of CTGV from conditions resembling it on radiographs.

Tomoda, H., Mitsumoto, H., Furuya, H., et al: Evaluation of intracardiac thrombus with computed tomography. Am. J. Cardiol., 49:972, 1982.

A series of patients were evaluated with CT scanning for the presence and resolution of intracardiac thrombi. The method presents excellent sensitivity and specificity for the diagnosis of intracardiac thrombi.

V ROLE OF MAGNETIC RESONANCE IMAGING IN CARDIOVASCULAR DIAGNOSIS

Robert J. Herfkens

Magnetic resonance (MR) imaging is a new imaging technique based on the discovery that the nuclei of some atoms have a magnetic moment. When placed in an external magnetic field, these nuclei tend to align with the magnetic field. When exposed to the proper radiofrequency, they absorb this radiofrequency energy and then return it in a form that can be detected. The basic technique of nuclear magnetic resonance (NMR) is not particularly new. The Nobel Prize was awarded in 1952 for the discovery of the NMR phenomenon. Until recently, the applications have mainly been for chemical analysis. In the 1970s, the development of large magnets capable of holding sizable subjects such as humans or animals, combined with the rapid development of relatively inexpensive computers, led to the development of the technique of MR imaging.

This new modality allows the imaging of atoms with odd-numbered protons by the complex interaction of a high magnetic field, magnetic gradients, and radiofrequencies. The specific advantage of this technique is that the individual components used in imaging are essentially noninvasive and do not have known biologic hazards. Once images are formed, the intrinsic contrast due to the changes in the local molecular environment of hydrogen in the body allows demonstration of normal and pathologic tissues. The differences in chemical behavior between tissues such as fat and normal water-containing structures such as the myocardium produce clear contrast. Additionally, the changes in water content that occur mainly in pathologic conditions such as edema in myocardial infarctions produce soft-tissue contrast. Because the intrinsic imaging process involves only radiofrequencies and magnetic field gradients and no moving parts, an image can be formed in almost any orientation or plane of the body. For example, sagittal, coronal, and oblique images can be obtained independently of the orientation of the body within the magnet.

Unlike traditional x-ray imaging modalities, which are based mainly on a singular factor known as absorption coefficient, the NMR signal is a complex relationship based not only on the presence of hydrogen atoms in the tissues but also on multiple complex factors known as relaxation times. These relaxation times, T1 and T2, or longitudinal and transverse relaxation times, depend on the specific chemical properties of the hydrogen ions within the tissues. These parameters—hydrogen content, T1, and T2—form the differences in image intensity in any NMR image. Specifically related to the cardiovascular system is one additional factor that strongly adds to its use in the evaluation of cardiovascular processes: the sensitivity to flow. Any tissue moving during the process has an altered signal that depends on its motion within the magnetic field. This strong sensitivity to motion, or flow-related signal, is an additional advantage in that rapidly moving protons such as those in blood may produce a signal that is sufficiently altered to add significant contrast to an image.

The motion sensitivity of the MR imaging technique is a complex phenomenon. The acquisition of MR images is affected by a number of factors. The complex application of radiofrequency pulses and gradient pulses is determined mainly by the relaxation times of the tissues. Therefore, acquisition of an MR image may require an exposure time of several minutes. Complex motion effects such as blood flow and cardiac structures must be coordinated with the acquisition to obtain a coherent image. When nuclei are moving during the imaging period there is a general reduction in the signal because of their movement. To obtain coherent images of cardiovascular structures, an acquisition coordinated to the cardiac cycle is necessary for the proper imaging of cardiovascular diseases.

To obtain satisfactory images of the heart itself, coordination of the imaging device is triggered by the patient's electrocardiogram or pulse signal, which poses a number of difficulties. To adequately visualize cardiovascular structures over a period of time, which routinely requires at least 128 or 256 heartbeats, requires a regular heart rhythm. The contrast in the image itself is dictated mainly by the patient's heart rate and the ability to routinely trigger from a consistently regular rhythm. Therefore, acquisition of cardiac images in patients with atrial fibrillation or frequent ventricular arrhythmias is difficult. Once a regular trigger is established by either the electrocardiogram or peripheral pulse gating, excellent images of the heart can be obtained. The soft-tissue contrast from spin-echo images is dictated, as mentioned earlier, by the relaxation times of the specific tissues. Images can be created in which the myocardium generates intermediate signal intensity; epicardial fat and pericardial fat produce very high signal intensity; and flowing blood, which is moving too rapidly to be imaged during the sequence, produces a greatly decreased signal or black area. This relationship of intrinsic contrast for specific tissues allows demonstration of both normal and pathologic features.

The spin-echo techniques, which generally produce images of high contrast in as little as 128 or 256 heartbeats, provide a favorable signal-to-noise ratio and high-contrast images. However, these techniques lack one specific element for studying cardiovascular diseases: They present images obtained at one particular point in the cardiac cycle. The dynamic nature of many cardiovascular processes cannot be evaluated with this technique. Thus, a number of additional techniques use *gradient-recalled echoes*. These techniques allow acquisition of images in a more rapid manner and change the essential imaging contrast so that flowing blood becomes the brightest portion of the image. This intrinsic relationship to flowing blood and gradient-recalled images is a significant addition to MR imaging abilities. These rapid imaging techniques can obtain images of the entire cardiac cycle at multiple levels with a high dependency of signal intensity in vascular structures on blood flow velocities. They represent a unique advantage in depicting pulsatile blood flow and contribute to spatial resolution and temporal resolution. The ability to acquire images at multiple anatomic levels with high spatial contrast up to 32 phases throughout the cardiac cycle provides a unique imaging situation for appraising cardiovascular processes. High spatial resolution is possible, along with the ability to evaluate physiologic processes in a time frame allowing analysis of a number of functional events that occur during the cardiac cycle.

ANATOMY

The relationship between relatively high signal from stationary structures and relatively decreased signal from rapidly flowing structures such as blood provides contrast for documenting normal and pathologic anatomic structures. By adding gradient-recalled techniques in which blood flow can be imaged throughout the cardiac cycle, high spatial and temporal resolution in combination with high-resolution tomographic imaging allows unrivaled images of cardiovascular processes (Fig. 31–54).

Because the MR device uses only radiofrequencies and superimposed magnetic field gradients, there are no moving parts in an MR scanner. The orientation of these magnetic gradients allows almost limitless orientation of the imaging plane to a normal or pathologic anatomic structure. Simple sagittal, axial, or coronal images can be obtained, or complex two-dimensional oblique planes can cross through cardiovascular structures to image the pathologic or normal anatomic structures advantageously (Fig. 31–55). The correct orientation of the slices depends on the specific anatomy or pathology that is to be imaged. In general, it is best that the image be chosen perpendicular to the pathologic process. For example, an aortic dissection is best viewed in the transverse plane, where the image itself is perpendicular to the aorta and the potential intimal flap.

The general contrast shown in MR imaging is secondary to the T1 and T2 relaxation times of the tissues. Certain tissues have slightly unusual characteristics. Fat, for example, has a relatively short T1 and long T2, distinguishing it from most other tissues because it remains relatively bright in most imaging sequences. This characteristic is advantageous for demonstrating pathologic processes involving the mediastinum. Most water-containing structures have a relatively long T1 and long T2 and in general imaging sequences have an intermediate signal intensity. Therefore, spin-echo imaging of blood flow within the major vascular structures produces a relatively decreased NMR signal. The decrease in signal within the bronchial tree is due to the lack of hydrogen nuclei within air. Fat, because of its typical characteristic, produces a relatively high signal intensity. MR imaging of the mediastinum therefore shows dark signals from bronchial and vascular structures and a high signal from mediastinal fat. Structures such as abnormal lymph nodes appear gray because of their intermediate water content. The pericardium, because of its fibrous nature and relative lack of hydrogen, has a decreased signal (Fig. 31–56). If the pericardium is inflamed or contains a soft-tissue structure such as tumor metastasis, there is a general increase in water content and an intermediate signal intensity. Pericardial fluid, although high in water content, is flowing much as blood is flowing within the myocardium and shows a greatly decreased signal on spin-echo imaging. This contrasted relationship then allows the differentiation of several pathologic processes simply on the basis of spin-echo imaging. The addition of gradient-recalled images allows demonstration of free-flowing pericardial fluid, which again shows increased signal intensity along with increased signal intensity from flowing blood. A combination of these two techniques

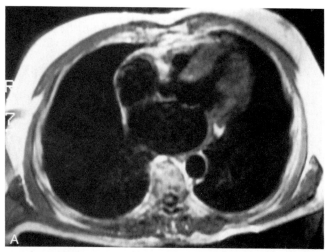

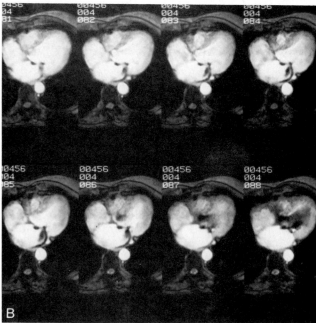

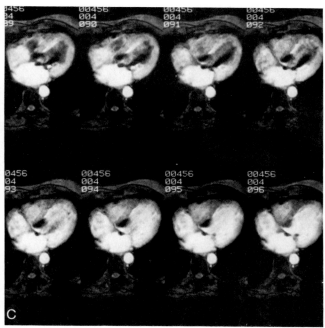

Figure 31–54. *A,* Transaxial spin-echo image gated to the patient's electrocardiogram through the midleft ventricle. Note the enlarged left atrium and thickened left ventricular wall. The reduction in signal within the vascular structures is typical of spin-echo images. *B* and *C,* A series of 16 cine-gradient-recalled images throughout the cardiac cycle obtained transaxially at the same level as in *A.* These gradient-recalled acquisitions change the image contrasts so that flowing blood is relatively bright and turbulence is relatively dark. Note the reduction in signal in the region of the mitral valve throughout all images, consistent with calcification in the mitral valve. During the diastolic phases of the cycle, images 9 to 96 show a decrease in signal originating from the mitral valve consistent with mitral stenosis. Additionally, medial to this area and anterior to the anterior leaflets of the mitral valve is also a decreased signal intensity, which conforms to aortic insufficiency. The dynamic information provided by cine gradient-recalled images can greatly improve the ability of MR imaging to show functional abnormalities as well as anatomic abnormalities.

sensitively differentiates several pathologic processes.

BASIC SCIENCE

The tomographic format of MR imaging allows delineation of several quantitative measurements. The ability to measure the myocardium in almost any plane permits sensitive calculations of myocardial mass (Fig. 31–57), volumes, and wall thickness. The addition of gradient-recalled imaging techniques allows relatively high temporal resolution and appraisal of sensitive measurements of ejection fraction and other dynamic measurements throughout the cardiac cycle.

The specific relationship between the NMR signal and the relaxation times of individual tissues was one of the strongest influences in the development of MR imaging techniques. Early studies demonstrated that neoplastic tissues typically had longer T1 and T2 relaxation times than normal tissues. Although this factor has not added significant specificity to the NMR image, it does allow differentiation of a number of pathologic processes. The increase in water content that occurs in the presence of acute myocardial infarction generates significant contrast in the NMR image. The increase in water content in a number of cystic structures also generates relatively specific imaging characteristics, allowing characterization of certain pathologic processes. In remote myocardial infarction, the evolution of the process of scarring of the myocardium leads to deposition of collagen and a relative decrease in the signal intensity of the involved myocardium. This scar shows a relative decrease in signal intensity and therefore can

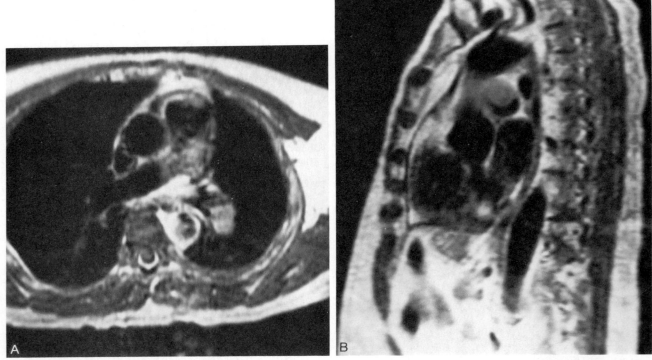

Figure 31–55. Spin-echo images through the midthorax show (A) the transaxial spin-echo gated image, a filling defect in the left pulmonary artery. On the sagittal image (B), a well-defined clot can be seen in the superior portion of the left pulmonary artery, occluding 75% of the lumen.

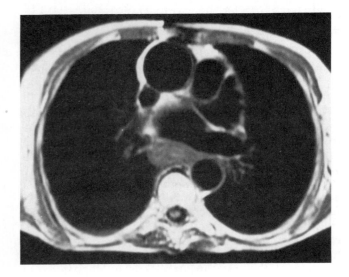

Figure 31–56. A gated transaxial image through the great vessels. The typical contrast on a spin-echo image shows decrease in signal where flowing blood exists in vascular lumina and increased signal intensity from fat from the mediastinum. The gray area represents abnormal soft tissue, in this case an esophageal carcinoma intimately associated with the descending aorta, eliminating the fat plane around the aorta and interposing itself on the posterior portion of the pulmonary arteries.

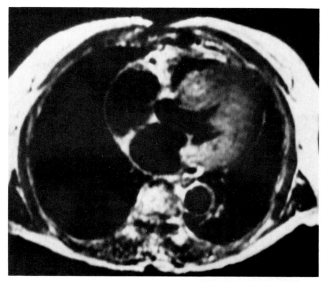

Figure 31–57. A transaxial spin-echo image through the upper left ventricle. The high contrast between flowing blood in the vascular chambers delineates well the endocardial border. The contrast between the decreased signal of surrounding air show the epicardial borders. Note in this patient with severe left ventricular hypertrophy the very thick wall and the mild heterogeneity of signal within the wall.

be characterized because of its overall behavior during the MR imaging process.

Certain other processes such as the deposition of iron-containing compounds (iron in hemosiderin or hemoglobin) alter the NMR signal significantly because of the paramagnetic and diamagnetic effects of these compounds. Acute thrombus generally has significantly decreased signal intensity. However, the specific paramagnetic effects of blood that is formed in a hematoma produce relatively increased signal intensity. Although the relationship of blood to the NMR signal is complex, the overall characteristics allow distinct contrast to be shown between acute thrombus, chronic thrombus, and hematoma.

CLINICAL IMPLICATIONS

Ischemic Heart Disease

The use of MR imaging for evaluating ischemic heart disease provides exciting new potentials. The ability to image in high contrast in a tomographic manner allows precise delineation of myocardial structures. Areas of altered water content due to capillary leakage can be visualized in acute myocardial infarction. This strong relationship between the evolution of edema and inflammation and eventually the resultant fibrosis in acute myocardial infarction provides a means of characterizing the age and size of infarction as well as the resultant damage. The sensitivity to wall motion presented by gradient-recalled imaging provides not only the ability to measure accurately the area of acute injury but also supplies additional information about the functional abnormalities. Gradient-recalled imaging techniques, with their high temporal resolution, also facilitate detection of subtle changes in wall thinning in a sensitive manner (Fig. 31–58).

The high-contrast relationship in spin-echo imaging serves as a means for quantitating patency of relatively small vessels or vascular structures such as coronary artery bypass grafts. This technique is extremely sensitive for appraising patency in small structures such as grafts; however, it is also sensitive to metallic structures such as surgical clips placed near the imaging volume. The overall sensitivity for graft patency is superior, but the interference from adjacent clips may limit clinical use (Fig. 31–59). The use of cine gradient-recalled imaging techniques that allow sensitive measurement of blood flow may ultimately aid in the noninvasive evaluation of coronary artery bypass graft function.

Congenital Heart Disease

The high-contrast tomographic images of MR imaging with minimal risk to the patient can be advantageously applied for evaluating congenital heart disease. The ability to differentiate endocardium, epicardium, and the integrity of the walls of the cardiac structures and vascular relationship by using MR imaging is particularly useful for documenting congenital heart disease (Fig. 31–60). Imaging planes can be oriented in almost any dimension, permitting not only demonstration of intrinsic anatomic abnormalities but also characterization of postoperative shunts. Echocardiography is an adequate method of screening younger children. In older patients, MR imaging can be used when there is difficulty in finding an appropriate acoustic window with echocardiography. The specific advantage of MR imaging in this older age group is the ability to image the great vessels in the upper mediastinum when postoperative shunt assessment may be necessary. MR imaging can be used to measure and characterize flow in these shunts in children. It has been shown

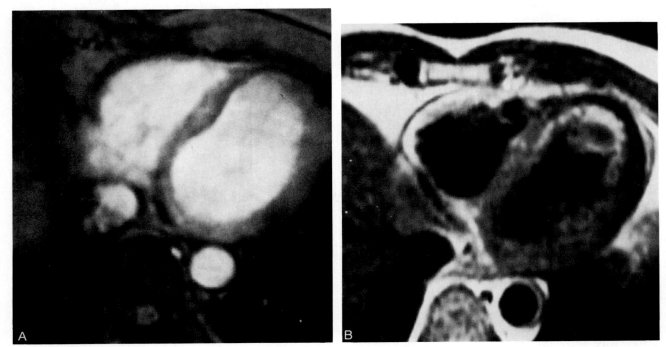

Figure 31–58. *A,* A single image from 16 images obtained throughout the cycle with the cine-gradient-recalled imaging techniques shows that the blood flow has relatively increased in signal intensity. Note in this particular individual that the anterior wall is very thin, with a relative decrease in signal intensity. The contrast by the cine-gradient-recalled images combined with the dynamic information provides a method of evaluating acute myocardial infarction. *B,* A transaxial spin-echo image at the same level of the chest as Figure 31–58*A.* Considerable thinning of the antral-apical portion of the left ventricle is again noted. The general increase in signal intensity in the left ventricular cavity represents very slow flow associated with this abnormal area of myocardium from a recent acute anterior wall myocardial infarction.

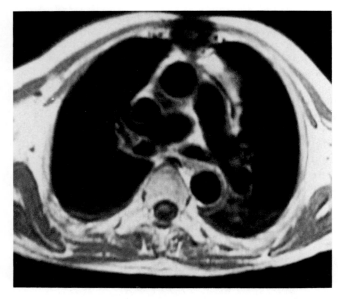

Figure 31–59. A transaxial image through the level of ascending and descending aorta shows the typical contrast of spin-echo images with decreased signal in the major vascular structures and prominent increased signal from mediastinal fat. Note in the anterior mediastinum an oblique area of decreased signal coursing from the aorta across the main pulmonary artery. This area is a bypass graft extending from the aorta toward the circumflex coronary artery. Patency of bypass grafts is identified by this decreased signal, whereas slow flow or no flow would be represented by a relative increase in signal intensity.

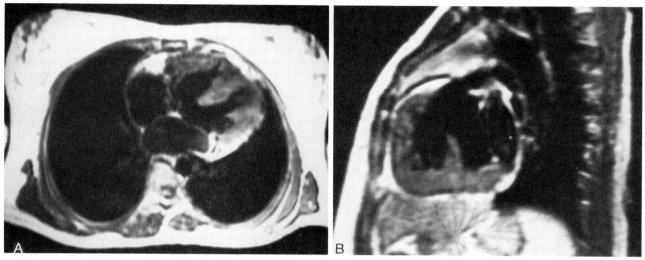

Figure 31–60. *A,* A transaxial gated spin-echo image through the midventricular level. Note the discontinuity of the basilar portion of the interventricular septum representing a large atrial septal defect. There also is right ventricular hypertrophy, with the right ventricular wall approximately 12 mm thick similar to that of the interventricular septum. *B,* A sagittal image through the right and left ventricles. The interventricular septum is interrupted in its basilar portion. Again note the prominent right ventricular thickening.

that the combination of echocardiography and MR imaging in older children can successfully be used to evaluate complex congenital heart disease and in many cases may obviate the necessity for cardiac catheterization.

Pericardial Disease

The general appearance of the pericardium, because of its fibrous nature, is one of relatively decreased signal on MR imaging. It is typically visualized between two relatively high signals of epicardial and pericardial fat. The normal thickness is considered to be less than 3 mm. In many pericardial diseases there is a general increase in the water content of the pericardium secondary to inflammatory processes such as those associated with acute pericarditis (Fig. 31–61). This increase in water content leads to an increase in signal intensity on T2-weighted images and allows visualization of these processes. MR imaging is relatively insensitive to the presence of calcification within the pericardium, however. Nodules within the pericardium associated with neoplastic or granulomatous disease can be easily shown because of the relatively high-contrast relationship. The use of gradient-recalled images has provided another sensitive method for evaluating the presence of free-flowing fluid within the pericardium and may be the most sensitive measure for identifying small amounts of pericardial fluid. The true sensitivity and specificity of this MR imaging technique have yet to be fully evaluated.

Figure 31–61. A spin-echo transaxial image through the midventricular level shows an area of abnormal signal lateral to the right atrium. This area is loculated pericardial effusion and shows the minor thickening associated with pericardial disease; free-flowing pericardial fluid may have a mild increase or decrease in signal intensity depending on the quality of the fluid.

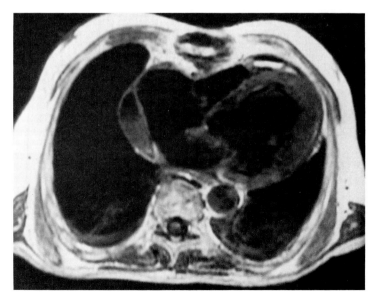

Myocardial Masses

The intrinsic relationship between relaxation times and the tomographic format of MR imaging facilitates study of pericardial and myocardial masses. The associated signal intensity changes of neoplastic lesions are relatively characteristic, with prolonged T1 and T2. Additionally, lesions with unusual characteristics, such as lipomas with their high fat content, can easily be differentiated on the basis of their signal characteristics. Because MR imaging can depict extracardiac structures, it is the procedure of choice for evaluating cardiac and pericardial masses.

Vascular Disease

Because MR imaging is sensitive to flow, it provides the necessary contrast for differentiating most pathologic processes mentioned. There is no area in which this technique can be more useful than in its ability to image vascular structures noninvasively. The superior spatial resolution and temporal resolution provided by the combination of spin-echo and gradient-recalled images supply the necessary elements for characterizing vascular pathology. Unlike echocardiography, which requires an acoustic window for visualization of structures, MR imaging can easily visualize the great vessels in almost any

imaging plane that may be necessary to show the pathology (Fig. 31–62). Furthermore, because MR imaging can detect thrombus within vascular lesions and estimate the relative age of these thrombi on the basis of signal intensity, the technique has additional benefits in the study of vascular pathology. MR imaging permits noninvasive routine follow-up of postoperative changes in entities such as dissections without posing risks to the patient. The tomographic nature and multiformat capabilities allow a high degree of accuracy in vascular measurements and reproducibility unobtainable by other imaging modalities.

Valvular Disease

Routine spin-echo images are relatively insensitive for identifying valvular disease. The introduction of gradient-recalled imaging techniques with relatively high temporal resolution and sensitivity to blood flow contributed to precise delineation of valvular structures. Regurgitant lesions can be seen as areas of relatively decreased signal intensity in the cavity as a result of turbulent blood flow surrounded by relatively high signal from normal laminar blood flow. Because gradient-recalled images can detect turbulent blood flow in a high spatial and temporal resolution format, they provide an effective and noninvasive means of documenting valvular heart

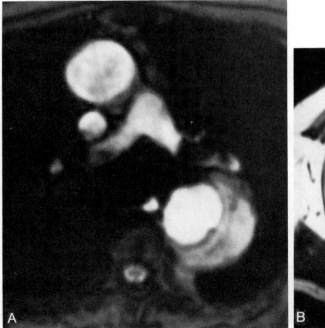
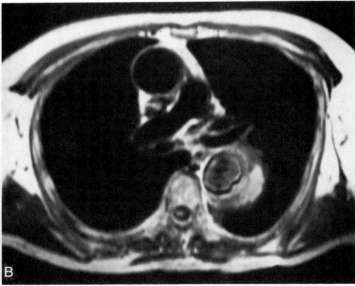

Figure 31–62. *A,* Transaxial cine-gradient-recalled image through the level of the ascending and descending aorta shows a prominent double lumen in the descending aorta filled mainly with intermediate signal intensity. Note that there are several different signal intensities in this area, which suggests the presence of thrombus of various ages. *B,* Again, two distinct areas are identified in the descending aorta; the intermediate signal intensity in the main lumen within the descending aorta is consistent with relatively slow flow. The moderate heterogeneous signal surrounding this represents thrombi of various ages in a false lumen of Type B dissection of the descending aorta.

disease (see Fig. 31–54). MR imaging can be used to evaluate almost any valvular lesion because it is reproducible, does not require an appropriate acoustic window, and is not subject to interference by calcification.

SUMMARY

Although it is in its infancy for the study of most structures, MR imaging has excelled for showing many cardiac and vascular pathologies. The high spatial resolution, high contrast resolution, and the high temporal resolution of the gradient-recalled imaging techniques are superior tools for appraising cardiovascular diseases. These techniques provide the ability to detect and monitor pathologic processes noninvasively. Improved techniques and further evaluation of MR imaging techniques undoubtedly lead to improved diagnostic methods for safer management of patients and follow-up.

Selected Bibliography

Bank, E. R., and Hernandez, R. J.: CT and MR of congenital heart disease. Radiol. Clin. North Am., 26:241, 1988.

CT scanning and MR imaging join echocardiography in the non-invasive evaluation of children with congenital heart disease. This article discusses the uses of these modalities in the assessment of the cardiovascular system in children.

Council on Scientific Affairs. Report of the Magnetic Resonance Imaging Panel: Magnetic resonance imaging of the cardiovascular system. Present state of the art and future potential. J.A.M.A., 8:259, 1988.

State-of-the-art MR imaging generates high-resolution images of the cardiovascular system. Conventional MR techniques provide images in 6 to 10 minutes per tomographic slice. New strategies have substantially improved the speed of imaging. The technology is relatively expensive, and its cost-effectiveness remains to be defined in relation to other effective, less expensive, and noninvasive technologies, such as echocardiography and nuclear medicine. The ultimate role of MR imaging depends on several factors, including the development of specific applications such as (1) noninvasive angiography, especially of the coronary arteries; (2) noninvasive, high-resolution assessment of regional myocardial blood flow distribution (e.g., using paramagnetic contrast agents); (3) characterization of myocardial diseases using proton-relaxation property changes; and (4) evaluation of in-vivo myocardial biochemistry. The three-dimensional imaging capability and the ability to image cardiovascular structures without contrast material give MR imaging a potential advantage over existing noninvasive diagnostic imaging techniques. This report analyzes current applications of MR imaging to the cardiovascular system and speculates on their future.

Freeberg, R. S., Kronzon, I., Rumancik, W. M., and Liebeskind, D.: The contribution of magnetic resonance imaging to the evaluation of intracardiac tumors diagnosed by echocardiography. Circulation, 77:96, 1988.

MR imaging was done in 14 patients with intracavitary cardiac tumors diagnosed by echocardiography. Except in the patients whose echocardiograms were diagnostic of atrial myxomas, this modality contributed important additional anatomic information regarding the tumor's relationship to the normal intracardiac structures or its extension to the adjacent vascular and mediastinal structures. The MR imaging findings correlated closely with the findings in all 12 patients who had surgical exploration or post-mortem examination, and in the other two patients, MR imaging guided the decision to obtain transvenous biopsy samples of their right-sided heart masses.

Gomes, A. S., Lois, J. F., Child, J. S., et al: Cardiac tumors and thrombus: Evaluation with MR imaging. A.J.R., 149:895, 1987.

Thirty patients with a suspected cardiac or pericardial mass had MR imaging. Twenty-six also had two-dimensional (2D) echocardiography, and three also had CT scanning; one patient had MR imaging only. Overall, 18 (60%) of the 30 patients had a mass lesion. The lesion was confirmed by biopsy, operation, or unequivocal demonstration on CT, 2D echocardiography, or MR imaging. Fourteen of the lesions were soft-tissue or tumor masses, and four were thrombi. The findings on 2D echocardiography and MR imaging were in agreement in 17 (65%) of 26 patients who had both studies. MR imaging was equivocal or in error in two patients (7%), and 2D echocardiography was nondiagnostic in seven (27%). In all seven patients with equivocal 2D echocardiography, the diagnosis was made by MR imaging. In the four patients who did not have 2D echocardiography, MR imaging showed the mass clearly. MR imaging is useful in the diagnosis of cardiac mass lesions. It can be used effectively in addition to 2D echocardiography to increase the certainty of diagnosis, and it is useful when 2D echocardiography is equivocal or inadequate.

Higgins, C. B.: MR of the heart: Anatomy, physiology, and metabolism. A.J.R., 151:239, 1988.

During the initial years of its use, MR imaging focused on the display of normal and abnormal cardiac anatomy. Electrocardiographic-gated spin-echo imaging provides high-quality static images that clearly depict cardiac anatomy and various anatomic abnormalities. However, it is now becoming clear that, with the addition of recent innovations, MR imaging also is capable of evaluating cardiovascular physiology. With the use of fast imaging techniques, images can be acquired with essentially high temporal resolution so that cardiac function can be quantitated. Moreover, the use of proton and ^{31}P MR spectroscopy provides additional information, which should enable the sequential monitoring of both cardiac function and metabolism.

Higgins, C. B., Holt, W., Pflugfelder, P., and Sechtem, U.: Functional evaluation of the heart with magnetic resonance imaging. Magn. Reson. Imaging, 6:121, 1988.

This review examines the capability of cine MR imaging for evaluating cardiovascular function and shows early results in valvular, ischemic, and congenital heart disease. MR imaging assessment of left and right ventricular volumes is independent of geometric models; dimensional values have been defined for normal individuals. Noninvasive measurement of peak and end-systolic pressure along with cine MR imaging can be used to calculate left ventricular meridional wall stress, which can be used for monitoring of myocardial disease and evaluation of therapeutic intervention. Cine MR imaging may be more accurate than angiography for identifying regional left ventricular dysfunction because it can measure wall thickening as well as inward wall motion. Regurgitant jets due to valvular lesions are readily seen, and their characteristics may be used to define the severity of aortic or mitral regurgitation. Calculation of the regurgitant volume across ventricular and atrial septal defects has been visualized in cine MR images and shunt flow calculated. Cine MR imaging serves as a 3D imaging technique with high temporal resolution. It extends the capability of MR imaging in cardiac disease beyond the depiction of anatomy and renders a comprehensive cardiac imaging technique for quantitation of cardiac anatomy and function.

Johnston, D. L., and Liu, P.: Evaluation of myocardial ischemia and infarction by nuclear magnetic resonance techniques. Can. J. Cardiol., 4:116, 1988.

Proton NMR imaging of myocardial ischemia without infarction requires the use of paramagnetic contrast agents. Even during the first few hours of infarction, imaging without contrast enhancement reveals only slight natural image contrast. Myocardial infarction, however, is more readily detected during the first few days and weeks after coronary occlusion; this is because of a sharp elevation in T2 during this period. Chronic infarction, several months after the acute event, does not demonstrate altered signal intensity but can be detected by visualizing myocardial wall thinning and aneurysm formation. Information regarding high-energy phosphate metabolism can be acquired in vivo in ischemic animal preparations; preliminary data have shown that it is possible to acquire similar information noninvasively in humans. Development of this technique will eventually permit the study of pharmacologic and mechanical interventions directed at preserving myocardium in the ischemic heart. Exogenous labeling of myocardial tissue with ^{13}C permits the study of the effects of substrates on cellular metabolism. The technique of chemical shift imaging ultimately will provide a method of spatially resolving valuable metabolic information in the form of an NMR image. With the gradual development of NMR technology, imaging and spectroscopy will eventually become important clinical measures in the investigation of ischemic heart disease.

Reed, J. D., Jr., and Soulen, R. L.: Cardiovascular MRI: Current role in patient management. Radiol. Clin. North Am., *26*:589, 1988.

The role of cardiovascular MR imaging in the management of patients is still evolving. Its capability to show anatomy without risk has made it an important supplement to ultrasonography and a replacement for CT scanning and angiography in many settings. In-vivo metabolic studies of congenital and acquired diseases may be the most important future developments.

Rees, R. S., Somerville, J., Underwood, S. R., et al: Magnetic resonance imaging of the pulmonary arteries and their systemic connections in pulmonary atresia: Comparison with angiographic and surgical findings. Br. Heart J., *58*:621, 1987.

Patients with pulmonary atresia require several investigations and operations. The role of MR imaging in assessing the anatomy of the central pulmonary arteries, the origin and course of systemic collateral arteries, and the patency of surgical shunts have been studied with the aim of reducing the need for invasive angiography. Transverse, coronal, and sagittal images were obtained in ten adult patients and assessed without knowledge of surgical and angiographic data. Central pulmonary artery anatomy varied from full development to complete absence. Transverse slices showed hypoplastic arteries particularly well, and the findings accorded with surgical and angiographic data in all patients. The origin and proximal course of 15 large collaterals were identified on the MR images, and 18 were identified by surgical and angiographic data. MR imaging did not show their distal connections; if this information is required, angiography is needed. Five surgical shunts were shown to be patent and two occluded at operation and angiography, and this was confirmed on the MR images. The patency of a further four shunts was uncertain, but they were not seen by MR and were presumed to be occluded.

Schaefer, S., Peshock, R. M., Malloy, C. R., et al: Nuclear magnetic resonance imaging in Marfan's syndrome. J. Am. Coll. Cardiol., *9*:70, 1987.

Detection and evaluation of aortic root and other cardiovascular abnormalities in patients with Marfan's syndrome are important in determining appropriate therapy and preventing premature mortality. To evaluate the role of NMR imaging in this syndrome, ten patients were evaluated using a 0.35-tesla commercial MR imaging system. Findings from these studies were compared with data from other noninvasive tests as well as surgical follow-up. Results from these examinations indicate that NMR-derived measurements of aortic root diameter agree closely with echocardiographic measurements. In addition, NMR provides more complete anatomic detail than does echocardiography and can be used to assess and monitor almost all patients with this syndrome.

Sechtem, U., Pflugfelder, P. W., Cassidy, M. M., et al: Mitral or aortic regurgitation: Quantification of regurgitant volumes with cine MR imaging. Radiology, *167*:425, 1988.

A new, rapid MR imaging method, cine MR imaging, was used to determine the regurgitant fraction (RF) in patients with left-sided regurgitant lesions. Right and left ventricular volumes were calculated using a modified Simpson formula in ten healthy volunteers and 23 patients known to have either predominant mitral (n = 17) or aortic (n = 6) regurgitation. RFs evaluated at cine MR imaging were compared in healthy persons and patients with mild, moderate, or severe regurgitation demonstrated at angiography (n = 10) and Doppler echocardiography (n = 13). Cine MR imaging showed regurgitant blood flow in all 29 regurgitant lesions in 23 patients as areas of low signal intensity within the regurgitant chamber. The RF was 4% ± 7% in healthy subjects and 12% ± 12% in those with mild, 35% ± 14% in those with moderate, and 63% ± 5% in those with severe regurgitation. The RFs determined by two observers were similar.

Sechtem, U., Pflugfelder, P. W., Gould, R. G., et al: Measurement of right and left ventricular volumes in healthy individuals with cine MR imaging. Radiology, *163*:697, 1987.

Cine MR imaging is a new, rapid MR pulse sequence that acquires up to 32 images per cardiac cycle at up to four levels of the heart within 4 minutes. In this study, the whole heart was encompassed by contiguous 10-mm transverse sections. Ventricular volumes were calculated by adding luminal areas determined in each section at end-diastole and end-systole. The left ventricular volume index was 57 ml/m^3 ± 9 at end diastole and 17 ml/m^3 ± 4 at end systole. The right ventricular volume index was 63 ml/m^3 ± 4 at end systole. The right ventricular volume index was 63 ml/m^3 ± 9 at end diastole and 22 ml/m^3 ± 6 at end systole. The left-to-right ventricular stroke volume ratio was 0.97 ± 0.06, which was not statistically different from the theoretically expected ratio of 1. Interobserver and intraobserver measurements were closely correlated. Volume measurements were validated with 2D echocardiography in five volunteers. Cine MR imaging allows reproducible 3D measurement of right and left ventricular volumes with short imaging time and good temporal resolution.

Soulen, R. L., Donner, R. M., and Capitanio, M.: Postoperative evaluation of complex congenital heart disease by magnetic resonance imaging. Radiographics, *7*:975, 1987.

This study suggests that the use of MR imaging together with echocardiography may reduce the need for serial cardiac catheterizations in the postoperative care of children with complex congenital heart disease.

Utz, J. A., Herfkens, R. J., Heinsimer, J. A., et al: Valvular regurgitation: Dynamic MR imaging. Radiology, *168*:91, 1988.

Cine MR imaging is a new technique that combines short repetition times, limited flip angles, gradient-refocused echoes, and cardiac gating. This technique has a temporal resolution of up to 32 time frames per cardiac cycle and accentuates signal from flowing blood. Cine MR images of 56 valves in 27 patients were evaluated and compared with either Doppler echocardiograms or cardiac catheterization images. An area of decreased signal that correlated spatially and temporally with regurgitant blood flow was seen in all instances in which valvular incompetence was shown on either Doppler echocardiograms or cardiac catheterization images (20 valves). This abnormality was seen in 9 of 36 cases without valvular incompetence. Cine MR imaging may be sensitive to turbulence and thus sensitive to valvular regurgitation.

White, R. D., Holt, W. W., Cheitlin, M. D., et al: Estimation of the functional and anatomic extent of myocardial infarction using magnetic resonance imaging. Am. Heart J., *115*:740, 1988.

This study assesses MR imaging for the evaluation of both the functional and anatomic extent of damage to the left ventricle (LV) from myocardial infarction. This was accomplished by blinded region-of-interest analysis of 36 MR examinations (orthogonal-transaxial, electrocardiographically gated, multiphasic, single spin-echo) for determination of ejection fraction (EF) and relative myocardial infarction volume (i.e., per cent of total LV myocardial volume). Comparison of the results was then made with a measure of global residual LV function (i.e., score quotient [SQ]) derived from segmental scoring of LV wall motion on a 2D echocardiogram (Echo) and with an EF value from a left ventriculogram (LVG), both done relatively concurrently with MR imaging. Significant (p < 0.01) overall correlations were noted between MR-EF and both Echo-SQ (r = 0.56) and LVG-EF (r = 0.78), and these relationships were relatively stronger when myocardial infarction was located in the right coronary artery (RCA) than when it was found in the left anterior descending (LAD) distribution (e.g., MR-EF compared with LVG-EF: r = 0.87, p <0.05 for RCA; abd r = 0.48, p = NS for LAD). The best expression of relative myocardial infarction volume appeared to be based on absolute volume of regionally thinned LV wall multiplied by a correction factor for its residual contractility and then the addition of a volume correcting for the amount of regional wall thinning by necrosis (i.e., "total-Fxn" myocardial infarction volume).

Winkler, M., and Higgins, C. B.: Suspected intracardiac masses: Evaluation with MR imaging. Radiology, 165:117, 1987.

Electrocardiographically gated MR imaging was used to examine 34 patients believed or known to have intracardiac masses on the basis of results of 2D echocardiography. Cardiac masses were confirmed in 15 patients on the basis of MR imaging results. In seven patients, MR imaging confirmed the absence of an intracardiac mass but showed an anatomic variant or other abnormality that had been interpreted as a possible mass on the echocardiogram. In 12 patients, MR imaging showed neither an intracardiac nor an anatomic variant that was likely to have been misinterpreted as a mass on the echocardiogram. Clinical follow-up in these patients at 10 months to 2 years and repeated 2D echocardiography have not revealed a definite mass. In six patients, tissue characterization of the mass with MR imaging added some specificity to the MR diagnosis. Thus, MR imaging can be used to verify intracardiac masses found on 2D echocardiograms and to exclude a mass as the cause of equivocal findings on 2D echocardiography.

VI RADIONUCLIDE IMAGING IN CARDIAC SURGERY

Robert H. Jones

The standard approach to evaluation of patients before cardiac procedures includes thorough clinical evaluation followed by cardiac catheterization with cineangiography. Newer cardiac imaging modalities, such as ultrasonography, color-flow Doppler, cine computed tomography (CT) scanning, and magnetic resonance (MR) imaging, offer less invasive characterization of cardiac anatomy that may require catheterization before cardiac operations in selected patients. Radionuclide images provide less spatial resolution of the heart than these other imaging techniques and rarely depict sufficient anatomic detail to replace cardiac catheterization before cardiac surgical procedures. However, radionuclide techniques characterize cardiac function in patients more simply and completely than techniques that excel in anatomic definition. Unique insight into physiologic abnormalities provided by radionuclide tests often aids in the selection and timing of operative therapy in individual patients with cardiac disorders. The simplicity of radionuclide procedures facilitates serial measurements before and after therapy to objectively document the outcome of operation. Widespread use of these modalities in modern cardiology requires that cardiac surgeons be familiar with the basic aspects of these techniques and their application in common cardiac surgical disorders.

RADIONUCLIDE TECHNIQUES FOR ASSESSMENT OF CARDIAC FUNCTION

The first use of radioactive tracers to assess any biologic process in humans was for evaluation of blood flow. More than 50 years ago, Blumgart and associates (1927) injected radon gas into veins of normal subjects and into patients with various cardiac disorders to measure transit times throughout the cardiovascular system. The crude technology then available for detecting radiation and lack of an apparent clinical use for these measurements caused this early insightful work to lapse into obscurity. In 1948, Prinzmetal and associates used newly developed single-probe detectors to quantitate the passage of a tracer bolus of radioactive sodium through the heart and they called this rediscovered procedure *radiocardiography*. This improvement in technology renewed interest in the use of radionuclide indicator-dilution curves for calculation of cardiac output and measurement of intracardiac shunts in patients (MacIntyre et al, 1951).

Soon after their development, gamma cameras were used to image individual cardiac chambers as tracer flowed through the heart (Bender and Blau, 1963). The potential was soon recognized for these instruments to be interfaced with computers to obtain data with sufficient anatomic resolution to provide indicator-dilution curves from individual cardiac chambers (Jones et al, 1967, 1972). Initial transit radionuclide angiocardiography evolved as a useful clinical modality applied primarily to measure left ventricular function (Jones et al, 1971; Scholz et al, 1980). This technique requires intravenous injection of a single bolus of radioactive tracer by using a high-sensitivity gamma camera for precordial counting at brief intervals, usually 25 msec. Dynamic counting images blood flow through the right side of the heart, lungs, and left side of the heart (Fig. 31–63). To construct left-sided ventriculograms, computerized processing combines phasically related counts from within the left ventricle during several cardiac cycles into an averaged cardiac beat, which has greater spatial and temporal resolution than the individual beats (Fig. 31–64). After subtraction of background counts arising outside the left ventricle, the remaining left ventricular count changes reflect relative left ventricular volume changes during the cardiac cycle (Fig. 31–65). Geometric assumptions commonly applied to contrast ventriculograms are applied to the radionuclide image to calculate absolute left ventricular end-diastolic volume. Radionuclide measurements of ejection fraction, cardiac chamber volumes, and volumetric cardiac output compare favorably with contrast ventriculogram measurements.

Technology for doing initial transit radionuclide angiocardiography has now been well standardized and is commercially available. Newer instrumentation, such as the Scinticor, is portable and can be taken into the operating room and intensive care units to measure cardiac function in surgical patients (Fig. 31–66). Moreover, the introduction of a high-fidelity micromanometer into the left ventricle to simultaneously record pressure during radionuclide volume measurement permits the construction of pressure-volume loops, which more completely characterize systolic and diastolic left ventricular function than the use of either pressure or volume parameters alone (Purut et al, 1988) (Fig. 31–67).

Standard gamma cameras do not have sufficient counting sensitivity to image the heart from data recorded during the five to ten cardiac beats when an injected tracer bolus first passes through the heart. An alternate approach of gated cardiac imaging acquires data after injected labeled red blood cells reach equilibrium within the blood pool. A simultaneous electrocardiogram synchronizes the acquisition of radionuclide data with the appropriate phase of each of the 100 to 300 heartbeats as counts are added to form a single averaged cardiac beat that is used to image cardiac motion and calculate ejection fraction. The advantage of gated equilibrium over initial transit cardiac imaging is that it does not require specific

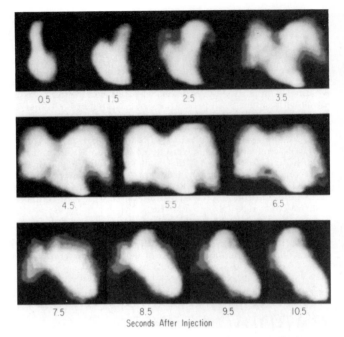

Figure 31–63. Serial 1-second images each composed of twenty 0.05-second data frames show the progression of the tracer bolus through the central circulation in the anterior view. The rapid transit through the heart is made apparent by the almost complete clearance of counts from the right ventricle during the time when count rates are maximal in the left ventricle.

instrumentation or a discrete bolus injection. However, the 2 to 3 minutes required to acquire the gated image make the approach less well suited than the initial transit technique for measuring cardiac function during periods of rapid change in cardiac function, such as during exercise or pharmacologic intervention. Moreover, cardiac volume calculations are less accurate and reproducible by using the gated technique because of higher background, which results when tracer is at equilibrium in the blood pool. Measurement of cardiac volumes by using the gated equilibrium technique also requires withdrawal of a blood sample at equilibrium to relate observed counts to absolute cardiac volumes. This step is not required when using the initial-transit approach.

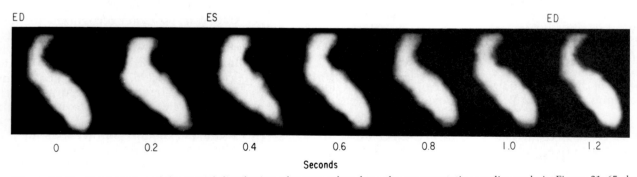

Figure 31–64. Serial images of the spatial distribution of counts taken from the representative cardiac cycle in Figure 31–65 show normal left ventricular wall motion.

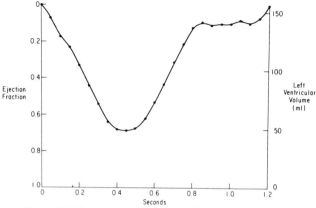

Figure 31–65. A representative cardiac cycle was constructed from radionuclide data obtained during several individual contractions during the initial passage of tracer through the left ventricle. The volume changes are expressed as fractional changes. In addition, planimetry of the end-diastolic image provides an end-diastolic volume in milliliters so that the volume curve can also be calibrated as an absolute change in volume relative to time. The rapid increase in volume during end-diastole reflects left atrial contraction.

RADIONUCLIDE TECHNIQUES FOR ASSESSMENT OF MYOCARDIAL PERFUSION AND METABOLISM

Radionuclide methods for noninvasive regional myocardial blood flow measurement are based on the observation of Sapirstein (1958) that the tissue content of any tracer with a high extraction rate during initial capillary transit is determined primarily by blood flow. This principle applies to potassium and the similar cationic tracers cesium, rubidium, and thallium, which accumulate in the myocardium proportional to blood flow after intravenous injection in a manner similar to particulate indicators injected directly into the coronary arteries. Love and Burch (1958) first reported use of ^{86}Rb in dogs and humans for estimation of myocardial perfusion. The potassium analogue ^{201}Tl, with a half-life of 73 hours, is currently the most widely used radionuclide for evaluation of regional myocardial perfusion. A large clinical experience with ^{201}Tl has documented the value and limitations of myocardial scintigraphy in patients with myocardial infarction and ischemia. Other promising myocardial perfusion agents with superior physical characteristics for imaging may soon replace ^{201}Tl for measurements of the distribution of coronary blood flow.

After intravenous injection, ^{201}Tl attains a high initial myocardial concentration as the initial bolus passes through the coronary circulation. The subsequent myocardial distribution changes continually as the intracellular tracer exchanges with that remaining in the blood pool. Therefore, the distribution of ^{201}Tl during the first few minutes after injection closely reflects regional myocardial blood flow, but several hours after injection it more closely resembles the amount of potassium in the heart. This characteristic of ^{201}Tl is used to obtain exercise and delayed redistribution images from a single tracer injection.

The interaction of specific radiopharmaceuticals with the heart may be used to study regional myo-

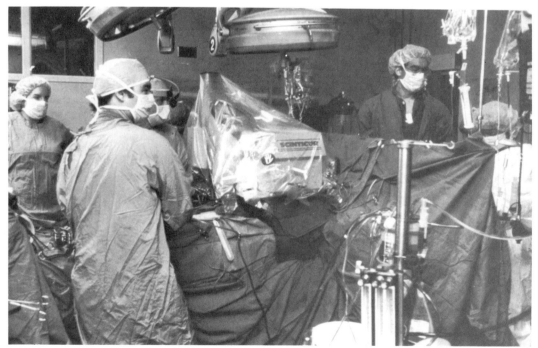

Figure 31–66. Newer computerized gamma cameras designed for doing first-pass radionuclide angiocardiography, such as the Scinticor, can be easily taken to the operating room or acute care environments for studies on patients.

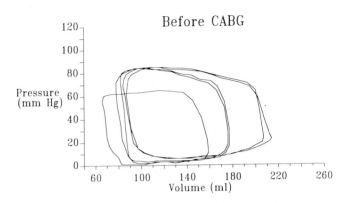

Before CABG

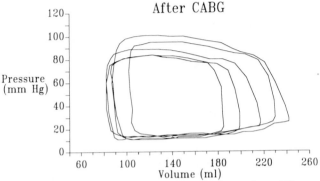

After CABG

Figure 31–67. Pressure-volume loops obtained at different levels of filling before and immediately after coronary artery bypass grafting obtained by David Harpole, M.D., of Duke University Medical Center, show minimal depression of left ventricular function immediately after myocardial revascularization.

cardial metabolism. During myocardial infarction, calcium ions accumulate within injured myocardial cells. The affinity of ^{99m}Tc pyrophosphate for calcium results in a high accumulation of this tracer in infarcted myocardium (Bonte et al, 1974). Labeled monoclonal antibodies that react with myosin and fibrin have been developed; they have shown promise for detecting myocardial cell breakdown and intravascular thrombosis (Haber, 1986). Cyclotron production of positron-emitting radiopharmaceuticals containing radioisotopes of carbon, oxygen, nitrogen, and fluorine now permit investigation of the full array of biochemical pathways in the myocardium (Schelbert and Buxton, 1988). In addition to measurement of blood flow, regional myocardial accumulation and utilization of glucose, fatty acids, and amino acids can be assessed. Future application of these techniques is certain to improve understanding of abnormal cardiac metabolism in patients with cardiac disorders.

RADIONUCLIDE IMAGING TECHNIQUES

Images of the distribution of a radioactive tracer in the heart detected by a gamma camera represent two-dimensional projections of counts arising from

three dimensions of the cardiac volume. Simultaneous interpretation of several images obtained from different projections offers reasonable approximation of the three-dimensional counts distribution in the heart (Fig. 31–68). The most quantitative approach now available for imaging three-dimensional cardiac counts is single-photon-emission computed tomography (SPECT) (Fig. 31–69). During SPECT imaging, the gamma camera detector encircles the patient, and data from these multiple projections are later reconstructed into a three-dimensional representation of counts. These count matrices can be quantitated by comparison with normal standards or can be visually interpreted as a series of heart slice images. The accurate regional quantitation of counts provided by SPECT imaging adds objectivity to radionuclide measurements of regional perfusion and metabolism.

Positron-emission tomography (PET) is a technique that also uses a number of detectors encircling a patient to image positron-emitting tracers. Positron decay emits high-energy photons in opposite directions simultaneously, and this characteristic is used to accurately position the three-dimensional location of the original event. PET requires more expensive and complicated technology than SPECT imaging, and present applications are primarily for cardiac metabolism research.

APPLICATIONS IN PATIENTS WITH CONGENITAL HEART DISORDERS

Definition of the path of blood flow through the central circulation may be useful in selected patients

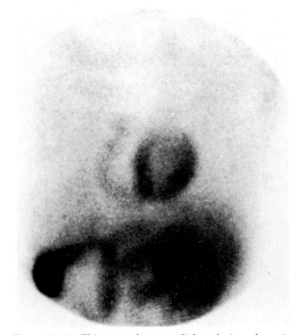

Figure 31–68. This normal myocardial perfusion planar image in the left anterior oblique projection was obtained after injection of ^{99m}Tc hexakis (methoxyisobutylisonitrile). This promising new agent has many advantages over ^{201}Tl as a perfusion agent.

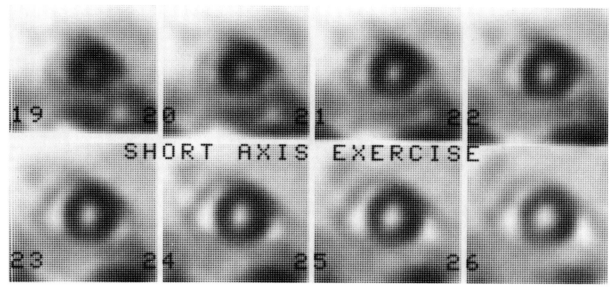

Figure 31-69. SPECT images of the exercise ^{99m}Tc hexakis (methoxyisobutylisonitrile) study of the normal patient in Figure 31-68 show the cross-sectional images of regional perfusion available by this method.

with congenital heart disorders (Jones et al, 1981a). Examples of these uses include demonstration of a persistent left superior vena cava in a patient with an atrial septal defect, evaluation of vena cava flow after Mustard repair of transposition of the great vessels, and definition of relative flow to each lung after Fontan correction of tricuspid atresia. In these and similar situations in which answers to simple questions of blood flow may influence decisions about the management of patients, radionuclide angiocardiography offers a quantitative assessment of hemodynamics with less anatomic definition, but also less risk than cardiac catheterization.

Initial-transit radionuclide angiocardiography permits recognition and quantitation of intracardiac shunts. Large right-to-left intracardiac shunts are apparent on radionuclide angiocardiogram images, but accurate recognition of small shunts requires quantitative analysis of curves generated from the heart and aorta (Fig. 31-70). Counts detected in the aorta soon after tracer appearance in the right side of the heart confirm the presence of right-to-left shunting. Data used to quantitate the shunt must be recorded from a site peripheral to the heart, such as the carotid arteries, because data recorded from more central sites such as the ascending aorta may include counts scattered from the adjacent pulmonary artery. Systemic radionuclide curves in patients with right-to-left shunting have configurations similar to those obtained with indicator-dilution methods (Fig. 31-71). Scattered radiation causes an early, relatively constant counting rate before the actual levophase in patients without a right-to-left shunt. In children with a right-to-left shunt, the early plateau is replaced by a definite increase in carotid counts, and the magnitude of this increase is greatest in the child with the largest shunt. In 20 children with cyanotic

heart disease studied by Peter and associates (1981a), shunt values calculated from radionuclide data correlated well with right-to-left shunts calculated from Fick data obtained at time of cardiac catheterization.

Left-to-right intracardiac shunts greater than 30% of the systemic blood flow can be recognized consistently on serial images by a more brisk than normal transit of tracer through the lungs and by reappearance of tracer in right-sided heart chambers distal to the site of the shunt. Shunts of smaller magnitude return less tracer to the right side of the heart and, therefore, prove to be more difficult to recognize by images alone. The most proximal site of left-to-right shunting can usually be located unless shunt flow is trivial. Further improvement in data processing techniques should permit localization of multiple sites of left-to-right shunting.

The curve configuration typical of left-to-right shunting shows an initial transit of tracer through sites distal to the shunt followed by an early reappearance of tracer returned by the shunt flow. Shunted tracer interrupts the exponential decline of counts and may actually increase counts sufficiently to cause a second curve peak. More commonly, the recirculated counts blend with the initial counts, and the multiple rapid recirculations cause the curve to break from an exponential decline and remain relatively flat with a high background. Curves over the right and left cardiac chambers may show typical alterations, with tracer entering the right heart chambers before transit through the lungs and again shortly after left-sided heart appearance. However, this typical curve configuration may also be erroneously produced by including counts from the left cardiac chambers within regions of interest designated as right atrium and right ventricle. Therefore, data recorded over the lung at a site remote from the

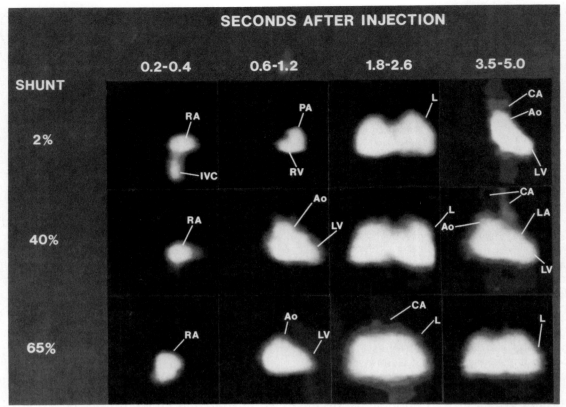

Figure 31–70. These images show tracer transit through the right side of the heart, lung (L), and left side of the heart in three of the children. The child with a 2% right-to-left shunt had a small ventricular septal defect. The 3-year-old boy with a 40% right-to-left shunt had tetralogy of Fallot. The child with a 65% right-to-left shunt was a 9-month-old boy with transposition of the great vessels. (RA = right atrium; IVC = inferior vena cava; PA = pulmonary artery; RV = right ventricle; CA = carotid artery; Ao = aorta; LV = left ventricle; and LA = left atrium.)

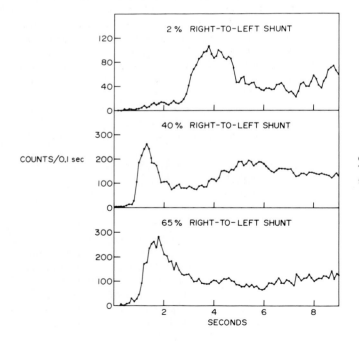

Figure 31–71. Carotid artery time-activity curves were recorded in the three children who were described in Figure 31–70. The ratio of the first to the second component reflects the size of the right-to-left shunt.

heart provide the most accurate quantitation of shunt flow. All approaches for quantitation of left-to-right shunts by using these curves require separation of the first passage of tracer from the subsequent transit of tracer through the lungs. Shunt calculation by radionuclide methods has been accurate even in very young children (Anderson et al, 1984).

The most important application of radionuclide methods of shunt detection is as a simple outpatient procedure to confirm the presence or absence of a left-to-right shunt without the risk and discomfort of cardiac catheterization. Functional cardiac murmurs are common in children and often raise the consideration of congenital heart disease. Even when the diagnosis of cardiac pathology appears highly unlikely in many of these patients, the objective documentation of the normal blood flow may provide worthwhile information to reassure the patient and the family. Moreover, many intracardiac defects associated with left-to-right shunting are not repaired surgically when the diagnosis is first recognized, and radionuclide angiocardiography can demonstrate the magnitude of shunting. In addition, postoperative studies may provide documentation of complete closure of septal defects (Fig. 31–72).

Surgical treatment of congenital heart disorders has progressed so that most patients who have these diseases and previously would have died now survive. Therefore, therapy is no longer evaluated by the survival of the patient alone, and attention has been focused on forms of treatment that minimize myocardial tissue loss and optimally preserve cardiac function. Studies in adults with cardiac disease have documented that many patients with normal resting ventricular function have depressed ejection fractions during exercise. Much of this change appears to be related to exercise-induced myocardial ischemia, but these changes have also been observed in patients with long-standing ventricular volume overload resulting from valvular regurgitation. Therefore, the definition of cardiovascular function should, ideally, describe the performance of the heart both at rest and during the maximal level of activity typical in the daily routine of individual patients. Children studied after Fontan and Mustard operations increased cardiac output during exercise as much as normal children (Peterson et al, 1984, 1988). However, cardiac volume changes were abnormal during exercise in both groups of patients, reflecting chronic adaptations to abnormal anatomy of the congenital abnormality altered surgically. These measurements of ventricular function during exercise provide valuable insight into myocardial reserve in children with surgically corrected congenital heart disorders.

APPLICATIONS IN PATIENTS WITH VALVULAR CARDIAC DISORDERS

Cardiac valvular abnormalities may alter left ventricular function either by the direct effect of the valve disorder on ventricular filling or emptying or by chronic changes within the myocardium in response to the long-standing hemodynamic alteration. Patients with mitral stenosis have restriction of left ventricular filling that becomes more prominent during exercise and limits forward cardiac output. Mitral valvulotomy or replacement eliminates the restriction to filling and returns cardiac function toward normal during both rest and exercise (Newman et al, 1979). Aortic stenosis restricts left ventricular emptying, and the decrease in left ventricular ejection fraction that occurs during exercise in these patients may result from the large afterload imposed by the stenosis. Also, myocardial ischemia may occur during exercise when myocardial work increases oxygen utilization above that supplied by the coronary blood flow, which is limited by the stenosis. Early in the course of aortic stenosis, left ventricular hypertrophy decreases the end-diastolic volume and results in an abnormally high left ventricular ejection fraction. Later in the natural history of aortic stenosis, the ejection fraction during exercise decreases, and the resting ejection fraction ultimately is also abnormally

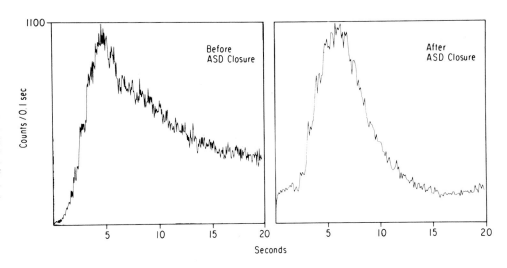

Figure 31–72. These lung curves obtained before (left) and after (right) closure of an atrial septal defect document change from a pattern typical of left-to-right shunting with early reappearance of tracer in the lung interrupting the expected exponential decline of counts. The study was done after closure of the atrial septal defect and provides a normal lung curve, documenting absence of shunting.

low. Patients who have aortic stenosis and who are permitted to progress to resting left ventricular dysfunction have a less favorable prognosis after aortic valve replacement.

Aortic and mitral valve regurgitation increases left ventricular end-diastolic and stroke volumes, and patients with incompetent left-sided valves commonly eject a normal forward cardiac output in addition to the amount of regurgitant blood. An ideal management strategy for patients with aortic and mitral regurgitation would be to withhold valve replacement until the time in the natural history of the disease when the ultimate prognosis for the patient would be adversely affected by further nonoperative therapy. Signs or symptoms of cardiac failure in these patients are a frequently used, but inconsistent, index of cardiac deterioration. The appearance of moderate resting left ventricular dysfunction identifies patients who have greater operative risk if operation is further delayed. Moreover, patients with clinical cardiac failure or left ventricular dysfunction before replacement or repair of an insufficient valve may not regain normal exercise tolerance or cardiac function after valve replacement (Peter et al, 1981b). Serial measurements of left ventricular function during rest and exercise by using radionuclide angiocardiography define the time of onset of exercise-induced left ventricular dysfunction that consistently appears before resting dysfunction (Peter and Jones, 1980). Patients with mild exercise-induced left ventricular dysfunction may be safely continued on medical treatment. Patients with more severe dysfunction should be carefully considered for valve replacement.

APPLICATIONS IN PATIENTS WITH CORONARY ARTERY DISEASE

Pathologic studies of victims of war or accidents and patients with noncardiac causes of death indicate a high prevalence of atherosclerotic change in coronary arteries, which is more common in men than women and more prevalent and severe with increasing age. This information, combined with the known annual mortality of only 3 to 5% in medically treated patients with documented coronary artery disease, characterizes coronary atherosclerosis as a chronic disease with a slowly progressive course spanning several decades in most patients. However, the sudden clinical symptoms that can acutely interrupt the chronic course of this disease preclude a leisurely attitude toward its management. Data from the Framingham study suggest that approximately 13% of newly symptomatic patients with coronary artery disease die at the onset of their first symptom (Oberman et al, 1977). The other newly symptomatic patients are evenly divided between those with a myocardial infarction and those with onset of angina pectoris.

Cardiac surgeons have ignored the large number of asymptomatic individuals who would probably have benefited from myocardial revascularization if they could have been identified before they died suddenly of coronary occlusion. Moreover, patients with end-stage complications of coronary artery disease, such as severe left ventricular dysfunction, left ventricular aneurysm with arrhythmias, or ventricular septal defects, who with much effort survive operation may be appropriately considered to be surgical triumphs but actually represent failures in the present ability of medical technology to recognize patients before these events. Until clinical studies are devised to detect and treat high-risk asymptomatic patients with coronary artery disease, cardiac surgeons should be optimistic about the likely effectiveness of myocardial revascularization in this setting and eager for any approach that improves the capability of predicting the future course of this disease in an individual patient.

Patients in whom coronary artery disease becomes apparent with myocardial infarction or angina continuously join the pool of approximately six million patients in the United States who receive medical treatment for this disorder. Even though the annual death rate is relatively low in this group, the population at risk is large, so that most patients who die each year with coronary artery disease will have interacted with a physician. The group of approximately 500,000 patients with coronary artery disease treated annually in the United States with bypass surgery or angioplasty represent a small subset of those for whom these therapies must be considered.

The major challenge in current management of symptomatic patients known to have coronary artery disease is a task of risk stratification. The large group of low-risk patients must be separated from the smaller subset of patients with a sufficiently high probability of a cardiac event in the future to require an evaluation for interventional therapy. Previous clinical studies of treatment of coronary artery disease have emphasized that the anatomic severity and extensiveness of coronary atherosclerosis is one of the most important predictors of natural history of the disease in an individual patient. The number, severity, and location of stenoses in coronary arteries dictate the amount of myocardium at jeopardy for ischemic events and identify patients with a higher incidence of myocardial infarction and cardiac death. Patients with the most extensive forms of disease, such as left main coronary artery stenosis, derive the greatest benefit from revascularization procedures. Despite the prognostic importance of coronary angiographic definition of extensiveness of disease, this single parameter does not contain all the information needed for risk stratification. For example, even in patients who have left main coronary artery stenosis and who are treated medically, 70% will survive at least for 5 years so that even this strong predictor of risk contains considerable uncertainty when applied to an individual patient.

Radionuclide tests appear particularly well suited for screening large groups of patients, and individuals with the most severe abnormalities can be selected for cardiac catheterization and possible further intervention, whereas those who are defined to be at very low risk would require catheterization in only special circumstances. Myocardial ischemia can be detected clinically by angina pectoris, electrocardiographically by ST segment depression, and functionally by regional perfusion abnormalities and segmental contraction abnormalities with associated hemodynamic alterations. Exercise-induced left ventricular dysfunction is a sensitive marker of ischemia that commonly occurs before an electrocardiographic abnormality as ischemia progressively increases in an individual patient (Upton et al, 1980). Radionuclide techniques measuring ventricular function and myocardial perfusion reflect similar biologic processes because of the close link between myocardial integrity and blood flow. Therefore, perfusion defects on myocardial scintigraphy done during exercise, which disappear after an interval adequate for ^{201}Tl redistribution, are also sensitive markers of ischemia. Myocardial infarction with subsequent fibrosis decreases resting regional and global ventricular function and also results in a resting perfusion defect because of loss of myocardial mass and the lower tissue blood flow rate of fibrotic myocardium.

Soon after radionuclide tests were introduced for detecting exercise-induced perfusion defects and functional abnormalities as indicators of myocardial ischemia, enthusiastic reports suggested that these procedures were highly accurate for diagnosis of coronary artery disease. Further experience with broader populations of patients shows that rest-exercise perfusion and function tests have an accuracy that ranges between 0.75 and 0.85 for the prediction of coronary disease (Jones et al, 1981b; Rozanski and Berman, 1987). Therefore, the severity of coronary artery disease reflected by the anatomic information from the coronary arteriogram correlates with that suggested by ischemia assessment of radionuclide stress tests in groups of patients. However, a consistent discrepancy occurs between the two approaches of assessment in 15 to 25% of patients with coronary artery disease. The early disappointment in the lack of complete agreement between radionuclide tests and coronary angiograms has been interpreted as being a benefit because the two forms of information appear to be complementary but independent.

^{201}Tl imaging provides higher diagnostic accuracy for detection of coronary artery disease than treadmill electrocardiography. The number and location of perfusion defects on ^{201}Tl scans relate to the extent of coronary artery disease, and the severity of perfusion defects relates to the degree of coronary artery stenosis. Brown and associates (1983) monitored 100 medically treated patients without previous myocardial infarction for a mean of 3.7 years and documented a cardiac event rate of 3% in patients with a normal thallium test and of 33% in patients with three or more defects. In 1,689 consecutive patients with suspected coronary artery disease followed for 1 year, Ladenheim and associates (1986) found three variables that provided independent prognostic information: (1) the number of reversible thallium defects, an extent variable; (2) the magnitude of initial reversible defect, a severity variable; and (3) the maximal heart rate achieved during exercise. Combining these variables into a prognostic model categorized risk of a cardiac event from a low cardiac event rate of less than 1% in patients with a normal exercise thallium study to a high event rate of 78% in patients developing severe and extensive reversible defects at a low achieved heart rate.

Reversible left ventricular dysfunction as an indicator of ischemia was first shown in humans by Herman and colleagues (1967), who studied patients with unstable angina during and after periods of spontaneous pain. Sharma and associates (1976) used contrast angiography to show reversible alterations of regional left ventricular function induced by exercise and cardiac pacing. Measurements of ventricular function obtained at rest and during exercise by using radionuclide angiocardiography provide a simple approach for assessing the extent of fibrosis and the quantity of potentially ischemic myocardium in individual patients (Rerych et al, 1978) (Fig. 31–73).

Pryor and associates (1984) used multivariate analysis of radionuclide variables to identify those that related to later myocardial infarction or cardiovascular death in 386 medically treated patients. The exercise ejection fraction was the most important radionuclide variable providing prognostic information in patients with coronary artery disease. This simple variable contained more than 70% of the prognostic information provided by combination of other important variables such as the coronary anatomy on arteriogram. The relationship between cardiac event and exercise ejection fraction was not linear, and patients with an exercise ejection fraction above 0.5 had few myocardial infarctions or cardiac deaths for 2 years after study (Fig. 31–74). In groups of patients with progressively lower ejection fractions, the number of cardiac events increased dramatically. These observations suggest that measurement of variables such as the exercise ejection fraction, which relates to the magnitude of ischemia, can be used to stratify the risk for individual patients with coronary artery disease. Patients recognized to have a low risk of cardiac event should receive medical treatment. Patients identified to have a high likelihood of myocardial infarction or death benefit most from bypass surgery or other interventional therapy. Jones (1987) reported an observational study of a group of 857 patients who had significant stenoses in one or more coronary arteries and who had been followed clinically for an average of 30 months after radionuclide measurement of rest and exercise left ventricular function. Selection of treatment was not randomized, and clinical and arteriographic criteria were used by the clinician responsible for each patient to recommend medical treatment to 473 pa-

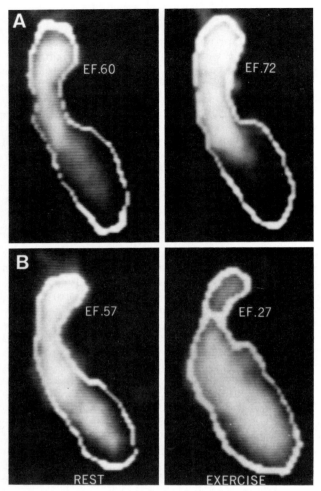

Figure 31–73. End-diastolic outlines and end-systolic images showing wall motion at rest and at exercise in a normal subject *(A)* and in a patient with coronary artery disease *(B)*. Patients with myocardial ischemia show cardiac dilatation and global hypokinesia with acute exercise.

nuclide angiocardiography, patients treated surgically had better survival and a higher incidence of pain relief than those treated medically (Fig. 31–77). Analysis of these patients by anatomic subgrouping shows that most of the survival benefit accrued to patients with three-vessel and left main coronary artery disease (Fig. 31–78). However, operation also appeared to improve survival in patients with two-vessel disease. A small number of patients in this group with single-vessel disease received bypass procedures so that the difference in survival was apparent between medical and surgical therapy. However, it appears reasonable to offer interventional therapy to any patient with severe physiologic ischemia during exercise regardless of the anatomic extent of disease.

Measurement of cardiac function during exercise, especially documentation of the exercise ejection fraction, appears to provide a very sensitive index of the magnitude of myocardial ischemia. The amount of potential myocardial ischemia is the main determinant of survival in individual patients with coronary artery disease. Interventional therapy that is devised to reverse ischemia can be expected to benefit only patients with a significant amount of ischemic potential. Definition of the pathologic anatomy of the coronary arterial tree by angiography is indispensable for planning the interventional procedures and provides some insight regarding the magnitude of myocardium at potential risk. However, radionuclide measurements of ventricular function during exercise provide important independent prognostic information useful in identifying patients who are likely to benefit from interventional therapy. Comparison of the selection of patients by different approaches used to assess individual patients for ischemic potential

tients and surgical therapy to 384 patients. Therefore, baseline characteristics differed between the two treatment groups, with a greater incidence of typical and progressive angina and more anatomically severe coronary artery disease in the surgical subgroup. Exercise-induced dysfunction occurred in 649 (76%) of the 857 patients. In the 208 patients without anatomically significant ischemia shown by radionuclide angiocardiography, no difference was apparent in survival or relief from pain between medical or surgical therapy (Fig. 31–75). When these groups of patients were further subdivided by the anatomic extensiveness of coronary artery disease on angiography, no statistical difference in survival was found in any subgroup (Fig. 31–76). Especially noteworthy were outcomes in the 51 patients with three-vessel and left main coronary artery disease but no demonstrable ischemia; their survival did not appear to be influenced by surgical therapy. In the 649 patients with physiologic ischemia documented by radio-

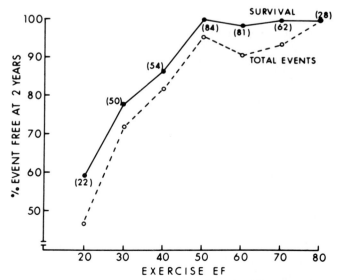

Figure 31–74. Two-year survival and total cardiac event-free rates as a function of the exercise ejection fraction (EF) rounded to the nearest 10. Numbers in parentheses are the numbers of patients within each exercise EF subgroup.

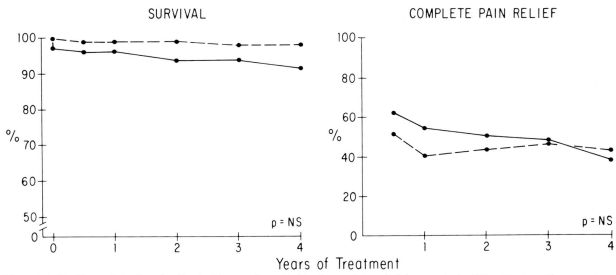

Figure 31–75. These data describe the incidence of survival and complete relief from pain in 208 patients with coronary artery disease documented by angiography but no ischemia on the exercise radionuclide angiocardiogram.

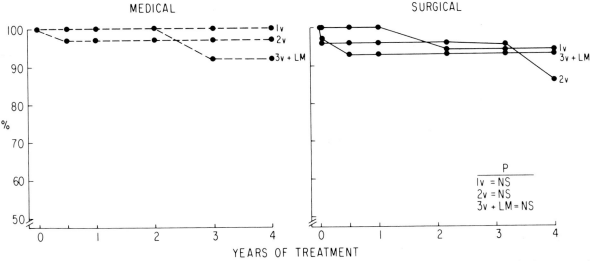

Figure 31–76. These data show the lack of influence of anatomic information in predicting survival after medical or surgical therapy in 208 patients without ischemia documented by radionuclide angiocardiogram. There were 94 patients with one-vessel (1v) stenosis, 63 patients with two-vessel (2v) stenosis, and 51 patients with three-vessel or left main coronary artery disease (3v + LM).

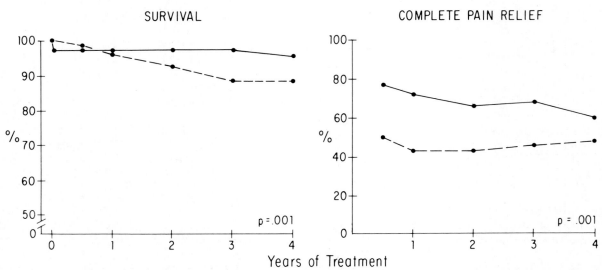

Figure 31–77. These data describe the incidence of survival and complete relief from pain in 649 patients with coronary artery disease documented by angiography and no ischemia on the exercise radionuclide angiocardiogram.

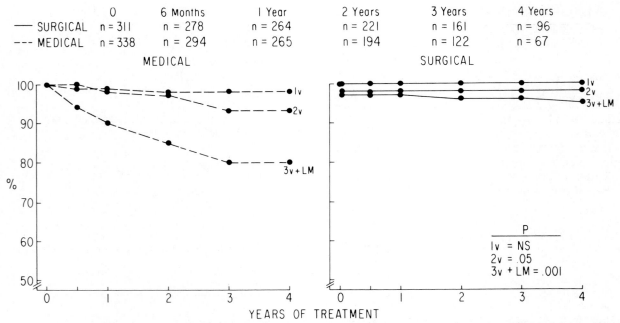

Figure 31–78. These data show the lack of influence of anatomic information in predicting survival after medical or surgical therapy in 649 patients with ischemia documented by radionuclide angiocardiogram. There were 159 patients with one-vessel (1v) disease, 208 patients with two-vessel (2v) disease, and 282 patients with three-vessel or left main coronary artery disease (3v + LM).

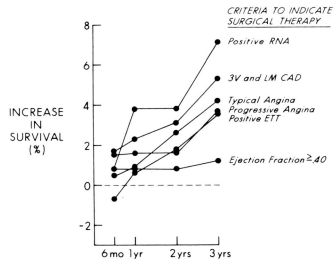

Figure 31–79. Data documenting the maximal per cent increase in survival of the total population that could be achieved at each time interval by using specific criteria to indicate surgical therapy and absence of those criteria to indicate medical therapy.

suggests that radionuclide angiocardiography is one of the most useful (Fig. 31–79) (Jones et al, 1983). The simplicity and low cost intrinsic in this radionuclide measurement also make it ideally suited as one of the first procedures to be done in patients evaluated for stable chronic coronary artery disease.

RADIONUCLIDE ANGIOCARDIOGRAPHY AFTER CORONARY ARTERY BYPASS GRAFTING

Not every patient who survives coronary artery bypass grafting has an optimal functional result. Even the absence of angina after bypass cannot be used as a valid end-point, because either denervation of the heart or perioperative infarction of myocardium previously ischemic may decrease or obliterate anginal pain.

Patients with good anatomic results documented by angiography after coronary bypass grafting also improve exercise-induced myocardial dysfunction and perfusion deficits after successful bypass. However, coronary blood flow at rest and the potential for flow augmentation during exercise cannot always be predicted from the coronary angiogram. Graft and vessel patency on arteriogram does not always correlate with improvements in regional function and perfusion. Therefore, as before operation, radionuclide tests provide important data that are complementary but do not always duplicate the information obtained from coronary angiography. Radionuclide procedures objectively document improvement in myocardial perfusion and function, and the end-

points are useful to judge effectiveness of operative outcome and predict the future clinical course of individual patients.

Radionuclide measurements of resting left ventricular function before and after bypass operation show that 10 to 20% of patients have a significant decrease in left ventricular function (Floyd et al, 1983a). This loss in function is permanent and often occurs without clinical symptoms or changes that suggest infarction on the electrocardiogram. A prospective study of 104 patients by Floyd and associates (1983b) showed a lack of relationship between QRS change on the electrocardiogram and left ventricular function after coronary artery bypass grafting. The loss of left ventricular function did not relate to the duration of hypothermic cardioplegic arrest, and the cause of this functional result probably relates to multiple factors that are now poorly understood. Approximately 10 to 20% of patients significantly improve resting function after myocardial revascularization, which suggests that reversible resting ischemic dysfunction was present before operation in the absence of resting pain. Although resting improvement in left ventricular function is modest in most patients, significant abnormal function observed before operation normalized dramatically after revascularization in some patients.

Physiologic improvement after myocardial revascularization is documented most consistently by radionuclide studies of myocardial function and perfusion during exercise. As early as 8 days after operation, patients have been shown to greatly improve exercise left ventricular ejection fraction and this improvement persists in later studies (Austin et al, 1983). This early documentation of reversal of myocardial ischemia provides a useful baseline for patients who later become symptomatic. Subsequent radionuclide studies can quantify the amount of return of ischemia associated with disease progression or graft occlusion and provide a rational basis for the selection of patients who might profit from repeated catheterization and consideration of another revascularization procedure.

Selected Bibliography

Blumgart, H. L., and Weiss, S.: Clinical studies on the velocity of blood flow. The pulmonary circulation time, the velocity of venous blood flow to the heart, and related aspects of the circulation in patients with cardiovascular disease. J. Clin. Invest., 4:343, 1927.

This series of related articles represents the first use of radioactive tracers in humans and is a model of early insightful clinical investigation.

Jones, R. H., Austin, E. H., Peter, C. A., and Sabiston, D. C., Jr.: Radionuclide angiocardiography in the diagnosis of congenital heart disorders. Ann. Surg., 193:710, 1981a.

This experience describes the use of radionuclide studies in 343 patients with congenital heart disorders.

Jones, R. H., Floyd, R. D., Austin, E. H., and Sabiston, D. C., Jr.: The role of radionuclide angiocardiography in the preoperative prediction of pain relief and prolonged survival following coronary artery bypass grafting. Ann. Surg., 197:743, 1983.

This report was the first to show that measurement of the magnitude of exercise-induced ischemia was an important variable in selecting patients who would benefit from coronary artery bypass grafting.

Pryor, D. B., Harrell, F. E., Jr., Lee, K. E., et al: Prognostic indicators from radionuclide angiography in medically treated patients with coronary artery disease. Am. J. Cardiol., 53:18, 1984.

This study emphasizes the prognostic information reflected by measurement of left ventricular ejection fraction during exercise in defining the natural history of medically treated patients with coronary artery disease. Data presented clearly document that patients with an exercise ejection fraction of 0.5 or more have a low incidence of subsequent myocardial infarction or cardiac death. This observation has important implications in screening large populations of patients to identify those with a low risk of untoward events.

Rozanski, A., and Berman, D. S.: The efficacy of cardiovascular nuclear medicine exercise studies. Semin. Nucl. Med., 17:104, 1987.

This review article summarizes the appropriate clinical uses of radionuclide studies in the evaluation and management of patients with cardiovascular disease.

Bibliography

Anderson, P. A., Bowyer, K. W., and Jones, R. H.: Effects of age on radionuclide angiographic detection and quantitation of left-to-right shunts. Am. J. Cardiol. 53:879, 1984.

Austin, E. H., Oldham, H. N., Jr., Sabiston, D. C., Jr., and Jones, R. H.: Early assessment of rest and exercise left ventricular function following coronary artery surgery. Ann. Thorac. Surg., 35:159, 1983.

Bender, M. A., and Blau, M.: The autofluoroscope. Nucleonics, 21:52, 1963.

Bonte, F. J., Parkey, R. W., Graham, K. D., et al: A new method for radionuclide imaging of myocardial infarcts. Radiology, 110:473, 1974.

Brown, K. A., Boucher, C. A., Okada, R. D., et al: Prognostic value of exercise thallium-201 imaging in patients presenting for evaluation of chest pain. J. Am. Coll. Cardiol., 4:146, 1983.

Floyd, R. D., Sabiston, D. C., Jr., Lee, K. L., and Jones, R. H.: The effect of duration of hypothermic cardioplegia on ventricular function. J. Thorac. Cardiovasc. Surg., 85:606, 1983a.

Floyd, R. D., Wagner, G. S., Austin, E. H., et al: Relation between QRS changes and left ventricular function after coronary artery bypass grafting. Am. J. Cardiol., 52:943, 1983b.

Haber, E.: In vivo diagnostic and therapeutic uses of monoclonal antibodies in cardiology. Ann. Rev. Med., 37:249, 1986.

Herman, M. V., Heinle, R. A., Klein, M. D., et al: Localized disorders in myocardial contraction: Asynergy and its role in congestive heart failure. N. Engl. J. Med., 277:222, 1967.

Jones, R. H.: Use of radionuclide measurements of left ventricular function for prognosis in patients with coronary artery disease. Semin. Nucl. Med., 17:95, 1987.

Jones, R. H., Floyd, R. D., Austin, E. H., and Sabiston, D. C., Jr.: The role of radionuclide angiocardiography in the preoperative prediction of pain relief and prolonged survival following coronary artery bypass grafting. Ann. Surg., 197:743, 1983.

Jones, R. H., Goodrich, J. K., and Sabiston, D. C., Jr.: Radioactive lung scanning in the diagnosis and management of pulmonary disorders. J. Thorac. Cardiovasc. Surg., 54:520, 1967.

Jones, R. H., Goodrich, J. K., and Sabiston, D. C., Jr.: Quantitative radionuclide angiocardiography in evaluation of cardiac function. Surg. Forum, 22:128, 1971.

Jones, R. H., McEwan, P., Newman, G. E., Port, S., et al: Accuracy of diagnosis of coronary artery disease by radionuclide measurement of left ventricular function during rest and exercise. Circulation, 64:585, 1981b.

Jones, R. H., Sabiston, D. C., Jr., Bates, B. B., et al: Quantitative radionuclide angiocardiography for determination of chamber-to-chamber cardiac transit times. Am. J. Cardiol., 30:855, 1972.

Ladenheim, M. L., Pollock, B. H., Ruzanski, A., and Berman, D. S.: Extent and severity of myocardial hypoperfusion as predictors of prognosis in patients with suspected coronary artery disease. J. Am. Coll. Cardiol., 7:464, 1986.

Love, W. D., and Burch, G. E.: Estimation of the rates of uptake of Rb-86 by the heart, liver and skeletal muscle of man with and without cardiac disease. Int. J. Appl. Radiat. Isot., 3:207, 1958.

MacIntyre, W. J., Pritchard, W. H., Eckstein, R. W., and Friedell, H. L.: The determination of cardiac output by a continuous recording system utilizing iodinated (I-131) human serum albumin. Circulation, 4:552, 1951.

Newman, G. E., Rerych, S. K., Bounous, P. E., et al: Noninvasive assessment of hemodynamic effects of mitral valve commissurotomy during rest and exercise in patients with mitral stenosis. J. Thorac. Cardiovasc. Surg., 78:750, 1979.

Oberman, A., Kouchoukos, N. T., Holt, J. H., Jr., and Russell, R. O., Jr.: Long-term results of the medical treatment of coronary artery disease. Angiology, 28:160, 1977.

Peter, C. A., Armstrong, B. E., and Jones, R. H.: Radionuclide quantitation of right-to-left intracardiac shunts in children. Circulation, 64:572, 1981a.

Peter, C. A., Austin, E. H., and Jones, R. H.: Effect of valve replacement for chronic mitral insufficiency on left ventricular function during rest and exercise. J. Thorac. Cardiovasc. Surg., 82:127, 1981b.

Peter, C. A., and Jones, R. H.: Radionuclide measurements of left ventricular function: Their use in patients with aortic insufficiency. Arch. Surg., 115:1348, 1980.

Peterson, R. J., Franch, R. H., Fajman, W. A., et al: Noninvasive determination of exercise cardiac function following Fontan operation. J. Thorac. Cardiovasc. Surg., 88:263, 1984.

Peterson, R. J., Franch, R. H., Fajman, F. A., and Jones, R. H.: Comparison of cardiac function in surgically corrected and congenitally corrected transposition of the great vessels. J. Thorac. Cardiovasc. Surg., 96:227, 1988.

Prinzmetal, M., Corday, E., Bergman, H. C., et al: Radiocardiography: A new method for studying the blood flow through the chambers of the heart in human beings. Science, 108:340, 1948.

Purut, C. M., Sell, T. L., and Jones, R. H.: A new method to determine left ventricular pressure-volume loops in the clinical setting. J. Nucl. Med., 29:1492, 1988.

Rerych, S. K., Scholz, P. M., Newman, G. E., et al: Cardiac function at rest and during exercise in normals and in patients with coronary heart disease: Evaluation by radionuclide angiocardiography. Ann. Surg., 187:449, 1978.

Sapirstein, L. A.: Regional blood flow by fractional distribution of indicators. Am. J. Physiol., 193:161, 1958.

Schelbert, H. R., and Buxton, D.: Insights into coronary artery disease gained from metabolic imaging. Circulation, 78:496, 1988.

Scholz, P. M., Rerych, S. K., Moran, J. F., et al: Quantitative radionuclide angiocardiography. Cathet. Cardiovasc. Diagn., 6:265, 1980.

Sharma, B., Goodwin, J. F., Raphael, M. J., et al: Left ventricular angiography on exercise: A new method of assessing left ventricular function in ischemic heart disease. Br. Heart J., 38:59, 1976.

Upton, M. T., Rerych, S. K., Newman, G. E., et al: Detecting abnormalities in left ventricular function during exercise before angina and ST-segment depression. Circulation, 62:341, 1980.

VII ULTRASOUND APPLICATIONS IN CARDIAC SURGERY: ECHOCARDIOGRAPHY

Peter K. Smith
Joseph A. Kisslo

In 1954, Edler and Hertz (Edler et al, 1954) introduced the use of ultrasound to image cardiac structures dynamically. A-mode echocardiography (Fig. 31–80) permitted the diagnosis of pericardial effusion in a noninvasive manner. The development of M-mode echocardiography provided a spatially limited, time-oriented view of the heart and resulted in the ability to assess cardiac valve motion (Fig. 31–81). Obtaining a satisfactory sonogram required a high degree of technical skill, however, and interpretation remained the domain of the trained echocardiographer. Despite these limitations, several investigators used this technology to study ventricular function during cardiac procedures in humans (Spotnitz et al, 1979) and in animals (Gaudiani et al, 1978). M-mode echocardiography was also used to assess the efficacy of mitral commissurotomy (Johnson et al, 1972; Mary et al, 1976) and to detect late cardiac tamponade after open heart procedures (Fernando et al, 1977).

Since that time, four technologic developments have significantly broadened the clinical and research applications of ultrasound.

1. Two-dimensional echocardiography
2. Pulsed and continuous-wave Doppler echocardiography
3. Color-flow Doppler echocardiography
4. Transesophageal echocardiography

These developments have made it mandatory that cardiothoracic surgeons understand ultrasound and its applications.

This chapter emphasizes the application of ultra-

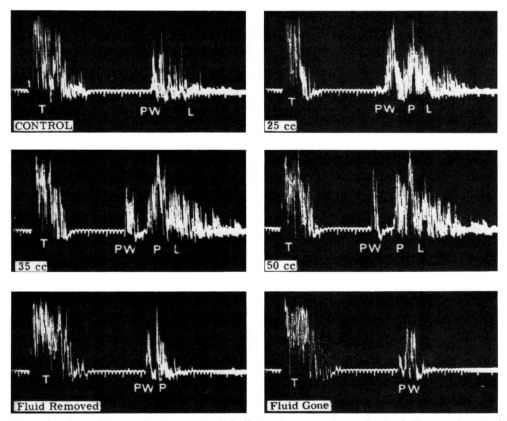

Figure 31–80. A-mode echocardiogram showing pericardial effusion in an experimental animal. The panels are individually labeled and progress from top left to bottom right. (T = transducer; PW = posterior wall of ventricle; P = pericardium; L = lung.) The control panel shows no echo-free space between the posterior ventricular wall and lung. Twenty-five ml of saline are infused into the pericardial space, permitting visual separation of the posterior ventricular wall and the pericardium. This space progressively increases as 35 ml and then 50 ml are infused. In the last two panels, the fluid is removed, obliterating the pericardial space. (From Feigenbaum, H., Waldhausen, J. A., and Hyde, L. P.: Ultrasound diagnosis of pericardial effusion. J.A.M.A., *191*:711–714. Copyright 1965, American Medical Association.)

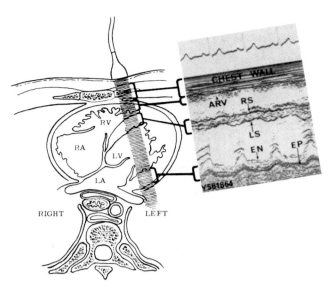

Figure 31–81. M-mode echocardiogram demonstrating an "ice-pick" view through the heart over time, with the transducer placed parasternally. (ARV = anterior right ventricle; RS = right side of ventricular septum; LS = left side of ventricular septum; EN = endocardium; EP = epicardium.) There is no pericardial effusion. (From Feigenbaum, H.: Echocardiography, 4th ed. Philadelphia, Lea & Febiger, 1986.)

sound techniques in the operating room. Perioperative ultrasound applications that offer *unique* diagnostic and therapeutic options for cardiac surgical patients are also discussed.

BASIC PRINCIPLES OF ULTRASOUND

Ultrasound is defined as sound with a frequency greater than 20,000 cycles per second (Kossoff et al,

1966). Sound is composed of a time-oriented series of compressed and rarefied air (Fig. 31–82). Frequencies in the range of 2.5 to 10 million cycles per second (mHz) are currently used for various medical diagnostic applications. Ultrasound is inaudible, is reflected at tissue interfaces, and can be directed into a relatively coherent beam. It is propagated well through a liquid medium and extremely poorly through a gaseous medium. Thus, to visualize cardiac structures, an acoustic window or pathway that is air-free must be found through which to direct the beam and its reflections appropriately. These features of ultrasound have limited its application in pulmonary medicine but have also led to the development of various microbubble echocardiographic contrast agents, which are discussed later.

The acquisition of an ultrasound image begins with the generation of a sound wave from an ultrasound transducer, which changes electrical to mechanical (sound) energy. This wave travels through soft tissue and blood at an average speed of 1,540 m/sec (Goldman et al, 1956). As it passes through tissue, the sound wave is attenuated and scattered in proportion to the acoustic impedance of each particular tissue (Gregg and Palogallo, 1969). When the sound wave encounters a boundary between two tissues of different acoustic impedance (Fig. 31–83), this mismatch causes reflection and refraction of the sound wave. The amount of reflection is directly proportional to the degree of acoustic impedance mismatch and the angle at which the sound wave intercepts the boundary (Fig. 31–84). Additional factors influencing reflection include the size of the medium traversed and the sound frequency.

Currently available commercial transducers spend approximately 0.1% of the time transmitting ultrasound and the remaining 99.9% of time receiving reflected sound waves. Transducer sensitivity allows

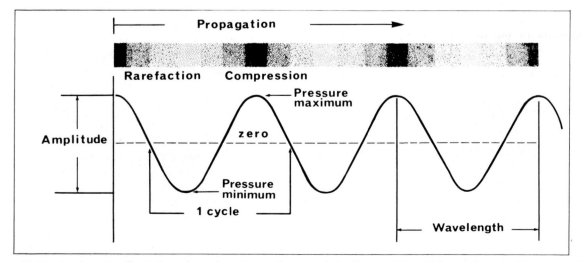

Figure 31–82. A schematic illustration of a coherent sound wave. A continuous sinusoidal waveform is demonstrated in the direction of propagation showing the amplitude on an arbitrary pressure scale. The cycle length and wave length are shown on an arbitrary time scale. The sound frequency is the reciprocal of wave length. (From Feigenbaum, H.: Echocardiography, 4th ed. Philadelphia, Lea & Febiger, 1986.)

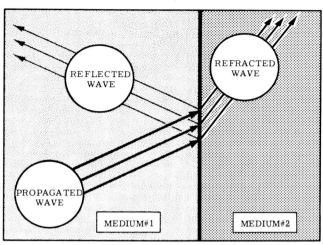

Figure 31–83. The relative reflection and refraction of a propagated ultrasound wave between two media of differing acoustic impedance are demonstrated. (From Feigenbaum, H.: Echocardiography, 4th ed. Philadelphia, Lea & Febiger, 1986.)

the detection of returning sound waves, which are reduced to less than 1% of the transmitted ultrasonic energy. The received signal is related in time to the transmitted signal, and that time is related to the speed of sound in tissue to determine the distance of the reflecting agent. In this way, various "echoes" are arrayed along the line of the ultrasound beam. An oscilloscope can show the relative intensity and timing of the returned signal (A mode) (Fig. 31–85). The intensity of returned ultrasound can alternately be converted into a varying display intensity, while the timing is recorded as distance on the oscilloscope screen (B mode) (see Fig. 31–85). In these modes, positional changes of the ultrasound reflector studied (*horizontal arrow* in Fig. 31–85) are shown instantly. By using the second dimension of the display as a time base, these positional changes can be shown continuously (M mode) (see Figs. 31–81 and 31–85). By sweeping this line throughout an arc, either mechanically or electronically (Fig. 31–86), a tomo-

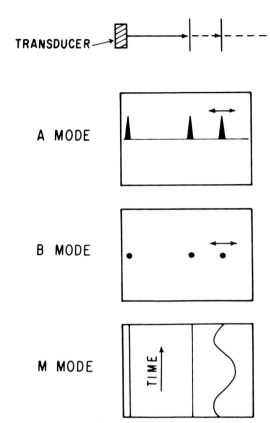

Figure 31–85. A schematic illustration relating the position of the transducer to two reflecting objects, the second varying in time (*horizontal arrow*). A-, B-, and M-mode echocardiography are illustrated (see text for description). (From DeBruijn, N. P., and Clements, F. M. [eds]: Transesophageal Echocardiography. Boston, Martinus Nijhoff Publishing, 1987, p. 22.)

gram of reflected sound can be obtained (Fig. 31–87). These methods and displays are approximately similar to those used in radar.

The depth and resolution of the tomogram are highly dependent on the frequency of ultrasound used. With increasing frequency, smaller objects and interfaces cause reflections. At the same time, as the acoustic pathway is traversed, less ultrasonic energy is available. Thus, increasing frequency leads to better resolution at the expense of penetration. A 2.25-mHz ultrasound wave can effectively penetrate to a depth of approximately 20 cm and yield a range resolution of approximately 1 mm.

PRINCIPLES OF DOPPLER ECHOCARDIOGRAPHY

The Doppler principle has been applied to ultrasound to quantify regional blood velocity either in the heart or great vessels. The physical principle was described originally by Doppler in reference to the effect of motion on the wavelength of light.

The Doppler shift in clinical ultrasound is created by motion of red blood cells (as ultrasound reflectors)

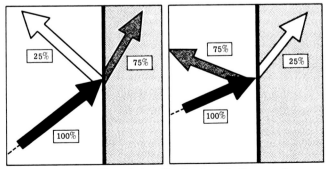

Figure 31–84. The relative distribution of ultrasound energy at the time of reflection and refraction is shown to be proportionate to the incidence angle when the acoustic impedance mismatch is held constant (propagated wave is shown as the *black arrow*). (From Feigenbaum, H.: Echocardiography, 2nd ed. Philadelphia, Lea & Febiger, 1976.)

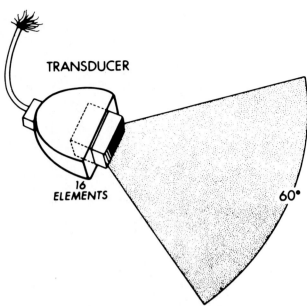

Figure 31–86. An early phased-array transducer capable of electronically transmitting ultrasound through a 60-degree arc. (From von Ramm, O. T., and Thurstone, F. L.: Cardiac imaging using a phased array ultrasound system. I: System design. Circulation, 53:258, 1976. By permission of the American Heart Association, Inc.)

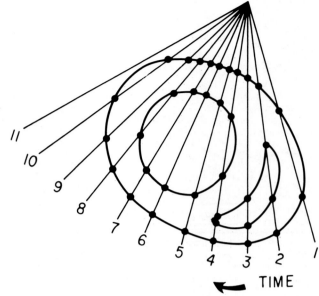

Figure 31–87. As the ultrasound beam is swept through a tomographic plane, the returning echo data (depicted as dots at the intersection of each discrete ultrasound wave and schematic endocardial and epicardial surfaces) are stored and displayed sequentially as numbered. The time of the return is displayed sequentially as numbered. The time of the return signal is used to determine range, and the time from signal transmission used to reconstruct the sweep angle. (From DeBruijn, N. P., and Clements, F. M. [eds]: Transesophageal Echocardiography. Boston, Martinus Nijhoff Publishing, 1987.)

either toward or away from the transducer (Fig. 31–88). Motion of red blood cells toward the transducer increases the frequency of the returned signal in proportion to their velocity, which is expressed by the Doppler equation (Fig. 31–89). The angle θ (the angle between the Doppler beam and the direction of blood flow) also affects the Doppler shift. Similarly, flow away from the transducer reduces the returning frequency. The Doppler equation can be solved for velocity by using the assumption that the angle θ is zero (which may not always be the case). Information about the Doppler shift is also converted into audible sounds, which are broadcast to the equipment operator.

Quantification of this information is accomplished by showing the distribution of velocities detected over time on the echocardiographic monitor (Fig. 31–90). This spectrum can be further analyzed by fast Fourier transformation to display the distribution of the various velocities encompassed by the acoustic pathway over time (Fig. 31–91) and to calculate various indices characterizing portions of the cardiac cycle (Fig. 31–92).

Continuous-wave Doppler echocardiography uses continuous, simultaneous ultrasound generation and reception with a two-crystal transducer (Fig. 31–93). Although this can determine high velocities, it cannot discriminate the location of any particular group of velocities shown. By using a single transducer that alternates between transmission and reception of ultrasound, it is possible to discriminate the depth at which velocity is determined, again by

knowing the speed of sound on average through tissues and blood (Fig. 31–94). This range gating, called pulsed-wave Doppler, can be superimposed on a stored two-dimensional (2D) echocardiographic image. This combination of geometric and velocity information permits detailed evaluation of valvular regurgitation, stenosis, and intracardiac defects. The main disadvantage of pulsed-wave Doppler is an inability to measure high blood flow velocities (above

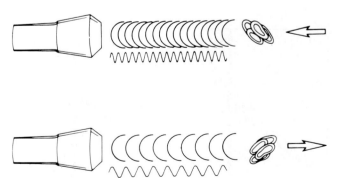

Figure 31–88. The Doppler shift showing an increase in the frequency of return sound from red blood cell reflectors moving toward the transducer *(top)* and a corresponding decrease in return frequency from red blood cells moving away from the transducer *(bottom)*. (From Kisslo, J., and Adams, D. B.: An Introduction to Doppler Echocardiography, Vol. 1. New York, Medi Cine Productions, 1987.)

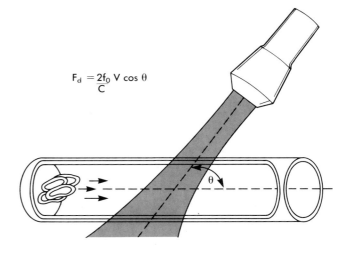

Figure 31–89. An illustration of the Doppler equation as applied to red blood cells moving toward the transducer within a blood vessel. The angle ø represents the angle of incidence between the ultrasound beam and the direction of flow. As this angle is minimized, cosine ø approaches 1 and the angle effect is removed from the equation. (From Kisslo, J., and Adams, D. B.: An Introduction to Doppler Echocardiography, Vol. 1. New York, Medi Cine Productions, 1987.)

$$F_d = \frac{2f_0 \, V \cos \theta}{C}$$

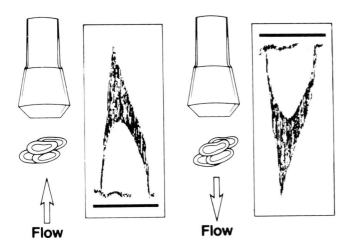

Flow   **Flow**

Figure 31–90. Flowing elements toward the transducer *(left)* are displayed with positive velocities above the baseline. In mid ejection, there is a relatively wide range of velocities present within the acoustic pathway, creating a broad band in the velocity spectrum. Similarly, flow away from the transducer *(right)* creates a spectrum of velocities presented below the baseline. (From Kisslo, J., and Adams, D. B.: An Introduction to Doppler Echocardiography, Vol. 1. New York, Medi Cine Productions, 1987.)

Figure 31–91. The velocity data detected by the Doppler instruments are processed by fast Fourier transform, and the resulting spectrum of velocities present is displayed. Laminar flows are uniform, whereas turbulent flow shows spectral broadening.

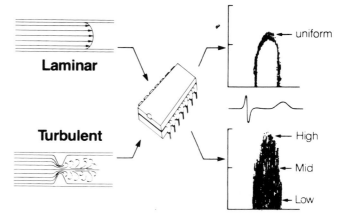

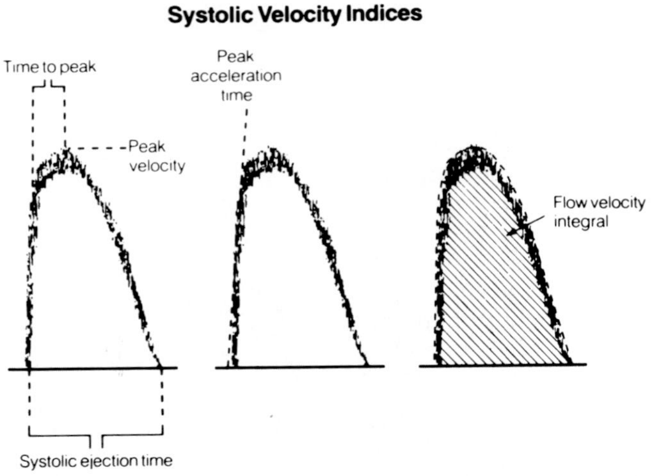

Systolic Velocity Indices

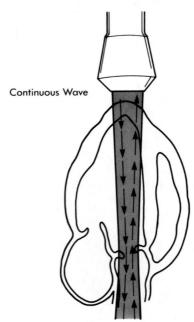

Figure 31–92. An idealized systolic aortic velocity profile and the derived indices, systolic ejection time, peak velocity, and time to peak velocity are shown on the left side of the panel. Peak acceleration time and the flow velocity integral can also be automatically derived. (From Kisslo, J., and Adams, D. B.: An Introduction to Doppler Echocardiography, Vol. 2. New York, Medi Cine Productions, 1987.)

1.5 to 2 m/sec). This limitation has practical implications because a modification of Bernoulli's equation $(P1 - P2 = 4 \; v^2)$ is used to relate blood flow velocity to the pressure differential across stenotic valvular

Figure 31–93. Continuous-wave Doppler positioned to interrogate blood velocity along a path from the left ventricular apex through the left ventricular outflow tract and into the aorta. Separate sending and receiving transducers analyze continuous ultrasound, which can be used to determine high velocities occurring along this pathway. As can be seen, these velocities are returned from any position within the acoustic pathway (outlined in gray), but the specific location of each discrete velocity subset cannot be determined. (From Kisslo, J., and Adams, D. B.: An Introduction to Doppler Echocardiography, Vol. 1. New York, Medi Cine Productions, 1987.)

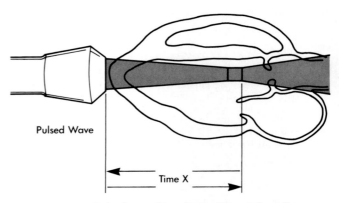

Figure 31–94. Pulsed-wave Doppler positioned along the same acoustic pathway uses a single transducer alternating between transmission and reception of ultrasound. The information can be range gated, in this case specifically interrogating the region of the left ventricular outflow tract for velocity information. (From Kisslo, J., and Adams, D. B.: An Introduction to Doppler Echocardiography, Vol. 1. New York, Medi Cine Productions, 1987.)

cardiac lesions. In practice, these velocities can exceed 6 m/sec and can only be absolutely quantified with continuous-wave Doppler technique.

COLOR-FLOW DOPPLER ECHOCARDIOGRAPHY

The returning ultrasound data from a conventional 2D echocardiography transducer also contain frequency-shift information resulting from encounters with moving structures and blood. The addition of a processor devoted to the analysis of this information, separate from that used to create the 2D echocardiographic image, is used to create color-flow images. Doppler information is obtained from multiple gates along each line and is then coded in color according to the direction of flow. By convention, *red hues* indicate flow *toward* the transducer and *blue hues* indicate flow *away* from the transducer. The brighter the color, the higher is the velocity. Additional circuitry compares the spectrum of velocities within each gated sample to the mean velocity. With great variance, indicating turbulent flow, green is added to the predominant red or blue in proportion to the variance.

Thus, the addition of color-flow imaging to 2D echocardiography permits simultaneous display of cardiac anatomy and physiology.

DEVELOPMENT AND APPLICATION: GENERAL ASPECTS

The development of real-time 2D echocardiography, initially termed "ultrasound cardiotomography," began in the mid-1960s (Ebina et al, 1967). The provision of spatial orientation and tomographic information greatly enhanced the value of the resultant image. By providing a frame of reference, it became easier to position the M-mode acoustic pathway, the tomogram providing a template of recognizable overall cardiac structure within which to work.

The introduction of 2D and color-flow devices has removed much of the mystery of echocardiographic interpretation and moved the technique into the surgeon's hands. In heart operations, the pathophysiology and anatomy are shown in a format that surgeons intuitively understand. As a result, more and more studies are done in the operating room, and the results are interpreted in real time. The first reported surgical case involved the intraoperative use of 2D echocardiography to localize and successfully remove an intracardiac bullet (Harrison et al, 1981). In early studies, the ultrasound transducer and cable were sterilized with gas before each procedure. More recently, it has been shown to be simple and safe to rinse the transducer in glutaraldehyde (Cidex) and place it in a commercially available, presterilized sheath for intraoperative use.

Transesophageal echocardiography is usually done by the anesthesiologist. The transesophageal approach improves the acoustic window available for cardiac visualization and permits the diagnostic procedure to be done unobtrusively. Satisfactory images can be obtained with the chest open or closed and can be useful in the immediate postoperative period.

TWO-DIMENSIONAL ECHOCARDIOGRAPHY: CLINICAL APPLICATIONS

Cardiac Function

Although echocardiography has been widely applied in the assessment of cardiac function, credit must be given to Omoto (Omoto, 1982) and to Spotnitz (1982) and associates (Spotnitz et al, 1979) for introducing this application to the operating room.

Global ventricular function has been assessed in many ways. Systolic global ventricular function can be approximated by measuring the ejection fraction. By using echocardiography, this can be determined as a relationship between end-systolic and end-diastolic areas in the short (or minor) axis of the heart, as follows:

EF = (EDA − ESA)/EDA
EF = ejection fraction
EDA = end-diastolic area
ESA = end-systolic area

End-diastolic area is determined by planimetry of the endocardial surface (usually excluding the papillary muscles). The simultaneously recorded electrocardiogram is used to synchronize these determinations over multiple cardiac cycles. End-systolic area is determined similarly at minimal area

during ventricular ejection. There are several potential inaccuracies in this determination. It is important that the ejection fraction be determined in the same plane throughout the cardiac cycle, both before and after any intervention. Intraoperatively, this can be accomplished by reference to external anatomic landmarks or by maintaining constant internal landmarks on the image. Spotnitz (1982) reported the use of the long-axis view of the left ventricle to determine the point at which the short-axis diameter would be maximal as a method to maintain consistency. Accurate determination of the ejection fraction also depends on symmetric global systolic function and minimal cardiac translational motion, neither of which can be assumed in patients having cardiac operations (Waggoner et al, 1982). Additionally, area measurements reflect volume changes only if one of a number of different models of global ventricular geometry is assured. Nonetheless, results obtained by using these methods in humans have consistently correlated with findings obtained in animal models. The ejection fraction has improved by aortic valve replacement for aortic stenosis (Spotnitz, 1982), but not for aortic insufficiency (Ren et al, 1985). Similarly, the ejection fraction falls after mitral valve replacement for mitral insufficiency (Ren et al, 1985; Spotnitz, 1982; Wong and Spotnitz, 1981). For unselected patients having coronary artery bypass grafting, the ejection fraction has been reported to change in either direction or to remain the same (Spotnitz, 1982).

Diastolic ventricular function has also been studied before and after cardioplegic arrest in patients. By relating left ventricular end-diastolic pressure to echocardiographically determined end-diastolic diameter, left ventricular compliance was unchanged by short periods of ischemia and decreased with longer periods of ischemia (Spotnitz et al, 1979).

The quantitation of regional myocardial wall motion abnormalities has been a very sensitive indicator of regional ischemia (Buda et al, 1986; Meltzer et al, 1979; Wyatt et al, 1981). Changes in regional systolic thickening have been closely correlated with regional blood flow in experimental preparations, although functional deficits tend to slightly overestimate infarct size (Buda et al, 1986). These regions, when identified at coronary operative procedures, have improved immediately after revascularization (Topol et al, 1984). This method may be more applicable in patients having coronary artery procedures, when nonuniform systolic function is expected (Heger et al, 1980; Omoto et al, 1982). However, translational artifacts can obscure the results (Waggoner et al, 1982).

The sensitivity of echocardiography in detecting regional wall motion abnormalities has been applied in the development of exercise echocardiography. With exercise, developed regional wall motion abnormalities have correlated with the number and location of coronary arterial stenoses (Armstrong et al, 1987). This noninvasive method may become a useful screening procedure and may become critical

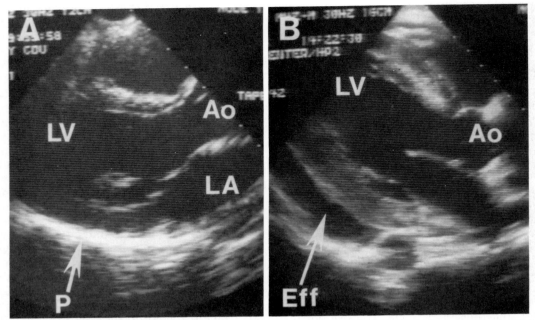

Figure 31–95. A long-axis parasternal, 2D echocardiogram. *A,* Normal cardiac structure and absence of pericardial effusion are noted. (LV = left ventricle; Ao = aorta; LA = left atrium; P = pericardium.) A large posterior pericardial effusion is shown in a similarly oriented 2D echocardiogram (Eff = effusion).

in identifying *physiologically significant* coronary disease.

Valvular insufficiency can also be detected by using an adjunctive echo-contrast agent and 2D echocardiography. Simple saline solutions, when agitated, produce relatively large microbubbles that are readily imaged. After intracardiac injection, regurgitant lesions are easily identified. This technique has been widely applied, particularly after valve reconstruction. It has been replaced mainly by the introduction of color-flow Doppler echocardiography.

Cardiac Structure

Two-dimensional echocardiography has been particularly useful in the recognition of abnormalities of intracardiac structure and is the method of choice for evaluation of pericardial effusion (Fig. 31–95), for intraoperative localization of foreign bodies (Figs. 31–96 and 31–97) (Hassett et al, 1986; Sakai et al, 1984), and for assessing cardiac tumors (Effert and Domanig, 1959).

Mural thrombi associated with myocardial in-

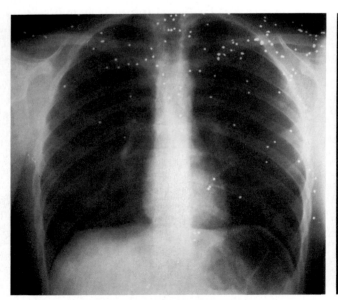
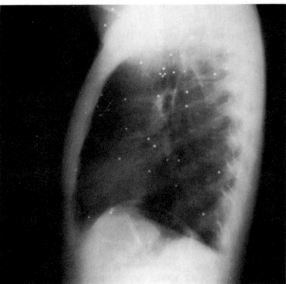

Figure 31–96. Posteroanterior and lateral chest films of a patient who sustained a shotgun wound to the thorax. Several of the projectiles appear to involve the heart.

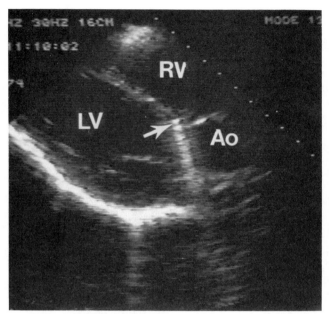

Figure 31–97. Two-dimensional echocardiography (same patient as Fig. 31–96) confirms the presence of a single pellet within the ventricular septum near the aortic valve, seen in the parasternal long-axis view. This patient had a newly developed conduction abnormality in association with this injury. (RV = right ventricle; LV = left ventricle; Ao = aorta.)

farction can be studied by using 2D echocardiography (Fig. 31–98). Applied transthoracically, the technique has a sensitivity of 77 to 92% and a specificity of 84 to 94% (Ezekowitz et al, 1982; Stratton et al, 1983; Visser et al, 1983), but an adequate study can be obtained in only 75% of patients (Ezekowitz et al, 1982). The relationship of echocardiographically identified mural thrombi and embolization is by no means certain, however (Ezekowitz, 1985). Further developments in the tissue characterization potential of ultrasound, combined with intraoperative studies during coronary bypass grafting for acute myocardial infarction, may clarify this relationship.

Two-dimensional echocardiography has been used extensively in congenital heart operations (Gussenhoven et al, 1987) and was initially applied to evaluate the degree of right ventricular outflow tract obstruction in tetralogy of Fallot (Spotnitz et al, 1978). In the pediatric age group, the small size of the subjects allows the use of higher-frequency transducers with consequent better resolution of the intracardiac structures. Direct measurements of pulmonary artery dimension have been used for prognostic information (Lappen et al, 1983; Snider et al, 1984), and even structures as small as a patent ductus arteriosus can be directly imaged in 90 to 100% of patients (Huhta et al, 1984; Sahn et al, 1978; Vick et al, 1985). When used intraoperatively, the technique often yields additional diagnostic information and permits an accurate assessment of the operative results at the time of weaning from cardiopulmonary bypass.

With the injection of intracavitary microbubbles, 2D echocardiography has been used to detect intracardiac shunts, confirm the preoperative diagnoses, and verify operative repair. In preoperative evaluation, microbubbles can be injected in an arm vein to detect right-to-left shunts or bidirectional shunts at the atrial and ventricular level. In addition, a left arm vein injection provides an easy method to show a persistent left superior vena cava.

Two-dimensional echocardiography permits a high-resolution evaluation of the intracardiac structures. In endocarditis, echocardiography has been particularly useful in the identification of valvular vegetations, valve destruction, and the development of intramyocardial or annular abscesses. The sensitivity for vegetations in endocarditis is 80 to 85% (Martin et al, 1980), but it does not necessarily follow that the presence of a vegetation is an indication for operative intervention or that the disappearance of vegetation is indicative of embolization. Only 32 to 50% of patients with echocardiographically demonstrated vegetations eventually require operation (Martin et al, 1980; Stewart et al, 1980). In complicated cases of endocarditis, it can provide detailed information regarding abscess and fistula formation that is not apparent at cardiac catheterization (Figs. 31–99 and 31–100) (Bardy et al, 1982; van Herwerden et al, 1987).

Two-dimensional echocardiography is sensitive in the detection of intracardiac air bubbles associated with cardiopulmonary bypass or with cardiotomy (Krebber et al, 1982). Air bubbles are identified within the cardiac chambers in 14 to 67% of patients having cardiopulmonary bypass for either coronary artery bypass grafting or valve replacement (Rodigas et al,

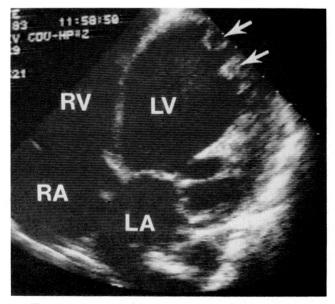

Figure 31–98. Apical long-axis echocardiogram that clearly demonstrates two large apical thrombi *(arrows)*. (LV = left ventricle; RV = right ventricle; RA = right atrium; LA = left atrium.)

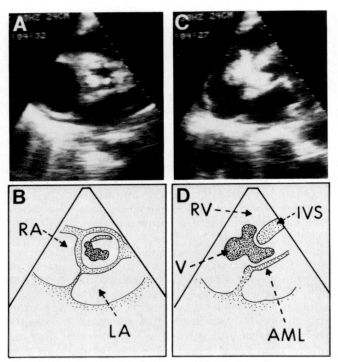

Figure 31–99. Two-dimensional echocardiographic image in the parasternal short-axis view of the aortic root (A) and accompanying schematic diagram (B). The vegetation (V) is heavily stippled and within the aortic root. C, A tangential view is obtained through the aortic root and proximal interventricular septum (IVS). As can be seen in the accompanying schematic (D), fistulous tracts surrounding the vegetation are suggested. (AML = anterior mitral leaflet; LA = left atrium; RA = right atrium; RV = right ventricle.) (From Bardy, G. H., Valenstein, P., Stack, R. S., et al: Two-dimensional echocardiographic identification of sinus of Valsalva-right heart fistula due to infective endocarditis. Am. Heart J., 103:1068, 1982.)

1982; Spotnitz, 1982). Although "echocardiographic bubbles" can cause concern, there has been no correlation between their presence and neurologic outcome (Diehl et al, 1987; Topol et al, 1985). Nonetheless, echocardiographic guidance can be used to assist in transcardiac or trans-septal needle aspiration in the operating room (Diehl et al, 1987).

The development of high-frequency transducers has improved resolution to the extent that human coronary arteries can be visualized directly in the operating room (Hiratzka et al, 1986a, 1986b, 1987; Johnson et al, 1988; Sahn et al, 1982) and even through the chest wall (Douglas et al, 1988; Weyman et al, 1976). A high degree of correlation (r = 0.91) between coronary arterial lumen size at echocardiography and at cardiac catheterization has been found (Sahn et al, 1982). The accurate characterization of stenotic lesions is more difficult when extensive calcification is present. By using a 12-mHz transducer, it is possible to show coronary bypass graft anastomotic defects that might not otherwise be recognized and later to confirm intraoperative correction. Additionally, these probes are capable of

locating intramyocardial coronary arteries that may otherwise be difficult to identify (Hiratzka et al, 1986a, 1986b, 1987; Johnson et al, 1988). It is possible that these methods may replace currently available, highly empiric methods to determine the effectiveness of myocardial revascularization intraoperatively.

The ease of application of this method and its relatively recent introduction have led to numerous isolated and promising applications that have not yet become incorporated into the standards of surgical care. For example, 2D echocardiography has been advanced as a method to evaluate the operative correction of idiopathic hypertrophic subaortic stenosis (Syracuse et al, 1978), and it has been used to

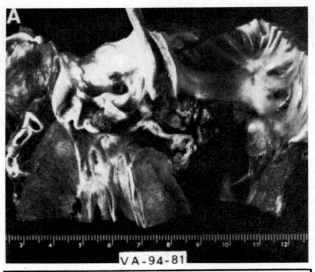

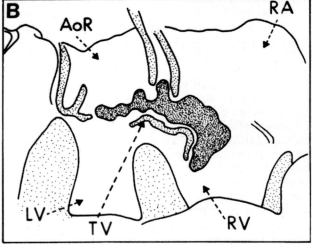

Figure 31–100. Gross pathologic specimen (A) showing the relationship of the large vegetation to the aortic root (AoR), right atrium (RA), right ventricle (RV), tricuspid valve (TV), and left ventricle (LV) in relation to a schematic drawing in B. The fistulous tracts surround the vegetation and extend through the interventricular system and aortic wall. (From Bardy, G. H., Valenstein, D., Stack, R. S., et al: Two-dimensional echocardiographic identification of sinus of Valsalva-right heart fistula due to infective endocarditis. Am. Heart J., 103:1068, 1982.)

evaluate prosthetic strut encroachment after mitral valve replacement (Spotnitz, 1982). In the latter case, both high- and low-profile prosthetic valves produce severe acoustic artifacts by effectively blocking a large portion of the ultrasound energy. Ventricular pseudoaneurysms secondary to myocardial infarction have been delineated noninvasively and appropriately treated surgically after ultrasound diagnosis (Adamick et al, 1986; Hamilton et al, 1985).

Echocardiography has been used to calculate the overall mass of the left ventricle (Wyatt et al, 1979). Ventricular mass has been monitored in cardiac transplant recipients and has been correlated with transplant rejection (Sagar et al, 1980). Nonetheless, this method has been no more specific than other noninvasive methods, and percutaneous transvenous endomyocardial biopsy has remained the standard method for post-transplant follow-up. Ultrasound may still have a role in this area because it is highly effective in guiding transvenous manipulation of the bioptome (French et al, 1983). By using 2D echocardiography instead of fluoroscopy, both the patient and the surgeon or cardiologist are protected from cumulative radiation hazard. Endomyocardial biopsy can then be accomplished in various locations with portable echocardiography and is not restricted to a specially equipped operating room. Additional attractive features of this method are the simultaneous determination of ventricular function, protection of the tricuspid valve apparatus from injury, and, as described later, noninvasive determination of pulmonary artery pressure and cardiac output. In a similar manner, echocardiography has been an effective aid in transvenous pacemaker placement (Ren et al, 1987) and in pericardiocentesis (Pandian et al, 1988).

PULSED AND CONTINUOUS-WAVE DOPPLER ECHOCARDIOGRAPHY: CLINICAL APPLICATIONS

The use of pulsed Doppler in combination with 2D echocardiography results in the ability to *quantitate* intracardiac blood velocity in a precisely defined anatomic location. Continuous-wave Doppler can then be used to extend the detectable velocity limit, accepting some ambiguity as to location of velocity along the acoustic pathway. Doppler echocardiography has become most accepted in congenital heart procedures in which it can be used to determine the patency of Blalock-Taussig shunts (Stevenson et al, 1983) and has been 96% sensitive and 100% specific for the presence of a patent ductus arteriosus (Stevenson et al, 1980).

As described earlier, blood velocity across a regurgitant valve can be used to estimate the transvalvular pressure gradient. The gradient in tricuspid regurgitation has been used to estimate right ventricular systolic pressure (and, in the absence of pul-

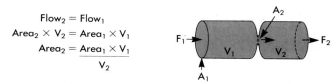

Continuity Equation

$$Flow_2 = Flow_1$$
$$Area_2 \times V_2 = Area_1 \times V_1$$
$$Area_2 = \frac{Area_1 \times V_1}{V_2}$$

Figure 31–101. The continuity equation assumes that total volume flow before and after a stenotic lesion are equal ($Flow_2 = Flow_1$). Flow is equal to area × velocity, assuming that the velocity profile is flat. In this example, Area 2 (A_2) represents a significant stenosis, and Area 1 (A_1) the area just preceding the stenosis. V_1 is the velocity just before reaching the stenosis (within Area 1), and V_2 represents the velocity within the zone of stenosis (A_2). Area 1 can be calculated using 2D echocardiography, and both velocities calculated using Doppler echocardiography. Solving the equation for Area 2 yields the effective stenotic orifice area, which may be too geometrically complex to determine by 2D echocardiography. (From Kisslo, J., and Adams, D. B.: An Introduction to Doppler Echocardiography, Vol. 2. New York, Medi Cine Productions, 1987.)

monic stenosis, systolic pulmonary artery pressure) by calculation with a clinical estimate of the central venous pressure (or right atrial pressure) (Chan et al, 1987; Masuyama et al, 1986).

By using the continuity equation, actual valve areas can also be estimated from multiple-gated Doppler velocities along the transvalvular blood path (Figs. 31–101 and 31–102) (Richards et al, 1986). These quantitative estimates have been used to evaluate numerous surgical conditions, such as aortic stenosis (Fig. 31–103), mitral stenosis, pulmonary hypertension, idiopathic hypertrophic subaortic stenosis, and congenital heart disease (Williams et al, 1987). Cardiac tamponade has been associated with a sharp increase in Doppler flow velocity across the pulmo-

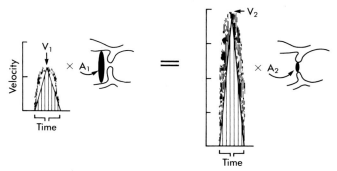

Continuity

Figure 31–102. In this example, continuity equation is used to calculate valvular stenotic area (A_2). A_1 is easily determined by 2D echocardiography, and V_1 and V_2 with pulsed Doppler. In practice, V_1 may be obtained with pulsed Doppler, and V_2 by continuous-wave Doppler. In this case, a nearly fourfold increase in velocity results from flow through the stenotic area. (From Kisslo, J., and Adams, D. B.: An Introduction to Doppler Echocardiography, Vol. 2. New York, Medi Cine Productions, 1987.)

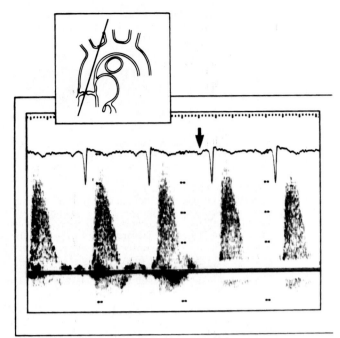

Figure 31–103. A typical continuous-wave Doppler recording from a patient with aortic stenosis. The ultrasound beam is directed from the suprasternal notch, and the acoustic pathway incorporates the ascending aorta, aortic valve orifice, and left ventricular outflow tract. The velocity profile shows a great degree of variance and high velocity (4 m/sec). A baseline filter *(arrow)* is turned on to remove low-velocity noise. (From Kisslo, J., and Adams, D. B.: An Introduction to Doppler Echocardiography, Vol. 1. New York, Medi Cine Productions, 1987.)

nary and tricuspid valves associated with inspiration, combined with a decrease in flow across the aortic and mitral valves. These transvalvular velocities, and the clinical syndrome, have been shown to reverse with therapy (Leeman et al, 1988).

Continuous cardiac output determination has also been made possible by measuring velocity in the ascending aorta and calculating its instantaneous diameter by using 2D echocardiography (Mark et al, 1986).

Specifically designed Doppler probes have been attached to the ascending aorta at the time of heart procedures and have been safely removed percutaneously. By using a single echocardiographic measure of aortic diameter, the velocity was converted to calculate flow continuously in the postoperative period in 20 patients (Svennevig et al, 1986).

Specific intraoperative applications of Doppler echocardiography include detection of postreparative valve area, determination of residual valvular regurgitation or residual shunts (when high-velocity residua are found, the defects are usually inconsequential), and precise localization of coronary arteriovenous fistulas (Miyatake et al, 1984).

Doppler velocitometry has been useful in the surgical management of coronary artery disease, both clinically and on a clinical research basis. Initially used transthoracically to determine left internal

mammary-coronary artery bypass graft patency (Benchimol et al, 1978), this method was introduced in the operating room by Marcus and co-workers (1981). These investigators developed a Doppler probe that can be reversibly attached to the epicardial surface of the heart by suction and that reliably measures coronary velocity in epicardial coronary arteries. In humans, this instrument was used to determine the reactive hyperemic response after occlusion (20 seconds) of both normal and diseased coronary arteries. This measure of physiologic significance correlated poorly with visual interpretation of the coronary arteriogram (Marcus et al, 1986; White et al, 1984). Even with a computer-assisted definition of the anatomic extent of coronary disease at cardiac catheterization, a poor correlation with reactive hyperemia has been found (Wilson et al, 1987), unless there is very limited coronary disease (Wilson et al, 1987). This method has also been applied to performance of coronary bypass grafting without angiography in a single case of severe adverse dye reaction (Wright et al, 1987). Other physicians have modified the Doppler system to permit multiple-channel pulsed Doppler velocities to be measured in coronary arteries, thus extending its application to lesions that create a nonuniform velocity profile (Kajiya et al, 1986). The major advantage of this technique is the ability to accurately determine the zero velocity level and the fact that it can be done on undissected native coronary arteries. The major disadvantages include difficulty in measuring coronary velocity on posterior coronary arteries and inability to determine actual blood flow. Recent developments have enabled automatic determination of vessel diameter, which, combined with velocity, yields actual blood flow. Thus far, this can only be applied to coronary bypass grafts (Payen et al, 1986).

COLOR-FLOW DOPPLER ECHOCARDIOGRAPHY: CLINICAL APPLICATIONS

The development of real-time display of tomographic blood velocity, direction, and degree of turbulence has perhaps been the single most significant recent advance in echocardiography. This information, color coded and displayed by superimposition on the 2D echocardiograph, is now called color-flow Doppler echocardiography and was introduced by Omoto and others with the development of a new autocorrelator (Bommer et al, 1982; Namekawa et al, 1982; Omoto et al, 1984). Their initial report on 72 patients with acquired valvular heart disease showed that color-flow imaging provides a useful estimate of valve dysfunction, particularly regurgitation (Omoto et al, 1984). Examples of aortic insufficiency (see Fig. 31–104, color plate) and mitral insufficiency (see Fig. 31–105, color plate) show the sensitivity of this technique.

This technique has been highly sensitive and specific in the accurate localization of valvular regurgitation and intracardiac shunts. In congenital heart disease, color-flow imaging has been routinely applied in the operating room at several institutions (Hagler et al, 1988; Takamoto et al, 1985), including Duke University Medical Center. The preoperative diagnosis of an atrial septal defect is shown in Figure 31–106 (see color plate).

In the Mayo Clinic series, 21 residual lesions were diagnosed intraoperatively in 30 patients. In Duke's series, the intraoperative color-flow findings were useful in modifying the preoperative diagnosis and in correcting significant residual defects at the time of the original operation (see Figs. 31–107 and 31–108, color plates).

Surgeons using reparative techniques for mitral regurgitation have found color-flow imaging to provide an accurate intraoperative evaluation both before and after repair. Analysis of the image by the operating surgeon often clarifies specific portions of the mitral valve apparatus that are defective and adds an important perspective to direct examination of the mitral valve during cardioplegic arrest. This technique has a sensitivity of 94% and specificity of 93% for detecting the presence or absence of mitral regurgitation (Czer et al, 1987), and it can be relied on to confirm valve repair. In addition, it has great promise for elucidating the mechanisms of mitral regurgitation associated with myocardial infarction and coronary artery disease (Izumi et al, 1987).

Recent specific uses of color-flow echocardiography presage wide application. It has been used in the identification of aortic root abscesses associated with fistulization (Fisher et al, 1987). Color-flow imaging has been applied in the diagnosis and management of aortic dissection (Iliceto et al, 1987; Omoto et al, 1987). Its value for precisely localizing the intimal flap at the time of operation may alter traditional operative approaches. Intraoperative confirmation of aortic valve sufficiency (see Figs. 31–109 and 31–110, color plates) and identification of anastomotic leaks have also been beneficial. The evolution of color-flow systems for transesophageal echocardiography may have a significant impact on current algorithms for preoperative diagnosis of this lesion.

Despite the numerous advantages of color-flow echocardiography, its clinical role is still rapidly evolving. The main drawbacks at this stage are the limitations in frame rate imposed by the sheer volume of data acquired (making examinations at fast heart rate difficult) and the fact that it is so sensitive. The differentiation between color-flow disorders and clinically significant disorders will require reference to pulsed or continuous-wave Doppler findings, as well as further experience.

TRANSESOPHAGEAL ECHOCARDIOGRAPHY: DEVELOPMENT AND CLINICAL APPLICATIONS

The development of transesophageal echocardiography has greatly increased the use of echocardiographic examinations in the operating room. By placing the transducer within the esophagus, the amount of tissue intervening between the transducer and the heart is greatly reduced, particularly in the supine position (Fig. 31–111). In addition, examinations can be done in patients with barrel chests, chronic obstructive pulmonary disease, or obesity, when transthoracic acoustic pathways are not available. By placing the ultrasound transducer at the tip of a flexible gastroscope, the image plane can be easily controlled (Fig. 31–112).

The reduction of transducer size, while maintaining state-of-the-art imaging features, has been critical to the development of transesophageal echocardiography. In 1976, Frazin and co-workers, by using a 19 × 13 × 6-mm transducer, obtained M-mode transesophageal echocardiograms. Initial real-time transesophageal 2D images were obtained by Hisanaga and associates (1980) by using a mechanically rotating transducer. This technique has mainly been replaced by the introduction of miniature phased-array ultrasound transducers (Schluter et al, 1982). Although the procedure was initially developed by cardiologists for use in awake patients, its predominant application today is in the operating room under the control of the anesthesiologist

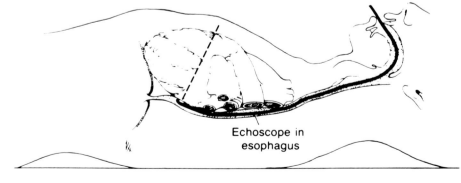

Figure 31–111. Transducer position for a short-axis view of the left ventricle during transesophageal echocardiography. (From DeBruijn, N. P., and Clements, F. M. [eds]: Transesophageal Echocardiography. Boston, Martinus Nijhoff Publishing, 1987, p. 6)

Echoscope in esophagus

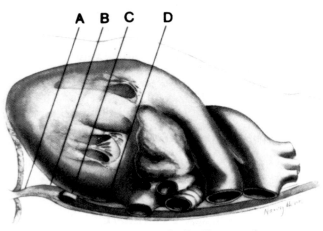

A. Apical

B. Low left ventricular

C. Papillary muscles

D. Mitral valve leaflets

Figure 31–112. In transesophageal echocardiography, the gastroscope can be manipulated along the length of the esophagus and the tip can be flexed to acquire these four typical short-axis views of the heart. (From DeBruijn, N. P., and Clements, F. M. [eds]: Transesophageal Echocardiography. Boston, Martinus Nijhoff Publishing, 1987, p. 36)

(DeBruijn et al, 1987a). In this setting, it has been safe in patients without manifestations of esophageal disease.

Although transesophageal echocardiography is useful for diagnostic purposes, its ability to display various cardiac dimensions continuously without intruding on the operation has provided a unique monitoring ability. Under the control of anesthesiologists, it has supplied information that was previously unavailable to them despite direct observation of the heart or communication with the surgeon. The addition of color-flow mapping to this equipment has provided physiologic information that was previously unavailable unless the cardiac surgeon was a devoted echocardiographer. These factors have led to a highly cooperative endeavor between operating and nonoperating physicians in the overall management of cardiac surgical patients and are certain to have a positive impact greater than the actual technology available to each.

The continuous monitoring of ventricular function is accomplished by several methods. Regional wall motion abnormalities indicative of ischemia can be directly observed by using transesophageal echocardiography (see Figs. 31–113 and 31–114, color plates) (DeBruijn et al, 1987a). This can be particularly helpful for identifying ventricular septal abnormalities (Corya et al, 1981) and appears to be a more effective monitoring technique than continuous electrocardiography (Smith et al, 1985). Although regional systolic thickening can be quantitatively analyzed fairly easily, simple observation by the anesthesiologist has been easily learned and relatively independent of interobserver variability (Clements et al, 1986). Regional wall motion abnormalities

thus detected have responded appropriately both to alterations in anesthetic management and to revascularization (DeBruijn et al, 1987b). Transesophageal echocardiography has also been used to optimize ventricular function as it is affected by preload and afterload. These aspects of the overall management of cardiac surgical patients are amenable to quantitation by determining atrial volume (Matsuzaki et al, 1985) and end-diastolic left ventricular area (DeBruijn et al, 1987b). In the setting of frequent alterations in left ventricular compliance, these data have provided useful supplemental information in the assessment of intracardiac pressures. The continuous availability of left ventricular global dimensions and wall thickness also permits calculation of wall stress (DeBruijn et al, 1987b). Thus, specific manipulations can be done to optimize preload and afterload and to monitor efficacy of therapy.

The addition of color-flow capabilities to the transesophageal transducer has added utility to this technique. All applications of transthoracic or epicardial color-flow echocardiography can be similarly made with transesophageal echocardiography, with minimal if any loss of image resolution. Images of the left atrium, mitral valve apparatus, and great vessels may be superior because of their proximity to the transducer. A large number of groups are now routinely applying transesophageal echocardiography during cardiac operations, to such an extent that equipment availability may become a limiting factor (Beaupre et al, 1984; DeBruijn et al, 1987a; Kyo et al, 1987; Smith et al, 1985). Transesophageal echocardiography has also been used to monitor cardiac function in patients having noncardiac procedures, particularly during vascular surgery when the thoracic or abdominal aorta must be occluded. The detection of regional wall motion abnormalities in response to increased wall stress has been shown to respond to specific modifications of anesthetic technique to the patient's benefit (DeBruijn et al, 1987b; Gewertz et al, 1987).

FUTURE DIRECTIONS
Tissue Characterization

Detailed analysis of the myocardial image holds promise for the specific detection and diagnosis of intrinsic structural damage. Early attempts to quantify these changes and associate them with pathologic material (Tanaka and Terasawa, 1979) were complicated by poor resolving capacity and the need to assess transmission rather than reflection of ultrasound (Stefan et al, 1972; Tanaka and Terasawa 1979; von Ramm and Thurstone, 1979; Weiss et al, 1981; Wyatt et al, 1979). Ultrasound was capable of showing only large differences, such as between normal myocardium and myocardium late after infarction. In addition, the images often represent tertiary data that have been log compressed, manipulated in order to enhance boundaries, and in general processed to "please the eye." The resultant data loss, which was beyond the control of clinical investigators, precluded vigorous interpretation. Computer analysis of the average gray level in animal preparations of coronary occlusion has shown great difficulty in distinguishing abnormal regions from normal regions under conditions that are approximate to those found clinically (Skorton et al, 1983).

In the laboratory, the measurement of ultrasonic integrated back scatter, which measures reflected rather than transmitted ultrasound, has been closely correlated with ischemia at 1 and 6 hours. This is thought to result from an increase in tissue fluid content and contributions of formed elements in the blood (Mimbs et al, 1981).

Methods using analysis of the raw radiofrequency signal, such as time-averaged integrated back scatter (Sagar et al, 1987), real-time integrated back scatter (Thomas et al, 1986), and the mean amplitude/standard deviation of the amplitude (Schnittger et al, 1985) have shown promise in the early identification of ischemic areas (Fig. 31–115). Internal calibration and the need for normal reference tissue often result in obstacles to clinical application (Rasmussen et al, 1984). Cyclic variations in the cardiac cycle ranging from 5 to 10 dB present obstacles to tissue characterization without enhancement (Thomas et al, 1986). The loss of cyclic variation during isometric contraction suggests that the physical arrangement of structures within the tissue may have an important role (Sagar et al, 1987; Wear et al, 1986). Cyclic back scatter power decreases with ischemia but returns toward normal within 5 hours, but it is unable to be used alone to distinguish normal from abnormal myocardium (Fitzgerald et al, 1987). The Fourier coefficient of the amplitude modulation

has been useful in analyzing the cardiac cycle-dependent changes in back scatter (Sagar et al, 1988). In addition to the assessment of myocardial ischemia, back scatter analysis has aided in the early recognition of cardiac transplant rejection in an animal model and may have a potential clinical role (Chandrasekaran et al, 1987).

Determination of Regional Perfusion

Advances in tissue characterization are dependent on similar advances in equipment to distinguish fine changes related to the cardiac cycle and to microscopic characteristics of the tissue. An alternative method is to provide enhancement of the tissue in relationship to its blood supply, which has been accomplished with the development of intravascular microbubbles to act as reflectors specific for regional perfusion. First noted by Gramiak and Shah (1968), contrast enhancement was initially obtained by the forceful injection of indocyanine green. A host of additional contrast agents have been used, such as hydrogen peroxide (Armstrong et al, 1984; Kemper et al, 1983), gelatin-encapsulated microbubbles (Armstrong et al, 1982), and hand-agitated saline or Renografin 76 (Maurer et al, 1984; Taylor et al, 1985). The main disadvantages of these agents have been their relatively short half-lives, large particle size resulting in embolization rather than true perfusion, and large variance in microbubble size. A significant advance in this area has been made by Feinstein and colleagues (1984), who developed a method to sonicate Renografin 76 to yield a uniform microbubble solution in which the average bubble size was less than that of a red blood cell. They have been able to show that these particles traverse the capillary network in a manner similar to red blood cells (Feinstein et al, 1984). They and others have investigated the use of this agent in myocardial perfusion studies in animal models (Lang et al, 1987; Tei et al, 1983) and have shown it to be safe in human application (Feinstein et al, 1986). The more recent development of a stable albumin microbubble with similar size distribution holds great promise for physiologic measurements with 2D echocardiography (Feinstein et al, 1986). This contrast agent is capable of transpulmonary passage and may enable investigators to examine regional myocardial perfusion after arm vein injection.

Through the use of intravascular agents, regional brightness changes over time after intravascular administration in relationship to regional perfusion. The enhanced back scatter related to the presence of microbubbles is more easily shown with commercially available equipment. Analysis of these images and the time domain provides a useful estimate of regional perfusion (Ong et al, 1984), although quantitation of that perfusion remains problematic. Despite this, there is abundant evidence that such contrast enhancement can be a useful method of

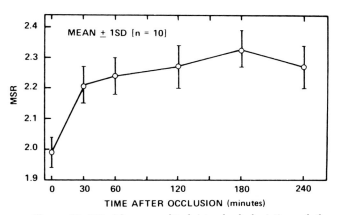

Figure 31–115. Mean amplitude/standard deviation of the amplitude (MSR) of the unprocessed ultrasound radiofrequency signal returned from myocardium supplied by the left anterior descending (LAD) coronary artery, showing a significant increase in this parameter over time after LAD occlusion. (From Schnittger, I., Vieli, A., Heiserman, J. E., et al: Ultrasonic tissue characterization: Detection of acute myocardial ischemia in dogs. Circulation, 72:193, 1985. By permission of the American Heart Association, Inc.)

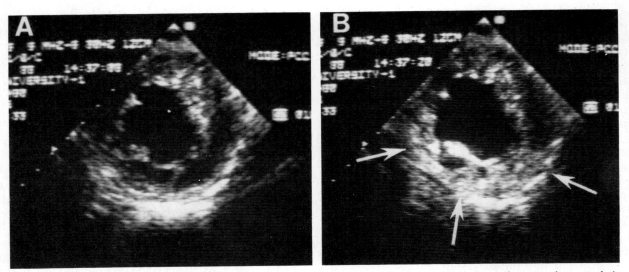

Figure 31–116. *A,* Intraoperative short-axis 2D echocardiogram done epicardially on cardiopulmonary bypass, after completion of three saphenous vein bypass grafts. *B,* After the injection of 2 ml of sonicated Renografin 76 into the graft supplying the dominant right coronary artery. Note the contrast enhancement of the posterior septum and posterior left ventricle *(arrows),* indicating excellent bypass graft function.

identifying the area at risk after coronary occlusion in animal preparations. In the operating room, it is a simple matter to inject sonicated Renografin into coronary artery bypass grafts before weaning from cardiopulmonary bypass. Two-dimensional echocardiography then reveals the tomographic region of the heart supplied by each graft, and a qualitative measure of the perfusion rate can be determined by observing the clearance rate of the agent (Fig. 31–116).

ECHOCARDIOGRAPHY: OPERATIVE PROCEDURES WITHOUT CARDIAC CATHETERIZATION

The advances in echocardiography described earlier, the anticipation of further improvement in resolution, and the development of contrast agents capable of peripheral venous injection raise the question of the degree to which echocardiography can be depended on to replace cardiac catheterization for preoperative evaluation of surgical patients. The broad institution of such an approach would be less expensive than cardiac catheterization and in some cases may reduce the overall risk to the patient of surgical correction.

This approach was initially undertaken in valvular heart disease (St. John Sutton, 1981) and was applied in approximately 75% of cases without adverse effects on the outcome for patients (Borow et al, 1983; Motro and Neufeld, 1980; St. John Sutton et al, 1981).

Through the use of a detailed clinical history and physical examination, as well as routine roent-

genographic and laboratory investigation, approximately 25% of patients with valvular heart disease still require cardiac catheterization preoperatively. Thus, at this time, it appears to be possible to select a population in which cardiac catheterization can be avoided.

In cases of cardiac trauma, the surgeon is often confronted with a critically ill patient requiring emergent operation. Intraoperative echocardiography has been used successfully to assess intracardiac trauma after life-threatening problems have been solved (see Fig. 31–117, color plate). Through intraoperative diagnosis, postoperative cardiac catheterization and delayed corrective procedures can be avoided.

In congenital heart disease, the policy of selective cardiac catheterization is becoming widespread, probably because of the increased risk of cardiac catheterization in this setting. The low incidence of coronary artery abnormalities in this age group also tends to make cardiac catheterization less often necessary (Krabill et al, 1987). A large variety of disorders, as outlined earlier, are suitable for definitive diagnosis by echocardiographic techniques with a high degree of specificity (Freed et al, 1984; Gutgesell et al, 1985); (Macartney, 1983; Rice et al, 1983; Stark et al, 1983). In a review of 100 patients operated on for congenital heart defects without cardiac catheterization, there was a trend toward lower mortality when cardiac catheterization could be avoided (Huhta et al, 1987). In some disorders, particularly left ventricular outflow tract obstruction, avoiding cardiac catheterization has definitely improved results. With the advent of more liberally applied intraoperative echocardiography, this diagnostic method can be used throughout the procedure to further refine its specificity and to guide the operative procedure in the absence of cardiac catheterization.

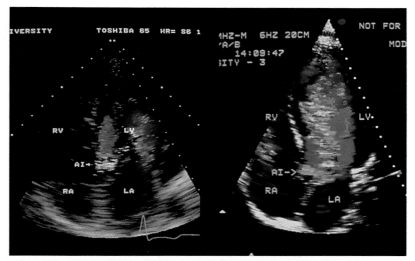

Figure 31-104

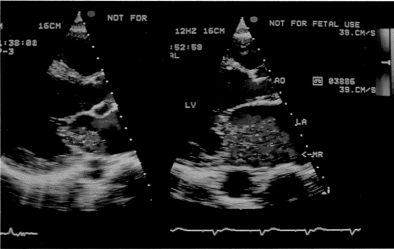

Figure 31-105

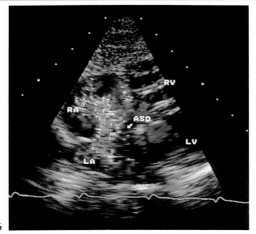

Figure 31-106

Figure 31-104. Two patients with aortic insufficiency. One is small in degree (left), and the other larger (right). The mosaic of colors indicates the regurgitant jet.

Figure 31-105. Two patients with mitral regurgitation. One is small in degree (left), and the other is large (right).

Figure 31-106. Subcostal view of all four cardiac chambers showing a massive interatrial flow communication.

PLATE 1

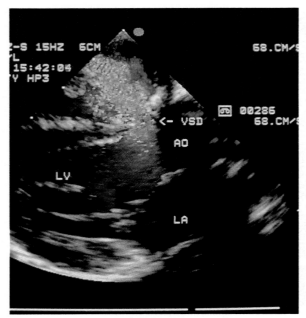

Figure 31–107

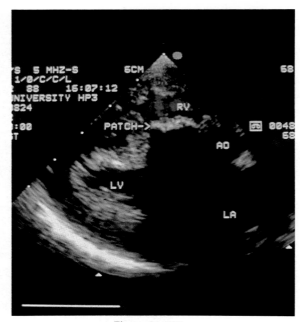

Figure 31–108

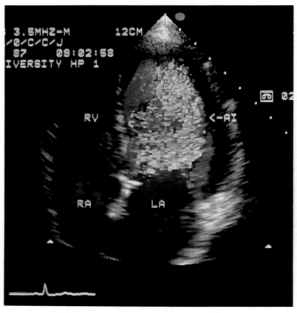

Figure 31–109

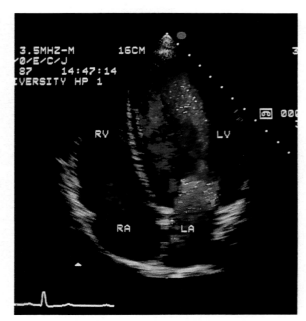

Figure 31–110

Figure 31–107. Pre-cardiopulmonary bypass evaluation of a child with a large ventricular septal defect. The study was done epicardially.

Figure 31–108. Postcardiopulmonary bypass epicardial scan showing the patch repair and no residual VSD.

Figure 31–109. Apical four-chamber image showing massive aortic insufficiency associated with an ascending aortic dissecting aneurysm.

Figure 31–110. Apical four-chamber image showing no aortic insufficiency after aortic valve resuspension.

PLATE 2

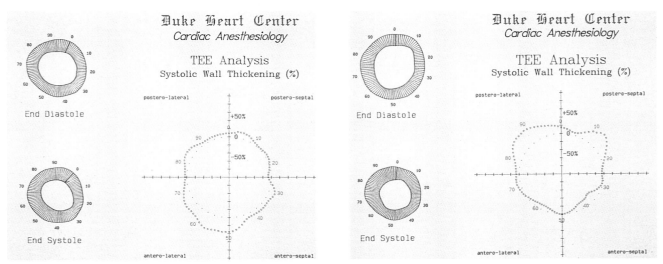

Figure 31–113

Figure 31–114

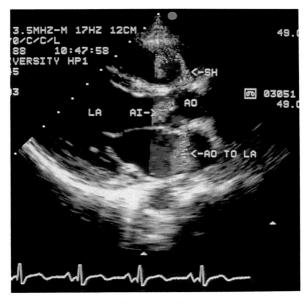

Figure 31–117

Figure 31–113. An example of transesophageal analysis of systolic wall thickening. Two hundred transmural chords are defined in end-diastole (upper left) and in end-systole (lower left). These results are normalized and graphically displayed for each chord on a polar coordinate system (right). A circle of unity (no change in chord length from diastole to systole) is marked by small dots and actual data points represented by small squares arrayed circumferentially as they would appear in a short-axis transesophageal view. In this example, most experimental data reside outside the circle of unity (green boxes), indicating systolic wall thickening. Systolic wall thinning (red boxes) is seen only in the mid-septum. (Courtesy of Dr. Thomas E. Stanley, III.)

Figure 31–114. In this example, there is anteroseptal and anterolateral systolic wall thinning, represented by data points (red boxes) falling within the circle of unity. Posteriorly, there appears to be a compensatory increase in systolic wall thickening (green boxes). (Courtesy of Dr. Thomas E. Stanley, III.)

Figure 31–117. Parasternal long axis view of a child shot in the chest at close range with an air gun. The child underwent emergency closure of a right ventricular perforation at another institution. No intraoperative or other evaluation was performed. The child was found to have a murmur following discharge. The echocardiogram shows an aorto–right ventricular shunt as well as an aorto–left atrial shunt. Aortic insufficiency from an aortic cusp perforation is also noted.

PLATE 3

SUMMARY

Recent advances in echocardiography have led to its more general application in the diagnosis and management of cardiac surgical problems. These developments have been technologic and have resulted in attitude changes that have made the technique valuable, if not essential, to surgeons.

With rapid advances in computer technology, it can be anticipated that this trend will continue. Three-dimensional echocardiography, digital image analysis, and automated data reduction to provide on-line indices of ventricular function and regional myocardial perfusion hold promise in increasing the clinical impact of ultrasound.

Selected Bibliography

DeBruijn, N. P., and Clements, F. M. (eds): Transesophageal Echocardiography. Boston, Martinus Nijhoff Publishing, 1987.

An excellent monograph that describes the historical aspects of the development of transesophageal echocardiography as well as its current application in the operating room. The monograph is extensively illustrated and contains an excellent description of the use of transesophageal echocardiography as a monitoring method in all types of operative procedures, particularly cardiac surgery.

Kisslo, J., and Adams, D. B. (eds): An Introduction to Doppler Echocardiography, Vols. 1–4. New York, Medi Cine Productions, 1987.

Vol. 1: Principles of Doppler Echocardiography and the Doppler Examination
Vol. 2: Doppler Evaluation of Valvular Regurgitation
Vol. 3: Doppler Evaluation of Valvular Stenosis
Vol. 4: Doppler Color-Flow Imaging

A series of monographs describing the principles of Doppler echocardiography. This series develops physical concepts of the Doppler effect as it is used in echocardiography in a comprehensive and easy-to-understand manner. There are numerous excellent illustrations (many in color) describing current applications of Doppler echocardiography. These monographs serve as an excellent resource for the novice, who can rapidly obtain a working knowledge of Doppler echocardiography in a short time.

Feigenbaum, H.: Echocardiography, 4th ed. Philadelphia, Lea & Febiger, 1986.

The comprehensive textbook on echocardiography. This excellent resource presents a full background on the physical properties of ultrasonography and reviews the historical development of all aspects of echocardiography. It is particularly strong in the area of two-dimensional echocardiography and covers early applications of color-flow echocardiography well.

Bibliography

Adamick, R., Sprecher, D., Coleman, R. E., and Kisslo, J.: Pseudoaneurysm of the left ventricle. Echocardiography, 3:237, 1986.
Armstrong, W. F., Mueller, T. M., Kinney, E. L., et al: Assessment of myocardial perfusion abnormalities with contrast-enhanced two-dimensional echocardiography. Circulation, 66:166, 1982.
Armstrong, W. F., O'Donnell, J., Ryan, T., and Feigenbaum, H.: Effect of prior myocardial infarction and extent and location of coronary disease on accuracy of exercise echocardiography. J. Am. Coll. Cardiol., 10:531, 1987.
Armstrong, W. F., West, S. R., Dillon, J. C., and Feigenbaum, H.: Assessment of location and size of myocardial infarction with contrast-enhanced echocardiography. II: Application of digital imaging techniques. J. Am. Coll. Cardiol., 4:141, 1984.
Bardy, G. H., Valenstein, P., Stack, R. S., et al: Two-dimensional echocardiographic identification of sinus of Valsalva-right heart fistula due to infective endocarditis. Am. Heart J., 103:1068, 1982.
Beaupre, P. N., Kremer, P. F., Cahalan, M. K., et al: Intraoperative detection of changes in left ventricular segmental wall motion by transesophageal two-dimensional echocardiography. Am. Heart J., 107:1021, 1984.
Benchimol, A., Reyns, P., Alvarez, S., et al: Non-invasive assessment of left internal mammary-coronary bypass patency using the external Doppler probe. Am. Heart J., 96:347, 1978.
Bommer, W., and Miller, L.: Real-time two-dimensional color-flow Doppler. Enhanced Doppler flow imaging in the diagnosis of cardiovascular diseases (Abstract). Am. J. Cardiol., 49:944, 1982.
Borow, K. M., Wynne, J., Sloss, L. J., et al: Noninvasive assessment of valvular heart disease: Surgery without catheterization. Am. Heart J., 106:443, 1983.
Buda, A. J., Zotz, R. J., and Gallagher, K. P.: Characterization of the functional border zone around regionally ischemic myocardium using circumferential flow-function maps. J. Am. Coll. Cardiol., 8:150, 1986.
Chan, K. L., Currie, P. J., Seward, J. B., et al: Comparison of three Doppler ultrasound methods in the prediction of pulmonary artery pressure. J. Am. Coll. Cardiol., 9:549, 1987.
Chandrasekaran, K., Bansal, R. C., Greenleaf, J. F., et al: Early recognition of heart transplant rejection by backscatter analysis from serial 2D echos in a heterotopic transplant model. J. Heart Transplant, 6:1, 1987.
Clements, F. M., Hill, R., Kisslo, J., and Orchard, R.: How easily can we learn to recognize regional wall motion abnormalities with 2-D transesophageal echocardiography? Proc. Soc. Cardiovasc. Anesthesiol. 7th Annual Meeting, Montreal, May 1986.
Corya, B. C., Phillips, J. F., Black, M. J., et al: Prevalence of regional left ventricular dysfunction in patients with coronary artery disease. Chest, 79:631, 1981.
Czer, L. S. C., Maurer, G., Bolger, A. F., et al: Intraoperative evaluation of mitral regurgitation by Doppler color flow mapping. Circulation, 76-III:108, 1987.
DeBruijn, N. P., and Clements, F. M.: Development of transesophageal echocardiography. In DeBruijn, N. P., and Clements, F. M. (eds): Transesophageal Echocardiography, Chapter 1. Boston, Martinus Nijhoff Publishing, 1987a.
DeBruijn, N. P. and Clements, F. M.: Clinical applications of 2D transesophageal echocardiography. In DeBruijn, N. P., and Clements, F. M. (eds): Transesophageal Echocardiography. Boston, Martinus Nijhoff Publishing, Chapter 4, 1987b.
Diehl, J. T., Ramos, D., Dougherty, F., et al: Intraoperative, two-dimensional echocardiography-guided removal of retained intracardiac air. Ann. Thorac. Surg., 43:674, 1987.
Douglas, P. S., Fiolkoski, J., Berko, B., and Reichek, N.: Echocardiographic visualization of coronary artery anatomy in the adult. J. Am. Coll. Cardiol., 11:565, 1988.
Ebina, T., Oka, S., Tanaka, M., et al: The ultrasono-tomography of the heart and great vessels in living human subjects by means of the ultrasonic reflection technique. Jpn. Heart J., 8:331, 1967.
Edler, I., and Hertz, C. H.: Use of ultrasonic reflectoscope for continuous recording of movement of heart walls. Kung Fysiogr Sallsk Lund Fordhandle, 24:40, 1954.
Effert, S., and Domanig, E.: The diagnosis of intra-atrial tumor and thrombi by the ultrasonic echo method. German Med. Mth., 4:1, 1959.
Ezekowitz, M. D.: Acute infarction, left ventricular thrombus and

systemic embolization: An approach to management. J. Am. Coll. Cardiol., 5:1281, 1985.

Ezekowitz, M. D., Wilson, D. A., Smith, E. O., et al: Comparison of indium-111 platelet scintigraphy and two-dimensional echocardiography in the diagnosis of left ventricular thrombi. N. Engl. J. Med., 306:1509, 1982.

Feigenbaum, H.: Echocardiography, 2nd ed. Philadelphia, Lea & Febiger, 1976.

Feigenbaum, H.: Echocardiography, 4th ed. Chapters 1 and 8. Philadelphia, Lea & Febiger, 1986.

Feigenbaum, H., Waldhausen, J. A., and Hyde, L. P.: Ultrasound diagnosis of pericardial effusion. J. Am. Coll. Cardiol., 191:107, 1965.

Feinstein, S. B.: Myocardial perfusion imaging: Contrast echocardiography today and tomorrow. J. Am. Coll. Cardiol., 8:251, 1986.

Feinstein, S. B., Lang, R. M., Dick, C., et al: Contrast echocardiographic perfusion studies in humans. Am. J. Cardiac Imaging, 1:29, 1986.

Feinstein, S. B., Shah, P. M., Bing, R. J., et al: Microbubble dynamics visualized in the intact capillary circulation. J. Am. Coll. Cardiol., 4:595, 1984.

Feinstein, S. B., Ten Cate, F. J., Zwehl, W., et al: 2D contrast echocardiography. I: In vitro development and quantitative analysis of echo contrast agents. J. Am. Coll. Cardiol., 3:14, 1984.

Fernando, H. A., Friedman, H. S., Lajam, F., and Sakurai, H.: Late cardiac tamponade following open-heart surgery: Detection by echocardiography. Ann. Thorac. Surg., 24:174, 1977.

Fisher, E. A., Estioko, M. R., Stern, E. H., and Goldman, M. E.: Left ventricular to left atrial communication secondary to a paraaortic abscess: Color flow Doppler documentation. J. Am. Coll. Cardiol., 10:222, 1987.

Fitzgerald, P. J., McDaniel, M. D., Rolett, E. L., et al: Two-dimensional ultrasonic tissue characterization: Backscatter power, endocardial wall motion, and their phase relationship for normal, ischemic, and infarcted myocardium. Circulation, 76:850, 1987.

Frazin, L., Talano, J. V., Stephanides, L., et al: Esophageal echocardiography. Circulation, 54:102, 1976.

Freed, M. D., Nadas, A. S., Norwood, W. I., and Castaneda, A. R.: Is routine preoperative cardiac catheterization necessary before repair of secundum and sinus venosus atrial septal defects? J. Am. Coll. Cardiol., 4:333, 1984.

French, J. W., Popp, R. L., and Pitlick, P. T.: Cardiac localization of transvascular bioptome using two-dimensional echocardiography. Am. J. Cardiol., 51:219, 1983.

Gaudiani, V. A., Shemin, R. J., Syracuse, D. C., et al: Continuous epicardial echocardiographic assessment of postoperative left ventricular function. J. Thorac. Cardiovasc. Surg., 76:64, 1978.

Gewertz, B. L., Kremser, P. C., Zarins, C. K., et al: Transesophageal echocardiographic monitoring of myocardial ischemia during vascular surgery. J. Vasc. Surg., 5:607, 1987.

Goldman, D. E., and Jueter, T. F.: Tabular data of the velocity and absorption of high-frequency sound in a million tissues. J. Acoust. Soc. Am., 28:35, 1956.

Goldman, M. E., Mora, F., Guarino, T., et al: Mitral valvuloplasty is superior to valve replacement for preservation of left ventricular function: An intraoperative two-dimensional echocardiographic study. J. Am. Coll. Cardiol., 10:568, 1987.

Gramiak, R., and Shah, P. M.: Echocardiography of the aortic root. Invest. Radiol., 3:356, 1968.

Gregg, E. C., and Palogallo, G. L.: Acoustic impedance of tissue. Invest. Radiol., 4:357, 1969.

Gussenhoven, E. J., vanHerwerden, L. A., Roelandt, J., et al: Intraoperative two-dimensional echocardiography in congenital heart disease. J. Am. Coll. Cardiol., 9:565, 1987.

Gutgesell, H. P., Huhta, J. C., Latson, L. A., et al: Accuracy of two-dimensional echocardiography in the diagnosis of congenital heart disease. Am. J. Cardiol., 55:514, 1985.

Hagler, D. J., Tajik, J., Seward, J. B., et al: Intraoperative two-dimensional Doppler echocardiography. A preliminary study for congenital heart disease. J. Thorac. Cardiovasc. Surg., 95:516, 1988.

Hamilton, K., Ellenbogen, K., Lowe, J. E., and Kisslo, J.: Ultrasound diagnosis of pseudoaneurysm and contiguous ventricular septal defect complicating inferior myocardial infarction. J. Am. Coll. Cardiol., 6:1160, 1985.

Harrison, L. H., Jr., Kisslo, J. A., Jr., and Sabiston, D. C., Jr.: Extraction of intramyocardial foreign body utilizing operative ultrasonography. J. Thorac. Cardiovasc. Surg., 82:345, 1981.

Hassett, A., Moran, J., Sabiston, D. C., and Kisslo, J.: Utility of echocardiography in the management of patients with penetrating missile wounds of the heart. J. Am. Coll. Cardiol., 7:1151, 1986.

Heger, J. J., Weyman, A. E., Wann, L. S., et al: Cross-sectional echocardiographic analysis of the extent of left ventricular asynergy in acute myocardial infarction. Circulation, 61:1113, 1980.

Hiratzka, L. F., McPherson, D. D., Lamberth, W. C., Jr., et al: Intraoperative evaluation of coronary artery bypass graft anastomoses with high-frequency epicardial echocardiography: Experimental validation and initial patient studies. Circulation, 73:1199, 1986a.

Hiratzka, L. F., McPherson, D. D., Brandt, B., III, et al: Intraoperative high-frequency epicardial echocardiography in coronary revascularization: Locating deeply embedded coronary arteries. Ann. Thorac. Surg., 42:S9, 1986b.

Hiratzka, L. F., McPherson, D. D., Brandt, B., III, et al: The role of intraoperative high-frequency epicardial echocardiography during coronary artery revascularization. Circulation, 76:V-33, 1987.

Hisanaga, K., Hisanaga, A., Hibi, N., et al: High speed rotating scanner for transesophageal cross-sectional echocardiography. Am. J. Cardiol., 46:837, 1980.

Huhta, J. C., Glascoe, P., Murphy, D. J., Jr., et al: Surgery without catheterization for congenital heart defects: Management of 100 patients. J. Am. Coll. Cardiol., 9:823, 1987.

Huhta, J. C., Gutgesell, H. P., Latson, L. A., and Huffines, F. D.: Two-dimensional echocardiographic assessment of the aorta in infants and children with congenital heart disease. Circulation, 70:417, 1984.

Iliceto, S., Nanda, N. C., Rizzon, P., et al: Color Doppler evaluation of aortic dissection. Circulation, 75:748, 1987.

Izumi, S., Miyatake, K., Beppu, S., et al: Mechanism of mitral regurgitation in patients with myocardial infarction: A study using real-time two-dimensional Doppler flow imaging and echocardiography. Circulation, 76:777, 1987.

Johnson, M. L., Holmes, J. H., Spangler, R. D., and Paton, B. C.: Usefulness of echocardiography in patients undergoing mitral valve surgery. J. Thorac. Cardiovasc. Surg., 64:922, 1972.

Johnson, M. R., McPherson, D. D., Fleagle, S. R., et al: Video-densitometric analysis of human coronary stenoses: Validation in vivo by intraoperative high-frequency epicardial echocardiography. Circulation, 77:328, 1988.

Kajiya, F., Ogasawara, Y., Tsujioka, K., et al: Evaluation of human coronary blood flow with an 80 channel 20 mHz pulsed Doppler velocimeter and zero-cross and Fourier transform methods during cardiac surgery. Circulation, 74-III:53, 1986.

Kemper, A. J., O'Boyle, J. E., Sharma, S., et al: Hydrogen peroxide contrast-enhanced two-dimensional echocardiography: Real-time in vivo delineation of regional myocardial perfusion. Circulation, 68:603, 1983.

Kisslo, J., and Adams, D. B.: An Introduction to Doppler Echocardiography. Vol. 1. Principles of Doppler Echocardiography and the Doppler Examination. New York, Medi Cine Productions, 1987a.

Kisslo, J., and Adams, D. B.: An Introduction to Doppler Echocardiography. Vol. 2. Doppler Evaluation of Valvular Regurgitation. New York, Medi Cine Productions, 1987b.

Kisslo, J., and Adams, D. B.: An Introduction to Doppler Echocardiography. Vol. 3. Doppler Evaluation of Valvular Stenosis. New York, Medi Cine Productions, 1987c.

Kisslo, J., and Adams, D. B.: An Introduction to Doppler Echocardiography. Vol. 4. Doppler Color-Flow Imaging. New York, Medi Cine Productions, 1987d.

Kossoff, G.: Diagnostic applications of ultrasound in cardiology. Aust. Radiol., 10:101, 1966.

Krabill, K. A., Ring, W. S., Foger, J. E., et al: Echocardiographic versus cardiac catheterization diagnosis of infants with congenital heart disease requiring cardiac surgery. Am. J. Cardiol., 60:351, 1987.

Krebber, H. J., Hanrath, P., Janzen, R., et al: Gas emboli during open heart surgery. Thorac. Cardiovasc. Surg., 30:401, 1982.

Kyo, S., Takamoto, S., Matsumura, M., et al: Immediate and early postoperative evaluation of results of cardiac surgery by transesophageal two-dimensional Doppler echocardiography. Circulation, 76:V-113, 1987.

Lang, R. M., Borow, K. M., Neumann, A., and Feinstein, S. B.: Echocardiographic contrast agents: Effect of microbubbles and carrier solutions on left ventricular contractility. J. Am. Coll. Cardiol., 9:910, 1987.

Lappen, R. S., Riggs, T. W., Lapin, G. D., et al: Two-dimensional echocardiographic measurement of right pulmonary artery diameter in infants and children. J. Am. Coll. Cardiol., 2:121, 1983.

Leeman, D. E., Levine, M. J., and Come, P. C.: Doppler echocardiography in cardiac tamponade: Exaggerated respiratory variation in transvalvular blood flow velocity integrals. J. Am. Coll. Cardiol., 11:572, 1988.

Macartney, F. J.: Cross-sectional echocardiographic diagnosis of congenital heart disease. Br. Heart J., 50:501, 1983.

Marcus, M., Wright, C., Doty, D., et al: Measurements of coronary velocity and reactive hyperemia in the coronary circulation of humans. Circ. Res., 49:877, 1981.

Marcus, M. L., Hiratzka, L. F., Doty, D. B., et al: Coronary obstructive lesions: Assessing their physiological significance in humans. Ann. Thorac. Surg., 42:S5, 1986.

Mark, J. B., Steinbrook, R. A., Gugino, L. D., et al: Continuous noninvasive monitoring of cardiac output with esophageal Doppler ultrasound during cardiac surgery. Anesth. Analg., 65:1013, 1986.

Martin, R. P., Meltzer, R. S., Chia, B. L., et al: Clinical utility of two-dimensional echocardiography in infective endocarditis. Am. J. Cardiol., 46:379, 1980.

Mary, D. A. S., Catchpole, L. A., and Ionescu, M. I.: Intraoperative echocardiographic studies of the mitral valve: Assessment of commissurotomy and repair. J. Clin. Ultrasound, 4:349, 1976.

Maurer, G., Ong, K., Haendchen, R., et al: Myocardial contrast two-dimensional echocardiography: Comparison of contrast disappearance rates in normal and underperfused myocardium. Circulation, 69:418, 1984.

Masuyama, T., Kodama, K., Kitabatake, A., et al: Continuous-wave Doppler echocardiographic detection of pulmonary regurgitation and its application to noninvasive estimation of pulmonary artery pressure. Circulation, 74:484, 1986.

Matsuzaki, M., Tohma, Y., Anno Y., et al: Esophageal echocardiographic analysis of atrial dynamics. Am. Heart J., 109:355, 1985.

Meltzer, R. S., Woythaler, J. N., Buda, A. J., et al: Two-dimensional echocardiographic quantification of infarct size alteration by pharmacologic agents. Am. J. Cardiol., 44:257, 1979.

Mimbs, J. W., Bauwens, D., Cohen, R. D., et al: Effects of myocardial ischemia on quantitative ultrasonic backscatter and identification of responsible determinants. Circ. Res., 49:89, 1981.

Miyatake, K., Okamoto, M., Kinoshita, N., et al: Doppler echocardiographic features of coronary arteriovenous fistula: Complementary roles of cross-sectional echocardiography and the Doppler technique. Br. Heart J., 51:508, 1984.

Motro, M., and Neufeld, H. N.: Should patients with pure mitral stenosis undergo cardiac catheterization? Am. J. Cardiol., 46:515, 1980.

Namekawa, K., Kasai, C., Tsukamoto, M., and Koyano, A.: Imaging of blood flow using autocorrelation. Ultrasound Med. Biol., 8:138, 1982.

Omoto, R.: Echocardiographic evaluation of left ventricular size, shape and function: Advantages and limitations of this method. Jpn. Circ. J., 46:1121, 1982.

Omoto, R., Takamoto, S., Kyo, S., and Yokote, Y.: The use of two-dimensional color Doppler sonography during the surgical management of aortic dissection. World J. Surg., 11:604, 1987.

Omoto, R., Yokote, Y., Takamoto, S., et al: The development of real-time two-dimensional Doppler echocardiography and its clinical significance in acquired valvular diseases. With special reference to the evaluation of valvular regurgitation. Jpn. Heart J., 25:325, 1984.

Ong, K., Maurer, G., Feinstein, S., et al: Computer methods for myocardial contrast two-dimensional echocardiography. J. Am. Coll. Cardiol., 3:1212, 1984.

Pandian, N. G., Brockway, B., Simonetti, J., et al: Pericardiocentesis under two-dimensional echocardiographic guidance in loculated pericardial effusion. Ann. Thorac. Surg., 45:99, 1988.

Payen, D., Bousseau, D., Laborde, F., et al: Comparison of perioperative and postoperative phasic blood flow in aortocoronary venous bypass grafts by means of pulsed Doppler echocardiography with implantable microprobes. Circulation, 74-III:61, 1986.

Rasmussen, S., Lovelace, D. E., Knoebel, S. B., et al: Echocardiographic detection of ischemia and infarcted myocardium. J. Am. Coll. Cardiol., 3:733, 1984.

Ren, J., Panidis, I. P., Kotler, M. N., et al: Effect of coronary bypass surgery and valve replacement on left ventricular function: Assessment by intraoperative two-dimensional echocardiography. Am. Heart J., 109:281, 1985.

Ren, J. Y., Gian, R. H., Huang, W. M., et al: Two-dimensional echocardiography in the guidance and evaluation of right intraventricular pacemaker implantation. J. Cardiovasc. Ultrason., 6:141, 1987.

Rice, M. J., Seward, J. B., Hagler, D. J., et al: Impact of 2-dimensional echocardiography on the management of distressed newborns in whom cardiac disease is suspected. Am. J. Cardiol., 51:288, 1983.

Richards, K. L., Cannon, S. R., Miller, J. F., and Crawford, M. H.: Calculation of aortic valve area by Doppler echocardiography: A direct application of the continuity equation. Circulation, 73:964, 1986.

Rodigas, P. C., Meyer, F. J., Haasler, G. B., et al: Intraoperative 2-dimensional echocardiography: Ejection of microbubbles from the left ventricle after cardiac surgery. Am. J. Cardiol., 50:1130, 1982.

Sagar, K. B., Hastillo, A., Wolfgang, T. C., et al: Echocardiographic left ventricular mass in the detection of acute rejection in cardiac transplantation (Abstract). Circulation, 62-III:235, 1980.

Sagar, K. B., Pelc, L. E., Rhyne, T. L., et al: Influence of heart rate, preload, afterload, and inotropic state on myocardial ultrasonic backscatter. Circulation, 77:478, 1988.

Sagar, K. B., Rhyne, T. L., Warltier, D. C., et al: Intramyocardial variability in integrated backscatter: Effects of coronary occlusion and reperfusion. Circulation, 75:436, 1987.

Sahn, D. J., and Allen, H. D.: Real-time cross-sectional echocardiographic imaging and measurement of the patent ductus arteriosus in infants and children. Circulation, 58:343, 1978.

Sahn, D. J., Barratt-Boyes, B. G., Graham, K., et al: Ultrasonic imaging of the coronary arteries in open-chest humans: Evaluation of coronary atherosclerotic lesions during cardiac surgery. Circulation, 66:1034, 1982.

Sakai, K., Hoshino, S., and Osawa, M.: Needle in the heart: Two-dimensional echocardiographic findings. Am. J. Cardiol., 53:1482, 1984.

Schluter, M., Langenstein, B. A., Polster, J., et al: Transesophageal cross-sectional echocardiography with a phased ray transducer system: Technique and initial clinical results. Br. Heart J., 48:67, 1982.

Schnittger, I., Vieli, A., Heiserman, J. E., et al: Ultrasonic tissue characterization: Detection of acute myocardial ischemia in dogs. Circulation, 72:193, 1985.

Skorton, D. J., Melton, H. E., Jr., Pandian, N. G., et al: Detection of acute myocardial infarction in closed-chest dogs by analysis of regional two-dimensional echocardiographic gray-level distributions. Circ. Res., 52:36, 1983.

Smith, J. S., Cahalan, M. K., Benefiel, D. J., et al: Intraoperative detection of myocardial ischemia in high-risk patients: Electrocardiography versus two-dimensional transesophageal echocardiography. Circulation, 72:1015, 1985.

Snider, A. R., Enderlein, M. A., Teitel, D. F., and Juster, R. P.: Two-dimensional echocardiographic determination of aortic and pulmonary artery sizes from infancy to adulthood in normal subjects. Am. J. Cardiol., 53:218, 1984.

Spotnitz, H. M.: Two-dimensional ultrasound and cardiac operations. J. Thorac. Cardiovasc. Surg., 83:43, 1982.

Spotnitz, H. M., Bregman, D., Bowman, F. O., Jr., et al: Effects of open heart surgery on end-diastolic pressure-diameter relations of the human left ventricle. Circulation, 59:662, 1979.

Spotnitz, H. M., Malm, J. R., King, D. L., et al: Outflow tract obstruction in tetralogy of Fallot: Intraoperative analysis by echocardiography. N.Y. State J. Med., 6:1100, 1978.

Stark, J., Smallhorn, J., Huhta, J., et al: Surgery for congenital heart defects diagnosed with cross-sectional echocardiography. Circulation, 68-II:129, 1983.

Stefan, G., and Bing, R. J.: Echocardiographic findings in experimental myocardial infarction of the posterior left ventricular wall. Am. J. Cardiol., 30:629, 1972.

Stevenson, J. G., Kawabori, I., and Bailey, W. W.: Noninvasive evaluation of Blalock-Taussig shunts: Determination of patency and differentiation from patent ductus arteriosus by Doppler echocardiography. Am. Heart J., 106:1121, 1983.

Stevenson, J. G., Kawabori, I., and Guntheroth, W. G.: Pulsed Doppler echocardiographic diagnosis of patent ductus arteriosus: Sensitivity, specificity, limitations, and technical features. Cathet. Cardiovasc. Diagn., 6:255, 1980.

Stewart, J. A., Silimperi, D., Harris, P., et al: Echocardiographic documentation of vegetative lesions in infective endocarditis: Clinical implications. Circulation, 61:374, 1980.

St. John Sutton, M. G.: Routine cardiac catheterization: A prerequisite for valve surgery? Int. J. Cardiol., 1:320, 1981.

St. John Sutton, M. G., St. John Sutton, M. B., Oldershaw, P. J., et al: Valve replacement without preoperative cardiac catheterization. N. Engl. J. Med., 305:1233, 1981.

Stratton, J. R., Tirchie, J. L., Hamilton, G. W., et al: Left ventricular thrombi: In vivo detection by indium-111 platelet imaging and two-dimensional echocardiography. Am. J. Cardiol., 47:874, 1983.

Svennevig, J. L., Grip, A., Lindberg, H., et al: Continuous monitoring of cardiac output postoperatively using an implantable Doppler probe. Scand. J. Thorac. Cardiovasc. Surg., 20:145, 1986.

Syracuse, D. C., Gaudiani, V. A., Kastl, D. G., et al: Intraoperative intracardiac echocardiography during left ventriculomyotomy and myectomy for hypertrophic subaortic stenosis. Circulation, 58:I-23, 1978.

Takamoto, S., Kyo, S., Adachi, H., et al: Intraoperative color flow mapping by real-time two-dimensional Doppler echocardiography for evaluation of valvular and congenital heart disease and vascular disease. J. Thorac. Cardiovasc. Surg., 90:802, 1985.

Tanaka, M., and Terasawa, Y.: Echocardiography evaluation of the tissue character in myocardium. Jpn. Circ. J., 43:367, 1979.

Taylor, A. L., Collins, S. M., Skorton, D. J., et al: Artifactual regional gray level variability in contrast-enhanced two-dimensional echocardiographic images: Effect on measurement of the coronary perfusion bed. J. Am. Coll. Cardiol., 6:831, 1985.

Tei, C., Sakamaki, T., Shah, P. M., et al: Myocardial contrast echocardiography: A reproducible technique of myocardial opacification for identifying regional perfusion deficits. Circulation, 67:585, 1983.

Thomas, L. J., III, Wickline, S. A., Perea, J. E., et al: A real-time integrated backscatter measurement system for quantitative cardiac tissue characterization. IEEE Trans. Ultrasonics, Ferroelectrics, and Frequency Control, UFFC-33, 1:27, 1986.

Topol, E. J., Humphrey, L. S., Borkon, A. M., et al: Value of intraoperative left ventricular microbubbles detected by transesophageal two-dimensional echocardiography in predicting neurologic outcome after cardiac operations. Am. J. Cardiol., 56:773, 1985.

Topol, E. J., Weiss, J. L., Guzman, P. A., et al: Immediate improvement of dysfunctional myocardial segments after coronary revascularization: Detection by intraoperative transesophageal echocardiography. J. Am. Coll. Cardiol., 4:1123, 1984.

van Herwerden, L. A., Gussenhoven, E. J., Roelandt, J. R. T. C., et al: Intraoperative two-dimensional echocardiography in complicated infective endocarditis of the aortic valve. J. Thorac. Cardiovasc. Surg., 93:587, 1987.

Vick, G. W., III, Huhta, J. C., and Gutgesell, H. P.: Assessment of the ductus arteriosus in preterm infants utilizing suprasternal two-dimensional/Doppler echocardiography. J. Am. Coll. Cardiol., 5:973, 1985.

Visser, C. A., Kan, G., David, G. K., et al: Two-dimensional echocardiography in the diagnosis of left ventricular thrombus: A prospective study of 67 patients with anatomic validation. Chest, 83:228, 1983.

von Ramm, O. T., and Smith, S. W.: Prospects and limitations of diagnostic ultrasound. Proceedings of the Society of Photooptical Instrumentation Engineers (SPIE) 206:6, 1979.

von Ramm, O. T., and Thurstone, F. L.: Cardiac imaging using a phased array ultrasound system. I. System design. Circulation, 53:258, 1976.

Waggoner, A. D., Shah, A. A., Schuessler, J. S., et al: Effect of cardiac surgery on ventricular septal motion: Assessment by intraoperative echocardiography and cross-sectional two-dimensional echocardiography. Am. Heart J., 104:1271, 1982.

Wear, K. A., Shoup, T. A., and Popp, R. L.: Ultrasonic characterization of canine myocardium contraction. IEEE Trans. Ultrasonics, Ferroelectrics, and Frequency Control, UFFC-33, 4:347, 1986.

Weiss, J. L., Bulkley, B. H., Hutchins, G. M., and Mason, S. J.: Two-dimensional echocardiographic recognition of myocardial injury in man: Comparison with post-mortem studies. Circulation, 63:401, 1981.

Weyman, A. E., Feigenbaum, H., Dillon, J. C., et al: Noninvasive visualization of the left main coronary artery by cross-sectional echocardiography. Circulation, 54:169, 1976.

White, C. W., Wright, C. B., Doty, D. B., et al: Does visual interpretation of the coronary arteriogram predict the physiologic importance of a coronary stenosis? N. Engl. J. Med., 310:819, 1984.

Williams, W. G., Wigle, E. D., Rakowski, H., et al: Results of surgery for hypertrophic obstructive cardiomyopathy. Circulation, 76:V-104, 1987.

Wilson, R. F., Marcus, M. L., and White, C. W.: Prediction of the physiologic significance of coronary arterial lesions by quantitative lesion geometry in patients with limited coronary artery disease. Circulation, 75:723, 1987.

Wong, C. Y. H., and Spotnitz, H. M.: Systolic and diastolic properties of the human left ventricle during valve replacement of chronic mitral regurgitation. Am. J. Cardiol., 47:40, 1981.

Wright, C. B., Melvin, D. B., Flege, J. B., et al: Coronary bypass without angiography: An unusual circumstance. J. Thorac. Cardiovasc. Surg., 93:936, 1987.

Wyatt, H. L., Heng, M. K., Meerbaum, S., et al: Cross-sectional echocardiography. I. Analysis of mathematical models for quantifying mass of the left ventricle in dogs. Circulation, 60:1104, 1979.

Wyatt, H. L., Meerbaum, S., Heng, M. K., et al: Experimental evaluation of the extent of myocardial dyssynergy and infarct size by two-dimensional echocardiography. Circulation, 63:607, 1981.

CHAPTER 32

CARDIOPULMONARY BYPASS FOR CARDIAC SURGERY

James K. Kirklin
John W. Kirklin

Cardiopulmonary bypass (CPB) is a technique by which the pumping action of the heart and the gas exchange functions of the lung are replaced temporarily by a mechanical device, the pump oxygenator, attached to a patient's vascular system. Although some temporary dysfunction of organs and systems are the sequelae of present techniques, CPB has become an indispensable technique for most cardiac surgical procedures. It has also been used in series with the patient's own heart and lungs for partial temporary CPB in patients with severe but potentially reversible respiratory distress, for patients having operations on the thoracic aorta, and for a few other purposes not discussed in this chapter.

The temporary provision of arterial blood flow by means of a pump oxygenator is an abnormal situation in which most if not all of the body's physiologic processes are affected. In *total CPB*, essentially all systemic venous blood returns to the pump oxygenator instead of to the heart. In *partial CPB*, some systemic venous blood returns to the heart and is ejected into the aorta.

Compared with the situation in intact humans, a number of physiologic variables are directly under external control during CPB. These variables include total systemic blood flow (cardiac output), input pressure waveform, systemic venous pressure, pulmonary venous pressure, hematocrit of the initial perfusate and its chemical composition, arterial oxygen and carbon dioxide (and nitrogen) levels, and temperature of the perfusate and the patient. Treatment decisions should therefore be based on all of these variables. Unfortunately, sometimes no formal decision is made, and a situation is merely accepted rather than actually chosen.

Another group of variables is determined in part by the externally controlled factors and in part by the patient. These variables include systemic vascular resistance, total body-oxygen consumption, mixed venous oxygen levels, lactic acidemia and pH, regional and organ blood flow, and regional and organ function.

A number of undesirable side effects occur to a greater or lesser degree with CPB. These side effects include blood coagulation abnormalities, changes in red blood cells and plasma proteins produced by their passage through the extracorporeal system, gaseous and particulate emboli, and liberation or production of various vasoactive and otherwise biologically active substances by contact of blood with foreign surfaces.

HISTORICAL ASPECTS

The historical aspects of CPB for cardiac procedures are not easily described, because it is not clear who originated the concept of diverting the circulation to an oxygenator outside the body and pumping it back to the patient's arterial system to allow surgical therapy within the heart.

References to extracorporeal gas exchange in blood date back to the last part of the 19th century. Frey and Gruber worked with an "oxygenator" in 1885. Scores of laboratory studies with oxygenators and pumps were subsequently reported. However, serious consideration of the use of pump oxygenators for cardiac procedures awaited the development of modern anesthesia and modern surgical methods and, particularly, scientific developments such as the discovery and use of heparin, plastic material, and the like. Without doubt, Gibbon's pioneering experimental work at the Massachusetts General Hospital in Boston in the late 1930s (Gibbon, 1939) contributed significantly to the advancement of CPB, proceeding from the concept to productive laboratory work and then to successful clinical application. When Gibbon went to Jefferson Medical School in Philadelphia, after his work was interrupted by military service in World War II, he resumed his work with CPB, its pathophysiology, and the equipment required for it. Most of the medical and surgical world took little note of his work and considered it unlikely to lead to any useful knowledge. However, Gibbon perse-

1107

vered. He did the first successful operation in which the patient was totally supported by CPB when he repaired an atrial septal defect in a young woman while using a pump oxygenator in 1953 (Gibbon, 1954). Unfortunately, his subsequent four patients died of various problems, and he became discouraged about the method (Gibbon, 1955).

During the late 1940s, others, including Dennis at the University of Minnesota, began to work with pump oxygenators for CPB. Dennis' laboratory studies led him to make what may have been the first attempt to use a pump oxygenator for clinical cardiac procedures (Dennis et al, 1951). Dennis and Varco operated on a patient who was thought to have an atrial septal defect and believed that they had completed a satisfactory repair, but the patient died. Autopsy showed that the lesion was a partial atrio-ventricular canal defect, and misinterpretation of the anatomy was a major factor in the patient's death. In Stockholm, Sweden, Bjork (1948) and Senning (1952) also worked with CPB in the late 1940s and early 1950s. Related to this is Crafoord's early use of this method for the removal of an atrial myxoma (Crafoord et al, 1957).

After Dennis' unsuccessful effort, Cohen and Lillehei (1954), at the University of Minnesota, began working in the laboratory with controlled cross-circulation, using another intact subject as the "oxygenator." Their experimental studies led them to adopt the "azygous flow principle" (Andreason and Watson, 1952), which was that only very small perfusion flow rates were needed. In April, 1954, they began a spectacular series of operations for congenital heart disease by using controlled cross-circulation and usually the mother as the oxygenator (Warden et al, 1954). Although this particular technique was ultimately abandoned, the work of Lillehei and colleagues (1955) brought into being the modern era of open heart surgery.

Kirklin began experimental work with pump oxygenators at the Mayo Clinic, in Rochester, Minnesota, in the early 1950s (Donald et al, 1955; Jones et al, 1955), leading to the first use of CPB with a pump oxygenator in March, 1955, in successfully repairing a ventricular septal defect. This initiated the world's first series of intracardiac operations by using a pump oxygenator (Kirklin et al, 1955). The field of intracardiac surgery by using a pump oxygenator for CPB began to expand rapidly, and it is now practiced in all parts of the world.

SURGICAL TECHNIQUES

Arterial Cannulation

The ascending aorta is usually cannulated directly when using CPB for cardiac procedures (exceptions, in which the femoral artery is cannulated, include, for example, patients having resection of aneurysms of the ascending aorta and those having closure of a previously constructed descending aorta–left pulmonary artery or Potts' anastomosis). The hemodynamic advantages of entrance of the arterial inflow into the ascending aorta compared with the femoral artery are controversial. Most studies indicate that regional blood flow, including cerebral blood flow, is the same no matter which site is chosen (Lees et al, 1971; Schenk et al, 1963). The aortic cannula should be inserted as proximal to the takeoff of the innominate artery as is surgically acceptable, and only a short length of cannula is introduced so that its tip cannot actually enter a brachiocephalic vessel or lie near its orifice.

The authors generally place two concentric purse-string sutures in the aortic adventitia and media at the proposed site of cannulation. The aorta is then incised by a stab wound within the purse-string suture, and the arterial cannula is directly inserted. Alternatively, this portion of the aorta can be exteriorized with a side-biting clamp such as a Derra or Cooley clamp, the exteriorized portion of the aorta can be incised, and a tapered plastic cannula can be inserted as the clamp is removed. The ends of the inner purse-string suture have previously been threaded through a long narrow rubber tube, and the tube is tucked down snugly and secured as a tourniquet and then tied to the cannula. After the cannula is connected to the arterial lines in such a way as to exclude or remove any air bubbles, the line and cannula are secured so that the end of the cannula lies freely within the aortic lumen and the beveled end faces downstream, the surgical field is uncluttered, and the line from the pump oxygenator is free of kinks.

As the cannula is removed after bypass, the outer purse-string suture is crossed by the assistant for hemostasis, and the surgeon ties the inner suture. The outer purse-string suture is then tied.

The tapered plastic cannula* is fitted for each patient, and a small collar is adjusted so that just the right short length of cannula is beyond the collar. The cannula is inserted up to the collar. A size of cannula across which the pressure gradient, at the highest flow rate that will be used, is less than 100 mm Hg is selected (Table 32–1) (Broadman et al, 1985). The authors use this relatively low gradient to minimize the turbulence as blood leaves the cannula tip and to keep the arterial line pressure (as measured by the arterial line manometer on the pump oxygenator) less than approximately 250 mm Hg to minimize the possibility of blowouts of the line or its connectors.

Venous Cannulation

The vena cava or the right atrium is usually cannulated to provide return of systemic venous

---

*THI Aortic Perfusion Cannula, Med-Science Electronics, Inc., St. Louis, MO.

TABLE 32–1. SELECTION OF CANNULA SIZE FOR CPB

Cannula Size in French Scale	Pressure Gradient (mm Hg)							
	0.5 l/min*	1.0 l/min	1.5 l/min	2.0 l/min	2.5 l/min	3.0 l/min	3.5 l/min	4.0 l/min
10	60	175	350	325				
12	40	100	225	240	350			
14	25	60	140	90	150	200	260	
16		25	50	60	80	120	150	200
18		20	40	40	60	80	100	120
20			25	40	50	60	75	90
22			25	40	50	60	70	80
24								

*Flow in l/min.

blood to the pump oxygenator. In infants and children, two angled, metal-tip venous cannulas (developed by Pacifico) (Fig. 32–1), which are inserted directly into each vena cava, are used for most operations, particularly if working through the right atrium or right ventricle. When the Kyoto-Barratt-Boyes technique of profound hypothermia, (Barratt-Boyes et al, 1971; Hikasa et al, 1967), limited CPB, and total circulatory arrest is used (selected infants and neonates), a single venous cannula is inserted into the right atrium. In adults, a single large cavo-atrial (two-stage) venous cannula (Bennett et al, 1983), with additional holes that lie in the right atrium while the tip is in the inferior vena cava, is generally used for coronary bypass grafting, aortic valve operations, left ventricular operations, and occasionally for mitral valve procedures. During procedures in the right atrium, two venous cannulas are used.

Whatever cannulation technique is used, the cannulas have relatively large internal diameters, and their exact size is determined by the maximal perfusion flow rate to be used for that patient (Table 32–2). This ensures as low a venous pressure as possible during bypass. When two or more venous cannulas are used, they are joined to the large single venous line to the pump oxygenator by a Y connector.

Intracardiac Suction Devices

Suction lines are required to aspirate blood from the opened heart, return it to the pump oxygenator as part of the venous return, and decompress the heart (particularly the left side) when needed. Therefore, just after establishing CPB for some operations, a right-angled catheter vent (2/16- or 3/16-inch internal diameter) is inserted into the left atrium through a small stab wound, protected by a purse-string suture, in the right side of the left atrium or in the anterior wall of the superior pulmonary vein near the left atrium. The venting catheter is generally advanced through the mitral valve into the left ventricle. In most pediatric open heart operations, the left atrium and left ventricle are decompressed by a small metal "infant sump" catheter passed through a patent foramen ovale or a stab wound in the atrial septum. Gentle suction is applied to the vent, ideally by a regulated vacuum system but in practice by a well-controlled occlusive pump.

For aspirating blood from the opened heart, a special sucker that has a guard over the tip is used to minimize the tendency of leaflet and other intracardiac tissue to be drawn up into it. This is used as a sump drain and therefore functions best when positioned in a pool of blood in a dependent portion of the opened heart. The sucker is attached to one of the intracardiac return lines, again activated by a well-controlled occlusive pump.

EXTERNALLY CONTROLLED VARIABLES DURING CARDIOPULMONARY BYPASS

Total Systemic Blood Flow (Perfusion Flow Rate)

During total CPB, the systemic blood flow (Q) is under the control of the perfusionist. It can be set at

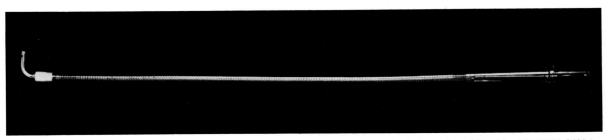

Figure 32–1. Thin-walled right-angled cannula for direct caval cannulation. (DLP, Inc., Grand Rapids, MI 49501-0409.)

TABLE 32–2. VENOUS CANNULA CHART

Total Flow (l/min)	Single Tygon Size (inches)	Single USCI* (French Size)	Two-Angled Metal (DLP†)	
			SVC (French Size)	IVC (French Size)
≤0.7	3/16	20	12	12
0.7–0.9			12	16
0.9–1.2	4/16	24	16	16
1.2–1.6			16	20
1.6–1.7			20	20
1.7–2.2		28	20	24
2.2–2.8	5/16		24	24
2.8–3.2			24	24
3.2–3.7	6/16		24	28
>3.7	8/16		28	28

*In adults, at UAB, a USCI "two-stage" single cannula is used (46 French, tapering to 34 French).
†DLP: Thin-walled right-angled cannula for direct caval cannulation (DLP, Inc., Grand Rapids, MI 49501-0409).

an arbitrary level or may be determined by the venous return from the patient ("pump back all that is received"). The authors believe it is rational to set it at an arbitrary flow rate.

The *optimal flow rate* during CPB is still being debated. A few facts are clear. Acidosis with increased lactic acid production, low oxygen consumption, and the other features of cardiogenic shock result from normothermic CPB at flows of less than approximately 1.6 l/min/m² (or less than approximately 50 ml/kg/min) (Diesh et al, 1957). Animal experiments and the authors' clinical data (Levin et al, 1960; Moffitt et al, 1962) and experience indicate that at normothermia flows more than 1.8 l/min/m² are acceptable with regard to total body-oxygen consumption, but that flows of 2.2 to 2.5 l/min/m² are more securely adequate. During hypothermic perfusions, adequate or acceptable flow rates are slightly lower (Fig. 32–2) (Hickey and Hoar, 1983; Kirklin and Barrett-Boyes, 1986).

The best criterion of acceptability or adequacy of flow rate at any temperature is the survival of the subject without structural or functional evidence or organ or system damage. The authors believe survival without damage is most likely to occur when the entire microcirculation is perfused at flow rates that maintain near-normal tissue oxygen levels. In patients on CPB, this probably pertains to when whole-body oxygen consumption ($\dot{V}O_2$) is near (±85% of) the asymptote of the temperature-specific curve relating flow to $\dot{V}O_2$ (represented by the x's in Fig. 32–2).

As might be expected, high flow is achieved at the expense of some loss of safety and convenience in other variables. Blood trauma in the oxygenator is probably greater when high blood flows pass through it, and with a bubble oxygenator, the risks of gaseous emboli are also greater. The pressure gradients across the arterial cannula are greater at high rates of flow. The higher pressure gradients increase cavitation, and thus blood trauma, and the risk of bubbles forming as blood emerges from the cannula.

In clinical practice, when body temperature is 28° C or higher, the authors usually choose a flow rate of 2.5 l/min/m² for infants and children less than about 4 years of age, and one of 2.2 l/min/m² for older patients. For very large adults with a body surface area of 2 m² or more, a flow rate of 1.8 to 2 l/min/m² is selected to avoid the disadvantage of high flow rates through the oxygenator. Lower flow rates are chosen when body temperature is lower (see Fig. 32–2).

Temperature of the Perfusate and the Patient

Since Brown and co-workers (1958) introduced an efficient heat exchanger for extracorporeal circulation, the temperature of the perfusate and, secondarily, that of the patient have been under the control of the perfusionist. Temperature has become one of the most important parameters to be selected for each patient having CPB. The potential surgical flexibility of CPB is achieved only when it is combined with hypothermia.

In choosing the temperature for the patient during CPB, several facts must be considered. Slightly lower CPB flow rates can be used at low temperatures. Because of the coronary collateral circulation, some of the perfusate reaches the heart and affects its temperature, even when the aorta is cross-clamped. Thus, after cold cardioplegia, the heart tends to return to the temperature of the body around it. The patient's body temperature is related to the "safe" total circulatory arrest time that is available. If the nasopharyngeal temperature is, for example, 28° C, circulatory arrest lasting 10 to 15 minutes is possible for repair of a split arterial pump tube or electrical or mechanical pump oxygenator failure or

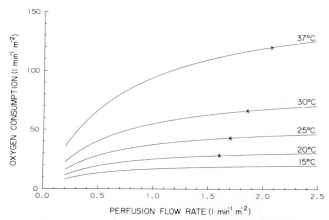

Figure 32–2. Nomogram of an equation, expressing the relation of oxygen consumption ($\dot{V}O_2$) to perfusion flow rate (Q) and temperature (T). The small x's represent the perfusion flow rates that the authors used at these temperatures. The equation is as follows:

$$1/\dot{V}O_2 = 0.168 \times 10^{-0.0387T} + 0.0378 \times Q^{-1} \times 10^{-0.0253T}$$

(From Kirklin, J. W., and Barratt-Boyes, B. G.: Cardiac Surgery. New York, John Wiley & Sons. Copyright 1986.)

to improve surgical exposure. Another fact to be considered is that longer rewarming time is required when hypothermia is profound. At the University of Alabama at Birmingham (UAB), moderate hypothermia is used (25° C) in most CPB procedures. If low-flow perfusion or total circulatory arrest is anticipated (particularly in small infants), temperatures of 16 to 20° C are usually used.

Arterial Input Pressure Waveform

The most commonly used type of arterial pump is the roller pump, originally used by DeBakey (1934) for blood transfusion. It generates a relatively *non-pulsatile flow*, and the relatively narrow orifice of the arterial cannula tends to depulse the inflow still further.

A *pulsatile arterial input* can be achieved in several ways. When the atrial pressures, and thus ventricular filling pressures, are increased by increasing the patient's blood volume (with no tapes around the caval cannulas, arterial inflow to the patient is temporarily increased over venous return from the patient. Alternatively, venous return is temporarily reduced below arterial input by partially occluding the venous line), and if cardiac function is adequate, left ventricular ejection augments systemic blood flow and produces a pulsatile arterial blood flow. In other words, pulsation is achieved by substituting partial CPB. The authors use this latter method during rewarming whenever possible. A pulsatile waveform can also be produced by using intra-aortic balloon pulsation during CPB or a pulsatile type of arterial pump.

The effect on the patient of using a system that results in a pulsatile (versus a nonpulsatile) arterial waveform during CPB has been controversial since clinical CPB began (Singh et al, 1980; Sink et al, 1980).

Systemic Venous Pressure

Systemic venous pressure in the patient during CPB is determined by the cannulation methods used (Kirklin and Theye, 1962), since

$$PV_{sys} = f \left(\frac{Q, \text{viscosity}}{\text{cannula size, venous line size, venous line suction}} \right) \quad (1)$$

where PV_{sys} = the mean systemic venous pressure and Q = the systemic blood flow. The cross-sectional area of the single or multiple venous cannulas and their length and, to a lesser extent (because it usually has a large diameter), that of the venous line to the pump oxygenator are the fixed factors determining venous pressure during total CPB. Thus, the largest venous cannulas that are compatible with the clinical situation are used. When smaller cannulas must be used, the other variables in equation 1 can be manip-

ulated (e.g., the systemic blood flow may be reduced) to ensure an acceptable venous pressure.

There is no apparent physiologic advantage in having a central venous pressure of more than zero during CPB. Raising the venous pressure requires more intravascular volume and often an additional priming volume. The authors prefer to maintain the venous pressure at close to zero, and certainly not above 10 mm Hg to minimize increases in extracellular fluid.

Pulmonary Venous (Left Atrial) Pressure

This pressure should ideally be at zero during total CPB, and not above 10 mm Hg. Undue rises are dangerous because they tend to produce increased extravascular pulmonary water and eventually pulmonary edema, according to Starling's law of transcapillary fluid exchange:

$$P_c - P_t = \pi_c - \pi_t \quad (2)$$

where P_c = "effective" blood pressure within the capillary; P_t = tissue turgor pressure (interstitial fluid pressure); π_c = osmotic pressure of the plasma (colloid) inside the capillary; and π_t = osmotic pressure of the extracellular fluid (tissue colloid osmotic pressure). The increase in extracellular pulmonary water is related to the duration of elevation of pulmonary venous or pulmonary capillary pressure, other things being equal.

Hematocrit of the Mixed Patient and Pump Oxygenator Blood Volume

Hematocrit of the mixed patient and pump oxygenator blood volume is determined by the composition and amounts of blood and fluids infused before and during CPB, the blood loss, and the amount and composition of the initial (priming) volume of the pump oxygenator. The hematocrit is also affected by patient interactions, primarily transcapillary movement of fluid from the intravascular to the interstitial space and into urine volume.

In intact patients at 37° C, the normal hematocrit of 0.4 to 0.5 is optimal for oxygen transport (Chien, 1972). This level provides sufficient oxygen delivery to maintain normal mitochondrial PO_2 levels of approximately 0.05 to 1 mm Hg and average intracellular PO_2 levels of approximately 5 mm Hg, which are reflected in normal oxygen levels ($P\bar{v}_{O_2}$ of approximately 40 mm Hg, SV_{O_2} of approximately 75% in mixed venous blood. The normal hematocrit is also optimal rheologically in intact persons (Chien, 1972). When the hematocrit is abnormally high, oxygen content is high, but the increased viscosity tends to decrease blood flow. Thus, the rate of oxygen transport varies directly with hematocrit (because oxygen content varies directly with hematocrit, assuming normal red blood cell hemoglobin concentrations and adequate oxygenation) and inversely with the blood's (apparent) viscosity (which is also determined primarily by hematocrit). Hypothermia increases the blood's (apparent) viscosity, so that at low temperatures, a lower hematocrit is more appropriate than that at 37° C. A hematocrit less than "normal" appears desirable during hypothermic CPB because of its association with lower apparent blood viscosity and low shear rates, thus presumably resulting in better perfusion of the microcirculation. Thus, a hematocrit of approximately 0.25 to 0.3 is desirable during hypothermic perfusions. During rewarming, a higher hematocrit ($\geq$0.30) is desirable because of the increased oxygen demands, and the higher apparent viscosity at these higher hematocrits is appropriate during normothermia. The body's autoregulatory mechanisms, including its capacity to recover from transient abnormalities in oxygen delivery, are so well developed that a considerable range ($\pm$0.05) of hematocrits around the desirable point are acceptable. This is fortunate; otherwise, the need for homologous blood, with its own economic and medical disadvantages, in the priming volume would be increased. Because at the UAB essentially all CPB procedures are done by using hypothermia (20 to 25° C), an initial hematocrit of 0.25 to 0.3 is accepted. Thus, the authors calculate the mixed patient-machine hematocrit that will result if the pump oxygenator is primed with an asanguineous solution, using equation (3), where Hct_{pm} = hematocrit of combined patient-machine blood volume, Hct_p = patient hematocrit, and BV = blood volume. Therefore, when no blood is in the priming volume,

$$Hct_{pm} = \frac{(\text{body weight [kg]} \times f \times 1,000)\, Hct_p}{(\text{body weight [kg]} \times f \times 1,000) + \text{machine BV}} \quad (3)$$

where f = 0.08 in infants and children ($\leq$ 12 years) and f = 0.065 in older patients ($\leq$ 12 years).* If the calculated hematocrit is in the desired range, the clear priming solution is used. Approximately 20% of the priming solution is 5% dextrose and 80% balanced salt solution with sufficient concentrated human albumin added to make it colloidally iso-osmotic. If the calculated hematocrit is too low, an appropriate amount of blood is added by using equation 4 to solve for the desired volume of packed red blood cells to be added to obtain the desired patient-machine hematocrit.

$$Hct_{pm} = \frac{\substack{\text{patient red blood cell volume (ml)} \\ + \text{machine red blood cell volume (ml)}}}{\text{patient BV} + \text{machine BV (ml)}} \quad (4)$$

Banked blood less than about 48 hours old is used, but older blood for adults is accepted when necessary. The blood has, of course, been rendered Ca^{++} free by the anticoagulant solution and is acidotic so that heparin, calcium, and buffer are added (Table 32–3).

Albumin Concentration in the Mixed Patient and Pump Oxygenator Blood Volume

Albumin concentration is also affected by the amount of hemodilution. Theoretically, according to equation 2, a reduction of albumin and thus of the colloidal osmotic pressure of the plasma accentuates movement of fluid out of the vascular space into the interstitial space, and it is believed that this does occur. Cohn and colleagues (1971) showed that the extracellular fluid volume increases more rapidly when hemodilution is used than when it is not. It is believed that during long periods of CPB with hemodilution, more volume additions are required when albumin is not added to produce more or less normal colloidal osmotic pressure than when it is added. This is presumably the result of transcapillary fluid loss (and, to some extent, urinary losses). However, most patients adapt and tolerate these transient abnormalities well.

Enough concentrated serum albumin is added to the balanced salt solution in the priming volume to make it approximately colloidally iso-osmotic. The authors believe that this is particularly important in infants.

Glucose Concentration

At UAB, where no mannitol is used in the priming solution, the glucose concentration (350 mg/dl) is deliberately raised to promote osmotic diuresis during and for a few hours after operation and to provide a source of energy.

Ionic Composition of the Perfusate

The perfusate should have an ionic composition similar to that of plasma. Thus, the vehicle for hemodilution is a balanced salt solution with a relatively normal pH.

TABLE 32–3. ADDITIVES TO A UNIT OF CPD* BLOOD FOR THE PUMP OXYGENATOR

Additive	Amount
CPD blood	500 ml
Heparin	3 ml (3,000 units; 6 units/ml of blood)
NaHCO₃ (8.4%)	10 ml
CaCl₂ (10%)	5 ml (added last)
	518 ml

*CPD = citrate-phosphate-dextrose.

---

*These are average values and provide a method of estimating blood volume. More complex regression equations are available for more precise estimates.

Arterial Oxygen Levels

With present-day bubble and membrane oxygenators, maintenance of an arterial oxygen pressure (Pa$_{O_2}$) of approximately 250 mm Hg is easily accomplished and can be considered to be optimal. A higher Pa$_{O_2}$ is unnecessary and theoretically subjects patients to the risk of oxygen toxicity and bubble formation. A Pa$_{O_2}$ lower than 85 mm Hg results in a rather rapidly declining arterial oxygen content (according to the oxygen dissociation curve of the blood) and a corresponding reduction of tissue and mixed venous oxygen levels. Shepard (1973) showed in dogs having normothermic CPB that total-body oxygen consumption fell when arterial oxygen saturation fell below 65%. This situation indicates hypoxic cell damage.

The temperature of the patient, related as it is to whole-body oxygen consumption ($\dot{V}o_2$), affects arterial oxygen levels with any given oxygenator at any given blood and gas flow rate. A reduction of the patient's body temperature reduces $\dot{V}o_2$ and increases P$\bar{v}_{O_2}$, both resulting, in this setting, in increased Pa$_{O_2}$. During rewarming by perfusion from the pump oxygenator, increasing $\dot{V}o_2$, due presumably in part to the oxygen debt that has accumulated, results in relatively low mixed venous oxygen levels and relatively high $\dot{V}o_2$ (Theye and Kirklin, 1963). This period, then, determines the requirements on the oxygenator with regard to oxygen transfer capacity for any particular patient (Levin et al, 1960; Theye et al, 1962a, 1962).

Arterial Carbon Dioxide Pressure

The authors believe that an arterial carbon dioxide pressure (Pa$_{CO_2}$) between 30 and 40 mm Hg (measured at 37° C) is desirable during CPB. As in the lungs of intact persons, this measurement is determined by the ratio of gas flow to blood flow in the oxygenator (Hallowell et al, 1967), higher ratios resulting in lower Pa$_{CO_2}$. Present-day bubble and membrane oxygenators ventilated appropriately give a Pa$_{CO_2}$ within this range.

Optimal Pa$_{CO_2}$ during profound hypothermia is controversial, in part because of the effect of Pa$_{CO_2}$ on arterial pH. Rahn and colleagues (1975), Reeves (1976), and Swan (1974) have emphasized that at low temperatures *neutrality* is associated with a higher pH than at normothermia because of the change in the dissociation constant of water. They contend that during CPB when the perfusate temperature and the patient's nasopharyngeal temperature are 20° C, the Pa$_{CO_2}$ measured at 37° C should be 30 to 40 mm Hg, which indicates a Pa$_{CO_2}$ of 14 to 20 mm Hg at 20° C (by the Reeves' correction [Reeves, 1976]) and that pH measured at 37° C should be approximately 7.38, which indicates a pH of approximately 7.6 at 20° C (by the Rosenthal correction [Rosenthal, 1948]) (the so-called alpha-stat concept) (Bove et al, 1987). When

carbon dioxide has been added to the ventilatory mixture during cooling for profound hypothermia (in the belief that brain cooling would be more rapid because of the assumed increase in cerebral blood flow), too acidotic a milieu develops, according to this concept. Instead, Rahn and associates (1975) believe that *relative* hyperventilation should be practiced during hypothermic CPB so that Pa$_{CO_2}$ will be below 40 mm Hg and the milieu alkalotic. This can be accomplished by maintaining the ratio of gas flow to blood flow constant during cooling and *not* adding carbon dioxide to the ventilatory mixture. Carbon dioxide production falls as the patient cools, and relative hyperventilation results. At UAB, these principles are followed.

PATIENT'S RESPONSES TO CARDIOPULMONARY BYPASS

The patient's response to CPB involves the entire body, is complex, and defies complete description because of gaps in our knowledge. Part of this response is to the damaging effects of CPB and is described later under that heading. Some aspects of the response become apparent only in the postoperative period. Some of the easily categorized responses during operation are described here.

Systemic Vascular Resistance

At the onset of normothermic or moderately hypothermic CPB, systemic vascular resistance usually falls abruptly. After that, it gradually rises throughout the period of CPB. There is considerable variation from one patient to another in the systemic vascular resistance, and thus in the systemic arterial blood pressure, during perfusion. Patients with coronary artery disease tend particularly to develop a high systemic vascular resistance during CPB (Wallach et al, 1980). When profound hyperthermia is produced during CPB, systemic vascular resistance usually falls more than during normothermic or moderately hypothermic bypass.

The advisability of pharmacologically manipulating the systemic vascular resistance during CPB has been extensively debated. Some evidence indicates that cerebral blood flow is lower than desirable when mean arterial blood pressure during normothermic or moderately hypothermic CPB falls below 55 mm Hg. Therefore, when it is lower than that for more than a few minutes during rewarming, the authors generally pharmacologically increase systemic vascular resistance and thus arterial blood pressure. More adequate coronary blood flow results. Increasing the perfusion flow rate above the usual values during rewarming is ineffective in increasing arterial pressure. When systemic vascular resistance during this phase of CPB becomes so high that mean arterial blood pressure rises above 100 mm Hg, the authors

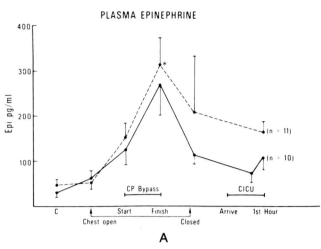
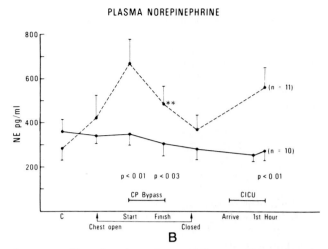

Figure 32–3. Studies in patients having CPB for coronary artery bypass grafting at various stages of the operation and early postoperative period. *A,* Plasma epinephrine levels (mean + standard error) in patients who were normotensive early postoperatively *(solid line)* and those who were hypertensive *(broken line). B,* Plasma norepinephrine levels *(solid* and *broken lines* represent same as in *A)* (C = control). (From Wallach, R., Karp, R. B., Reves, J. G., et al: Pathogenesis of paroxysmal hypertension developing during and after coronary artery bypass surgery: A study of hemodynamic and humeral factors. Am. J. Cardiol., 46:559, 1980.)

believe that it is wise to reduce it pharmacologically below that level.

Total Body-Oxygen Consumption

Although $\dot{V}O_2$ is mainly determined by the perfusion flow rate and the patient's temperature during CPB, the patient's biologic response is also a factor. Its exact nature has not been completely determined.

Mixed Venous Oxygen Levels

Although mixed venous oxygen levels are related to the controlled variables of perfusion flow rate, the hemoglobin concentration of the perfusate, and the arterial oxygen tension, they are also related to the patient's response in terms of $\dot{V}O_2$. In addition, they are related to some partially controlled variables that probably affect $\dot{V}O_2$, such as 2,3-diphosphoglycerate levels in the red blood cells and pH. These former inter-relations are expressed by the Fick equation.

When most of the microcirculation is known to be perfused, mixed venous oxygen levels reflect some sort of mean value for tissue oxygen levels. Thus, the assumption can be made that when mixed venous oxygen levels during CPB are relatively normal ($P\bar{V}_{O_2}$ of 30 to 40 mm Hg, $S\bar{V}_{O_2}$ of 60 to 70%) and $\dot{V}O_2$ is relatively normal, tissue oxygen levels are relatively normal and the total body perfusion is meeting the patient's metabolic demands.

Metabolic Acidosis

Metabolic acidosis, primarily from lactic acidemia, is well known to complicate many situations characterized by acute reductions of systemic blood flow rate, including CPB. There is always a steady

and significant increase in blood lactate concentration during an operation using CPB, but when the recommended criteria are followed in setting perfusion flow rates, this concentration generally does not exceed 5 mmol/l (Harris et al, 1970).

Catecholamine Response

The response of circulating catecholamines to CPB has been studied by many groups and has slightly conflicting results (Hine et al, 1976; Philbin et al, 1979; Turley et al, 1979). It now appears clear that CPB is associated with a large release of epinephrine (primarily from the adrenal medulla). Plasma epinephrine levels rise shortly after the onset of CPB and begin to fall after CPB (Wallach et al, 1980) (Fig. 32–3). Norepinephrine levels apparently rise only in patients who develop hypertension early after operation (the rise resulting presumably from generalized sympathetic nervous system discharge) (Fig. 32–3B). The increased blood norepinephrine levels may partly result from reduced blood flow through the lungs during CPB, where norepinephrine is mainly inactivated (Reves et al, 1982; Pitt et al, 1984).

DAMAGING EFFECTS OF CARDIOPULMONARY BYPASS

Safe CPB is characterized by the absence of structural or functional damage after the perfusion. Paradoxically, detailed information about these parameters is currently more complete after profound hypothermic circulation arrest procedures than after conventional CPB. It is known, of course, that thousands of patients have no apparent ill effects from CPB, but few specific studies of organ function have been made. Walker and colleagues (unpublished data), at UAB, have found no change in the intelligence quotient and intellectual performance tests before and 1 week after coronary artery bypass grafting using CPB. In general, however, the conclusion that CPB is safe has not been rigorously supported. Despite the normal convalescence of most patients, it is likely that all patients have a rather specific physiologic response to CPB, which in an occasional patient will have very deleterious effects. In its most severe form, this adverse response to CPB has been called the postperfusion syndrome, and it may to a greater or lesser extent include clinical signs of pulmonary dysfunction, renal dysfunction, an abnormal bleeding diathesis, increased susceptibility to infection, increased interstitial fluid, leukocytosis, fever, vasoconstriction, and hemolysis.

Unfortunately, most studies of the adverse effects of CPB merely document that these effects exist without elucidating the basic mechanisms involved. As a result, both prevention and treatment remain mainly empiric. During clinical CPB, the most obvious possible mechanisms for damage are exposure of blood to various abnormal events and altered arterial blood flow patterns. The complexity of the situation is aggravated by the interactions between these. The authors believe that the first of these, the exposure of blood to abnormal events (Fig. 32–4), is the most generalized and the most powerful in its effects on the patient, and it is therefore the one that is discussed.

Exposure of Blood to Abnormal Events

Blood is a complex substance containing formed elements (red blood cells, white blood cells, and platelets) and unformed elements. Among the latter, the plasma proteins are particularly vulnerable. They can be divided into those with *primarily osmotic effects* (albumin), those that are *carrier vehicles* for other bloodborne substances (e.g., albumin, lipoproteins, immunoglobulins), and those that are part of the *humoral amplification systems** (e.g., coagulation, fibrinolytic, complement, and kallikrein-bradykinin cascades).

Nonbiologic effects on the blood during CPB are due to exposure to nonendothelial surfaces, exposure to shear stresses, and incorporation of abnormal substances such as bubbles, fibrin particles, and aggregates of platelets. Other things being equal, the damage produced by contact of blood with a nonendothelial surface is greater when the proportion of blood in the boundary layer where surface effects occur is larger. Thus, the most critical surfaces are

---

Humoral amplification systems are those in which a small stimulus results in a self-perpetuating and ever widening response in the system. Generally, in intact persons, these are triggered and are active in a localized area, such as a burn, an area of peritonitis, or a wound. CPB is perhaps the only situation in which the whole body is directly exposed to the results of activation of these substances. In hemodialysis, in which the blood is returned to a large vein, only the heart and lungs are exposed directly.

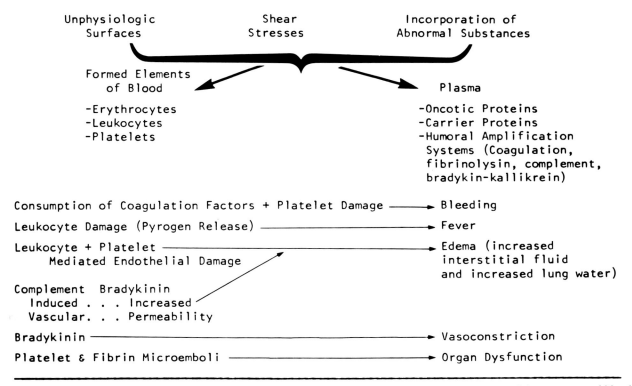

Figure 32–4. Schematic representation of a current concept of the damaging effects of CPB in terms of the exposure of blood to abnormal events. (From Kirklin, J. K., Kirklin, J. W., and Pacifico, A. D.: Cardiopulmonary bypass. *In* Arcinegas, E. [ed]: Pediatric Cardiac Surgery. Chicago, Year Book Medical Publishers. Copyright © 1985. Reproduced with permission.)

those of the oxygenating area, where a relatively large proportion of blood is deliberately maneuvered into the boundary layer for gas exchange. In bubble, disk, and screen oxygenators, the nonbiologic surface is gas (generally 100% oxygen). In membrane oxygenators, the surface is generally the membrane. However, studies (Ward et al, 1974) have shown that microbubbles of air have a strong tendency to cling to the membrane surface so that the nonbiologic surface is more complex than expected. Next are the nonbiologic surfaces of the heat exchanger, where a large proportion of blood is present in the boundary layer for heat exchange, and those of the various defoaming, debubbling, and filtering devices. The proportion of blood in the boundary layer is small in the reservoirs, tubes, and cannulas, and thus these surfaces should be expected to be the least critical.

The nonbiologic surfaces have direct and indirect effects on *platelets*, resulting in platelet clumps that may embolize, a reduction in the number of platelets, and a reduction simultaneously in their important adhesive and aggregating properties (as measured by their response to adenosine diphosphate [ADP], epinephrine, or collagen). Platelet thrombi have been shown in membrane oxygenators by Edmunds and colleagues (1978). Many studies have documented the reduction in the number of circulating platelets after CPB. For example, Kalter and colleagues (1979), by using a bubble oxygenator, observed a decrease from a mean preoxygenation platelet count of 222,100/mm³ to a postoxygenation count of 85,000/mm³. The decrease does not correlate with the duration of CPB (Han et al, 1980). Other workers (Addonizio et al, 1979b; Friedenberg et al, 1978) have shown a significant deterioration in function in the platelets that remain, as shown by a decrease in platelet aggregation in response to ADP (Bharadwaj and Chong, 1980). The systemic synthesis of prostanoids such as thrombrane B₂ during CPB (Fleming et al, 1986; Kobinia et al, 1986; Teoh et al, 1987) may result from platelet aggregation and deposition. The development of selective inhibitors of thromboxane B₂ production may reduce the deleterious vasoconstrictive effects of thromboxane during and after CPB (DeCampli et al, 1986).

Platelets are apparently not reduced in either number or function by shear stresses per se (Addonizio et al, 1979a; Solen et al, 1978; Tamari et al, 1975). There is no evidence to indicate that platelets are destroyed in any significant quantity during CPB. Rather, the decrease in their number is due to clumping on the foreign surfaces in response to the "invasion" of the body's integrity (Addonizio et al, 1980) and to the finite number of replacement platelets that are available. The severe reduction in the number of normally functioning platelets is probably the most important factor in the postoperative bleeding diathesis produced by CPB.

Platelet damage and depletion could theoretically be prevented by reducing the platelet-stimulating properties of the nonbiologic surface or by mak-

ing the platelets reversibly nonfunctional during CPB so that they do not adhere and aggregate. Addonizio and colleagues (1979a) have shown that the former can to some extent be accomplished by "coating" the membrane oxygenator surfaces with albumin. They and others have also conducted investigations suggesting the feasibility and usefulness of rendering the platelets reversibly nonfunctional by infusing prostaglandins (prostaglandin E₁ and prostacyclins) during CPB (Addonizio et al, 1978, 1979).

Exposure of the blood to nonbiologic surfaces probably has some effect on white blood cells, but shear stresses probably have the most significant effect.

Damage to red blood cells, either from direct cell fragmentation or from alterations of the cellular membrane and later cell fragmentation, results in liberation of hemoglobin into the plasma. This is generally estimated by measuring serum hemoglobin levels. The damage is produced mainly by shear forces, but also to some extent by exposure of blood in the boundary layer to nonbiologic surfaces (Solen et al, 1978).

The *carrier proteins* are significantly damaged by exposure of blood to nonbiologic surfaces. Lee and colleagues (1961) showed many years ago that protein denaturation occurred in oxygenators, with the lipoproteins liberating free fat in the process. Fat microemboli result. During CPB for cardiac procedures, the large globules of free fat seen on the surface of the intracardiac or intrapericardial blood pool result from this change. Because of protein denaturation, plasma viscosity is increased; no doubt there are other widespread effects. The denatured proteins are also believed to increase the clumping of red blood cells, making them more likely to be traumatized by shear forces.

The carrier gamma globulins are denatured at the foreign interface, especially when it is a blood-gas interface (Pruit et al, 1971; Scott, 1970). The magnitude of denaturation is related to the proportion of the plasma in the boundary layer and also to the concentration of gamma globulin. In addition to the mechanical effects, denaturation of gamma globulins may contribute to the humoral and cellular immune defects that appear to be present after CPB.

Damage to the proteins that are part of the humoral amplification systems has more complex and widespread results, involving all four components of the systems. No doubt, the protein called *Hageman's factor* (Factor XII) is activated (denatured or uncoiled) almost immediately after initiation of CPB by the massive contact of blood in the boundary layers with nonbiologic surfaces (Feijen, 1977; Verska, 1977). (Most of the evidence for this effect is indirect and includes the demonstration of fibrinopeptide A, a product of fibrinogen activation, during CPB [Davies et al, 1980] and the demonstration of the presence of bradykinin and plasmin during CPB, both of which are byproducts of the activation of Hageman's factor.) The cascade of the coagulation system begins, possibly followed in sequence by the other three amplification systems. Thus, even in the presence of adequate heparin levels during CPB, microcoagulation is continuing, generating fibrin and consuming the coagulation factors to various degrees (Davies et al, 1980; Kalter et al, 1979). The demonstrated reduction of essentially all of these (except Hageman's factor) is believed to be a result of this consumption, rather than of denaturation at contact with nonendothelial surfaces. The relative degree to which various nonbiologic surfaces, including an air-blood interface, activate the coagulation cascade has not been determined in detail. Microcoagulation and consumption of coagulation factors are further aggravated by platelet adhesion, aggregation, and granule release.

The *fibrinolytic cascade*, a second humoral amplification system, is probably activated to some extent in all operations in which CPB is used (and perhaps in many in which it is not). Thus, many studies have shown an important incidence of fibrinolysis after CPB. For example, hyperfibrinolysis has been present in 159 of 774 patients (20%) having coronary artery bypass grafting (Lambert et al, 1979). Naturally occurring plasminogen (which normally is incorporated within thrombi) can be transformed into the active fibrinolytic agent plasmin, and measurable blood plasmin levels have been shown in patients shortly after initiation of CPB (Backman et al, 1975). This is believed to be in response to the disseminated microcoagulation mentioned earlier. Because the conversion of plasminogen to plasmin is facilitated by kallikrein, which also results from the activation of Hageman's factor, the fibrinolytic cascade may be initiated also by the activation of Factor XII. Moreover, because plasmin also serves as an activator of complement, prekallikrein, and possibly Hageman's factor, the widespread activation of plasminogen into plasmin (which in intact persons is usually a circumscribed and localized phenomenon) may initiate the cascades of all the humoral amplification systems.

A third humoral amplification system involves kallikrein and bradykinin. Contact activation of Hageman's factor initiates the kallikrein-bradykinin system. Bradykinin increases vascular permeability, dilates arterioles, initiates smooth-muscle contraction, and elicits pain. Kallikrein activates Hageman's factor and activates plasminogen to form plasmin, demonstrating again the complex interactions between the various reactions of blood to a nonphysiologic experience.

Several studies using appropriate methodology have shown that important amounts of bradykinin are present during CPB (Ellison et al, 1980; Friedli et al, 1973; Pang et al, 1979). Hypothermia itself apparently results in production of bradykinin, and immaturity such as is present in young infants results in less effective means of elimination of bradykinin (Friedli et al, 1973). Exclusion of the pulmonary circulation probably also reduces the patient's ability to cope with circulating bradykinin, because the lungs are the main site of elimination of bradykinin.

Nagaoka and Katori (1975) showed a reduction in peripheral resistance and in fluid requirement during CPB with the administration of aprotinin (Trasylol), an agent that neutralizes the kallikrein-bradykinin system.

A fourth amplification system involves complement, a group of circulating glycoproteins that forms the basic matrix of the body's response to immunologic injury, infections, or traumatic insult. Two pathways exist for complement activation. The classical pathway is usually initiated by interaction with antigen-antibody complexes, whereas the alternative or properdin pathway is generally activated by exposure of blood to foreign surfaces (Goldstein, 1980). The complement cascade, once activated, also results in the production of powerful *anaphylatoxins* (Hugli, 1978) called C3a, C4a and C5a, which increase vascular permeability, cause smooth-muscle contraction, mediate white blood cell chemotaxis, and facilitate aggregation of white blood cells and enzyme release (Bjork et al, 1985; Goldstein et al, 1980; Grant et al, 1975).

Although earlier studies (Parker, 1972) have shown complement consumption during CPB and even hypothesized a relationship between complement activation and increased capillary permeability after CPB, Chenoweth and colleagues (1981) at the UAB and Scripps Institute first showed that complement anaphylatoxin C3a is released shortly after initiation of CPB, with continued production throughout the duration of bypass (Fig. 32–5). Although some controversy exists, it is generally acknowledged that complement is activated predominantly by the alternative (properdin) pathway at the initiation of CPB (Cavarocchi et al, 1985; Kirklin et al, 1986).

Although complement activation has been shown during operative procedures without CPB,

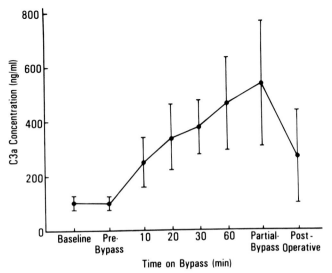

Figure 32–5. Plasma levels of C3a in patients having CPB. (Reprinted with permission from The New England Journal of Medicine, Vol. 304, p. 497, 1981.)

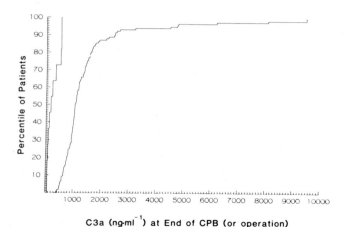

Figure 32–6. C3a levels (ng/ml^{-1}) at the end of CPB, expressed in a cumulative percentile plot. The steep *vertical line* on the left represents closed heart patients, 100% of whom had normal or almost normal levels. The curve on the right represents open heart patients, almost all of whom had increased levels. Fifty per cent had levels above 1,000 (ng/ml^{-1}), and 25% had levels above 1,600. (From Kirklin, J. K., Westaby, S., Blackstone, E. H., et al: Complement and the damaging effects of coronary bypass. J. Thorac. Cardiovasc. Surg. *86*:845, 1983.)

the magnitude of activation is very small compared with activation during CPB. In cardiac operations without CPB, for example, levels of C3a are essentially normal at the completion of the procedure (Kirklin et al, 1983) (Fig. 32–6). Fosse and colleagues (1987) have also shown increased levels of the terminal complement complex (TCC) shortly after the initiation of CPB (Fig. 32–7). TCC represents the end-product of complement activation and requires splitting of C5 into C5a and C5b. However, patients having thoracotomy without CPB showed no increase in TCC levels (Fosse et al, 1987).

A prospective clinical study at UAB examined variables related to CPB and their relationship to morbidity after cardiac procedures (Kirklin et al, 1983). Cardiac dysfunction (first 24 hours) after op-

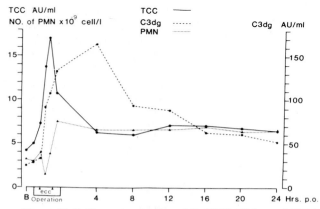

Figure 32–7. The concentration of the TCC, C3dg, and PMNs in the blood of 10 patients having aortocoronary bypass operations during ecc (median values). (B = baseline; ecc = extracorporeal circulation; PMN = polymorphonuclear leukocyte; TCC = terminal complement complex.) (From Fosse, E., Mollnes, T. E., and Ingvaldsen, B.: Complement activation during major operations without cardiopulmonary bypass. J. Thorac. Cardiovasc. Surg., *93*:860, 1987.)

eration was significantly related to higher C3a levels 3 hours after CPB, longer duration of CPB, and younger age at operation. Similarly, postoperative pulmonary dysfunction was related to the same risk factors. Risk factors specific for postoperative renal dysfunction included higher C3a levels 3 hours after CPB and younger age. An overall index of morbidity was also determined, and it related significantly to higher levels of C3a, longer duration of CPB, and younger age at operation. This relationship between morbidity following CPB and complement activation is particularly interesting, because the anaphylatoxins C5a and C3a have physiologic effects similar to those observed in many patients after CPB, including vasoconstriction and increased capillary permeability (Muller-Eberhard, 1975).

Salama and colleagues (1988), from West Germany, also showed deposition of the terminal C5b,9 complement complexes on red blood cells and neutrophils during CPB. Intravascular hemolysis was observed in all patients, and C5b,9 was shown on red blood cell ghosts but not on intact red blood cells, inferring a relationship between complement activation on red blood cells and hemolysis during CPB. In addition, granulocytes were almost uniformly found to carry C5b,9 complexes during CPB and transiently afterward (less than 24 hours).

Alterations in Microvascular Permeability

Accumulation of extravascular fluid has often been described after CPB, with clinical manifestations that include increased pulmonary interstitial fluid without a rise in left atrial pressure, increased tissue and peripheral edema, and ascites. Cleland and colleagues (1966), at the Mayo Clinic, noted that progressive increases in extravascular fluid after cardiac operations were directly related to the duration of CPB. Studies by Royston and colleagues (1985) on the clearance of ^{99m}Tc-labeled diethylenetriamine-penta-acetate (DTPA) suggest an increased permeability of the pulmonary alveolar-capillary barrier associated with CPB. Despite these and many other studies documenting alterations in the distribution of fluid after CPB, direct evidence of alterations in capillary permeability was lacking. Smith and colleagues (1987) provided the first direct evidence that microvascular permeability is increased after CPB. By using ultrafiltration techniques in a dog, a segment of small intestine was isolated, its lymphatic drainage was cannulated, and the segment's venous pressure progressively increased during a 3-hour period to augment lymphatic flow. The colloid osmotic sieving ratio is determined by the minimal lymph-plasma protein concentration and was used as a measure of microvascular permeability (Granger and Taylor, 1980). The permeability to each of six sizes of plasma proteins measured by density gradient gel electrophoresis was determined. A systematic increase in permeability to proteins by 2 hours of normothermic

CPB was shown, and larger molecules were proportionately more affected (Fig. 32–8).

Protamine-Complement Interaction

The deleterious response to CPB may be further complicated by accompanying pharmacologic interventions. This is particularly true with protamine sulfate, which is routinely used to reverse the anticoagulation effect of heparin after CPB. The protamine reversal after CPB may be associated occasionally with raised systemic hypotension and low left atrial pressure secondary to raised peripheral vasodilation. Rarely, there is accompanying intense and potentially fatal pulmonary vasoconstriction that produces acute right ventricular failure (Lowenstein et al, 1983). The protamine-heparin complex may also have a direct myocardial depressant effect (Fiser et al, 1985; Hendry et al, 1987). The classical pathway of complement is activated by protamine-heparin interaction, which is indicated by the generation of the anaphylatoxin C4a in addition to C3a and C5a (Cavarocchi et al, 1985; Kirklin et al, 1986) (Fig. 32–9). Thus, CPB is associated with predominant activation of the alternative complement pathway, whereas protamine administration at the end of bypass further activates complement by the classical pathway. The physiologic effects of the anaphylatoxins C3a, C4a, and C5a include peripheral vasodilation, which is encountered occasionally with administration of protamine. Although left atrial administration of protamine has been reported to eliminate the adverse hemodynamic effects (Frater et al, 1984), the authors have found that this is unreliable. When a serious reaction to protamine administration occurs after CPB, volume administration, alpha-adrenergic agents, and possibly steroid administration

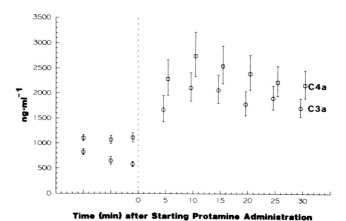

Figure 32–9. Levels of C3a and C4a after CPB and the initiation of protamine sulfate administration. Zero and the *broken vertical line* indicate the beginning of protamine administration, which was 10 minutes after discontinuation of CPB. Protamine was infused during a 5-minute period. The *vertical bars* represent the 70% confidence limits. The mean normal value of C3a is 76 $ng·ml^{-1}$ and for C4a, 1,200 $ng·ml^{-1}$. (From Kirklin, J. K., Chenoweth, D. E., Naftel, D. C., et al: Effects of protamine administration after cardiopulmonary bypass on complement, blood elements, and the hemodynamic state. Ann. Thorac. Surg., 41:193, 1986.)

have been noted clinically to be of benefit. Readministration of heparin occasionally appears to ameliorate the adverse hemodynamic effects. If these measures are unsuccessful, it is advisable to re-establish CPB promptly and regain hemodynamic stability. When the hemodynamic condition is again stable, CPB can be discontinued without further administration of protamine.

PUMP OXYGENATOR

Although the apparatus available for CPB changes continually, some components are common to all types and warrant discussion.

A *venous reservoir* is generally incorporated and is positioned to provide adequate siphonage from gravity (Paneth et al, 1947). Such a reservoir allows the escape of any air returning with the venous blood and the storage of excess volume. Bubble oxygenators can act as a venous reservoir. A venous pump, instead of gravity drainage, can be used to move blood directly from the venae cavae into the oxygenator, but such a system requires precise control.

Bubble oxygenators and *membrane oxygenators* are essentially the only pump oxygenators currently used for clinical CPB. Membrane oxygenators probably reduce blood trauma without production of emboli and in addition facilitate control of Pa_{O_2} and Pa_{CO_2} during hypothermia. However, no clear-cut advantage of membrane over bubble oxygenators has been shown, even in children (Sade et al, 1980). Perhaps this is partly because of platelet adhesion despite absence of a blood-gas interface (Sade et al, 1980).

There is also no clear evidence that the type of oxygenator used affects the magnitude of the inflam-

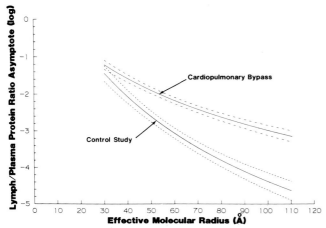

Figure 32–8. Nomogram relating the asymptote of the lymph-plasma protein ratio (permeability ratio) to the effective molecular radius of the proteins and to the conditions of the experiments (CPB or sham procedure). The vertical axis is in logarithmic units. (From Smith, E. E. J., Naftel, D., Blackstone, E. H., and Kirklin, J. W.: Microvascular permeability after cardiopulmonary bypass. J. Thorac. Cardiovasc. Surg., 94:225, 1987.)

TABLE 32–4. OXYGEN CONSUMPTION AT DIFFERENT PERFUSION FLOW RATES (0.5–1.5 l/min^{-1}/m^{-2}) DURING PROFOUNDLY HYPOTHERMIC (20° C), NONPULSATILE, HEMODILUTED CPB IN THE MONKEY*

| Organ | Oxygen Consumption (ml/min^{-1}/100 g^{-1}) | | | p Value |
	1.5	1.0	0.5	
Whole body	0.119 ± 0.0077	0.086 ± 0.0045	0.57 ± 0.0029	<0.0001
Brain	0.5 ± 0.095	0.47 ± 0.076	0.45 ± 0.113	0.5
Whole body minus brain	0.114 ± 0.0074	0.081 ± 0.0085	0.0518 ± 0.001	<0.0001

*From Fox, L. S., Blackstone, E. H., Kirklin, J. W., et al: Relationship of brain blood flow and oxygen consumption to perfusion flow rate during hypothermic cardiopulmonary bypass. J. Thorac. Cardiovasc. Surg., 87:658, 1984.

matory response (Oeveren et al, 1985). In a porcine model, similar and marked complement activation with elaboration of C3a was observed with both a membrane and a bubble oxygenator system (Kirklin et al, 1987). A clinical study by Cavarocchi and colleagues (1986), however, indicated a potentially favorable effect of the membrane oxygenator. In this study, a bubble oxygenator was associated with greater C3a generation at the end of CPB and greater transpulmonary white blood cell sequestration when compared with a membrane oxygenator. These differences were, however, eliminated when patients in the bubble oxygenator group received methylprednisolone (30 mg/kg) 20 minutes before CPB (Fig. 32–10).

The *arterial pump* is most commonly a roller pump. It should be adjusted before each perfusion so that it is slightly nonocclusive. The pump tubing should be Silastic or latex, because neither will become stiff at low temperatures. Other plastic tubing stiffens at low temperatures, and the recoil and thus the stroke volume of the pump and perfusion flow rate are reduced during hypothermia. The arterial pump should be calibrated at frequent intervals so that the perfusion flow rate can be accurately established.

The *arterial line pressure* in the pump oxygenator must be continuously monitored. When this pressure becomes greater than 250 to 300 mm Hg, the risk of disruption of the arterial line and of cavitation in the region of the arterial cannula increases. These risks are prevented by a properly positioned, adequately sized cannula.

An *arterial bubble trap* may be used as a safety device to remove air that has inadvertently entered the arterial line. An arterial line filter has been recommended by some surgeons, but its benefit is questionable (Aris et al, 1986).

The CPB circuit should contain at least two *cardiotomy suction lines* for return of blood from the opened heart. This blood contains particulate matter and air and must be passed through a low-porosity filter and defoamed in a separate chamber that is open to air before it is returned to the circuit. If this blood remains for a long time in the pericardial space, it is a powerful source of hemolysis. This part of the extracorporeal apparatus is the most damaging to blood (Osborn et al, 1962). Ideally, these lines should be activated by a continuously and rapidly variable high-capacity vacuum system; however, this has proved to be impractical, and roller pumps are there-

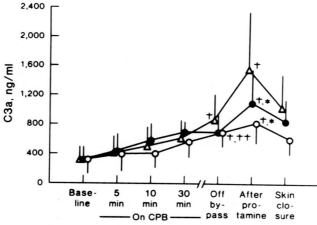

Figure 32–10. Plasma levels of C3a in patients having CPB. Compared with the bubble oxygenator group (△), C3a levels in the bubble oxygenator group with Solu-Medrol (●) and the membrane oxygenator group (○) were significantly lower after bypass. Each point represents mean ± standard deviation. († = p<0.001 versus baseline; †† = p<0.02 versus bubble oxygenation group; * = p<0.001 versus bubble oxygenation group.) (From Cavarocchi, N. C., Pluth, J. R., Schaff, H. V., et al: Complement activation during cardiopulmonary bypass. J. Thorac. Cardiovasc. Surg., 91:252, 1986.)

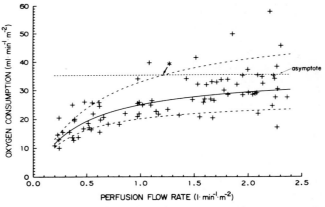

Figure 32–11. Relationship of oxygen consumption and perfusion flow rate during nonpulsatile CPB at 20° C (n=17). The (+) signs represent individual measurements. The *solid line* is the nomogram of a hyperbolic equation fitted to the data. The *dashed lines* are the 70% confidence limits (CL) for the observations. The *broken line* is the estimated asymptote, and the asterisk (*) indicates the flow rate above which the upper 70% CL overlaps the asymptote. (From Fox, L. S., Blackstone, E. H., Kirklin, J. W., et al: Relationship of whole body-oxygen consumption to perfusion flow rate during hypothermic bypass. J. Thorac. Cardiovasc. Surg., 83:239, 1982.)

TABLE 32–5. BRAIN AND BODY MINUS THE BRAIN BLOOD FLOW RESISTANCES AT VARIOUS PERFUSION FLOW RATES ($0.25-1.75$ l/min/m^{-2}) IN THE MONKEY DURING CARDIOPULMONARY BYPASS AT 20° C*

Organ	Resistance (units/100 g)							p Value
	1.75	1.5	1.25	1.0	0.75	0.5	0.25	
Brain	1.2 ± 0.51	0.80 ± 0.080	0.8 ± 0.22	0.78 ± 0.126	1.05 ± 0.165	0.80 ± 0.117	1.02 ± 0.173	0.4
Whole body minus brain	2.8 ± 0.157	3.3 ± 0.22	3.3 ± 1.21	3.9 ± 0.24	4.6 ± 0.077	5.1 ± 0.49	9.5 ± 0.70	<0.0001

*From Fox, L. S., Blackstone, E. H., Kirklin, J. W., et al: Relationship of brain blood flow and oxygen consumption to perfusion flow rate during hypothermic cardiopulmonary bypass. J. Thorac. Cardiovasc. Surg., *87*:658, 1984.

fore used. With this system, when the end of the line is obstructed, the suction rapidly increases, possibly damaging either the tissue or the blood. Constant supervision of the open heart roller pump rates is mandatory.

The pump-oxygenator should be designed to *minimize priming volume*. This parameter is most critical in infants, in whom the priming volume can be greatly in excess of blood volume. Almost all infant circuits are less than optimal in this regard (Turina et al, 1972).

STRATEGIES IN THE APPLICATION OF CARDIOPULMONARY BYPASS AS A SUPPORT TECHNIQUE FOR NEONATAL AND INFANT INTRACARDIAC THERAPY

CPB can be used effectively as a flexible technique during open heart operations in small infants and neonates, not only as a support device, but also as a method for generating optimal exposure for intracardiac repairs. Two techniques that are most commonly used for neonatal and infant intracardiac operations are low-flow perfusion and deep hypothermic total circulatory arrest.

Low-Flow Perfusion

In a clinical study of CPB at 20° C, Fox and colleagues (1982) noted a continuous relationship between $\dot{V}O_2$ and perfusion flow rates, such that $\dot{V}O_2$ at 20° C remains fairly constant as flow rates are reduced to approximately 1.2 l/min/m^2, but further reductions in flow rate are accompanied by a progressive fall in $\dot{V}O_2$ (Fig. 32–11). The authors interpret this data to indicate that during clinical CPB at 20° C, most of the microcirculation is perfused at flow rates of 1.2 l/min/m^2 and greater. Below that level, decrease in flow rates results in a decrease of effective body mass participating in microvascular oxygen exchange.

The brain is probably the organ that is most sensitive to reductions in oxygen supply. The effects of altered flow rates on brain blood flow and oxygen

consumption have been studied in monkeys during CPB at 20° C (Fox et al, 1984). Oxygen consumption of the brain was well maintained as flow was reduced from 1.5 to 0.5 l/min/m^2 on bypass at 20° C (Table 32–4). The resistance to blood flow in the brain remained unchanged, whereas that of the remaining body increased as the flow rate was reduced (Table 32–5). Even at the lowest perfusion flow rate (0.25 l/min/m^2), all areas of the brain were perfused. It thus appears that the brain, the resistance of which does not change, becomes the passive recipient of proportionally more blood flow during low-flow, hypothermic CPB. In addition to these experimental studies, a large clinical experience indicates that perfusion flow rates can be safely reduced to 0.5 l/min/m^2 for 30 to 45 minutes at 20° C. By using separate caval cannulation (see Fig. 32–1 and Table 32–2), low-flow perfusion can be used when necessary to optimize exposure during transatrial or transventricular intracardiac repairs.

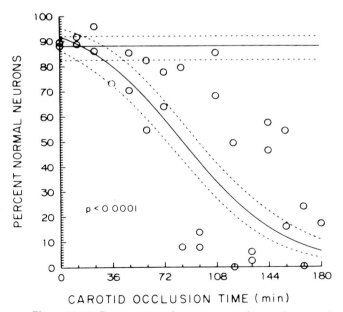

Figure 32–12. Per cent normal neurons according to the carotid occlusion time at 18 to 19° C in gerbils (each gerbil is represented by a *circle*). The *solid line* is the nomogram of the equation fitted to the data, with its 70% CL (±1 SD, *dashed lines*). The *transverse lines* are the mean value with its 70% CL for normal gerbils. (From Treasure, T., Naftel, D. C., Conger, K. A., et al: The effect of hypothermic circulatory arrest time on cerebral function morphology and biochemistry. J. Thorac. Cardiovasc. Surg., *86*:761, 1983.)

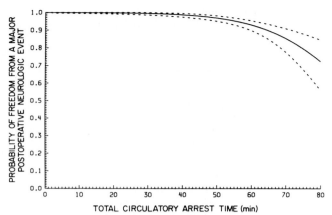

Figure 32–13. The relation between the probability of a major neurologic event occurring postoperatively and the total circulatory arrest (TCA) time in 219 patients (eight events) having open intracardiac operations at UAB. Among the 211 without these events, TCA time was 42 ± 14.0 (SD) minutes versus 59 ± 10.2 for the eight with such events (p = 0.0008). The logistic equation for the nomogram is as follows:

$$Z = -7.3 + 0.08 \times TCA, \text{ where TCA is TCA time in minutes}$$

(From Kirklin, J. K., Kirklin, J. W., and Pacifico, A. D.: Deep hypothermia and total circulatory arrest. *In* Arcinegas, E. [ed]: Pediatric Cardiac Surgery. Chicago, Year Book Medical Publishers. Copyright © 1985. Reproduced with permission.)

Deep Hypothermic Total Circulatory Arrest

For some operations, particularly in very small neonates, the technique of deep hypothermia and total circulatory arrest provides elegant exposure with a bloodless, uncluttered operative field for the intracardiac repair. The cannulation technique for CPB is simplified by using a single venous cannula in the right atrium for cooling and rewarming. Despite the use of total circulatory arrest clinically for more than 25 years and a number of clinical and experimental studies (Clarkson et al, 1980; Haka-Ikse et al, 1978; Stevenson et al, 1974) there continues to be controversy regarding the safe duration of total circulatory arrest and the presence of neurologic damage associated with its use and duration. Treasure and colleagues (1983), using gerbils, indirectly examined the safe period of total circulatory arrest during cardiac operations by studying the effects of periods of 0 to 180 minutes of profoundly hypothermic (20° C) cerebral circulatory arrest produced by bilateral carotid artery occlusion. Gerbils are uniquely suited for these studies because of an incomplete circle of Willis, such that bilateral carotid occlusion reliably produces global cerebral ischemia. Abnormal neurologic function and a decrease in the proportion of normal neurons (Fig. 32–12) became evident when the occlusion time exceeded 45 minutes. These changes were accompanied by a sharp reduction of high-energy phosphates. It can be inferred from these studies that the safe period of total circulatory arrest at 20° C is likely to be approximately 45 minutes.

Studies in humans after total circulatory arrest have focused on electroencephalographic changes during and after total circulatory arrest, development of postoperative choreoathetosis and seizures, and late studies of motor development. It is generally acknowledged that uniform cooling of any organ, and in this case the brain, requires an adequate time for caloric exchange to occur. More uniform cooling would be expected to provide greater safety during periods of total circulatory arrest. Studies of patients having total circulatory arrest at UAB showed an increased incidence of choreoathetosis in patients with core cooling (compared with preliminary surface cooling combined with core cooling) (Kirklin et al, 1983). The probability of freedom from a major postoperative neurologic event decreased rapidly when the arrest time exceeded 50 minutes at 18 to 20° C (Fig. 32–13). Most available clinical studies indicate that intellectual and psychomotor development are usually not impaired when circulatory arrest time is less than approximately 60 minutes at 18 to 20° C (Clarkson et al, 1980; Messmer et al, 1976; Wells et al, 1983).

Clinical studies in adult patients with circulatory arrest (Coselli et al, 1988) have suggested that the safe period of total circulatory arrest may be further prolonged by more complete cooling of the brain (as judged by electrocerebral silence on detailed intraoperative electroencephalography) to temperatures of 12 to 16° C (nasopharyngeal).

Selected Bibliography

Chenoweth, D. E., Cooper, S. W., Hugli, T. E., et al: Complement activation during cardiopulmonary bypass: Evidence for generation of C3a and C5a anaphylatoxins. N. Engl. J. Med., *304*:497, 1981.

CPB is currently a safe support system for most patients having cardiac surgical procedures. An occasional patient, particularly if seriously ill, very young, or very old, suffers additional morbidity related to CPB. Chenoweth and colleagues provided the first direct quantitative evidence for activation of the alternative complement pathway during CPB, resulting from exposure of blood to nonbiologic surfaces. This and other techniques for studying the damaging effects of bypass may ultimately lead to safer support systems for cardiac surgical procedures.

Coselli, J. S., Crawford, E. S., Beall, A. C., Jr., et al: Determination of brain temperatures for safe circulatory arrest during cardiovascular operation. Ann. Thorac. Surg., *45*:638, 1988.

Profound hypothermia and temporary circulatory arrest have been the basic technique for intracardiac surgical procedures in neonates. A safe period of circulatory arrest of 45 to 60 minutes has generally been accepted, with deep hypothermia to 18 to 20° C. The authors report superb results with the technique of deep hypothermic circulatory arrest in adult patients having aortic procedures. By using detailed intraoperative electroencephalography, electrocerebral silence was frequently not achieved until the nasopharyngeal temperature was reduced to 16° C or less. This experience suggests that more complete and profound brain cooling could provide longer periods of safe circulatory arrest than have traditionally been accepted.

Gibbon, J. H.: Application of a mechanical heart and lung apparatus to cardiac surgery. Minn. Med., *37*:171, 1954.

This classic paper describes the first successful use of a heart-lung machine in humans to entirely support the circulation during open heart surgery, with the closure of an atrial septal defect. The author discusses the physiologic response to CPB, including hemolysis, adequate tissue perfusion, and the problems of cardiac distention and air emboli. Gibbon concluded, "It seems to me that there will always be a place for an extracorporeal blood circuit because it permits a longer safe interval for opening the heart than can ever be obtained by any of the hypothermic methods."

Kirklin, J. W., Dushane, J. W., Patrick, R. T., et al: Intracardiac surgery with the aid of a mechanical pump-oxygenator (Gibbon type): Report of eight cases. Proc. Staff Meet. Mayo Clin., *30:*201, 1955.

This is the first report of a series of patients successfully having cardiac surgery with the use of a mechanical pump oxygenator. Four patients had ventricular septal defects, and two survived postoperatively. Two patients had atrioventricular canal defects, and one survived. One patient had tetralogy of Fallot, and he died. One patient had closure of an atrial septal defect and survived. At the time of this report, it was widely believed that a totally mechanical support system would not allow successful cardiac surgical procedures.

Kirklin, J. K., Westaby, S., Blackstone, E. H., et al: Complement and the damaging effects of cardiopulmonary bypass. J. Thorac. Cardiovasc. Surg., *86:*845, 1983.

This prospective clinical study is one of the first rigorous attempts to identify those factors associated with CPB that contribute to organ system dysfunction after cardiac surgical procedures. Complement levels remained normal in patients having cardiac operations without CPB, compared with the marked complement activation that occurred during CPB. Cardiac, renal, pulmonary, and hemostatic dysfunction increased with higher levels of the complement anaphylatoxin C3a after bypass, younger age at operation, and longer time on bypass. The authors suggest that a more complete understanding of the biologic response to CPB may eventually lead to the neutralization of these damaging effects.

Lillehei, C. W., Cohen, M., Warden, H. E., and Varco, R. L.: The direct vision intracardiac correction of congenital anomalies by controlled cross circulation. Surgery, *38:*11, 1955.

The authors report the first successful series of intracardiac operations using CPB. The experimental and physiologic bases for the use of another human being as the source of oxygenation and perfusion are discussed. Twenty-two patients had repair of a ventricular septal defect (18 survivors), 6 had tetralogy of Fallot (3 survivors), 2 had an atrioventricular canal defect (1 survivor), and 2 had pulmonary stenosis (1 survivor).

Smith, E. E. J., Naftel, D. C., Blackstone, E. H., and Kirklin, J. W.: Microvascular permeability after cardiopulmonary bypass. J. Thorac. Cardiovasc. Surg., *94:*225, 1987.

Since its inception, CPB has been presumed to produce increases in microvascular permeability, but this had not been directly shown. In this controlled experimental study of the small intestinal microvasculature of the dog, the authors provided the first direct evidence that CPB produces an increase in microvascular permeability, particularly for large molecules.

Bibliography

Addonizio, V. P., Jr., Macarak, E. J., Nicolaou, K. C., et al: Effects of prostacyclin and albumin on platelet loss during in vitro simulation of extracorporeal circulation. J. Am. Soc. Hematol., *53:*1033, 1979a.

Addonizio, V. P., Jr., Smith, J. B., Strauss, J. F., III, et al: Thromboxane synthesis and platelet secretion during cardiopulmonary bypass with bubble oxygenator. J. Thorac. Cardiovasc. Surg., *79:*91, 1980.

Addonizio, V. P., Jr., Strauss, J. F., III, Colman, R. W., and Edmunds, L. H., Jr.: Effects of prostaglandin E_1 on platelet loss during in vivo and in vitro extracorporeal circulation with a bubble oxygenator. J. Thorac. Cardiovasc. Surg., *77:*119, 1979b.

Addonizio, V. P., Jr., Strauss, J. F., III, Macarak, E. J., et al: Preservation of platelet number and function with prostaglandin E_1 during total cardiopulmonary bypass in rhesus monkeys. Surgery, *83:*619, 1978.

Andreason, A. T., and Watson, F.: Experimental cardiovascular surgery, "the azygos factor." Br. J. Surg., *39:*548, 1952.

Aris, A., Solanes, H., Camara, M. L., et al: Arterial line filtration during cardiopulmonary bypass. J. Thorac. Cardiovasc. Surg., *91:*526, 1986.

Backmann, F., McKenna, R., Cole, E. R., and Najafi, H.: The hemostatic mechanism after open-heart surgery. I. Studies on plasma coagulation factors and fibrinolysis in 512 patients after extracorporeal circulation. J. Thorac. Cardiovasc. Surg., *70:*76, 1975.

Barratt-Boyes, B. G., Simpson, M., and Neutze, J. M.: Intracardiac surgery in neonates and infants using deep hypothermia with surface cooling and limited cardiopulmonary bypass. Circulation, *43,44*(Suppl. 1):25, 1971.

Bennett, E. V., Jr., Fewel, J. G., Ybarra, J., et al: Comparison of flow differences among venous cannulas. Ann. Thorac. Surg., *36:*59, 1983.

Bharadwaj, B. B., and Chong, G.: Effects of extracorporeal circulation on structure, function, and population distribution of canine blood platelets. Presented at the Combined Meeting of the Royal Australasian College of Surgeons and Royal Australasian College of Physicians, Sydney, Australia, February 24–29, 1980.

Bjork, J., Hugli, T. E., and Smedegard, G.: Microvascular effects of anaphylatoxins C3a and C5a. J. Immunol. *134:*2, 1115, 1985.

Bjork, V. O.: Brain perfusions in dogs with artificially oxygenated blood. Acta Chir. Scand., *96*(Suppl. 137):1, 1948.

Bove, E. L., West, H. L., and Paskanik, A. M.: Hypothermic cardiopulmonary bypass: A comparison between alpha and pH stat regulation in the dog. J. Surg. Res., *42:*66, 1987.

Broadman, R., Siegel, H., Lesser, M., and Frater, R.: A comparison of flow gradients across disposable arterial perfusion cannulas. Ann. Thorac. Surg., *39:*225, 1985.

Brown, I. W., Smith, W. W., and Emmons, W. O.: An efficient blood heat exchanger for use with extracorporeal circulation. Surgery, *44:*372, 1958.

Cavarocchi, N. C., Pluth, J. R., Schaff, H. V., et al: Complement activation during cardiopulmonary bypass. J. Thorac. Cardiovasc. Surg., *91:*252, 1986.

Cavarocchi, N. C., Schaff, H. V., Orszulak, T. A., et al: Evidence for complement activation by protamine-heparin interaction after cardiopulmonary bypass. Surgery, *98:*525, 1985.

Chenoweth, D. E., Cooper, W. W., Hugli, T. E., et al: Complement activation during cardiopulmonary bypass: Evidence for generation of C3a and C5a anaphylatoxins. N. Engl. J. Med., *304:*497, 1981.

Chien, S.: Present state of blood rheology. *In* Messmer, K., and Schmid-Schonbein, H. (eds): Hemodilution: Theoretical Basis and Clinical Application. New York, Karger, 1972, pp. 1–45.

Clarkson, P. M., MacArthur, B. A., Barratt-Boyes, B., et al: Development progress after cardiac surgery in infancy using profound hypothermia and circulatory arrest. Circulation, *62:*855, 1980.

Cleland, J., Pluth, J. R., Tauxe, W. N., and Kirklin, J. W.: Blood volume and body fluid compartment changes soon after closed and open intracardiac surgery. J. Thorac. Cardiovasc. Surg., *52:*698, 1966.

Cohen, M., and Lillehei, C. W.: A quantitative study of the "azygos factor" during vena caval occlusion in the dog. Surg. Gynecol. Obstet., *98:*225, 1954.

Cohn, L. H., Angell, W. W., and Shumway, N. E.: Body fluid shifts after cardiopulmonary bypass. I: Effects of congestive heart failure and hemodilution. J. Thorac. Cardiovasc. Surg., *62:*423, 1971.

Coselli, J. S., Crawford, E. S., Beall, A. C., Jr., et al: Determination of brain temperatures for safe circulatory arrest during cardiovascular operation. Ann. Thorac. Surg., 45:638, 1988.

Crafoord, C., Norberg, B., and Senning, A.: Clinical studies in extracorporeal circulation with a heart-lung machine. Acta Chir. Scand., 112:200, 1957.

Davies, G. C., Sobel, M., and Salzman, E. W.: Elevated plasma fibrinopeptide A and thromboxane B₂ levels during cardiopulmonary bypass. Circulation, 61:808, 1980.

DeBakey, M. D.: Simple continuous flow blood transfusion instrument. New Orleans Med. Surg. J., 87:386, 1934.

DeCampli, W. M., Goodwin, D., Kosek, J. C., et al: Pharmacological, hematological, and physiological effects of a new thromboxane synthetase inhibitor (CGS-13080) during cardiopulmonary bypass in dogs. Ann. Thorac. Surg., 42:690, 1986.

Dennis, C., Spreng, D. S., Jr., Nelson, G. E., et al: Development of a pump-oxygenator to replace the heart and lungs: An apparatus applicable to human patients, and application to one case. Ann. Surg., 134:709, 1951.

Diesh, G., Flynn, P. J., Marable, S. A., et al: Comparison of low (azygos) flow and high flow principles of extracorporeal circulation employing a bubble oxygenator. Surgery, 42:67, 1957.

Donald, D. E., Harshbarger, H. G., Hetzel, P. S., et al: Experiences with a heart-lung bypass (Gibbon type) in the experimental laboratory: Preliminary report. Proc. Staff Meet. Mayo Clin., 30:113, 1955.

Edmunds, L. H., Jr., Saxena, N. C., Hillyer, P., and Wilson, T. J.: Relationship between platelet count and cardiotomy suction return. Ann. Thorac. Surg., 25:306, 1978.

Ellison, N., Behar, M., MacVaugh, H., III, and Marshall, B. E.: Bradykinin, plasma protein fraction and hypotension. Ann. Thorac. Surg., 29:15, 1980.

Feijen, J.: Thrombogenesis caused by blood-foreign surface interaction. In Kenedi, R. M., Courtney, J. M., Gaylor, J. D. S., and Gilchrist, T.: Artificial Organs. Baltimore, University Park Press, 1977, pp. 235–247.

Fiser, W. P., Fewell, J. E., Hill, D. E., et al: Cardiovascular effects of protamine sulfate are dependent on the presence and type of circulating heparin. J. Thorac. Cardiovasc. Surg., 89:63, 1985.

Fleming, W. H., Sarafian, L. B., Leuschen, M. P., et al: Serum concentrations of prostacyclin and thromboxane in children before, during, and after cardiopulmonary bypass. J. Thorac. Cardiovasc. Surg., 92:73, 1986.

Fosse, E., Mollnes, T. E., and Ingvaldsen, B.: Complement activation during major operations without cardiopulmonary bypass. J. Thorac. Cardiovasc. Surg., 93:860, 1987.

Fox, L. S., Blackstone, E. H., Kirklin, J. W., et al: Relationship of brain blood flow and oxygen consumption to perfusion flow rate during hypothermic cardiopulmonary bypass. J. Thorac. Cardiovasc. Surg., 87:658, 1984.

Fox, L. S., Blackstone, E. H., Kirklin, J. W., et al: Relationship of whole-body oxygen consumption to perfusion flow rate during hypothermic bypass. J. Thorac. Cardiovasc. Surg., 83:239, 1982.

Frater, R. W. M., Oka, Y., Hong, Y., et al: Protamine-induced circulatory changes. J. Thorac. Cardiovasc. Surg., 87:687, 1984.

Frey, M. V., and Gruber, M.: Untersuchungen Über den Staffwechsel Isolierter Organe: Ein Respirations Apparat Fur Isolierte Organe. Arch. F. Physiol., 9:519, 1885.

Friedenberg, W. R., Myers, W. O., Plotka, E. D., et al: Platelet dysfunction associated with cardiopulmonary bypass. Ann. Thorac. Surg., 25:298, 1978.

Friedli, B., Kent, G., and Olley, P. M.: Inactivation of bradykinin in the pulmonary vascular bed of newborn and fetal lambs. Circ. Res., 33:421, 1973.

Gibbon, J. H., Jr.: The maintenance of life during experimental occlusion of the pulmonary artery followed by survival. Surg. Gynecol. Obstet., 69:602, 1939.

Gibbon, J. H., Jr.: Application of a mechanical heart and lung apparatus to cardiac surgery. Minn. Med., 37:171, 1954.

Gibbon, J. H., Jr.: Personal communication, 1955.

Goldstein, I. M.: Current Concepts: Complement in Infectious Diseases. Kalamazoo, MI, The Upjohn Company, 1980, p. 7.

Granger, D. N., and Taylor, A. E.: Permeability of intestinal capillaries to endogenous macromolecules. Am. J. Physiol., 238:H457, 1980.

Grant, J. A., Dupree, E., Goldman, A. S., et al: Complement-mediated release of histamine from human leukocytes. J. Immunol., 114:1101, 1975.

Haka-Ikse, K., Blackwood, M. J. A., and Steward, D. J.: Psychomotor development of infants and children after profound hypothermia during surgery for congenital heart disease. Devel. Med. Child Neurol., 29:62070, 1978.

Hallowell, P., Austen, W. G., and Laver, M. B.: Influence of oxygen flow rate on arterial oxygenation and acid-base balance during cardiopulmonary bypass with use of a disc oxygenator. Circulation, 35(Suppl. 1):199, 1967.

Han, P., Turpie, A. G. G., Butt, R., et al: The use of β-thromboglobulin release to assess platelet damage during cardiopulmonary bypass. Presented at the Combined Meeting of the Royal Australasian College of Surgeons and Royal Australasian College of Physicians, Sydney, Australia, February 24–29, 1980.

Harris, E. A., Seelye, E. R., and Barratt-Boyes, B. G.: Respiratory and metabolic acid-base changes during cardiopulmonary bypass in man. Br. J. Anaesth., 42:912, 1970.

Hendry, P. J., Taichman, G. C., and Keon, W. J.: The myocardial contractile responses to protamine sulfate and heparin. Ann. Thorac. Surg., 44:263, 1987.

Hickey, R. F., and Hoar, P. F.: Whole-body oxygen consumption during low-flow hypothermic cardiopulmonary bypass. J. Thorac. Cardiovasc. Surg., 86:903, 1983.

Hikasa, Y., Shirotani, H., Satomura, K., et al: Open heart surgery in infants with the aid of hypothermic anesthesia. Arch. Jpn. Chir., 36:495, 1967.

Hine, I. P., Wood, W. G., Mainwaring-Buton, R. W., et al: The adrenergic response to surgery involving cardiopulmonary bypass, as measured by plasma and urinary catecholamine concentrations. Br. J. Anaesth., 48:355, 1976.

Hugli, T.: Chemical aspects of the serum anaphylatoxins. Contemp. Top. Mol. Immunol., 7:181, 1978.

Jones, R. E., Donald, D. E., Swan, H. J. C., et al: Apparatus of the Gibbon type of mechanical bypass of the heart and lungs: Preliminary report. Proc. Staff Meet. Mayo Clin., 30:105, 1955.

Kalter, R. D., Saul, C. M., Wetstein, L., et al: Cardiopulmonary bypass: Associated hemostatic abnormalities. J. Thorac. Cardiovasc. Surg., 77:428, 1979.

Kirklin, J. K., Blackstone, E. H., and Kirklin, J. W.: Cardiopulmonary bypass: Studies on its damaging effects. Blood Purif., 5:168, 1987.

Kirklin, J. K., Chenoweth, D. E., Naftel, D. C., et al: Effects of protamine administration after cardiopulmonary bypass on complement, blood elements, and the hemodynamic state. Ann. Thorac. Surg., 41:193, 1986.

Kirklin, J. K., Kirklin, J. W., and Pacifico, A. D.: Cardiopulmonary bypass. In Arcinegas, E. (ed): Pediatric Cardiac Surgery. Chicago, Year Book Medical Publishers, 1985a, pp. 67–77.

Kirklin, J. K., Kirklin, J. W., and Pacifico, A. D.: Deep hypothermia and total circulatory arrest. In Arcinegas, E. (ed): Pediatric Cardiac Surgery. Chicago, Year Book Medical Publishers, 1985b, pp. 67–77.

Kirklin, J. K., Westaby, S., Blackstone, E. H., et al: Complement and the damaging effects of cardiopulmonary bypass. J. Thorac. Cardiovasc. Surg., 86:845, 1983.

Kirklin, J. W.: A letter to Helen. J. Thorac. Cardiovasc. Surg., 78:643, 1979.

Kirklin, J. W., Barratt-Boyes, B. G.: Cardiac Surgery. New York, John Wiley and Sons, 1986.

Kobinia, G. S., LaRaia, P. J., D'Ambra, M. N., et al: Effect of experimental cardiopulmonary bypass on systemic and transcardiac thromboxane B₂ levels. J. Thorac. Cardiovasc. Surg., 91:852, 1986.

Lambert, C. J., Marengo-Rowe, A. J., Leveson, J. E., et al: The treatment of postperfusion bleeding using ε-aminocaproic acid, cryoprecipitate, fresh-frozen plasma, and protamine sulfate. Ann. Thorac. Surg., 28:440, 1979.

Lee, W. H., Jr., Krumbhoar, D., Fonkalsrud, E. W., et al: Denaturation of plasma proteins as a cause of morbidity and death after intracardiac operations. Surgery, 50:29, 1961.

Cardiopulmonary Bypass for Cardiac Surgery / 1125

Lees, M. H., Herr, R. H., Hill, J. D., et al: Distribution of systemic blood flow of the rhesus monkey during cardiopulmonary bypass. J. Thorac. Cardiovasc. Surg., 61:570, 1971.

Levin, M. B., Theye, R. A., Fowler, W. S., and Kirklin, J. W.: Performance of the stationary vertical-screen oxygenator (Mayo-Gibbon). J. Thorac. Cardiovasc. Surg., 39:417, 1960.

Lillehei, C. W., Cohen, M., Warden, H. E., and Varco, R. L.: The direct-vision intracardiac correction of congenital anomalies by controlled cross circulation. Surgery, 38:11, 1955.

Lowenstein, E., Johnston, W. E., Lappas, D. G., et al: Catastrophic pulmonary vasoconstriction associated with protamine reversal of heparin. Anesthesiology, 59:470, 1983.

Messmer, B. J., Schallberger, U., Gattiker, R., et al: Psychomotor and intellectual development after deep hypothermia and circulatory arrest in early infancy. J. Thorac. Cardiovasc. Surg., 72:495, 1976.

Moffitt, E. A., Kirklin, J. W., and Theye, R. A.: Physiologic studies during whole-body perfusion in tetralogy of Fallot. J. Thorac. Cardiovasc. Surg., 44:180, 1962.

Muller-Eberhard, H. J.: Complement. Am. Rev. Biochem., 44:697, 1975.

Nagaoka, H., and Katori, M.: Inhibition of kinin formation by a kallikrein inhibitor during extracorporeal circulation in open-heart surgery. Circulation, 52:325, 1975.

Oeveren, W. V., Kazatchkine, M. D., Descamps-Latscha, B., et al: Deleterious effects of cardiopulmonary bypass. J. Thorac. Cardiovasc. Surg., 89:888, 1985.

Osborn, J. J., Cohn, K., Hait, M., et al: Hemolysis during perfusion: Sources and means of reduction. J. Thorac. Cardiovasc. Surg., 43:459, 1962.

Paneth, M., Sellers, R., Gott, V. L., et al: Physiologic studies upon prolonged cardiopulmonary bypass with the pump oxygenator with particular reference to (1) acid-base balance, (2) siphon canal drainage. J. Thorac. Surg., 34:570, 1947.

Pang, L. M., Stalcup, S. A., Lipset, J. S., et al: Increased circulating bradykinin during hypothermia and cardiopulmonary bypass in children. Circulation, 60:1503, 1979.

Parker, D. J., Cantrell, J. W., Karp, R. B., et al: Changes in serum complement and immunoglobulins following cardiopulmonary bypass. Surgery, 71:824, 1972.

Philbin, D. M., Levine, F. H., Emerson, C. W., et al: The renin-catecholamine vasopressor response to cardiopulmonary bypass with pulsatile flow (Abstract). Circulation, 59,60(Suppl. 2):34, 1979.

Pitt, B. R., Gillis, C. N., and Hammond, G. L.: Depression of pulmonary metabolic function by cardiopulmonary bypass procedures increases levels of circulating norepinephrine. Ann. Thorac. Surg., 38:508, 1984.

Pruitt, K. M., Stroud, R. M., and Scott, J. W.: Blood damage in the heart-lung machine (35651). Proc. Soc. Exp. Biol. Med., 137:714, 1971.

Reves, J. G., Karp, R. B., Buttner, E. E., et al: Neuronal and adrenomedullary catecholamine release in response to cardiopulmonary bypass in man. Circulation, 66:48, 1982.

Rahn, H., Reeves, R. B., and Howell, B. J.: Hydrogen ion regulation, temperature, and evolution. Am. Rev. Respir. Dis., 112:165, 1975.

Reeves, R. B.: Temperature-induced changes in blood acid-base status: pH and P_{CO_2} in a binary buffer. J. Appl. Physiol., 40:752, 1976.

Rosenthal, T. B.: The effect of temperature on the pH of blood and plasma in vitro. J. Biol. Chem., 173:23, 1948.

Royston, D., Minty, B. D., Tiol, M. I., et al: The effect of surgery with cardiopulmonary bypass on alveolar-capillary barrier function in human beings. Ann. Thorac. Surg., 40:1139, 1985.

Sade, R. H., Bartles, D. M., Dearing, J. P., et al: A prospective randomized study of membrane vs. bubble oxygenators in children. Ann. Thorac. Surg., 29:502, 1980.

Salama, A., Ferdinand, H., Dieter, H., et al: Deposition of terminal C5b-9 complement complexes on erythrocytes and leukocytes during cardiopulmonary bypass. N. Engl. J. Med., 318:408, 1988.

Schenk, W. G., Jr., Pollock, L. A., Kjarstansson, K. B., and Delin, N. A.: Influence of aortic perfusion on regional blood flow. Arch. Surg., 87:1059, 1963.

Scott, J.: Mechanism of gamma globulin denaturation. Doctoral Dissertation, University of Alabama at Birmingham, 1970.

Senning, A.: Ventricular fibrillation during extracorporeal circulation: Used as a method to prevent air-embolisms and to facilitate intracardiac operations. Acta Chir. Scand., 171(Suppl.):1, 1952.

Shepard, R. B.: Whole body oxygen consumption during hypoxic hypoxemia and cardiopulmonary bypass circulation. Proc. Tenth Int. Symp. Space Technol. Sci. Tokyo, 1973, pp. 1307–1318.

Singh, R. K. K., Barratt-Boyes, B. G., and Harris, E. A.: Does pulsatile flow improve perfusion during hypothermic cardiopulmonary bypass? J. Thorac. Cardiovasc. Surg., 79:827, 1980.

Sink, J. D., Chitwood, R., Jr., Hill, R. C., et al: Comparison of nonpulsatile and pulsatile extracorporeal circulation on renal cortical blood flow. Ann. Thorac. Surg., 29:57, 1980.

Smith, E. E. J., Naftel, D. C., Blackstone, E. H., and Kirklin, J. W.: Microvascular permeability after cardiopulmonary bypass. J. Thorac. Cardiovasc. Surg., 94:225, 1987.

Solen, K. A., Whiffen, J. D., and Lightfoot, E. N.: The effect of shear, specific surface, and air interface on the development of blood emboli and hemolysis. J. Biomed. Mater. Res., 12:381, 1978.

Stevenson, J. G., Stone, E. F., Dillard, D. H., and Morban, B. C.: Intellectual development of children subjected to prolonged circulatory arrest during hypothermic open heart surgery in infancy. Circulation, 49/50(Suppl. 2):54, 1974.

Swan, H.: Thermoregulation and Bioenergetics: Patterns for Vertebrate Survival. New York, American Elsevier Publishers, 1974, pp. 183–187.

Tamari, Y., Aledort, L., Puszkin, E., et al: Functional changes in platelets during extracorporeal circulation. Ann. Thorac. Surg., 19:639, 1975.

Teoh, K. H., Fremes, S. E., Weisel, R. D., et al: Cardiac release of prostacyclin and thromboxane A_2 during coronary revascularization. J. Thorac. Cardiovasc. Surg., 93:120, 1987.

Theye, R. A., and Kirklin, J. W.: Vertical film oxygenator performance at 30° C and oxygen levels during rewarming. Surgery, 54:569, 1963.

Theye, R. A., Kirklin, J. W., and Fowler, W. S.: Performance and film volume of sheet and screen vertical film oxygenators. J. Thorac. Cardiovasc. Surg., 43:381, 1962.

Treasure, T., Naftel, D. C., Conger, K. A., et al: The effect of hypothermic circulatory arrest time on cerebral function morphology and biochemistry. J. Thorac. Cardiovasc. Surg., 86:761, 1983.

Turina, M., Housman, L. B., Intaglietta, M., et al: An automatic cardiopulmonary bypass unit for use in infants. J. Thorac. Cardiovasc. Surg., 63:263, 1972.

Turley, K., Graham, B., Roizen, M., and Ebert, P. A.: Catecholamine response to deep hypothermia and total circulatory arrest (Abstract). Circulation, 59,60(Suppl. 2):169, 1979.

Verska, J. J.: Control of heparinization by activated clotting time during bypass with improved postoperative hemostasis. Ann. Thorac. Surg., 24:170, 1977.

Wallach, R., Karp, R. B., Reves, J. G., et al: Pathogenesis of paroxysmal hypertension developing during and after coronary artery bypass surgery: A study of hemodynamic and humoral factors. Am. J. Cardiol., 46:559, 1980.

Ward, C. A., Ruegsegger, B., Stanga, D., and Zingg, W.: Reduction in platelet adhesion to biomaterials by removal of gas nuclei. Trans. Am. Soc. Artif. Intern. Organs, 20:77, 1974.

Warden, H. E., Cohen, M., Read, R. C., and Lillehei, C. W.: Controlled cross circulation for open intracardiac surgery. J. Thorac. Surg., 28:331, 1954.

Wells, F. C., Coghill, S., Caplan, H. L., et al: Duration of circulatory arrest does influence the psychological development of children after cardiac operations in early life. J. Thorac. Cardiovasc. Surg., 86:823, 1983.

CHAPTER 33

THE AORTA
I AORTIC GRAFTS AND PROSTHESES

Robert B. Peyton
O. Wayne Isom

Aortic grafts and prostheses were developed to replace or bypass diseased segments of the aorta; early experimental attempts by Jaboulay and Briau (1896), Exner (1903), and Ward (1908) were unsuccessful. In 1949, Gross and associates reported the first use of human arterial homografts for correcting aortic defects. These grafts were removed from trauma victims and stored in a balanced salt solution of 10% human serum at 4° C. The increased demands for homografts led to the development of blood vessel banks and various techniques for collecting, sterilizing, preserving, and storing homografts. Dubost (1952) described the first successful resection of an abdominal aneurysm and insertion of a homograft. DeBakey and Cooley (1953) successfully resected an aneurysm of the thoracic aorta and restored continuity with an aortic homograft. Although the initial experiments with homografts seemed promising, it became apparent by the mid-1950s that results were disappointing (Linton, 1958; Szilagyi et al, 1957). The failure rate of aortic homografts, their limited supply, and difficulties associated with harvesting, sterilization, and preservation provided the impetus to find suitable synthetic substitutes for arteries (Wesolowski et al, 1963).

Experimental arterial synthetic substitutes included cylinders of glass, aluminum, plated gold, paraffin-lined silver, methyl methacrylate, and polyethylene plastics (Carrel, 1912; Hufnagel, 1947; McGee et al, 1987; Sawyer, 1987). These materials were associated with thrombus formation and resulted in distal embolization. Voorhees noted that silk within the right ventricle of a dog became coated with an endothelial surface. He reasoned that a cylindrical prosthesis of fine-mesh synthetic fibers might be useful to restore arterial defects (Sawyer, 1987). In 1942, Voorhees and colleagues reported successful use of Vinyon "N" cloth tube as an aortic substitute in mongrel dogs and are credited with stimulating the present era of reconstructive arterial therapy with synthetic fiber conduits.

Numerous substances including Vinyon "N," nylon, Teflon, Orlon, and Dacron have been used to construct vascular grafts in a knitted (highly porous) or woven (tight) weave, with or without velour (Mathisen et al, 1986). Velour is a warp knitted cloth with a surface resembling velvet. Small loops of yarn extend perpendicularly from the fabric surface. The addition of a double velour surface is reported to provide a superior matrix for improved luminal healing and a decreased incidence of thromboembolic episodes (Lindenauer et al, 1984; Mitchell et al, 1980; Muto et al, 1988; Scott et al, 1985; Zammit et al, 1986). Based on experimentation with numerous synthetics, Wesolowski and colleagues (1961) defined characteristics of an "ideal" vascular graft: (1) durability, (2) nontoxicity, (3) minimal implantation porosity, (4) maximal tissue permeability, and (5) ease of mechanical handling.

The healing of implanted synthetic grafts has been well described (Berger et al, 1972; Burkel et al, 1981; Goldman et al, 1982b; Graham et al, 1980; Noishiki, 1978; Sawyer, 1987; Scott et al, 1985). The lumen becomes coated with fibrinogen, albumin, and other plasma proteins. If the patient is heparinized, a white thrombus of platelets and leukocytes forms on the graft surface, and the prosthesis is converted gradually to a fibrin-coated tube. Healing is characterized by slow cellular infiltration (fibroblasts) and capillary formation. For optimal healing, the neointima should be thin and have an excellent blood supply, and endothelial cells gradually cover the luminal surface.

It was recognized early that the degree of porosity of the prosthesis was an important determinant of luminal surface thrombogenicity (Goldman et al, 1982a; Harrison and Davalos, 1961; Wesolowski et al, 1961). The larger interstices of the more porous knitted grafts provide less resistance to the ingrowth of fibrous tissues and neointima from the surrounding tissues and thus give more complete healing. The more porous knitted grafts are reported to be less thrombogenic, more durable, and more resistant to ulceration and degeneration (Haverich et al, 1984).

Complex proximal aortic reconstruction requires full heparinization and cardiopulmonary bypass. Tightly woven low-porosity Dacron grafts preclotted with the standard technique frequently "declot," and operative blood loss can be excessive. Additional preclotting techniques have been proposed, consisting of autoclaving the graft previously soaked in heparinized blood (Bethea and Reemtsma, 1979), using autogenous platelet-rich plasma (Cooley et al, 1981) or albumin (Gloviczki et al, 1984; Glynn and Williams, 1980; McGee et al, 1987; Rumisek et al, 1986; Thurer et al, 1982). Preclotted tightly woven Dacron prostheses are still the graft most commonly used (Cabrol et al, 1986; Crawford et al, 1981; Kouchoukos et al, 1980). Dacron is durable, is relatively inert in the body, and is well incorporated into the tissues. Tightly woven Dacron prostheses have been reported to be associated with early and late thromboembolic complications (Agarwal et al, 1982; Makin, 1988; Stratton and Hall, 1979).

With the advent of "biologic sealants," knitted Dacron grafts are now being implanted in the thoracic aorta. Dacron knitted grafts are reported to have superior tissue ingrowth, minimal intimal dissection, and minimal luminal thrombogenicity (McGee et al, 1987; Tanabe et al, 1980). The Dacron knitted grafts are made leak-proof by albumin impregnation (Guidoin et al, 1984; McGee et al, 1987), collagen coating (Quinones-Baldrich et al, 1986), or fibrin gluing (Borst et al, 1982; Haverich et al, 1984; Zammit et al, 1985).

None of the aortic prostheses developed is totally free of complications and deterioration (Berger and Sauvage, 1981; Kinley and Marble, 1980; Sawyer, 1987). The ideal vascular graft has the following characteristics: durability, nontoxicity, minimal implantation porosity, maximal tissue permeability, ease of mechanical handling, minimal luminal surface thrombogenicity, no intimal dissection, and complete luminal endothelial coverage.

Bibliography

Agarwal, K. C., Edwards, W. D., and Feldt, R. H.: Pathogenesis of nonobstructive fibrous peels in right-sided porcine-valved extracardiac conduits. J. Thorac. Cardiovasc. Surg., 83:584, 1982.

Berger, K., and Sauvage, L. R.: Late fiber deterioration in Dacron arterial grafts. Ann. Surg., 193:477, 1981.

Berger, K., Sauvage, L. R., Rao, A. M., and Wood, S. J.: Healing of arterial prostheses in man: Its incompleteness. Ann. Surg., 175:118, 1972.

Bethea, M. C., and Reemtsma, K.: Graft hemostasis: An alternative to preclotting. Ann. Thorac. Surg., 27:374, 1979.

Borst, H. G., Haverich, A., Walterbusch, G., and Maatz, W.: Fibrin adhesive: An important hemostatic adjunct in cardiovascular operations. J. Thorac. Cardiovasc. Surg., 84:549, 1982.

Burkel, W. E., Vinter, D. W., Ford, J. W., et al: Sequential studies of healing in endothelial seeded vascular prostheses: Histologic and ultrastructure characteristics of graft incorporation. J. Surg. Res., 30:305, 1981.

Cabrol, C., Pavie, A., Mesnildrey, P., et al: Long-term results with total replacement of the ascending aorta and reimplan-

tation of the coronary arteries. J. Thorac. Cardiovasc. Surg., 91:17, 1986.

Carrel, A.: Permanent intubation of the thoracic aorta. J. Exp. Med., 16:17, 1912.

Cooley, D. A., Romagnoli, A., Milam, J. D., and Bossart, M. I.: A method of preparing woven Dacron aortic grafts to prevent interstitial hemorrhage. Cardiovasc. Dis. Bull. Tex. Heart Inst., 8:48, 1981.

Crawford, E. S., Walker, H. S. J., Saleh, S. A., and Normann, N. A.: Graft replacement of aneurysm in descending thoracic aorta: Results without bypass or shunting. Surgery, 89:73, 1981.

Crawford, E. S., Stowe, C. L., Crawford, J. L., et al: Aortic arch aneurysm: A sentinel of extensive aortic disease requiring subtotal and total aortic replacement. Ann. Surg., 199:742, 1984.

DeBakey, M. E., and Cooley, D. A.: Successful resection of aneurysm of the thoracic aorta and replacement by graft. J.A.M.A., 152:673, 1953.

Dubost, C., Allary, M., and Oeconomos, N.: Resection of an aneurysm of the abdominal aorta. Arch. Surg., 64:405, 1952.

Exner, A.: Einige Tierversuche über Vereinigung und Transplantation von Blutgefaden. Wien. Klin. Wochenschr., 16:273, 1903.

Gloviczki, P., Hollier, L. H., Hoffman, E. A., et al: The effect of preclotting on surface thrombogenicity and thromboembolic complications of Dacron grafts in the canine aorta. J. Thorac. Cardiovasc. Surg., 88:253, 1984.

Glynn, M. F. X., and Williams, W. G.: A technique for preclotting vascular grafts. Ann. Thorac. Surg., 29:182, 1980.

Goldman, M., McCollum, C. N., Hawker, R. J., et al: Dacron arterial grafts: The influence of porosity, velour, and maturity on thrombogenicity. Surgery, 92:947, 1982a.

Goldman, M., Norcott, H. C., Hawker, R. J., et al: Platelet accumulation on mature Dacron grafts in man. Br. J. Surg., 69(Suppl.):38, 1982b.

Graham, L. M., Vinter, D. W., Ford, J. W., et al: Endothelial cell seeding of prosthetic vascular grafts: Early experimental studies with cultured autologous canine endothelium. Arch. Surg., 115:929, 1980.

Gross, R. E., Bill, A. H., and Pierce, E. C.: Methods for preservation and transplantation of arterial grafts. Observations on arterial grafts in dogs: Report of transplantation of preserved arterial grafts in nine human cases. Surg. Gynecol. Obstet., 88:689, 1949.

Gross, R. E., Hurwitt, E. S., Bill, A. H., and Pierce, E. C.: Preliminary observations on the use of human arterial grafts in the treatment of certain cardiovascular defects. N. Engl. J. Med., 239:578, 1948.

Guidoin, R., Snyder, R., Martin, L., et al: Albumin coating of a knitted polyester arterial prosthesis: An alternative to preclotting. Ann. Thorac. Surg., 37:457, 1984.

Harrison, J. H., and Davalos, P. A.: Influence of porosity on synthetic grafts: Fate in animals. Arch. Surg., 82:28, 1961.

Haverich, A., Oelert, H., Maatz, W., and Borst, H. G.: Histopathological evaluation of woven and knitted Dacron grafts for right ventricular conduits: A comparative experimental study. Ann. Thorac. Surg., 37:404, 1984.

Haverich, A., Walterbusch, G., and Borst, H. G.: The use of fibrin glue for sealing vascular prosthesis of high porosity. Thorac. Cardiovasc. Surg., 29:252, 1981.

Hufnagel, C. A.: Permanent intubation of the thoracic aorta. Arch. Surg., 54:382, 1947.

Jaboulay, M., and Briau, E.: Recherches expérimentales sur la suture greffe arterielles. Lyon Med., 81:97, 1896.

Kinley, C. E., and Marble, A. E.: Compliance: A continuing problem with vascular grafts. J. Cardiovasc. Surg., 21:163, 1980.

Kouchoukos, N. T., Karp, R. B., Blackstone, E. H., et al: Replacement of the ascending aorta and aortic valve with a composite graft. Results in 86 patients. Ann. Surg., 3:403, 1980.

Lindenauer, S. M., Stanley, J. C., Zelenock, G. B., et al: Aorto-iliac reconstruction with Dacron double velour. J. Cardiovasc. Surg., 25:36, 1984.

Linton, R. R.: Discussion of paper by DeBakey, M. E., Crawford,

E. S., Cooley, D. A., and Morris, G. C.: Surgical considerations of occlusive disease of the abdominal aorta and iliac and femoral arteries: Analysis of 803 cases. Ann. Surg., *148*:306, 1958.

Makin, G. S.: Peripheral emboli following aortic grafting. Br. J. Surg., *54*:650, 1988.

Mathisen, S. R., Wu, H. D., Sauvage, L. R., et al: An experimental study of eight current arterial prostheses. J. Vasc. Surg., *4*:33, 1986.

McGee, G. S., Shuman, T. A., Atkinson, J. B., et al: Experimental evaluation of a new albumin-impregnated knitted Dacron prosthesis. Am. Surg., *53*:69, 1987.

Mitchell, R. S., Miller, D. C., Billingham, M. E., et al: Comprehensive assessment of the safety, durability, clinical performance, and healing characteristics of a double velour knitted Dacron arterial prosthesis. Vasc. Surg., *14*:197, 1980.

Muto, Y., Miyazaki, T., Eguchi, H., et al: Aneurysm in a double velour knitted Dacron graft. J. Cardiovasc. Surg., *28*:723, 1988.

Noishiki, Y.: Pattern of arrangement of smooth muscle cells in neointima of synthetic vascular prostheses. J. Thorac. Cardiovasc. Surg., *75*:894, 1978.

Quinones-Baldrich, W. J., Moore, W. S., Ziomek, S., and Chvapil, M.: Development of a "leak-proof," knitted Dacron vascular prosthesis. Vasc. Surg., *3*:895, 1986.

Rumisek, J. D., Wade, C. E., Brooks, D. E., et al: Heat-denatured albumin-coated Dacron vascular grafts: Physical characteristics and in vivo performance. J. Vasc. Surg., *4*:136, 1986.

Sawyer, P. N.: Patency of small-diameter negatively charged glutaraldehyde-tanned (St. Jude Medical Biopolymeric) Grafts. In: Sawyer, P. N. (ed): Modern Vascular Grafts. New York, McGraw-Hill Book Company, 1987.

Scott, S. M., Hoffman, H., Gaddy, L. R., et al: A new woven double velour vascular prosthesis. J. Cardiovasc. Surg., *26*:175, 1985.

Stratton, J. W., and Hall, R. V.: Pseudointimal embolism from a woven Dacron graft. Surgery, *86*:772, 1979.

Szilagyi, D. E., McDonald, R. T., Smith, R. F., and Whitcomb, J. G.: Biological fate of human arterial homografts. Arch. Surg., *75*:506, 1957.

Tanabe, T., Kubo, Y., Hashimoto, M., et al: Wall reinforcement with highly porous Dacron mesh in aortic surgery. Ann. Surg., *191*:452, 1980.

Thurer, R. L., Hauer, J. M., and Weintraub, R. M.: A comparison of preclotting techniques for prosthetic aortic replacement. Circulation, *66*(Suppl. I):143, 1982.

Voorhees, A. B., Jaretzki, A., and Blakemore, A. H.: The use of tubes constructed from Vinyon "N" cloth in bridging arterial defects. Ann. Surg., *135*:332, 1942.

Ward, W.: Blood vessel anastomosis by means of rubber tubing. N. Y. Med. Rec., *74*:671, 1908.

Wesolowski, S. A., Fries, C. C., Domingo, R. T., et al: The compound prosthetic vascular graft: A pathologic survey. Surgery, *53*:19, 1963.

Wesolowski, S. A., Fries, C. C., Karlson, K. E., et al: Porosity: Primary determinant of ultimate fate of synthetic vascular grafts. Surgery, *50*:91, 1961.

Zammit, M., and Wu, H.-D.: A comparison of external velour and double velour Dacron grafts in the canine thoracic aorta. Am. Surg., *51*:637, 1985.

Zammit, M., Wu, H.-D., Mathisen, S. R., and Sauvage, L. R.: Influence on healing in the canine thoracic aorta of three substances used to close the interstices of macroporous Dacron grafts. Am. Surg., *52*:667, 1986.

II PATENT DUCTUS ARTERIOSUS, COARCTATION OF THE AORTA, AORTOPULMONARY WINDOW, AND ANOMALIES OF THE AORTIC ARCH

J. William Gaynor
David C. Sabiston, Jr.

PATENT DUCTUS ARTERIOSUS

Nature is neither lazy nor devoid of foresight. Having given the matter thought, she knew in advance that the lung of the fetus, a lung still contained in the uterus and in the process of formation and spared continual motion, does not require the same arrangements of a perfected lung endowed with motion. She has, therefore, anastomosed the pulmonary artery to the aorta.

GALEN

Galen was the first to describe the ductus arteriosus. Harvey, in 1628, demonstrated the role of the ductus arteriosus in the fetal circulation (Boyer, 1967). The eponym *ductus Botalli* is a misnomer resulting from a mistranslation of Botallo's work (Boyer, 1967). During the 19th century, the morbidity associated with patent ductus arteriosus (PDA) was recognized, and Gibson (1900) described the characteristic murmur. Munro (1907) first proposed surgical correction by ligating or crushing the ductus. Surgical intervention was attempted unsuccessfully by Graybiel and colleagues (1938) in a patient with bacterial endocarditis. Because of the friable tissues, they were unable to successfully ligate the ductus and attempted to obliterate it with plicating sutures. The patient survived the operation but with a persistent murmur and died 4 days postoperatively of gastric dilatation and aspiration. In 1938, Gross successfully ligated a PDA in a 7-year-old girl, initiating the modern era (Gross and Hubbard, 1939). Touroff and Vesell (1940) successfully divided the ductus in a patient with bacterial endocarditis and cured the infection. An increased incidence of PDA in premature infants was reported by Burnard (1959). Powell (1963) and Decancq (1963) independently reported ligation of a

PDA in premature infants. In 1966, Porstmann and colleagues first described a nonoperative catheter technique for closure of a PDA using an Ivalon plug (Porstmann et al, 1971). Successful closure of PDA in premature infants by pharmacologic methods was reported independently in 1976 by Friedman and associates and by Heymann and co-workers. Rashkind and Cuaso (1979) reported the use of a transcatheter device to close a PDA in an infant. Wessel and co-workers (1988) recently reported the use of this device for closure of PDA as an outpatient procedure.

Embryology and Pathologic Anatomy

The ductus arteriosus is derived from the sixth aortic arch and normally extends from the main or left pulmonary artery to the descending aorta just distal to the origin of the left subclavian artery. The ductus is usually 5 to 10 mm long but is variable, and the diameter varies from a few millimeters to 1 to 2 cm (Oldham et al, 1964). The aortic orifice is usually larger than the pulmonary orifice. Rarely the ductus may be right-sided, bilateral, or completely absent. In utero, blood ejected by the right ventricle flows almost exclusively through the ductus to the lower extremities and placenta, bypassing the high-resistance pulmonary circulation. The relationship of the ductus and the ascending aorta is determined by the presence or absence of associated anomalies. In pulmonary atresia, the pulmonary circulation is ductus dependent; blood flows from the aorta to the pulmonary artery, and the ductus may appear to be a downward-directed branch of the aorta. In isthmic hypoplasia or interruption of the aortic arch, the descending aorta may appear to be a continuation of the ductus.

Closure of the ductus occurs at birth during the transition from the fetal to the adult circulation. The lungs expand with the first breath, decreasing the pulmonary vascular resistance, resulting in increased pulmonary blood flow and arterial oxygen concentration. In normal full-term neonates, functional closure of the ductus occurs within the first 10 to 15 hours of life (Moss et al, 1963). Closure occurs after constriction of the smooth-muscle layer, causing apposition of intimal cushions in the wall of the ductus, and is mediated by various substances that constrict or dilate ductal smooth muscle. There is proliferation of the intima and media resulting in mounds, mucoid-filled spaces, and disruption of the internal elastic membrane (Ho and Anderson, 1979). Two-dimensional Doppler echocardiography shows intraluminal protrusions in the ductus of 30% of normal full-term infants within 1 hour of birth and in 96% by 8 hours (Hiraishi et al, 1987). Closure by Doppler echocardiography is complete in 96% of full-term infants by 48 hours (Gentile et al, 1981). The sensitivity of the ductal smooth muscle to these substances is dependent on gestational age. In full-term infants,

rising arterial oxygen tension causes constriction of the muscle fibers in the wall of the ductus. Prostaglandins of the E series dilate the ductus; therefore, the lower concentrations after birth potentiate closure. Ductal smooth muscle in premature infants is less sensitive to oxygen-induced constriction and more sensitive to the vasodilatory effects of certain prostaglandins. Various other substances may also be mediators of ductal closure. Anatomic closure by fibrosis is usually complete by 2 to 3 weeks postnatally and produces the ligamentum arteriosum connecting the pulmonary artery to the aorta. Closure is complete in 88% of newborns by the age of 8 weeks (Christie, 1930).

Delayed closure of the ductus is called prolonged patency, and failure of closure results in persistent patency. Final closure may occur at any age but is uncommon after 6 months. Intermittent closure and reopening of the ductus may also occur. Persistent patency of the ductus may occur as an isolated lesion or may be associated with a variety of other congenital defects. Histologic examination of the wall of a persistently patent ductus reveals significant differences in the subendothelial elastic lamina when compared with a ductus that closes normally, suggesting that a primary defect in the composition of the ductal wall may be responsible for failure of closure (Gittenberger-deGroot, 1977). In infants with complex congenital heart disease, pulmonary or systemic blood flow may be dependent on the patency of the ductus, and these infants may suddenly decompensate as the ductus closes. Infusion of prostaglandins to dilate the ductus often results in dramatic improvement and allows stabilization before surgical intervention.

Prolonged or persistent patency of the ductus results in a left-to-right shunt of blood, with pulmonary congestion and left ventricular volume overload. The magnitude of this shunt depends on the size of the ductus. With a large, nonrestrictive ductus, the level of pulmonary vascular resistance is important in determining the severity of shunting. Shunting occurs throughout systole and diastole and results in diastolic hypotension and possibly impaired perfusion of the brain, lower extremities, and abdominal organs. ST-T wave changes suggestive of subendocardial ischemia have been reported in infants with PDA. Myocardial dysfunction may result and lead to increasing left ventricular failure.

Incidence, Mortality, and Morbidity

Isolated PDA occurs approximately once in 2,500 to 5,000 live births. The incidence increases greatly with prematurity and with decreasing birth weight. The incidence may be more than 80% in infants weighing less than 1,000 g and is related to several factors including decreased smooth muscle in the ductal wall, diminished responsiveness of the ductal smooth muscle to oxygen, and possibly elevated circulating levels of vasodilatory prostaglandins. Persistent patency of the ductus occurs more commonly in females than males, with a 2:1 ratio. Genetic factors may be involved, and there is an association with maternal rubella.

PDA is not a benign entity, although prolonged survival has been reported. The mortality of infants with untreated PDA may be as high as 30%. In her classic series, Abbott (1928) reported an average age at death of 24 years. In a study of the natural history of untreated PDA, Shapiro and Keys (1943) found that 80% of patients with PDA would eventually die of their cardiac disease. In their series, the life expectancy of patients alive at 17 years of age was a mean of 18 years. Forty per cent of patients with PDA died of bacterial endocarditis in the preantibiotic era, and most of the remainder died of congestive heart failure. Campbell (1968) calculated that 42% of patients with untreated PDA are dead by 45 years of age. Patients surviving to adulthood may develop congestive heart failure or pulmonary hypertension, with reverse shunting through the ductus. Premature infants with PDA often have associated problems of prematurity that are aggravated by the left-to-right shunting and abnormal hemodynamics. These problems include respiratory distress syndrome, necrotizing enterocolitis, and intraventricular hemorrhage. Congestive heart failure often results and may respond poorly to medical management. The incidence of long-term sequelae of prematurity such as bronchopulmonary dysplasia may be increased by the presence of a PDA. Young children with persistent patency of the ductus may show growth retardation. Infants with a large PDA may develop severe pulmonary hypertension at an early age. Calcification is often encountered in older patients and may complicate surgical repair.

Clinical Manifestations and Diagnosis

The signs and symptoms of PDA depend on the size of the ductus, the pulmonary vascular resistance, the age at presentation, and associated anomalies. Full-term infants do not usually become symptomatic until the pulmonary vascular resistance decreases at 6 to 8 weeks of life, allowing a significant left-to-right shunt. Because premature infants have less smooth muscle in the pulmonary arterioles, vascular resistance decreases earlier and symptoms may develop during the first week of life. In very low-birth-weight infants (less than 1,000 g), as many as 60% may show ductal shunting echocardiographically at 2 to 3 days of life without the presence of a murmur or other clinical signs of a PDA (Dudell and Gersony, 1984; Hammerman et al, 1986). Approximately 40% of these infants eventually develop a hemodynamically significant left-to-right shunt. Infants with a birth weight greater than 1,000 g have a much lower risk of developing a clinically significant shunt even if a murmur is present (Clyman and Campbell, 1987).

A large hemodynamically significant PDA usu-

ally presents in infancy with congestive heart failure. Afflicted infants are irritable, tachycardic, and tachypneic and take feedings poorly. Physical examination usually reveals evidence of a hyperdynamic circulation, with a hyperactive precordium and bounding peripheral pulses. The systolic blood pressure is usually normal, but diastolic hypotension may be present secondary to the large left-to-right shunt. Auscultation reveals a systolic or continuous murmur, often called a machinery murmur, which is heard best in the pulmonic area and radiates toward the middle third of the clavicle. The classic description of this murmur was provided by Gibson (1900):

. . . a murmur which may be regarded as almost pathognomonic. Beginning distinctly after the first sound, it accompanies the latter part of that sound, occupies the short pause, accompanies the second sound, which may be accentuated in the pulmonary area, or may be, and often is, doubled, and finally dies away during the long pause.

Absence of the characteristic murmur does not, however, exclude the presence of a PDA, especially in premature infants. A mid-diastolic apical rumble may result from increased flow across the mitral valve. If cardiac failure is present, a gallop may also be heard. Hepatomegaly is frequently present. Cyanosis is not present in uncomplicated isolated PDA.

The diagnosis of PDA can often be made non-invasively, and the physical examination alone may be almost diagnostic. The chest film often shows cardiomegaly, and if cardiac failure is present, pulmonary congestion may be seen. In older infants, children, and adults, the electrocardiogram (ECG) may show left ventricular hypertrophy. Two-dimensional echocardiography demonstrates the ductus and associated anomalies. The left atrial and aortic root diameters can be measured, and if their ratio is greater than 1.4 to 1.5, a left-to-right shunt is likely. However, the ratio may be normal in infants who have PDA and who have been fluid restricted and treated with diuretics. Contrast echocardiography with agitated saline injected via an umbilical artery catheter may also demonstrate the shunt. Continuous-wave and pulsed Doppler echocardiography documents abnormal aortic flow patterns and estimates the magnitude of ductal flow. Echocardiography may provide evidence of significant left-to-right shunting before it becomes clinically apparent. Color-flow Doppler imaging also shows flow in a PDA and reveals the direction of shunting (see Fig. 33–1, color plate). Retrograde aortography to visualize the PDA may be done in infants with an umbilical artery catheter. Formal cardiac catheterization is not required in children and young adults with classic findings and should be reserved for older patients or those with atypical findings, suspicion of associated anomalies, or pulmonary hypertension. Echocardiography is especially useful to exclude associated anomalies.

Patients with a moderate-sized PDA may remain

asymptomatic until the second or third decade of life when left ventricular failure occurs. The earliest symptom is usually dyspnea on exertion, followed by signs and symptoms of increasing congestive heart failure. Auscultation reveals the typical murmur. The ECG and chest film may show evidence of left ventricular enlargement and hypertrophy. A small PDA usually causes no symptoms or growth retardation. A systolic or continuous murmur is present. The ECG and chest film usually appear to be normal. Some patients with PDA present with bacterial endocarditis as the first clinical manifestation of their disorder. Bacterial endocarditis usually develops at the pulmonary orifice of the ductus.

Aneurysmal dilatation and rupture of the ductus arteriosus, although rare, may occur in infants or adults. Ductal aneurysm was first described by Martin in 1827 (Falcone et al, 1972). Closure of the pulmonary orifice with delayed closure of the aortic orifice of the ductus, exposing the ductal tissue to systemic blood pressure, was proposed as the most likely etiology by Taussig in 1947 (Kirks et al, 1980). Degenerative changes in the ductal wall may also be a factor. Neonatal aneurysm of the ductus must be differentiated from the "ductus bump." This transient dilatation of the ductus seen on the chest film is a benign finding that usually resolves by 48 hours of age, but may persist into adulthood. Aneurysmal dilatation of a PDA has also been described. Ductal aneurysm may present as an asymptomatic mediastinal mass on the chest film, or if significant enlargement has occurred, respiratory distress may occur secondary to airway compression and hoarseness may be present secondary to recurrent nerve involvement. Calcification of the wall and thrombus within the aneurysm are seen frequently. Because of a risk of progressive enlargement and rupture, surgical therapy should be undertaken at the time of diagnosis. Frequently, a discrete neck is present and aneurysmorrhaphy is indicated rather than resection and grafting of the aorta.

The development of pulmonary hypertension in a patient with PDA is a serious prognostic sign. Pulmonary hypertension may be encountered in children who are under 2 years of age and have a nonrestrictive ductus and greatly increased pulmonary blood flow; however, significant pulmonary hypertension is usually noted in older patients with PDA. The elevated pulmonary pressures may be secondary to the increased blood flow and may become normal after surgical closure of the PDA. In some patients, irreversible pulmonary vascular changes occur and pulmonary hypertension persists after closure of the PDA. These patients usually have pulmonary artery pressures that approach systemic levels and show evidence of Eisenmenger's physiology, with a bidirectional or right-to-left shunt resulting in cyanosis. Closure of the PDA in these patients is hazardous and may not lower pulmonary artery pressures.

Management

The presence of a persistent PDA in a child or adult is sufficient indication for surgical closure because of the increased mortality and risk of endocarditis. In symptomatic patients, closure should be performed when the diagnosis is made. In asymptomatic children, intervention can be postponed if desired, but should be done in the preschool years. Older patients should have the ductus closed when the diagnosis is made. However, if severe pulmonary hypertension has occurred with reversal of the ductal shunt, closure is associated with a higher mortality and may not improve symptoms. The management of PDA in premature infants remains controversial.

Surgical Procedures

Gross initially used simple ligation to interrupt the PDA (Gross and Hubbard, 1939). Because of difficulties with recanalization, he attempted ligation and wrapping with cellophane to induce fibrosis; however, recanalization still occurred. Touroff and Vesell (1940) were the first to report division of a PDA. They were attempting to ligate a PDA in a patient with bacterial endocarditis and, when significant hemorrhage occurred, successfully divided the ductus to control the bleeding. Gross (1944) pioneered division of the PDA as the therapy of choice because of difficulties with recanalization. Blalock (1946) suggested ligation with multiple transfixion sutures as the preferred method because of concern about the safety of ductal division. In children, either division or multiple suture ligation of the ductus is appropriate. Ligation is usually done in neonates because of its simplicity and rare, if any, recurrences. In adults with a large ductus (10 mm or more) or patients with pulmonary hypertension, division is indicated.

The operation may be done through either a left anterior or posterior thoracotomy. The lung is retracted, and an incision is made in the pleura overlying the pulmonary artery between the phrenic and vagus nerves. The ductus is exposed, taking care to avoid damage to the recurrent laryngeal nerve. After the ductus has been mobilized, it may be obliterated with multiple suture ligation (Fig. 33–2) or divided (Fig. 33–3). If division is planned, vascular clamps are placed across the ductus, which is then divided. Closure of each end is accomplished with two rows of nonabsorbable suture. If the ductus is particularly short and wide, it may be necessary to cross-clamp the aorta above and below the ductus as in a coarctation repair. The pulmonary end of the ductus is clamped and the ductus is divided at the aorta, leaving a sufficient margin for closure. The opening in the aorta is closed and the cross-clamps are removed. The pulmonary end of the ductus is closed and the clamp is removed.

A calcified ductus in older patients presents a difficult surgical problem. Simple ligation or division

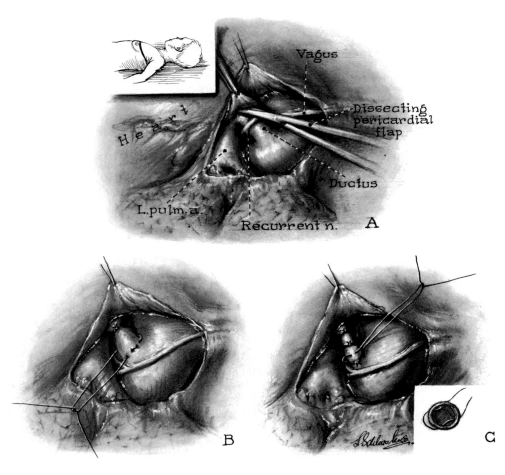

Figure 33–2. Operative treatment of PDA by ligation. Incision is anterolateral in the third interspace. In females, the incision circles beneath the breast. Elevation of pericardial lappet exposes the ductus. A purse-string suture, which does not enter the lumen, is placed at each end, and perforating mattress sutures are placed in between. The ductus should be obliterated over an 8- to 10-mm distance.

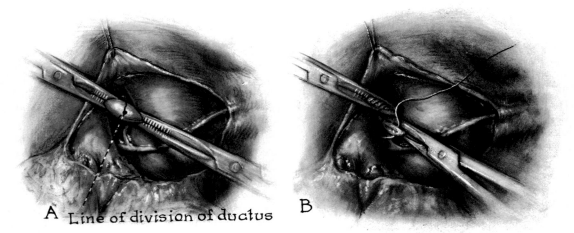

Figure 33–3. Treatment of PDA by division. Anterolateral third interspace incision is used with exposure, as for ligation. A thin occluding clamp is placed at each end, and the ductus is divided. Pressing the clamp against the pulmonary artery or aorta after division reduces the likelihood of slipping. Suture of the ductus is by a continuous mattress suture adjacent to clamp, followed by whipstitch backup over the free edge. Suture of the pulmonary artery is easier when done from the patient's right side.

and oversewing are not possible in patients with a PDA with diffuse circumferential calcification. Several techniques using cardiopulmonary bypass and closure from within the aorta or pulmonary artery have been described (Goncalves-Estella et al, 1975). A median sternotomy is done and cardiopulmonary bypass is instituted. As the patient is cooled, the ductus is occluded by finger compression of the left pulmonary artery to prevent overdistention of the pulmonary vasculature. The aorta is cross-clamped, and cardioplegia is infused. Pump flow is reduced and a pulmonary arteriotomy is done. The pulmonary orifice of the ductus is closed by using direct sutures, followed by the repair of the pulmonary arteriotomy. Patch closure of the aortic orifice of a PDA has also been described. This repair may be done by using either cardiopulmonary bypass or a heparin-bonded shunt. The aorta is cross-clamped above and below the ductus arteriosus and an aortotomy is performed (Wernly and Ameriso, 1980). The ductus is occluded by using a balloon catheter and a Dacron patch to close the aortic orifice. A similar technique has been reported without the use of shunts or bypass (Johnson and Kron, 1988). In patients with a noncalcified ductus arteriosus and associated cardiac anomalies that require correction, the ductus arteriosus may be ligated via a median sternotomy before instituting cardiopulmonary bypass. If aneurysmal dilatation has occurred, the ductus should be excised and the aorta and pulmonary artery should be repaired.

In neonates, single or double ligation is usually the procedure of choice. Closure of the ductus in neonates by applying one or two surgical clips has also been described (Adzick et al, 1986; Kron et al, 1983). In recent years, several authors have advocated surgical closure of the ductus in the neonatal intensive care unit rather than transporting critically ill neonates to the operating room (Pate et al, 1981).

Closure of a PDA in patients with pulmonary hypertension presents special difficulties. In patients with pulmonary vascular changes, closure may cause further elevation of the pulmonary pressures, with right ventricular failure and decline in systemic pressures. Ellis and associates (1956) reported closure of a PDA in 72 patients with pulmonary hypertension; overall mortality was 18% and was 56% in patients with a right-to-left shunt. John and co-workers (1981) reported five deaths after PDA closures in 22 patients with pulmonary artery pressures greater than 70 mm Hg. Patients who have marked pulmonary hypertension and right-to-left shunt and who survive closure may not improve and may develop progressive cor pulmonale.

Surgical closure of a PDA may be complicated by hemorrhage, pneumothorax, chylothorax, left recurrent nerve damage (Davis et al, 1988), and infection. Phrenic nerve paralysis has also been reported after closure of a PDA. Great care must be exercised when dissecting or placing clamps on the ductus, because the ductal tissue may be friable and a tear may result in hemorrhage that is difficult to control. Inadvertent ligation or division of the left pulmonary artery has been reported after attempted ductal ligation (Pontius et al, 1981). Ligation of the left pulmonary artery should be considered if the child fails to improve postoperatively, the chest film shows decreased pulmonary vascular markings of the left lung, and there is continued evidence of a PDA. The diagnosis can be confirmed by perfusion scan (Orzel and Monaco, 1986) or pulmonary arteriography. Removal of the ligature or reanastomosis usually results in reperfusion of the lung (Fleming et al, 1983). In the early days of surgical closure of PDA, recanalization constituted a major problem; however, the incidence of recurrent ductal patency should approach zero after division or multiple suture ligation.

Nonoperative Therapy

In recent years there has been increasing interest in the nonoperative closure of PDA in high-risk patients. Porstmann, in 1966, successfully used a transcatheter technique to block the PDA with an Ivalon plug (Porstmann et al, 1971). Rashkind and Cuaso (1979) used a double umbrella device inserted via a right-sided catheter to close the ductus. Porstmann, in 1986, reported long-term follow-up on 208 patients who had closure of a PDA with an Ivalon plug (Wierny et al, 1986). Ductal closure was successful in 94.7% of the patients. There were no deaths, and no patient required thoracotomy for retrieval of the plug after dislodgment. Arterial complications occurred in 16 patients, 9 of whom required surgical intervention. Rashkind and colleagues (1987) reported attempted ductal closure by using a double umbrella device in 146 patients. Closure was successful in 94 patients. Embolization occurred after release in 19 patients, one of whom required emergency operation. Wessel and co-workers (1988) reported transcatheter closure by using Rashkind's device in 23 children, 19 of whom were discharged on the day of the procedure. Transcatheter techniques are potentially useful in patients who are poor candidates for operation. However, these techniques are still being investigated, and the exact role of transcatheter closure of PDA has not been determined.

Management of PDA in Premature Infants

Premature infants face many problems, including immature lungs and hyaline membrane disease. These infants often require mechanical ventilation and oxygen therapy. The increased incidence of PDA in these infants correlates with increasing prematurity and decreasing birth weight. The additional burden on the heart and lungs imposed by the left-to-right shunt may be poorly tolerated. The increased pulmonary blood flow causes increased pulmonary arterial pressures, decreased lung compliance, hypercarbia, and hypoxia, often necessitating prolonged mechanical ventilation, which may result in an increased incidence of bronchopulmonary dysplasia (Brown, 1979) and retrolental fibroplasia. The abnormal hemodynamics may potentiate other problems of prematurity such as necrotizing enterocolitis and intraventricular hemorrhage. It is sometimes difficult to differentiate the effects of a PDA from the underlying pulmonary disease. If the pulmonary disease is severe, ligation of the PDA may result in little or no improvement. A hemodynamically significant PDA is suggested by the presence of a hyperactive precordium, a continuous murmur, and bounding pulses. The chest film usually shows cardiomegaly, pulmonary congestion, and the changes of hyaline membrane disease. Echocardiography is very useful in these patients in determining the presence of a significant left-to-right shunt.

Management of PDA in premature infants is controversial because the ductus may close as the child matures. There is an increased incidence of PDA in neonatal units in which fluids are not restricted (Bell et al, 1980; Stevenson, 1977). Some infants can be managed satisfactorily with fluid restriction and diuretics. Anemia increases the heart failure, and transfusion of packed red blood cells is indicated as being necessary. Digitalis is rarely used in these infants because there is little evidence of therapeutic benefit and a high incidence of toxicity (Berman et al, 1978).

In some infants, conservative therapy fails. If a child with evidence of left-to-right shunting shows persistent congestive heart failure, need for continuing mechanical ventilation, or inability to receive adequate nutrition secondary to fluid restriction, further intervention is indicated. Two therapeutic options exist at this point. Pharmacologic closure can be attempted with prostaglandin inhibitors such as indomethacin. Final closure may be achieved in more than 70% of infants, although the ductus may reopen transiently in some children. Reopening occurs most frequently in the most premature infants and may be treated with a second course of indomethacin, but the success rate is lower. The success of therapy with indomethacin is related to the birth weight and postnatal age of the infant (Achanti et al, 1986). Side effects of indomethacin include renal dysfunction, hyponatremia, impaired platelet function, and gastrointestinal hemorrhage. Impaired left ventricular diastolic function has been reported following administration of indomethacin and may worsen pulmonary edema (Appleton et al, 1988). No adverse long-term sequelae of successful indomethacin therapy have been identified. Surgical closure can be used if there is a contraindication to indomethacin or failure of the PDA to close. In some centers, surgical intervention is the primary therapy after conservative medical therapy fails. A national collaborative trial (Gersony et al, 1983) was done to compare methods of treatment. Indomethacin as primary therapy was compared with indomethacin as reserve therapy for conventional medical treatment and with

operation as primary therapy. The use of indomethacin significantly reduced the need for surgical closure of the PDA. There was an increased incidence of bleeding other than intraventricular hemorrhage in infants receiving indomethacin as primary therapy, but no other adverse results. The incidence of retinopathy of prematurity was higher in the group having primary surgical closure. There was no difference in outcome if the indomethacin was given as first-line therapy or after failure of conservative medical therapy.

Early closure of a PDA in premature infants has been shown to decrease the need for mechanical ventilation and to decrease complications such as bronchopulmonary dysplasia, necrotizing enterocolitis, and intolerance of enteral feeding. Closure with indomethacin is as effective as surgical ligation is in preventing these complications. There has been a trend toward earlier intervention in premature infants, and the prophylactic use of indomethacin before the development of a hemodynamically significant shunt has been suggested. Studies suggest that indomethacin is indicated in very low-birth-weight infants (less than 1,000 g) when clinical signs of a PDA first appear, because most of these infants develop significant shunting. In infants with a birth weight more than 1,000 g, there is no benefit to initiation of therapy before the development of significant shunting (Clyman and Campbell, 1987). If indomethacin fails to close the ductus or if the ductus closes and reopens, surgical ligation is indicated. One study has reported a 42% failure rate with indomethacin in infants of very low birth weight and suggested that primary surgical closure is more predictable with minimal morbidity (Palder et al, 1987).

Results

Surgical closure of an isolated PDA has become a very safe procedure. Operative mortality approaches zero even in critically ill neonates. In premature infants, hospital mortality and long-term results depend primarily on associated pulmonary disease, coexistent anomalies, and the degree of prematurity. Mortality is increased and long-term results are poor in older patients with a calcified ductus and are poorer in those patients with severe pulmonary hypertension and reverse shunting. Most patients with PDA become functionally normal and have a normal life expectancy after closure.

COARCTATION OF THE AORTA

Coarctation is derived from the Latin *coarctatio* (a drawing or pressing together). Coarctation of the aorta is defined as a narrowing that diminishes the lumen and produces an obstruction to the flow of blood. The lesion may be a definite, localized obstruction or may be a diffusely narrowed segment, which

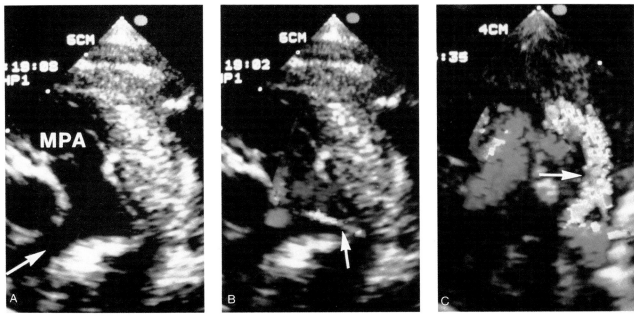

Figure 33–1 ABC

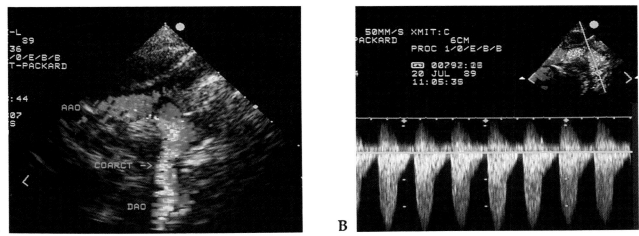

Figure 33–5 A & B

Figure 33–1. *A,* Two-dimensional echocardiogram in an infant with a small PDA showing main pulmonary artery (MPA), right pulmonary artery *(arrow),* and left pulmonary artery. *B,* Same patient with color Doppler image *(arrow)* of turbulent flow in pulmonary artery secondary to the PDA. *C,* Infant with large PDA. Color Doppler image shows large left-to-right shunt with turbulent flow in the main pulmonary artery *(arrow).* (Courtesy of Dr. Joseph Kisslo.)

Figure 33–5. *A,* Freeze frame two-dimensional color Doppler echocardiogram of the aortic arch in a child with coarctation of the aorta. This is a suprasternal view showing the ascending aorta (AAO) at the left and the descending aorta (DAO) at the bottom. Note the coarctation (coarct) with narrowing of the aorta and turbulent flow. *B,* Steerable continuous wave spectral velocity recording from the child shown in *A.* The two-dimensional image in the upper right-hand corner shows the location and the direction of the continuous wave Doppler beam. The flow is away from the transducer and therefore is represented below the baseline. The velocity is proportional to the degree of stenosis in most cases. Peak velocity in this patient is 3 m/sec. (Courtesy of Dr. Joseph Kisslo.)

PLATE 4

is called tubular hypoplasia. Localized coarctation of the aorta and tubular hypoplasia may occur separately or may coexist. Isolated coarctation may occur at any site in the aorta, but the most common location is at the site of the insertion of the ductus (or ligamentum) arteriosus. Externally the aorta appears to be sharply indented or constricted, and internally the obstructing diaphragm on the posterior wall (located preductally, postductally, or paraductally) is usually more marked than is apparent by external appearance. The "shelf" consists of an infolding of the aortic media with a ridge of intimal hyperplasia. Tubular hypoplasia most often occurs in the aortic isthmus (the segment of aorta between the left subclavian artery and the insertion of the ductus arteriosus). Localized coarctation of the aorta and tubular hypoplasia are part of a spectrum of disorders ranging from pseudocoarctation (a kinking or buckling of the aorta without producing obstruction to flow) to complete interruption of the aorta. Aortic atresia occurs when the lumen is totally obliterated and a fibrous connection remains between the proximal and distal segments.

Historical Aspects

Paris (1791) provided the first accurate description of coarctation of the aorta. Meckel in 1750 and Morgagni in 1760 had reported finding aortic narrowing at autopsy (Jarcho, 1961). Throughout the 19th century, coarctation of the aorta was considered a rare disorder. Legrand, in 1835, made the first premortem diagnosis of obstruction of the thoracic aorta (Jarcho, 1962b). In 1903 Bonnet published an extensive review and distinguished between preductal coarctation (infantile) and postductal coarctation (adult). In 1928, Abbott documented 200 cases of coarctation in patients over 2 years of age. This historic report stimulated much interest in the disorder, and in 1944, Blalock and Park proposed anastomosis of the left subclavian artery to the descending aorta to bypass the obstruction. In the same year, Crafoord and Nylin (1945) performed the first surgical correction with resection of the coarctation and end-to-end anastomosis. Gross and Hufnagel independently performed a similar procedure in 1945. Subsequently, Gross (1951) was the first to use aortic homografts to replace the narrowed segment of aorta. Lynxwiler and colleagues (1951) reported the first successful repair of coarctation in an infant. The use of prosthetic onlay grafts was reported by Vossschulte in 1957 (Vossschulte, 1961), and in 1966 Waldhausen and Nahrwold described the subclavian flap aortoplasty. In recent years there has been increasing interest in the use of percutaneous transluminal angioplasty for native and recurrent coarctation.

Embryology and Pathologic Anatomy

The cause of coarctation of the aorta and tubular hypoplasia is still controversial. Two major theories have been proposed to explain the embryonic development of aortic narrowing; each may be important in different clinical situations. It has been proposed that in some patients tissue from the ductus arteriosus extends circumferentially into the aortic wall; contraction and fibrosis of this tissue at the time of ductal closure could lead to a localized narrowing. Extension of ductal tissue into the aortic wall has been shown histologically by Wielenga and Dankmeijer (1968) and by Ho and Anderson (1979). Other investigators have not found this abnormal tissue and hypothesize that coarctation results from abnormal fetal blood flow patterns (Rudolph et al, 1972; Shinebourne and Elseed, 1974). In the normal fetus, blood flow across the aortic isthmus is much less than flow in either the ascending aorta or the descending aorta (which receives ductal blood flow), and thus the diameter of the isthmus is less than that of either the ascending or descending aorta. An increased incidence of coarctation is found with certain ventricular septal defects (those producing left ventricular outflow tract obstruction), aortic stenosis, and mitral valve anomalies, which diminish ascending aortic flow and increase ductal flow. The resultant decrease in flow across the isthmus leads to abnormal narrowing of the isthmus. Coarctation is rarely associated with anomalies that decrease ductal flow and increase ascending aortic and isthmic flow (e.g., tetralogy of Fallot). The exact cause is important in the choice of appropriate surgical therapy; if abnormal ductal tissue is present, failure to completely excise the constricting shelf may allow further contraction and recurrent coarctation. There is evidence of an increased incidence of cystic medial necrosis in patients with coarctation (Lindsay, 1988). It is uncertain whether this is a primary weakness of the aortic wall or is secondary to the stresses produced by the coarctation. This increased fragility may lead to aneurysmal dilatation, aortic dissection, or rupture of the aorta.

Incidence and Associated Anomalies

Coarctation of the aorta represents 5 to 10% of congenital heart disease, and the autopsy incidence is 1 in 3,000 to 4,000 autopsies. With isolated coarctation, males predominate, but there is no sex predisposition in patients with more complex lesions. Several anomalies occur commonly in patients with coarctation of the aorta (Becker et al, 1970): bicuspid aortic valve, ventricular septal defect, PDA, and various mitral valve disorders. Congenital aortic stenosis, aortic atresia, and the hypoplastic left heart syndrome may occur with coarctation, in addition to bicuspid aortic valves. Ventricular septal defects that occur with coarctation often result from septal malalignment, which compromises the left ventricular outflow tract and thus might be an etiologic factor in the development of the coarctation. A study by Moene and associates (1987) revealed that up to 70% of ventricular septal defects occurring in association with coarctation are of types characterized by frequent spontaneous closure. Shone's syndrome is the complex of parachute mitral valve, cor triatriatum, subaortic stenosis, and coarctation (Shone et al, 1963). Mitral stenosis and regurgitation frequently occur secondary to abnormalities of the chordae tendineae and papillary muscles (Celano et al, 1984; Freed et al, 1974; Rosenquist, 1974). Coarctation of the aorta may occasionally be noted in patients with transposition of the great arteries (Vogel et al, 1984) and usually occurs in patients who have transposition with associated right ventricular outflow tract obstruction (Moene et al, 1985). Coarctation may be encountered in up to 50% of patients with the Taussig-Bing anomaly (Parr et al, 1983; Sadow et al, 1985). Genetic factors may have a role, because there are reports of familial occurrences and 15 to 36% of patients with Turner's syndrome have a coarctation (Ravelo et al, 1980). There is also an increased incidence of aortic arch anomalies, especially interrupted arch, in patients with DiGeorge's syndrome. Patients with severe associated defects tend to have tubular hypoplasia rather than isolated coarctation.

Clinical Manifestations

The age at presentation and the mode of presentation depend mainly on the location of the coarctation and the associated anomalies. When the obstruction is preductal, there is an increased incidence of other cardiac defects and the patients usually present in infancy with congestive heart failure. Preductal coarctation usually consists of tubular hypoplasia that terminates in an obstructing shelf. Paraductal and postductal coarctation are usually isolated obstructions and have a low incidence of associated defects. Preductal coarctation was considered by Bonnet to be the infantile form because of its usual presentation in infancy. However, the terms *infantile* and *adult* are inappropriate descriptions of preductal and postductal coarctation because patients with the so-called infantile form can survive to adulthood and some patients with the so-called adult type develop clinical manifestations in infancy.

Preductal coarctation and even interruption of the aortic arch may not seriously alter the normal fetal circulation and therefore do not provide a stimulus to the development of collateral circulation in utero. Infants with severe narrowing may appear normal at birth and have palpable femoral pulses, because a PDA allows blood to flow past the obstructing shelf. Symptoms usually develop as the PDA closes, which results in significant aortic obstruction. The infant becomes irritable, tachypneic, and disinterested in feeding. A systolic murmur may be present over the left precordium and posteriorly between the scapulae. Although the blood pressure is difficult to record accurately in neonates, moderate upper-extremity hypertension and an arm-leg systolic pressure gradient are usually present. These findings may be absent in critically ill infants with a

low cardiac output. Hypotension, oliguria, and severe metabolic acidosis may be present in severely ill infants. In severe obstruction or complete aortic interruption, a pulmonary artery pulse may be felt in the femoral arteries when the ductus is open and may obscure the diagnosis. Differential cyanosis may be present between the upper and lower extremities. Left-to-right shunting may occur through a patent foramen ovale. In neonates, there are no signs of collateral circulation because this becomes clinically apparent only with time.

Older children and adults often present with unexplained hypertension or complications of hypertension, and some may be entirely asymptomatic for many years and lead an active life. Presenting complaints include headache, epistaxis, visual disturbances, and exertional dyspnea. Some patients present with a cerebrovascular accident (secondary to an aneurysm of the circle of Willis), aortic rupture, dissecting aneurysm, or bacterial endocarditis (Shearer et al, 1970). Many cases are discovered during evaluation of hypertension or of a murmur heard on routine examination.

Diagnosis

The diagnosis of coarctation can usually be made clinically and depends on evidence of obstruction to blood flow in the thoracic aorta. The findings include hypertension, a systolic pressure gradient between the arms and legs, a systolic murmur heard over the left precordium and posteriorly between the scapulae, and diminished or absent femoral pulses with a delayed upstroke. Presence of an anterior diastolic murmur may indicate aortic regurgitation secondary to a bicuspid aortic valve. Anomalous origin of the right subclavian artery can occur with the orifice distal to the coarctation. The blood pressure must be obtained in both arms because the orifice of either subclavian artery may be involved in the coarctation. There may be evidence of collateral circulation in older children and adults. The collateral circulation involves branches of the subclavian arteries that are proximal to the obstruction, including the internal mammary, vertebral, thyrocervical, and costocervical arteries. These vessels anastomose with intercostals and other arteries below the obstruction. Enlarged collateral vessels may be seen or palpated in the infrascapular region; bruits may be audible as well. Aneurysmal dilatation of the intercostal arteries can occur and may complicate surgical reconstruction. Poststenotic dilatation of the descending aorta is common, and, rarely, an aneurysm of the ascending or descending aorta may occur.

The ECG in infancy may show right, left, or biventricular hypertrophy. In older children and adults, it may be normal or show evidence of left ventricular hypertrophy, often with a "strain" pattern. The chest film is usually helpful, showing cardiomegaly with left ventricular hypertrophy. In infants with heart failure, extreme cardiomegaly and pulmonary congestion may be present. Rib notching secondary to the enlarged, tortuous intercostal vessels is almost pathognomonic (Fig. 33–4) and was first described by Meckel in 1827 (Jarcho, 1962a). Rosler, in 1928 (Christiansen, 1948), and Railsback and Dock (1929) emphasized the presence of rib notching roentgenographically. These erosions occur on the underside of the rib and may be unilateral if the orifice of the left subclavian artery is narrowed by the coarctation, arises distal to the obstruction, or if there is anomalous origin of the right subclavian artery distal to the coarctation. Absence of rib notching in older patients may indicate a poor collateral circulation. The "3" sign may be present, consisting of proximal enlargement of the aorta, aortic constriction, and poststenotic dilatation (see Fig. 33–4).

Angiocardiography is still the most objective method of showing the coarctation, providing evidence of the location and extent of narrowing, the involvement of the great vessels, and the extent of collateral circulation. The pressure gradient can be measured, and associated cardiac defects can be evaluated by cardiac catheterization. Newer methods of noninvasive imaging also provide valuable information. Two-dimensional echocardiography with spectral and color-flow Doppler echocardiography may show the site of obstruction, suggest or exclude associated anomalies, and provide an estimate of the arterial pressure gradient (see Fig. 33–5, color plate). Computed tomography (CT), digital subtraction angiography, and magnetic resonance imaging (MRI) are also helpful and can be used postoperatively to assess the result (Fig. 33–6).

Natural History

The natural history of untreated coarctation of the aorta depends on the age at presentation and associated anomalies. Symptomatic infants have a high mortality, depending on the severity of the coarctation and the presence of associated defects. Patients surviving until adulthood have a greatly decreased life expectancy. In 1928, before the development of antibiotics and surgical correction of coarctation, Abbott reviewed 200 cases of coarctation confirmed at autopsy in patients older than 2 years of age. Death occurred in 74% of the patients by 40 years of age, and the average age at death was 32 years. However, the lesion does not preclude prolonged survival, because one patient lived to the age of 92. The most common causes of death were spontaneous rupture of the aorta, bacterial endocarditis, and cerebral hemorrhage. Reifenstein and colleagues reported 104 cases of coarctation in 1947. The average age at death was 35 years; 23% of the patients died of aortic rupture, 22% of bacterial endocarditis or aortitis, 18% of congestive heart failure, and 11% of cerebrovascular accident. Rupture of the aorta or an intracranial aneurysm occurred usually in the second or third decade of life. Endocarditis was most commonly associated with a bicuspid aortic valve. Campbell (1970) calculated that of patients with coarctation surviving the first 2 years of life 25% would die by 20 years of age, 50% by 32 years of age, 75% by 46 years of age, and 90% by 58 years of age. The coronary arteries in patients with untreated coarctation show striking changes, with intimal degeneration, medial thickening, and increased mineralization. These changes can be shown even in young children and may predispose patients to early atherosclerosis. Hypertension secondary to the coarctation is thought to be the most important factor in the pathogenesis of these changes. The advent of surgical therapy has significantly increased the life expectancy of patients with coarctation, although they do not become fully normal.

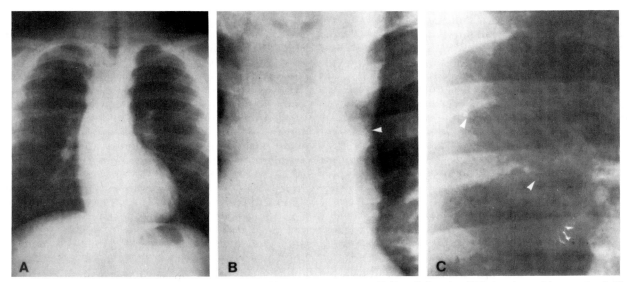

Figure 33–4. Patient with coarctation of the aorta. *A,* Chest roentgenogram. *B,* Detail showing "3" sign formed by proximal dilated aorta, area of constriction (*arrow*), and distal dilated aorta. *C,* Detail showing rib notching (*arrows*) secondary to dilated intercostal vessels. (Courtesy of Dr. James Chen.)

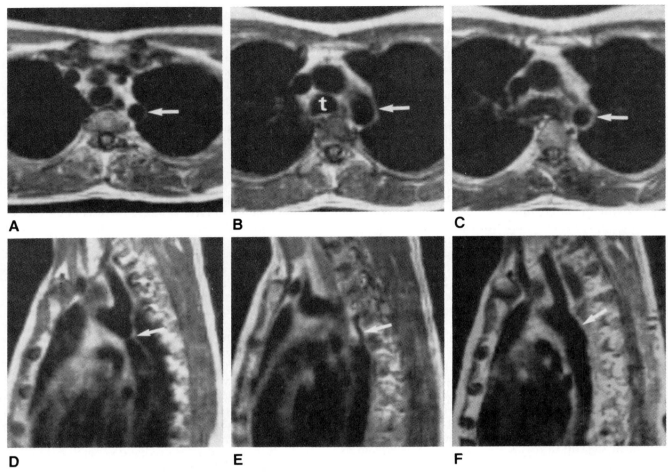

Figure 33–6. Magnetic resonance images. *A,* Transaxial section above arch. Dilated left subclavian artery *(arrow). B,* More caudal section. Posterior aortic arch immediately proximal to coarctation *(arrow).* (t = trachea.) *C,* 1 cm below *B.* Reduction in caliber of descending aorta *(arrow). D,* Parasagittal section. Coarctation distal to dilated left subclavian artery *(arrow).* Diaphragm-like stricture is better appreciated than on transaxial sections. *E,* Parasagittal section through the distal descending aorta. Dilated collateral artery *(arrow). F,* Postoperative parasagittal section through distal descending aorta. Dilated collateral artery *(arrow).* Widely patent lumen at the previous site of coarctation. (From Amparo, E. G., Higgins, C. B., and Shafton, E. P.: Demonstration of coarctation of the aorta by magnetic resonance imaging. Am. J. Roentgenol., *143:*1192–1194. Copyright © 1984 by Williams & Wilkins Company.)

Pseudocoarctation

Pseudocoarctation, first reported by Souders and associates (1951), is a buckling or kinking of the aorta that does not produce an obstruction to flow. The term "pseudocoarctation" was introduced by Dotter and Steinberg (1952). The chest film usually reveals an abnormal aortic contour mimicking a left superior mediastinal mass. There is no evidence of collateral circulation, and the diagnosis is confirmed by aortography showing a tortuous, kinked aorta with no measurable pressure gradient. Pseudocoarctation was thought to be a benign entity; however, aneurysmal dilatation can occur in the segment of aorta distal to the buckled area. Gay and Young (1969) reported a patient who had pseudocoarctation and who died secondary to aortic rupture. They recommended careful evaluation of all patients with pseudocoarctation for aneurysmal formation. Surgical intervention should be undertaken in patients developing aortic dilatation.

Physiology of Hypertension

The pathogenesis of hypertension in coarctation is multifactorial, and the most prominent causes appear to be mechanical and renal factors. Abbott (1928) and Lewis (1933) emphasized the importance of hypertension in coarctation of the aorta. Rytand (1938) and others noted an increase in vascular resistance proximal and distal to the narrowed segment resulting in diastolic hypertension and suggested that coarctation might be analogous to Goldblatt's model of hypertension. Gupta and Wiggers (1951) showed that it was necessary to diminish the aortic lumen by 45 to 55% to cause an elevation in the blood pressure and suggested that mechanical factors alone were responsible for the hypertension. Scott and Bahnson (1951) were the first to definitely demonstrate the role of the kidneys in the pathogenesis of the hypertension of coarctation. In experimental coarctation, they showed that hypertension could be eliminated by transplanting one kidney to the neck (proximal to the obstruction) with contralateral nephrectomy. Young and co-workers (1969) later found normal renal blood flow in experimental coarctation. Renal blood flow is usually normal in patients with coarctation, and studies of the renin-angiotensin system have yielded conflicting results. Renin and angiotensin levels have been reported to be normal in both experimental animals and patients with coarctation. However, Bagby and co-workers (1975, 1980), using a canine model of coarctation, were able to show greater than expected elevation of plasma renin during sodium restriction. During low, normal, and high sodium intake, plasma volume, extracellular volume, and plasma renin activity were higher in coarcted animals than in control animals. Alpert and colleagues (1979) showed significant increases in plasma renin activity during volume depletion in children with coarctation compared with normal persons or patients with essential hypertension. These findings suggest that coarctation is similar to a one-kidney Goldblatt model of hypertension. Plasma renin activity is initially elevated and leads to an increase in plasma volume that restores renal perfusion to normal levels. The stimulus for increased renin secretion is thus diminished, plasma renin activity returns to normal levels, and the hypertension is maintained by volume expansion (Parker et al, 1980). Angiotensin blockade has not been consistently useful in treating the hypertension of coarctation. Ferguson and co-workers (1977), by using a model of coarctation similar to that of Scott and Bahnson, showed that animals with coarctation developed generalized hypertension, but when a graft was used to re-establish renal blood flow, hypertension developed only proximal to the stenosis. Other investigators have shown abnormal rigidity of the prestenotic aortic wall (Sehested et al, 1982) and abnormal baroreceptor function (Beekman et al, 1983). Both mechanical and renal factors are important in the development of hypertension in patients with coarctation.

Management

Nonsurgical therapy has only a small role in the management of patients with coarctation, and the presence of coarctation is generally sufficient indication for surgical correction. The major questions are the timing and method of repair. Symptomatic infants usually require intervention, although a few improve with conservative medical treatment of congestive heart failure and can then undergo elective surgical correction. A major advance in the treatment of critically ill neonates with coarctation and interrupted arch has been the introduction of prostaglandin E_1 therapy (Leoni et al, 1984). Infusion of prostaglandin E_1 can reopen and maintain patency of the ductus arteriosus in many neonates and allow perfusion of the lower body with correction of the severe metabolic acidosis and oliguria that are often present (Heymann et al, 1979). Stabilization of these severely ill patients allows surgical correction to be accomplished under more optimal conditions with decreased mortality.

The timing of elective repair of coarctation of the aorta is perhaps the most important determinant of surgical outcome. Repair in late childhood or adulthood, although providing relief of some symptoms, has an increased incidence of persistent hypertension with its associated morbidity. Repair in infancy using the classic method of resection and end-to-end anastomosis was reported to result in a high incidence (up to 60%) of residual or recurrent stenosis, although recent series report a much lower occurrence. Alternative techniques of repair were developed to allow repair at an earlier age with fewer recoarctations. The current trend is for elective repair at an early age, and some authors believe that repair should be made at the time of diagnosis in symptomatic and asymptomatic infants to prevent development of complications (Waldhausen et al, 1981). Others prefer elective repair in asymptomatic children at the age of 1 to 6 years to decrease the recoarctation rate.

Surgical Procedures

The classic method of repair used by Crafoord and by Gross is resection of the area of obstruction with primary end-to-end anastomosis. A left thoracotomy is done, and an incision is made in the pleura overlying the coarctation. The proximal aorta, left subclavian artery, area of coarctation, and the ligamentum (or ductus) arteriosum are dissected first, avoiding damage to the recurrent laryngeal nerve (Fig. 33–7). Abbott's artery, an anomalous branch sometimes originating from the isthmus, which may be a remnant of the fifth aortic arch, is occasionally present and should be divided. The ductus or ligamentum is divided, greatly increasing the mobility of the aorta. Care is taken not to injure any enlarged intercostal arteries during the dissection. It may be necessary to divide these arteries, especially if aneurysmal dilatation has occurred, but it is preferable to preserve all collaterals. The aorta is cross-clamped proximally and distally and the area of constriction is excised. To obtain an optimal result, it is absolutely necessary to resect the entire constricted segment and construct the anastomosis without tension (Fig. 33–8). Even in infants with tubular hypoplasia, the aorta is elastic and can usually be mobilized sufficiently to allow primary repair. The earliest repairs used a continuous silk suture. An unacceptable rate of restenosis resulted, probably secondary to failure of the anastomosis to grow. Many surgeons currently use interrupted sutures, fine nonabsorbable monofilament sutures (polypropylene), or fine absorbable monofilament sutures (polydioxanone) to improve results. Several groups have recently reported excellent results with resection and primary anastomosis even in neonates. Cobanoglu and associates (1985)

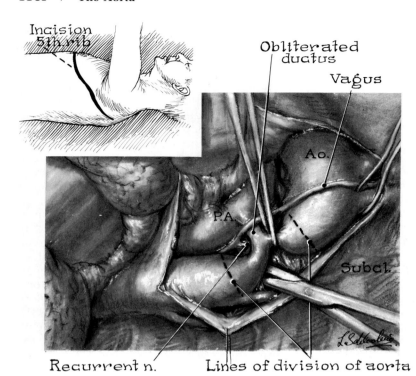

Incision 5th rib

Obliterated ductus

Vagus

Ao.

P.A.

Subcl.

Recurrent n.   Lines of division of aorta

Figure 33–7. Operative exposure for resection of coarctation of the aorta is through the bed of the fifth rib. The entire rib is removed from neck to cartilage. The constricted segment is usually held medially by an obliterated ductus, division of which allows considerable mobility. The coarctation is held forward to facilitate dissection posteriorly. Large intercostal arteries must be carefully avoided. Division of the aorta should be through a point of normal diameter.

reported a 5-year reoperation-free rate of 92% in neonates with coarctation after resection and primary anastomosis. Korfer and co-workers (1985) reported 55 infants under 3 months of age who had resection with end-to-end anastomosis with a hospital mortality of 3.6%. At a mean follow-up of 5 years, only three showed evidence of significant restenosis. Harlan and colleagues (1984) reported a significantly decreased rate of restenosis in infants whose repair was done with polypropylene as compared with silk. Experimental work (Chiu et al, 1988) has shown that the use of the absorbable monofilament suture for end-to-end anastomosis permits significant growth of the suture line. Advantages of the classic repair include complete resection of abnormal tissue, preservation of normal vascular anatomy, and no requirement for prosthetic material.

In some patients with tubular hypoplasia and some older patients with inelastic aortas, it is not possible to resect the narrowed segment completely and restore aortic continuity by primary anastomosis. Gross pioneered the use of aortic homografts to bridge the gap in these patients. In 1961, he reported follow-up of 70 patients who had had homograft insertion (Schuster and Gross, 1962). No complications other than calcification of the graft (which was present in less than 50% of the patients) were reported, and there were no cases of aneurysm formation. Morris, Cooley, DeBakey, and Crawford introduced the use of prosthetic interposition grafts in 1960. Tube grafts are rarely indicated but may be useful in patients with complex coarctation, recurrent coarctation, or aneurysm formation.

Because of early unsatisfactory results, especially in infants, other techniques were developed. In 1957, Vossschulte (Vossschulte, 1961) introduced the prosthetic patch onlay graft technique (Fig. 33–9). The area of constriction is incised longitudinally, the obstructing shelf is excised, and a Dacron patch is used to enlarge the lumen. Yee and associates (1984) reported the use of Gore-Tex patches and emphasized the advantages of the technique, including decreased operative time, decreased dissection, maximal augmentation of the area of stenosis, preservation of the collateral vessels, and no need for sacrifice of normal vascular structures. A thoracotomy incision has commonly been used for synthetic patch aortoplasty. However, Ungerleider and Ebert (1987) showed the applicability of patch aortoplasty via a median sternotomy in selected infants who require simultaneous correction of coarctation and intracardiac defects. Sade and co-workers (1984) have documented growth of the posterior wall of the aorta after patch aortoplasty. Patch aortoplasty is highly effective in relieving the aortic obstruction (Sade et al, 1979), with a low incidence of restenosis and persistent hypertension (at rest and following exercise) (Smith et al, 1984). However, the use of prosthetic material may predispose to infection, and there are increasingly frequent reports of the formation of aneurysms and pseudoaneurysms (Bergdahl and Ljungquist, 1980). Aneurysmal dilatation of the posterior aortic wall opposite the prosthetic patch has been reported with increasing frequency (up to 38% of patients followed long term) (Clarkson et al, 1985), but the true incidence is unknown. An experimental study suggested that damage to the posterior wall during excision of the obstructing shelf may predis-

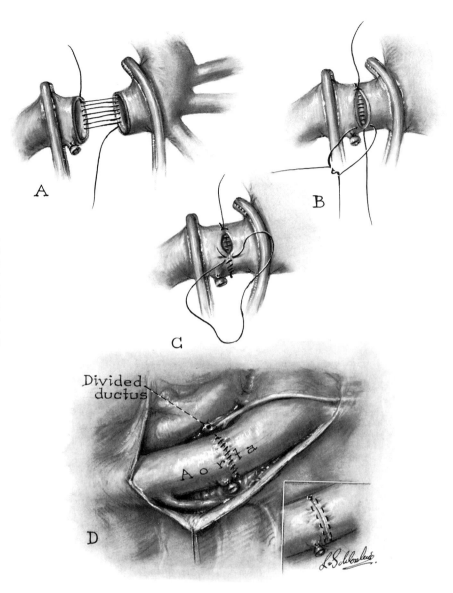

Figure 33–8. Anastomosis after excision of coarctation. *A,* An everting mattress suture is placed over about one-third of the posterior row before the vessels are approximated and the suture is pulled up (*B*). *C,* The anastomosis is completed with continuous over-and-over suture. *Inset* in *D* shows the everting mattress suture sometimes used. In children, interrupted mattress sutures are used for the entire anterior row.

pose to aneurysm formation (DeSanto et al, 1987). In 15 patients who developed aneurysmal dilatation following patch aortoplasty with resection of the posterior ridge, microscopic examination of the aneurysm wall demonstrated degeneration of the media in greater than 50% of the patients (Hehrlein et al, 1986). Differences in tensile strength between the prosthetic patch and native aortic wall may be a factor in the formation of true and false aneurysms. If patch aortoplasty is done without excision of the obstructing shelf, it is possible to achieve excellent enlargement of the stenotic area if a sufficiently large patch is used. This modification may decrease the incidence of posterior wall aneurysms. Patch aortoplasty is very useful in surgical therapy of recurrent coarctation. All patients who have had patch aortoplasty must be followed closely to monitor development of an aneurysm (del Nido et al, 1986).

The subclavian flap aortoplasty was introduced by Waldhausen and Nahrwold in 1966 (Fig. 33–10). A left thoracotomy is done and the pleura overlying the aorta is incised. The left subclavian artery is dissected free and ligated at its first branch. The vertebral artery should be ligated to prevent a subclavian steal phenomenon. A longitudinal incision is made through the region of coarctation and continued onto the subclavian artery, creating a flap. The posterior obstructing shelf is resected, and the flap of subclavian artery is turned down to enlarge the constriction. It is important that the flap be of sufficient length to bridge the obstruction completely. Advantages of this technique include avoidance of prosthetic material, decreased dissection, decreased aortic cross-clamp period, and increased anastomotic growth because there is no circumferential suture line. If the area of narrowing occurs proximal to the left subclavian artery, the flap may be directed proximally and a reversed subclavian flap aortoplasty

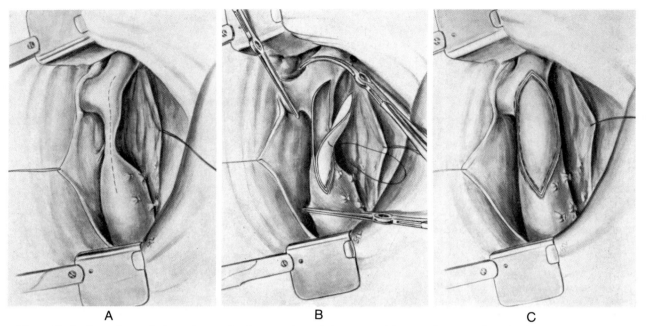

Figure 33–9. Operative technique for repair of coarctation of the aorta with a synthetic patch aortoplasty. *A*, Operative view showing the line of incision across coarctation. *B*, Placement of patch to enlarge area of constriction. *C*, Completed repair. (From Vossschulte, K.: Surgical correction of coarctation of the aorta by an "isthmusplastic" operation. Thorax, *16*:338, 1961.)

should be done to enlarge the aortic arch. Campbell and associates (1984) reported the use of the subclavian flap repair in 53 patients under 1 year of age. Operative mortality was 4%, and follow-up revealed no pressure gradient greater than 20 mm Hg. Hamilton and co-workers (1978) reported 45 infants who underwent subclavian flap aortoplasty, with an overall mortality of 24%; all deaths occurred in children who had associated anomalies and who had opera-

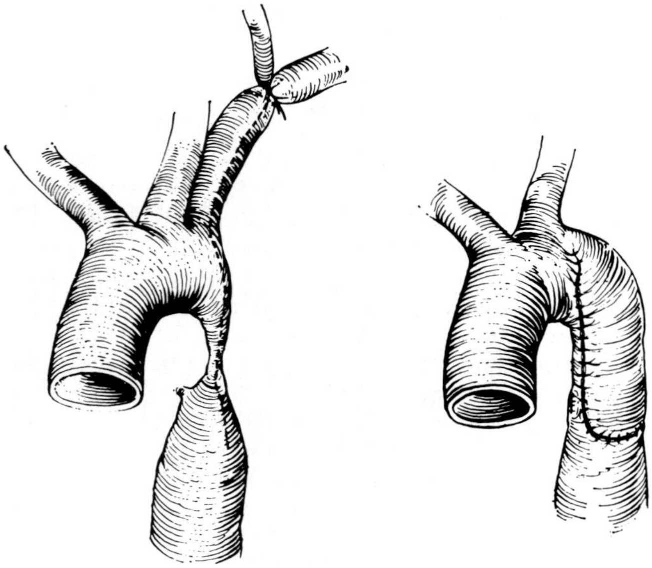

Figure 33–10. The operative technique of repair of coarctation with a subclavian flap. (From Waldhausen, J. A., and Nahrwold, D. L.: Repair of coarctation of the aorta with a subclavian flap. J. Thorac. Cardiovasc. Surg., *51*:532, 1966.)

tion before 2 months of age. There was no evidence of residual or recurrent coarctation in the survivors.

The subclavian flap aortoplasty has commonly been recommended for use in infants, although it is occasionally done in older children as well. However, there has been concern that subclavian flap aortoplasty may not be the optimal method for coarctation repair in very young infants. Cobanoglu and co-workers (1985) reported an increased incidence of early recoarctation in infants under 3 months of age after subclavian flap aortoplasty when compared with resection and primary anastomosis. They proposed that the cause was inadequate resection of ductal tissue in the aortic wall, which continued to involute and fibrose. Sanchez and colleagues (1986) reported a 22% incidence of early recoarctation secondary to a posterior shelf in infants less than 3 months old. Restenosis was strongly correlated with younger age at the time of surgical correction and was thought to be secondary to the presence of ductal tissue in the aortic wall.

In addition to the possibility of early recoarctation in very young neonates, there is concern about sacrifice of the major vascular supply to the left upper extremity. The subclavian artery is frequently divided for creation of systemic-to-pulmonary shunts, and adverse sequelae have been rare. There is some evidence of decreased growth of the extremity resulting in decreased length and mass (Todd et al, 1983), and rare reports of vascular insufficiency and gangrene of the arm (Geiss et al, 1980; Mellgren et al, 1987; Webb and Burford, 1952), especially if branches of the subclavian artery distal to the vertebral artery are ligated.

In some infants with tubular hypoplasia, it is difficult to excise the narrowed segment completely and create a satisfactory anastomosis. Amato and associates (1977) proposed anastomosis of the distal aorta to the inferior aspect of the arch with anastomosis of the contiguous walls of the left carotid and subclavian arteries if necessary to relieve the obstruction (Amato et al, 1977). Lansman and colleagues (1986) proposed an extended resection with primary anastomosis (Fig. 33–11). The coarcted segment is excised and the distal aorta anastomosed to an incision on the inferior aspect of the arch. A more extensive procedure has been described by Elliott (1987): The arch is completely dissected, the descending aorta is mobilized to the diaphragm, an incision is made on the inferior aspect of the arch as proximal as possible, and the anastomosis completed. There have been no reports of neurologic complications. These techniques have not been widely applied, but the reported mortality is low.

Various other surgical repairs have been proposed to correct coarctation. The Blalock-Park anastomosis involves division of the left subclavian artery with anastomosis to the descending aorta to bypass the obstruction (Blalock and Park, 1944). Ascending aorta to descending aorta bypass grafts have been used and may be useful at the time of reoperation.

Management of Associated Anomalies

Outcome after surgical correction depends on the age at the time of operation, the method of repair chosen, and especially the presence of associated anomalies. The optimal management of infants with associated anomalies is still controversial. A PDA is frequently present and should be divided or ligated.

A bicuspid aortic valve may be present but often requires no intervention at the time of correction of the coarctation. Appropriate management of associated ventricular septal defects is less clear. Several therapeutic options are available. In the past, the pulmonary artery was often banded at the time of repair of the coarctation in infants with a nonrestrictive ventricular septal defect. However, ventricular septal defects associated with coarctation are often of a type with a high incidence of spontaneous closure. In infants with coarctation, a ventricular septal defect, and no other associated anomalies, some experts advocate repair of the coarctation alone. If the congestive heart failure does not resolve, the septal defect is closed at a second operation. Hammon and associates (1985) reported improved survival with pulmonary artery banding at the time of coarctation repair and later closure of the ventricular septal defect. Leanage and colleagues (1981) suggest that the banding should be done only in infants with an associated large ventricular septal defect. Goldman and co-workers (1986) found no survival benefit to pulmonary artery banding even in infants with a large ventricular septal defect. They did, however, report decreased mortality with the use of pulmonary artery banding in patients with coarctation, ventricular septal defect, and associated intracardiac anomalies. If pulmonary artery banding is to be done, some experts advocate banding before clamping the aorta to prevent increased shunting due to the increased left ventricular afterload; others contend that the timing of banding is not critical. Children with associated complex anomalies may improve sufficiently after coarctation repair to allow elective repair or palliation at a later date. Some authors advocate that a one-stage repair of the coarctation and associ-

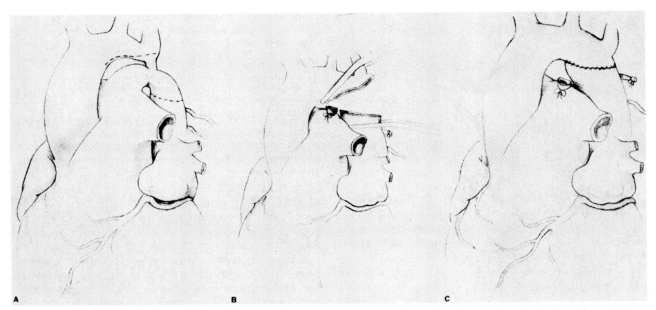

Figure 33–11. The operative technique for extended aortic arch anastomosis for repair of coarctation. *A*, Region of coarctation to be excised. *B*, The aortic arch and descending aorta have been mobilized and the PDA ligated. The entire segment of abnormal aorta has been resected with extension of the incision onto the inferior aspect of the arch. *C*, Completed repair. (From Lansman, S., Shapiro, A. J., Schiller, M. S., et al: Extended aortic arch anastomosis for repair of coarctation in infancy. Circulation, *74*(Suppl. I):I-37, 1986.)

ated defects and a median sternotomy may be the optimal approach.

Nonoperative Therapy

In recent years, percutaneous transluminal balloon angioplasty has been introduced as an alternative therapy for coarctation. Initial results were encouraging; however, reports soon appeared of aneurysmal dilatation after balloon angioplasty of previously unoperated coarctations. Dilatation of recurrent stenosis has been more successful, and there have been fewer reports of aneurysm formation, presumably secondary to surrounding scar tissue (Fig. 33–12). Several centers have continued to use balloon angioplasty for native coarctation (Beekman et al, 1987). Morrow and co-workers (1988) reported successful angioplasty in 31 of 33 patients with native coarctation. Follow-up angiography in ten patients showed no significant restenosis; however, aneurys-

mal dilatation was present in two patients. Cystic medial necrosis has been described as a consistent histologic finding in patients with coarctation (Lindsay, 1988), suggesting that balloon-induced tears into an abnormal media may provide the substrate for aneurysm formation (Isner et al, 1987). The long-term results of balloon angioplasty for native coarctation in terms of recoarctation and especially aneurysm formation are unknown, and the technique must be considered investigational. The results of angioplasty of postoperative recoarctation appear to be better, and angioplasty may be associated with less mortality and morbidity than reoperation; however, long-term follow-up is necessary (Saul et al, 1987).

Complications

Correction of coarctation may be complicated by hemorrhage, chylothorax, recurrent nerve paralysis, infection, and suture line thrombosis. It has been suggested that patients with Turner's syndrome may be at increased risk for hemorrhage because of their friable tissues (Brandt et al, 1984; Ravelo et al, 1980). Several unique problems may develop in the postoperative period. Paradoxical elevation of the blood pressure to greater than preoperative levels may occur. This is a two-phase phenomenon characterized by a rise in the systolic blood pressure during the first 24 to 36 hours after operation and a later increase in the diastolic pressure. The first phase is characterized by activation of the sympathetic nervous system with elevation of serum catecholamines (Benedict et al, 1978). The late phase is characterized by elevation of plasma renin and angiotensin levels (Fox et al, 1980). Postoperative elevation of blood pressure has not been described in children having thoracotomy for repair of other cardiac lesions. Paradoxical hypertension may be associated with the postcoarctectomy syndrome of abdominal pain and distention first reported by Sealy in 1953 (Sealy et al, 1957, 1967). Up to 20% of patients having repair of coarctation experience abdominal pain and distention postoperatively. Laparotomy is occasionally indicated and may reveal evidence of mesenteric ischemia (Downing et al, 1958); rarely, bowel resection may be necessary. Arteriography shows changes in the mesenteric vessels, and pathologic examination reveals necrotizing mesenteric arteritis (Kawauchi et al, 1985). The syndrome is possibly related to elevated renin levels. Aggressive therapy of hypertension appears to prevent full manifestation of the postcoarctectomy syndrome. Many drugs have been successfully used to control the postoperative hypertension, including sodium nitroprusside, propranolol, and reserpine (Will et al, 1978). Interestingly, a small series suggested that paradoxical hypertension does not occur after balloon angioplasty of the obstructing lesion (Choy et al, 1987). This may be related to less-effective relief of the stenosis or lack

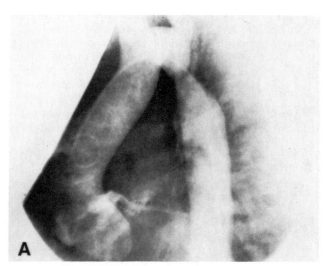

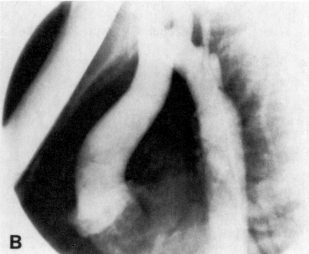

Figure 33–12. *A,* Aortogram showing recurrent stenosis after surgical correction of coarctation of the aorta. *B,* Aortogram after balloon angioplasty of the recoarctation. (Courtesy of Dr. Bennett Pearce.)

of surgical manipulation of the aorta and periaortic neural fibers.

A dreaded complication of coarctation repair is paraplegia, which occurs in 0.5 to 1% of patients. Poor collaterals, anomalous origin of the right subclavian artery, distal hypotension during the period of aortic cross-clamping, reoperation, or hyperthermia may predispose to paraplegia during the procedure. Brewer and colleagues (1972) reviewed 66 cases of paraplegia after 12,532 procedures for repair of coarctation, an incidence of 0.41%. In this study, neither sacrifice of intercostals nor duration of aortic cross-clamping could be related to the occurrence of paraplegia. Brewer emphasized the marked variation in spinal cord blood supply and suggested that measurement of distal pressure after cross-clamping of the aorta be done to assess adequacy of the collateral circulation. Hughes and Reemtsma (1971), based on results in two patients, suggested monitoring distal perfusion pressure with use of bypass if the pressure fell below 50 mm Hg. Others have recommended monitoring of cerebrospinal fluid pressure with the use of bypass and drainage of spinal fluid if necessary to maintain adequate perfusion pressure of the spinal cord. Krieger and Spencer (1985) have extensively investigated the use of somatosensory evoked potentials to assess adequacy of spinal cord perfusion, as have others (Laschinger et al, 1987). Loss of somatosensory evoked potentials was a sensitive indicator of spinal cord ischemia. Maintenance of distal aortic pressure during aortic cross-clamping above 60 mm Hg correlated with preservation of the somatosensory evoked potentials. Distal hypotension with loss of somatosensory evoked potentials for more than 30 minutes was associated with a greater than 70% incidence of paraplegia (Cunningham et al, 1987). Distal aortic pressure should be measured during repair of coarctation and maintained above 60 mm Hg with shunt or bypass techniques as necessary.

Results

The results of surgical correction depend on the age at repair, the type of repair used, and the associated anomalies. Operative mortality in neonates has decreased to 5 to 10% and is lower in older children. It is very low in patients with isolated coarctation and no associated anomalies. Classically, in patients who had resection and end-to-end anastomosis in infancy, the rate of recoarctation was as high as 60%. There is a decreased incidence of recurrent coarctation with the subclavian patch aortoplasty and the prosthetic patch graft repair compared with historical series. The most recent series using resection and end-to-end anastomosis show, even in neonates, results that compare very favorably with other methods in terms of mortality and recoarctation. Trinquet and associates (1988) reported a follow-up on 178 infants undergoing coarctation re-

pair at less than 3 months of age. Sixty-three infants had isolated coarctation, 47 had associated ventricular septal defects, and 68 had other associated anomalies. Actuarial survival at 5 years was 90% for infants with isolated coarctation, 84% for those with associated ventricular septal defects, and 40% for those with complex anomalies. The rate of restenosis was the same for subclavian flap angioplasty, resection with primary anastomosis, and extended resection with anastomosis.

Any comparison of techniques for repair of coarctation must consider the historical time frame (Ziemer et al, 1986). Advances in the care of critically ill infants such as the introduction of neonatal intensive care units and prostaglandin therapy have resulted in dramatic improvements in the preoperative condition of patients, which may affect mortality as much as the choice of repair. Advances in suture materials and vascular surgical technique also make it difficult to compare results from different time periods. Circumferential arterial suture lines have been effectively used in the arterial switch operation for transposition of the great arteries (Arensman et al, 1985) and should be as successful in coarctation repair. Since a prospective, randomized trial of the various repair techniques has not been done, long-term results cannot be accurately compared. The optimal method for coarctation repair is unknown, and therapy should be individualized on the basis of each patient's anatomy, clinical condition, and associated anomalies.

Recoarctation usually manifests as persistent hypertension or arm-leg gradient. The arm-leg pressure gradient should be measured in the immediate postoperative period to differentiate residual stenosis secondary to an inadequate repair from true recoarctation. The causes of recoarctation include failure of growth of the anastomosis, inadequate resection of the narrowed segment, residual abnormal ductal tissue, and suture line thrombosis. Exercise testing with measurement of the arm-leg gradient should be done to evaluate postoperative patients (Connors, 1979). Many patients who are normotensive at rest and do not have an arm-leg gradient develop severe hypertension and a gradient after exercise. They may have significant restenosis. It is important to measure arm and leg pressures simultaneously to assess the gradient accurately. This can easily be done by using Doppler pressure measurements at rest and immediately after exercise. In infants, the arm-leg gradient should be assessed before and after a noxious stimulus. The long-term consequences of exercise-induced hypertension after correction of coarctation are unknown but may adversely affect the prognosis (Freed et al, 1979; Markel et al, 1986).

Reoperation is indicated if significant hypertension or other symptoms occur and a pressure gradient can be shown (Foster, 1984). Reoperation is more difficult when there is scarring, and there is an increased morbidity and mortality. Lack of collaterals may result in an increased incidence of paraplegia.

In patients who have had previous resection and end-to-end anastomosis, subclavian flap aortoplasty or prosthetic patch onlay grafting is an appropriate method for repair of the recoarctation (Pollack et al, 1983). Sweeney and associates (1985) reported follow-up of 53 patients who required reoperation. Patch aortoplasty was used in 26 patients; bypass grafting was used in 16 patients; and interposition grafts were used in 8 patients; and three patients underwent resection with end-to-end anastomosis. Temporary shunts and bypass techniques were not used. There were no operative deaths and no neurologic complications. Balloon angioplasty has become a frequently used technique in patients with recoarctation and may be the optimal initial therapy for recoarctation (Kan et al, 1983). Jacob and associates reported the use of ascending aorta—descending aorta bypass in 10 patients with recoarctation without mortality, paraplegia, or residual hypertension. They utilize a two-incision approach via a left thoracotomy and median sternotomy, without cardiopulmonary bypass (Jacob et al, 1988).

Some patients who have had a technically excellent repair may not have complete resolution of the elevated blood pressure (Nanton and Olley, 1976). The cause of this persistent hypertension is unclear, but it is related to the age at repair and the duration of the preoperative hypertension. Follow-up of surgical patients indicates that they are not rendered entirely normal (Simon and Zloto, 1974). Maron and associates (1973), reporting long-term follow-up of 248 patients who had correction of aortic coarctation, found an increased incidence of premature death usually secondary to cardiovascular disease and related this to the duration of preoperative hypertension. There is evidence of increased coronary atherosclerosis secondary to coarctation (Cokkinos et al, 1979). Koller and colleagues (1987) found that patients operated on between the ages of 2 and 4 years had the lowest risk for restenosis and persistent hypertension. There is evidence of abnormal left ventricular function despite relief of the obstruction (Carpenter et al, 1985). Kimball and associates (1986a) showed a persistent increase in ventricular contractility after successful coarctation repair, possibly secondary to cardiac ultrastructural changes resulting from congenital pressure overload. They have also documented abnormal thallium scans after successful coarctation repair, suggesting persistent changes in the coronary arteries (Kimball et al, 1986b). Aortic stenosis or regurgitation secondary to a bicuspid aortic valve may develop and necessitate valve replacement. As has been emphasized, the long-term prognosis of many patients is determined primarily by the associated anomalies.

INTERRUPTION OF THE AORTIC ARCH

Complete absence of a segment of the aortic arch without any anatomic connection between the prox-imal and distal segments is termed interruption of the aortic arch. If a fibrous strand connects the segments, the condition is termed aortic atresia. Interruption of the aortic arch at the aortic isthmus was first described by Steidele (1778). Seidel (1818) reported absence of the segment between the left subclavian and left common carotid arteries. Interruption of the aortic arch between the left common carotid and the innominate arteries was reported by Weisman and Kesten (1948). Samson and colleagues reported the first successful correction in 1955 (Merrill et al, 1957). Sirak and associates (1968) were the first to successfully correct an interrupted aortic arch in a neonate. Barratt-Boyes and colleagues (1972) reported the first simultaneous correction of interrupted aortic arch and all associated anomalies. In 1976, the introduction of prostaglandin therapy to maintain ductal patency allowed preoperative stabilization of infants with interrupted arch and greatly improved surgical results.

Incidence

Interruption of the aortic arch is a rare anomaly constituting less than 1.5% of congenital heart disease. Interrupted arch may be an isolated defect but is usually associated with other anomalies. Everts-Suarez and Carson (1959) noted the frequent association of interrupted arch, PDA, and ventricular septal defect. Interruption of the arch may be associated with a wide variety of cardiac anomalies and is often found coexistent with truncus arteriosus or aortopulmonary window. As with coarctation, interrupted arch is infrequently encountered in association with right ventricular outflow tract obstruction.

Embryology and Pathologic Anatomy

Celoria and Patton (1959) classified interrupted aortic arch based on the absent segment. In Type A, the interruption occurs distal to the left subclavian artery; in Type B, the interruption occurs between the left subclavian and left common carotid arteries; and with Type C, the interruption occurs between the left common carotid and innominate arteries (Fig. 33–13). These classifications may be further subdivided by the presence or absence of anomalous origin of the right subclavian artery from the distal aorta segment and are designated A_1, B_1, C_1 if an anomalous origin is present. In a review of 165 cases of interrupted aortic arch, Van Praagh and associates (1971) found that 43% were Type A, 53% were Type B, and 4% were Type C.

The cause of interrupted arch is unclear. As with coarctation, there is an association with defects that decrease ascending aortic flow and increase ductal flow, implying that abnormal fetal blood flow patterns are an etiologic factor. Type B interrupted arch is frequently found in association with DiGeorge's syndrome (absence of the third and fourth pharyngeal pouches) (Van Mierop and Kutsche, 1984). In

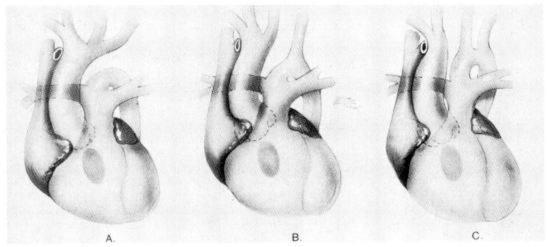

Figure 33–13. Three types of interrupted arch. Type A is between the left subclavian artery and descending aorta; Type B is between the left carotid and left subclavian arteries; and Type C is between the innominate and left carotid arteries. Incidence is 43% for Type A; 53% for Type B; and 4% for Type C. (From Turley, K., Yee, E. S., and Ebert, P. A.: The total repair of interrupted arch complex in infants: The anterior approach. Circulation, *70*(Suppl. I):I-16, 1984.)

DiGeorge's syndrome, the thymus and parathyroid glands are absent and patients are hypocalcemic and suffer from defects in cellular immunity. Defects in the development of neural crest may be responsible for DiGeorge's syndrome and Type B interrupted arch.

Natural History and Clinical Manifestations

The prognosis of uncorrected interruption of the aortic arch is poor. The mean age at death has been reported to be 4 to 10 days. Ninety per cent of infants with interrupted arch die in the first year of life unless they undergo surgical intervention. Only in the rare case of interrupted arch with no associated anomalies is prolonged survival possible, presumably because of the development of a collateral circulation in utero (Dische et al, 1975).

Diagnosis and Management

Most infants with interrupted aortic arch present with congestive heart failure secondary to left-to-right shunting through a ventricular septal defect and increased left ventricular afterload. Lower body perfusion is maintained by right-to-left shunting through a PDA. When the ductus closes, perfusion of the lower body essentially ceases and the infants become anuric, severely acidotic, and the femoral pulses become nonpalpable. The congestive heart failure and acidosis are resistant to medical therapy, and death occurs within a few days. Since the advent of prostaglandin E_1 therapy, however, it is possible to maintain ductal patency, improve lower body perfusion, reverse the acidosis, and increase urinary output (Zahka et al, 1980). The physical examination is not specific for interrupted arch, and there are no characteristic murmurs. The ECG is not useful, and

the chest film reveals an enlarged heart with pulmonary congestion. Cardiac catheterization with angiography is essential for accurate diagnosis. Contrast injection must be done in both the proximal and distal segments to define the anatomy adequately. When the diagnosis has been made and the infant is stabilized with prostaglandin therapy, surgical correction is done. In infants with Type B interrupted arch, there is a high incidence of DiGeorge's syndrome and great care must be taken to avoid hypocalcemia. Because of their immunologic defect, these patients should receive irradiated blood products to prevent the development of graft-versus-host disease.

Various procedures have been used to either palliate or correct interrupted arch. The ultimate goal is restoration of aortic continuity and correction of associated anomalies. Aortic continuity may be restored by distal anastomosis of the aortic segments, end-to-side anastomosis of an arch vessel to either the proximal or distal segment, division of the ductus with anastomosis to the proximal segment, or use of an interposition graft.

If palliation is planned, a left thoracotomy may be done and aortic continuity restored by using one of the arch vessels as a conduit. In Type A interrupted arch, a Blalock-Park anastomosis is used; in Type B, the left common carotid artery is anastomosed to the distal segment or a "reversed" Blalock-Park anastomosis may be created; and in Type C, the left common carotid artery may be anastomosed to the ascending aorta. The use of ductal tissue in the anastomosis should be avoided because obstruction may occur if the tissue contracts and fibroses. Alternatively, interposition of a Dacron or Gore-Tex graft may be done to restore continuity. Simultaneous correction of intracardiac anomalies is not possible through a left thoracotomy; however, pulmonary artery banding may be done if indicated. Repair of a ventricular septal defect and other anomalies may be done at a later date through a median sternotomy.

Norwood and associates (1983) reported improved survival after primary correction of interrupted arch. A tube graft is used to restore aortic continuity, and the distal anastomosis is performed via a left thoracotomy after ductal division. A median sternotomy is then done, the proximal anastomosis is completed, and cardiopulmonary bypass is instituted for closure of the ventricular septal defect. Ten of 13 patients survived the reparative operation with good results despite the eventual development of subaortic stenosis in several patients. Turley and colleagues (1984) reported total correction via an anterior approach (Fig. 33–14). Cardiopulmonary bypass with biaortic cannulation is used for cooling, with profound hypothermia and circulatory arrest during the arch repair. The ductus is divided, the aorta is mobilized to the diaphragm, and aortic continuity is restored by direct anastomosis of the proximal and distal aortic segments. The ventricular septal defect is repaired through a right ventriculotomy. Early mortality was 20%, compared with 33 to 43% mortality for staged procedures at the same institution. Development of subaortic stenosis has been reported after successful repair of interrupted aortic arch and may necessitate further surgical intervention.

Sell and associates reported 71 patients seen with interrupted aortic arch between 1974 and 1987. In the early years, tube graft repair was done. More recently, direct anastomosis with repair of the VSD has been performed. Actuarial survival at 10 years was 47% and mortality declined with increasing experience. Recurrent arch obstruction was managed with reoperation or balloon angioplasty. Left ventricular outflow tract obstruction occurred in approximately 50% of patients undergoing repair (Sell et al, 1988). Improved results with direct anastomosis have also been reported by Scott and colleagues (1988).

Interrupted aortic arch remains a difficult surgical problem. Advances in surgical techniques, neonatal intensive care, and the introduction of prostaglandin E₁ therapy have greatly improved survival. After stabilization of these critically ill infants, total correction of the interrupted arch and associated anomalies should be undertaken via a median sternotomy.

AORTOPULMONARY WINDOW

Aortopulmonary window is a rare congenital heart defect resulting from abnormal septation of the truncus arteriosus into the aorta and pulmonary artery. Various terms have been applied to this anomaly: aortopulmonary fistula, aortic septal defect, aorticopulmonary septal defect, and aortopulmonary fenestration. Elliotson first described aortopulmonary window in 1830. Abbott was able to include only ten cases of aortopulmonary window in her classic re-

view of 1,000 cases of congenital heart disease (Gross, 1952). Gross and Neuhauser (1948) successfully ligated an aortopulmonary window, but noted that this method would be dangerous in many patients because of the friability of the tissues. In 1951, Gasul and colleages reported the use of retrograde aortography for preoperative diagnosis of aortopulmonary window. Scott and Sabiston described a closed method for division of an aortopulmonary window in 1953. Cooley and associates (1957) reported successful division of an aortopulmonary window by using cardiopulmonary bypass. In 1966, Putnam and Gross suggested a transpulmonary approach for closure of the defect. In 1968, Wright and associates reported direct suture closure of an aortopulmonary window via a transaortic approach. Deverall and colleages (1969) subsequently described patch closure of the defect by using a transaortic approach.

A closely related defect is anomalous origin of the right pulmonary artery from the aorta, which was first reported by Fraentzel in 1868 (Fontana et al, 1987). Caro and associates (1957) first attempted surgical correction with an interposition graft in 1957, but the patient died shortly after the operation. Armer and colleagues (1961) reported the first successful correction by using an interposition graft. Kirkpatrick and associates (1967) reported successful direct anastomosis of the right pulmonary artery to the main pulmonary artery. Aortic origin of the left pulmonary artery or both pulmonary arteries from the aorta occurs less commonly. Herbert and associates (1973) reported correction of aortic origin of the left pulmonary artery.

Embryology and Pathologic Anatomy

In the truncus arteriosus, two conotruncal ridges form proximally and fuse to create the septum between the aorta and the pulmonary artery. More distally, the right and left sixth aortic arches fuse with the main pulmonary artery to form the right and left pulmonary arteries and complete formation of the aortopulmonary septum. Failure of fusion or malalignment of the conotruncal ridges may result in a defect in the aortopulmonary septum. Abnormal migration of the sixth aortic arches may result in aortic origin of a pulmonary artery. It is important to note that the aortic and pulmonic valves are normally formed, distinguishing these defects from persistent truncus arteriosus. Unlike persistent truncus arteriosus and Type B interrupted aortic arch, there is no association between aortopulmonary window and DiGeorge's syndrome.

An aortopulmonary window is usually a single large defect beginning a few millimeters above the aortic valve on the left lateral wall of the aorta (Fig. 33–15). Multiple defects have been rarely reported. The defect may occasionally be found more distally overlying the origin of the right pulmonary artery, and rarely absence of the entire aortopulmonary septum may be encountered. Origin of the right

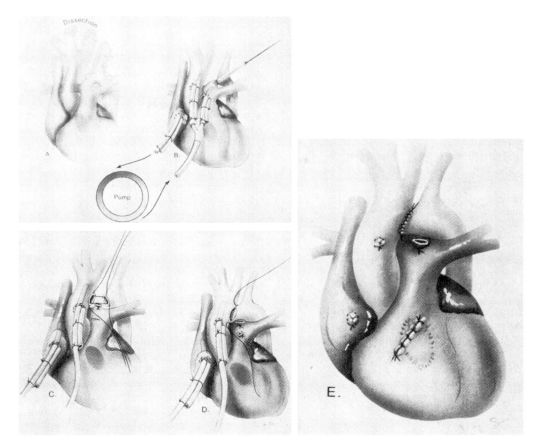

Figure 33–14. *A,* Dissection. The arch vessels are dissected to the thoracic outlet laterally, carotid bifurcations superiorly, and the descending aorta inferiorly with the use of electrocautery to the diaphragm. This dissection maximizes anterior-posterior displacement of both vessels, minimizing anastomotic tension not possible when mobilization of the descending aorta alone from the lateral approach is used. *B,* Single atrial-to-biaortic cannulation. Ascending aortic and transductal descending aortic cannulation is used, and a tourniquet is used to isolate the pulmonary circulation, preventing flooding of the lungs during bypass and affording continued total perfusion of the entire body until deep hypothermia is achieved. *C* and *D,* Removal of the descending aortic cannula after total circulatory arrest affords a bloodless field for precise repair and maximal anastomotic size when the descending aorta is anastomosed to the posterior aspect of the ascending aorta: The pulmonary arteriotomy and ductus are simultaneously repaired. *E,* During rewarming with single atrial-to-ascending aortic cannulation the aortic anastomosis can be assessed, and through a right ventriculotomy (outflow tract) the ventricular septal defect is repaired. (From Turley, K., Yee, E. S., and Ebert, P. A.: The total repair of interrupted arch complex in infants: The anterior approach. Circulation, *70*(Suppl. I):I-16, 1984.)

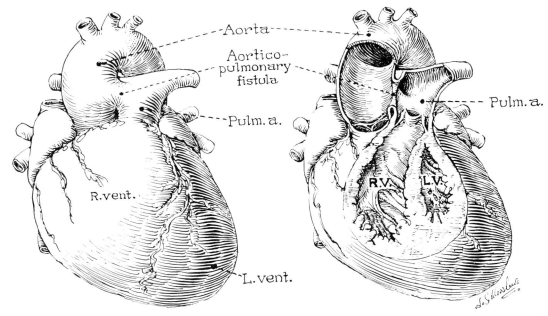

Figure 33–15. Aortopulmonary window. The size of the fistula and its relation to the semilunar valves vary. (From Scott, H. W., Jr., and Sabiston, D. C., Jr.: Surgical treatment for congenital aorticopulmonary fistula. J. Thorac. Surg, 25:26, 1953.)

coronary artery (Luisi et al, 1980) and rarely the left (Agius et al, 1970) from the pulmonary artery can complicate surgical correction. Associated anomalies include Type A interrupted aortic arch, ventricular septal defect, tetralogy of Fallot, and PDA.

Aortopulmonary window allows a large left-to-right shunt, resulting in pulmonary hypertension and congestive heart failure. As with a nonrestrictive ventricular septal defect, irreversible pulmonary vascular disease may occur at an early age. In patients with aortic origin of the right pulmonary artery, pulmonary hypertension is encountered in the left lung. The cause of this contralateral pulmonary hypertension is uncertain, and a reflex mechanism has been postulated.

Natural History

Aortopulmonary window and aortic origin of a pulmonary artery are rare defects, and thus the natural history is not well defined. Patients with a large aortopulmonary window usually do not survive infancy. Children or young adults with an aortopulmonary window are encountered occasionally and usually have developed significant pulmonary vascular disease. The clinical course is thought to be similar to that in untreated patients with a large ventricular septal defect.

Diagnosis

Infants with aortopulmonary window usually present with congestive heart failure early in life (Blieden and Moller, 1974). They often have growth retardation and recurrent pulmonary infections. Physical examination reveals a systolic murmur and occasionally a continuous murmur suggestive of PDA. The chest film shows cardiomegaly, with pulmonary vascular engorgement or congestive heart failure. Aortopulmonary window must be differentiated from PDA, persistent truncus arteriosus, ventricular septal defect with aortic regurgitation, and ruptured aneurysm of the sinus of Valsalva.

Two-dimensional echocardiography can be used to show the defect. Cardiac catheterization reveals an oxygen saturation step-up at the level of the pulmonary artery, and the course of the catheter may suggest the diagnosis. Retrograde aortography provides accurate visualization of the defect. It is necessary to document the presence of normal aortic and pulmonic valves to confirm the diagnosis, and the location of coronary ostia must be carefully demonstrated before surgical intervention. Catheterization and angiography are also necesssary for the diagnosis of aortic origin of a pulmonary artery.

Method of Surgical Correction

The presence of an aortopulmonary window is sufficient indication for repair unless severe pulmonary vascular disease has occurred. The preferred technique for repair is transaortic closure either by direct suture or patch closure (Doty et al, 1981). Simple ligation should not be done because of the risk of hemorrhage from the friable tissues. Division and primary closure may result in narrowing of the vessels. The transaortic approach is preferred to the transpulmonary method because it allows better visualization of the defect and the coronary ostia. The operation is done via a median sternotomy, and either cardiopulmonary bypass or hypothermic circulatory arrest may be used.

A transverse aortotomy at the level of the window is done and the anatomy is carefully defined. Particular attention should be given to the location of the coronary ostia and the origin of the right pulmonary artery. Small defects may be closed by direct suture. Larger defects should be closed with a Dacron patch. Care must be taken to place the patch so that the coronary ostia are on the aortic side. If the defect involves the origin of the right pulmonary artery, a teardrop-shaped patch extending along the right pulmonary artery may be used to repair the defect. Johansson and colleagues (1978) described a method of repair by opening the anterior wall of the defect, suturing a patch to the posterior wall, and continuing this suture to close the incision incorporating the patch with the suture line. Aortic origin of the right pulmonary artery is best repaired by division of the right pulmonary artery and direct reanastomosis to the main pulmonary artery. The optimal management of associated anomalies is uncertain and must be individualized. Total correction may be done, although in critically ill neonates a two-stage procedure may be advisable.

Operative mortality is low for repair of isolated aortopulmonary window or aortic origin of a pulmonary artery in infancy. Long-term results are good if there are no associated anomalies. In older infants and children, the results depend on the severity and reversibility of the pulmonary vascular disease.

ANOMALIES OF THE AORTIC ARCH

At length, by mere accident I discovered an extraordinary lusus naturae in the disposition of the right subclavian artery. . . .

DAVID BAYFORD

Vascular rings are developmental anomalies of the aorta and great vessels that encircle and may constrict the esophagus and trachea. In 1735, Hunauld reported the necropsy finding of anomalous origin of the right subclavian artery from the descending aorta. A persistent double aortic arch was described in 1737 by Hommel. In a case report read before the Medical Society of London in 1787 and published in 1794, Bayford presented the case history and autopsy findings of a 62-year-old woman who died of starvation secondary to severe dysphagia. An anomalous origin of the right subclavian artery from the descending aorta was present, and he attributed the woman's dysphagia to this anomaly, although the artery coursed between the trachea and esophagus rather than posterior to the esophagus. He called the finding a *lusus naturae*, or "prank of nature," and coined the term *dysphagia lusoria*. Throughout the 19th century, aortic arch anomalies remained anatomic curiosities. Congdon (1922) greatly clarified the embryology of the aortic arches. Kommerell (1936) described origin of the right subclavian artery from a diverticulum of the descending aorta. The clinical syndrome of stridor and dysphagia in early infancy secondary to persistent double aortic arch was clearly delineated by Wolman (1939). Surgical correction of constricting vascular rings was not done until 1945, when Gross (1945b) successfully divided a double aortic arch and an aberrant right subclavian artery (Gross, 1946). Neuhauser (1946) later pioneered the use of the barium esophagogram for diagnosis of vascular rings (Gross and Neuhauser, 1951). Edwards (1948) presented the concept of a hypothetical double arch to allow classification of the multiple possible arch anomalies, forming the basis for subsequent classification.

Embryology and Pathologic Anatomy

In the embryo, six pairs of aortic arches arise sequentially from the truncus arteriosus and join paired dorsal aortas. Persistence or regression of various segments of these arches results in the normal pattern of the aorta, pulmonary artery, and great vessels. In normal development, the third pair of arches form parts of the common carotid arteries. The left fourth arch forms the adult aortic arch, and the proximal portion of the right fourth arch persists as the innominate artery. The pulmonary arteries develop from the proximal right and left sixth aortic arches. The distal left sixth arch develops into the ductus arteriosus, whereas the distal right sixth arch normally regresses. Failure of a segment to regress normally may result in a vascular ring.

Various anomalies occur and may be easily visualized by using the hypothetical scheme of Edwards, consisting of an ascending aorta, right and left aortic arches, a descending aorta on either the right or left, and bilateral ductus arteriosi. Theoretically, involution of the ring at only one point allows 36 possible configurations, although not all have appeared in humans (Blake and Manion, 1962b). Involution at two or more points would produce a greater number of possibilities. Some of the possible configurations are shown in Figures 33–16 and 33–17. Associated cardiac defects may be encountered, especially in patients with a persistent right aortic arch, frequently tetralogy of Fallot.

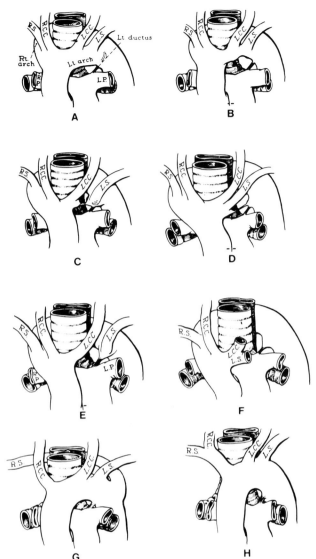

Figure 33–16. Aortic arch anomalies (left descending aorta and ligamentum arteriosum). *A*, Double aortic arch with equal anterior and posterior arches. *B*, Double aortic arch with smaller anterior (left) arch. *C*, Double aortic arch with atresia of anterior arch between the carotid and subclavian arteries. *D*, Double aortic arch with atresia of anterior arch distal to subclavian artery. *E*, Right aortic arch with retroesophageal segment and anomalous origin of the left subclavian artery from Kommerell's diverticulum. *F*, Right aortic arch with retroesophageal segment and mirror image branching. (Note the ligamentum arteriosum inserting onto diverticulum of the descending aorta.) *G*, Left aortic arch with anomalous origin of the right subclavian artery. *H*, Normal pattern. (From Edwards, J. E.: Anomalies of the derivatives of the aortic arch system. Med. Clin. North Am., [July] 925, 1948.)

Clinical Manifestations and Natural History

The natural history of vascular rings is obscured by the wide spectrum of anomalies and the range of symptoms. Vascular rings should be suspected in any infant with stridor, dysphagia, recurrent respiratory tract infections, difficult feeding, or failure to thrive. Vascular rings are not necessarily inconsistent

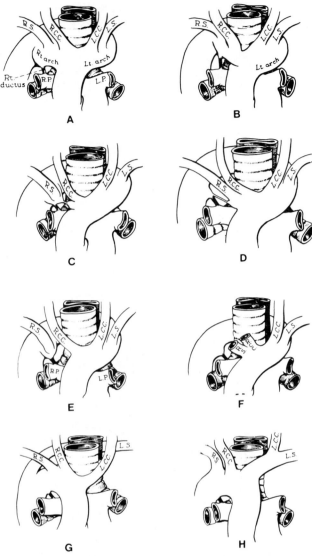

Figure 33–17. Aortic arch anomalies (right descending aorta and ligamentum arteriosum). *A,* Double aortic arch with equal anterior and posterior arches. *B,* Double aortic arch with smaller anterior (right) arch. *C,* Double aortic arch with atresia of anterior arch between carotid and subclavian arteries. *D,* Double aortic arch with atresia of anterior arch distal to subclavian artery. *E,* Left aortic arch with retroesophageal segment and anomalous origin of right subclavian artery from Kommerell's diverticulum. *F,* Left aortic arch with retroesophageal segment (note the insertion of the ligamentum arteriosum onto the diverticulum of the descending aorta). *G,* Right aortic arch with mirror image branching. (From Edwards, J. E.: Anomalies of the derivatives of the aortic arch system. Med. Clin. North Am., [July] 925, 1948.)

with prolonged survival, and many patients are totally asymptomatic. Anomalies that become symptomatic usually appear by 6 months of age, although some adults present when atherosclerosis results in dilatation of the aorta and increasing constriction. Children with mild symptoms may show marked improvement as they grow (Godtfredsen et al, 1977).

Afflicted infants most commonly present with respiratory difficulties; the breathing is stridorous

and may be exacerbated by feeding. Hyperextension of the neck tends to reduce the constriction, and marked respiratory difficulties may occur if the neck is flexed. The physical examination is usually nonrevealing, although signs of associated cardiovascular defects may be found.

The plain chest film may be normal, may show pneumonia, or occasionally may show compression of the air-filled trachea. A right aortic arch is seen in some anomalies. The barium esophagogram is a particularly valuable study. The combination of posterior compression of the esophagus on barium swallow and anterior tracheal compression is almost pathognomonic for a vascular ring. Angiocardiography accurately delineates the anatomy of vascular rings and allows evaluation of associated anomalies. Although most vascular rings can be divided without preoperative catheterization, many centers routinely perform catheterization because misdiagnosis can occur.

Various other diagnostic modalities may occasionally be useful, including echocardiography, MRI, and digital subtraction angiography. Bronchoscopy is indicated in some patients, especially those with suspected anomalous origin of the innominate artery.

Management

Although a few patients with constricting vascular rings improve with growth, the long-term prognosis of medical therapy is poor in most symptomatic patients. Despite the wide spectrum of anomalies, the principles of surgical therapy are simple (Arciniegas et al, 1979; Backer et al, 1989; Binet and Langlois, 1977). Surgical intervention should be undertaken at the time of diagnosis and is designed to divide the vascular ring, relieve the constriction, and preserve circulation to the aortic branches. Adequate exposure is an absolute necessity. Gross stated that all vascular rings could be safely divided through a left thoracotomy; however, a few anomalies require approach via a right-sided thoracotomy (McFaul et al, 1981).

Double Aortic Arch

The most common anomaly resulting in a true vascular ring is persistence of the right and left fourth aortic arch, forming a double aortic arch. The right or posterior arch is usually larger, and there is a left descending aorta and a left ductus arteriosus (see Fig. 33–16B). However, occasionally the arches are of equal size (see Fig. 33–16A) or the anterior (left) arch is larger. Rarely, a right descending aorta is encountered in which case the right arch is anterior (see Fig. 33–17A). Partial atresia of an arch may be noted, usually in the smaller anterior arch (see Fig. 33–16C and D). The right carotid and subclavian arteries arise from the right arch, and the left carotid and subclavian arteries arise from the left arch. Patients with double aortic arch usually present early in infancy and are severely symptomatic. The diagnosis of double aortic arch can be made easily from the barium esophagogram. In the common situation, the anterior-posterior projection shows right- and left-sided indentation of the barium-filled esophagus, with the right indentation being higher and larger (Fig. 33–18). The lateral projection shows posterior esophageal compression from the retroesophageal posterior arch. Arteriography may also be used to make the diagnosis (see Fig. 33–18), although atretic segments will not be visualized. Surgical division is indicated at the time of diagnosis.

In the common situation, a left-sided thoracotomy is done and the smaller anterior arch divided and oversewn at its junction with the descending aorta so that the left carotid and subclavian arteries arise from the ascending aorta or are divided at an atretic segment, if present (Fig. 33–19). The ligamentum arteriosum is also divided, and the constricting vessels dissected are away from the trachea and esophagus. If necessary, the divided left arch may be suspended from the posterior surface of the sternum to further relieve the constriction (Fig. 33–20). In patients with atresia of the posterior (right) arch, a right-sided thoracotomy would provide optimal exposure.

Left Aortic Arch with Anomalous Right Subclavian Artery

Aberrant origin of the right subclavian artery is a common anomaly but rarely causes symptoms (see Fig. 33–16G). This defect results from regression of the right fourth aortic arch between the carotid and subclavian arteries rather than distal to the subclavian. The artery may appear to arise from a diverticulum of the descending aorta (Kommerell's diverticulum), which is actually a remnant of the distal right fourth arch (Shannon, 1961). The artery most often courses posterior to the esophagus but may pass between the trachea and esophagus or anterior to the trachea. Anomalous origin of the right subclavian artery is not a true vascular ring encircling the trachea and esophagus. However, the aberrant artery or occasionally the diverticulum may compress the esophagus, resulting in dysphagia, the so-called dysphagia lusoria. If a right ligamentum arteriosum is present, connecting the right subclavian artery to the right pulmonary artery, a true vascular ring is formed. Aneurysmal dilatation of Kommerell's diverticulum was first reported by Schaff in 1950. The diagnosis of aberrant origin of the right subclavian artery can be made by a barium swallow. The lateral esophagogram shows an oblique posterior impression coursing upward from left to right, and arterial pulsations may be seen. This anomaly may be an incidental finding at the time of barium swallow for other indications.

Gross (1946) pioneered surgical therapy for anomalous origin of the right subclavian artery. In children, the artery may be simply ligated and divided without sequelae. In adults, a subclavian steal syndrome may result after simple division, and re-

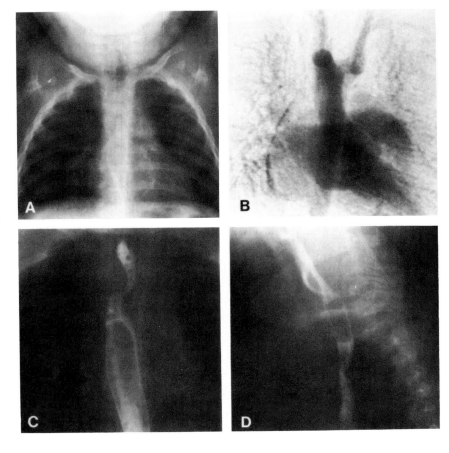

Figure 33–18. Infant with double aortic arch. *A,* Plain chest film. (Note the increased width of mediastinal soft tissue to the right of the trachea.) *B,* Digital subtraction angiogram showing double aortic arch. (Note the larger right arch to the right and posterior to trachea.) *C,* Barium esophagogram (AP) showing double indentation characteristic of double aortic arch. (Note the higher, deeper indentation on the right caused by the larger right posterior arch.) *D,* Barium esophagogram (lateral) showing posterior indentation of the esophagus. (Courtesy of Dr. Eric Effman.)

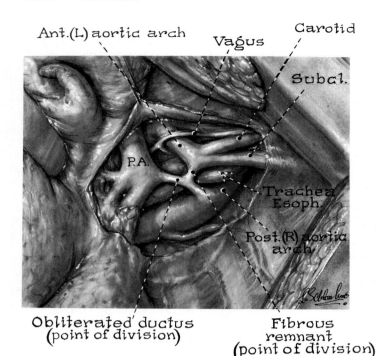

Ant.(L) aortic arch Vagus Carotid

Subcl.

P.A.

Trachea
Esoph.

Post.(R) aortic
arch

Obliterated ductus
(point of division)

Fibrous
remnant
(point of division)

Figure 33–19. Operative view of tracheal ring completed by obliterated remnant of distal left arch and ligamentum arteriosum. After complete exposure of the vascular components, the proper point of division of the ligaments can easily be determined.

anastomosis to the aorta may be necessary. A large or aneurysmal aortic diverticulum may require excision with grafting of the subclavian artery (Austin and Wolfe, 1985; Esposita et al, 1988).

Left Aortic Arch with Right Descending Aorta

Left aortic arch with a retroesophageal segment and a right descending aorta is a rare arch anomaly that was first reported by Paul (1948) (see Fig. 33–17E). The right subclavian artery arises from the descending aorta, and the ring is completed by a right ligamentum arteriosum. Most of the patients reported to have this anomaly have had minimal symptoms (de Balsac, 1960); however, a short ligamentum may result in a symptomatic constricting ring. The diagnosis may be suspected on the plain chest film and confirmed by barium swallow or arteriography. Surgical therapy consists of division

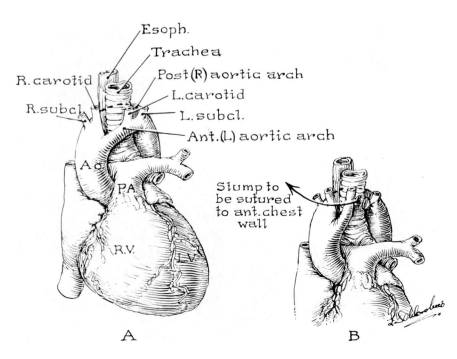

Esoph.

Trachea

R. carotid

Post (R) aortic arch

L. carotid

R. subcl.

L. subcl.

Ant.(L) aortic arch

Ao

P.A.

Stump to
be sutured
to ant. chest
wall

R.V.

L.V.

A

B

Figure 33–20. Double aortic arch. *A,* The larger channel is usually posterior and on the right. Branches of the arch arise independently. In almost all cases, the descending thoracic aortic arch is on the left as shown. *B,* Point of division of the smaller arch is selected to preserve circulation to the branches. The left common carotid artery is then tacked to the anterior chest wall to further relieve tracheal compression.

of the ligamentum arteriosum through a right-sided thoracotomy.

Anomalous Origin of the Innominate Artery

Compression of the anterior trachea by an innominate artery originating farther to the left on the aortic arch than usual was first described by Gross and Neuhauser (1948) (Fig. 33–21). Fearon and Shortreed (1963) described 69 patients with compression of the airway by an anomalous innominate artery. They emphasized the importance of endoscopy as a diagnostic modality and described "reflex apnea" or respiratory arrest following stimulation of the compressed area of the trachea. Mustard and associates (1969) reported 285 cases of innominate artery compression. Less than 14% of the patients required surgical intervention, and reflex apnea was the major indication for operation.

Children with anomalous origin of the innominate artery present with respiratory distress, stridor, and occasionally respiratory arrest. Dysphagia does not occur because the esophagus is not obstructed. Reflex apnea may result from irritation of the trachea by accumulated secretions or from further compression of the trachea by a bolus of food in the esophagus (see Fig. 33–21). Recurrent pneumonia and atelectasis may also occur because of innominate artery compression. The physical examination is not helpful in the diagnosis of innominate artery compression. The chest film may show only pneumonia or atelectasis, and the barium esophagogram is normal. Arteriography may show an abnormally leftward origin of the innominate artery, but this finding is not diagnostic of tracheal compression. Bronchoscopy is the optimal method for confirming tracheal compression and shows buckling of the tracheal cartilages in affected patients (Filston et al, 1987). Many infants with innominate artery compression

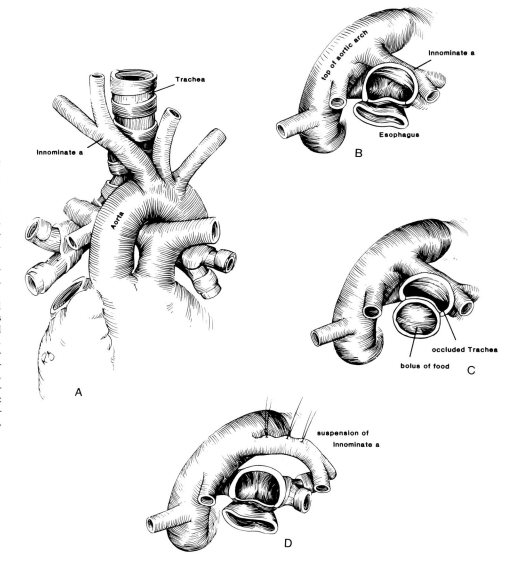

Figure 33–21. *A*, Depiction of the normal relationships of the aorta and its major branches to the trachea showing the innominate artery crossing the lower trachea, producing compression of the trachea and buckling of the cartilages. *B*, "Endoscopic view" of these relationships shows the buckled arch impinging on the lumen of the distal trachea. *C*, A bolus of food in the esophagus forces the posterior membranous portion of the trachea into the tracheal lumen, causing almost complete airway obliteration by the anterior compression and the posterior bulge. *D*, Suspension of the aorta and the innominate artery eliminates the anterior compression and buckling of the tracheal rings, increasing the cross-sectional diameter of the trachea. (From Filston, H. C., Ferguson, T. B., Jr., and Oldham, H. N.: Airway obstruction by vascular anomalies: Importance of telescopic bronchoscopy. Ann. Surg., *205*:541, 1987.)

have mild symptoms and improve as they grow. The primary indication for surgical intervention is reflex apnea.

Aortopexy may be done via a median sternotomy or a right-sided anterior thoracotomy. By using multiple adventitial sutures, the aorta and innominate artery are suspended from the posterior aspect of the sternum (see Fig. 33–21). The innominate artery is not dissected free from the trachea but suspended and allowed to exert traction on the buckled tracheal cartilages.

Right Aortic Arch

Fiorratti and Aglietta reported a right aortic arch in 1763, and Corvisart described a right aortic arch in a patient with tetralogy of Fallot in 1818. Persistence of the right aortic arch occurs commonly, but a vascular ring cannot result unless there is a retroesophageal segment or aberrant vessel (Knight and Edwards, 1974). The right aortic arch with a mirror image origin of the branches frequently accompanies tetralogy of Fallot (see Fig. 33–17H). In some patients, the left subclavian artery arises aberrantly from the descending aorta and courses posterior to the esophagus (see Fig. 33–17G); a Kommerell's diverticulum may be present, representing the distal left arch. This anomaly may result in dysphagia, and if a left ligamentum arteriosum connects to the aberrant subclavian artery, a true vascular ring is formed. In some patients, a right aortic arch is found with a retroesophageal segment and a left descending aorta, the branches may arise in mirror image fashion (see Fig. 33–16F), or the left subclavian may arise from a diverticulum of the descending aorta (see Fig. 33–16E). In either case, the presence of a left ligamentum arteriosum that attaches to the descending aorta constitutes a true vascular ring. There have been rare reports of right aortic arches with a retroesophageal left innominate artery and rare reports of right aortic arch with isolation of the left subclavian artery. The latter defect requires involution of the left arch at two sites. The subclavian artery arises from the ductus or ligamentum arteriosum, and a subclavian steal syndrome may occur.

In a symptomatic patient with a right aortic arch, retroesophageal segment, and left descending aorta or an aberrant left subclavian artery, a left ligamentum arteriosum usually must be present for significant tracheal and esophageal compression to occur. Surgical therapy would be division of the ligamentum arteriosum through a left-sided thoracotomy. Patients occasionally may develop dysphagia secondary to an anomalous left subclavian artery or an enlarged Kommerell's diverticulum. In these patients, the aberrant artery may be divided via a left-sided thoracotomy, or a right-sided thoracotomy may be necessary to excise the diverticulum.

Cervical Aortic Arch

Cervical aortic arch is a rare anomaly in which the aortic arch rises to a point above the clavicle.

Bevan and Fatti (1947) reported the first case in a 9-year-old girl, who rapidly expired after ligation of a presumed carotid artery aneurysm. Cervical aortic arch is thought to represent persistence of the third rather than the fourth aortic arch. Cervical aortic arch may be an isolated finding or may occur in association with other arch anomalies. Presence of a cervical aortic arch can be confirmed if compression of a pulsatile neck mass results in loss of the femoral pulses. No intervention is indicated unless another symptomatic anomaly is present (Mullins et al, 1973).

Results

Results in terms of both survival and relief of symptoms of surgical therapy are good in infants with isolated vascular rings. Operative mortality is low but not zero. Postoperative morbidity is often related to tracheomalacia secondary to the vascular compression (Roesler et al, 1983). The infants may continue to have residual obstruction leading to recurrent respiratory distress and infection. These problems usually diminish as the child grows. In children with associated cardiac anomalies, the long-term outcome is related to the severity of the cardiac defect.

PULMONARY ARTERY SLING

Pulmonary artery sling is a rare cardiac anomaly occurring when the left pulmonary artery arises aberrantly from the right pulmonary artery and courses between the trachea and esophagus. A true vascular ring is not present; however, compression of the distal trachea and mainstem bronchi usually occurs. Glaevecke and Doehle (1897) first described pulmonary artery sling. Scheid (1938) reported a pulmonary artery sling with associated tracheal stenosis and complete cartilaginous rings. Welsh and Munro (1954) reported a patient with aberrant left pulmonary artery and suggested that this anomaly would produce an anterior defect in the barium esophagogram, a finding that was later described by Wittenborg and colleagues (1956).

Potts and associates (1954) performed a thoracotomy in a child with a suspected vascular ring and discovered a pulmonary artery sling. They divided the anomalous left pulmonary artery and reanastomosed the artery to the proximal portion of the artery anterior to the trachea. A similar procedure was reported by Hiller and MacLean (1957); however, they anastomosed the left pulmonary artery to the main pulmonary artery rather than to the proximal left pulmonary artery. Other suggested procedures include division of the ligamentum arteriosus and division of the right mainstem bronchus with reanastomosis in front of the aberrant left pulmonary artery, although these procedures are not recommended currently.

Embryology and Pathologic Anatomy

The aberrant left pulmonary artery arises from the posterior aspect of the right pulmonary artery (Fig. 33–22). It then courses posteriorly over the right mainstem bronchus and passes between the trachea and esophagus. The hilum of the left lung is lower than normal. Tracheal stenosis with complete cartilaginous rings and absence of the membranous portion of the trachea occurs frequently. Tracheal stenosis may extend proximally, may also include the left mainstem bronchus, and may be present in segments not actually compressed by the anomalous vessel. Tracheomalacia and origin of the right mainstem bronchus from the trachea (bronchus suis) are also commonly associated with pulmonary artery sling.

The proximal pulmonary arteries normally develop from the proximal portion of the right and left sixth aortic arches (Bamman et al, 1977). The distal portions of the pulmonary arteries develop from the vascular plexus of the lung buds. If the sixth aortic arch develops abnormally, the lung bud may establish a vascular connection with any nearby artery. If a connection is established with a systemic artery, complete absence of a pulmonary artery occurs. If a connection is established across the midline to the right sixth aortic arch and posterior to the trachea, a pulmonary artery sling results. The ductus arteriosus arises from the main pulmonary artery and passes anterior to the trachea to connect with the aorta in the usual manner. The etiology of the tracheobronchial anomalies is unclear but may be related to compression by the aberrant vessel. Various associated cardiac anomalies have been reported, including PDA, persistent left superior vena cava, atrial septal defect, ventricular septal defect, and aortic arch anomalies.

Clinical Findings and Diagnosis

Infants with pulmonary artery sling often present with respiratory symptoms at birth, and most are symptomatic by 1 month. It is impossible to estimate the number of asymptomatic patients with pulmonary artery sling (Dupuis et al, 1988). The most common findings are respiratory distress, wheezing, and expiratory stridor. Acute respiratory failure secondary to obstruction may occur, requiring intubation. Signs and symptoms of esophageal obstruction are rare. Repeated respiratory tract infections may occur.

The physical examination is not helpful in the diagnosis of pulmonary artery sling. The chest film may be normal or may show a number of findings suggestive of pulmonary artery sling, including hyperinflation of one lung (most commonly the right, but occasionally the left), anterior bowing of the tracheal air column, and a low hilum of the left lung (see Fig. 33–22). Infants may present at birth with

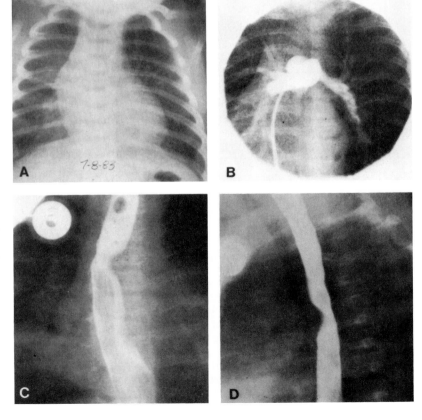

Figure 33–22. Infant with pulmonary artery sling. A, Plain chest film that shows hyperaeration of the left lung. B, Pulmonary arteriogram that shows anomalous origin of the left pulmonary artery from the right pulmonary artery. (Note the course of the left pulmonary artery around the tracheal air column.) C, Barium esophagram (AP) showing compression of the esophagus. D, Barium esophagogram (lateral) showing characteristic anterior indentation of the esophagus behind the distal trachea. (Courtesy of Dr. Eric Effman and Dr. Bennett Pearce.)

opacification of one lung secondary to retention of fetal fluid (Zumbro et al, 1974). Pulmonary artery sling may present in adults as a mediastinal or paratracheal mass. The barium esophagogram is particularly useful and shows anterior pulsatile compression of the esophagus (see Fig. 33–22). This finding strongly suggests a pulmonary artery sling but can be seen if an anomalous subclavian artery courses between the trachea and esophagus or if a so-called ductus anteriosus sling is present (Binet et al, 1978). Mediastinal tumors, cysts, or lymph nodes may occasionally cause anterior esophageal compression, but these lesions are nonpulsatile. Angiocardiography is useful to show the aberrant vessel and evaluate associated anomalies (see Fig. 33–22). Newer techniques including digital subtraction angiography, two-dimensional echocardiography, CT, and MRI are proving useful in the diagnosis of pulmonary artery sling. Bronchoscopy is particularly useful in these patients for evaluation of associated tracheobronchial anomalies. Bronchography is now rarely used.

Natural History

The exact incidence of pulmonary artery sling is unknown. Patients may present with severe symptoms in infancy, but survival to an advanced age is also possible. The oldest reported patient was 78 years old, and he was asymptomatic until a few months before his death. There are increasing reports of children and adults who have pulmonary artery sling but minimal or no symptoms; the anomaly is discovered during evaluation for unrelated complaints (Dupuis et al, 1988).

The natural history of patients with pulmonary artery sling depends on the degree of respiratory obstruction and associated tracheobronchial and cardiac anomalies (Sade et al, 1975). Infants who present with respiratory obstruction may succumb to the acute event; if they survive, their prognosis is poor without surgical intervention. Phelan and Venables (1978) reported nonsurgical management in five patients (one patient had division of a ligamentum arteriosum), with resolution or marked diminution of symptoms in all of the patients. Three of these patients had associated tracheobronchial stenosis, which was thought to contribute to the residual symptoms.

Management

Surgical intervention is indicated in any patient with a pulmonary artery sling and symptoms of significant respiratory obstruction. Nonsurgical management may be possible in patients with minor symptoms. The recommended procedure is division of the anomalous artery with anastomosis to the main pulmonary artery rather than to the proximal left pulmonary artery to avoid kinking. This may be done by using either a left-sided thoracotomy or a median sternotomy with cardiopulmonary bypass. A right-sided thoracotomy was occasionally used in the past, but the approach should not be used because patients usually do not tolerate collapse of the right lung with simultaneous interruption of the vascular supply to the left lung.

A left-sided thoracotomy is performed through the fourth interspace, and the ligamentum arteriosum is divided. The anomalous pulmonary artery is dissected free from the trachea and surrounding mediastinal structure (Fig. 33–23). Heparin is administered, the left pulmonary artery is divided between clamps, and the proximal portion is doubly oversewn with a continuous nonabsorbable suture. The pericardium is opened, and the left pulmonary artery is passed through a second pericardial incision posterior to the phrenic nerve. The artery is positioned so that the anastomosis may be constructed without kinking or tension. A partial occlusion clamp is placed on the main pulmonary artery, and an ellipse of arterial wall is excised. An end-to-side anastomosis is done by using a continuous fine monofilament suture. Alternatively, the posterior wall may be a continuous suture and the anterior anastomosis may be done with interrupted sutures.

A median sternotomy with or without cardiopulmonary bypass may be used for repair of pulmonary artery sling. After cannulation and the initiation of cardiopulmonary bypass, the left pulmonary artery is dissected free and divided at the right pulmonary artery. The proximal defect is closed, and the left pulmonary artery is passed anteriorly to the trachea and through the pericardium posterior to the phrenic nerve. An ellipse of the main pulmonary artery is excised and the anastomosis is done so that the left pulmonary artery lies without kinking or tension (see Fig. 33–23).

The management of associated tracheobronchial anomalies continues to be a difficult problem. If significant obstruction remains after correction of the pulmonary artery sling, resection of the stenotic segment of the trachea or bronchi may be necessary. If complete tracheal rings are present, an anterior tracheoplasty with autologous pericardium may be used to relieve the stenosis (Idriss et al, 1984). Hickey and Wood reported single-stage correction of pulmonary sling by reimplantation of the left pulmonary artery and tracheal resection using cardiopulmonary bypass (Hickey and Wood, 1987). Jonas and associates reported single-stage correction without a vascular anastomosis by performing a resection of the stenotic area, mobilizing the left pulmonary artery anteriorly, and reanastomosing the bronchus posterior to the artery (Jonas et al, 1989).

Results

Results of surgical therapy for pulmonary artery sling have been somewhat disappointing. Potts' first patient in 1953 fared very well and was discharged on the 11th postoperative day. Follow-up 24 years

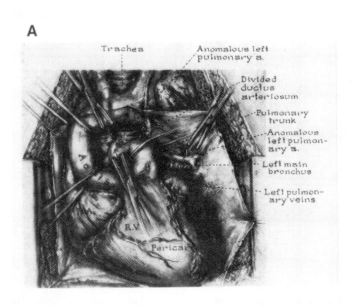
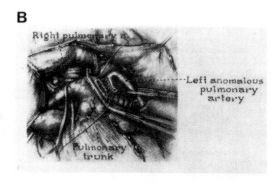
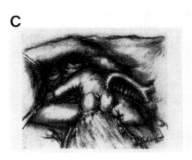

Figure 33–23. Surgical repair of pulmonary artery sling. *A*, The ligamentum is divided, and the anomalous vessel is transected and transferred anterior to the trachea. *B*, The left pulmonary artery is anastomosed in an end-to-side manner to the main pulmonary artery. *C*, Completed repair. (From Campbell, C. D., Wernly, J. A., Koltip, P. C., et al: Aberrant left pulmonary artery [pulmonary artery sling]: Successful repair and 24 year follow-up report. Am. J. Cardiol., *45*:316, 1980.)

later showed that the child had developed normally and had normal exercise tolerance (Campbell et al, 1980). However, a ventilation-perfusion scan showed minimal perfusion of the left lung. Sade and associates (1975) reviewed 40 cases of pulmonary artery sling that were treated surgically and had a 50% mortality. The survivors were generally asymptomatic; however, nine of ten patients studied had occluded left pulmonary arteries. Dunn and colleagues (1979) reported four patients who had repair of pulmonary artery sling. Patency of the left pulmonary artery was documented in all patients. Mortality is usually related to the severity of the tracheobronchial stenosis and associated defects. Survivors generally have a benign course despite occlusion of the left pulmonary artery, and residual symptoms tend to decrease as the patients grow. Although there has been concern that patients with an occluded left pulmonary artery might develop pulmonary hypertension in the right lung or hemoptysis secondary to bronchial collaterals, neither has been encountered. Attempts to restore patency to occluded pulmonary arteries have not met with success and are not generally recommended.

Selected Bibliography

Abbott, M. E.: Coarctation of the aorta of the adult type II: A statistical study and historical retrospect of 200 recorded cases, with autopsy of stenosis or obliteration of the descending arch in subjects above the age of two years. Am. Heart J., 3:574, 1928.

A classic series reporting the mechanical history, physical examination, and natural history of patients with coarctation of the aorta.

Brewer, L. A., III, Fosburg, R. G., Mulder, G. A., and Verska, J. J.: Spinal cord complications following surgery for coarctation of the aorta: A study of 66 cases. J. Thorac. Cardiovasc. Surg., 64:368, 1972.

An extensive review encompassing 12,532 cases of repair of coarctation of the aorta delineating the incidence and possible contributing factors.

Edwards, J. E.: Anomalies of the derivatives of the aortic arch system. Med. Clin. North Am., p. 925, July, 1948.

First description of the hypothetical double aorta arch that forms the basis for classification of vascular rings.

Sade, R. M., Rosenthal, A., Fellows, K., and Castaneda, A. R.: Pulmonary artery sling. J. Thorac. Cardiovasc. Surg., 69:333, 1975.

Excellent review of embryology, natural history, and surgical correction of pulmonary artery sling.

Schuster, S. R., and Gross, R. E.: Surgery for coarctation of the aorta: A review of 500 cases. J. Thorac. Cardiovasc. Surg., 43:54, 1962.

A report by Gross, a pioneer in cardiac surgery, of his extensive experience with coarctation of the aorta.

Scott, H. W., Jr., and Bahnson, H. T.: Evidence for a renal factor in the hypertension of experimental coarctation of the aorta. Surgery, 30:206, 1951.

Classic experimental demonstration of the role of the kidney in the hypertension of coarctation.

Waldhausen, J. A., and Nahrwold, D. L.: Repair of coarctation of the aorta with a subclavian flap. J. Thorac. Cardiovasc. Surg., 51:532, 1966.

First report of the subclavian flap technique for repair of coarctation that is currently one of the most commonly used repairs.

Yee, E. S., Turley, K., Soifer, S., and Ebert, P. A.: Synthetic patch aortoplasty: A simplified approach for coarctation in repair during early infancy and thereafter. Am. J. Surg., 148:240, 1984.

Review of the advantages of the prosthetic flap aortoplasty including decreased operative time, decreased need for dissection, and excellent hemodynamic result.

Bibliography

Aaron, B. L., Loew, A. G., Jr, and Mullen, J. T.: Coarctation of the aorta with spontaneous quadriparesis: A case report. J. Thorac. Cardiovasc. Surg., 68:76, 1974.

Abbott, M. E.: Coarctation of the aorta of the adult type. Am. Heart J., 3:574, 1928.

Acevedo, R. E., Thilenius, O. G., Moulder, P. V., and Cassels, D. E.: Kinking of the aorta (pseudocoarctation) with coarctation. Am. J. Cardiol., 21:442, 1968.

Achanti, B., Yeh, T. F., and Pildes, R. S.: Indomethacin therapy in infants with advanced postnatal age and patent ductus arteriosus. Clin. Invest. Med., 9:250, 1986.

Adkins, R. B., Jr., Maples, M. D., Graham, B. S., et al: Dysphagia associated with an aortic arch anomaly in adults. Am. Surg., 52:238, 1986.

Adzick, W. S., Harrison, M. R., and Delorimier, A. A.: Surgical clip ligation of patent ductus arteriosus in premature infants. J. Pediatr. Surg. 21:158, 1986.

Agius, P. V., Rushworth, A., and Connolly, N.: Anomalous origin of left coronary artery from pulmonary artery associated with an aorto-pulmonary septal defect. Br. Heart J., 32:708, 1970.

Allard, J. R., William, R. L., and Dobell, A. R. C.: Interrupted aortic arch: Factors influencing prognosis. Ann. Thorac. Surg., 21:243, 1976.

Allen, H. D., Marx, G. R., Ovitt, T. W., and Goldberg, S. J.: Balloon dilatation angioplasty for coarctation of the aorta. Am. J. Cardiol., 57:828, 1986.

Alpert, B. S., Bain, H. H., Balfe, J. W., et al: Role of the renin-angiotensin-aldosterone system in hypertensive children with coarctation of the aorta. Am. J. Cardiol., 43:828, 1979.

Amato, J. J., Rheinlander, H. F. and Cleveland, R. J.: A method of enlarging the distal transverse arch in infants with hypoplasia and coarctation of the aorta. Ann. Thorac. Surg., 23:261, 1977.

Amsterdam, E. A., Albers, W. H., Christlieb, A. R., et al: Plasma renin activity in children with coarctation of the aorta. Am. J. Cardiol., 23:396, 1969.

Anderson, R. H.: Coarctation, the arterial duct and aortic atresia. Int. J. Cardiol., 8:391, 1985.

Anyanwu, E., Dittrich, H., Jelesijevic, V., et al: Coarctation of the aorta: A risk factor for children for the development of arteriosclerosis. Atherosclerosis, 39:367, 1981.

Appleton, R. S., Graham, T. P., Cotton, R. B., et al: Decreased early diastolic function after indomethacin administration in premature infants. J. Pediatr., 112:447, 1988.

Arciniegas, E., Hakimi, M., Hertzler, J. H., et al: Surgical management of congenital vascular rings. J. Thorac. Cardiovasc. Surg., 77:721, 1979.

Ardito, J. M., Tucker, G. F., Jr., Ossoff, R. H., and DeLeon, S. Y.: Innominate artery compression of the trachea in infants with reflex apnea. Ann. Otolaryngol., 89:401, 1980.

Arensman, F. W., Sievers, H., Lange, P., et al: Assessment of coronary and aortic anastomoses after anatomic correction of transposition of the great arteries. J. Thorac. Cardiovasc. Surg., 90:597, 1985.

Armer, R. M., Shumacker, H. B., and Klatte, E. C.: Origin of the

right pulmonary artery from the ascending aorta: Report of a surgically correlated case. Circulation, 24:662, 1961.

Austin, E. H., and Wolfe, W. G.: Aneurysm of aberrant subclavian artery with a review of the literature. J. Vasc. Surg., 2:511, 1985.

Aytac, A., Ozme, S., Sarikayalar, F., and Saylam, A.: Pulmonary artery sling. Ann. Thorac. Surg., 22:596, 1976.

Backer, C. I., Ilbawi, M. N., Idriss, P. S., and DeLeon, S. Y.: Vascular anomalies causing tracheoesophageal compression. J. Thorac. Cardiovasc. Surg., 97:725, 1989.

Bagby, S. P., and Mass, R. D.: Abnormality of the renin/body-fluid-volume relationship in serially-studied inbred dogs with neonatally-induced coarctation hypertension. Hypertension, 2:631, 1980.

Bagby, S. P., McDonald W. J., Strong, D. W., et al: Abnormalities of renal perfusion and the renal pressor system in dogs with chronic aortic coarctation. Circ. Res., 37:615, 1975.

Bahabozorgui, S., Bernstein, R. G., and Frater, F. W. M.: Pseudocoarctation of aorta associated with aneurysm formation. Chest, 60:616, 1971.

Bahn, R. C., Edwards, J. E., and DuShane, J. W.: Coarctation of the aorta as a cause of death in early infancy. J. Pediatr., 8:192, 1951.

Bahnson, H. T.: Coarctation of the aorta and anomalies of the aortic arch. Surg. Clin. North Am., 32:1313, 1952.

Bailie, M. D., Donoso, V. S., and Gonzalez, N. C.: Role of the renin-angiotensin system in hypertension after coarctation of the aorta. J. Lab. Clin. Med., 104:553, 1984.

Bamman, J. L., Ward, B. H., and Woodrum, D. W.: Aberrant left pulmonary artery: Clinical and embryologic factors. Chest, 72:67, 1977.

Barratt-Boyes, B. G., Nicholls, T. T., Brandt, P. W. T., and Neutze, J. M.: Aortic arch interruption associated with patent ductus arteriosus, ventricular septal defect, and total anomalous pulmonary venous connection. Total correction in an 8-day-old infant by means of profound hypothermia and limited cardiopulmonary bypass. J. Thorac. Cardiovasc. Surg., 63:367, 1972.

Barry, A.: The aortic arch derivatives in the human adult. Anat. Rec., 111:221, 1951.

Bayford, D.: An account of a singular cafe of obstructed deglutition. Memoirs of the Medical Society of London, 2:275, 1794.

Baylen, B., Meyer, R. A., Korfhagen, J., et al: Left ventricular performance in the critically ill premature infant with patent ductus arteriosus and pulmonary disease. Circulation, 55:182, 1977.

Beavan, T. E. D.: Ligature of aortic arch in the neck. Br. J. Surg., 34:414, 1947.

Becker, A. E., Becker, M. J., and Edwards, J. E.: Anomalies associated with coarctation of aorta: Particular reference to infancy. Circulation, 41:1067, 1970.

Beekman, R. H., Katz, B. P., Moorehead-Steffens, C., and Rocchini, A. P.: Altered baroreceptor function in children with systolic hypertension after coarctation repair. Am. J. Cardiol., 52:112, 1983.

Beekman, R. H., and Robinow, M.: Coarctation of the aorta inherited as an autosomal dominant trait. Am. J. Cardiol., 56:818, 1985.

Beekman, R. H., Rocchini, A. P., MacDonald, D., II, et al: Percutaneous balloon angioplasty for native coarctation of the aorta. J.A.C.C., 10:1078, 1987.

Bell, E. F., Warburton, D., Stonestreet, B. S., and Oh, W.: Effect of fluid administration on the development of symptomatic patent ductus arteriosus and congestive heart failure in premature infants. N. Engl. J. Med., 302:598, 1980.

Bell-Thomson, J., Jewell, E., Ellis, F. H., Jr., and Schwaber, J. R.: Surgical techniques in the management of patent ductus arteriosus in the elderly patient. Ann. Thorac. Surg., 30:80, 1980.

Benedict, C. R., Phil, D., Grahame-Smith, D. G., and Fisher, A.: Changes in plasma catecholamines and dopamine beta-hydroxylase after corrective surgery for coarctation of the aorta. Circulation, 57:598, 1978.

Berendes, J. N., Bredee, J. J., Schipperheyn J. J., and Mashhour, T. A. S.: Mechanisms of spinal cord injury after cross-clamping of the descending thoracic aorta. Circulation, 66(Suppl. I):112, 1982.

Bergdahl, L., Bjork, V. O., and Jonasson, R.: Surgical correction of coarctation of the aorta: influence of age on late results. J. Thorac. Cardiovasc. Surg., 85:532, 1983.

Bergdahl, L., and Ljungqvist, A.: Long-term results after repair of coarctation of the aorta by patch grafting. J. Thorac. Cardiovasc. Surg., 80:177, 1980.

Bergdahl, L. A. L., Blackstone, E. H., Kirklin, J. W., et al: Determinants of early success in repair of aortic coarctation in infants. J. Thorac. Cardiovasc. Surg., 83:735, 1982.

Berlind, S., Bojs, G., Krosgren, M., and Varnauskas, E.: Severe pulmonary hypertension accompanying patent ductus arteriosus. Am. Heart J., 73:460, 1967.

Berman, W., Jr., Dubynsky, O., Whitman, V., et al: Digoxin therapy in low-birth-weight infants with patent ductus arteriosus. J. Pediatr., 93:652, 1978.

Berman, W., Jr., Yabek, S. M., Dillon, T., et al: Vascular ring due to left aortic arch and right descending aorta. Circulation, 63:458, 1981.

Bernatz, P. E., Lewis, D. R., and Edwards, J. E.: Division of the posterior arch of a double aortic arch for relief of tracheal and esophageal obstruction. Proc. Staff Meet. Mayo Clin., 34:1973, 1959.

Berry, T. E., Bharati, S., Muster, A. J., et al: Distal aortopulmonary septal defect, aortic origin of the right pulmonary artery, intact ventricular septum, patent ductus arteriosus and hypoplasia of the aortic isthmus: A newly recognized syndrome. Am. J. Cardiol., 49:108, 1982.

Bertrand, J. M., Chartrand, C., Lamarre, A., and Lapierre, J. G.: Vascular ring: Clinical and physiological assessment of pulmonary function following surgical correction. Pediatr. Pulmonol., 2:378, 1986.

Bessinger, F. B., Jr., Blieden, L. C., and Edwards, J. E.: Hypertensive pulmonary vascular disease associated with patent ductus arteriosus: Primary or secondary? Circulation, 52:157, 1975.

Binet, J. P., Consco, J. F., Losay, J., et al: Ductus arteriosus sling: Report of a newly recognised anomaly and its surgical correction. Thorax, 33:72, 1978.

Binet, J. P., and Langlois, J.: Aortic arch anomalies in children and infants. J. Thorac. Cardiovasc. Surg., 73:248, 1977.

Bing, R. J., Handelsman, J. C., Campbell, J. A., et al: The surgical treatment and the physiopathology of coarctation of the aorta. Ann. Surg., 128:803, 1948.

Black, L. L., and Goldman, B. S.: Surgical treatment of the patent ductus arteriosus in the adult. Ann. Surg., 175:290, 1972.

Blake, H. A., and Manion, W. C.: Atresia or absence of the aortic isthmus. J. Thorac. Cardiovasc. Surg., 43:607, 1962a.

Blake, H. A., and Manion, W. C.: Thoracic arterial arch anomalies. Circulation, 26:251, 1962b.

Blalock, A.: Operative closure of the patent ductus arteriosus. Surg. Gynecol. Obstet., 82:113, 1946.

Blalock, A., and Park, E. A.: The surgical treatment of experimental coarctation (atresia) of the aorta. Ann. Surg., 119:445, 1944.

Blatchford, J. W., III, Franciosi, R. A., Singh, A., and Edwards, J. E.: Vascular ring in interruption of the aortic arch with bilateral patent ductus arteriosus. J. Thorac. Cardiovasc. Surg., 94:596, 1987.

Blieden, L. C., and Moller, J. H.: Aorticopulmonary septal defect: An experience with 17 patients. Br. Heart J., 36:630, 1974.

Bonnett, L. M.: Stenose congenitale de l'aorte. Rev. Med. Paris, 23:108, 1903.

Boone, M. L., Swenson, B. W., and Felson, B.: Rib notching: Its many causes. Am. J. Roentgenol., 91:1075, 1964.

Borow, K. M., Colan, S. D., and Neumann, A.: Altered left ventricular mechanics in patients with valvular aortic stenosis and coarctation of the aorta: Effects on systolic performance and late outcome. Circulation, 72:515, 1985.

Bosher, L. H., Jr., and McCue, C. M.: Diagnosis and surgical treatment of aortopulmonary fenestration. Circulation, 25:456, 1962.

Boyer, N. H.: Patent ductus arteriosus: Some historical highlights. Ann. Thorac. Surg., 4:570, 1967.

Bradham, R., Sealy, W. C., and Young, W. G.: Respiratory distress associated with anomalies of the aortic arch. Surg. Gynecol. Obstet. 126:9, 1968.

Brandt, B., III, Heintz, S. E., Rose, E. F., et al: Repair of coarctation of the aorta in children with Turner's syndrome. Pediatr. Cardiol., 5:175, 1984.

Brandt, B., III, Marvin, W. J., Ehrenhaft, J. L., et al: Ligation of patent ductus arteriosus in premature infants. Ann. Thorac. Surg., 32:167, 1981.

Brandt, B., III, Marvin, W. J., Jr., Rose, E. F., and Mahoney, L. T.: Surgical treatment of coarctation of the aorta after balloon angioplasty. J. Thorac. Cardiovasc. Surg., 94:715, 1987.

Braunlin, E. A., Lock, J. E., and Foker, J. E.: Repair of type B interruption of the aortic arch: Results and follow-up. J. Thorac. Cardiovasc. Surg., 86:920, 1983.

Brewer, L. A., III, Fosburg, R. G., Mulder, G. A., and Verska, J. J.: Spinal cord complications following surgery for coarctation of the aorta: A study of 66 cases. J. Thorac. Cardiovasc. Surg., 64:368, 1972.

Brom, A. G.: Narrowing of the aortic isthmus and enlargement of the mind. J. Thorac. Cardiovasc. Surg., 50:167, 1965.

Brown, E. R.: Increased risk of bronchopulmonary dysplasia in infants with patent ductus arteriosus. J. Pediatr., 95:865, 1979.

Brown, J. W., Fiore, A. C., and King, H.: Isthmus flap aortoplasty: An alternative to subclavian flap aortoplasty for long-segment coarctation of the aorta in infants. Ann. Thorac. Surg., 40:274, 1985.

Bruins, C.: Competition between aortic isthmus and ductus arteriosus; reciprocal influence of structure and flow. Eur. J. Cardiol., 8:87, 1978.

Buchler, J. R., Braga, S. L. N., Fontes, V. F., and Sousa, J. E. M. R.: Angioplasty for primary treatment of aortic coarctation: Immediate results in two adult patients. Int. J. Cardiol., 17:7, 1987.

Buhlmeyer, J., Schober, J. G., Lorenz, H. P., et al: Early diagnosis and medical treatment of the persistent ductus arteriosus in infants. Cardiovasc. Intervent. Radiol., 9:273, 1986.

Bullock, L. T., Jones, J. C., and Dolley, F. S.: The diagnosis and the effects of ligation of the patent ductus arteriosus: A report of eleven cases. J. Pediatr., 126:786, 1939.

Burnard, E. D.: Discussion on the significance of continuous murmurs in the first days of life. Proc. R. Soc. Med., 52:77, 1959.

Burroughs, J. T., Schmutzer, K. J., Linder, F., and Neuhaus, G.: Anomalous origin of the right coronary artery with aortico-pulmonary window and ventricular septal defect. J. Cardiovasc. Surg., 3:142, 1922.

Calodney, M. M., and Carson, M. J.: Coarctation of the aorta in early infancy. J. Pediatr., 37:46, 1950.

Campbell, C. D., Wernly, J. A., Koltip, P. C., et al: Aberrant left pulmonary artery (pulmonary artery sling): Successful repair and 24 year follow-up report. Am. J. Cardiol., 45:316, 1980.

Campbell, C. F.: Repair of an aneurysm of an aberrant retro-esophageal right subclavian artery arising from Kommerell's diverticulum. J. Thorac. Cardiovasc. Surg., 62:330, 1971.

Campbell, D. B., Pae, W. E., Jr., and Waldhausen, J. A.: Coarctation of the aorta: Current surgical management. World J. Surg., 9:543, 1985.

Campbell, D. B., Waldhausen, J. A., Pierce, W. S., et al: Should elective repair of coarctation of the aorta be done in infancy? J. Thorac. Cardiovasc. Surg., 88:979, 1984.

Campbell, D. N., Paton, B. C., Wiggins, J. W., et al: Infant coarctation of the aorta: Alternatives to subclavian flap repair. Pediatr. Cardiol., 3:139, 1982.

Campbell, J., Delorenzi, R., Brown, J., et al: Improved results in newborns undergoing coarctation repair. Ann. Thorac. Surg., 30:273, 1980.

Campbell, M.: Natural history of coarctation of the aorta. Br. Heart J., 32:633, 1970.

Campbell, M.: Natural history of persistent ductus arteriosus. Br. Heart J., 30:4, 1968.

Caro, C., Lermanda V. C., and Lyons, H. A.: Aortic origin of the right pulmonary artery. Br. Heart J., 19:345, 1957.

Carpenter, M. A., Dammann, J. F., Watson, D. D., et al: Left ventricular hyperkinesia at rest and during exercise in normotensive patients 2 to 27 years after coarctation repair. J. Am. Coll. Cardiol., 6:879, 1985.

Castaneda, A. R.: Patent ductus arteriosus: A commentary. Ann. Thorac. Surg., 31:92, 1981.

Castaneda, A. R.: Pulmonary artery sling. Ann. Thorac. Surg., *28*:210, 1979.

Castaneda, A. R., and Kirklin, J. W.: Tetralogy of Fallot with aorticopulmonary window: Report of two surgical cases. J. Thorac. Cardiovasc. Surg., *74*:467, 1977.

Celano, V., Pieroni, D. R., Morera, J. A., et al: Two-dimensional echocardiographic examination of mitral valve abnormalities associated with coarctation of the aorta. Circulation, *69*:924, 1984.

Celoria, G. C., and Patton, R. B.: Congenital absence of the aortic arch. Am. Heart J., *58*:408, 1959.

Chang, J.-P., Chang, C.-H., and Sheih, M.-H.: Aneurysmal dilatation of patent ductus arteriosus in a case of Ehlers-Danlos syndrome. Ann. Thorac. Surg., *44*:656, 1987.

Cheng, T. O.: Pseudocoarctation of the aorta: An important consideration in the differential diagnosis of superior mediastinal mass. Am. J. Med., *49*:551, 1970.

Chiu, I.-S., Hung, C.-R., Chao, S.-F., et al: Growth of the aortic anastomosis in pigs. J. Thorac. Cardiovasc. Surg., *95*:112, 1988.

Choy, M., Rocchini, A. P., Beekman, R. H., et al: Paradoxical hypertension after repair of coarctation of the aorta in children: Balloon angioplasty versus surgical repair. Circulation, *75*:1186, 1987.

Christiansen, N. A.: Coarctation of the aorta: Historical review. Proc. Staff Meet. Mayo Clin., *23*:322, 1948.

Christie, A.: Normal closing time of the foramen ovale and the ductus arteriosus: Anatomic and statistical study. Am. J. Dis. Child., *40*:323, 1930.

Clarke, C. P., and Richardson, J. P.: The management of aortopulmonary window: Advantages of transaortic closure with a Dacron patch. J. Thorac. Cardiovasc. Surg., *72*:48, 1976.

Clarkson, P. M., Brandt, P. W. T., Barratt-Boyes, B. G., et al: Prosthetic repair of coarctation of the aorta with particular reference to Dacron onlay patch grafts and late aneurysm formation. Am. J. Cardiol., *56*:342, 1985.

Clarkson, P. M., Nicholson, M. R., Barratt-Boyes, B. G., et al: Results after repair of coarctation of the aorta beyond infancy: A 10 to 28 year follow-up with particular reference to late systemic hypertension. Am. J. Cardiol., *51*:1481, 1983.

Clarkson, P. M., Ritter, D. G., Rahimtoola, S. H., et al: Aberrant left pulmonary artery. Am. J. Dis. Child., *113*:373, 1967.

Clyman, R. I., and Campbell, D.: Indomethacin therapy for patent ductus arteriosus: When is prophylaxis not prophylactic? J. Pediatr., *111*:718, 1987.

Cobanoglu, A., Teply, J. F., Grunkemeier, G. L., et al: Coarctation of the aorta in patients younger than three months. J. Thorac. Cardiovasc. Surg., *89*:128, 1985.

Cokkinos, D. V., Leachman, R. D., and Cooley, D. A.: Increased mortality rate from coronary artery disease following operation for coarctation of the aorta at a late age. J. Thorac. Cardiovasc. Surg., *77*:315, 1979.

Congdon, E. D.: Transformation of the aortic-arch system during the development of the human embryo. Contrib. Embryol. *68*:47, 1922.

Connors, J. P., Hartmann, A. F., Jr., and Weldon, C. S.: Considerations in the surgical management of infantile coarctation of aorta. Am. J. Cardiol., *36*:489, 1975.

Connors, T. M.: Evaluation of persistent coarctation of aorta after surgery with blood pressure measurement and exercise testing. Am. J. Cardiol., *43*:75, 1979.

Contro, S., Miller, R. A., White, H., and Potts, W. J.: Bronchial obstruction due to pulmonary artery anomalies. Circulation, *17*:418, 1958.

Cooley, D. A., McNamara, D. G., and Latson, J. R.: Aorticopulmonary septal defect: Diagnosis and surgical treatment. Surgery, *42*:101, 1957.

Cooper, R. S., Ritter, S. B., and Golinko, R. J.: Balloon dilatation angioplasty: Nonsurgical management of coarctation of the aorta. Circulation, *70*:903, 1984.

Cotton, R. B., Stahlman, M. T., Kovar, I., and Catterton, W. Z.: Medical management of small preterm infants with symptomatic patent ductus arteriosus. J. Pediatr., *92*:467, 1978.

Crafoord, C.: Correction of aortic coarctation. Ann. Thorac. Surg., *30*:300, 1980.

Crafoord, C., and Nylin, G.: Congenital coarctation of the aorta and its surgical treatment. J. Thorac. Cardiovasc. Surg., *14*:347, 1945.

Crawford, F. A., Jr., and Sade, R. M.: Spinal cord injury associated with hyperthermia during aortic coarctation repair. J. Thorac. Cardiovasc. Surg., *87*:616, 1984.

Cucci, C. E., Doyle, E. F., and Lewis, E. W., Jr.: Absence of a primary division of the pulmonary trunk: An ontogenetic theory. Circulation, *29*:124, 1964.

Cunningham, H. N., Jr., Laschinger, J. C., and Spencer, F. C.: Monitoring of somatosensory evoked potentials during surgical procedures on the thoracoabdominal aorta. IV: Clinical observations and results. J. Thorac. Cardiovasc. Surg., *94*:275, 1987.

Currarino, G., and Engle, M. A.: The effects of ligation of the subclavian artery on the bones and soft tissues of the arms. J. Pediatr., *67*:808, 1965.

Daniels, S. R., Reller, M. D., and Kaplan, S.: Recurrence of patency of the ductus arteriosus after surgical ligation in premature infants. Pediatrics, *73*:56, 1984.

Davis, J. T., Baciewicz, F. A., Suriyapa, S., et al: Vocal cord paralysis in premature infants undergoing ductal closure. Ann. Thorac. Surg., *46*:214, 1988.

de Balsac, R. H.: Left aortic arch (posterior or circumflex type) with right descending aorta. Am. J. Cardiol., *5*:546, 1960.

Decancq, H. G. Jr.: Repair of patent ductus arteriosus in a 1417 gram infant. Am. J. Dis. Child., *106*:402, 1963.

DeLeon, S. Y., Idriss, F. S., Ilbasi, M. N., et al: Transmediastinal repair of complex coarctation and interrupted aortic arch. J. Thorac. Cardiovasc. Surg., *82*:98, 1981.

del Nido, P. J., Wiliams, W. G., Wilson, G. J., et al: Synthetic patch angioplasty for repair of coarctation of the aorta: Experience with aneurysm formation. Circulation, *74*(Suppl. I):32, 1986.

DeSanto, A., Bills, R. G., King, H., et al: Pathogenesis of aneurysm formation opposite prosthetic patches used for coarctation repair: An experimental study. J. Thorac. Cardiovasc. Surg., *94*:720, 1987.

Deverall, P. B., Lincoln, J. C. R., Aberdeen, E., et al: Aortopulmonary window. J. Thorac. Cardiovasc. Surg., *57*:479, 1969.

Dische, M. R., Tsai, M., and Baltaxe, H. A.: Solitary interruption of the arch of the aorta: Clinicopathologic review of eight cases. Am. J. Cardiol., *35*:271, 1975.

Doty, D. B., Richardson, J. V., Falkovsky, G. E., et al: Aortopulmonary septal defect: Hemodynamics, angiography, and operation. Ann. Thorac. Surg., *32*:244, 1981.

Downing, D. F., Grotzinger, P. J., and Weller, R. W: Coarctation of the aorta: The syndrome of necrotizing arteritis of the small intestine following surgical therapy. Am. J. Dis. Child., *96*:711, 1958.

Drucker, M. H., and Symbas, P. N.: Right aortic arch with aberrant left subclavian artery: Symptomatic in adulthood. Am. J. Surg., *139*:432, 1980.

Dudell, G. G., and Gersony, W. M.: Patent ductus arteriosus in neonates with severe respiratory disease. J. Pediatr., *104*:915, 1984.

Dumler, M. P.: A rare cause of dysphagia: Anomalous left pulmonary artery. J.A.M.A., *197*:233, 1966.

Dunn, J. M., Gordon, I., Chrispin, A. R., et al: Early and late results of surgical correction of pulmonary artery sling. Ann. Thorac. Surg., *28*:230, 1979.

Dupuis, C., Vaksmann, G., Pernot, C., et al: Asymptomatic form of left pulmonary artery sling. Am. J. Cardiol., *61*:177, 1988.

Edmunds, L. H., Jr.: Operation or indomethacin for premature ductus. Ann. Thorac. Surg., *26*:586, 1978.

Edmunds, L. H., Jr., McClenathan, J. E., and Hufnagel, C. A.: Subclinical coarctation of the aorta. Ann. Surg., *156*:180, 1962.

Edwards, B. S., Edwards, W. D., Connolly, D. C., and Edwards, J. E.: Arterial-esophageal fistulae developing in patients with anomalies of the aortic arch system. Chest, *86*:732, 1984.

Edwards, J. E.: Anomalies of the aortic arch system. Birth Defects: Original Article Series, *13*:47, 1977.

Edwards, J. E.: Anomalies of the derivatives of the aortic arch system. Med. Clin. North Am., July:925, 1948.

Edwards, J. E.: Retro-esophageal segment of the left aortic arch, right ligamentum arteriosum and right descending aorta causing a congenital vascular ring about the trachea and esophagus. Proc. Staff Meet. Mayo Clin., March:108, 1948.

Elliott, M. J.: Coarctation of the aorta with arch hypoplasia: Improvements on a new technique. Ann. Thorac. Surg., 44:321, 1987.

Elliotson, J.: Case of malformations of the pulmonary artery and aorta. Lancet, 1:247, 1830.

Ellis, F. H., Jr., Kirklin, J. W., Callahan, J. A., and Wood, E. H.: Patent ductus arteriosus with pulmonary hypertension. J. Thorac. Surg., 31:268, 1956.

Elzenga, N. J., and Gittenberger-deGroot, A. C.: Localised coarctation of the aorta: An age dependent spectrum. Br. Heart J., 49:317, 1983.

Elzenga, N. J., and Gittenberger-deGroot, A. C.: Coarctation and related aortic arch anomalies in hypoplastic left heart syndrome. Int. J. Cardiol., 8:379, 1985.

Elzenga, N. J., Gittenberger-deGroot, A. C., and Oppenheimer-Dekker, A.: Coarctation and other obstructive aortic arch anomalies: Their relationship to the ductus arteriosus. Int. J. Cardiol., 13:289, 1986.

Engle, M. A.: A long look at surgery for coarctation of aorta. J. Am. Coll. Cardiol., 6:887, 1985.

Ergin, M. A., Jayaram, N., and LaCorte, M.: Left aortic arch and right descending aorta: Diagnostic and therapeutic implications of rare type of vascular ring. Ann. Thorac. Surg., 31:82, 1981.

Esposito, R. A., Khalil, F., Galloway, A. C., and Spencer, F. C.: Surgical treatment for aneurysm of aberrant subclavian artery based on a case report and a review of the literature. J. Thorac. Cardiovasc. Surg., 95:888, 1988.

Everts-Suarez, E. A., and Carson, C. P.: The triad of congenital absence of aortic arch (isthmus aortae), patent ductus arteriosus, and interventricular septal defect—a trilogy. Ann. Surg., 150:153, 1959.

Falcone, M. W., Perloff, J. K., and Roberts, W. C.: Aneurysm of the nonpatent ductus arteriosus. Am. J. Cardiol., 29:422, 1972.

Fallo, F., Maragno, I., and Mantero, F: Resistance to captopril in hypertension of coarctation of the aorta. Int. J. Cardiol., 9:111, 1985.

Fearon, B., and Shortreed, R.: Tracheobronchial compression by congenital cardiovascular anomalies in children: Syndrome of apnea. Ann. Otol. Rhinol. Laryngol., 72:949, 1963.

Ferguson, J. C., Barrie, W. W., and Schenk, W. G., Jr.: Hypertension of aortic coarctation: The role of renal and other factors. Ann. Surg., 185:423, 1977.

Ferlic, R. M., Hofschire, P. J., and Mooring, P. K.: Ruptured ductus arteriosus aneurysm in an infant. Ann. Thorac. Surg., 20:456, 1975.

Filston, H. C., Ferguson, T. B., Jr., and Oldham, H. N.: Airway obstruction by vascular anomalies: Importance of telescopic bronchoscopy. Ann. Surg., 205:541, 1987.

Fineberg, C., and Stofman, H. C.: Tracheal compression caused by an anomalous innominate artery arising from a brachiocephalic trunk. J. Thorac. Surg., 37:214, 1959.

Finley, J. P., Beaulieu, R. G., Nanton, M. A., and Roy, D. L.: Balloon catheter dilatation of coarctation of the aorta in young infants. Br. Heart J., 50:411, 1983.

Fisher, E. A., DuBrow, I. W., Eckner, F. A. O., and Hastreiter, A. R.: Aorticopulmonary septal defect and interrupted aortic arch: A diagnostic challenge. Am. J. Cardiol., 34:356, 1974.

Fisher, R. G., Moodie, D. S., Sterba, R., and Gill, C. C.: Patent ductus arteriosus in adults—long-term follow-up: Nonsurgical versus surgical treatment. J. Am. Coll. Cardiol., 8:280, 1986.

Fishman, N. H., Bronstein, M. H., Berman, W., Jr., et al: Surgical management of severe aortic coarctation and interrupted aortic arch neonates. J. Thorac. Cardiovasc. Surg., 71:35, 1976.

Flege, J. B., Durnin, R. E., and Rossi, N. P.: Aortic origin of the right pulmonary artery and ventricular septal defect. J. Thorac. Cardiovasc. Surg., 59:469, 1970.

Fleming, W. H., Sarafian, L. B., Clark, E. B., et al: Critical aortic coarctation: Patch aortoplasty in infants less than age 3 months. Am. J. Cardiol., 44:687, 1979.

Fleming, W. H., Sarafian, L. B., Kugler, J. D., and Nelson, R. M., Jr.: Ligation of patent ductus arteriosus in premature infants:

Importance of accurate anatomic definition. Pediatrics, 71:373, 1983.

Fontana, G. P., Spach, M. S., Effmann, E. L., and Sabiston, D. C., Jr.: Origin of the right pulmonary artery from the ascending aorta. Ann. Surg., 206:102, 1987.

Foster, E. D.: Reoperation for aortic coarctation. Ann. Thorac. Surg., 38:81, 1984.

Fowler, B. N., Lucas, S. K., Razook, J. D., et al: Interruption of the aortic arch: Experience in 17 infants. Ann. Thorac. Surg., 37:25, 1984.

Fox, S., Pierce, W. S., and Waldausen, J. A.: Pathogenesis of paradoxical hypertension after coarctation repair. Ann. Thorac. Surg., 29:135, 1980.

Freed, M. D., Keane, J. F., Van Praagh, R., et al: Coarctation of the aorta with congenital mitral regurgitation. Circulation, 49:1175, 1974.

Freed, M. D., Rocchini, A., Rosenthal, A., et al: Exercise-induced hypertension after surgical repair of coarctation of the aorta. Am. J. Cardiol., 43:253, 1979.

Freedom, R. M., Moes, C. A. F., Pelech, A., et al: Bilateral ductus arteriosus (or remnant): An analysis of 27 patients. Am. J. Cardiol., 53:884, 1984.

Freedom, R. M., Rosen, F. S., and Nadas, A. S.: Congenital cardiovascular disease and anomalies of the third and fourth pharyngeal pouch. Circulation, 46:165, 1972.

Friedberg, D. Z., Gallen, W. J., Oechler, H. W., and Glicklich, M.: Ivemark syndrome with aortic atresia. Am. J. Dis. Child., 126:106, 1973.

Friedman, W. F., Hirschklau, M. J., Printz, M. P., et al: Pharmacologic closure of patent ductus arteriosus in the premature infant. N. Engl. J. Med., 295:526, 1976.

Fripp, R. R., Whitman, V., Werner, J. C., et al: Blood pressure response to exercise in children following the subclavian flap procedure for coarctation of the aorta. J. Thorac. Cardiovasc. Surg., 85:682, 1983.

Furzan, J. A., Reisch, J., Tyson, J. E., et al: Incidence and risk factors for symptomatic patent ductus arteriosus among inborn very-low-birth-weight infants. Early Hum. Dev., 12:39, 1985.

Fyler, D. C.: Report of the New England Regional Infant Cardiac Program. Pediatrics, 65:431, 1980.

Galla, J. D., Lansman, S. L., Lowery, R. C., et al: Primary reconstruction of interrupted aortic arch by total aortic outflow obstruction. J. Thorac. Cardiovasc. Surg., 91:200, 1986.

Gann, D., Gadgil, U. D., Samet, P., and Rabinowitz, H.: Severe pulmonary hypertension with patent ductus arteriosus. South. Med. J., 73:668, 1980.

Garti, I. J., Aygen, M. M., and Vidne, B.: Type C double aortic arch: Double aortic arch with aberrant left subclavian artery. Cardiovasc. Radiol., 1:143, 1978.

Garti, I. J., Aygen, M. M., Vidne, B., and Levy, M. J.: Right aortic arch with mirror-image branching causing vascular ring. A new classification of the right aortic arch patterns. Br. J. Radiol., 46:115, 1973.

Gasul, B. M., Fell, E. H., and Casas, R.: The diagnosis of aortic septal defect by retrograde aortography: Report of a case. Circulation, 4:251, 1951.

Gay, W. A., Jr., and Young W. G., Jr.: Pseudocoarctation of the aorta: A reappraisal. J. Thorac. Cardiovasc. Surg., 58:739, 1969.

Geiss, D., Williams, W. G., Lindsay, W. K., and Rowe, R. D.: Upper extremity gangrene: A complication of subclavian artery division. Ann. Thorac. Surg., 30:487, 1980.

Gentile, R., Stevenson, G., Dooley, T., et al: Pulsed doppler echocardiographic determination of time of ductal closure in normal newborn infants. J. Pediatr., 98:443, 1981.

Gersony, W. M.: Patent ductus arteriosus in the neonate. Pediatr. Clin. North Am., 33:545, 1986.

Gersony, W. M., Peckham, G. H., Ellison, R. C., et al: Effects of indomethacin in premature infants with patent ductus arteriosus: Results of a national collaborative study. J. Pediatr., 102:895, 1983.

Ghosh, P. K., Lubliner, J., Mogilnar, M., et al: Ligation of patent ductus arteriosus in very low birth-weight premature neonates. Thorax, 40:533, 1985.

Gibson, G. A.: Clinical lectures on circulatory affections. Lecture I. Persistence of the arterial duct and its diagnosis. Edinb. Med. J., 8:1, 1900.

Gidding, S. S., Rocchini, A. P., Moorehead, C., et al: Increased forearm vascular reactivity in patients with hypertension after repair of coarctation. Circulation, 71:495, 1985.

Gittenberger-deGroot, A. C.: Persistent ductus arteriosus: Most probably a primary congenital malformation. Br. Heart J., 39:610, 1977.

Gittenberger-deGroot, A. C., Moulaert, A. J., Harinck, E., and Becker, E.: Histopathology of the ductus arteriosus after prostaglandin E₁ administration in ductus dependent cardiac anomalies. Br. Heart J., 40:215, 1978.

Gittenberger-deGroot, A. C., van Ertbruggen, I., Moulaert, A. J. M. G., and Harinck, E.: The ductus arteriosus in the preterm infant: Histologic and clinical observations. J. Pediatr. 96:88, 1980.

Glaevecke, H., and Doehle, H.: Ueber eine saltene angeborne anomolie des pulmonalarterie. Munchen Med. Wschr., 44:950, 1897.

Glancy, D. L., Morrow, A. G., Simon, A. L., and Roberts, W. C.: Juxtaductal aortic coarctation: Analysis of 84 patients studied hemodynamically, angiographically, and morphologically after age 1 year. Am. J. Cardiol., 51:537, 1983.

Godtfredsen, J., Wennenvold, A., Efsen, F., and Lauridsen, P. P.: Natural history of vascular ring with clinical manifestations: A follow-up study of eleven unoperated cases. Scand. J. Thorac. Cardiovasc. Surg., 11:75, 1977.

Goldman, S., Hernandez, J., and Pappas, G.: Results of surgical treatment of coarctation of the aorta in the critically ill neonate, including the influence of pulmonary artery banding. J. Thorac. Cardiovasc. Surg., 92:732, 1986.

Goncalves-Estella, A., Perez-Villoria, J., Gonzalez-Reoyo, F., et al: Closure of a complicated ductus arteriosus through the trans-pulmonary route using hypothermia: Surgical considerations in one case. J. Thorac. Cardiovasc. Surg., 69:698, 1975.

Goodall, McC., and Sealy, W. C.: Increased sympathetic nerve activity following resection of coarctation of the thoracic aorta. Circulation, 39:345, 1969.

Graybiel, A., Strieder, J. W., and Boyer, N.: An attempt to obliterate the patent ductus arteriosus in a patient with subacute bacterial endarteritis. Am. Heart J., 15:621, 1938.

Green, T. P., Thompson, T. R., Johnson, D. E., and Lock, J. E.: Furosemide promotes patent ductus arteriosus in premature infants with the respiratory-distress syndrome. N. Engl. J. Med., 308:743, 1983.

Griffiths, S. P., Levine, O. R., and Andersen, D. H.: Aortic origin of the right pulmonary artery. Circulation, 25:73, 1962.

Gross, R. E.: Complete division for the patent ductus arteriosus. J. Thorac. Surg., 16:314, 1947.

Gross, R. E.: Complete surgical division of the patent ductus arteriosus: A report of fourteen successful cases. Surg. Obstet. Gynecol., 78:36, 1944.

Gross, R. E.: Surgical closure of an aortic septal defect. Circulation, 5:858, 1952.

Gross, R. E.: Surgical correction for coarctations of the aorta. Surgery, 18:673, 1945a.

Gross, R. E.: Surgical relief for tracheal obstruction from a vascular ring. N. Engl. J. Med., 233:586, 1945b.

Gross, R. E.: Surgical treatment for dysphagia lusoria. Ann. Surg., 124:532, 1946.

Gross, R. E.: Treatment of certain aortic coarctations by homolo-gous grafts. Ann. Surg., 134:753, 1951.

Gross, R. E., and Hubbard, J. P.: Surgical ligation of a patent ductus arteriosus: Report of first successful case. J.A.M.A., 112:729, 1939.

Gross, R. E., and Hufnagel, C. A.: Coarctation of the aorta: Experimental studies regarding its surgical corrections. N. Engl. J. Med., 233:287, 1945.

Gross, R. E., and Neuhauser, E. B. D.: Compression of the trachea by an anomalous innominate artery: An operation for its relief. Am. J. Dis. Child., 75:570, 1948.

Gross, R. E., and Neuhauser, E. B. D.: Compression of the trachea or esophagus by vascular anomalies. J. Pediatr., 7:69, 1951.

Gross, R. E., and Ware, P. F.: The surgical significance of aortic arch anomalies. Surg. Gynecol. Obstet., 83:435, 1946.

Grossman, L. B., Buonocore, E., Modic, M. T., and Meaney, T. F.: Digital subtraction angiography of the thoracic aorta. Radiology, 150:323, 1984.

Grover, F. L., Norton, J. B., Webb, G. E., and Trinkle, J.: Pulmonary sling: Case report and collective review. J. Thorac. Cardiovasc. Surg., 69:295, 1975.

Gula, G., Chew, C., Radley-Smith, R., and Yacoub, M.: Anoma-lous origin of the right pulmonary artery from the ascending aorta associated with aortopulmonary window. Thorax, 33:265, 1978.

Gumbiner, C. H., Mullins, C. E., and MacNamara, D. G.: Pul-monary artery sling. Am. J. Cardiol., 45:311, 1980.

Gupta, T. C., and Wiggers, C. J.: Basic hemodynamic changes produced by aortic coarctation and different degrees. Circu-lation, 3:17, 1951.

Hallett, J. W., Jr., Brewster, D. C., Darling, R. C., and O'Hara, P. J.: Coarctation of the abdominal aorta: Current options in surgical management. Ann. Surg., 191:430, 1980.

Hallman, G. L., and Cooley, D. A.: Congenital aortic vascular ring. Arch. Surg., 88:666, 1964.

Hallman, G. L., Yashar, J. J., Bloodwell, R. D., and Cooley, D. A.: Surgical correction of coarctation of the aorta in the first year of life. Ann. Thorac. Surg., 4:106, 1967.

Hamilton, D. I., Di Eusanio, G., Sandrasagra, F. A., and Donnelly, R. J.: Early and late results of aortoplasty with a left subclavian flap for coarctation of the aorta in infancy. J. Thorac. Cardio-vasc. Surg., 75:699, 1978.

Hamilton, D. I., Medici, D., Oyonarte, M., and Dickinson, D. F.: Aortoplasty with left subclavian flap in older children. J. Thorac. Cardiovasc. Surg., 82:103, 1981.

Hamilton, W. F., and Abbott, M. E.: Coarctation of the aorta of the adult type. Am. Heart J., 3:381, 1928.

Hammerman, C., Strates, E., and Valaitis, S.: The silent ductus: Its precursors and its aftermath. Pediatr. Cardiol., 7:121, 1986.

Hammon, J. W., Jr., Graham, T. P., Jr., Boucek, R. J., Jr., and Bender, H. W., Jr.: Operative repair of coarctation of the aorta in infancy: Results with and without ventricular septal defect. Am. J. Cardiol., 55:1555, 1985.

Hanson, E., Eriksson, B. O., and Sorensen, S. E.: Intra-arterial blood pressures at rest and during exercise after surgery for coarctation of the aorta. Eur. J. Cardiol., 11:245, 1980.

Harlan, H. L., Doty, D. B., Brandt, B., III, and Ehrenhaft, J. L.: Coarctation of the aorta in infants. J. Thorac. Cardiovasc. Surg., 88:1012, 1984.

Harley, H. R. S.: The development and anomalies of the aortic arch and its branches. Br. J. Surg., 56:36, 1959.

Hastreiter, A. R., D'Cruz, I. A., and Cantez, T.: Right-sided aorta. Part I: Occurrence of right aortic arch in various types of congenital heart disease. Part II: Right aortic arch, right descending aorta, and associated anomalies. Br. Heart J., 28:722, 1966.

Hatten, H. P., Jr., Lorman, J. G., and Rosenbaum, H. D.: Pul-monary sling in the adult. Am. J. Roentgenol., 128:919, 1977.

Haughton, V. M., Fellows, K. E., and Rosenbaum, A. E.: The cervical aortic arches. Radiology, 114:675, 1975.

Hays, J. T.: Spontaneous aneurysm of a patent ductus arteriosus in an elderly patient. Chest, 88:918, 1985.

Heinrich, W. D., and Tamayo, R. P.: Left aortic arch and right descending aorta. Case report. Am. J. Roentgenol., 76:762, 1956.

Hellerbrand, W. E., Kelley, M. J., Talner, N. S., et al: Cervical aortic arch with retroesophageal aortic obstruction: Report of a case with successful surgical intervention. Ann. Thorac. Surg., 26:86, 1978.

Herbert, W. H., Rohman, M., Farnsworth, P., and Saraswathi, S.: Anomalous origin of left pulmonary artery from ascending aorta, right aortic arch and right patent ductus arteriosus. Chest, 63:459, 1973.

Herrmann, V. M., Laks, H., Fagan, L., et al: Repair of aortic coarctation in the first year of life. Ann. Thorac. Surg., 25:57, 1978.

Hesslein, P. S., McNamara, D. G., Morriss, M. J. H., et al: Comparison of resection versus patch aortoplasty for repair of coarctation in infants and children. Circulation, 64:164, 1981.

Hewitt, R. L., Brewer, P. L., and Drapanas, T.: Aortic arch anomalies. J. Thorac. Cardiovasc. Surg., 60:746, 1970.

Heymann, M. A., Berman, W., Jr., Rudolph, A. M., and Whitman, V.: Dilatation of the ductus arteriosus by prostaglandin E₁ in aortic arch abnormalities. Circulation, 59:169, 1979.

Heymann, M. A., Rudolph, A. M., and Silberman, N. H.: Closure of the ductus arteriosus in premature infants by inhibition of prostaglandin synthesis. N. Engl. J. Med., 295:530, 1976.

Hickey, M. St. J., and Wood, A. E.: Pulmonary artery sling with tracheal stenosis. Ann. Thorac. Surg., 44:416, 1987.

Higgins, C. B., French, J. W., Silverman, J. F., and Wexler, L.: Interruption of the aortic arch: Preoperative and postoperative clinical, hemodynamic and angiographic features. Am. J. Cardiol., 39:563, 1977.

Hiller, H. G., and MacLean, A. D.: Pulmonary artery ring. Acta Radiol., 48:434, 1957.

Hiraishi, S., Misawa, H., Oyuchi, K., et al: Two dimensional Doppler echocardiographic assessment of closure of the ductus arteriosus in normal newborn infants. J. Pediatr., 111:755, 1987.

Hirschklau, M. J., DiSessa, T. G., Higgins, C. B., and Friedman, W. F.: Echocardiographic diagnosis: Pitfalls in the premature infant with a large patent ductus arteriosus. J. Pediatr., 92:474, 1978.

Ho, S. Y., and Anderson, R. H.: Anatomical closure of the ductus arteriosus: A study in 35 specimens. J. Anat., 128:829, 1979.

Ho, S. Y., and Anderson, R. H.: Coarctation, tubular hypoplasia, and the ductus arteriosus: Histological study of 35 specimens. Br. Heart J., 41:268, 1979.

Hoeffel, J. C., Henry, M., Mentre, B., et al: Pseudocoarctation or congenital kinking of the aorta: Radiologic considerations. Am. Heart J., 89:428, 1975.

Holman, E., Gerbode, F., and Purdy, A.: The patent ductus: A review of seventy-five cases with surgical treatment including an aneurysm of the ductus and one of the pulmonary artery. J. Thorac. Surg., 25:1, 1953.

Hubbell, M. M., Jr., O'Brien, R. G., Krometz, L. J., et al: Status of patients 5 or more years after correction of coarctation of the aorta over age 1 year. Circulation, 60:74, 1979.

Hughes, R. K., and Reemtsma, K.: Correction of coarctation of the aorta. Manometric determination of safety during test occlusion. J. Thorac. Cardiovasc. Surg., 62:31, 1971.

Huhta, J. C., Gutgesell, H. P., Latson, L. A., and Huffines, F. D.: Two-dimensional echocardiographic assessment of the aorta in infants and children with congenital heart disease. Circulation, 70:417, 1984.

Ibarra-Perez, C., Castaneda, A. R., Varco, R. L., and Lillehei, C. W.: Recoarctation of the aorta: Nineteen year clinical experience. Am. J. Cardiol., 23:778, 1969.

Idriss, F. S., DeLeon, S. Y., Ilbawi, M. N., et al: Tracheoplasty with pericardial patch for extensive tracheal stenosis in infants and children. J. Thorac. Cardiovasc. Surg., 88:527, 1984.

Isner, J. M., Donaldson, R. F., Fulton, D., et al: Cystic medial necrosis in coarctation of the aorta: A potential factor contributing to adverse consequences observed after percutaneous balloon angioplasty of coarctation sites. Circulation, 75:689, 1987.

Ito, K., Kohguchi, N., Ohkawa, Y., et al: Total one-stage repair of interrupted aortic arch associated with aortic septal defect and patent ductus arteriosus. J. Thorac. Cardiovasc. Surg., 74:913, 1977.

Ivey, H. H., Kattwinkel, J., Park, T. S., and Krovetz, L. J.: Failure of indomethacin to close persistent ductus arteriosus in infants weighing under 1000 grams. Br. Heart J., 41:304, 1979.

Jacob, T., Cobanoglu, A., and Starr, A: Late results of ascending aorta—descending aorta bypass grafts for recurrent coarctation of the aorta. J. Thorac. Cardiovasc., Surg., 95:782, 1988.

Jacobs, J., Gluck, L., DiSessa, T., et al: The contribution of PDA in the neonate with severe RDS. J. Pediatr., 96:79, 1980.

Jacobsen, J. R., Wennevold, A., and Boesen, I.: Coarctation of the aorta operated upon in infancy: Long-term follow-up. Eur. J. Cardiol., 10:123, 1979.

Jacobson, J. H., II, Morgan, B. C., Andersen, D. H., and Humphrey, G. H., II: Aberrant left pulmonary artery: A correctable cause of respiratory obstruction. J. Thorac. Cardiovasc. Surg., 39:602, 1960.

James, F. W., and Kaplan, S.: Systolic hypertension during submaximal exercise after correction of coarctation of aorta. Circulation, 49 and 50(Suppl. II):27, 1974.

Japko, L., Skolnick, L., Morecki, R., and Gartner, L.: Saccular aneurysm of ductus arteriosus. N.Y. State J. Med., December, p. 180, 1971.

Jarcho, S.: Coarctation of the aorta (Meckel, 1750; Paris, 1791). Am. J. Cardiol., 7:844, 1961.

Jarcho, S.: Coarctation of the aorta (Albrecht Meckel, 1827). Am. J. Cardiol., 9:307, 1962a.

Jarcho, S.: Coarctation of the aorta (Legrand, 1833). Am. J. Cardiol., 10:266, 1962b.

Jesseph, J. M., Mahony, L., Girod, D. A., and Brown, J. W.: Ductus arteriosus aneurysm in infancy. Ann. Thorac. Surg., 40:622, 1985.

Johansson, L., Michaelsson, M., Westerholm, C.-J., and Aberg, T.: Aortopulmonary window: A new operative approach. Ann. Thorac. Surg., 25:564, 1978.

John, S., Muralidharan, S., Jairaj, P. S., et al: The adult ductus: Review of surgical experience with 131 patients. J. Thorac. Cardiovasc. Surg., 82:314, 1981.

Johnson, A. M., and Kron, I. L.: Closure of the calcified patent ductus in the elderly: Avoidance ductal clamps and shunts. Ann. Thorac. Surg., 45:572, 1988.

Johnson, G. L., Breart, G. L., Gewitz, M. H., et al: Echocardiographic characteristics of premature infants with patent ductus arteriosus. Pediatrics, 72:864, 1983.

Jonas, R. A., Spevak, P. T., McGill, T., and Castenada, A. R.: Pulmonary artery sling: Primary repair by tracheal resection in infancy. J. Thorac. Cardiovasc. Surg., 97:548, 1989.

Jones, J. C.: Twenty-five years' experience with the surgery of patent ductus arteriosus. J. Thorac. Cardiovasc. Surg., 50:149, 1965.

Jones, J. C., Dolley, F. S., and Bullock, L. T.: The diagnosis and surgical therapy of patent ductus arteriosus. J. Thorac. Surg., 9:413, 1940.

Julsrud, P. R., and Ehman, R. L.: Magnetic resonancy imaging of vascular rings. Mayo Clin. Proc., 61:181, 1986.

Jung, J. Y., Almond, C. H., Saab, S. B., and Lababidi, Z.: Surgical repair of right aortic arch with aberrant left subclavian artery and left ligamentum arteriosum. J. Thorac. Cardiovasc. Surg., 75:237, 1978.

Kale, M. K., Rafferty, R. E., and Carton, R. W.: Aberrant left pulmonary artery presenting as a mediastinal mass: Report of a case in an adult. Arch. Intern. Med., 125:121, 1970.

Kamau, P., Miles, V., Toews, W., et al: Surgical repair of coarctation of the aorta in infants less than six months of age: Including the question of pulmonary artery banding. J. Thorac. Cardiovasc. Surg., 81:171, 1981.

Kan, J. S., White, R. I., Jr., Mitchell, S. E., et al: Treatment of restenosis of coarctation by percutaneous transluminal angioplasty. Circulation, 68:1087, 1983.

Kawauchi, M., Tada, Y., Asano, K., and Sudo, K.: Angiographic demonstration of mesenteric arterial changes in postcoarctectomy syndrome. Surgery, 98:602, 1985.

Keane, J. F., Maltz, D., Bernhard, W. F., et al: Anomalous origin of one pulmonary artery from the ascending aorta. Circulation, 50:588, 1974.

Keys, A., and Shapiro, M. J.: Patency of the ductus arteriosus in adults. Am. Heart J., 25:158, 1943.

Kimball, B. P., Shurvell, B. L., Houle, S., et al: Persistent ventricular adaptations in postoperative coarctation of the aorta. J. Am. Coll. Cardiol., 8:172, 1986a.

Kimball, B. P., Shurvell, B. L., Mildenberger, R. R., et al: Abnormal thallium kinetics in postoperative coarctation of the aorta: Evidence for diffuse hypertension-induced vascular pathology. J. Am. Coll. Cardiol., 7:538, 1986b.

Kirklin, J. W.: Vascular "rings" producing respiratory obstruction in infants. Staff Meet. Mayo Clin., 25:360, 1950.

Kirklin, J. W., Burchell, H. B., Pugh, D. G., et al: Surgical treatment of coarctation of the aorta in a ten-week old infant: Report of a case. Circulation, 6:411, 1952.

Kirkpatrick, S. E., Girod, D. A., and King, H.: Aortic origin of the right pulmonary artery. Circulation, 36:771, 1967.

Kirks, D. R., McCook, T. A., Serwer, G. A., and Oldham, H. N.,

Jr.: Aneurysm of the ductus arteriosus in the neonate. A.J.R., *134*:573, 1980.

Kirsh, M. M., Perry, B., and Spooner, E.: Management of pseudoaneurysms following patch grafting for coarctation of the aorta. J. Thorac. Cardiovasc. Surg., *74*:636, 1977.

Kitterman, J. A., Edmunds, H. L., Jr., Gregory, G. A., et al: Patent ductus arteriosus in premature infants: Incidence, relation to pulmonary disease and management. N. Engl. J. Med., *287*:473, 1972.

Kittle, C. F., and Schafer, P. W.: Gangrene of the forearm after subclavian arterio-aortostomy for coarctation of the aorta. Thorax, *8*:319, 1953.

Knight, L., and Edwards, J. E.: Right aortic arch: Types and associated cardiac anomalies. Circulation, *50*:1047, 1974.

Koller, M., Rothlin, M., and Sinning, A.: Coarctation of the aorta: Review of 362 operated patients. Long-term follow-up and assessment of prognostic variables. Eur. Heart J., *8*:670, 1987.

Koopot, R., Nikaidoh, H., and Idriss, F. S.: Surgical management of anomalous left pulmonary artery causing tracheobronchial obstruction: Pulmonary artery sling. J. Thorac. Cardiovasc. Surg., *69*:239, 1975.

Kopf, G. S., Hellenbrand, W., Kleinman, C., et al: Repair of aortic coarctation in the first 3 months of life: Immediate and long-term results. Ann. Thorac. Surg., *41*:425, 1986.

Korfer, R., Meyer, H., Kleikamp G., and Bircks, W.: Early and late results after resection and end-to-end anastomosis of coarctation of the thoracic aorta in early infancy. J. Thorac. Cardiovasc. Surg., *89*:616, 1985.

Krieger, K. H., and Spencer, F. C.: Is paraplegia after repair of coarctation of the aorta due principally to distal hypotension during aortic cross-clamping? Surgery, *2*:97, 1985.

Kron, I. L., Mentzer, R. M., Jr., Rheuban, K. S., and Nolan, S. P.: A simple, rapid technique for operative closure of patent ductus arteriosus in the premature infant. Ann. Thorac. Surg., *37*:422, 1984.

Kron, I. L., Rheuban, K. S., Carpenter, M. S., and Nolan, S. P.: Interrupted aortic arch: A conservative approach for the sick neonate. J. Thorac. Cardiovasc. Surg., *86*:37, 1983.

Krovetz, L. J., and Kattwinkel, J.: Commentary on patent ductus arteriosus complicating the respiratory distress syndrome. J. Pediatr., *90*:262, 1977.

Krueger, E., Mellander, M., Bratton, D., and Cotton, R.: Prevention of symptomatic patent ductus arteriosus with a single dose of indomethacin. J. Pediatr., *111*:749, 1987.

Kutsche, L. M., and Van Mierop, L. H. S.: Anomalous origin of a pulmonary artery from the ascending aorta: Associated anomalies and pathogenesis. Am. J. Cardiol., *61*:850, 1988.

Kutsche, L. M., and Van Mierop, L. H. S.: Cervical origin of the right subclavian artery in aortic arch interruption: Pathogenesis and significance. Am. J. Cardiol., *53*:892, 1984.

Lababidi, Z. A.: Neonatal transluminal balloon coarctation angioplasty. Am. Heart J., *1016*:752, 1983.

Lababidi, Z. A., Daskalopoulos, D. A., and Stoeckle, H., Jr.: Transluminal balloon coarctation angioplasty: Experience with 27 patients. Am. J. Cardiol., *54*:1288, 1984.

Lam, C. R.: The choice of the side for approach in operations for pulmonary stenosis. J. Thorac. Surg., *18*:661, 1949.

Lam, C. R.: A safe technique for closure of the recurrent patent ductus arteriosus. J. Thorac. Cardiovasc. Surg., *72*:232, 1976.

Lam, C. R., and Arciniegas, E.: Surgical management of coarctation of the aorta with minimal collateral circulation. Ann. Surg., *178*:693, 1973.

Lam, C. R., Kabbani, S., and Arciniegas, E.: Symptomatic anomalies of the aortic arch. Surg. Gynecol. Obstet., *147*:673, 1978.

Lansman, S., Shapiro, A. J., Schiller, M. S., et al: Extended aortic arch anastomosis for repair of coarctation in infancy. Circulation, *74*(Suppl. I):37, 1986.

Laschinger, J. C., Cunningham, J. N., Baumann, F. G., et al: Monitoring of somatosensory evoked potentials during surgical procedures on the thoracoabdominal aorta. II: Use of somatosensory evoked potentials to assess adequacy of distal aortic bypass and perfusion after thoracic aortic cross-clamping. J. Thorac. Cardiovasc. Surg., *94*:266, 1987.

Laschinger, J. C., Cunningham, J. N., Baumann, F. G., et al: Monitoring of somatosensory evoked potentials during sur-

gical procedures on the thoracoabdominal aorta. III. Intraoperative identification of vessels critical to spinal cord blood supply. J. Thorac. Cardiovasc. Surg., *94*:271, 1987.

Laschinger, J. C., Cunningham, J. N., Jr., Cooper, M. M., et al: Monitoring of somatosensory evoked potentials during surgical procedures on the thoracoabdominal aorta. I: Relationship of aortic cross-clamp duration, changes in somatosensory evoked potentials, and incidence of neurologic dysfunction. J. Thorac. Cardiovasc. Surg., *94*:260, 1987.

Lavin, N., Mehta, S., Liberson, M., and Pouget, J. M.: Pseudocoarctation of the aorta: An unusual variant with coarctation. Am. J. Cardiol., *24*:584, 1969.

Leanage, R., Taylor, J. F. N., DeLeval, M., et al: Surgical management of coarctation of aorta with ventricular septal defect. Br. Heart J., *46*:269, 1981.

Leenen, F. H. H., Balfe, J. A., Pelech, A. N., et al: Postoperative hypertension after repair of coarctation of aorta in children: Protective effect of propranolol? Am. Heart J., *113*:1164, 1987.

Lenox, C. C., Crisler, C., Zuberbuhler, J. R., et al: Anomalous left pulmonary artery: Successful management. J. Thorac. Cardiovasc. Surg., *77*:748, 1979.

Leonardi, H. K., Naggar, C. Z., and Ellis, F. H., Jr.: Dysphagia due to aortic arch anomaly. Arch. Surg., *115*:1229, 1980.

Leoni, F., Huhta, J. C., Douglas, J., et al: Effect of prostaglandin on early surgical mortality in obstructive lesions of the systemic circulation. Br. Heart J., *52*:654, 1984.

Lerberg, D. B., Hardesty, R. L., Stewers, R. D., et al: Coarctation of the aorta in infants and children: 25 years of experience. Ann. Thorac. Surg., *33*:159, 1982.

Lewis, T.: Material relating to coarctation of the aorta of the adult type. Heart, *16*:205, 1933.

Lima, J. A., Rosenblum, B. N., Reilly, J. S., et al: Airway obstruction in aortic arch anomalies. Otolaryngol. Head Neck Surg., *91*:605, 1983.

Lincoln, J. C. R., Deverall, P. B., Stark, J., et al: Vascular anomalies compressing the oesophagus and trachea. Thorax, *24*:295, 1969.

Lindsay, J., Jr.: Coarctation of the aorta, bicuspid aortic valve and abnormal ascending aortic wall. Am. J. Cardiol., *61*:182, 1988.

Litwin, S. B., VanPraagh, R., and Bernhard, W. F.: A palliative operation for certain infants with aortic arch interruption. Ann. Thorac. Surg., *14*:369, 1972.

Lock, J. E.: Now that we can dilate, should we? Am. J. Cardiol., *54*:1360, 1984.

Lock, J. E., Bass, J. L., Amplatz, K., et al: Balloon dilatation angioplasty of aortic coarctations in infants and children. Circulation, *68*:109, 1983.

Lock, J. E., Cockerham, J. T., Keane, J. F., et al: Transcatheter umbrella closure of congenital heart defects. Circulation, *75*:593, 1987.

Lodge, F. A., Lamberti, J. J., Goodman, A. H., et al: Vascular consequences of subclavian artery transection for treatment of congenital heart disease. J. Thorac. Cardiovasc. Surg., *86*:18, 1983.

Luisi, S. V., Ashraf, M. H., Gula, G., et al: Anomalous origin of the right coronary artery with aortopulmonary window: Functional and surgical considerations. Thorax, *35*:446, 1980.

Lynxwiler, C. P., Smith, S., and Babich, J.: Coarctation of the aorta. Arch. Pediar., *68*:203, 1951.

Macmanus, Q., Starr, A., Lambert, L. E., and Grunkemeier, G.: Correction of aortic coarctation in neonates: Mortality and late results. Ann. Thorac. Surg., *24*:544, 1977.

Mahoney, L., Carnero, V., Brett, C., et al: Prophylactic indomethacin therapy for patent ductus arteriosus in very-low-birth-weight infants. N. Engl. J. Med., *206*:506, 1982.

Maier, H. C., and Van der Woude, R.: Right-sided patent ductus arteriosus with right aortic arch. J. Thorac. Cardiovasc. Surg., *56*:401, 1968.

Malm, J. R., Bulmenthal, S., Jameson, A. G., and Humphreys, G. H., II: Observations on coarctation of the aorta in infants. Arch. Surg., *86*:110, 1963.

Markel, H., Rocchini, A. P., Beekman, R. H., et al: Exercise-induced hypertension after repair of coarctation of the aorta: Arm versus leg exercise. J. Am. Coll. Cardiol., *8*:165, 1986.

Markiewicz, A., Wojczuk, D., Kokot, F., and Cicha, A.: Plasma renin activity in coarctation of aorta before and after surgery. Br. Heart J., 37:721, 1975.

Marmon, L. M., Bye, M. R., Haas, J. M., et al: Vascular rings and slings: Long-term follow-up of pulmonary function. J. Plast. Surg., 19:683, 1984.

Maron, B. J., Humphries, J. O., Rowe, R. D., and Mellits, E. D.: Prognosis of surgically corrected coarctation of the aorta: A 20-year postoperative appraisal. Circulation, 47:119, 1973.

Marx, G. R., and Allen, H. D.: Accuracy and pitfalls of Doppler evaluation of the pressure gradient in aortic coarctation. J. Am. Coll. Cardiol., 7:1379, 1986.

Matsuda, H., Zavanella, C., Lee, P., and Subramanian, S.: Aortic origin of the right pulmonary artery. Ann. Thorac. Surg., 24:374, 1977.

Matsuyama, K., Sonoda, E., Nakoa, K. et al: Baroreceptor reflex in a patient with coarctation of the aorta. Clin. Cardiol., 10:535, 1987.

Mavroudis, C., Cook, L. N., Fleischaker, J. W., et al: Management of patent ductus arteriosus in the premature infant: Indomethacin versus ligation. Ann. Thorac. Surg., 36:561, 1983.

Mayer, J. E., Joyce, L. D., Reinke, D., et al: Aberrant left pulmonary artery presenting as a right paratracheal mass in an adult. J. Thorac. Cardiovasc. Surg., 72:571, 1976.

Mays, E. T., and Sergeant, C. K.: Postcoarctectomy syndrome. Arch. Surg., 91:58, 1965.

McCallen, A. M., and Schaff, B.: Aneurysm of an anomalous right subclavian artery. Radiology, 66:561, 1956.

McCarthy, J. S., Zies, L. G., and Gelband, H.: Age-dependent closure of the patent ductus arteriosus by indomethacin. Pediatrics, 62:706, 1978.

McFaul, R., Millard, P., and Nowicki, E.: Vascular rings necessitating right thoracotomy. J. Thorac. Cardiovasc. Surg., 82:306, 1981.

Mellander, M., Leheup, B., Lindstrom, D. P., et al: Recurrence of symptomatic patent ductus arteriosus in extremely premature infants, treated with indomethacin. J. Pediatr. 105:138, 1984.

Mellgren, G., Friberg, L. G., Eriksson, B. O., et al: Neonatal surgery for coarctation of the aorta. Scand. J. Thorac. Cardiovasc. Surg., 21:193, 1987.

Merrill, D. L., Webster, C. A., and Samson, P. C.: Congenital absence of the aortic isthmus. J. Thorac. Surg., 33:311, 1957.

Merritt, T. A., DiSessa, T. G., Feldman, B. H., et al: Closure of the patent ductus arteriosus with ligation and indomethacin: A consecutive experience. J. Pediatr., 93:639, 1978.

Merritt, T. A., White, C. L., Jacob, J., et al: Patent ductus arteriosus treated with ligation or indomethacin: A follow-up study. J. Pediatr., 95:588, 1979.

Metzdorff, M. T., Cobanoglu, A., Grunkemeier, G. L., et al: Influence of age at operation on late results with subclavian flap aortoplasty. J. Thorac. Cardiovasc. Surg., 89:235, 1985.

Midgley, F. M., Scott, L. P., Perry, L. W., et al: Subclavian flap aortoplasty for treatment of coarctation of early infancy. J. Pediatr. Surg., 13:265, 1978.

Mikhail, M., Lee, W., Toews, W., et al: Surgical and medical experience with 734 premature infants with patent ductus arteriosus. J. Thorac. Cardiovasc. Surg., 83:349, 1982.

Minami, K., Sagoo, K. S., Matthies, W., et al: Left aortic arch, retro-esophageal aortic segment, right descending aorta and right patent ductus arteriosus—a very rare "vascular ring" malformation. Thorac. Cardiovasc. Surg., 34:395, 1986.

Mitchell, R. S., Seifert, F. C., Miller, D. C., et al: Aneurysm of the diverticulum of the ductus arteriosus in the adult. J. Thorac. Cardiovasc. Surg., 86:400, 1983.

Moene, R. J., Gittenberger-DeGroot, A. C., Oppenheimer-Dekker, A., and Bartelings, M. M.: Anatomic characteristics of ventricular septal defect associated with coarctation of the aorta. Am. J. Cardiol., 59:952, 1987.

Moene, R. J., Oppenheimer-Dekker, A., and Wenink, A. C. G.: Relation between aortic arch hypoplasia of variable severity and central muscular ventricular septal defects: Emphasis on associated left ventricular abnormalities. Am. J. Cardiol., 48:111, 1981.

Moene, R. J., Ottenkamp, J., Oppenheimer-Dekker, A., and Bartelings, M. M.: Transposition of the great arteries and narrowing of the aortic arch: Emphasis on right ventricular characteristics. Br. Heart J., 53:58, 1985.

Monro, J. L., Brawn, W., and Conway, N.: Correction of type B interrupted aortic arch with ventricular septal defect in infancy. J. Thorac. Cardiovasc. Surg., 74:618, 1977.

Moor, C. G., Ionescu, M. I., and Ross, D. N.: Surgical repair of coarctation of the aorta by patch grafting. Ann. Thorac. Surg., 14:626, 1972.

Moore, G. W., and Hutchins, G. M.: Association of interrupted aortic arch with malformations producing reduced blood flow to the fourth aortic arches. Am. J. Cardiol., 42:467, 1978.

Moreno, N. N., de Campo, T., Kaiser, G. A., and Pallares, V. S.: Technical and pharmacologic management of distal hypotension during repair of coarctation of the aorta. J. Thorac. Cardiovasc. Surg., 80:182, 1980.

Morgan, J. R.: Left pulmonary artery from ascending aorta in tetralogy of Fallot. Circulation, 45:653, 1972.

Mori, K., Ando, M., Tako, A, et al: Distal type of aortopulmonary window: Report of four cases. Br. Heart J. 40:681, 1978.

Morrow, A. G., Greenfield, L. J., and Braunwald, E.: Congenital aortopulmonary septal defect: Clinical and hemodynamic findings, surgical technic, and results of operative correction. Circulation, 25:463, 1962.

Morrow, W. R., Vick, G. W., Nihill, M. R., et al: Balloon dilatation of unopened coarctation of the aorta: Short- and intermediate-term results. J. Am. Coll. Cardiol., 11:113, 1988.

Morse, H. R., and Gladdings, S.: Bronchial obstruction due to misplaced left pulmonary artery. Am. J. Dis. Child., 89:351, 1955.

Moss, A. J.: Coarctation of the aorta: Current status. J. Pediatr., 102:253, 1983.

Moss, A. J., Emmonoulides, G., and Duffie, E. R.: Closure of the ductus arteriosus in the newborn infant. Pediatr., 32:25, 1963.

Moulaert, A. J., Bruins, C. C., and Oppenheimer-Dekker, A.: Anomalies of the aortic arch and ventricular septal defects. Circulation, 53:1011, 1976.

Moulton, A. L., and Bowman, F. O., Jr.: Primary definitive repair of type B interrupted aortic arch, ventricular septal defect, and patent ductus arteriosus. J. Thorac. Cardiovasc. Surg., 82:501, 1981.

Moulton, A. L., Brenner, J. I., Roberts, G., et al: Subclavian flap repair of coarctation of the aorta in neonates. J. Thorac. Cardiovasc. Surg., 87:220, 1984.

Mullins, C. E., Gillette, P. C., and McNamara, D. G.: The complex of cervical aortic arch. Pediatrics, 51:210, 1973.

Munro, J. C.: Surgery of the vascular system: I: Ligation of the ductus arteriosus. Ann. Surg., 46:335, 1907.

Murphy, D. A., Lemire, G. G., Tessler, I., and Dunn, G. L.: Correction of type B aortic arch interruption with ventricular and atrial septal defects in a 3-day-old infant. J. Thorac. Cardiovasc. Surg., 65:882, 1973.

Murthy, K., Mattioli, L., Diehl, A., and Holder, T. M.: Vascular ring due to left aortic arch, right descending aorta, and right patent ductus arteriosus. J. Pediatr. Surg., 5:550, 1970.

Mustard, W. T., Bayliss, C. E., Fearon, B., et al: Tracheal compression by the innominate artery in children. Ann. Thorac. Surg., 8:312, 1969.

Mustard, W. T., Rowe, R. D., Keith, J. D., and Sirek, A.: Coarctation of the aorta with special reference to the first year of life. Ann. Surg., 141:429, 1955.

Mustard, W. T., Trimble, A. W., and Trusler, G. A.: Mediastinal vascular anomalies causing tracheal and esophageal compression and obstruction in childhood. Can. Med. Assoc. J., 87:1301, 1962.

Nagle, M. G., Peyton, M. D., Harrison, L. H., Jr., and Elkins, D. C.: Ligation of patent ductus arteriosus in very low birth weight infants. Am. J. Cardiol., 142:681, 1981.

Nair, U. R., Jones, O., and Walker, D. R.: Surgical management of severe coarctation of the aorta in the first month of life. J. Thorac. Cardiovasc. Surg., 86:587, 1983.

Nanton, M. A., and Olley, P. M.: Residual hypertension after coarctectomy in childen. Am. J. Cardiol., 37:769, 1976.

Nashef, S. A. M., Jamieson, M. P. G., Pollock, J. C. S., and Houston, A. B.: Aortic origin of right pulmonary artery: Successful correction in three consecutive patients. Ann. Thorac. Surg., 44:536, 1987.

Nasser, W. K., and Helmen, C.: Kinking of the aortic arch

(pseudocoarctation): Clinical, radiographic, hemodynamic, and angiographic findings in eight cases. Ann. Intern. Med., 64:971, 1966.

Naulty, C. M., Horn, S., Conry, J., and Avery, G. B.: Improved lung compliance after ligation of patent ductus arteriosus in hyaline membrane disease. J. Pediatr., 93:682, 1978.

Neal, W. A., Bessinger, F. B., Jr., Hunt, C. E., and Lucas, R. V., Jr.: Patent ductus arteriosus complicating respiratory distress syndrome. J. Pediatr., 86:127, 1975.

Neal, W. A., and Mullett, M. D.: Patent ductus arteriosus in premature infants: A review of current management. Pediatr. Cardiol., 3:59, 1982.

Neches, W. H., Park, S. C., Lenox, C. C., et al: Coarctation of the aorta with ventricular septal defect. Circulation, 55:189, 1977.

Nelson, D. J., Thiebeault, D. W., Emmanouilides, G. C., and Lippmann, M.: Improving the results of ligation of patent ductus arteriosus in small preterm infants. J. Thorac. Cardiovasc. Surg., 2:169, 1976.

Neufeld, H. N., Lester, R. G., Adams, P., Jr., et al: Aorticopulmonary septal defect. Am. J. Cardiol., 9:12, 1962.

Neuhauser, E. B. D.: The roentgen diagnosis of double aortic arch and other anomalies of the great vessels. Am. J. Roentgenol. Rad. Ther. 56:1, 1946.

Newcombe, C. P., Ongley, P. A., Edwards, J. E., and Wood, E. H.: Clinical, pathologic, and hemodynamic considerations in coarctation of the aorta associated with ventricular septal defect. Circulation, 24:1356, 1961.

Ng, A. S.-H., Vlietstra, R. E., Danielson, G. K., et al: Patent ductus arteriosus in patients more than 50 years old. Int. J. Cardiol., 11:277, 1986.

Nikaidoh, H., Idriss, F. S., and Riker, W. L.: Aortic rupture in children as a complication of coarctation of the aorta. Arch. Surg., 107:838, 1973.

Norton, J. B., Jr., Ullyot, D. J., Stewart, E. T., et al: Aortic arch atresia with transposition of the great vessels: Physiologic considerations and surgical management. Surgery, 67:1011, 1970.

Norwood, W. I., Lang, P., Castaneda, A. R., and Hougen, T. J.: Reparative operations for interrupted aortic arch with ventricular septal defect. J. Thorac. Cardiovasc. Surg., 86:832, 1983.

Norwood, W. I., and Stellin, G. J.: Aortic atresia with interrupted aortic arch: Reparative operation. J. Thorac. Cardiovasc. Surg., 82:239, 1981.

O'Donovan, T. G., and Beck, W.: Closure of the complicated patent ductus arteriosus. Ann. Thorac. Surg., 25:463, 1978.

Ohtsuka, S., Kakihana, M., Ishikawa, T., et al: Aneurysm of patent ductus arteriosus in an adult case: Findings of cardiac catheterization, angiography, and pathology. Clin. Cardiol., 10:537, 1987.

Oldham, H. N., Jr., Collins, N. P., Pierce, G. E., et al: Giant patent ductus arteriosus. J. Thorac. Cardiovasc. Surg., 47:331, 1964.

Olley, P. M., Coceani, F., and Bodach, E.: E-type prostaglandins: A new emergency therapy for certain cyanotic congenital heart malformations. Circulation, 53:728, 1976.

Orzel, J. A., and Monaco, M. P.: Inadvertent ligation of the left pulmonary artery instead of patent ductus arteriosus: Noninvasive diagnosis by pulmonary perfusion imaging. Clin. Nucl. Med., 11:629, 1986.

Ostermiller, W. E., Jr., Somerndike, J. M., Hunter, J. A., et al: Coarctation of the aorta in adult patients. J. Thorac. Cardiovasc. Surg., 61:125, 1971.

Otero-Cagide, M., Moodie, D. S., Sterba, R., and Gill, C. C.: Digital subtraction angiography in the diagnosis of vascular rings. Am. Heart J., 112:1304, 1986.

Oxnard, S. C., McGough, E. C., Jung, A. L., and Ruttenberg, H. D.: Ligation of the patent ductus arteriosus in the newborn intensive care unit. Ann. Thorac. Surg., 23:564, 1977.

Palatianos, G. M., Kaiser, G. A., Thurer, R. J., and Garcia, O.: Changing trends in the surgical treatment of coarctation of the aorta. Ann. Thorac. Surg., 40:41, 1985.

Palder, S. B., Schwartz, M. Z., Tyson, K. R. T., and Marr, C. C.: Management of patent ductus arteriosus: A comparison of operative vs pharmacologic treatment. J. Pediatr. Surg., 22:1171, 1987.

Paris, M.: Anatomie pathologique: Retrecissement considerable de l'aorte pectorale, observe a l'Hôtel-Dieu de Paris. J. Chir. DeSault, 2:107, 1791.

Park, S. C., Siewers, R. D., Neches, W. H., et al: Left aortic arch with right descending aorta and right ligamentum arteriosum: A rare form of vascular ring. J. Thorac. Cardiovasc. Surg., 71:779, 1976.

Parker, F. B., Farrell, B., Streeten, D. H. P., et al: Hypertensive mechanisms in coarctation of the aorta: Further studies of the renin-angiotensin system. J. Thorac. Cardiovasc. Surg., 80:568, 1980.

Parr, G. V. S., Waldhausen, J. A., Bharati, S., et al: Coarctation of Taussig-Bing malformation of the heart. J. Thorac. Cardiovasc. Surg., 86:280, 1983.

Pate, J. W., Korones, S., and Sarasohn, C.: Surgical closure of patent ductus arteriosus outside the operating theater. World J. Surg., 5:873, 1981.

Paul, R. N.: A new anomaly of the aorta: Left aortic arch with right descending aorta. J. Pediatr., 32:19, 1948.

Peckham, G. J., Miettinen, O. S., Ellison, R. C., et al: Clinical course to 1 year of age in premature infants with patent ductus arteriosus: Results of a multicenter randomized trial of indomethacin. J. Pediatr., 105:285, 1984.

Pellegrino, A., Deverall, P. D., Anderson, R. H., and Smith, A.: Aortic coarctation in the first 3 months of life: An anatomopathological study with respect to treatment. J. Thorac. Cardiovasc. Surg., 89:121, 1985.

Penkoske, P. A., Castaneda, A. R., Fyler, D. C., and Van Praagh, R.: Origin of pulmonary artery branch from ascending aorta. J. Thorac. Cardiovasc. Surg., 85:537, 1983.

Penkoske, P. A., Williams, W. G., Olley, P. M., and LaBlanc, J.: Subclavian arterioplasty: Repair of coarctation of the aorta in the first year of life. J. Thorac. Cardiovasc. Surg., 87:894, 1984.

Pennington, D. G., Liberthson, R. R., Jacobs, M., et al: Critical review of experience with surgical repair of coarctation of the aorta. J. Thorac. Cardiovasc. Surg., 77:217, 1979.

Peterson, A. C., Behrendt, D. M., Kirsch, M. M., and Rocchini, A. P.: Surgical management of neonates with complex preductal aortic coarctation. Ann. Thorac. Surg., 32:100, 1981.

Phelan, P. D., and Venables, A. W.: Management of pulmonary artery sling (anomalous left pulmonary artery arising from right pulmonary artery): A conservative approach. Thorax, 33:67, 1978.

Pierpont, M. E. M., Zollikofer, C. L., Moller J. H., and Edwards, J. E.: Interruption of the aortic arch with right descending aorta. Pediatr. Cardiol., 2:153, 1982.

Pifarre, R., Dieter, R. A., Jr., and Niedballa, R. G.: Definitive surgical treatment of the aberrant retroesophageal right subclavian artery in the adult. J. Thorac. Cardiovasc. Surg., 61:154, 1971.

Pifarre, R., Rice, P. L., and Nemickas, R.: Surgical treatment of calcified patent ductus arteriosus. J. Thorac. Cardiovasc. Surg., 65:635, 1973.

Pigott, J. D., Chin, A. J., Weinberg, P. M., et al: Transposition of the great arteries with aortic arch obstruction. J. Thorac. Cardiovasc. Surg., 94:82, 1987.

Pollack, P., Freed, M. D., Castaneda, A. R., and Norwood, W. I.: Reoperation for isthmic coarctation of the aorta: Follow-up of 26 patients. Am. J. Cardiol., 51:1690, 1983.

Pollock, J. C., Jamieson, M. P., and McWilliam, R.: Somatosensory evoked potentials in the detection of spinal cord ischemia in aortic coarctation repair. Ann. Thorac. Surg., 41:251, 1986.

Pontius, R. G.: Bronchial obstruction of congenital origin. Am. J. Surg., 106:8, 1963.

Pontius, R. G., Danielson, G. K., Noonan, J. A., and Judson, J. P.: Illusions leading to surgical closure of the distal left pulmonary artery instead of the ductus arteriosus. J. Thorac. Cardiovasc. Surg., 82:107, 1981.

Portsmann, W., Hieronymi, K., Wierny, L., and Warnke, H.: Nonsurgical closure of oversized patent ductus arteriosus with pulmonary hypertension: Report of a case. Circulation, 50:376, 1974.

Portsmann, W., Wierny, L., Warnke, H., et al: Catheter closure of patent ductus arteriosus: 62 cases treated without thoracotomy. Radiol. Clin. North Am. 9:203, 1971.

Porter, D. D., Canent, R. V., Jr., Spach, M. S., and Baylin, G. J.: Origin of the right pulmonary artery from the ascending aorta: Unusual cineangiocardiographic and pathologic findings. Circulation, 27:589, 1963.

Potts, W. J., Holinger, P. H., and Rosenblum, A. H.: Anomalous left pulmonary artery causing obstruction to right main bronchus: Report of a case. J.A.M.A., 155:1409, 1954.

Powell, M. L.: Patent ductus arteriosus in premature infants. Med. J. Aust., 2:58, 1963.

Presbitero, P., Demarie, D., Villani, M., et al: Long-term results (15–30 years) of surgical repair of aortic coarctation. Br. Heart J., 57:462, 1987.

Putnam, T. C., and Gross, R. E.: Surgical management of aortopulmonary fenestration. Surgery, 59:727, 1966.

Railsback, O. C., and Dock, W.: Erosion of the ribs due to stenosis of the isthmus (coarctation) of the aorta. Radiology, 12:58, 1929.

Rajaram, P. C., Hussain, A. T., Lakshmikanthan, C., et al: Type D double aortic arch: Double aortic arch with interruption of its left component proximal to the site of origin of left common carotid artery. J. Vasc. Dis., September:59, 1983.

Rao, P. S.: Balloon angioplasty for coarctation of the aorta in infancy. J. Pediatr. 110:713, 1987.

Rashkind, W. J., and Cuaso, C. C.: Transcatheter closure of patent ductus arteriosus: Successful use in a 3.5-kilogram infant. Pediatr. Cardiol., 1:3, 1979.

Rashkind, W. J., Mullins, C. E., Hellenbrand, W. E., and Tait, M. A.: Nonsurgical closure of patent ductus arteriosus: Clinical application of the Rashkind PDA occluder system. Circulation, 75:583, 1987.

Ravelo, H. R., Stephenson, L. W., Friedman, S., et al: Coarctation resection in children with Turner's syndrome: A note of caution. J. Thorac. Cardiovasc. Surg., 80:427, 1980.

Redo, S. F., Foster, H. R., Jr., Engle, M. A., and Ehlers, K. H.: Anomalous origin of the right pulmonary artery from the ascending aorta. J. Thorac. Cardiovasc. Surg., 50:726, 1955.

Reid, D. A., Foster, E. D., Stubberfield, J., and Alley, R. D.: Anomalous right subclavian artery arising proximal to a postductal thoracic aortic coarctation. Ann. Thorac. Surg., 32:85, 1981.

Reifenstein, G. H., Levine, S. A., and Gross, R. E.: Coarctation of the aorta: A review of 104 autopsied cases of the "adult type" 2 years of age or older. Am. Heart J., 33:146, 1947.

Reul, G. J., Jr., Kabbani, S. S., Sandiford, K. M., et al: Repair of coarctation of the thoracic aorta by patch graft aortoplasty. J. Thorac. Cardiovasc. Surg., 68:696, 1974.

Rheuban, K. S., Ayres, N., Still, J. G., and Alford, B.: Pulmonary artery sling: A new diagnostic tool and clinical review. Pediatrics, 69:472, 1982.

Ribeiro, A. B., and Krakoff, L. R.: Angiotensin blockade in coarctation of the aorta. N. Engl. J. Med., 295:148, 1976.

Richardson, J. V., Doty, D. B., Rossi, N. P., and Ehrenhaft, J. L.: The spectrum of anomalies of aortopulmonary septation. J. Thorac. Cardiovasc. Surg., 78:21, 1979.

Richardson, J. V., Doty, D. B., Rossi, N. P., and Ehrenhaft, J. L.: Operation for aortic arch anomalies. Ann. Thorac. Surg., 31:426, 1981.

Ring, D. M., and Lewis, F. J.: Abdominal pain following surgical correction of coarctation of the aorta: A syndrome. J. Thorac. Surg., 31:718, 1956.

Rittenhouse, E. A., Doty, D. B., Lauer, R. M., and Ehrenhaft, J. L.: Patent ductus arteriosus in premature infants: Indications for surgery. J. Thorac. Cardiovasc. Surg., 71:187, 1976.

Rocchini, A. P., Rosenthal, A., Barger, A. C., et al: Pathogenesis of paradoxical hypertension after coarctation resection. Circulation, 54:382, 1976.

Roesler, M., deLeval, M., Chrispin, A., and Stark, J.: Surgical management of vascular ring. Ann. Surg., 197:129, 1983.

Rosenberg, H. S., Hallman, G. L., Wolfe, R. R., and Latson, J. R.: Origin of the right pulmonary artery from the aorta. Am. Heart J., 72:106, 1966.

Rosenquist, G. C.: Congenital mitral valve disease associated with coarctation of the aorta. Circulation, 49:985, 1974.

Rosenquist, G. C., Taylor, J. F. N., and Stark, J.: Aortopulmonary fenestration and aortic atresia. Br. Heart J., 36:1146, 1974.

Ross, J. K., Monro, J. L., and Sbokos, C. G.: Late complications of surgery for coarctation of the aorta. Thorax, 30:31, 1975.

Rudolph, A. M., Heymann, M. A., and Spitznas, U.: Hemodynamic considerations in the development of narrowing of the aorta. Am. J. Cardiol., 30:514, 1972.

Rytand, D. A.: The renal factor in arterial hypertension with coarctation of the aorta. J. Clin. Invest., 17:391, 1938.

Saalouke, M. G., Perry, L. W., Breckbill, D. L., et al: Cerebrovascular abnormalities in postoperative coarctation of aorta: Four cases demonstrating left subclavian steal on aortography. Am. J. Cardiol., 42:97, 1978.

Sade, R. M., Crawford, F. A., Hohn, A. R., et al: Growth of the aorta after prosthetic patch aortoplasty for coarctation in infants. Ann. Thorac. Surg. 38:21, 1984.

Sade, R. M., Rosenthal, A., Fellows, K., and Castaneda, R.: Pulmonary artery sling. J. Thorac. Cardiovasc. Surg., 69:333, 1975.

Sade, R. M., Taylor, A. B., and Chariker, E. P.: Aortoplasty compared with resection for coarctation of the aorta in young children. Ann. Thorac. Surg., 28:346, 1979.

Sadow, S. H., Synhorst, D. P., and Pappas, G.: Taussig-Bing anomaly and coarctation of the aorta in infancy: Surgical options. Pediatr. Cardiol., 6:83, 1985.

Sahn, D. J., Allen, H. D., McDonald, G., and Goldberg, S. J.: Real-time cross-sectional echocardiographic diagnosis of coarctation of the aorta. Circulation, 56:762, 1977.

Sahn, D. J., Valdes-Cruz, L. M., Ovitt, T. W., and Pond, G.: Two-dimensional echocardiography and intravenous digital video subtraction angiography for diagnosis and evaluation of double aortic arch. Am. J. Cardiol., 50:342, 1982.

Samanek, M., Goetzova, J., Fiserova, J., and Svovranek, J.: Differences in muscle blood flow in upper and lower extremities of patients after correction of coarctation of the aorta. Circulation, 54:377, 1976.

Sampath, R., O'Connor, W. N., Noonan, J. A., and Todd, E. P.: Management of ascending aortic aneurysm complicating coarctation of the aorta. Ann. Thorac. Surg., 34:125, 1982.

Sanchez, G. R., Balsara, R. K., Dunn, J. M., et al: Recurrent obstruction after subclavian flap repair of coarctation of the aorta in infants. J. Thorac. Cardiovasc. Surg., 91:738, 1986.

Sanger, P. W., Taylor, F. H., Robicsek, F., and Najib, A.: Aortic origin of the right pulmonary artery with patent ductus arteriosus. Ann. Thorac. Surg., 1:179, 1965.

Santos, M. A., Moll, J. N., Drumond, C., et al: Development of the ductus arteriosus in right ventricular outflow tract obstruction. Circulation, 62:818, 1980.

Saul, J. P., Keane, J. F., Fellows, K. E., and Lock, J. E.: Balloon dilatation angioplasty of postoperative aortic obstructions. Am. J. Cardiol., 59:943, 1987.

Scheid, P.: Missbildung des tracheal skelettes un der linken arteria pulmonalis mit erstickangstad bei 2 monate alten Kind. Z. Path., 52:114, 1938.

Schlamowitz, S. T., diGiorgi, S., and Gensini, G. G.: Left aortic arch and right descending aorta. Am. J. Cardiol., 10:132, 1962.

Schmacher, G., Schreiber, R., Meisner, H., et al: Interrupted aortic arch: Natural history and operative results. Pediatr. Cardiol., 7:89, 1986.

Schuster, S. R., and Gross, R. E.: Surgery for coarctation of the aorta: A review of 500 cases. J. Thorac. Cardiovasc. Surg., 43:54, 1962.

Scott, H. W., and Sabiston, D. C., Jr.: Surgical treatment for congenital aorticopulmonary fistula. J. Thorac. Surg., 25:26, 1953.

Scott, H. W., Jr., and Bahnson, H. T.: Evidence for a renal factor in the hypertension of experimental coarctation of the aorta. Surgery, 30:206, 1951.

Scott, H. W., Jr., Dean, R. H., Boerth, R., et al: Coarctation of the abdominal aorta. Ann. Surg., 189:746, 1979.

Scott, W. A., Rocchini, A. P., Bove, E. L., et al: Repair of interrupted aortic arch in infancy. J. Thorac. Cardiovasc. Surg., 96:564, 1988.

Sealy, W. C.: Coarctation of the aorta and hypertension. Ann. Thorac. Surg., 3:15, 1967.

Sealy, W. C.: Indications for surgical treatment of coarctation of the aorta. Surg. Gynecol. Obstet., 97:301, 1953.

Sealy, W. C., DeMaria, W., and Harris, J.: Studies of the development and nature of the hypertension in experimental coarctation of the aorta. Surg. Gynecol. Obstet., 97:193, 1950.

Sealy, W. C., Harris, J. S., Young, W. G., Jr., and Callaway, H. A.: Paradoxical hypertension following resection of coarctation of aorta. Surgery, 42:135, 1957.

Sealy, W. C., Panijayanond, P., Alexander, J., and Seaber, A. V.: Activity of plasma angiotension II in experimental coarctation of the aorta. J. Thorac. Cardiovasc. Surg., 65:283, 1973.

Sehested, J., Baandrup, U., and Mikkelsen, E.: Different reactivity and structure of the prestenotic and poststenotic aorta in human coarctation. Circulation, 65:1060, 1982.

Sell, J. E., Jonas, R. A. Mayer, J. E., et al: The results of a surgical program for interrupted aortic arch. J. Thorac. Cardiovasc. Surg., 96:864, 1988

Seidel, J. F.: Inedx Musei Anatomici Killiensis. C. F. Mohr, 1818, p. 61.

Shaddy, R. E., Snider, A. R., Silverman, R. H., and Lutin, W.: Pulsed Doppler findings in patients with coarctation of the aorta. Circulation, 73:82, 1986.

Shannon, J. M.: Aberrant right subclavian artery with Kommerell's diverticulum: Report of a case. J. Thorac. Cardiovasc. Surg., 41:408, 1961.

Shapiro, M. J., and Keys, A.: The prognosis of untreated patent ductus arteriosus and the results of surgical intervention. Am. J. Med. Sci., 206:174, 1943.

Shearer, W. T., Rutman, J. Y., Weinberg, W. A., and Goldring, D.: Coarctation of the aorta and cerebrovascular accident: A proposal for early corrective surgery. J. Pediatr., 77:1004, 1970.

Shepherd, S. G., Park, F. R., and Kitchell, J. R.: A case of aortopulmonic communication incident to a congenital aortic septal defect: Discussion of embryologic changes involved. Am. Heart J., 27:733, 1944.

Shinebourne, E. A., and Elseed, A. M.: Relation between fetal flow patterns, coarctation of the aorta, and pulmonary blood flow. Br. Heart J., 36:492, 1974.

Shone, J. D., Sellers, R. D., Anderson, R. C., et al: The developmental complex of "parachute mitral valve" supravalvular ring of left atrium, subaortic stenosis, and coarctation of aorta. Am. J. Cardiol., 11:714, 1963.

Shuford, W. H., Sybers, R. G., and Edwards, F. K.: The three types of right aortic arch. Am. Heart J., 109:67, 1970.

Shuford, W. H., Sybers, R. G., and Schlant, R. C.: Right aortic arch with isolation of the left subclavian artery. Am. Heart J., 109:75, 1970.

Shuford, W. H., Sybers, R. G., and Schlant, R. C.: Subclavian steal syndrome in right aortic arch with isolation of the left subclavian artery. Am. Heart J., 82:98, 1971.

Shumway, N. E., and Lewis, F. J.: The closure of experimental aortic septal defects under direct vision and hypothermia. Surgery, 39:604, 1956.

Silver, M. M., Freedom, R. M., Silver, M. D., and Olley, P. M.: The morphology of the human newborn ductus arteriosus. Hum. Pathol., 12:1123, 1981.

Silverman, N. H., Lewis, A. B., Heymann, M. A., and Rudolph, A. M.: Echocardiographic assessment of ductus arteriosus shunt in premature infants. Circulation, 50:821, 1974.

Simon, A. B., and Zloto, A. E.: Coarctation of the aorta: Longitudinal assessment of operated patients. Circulation, 50:456, 1974.

Sinha, S. N., Kardatzke, M. L., Cole, R. B., et al: Coarctation of the aorta in infancy. Circulation, 40:385, 1969.

Sirak, H. D., Ressahat, M., Hosier, D. M., and Delorimer, A. A.: A new operation for repairing aortic arch atresia in infancy: Report of 3 cases. Circulation, 37:II43, 1968.

Smallhorn, J. F., Anderson, R. H., and MacCartney, F. J.: Two-dimensional echocardiographic assessment of communications between ascending aorta and pulmonary trunk or individual pulmonary arteries. Br. Heart J., 47:563, 1982.

Smith, R. T., Jr., Sade, R. M., Riopel, D. A., et al: Stress testing for comparison of synthetic patch aortoplasty with resection and end-to-end anastomosis for repair of coarctation in childhood. J. Am. Coll. Cardiol., 4:765, 1984.

Smyth, P. T., and Edwards, J. E.: Pseudocoarctation, kinking, or buckling of the aorta. Circulation, 46:1027, 1972.

Souclers, C R., Pearson, C. M., and Adams, H. D.: An aortic deformity simulating mediastinal tumor: A subclinical form of coarctation. Dis. Chest, 20:35, 1951.

Soulen, R. L., Kan, J., Mitchell, S., and White, R. I., Jr.: Evaluation of balloon angioplasty of coarctation restenosis by magnetic resonance imaging. Am. J. Cardiol., 60:343, 1987.

Sperling, D. R., Dorsey, T. J., Rowen, M., and Gazzaniga, A. B.: Percutaneous transluminal angioplasty of congenital coarctation of the aorta. Am. J. Cardiol., 51:562, 1983.

Sprong, D. H., and Cutler, N. L.: A case of human right aorta. Anat. Rec., 45:366, 1930.

Stauffer, H. M., and Pote, H. H.: Anomalous right subclavian artery originating on the left as the last branch of the aortic arch. Am. J. Roentgenol., 56:13, 1946.

Steele, J. M.: Evidence for general distribution of peripheral resistance in coarctation of the aorta: Report of three cases. J. Clin. Invest., 20:473, 1941.

Steidele, R. V.: Chir. Med. Beob. Vienna., 2:114, 1778.

Steinberg, I.: Anomalous (nonconstricting) left pulmonary artery. Circulation, 29:897, 1964.

Stevenson, J. G.: Fluid administration in the association of patent ductus arteriosus complicating respiratory distress syndrome. J. Pediatr., 90:257, 1977.

Stone, D. N., Bein, M. E., and Garris, J. B.: Anomalous left pulmonary artery: Two new adult cases. A.J.R., 135:1259, 1980.

Strange, M. J., Myers, G., Kirklin, J. K., et al: Surgical closure of patent ductus arteriosus does not increase the risk of intraventricular hemorrhage in the preterm infant. J. Pediatr., 107:602, 1985.

Sturm, J. T., vanHeeckeren, D. W., and Borkat, G.: Surgical treatment of interrupted aortic arch in infancy with expanded polytetrafluoroethylene grafts. J. Thorac. Cardiovasc. Surg., 81:245, 1981.

Sweeney, M. S., Walker, W. E., Duncan, J. M., et al: Reoperation for aortic coarctation: Techniques, results, and indications for various approaches. Ann. Thorac. Surg., 40:48, 1985.

Sweet, R. H., Findlay, C. W., Jr., and Reyersbach, C. G.: The diagnosis and treatment of tracheal and esophageal obstruction due to congenital vascular ring. J. Pediatr., 30:1, 1947.

Swensson, R. E., Valdes-Criz, L. M., Sahn, D. J., and Sherman, F. S.: Real-time Doppler color flow mapping for detection of patent ductus arteriosus. J. Am. Coll. Cardiol., 8:1105, 1986.

Symbas, P. N., Shuford, W. H., Edwards, F. K., and Sehdeva, J. S.: Vascular ring: Persistent right aortic arch, patent proximal left arch, obliterated distal left arch, and left ligamentum arteriosum. J. Thorac. Cardiovasc. Surg., 61:149, 1971.

Tabak, C., Moskowitz, W., Wagner, H., et al: Aortopulmonary window and aortic isthmic hypoplasia. J. Thorac. Cardiovasc. Surg., 86:273, 1983.

Talner, N. S., and Berman, M. A.: Postnatal development of obstruction in coarctation of the aorta: Role of the ductus arteriosus. Pediatrics, 56:562, 1975.

Tandon, R., da Silva, C. L., Moller, J. H., and Edwards, J. E.: Aorticopulmonary septal defect coexisting with ventricular septal defect. Circulation, 50:188, 1974.

Tawes, R. L., Jr., Aberdeen, E., Waterston, D. J., and Carter, R. E. B.: Coarctation of the aorta in infants and children: A review of 333 operative cases, including 179 infants. Circulation, 39 and 40:173, 1969.

Tawes, R. L., Jr., Bull, J. D., and Roe, B. B.: Hypertension and abdominal pain after resection of aortic coarctation. Ann. Surg., 171:409, 1979.

Tawes, R. L., Jr., Panogopoulos, P., Aberdeen, E., et al: Aortic arch atresia and interruption of the aortic arch: Experience in 11 cases of operation. J. Thorac. Cardiovasc. Surg., 58:492, 1969.

Taylor, R. L., Grover, F. L., Harman, P. K., et al: Operative closure of patent ductus arteriosus in premature infants in the neonatal intensive care unit. Am. J. Surg., 152:704, 1986.

Tesler, U. F., Balsara, R. H., and Niguidula, F. N.: Aberrant left pulmonary artery (vascular sling): Report of five cases. Chest, 66:4, 1974.

Thibault, W. N., Sperling, D. R., and Gazzaniga, A. B.: Subclavian artery patch angioplasty: Treatment of infants and young children with aorta coarctation. Arch. Surg., 110:1095, 1975.

Thibeault, D. W., Emmanouilides, G. C., Nelson, R. J., et al: Patent ductus arteriosus complicating the respiratory distress syndrome in preterm infants. J. Pediatr., *86*:120, 1975.

Timmis, G. C., and Gordon, S.: A renal factor in hypertension due to coarctation of the aorta. N. Engl. J. Med., *270*:814, 1964.

Tiraboschi, R., Salomone, G., Crupi, G., et al: Aortopulmonary window in the first year of life: Report on 11 surgical cases. Ann. Thorac. Surg., *46*:438, 1988.

Todd, P. J., Dangerfield, P. H., Hamilton, D. I., and Wilkinson, J. L.: Late effects on the left upper limb of subclavian flap aortoplasty. J. Thorac. Cardiovasc. Surg., *85*:678, 1983.

Touroff, A. S. W., and Vesell, H.: Subacute *Streptococcus viridans* endarteritis complicating patent ductus arteriosus. J.A.M.A., *115*:1270, 1940.

Traugott, R. C., Will, R. J., Schuchmann, G. F., and Treasure, R. L.: A simplified method of ligation of patent ductus arteriosus in premature infants. Ann. Thorac. Surg., *29*:263, 1980.

Trinquet, F., Vouhe, P. R., Vernant, F., et al: Coarctation of the aorta in infants: Which operation? Ann. Thorac. Surg., *45*:186, 1988.

Trusler, G. A., and Izukawa, T.: Interrupted aortic arch and ventricular septal defect. J. Thorac. Cardiovasc. Surg., *69*:125, 1975.

Tsuji, H., Shapiro, M., Magidson, O., et al: Surgical treatment of high-pressure patent ductus arteriosus. Circulation, *27*:652, 1963.

Turley, K., Yee, E. S., and Ebert, P. A.: The total repair of interrupted arch complex in infants: The anterior approach. Circulation, *70*:16, 1984.

Tyson, K. R., Harris, L. C., and Nghiem, Q. X.: Repair of aortic arch interruption in the neonate. Surgery, *67*:1006, 1970.

Ungerleider, R. M., and Ebert, P. E.: Indications and techniques for midline approach to aortic coarctation in infants and children. Ann. Thorac. Surg., *44*:517, 1987.

Vaccaro, P. S., Myers, J. C., and Smead, W. L.: Surgical correction of abdominal aortic coarctation and hypertension. J. Vasc. Surg., *3*:643, 1986.

van der Horst, R., Fisher, E. A., DuBrow, I. W., and Hastreiter, A. R.: Right aortic arch, right patent ductus arteriosus, and mirror-image branching of the brachiocephalic vessels. Cardiovasc. Radiol., *1*:147, 1978.

Van Mierop, L. H. S., and Kutsche, L. M.: Cardiovascular anomalies in DiGeorge syndrome and importance of neural crest as a possible pathogenetic factor. Am. J. Cardiol., *58*:133, 1986.

Van Mierop, L. H. S., and Kutsche, L. M.: Interruption of the aortic arch and coarctation of the aorta: Pathogenetic relations. Am. J. Cardiol., *54*:829, 1984.

Van Praagh, R., Bernard, W. F., Rosenthal, A., et al: Interrupted aortic arch: Surgical treatment. Am. J. Card., *27*:200, 1971.

Van Way, C. W., Michelakis, A. M., Anderson, W. J., et al: Studies of plasma renin activity in coarctation of the aorta. Ann. Surg., *183*:229, 1975.

Ventemiglia, R., Oglietti, J., Wukasch, D. C., et al: Interruption of the aortic arch: Surgical considerations. J. Thorac. Cardiovasc. Surg., *72*:235, 1976.

Verska, J. J., De Quattro, V., and Woolley, M. M.: Coarctation of the aorta: The abdominal pain syndrome and paradoxical hypertension. J. Thorac. Cardiovasc. Surg., *58*:746, 1969.

Vlodaver, Z., and Neufeld, H. N.: Coronary arteries in coarctation of the aorta. Circulation, *37*:449, 1968.

Vogel, M., Freedom, R. M. Smallhorn, J. F., et al: Complete transposition of the great arteries of coarctation of the aorta. Am. J. Cardiol., *53*:1627, 1984.

von Schulthess, G. K., Higashino, S. M., Higgins, S. S., et al: Coarctation of the aorta: MR imaging. Radiology, *158*:469, 1986.

Vossschulte, K.: Surgical correction of coarctation of the aorta by an "isthmusplastic" operation. Thorax, *16*:338, 1961.

Vouhe, P. R., Trinquet, F., Lecompte, Y., et al: Aortic coarctation with hypoplastic aortic arch: Results of extended end-to-end aortic arch anastomosis. J. Thorac. Cardiovasc. Surg., *96*:557, 1988.

Wagenvoort, C. A., Neufeld, H. N., Birge, R. F., et al: Origin of right pulmonary artery from ascending aorta. Circulation, *23*:84, 1961.

Wagner, H. R., Ellison, R. C., Zierler, S., et al: Surgical closure of patent ductus arteriosus in 268 preterm infants. J. Thorac. Cardiovasc. Surg., *87*:870, 1984.

Waldhausen, J. A., King, H., Nahrwold, D. L., et al: Management of coarctation in infancy. J.A.M.A., *187*:270, 1964.

Waldhausen, J. A., and Nahrwold, D. L.: Repair of coarctation of the aorta with a subclavian flap. J. Thorac. Cardiovasc. Surg., *51*:532, 1966.

Waldhausen, J. A., Whitman, V., Werner, J. C., and Pierce, W. S.: Surgical intervention in infants with coarctation of the aorta. J. Thorac. Cardiovasc. Surg., *81*:323, 1981.

Waldman, J. D., Goodman, A. H., Lamberti, J. J., and Turner, S. W.: Coarctation of the aorta. J. Thorac. Cardiovasc. Surg., *80*:187, 1980.

Waldman, J. D., Lamberti, J. J., Goodman, A. H., et al: Coarctation in the first year of life: Patterns of postoperative effect. J. Thorac. Cardiovasc. Surg., *86*:9, 1983.

Wallace, R. B., and Nast, E. P.: Postcoarctation mycotic intercostal arterial pseudoaneurysm. Am. J. Cardiol., *59*:1014, 1987.

Warren, J., Smith, R. S., and Naik, R. B.: Inappropriate renin secretion and abnormal cardiovascular reflexes in coarctation of the aorta. Br. Heart J., *45*:733, 1981.

Webb, W. R., and Burford, T. H.: Gangrene of the arm following use of the subclavian artery in a pulmonosystemic (Blalock) anastomosis. J. Thorac. Surg., *23*:199, 1952.

Weesner, K. M., Dillard, R. G., Boyle, R. J., and Block, S. M.: Prophylactic treatment of asymptomatic patent ductus arteriosus in premature infants with respiratory distress syndrome. South. Med. J., *80*:706, 1987.

Weisman, D., and Kesten, H. D.: Absence of the transverse aortic arch with defects of cardiac septums: Report of a case simulating acute abdominal disease in a newborn infant. Am. J. Dis. Child., *76*:326, 1948.

Welsh, T. M., and Munro, I. B.: Congenital stridor caused by an aberrant pulmonary artery. Arch. Dis. Child., *29*:101, 1954.

Werning, C., Schoenbeck, M., Weidmann, P., et al: Plasma renin activity in patients with coarctation of the aorta. Circulation, *50*:731, 1969.

Wernly, J. A., and Ameriso, J. L.: Intra-aortic closure of the calcified patent ductus. J. Thorac. Cardiovasc. Surg., *80*:206, 1980.

Wessel, D. L., Keane, J. F., Parness, I., and Lock, J. E.: Outpatient closure of the patent ductus arteriosus. Circulation, *77*:1068, 1988.

White, P. D., Mazurkie, S. J., and Boschetti, A. E.: Patency of the ductus arteriosus at 90. N. Engl. J. Med., *280*:146, 1969.

Whitman, G., Stephenson, L. W., and Weinberg, P.: Vascular ring: Left cervical aortic arch, right descending aorta, and right ligamentum arteriosum. J. Thorac. Cardiovasc. Surg., *83*:311, 1982.

Wielenga, G., and Dankmeijer, J.: Coarctation of the aorta. J. Pathol. Bacteriol., *95*:265, 1986.

Wierny, L., Plass, R., and Porstmann, W.: Transluminal closure of patent ductus arteriosus: Long-term results of 208 cases treated without thoracotomy. Cardiovasc. Intervent. Radiol., *9*:279, 1986.

Wilcox, B. R., and Croom, R. D., III: Aortic origin of the right pulmonary artery. Ann. Thorac. Surg., *5*:165, 1968.

Wilkerson, S. A., Feischaker, J., Mavroudis, C., and Cook, L. N.: Developmental sequelae in premature infants undergoing ligation of patent ductus arteriosus. Ann. Thorac. Surg., *39*:542, 1985.

Will, R. J., Walker, O. M., Traugott, R. C., and Treasure, R. L.: Sodium nitroprusside and propranolol therapy for management of postcoarctectomy hypertension. J. Thorac. Cardiovasc. Surg., *75*:722, 1978.

Williams, R. G., Jaffe, R. B., Condon, V. R., and Nixon, G. W.: Unusual features of pulmonary sling. A.J.R., *133*:1065, 1979.

Williams, W. G., Shindo, G., Trusler, G. A., et al: Results of repair of coarctation of the aorta during infancy. J. Thorac. Cardiovasc. Surg., *79*:603, 1980.

Wittenborg, M. H., Tantiwongse, T., and Rosenberg, B. F.: Anomalous course of left pulmonary artery with respiratory obstruction. Radiology, *67*:339, 1956.

Wolfe, W. G., Anderson, R. W., and Sealy, W. C.: Hyperlucent lung: Pathophysiology and surgical management. Ann. Thorac. Surg., 18:172, 1974.

Wolman, I. J.: Syndrome of constricting double aortic arch in infancy. J. Pediatr., 14:527, 1939.

Wolman, I. J.: Congenital stenosis of the trachea. Am. J. Dis. Child., 61:1231, 1941.

Woodruff, W. W., III, Gabliani, G., and Grant, A. O.: Patent ductus arteriosus in the elderly. South. Med. J., 76:1436, 1983.

Wright, J. S., Freeman, R., and Johnston, J. B.: Aorto-pulmonary fenestration: A technique of surgical management. J. Thorac. Cardiovasc. Surg., 55:280, 1968.

Wright, J. S., and Newman, D. C.: Ligation of the patent ductus: Technical considerations at different ages. J. Thorac. Cardiovasc. Surg., 75:695, 1978.

Wychulis, A. R., Kincaid, O. W., Weidman, W. H., and Danielson, G. K.: Congenital vascular ring: Surgical considerations and results of operation. Mayo Clin. Proc., 46:182, 1971.

Yasui, H., Kado, H., Nakano, E., et al: Primary repair of interrupted aortic arch and severe aortic stenosis in neonates. J. Thorac. Cardiovasc. Surg., 93:539, 1987.

Yee, E. S., Turley, K., Soifer, S., and Ebert, P. A.: Synthetic patch aortoplasty. Am. J. Surg., 148:240, 1984.

Yeh, T. F., Goldbarg, H. R., Henek, T., et al: Intravenous indo-methacin therapy in premature infants with patent ductus arteriosus. Am. J. Dis. Child., 136:803, 1982.

Yeh, T. F., Luken, J. A., Thalji, A., et al: Intravenous indomethacin therapy in premature infants with persistent ductus arteriosus—a double-blind controlled study. J. Pediatr., 98:137, 1981.

Yeh, T. F., Wilks, A., Luken, J., and Pildes, R. S.: Indomethacin therapy in premature infants with patent ductus arteriosus and oliguria. Dev. Pharmacol. Ther., 9:369, 1986.

Young, M. W., Lau, S. H., Stein, E., and Damato, A. N.: Pseudocoarctation of the aorta. Am. Heart J., 77:259, 1969.

Zahka, K. G., Roland, J. M., Cutilletta, A. F., et al: Management of aortic arch interruption with prostaglandin E₁ infusion and microporous expanded polytetrafluoroethylene grafts. Am. J. Cardiol., 46:1001, 1980.

Zielinsky, P., Rossi, M., Haertel, J. C., et al: Subaortic fibrous ridge and ventricular septal defect: Role of septal malalignment. Circulation, 75:1124, 1987.

Ziemer, G., Jonas, R. A., Perry, S. B., et al: Surgery for coarctation of the aorta in the neonate. Circulation, 74(Suppl. I):25, 1986.

Zumbro, G. L., Treasure, R. L., and Geiger, J. P.: Respiratory obstruction in the newborn associated with increased volume and opacification of the hemithorax. Ann. Thorac. Surg., 18:622, 1974.

III ANEURYSMS OF THE SINUSES OF VALSALVA

William L. Holman

The three sinuses of Valsalva are slight protuberances in the aortic root that arise immediately distal to the aortic valve. The sinuses of Valsalva are named either by their anatomic position (anterior, left posterior, and right posterior) or, more commonly, according to the coronary artery ostia that arise from the sinuses of Valsalva (right, left, and noncoronary). The first description of aneurysmal enlargement of a sinus of Valsalva with intracardiac rupture has been attributed to Hope (1839). Subsequently, Thurnam (1840) published a series of six cases including the one described by Hope and noted the importance of the anatomic relationship of these aneurysms to the chambers of the heart. The syphilitic etiology of sinus of Valsalva aneurysms was initially emphasized (Smith, 1914); however, the work of Abbott (1919) clearly established a congenital cause of sinus of Valsalva aneurysms. Abbott's concept of the congenital cause was subsequently furthered by Edwards and Burchell (1957), who histologically demonstrated the deficiency of elastic and muscular tissue at the site of congenital sinus of Valsalva aneurysms, and by Sakakibara and Konno (1962), who developed a classification system for congenital sinus of Valsalva aneurysms.

The advent of invasive cardiac diagnostic procedures and the development of cardiac surgical procedures in the first half of the 20th century led eventually to successful operative treatment of sinus of Valsalva aneurysms. Ingenious methods were devised for the direct closure of ruptured sinus of Valsalva aneurysms using hypothermia with inflow occlusion (Bigelow and Barnes, 1959; Morrow et al, 1957); however, the open approach supported by extracorporeal circulation as first described by McGoon and associates (1958) and by Lillehei and colleagues (1957) eventually became the accepted method of treatment.

ANATOMY, PATHOPHYSIOLOGY, AND NATURAL HISTORY

An aneurysm of the sinus of Valsalva represents the pathologic enlargement of the sinus into a thin-walled sac. The aneurysm may be entirely asymptomatic or it can produce symptoms by becoming infected, impinging on adjacent structures, or rupturing. The sinuses of Valsalva lie immediately distal to the aortic valve and its annulus within the aortic root (Sud et al, 1984). The right and left coronary arteries arise from the corresponding sinus of Valsalva before the narrowing of the sinuses distally to form the ascending aorta. The sinuses of Valsalva lie in a central region of the heart, and a consideration of the anatomic relations of the aortic root (Figs. 33–24 and 33–25) is crucial to the subsequent understanding of the pathophysiology associated with sinus of Valsalva aneursyms, as well as their operative treatment.

Sinus of Valsalva aneurysms are fairly rare, being described in 7 of 8,138 autopsies (Smith, 1914) and in 0.43 and 0.14% of open heart operations done at

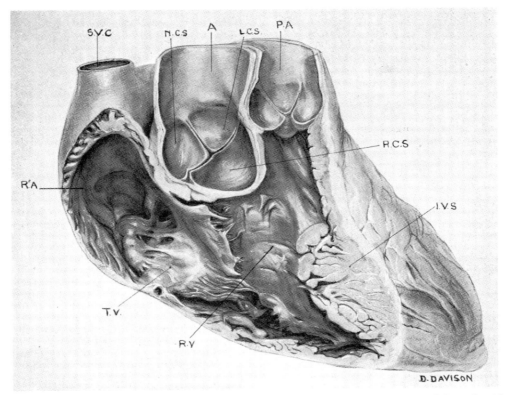

Figure 33–24. The relationship of the sinuses of Valsalva within the aortic root to the structures of the right side of the heart is shown. The anatomic distribution of fistulas resulting from the intracardiac rupture of sinus of Valsalva aneurysms can be understood by studying these anatomic relationships. (SVC = superior vena cava, RA = right atrium, TV = tricuspid valve, RV = right ventricle, NCS = noncoronary sinus, RCS = right coronary sinus, LCS = left coronary sinus, A = aorta, PA = pulmonary artery, IVS = intraventricular septum.) (From Jones, A. M., and Langley, F. A.: Aortic sinus aneurysms. Br. Heart J., *11*:325, 1949.)

two major cardiac surgical centers (Henze et al, 1983; Meyer et al, 1975). The variations in the anatomy of congenital and acquired sinus of Valsalva aneurysms derive from their different causes. Congenital aneurysms are due to a deficiency or absence of muscular and elastic tissue at the base of the aorta, which was shown earlier by Edwards and Burchell (Fig. 33–26). This structural deficiency may be related to an abnormality in the development of the distal bulbar septum (Abbott, 1919), a concept that is strengthened by the frequent (30 to 60%) association of ventricular septal defects and congenital sinus of Valsalva aneurysms (Bonfils-Roberts et al, 1971; Chih et al, 1981; Nowicki et al, 1977). The frequency of congenital aneurysms of the sinus of Valsalva is therefore highest in the right coronary cusp, because this cusp abuts the largest portion of the septum. There is less frequent occurrence in the noncoronary cusp, and only rare congenital aneurysms are reported in the left coronary cusp (Jones and Langley, 1949; Meyer et al, 1975; Nowicki et al, 1977) (Table 33–1). The anatomic classification system established by Sakakibara and Konno (1963) defines congenital sinus of Valsalva aneurysms according to their exact position relative to each aortic valve cusp. Direct extension of aneurysms from the left or midportion of the right coronary sinus (Types I and II) direct the aneurysm into the right ventricle (see Figs. 33–24 and 33–25), whereas an aneurysm originating in the right portion

of the right coronary sinus may penetrate either the right atrium or the right ventricle (Types III to V and III-A). Aneurysms from the noncoronary sinus (Type IV) extend into the right atrium immediately above the septal leaflet of the tricuspid valve. The rare left coronary sinus aneurysms were not classified by Sakakibara and Konno, but have been reported to pass into the right atrium, right ventricle, left atrium, and left ventricle. In addition to ventricular septal defects, other congenital cardiac lesions less commonly associated with sinus of Valsalva aneurysms include aortic valve abnormalities (prolapsing cusp, bicuspid valve, or other valve deformity) in approximately 10% of patients, and rarely pulmonary stenosis or regurgitation, atrial septal defects, or a patent ductus arteriosus (Bonfils-Roberts et al, 1971; Chih et al, 1981; Nowicki et al, 1977).

Acquired sinus of Valsalva aneurysms can be caused by several pathologic processes, including luetic degeneration (Smith, 1914), bacterial endocarditis (Bardy et al, 1982; Qizilbash, 1974; Shumacker, 1972), trauma (Morris et al, 1958), cystic medial necrosis (DeBakey et al, 1967), and atherosclerosis (DeBakey and Lawrie, 1979). The acquired aneurysms are more evenly distributed between the three sinuses, with 44% of reported cases arising from the right coronary sinus, 23% from the noncoronary sinus, 23% from the left coronary sinus, and 10% from multiple sinuses. Compared with those of con-

Back

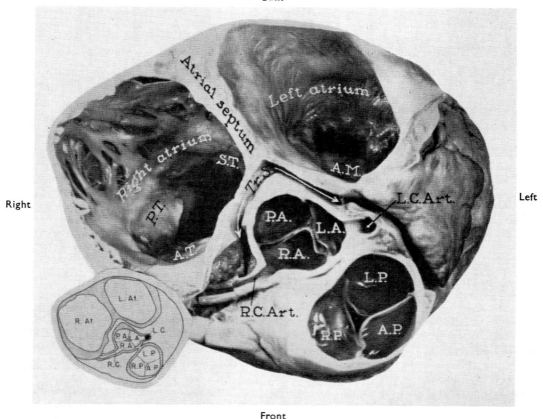

Right

Left

Front

Figure 33–25. On coronal section, the aortic root is seen within the central portion of the heart. The relationship of the sinuses of Valsalva to the right and left main coronary arteries is also emphasized. (PT, ST, AT = posterior, septal, and anterior tricuspid leaflets; AM = anterior mitral leaflet; TrS = transverse sinus; RA, PA, LA = right, posterior and left aortic valve leaflets; LCArt = left main coronary artery; RCArt = right coronary artery; AP, RP, LP = anterior, right, and left pulmonary valve leaflets.) (From Edwards, J. E., and Burchell, H. B.: The pathological anatomy of deficiencies between the aortic root and the heart, including aortic sinus aneurysms. Thorax, 12:125, 1957.)

genital origin, the acquired aneurysms tend to occupy more extensive regions of the aortic root and, as mentioned earlier, may involve multiple sinuses of Valsalva and even the ascending aorta. Compared with congenital aneurysms, the site of the acquired aneurysmal rupture is less frequently intracardiac (26% of reported cases) and is more often a catastrophic hemorrhage into the pericardium, pleural space, or externally (13% of reported cases) (DeBakey and Lawrie, 1979; Jones et al, 1949; Qizilbash, 1974).

Most patients with unruptured sinus of Valsalva aneurysms are asymptomatic, and diagnosis is made incidentally after diagnostic tests are done to evaluate other cardiac disorders. However, unruptured aneurysms may produce symptoms when infected (Abbott, 1919) or with impingement on other structures. Aneurysmal extension into the right ventricular outflow tract may produce obstruction (Desai et al, 1985; Warnes et al, 1984), and extension into the ventricular septum can cause medically refractory ventricular tachycardia (Raizes et al, 1979) or other conduction abnormalities (Heydorn et al, 1976; Mayer et al, 1986). Enlargement of the sinus and intramural thrombus formation can result in deformation or obstruction of

the left or right coronary arteries at their ostia, which then leads to myocardial ischemia (Hiyamuta et al, 1983) or infarction (Brandt et al, 1985; Faillace et al, 1985).

Expansion of a sinus of Valsalva aneurysm into an adjacent cardiac chamber may also be followed by rupture of the aneurysm. On gross inspection, this communication may appear either as a simple fistulous tract or as a thin-walled wind sock protrusion into a cardiac chamber with distal perforation of the wind sock (Fig. 33–27). The fistulous tract formed after aneurysmal rupture allows blood to flow from the aorta into the affected cardiac chamber, and if the recipient chamber is the right atrium, right ventricle, or pulmonary artery, a net left-to-right shunting of blood occurs. As well described by Morch and Greenwood (1966), the murmur associated with the most commonly ruptured sinus of Valsalva aneurysms (aorta to right ventricle or right atrium) is a harsh continuous murmur that for diagnostic purposes must be distinguished from the murmur of a patent ductus arteriosus, ventricular septal defect associated with aortic insufficiency, aortopulmonary window, coronary arteriovenous malformation, or

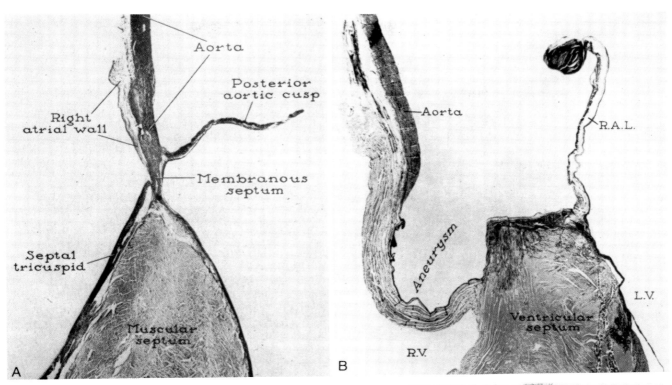

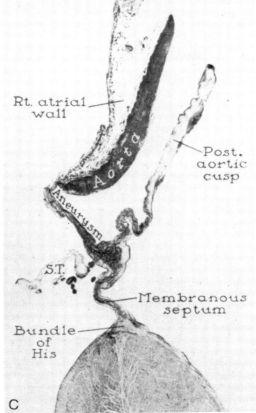

Figure 33–26. *A,* Longitudinal section of a normal heart taken through noncoronary sinus of Valsalva; *B,* Longitudinal section of the heart taken through an aneurysm of the right sinus of Valsalva. Note the attenuated wall of the aneurysm descending along the right side of the ventricular septum toward the right ventricle. (RV = right ventricle, LV = left ventricle, RAL = right aortic valve leaflet.) *C,* Longitudinal section of aorta taken through the noncoronary cusp. A thin-walled sinus of Valsalva aneurysm is protruding into the right atrium immediately above the septal leaflet of the tricuspid valve. (ST = septal leaflet of tricuspid valve; post. aortic cusp = posterior (noncoronary) aortic valve cusp.) (From Edwards, J. E., and Burchell, H. B.: The pathological anatomy of deficiencies between the aortic root and the heart, including aortic sinus aneurysms. Thorax, *12:*125, 1957.)

TABLE 33–1. ANEURYSMS OF THE SINUS OF VALSALVA*

Site of Origin	No. (% of Total)	Non-ruptured	Number of Ruptured Aneurysms†						
			RA	*RV*	*RA + RV*	*LA*	*LV*	*PA*	*Pericardium*
RCS	128 (65%)	13 (10%)	19 (14%)	86 (67%)	2 (2%)	0 (0%)	5 (4%)	2 (2%)	1 (1%)
NCS	54 (28%)	15 (28%)	28 (51%)	7 (13%)	0 (0%)	2 (4%)	1 (2%)	0 (0%)	1 (2%)
LCS	14 (7%)	5 (36%)	4 (29%)	3 (21%)	0 (0%)	1 (7%)	1 (7%)	0 (0%)	0 (0%)

A summary describing the anatomy of both ruptured and nonruptured congenital sinus of Valsalva aneurysms. The number of nonruptured sinus of Valsalva aneurysms is probably underestimated because they are frequently asymptomatic and therefore undetected.

*From Jones, A. M., and Langley, F. A.: Aortic sinus aneurysms. Br. Heart J., *11*:325, 1949; Mayer, E. D., Ruffman, K., Saggau, W., et al: Ruptured aneurysms of the sinus of Valsalva. Ann. Thorac. Surg., *42*:81, 1986; and Nowicki, E. R., Aberdeen, E., Friedman, S., et al: Congenital left aortic sinus–left ventricle fistula and review of aortocardiac fistulas. Ann. Thorac. Surg., *23*:378, 1977.

†Sites of rupture: LA = left atrium; LCS = left coronary sinus; LV = left ventricle; NCS = noncoronary sinus; PA = pulmonary artery; RA = right atrium; RCS = right coronary sinus; RV = right ventricle.

pulmonary arteriovenous malformation. In the classic descriptions, the regurgitation of aortic blood into the heart and left-to-right shunting immediately after the rupture of a sinus of Valsalva aneurysm into the right heart produces acute dyspnea and substernal

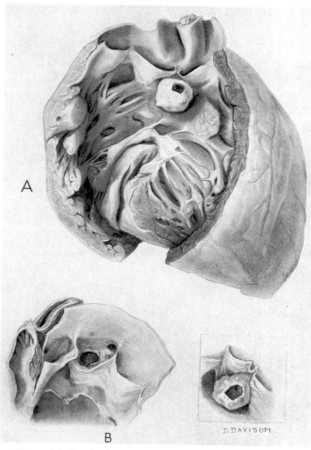

Figure 33–27. *A,* Gross appearance of the ruptured sinus of Valsalva aneurysm lying immediately beneath the pulmonary valve in the right ventricular outflow tract. *B,* Transaortic view of right coronary sinus of Valsalva aneurysm. The *insert* provides a detailed appearance of ruptured sinus of Valsalva aneurysm. (From Jones, A. M., and Langley, F. A.: Aortic sinus aneurysms. Br. Heart J., *11*:325, 1949.)

chest pain often associated with epigastric or right upper quadrant abdominal pain. These acute symptoms are in fact observed in only one-third of patients, whereas half of the patients note the gradual onset of dyspnea, fatigue, chest pain, and peripheral edema over several months or even years. The remainder of patients remain asymptomatic at the time of diagnosis (Bonfils-Roberts et al, 1971; Mayer et al, 1986; Nowicki et al, 1977). On physical examination, the patient with a ruptured sinus of Valsalva aneurysm is most commonly a man (two-thirds of patients) in the third or fourth decade of life (50 to 60% of patients), although infants and elderly patients have been reported. A continuous murmur along the left sternal border is almost always audible (90 to 95% of patients), and in approximately half the patients physical signs of congestive heart failure, including rales, peripheral edema, ascites, and hepatomegaly, are present (Mayer et al, 1986; Nowicki et al, 1977). The natural history of unruptured sinus of Valsalva aneurysms is impossible to define accurately, because most unruptured aneurysms are asymptomatic and probably remain undiagnosed. However, there is at least one report of an asymptomatic congenital sinus of Valsalva aneurysm that was monitored without operative intervention for 19 years (Martin et al, 1986). Rupture of a sinus of Valsalva aneurysm usually produces serious pathologic changes. Extracardiac rupture is generally fatal, although there is a reported survivor of an intrapericardial rupture (Killen et al, 1987). Intracardiac rupture of a sinus of Valsalva aneurysm may produce symptoms that improve spontaneously after the event; however, cardiac decompensation occurs over time, with cardiac failure that is eventually fatal without operative intervention. In addition, the associated problems of bacterial endocarditis and aortic insufficiency due to weakening of the annulus with prolapse of the cusp may occur and cause important additional morbidity and mortality. In patients not operatively treated, the mean survival time after diagnosis of a ruptured sinus of Valsalva aneurysm has been reported to be 3.9 years, although if two unusual patients who survived for 10 and 15 years are excluded from this series of 45 cases, the mean survival time would then be approximately 1 year (Sawyers et al, 1957).

The diagnosis of ruptured sinus of Valsalva aneurysm is generally made by history and physical examination, combined with echocardiography and angiography (Figs. 33–28 and 33–29) to define the precise anatomy of the aneurysm. Some of the points to be considered and clearly defined preoperatively include the following: The ventricular septal defects associated with sinus of Valsalva aneurysms generally lie immediately below the aneurysm. Without careful attention, these ventricular septal defects may not be diagnosed, particularly if the wall of the aneurysm descends to partially occlude the flow through the ventricular septal defect (Sakakibara and Konno, 1963). Aortic valve abnormalities, primarily abnormalities that lead to aortic insufficiency, are common. The degree of aortic insufficiency and an assessment of its effect on left ventricular function are therefore important. The position and patency of the coronary arteries should also be confirmed, particularly in larger aneurysms.

SURGICAL TREATMENT AND RESULTS

The repair of congenital sinus of Valsalva aneurysms may be accomplished by approaching the lesion from either the chamber of origin (i.e., the aorta) or the chamber of termination. The exact approach chosen depends on several factors, including whether the aneurysm has ruptured and whether there is associated aortic valvular insufficiency or a ventricular septal defect. The goal is to close the aneurysm securely and obliterate or excise the aneurysmal sac, while avoiding the creation of aortic valve dysfunction by the placement of sutures or the creation of heart block when closing an associated ventricular septal defect. Standard dual-venous cannulation and aortic cannulation are done, and the left ventricle can be vented via the right superior pulmonary vein. Systemic hypothermia is induced on bypass, then before ventricular fibrillation the aorta is cross-clamped, an aortotomy is created, and hypothermic cardioplegic solution is infused directly into the coronary ostia. If aortic insufficiency is not present and rupture of the aneurysm has not occurred or if the fistula is digitally occluded, then the cardioplegic solution may be infused directly into the aortic root. The aortic valve and annulus are inspected to assess valvular competence and the severity of pathologic changes in the structure of the aortic valve. The ventricular septum is then examined carefully for defects. The position and patency of the coronary artery ostia are also inspected. If the aneurysm is reasonably small and has not ruptured, closure of the aneurysm via a transaortic exposure of the sinus of Valsalva alone is sufficient (Henze et al, 1983; Meyer et al, 1975; Shumacker et al, 1965) (Fig. 33–30). Closure of the aortic aspect of the aneurysm can occasionally be accomplished with interrupted sutures with or without buttressing with Teflon felt.

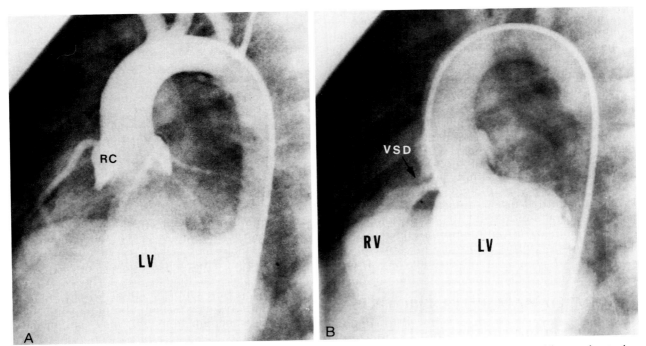

Figure 33–28. *A,* Aortic root injection, left lateral projection of right coronary sinus of Valsalva aneurysm with a moderate degree of aortic insufficiency. *B,* Left ventriculogram in the same patient showing a ventricular septal defect in proximity to the nonruptured sinus of Valsalva aneurysm. (RC = right coronary cusp; LV = left ventricle; RV = right ventricle; VSD = ventricular septal defect.) (Courtesy of Dr. Benigno Soto, University of Alabama at Birmingham.)

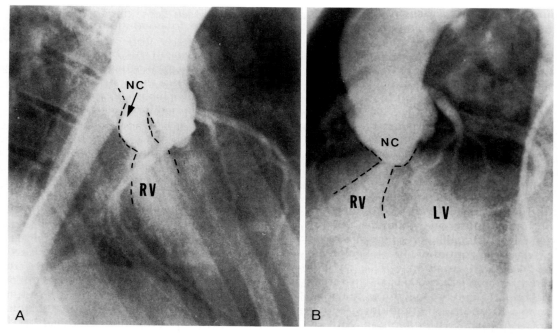

Figure 33–29. *A*, Aortic root injection, right anterior oblique projection during systole showing ruptured noncoronary sinus of Valsalva aneurysm terminating in the right ventricle. *B*, Left anterior oblique projection, aortic root injection during diastole in the same patient showing regurgitation of aortic blood into the right ventricle via the sinus of Valsalva aneurysm, and regurgitation into the left ventricle related to mild aortic insufficiency. (NC = noncoronary cusp; RV = right ventricle; LV = left ventricle.) (Courtesy of Dr. Benigno Soto, University of Alabama at Birmingham.)

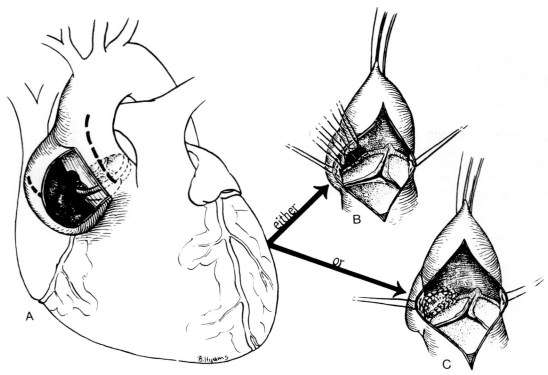

Figure 33–30. Transaortic repair of sinus of Valsalva aneurysm may be accomplished either by direct closure of the mouth of the aneurysm with interrupted sutures or by patching of the orifice of the aneurysm. (Reprinted with permission from The Society of Thoracic Surgeons [The Annals of Thoracic Surgery, Vol. 19, 1975, pp. 170–179].)

However, this closure is best accomplished by using a Dacron patch, possibly with an added layer of pericardium, to avoid deforming the normal coaptation of the aortic valve and to diminish stress on the suture line. If the aneurysm has ruptured, the chamber of termination (usually the right atrium, right ventricle, or pulmonary artery) should also be opened to expose the fistulous tract (Bonfils-Roberts et al, 1971; Chih et al, 1981; DeBakey et al, 1967; Lillehei et al, 1957; Mayer et al, 1986; McGoon et al, 1958). If a wind sock deformity is present, it is excised, and the terminal orifice of the fistula is occluded with sutures or a patch. The ventricular surface is also closely examined for a ventricular septal defect. If one is found, both the sinus of Valsalva aneurysm and the ventricular septal defect orifices may be occluded with a single patch (Fig. 33–31). Transaortic repair of the ventricular septal defect has been reported (Henze et al, 1983); however, because of the risk of injury to the His bundle and the risk of complete heart block, the right-sided approach is usually preferable.

If aortic valve insufficiency due to cusp prolapse is present, the native valve may be salvaged by using the technique of aortic valvuloplasty described by Trusler (1973). If there is other valvular pathology that does not lend itself to correction via this technique, valve replacement by using the standard criteria for aortic valve replacement is done. All valve procedures should be done after the sinus of Valsalva aneurysm repair has been completed. Compared with congenital sinus of Valsalva aneurysms, acquired aneurysms are a more heterogeneous group with regard to etiology and anatomic extent of disease. Sinus of Valsalva aneurysms due to syphilitic degeneration or cystic medial necrosis may be confined to a single sinus, but often the entire aortic root is affected with aneurysmal enlargement of the ascending aorta distally and severe aortic valvular insufficiency proximally. As described by DeBakey and colleagues (1967), some of these lesions can be managed by excision of the aneurysmal region and primary closure or Dacron patching with reimplantation of coronary arteries as necessary (Fig. 33–32). More extensive aneurysms may require replacement of the ascending aorta with a tube graft and coronary reimplantation, or even complete replacement of the aortic root with a composite graft.

Sinus of Valsalva aneurysms due to advanced bacterial endocarditis are often associated with extensive burrowing abscesses and destruction of tissue in the region of the aortic annulus. Debridement with reconstruction of these lesions is usually the only therapeutic option and is attempted despite the attendant risks of reinfection and high operative mortality (Bardy et al, 1982; Qizilbash, 1974; Shumacker, 1972).

Aneurysms of the sinus of Valsalva have been reported in association with both atherosclerotic coronary artery disease and atherosclerotic degeneration of the aorta (DeBakey and Lawrie, 1979). These aneurysms have been managed successfully by excision and patching of the aneurysmal region and coronary artery bypass grafting done in place of coronary reimplantation.

Management of unruptured asymptomatic sinus of Valsalva aneurysms remains an unresolved controversy. The importance of this controversy is increasing as noninvasive cardiac diagnostic procedures become more accurate and widely available. Some experts believe that this subgroup of aneurysms can be monitored by serial observations and contend that if the aneurysm enlarges, ruptures, or begins to cause symptoms related to impingement on adjacent structures, then surgical therapy can be initiated with no additional risk (Martin et al, 1986; Meyer et al, 1975). The one report of a patient successfully monitored for 19 years would support this contention. However, most surgeons reporting sinus of Valsalva aneurysms believe that the risks of correction are acceptable in light of the many serious potential complications of unruptured sinus of Valsalva aneurysms, including right ventricular outflow tract obstruction, infection, malignant arrhythmias, or acute ostial coronary artery obstruction (Faillace et al, 1985; Heydorn et al, 1976; Mayer et al, 1975). When symptoms related to a sinus of Valsalva aneurysm are identified or rupture of the aneurysm has occurred, operative repair is advised. Sinus of Valsalva aneurysms that are discovered incidentally at the time of operation for other cardiac pathology should also be repaired unless specific contraindications exist.

The results of repair reported for a small number of asymptomatic patients are excellent, at least in terms of operative mortality. However, both the short- and long-term results of operative therapy for sinus of Valsalva aneurysms associated with bacterial endocarditis have been poor (Bardy et al, 1982; Qizilbash, 1974; Shumacker, 1972). The early mortality after repair in patients with congenital sinus of Valsalva aneurysms has ranged from zero (Bonfils-Roberts et al, 1971; Mayer et al, 1986), to 10 to 12% (Chih et al, 1981; Nowicki et al, 1977). The perioperative deaths were related primarily to low postoperative cardiac output and often occurred in patients having simultaneous correction of coexisting cardiac anomalies. Longer postoperative follow-up has been reported by several groups (Bonfils-Roberts et al, 1971; Chih et al, 1981; DeBakey et al, 1967; Meyer et al, 1975; Nowicki et al, 1977) and ranges up to 20 years in one series. Recurrence of the aneurysm after repair is rare and has led to death in only one reported case. Persistent improvement in symptoms as determined by assessment of New York Heart Association functional class after closure of a ruptured sinus of Valsalva aneurysm has been shown to occur in 80 to 90% of patients. Late cardiovascular morbidity and mortality are uncommon in these series, but include native valve endocarditis, recurrence of previously repaired ventricular septal defects, and problems associated with prosthetic aortic valve replacement

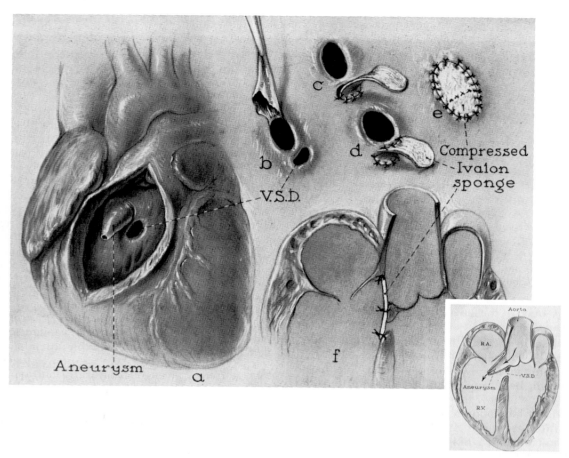

Figure 33–31. A schematic diagram of the right sinus of Valsalva aneurysm, which terminates in the right ventricle (*inset*). *A,* Wind-sock appearance of ruptured sinus of Valsalva aneurysm, which orginates immediately above a ventricular septal defect. *B–F,* Resection of wind-sock with repair of the VSD and sinus of Valsalva aneurysm with a single prosthetic patch. Dacron is the prosthetic material of choice. (VSD = ventricular septal defect; RA = right atrium; RV = right ventricle.) (From McGoon, D. C., Edwards, J. E., and Kirklin, J. W.: Surgical treatment of ruptured aneurysm of aortic sinus. Ann. Surg., *147*:387, 1958.)

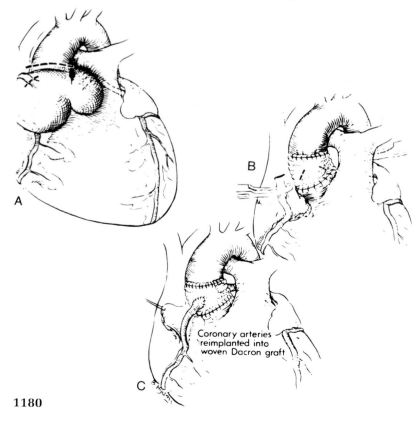

Figure 33–32. *A,* Acquired sinus of Valsalva aneurysm involving multiple sinuses. *B,* Resection of sinuses of Valsalva aneurysm with prosthetic tube graft. *C,* Coronary reimplantation to restore coronary arterial flow. (Reprinted with permission from The Society of Thoracic Surgeons [The Annals of Thoracic Surgery, vol. 19, 1975, pp. 170–179].)

(e.g., thrombosis, dehiscence, infection, degeneration, and embolization). Residual mild-to-moderate postoperative aortic insufficiency during the reported period of follow-up was generally not progressive, although in one case there was progression over a period of 8 years to severe insufficiency requiring valve replacement. In summary, the ultimate prognosis for patients having repair of sinus of Valsalva aneurysms is generally excellent unless their condition is complicated by extensive involvement of the aortic root and ascending aorta, infection, aortic valve dysfunction requiring valve replacement, or impaired ventricular function from chronic aortic insufficiency or other coexisting cardiac disorders.

Selected Bibliography

DeBakey, M. E., Dietrich, E. B., Liddicoat, J. E., et al: Abnormalities of the sinuses of Valsalva. J. Thorac. Cardiovasc. Surg., 54:312, 1967.

This is a summary of the management of 35 patients with sinus of Valsalva aneurysms, both with and without intracardiac fistulas. The clinical features are defined, as are several roentgenographic studies showing sinus of Valsalva aneurysms. The operative methods used on these patients include various procedures on the aortic root and ascending aorta.

Jones, A. M., and Langley, F. A.: Aortic sinus aneurysms. Br. Heart J., 11:325, 1949.

In this beautifully written and illustrated article, the authors define the anatomy of the aortic root as it relates to sinus of Valsalva aneurysms and carefully describe the clinical features and pathophysiology of this condition. The distinction between congenital and acquired sinus of Valsalva aneurysms is emphasized, and a collected review of patients illustrates the natural history of this condition.

Mayer, E. D., Ruffmann, K., Saggau, W., et al: Ruptured aneurysms of the sinus of Valsalva. Ann. Thorac. Surg., 42:81, 1986.

This review of 15 patients treated for both congenital and acquired sinus of Valsalva aneurysms includes a summary of the incidence and clinical features of this disorder. All patients underwent repair, and there were no early or late postoperative deaths. The clinical condition of the patients is described in a follow-up period averaging 7.9 years, with a range of 10 months to 20 years.

Nowicki, E. R., Aberdeen, E., Friedman, S., and Rashkind, W. J.: Congenital left aortic sinus-left ventricle fistula and review of aortocardiac fistulas. Ann. Thorac. Surg., 23:378, 1977.

This review summarizes the findings in 175 cases of aortocardiac fistulas previously published in the English literature from 1839 to 1972. There is an excellent summary of the clinical syndrome resulting from the formation of an aortocardiac fistula, and the principles of operative treatment are well reviewed.

Sakakibara, S., and Konno, S.: Congenital aneurysm of the sinus of Valsalva. Anatomy and classification. Am. Heart J., 63:405, 1962.

The authors draw on their extensive experience, as well as an excellent review of previous literature, to summarize the anatomy of congenital sinus of Valsalva aneurysms and to classify these aneurysms into a system that defines four basic groups. The etiology and development of sinus of Valsalva aneurysms and the relationship of these aneurysms to ventricular septal defects are discussed.

Bibliography

Abbott, M. E.: Clinical and developmental study of a case of ruptured aneurysm of the right anterior aortic sinus of Valsalva, leading to communication between the aorta and base of the right ventricle, diagnosed during life, opening in anterior interventricular septum (probably bulbar septal defect). Malignant endocarditis. In Contributions to Medical and Biological Research. New York, Paul B. Hoeber, 1919, p. 899.

Bardy, G. H., Valenstein, P., Stack, R. S., et al: Two-dimensional echocardiographic identification of sinus of Valsalva–right heart fistula due to infective endocarditis. Am. Heart J., 103:1068, 1982.

Bigelow, W. G., and Barnes, W. T.: Ruptured aneurysm of aortic sinus. Ann. Surg., 150:117, 1959.

Bonfils-Roberts, E. A., DuShane, J. W., McGoon, D. C., et al: Aortic sinus fistula—surgical considerations and results of operation. Ann. Thorac. Surg., 12:492, 1971.

Brandt, J., Jogi, P., and Luhrs, C.: Sinus of Valsalva aneurysm obstructing coronary arterial flow: Case report and collective review of the literature. Eur. Heart J., 6:1069, 1985.

Chih, P., Heng, T. C., Chun, C., et al: Surgical treatment of the ruptured aneurysm of the aortic sinuses. Ann. Thorac. Surg., 32:162, 1981.

DeBakey, M. E., Diethrich, E. B., Liddicoat, J. E., et al: Abnormalities of the sinuses of Valsalva: Experience with 35 patients. J. Thorac. Cardiovasc. Surg., 54:312, 1967.

DeBakey, M. E., and Lawrie, G. M.: Aneurysm of sinus of Valsalva with coronary atherosclerosis. Successful surgical correction. Ann. Surg., 189:303, 1979.

Desai, A. G., Sharma, S., Kumar, A., et al: Echocardiographic diagnosis of unruptured aneurysm of right sinus of Valsalva: An unusual cause of right ventricular outflow obstruction. Am. Heart J., 109:363, 1985.

Edwards, J. E., and Burchell, H. B.: The pathological anatomy of deficiencies between the aortic root and the heart, including aortic sinus aneurysms. Thorax, 12:125, 1957.

Faillace, R. T., Greenland, P., and Nanda, N. C.: Rapid expansion of a saccular aneurysm on the left coronary sinus of Valsalva: A role for early surgical repair? Br. Heart J., 54:442, 1985.

Henze, A., Huttunen, H., and Bjork, V. O.: Ruptured sinus of Valsalva aneurysms. Scand. J. Thorac. Cardiovasc. Surg., 17:249, 1983.

Heydorn, W. H., Nelson, W. P., Fitterer, J. D., et al: Congenital aneurysm of the sinus of Valsalva protruding into the left ventricle. Review of diagnosis and treatment of the unruptured aneurysm. J. Thorac. Cardiovasc. Surg., 71:839, 1976.

Hiyamuta, K., Ohtsuki, T., Shimamatsu, M., et al: Aneurysm of the left aortic sinus causing acute myocardial infarction. Circulation 67:1151, 1983.

Hope, J. A Treatise on the Diseases of the Heart and Great Vessels, 3rd ed. Philadelphia, Lea & Blanchard, 1839, pp. 466–471.

Jones, A. M., and Langley, F. A.: Aortic sinus aneurysms. Br. Heart J., 11:325, 1949.

Killen, D. A., Wathanacharoen, S., and Pogson, G. W., Jr.: Repair of intrapericardial rupture of left sinus of Valsalva aneurysm. Ann. Thorac. Surg., 44:310, 1987.

Lillehei, C. W., Stanley, P., and Varco, R. L.: Surgical treatment of ruptured aneurysms of the sinus of Valsalva. Ann. Surg., 146:459, 1957.

Martin, L. W., Hsu, I., Schwartz, H., et al: Congenital aneurysm of the left sinus of Valsalva: Report of a patient with 19-year survival without surgery. Chest, 90:143, 1986.

Mayer, E. D., Ruffmann, K., Saggau, W., et al: Ruptured aneurysms of the sinus of Valsalva. Ann. Thorac. Surg., 42:81, 1986.

Mayer, J. H., III, Holder, T. M., and Canent, R. V.: Isolated, unruptured sinus of Valsalva aneurysm: Serendipitous detection and correction. J. Thorac. Cardiovasc. Surg., 69:429, 1975.

McGoon, D. C., Edwards, J. E., and Kirklin, J. W.: Surgical treatment of ruptured aneurysm of aortic sinus. Ann. Surg., 147:387, 1958.

Meyer, J., Wukasch, D. C., Hallman, G. L., and Cooley, D. A.: Aneurysm and fistula of the sinus of Valsalva: Clinical considerations and surgical treatment in 45 patients. Ann. Thorac. Surg., 19:170, 1975.

Morch, J. E., and Greenwood, W. F.: Rupture of the sinus of Valsalva: A study of eight cases with discussion on the differential diagnosis of continuous murmurs. Am. J. Cardiol., 18:827, 1966.

Morris, G. C., Jr., Foster, R. P., Dunn, J. R., et al: Traumatic aortico-ventricular fistula: Report of two cases successfully repaired. Am. Surg., 24:883, 1958.

Morrow, A. G., Baker, R. R., Hanson, H. E., et al: Successful surgical repair of a ruptured aneurysm of the sinus of Valsalva. Circulation, 16:533, 1957.

Norwicki, E. R., Aberdeen, E., Friedman, S., et al: Congenital left aortic sinus–left ventricle fistula and review of aortocardiac fistulas. Ann. Thorac. Surg., 23:378, 1977.

Qizilbash, A. H.: Mycotic aneurysm of the aortic sinus of Valsalva with rupture. Arch. Pathol., 98:414, 1974.

Raizes, G. S., Smith, H. C., Vlietstra, R. E., et al: Ventricular tachycardia secondary to aneurysm of sinus of Valsalva. J. Thorac. Cardiovasc. Surg., 78:110, 1979.

Sakakibara, S., and Konno, S.: Congenital aneurysm of the sinus of Valsalva. Anatomy and classification. Am. Heart J., 63:405, 1962.

Sakakibara, S., and Konno, S.: Congenital aneurysm of the sinus of Valsalva: Criteria for recommending surgery. Am. J. Cardiol., 12:100, 1963.

Sawyers, J. L., Adams, J. E., and Scott, H. W., Jr.: Surgical treatment for aneurysms of the aortic sinuses with aorticoatrial fistula: Experimental and clinical study. Surgery, 41:26, 1957.

Shumacker, H. B, Jr.: Aneurysms of the aortic sinuses of Valsalva due to bacterial endocarditis, with special reference to their operative management. J. Thorac. Cardiovasc. Surg., 63:896, 1972.

Shumacker, H. B., Jr., King, H., and Waldhausen, J. A.: Transaortic approach for the repair of ruptured aneurysms of the sinuses of Valsalva. Ann. Surg., 161:946, 1965.

Smith, W. A.: Aneurysm of the sinus of Valsalva, with report of two cases. J.A.M.A., 62:1878, 1914.

Sud, A., Parker, F., and Magilligan, D. J., Jr.: Anatomy of the aortic root. Ann. Thorac. Surg., 38:76, 1984.

Thurnam, J.: On aneurisms, and especially spontaneous varicose aneurisms of ascending aorta and sinus of Valsalva, with cases. Medico-chir. Trans., 23:323, 1840.

Trusler, G. A., Moes, C. A. F., and Kidd, B. S. L.: Repair of ventricular septal defect with aortic insufficiency. J. Thorac. Cardiovasc. Surg., 66:394, 1973.

Warnes, C. A., Maron, B. J., Jones, M., et al: Asymptomatic sinus of Valsalva aneurysm causing right ventricular outflow obstruction before and after rupture. Am. J. Cardiol., 54:1383, 1984.

IV THORACIC AORTIC ANEURYSMS AND AORTIC DISSECTION

Lawrence H. Cohn

THORACIC AORTIC ANEURYSMS

An aneurysm of the aorta is a localized enlargement of the aorta contained by all layers of a normal aortic wall. A false aneurysm of the aorta consists of aortic adventitia and periaortic fibrous tissue. The intrathoracic aorta may have an aneurysm extending from the ascending aorta above the aortic valve to the diaphragm and into the abdomen, forming a thoracoabdominal aneurysm. Approximately one-fourth of all arteriosclerotic aneurysms involve the thoracic aorta (Crisler, 1972; Joyce et al, 1964; Lindsay, 1979b). The degenerative process that causes an aneurysm includes weakening of the aortic wall, medial degeneration, and increased local dilatation. Other causes of aneurysms of the thoracic aorta include syphilis (ascending only), bacterial infections, congenital abnormalities, trauma, and annuloaortic ectasia usually associated with Marfan's syndrome. Although all the pathologic processes may differ microscopically and etiologically, the fundamental process of dilatation, continued expansion, and eventual rupture or symptoms of pressure is the same.

The ultimate therapy for aneurysmal disease of the thoracic aorta is excision and grafting. Within that context are a wide variety of surgical approaches to the various anatomic segments of the aorta: the ascending aorta, the arch of the aorta, the descending thoracic aorta, and the thoracoabdominal aorta.

Surgical treatment of thoracic aneuryms began in the early 1950s after repair of aortic coarctation by Gross and colleagues (1948). Lam and Aram (1951) introduced homografts for descending thoracic aneurysms; DeBakey and Cooley (1953) pioneered the use of artificial grafts, and Bahnson (1953) introduced aneurysmorrhaphy. After the initial operations by DeBakey and Cooley, the surgical treatment of thoracic aneurysms increased when artificial grafts became available.

The ascending aorta (Cooley and DeBakey, 1956) and arch of the aorta (DeBakey et al, 1957) were first successfully approached by the Texas group in sequential stages by using modern cardiopulmonary bypass (CPB) techniques, and continuing technical modifications have improved the surgical treatment of ascending, arch, and descending aortic aneurysms by various new prostheses and conceptual advances. The one-piece valve graft conduit first proposed by Bentall and deBono (1968) and Edwards and Kerr (1979) was an important advance in the treatment of Marfan's syndrome and annuloaortic ectasia. Considerable improvement in survival after ARCH aneurysms has resulted from technical advances by using a single anastomosis for the head vessels (Bloodwell et al, 1968), profound hypothermia, and circulatory arrest with new support techniques (Griepp et al, 1975) and graft technology (Crawford and Crawford, 1984).

Natural History

The natural history of thoracic aortic aneurysms is not nearly as well documented as for abdominal aneurysms, but it appears that it is similar to the natural history of any arterial aneurysm—that is, the signs, symptoms, and prognosis in a patient with an aneurysm are related to the size of the aneurysm. The law of Laplace states that as a sphere increases in size, the wall tension of that sphere increases. Thus, thoracic aneurysms larger than 6 cm are more prone to rupture than are smaller ones (Lindsay, 1979b). The natural history of thoracic aneurysms has been difficult to document because so many patients have generalized arteriosclerosis that more than half with a diagnosed thoracic aneurysm will not be alive in 5 years. In a classic study by Joyce and colleagues (1964), the 5-year survival was 27% for symptomatic aneurysms, whereas 58% survived for 5 years with an asymptomatic aneurysm. One-third of the deaths were attributed to aneurysm rupture, and more than half of the mortality was due to the effects of generalized arteriosclerosis. Bickerstaff and co-workers (1982) showed a 5-year survival of only 19% after diagnosis of a thoracic aneurysm. In this study, rupture of the thoracic aneurysm occurred in 74% of patients. Rupture was also the most common cause of death in a large study by Pressler and colleagues (1985). In their series, rupture accounted for 44% of the deaths, and the surgical mortality for aneurysm resection was significantly less than the risk of late death in untreated patients.

Pathophysiologic Anatomic Correlations

Arteriosclerotic Aneurysms

Arteriosclerosis, the most common cause of thoracic aortic aneurysm, causes a degenerative process in the aortic wall. Approximately half of the aneurysms that require surgical therapy are related to this particular diagnosis (Crawford and Crawford, 1984). These aneurysms are usually fusiform but may be saccular. They are more common in the lower thoracic aorta than in the ascending aorta, possibly because of other degenerative processes. The lowest incidence of thoracic aneurysms is in the aortic arch (Bickerstaff et al, 1982).

Annuloaortic Ectasia

Annuloaortic ectasia in the ascending aorta is commonly associated with cystic medial necrosis (Lemon and White, 1978; Lindsay, 1979a; Pyeritz and McKusick, 1979). These changes include necrosis and

absence of muscle cells in the elastic laminar and cystic spaces filled with the mucoid material (Fig. 33–33). The resultant aneurysm is fusiform and has an equal circumference on all sides. Marfan's syndrome is commonly associated with severe aortic valvular incompetence. Many patients without classic Marfan's syndrome also have annuloaortic ectasia, whereas many patients with aortic regurgitation and annuloaortic ectasia have some stigmata of Marfan's syndrome (Emmanuel et al, 1977). As the media degenerates, the aorta widens, the root is involved, and the annulus dilates. The aortic leaflets are divided and do not coapt, and aortic regurgitation results. Dissection of the aorta is the most common cause of death of these individuals.

Traumatic Aneurysm

Severe deceleration injuries may cause disruption of the ascending aorta, but these patients rarely live to obtain surgical treatment. Trauma most commonly causes treatable aneurysms in the descending thoracic aorta at the level of the ligamentum arteriosum because of the hinge point of the ligamentum. A partial tear through the intima results. In the most

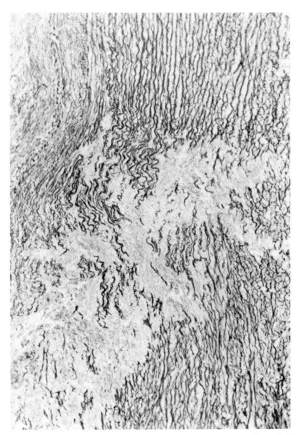

Figure 33–33. Medial degeneration of the aorta. Focal disintegration and disruption of the elastic lamina characterize the elastic-tissue type of medial degeneration. (From Gore, I.: Lesions of the aorta. *In* Gould, S. E. [ed]: Pathology of the Heart, 2nd ed. Springfield, IL, Charles C Thomas Publishers, 1960.)

serious situation, a traumatic transection of the descending aorta may result. In this case, blood remains in communication with the descending aorta only because a periadventitial hematoma forms a false aneurysm and requires immediate repair. A false aneurysm, if diagnosed late, may enlarge and form a typical thoracic aneurysm. Repair is required when the manifestations of the thoracic aneurysm become apparent either by diagnostic techniques or by symptoms of pressure. Kirklin and Barratt-Boyes (1986) have estimated that approximately 10% of descending thoracic aneurysms result from trauma. Tears may occur throughout the entire thoracic aorta with decreasing frequency, those of the descending aorta being more common than those in the ascending aorta, which are more common than those in the arch.

Infection

The term *mycotic aneurysm* was first used by Osler to define any localized dilatation caused by sepsis in the aortic wall. Mycotic aneurysms may result from various bacterial infections and are often localized saccular lesions with culture-positive organisms in the aortic wall. The pathogenesis is septic embolism from bacterial endocarditis to the normal or atherosclerotic aorta; contiguous spread from recent abscesses, infected lymph nodes, or empyema; and sepsis as a result of trauma, intravenous injections, or surgical procedure (Bakker-de Wekker et al, 1984; Crawford and Crawford, 1984; Jarrett et al, 1975). Any organism may invade the arterial wall, but *Salmonella* particularly appears to infect arteriosclerotic aneurysms. Granulomatous aortitis, tuberculosis, and syphilis may occasionally be encountered in aneurysms of the ascending aorta.

Clinical Signs and Symptoms

Most patients are men, and most report a history of hypertension. The symptoms of thoracic aneurysm are usually due to local pressure or obstruction of adjacent thoracic structures. In the ascending aorta, until the aneurysm increases to large dimensions, it may be asymptomatic and may be found only by chest films. Without annuloaortic ectasia and aortic regurgitation, a large aneurysm of the ascending aorta may obstruct the superior vena cava, producing the superior vena caval syndrome, or may exert pressure on the posterior table of the sternum, causing compression necrosis of parts of the sternum and erosion of ribs.

In the arch of the aorta, compression of adjacent structures, including the trachea (tracheal tug), as well as protrusion above the supersternal notch may be the only symptom and sign noted. Enlarging size may compress one of the cerebral arch vessels, producing cerebral ischemia.

The descending thoracic aorta may show a number of signs and symptoms related to enlarging size and stretching of various nerves. A common complaint is hoarseness due to compression and stretching of the left vagus and recurrent laryngeal nerve as it courses over and under the enlarged descending thoracic aorta. Phrenic paralysis may produce an elevated, nonfunctional left hemidiaphragm. Pressure on the esophagus, causing dysphagia, or on the bronchial tree, causing wheezing, may also be noted. In terminal or exaggerated situations, an aneurysm may leak into the pulmonary parenchyma, causing hemoptysis (St. Cyr et al, 1987). Erosion of the aortic aneurysm posteriorly into ribs and vertebrae can produce severe pain.

Diagnosis

Most thoracic aortic aneurysms are readily visible on the chest film, and fluoroscopy often differentiates an aneurysm from other types of neoplastic masses in the mediastinum or lung. The chest films, as shown in the accompanying illustrations, may show a convex shadow to the right of the cardiac shadow for ascending aneurysms (Fig. 33–34*A*), left-sided shadow in aneurysms of the transverse arch (Fig. 33–34*B*), and a shadow to the left and posterior in aneurysms of the descending thoracic aorta (Fig. 33–34*C*). The main differential diagnosis of the mass, particularly in the descending thoracic aorta, is a tortuous aorta.

The *standard* of radiologic diagnosis is the contrast thoracic aortogram. Aortography often differentiates the diameter of the total thoracic shadow from clot, outlines the extent of dilatation of the aorta and blood-filled space, characterizes the type of aortic morphology with annuloaortic ectasia, and denotes takeoff of various important vessels (Fig. 33–35).

Computed tomography (CT) of thoracic aneurysms is increasing in popularity. Without contrast material, the CT scan is a useful method of monitoring patients with thoracic aortic aneurysms (Godwin et al, 1980), particularly those of the descending thoracic aorta. CT scan is less reliable for visualizing ascending aneurysms, but in patients with annuloaortic ectasia and aneurysm, the echocardiogram can show the aortic regurgitation. Doppler echocardiography can semiquantitate the amount of regurgitation and estimate the size of the ascending aorta.

Surgical Treatment

Excision with graft replacement of thoracic aneurysms is the standard therapy and treatment of choice. Excision of aneurysms depends on their location and whether they are saccular or fusiform. Before operative therapy, however, the necessary preparations must be accomplished to ensure maximal safety for the patient during operation. Arterial pressure monitoring, multiple intravenous lines, uri-

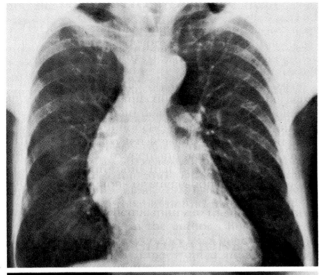

A

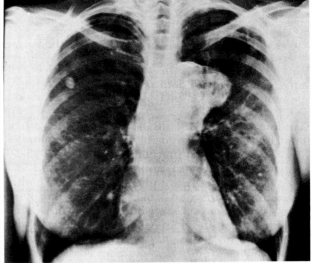

B

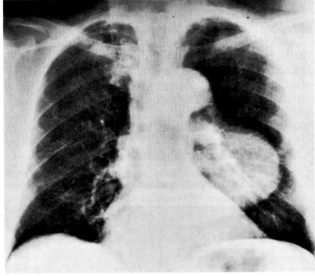

C

Figure 33–34. *A*, Chest film of a patient with an aneurysm of the ascending aorta, which shows the typical convex deformity to the right in the frontal view. *B*, Chest film of a patient with a large aneurysm of the transverse portion of the aortic arch. In the frontal view, the chest film shows the calcified aneurysm projecting to the left. *C*, Chest film of a patient with a large but well-localized aneurysm of the mid-descending thoracic aorta. (From Kirklin, J., and Barratt-Boyes, B.: Cardiac Surgery. New York, John Wiley & Sons, 1986. By permission.)

nary catheters, right and left atrial pressure lines, and a pulmonary artery catheter for the measurement of wedge pressure are important. For left-sided thoracotomy incisions, a double-lumen endotracheal tube to produce anesthesia of one lung is helpful so that the left lung is deflated during operation. Blood salvage systems are essential for all thoracic aortic operations. Appropriate shunts or CPB or both may be needed, depending on the location of the aneurysm, and are discussed later in the section on aneurysm repair. Careful evaluation of all organ subsystems, especially renal and pulmonary, should be done preoperatively, particularly on individuals with aneurysms of the descending thoracic aorta.

Sutures that are used for aneurysm repair are now exclusively monofilament polypropylene to minimize tissue resistance. Preclotting of grafts is sometimes appropriate, but increasingly popular is the technique of soaking synthetic grafts in albumin and autoclaving them to decrease blood leakage

through the graft pores after anastomosis (Cooley et al, 1981). Heparin is used for patients on CPB and may be used for patients with shunts for the descending thoracic aorta.

Ascending Aortic Aneurysm Repair

Right atrial and femoral arterial cannulation is the preferred technique to manage CPB for ascending aneurysms. The femoral artery is preferred to maximize working area at the distal aorta. Systemic and local hypothermia is used to cool the heart. During the interruption of the circulation to the heart by the distal ascending aortic clamp, intracoronary crystalloid or blood cardioplegia is administered because of aortic regurgitation. A left ventricular vent is placed in the right superior pulmonary vein, with or without aortic valve replacement.

The extent of the aneurysm resection requires

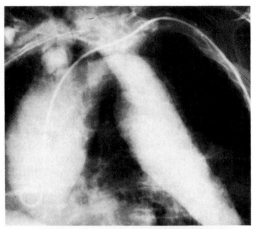
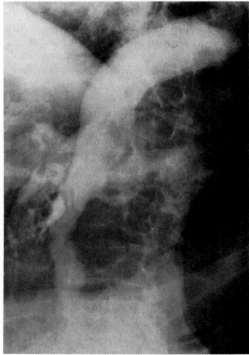

Figure 33–35. Aneurysm of the ascending aorta and aortic arch, the descending thoracic aorta, and dilatation of entire distal aorta in a 69-year-old woman. (From Crawford, E. S., and Crawford, J. L.: Diseases of the Aorta. © 1984. Reproduced with permission from Williams & Wilkins, Baltimore.)

considerable judgment. For example, patients with a large aneurysm extending into the aortic arch pose a more complex problem with a higher operative mortality. Therefore, the surgeon must be prudent in extending into the arch when the primary pathology is in the ascending aorta. The type of graft replacement relates to the pathology in the lower aspect of the ascending aorta, specifically whether the sinuses of Valsalva are involved or whether the patient has severe aortic regurgitation requiring valve replacement. If the aneurysm is confined to the ridge of the aorta above the coronary arteries, which is the case with most arteriosclerotic aneurysms, simple excision

and grafting of the aneurysm are satisfactory (Fig. 33–36). The inclusion technique for anastomosis of the graft into the ascending aorta is shown in Figure 33–37. The technique is adapted from the abdominal aneurysm technique first reported by Creech (1966) in which the back wall of the aorta distally and proximally is left completely intact. This technique is the subject of controversy because of its higher incidence of false aneurysms (Crawford, 1983), and some surgeons prefer not to use it (Fig. 33–38). If the aneurysm is not a result of dissection, the inclusion technique should be satisfactory. If the aneurysm is the result of a chronic dissection, it should be managed in a different manner, as discussed in the next section.

If the aortic sinuses are involved within the annuloaortic ectasia process and greatly dilated with aortic regurgitation, a composite valve graft conduit technique is often required. The applications for this operation vary, depending on the extent of pathology. Annuloaortic ectasia secondary to Marfan's syndrome is an absolute indication for the use of this technique, and replacement of the Marfan's ascending aorta is indicated when the echocardiographic dimensions of the ascending aorta exceed 5.5 cm (Gott, 1986) (Fig. 33–39). In other pathologic states, there are relative indications for this operation depending on coronary displacement. The technique for replacing the ascending aorta with a valve conduit

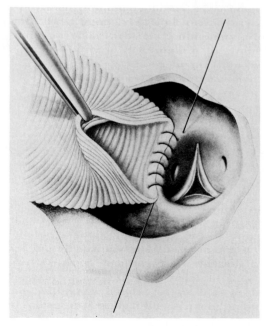

Figure 33–36. Replacement of the suprabulbar aorta. The graft is anastomosed to the aorta above the level of the aortic commissures, suturing entirely within the lumen. (From Borst, H. G.: Ascending aortic aneurysms. *In* Cohn, L. H. [ed]: Modern Technics in Surgery/Cardiac Thoracic Surgery. Mt. Kisco, NY, Futura Publishing Co., 1984.)

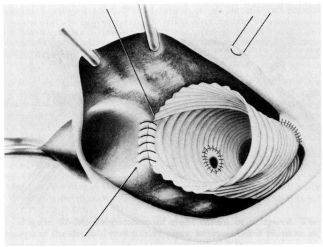

Figure 33–37. Distal graft-to-aorta inclusion anastomosis. The over-and-over suture begins posteriorly and proceeds anteriorly on both sides, suturing entirely from within the aortic lumen. (From Borst, H. G.: Ascending aortic aneurysms. *In* Cohn, L. H. [ed]: Modern Technics in Surgery/Cardiac Thoracic Surgery. Mt. Kisco, NY, Futura Publishing Co., 1984.)

in patients with annuloaortic ectasia, with or without aortic regurgitation, is shown in Figure 33–40. The operation consists of placing the proximal end first with a series of interrupted sutures around the annulus. All of these should have Teflon pledgets, because the strength of the tissue in the Marfan's aortic annulus is relatively poor. After completion of the proximal anastomosis, the graft should be stretched to the appropriate length and a coronary anastomosis should be done. The graft orifices for the coronary arteries are created with a cautery. In annuloaortic ectasia, the coronary arteries are usually displaced a considerable distance from the annulus. The graft orifices for coronary implantation are made so that they are much larger than the actual coronary orifices, leaving considerable pericoronary tissue for the 4-0 prolene sutures used in the running anastomoses. The coronary implantation is the major risk

factor of this operation, and if coronary displacement is not great (<5 mm), other techniques may be necessary. In Cabrol's technique (Cabrol et al, 1986), the graft is sewn to both coronary orifices and then side to side to the ascending aorta (Fig. 33–41). Direct extension of a saphenous vein or Gore-Tex graft from the coronary orifice directly to the graft itself can also be used (Piehler and Pluth, 1982). The coronary arteries can also be reimplanted by excising a button of aortic-coronary tissue and suturing this button to the graft (Fig. 33–42). The left coronary artery is reimplanted first, followed by the right coronary artery. The distal aortic anastomosis is then done in the usual manner using the inclusion or exclusion technique. As the last anastomotic suture is being completed, rewarming is begun and air is aspirated from the ascending aortic graft and left ventricle.

Some controversy exists about the use of the

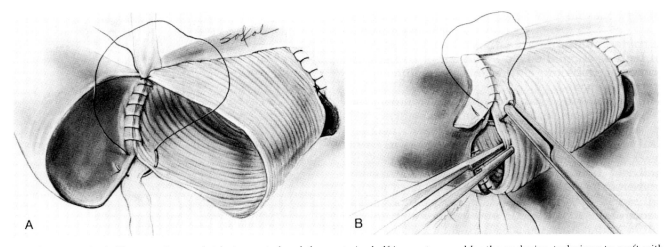

Figure 33–38. *A*, The aorta is completely transected and the posterior half is anastomosed by the exclusion technique to graft with 3-0 polypropylene sutures. The suture line is reinforced with strips of Teflon felt. *B*, The anterior half of the anastomosis is then completed. (From Kouchoukos, N. T., and Marshall, W. G.: Treatment of ascending aortic dissection in Marfan's syndrome. J. Cardiac. Surg., *1*:341, 1986.)

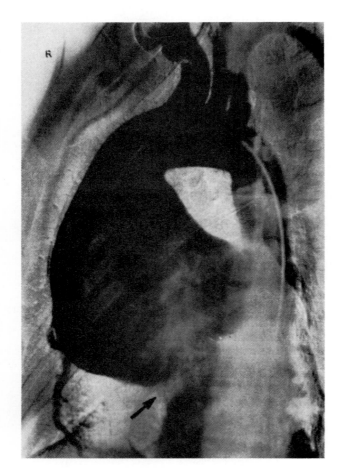

Figure 33–39. Aortogram of massive annuloaortic ectasia secondary to Marfan's syndrome in a 21-year-old woman. The *arrow* indicates the level of aortic valve. (From Cohn, L. H.: The long-term results of aortic valve replacement. Chest, *85*:389, 1984.)

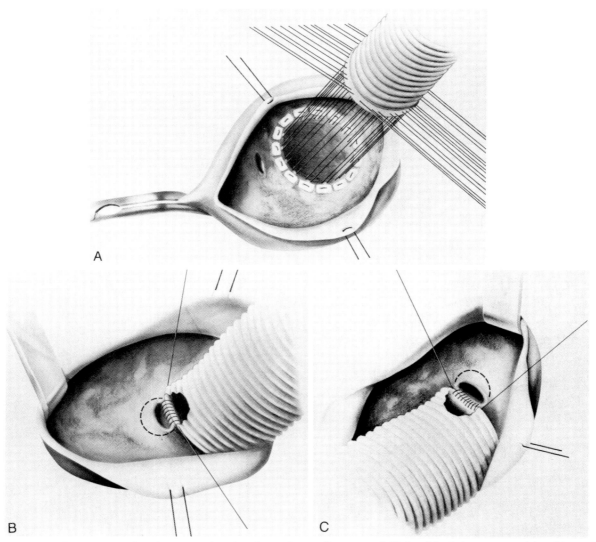

Figure 33–40. Composite graft replacement of aortic valve and ascending aorta. *A*, Teflon felt pledgets are used to achieve a blood-tight seal of the conduit against the aortic valve ring *(A)*. Anastomosis of the left *(B)* and right *(C)* coronary ostium appropriate to apertures made in the graft. The ostia are not excised from the aortic wall. Suturing proceeds from outside of the graft to periosteal tissue. (From Borst, H. G.: Ascending aortic aneurysms. *In* Cohn, L. H. [ed]: Modern Technics in Surgery/Cardiac Thoracic Surgery. Mt. Kisco, NY, Futura Publishing Co., 1984.)

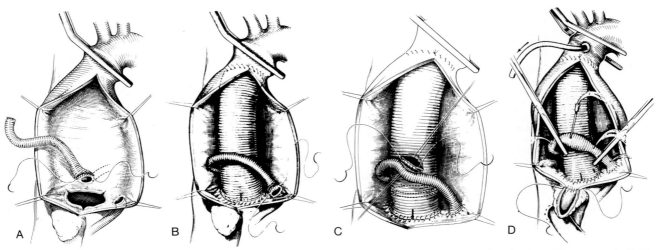

Figure 33–41. *A,* After excision of the aortic valve, the left coronary artery ostia is anastomosed to the 8-mm Dacron graft. *B,* The right coronary artery ostia is anastomosed to the 8-mm Dacron graft. *C,* The Dacron coronary graft is anastomosed side-to-side to the valved conduit above the aortic valvular prosthesis. *D,* The aorta is unclamped; air is evacuated carefully from the aortic graft and from both segments of the coronary graft. (From Cabrol, C., Gandjbakhch, I., and Pavie, A.: Surgical treatment of ascending aortic pathology. J. Cardiac Surg., 3:167, 1988.)

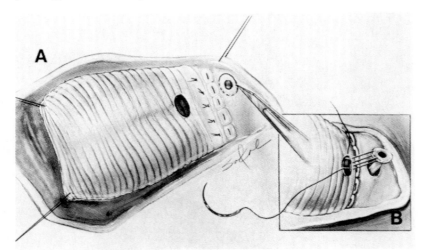

Figure 33–42. *A,* Technique for excision of a full-thickness button of aortic wall adjacent to coronary ostium. *B,* Mobilization and direct anastomosis to aortic graft. (From Kouchoukos, N. T., and Marshall, W. G.: Treatment of ascending aortic dissection in Marfan's syndrome. J. Cardiac Surg., 1:340, 1986.)

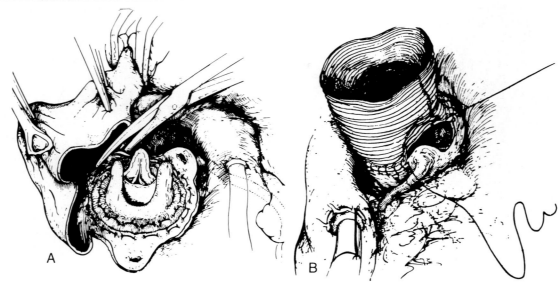

Figure 33–43. *A,* Using the scalloping technique (which entails insertion of the aortic valve prosthesis and the tubular synthetic graft separately), essentially the entire aortic root is either excised or obliterated. If aortic valve replacement (AVR) is not necessary, the sinuses of Valsalva are not resected. *B,* Completion of the anterior aspect of the proximal anastomosis; care is necessary to ensure that the right coronary artery (lying in the proximal right atrioventricular groove, not at the ostium) is not inadvertently compromised. (From Frist, W. H., and Miller, D. C.: Repair of ascending aortic aneurysms and dissections. J. Cardiac Surg., 1:33, 40, 1986.)

valve-graft conduit, even in Marfan's syndrome. Miller and colleagues (1984) have suggested that careful scalloping of the aorta and meticulous suturing around the coronary orifices may be as successful as the combined valve-graft conduit concept (Frist et al, 1986) (Fig. 33–43). Leaving even a centimeter of sinus tissue in a patient with Marfan's syndrome may cause recurrence of a false aneurysm, which is a difficult entity to treat. If the inclusion technique is used, the aortic wall is wrapped around the aneurysm and sutured closed to promote hemostasis. The common association of mitral valve prolapse and insufficiency may also allow mitral valve replacement via the aortic root (Crawford et al, 1988).

Another technique for ascending aortic aneurysms, particularly in elderly patients who are critically ill, is aortoplasty for the greatly dilated ascending aorta. This procedure involves tailoring the aortic size to prevent rupture by reducing wall stress in the relatively normal aorta and external graft wrapping (Robicsek, 1982).

The results of aneurysm repair, including operative mortality, are summarized in Table 33–2. The operative mortality is from 5 to 15% (Borst, 1984; Egloff et al, 1982; Grey et al, 1983; Kouchoukos and Marshall, 1986; Moreno-Cabral et al, 1984). Late results are shown in the actuarial curves in Figure 33–44.

Transverse Arch Aortic Aneurysms

Transverse arch aortic aneurysms are more complex clinically because resection involves preservation of the integrity of the blood supply to the central nervous system and protection of cerebral function during resection while cerebral blood flow is interrupted. Early techniques involved separate cannulation of the individual cerebral vessels, but more recent procedures have emphasized simplicity of repair and have used deep hypothermic circulatory arrest or very low CPB flow or both (Crawford and Crawford, 1984; Ergin and Griepp, 1981; Ergin et al, 1982; Kay, 1986; Livesay, 1983). The basic principles of arch resection are shown in Figure 33–45. The brachiocephalic vessels are occluded, and flow from the CPB machine is either totally interrupted or maintained minimally. At temperatures of 15 to 20° C, it is usually safe to arrest the circulation for as long as 60 minutes, clamp the brachiocephalic vessels, and remove the aneurysm by using all the cerebral vessel extensions from the aorta as a button

TABLE 33–2. ASCENDING AORTIC ANEURYSMS

Study	Operative Mortality
Grey et al, 1983	12/140
Kouchoukos et al, 1986	6/127
Moreno-Cabrol et al, 1984	8/124
Borst, 1984	6/54

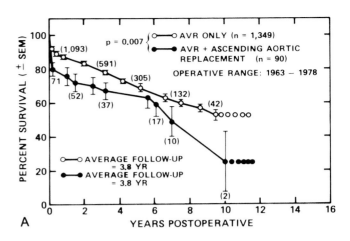

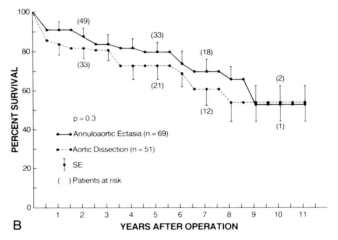

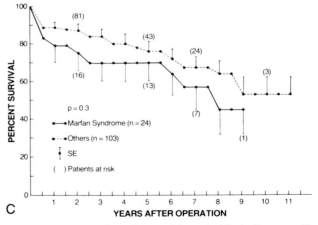

Figure 33–44. *A,* Overall actuarial survival including operative deaths. (From Miller, D. C., Stinson, E. B., Oyer, P. E., et al: Concomitant resection of ascending aortic aneurysm and replacement of the aortic valve. J. Thorac. Cardiovasc. Surg., 79:396, 1980.) *B,* Actuarial survival of 69 patients with annuloaortic ectasia and 51 patients with aortic dissection. (From Kouchoukos, N. T., Marshall, W. G., Jr., and Wedige-Stecher, T. A.: Eleven-year experience with composite graft replacement of the ascending aorta and aortic valve. J. Thorac. Cardiovasc. Surg., 92:696, 1986.) *C,* Actuarial freedom from reoperation on the ascending aorta or aortic valve for 127 patients. Early reoperations for hemorrhage are excluded. (From Kouchoukos, N. T., Marshall, W. G., Jr., and Wedige-Stecher, T. A.: Eleven-year experience with composite graft replacement of the ascending aorta and aortic valve. J. Thorac. Cardiovasc. Surg., 92:691, 1986.)

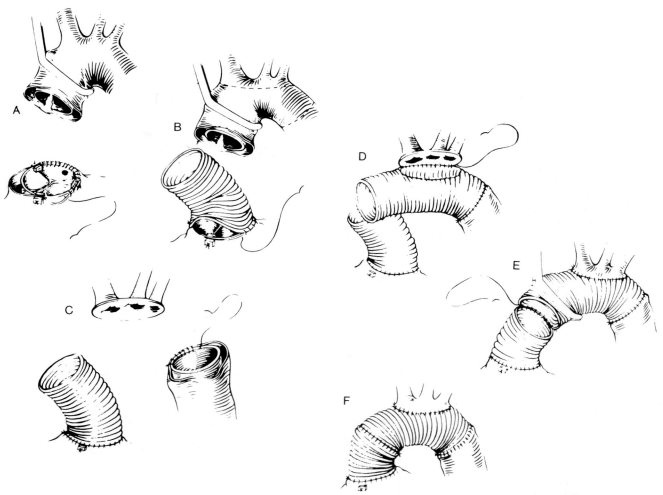

Figure 33–45. *A*, Techniques for replacement of arch of the aorta using a cerebrovascular button (*B*). The anastomosis is first made to the graft in the ascending aorta (C). The cerebral button, which contains the orifices of all three cerebral vessels, is then anastomosed to the apex of the transverse aortic arch graft (D). *E*, Shows the final step, which is anastomosis of the transverse arch graft to the ascending aortic graft. (From Ergin, M. A., and Griepp, R. B.: Progress in treatment of aneurysms of the aortic arch. World J. Surg., 4:535, 1980.)

of aorta. When the aneurysm is opened, various different techniques may be used. If the entire aorta is aneurysmal and the cerebral vessels require implantation, a graft is sutured to the descending and proximal aorta, and the button is sewn in as a patch graft. If there is an inferior aneurysm, however, a graft may be placed excluding an anastomosis into the descending aorta but basically into the underside of the arch. If there is simply an opening into a saccular aneurysm, it may be repaired by Dacron patch (Fig. 33–46). Occasionally, if the aneurysm is saccular, a clamp may be placed across the inferior margin of the aorta with no cross-clamping, circulatory arrest, or CPB.

Failure to remove air from the circulation when there is circulatory arrest is, of course, one of the major risk factors. After completion of the anastomosis, the patient is placed in Trendelenberg's position, bypass is slowly begun, and air is removed

from the ascending aorta and the cerebral vessels. When the cerebral vessel button is in position, the aorta is clamped proximally and perfusion is restarted with air evacuation. Completion of the ascending graft portion is accomplished, air is evacuated from this segment of aorta, and the patient is resuscitated and taken off bypass. Intraoperatively, embolic air or particulate material in the cerebral circulation, coagulation problems, and respiratory problems are many of the perioperative difficulties. Some surgeons have reported (Kay et al, 1986) that aneurysms of the left common carotid and the subclavian may be repaired only with perfusion of the innominate artery with excellent results. Although the median approach is the standard incision with CPB, some of these can be done by a posterolateral incision with partial CPB (Crawford et al, 1987).

With the advent of the technique using hypothermia and cerebral button, mortality has declined

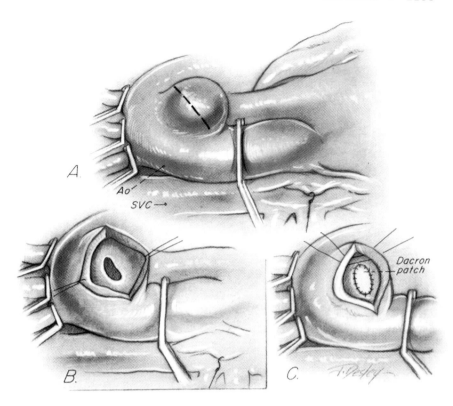

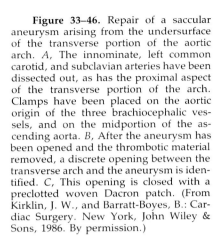

Figure 33–46. Repair of a saccular aneurysm arising from the undersurface of the transverse portion of the aortic arch. *A*, The innominate, left common carotid, and subclavian arteries have been dissected out, as has the proximal aspect of the transverse portion of the arch. Clamps have been placed on the aortic origin of the three brachiocephalic vessels, and on the midportion of the ascending aorta. *B*, After the aneurysm has been opened and the thrombotic material removed, a discrete opening between the transverse arch and the aneurysm is identified. *C*, This opening is closed with a preclotted woven Dacron patch. (From Kirklin, J. W., and Barratt-Boyes, B.: Cardiac Surgery. New York, John Wiley & Sons, 1986. By permission.)

(Table 33–3) from prohibitive levels to approximately 10 to 30%. The age of the patient and concomitant subsystem organ failure are important preoperative risk factors, and surgical treatment should be individualized for each patient.

Descending Thoracic Aortic Aneurysms

Aneurysms distal to the left subclavian artery are the most commonly encountered thoracic aortic aneurysms. Operation is indicated for aneurysms greater than 6 cm or their documented enlargement, or chest or back pain indicating expansion. Aneurysms of this area of the aorta are second in incidence only to infrarenal abdominal aortic aneurysms. Traumatic aneurysms are generally found at this location, because the ligamentum arteriosum offers some anchoring point of the thoracic aorta. At this site, shear forces often create a tear producing a traumatic aneurysm, which is sometimes evident many years after its production. Chronic dissections from aortic

TABLE 33–3. TRANSVERSE AORTIC ARCH ANEURYSMS

Study	Operative Mortality
Griepp et al, 1975	6/21
Crawford et al, 1985	7/93
Livesay et al, 1983	14/60
Kirklin and Barratt-Boyes, 1986	8/18

degeneration may occur. Patients with aneurysm of the descending aorta are older and often have complicated multisystem disease including pulmonary and renal disease, which must be properly controlled before operative intervention to reduce risk.

These aneurysms are approached through a left-sided thoracotomy with one-lung anesthesia. The fourth interspace generally provides the best exposure of the upper thoracic aortic aneurysm, but if the aneurysm is located in the lower part of the thoracic aorta, which is uncommon, an appropriately placed lower incision is necessary.

The parasympathetic nerves in this region complicate aneurysm repair and include the left phrenic, the vagus, and the recurrent laryngeal nerves. Identification of these structures during the course of aneurysm resection is mandatory. The lung is often adherent to the aneurysm, and resection of the lung must occasionally be undertaken before the aneurysm can be exposed.

Debate continues about the best way to protect the lower half of the body when the thoracic aorta is clamped. A major risk factor of these operations is paraplegia due to spinal cord ischemia. The protective methods vary from complete heparinization and femorofemoral bypass with a pump oxygenator to simple cross-clamping of the aorta and manipulation of the upper circulatory afterload increase by vasodilators, usually nitroprusside, and rapid restoration of the blood volume with bicarbonate after removal of the aortic cross-clamp. In addition to organ perfusion below the aneurysm, bleeding from the inserted grafts is a serious consideration, sometimes prohibiting use of heparin in patients with a descending thoracic aortic graft. Crawford and colleagues (1981) and Najafi and associates (1980) suggested that bypass shunts were not necessary but that simple clamping with performance of the aortic anastomosis under pharmacologic control was satisfactory. This technique poses pressure on the surgeon to accomplish this within a relatively short time (< 30 minutes) and does not take into account the more anatomically complicated aneurysms. Many surgeons have disagreed with the no-shunt approach, and have advocated some form of aortic bypass (Carlson et al,

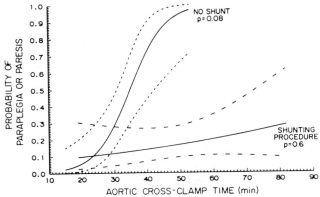

Figure 33–48. Nomogram of the logistic equations relating the probability of evidence for spinal cord injury (paraplegia or paresis) to aortic cross-clamp time (minutes) for patients in whom no shunting procedure was used and for those in whom it was used. The *broken lines* are the 70% confidence limits. (From Katz, N. M., Blackstone, E. H., Kirklin, J. W., and Karp, R. B.: Incremental risk factors for spinal cord injury following operation for acute traumatic aortic transection. J. Thorac. Cardiovasc. Surg., 81:672, 1981.)

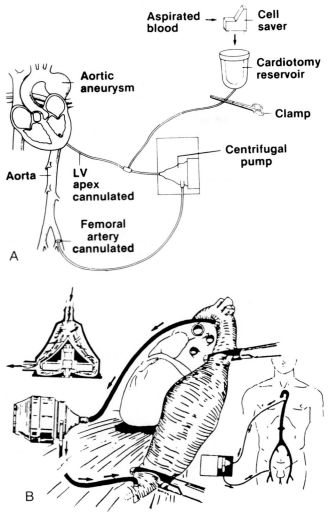

Figure 33–47. *A,* This is an example of left ventricular-femoral artery bypass graft for the protection of the lower half of the body during resection of a descending thoracic aortic aneurysm. (From Griepp, R. B., Stinson, E. B., Hollingsworth, J. F., and Buehler, D.: Prosthetic replacement of the aortic arch. J. Thorac. Cardiovasc. Surg., 70:1051, 1975.) *B,* Cannula placement for arterial bypass of the descending thoracic aorta. Aortoaortic bypass or aortofemoral bypass may be used in conjunction with the Biomedicus pump. *Inset* of pump head shows the vortex, which is the basis of the kinetic pump. *Arrows* indicate the direction of flow. (From Diehl, J. T., Payne, D. D., Rastegar, H., and Cleveland, R. J.: Arterial bypass of the descending thoracic aorta with the Biomedicus centrifugal pump. Ann. Thorac. Surg., 44:422, 1987.)

1983; Culliford et al, 1983; Diehl et al, 1987). It appears that the trend now is toward a shunt or bypass with albumin-preclotted grafts (Fig. 33–47).

Monitoring of spinal cord ischemia is now possible with somatosensory potential measurement, a technique popularized by Laschinger and colleagues (1982). In this technique, ischemia of the cord can be recognized by the decrease in the somatosensory potential of the lower extremities, and techniques to provide more blood to the lower aorta must be used. No technique can guarantee that paraplegia will not occur, but it now appears that the shunt techniques or femorofemoral bypass leads to a lower incidence of paraplegia, which occurs in approximately 5% of cases of descending thoracic aortic aneurysmectomy. The probability of paraplegia with and without shunts is shown in Figure 33–48. If large lateral intercostal arteries are identified within the aneurysm, these should be preserved and inserted into the graft with the patch angioplasty technique (Fig. 33–49). The basic technique for graft replacement using graft inclusion is shown in Figure 33–50. In unusual circumstances, particularly with various forms of traumatic aneurysms and chronic dissection, there may be small entry points from the lumen to the exterior, and these may be closed with a patch and the false lumen may be obliterated (Fig. 33–51). The sutureless graft, particularly effective for descending aneurysms, is discussed later.

The operative mortality after resection of a descending aneurysm varies from 5 to 15%, depending on the acuity and the demography of the groups of patients. Small midthoracic aortic aneurysms of an arteriosclerotic nature should be operated electively with a risk of no more than 5%, whereas large proximal descending aneurysms in elderly patients with multiple subsystem organ failure have a strik-

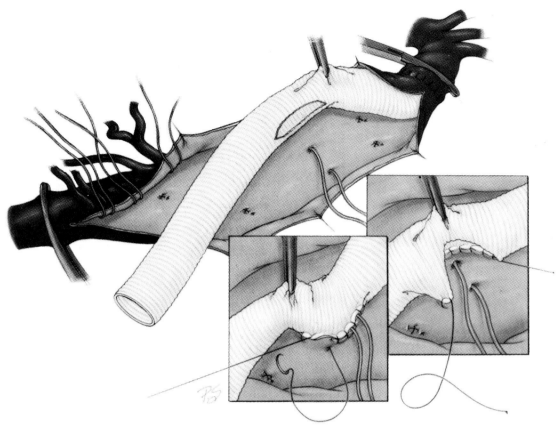

Figure 33–49. Steps in descending thoracic aortic aneurysm resection incorporating intercostal arteries. The graft is placed under tension, and an oval opening is made in it opposite to the intercostal arteries to be reattached. *K*, This opening is sutured around the origin of these arteries. The inside or medial part of the anastomosis is done first for convenience (*K*). *L*, The other side is then done, completing the anastomosis over the balloon catheters. (From Crawford, E. S., and Crawford, J. L.: Diseases of the Aorta. © 1984. Reproduced with permission from Williams & Wilkins, Baltimore.)

ingly higher risk. Long-term results comparing traumatic to arteriosclerotic aneurysms are shown in Figure 33–52, and descending to ascending aneurysms are shown in Figure 33–53.

Thoracoabdominal Aortic Aneurysms

Thoracoabdominal aortic aneurysms are perhaps the most complex to repair because they require reimplantation of all the abdominal visceral arterial supply and may involve serious injury to subsystem organ function, particularly the kidneys. DeBakey and colleagues (1956) were the first to treat this disease in large numbers of patients. These aneurysms are approached through a posterior thoracoabdominal incision, retroperitoneally, beginning in the seventh intercostal space and extending to the pubis. The aorta is approached retroperitoneally and the diaphragm is incised (Fig. 33–54). The thoracic portion is removed, and the proximal aortic graft is anastomosed. If intercostal arteries are encountered, they may be reimplanted into the main channel

thoracic aortic graft as a patch graft. This patch graft may include a significant spinal accessory artery to provide the best possible blood supply to the spinal cord. Left ventricular-left femoral artery shunts or atrial femoral artery shunts are rarely used. The entire abdominal visceral artery supply is anastomosed as a large patch graft to the aorta. One-lung anesthesia with meticulous hemodynamic monitoring is critical, and afterload manipulation by nitroprusside is necessary. As with other thoracic aortic aneurysms, the aneurysmal sac is usually placed over the aortic graft and oversewn. The inclusion technique for graft replacement is generally used.

The largest series and best results are attributed to Crawford and colleagues (1978), who have reimplanted the abdominal visceral arteries with minimal morbidity. Operative mortality is from 10 to 40%. Paraplegia is a major risk factor with repair of these aneurysms and is higher than with thoracic aneurysms (10%) (Crawford and Crawford, 1984). Actuarial survival of patients after chronic thoracoabdominal aneurysm surgery is approximately 60% at 5 years.

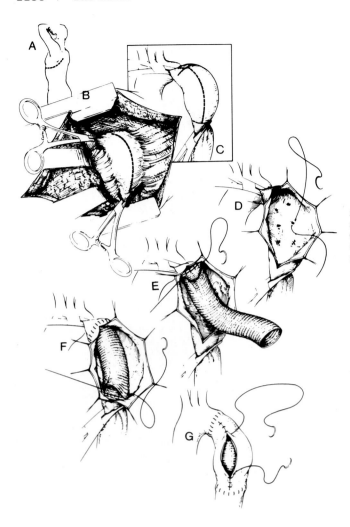

Figure 33–50. Illustrations of method for graft replacement of fusiform aneurysm of descending thoracic aorta using graft inclusion technique. (From Crawford, E. S., Snyder, D. M., and Graham, J. M.: Aneurysm of the descending thoracic aorta. *In* Cohn, L. H. [ed]: Modern Technics in Surgery/Cardiac Thoracic Surgery. Mt. Kisco, NY, Futura Publishing Co., 1982.)

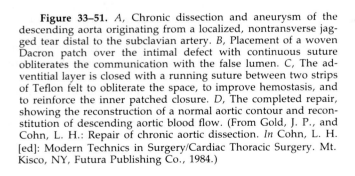

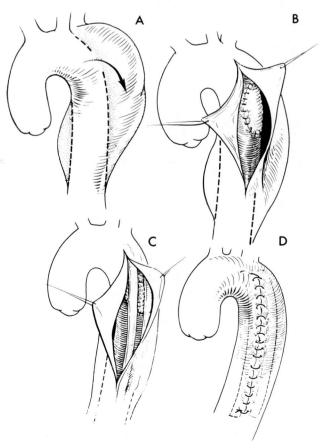

Figure 33–51. *A,* Chronic dissection and aneurysm of the descending aorta originating from a localized, nontransverse jagged tear distal to the subclavian artery. *B,* Placement of a woven Dacron patch over the intimal defect with continuous suture obliterates the communication with the false lumen. *C,* The adventitial layer is closed with a running suture between two strips of Teflon felt to obliterate the space, to improve hemostasis, and to reinforce the inner patched closure. *D,* The completed repair, showing the reconstruction of a normal aortic contour and reconstitution of descending aortic blood flow. (From Gold, J. P., and Cohn, L. H.: Repair of chronic aortic dissection. *In* Cohn, L. H. [ed]: Modern Technics in Surgery/Cardiac Thoracic Surgery. Mt. Kisco, NY, Futura Publishing Co., 1984.)

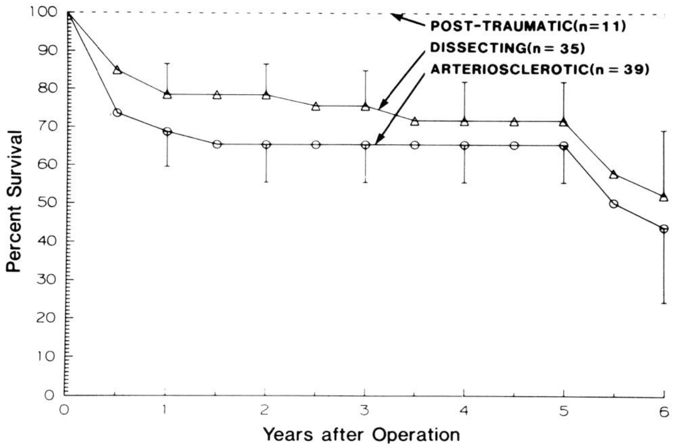

Figure 33–52. Actuarial survival after resection of aneurysm of the descending thoracic aorta (UAB, 1967–1980). The vertical bars indicate the 70% confidence limits. (From Kirklin, J. W., and Barratt-Boyes, B.: Cardiac Surgery. New York, John Wiley & Sons, 1986. By permission.)

Special Features

Surgical Glue

Fibrin glue (Walterbusch et al, 1982) may be used in the suture lines of a friable aorta in aneurysm repair to minimize hemorrhage and promote tissue ingrowth in porous grafts by producing a neointima. Use of this material is increasing, and the Food and Drug Administration is considering its approval.

Sutureless Intraluminal Grafts

Sutureless intraluminal grafts were first adopted by Ablaza and colleagues (1978) and popularized by Spagna and associates (1985). They have been increasingly used for complex ascending and descending aneurysms and aortic dissections when rapid operating time is desirable. The sutureless intraluminal graft is anchored with two sutures, and a very strong circumferential umbilical tape is placed around the aneurysm and tied down on the ring of the intraluminal graft. In some cases, one end of the ring may be used while the other end is sutured to the aorta, especially in the ascending aorta. The long-term results of these grafts are unknown, and false aneurysms occasionally occur when the umbilical tapes slip or loosen and blood permeates the ring inside the aorta. This important graft adjunct will be used more in future years for more complex aneu-

rysm operations, especially in elderly, seriously ill patients needing urgent, efficient operations.

Stapling

Excluding large thoracic aneurysms and placement of bypass, shunts may be necessary in some debilitated patients who cannot have conventional procedures. Ergin and colleagues (1983) have used TA stapling in seven patients, reporting long-term success and no recurrence. These patients had exclusion of aneurysm and bypass Dacron/Teflon grafts around the aneurysm site without disturbing the aneurysms. Carpentier and associates (1981) have also used a stapling technique for thrombus exclusion for large aneurysms in high-risk patients.

AORTIC DISSECTION AND DISSECTING AORTIC ANEURYSMS

Acute aortic dissection is a sudden catastrophic event in which a tear in the intima allows blood to escape from the true lumen of the aorta, rapidly dissecting the inner from the outer layer of the media. This column of blood is driven by the force of the arterial pressure, which strips the intima from the adventitia for various distances along the length of the aorta. The process is considered to be acute when

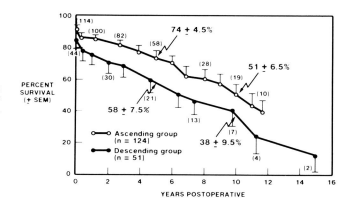

Figure 33–53. Actuarial survival rates for patients with thoracic aortic aneurysms, excluding dissection. (SEM = standard error of the mean.) (From Moreno-Cabral C. E.: Degenerative and atherosclerotic aneurysms of the thoracic aorta. J. Thorac. Cardiovasc. Surg., 88:1025, 1984.)

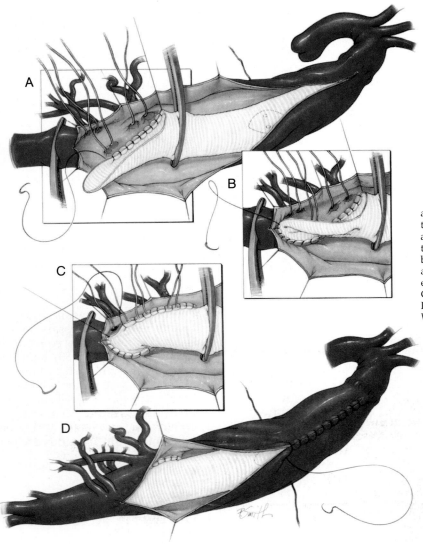

Figure 33–54. Steps in thoracoabdominal aneurysm resection and visceral artery reattachment. The distal end of the graft is beveled and attached to restore aortic continuity and to replace the involved aortic circumference behind the visceral artery openings (*A,B*). The anastomosis is completed by suturing the lateral margin (*C,D*). (From Crawford, E. S., and Crawford, J. L.: Diseases of the Aorta. © 1984. Reproduced with permission from Williams & Wilkins, Baltimore.)

it is less than 14 days old. It is actually unclear whether the rupture of the intima is primarily caused by hemorrhage occurring within a diseased media followed by disruption of the intima or whether it is a dissecting hematoma into the intimal tear. The clinical and pathologic manifestations of the aortic dissection are determined by the path that is taken by the dissecting hematoma as it progresses between the layers of aorta around its entire length. The circulation in any major artery that arises from the aorta may be compromised, and disruption of the aortic root and actual rupture through the adventitia anywhere along the aorta may result in a fatal hemorrhage.

Aortic dissection has been recognized for centuries. The term *dissecting aneurysm* was introduced by Laënnec (1826), but until the classic medical studies by Shennan (1934) and by Hirst and colleagues

(1958), there was little evidence that the entity was more common than previously realized and that it predisposes the patient to acute catastrophic cardiovascular events. Early operations for dissection were tailored toward the production of distal internal fenestration to cause downstream decompression in the aorta such as that proposed by Shaw (1955). Debakey and associates (1955) first successfully repaired acute dissection of the descending thoracic aorta with resection of both dissected ends and placement of an interposition graft. Spencer and Blake (1962) first repaired a chronic ascending aortic dissection, and Morris and co-workers (1963) first successfully repaired an acute ascending dissection. Wheat and associates (1965) advocated a major advance in the general management of acute aortic dissection by correlating and integrating medical as well as surgical treatment in various anatomic locations.

Etiology and Pathogenesis

The most common cause was once believed to be degeneration of the aortic media associated with cystic changes from which were derived the term *cystic medial necrosis*, which was encountered in patients with Marfan's syndrome and other inherited connective tissue disorders. Only a few patients with dissection show these classic changes (Larson and Edwards, 1984), but all patients probably have some inherent anatomic weakness of the aortic wall. A number of predisposing conditions are associated with aortic dissection. Hypertension is the most common factor contributing to aortic dissection and is found in approximately 70 to 90% of all dissections, more commonly in distal than in proximal dissections. Although many patients do have cystic medial necrosis and Marfan's syndrome, many simply have a normal aorta and may not have associated hypertension. Pregnancy has been associated with acute aortic dissection, but the number of patients reported is small and may reflect the hypertension of pregnancy (Pumphrey et al, 1986). Iatrogenic aortic dissection has become increasingly frequent as more patients have had cardiac operations. It may occur at the aortic cannulation site, from aorta-saphenous vein bypass, during the course of aortic valve replacement, or from retrograde femoral artery perfusion (Dabir and Serry, 1988; Murphy et al, 1983; Najafi, 1979) and also as a late consequence of aortic valve replacement (Derkac et al, 1974; Muna et al, 1977; Orszulak et al, 1982). Bicuspid aortic valves are more frequently associated with aortic dissection (Roberts, 1970), and aortic coarctation is associated with acute dissection in some patients, but this may again be attributed to the long-standing systemic hypertension (Roberts, 1981). Closed chest trauma may also be a cause of dissection, especially in the descending thoracic aorta (Wilson and Hutchins, 1982).

Pathoanatomy

In approximately 95% of patients, dissections of the thoracic aorta arise in one of two locations: (1) in the ascending aorta within several centimeters of the aortic valve (approximately 66%) and (2) in the descending thoracic aorta just beyond the origin of the left subclavian at the site of the ligamentum arteriosum. In a small percentage of patients, the intimal laceration begins in the aortic arch or in the distal descending thoracic aorta. The tear is usually transverse and separates the aortic media for various lengths. Ascending dissection may extend into the descending aorta, but retrograde extension is relatively uncommon. Controversy has centered on the rapidity of dissection. Most experts now believe that in the immediate period after dissection occurs in the media, blood rushes into the dissected area between the two layers of the aorta and the pathology is established. According to Najafi (Najafi, 1983), evidence for this theory is confirmed by the events after retrograde aortic dissections during CPB, when the dissection of the entire aorta occurs almost instantaneously. Blood in the false lumen in dissections is separated from the exterior by the thin outer media and adventitia, and unless pressure is controlled, rupture may ensue. Several days after the onset of dissection, necrosis of the aortic wall may develop, causing the aorta to rupture (see Fig. 33–53). Aortic wall necrosis was observed in 62% of dissections (Barsky and Rosen, 1978), and clinical complications of dissection include aortic rupture through the false lumen, obstruction, and occlusion of aortic branches, producing major clinical sequelae (Fig. 33–55).

Clinical Classification of Aortic Dissections

Two basic clinical classifications of aortic dissections exist. DeBakey's classification (Fig. 33–56) is perhaps the more widely known and accepted. Type I is in the ascending aorta, the transverse arch, and the descending aorta. The intimal tear occurs in the anterior wall of the ascending aorta, but in some patients with intimal tears in the left subclavian the dissection may evolve into the ascending aorta, thus providing an anatomic DeBakey's Type I. In the DeBakey's Type II, the ascending aorta only is involved and the dissection stops proximal to the innominate artery. In DeBakey's Type III, the aortic dissection involves the descending thoracic aorta from a tear at the left subclavian but most commonly extends into the abdominal aorta.

The other commonly used clinical classification is that proposed by Dailey and colleagues (1970) (Fig. 33–57), which categorizes the dissection tear as beginning in the ascending aorta (Type A) or the descending aorta (Type B). This simplified classification does not provide as much detail about the pathoanatomic involvement as does that of DeBakey, but it is more usable clinically.

Clinical Signs and Symptoms

Acute aortic dissection affects more men than women by a ratio of 3:1 (although it is as high as 7:1 in some series (Wolfe et al, 1983), and the most common age of presentation is in the sixth or seventh decade of life (Doroghazi et al, 1984). Patients who present with dissection of the ascending aorta are about 10 years younger than the average age of patients presenting with a descending dissection. The most common manifestation is sudden severe chest pain, which signifies the onset of the dissection and the formation of the false channel. The chest pain usually is described as a tearing sensation that is felt in the front of the chest for ascending thoracic

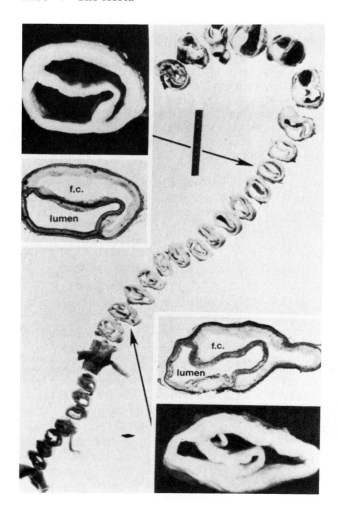

Figure 33–55. Dissection involving the entire length of the aorta in a 66-year-old woman. She suffered this serious complication 3 days after a seemingly uneventful aortic valve replacement. (f.c. = false channel.) (From Roberts, W. C.: Aortic dissection: Anatomy, consequences, and causes. Am. Heart J., *101*:195, 1981.)

aortic dissections and in the back between the scapulae for descending thoracic aortic dissections. The absence of posterior scapular pain is a strong indication that a posterior dissection is not present. The pain may often be in the jaw or neck, or it may simulate upper esophageal pain. Pain occurs in al-

most every patient (Slater and DeSanctis, 1976), although tiny painless dissections have been reported (Greenwood, 1986). With the onset of pain, hypovolemic shock of various degrees may result from loss of blood into the false channel from acute aortic valve regurgitation secondary to cardiac tamponade

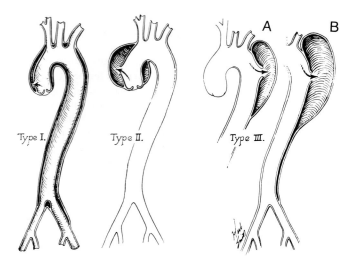

Figure 33–56. Illustration of surgical classification of dissecting aneurysm of the aorta into three basic types in accordance with the origin and extent of the dissecting process. (From DeBakey, M. E., Henly, W. S., Cooley, D. A., et al: Surgical management of dissecting aneurysms of the aorta. J. Thorac. Cardiovasc. Surg., *49*:131, 1965.)

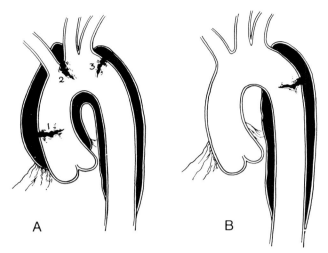

Figure 33–57. Classification of aortic dissections (Stanford). In Type A, the ascending aorta is dissected (*A*). The intimal tear has always been at position 1, but it can occur at position 2 or 3. In Type B dissection, the dissection is limited to the descending aorta (*B*), and the intimal tear is usually within 2 to 5 cm of the left subclavian artery. (From Daily, P. O., Trueblood, H. W., Stinson, E. B., et al.: Management of acute aortic dissections. Ann. Thorac. Surg., *10*:244, 1970.)

when the dissected aorta tears into the pericardial space below the pericardial reflection. Sudden death may occur from dissection of the right or left coronary artery.

Rarely, a patient with dissection may present with severe neurologic complications as the dissection immediately shears off one of the major cerebral arteries, such as the innominate or the left common carotid, producing stroke. Paraplegia may develop as the intercostal arteries are separated from the aortic lumen, or ischemic neuropathy may result from limb ischemia. Similarly, occlusion of the arteries in the lower leg may indicate acute obstruction of the arterial supply of the lower leg, stimulating embolism or thrombotic occlusion. Occlusion of the renal arteries may be associated with acute hypertension or renal shutdown (Gott et al, 1986). Thus, the clinical manifestations of acute aortic dissection depend on the variation in flow of blood in the false channel and the extent of peripheral or central arterial occlusion.

Diagnostic Tests

Chest Films

Patients with acute aortic dissection usually have a widened mediastinum, particularly in the upper part and toward the left thorax. In dissection of the ascending aorta, concomitant cardiomegaly may be secondary to pericardial effusion. There may be successive changes in the configuration of the aorta such as displacement of intimal calcification, a localized hump in the aortic arch, disparity of size in the ascending versus the descending aorta, and often a left pleural effusion (Smith and Jang, 1983).

Electrocardiogram

Electrocardiography helps to exclude the most common differential diagnosis—acute myocardial infarction. Absence of an acute injury pattern, together with negative serum cardiac enzyme elevation, supports the diagnosis of dissection, although if an ascending dissection separates the coronary arteries, the distinction may be impossible to make.

Contrast Radiographic Techniques

The contrast aortic angiogram is also a standard method for identifying patients suspected of having an acute aortic dissection, as it is for thoracic aneurysms, and is almost always done before operation (Fig. 33–58). The accuracy of this test is approximately 95% (Eagle et al, 1986; Slater and DeSanctis, 1976). The angiogram should (1) establish the diagnosis of dissection, (2) determine the site of the tear, and (3) delineate the extent of the dissection distally. In every case, unless the patient has absolutely classic historical and local findings and is in dire hemodynamic straits, aortography should be done. CT scanning may be helpful in the diagnosis of acute aortic dissection. A double aortic channel can usually be seen with an accuracy of almost 90% (Singh et al, 1986; White et al, 1986). The aortogram is still necessary to differentiate the exact location of the origin of the intimal tear. The main purpose of the CT scan is to differentiate a myocardial infarction from the dissection and to allow immediate progression to aortography to determine the intimal tear site. Magnetic resonance imaging (MRI) is also approximately 90% accurate in diagnosing aortic dissection and origins of main arterial trunks, but arguing against its routine use is the logistical preparation. CT scan, MRI, and echocardiography may often establish the diagnosis when aortograms are negative (Goldman et al, 1986).

Therapy

Natural History

The overall survival of patients with acute aortic dissection is difficult to predict because many patients die acutely, particularly with ascending dissection by aortic rupture into the pericardial cavity (Joyce et al, 1964) or into a main coronary artery. Without treatment, approximately only 8% of patients with ascending dissection survive for more than 1 month, whereas more than 75% may survive after dissection of the descending aorta (Kay et al, 1986). The accompanying data (Fig. 33–59) show the estimates of survival without surgical treatment of acute dissection of both the ascending and descending aorta, 5 and 70% at 1 year, respectively.

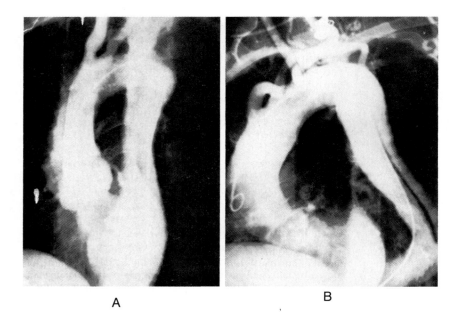

A   B

Figure 33–58. *A,* Thoracic aortogram in the left anterior oblique projection showing a dissection beginning in the ascending aorta and spiraling through the aortic arch into the descending aorta. The false lumen can be faintly seen. *B,* Left oblique anterior view of the aorta outlined angiographically showing a distal aortic dissection in a 63-year-old man. The true and false channels are clearly seen. The false channel is heavily opacified. (From Braunwald, E. [ed]: Heart Disease: A Textbook of Cardiovascular Medicine. Philadelphia, W. B. Saunders Company, 1984.)

Medical Therapy

Patients suspected of having aortic dissection should immediately be admitted to an intensive care unit for monitoring of arterial, central, and pulmonary artery pressures as well as urinary volume and electrocardiographic changes. The arterial blood pressure is immediately lowered with primary vasodilators such as sodium nitroprusside, trimethaphan, or reserpine (Wheat et al, 1965).

The drug most commonly used is sodium nitroprusside, 50 to 100 mg in 500 ml of saline infused at 25 to 50 μg/min to reduce the systolic blood pressure to the lowest level that still allows normal function of the cerebral, cardiac, and renal organs. The side

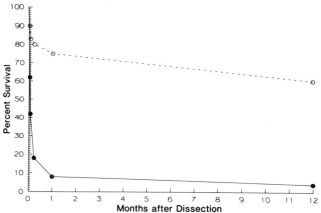

Figure 33–59. Estimate of survival without surgical treatment after acute aortic dissection. (Solid circles = patients with ascending aortic involvement; open circles = patients with only descending aortic involvement with or without abdominal aortic extension.) The estimate is based on data from the literature. (From Kirklin, J. W., and Barratt-Boyes, B.: Cardiac Surgery. New York, John Wiley & Sons, 1986. By permission.)

effects of prolonged use of nitroprusside may include cyanide toxicity developing after 48 hours of intensive use. Routine simultaneous beta-blockade is particularly important when sodium nitroprusside is used, because the latter may cause an increase in DV/DT (DeSanctis et al, 1987). If nitroprusside is insufficient or contraindicated, trimethaphan, 1 to 2 mg/min, can be used.

To reduce DV/DT, beta-blockade is used. Propranolol (1 mg every 5 minutes) is administered until there is evidence of beta-blockade, which is indicated by a slowing pulse rate. Beta blockade with an ultra-short-acting intravenous agent, esmolol, has been suggested for control of hypertension. It may be more effective because of its more rapid action (Gray, 1988). When the patient is stabilized, preparations are made for immediate CT scan or emergency aortic angiography or both (Fig. 33–60).

Medical therapy is generally considered to be the primary treatment for descending thoracic aneurysms, and operation is usually indicated only when there is a complication. Surgical repair is the treatment of choice for all ascending dissections, and medical therapy is only preparatory for operation. Medical therapy may also be used in patients with an ascending dissection if there are serious associated medical problems prohibiting operation. Although aortic arch dissection is rare and is reported to be treated successfully by operative intervention with decreasing risk, many prefer to treat aortic arch dissection primarily with medical therapy at least initially. Long-term therapy with antihypertensives, oral beta-blockade, diuretics, salt restriction, and careful re-examination by echocardiographic studies (ascending or descending) to note an increase in diameter of the aorta are necessary in the follow-up of aortic dissection.

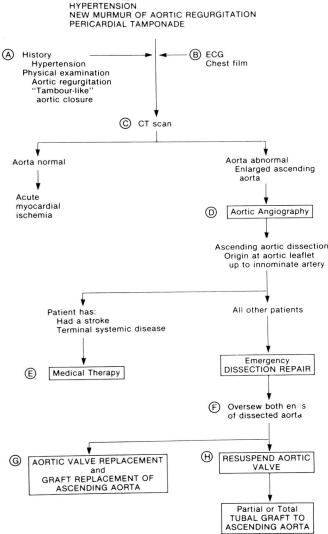

ANTERIOR CHEST PAIN
HYPERTENSION
NEW MURMUR OF AORTIC REGURGITATION
PERICARDIAL TAMPONADE

Ⓐ History
Hypertension
Physical examination
Aortic regurgitation
"Tambour-like"
aortic closure
Ⓑ ECG
Chest film

Ⓒ CT scan

Aorta normal
Aorta abnormal
Enlarged ascending
aorta

Acute
myocardial
ischemia

Ⓓ Aortic Angiography

Ascending aortic dissection
Origin at aortic leaflet
up to innominate artery

Patient has:
Had a stroke
Terminal systemic disease
All other patients

Ⓔ Medical Therapy
Emergency
DISSECTION REPAIR

Ⓕ Oversew both ends
of dissected aorta

Ⓖ AORTIC VALVE REPLACEMENT
and
GRAFT REPLACEMENT OF
ASCENDING AORTA
Ⓗ RESUSPEND AORTIC
VALVE

Partial or Total
TUBAL GRAFT TO
ASCENDING AORTA

Figure 33–60. Algorithm for decision making in acute aortic dissection. (From Cohn, L. H., Doty, D. B., and McElvein, R. B.: Decision Making in Cardiothoracic Surgery. Toronto, B. C. Decker, 1987.)

Surgical Therapy

DISSECTION OF THE ASCENDING AORTA

The optimal therapy for acute ascending dissections is early surgical therapy. The purpose of surgical treatment is to prevent exsanguination due to rupture and to re-establish blood flow in areas that may be occluded by the development of the intimal flap and false lumen. Operation is indicated even with serious complications related to the dissection. Obviously, considerable surgical judgment is indicated regarding surgical intervention in patients with an evolving stroke. Immediate repair of ascending dissections was suggested by retrospective analyses of a number of medical and surgically treated cases in the 1960s and 1970s (Appelbaum et al, 1976; Daily et al, 1970; Dalen et al, 1974). In the early repair of

ascending dissection, high mortality was associated with complications. However, in the 1960s and 1970s, when a limited number of surgical operations were done, repair of ascending aortic dissection proved to be more successful than medical therapy. These data have been duplicated by several other investigators and apply to any patient with any form of acute or chronic dissection of the ascending aorta (Crawford and Crawford, 1984; DeBakey and McCollum, 1982; DeSanctis et al, 1987; Miller et al, 1984; Wolfe et al, 1983).

The objectives of repair of the acute dissection of the ascending aorta are obliteration of the intimal tear and the false lumen, proximally and distally, and reapproximation of the edges of the dissected aorta proximally and distally by a prosthetic interposition graft (Fig. 33–61). Controversy exists, however, about the treatment of the regurgitant aortic valve in acute proximal dissections. Many surgeons have suggested aortic valve replacement with proximal dissection if there is aortic regurgitation, including a valve conduit for acute and chronic dissection (Cabrol et al, 1986; Crawford, 1983; Gott et al, 1986; Kouchoukos and Marshall, 1986; Kouchoukos et al, 1986). Others prefer reconstructive procedures when possible, preserving the native aortic valve by tacking the commissures with pledgeted sutures (see Fig. 33–61A) to preserve the valve, yet obliterating the aortic dissection (Kirklin and Barrett-Boyes, 1986; Koster et al, 1978, Meng et al, 1981).

In chronic dissection (> 14 days), a more studied angiographic and diagnostic approach may be taken because these patients have survived the acute episode. Results are excellent, because most have associated aneurysms (DeBakey et al, 1982; Miller et al, 1984). In chronic dissection, patients are operated on for specific indications such as expanding aortic aneurysm associated with the false aneurysm or, most commonly, severe aortic regurgitation (Fig. 33–62). In some patients, primary repair without an interposition graft has been reported (Olinger et al, 1987) to be successful, but long-term follow-up is necessary before this can be widely accepted. Another technique for repair of ascending aortic dissections that has received increased attention is use of the intraluminal graft, developed because of the hemorrhagic complications in the friable aortic suture lines. Reports by Spagna and colleagues (1985) and Berger and associates (1983) indicate favorable results and a decrease in the incidence of hemorrhagic complications (Fig. 33–63).

Bachet and colleagues (1982) have reported use of gelatin-resorcine-formol (GRF) adhesive to literally "glue" the edges of the dissected aorta together and also to toughen and tan the aorta at the point of dissection. This glue has been used extensively in France and Argentina, and the experience suggests that there is considerable improvement in results, because proximal and distal suture lines are not necessary if the layers are sealed. More investigation of these techniques is critical before they can be widely used, but they are of great interest.

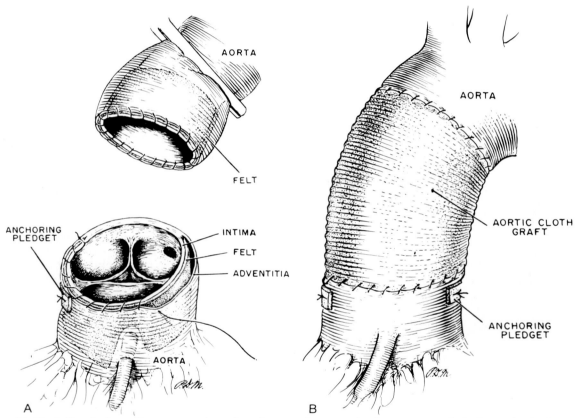

Figure 33–61. *A*, Prosthetic media reconstruction when the ascending aorta has been transected. *B*, Circumferential woven cloth graft to replace excised ascending aorta. (From Koster, J. K., Jr., Cohn, L. H., Mee, R. B. B., and Collins, J. J., Jr.: Late results of operation for acute aortic dissection producing aortic insufficiency. Ann. Thorac. Surg., 26:463, 1978.)

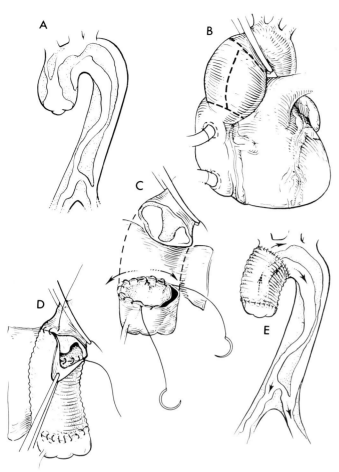

Figure 33–62. *A,* Chronic dissection of the entire aorta with a fragmented intima-medial flap. *B,* Limited transverse aortic root incision followed by "H" extension to facilitate graft replacement of the ascending aorta. *C,* Whipstitch used to obliterate the proximal false lumen and resuspend the aortic valve. The chronic false lumen is visible at the distal cut margin. *D,* A woven Dacron graft is interposed between the oversewn ends of the aorta and is sewn into place with a continuous suture. *E,* Completed repair shows perforation of both the true lumen and false lumen distally, thus reconstituting aortic blood flow. (From Gold, J. P., and Cohn, L. H.: Repair of chronic aortic dissection. *In* Cohn, L. H. [ed]: Modern Technics in Surgery/Cardiac Thoracic Surgery. Mt. Kisco, NY, Futura Publishing Co., 1984.)

DESCENDING DISSECTION

Controversy still exists about the exact timing of surgical intervention for dissection of the descending thoracic aorta. In some series, medically treated patients have fared better than surgically treated patients. Repair of dissecting aortic aneurysms in most clinics is reserved for those who have had distal dissection with leakage of blood from the aorta, compromise of arterial supply to a specific organ or limb, continued thoracic pain, or extension of the dissection while the patient is receiving satisfactory medical treatment. Inability to treat hypertension by maximal medical therapy is also an indication for repair. Some centers have excellent results with operative intervention, however, and believe that most patients at some time during the first year after the

acute event will require operation for acute dissection of the thoracic descending aorta (Ergin et al, 1985; Jex et al, 1986; Miller, 1983; Miller et al, 1984) unless the false lumen is clotted. Acute dissection of the descending thoracic aorta should be aggressively treated medically if no complications exist. The patient is stabilized for approximately 4 to 6 weeks after treatment of the acute event in preparation for definitive resection. At this time, edema of the aortic wall has resolved and the patient is better prepared to survive the repair.

The technical aspects of surgical intervention for descending thoracic aortic dissection are similar to those for the ascending aorta. Grafts are sewn in with the inclusion technique or intraluminal graft techniques by using one-lung anesthesia and intensive monitoring. For repair of the descending thoracic aorta, various techniques may be used to protect the

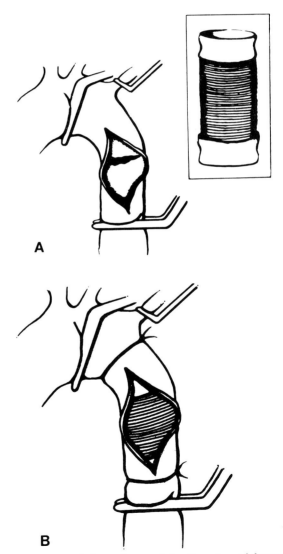

Figure 33–63. *A,* Sutureless graft for dissection of descending aorta—the tear and graft. *B,* The graft in place secured by heavy ties. (From Ergin, M. A., Lansmann, S., and Griepp, R. B.: Acute dissections of the aorta. Cardiac Surgery: State of the Art Reviews, *1:*377, 1987.)

spinal cord, as for descending aortic aneurysm: femorofemoral bypass, left atrial-femoral bypass, or left ventricular-femoral bypass. In acute dissections, the aorta is very friable and insertion of bypass shunts or cannulas into the thoracic aorta is contraindicated. The incidence of paraplegia is approximately 5 to 10% (Jex et al, 1986).

DISSECTION OF THE AORTIC ARCH

Dissection of the arch of the aorta is a formidable problem that until recently has been treated medically unless there has been rapid expansion or rupture. Some investigators have reported reasonable success with profound hypothermia and circulatory arrest (Ergin et al, 1982; Livesay et al, 1983) or low flow and moderate hypothermia with cerebral perfusion (Frist et al, 1986). With emergency operation, the risk is still 25 to 40% (Ergin et al, 1987). A simplified technique to reimplant cerebral vessels and obliterate arch dissection is shown in Figure 33–64.

Dissections that begin distally and extend prox-

imally and the development of late false aneurysms requiring reoperation represent another problem. Although surgical attempts are used to obliterate the false channel, an intimal tear may extend beyond the cross-clamp of the aorta or may not be detected at the time of the exploration. Haverich and colleagues (1985), Crawford and associates (1985), and Ergin and co-workers (1987) believe that the total extent of the intimal tear should be identified. Repair of the arch of the aorta may be required. Similarly, in dissection of the ascending aorta, when the spiral tear in an acute dissection extends into the arch beyond the clamp, techniques to do arch repair should be available and the tear should be repaired.

Results of Surgical Therapy for Dissection

Operative mortality for ascending dissection is 5 to 20%, and chronic dissections have lower mortality with a range of 5 to 10%. In the descending thoracic aorta, acute operations for dissection have an operative mortality of approximately 10 to 20%, mainly

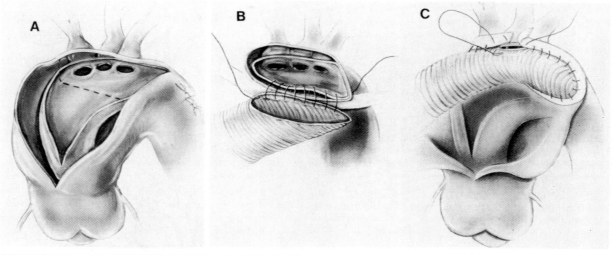

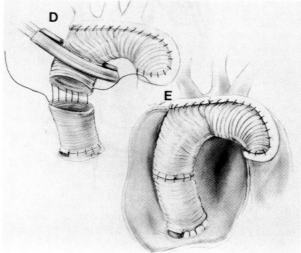

Figure 33–64. Repair of dissection of the aortic arch. *A*, Line of incision for distal aortic anastomosis when dissection extends into the aortic arch. *B* and *C*, The aorta is completely transected and anastomosed to the tube graft using an outer strip of Teflon felt. *D*, The tube graft is clamped proximal to the innominate artery after re-establishing bypass and evacuating air. *E*, The tube graft is sutured to the composite graft with 3-0 polypropylene. (From Kouchoukos, N. T., and Marshall, W. G.: Treatment of ascending aortic dissection in the Marfan syndrome. J. Cardiac. Surg., 1:342, 1986.)

because most operations are not done unless there is a complication. Chronic dissection aneurysms, in comparison, have much lower mortality, approximately 5 to 10%. Miller and colleagues (1984) analyzed 175 patients with aortic dissection by logistic descriptive analysis to identify high operative risk factors. After univariant screening, most predictive factors of operative mortality for Type A patients were renal dysfunction, tamponade, ischemia, and the time of operation. In Type B (descending) rupture, renal or visceral ischemia and age were the significant risk factors. Hemorrhage due to bleeding through and around the grafts from suture lines in the friable aorta has been the most common cause of operative mortality. The largest series in the literature of surgically treated patients with dissection is that of DeBakey, with 527 patients (DeBakey et al, 1982). The most common cause of late death in this series was rupture of false aneurysms and vascular events including myocardial infarction and stroke. Actuarial curves comparing medical (916 patients) and surgical treatment (527 patients) during a 20-year period are shown in Figures 33–65 and 33–66; 10-year survival is approximately 40%. Others have reported a 10-year survival of 60% in patients who leave the hospital (Kirklin and Barrett-Boyes, 1986). DeSanctis and associates (1987) found that 40% of late deaths among 119 survivors were due to complications of the dissection.

Redissection is an important consideration in therapy of aortic dissection. Patients with chronic untreated dissections and those who are postoperative must have continual long-term follow-up with chest films and noninvasive imaging to detect redissection. Reoperations pose an additional risk and are approached for expansion or leakage or recurrent aortic insufficiency in patients treated by valve resuspension. In Crawford and associates' experience (1985), the interval between operations varied from 2 months to 11 years in acute dissection in 12 patients

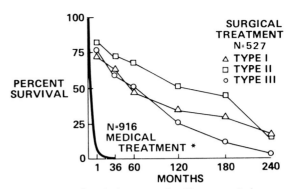

Figure 33–66. Survival curves of a 20-year period comparing medical and surgical treatment of 527 patients with dissecting aneurysms of the aorta, according to type. (From DeBakey, M. E., McCollum, C. H., Crawford, E. S., et al: Dissection and dissecting aneurysms of the aorta: 27-year follow-up of 527 patients treated surgically. Surgery, 92:1129, 1982.)

treated initially for Type I aortic dissection. Recurrent false aneurysms have been prevented in many patients by new suturing techniques by using more reinforced Teflon strips and GRF glue. In reoperations, CPB reduction of body temperature to deep hypothermic levels of 12 to 14° C is standard therapy. The circulation may be arrested and the patient's aneurysm repaired during the period of hypothermic arrest (Crawford et al, 1985).

Selected Bibliography

Crawford, E. S., and Crawford, J. L.: Diseases of the Aorta Including an Atlas of Angiographic Pathology and Surgical Technique. Baltimore, Williams & Wilkins, 1984.

This is a comprehensive atlas and treatise on surgical technique and a summary of results of one of the leading aortic surgeons in the world. The illustrations are magnificient, and the philosophy of the surgeon permeates the entire volume, which includes sections on all forms of aortic pathology, including arteriosclerosis, Marfan's syndrome, inflammatory diseases, dissections, and so on. There is also a concomitant wealth of angiographic anatomy.

DeBakey, M. E., McCollum, C. H., Crawford, E. S., et al: Dissection and dissecting aneurysms of the aorta: Twenty-year follow-up of five hundred twenty-seven patients treated surgically. Surgery, 92:1118, 1982.

This important article discusses the long-term effects of surgical treatment of dissection of the aorta. It includes the largest series of surgically treated patients with dissection of the aorta in the literature. The 20-year follow-up of 527 patients presents an enormous amount of important data and is a classic paper in the surgical era of treatment of aortic dissection.

DeSanctis, R. W., Doroghazi, R. M., Austen, W. G., and Buckley, M. J.: Aortic dissection. N. Engl. J. Med., 317:1060, 1987.

This is the most recent overview of the current diagnostic and therapeutic advances in the treatment of aortic dissection. The article is comprehensive and discusses many of the current diagnostic techniques, including MRI.

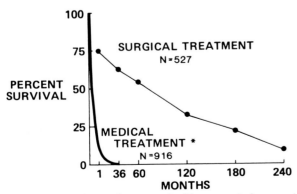

Figure 33–65. Survival curves of a 20-year period comparing medical and surgical treatment of 527 patients with dissecting aneurysms of the aorta. (From DeBakey, M. E., McCollum, C. H., Crawford, E. S., et al: Dissection and dissecting aneurysms of the aorta: 27 year follow-up of 527 patients treated surgically. Surgery, 92:1129, 1982.)

Gott, V. J., Pyeritz, R. E., Magovern, G. J., Jr., et al: Surgical treatment of aneurysms of the ascending aorta in the Marfan syndrome: Results of composite graft repair in 50 patients. N. Engl. J. Med., *314*:1070, 1986.

This is a superb article on pathophysiology and surgical technique. In their medical genetics clinic, the authors have studied connective tissue disorders, including Marfan's syndrome, as thoroughly as any service in the world. This is an excellent article on the guidelines for surgical intervention in patients with symptomatic and asymptomatic Marfan's syndrome. It provides superb long-term follow-up of the valve-graft conduit concept for replacement of the ascending aorta in Marfan's syndrome.

Hirst, A. E., Jr., Johns, V. J., Jr., and Kime, S. W., Jr.: Dissecting aneurysm of the aorta: A review of 505 cases. Medicine, *37*:217, 1958.

This article is a description of the natural history and pathology of acute aortic dissection. It represents one of the largest series in the literature and is well worth reading for its historical value. Now that operative connection is available, the series has become a classic.

Bibliography

Ablaza, S. G., Ghosh, S. C., and Grana, V. P.: Use of a ringed intraluminal graft in the surgical treatment of dissecting aneurysms of the thoracic aorta. J. Thorac. Cardiovasc. Surg., *76*:390, 1978.

Amparo, E. G., Higgins, C. B., Hricak, H., and Solitto, R.: Aortic dissection: Magnetic resonance imaging. Radiology, *155*:399, 1985.

Appelbaum, A., Karp, R. B., and Kirklin, J. W.: Ascending vs. descending aortic dissections. Ann. Surg., *183*:296, 1976.

Bachet, J., Gigou, F., Laurian, C., et al.: Four-year clinical experience with the gelatin-resorcine-formol biological glue in acute aortic dissection. J. Thorac. Cardiovasc. Surg., *83*:212, 1982.

Bahnson, H. T.: Definitive treatment of saccular aneurysms of the aorta with excision of sac and aortic suture. Surg. Gynecol. Obstet., *96*:383, 1953.

Bakker-de Wekker, P., Alfuri, O., Vermeulen, F., et al: Surgical treatment of infected pseudoaneurysm. J. Thorac. Cardiovasc. Surg., *88*:447, 1984.

Barsky, S. H., and Rosen, S.: Aortic infarction following dissecting aortic aneurysm. Circulation, *58*:876, 1978.

Bentall, H., and deBono, A.: A technique for complete replacement of the ascending aorta. Thorax, *23*:338, 1968.

Berger, R. L., Romero, L., Chaudry, A. G., and Dobnik, D. B.: Graft replacement of the thoracic aorta with a sutureless technique. Ann. Thorac. Surg., *35*:231, 1983.

Bickerstaff, L. K., Pairolero, P. C., Hollier, L. H., et al: Thoracic aortic aneurysms: A population-based study. Surgery, *92*:1103, 1982.

Bloodwell, R. D., Hallman, G. L., and Cooley, D. A.: Total replacement of the aortic arch and the "subclavian steal" phenomenon. Ann. Thorac. Surg., *5*:236, 1968.

Borst, H. G.: Ascending aortic aneurysms. *In* Cohn, L. H. (ed): Modern Techniques in Surgery/Cardiac Thoracic Surgery. Mt. Kisco, NY, Futura Publishing Company, 1984.

Cabrol, C., Pavie, A., Mesnildrey, P., et al: Long-term results with total replacement of the ascending aorta and reimplantation of the coronary arteries. J. Thorac. Cardiovasc. Surg., *91*:17, 1986.

Carlson, D. E., Karp, R. B., and Kouchoukos, N. T.: Surgical treatment of aneurysms of the descending thoracic aorta: An analysis of 85 patients. Ann. Thorac. Surg., *35*:58, 1983.

Carpentier, A., Deloche, A., Fabiani, J. N., et al: New surgical approach to aortic dissection: Flow reversal and thromboexclusion. J. Thorac. Cardiovasc. Surg., *81*:659, 1981.

Cooley, D. A., and DeBakey, M. E.: Resection of entire ascending aorta in fusiform aneurysm using cardiac bypass. J.A.M.A., *162*:1158, 1956.

Cooley, D. A., Romagnoli, A., and Milani, J. D.: A method of preparing woven Dacron grafts to prevent interstitial hemorrhage. Bull. Tex. Heart Inst., *8*:48, 1981.

Crawford, E. S.: Marfan's syndrome: Broad spectral surgical treatment of cardiovascular manifestations. Ann. Surg., *198*:487, 1983.

Crawford, E. S., and Coselli, J. S.: Marfan's syndrome: Combined composite valve graft replacement of the aortic root and transaortic mitral valve replacement. Ann. Thorac. Surg., *45*:296, 1988.

Crawford, E. S., Coselli, J. S., and Safi, H. T.: Partial cardiopulmonary bypass, hypothermic circulatory arrest and posterolateral exposure for thoracic aortic aneurysm operation. J. Thorac. Cardiovasc. Surg., *94*:824, 1987.

Crawford, E. S., and Crawford, J. L.: Diseases of the Aorta Including an Atlas of Angiographic Pathology and Surgical Technique. Baltimore, Williams & Wilkins, 1984.

Crawford, E. S., Crawford, J. L., Safi, H. J., and Coselli, J. S.: Redo operations for recurrent aneurysmal disease of the ascending aorta and transverse aortic arch. Ann. Thorac. Surg., *40*:439, 1985.

Crawford, E. S., Snyder, D. M., Cho, G. C., and Roehm, J. O. F., Jr.: Progress in treatment of thoraco-abdominal and abdominal aortic aneurysms involving celiac, superior mesenteric, and renal arteries. Ann. Surg., *188*:404, 1978.

Crawford, E. S., Walker, H. S. J., Saleh, S. A., and Normann, N. A.: Graft replacement of aneurysm in descending thoracic aorta: Results without bypass or shunting. Surgery, *89*:73, 1981.

Creech, O., Jr.: Endo-aneurysmorrhaphy and treatment of aortic aneurysm. Ann. Surg., *164*:935, 1966.

Crisler, C., and Bahnson, H. T.: Aneurysm of the aorta. Curr. Probl. Surg., *1*:64, 1972.

Culliford, A. T., Ayvaliotis, B., Shemin, R., et al: Aneurysms of the descending aorta. J. Thorac. Cardiovasc. Surg., *85*:98, 1983.

Dabir, R., and Serry, C.: Mycotic disruption of aortic cannulation site. J. Cardiovasc. Surg., *3*:77, 1988.

Daily, P. O., Trueblood, W., Stinson, E. B., et al: Management of acute aortic dissections. Ann. Thorac. Surg., *10*:237, 1970.

Dalen, J. E., Alpert, J. S., Cohn, L. H., et al: Dissection of the thoracic aorta: Medical or surgical therapy? Am. J. Cardiol., *34*:803, 1974.

DeBakey, M. E., and Cooley, D. A.: Successful resection of aneurysm of thoracic aorta and replacement by graft. J.A.M.A., *152*:673, 1953.

DeBakey, M. E., Cooley, D. A., and Creech, O., Jr.: Surgical considerations of dissecting aneurysm of the aorta. Ann. Surg., *142*:586, 1955.

DeBakey, M. E., Crawford, E. S., Cooley, D. A., and Morris, G. C., Jr.: Successful resection of fusiform aneurysm of aortic arch with replacement by homograft. Surg. Gynecol. Obstet., *105*:657, 1957.

DeBakey, M. E., Creech, O., Jr., and Morris, G. C., Jr.: Aneurysm of thoraco-abdominal aorta involving the celiac, superior mesenteric, and renal arteries: Report of four cases treated by resection and homograft replacement. Ann. Surg., *144*:549, 1956.

DeBakey, M. E., Henly, W. S., Cooley, D. A., et al: Surgical management of dissecting aneurysms of the aorta. J. Thorac. Cardiovasc. Surg., *49*:130, 1965.

DeBakey, M. E., McCollum, C. H., Crawford, E. S., et al: Dissection and dissecting aneurysms of the aorta: Twenty-year follow-up of five hundred twenty-seven patients treated surgically. Surgery, *92*:1118, 1982.

Derkac, W., Laks, H., Cohn, L. H., and Collins, J. J., Jr.: Dissecting aneurysm after aortic valve replacement. Arch. Surg., *109*:388, 1974.

DeSanctis, R. W., Doroghazi, R. M., Austen, W. G., and Buckley, M. J.: Aortic dissection. N. Engl. J. Med., *317*:1060, 1987.

Diehl, J. T., Payne, D. D., Rastegar, H., and Cleveland, R. J.: Arterial bypass of the descending thoracic aorta with the

Biomedicus centrifugal pump. Ann. Thorac. Surg., 44:422, 1987.

Doroghazi, R. M., Slater, E. E., DeSanctis, R. W., et al: Long-term survival of patients with treated aortic dissection. J. Am. Coll. Cardiol., 3:1026, 1984.

Eagle, K. A., Quertermous, T., Kritzer, G. A., et al: Spectrum of conditions initially suggesting aortic dissection but with negative aortograms. Am. J. Cardiol., 57:322, 1986.

Edwards, W. S., and Kerr, A. R.: A safer technique for replacement of the entire ascending aorta and aortic valve. J. Thorac. Cardiovasc. Surg., 59:837, 1970.

Egloff, L., Rothlin, M., Kugelmeier, J., et al: The ascending aortic aneurysm: Replacement or repair? Ann. Thorac. Surg., 34:117, 1982.

Emmanuel, R., Ng, R. A. L., Marcomichelakis, J., et al: Formes frustes of Marfan's syndrome presenting with severe aortic regurgitation: Clinicogenetic study of 18 families. Br. Heart J., 39:190, 1977.

Ergin, M. A., Galla, J. D., Lansmann, S., and Griepp, R. B.: Acute dissection of the aorta: Current surgical treatment. Surg. Clin. North Am., 65:721, 1985.

Ergin, M. A., and Griepp, R. B.: Surgical management of aortic arch aneurysms. In Cohn, L. H. (ed): Modern Technics in Surgery/Cardiac Thoracic Surgery. Mt. Kisco, NY, Futura Publishing Company, 1981.

Ergin, M. A., Lansmann, S. L., and Griepp, R. B.: Acute Dissections of the Aorta. Cardiac Surgery: State of the Art Reviews. Vol. 1, 1987.

Ergin, M. A., O'Connor, J. V., Blanche, C., and Griepp, R. B.: Use of stapling instruments in surgery for aneurysms of the aorta. Ann. Thorac. Surg., 36:161, 1983.

Ergin, M. A., O'Connor, J., Guinto, R., and Griepp, R. B.: Experience with profound hypothermia and circulatory arrest in the treatment of aneurysms of the aortic arch. J. Thorac. Cardiovasc. Surg., 84:649, 1982.

Frist, W. H., Baldwin, J. C., Starnes, V. A., et al: Reconsideration of cerebral perfusion in aortic arch replacement. Ann. Thorac. Surg., 42:273, 1986.

Frist, W. H., and Miller, D. C.: Repair of ascending aortic aneurysms and dissections. J. Cardiovasc. Surg., 1:33, 1986.

Geisinger, M. A., Risius, B., O'Donnell, J. A., et al: Thoracic aortic dissections: Magnetic resonance imaging. Radiology, 155:407, 1985.

Godwin, J. D., Herfkens, R. H., Skioldebrand, C. G., et al: Evaluation of dissections and aneurysms of the thoracic aorta by conventional and dynamic CT scanning. Radiology, 136:125, 1980.

Goldman, A. P., Kotler, M. N., Scanlon, M. H., et al: The complementary role of magnetic resonance imaging, Doppler echocardiography, and computed tomography in the diagnosis of dissecting thoracic aneurysm. Am. Heart J., 111:970, 1986.

Gott, V. L., Pyeritz, R. E., Magovern, G. J., Jr., et al: Surgical treatment of aneurysms of the ascending aorta in the Marfan syndrome: Results of composite graft repair in 50 patients. N. Engl. J. Med., 314:1070, 1986.

Gray, R. J.: Managing critically ill patients with esmolol, an ultra short-acting adrenergic blocker. Chest, 93:398, 1988.

Greenwood, W. R., and Robinson, M. D.: Painless dissection of the thoracic aorta. Am. J. Emerg. Med., 4:330, 1986.

Grey, D. P., Ott, D. A., and Cooley, D. A.: Surgical treatment of aneurysm of the ascending aorta with aortic insufficiency. J. Thorac. Cardiovasc. Surg., 86:864, 1983.

Griepp, R. B., Stinson, E. B., Hollingsworth, J. F., and Buehler, D.: Prosthetic replacement of the aortic arch. J. Thorac. Cardiovasc. Surg., 70:1051, 1975.

Gross, R. E., Hurwitt, E. S., Bill, A. H., Jr., and Peirce, E. C.: Preliminary observations on the use of human arterial grafts in the treatment of certain cardiovascular defects. N. Engl. J. Med., 239:578, 1948.

Haverich, A., Miller, D. C., Scott, W. C., et al: Acute and chronic aortic dissections—determinants of long-term outcome for operative survivors. Circulation, 72(Suppl. II):22, 1985.

Hirst, A. E., Jr., Johns, V. J., Jr., and Kime, S. W., Jr.: Dissecting

aneurysm of the aorta: A review of 505 cases. Medicine, 37:217, 1958.

Jarrett, F., Darling, R. C., Mundth, E. D., and Austen, W. G.: Experience with infected aneurysms of the abdominal aorta. Arch. Surg., 110:1281, 1975.

Jex, R. K., Schaff, H. V., Piehler, J. M., et al: Early and late results following repair of dissections of the descending thoracic aorta. J. Vasc. Surg., 3:226, 1986.

Joyce, J. W., Fairbairn, J. F., Kincaid, O. W., and Juergens, J. L.: Aneurysms of the thoracic aorta—a clinical study with special reference to prognosis. Circulation, 29:176, 1964.

Kay, G. L., Cooley, D. A., Livesay, J. J., et al: Surgical repair of aneurysms involving the distal aortic arch. J. Thorac. Cardiovasc. Surg., 91:397, 1986.

Kirklin, J., and Barratt-Boyes, B.: Cardiac Surgery. New York, John Wiley & Sons, 1986, p. 1497.

Koster, J. K., Jr., Cohn, L. H., Mee, R. B. B., and Collins J. J., Jr.: Late results of operation for acute aortic dissection producing aortic insufficiency. Ann. Thorac. Surg., 26:461, 1978.

Kouchoukos, N. T., and Marshall, W. G., Jr.: Treatment of ascending aortic dissection in Marfan's syndrome. J. Cardiac Surg., 1:333, 1986.

Kouchoukos, N. T., Marshall, W. G., and Wedige-Stecher, T. A.: Eleven-year experience with composite graft replacement of the ascending aorta and aortic valve. J. Thorac. Cardiovasc. Surg., 92:691, 1986.

Laënnec, R. T. H.: Traite de l'auscultation mediate et des maladies des poumons et du coeur, 2nd ed., Vol. 2. Paris, J. J. Chand, 1826, p. 696.

Lam, C. R., and Aram, H. H.: Resection of the descending thoracic aorta for aneurysm: A report of the use of a homograft in a case and an experimental study. Ann. Surg., 134:743, 1951.

Larson, E. W., and Edwards, W. D.: Risk factors for aortic dissection: A necropsy study of 161 cases. Am. J. Cardiol., 53:849, 1984.

Laschinger, J. C., Cunningham, J. N., Catinella, F. P., et al: Detection and prevention of intraoperative spinal cord ischemia after cross-clamping of the thoracic aorta: Use of somatosensory evoked potentials. Surgery, 92:1109, 1982.

Lemon, D. K., and White, C. W.: Annuloaortic ectasia: Angiographic, hemodynamic, and clinical comparison with aortic valve insufficiency. Am. J. Cardiol., 41:482, 1978.

Leonard, J. C., and Hasleton, P. S.: Dissecting aortic aneurysms: A clinicopathological study. Q. J. Med., 48:55, 1979.

Lindsay, J., Jr.: The Marfan syndrome and idiopathic cystic medial degeneration. In Lindsay, J., Jr., and Hurst, J. W. (eds): The Aorta. New York, Grune & Stratton, 1979b, p. 263.

Lindsay, J., Jr.: Thoracic aneurysms. In Lindsay, J., Jr., and Hurst, J. W. (eds): The Aorta. New York, Grune & Stratton, 1979a, p. 121.

Lindsay, J., Jr., and Hurst, J. W.: Clinical features and prognosis in dissecting aneurysm of the aorta: A re-appraisal. Circulation, 35:880, 1967.

Livesay, J. J., Cooley, D. A., Reul, G. J., et al: Resection of aortic arch aneurysms: A comparison of hypothermic techniques in 60 patients. Ann. Thorac. Surg., 36:19, 1983.

Meng, R. L., Najafi, H., Javid, H., et al: Acute ascending aortic dissection: Surgical management. Circulation, 64(Suppl. II):231, 1981.

Miller, D. C.: Surgical management of aortic dissections: Indications, perioperative management, and long-term results. In Doroghazi, R. M., and Slater, E. E. (eds): Aortic Dissection. New York, McGraw-Hill, 1983, pp. 193–243.

Miller, D. C., Mitchell, R. S., Oyer, P. E., et al: Independent determinants of operative mortality for patients with aortic dissections. Circulation, 70(Suppl. 1):153, 1984.

Moreno-Cabral, C. E., Miller, D. C., Mitchell, R. S., et al: Degenerative and atherosclerotic aneurysms of the thoracic aorta. J. Thorac. Cardiovasc. Surg., 88:1020, 1984.

Morris, G. C., Jr., Henly, W. S., and DeBakey, M. E.: Correction of acute dissecting aneurysm of aorta with valvular insufficiency. J.A.M.A., 184:63, 1963.

Muna, W. F., Spray, T. L., Morrow, A. G., and Roberts, W. C.: Aortic dissection after aortic valve replacement in patients with valvular aortic stenosis. J. Thorac. Cardiovasc. Surg., 74:65, 1977.

Murphy, D. A., Craver, J. M., Jones, E. L., et al: Recognition and management of ascending aortic dissection complicating cardiac surgical operations. J. Thorac. Cardiovasc. Surg., 85:247, 1983.

Najafi, H.: Vascular complications of extracorporeal circulation. In Cordell, A. R., and Ellison, R. G. (eds): Complications of Intrathoracic Surgery. Boston, Little, Brown & Company, 1979, p. 78.

Najafi, H.: Aortic dissection. In Sabiston, D. C., Jr., and Spencer, F. C. (eds): Gibbon's Surgery of the Chest. Philadelphia, W. B. Saunders Company, 1983, pp. 956–967.

Najafi, H., Javid, H., Hunter, J., et al: Descending aortic aneurysmectomy without adjuncts to avoid ischemia. Ann. Thorac. Surg., 30:326, 1980.

Olinger, G. N., Schweiger, J. A., and Galbraith, T. A.: Primary repair of acute ascending aortic dissection. Ann. Thorac. Surg., 44:389, 1987.

Orszulak, T. A., Pluth, J. R., Schaff, H. V., et al: Results of surgical treatment of ascending aortic dissections occurring late after cardiac operation. J. Thorac. Cardiovasc. Surg., 83:538, 1982.

Piehler, J. M., and Pluth, J. R.: Replacement of the ascending aorta and aortic valve with a composite graft in patients with non-displaced coronary ostia. Ann. Thorac. Surg., 33:406, 1982.

Pressler, V., and McNamara, J. J.: Aneurysm of the thoracic aorta. Review of 260 cases. J. Thorac. Cardiovasc. Surg., 89:50, 1985.

Pumphrey, C. W., Fay, T., and Weir, I.: Aortic dissection during pregnancy. Br. Heart J., 55:106, 1986.

Pyeritz, R. E., and McKusick, V. A.: The Marfan syndrome: Diagnosis and management. N. Engl. J. Med., 300:772, 1979.

Roberts, W. C.: Aortic dissection: Anatomy, consequences, and causes. Am. Heart J., 101:195, 1981.

Roberts, W. C.: The congenitally bicuspid aortic valve: A study of 85 autopsy cases. Am. J. Cardiol., 26:72, 1970.

Robicsek, F.: A new method to treat fusiform aneurysms of the ascending aorta associated with aortic valve disease: An alternative to radical resection. Ann. Thorac. Surg., 34:92, 1982.

Shaw, R. S.: Acute dissecting aortic aneurysm: Treatment by fenestration of the internal wall of the aneurysm. N. Engl. J. Med., 253:331, 1955.

Shennan, T.: Dissecting aneurysms. Medical Research Clinical Special Report Series No. 193. London, H.M.S.O., 1934.

Singh, H., Fitzgerald, E., and Ruttley, M. S.: Computed tomography: The investigation of choice for aortic dissection? Br. Heart J., 56:171, 1986.

Slater, E. E., and DeSanctis, R. W.: The clinical recognition of dissecting aortic aneurysm. Am. J. Med., 60:625, 1976.

Smith, D. C., and Jang, G. C.: Radiological diagnosis of aortic dissection. In Doroghazi, R. M., and Slater, E. E. (eds): Aortic dissection. New York, McGraw-Hill, 1983, pp. 71–132.

Spagna, P. M., Lemole, G. M., Strong, M. D., and Karmilowicz, N. P.: Rigid intraluminal prostheses for replacement of thoracic or abdominal aorta. Ann. Thorac. Surg., 39:47, 1985.

Spencer, F. C., and Blake, H.: A report of the successful surgical treatment of aortic regurgitation from a dissecting aortic aneurysm in a patient with the Marfan syndrome. J. Thorac. Cardiovasc. Surg., 44:238, 1972.

St. Cyr, J. A., Ward, H. B., and Molena, J. E.: Correction of thoracic aortic aneurysm-bronchial fistula. J. Cardiovasc. Surg., 2:109, 1987.

Walterbusch, G., Haverich, A., and Borst, H. G.: Clinical experience with fibrin glue for local bleeding control and sealing of vascular prostheses. Thorac. Cardiovasc. Surg., 30:234, 1982.

Wheat, M. W., Jr., Palmer, R. F., Bartley, T. D., and Seelman, R. C.: Treatment of dissecting aneurysms of the aorta without surgery. J. Thorac. Cardiovasc. Surg., 50:364, 1965.

White, R. D., Lipton, M. J., Higgins, C. B., et al: Noninvasive evaluation of suspected thoracic aortic disease by contrast-enhanced computed tomography. Am. J. Cardiol., 57:282, 1986.

Wilson, S. K., and Hutchins, G. M.: Aortic dissecting aneurysms: Causative factors in 204 subjects. Arch. Pathol. Lab. Med., 206:175, 1982.

Wolfe, W. G., Oldham, H. N., Rankin, J. S., and Moran, J. F.: Surgical treatment of acute ascending aortic dissection. Ann. Surg., 197:738, 1983.

V HEPARINIZED SHUNTS FOR THORACIC VASCULAR OPERATIONS

Vincent L. Gott

Most cardiothoracic surgeons agree that some type of temporary vascular bypass is required for major operative procedures involving the thoracic aorta. Aneurysms of the ascending aorta or proximal arch of the aorta require total cardiopulmonary bypass. For resection of segments of the distal arch of the aorta or descending thoracic aorta, several different bypass techniques are available. From a historical standpoint, the most common bypass technique used for aneurysms of the descending thoracic aorta during the 1960s and early 1970s was the left atrial–femoral artery bypass. This technique uses a pump to transfer approximately half of the cardiac output from the left atrium to the femoral artery while the descending thoracic aorta is cross-clamped. A second technique, which became popular 15 years ago, uses femoral vein–femoral artery bypass with an interposed pump oxygenator. This technique is advantageous because it does not require cardiac cannulation. It does, however, require the use of a heart-lung machine. Both of these bypass techniques require some systemic heparinization.

Because of problems with generalized bleeding from a large operative field in a heparinized patient, a technique that uses a simple temporary shunt around a thoracic aneurysm is appealing. This technique is advantageous because it eliminates the need for systemic heparinization and also obviates the need for an interposed blood pump. Actually, some of the earliest resections of aneurysms of the descending thoracic aorta were done with either a temporary internal plastic shunt (Johnson et al, 1955) or a temporary external shunt (Chamberlain et al, 1956; Stranahan et al, 1955). With the availability of suitable blood pumps, the simple tube-shunt techniques were abandoned for the left atrial–femoral artery bypass.

The introduction of polymers with wall-bonded heparin (Gott et al, 1963) allowed reintroduction of a temporary tube-shunt system that can be used safely. The first bypass shunts with wall-bonded heparin (Valiathan et al, 1968) used polyvinyl tubing with a graphite surface that was later immersed in benzalkonium chloride (a cationic surfactant) and then in heparin. The graphite, because of its absorptive properties, firmly bonded the positively charged surfactant. Then, with immersion in heparin, a strong electrochemical bond developed because heparin has a high negative charge. This surface permitted the bonding of heparin to the polyvinyl shunt and thus eliminated the need for systemic heparinization for patients with aneurysms of the descending thoracic aorta. The graphite-benzalkonium-heparin (GBH)-coated shunts were used initially as a bypass conduit for patients with thoracic aneurysms. Subsequently, an improved heparinized surface, the tridodecylmethylammonium chloride (TDMAC) heparin surface, was developed by the polymer chemists at the Battelle Columbus Laboratories (Grode et al, 1969). For several years, the Battelle chemists performed extensive studies on this TDMAC-heparin surface, which demonstrated firm bonding of high concentrations of heparin to the polymer (10 μg/cm^2).

An aortic bypass shunt made of polyvinylchloride and tapered at each end to facilitate proximal and distal cannulation has been designed* (Fig. 33–67). The central portion of this unitized shunt has a larger diameter to reduce the overall resistance to blood flow. This shunt is then coated with the transparent TDMAC-heparin coating. After sterilization with

*Available from Sherwood Medical Industries, Inc., 1831 Oliver Street, St. Louis, MO 63103

ethylene oxide, it has an indefinite shelf-life, and the wall-bonded heparin does not deteriorate.

Several excellent hemodynamic studies have been done on the use of the tapered heparinized shunt. One study (Frantz et al, 1981) showed that in adult sheep the mean left ventricular pressure rose by 64 ± 15 mm Hg when the descending thoracic aorta was cross-clamped. At the same time, the mean femoral artery pressure was only 28 ± 4 mm Hg. With the cross-clamp on the descending thoracic aorta, the left ventricular end-diastolic pressure rose to an average of 31 ± 8 mm Hg and v waves developed in the left atrium. At the same time, the left ventricle showed evidence of cardiac decompensation, and ventricular fibrillation frequently occurred after 15 to 20 minutes. When the tapered heparinized shunt was inserted from the apex of the left ventricle to the left common iliac artery, the mean left ventricular pressure rose by only 23 ± 9 mm Hg; the mean femoral artery pressure was 62 ± 15 mm Hg, and the left ventricular end-diastolic pressure and mean left atrial pressure were within normal range. Shunt flow averaged 1.6 ± 0.49 l/min, which was approximately one-third of the cardiac output. In these animals with left ventricular–common iliac bypass, the overall cardiac output was essentially normal. This technique of placing a vascular shunt between the left ventricular apex and the common iliac artery was first suggested by English (1965), of Guy's Hospital, London. These original shunts were constructed of simple polymer tubing without wall-bonded heparin. Murray and Young (1976) first used the heparinized shunt as a left ventricular–common iliac conduit. Murray (1974) has also shown that although there is no valve in the tapered shunt, the reverse flow in the shunt is less than 10% of the forward flow.

An excellent study (Verdant et al, 1988) reported the use of the heparinized shunt in 173 patients with

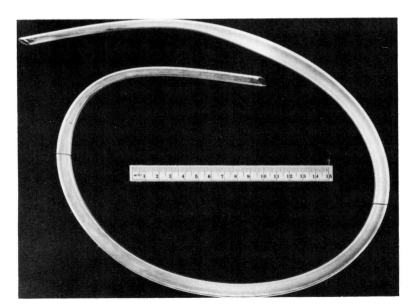

Figure 33–67. Unitized polyvinylchloride catheter with a heparinized coating for bypass of the descending thoracic aorta. The catheter is tapered at each end to facilitate proximal and distal cannulation. The central portion of the shunt has a larger diameter to reduce resistance to blood flow. (From Murray, G. F., Brawley, R. K., and Gott, V. L.: Reconstruction of the innominate artery by means of a temporary heparin-coated shunt bypass. J. Thorac. Cardiovasc. Surg., 62:34, 1971.)

descending thoracic aortic aneurysms. The authors of this study placed a flowmeter in the shunt and noted flow rates as high as 4000 ml/min and a mean proximal aortic pressure of 140 mm Hg. They recorded an average shunt flow of 2,500 ml/min and also noted an average distal aortic pressure of 62 mm Hg.

A number of laboratory and clinical studies have emphasized the importance of maintaining a distal perfusion pressure of more than 60 mm Hg to minimize the problems of spinal cord injury during thoracic aortic surgery. The most important work in this area of research was done by Cunningham and colleagues (1987), who monitored somatosensory evoked potentials during operative procedures on the thoracic aorta. By using this system, the authors stimulated the posterior tibial nerves with a bipolar input channel. Impulses conducted by the dorsal spinal column are recorded from midline scalp electrodes. Two parameters are usually monitored: latency of onset and amplitude of generated response. The studies in both animals and patients have shown close relationship between the decay and loss of these somatosensory evoked potentials and the development of spinal cord ischemia. An excellent clinical study by this group (Cunningham et al, 1987) correlated the changes in somatosensory evoked potentials in 33 patients having operations on the descending thoracic or thoracoabdominal aorta. The authors showed that when the distal aortic perfusion pressure could be maintained at greater than 60 mm Hg by either a shunt or bypass technique, the somatosensory evoked potentials were preserved and postoperative neurologic status was normal irrespective of the interval of thoracic aorta cross-clamp time. Also, if spinal cord injury is to be avoided, it is obviously imperative that the arterial blood supply to the cord not be permanently interrupted during the course of the operative procedure.

It should be emphasized that a number of thoracic aneurysms have been resected with simple cross-clamping and no protective shunting. Cross-clamping of the thoracic aorta appears to be tolerated reasonably well for as long as 30 minutes, but longer cross-clamping is associated with a fairly high risk of spinal cord injury. Katz and colleagues (1981) clearly showed the importance of some type of shunt bypass when the thoracic aorta is cross-clamped for more than 30 minutes. In their study, 35 patients had resection of a portion of the descending thoracic aorta for acute trauma. In 15 patients, no shunt was used and there was no paresis or paralysis in patients with the cross-clamp placed for less than 30 minutes. However, five of seven patients (71%) with cross-clamp times of 32 to 53 minutes did show evidence of spinal cord injury. Twenty additional patients had either a simple tube shunt or femoral-femoral bypass, and only three of these patients showed paresis or paralysis in the postoperative period. The cross-clamping times for these three patients were 34, 40, and 82 minutes. This study clearly showed that if

the thoracic aorta is cross-clamped for more than 30 minutes, some type of shunt or pump bypass should be used. A similar study from the Mayo Clinic (Jex et al, 1986) of patients having operative repair for dissections of the descending thoracic aorta provides similar data. In this study, the authors showed that the risk of spinal cord ischemia was significantly lower in patients who had protection of the distal circulation during operative repair: 8% incidence of spinal cord ischemia in those with protection compared with 44% in those without protection. The Mayo Clinic study also described a significant increase in risk of spinal cord injury after 45 minutes of aortic occlusion for patients who did not have protection of the distal circulation. No relationship between the probability of spinal cord injury and the length of aortic occlusion was noted for patients who had protection of the distal circulation.

HEPARINIZED SHUNTS FOR ANEURYSMS OF THE DESCENDING THORACIC AORTA

Selection of Patients

Heparinized shunts for temporary bypass of the descending thoracic aorta appear to be satisfactory for any patient who has a nonrupturing atherosclerotic aneurysm within any portion of the descending thoracic aorta. The ideal patient for shunt bypass has an aneurysm that begins just distal to the left subclavian artery and terminates several centimeters above the diaphragm. This type of aneurysm permits easy cannulation of the subclavian artery proximally or of the distal aortic arch. If the aneurysm involves the distal arch of the aorta, the shunt can be used with proximal cannulation in the ascending aorta or with proximal cannulation of the left ventricular apex, which was reintroduced by Murray and Young (1976).

Heparinized shunts have been used successfully in patients with a rupturing atherosclerotic aneurysm of the descending thoracic aorta. However, in the author's opinion, femoral vein–femoral artery bypass with a pump oxygenator is preferable for these patients because this system allows the retrieval of free blood from the chest cavity by means of a cardiotomy sucker system. If a pump oxygenator system is not available for a patient who has a rupturing atherosclerotic aneurysm of the descending thoracic aorta, the heparinized shunt bypass combined with an autotransfusion system can be a satisfactory alternative.

Surgical Technique

Several different methods exist for bypassing aneurysms of the descending thoracic aorta with the heparinized shunt. The original technique (Valiathan et al, 1968) used an approach in which the subclavian artery was cannulated proximally and the left common femoral artery was cannulated distally (Fig. 33–68). This particular bypass technique works well when the proximal portion of the aneurysm is 3 or 4 cm distal to the left subclavian artery. A thoracotomy is usually made through the fourth interspace or through the bed of the fifth rib. In the patient shown in Figure 33–68, because the aneurysm extended to the diaphragm, a second incision was made in the seventh interspace to facilitate cross-clamping of the aorta below the aneurysm. Generally, for the more standard-sized aneurysms of the descending thoracic aorta, the total procedure can be done through the bed of the fifth rib. After the thoracotomy is completed, the aorta is encircled with umbilical tapes above and below the aneurysm at the sites for eventual application of the vascular clamps.

The distal cannulation site most commonly selected is the left common femoral artery (see Fig. 33–68). It is possible, of course, to use the left common iliac site or, with a smaller aneurysm not extending

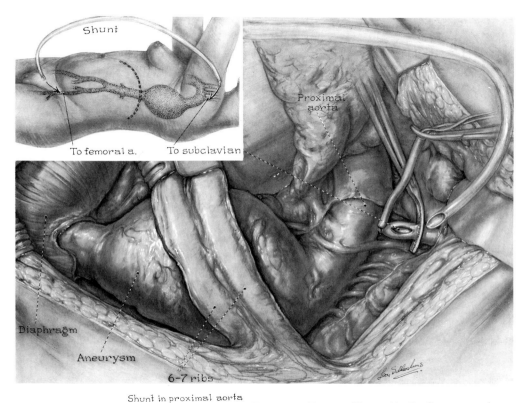

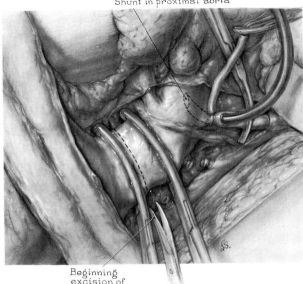

Figure 33–68. One type of surgical approach using the heparinized shunt during the resection of a large arteriosclerotic aneurysm of the descending thoracic aorta. *A*, Excellent exposure obtained through the bed of the fifth rib with a second incision through the seventh interspace. In this patient, the proximal cannulation is being done through the left subclavian artery and the distal cannulation is being done through the left common femoral artery. *B*, The aorta is prepared for proximal transection. *C*, Placement of the prosthetic graft with the heparinized shunt in position (From Valiathan, M. S., Weldon, C. S., Bender, H. W., Jr., et al: Resection of aneurysms of the descending thoracic aorta using a GBH-coated shunt bypass. J. Surg. Res., *8*:197, 1968.)

to the diaphragm, the distal cannulation site may be placed in the descending thoracic aorta just above the diaphragm.

If the aneurysm involves the aorta at the takeoff of the left subclavian artery, the proximal cannulation site can be placed in the distal transverse arch or in the ascending aorta. If the ascending aorta is used, generally the thoracotomy incision is extended across the sternum into the right side of the chest. For the latter type of aneurysm, the author prefers to cannulate the ventricular apex, a method popularized by Murray and Young (1976). This technique (Fig. 33–69) has the advantage of not requiring extensive dissection either in the transverse arch or in the area of the ascending aorta, which can be difficult through a left thoracotomy. Most cardiac surgeons are familiar with the placement of left ventricular vents in the apex, and the proximal end of the shunt is placed in a similar manner. As mentioned earlier, the hemodynamic parameters determined by Murray with this type of cannulation were satisfactory, and there was a less than 10% reversal of flow, even though there was no valve in the shunt.

Although the TDMAC-heparin surface has an indefinite shelf-life in terms of its anticoagulant properties, it is advisable to moisten the surface of the catheter in heparinized saline before use (5,000 units of heparin in 100 ml of saline). The author prefers to divide the shunt and do the proximal cannulation initially, followed by the distal cannulation, and then to re-establish continuity by using a highly polished stainless-steel connector. The aneurysm is then isolated with vascular clamps, and resection of the aneurysm and insertion of a prosthetic graft can be done without haste. A woven Dacron prosthesis is preferred, but a preclotted, knitted Dacron graft can be used because systemic heparinization is not used. The aortic anastomoses are ordinarily done with 4-0 monofilament polypropylene suture material. After the graft is in place and the clamps have been removed, the heparinized shunt is removed and the cannulation sites are repaired.

Results

During the last 15 years, a number of reports from several different institutions have described the use of the heparinized shunt for aneurysms of the descending thoracic aorta. Because this is not a particularly common cardiovascular problem, no single institution has had extensive experience. One of the best early reports in the literature was a survey of the experience of the members of the Samson Thoracic Surgery Society regarding repair of aneurysms of the descending thoracic aorta (Lawrence et

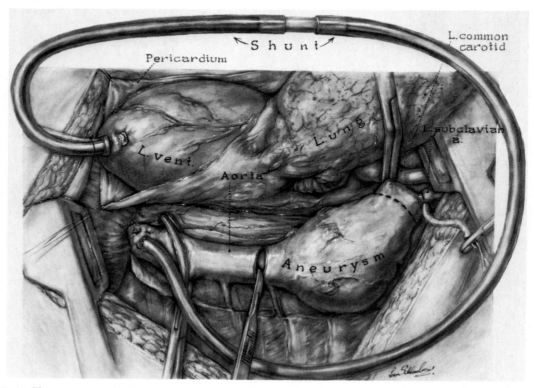

Figure 33–69. The newer cannulation technique using the heparin-coated shunt for resection of a thoracic aneurysm. The use of the left ventricle–to–aorta or iliac artery shunting technique has been made popular by Murray and Young (1976). The procedure is done through the bed of the fifth rib. The shunt has been divided to facilitate cannulation of the left ventricular apex proximally and the descending thoracic aorta distally.

al, 1977). In this report, 29 patients had shunt bypass of nontraumatic thoracic aneurysms; four deaths (13.8%) resulted, and no cases of paraplegia. In the same report, 127 patients had bypass of thoracic aneurysms by using a pump system with systemic heparinization. Fourteen patients had resection of thoracic aneurysms without any type of shunt protection, and there were two deaths (14.3%) and one case of paraplegia (7.1%). Nine of 61 respondents did 82% of the operations, and the 17 other surgeons who did the remaining operations performed an average of only 3.5 operations per decade. These data show that the average cardiothoracic surgeon deals with the problem of thoracic aneurysm rather infrequently, and therefore, a technique that protects the spinal cord should be used so that resection and repair can be done in a careful and unhurried manner.

At Johns Hopkins Hospital, 27 patients have had resection of nontraumatic aneurysms of the descending thoracic aorta by use of the heparinized shunt. The ten patients who had elective resection of an atherosclerotic aneurysm of the descending aorta survived and had satisfactory long-term results. Of the three patients who had acute rupturing atherosclerotic aneurysms of the descending thoracic aorta and who were operated on, only one survived. Although the results in these critically ill patients might not have been improved by using femoral vein–femoral artery bypass, this approach is currently preferred for rupturing thoracic aneurysms because of the availability of a cardiotomy suction unit in combination with the pump oxygenator. The operative results of resection for Type III dissections of the descending thoracic aorta have not been as good, particularly in individuals with acute dissections. Five of eight patients operated on for a chronic Type III dissection survived, whereas only two of six patients with an acute Type III dissection survived. Two of these six patients had a rupturing process at the time of operation, and three of the remaining patients had preoperative leg ischemia or bowel necrosis secondary to the dissecting process. None of the latter three patients survived. In this series of 27 patients with nontraumatic aneurysms, there were two cases of paraplegia, both in patients with rupturing atherosclerotic aneurysms. Both patients had resection of long segments of descending thoracic aorta; one patient survived, and the other died of a myocardial infarction 3 weeks postoperatively.

Other reports with the heparinized shunt for aneurysms of the descending thoracic aorta include 39 patients from Duke University (Wolfe et al, 1977). Thirty-four of these patients (87%) survived. The proximal end of the shunt was placed in the subclavian artery in 17 patients, in the left ventricle in 10 patients, and in the ascending or transverse aortic arch in 12 patients. These authors believe that if the site of proximal insertion of the shunt can be selected, it should be distal to the aortic valve, because that site allowed slightly better hemodynamics than did the proximal cannulation in the left ventricular apex.

Frantz and associates (1981) reported the clinical experience from the University of North Carolina. These investigators used the ventriculoiliac bypass technique with the heparinized shunt in 33 patients and found excellent hemodynamic parameters. Six deaths occurred in this group of 33 patients; three deaths occurred in six patients who were being operated on for dissection of the thoracic aorta. One patient was rendered paraplegic after resection of a long segment of thoracic aorta from the left subclavian artery to the diaphragm.

The largest series of patients having resection of aneurysm of the descending thoracic aorta by using the heparinized shunt was published from Montreal (Verdant et al, 1988). In this series, 173 patients had resection of a descending thoracic aortic aneurysm with use of the heparinized shunt. The cause of the aneurysms was atherosclerotic or medial degeneration in 83 patients, dissection in 34 patients, congenital malformation in 6 patients, and trauma in 50 patients. The overall operative mortality was 15% (26 patients), but of those patients operated on electively, the operative mortality was only 5%. Of greatest significance is the fact that although the aortic cross-clamp time was as long as 105 minutes, no paraplegia or other spinal cord ischemic deficit occurred in any of the 168 patients who survived long enough to allow an accurate postoperative evaluation of the function of the spinal cord. Only one patient developed renal failure requiring hemodialysis after resection of a ruptured false aneurysm into the left upper lobe.

HEPARINIZED SHUNTS FOR TRAUMA OF THE THORACIC AORTA

At the time the heparinized shunt was first developed in 1966, the only alternative method for spinal cord protection involved a pump and systemic heparinization (left atrial bypass). With systemic heparinization, one of the principal causes of death and morbidity was the significant bleeding that could occur, particularly through the interstices of the prosthetic graft and at the anastomotic sites. The ability to use a bypass system, such as the heparinized shunt, which did not necessitate systemic heparinization, appeared to offer a distinct advantage for some of these patients having thoracic aortic repair. During the last 20 years, prosthetic grafts have greatly improved, as have the techniques for anastomosing the grafts and controlling intraoperative bleeding as a result of systemic heparinization. The technique of femoral vein–femoral artery bypass using a pump oxygenator has been widely adopted, with currently a low morbidity and mortality related to intraoperative bleeding from systemic heparinization. The femoral vein–femoral artery bypass system also allows easy retrieval of blood from the operative field by using the cardiotomy suction device. The author is in agreement with those surgeons who prefer to use femoral-femoral bypass for resection of most thoracic aneurysms. The heparinized shunt may still be the bypass technique of choice in one situation—when an individual has sustained trauma to the thoracic aorta. This type of patient, particularly if additional head injury or soft-tissue injury is present, would ordinarily not be a candidate for systemic heparinization, and the surgeon would choose either simple clamping if the cross-clamp time can be limited to 30 minutes or possibly the use of a heparinized shunt if a cross-clamp time longer than 30 minutes is anticipated.

It should be emphasized that the availability of new centrifugal pumps that do not require systemic heparinization has allowed surgeons to return to the older technique of left atrial bypass and avoid some of the problems related to systemic heparinization, particularly in traumatized patients (Oliver et al, 1984). This type of system, which bypasses the left side of the heart and uses a centrifugal pump, would therefore be suitable for patients with thoracic aorta trauma and a head injury or soft-tissue injury. However, the heparinized shunt bypass technique may be simpler to use than the centrifugal pump because of the required left atrial cannulation and the potential problem of air embolism or thromboembolic complications from the pump.

Selection of Patients with Trauma of the Thoracic Aorta

Most patients sustaining major trauma to the thoracic aorta do not survive long enough to reach the operating room. This is particularly true for patients with penetrating wounds of the thoracic aorta. If a patient is alive on arrival at the hospital after suffering a penetrating injury of the aorta, it is imperative that he or she be moved quickly to the operating suite. A patient with this type of injury can occasionally be stabilized briefly before the operative procedure, and in this case, an aortogram should be obtained. Sometimes it is not possible to set up a heart-lung machine for immediate bypass of the aorta, and the surgeon can proceed with emergency operative intervention by using the heparinized shunt. In some cases, a heart-lung machine is not even available at the hospital, and for these patients, the use of the temporary shunt may permit immediate surgical intervention and successful correction of an otherwise hopeless clinical problem.

A relatively common injury of the aorta occurs as the result of an automobile collision: The descending thoracic aorta is almost transected at the level of the ligamentum ductus. In these patients with a blunt injury of the aorta, more time can be taken to prepare for operation than in patients with a penetrating

injury of the aorta. However, as stated earlier, these patients frequently have associated head and soft-tissue injuries that contraindicate systemic heparinization. The use of the heparinized shunt does appear to have considerable value in these cases.

Surgical Technique

The same shunting techniques that were described earlier for resection of thoracic aortic aneurysms can be used for traumatic injuries of the aorta. One of the advantages of the heparinized shunt in these cases is that it can be used in hospitals in which there is no pump oxygenator or when the urgency of the procedure dictates that the surgeon proceed quickly and not wait for the pump team. A case of this type has been reported earlier from Johns Hopkins (DeMeester et al, 1973) and is shown in Figure 33–70. This patient was admitted at 2:00 a.m. with a gunshot wound of the left side of the chest. The entrance wound was located over the second rib near the midclavicular line, and no exit wound could be found in the skin. The left carotid pulse was absent, and a progressive right-sided hemiparesis (face and trunk) was observed. The peripheral systolic blood pressure was 65 mm Hg. A chest film showed a widened superior mediastinum, with extension of the opacification into the left side of the chest. A metallic foreign body could be seen in the vicinity of the great vessels.

The patient was taken directly to the operating room, and a median sternotomy was made. Massive bleeding occurred from the anterior mediastinal hematoma. Cardiac massage was done while the descending thoracic aorta was exposed and cross-clamped distal to the innominate artery. A left anterior thoracotomy incision was made in the third intercostal space, and the descending thoracic aorta was isolated and cross-clamped. The heparinized shunt was then inserted between the ascending aorta and the left femoral artery for perfusion of the distal aorta, as shown in Figure 33–70. The aortic arch was dissected out to localize the injury. This injury consisted of avulsion of the left carotid artery at its origin and a linear laceration on the underside of the aortic arch (wound of exit) just above the left pulmonary artery. The bullet was found resting between the latter two structures. Retrograde bleeding from the left subclavian artery and the avulsed left carotid artery was controlled by cross-clamping these vessels, and the linear laceration of the underside of the aortic arch was then closed. The avulsed orifice of the left carotid artery on the arch was oversewn. The distal left carotid artery was then anastomosed end to side to the left subclavian artery. During the repair, the patient had two cardiac arrests and responded both times to massage and intracardiac epinephrine. Neurologic examination on the first postoperative day confirmed the presence of a right-sided hemiparesis, but at the time of discharge the patient's

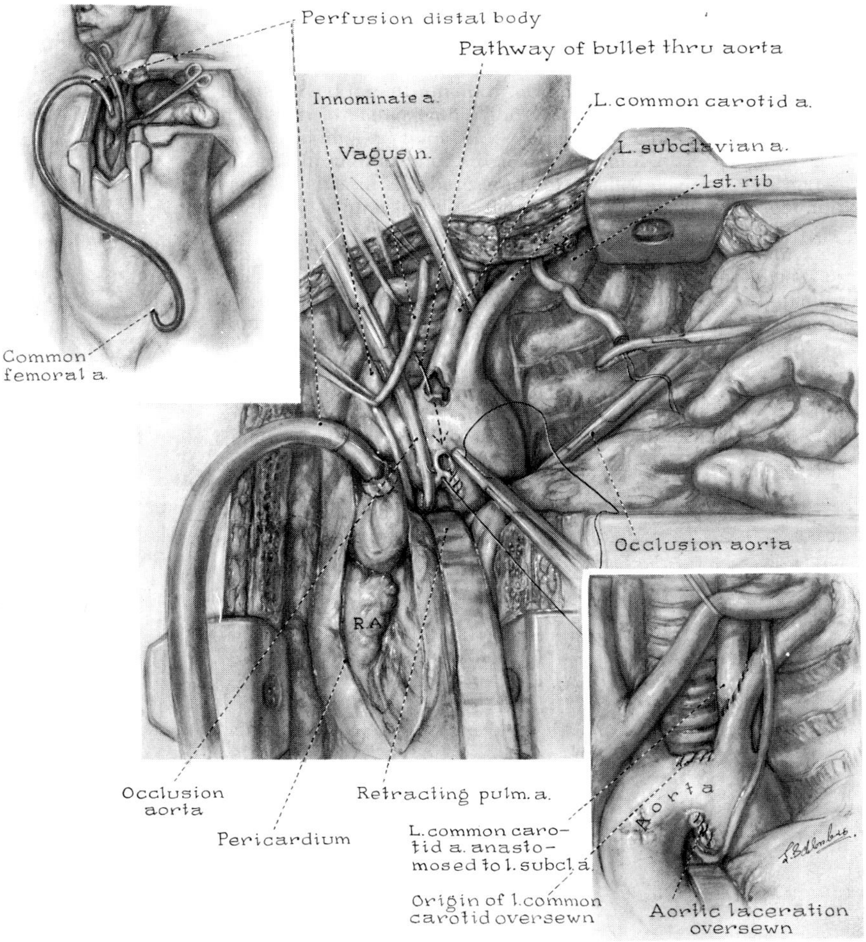

Figure 33–70. The operative approach for a through-and-through gunshot wound of the arch of the aorta by using a heparinized shunt. The wound has been isolated by cross-clamping the arch of the aorta just distal to the innominate artery and also clamping the proximal descending thoracic aorta, the left carotid artery, and the left subclavian artery. During the operative repair, blood is being shunted to the lower portion of the body through the heparinized shunt from the ascending aorta to the common femoral artery. (Reported with permission from The Society of Thoracic Surgeons [The Annals of Thoracic Surgery, Vol. 16, 1973, p. 193].)

right arm had begun to function again. With continued physical therapy, he regained total function of his right arm except for fine movement of the right hand.

Results

Most patients with major trauma of the thoracic aorta do not survive long enough to reach a hospital for definitive repair. Therefore, no single institution has reported a large number of patients operated on by using the heparinized shunt for traumatic lesions of the thoracic aorta. Again, one of the best early reports on this topic is the summary of the experience of the members of the Samson Society of Thoracic Surgeons (Lawrence et al, 1977). Those researchers reported their own personal experience with 16 traumatic aneurysms of the thoracic aorta treated with the use of the heparinized shunt. They reported two deaths (12%) and one case of paraplegia (6%). In addition, they summarized the experience of the 26 respondents to a questionnaire. These 26 surgeons had used the heparinized shunt in 39 patients with trauma of the thoracic aorta, and no deaths and no paraplegia were reported. Their experience with

pump bypass and systemic heparinization for traumatic injury of the thoracic aorta totaled 134 cases, with 11 deaths (8%) and three patients with paraplegia (2%).

The largest single series of patients having repair of thoracic aorta trauma by using the heparinized shunt is the Montreal experience (Verdant et al, 1988). Of this group of 173 patients who had thoracic aorta repair with the heparin shunt bypass, 50 were operated on for a traumatic injury of the aorta. The overall operative mortality was 4%; four hospital deaths occurred in 26 patients (15%) who were operated on for an acute injury to the aorta, and no deaths occurred in the remaining 24 patients with a chronic aortic injury. These authors reported no case of paraplegia among the 50 patients having operation for thoracic aorta trauma with the use of the heparin shunt.

Ten patients who suffered trauma to the thoracic aorta and who had operative repair by using the heparinized shunt have been seen at the Johns Hopkins Hospital. Six patients were operated on for acute traumatic damage and four for chronic traumatic problems. No deaths occurred in this group of patients with trauma, and no paraplegia resulted.

HEPARINIZED SHUNTS FOR RECONSTRUCTION OF THE INNOMINATE ARTERY

Selection of Patients

Vascular reconstruction for innominate artery lesions has become possible only during the last 30 years. Successful excision of a saccular aneurysm of the innominate artery with preservation of arterial continuity was first reported in 1953 (Bahnson, 1953). In addition, a 10-year experience with reconstruction for arteriosclerotic occlusive disease of the innominate artery has been reported (Crawford et al, 1969).

Provision for perfusion of the central nervous system must be considered in the correction of any innominate artery lesion. The common technique previously used for repair of traumatic lesions or aneurysms of the innominate artery was cardiopulmonary bypass with perfusion of the cerebral vessels. Although this technique of innominate artery bypass is satisfactory for supporting the cerebral circulation, the overall procedure can be simplified considerably by using the heparinized shunt (Murray et al, 1971).

A number of operative procedures have been done on the innominate artery with simple occlusion of this vessel during the operative procedure. Catlin (1960) reported a patient who survived bilateral carotid artery ligation. The reported incidence of hemiplegia after ligation of the common carotid artery was from 25 to 70% (Watson and Silverstone, 1939). Similarly, the ability of patients to tolerate periods of innominate artery occlusion was inconsistent (De-Bakey and Crawford, 1957; Kirby and Johnson, 1953).

Surgical Technique

The application of the heparinized shunt for innominate artery repair is shown in Figure 33–71. The patient was a 47-year-old man who was brought to the hospital after an automobile accident. He had had severe head injuries with a scleral rupture of his left globe and had also a flail right-sided chest with an associated hemopneumothorax. X-ray films of the skull and facial bones showed multiple facial fractures. A retrograde aortogram revealed avulsion injuries of the innominate and left subclavian arteries (see Fig. 33–71).

The patient was taken to the operating room 5 hours after admission, and the ascending aorta and great vessels were exposed through a median sternotomy incision (Fig. 33–72). A GBH-coated shunt was placed between the proximal aorta and the right common carotid artery to bypass the innominate artery injury. A partial occluding clamp was placed across the arch of the aorta, sparing the left carotid artery. The innominate artery was occluded distally and the false aneurysm was entered. A complete avulsion of the innominate artery from the aortic

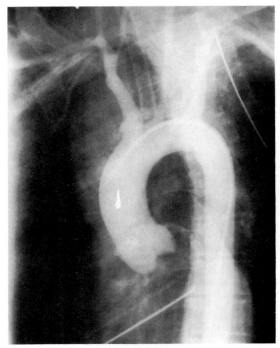

Figure 33–71. Thoracic aortogram of a patient who sustained blunt trauma to the chest. Disruption of the innominate artery near its origin and of the left subclavian artery in its second portion can be seen. (From Murray, G. F., Brawley, R. K., and Gott, V. L.: Reconstruction of the innominate artery by means of a temporary heparin-coated shunt bypass. J. Thorac. Cardiovasc. Surg., 62:34, 1971.)

arch was found. The defect in the aorta was oversewn, and the vessel was reconstructed with a Dacron prosthesis. A complete circumferential tear in the left subclavian artery just distal to the vertebral artery was repaired through a separate supraclavicular incision. The scleral rupture was repaired, and exploratory laparotomy showed bleeding from a small mesenteric vessel. The patient had a difficult postoperative course but later improved. However, several months after discharge from the hospital, he became jaundiced and had evidence of homologous serum hepatitis. His condition then deteriorated, and death was precipitated by pneumonia 10 months after operation.

This type of patient with an avulsion injury of the innominate artery and multiple head and abdominal injuries does not tolerate systemic heparinization for total cardiopulmonary bypass, and the use of the heparinized shunt may therefore be a determining factor in achieving successful results.

Results

Heparinized shunts have not been widely used for innominate artery operations, but in the few reported cases the results have been favorable. A total of seven patients have had innominate artery

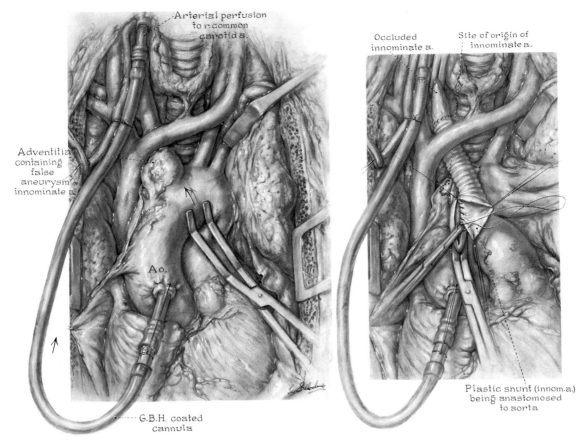

Figure 33–72. Bypass of the traumatic aneurysm shown in Figure 33–71, with a GBH-coated shunt. Entry into the false aneurysm revealed complete avulsion of the innominate artery from the arch. As shown, the defect in the aorta was oversewn and the innominate artery was reconstructed with a Dacron prosthesis. (From Murray, G. F., Brawley, R. K., and Gott, V. L.: Reconstruction of the innominate artery by means of a temporary heparin-coated shunt bypass. J. Thorac. Cardiovasc. Surg., 62:34, 1971.)

reconstruction by using the heparinized shunt at the Johns Hopkins Hospital. In addition to the patient shown in Figure 33–72, four other patients at Johns Hopkins have had innominate artery endarterectomy for arteriosclerotic disease and the results have been excellent. A fifth patient had a successful repair of a penetrating injury of the innominate artery, and another had successful repair of a large luetic aneurysm of the innominate artery.

OTHER APPLICATIONS FOR HEPARINIZED VASCULAR SHUNTS

Although the primary application of this type of heparinized shunt has been in patients with either aneurysms or trauma involving the descending thoracic aorta or in patients requiring an operative procedure on the innominate artery, other vascular procedures have been done by using this bypass system. Murray (1974) reported the use of the heparin-coated shunt in two patients with atypical coarctation of the aorta. In both patients, coarctation of the aorta involved the left subclavian artery or occurred proximal

to it. At the time of cross-clamping of the aorta for the coarctation repair, collateral flow to the distal aorta was inadequate, with a virtual collapse of this vessel beyond the vascular clamps. In both cases, bypass was established with the heparinized shunt and a satisfactory repair of the coarctation was achieved. This type of heparinized shunt has also been used for resecting an aneurysm of the upper aspect of the abdominal aorta (Edwards, 1973). The aneurysm in this patient was secondary to an earlier gunshot wound, and the operating surgeon reported that the procedure was considerably simplified by using the heparinized shunt bypass.

An additional nonthoracic application of the heparinized shunt has been in carotid endarterectomy. Standard carotid artery plastic shunts have been prepared with the TDMAC-heparin coating, which requires systemic heparinization. In these patients, the operative field is much smaller than in patients having resection of a thoracic aneurysm, and the advantage of eliminating systemic heparinization would not be as great as in the thoracic cases. Finally, the standard heparinized shunts for thoracic aorta bypass are now being used widely in combination with the centrifugal blood pump for venous-venous bypass in transplantation of the liver (Griffith et al, 1985).

Selected Bibliography

Frantz, P. T., Murray, G. F., Shallal, J. A., and Lucas, C. L.: Clinical and experimental evaluation of left ventriculoiliac shunt bypass during repair of lesions of the descending thoracic aorta. Ann. Thorac. Surg., 31:551, 1981.

This article reports a thorough hemodynamic evaluation of the heparinized shunt in adult sheep by using left ventriculoiliac shunt bypass. When compared with control animals with total occlusion of the thoracic aorta, aortic pressure above and below the clamped aorta returned almost to normal with the use of the interposed shunt. No significant changes occurred in cardiac output, left ventricular end-disastolic pressure, or left atrial pressure with the use of the shunt and a cross-clamped thoracic aorta. In addition, reversed flow through the shunt was less than 10%, despite the fact that there was no valve in the shunt.

Gott, V. L., Whiffen, J. D., and Dutton, R. C.: Heparin bonding on colloidal graphite surfaces. Science, 142:1297, 1963.

This is the first report of a surface that appears to have significant thromboresistance. Both in-vitro and in-vivo studies showed that a surface coated with graphite, benzalkonium, and heparin is superior to plain polymer and silicone surfaces. The in-vitro studies were done by using standard Lee-White clotting times, and the in-vivo studies were done by using small conduits placed in the canine vena cava.

Grode, G. A., Anderson, S. J., Grotta, H. M., and Falb, R. D.: Nonthrombogenic materials via a simple coating process. Trans. Am. Soc. Artif. Intern. Organs, 15:1, 1969.

This important article presents an improved method for heparinizing the surface of polymers by using the cationic surfactant TDMAC as the bonding substance for the heparin. The TDMAC-heparin coating allows bonding of a greater quantity of heparin than does the GBH coating, and the surface is transparent and has excellent mechanical durability.

Murray, G. F., and Young, W. G., Jr.: Thoracic aneurysmectomy utilizing direct left ventriculofemoral shunt (TDMAC-heparin) bypass. Ann. Thorac. Surg., 21:26, 1976.

In this article, the authors describe the first reported use of the heparinized shunt with proximal cannulation in the left ventricular apex and distal cannulation in the femoral artery. They report successful use of this technique in two patients with traumatic aneurysms of the descending thoracic aorta. This particular shunting technique has now become a popular method of bypassing the thoracic aorta, and for some patients it is simpler than cannulating the arch of the aorta or the left subclavian artery. This technique of left ventriculofemoral shunting was first described by English (1965) and used a non-heparin-coated shunt resection of a coarctation of the aorta.

Valiathan, M. S., Weldon, C. S., Bender, H. W., Jr., et al: Resection of aneurysms of the descending thoracic aorta using a GBH-coated shunt bypass. J. Surg. Res., 8:197, 1968.

This is the first report of the use of a shunt with wall-bonded heparin for the resection of aneurysms of the descending aorta. Four patients had elective resection of an aneurysm of the descending thoracic aorta, and all four patients had an excellent recovery. Two patients were operated on with rupturing aneurysms of the descending aorta, and long-term survival was not achieved in these patients.

Verdant, A., Mercier, C., Page, A., et al: Surgery of the descending thoracic aorta: Spinal cord protection with the Gott shunt. Ann. Thorac. Surg., 46:147, 1988.

This is the largest series of patients having repair of the descending thoracic aorta by using the heparinized shunt. The authors have exclusively used the heparinized shunt for all patients having operation on the descending thoracic aorta. Their series consists of 173 unselected patients who had descending thoracic aortic resection since 1974. Fifty patients had traumatic aneurysms, 83 had degenerative arteriosclerotic aneurysms, 34 had Type III dissecting aneurysms, and 6 had congenital aneurysms. There were 26 deaths related to resection, an overall operative mortality of 15%. The operative mortality was only 5.4% for patients having elective aortic surgery with the heparin shunt bypass. Of the 173 patients, 168 survived long enough to allow an accurate postoperative evaluation of the function of the spinal cord. No paraplegia and no other spinal cord ischemic deficits were noted in any of the 168 patients.

Bibliography

Bahnson, H. T.: Definitive treatment of saccular aneurysms of the aorta with excision of sac and aortic suture. Surg. Gynecol. Obstet., 96:383, 1953.

Catlin, D.: A case of carcinoma of the larynx surviving bilateral carotid artery ligation. Ann. Surg., 153:809, 1960.

Chamberlain, J. M., Klopstock, R., Parnassa, P., et al: The use of shunts in surgery of the thoracic aorta. J. Thorac. Surg., 31:251, 1956.

Crawford, E. S., DeBakey, M. E., Morris, G. C., Jr., and Howell, J. F.: Surgical treatment of occlusion of the innominate, common carotid and subclavian arteries: A 10-year experience. Surgery, 65:17, 1969.

Cunningham, J. N., Jr., Laschinger, J. C., and Spencer, F. C.: Monitoring of somatosensory evoked potentials during surgical procedures in the thoracoabdominal aorta. IV: Clinical observations and results. J. Thorac. Cardiovasc. Surg., 94:275, 1987.

DeBakey, M. E., and Crawford, E. S.: Resection and homograft replacement of innominate and carotid arteries with the use of shunt to maintain circulation. Surg. Gynecol. Obstet., 105:129, 1957.

DeMeester, T. R., Cameron, J. L., and Gott, V. L.: Repair of a through-and-through gunshot wound of the aortic arch using a heparinized shunt. Ann. Thorac. Surg., 16:193, 1973.

Edwards, W. S.: Personal communication, 1973.

English, T. A. H.: Direct left ventriculofemoral bypass during resection of coarctation of the aorta with anomalous subclavian arteries. Thorax, 20:36, 1965.

Frantz, P. T., Murray, G. F., Shallal, J. A., and Lucas, C. L.: Clinical and experimental evaluation of left ventriculoiliac shunt bypass during repair of lesions of the descending thoracic aorta. Ann. Thorac. Surg., 31:551, 1981.

Gott, V. L., Whiffen, J. D., and Dutton, R. C.: Heparin bonding on colloidal graphite surfaces. Science, 142:1297, 1963.

Griffith, B. P., Shaw, B. W., Jr., Hardesty, R. L., et al: Veno-venous bypass without systemic anticoaguation for transplantation of the human liver. Surg. Gynecol. Obstet., 169:271, 1985.

Grode, G. A., Anderson, S. J., Grotta, H. M., and Falb, R. D.: Nonthrombogenic materials via a simple coating process. Trans. Am. Soc. Artif. Intern. Organs, 15:1, 1969.

Jex, R. K., Schaff, H. V., Piehler, J. M., et al: Early and late results following repair of dissections of the descending thoracic aorta. J. Vasc. Surg., 3:226, 1986.

Johnson, J., Kirby, C. K., and Lehr, H. B.: A method of maintaining adequate blood flow through the thoracic aorta while inserting an aorta graft to replace an aortic aneurysm. Surgery, 37:54, 1955.

Katz, N. M., Blackstone, E. H., Kirklin, J. W., and Karp, R. B.: Incremental risk factors for spinal cord injury following operation for acute traumatic aortic transection. J. Thorac. Cardiovasc. Surg., *81*:669, 1981.

Kirby, C. K., and Johnson, J. J.: Innominate artery aneurysm treated by resection and end-to-end anastomosis. Surgery, *33*:562, 1953.

Lawrence, G. H., Hessel, E. A., Sauvage, L. R., and Krause, A. H.: Results of the use of the TDMA-heparin shunt in the surgery of aneurysms of the descending thoracic aorta. J. Thorac. Cardiovasc. Surg., *73*:393, 1977.

Murray, G. F.: Atypical proximal coarctation of the aorta: Reconstruction by means of a heparin-coated temporary shunt bypass. Ann. Surg., *180*:309, 1974.

Murray, G. F., Brawley, R. K., and Gott, V. L.: Reconstruction of the innominate artery by means of a temporary heparin-coated shunt bypass. J. Thorac. Cardiovasc. Surg., *62*:34, 1971.

Murray, G. F., and Young, W. G., Jr.: Thoracic aneurysmectomy utilizing direct left ventriculofemoral shunt (TDMAC-heparin) bypass. Ann. Thorac. Surg., *21*:26, 1976.

Oliver, H. F., Jr., Maher, T. D., Liebler, G. A., et al: Use of the Biomedicus centrifugal pump in traumatic tears of the thoracic aorta. Ann. Thorac. Surg., *38*:586, 1984.

Stranahan, A., Alley, R. D., Sewell, W. H., and Kausel, H. W.: Aortic arch resection and grafting for aneurysm employing an external shunt. J. Thorac. Surg., *29*:54, 1955.

Valiathan, M. S., Weldon, C. S., Bender H. W., Jr., et al: Resection of aneurysms of the descending thoracic aorta using a GBH-coated shunt bypass. J. Surg. Res., *8*:197, 1968.

Verdant, A., Page, A., Cossette, R., et al: Surgery of the descending thoracic aorta: Spinal cord protection with the Gott shunt. Ann. Thorac. Surg., *46*:147, 1988.

Watson, W. L., and Silverstone, S. M.: Ligature of the common carotid artery in cancer of the head and neck. Ann. Surg., *109*:1, 1939.

Wolfe, W. G., Kleinman, L. H., Wechsler, A. S., and Sabiston, D. C., Jr.: Heparin-coated shunts for lesions of the descending thoracic aorta: Experimental and clinical observations. Arch. Surg., *112*:1481, 1977.

VI OCCLUSIVE DISEASE OF BRANCHES OF THE AORTA

Robert B. Peyton
O. Wayne Isom

Occlusive disease of the arch vessels presents as ischemic disturbances of the head, neck, and upper extremities with absent or decreased pulses. Savory (1856) first described this condition in a young woman whose main arteries of both upper extremities and left carotid artery were completely occluded. Aortic arch syndrome (Ross and McKusick, 1953), Takayasu's disease (Takayasu, 1908), pulseless disease (Davis et al, 1956), reverse coarctation (Crawford et al, 1962), Martorell's syndrome (Davis et al, 1956) thrombotic obliteration of the branches of the aortic arch (Crawford et al, 1962), and aortic dome syndrome (Thevenet, 1979) are other names for this condition (Crawford et al, 1983).

In early reports, most patients had advanced clinical manifestations with extensive arterial occlusion, and their affliction was considered to be rare and incurable. With the advent of cerebral angiography, this disease has been recognized with increasing frequency and is often segmental and well localized, and proximal and distal arterial segments are relatively normal. This form of the disease has been treated successfully with numerous operative techniques during the last 30 years.

PATHOLOGY

Occlusive lesions in the branches of the aortic arch have been reported to represent only 5 to 15% of extracranial lesions producing cerebral symptoms, (Fields and Lemak, 1972; Hass et al, 1968; Zelenock et al, 1985). Most of these obstructive lesions are caused by atherosclerosis. Atherosclerosis of the aortic arch branches is usually a multifocal disease, with some degree of lesion at the origins of all three branches, and the superior wall of the aortic arch may also be involved.

Stenotic and occlusive lesions of the aortic arch are more common in men and are found predominately in patients older than 50 years of age. These patients have associated risk factors of smoking, hypertension, hyperlipidemia, cardiovascular disease, and diabetes (Brewster et al, 1985). In young women, the syndrome of multiple occlusions of the aortic arch vessels, rather than stenosis (Takayasu's arteritis), is due to a nonspecific arteritis (Fig. 33–73) (Takayasu, 1908). The arteritis involves all layers of the aortic wall, with degeneration of the elastic fibers and proliferation of connective tissue. Takayasu's disease represents a specific entity and is different from the atherosclerotic lesions of the arch vessels treated surgically in the literature. Surgical therapy for Takayasu's arteritis is usually disappointing, because endarterectomy sites and grafts are prone to reocclusion. Patients with Takayasu's disease who have disabling symptoms are occasionally offered surgical therapy (Bloss et al, 1979; Ekestrom et al, 1983; Langneau et al, 1987).

Other causes of occlusive disease of the branches of the aorta include syphilis, tuberculosis, periarteritis nodosa, collagen-vascular disease, rheumatic fever, trauma, congenital malformations, radiation injury, fibromuscular dysplasia (Manns et al, 1987; McCready et al, 1982), aneurysmal disease, aortic dissection, and tumor and scar (Brewster et al, 1985; Harris et al, 1984; Najafi et al, 1979).

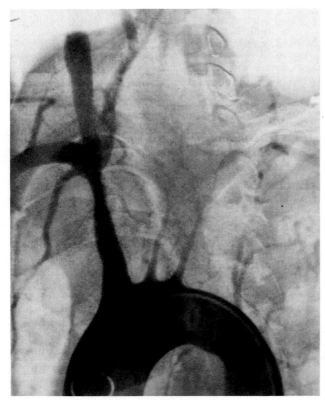

Figure 33–73. Arch arteriogram of a 32-year-old woman with Takayasu's disease.

CLINICAL MANIFESTATIONS— PATHOPHYSIOLOGY

Atherosclerotic disease at the origin of the arch vessels rarely causes irreversible neurologic changes, but symptoms of disability occur. The signs and symptoms depend on the location, the nature of the lesion (ulcerative versus obstructive), the extent of obstruction, and the degree of collateral circulation. The collateral circulation across the thoracic outlet, neck, and face is so extensive that the overall result of single or multiple lesions is often one of symptoms secondary to reduction of total cerebral perfusion rather than to lack of perfusion of one area of the brain (Wylie et al, 1980).

As observed in several large series of aortic arch and brachiocephalic arteriograms, occlusive lesions of the arch vessels occurring near the origin are relatively common in patients older than 65 years of age, but uncommon in younger patients. Most of these lesions are asymptomatic because they are associated with either minimal obstruction, usually the left subclavian, or have extensive collateral circulation. Patients with symptoms tend to have ulcerative lesions, multiple proximal arch vessel obstruction, or associated obstructions in one or more distal vessels, including the internal carotid or vertebral arteries (Crawford et al, 1983) (Tables 33–4 and 33–5).

Three pathophysiologic mechanisms are responsible for the development of the wide range of clinical features found with these lesions. The first is the diminished forward flow through the involved vessel; the second is the reversal of cerebral blood flow away from the brain; and the third is ulcerative lesions that discharge emboli into the involved vessel.

Symptoms of inadequate cerebral circulation include unilateral impairment of motor or sensory functions, syncope, headaches, confusion, speech disorders, tinnitus, impaired vision, and sometimes convulsions and paralysis. These symptoms tend to be intermittent and transient (Campbell and Simons, 1987; Carlson et al, 1977). Cerebellar transient ischemic attacks or basal artery hypoperfusion is the result of diminished or reversed vertebral artery blood flow. These symptoms include episodic vision loss, vertigo, ataxia, dizziness, syncope, visual hallucinations, and "drop" attacks (Edwards and Muhlerin, 1983). Upper-extremity ischemic symptoms are usually mild because of the abundance of collaterals to the arms and the small muscle mass affected. Patients may feel weak and tire easily. They may describe intermittent claudication and may occasionally have ischemic changes in the fingers produced by microemboli. Patients with more advanced disease may develop rest pain or gangrene (Gross et al, 1978; Harris et al, 1984; Rapp et al, 1986). Other clinical manifestations of aortic occlusive disease include facial atrophy, inequality of pulses of the cervical arteries and arms, optic atrophy without papilledema, and presenile cataracts (Davis et al, 1956; Najafi et al, 1979).

TABLE 33–4. LOCATION OF GREAT VESSEL LESION AND PREOPERATIVE SYMPTOMS

Location	No. of Patients	No. of Symptoms				
		Carotid	Vertebrobasilar	Extremity Ischemia	Multiple	None
Subclavian	80	6	22	24	24	4
Innominate	18	2	8	4	4	0
Common carotid	8	2	3	0	3	0
Multiple proximal lesions	36	5	17	2	11	1
Total	142	15	50	30	42	5

*From Crawford, E. S., Stowe, C. L., and Powers, R. W., Jr.: Occlusion of the innominate, common carotid, and subclavian arteries: Long-term results of surgical treatment. Surgery, *94*:781, 1983.

**TABLE 33–5. INCIDENCE AND LOCATION OF DISTAL DISEASE
ACCORDING TO LOCATION OF PROXIMAL LESION***

Proximal Lesion	Total No. of Patients	No. (%) with Distal Disease	No. with Distal Disease at			
			Internal Carotid	*Vertebral*	*Intracranial*	*Mixed*
Subclavian	80	28 (35)	12	8	0	8
Innominate	18	3 (17)	1	1	0	1
Common carotid	8	4 (50)	2	2	0	0
Multiple lesions	36	23 (64)	11	4	0	8
Total	142	58 (41)	26	15	0	17

*From Crawford, E. S., Stowe, C. L., and Powers, R. W., Jr.: Occlusion of the innominate, common carotid, and subclavian arteries: Long-term results of surgical treatment. Surgery, *94*;781, 1983.

DIAGNOSIS

The symptoms described earlier, together with bruits, pulse deficits, and upper-extremity pressure gradients on physical examination, facilitate the diagnosis in most patients. Arch arteriography by the digital method is the diagnostic roentgenographic technique used to visualize stenotic arch and cerebrovascular lesions. The addition of selective cerebral angiography further delineates the cerebroarteriographic anatomy and is necessary to observe ulcerative or stenotic lesions and distal disease (Heinz, 1988). Computed tomography and magnetic resonance imaging are being evaluated as an adjunct to aortography in patients with complex aortic problems (Dooms and Higgins, 1986; Williams et al, 1986).

SURGICAL THERAPY

The technique of arterial reconstruction of branches of the aortic arch has advanced considerably since it was first described by DeBakey and associates (1959) and Cate and Scott (1959). The branches of the aortic arch are particularly prone to a wide spectrum of obstructive lesions. The various surgical approaches to the lesions are summarized in Table 33–6. Brachiocephalic disease sufficiently severe to require surgical correction is relatively uncommon when compared with atherosclerosis of the carotid bifurcation. This is exemplified by the report by the Cleveland Clinic that studied patients from 1965 to 1980, when 1,500 carotid endarterectomies were done. During the same period, only 100 reconstructive brachiocephalic procedures were done (Vogt et al, 1982; Zelenock et al, 1985).

Most aortic arch lesions can readily be managed by one of three surgical techniques: (1) extrathoracic carotid-subclavian bypass (Fig. 33–74); (2) extrathoracic or intrathoracic endarterectomy (Fig. 33–75); or (3) intrathoracic aorta-distal artery bypass (Fig. 33–76). The most commonly used method for restoration of blood flow in arch vessel occlusions is implantation of a synthetic bypass graft. Most lesions can be bypassed by a graft (Dacron, Gore-Tex, saphenous vein) from the carotid to the unilateral distal subcla-

vian artery (Otis et al, 1984). Most surgeons implant unilateral short grafts that avoid crossing the midline because of the possibility of tracheal compression-erosion or future interference with a tracheostomy or median sternotomy. Much controversy exists about the use of extrathoracic versus intrathoracic procedures. In early reports, intrathoracic procedures were associated with 20 to 40% mortality. However, contemporary experience using better selection of patients and improved surgical and anesthetic techniques has lowered this mortality to less than 5% (Brewster et al, 1985).

Innominate Artery

Atherosclerotic lesions of the innominate artery are most prominent in the proximal third of the vessel. These lesions usually involve the full circumference of the vessel origin and then taper into a posterior plaque extending into the subclavian, sparing the common carotid artery (Ehrenfeld and Rapp, 1985).

Multiple surgical approaches to occlusive innominate artery disease are well described (see Table 33–6). For several reasons, the trans-sternal approach is now preferred over the various extrathoracic procedures that are available: (1) median sternotomy is well tolerated, with minimal postoperative pain or respiratory difficulties; (2) anatomic trans-sternal repair provides superior long-term patency and relief of symptoms; (3) endarterectomy or anatomic graft reconstruction eliminates the embolic potential of innominate lesions; and (4) the most reliable extrathoracic graft—ipsilateral carotid subclavian bypass—is not applicable for innominate lesions (Brewster et al, 1985). Trans-sternal innominate endarterectomy has been well described as the most simple and satisfactory operation for managing innominate occlusive disease (see Fig. 33–75). Aorta-distal artery bypass is also accepted as a technically easy, well-tolerated procedure providing excellent relief of symptoms and long-term patency (see Fig. 33–76). Extrathoracic grafts are used selectively when anticipating technical problems. Patients with prior mediastinal operations, aortic dissection, mediastinal infections, or complex anatomic problems or high-

TABLE 33–6. MULTIPLE SURGICAL APPROACHES TO VASCULAR LESIONS

Arterial Lesion	Surgical Therapy	Figure	Study
Single Vessel			
Innominate	Aorta-distal artery bypass	Figure 33–76	Brewster et al, 1985; Crawford et al, 1983; Deriu and Ballotta, 1981; Thevenet, 1979; Vogt et al, 1982; Zelenock et al, 1985
	Endarterectomy	Figure 33–75	Brewster et al, 1985; Carlson et al, 1977; Crawford et al, 1983; Ehrenfeld, 1985; Ekestrom et al, 1983; Thevenet, 1984; Vogt et al, 1982; Zelenock et al, 1985
	Axilloaxillary bypass		Brewster et al, 1985; Moore, 1988
	Subclavian-subclavian bypass		Brewster et al, 1985
	Carotid-carotid bypass		Brewster et al, 1985; Moore, 1988
Carotid			
Right	Carotid-subclavian bypass		Brown et al, 1983; Crawford et al, 1983; Maggisano and Provan, 1981; Thompson et al, 1980
	Endarterectomy (patch)		Najafi et al, 1979
Left	Carotid-subclavian bypass	Figure 33–74	Brown et al, 1983; Crawford et al, 1983; Gerety et al, 1981; Moore, 1988; Vogt et al, 1982
	Endarterectomy		Moore, 1988; Najafi et al, 1979; Thevenet, 1984; Vogt et al, 1982; Zelenock et al, 1985
	Carotid-subclavian implantation		Vogt et al, 1982
	Carotid-innominate implantation		Ehrenfeld, 1985
Subclavian			
Right	Carotid-subclavian bypass		Crawford et al, 1983; Raithel, 1980; Vogt et al, 1982
	Carotid-subclavian implantation		Edwards and Mulherin, 1983; Moore, 1988; Vogt et al, 1982
Left	Carotid-subclavian bypass		Posner et al, 1983; Vogt et al, 1982
	Axilloaxillary bypass		Posner et al, 1983; Schanzer et al, 1987; Vogt et al, 1982
	Endarterectomy		Ehrenfeld, 1985; Thevenet, 1984; Vogt et al, 1982
Vertebral	Endarterectomy		Edwards and Mulherin, 1983; Ehrenfeld, 1985
	Vertebral-carotid implantation		Imparato, 1985; Thevenet, 1983; Vogt et al, 1982
	Internal mammary-vertebral artery bypass		Baker et al, 1986
Multivessel			
	Aorta-distal artery bypass		Crawford, 1983

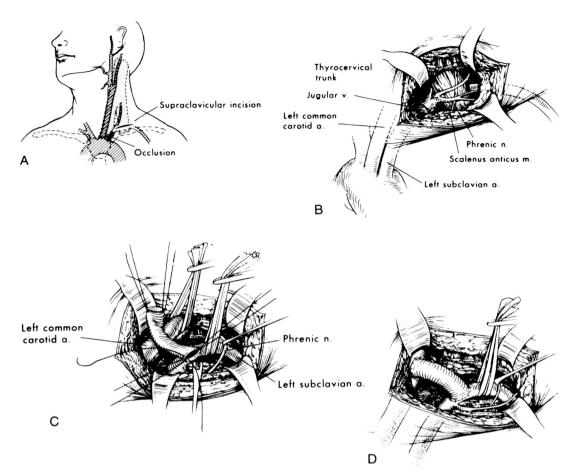

Figure 33–74. *A,* Demonstration of the placement of the supraclavicular incision. It is centered over the clavicular head of the sternomastoid muscle. *B,* After division of the clavicular head of the sternomastoid muscle, the relationships of the phrenic nerve, scalenus anticus, and subclavian artery are shown. *C,* After mobilization of the carotid and subclavian arteries, preparation is made for a graft connection. *D,* Completion of the subclavian-carotid artery bypass is shown and denotes the proximity of the two arteries and the short length of graft that is required. (From Moore, W. S., Malone, J. M., and Goldstone, J.: Extrathoracic repair of branch occlusions of the aortic arch. Am. J. Surg., *132*:249, 1976.)

risk patients may be treated with one of the available extrathoracic graft procedures (Brewster et al, 1985).

Common Carotid Artery

The most common cause of common carotid artery occlusion is retrograde thrombosis after progression of atheromatous plaque of the common carotid bifurcation (Moore et al, 1976). Proximal carotid lesions that cause prograde thrombosis are rare, and midcarotid occlusions are usually due to previous neck irradiation (Ehrenfeld and Rapp, 1985; Rapp et al, 1986). Treatment of left common carotid occlusions includes various approaches. Some surgeons prefer a carotid bifurcation endarterectomy followed by a retrograde thrombectomy (Moore et al, 1976); common carotid transection caudal to the clavicle followed by thrombectomy and end-to-side anastomosis to the left subclavian artery; median

sternotomy with common carotid thrombectomy; median sternotomy with proximal common carotid transection anastomosed into the innominate artery (Ehrenfeld and Rapp, 1985; Rapp et al, 1986); and carotid subclavian bypass (Brown et al, 1983; Crawford et al, 1983; Vogt et al, 1982).

Subclavian Artery

The left subclavian artery is the most common arch vessel involved with occlusive disease, and many afflicted individuals are asymptomatic (Thompson et al, 1980). Symptomatic subclavian occlusions are uncommon without concomitant carotid disease. The relief of vertebral basal insufficiency is the most common indication for subclavian-vertebral operations. Four principal extrathoracic construction options are available: (1) a bypass graft, placed between the ipsilateral carotid artery and the subclavian artery

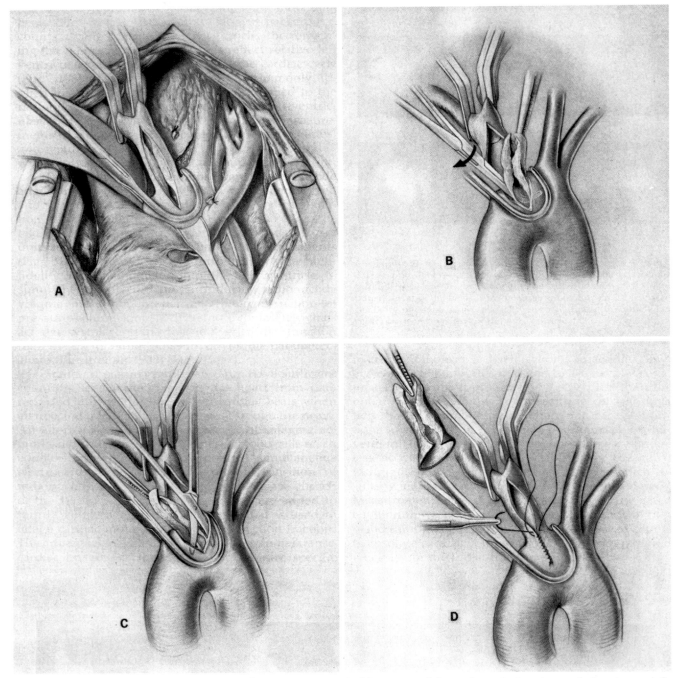

Figure 33–75. A full-length sternotomy and upper cutaneous incision are used for an innominate artery endarterectomy. A J-shaped clamp is used to occlude the side of the aorta adjacent to the innominate orifice, and the endarterectomy is completed. (From Carlson, R. E., Ehrenfeld, W. K., Stoney, R. J., and Wylie, E. J.: Innominate artery endarterectomy. Arch. Surg., 112:1389–1393. Copyright 1977, American Medical Association.)

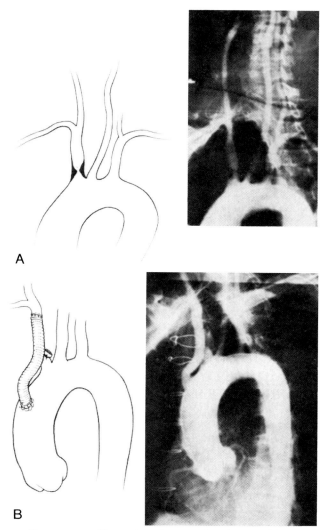

A

B

Figure 33–76. Illustration of proximal occlusion of the innominate artery causing amaurosis fugax, which is treated by bypass grafting of the ascending aorta to the distal end of the innominate artery. *A,* Drawing and aortogram made before operation show the location and the extent of occlusion. *B,* Drawing and aortogram made after operation show the location and method of operation. (From Crawford, E. S., Stowe, C. L., and Powers, R. W.: Occlusion of the innominate, common carotid, and subclavian arteries: Long-term results of surgical treatment. Surgery, *94:*781, 1983.)

distal to its obstruction (see Fig. 33–74); (2) detachment of the subclavian artery proximal to the takeoff of the vertebral artery with reconstruction to the ipsilateral carotid in an end-to-side manner; (3) a bypass graft from the contralateral axillary artery passed subcutaneously across the sternum and anastomosed end to side into the ipsilateral artery, providing bidirectional flow (Moore et al, 1976; Posner et al, 1983; Schanzer et al, 1987); and (4) transposition of the left vertebral artery to the side of the left common carotid artery (Ehrenfeld and Rapp, 1985; Moore et al, 1976).

Intrathoracic procedures preferred by other surgeons consist of subclavian and vertebral endarterectomies (Ehrenfeld and Rapp, 1985).

PERCUTANEOUS TRANSLUMINAL ANGIOPLASTY

The safety and efficacy of percutaneous transluminal angioplasty differ significantly with the vessels involved, the expertise of the physician doing the procedure, and the criteria used for selecting patients. Data are now available regarding the safety of this technique in coronary, iliac, femoral, popliteal, and renal arteries. There are few data concerning the safety of percutaneous transluminal angioplasty in the aortic arch arteries (Fallon, 1980; Health and Public Policy Committee, 1983; Srur et al, 1985; Vitek et al, 1986). Use of this technique in the carotid, vertebral, and subclavian arteries must be considered investigational at this time.

RESULTS

The results of surgical therapy are excellent. Most large series report an operative mortality of 2 to 5%, with a postoperative stroke rate of 2 to 5%. Ninety-five per cent of patients have early relief of symptoms, and 85% remain asymptomatic on long-term follow-up. Graft patency at 6.5 years is reported to be 88%. Actuarial survival curves show an 85% 5-year survival and a 50% 10-year survival (Brewster et al, 1985; Crawford et al, 1983; Deriu and Ballotta, 1981; Edwards and Mulherin, 1980; Maggisano and Provan, 1981; Schroeder and Hansen, 1980; Vogt et al, 1982).

Selected Bibliography

Brewster, D. C., Moncure, A. C., Darling, C., et al: Innominate artery lesions: Problems encountered and lessons learned. J. Vasc. Surg., 2:99, 1985.

The authors review the problems, approaches, and principles of management of patients with innominate artery lesions. A series of 71 patients during a 20-year period are reviewed retrospectively. Direct repair by median sternotomy gave the best long-term results, with a mortality of 3.4%. Extrathoracic grafting proved to be safe but less durable and should be reserved for high-risk patients or special circumstances.

Crawford, E. S., Stowe, C. L., and Powers, R. W.: Occlusion of the innominate, common carotid, and subclavian arteries: Long-term results of surgical treatment. Surgery, 94:781, 1983.

The authors present a comprehensive review of their 23 years of experience with brachiocephalic occlusive disease. One hundred forty-two patients are reviewed, with an operative mortality of 2% and a relief of symptoms in 94% of patients. A mean follow-up of 7.5 years showed that 83% of patients were asymptomatic, with a 5-year survival of 85% and 10-year survival of 58%.

Vogt, D. P., Hertzer, N. R., O'Hara, P. J., and Beven, E. G.: Brachiocephalic arterial reconstruction. Ann. Surg., 196:541, 1982.

This report summarizes the authors' experience from 1965 through 1980 with 100 patients with occlusive disease of branches of the aorta. Extrathoracic reconstruction (69%) was the most common approach. Late results (mean of 52 months) showed that 82% of patients were asymptomatic and 5- and 10-year survival was 85% and 45%, respectively.

Bibliography

Baker, N. H., Ewy, H. G., Moore, P. J., et al: Direct internal mammary-vertebral artery anastomosis: An 18-year follow-up. J. Thorac. Cardiovasc. Surg., 92:1103, 1986.

Bloss, R. S., Duncan, J. M., Cooley, D. A., et al: Takayasu's arteritis: Surgical considerations. Ann. Thorac. Surg., 27:574, 1979.

Brewster, D. C., Moncure, A. C., Darling, C., et al: Innominate artery lesions: Problems encountered and lessons learned. J. Vasc. Surg., 2:99, 1985.

Brown, O. W., Hollier, L. H., and Pairolero, P. C.: Amaurosis fugax and transient ischemic attacks secondary to proximal carotid artery lesions. Am. Surg., 49:18, 1983.

Campbell, J. B., and Simmons, R. M.: Brachiocephalic artery stenosis presenting with objective tinnitus. J. Laryngol. Otol., 101:718, 1987.

Carlson, R. E., Ehrenfeld, W. K., Stoney, R. J., and Wylie, E. J.: Innominate artery endarterectomy. Arch. Surg., 112:1389, 1977.

Cate, W. R., and Scott, H. W., Jr.: Cerebral ischemia of central origin: Relief by subclavian-vertebral artery thromboendarterectomy. Surgery, 45:19, 1959.

Crawford, E. S., DeBakey, M. E., Morris, G. C., and Cooley, D. A.: Thrombo-obliterative disease of the great vessels arising from the aortic arch. J. Thorac. Cardiovasc. Surg., 43:38, 1962.

Crawford, E. S., DeBakey, M. E., Morris, G. C., Jr., and Howell, J. F.: Surgical treatment of occlusion of the innominate, common carotid, and subclavian arteries: A 10-year experience. Surgery, 65:17, 1969.

Crawford, E. S., Stowe, C. L., and Powers, R. W., Jr.: Occlusion of the innominate, common carotid, and subclavian arteries: Long-term results of surgical treatment. Surgery, 94:781, 1983.

Davis, J. B., Grove, W. J., and Julian, O. C.: Thrombic occlusion of the branches of the aortic arch, Mortorell's syndrome: Report of a case treated surgically. Ann. Surg., 144:124, 1956.

DeBakey, M. E.: Successful carotid endarterectomy for cerebrovascular insufficiency: Nineteen-year follow-up. J.A.M.A., 233:1083, 1958.

DeBakey, M. E., Crawford, E. S., and Cooley, D. A.: Surgical considerations of occlusive disease of innominate, carotid, subclavian, and vertebral arteries. Ann. Surg., 149:690, 1959.

Deriu, G. P., and Ballotta, E.: The surgical treatment of atherosclerotic occlusion of the innominate and subclavian arteries. J. Cardiovasc. Surg., 22:532, 1981.

Dooms, C., and Higgins, C. B.: The potential of magnetic resonance imaging for the evaluation of thoracic arterial diseases. J. Thorac. Cardiovasc. Surg., 92:1088, 1986.

Edwards, W. H., and Mulherin, J. L., Jr.: The management of brachiocephalic occlusive disease. Am. Surg., 49:465, 1983.

Edwards, W. H., and Mulherin, J. L., Jr.: The surgical approach to significant stenosis of vertebral and subclavian arteries. Surgery, 87:20, 1980.

Ehrenfeld, W. K., Chapman, R. D., and Wylie, E. J.: Management of occlusive lesions of the branches of the aortic arch. Am. J. Surg., 118:236, 1969.

Ehrenfeld, W. K., and Rapp, J. H.: Direct revascularization for occlusion of the trunks of the aortic arch. J. Vasc. Surg., 2:228, 1985.

Ekestrom, S., Liljeqvist, L., and Nordhus, O.: Surgical management of obliterative disease of the brachiocephalic trunk: Experience from 24 cases. Scand. J. Thorac. Cardiovasc. Surg., 17:305, 309, 1983.

Fallon, J. T.: Pathology of arterial lesions amenable to percutaneous transluminal angioplasty. A.J.R., 135:913, 1980.

Fields, W. S., and Lemak, N. A.: Joint study of extracranial arterial occlusion. VII: Subclavian steal: A review of 168 cases. J.A.M.A., 222:1130, 1972.

Gerety, R. L., Andrus, C. H., May, A. G., et al: Surgical treatment of occlusive subclavian artery disease. Circulation, 64(Suppl. II):228, 1981.

Gross, W. S., Flanigan, P., Kraft, R. O., and Stanley, J. C.: Chronic upper extremity arterial insufficiency: Etiology, manifestations, and operative management. Arch. Surg., 113:419, 1978.

Harris, R. W., Andros, G., Dulawa, L. B., et al: Large-vessel arterial occlusive disease in symptomatic upper extremity. Arch. Surg., 119:1277, 1984.

Hass, W. K., Field, W. S., North, R. R., et al: Joint study of extracranial arterial occlusion. II: Arteriography, techniques, sites, and complications. J.A.M.A., 203:159, 1968.

Health and Public Policy Committee, American College of Physicians: Percutaneous transluminal angioplasty. 99:864, 1983.

Heinz, E. R.: Personal communication, 1988.

Imparato, A. M.: Vertebral arterial reconstruction: A nineteen-year experience. J. Vasc. Surg., 2:626, 1985.

Ishikawa, K.: Natural history and classification of occlusive thromboaortopathy (Takayasu's disease). Circulation, 57:27, 1978.

Lagneau, P., Michel, J. B., and Vuong, P. N.: Surgical treatment of Takayasu's disease. Ann. Surg., 205:157, 1987.

Maggisano, R., and Provan, J. L.: Surgical management of chronic occlusive disease of the aortic arch vessels and vertebral arteries. CMA Journal, 124:972, 1981.

Manns, R. A., Nanda, K. K., and Mackie, G.: Case Report: Fibromuscular dysplasia of the cephalic and renal arteries. Clin. Radiol., 38:427, 1987.

McCready, R. A., Pairolero, P. C., Hollier, L. H., et al: Fibromuscular dysplasia of the right subclavian artery. Arch. Surg., 117:1243, 1982.

Moore, W. S.: Extra-anatomic bypass for revascularization of occlusive lesions involving the branches of the aortic arch. J. Vasc. Surg., 2:230, 1988.

Moore, W. S., Malone, J. M., and Goldstone, J.: Extrathoracic repair of branch occlusions of the aortic arch. Am. J. Surg., 132:249, 1976.

Najafi, H., Javid, H., Hunter, J. A., et al: Occlusive disease of the branches of the aortic arch. In Bergan, J. J., and Yao, J. S. T. (eds): Surgery of the Aorta and Its Body Branches. New York, Grune & Stratton, 1979.

Otis, S., Rush, M., Thomas, M., and Dilley, R.: Carotid steal syndrome following carotid subclavian bypass. J. Vasc. Surg., 1:649, 1984.

Posner, M. P., Riles, T. S., Ramirez, A. A., et al: Axillo-axillary bypass for symptomatic stenosis of the subclavian artery. Am. J. Surg., 145:644, 1983.

Raithel, D.: Our experience of surgery for innominate and subclavian lesions. J. Cardiovasc. Surg., 21:423, 1980.

Rapp, J. H., Reilly, L. M., Goldstone, J., et al: Ischemia of the upper extremity: Significance of proximal arterial disease. Am. J. Surg., 152:122, 1986.

Ross, R. S., and McKusick, V. A.: Aortic arch syndromes. Arch. Intern. Med., 92:701, 1953.

Savory, W. S.: Case of a young woman in whom the main arteries of both upper extremities and of the left side of the neck were throughout completely obliterated. Trans. Med. Soc. Lond., 39:205, 1856.

Schanzer, H., Chung-Loy, H., Kotok, M., et al: Evaluation of axillo-axillary artery bypass for the treatment of subclavian or innominate artery occlusive disease. J. Cardiovasc. Surg., 28:258, 1987.

Schroeder, T., and Hansen, H. J. B.: Arterial reconstruction of the brachiocephalic trunk and the subclavian arteries: Ten years' experience with a follow-up study. Acta Chir. Scand., 502:122, 1980.

Srur, M. F., Sos, T. A., Saddekni, S., et al: Intimal fibromuscular dysplasia and Takayasu arteritis: Delayed response to percutaneous transluminal renal angioplasty. Radiology, 157:657, 1985.

Takayasu, M.: Case of queer changes in central blood vessels of retina. Acta Soc. Ophthalmol. Jpn., *12*:2554, 1908.

Thevenet, A.: Surgical management of the aortic dome and origin of supra-aortic trunks. World J. Surg., *3*:187, 1979.

Thevenet, A., and Ruotolo, C.: Surgical repair of vertebral artery stenosis. J. Cardiovasc. Surg., *25*:101, 1984.

Thompson, B. W., Read, R. C., and Campbell, G. S.: Operative correction of proximal blocks of the subclavian or innominate arteries. J. Cardiovasc. Surg., *21*:125, 1980.

Vitek, J. J., Keller, F. S., Duvall, E. R., et al: Brachiocephalic artery dilation by percutaneous transluminal angioplasty. Radiology, *158*:779, 1986.

Vogt, D. P., Hertzer, N. R., O'Hara, P. J., and Beven, E. G.: Brachiocephalic arterial reconstruction. Ann. Surg., *196*:541, 1982.

Williams, L. R., Flinn, W. R., Yao, J. S. T., et al: Extended use of computed tomography in the management of complex aortic problems: A learning experience. J. Vasc. Surg., *4*:264, 1986.

Wylie, E. J., Stoney, R. J., and Ehrenfeld, W. K.: Manual of Vascular Surgery. New York, Springer-Verlag, 1980, pp. 85–106.

Zelenock, G. B., Cronenwett, J. L., Graham, L. M., et al: Brachiocephalic arterial occlusions and stenoses: Manifestations and management of complex lesions. Arch. Surg., *120*:370, 1985.

CHAPTER 34

THE PERICARDIUM

Paul A. Ebert
Hassan Najafi

HISTORICAL ASPECTS

The pericardium was described by Hippocrates (460 B.C.) as "a smooth tunic which envelops the heart and contains a small amount of fluid resembling urine." Galen (130 A.D.) observed pericardial effusion in a monkey and scirrhous thickening of the pericardium in a cock and surmised that the same conditions might occur in humans.

Lower (1631 to 1691) should receive credit for the first satisfactory account of pericardial disease in humans. He accurately described cardiac tamponade:

It sometimes happens that a profuse effusion oppresses and inundates the heart. This envelope becomes filled in hydrops of the heart; the walls of the heart are compressed by the fluid settling everywhere so that they cannot dilate sufficiently to receive blood, then the pulse becomes exceedingly small, until finally it becomes utterly suppressed by the great inundation of fluid, whence succeed syncope and death itself.

In 1649, Riolan suggested doing a pericardiotomy for an effusion compressing the heart by trephining the sternum, a technique that was not adopted until two centuries later. Vieussens reported cases in 1679 and 1715 and insisted that pericardial adhesions were inflammatory and not congenital.

Lancisi (1728) correlated the clinical picture of constrictive pericarditis with the necropsy findings. Morgagni (1761) reported seven cases of constrictive pericarditis and recognized the danger of cardiac compression by describing the heart as "so constricted and confined that it could not receive a proper quantity of blood to pass on." He also recognized that most of these cases were incommoded little or not at all even shortly before death. Senac (1749) recognized clinical symptoms of "hydropsia pericardii." Laennec (1819) further emphasized the few symptoms that were often associated with pericardial constriction and noted the "bread and butter" appearance of the pericardial and epicardial surfaces in pericarditis.

Romero (1819), through an approach in the fifth interspace on the left, incised the pericardium in three patients, two of whom recovered. Schuh (1840) did a blind insertion of a trocar into the pericardial sac for relief of effusion. Karanaeff (1840) did pericardiocentesis for hemorrhagic effusion accompanying an outbreak of scurvy. Seven of his 30 patients survived.

Cheevers (1842), under the title of *Observations on the Diseases of the Orifice and Valves of the Aorta*, gave a clear clinical picture of chronic constrictive pericarditis and concluded that "the principal cause of dangerous symptoms appears to rise from the occurrence of gradual contraction in the layer of adhesive matter which has been deposited around the heart, compressing its muscular tissue and embarrassing its systolic and diastolic movements, but more particularly the latter." Wilkes (1870) observed in constrictive pericarditis that "the predominant thickening was in front so as to involve the right ventricle and auricle." Kussmaul (1873) gave the first critical exposition of the paradoxical pulse and the rise in venous pressure on inspiration in constrictive pericarditis. In 1877, Cohnheim did classic experiments to show that, as oil was injected into the pericardial sac, the venous pressure rose and the arterial pressure fell with a reduction in cardiac output. Rose (1884) described the deleterious effects of an effusion or hemorrhage on the heart and presented the term "herz tamponade."

In 1896, Pick presented a paper entitled "Concerning Chronic Pericarditis Running Its Course Under the Guise of Cirrhosis of the Liver (pericarditis pseudocirrhosis of the liver) with Observations on the Frosted Liver." Weill (1895) and Délorme (1898) proposed the excision of the thickened fibrous pericardium in constrictive pericarditis. Pericardial resection was introduced independently by Rehn and by Sauerbruch in 1913. Schmieden and Fischer (1926) reported seven cases of pericardial resection with pertinent descriptions of the operative technique. Many English and American authors have contributed to our understanding and treatment of pericardial disease, including the internists Wood (1956) and White (1951). Sellors (1946) considered that tuberculosis was the primary agent in constrictive pericarditis; Churchill (1929) did the first successful pericardiectomy for constrictive pericarditis in the United States; Beck (1937) was a pioneer in the experimental production of pericarditis; Blalock and Levy (1937), Burwell and Blalock (1938), Bloomfield and associates (1946), and McKusick (1952) have clarified both the clinical and the physiologic picture of pericardial disease. Mannix and Dennis (1955) and Blakemore and associates (1960) extended the usefulness of pericardiectomy by advocating its early application to chronic, massive effusions producing symptoms of cardiac compression and to a relapsing type of chronic pericarditis with effusion.

Parsons and Holman (1951 and 1955) and Isaacs and colleagues (1952) did classic experimental studies that clarified the physiologic effects of segmental compressions of the heart. Bigelow and associates (1956), Schumacker and Roshe (1960), and Fitzpatrick and associates (1962) have emphasized the necessity of radical pericardiectomy as the only method by which recurrence of pericardial constriction requiring secondary operations can be avoided.

Fowler (1970) re-emphasized the importance of understanding the hemodynamics of cardiac tamponade and constrictive pericarditis to provide the proper treatment. Bush and associates (1977) identified occult constrictive pericardial disease as that which impaired cardiac performance without actual adherence to the epicardium. Advancements in the diagnosis and management of the disease processes of the pericardium continue to improve the prognosis.

FUNCTIONS OF THE PERICARDIUM

The pericardium is presumed to serve a useful purpose because it is present in most mammals. Yet there is little, if any, disability noted after operative removal of the pericardium or in patients with congenital absence of the structure. The pericardium provides a smooth serous sac with secreted fluid that allows the heart a frictionless chamber in which to function. The pericardium is a strong fibrous sac that provides a restraining influence over overdilatation of the heart, a condition that might lead to the destruction of myocardial cells and the degeneration of cardiac musculature. Enlargement of the heart over a period of time results in stretching and enlargement of the pericardial sac, but sudden changes in the size of the heart are restricted by this structure. This restraining influence also tends to support the heart and limit its displacement with changes in body position. It prevents kinking and torsion of the great vessels and vena cava.

The unusual strength of the pericardium has made it an excellent tissue to use to close intracardiac defects, reconstruct the pulmonary artery and right ventricular outflow, and serve as a material to reconstruct the major veins. The strength of this tissue protects the heart from extension of infection from neighboring structures, such as the lungs, mediastinal glands, and esophagus and from infradiaphragmatic abscesses, which frequently rupture into the pleural spaces.

The pericardium clearly limits cardiac dimensions and prevents acute distention. The pericardium appears to contribute more to prevention of distention of the right side of the heart in patients with existing severe left ventricular disease. In some of these cases, right ventricular performance may be impaired by bulging of the ventricular septum into the right ventricle in a setting in which the pericardium limits outward distention of the right ventricular wall. In some settings dilatation of the left ventricle, because of its larger mass, increases intrapericardial pressure and thus limits right ventricular filling. Thus, the pericardium can evoke reciprocal shifts of the Frank-Starling curves of the two ventricles. The pericardium may have a more major role in cardiac performance in patients with the acute development of left ventricular or right ventricular failure.

CONGENITAL PERICARDIAL DEFECTS

Congenital Absence

Congenital absence of the entire pericardium has been reported, but more commonly small segments may be missing. Absence of small portions of the pericardium on the left side is most often seen. This absence results from a defect that occurs during the fifth week of fetal life. Premature obliterations of the left duct of Cuvier may produce deficiency of the blood supply to the pleuropericardial membrane and result in failure of formation or incomplete formation. No clinical symptoms are known to result from congenital absence of the pericardium. Ronka and Tessmer (1944) studied 74 recorded clinical cases; all patients led active, strenuous lives, and in no case was the defect associated with symptoms or related ultimately to the cause of death. Studies in the experimental animal have substantiated the clinical impression, because complete excision of the pericardium in the adult results in no obvious deleterious effects. Beck and Moore (1925) showed that vigorous swimming for 30 to 60 minutes was tolerated without signs of fatigue or abnormal cardiac rhythm. If an animal is subjected to acute hydremic plethora by intravenous infusion of blood and salt solution (Holman and Beck, 1925) and the pericardium is incised widely, sharp dilatation of the heart occurs, the pulse rate doubles, and the cardiac output is temporarily greatly increased. Barnard (1898) found that without its pericardium, the heart ruptures under an intracardiac pressure of 1 atm, whereas with an intact pericardium, 1.75 atm of pressure is required to rupture the heart.

Cysts

The pericardium has been postulated to form from a series of disconnected lacunae that appear early in fetal life (Lambert, 1940). For a brief period, these lacunae remain as individual spaces in the mesenchyme, but they eventually coalesce to form the pericardial coelom. Occasionally, the communication with the pericardium in these cysts persists and is called a diverticulum. If one or any of these lacunar cavities fail to fuse, it may either atrophy or persist as a separate pericardial space or cyst. In general, these cysts do not cause symptoms and are usually discovered on routine chest film or at necropsy (Craddock, 1950). A mass lying anteriorly in the chest in either cardiophrenic sulcus is the classic description of a pericardial coelomic cyst given by radiologists (Bates and Leaver, 1951). Exploratory thoracotomy is usually recommended to establish a definitive diagnosis. Pericardial cysts can be confused radiographically with tumors in the lung, thymomas, and other mediastinal lesions.

Occasionally, a pericardial cyst can be incapacitating and life-threatening. Shidler and Holman (1952) reported such a case in an infant with marked respiratory distress requiring oxygen for the first 3 months of life. The symptoms were marked dyspnea, fluctuating cyanosis, wheezing, and difficulty in swallowing. Two operations were required to remove this intrapericardial "spring-water" cyst that was located between the aorta and superior vena cava. A similar case in an adult had been reported by Lam in 1947. This patient was incapacitated by dyspnea, fatigue, and angina and was bedridden for 1 year. A large cyst was present in the anterior chest in close association with the pericardium. The patient recovered after the cyst was removed.

Diverticula

The literature reflects the considerable difficulty in defining the difference between pericardial cysts and diverticula. The latter are described as protrusions of the pericardial sac at points of weakness. The diverticula vary greatly from 0.5 to 12 cm in size and occur more frequently on the right side. These lesions may be confused on routine chest films with aneurysm of the ascending aorta or dermoid cysts of the mediastinum, and, by definition, communicate with the pericardial sac. Areas of congenital weakness, such as the point at which the fibrous pericardial layer emerges along the great vessels, are common locations for diverticula. The structure may not have a normal absorptive surface, but communication with the pericardium prevents accumulation of fluid. However, mechanical kinking of the communicating isthmus can result in distention of the diverticulum either by fluid being formed by its own membrane or by pericardial fluid being forced into the sac by the massaging action of the heart beat. It is conceiv-able that after the communicating tract is kinked, atrophy of the tract would occur and the lesion would, by definition, be considered to be a cyst. These diverticula are rarely symptomatic, and excision is advised to establish a definitive diagnosis.

ACQUIRED PERICARDIAL DEFECTS

Neoplasms

Primary neoplasms of the pericardium are rare. Benign tumors, such as lipomas, lobulated fibrous polyps, and hemangiomas, have been reported. Several cases of primary mesotheliomas have been described, which apparently arise from the lining endothelium. Sarcomas and teratomas occasionally arise from the pericardium, and successful removal of these lesions has rarely been reported. The pericardium is commonly infiltrated by primary myocardial tumors and by infiltrating lung cancer.

Cardiac Tamponade

In cardiac tamponade, the heart is limited during diastole by increased pressure from the pericardium or from fluid or blood filling the pericardial space. Systolic contraction is rarely limited, but during diastole the filling of the ventricles requires a greater venous pressure owing to the force applied against the surface of the heart. Tamponade may occur after penetrating injuries to the heart in which blood escapes into the pericardial sac. If the blood or fluid cannot escape through the laceration in the pericardium, tamponade ensues. In acute injuries, a relatively small amount of blood, 150 to 250 ml, may be sufficient to cause tamponade, whereas in cases of chronic effusion, the pericardium becomes stretched during a period of time and may have the capacity to contain several liters of fluid with minimal cardiodynamic effects. The fluid or blood around the heart ultimately stretches the pericardium to a critical point. Before this occurs, cardiac output is minimally reduced, but when this stage is reached, the addition of a small volume may reduce cardiac output and death may ensue. Treatment may be equally dramatic when a small volume of blood or fluid is removed and the blood pressure and cardiac output are allowed to return almost to normal ranges.

As pressure in the pericardial sac increases, diastolic filling pressure rises and the stroke volume is reduced. Compensatory mechanisms attempt to maintain circulatory dynamics. Increased sympathetic activity causes vasoconstriction, which tends to maintain systemic arterial pressure. The heart rate increases, and systolic ejection becomes more vigorous. These increase the ejection fraction so that a greater portion of blood present in the heart at the end of diastole is expelled. Venous pressure rises as a result of compression of the heart during diastole.

No gradients have been shown between the great veins and the right atrium during experimental cardiac tamponade. Coronary blood flow may be affected because of the reduction of cardiac output and of the pressure gradient between the aorta and coronary circulation. Myocardial failure can result from reduced coronary flow.

In acute cardiac tamponade, clinical shock is evident. The patient has cool and moist skin, heart sounds are distant, pulse is rapid, and blood pressure may be normal or low. The striking clinical manifestation is venous distention at a time when other signs suggest peripheral circulatory failure similar to that in hemorrhagic shock. Cyanosis may be present as a result of venous stasis. Martin and Schenk (1960) have emphasized the importance of using the venous pressure, rather than the arterial pressure, as a guide to treatment, because the latter may be artificially maintained by a raised peripheral resistance.

Treatment of acute tamponade must not be delayed because it is a life-threatening situation. Venous pressure should be obtained immediately in any patient who is suspected of having cardiac tamponade. Further elevation of venous pressure by infusion of blood or colloid solution temporarily improves cardiac output by increasing diastolic filling pressure. Pericardial aspiration should be done with an electrocardiogram lead attached to the needle to identify contact with the surface of the heart and may be a life-saving procedure (Fig. 34–1). Repeated aspirations have been successful in treating traumatic tamponade, but the patient requires careful observation of arterial and venous pressures by skilled personnel. Thoracotomy with direct repair of the cardiac injury is preferable to repeated pericardial aspirations. Aspiration of a few milliliters of blood may restore cardiac output and reduce venous pressure, but because reaccumulation of such a small volume can cause such marked hemodynamic consequences, early operative treatment should be started in most cases. In some cases of chronic effusion, a small plastic catheter may be passed percutaneously into the pericardial sac. Pericardiotomy is often indicated in chronic effusion and may be necessary as an emergency procedure if repeated aspirations do not relieve the tamponade.

Cardiac Tamponade After Cardiac Operations

Cardiac tamponade is a rare but major complication of open heart procedures. It should always be included in the differential diagnosis if the low cardiac output syndrome develops postoperatively. Bleeding is often excessive (more than 150 to 200 ml/hr) before tamponade develops. Sudden cessation of bleeding followed by progressive hypotension and oliguria that do not respond to volume restoration and cardiotonic drugs should raise a strong suspicion that tamponade is the cause of hemodynamic deterioration. If this deterioration is not reversed, jugular venous distention accompanied by central venous pressure exceeding 20 cm, narrowed pulse pressure, acrocyanosis, agitation, poor gas exchange, and acidosis may develop and ultimately lead to cardiac arrest. The compensatory mechanisms maintaining the patient in a marginal circulatory state suddenly fail and tamponade precipitates a state of profound shock.

The physician must be able to recognize when tamponade is developing and must avoid rapid catastrophic cardiopulmonary deterioration. Because rising venous pressure accompanied by falling systemic pressure and urine output are frequently manifestations of myocardial disability, the differential diagnosis demands considerable clinical judgment. The diagnostic signs favoring tamponade include an abrupt change in the character and volume of mediastinal bloody drainage, excessively high venous pressure associated with normal or low pulmonary capillary wedge or left atrial pressure, poor response to vasopressor drugs and diuretics, and enlarging cardiac silhouette on repeated chest films. A flow-directed balloon-tip pulmonary artery catheter (Swan-Ganz) is very helpful both as a diagnostic method and as a monitoring device to judge the efficacy of continuing treatment. This catheter provides valuable information such as pulmonary capillary wedge pressure (an indirect measurement of left atrial pressure, or, in the absence of mitral valve disease, a reflection of left ventricular end-diastolic pressure), central venous pressure, and an opportunity to measure cardiac output. The device is used frequently to adjust the dosage of drugs and fluid volumes to achieve maximal cardiac output.

In pericardial tamponade, the most significant aspect of treatment is the release of tension and restoration of permanent hemostasis. Not infrequently, an indecisive attitude or inappropriate passiveness may require reopening the sternum before operative intervention. In the absence of myocardial disability, a high index of suspicion should be sufficient to proceed with mediastinal exploration before catastrophic disturbance of the patient's cardiopulmonary function demands or forces opening the wound in the intensive care unit.

Hydropneumopericardium

Bricheteau (1844) reported a case of air in the pericardium. This rare phenomenon was reviewed by Shackelford (1931), and 77 cases were recorded in the world literature. The characteristic signs are precordial tympany and metallic splashing sounds that may be heard several feet away and may keep the patient awake. A chest film provides conclusive evidence. Small amounts of air in or about the pericardial sac are common findings after severe chest trauma.

The prognosis is generally good if the disease is

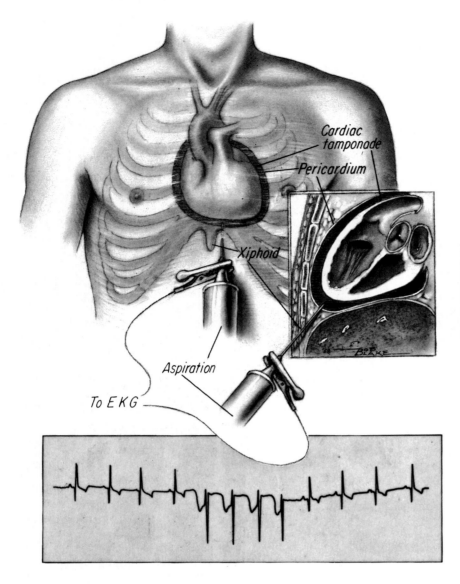

Figure 34–1. The needle is inserted to the left of the xiphoid and directed toward the midscapular area. The electrocardiogram is attached to the needle, and the negative deflection of the QRS complex represents contact with the surface of the heart. The needle is slowly withdrawn, and the electrocardiogram reverts to normal when the needle loses contact with the myocardium.

limited to a pneumopericardium, because air itself is not deleterious. If infection is present, the organisms must be identified by pericardial aspiration and the proper systemic antibiotics must be administered. Pericardiotomy is indicated if prompt improvement is not obtained with systemic antibiotics.

Acute Necrosis of Pericardial Fat

Precordial or pleuritic pain in the left side of the lower chest associated with a soft-tissue mass that cannot be distinguished from the pericardium on a chest film is the classic description of acute necrosis of pericardial fat. Histologic study of the excised tissue shows that necrosis is due to a vascular accident with extravasation of blood, formation of a hematoma, and intravascular thrombosis. Surgical removal provides prompt relief (Chester and Tully, 1959; Jackson et al, 1957).

Pericarditis

Pericarditis occurs as a primary disease process without systemic illness, as a secondary manifestation of a systemic disease, and as the only area of involvement of a normally systemic disease process. It has been given many names, such as acute, chronic, dry, fibrinous, transudative, hemorrhagic, exudative, or purulent. In its simplest and most common form, pericarditis is an acute, self-limiting inflammation, due probably to a diversity of etiologic agents, among which viruses are included. Coxsackie viruses A and B and influenza viruses A and B have been identified by culture and neutralization tests from pericardial fluid (Gillett, 1959). This disease may occur in any age group but is often seen in young, otherwise healthy individuals.

Nonspecific Pericarditis. Nonspecific pericarditis, or so-called "benign pericarditis," is seen preceded by an upper respiratory tract infection. The symptoms are not always specific, but findings of fever, usually about 38.3° C (101° F) but sometimes as high as 40 to 40.5° C (104 to 105° F), substernal or precordial pain, and a pericardial friction rub are classic. All degrees of severity are found. Frequently the disease is minimal, and symptoms may persist for weeks before medical advice is sought. Shortness of breath, grunting respirations, dry cough, and orthopnea with a tendency to lean forward are characteristic symptoms. The pain may be sharp or dull with radiation to the right or left shoulder, arm, or back. It can be accentuated by coughing, respiration, or activity, exaggerated by lying down, or relieved by sitting up. Leukocytosis, with a predominant lymphocyte increase, is usually present. A chest film may show mild cardiac enlargement due to pericardial effusion. These symptoms sometimes may be difficult to distinguish from pain due to myocardial ischemia. Marked ST segment elevation of the electrocardiogram, with absence of Q waves in the presence of a pericardial friction rub, strongly suggests pericarditis. Arrhythmias are uncommon, usually atrial in origin, and are more frequent in patients who have pre-existing heart disease.

Laparotomy has been done unnecessarily for abdominal symptoms, including epigastric pain, cramps, distention, and vomiting, that simulated acute abdominal catastrophe (Powers et al, 1955). This has been ascribed to peritoneal serositis, a local manifestation of a more generalized polyserositis.

The diagnosis of nonspecific pericarditis is usually made by excluding the more specific forms, such as the rheumatic, purulent, and traumatic forms. The disease process is usually self-limiting, and complications are rare, although recurrences have been noted. Infrequently, pericardial effusion occurs, and cardiac tamponade may result. There have been isolated reports of constrictive pericarditis developing after the inflammatory process had subsided (Krook, 1954). Many cases of constrictive pericarditis in which the etiology remains obscure are likely to be a result of benign idiopathic pericarditis, which may have been present with few, if any, symptoms.

Treatment is usually supportive and consists of bed rest for 2 to 3 weeks and analgesics. Salicylates have been successful in relieving pain, although morphine may be required. Occasionally in patients who do not respond to supportive treatment, steroids have been used to control the inflammatory process. Relief of symptoms is prompt, but routine use is discouraged because the disease may recur when the steroids are withdrawn. A distressing factor of this disease is that pain, fever, friction rub, and even pericardial effusion frequently recede and recur in a short period of time. These remissions and exacerbations may continue and the whole attack may last for several months. Heart failure is an infrequent finding, but when present, digitalis is indicated. Arrhythmias, such as ectopic ventricular activity, can be controlled with quinidine or lidocaine. Atrial fibrillation occasionally develops, but spontaneous reversal to sinus rhythm may occur after the inflammatory process subsides.

Pericarditis may occur as a result of many systemic diseases. When pericardial effusion or inflammation accompanies rheumatic arthralgia, the prognosis is worse. It frequently accompanies other collagen diseases, such as scleroderma, rheumatic fever, and lupus erythematosus. Sarcoidosis commonly involves the pericardium and heart but is rarely responsible for isolated pericarditis. It may be a manifestation of tertiary syphilis. Hypersensitivity states, such as serum sickness, autoimmune reactions, and various drug reactions, result in either pericarditis or effusion.

Less than 2% of patients with amebic abscesses in the liver develop pericarditis. It is thought to result from direct extension of the abscess, usually from the left lobe of the liver. Rupture of the abscess into the pericardium is accompanied by severe pain, dyspnea, and collapse. Cardiac tamponade associated with suppurative pericarditis requires immediate pericardial aspiration. Echinococcus cysts are rare in the pericardium. The majority are primarily in the heart and rupture into the pericardium. Rupture may cause only a localized reaction about the contents of the cyst, or rapid multiplication can occur, with involvement of the entire pericardial sac. Hepatic hydatid cysts rarely rupture into the pericardial sac.

Cholesterol Pericarditis. In cholesterol pericarditis, the pericardial fluid has a characteristic "gold paint" color. Diagnosis is usually confirmed by pericardial aspiration and by demonstration of cholesterol crystals. Hypothyroidism is frequently present, and in many cases, the pericarditis disappears with administration of thyroid extract (Brawley et al, 1966). Cholesterol turnover in the pericardium has been approximately 12 times longer in this disease (Doherty and Jenkins, 1966). If effusion persists, pericardiectomy is indicated (Creech et al, 1955).

Acute Pyogenic Pericarditis. Acute pyogenic pericarditis can occur as a result of direct contamination of the pericardium after a penetrating injury. It may also result from septicemia or pyemia or follow the bacteremia of osteomyelitis or pneumonia. Hepatic or subphrenic abscesses can rupture into the pericardial sac, or acute pyogenic pericarditis may be a complication of an operation on the heart, lungs, or esophagus.

Severe chest pain and fever are the usual clinical signs. It is difficult to differentiate pyogenic pericarditis from the more common benign form in the early stages. A pericardial effusion can occur more rapidly, and cardiac tamponade must be expected because the fluid accumulates quickly from the severely inflamed pericardium.

In the past, the most common cause of acute pyogenic pericarditis was pneumococcus, which was usually associated with pneumonia. Currently, in children, the more common cause is staphylococcus (Weir and Joffe, 1977), and in adults, it is either staphylococcus or gram-negative bacteria (Klacsmann et al, 1977). The diagnosis is confirmed by pericardial aspiration, with the finding of organisms on smear and subsequent culture. Treatment with systemic antibiotics is indicated, and open drainage usually results in a more rapid convalescence. Systemic antibiotics penetrate the pericardium with difficulty, and it is usually preferable to make a small subxiphoid incision and place a drainage catheter behind the heart with a second catheter placed on the anterior surface of the heart. Thus, irrigation of the posterior catheter results in drainage from the anterior catheter, and the purulent material can be evacuated more easily. Drainage usually results in rapid cessation of fever and symptoms.

Tuberculous Pericarditis. Tuberculous pericarditis is usually considered to be secondary to tuberculosis elsewhere, and the disease spreads to the pericardial sac by direct extension from the pleura or lung, from mediastinal lymph nodes, or through the blood or lymphatics. The onset of clinical symptoms may be so insidious that the patient cannot date the inception. The patient is not usually known to have pulmonary tuberculosis, and pericarditis is not suspected from the early nonspecific symptoms. Tuberculous pericarditis can be accompanied by malaise, fever, sweats, pleural pain, cough, and a pericardial friction rub. In this situation, the diagnosis of pericarditis is more evident. Pericardial effusion develops slowly and distention of the pericardium is allowed to occur without cardiac tamponade. The fluid may be clear, straw-colored, or sanguineous. Early pericardiocentesis may establish the diagnosis by the finding of acid-fast bacilli in the fluid. In some cases, the skin test may be negative even though acid-fast bacilli are present in the pericardium and should not be used to exclude the diagnosis. Occasionally, the large cardiac area must be differentiated from cardiac dilatation. If the patient is not treated, the course may be prolonged and progressive emaciation, toxemia, and death may occur. Patients who are not treated may die of cardiac failure, but the more common cause is widespread tuberculosis (Carroll, 1951).

Early treatment of tuberculous pericarditis is important because the fibrous scarring prevents effective concentrations of antituberculosis drugs from reaching the tubercle bacilli. The fibrotic process of healing, beneficial in pulmonary tuberculosis, is associated with the threat of pericardial contracture and constriction. There seems to be a direct relationship between the development of pericardial constriction and the length of time that the disease is present before treatment is begun. Wood (1956) emphasized that pericardial constriction was the rule if treatment was delayed for more than 4 months from the recognized onset of the disease, which again emphasizes the value of pericardial aspiration in determining specific causes of pericardial effusion.

Treatment with antituberculosis drugs should be started as soon as the diagnosis is established. In some cases, confirmation of the diagnosis of tuberculous pericarditis by laboratory techniques can be most difficult, and, if the clinical picture is convincing, it is probably best to administer antituberculosis therapy even though the diagnosis is not confirmed. Use of a single drug is ineffective, and only combination therapy should be done. In most patients who are treated promptly, clinical signs of improvement appear in 2 to 3 weeks. Increased heart size, raised venous pressure, and the quantity of effusion disappear more slowly and usually require 2 months before significant changes are noted.

It is predictable that a significant number of patients with massive effusion due to tuberculous pericarditis will suffer the effects of pericardial constriction (Sellors, 1946). As the fluid is absorbed, it becomes more viscid and is more irritating to the surrounding structures. It is postulated that the fluid then gravitates toward the diaphragmatic pericardium, because the majority of these patients are ambulatory. This area is subjected to longer periods of irritation and thus to a greater deposition of fibrous tissue. At operation, the diaphragmatic surface of the heart is found to have a thicker, more fibrous, and more calcified pericardial covering. The anterior pericardium over the right side of the heart is also found to be more severely involved, which is ascribed to the more forceful pulsations of the left ventricle that displace the exudate during the preconstrictive period into the less active and quieter areas over the right ventricle. This concept is questioned because the great vessels and atria have minimal movement and yet are rarely heavily calcified.

No concrete statement can be made concerning the stage in tuberculous pericarditis in which surgical therapy is best undertaken. It is futile to operate on febrile, acutely ill, toxic patients with active tuberculous pericarditis. However, it is also equally unwise to wait for a period of relative inactivity, a time when the operation is most difficult. Although some physicians believe that these patients should not be operated on until the disease has been present for 2 years or more (Sellors, 1956), this appears to lead to prolonged and needless suffering and probably to deaths that could have been prevented. The period in the early phase when the patient is clinically well appears to be the optimal time for intervention. These patients should receive antituberculosis therapy with two drugs; the addition of a third drug approximately 10 days before the operation is common practice.

Chronic Pericardial Effusion. The patient with a large heart shadow on the chest film presents the differential diagnosis of heart failure with marked cardiomegaly or chronic pericardial effusion. Physical findings of heart murmurs, gallop rhythm, or vigorous precordial pulsations indicate myocardial disease. Distant heart sounds, absence of murmurs, and shifting intensity of heart sounds are more likely seen in pericardial effusion; a pericardial splash or friction rub is rarely heard.

The electrocardiogram in effusion may show low voltage, ST segment elevation, and electrical alternans of the QRS complex. These QRS complexes are regular in time but alternate in height or direction of the major deflection, which is not affected by respiration. The explanation for this electrical alternans is that the heart, floating freely in abundant fluid, is no longer under normal mediastinal and pulmonary restraints; a periodic rotary oscillation can be established similar to that of the pendulum of a clock. ST segment elevation is seen in acute tamponade and results from compression and consequent myocardial ischemia.

Various diagnostic techniques have been used to differentiate effusion from cardiomegaly. Wood (1951) used cardiac catheterization and pressure measurements to identify cardiac failure. Soulen and associates (1966) have had good results by using echocardiography, and this seems to be the best current technique. Turner and associates (1966) used an intravenous carbon dioxide injection with the patient lying on the left side and differentiated the right atrial wall and pericardium. Routine angiocardiography similarly outlines the heart in reference to the cardiac silhouette (Holman and Steinberg, 1958). Pericardiocentesis, by using the electrocardiogram to identify contact with the heart, is the most direct method of confirming the diagnosis (see Fig. 34–1). Fluid removed should be examined for bacteria and fungi; cytologic studies should be done and serology and cell counts should be taken.

Repeated pericardiocentesis may provide temporary relief from effusion, but surgical therapy offers the best prognosis. The creation of a window between the pericardial sac and the pleural space to drain fluid into the pleural space for absorption has produced good results (Effler and Proudfit, 1957). However, whenever resection of the pericardium can be accomplished at a comparable risk, it should be done, because relief of effusion is most certain.

Most surgeons prefer to resect the pericardium in cases of chronic effusion because this is a more definitive procedure than the creation of a simple pleuropericardial window. The chance of recurrence is less, and the possibility of developing constrictive pericarditis is almost eliminated. Operative resection can be done easily in this situation, and fluid formed by the pericardial remnant drains into either pleural space. Excellent results have been reported in children with chronic effusion and tamponade treated with pericardiectomy (Shumacker and Harris, 1956; Roshe and Shumacker, 1959).

Bloody pericardial effusion commonly occurs in uremia and in patients receiving chronic hemodialysis. This effusion has not responded well to aspiration, and repeated aspirations are contraindicated because these patients may be prone to profuse bleeding from injury by the needle. Although the uremic patient may be desperately ill, an excellent response to creation of a simple pleuropericardial window has been noted. This should be done early after diagnosis, because tamponade and death are common from intrapericardial bleeding.

The diagnosis of chronic low-grade tamponade in the first several days after open heart procedures may be elusive. A persistent rise in venous pressure, often 15 to 20 cm H_2O, is the most uniform finding. Differential diagnosis includes heart failure, hypervolemia, and pulmonary embolism. There are no certain diagnostic techniques for excluding the diagnosis, such as pericardial scan, ultrasound, or echocardiography. A high degree of clinical suspicion accompanied by these diagnostic techniques can usually identify accumulations of intrapericardial fluid. Pericardial aspiration has been advocated by Borkon and associates (1981), and the role of anticoagulants and the postpericardiotomy syndrome that causes pericardial effusion has been emphasized by Ofori-Krakye and associates (1981). A diagnostic subxiphoid exploration of the pericardial cavity is the most certain way to confirm the diagnosis, and placement of drainage catheters into the pericardial space will resolve the diagnostic dilemma and result in rapid clearing of the effusion.

Chronic Constrictive Pericarditis. Constrictive pericarditis is the end stage of a chronic inflammatory process that produces a fibrous, thick, constricting pericardium surrounding the heart with a limitation of diastolic ventricular filling. As the encompassing scar shrinks, the heart is compressed further, especially the right side of the heart and great veins. This thickened and scarred pericardium is densely adherent to the heart, thus limiting systolic ejection as well as restricting diastolic filling. This results in a raised venous pressure and a reduced cardiac output, usually with a low systemic blood pressure. The rise in venous pressure is particularly interesting because a further rise by infusion of blood or plasma results in no change in cardiac output. Similar observations have been noted when paracentesis or phlebotomies were done. In these cases, venous pressure was reduced with no change in cardiac output. Obviously, these measures cannot be carried to extremes because reduction of venous pressure below a critical value lowers cardiac output. However, in contradistinction to acute cardiac tamponade, raising venous pressure does not result in an increase in cardiac output. This finding is due to more rigid restriction of diastolic filling imposed by the fibrous or calcified pericardium compared with that imposed by fluid or blood.

The reduced cardiac output results in less effective perfusion of the liver and kidney. The tendency toward salt and water accumulation accounts for an expansion of blood volume and further increases venous pressure. Thus, the kidney actually worsens the condition and increases venous pressure and blood volume even though these measures do not increase cardiac output. Ganglionic blocking agents may reduce venous pressure 35 to 50% without effecting a change in cardiac output (Lange, 1967). These patients may have diuresis with reduction of venous pressure and diastolic pressure in both the left and right sides of the heart while still maintaining an adequate cardiac output. These considerations suggest that some of the secondary manifestations

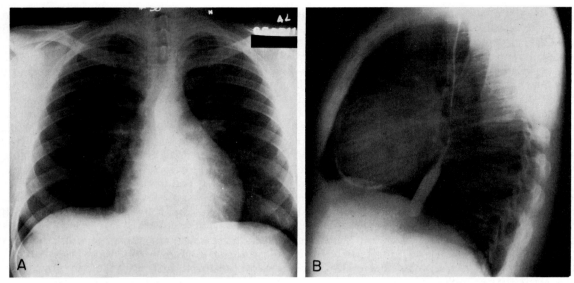

Figure 34–2. Chest films of a 45-year-old man with calcific constrictive pericarditis. The rim of calcium is clearly visible encircling the heart on the lateral film *(B)* but is not identifiable on the anterior view *(A)*.

of constrictive pericarditis can be improved by methods that do not attack the primary disorder.

Patients complain of weakness, easy fatigability, and shortness of breath with exertion that clears with rest. Formation of ascites without peripheral edema is a common finding. The ascites can be profound, and there may be no evidence of pedal edema, despite a venous pressure of 30 to 45 cm of water. Syncopal attacks may occur in association with activity and are thought to be due to the inability of the heart to increase its output to meet demands. Abdominal pain and tenderness may accompany enlargement of the liver. The feeling of fullness is due at first to the liver and then to formation of ascites. The ascites becomes excessive, and there is no evidence of peripheral edema. The opposite is true in congestive heart failure.

Physical findings vary considerably, depending on the stage of the disease. The patient may present a grotesque appearance with a puffy face and protuberant abdomen, although dyspnea may be present only with exercise. The heart is quiet, the apex beat may not be felt, and there is no right ventricular lift. A distinct diastolic shock may be palpated at the time of rapid filling, with a raised venous pressure. A rapid diastolic heart sound, coinciding with the rapid filling, has been described (Mounsey, 1955; Potain, 1856). Murmurs are usually absent. The liver is usually enlarged and is tender, and ascites may be present. Pedal edema, if present, is not marked. The disease is found more commonly in younger patients, 25 to 45 years old.

The hepatojugular reflex is prominent, and venous pressure increases momentarily during inspiration in patients with constrictive pericarditis (Kussmaul, 1873). Atrial fibrillation is present in approximately one-third of the patients. The peripheral pulse may be paradoxical and may disappear during inspiration even though cardiac rate and the apical pulse remain unchanged. Explanations of the mechanisms of the paradoxical pulse are that blood is sequestered in the pulmonary bed during inspiration (Hitzig, 1942) or that the thickened pericardium anchors the heart rigidly to the diaphragm. As the latter descends in inspiration, it further tenses the pericardium, which interferes with ventricular filling (Lower, 1669; Wood, 1956). Arterial blood pressure is usually low with a narrowed pulse pressure. Arm-to-tongue circulation time is prolonged.

The heart is usually normal or mildly enlarged on the chest film. Calcium deposits may be seen more commonly on the lateral film (Fig. 34–2). The superior vena cava may be prominent. The pulsation of the heart is reduced on fluoroscopic examination. The electrocardiogram shows a low voltage in the QRS complexes, the reason for which is not clear. T waves are flat and often inverted. The P wave may be broad and bifid, and the second wave may be taller than the first. The serum proteins may be low because of a loss of protein throughout the gastrointestinal tract. The increased portal pressure may cause an increase in lymph production and an increased rate of thoracic duct flow (Wilkinson et al, 1965). Lymphatic dilatation causes chylous effusions in the chest and abdomen. Intestinal lymphangiectasis is thought to result from increased pressure in the capillaries and lymphatics. The resultant congestion of the intestinal wall and the mucosal surface of the small bowel causes diminished absorption of ingested protein accompanied by an actual loss of protein from the congested lymphatics. Studies of thoracic duct lymph showed an increased production with a low protein content. Fat transport is reduced after ingestion. The loss of protein, especially albumin, probably results from the increased intestinal capillary pressure, which causes increased lymph

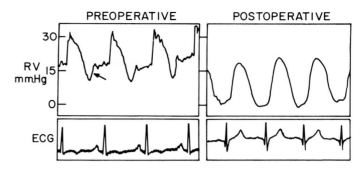

Figure 34–3. The right ventricular pressure tracing of a patient with constrictive pericarditis. The early rapid diastolic pressure elevation *(arrow)* with a plateau throughout the remainder of diastole is characteristic. Atrial contraction results in minimal pressure change in late diastole. The right ventricular pressure is normal at the time of catheterization 6 months after pericardiectomy.

production and secondary dilation of the lymphatics. Fat and protein are lost by transudation under high pressure or by rupture of these dilated lymphatics. This process is reversed after relief of pericardial constriction.

Establishing the diagnosis in constrictive pericarditis is not always simple, because the entity is often confused with hepatic cirrhosis or cardiac disease. Various forms of familial and acquired myocardiopathy are easily confused clinically with constrictive pericarditis. Catheterization of the heart has been the most satisfactory technique for differentiating between myocardial and pericardial disease. In constrictive pericarditis, the diastolic pressure in the right ventricle rises rapidly during early filling with a plateau effect and a small A wave (Fig. 34–3). The systolic pulmonary artery pressure is not above 45 mm Hg. Right atrial pressure is always greatly elevated. The left ventricular end-diastolic pressure is not much greater than the right end-diastolic pressure (average of 4 mm Hg), whereas in myocardiopathies, it was usually greater, with an average of 17 mm Hg (Conti and Friesinger, 1967). Angiocardiography is helpful in outlining the thickness of the atrial wall, the stiffness of the atrium, and the quality of atrial contraction. In constrictive pericarditis, the thin atrial wall is fixed to the scarred pericardium and contracts poorly, whereas atrial activity is usually vigorous in myocardial disease. In approximately three-fourths of the patients the correct diagnosis is obtained by these techniques. In some patients the diagnosis is elusive and can be accurately defined only by pericardial biopsy. This can be followed by an immediate extension of the thoracotomy or by a sternal splitting approach if pericardial constriction is confirmed.

In many patients the cause of constrictive pericarditis is unknown and can follow suppurative pericarditis. Tuberculosis was previously a common cause, but any type of infectious process may initiate dense pericardial scarring. Hemopericardium resulting from a penetrating injury has been a rare cause of chronic pericardial constriction (McKusick et al, 1955). Blunt trauma to the chest, such as a kick, automobile accident, or athletic injury that results in hemopericardium, may precipitate chronic scarring. The time interval between injury and pericardial disease may be considerable (Schneider and Rivier, 1960). The process may be rapid, such as in the case of a 25-year-old man who was stabbed in the chest with a penknife. Pericardiocentesis with removal of 200 ml of blood was required to control tamponade, but no subsequent aspirations were necessary. Pericardial calcification and symptoms of constrictive heart disease were present 4 months later, and pericardiectomy was done.

Pericardial constriction has been reported after cardiac operation, but the incidence is low, probably less than 1%. In some cases, the constriction has occurred within 2 weeks after operation, which suggests an acute inflammatory response with immediate adherence of the pericardium to the heart. Similarly, constrictive pericarditis occurs after Dressler's syndrome following myocardial infarction.

TECHNIQUE OF PERICARDIAL ASPIRATION

Pericardial aspiration can be a life-saving therapeutic technique for cardiac tamponade or a diagnostic method for pericarditis or effusion. Serous fluid is usually found in nonspecific pericarditis. Characteristic gold-colored, thick fluid can be obtained in cholesterol pericarditis or in pericardial effusion after myocardial infarction. Frank pus or cloudy, milky fluid may be aspirated in pyogenic pericarditis. Blood or serosanguineous fluid may be seen in cases of neoplasm and also of idiopathic pericarditis. Blood aspirated from the pericardial sac does not clot because it has been rapidly defibrinated by the movement of the heart. Aspiration of blood that later clots usually means that it was obtained from a chamber in the heart.

Pericardial aspiration is done routinely by either the left parasternal approach (in the fourth and fifth intercostal spaces) or the subxiphoid route under local anesthesia. A long needle (12 to 18 cm) is attached to a stopcock and syringe and is inserted just beneath the xiphoid process. A precordial electrocardiogram lead is attached to the needle by a small clip (see Fig. 34–1). The needle is inserted at a 45-degree angle directed posteriorly toward a point midway between the scapulas. The needle should be advanced until fluid is encountered or the electrocardiogram shows contact with the surface of the heart.

This is easily detected by the sharp negative deflection seen on the electrocardiogram (see Fig. 34–1). If the needle is in contact with the heart, it should be withdrawn slowly to a point proximal to cardiac contact, which should place the needle tip in the pericardium. Fluid aspirated should be saved for bacteriologic and cytologic examinations. The protein content should be determined. If a large volume of fluid is removed, the insertion of 100 to 200 ml of air into the pericardial sac is helpful to determine the thickness of the pericardium (Fig. 34–4). Immediate roentgenographic studies after air injection reveal not only the pericardial thickness but also the size of the heart and any masses projecting into the pericardial space.

Certain complications must be considered in needle aspiration in either the parasternal or the subxiphoid approach: laceration of the heart or a coronary artery, laceration of the internal mammary artery, penetration and possible contamination of the pleural cavity in purulent pericarditis, laceration or puncture of the lung with resultant pneumothorax, aspiration of blood from the intracardiac chambers, and, rarely, a shock-like reaction to the penetration of the pericardium by the needle. In addition, in the subxiphoid approach, perforation of abdominal organs and laceration of the liver may occur. These complications are unusual, however.

In large effusions or cardiac tamponade from penetration of the heart, a larger bore, thin-walled needle can be positioned in the pericardial space and a polyethylene catheter can be passed through the needle into the pericardial sac. A reasonable estimation of continued bleeding into the pericardial sac can be obtained because the blood rarely clots in the catheter owing to the defibrinating effect of the heart. These catheters can be left in place for several hours without fear of infection and may alleviate the necessity for repeated pericardiocentesis.

Some surgeons prefer open pericardiocentesis. In this procedure, the pericardium is exposed under local anesthesia through a small incision in the fourth or fifth interspace 1 cm to the left of the sternum. The needle is then passed through the pericardium under direct vision. A similar approach can be made by a small subxiphoid incision that bluntly frees the diaphragm from the anterior abdominal wall. Thus, the pericardium can be exposed superiorly to the diaphragm without entering either the abdominal or the thoracic cavity. Direct aspiration of the pericardial sac can be accomplished.

Unfortunately, pericardiocentesis may result occasionally in sudden death due to laceration of a coronary artery or to ventricular fibrillation. Pericardial tapping must be considered to be a serious procedure and must be done carefully. The use of the electrocardiogram to detect contact with the heart greatly reduces the risk of myocardial or coronary artery injury and has significantly reduced the dangers of this procedure.

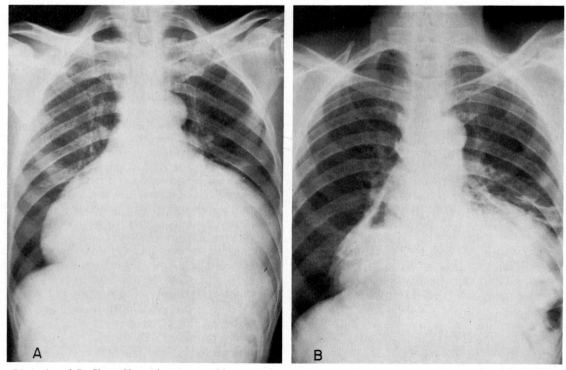

Figure 34–4. A and B, Chest films of a 48-year-old man with massive pericardial effusion. By doing pericardiocentesis 1500 ml of fluid was removed and a small quantity of air was injected into the pericardial sac. Film B shows the thin line of pericardium that is not adherent to the heart. An additional liter of fluid was removed after film B was taken.

PERICARDIOTOMY

Open drainage of the pericardium is usually done in cases of purulent pericarditis in which adequate drainage of pus is as important as in any type of purulent collection. Repeated needle aspiration of thick purulent material is often unsatisfactory in controlling infection. Originally, pericardiotomy was done by trephining an opening 2 to 3 cm in diameter in the sternum, but this procedure is now obsolete.

A subxiphoid approach by an incision to the left of the xiphoid process is carried through the rectus muscles to the transversus abdominis fibers. The dissection remains above this muscle and proceeds superiorly beneath the costal margin so that it enters the pericardial sac without encountering peritoneum, diaphragm, or pleura. Excellent drainage is obtained through this approach because the most dependent area of the pericardial sac is opened.

The anterior approach is most commonly used when the cartilages of the fifth and sixth ribs are resected. The entire cartilage between rib and sternum must be resected to avoid chondritis. Some physicians advocate excision of the seventh cartilage to obtain more dependent drainage. The mammary artery is divided, and the pleura is displaced laterally. A section of exposed pericardium is excised and is sent for histologic examination and culture.

For best drainage, two catheters should be placed in the pericardium—one anterior and one posterior to the heart. By this method, the posterior catheter may be irrigated, and the fluid rising can exit via the anterior catheter. Thus, the thick pus and loculations are more likely to be broken down and a more complete drainage of the pericardial space is accomplished.

PERICARDIAL BIOPSY

Biopsy of the pericardium is frequently the best approach to establish an exact and early diagnosis (Effler and Proudfit, 1957). Under general anesthesia, the pericardium is exposed through the fourth left interspace. A round segment of pericardium is excised for examination. Pericardial fluid may be examined microscopically and bacteriologically. In the case of chronic pericardial fluid, the defect may be drained into the pleural space from which it may be evacuated by an indwelling catheter. In some cases, the catheter can be left directly in the pericardial space for drainage of the chronic effusion. This is most useful when the effusion is likely to be self-limiting, such as in nonmalignant conditions.

An alternate method of pericardial biopsy is to resect the fifth costal cartilage on the left. All cartilage is removed, and the pericardium is exposed through the bed of the cartilage (Fig. 34–5). This technique is preferred when the differential diagnosis is between constrictive pericarditis and myocardiopathy, because the pleural space need not be entered. If constrictive pericarditis is present, the incision may be closed and a median sternotomy approach may be used, or the transverse incision can be extended to a left anterior thoracotomy and the sternum can be transected to gain exposure to the right ventricle and atrium.

PERICARDIECTOMY

By definition, constrictive pericarditis is a mechanical limitation of cardiac filling. Taking into account that myocardial atrophy may result from long-standing constrictive pericarditis, excision of the constricting tissue should offer definite improvement. Surgical results must be evaluated in reference to the period in which the operation was done (Kloster et al, 1965). Operative removal of the pericardium from the anterior and posterior surfaces of the heart is more extensive than the original surgical procedures. Pericardial resections formerly were inadequate and the clinical results were disappointing (Shumacker and Roshe, 1960). Operative mortality has been reduced by improved anesthesia, blood replacement, antibiotics, and management of cardiac arrhythmias.

Preoperative Preparation

Pericardiectomy is usually not done as an emergency operation, although there have been cases in which very ill patients benefited by emergency resection (Bigelow et al, 1956). The patients are usually hospitalized and brought into a better nutritional and cardiovascular state while diagnostic studies are being done. Vigorous efforts to correct ascites and cardiac failure should be made by salt restriction, control of arrhythmias, and adequate digitalization. Antituberculosis therapy should be started in any patient suspected of having tuberculous pericarditis.

Operative Technique

If the diagnosis of constrictive pericarditis has been ensured by preoperative studies, a definitive surgical approach should be made. Radical pericardiectomy is preferred by Holman and Willett (1949), Johnson and Kirby (1951), Bigelow and associates (1956), and Shumacker and Roshe (1960). Inadequate exposure does not allow complete removal of the pericardium and does not permit the surgeon to manage effectively any emergency, such as penetration of the thin-walled right ventricle or right atrium. The extent of pericardial resection should be determined by the operative findings, but most errors have been made by removal of insufficient pericardium.

A median sternotomy incision is frequently used (Holman and Willett, 1949). This incision provides

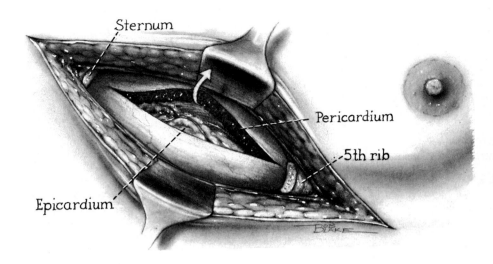

Figure 34–5. The left fifth costal cartilage is resected and the pericardium is exposed. A section of pericardium can be excised for histologic examination. The surface of the heart must be identified because a thick granular layer, loosely attached to the pericardium and more firmly adherent to the epicardium, can be present.

Figure 34–6. The pericardium is exposed through a midline sternal splitting incision. A longitudinal incision is made in the pericardium and a plane of dissection is established so that the thickened pericardium can be removed from the left ventricle.

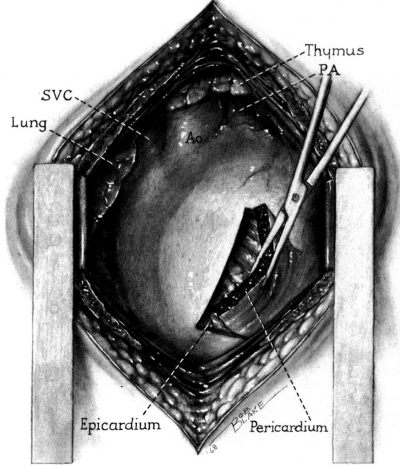

good exposure of the left ventricle, although the area posterior to the left phrenic nerve is difficult to visualize. Exposure of the right side of the heart and great vessels is excellent. Laceration of the thin-walled right ventricle commonly occurs. This complication is dangerous only if the exposure is inadequate to simply suture the raised pericardial flap back to the right ventricle and thus effectively close the hole.

A vertical skin incision is made from the manubrium to below the xiphoid. The sternum is divided by use of an electric bone saw. The two edges are separated and the mediastinum is exposed. On initial examination, it may appear that the heart is not beating because of the thickness and immobility of the diseased pericardium. The pleura is freed laterally and the thymus is raised off the pericardium. The pericardium is continuously incised longitudinally just anterior to the left border of the heart (Fig. 34–6). When cardiac musculature is identified, a plane is selected exterior to the muscle for the mobilization of the pericardium. The correct plane of dissection is anterior to the epicardium, and the organized pericardial exudate and the pericardium are removed. This plane may initially be difficult to find. Bleeding usually indicates that the surgeon has dissected too deeply through the epicardium into the myocardium.

If the correct plane can be followed, blood loss may be small. Care is taken to avoid injury to the coronary vessels because many of the arrhythmias encountered at the time of operation may be due to small infarcts created by injury to coronary vessels. Bleeding from the heart muscle should be controlled by finely placed sutures. The dissection is extended laterally over the left ventricle and apex. It may be important to free the left ventricle first so that pulmonary congestion does not occur when the right ventricular output increases. The heart is raised to the right so that the posterior surface of the left ventricle can be freed and the pericardium can be excised (Fig. 34–7). The phrenic nerve should be mobilized from the pericardium to avoid damage to this structure and to allow resection of the left posterior pericardium.

Care is taken while excising the pericardium from the thin-walled right ventricle and right atrium. The resection is continued laterally to include the great veins and superiorly onto the aorta and pulmonary artery (Fig. 34–8). The unusually thickened pericardium, extending from the inferior vena cava to the diaphragm and the apex of the heart, is excised (Fig. 34–9). Pockets of localized pus may be encountered between the epicardium and the thickened pericardium. Emphasis has been placed on the fact

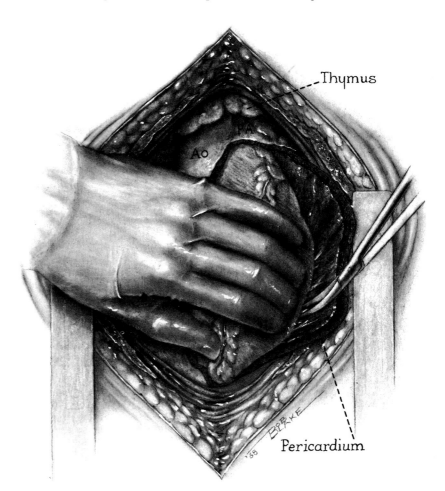

Figure 34–7. The heart is held to the right so that the posterior left ventricle can be freed. The phrenic nerve must be isolated to avoid injuring this structure. The large pericardial flap will be excised.

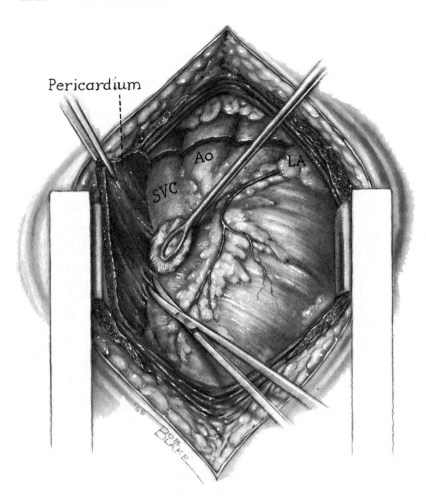

Figure 34–8. The pericardium is freed from the right atrium and venae cavae. These thin-walled structures are easily torn, and adequate exposure is mandatory for this part of the dissection.

Figure 34–9. The thick pericardium attached between the apex of the heart and the diaphragm must be excised to prevent recurrent adherent bands and inferior vena cava obstruction.

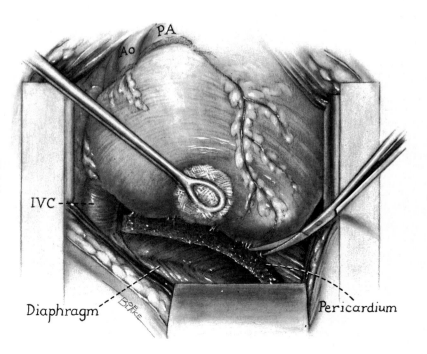

that the epicardial lining of these pockets should be removed to reduce the risk of later scarring (Churchill, 1936). Oozing from the surface of the heart usually ceases with gentle pressure. Overzealous suturing of bleeders on the surface of the heart should be discouraged to reduce the risk of injuring coronary vessels. The large area of denuded tissue resulting from the pericardiotomy can cause an outpouring of fluid. The pleura is opened widely into both pleural spaces, and catheter drainage of each is instituted by using gentle suction with the usual water-seal technique. Hemostasis is again observed to be certain that the accumulation of blood about the heart is minimized; this reduces the chance of recurrent fibrosis or of the formation of narrow bands that can again compress the heart. The edges of the sternum are approximated with encircling, interrupted stainless-steel wire sutures. The fascia, subcutaneous tissues, and skin are closed with interrupted silk sutures. Cardiopulmonary bypass has been used to facilitate removal of the thickened pericardium because of the ability to control hemorrhage in manipulation of the heart (Copeland et al, 1975). Bleeding is increased, however, from the required use of heparin; thus, bypass should be used only when simpler measures are inadequate.

The disadvantage of median sternotomy is the need for extensive manipulation of the heart to reach the areas of the pericardium that cover the posterolateral and diaphragmatic aspects of the left ventricle. Left anterolateral thoracotomy (fifth intercostal space) with transverse section of the sternum without entering into the right side of the chest is preferred by the authors. The patient is in a supine position with the left side of the chest slightly raised and the left arm carefully suspended from the anesthesia screen. The incision is restricted laterally to the midaxillary line, but the intercostal space is opened all the way to the spine. This and the transverse division of the sternum allow generous retraction and provide ample exposure to almost the entire pericardium. If necessary, partial cardiopulmonary bypass can be done by using the common femoral vessels.

Extensive pericardiectomy is possible with minimal manipulation of the heart. Exposure is optimal for left ventricular decortication, and, often, this part of the operation leads to better cardiac hemodynamics. Gradually, pericardiectomy is extended to the right cardiac chambers and terminates the line of resection anterior to the right phrenic nerve.

In a comprehensive review of pericardiectomy at the Mayo Clinic encompassing 46 years and 231 patients, left anterolateral thoracotomy used in 78 patients was considered to be the preferred incision. In respect to the extent of resection, fewer surgeons consider that pericardiectomy is satisfactory only if the entire pericardium covering all surfaces of the heart and major vascular structures within the pericardium is removed. They refer to this procedure as a radical pericardiectomy. Most surgeons advocate extensive pericardiectomy consisting of resection of

the pericardium covering the ventricles. Occasionally, decortication is necessary down to the myocardium if the epicardium has altered enough to act as a constricting mechanism. After successful pericardiectomy, the heart becomes larger and contracts more vigorously. The coronary arteries, which were initially obscured, assume their normal texture. Early hemodynamic responses may not be dramatic, but consistently good results have been achieved in most series (McCaughan et al, 1985).

Arrhythmias can cause concern during the course of operation because of manipulation of the heart and the small areas of infarction that can result from injury to small coronary vessels. Usually the patients have been receiving digitalis; this treatment reduces the likelihood of a rapid ventricular response to atrial arrhythmias, such as fibrillation and flutter. Ectopic ventricular activity is best controlled by a slow intravenous drip of 0.1% solution of lidocaine hydrochloride, which usually controls ectopic ventricular beats without depressing myocardial function. Care must be taken not to overtransfuse these patients during the operation or in the early postoperative period, because the thin-walled right ventricle can overdilate.

Postoperative Care

Although the hemodynamic improvements from pericardiectomy are dramatic, cardiac function may not return to normal owing to chronic myocardial injury from the pericardial constriction. Measurement of ventricular filling pressures is useful to prevent overdistention of the thin-walled right and left ventricles. Myocardial stimulants may be needed if cardiac contractility decreases. A slow infusion of dopamine is preferable because it is an agent that is least likely to produce ventricular irritability. Antibiotics are usually administered, and if tuberculosis is suspected, chemotherapy should be continued for several months until the culture reports on the pericardial material are returned. Daily maintenance fluid is kept at a low level until the cardiac status is stable and renal function is established. Digitalis may be necessary for several months postoperatively to help strengthen the damaged myocardium. Ambulation and exercise are gradually increased, depending on symptoms, but should be limited for at least the first month. Ascites and edema as well as hepatic enlargement usually subside after operation.

Some surgeons have thought it unnecessary to free the vena cava and right atrium; they contend that only liberation of the ventricles is important, but failure to completely liberate the right side of the heart has necessitated operations later on. Constriction of the great veins as they enter the heart has been shown at cardiac catheterization after incomplete excision of the pericardium. Operative removal of the remaining pericardium over the right atrium and great veins lowered venous pressure and cured the patient's ascites.

It has been shown with animals that, in experimentally produced generalized pericardial constriction, removal of the scar over the right side of the heart resulted in the disappearance of the high venous pressure and ascites, but the animals died in congestive heart failure (Isaacs et al, 1952). In other animals, the scar was removed from the left side of the heart with no reduction in venous pressure or loss of ascites. Thus, a complete pericardiectomy is necessary before failure to relieve a high venous pressure or to clear ascites is attributed to myocardial atrophy. Similarly, emphasis has also been placed on the importance of removing the pericardium from the right side of the heart and vena cava to relieve ascites and venous hypertension (Parsons and Holman, 1951, 1955).

POSTPERICARDIOTOMY SYNDROME

An unusual syndrome, which may be characterized by fever, pericardial pain, pleural pain, pulmonary infiltrates, arthralgias, dyspnea, pericardial effusion, pleural effusion, pericardial friction rub, or any combination of these signs and symptoms, occurs in approximately 10 to 40% of patients having cardiac procedures. The actual incidence is probably higher because mild cases remain unrecognized. The sedimentation rate is elevated; leukocytosis with an increase in lymphocytes is usually present; and occasionally the electrocardiogram shows changes of pericarditis. The syndrome must be differentiated from these postoperative conditions as incisional pain, myocardial infarction, pulmonary embolus, bacterial endocarditis, pneumonia, and atelectasis.

This syndrome was first described by Cox (1928) and Koucky and Milles (1935). It was initially described after wounds of the heart and was referred to as "polyserositis." It was called the "postcommissurotomy syndrome" in the early 1950s because of being observed after mitral commissurotomy. At this time, it was postulated to be due to a reactivation of rheumatic fever. The syndrome was observed after a pericardiotomy and was called the "postpericardiotomy syndrome" (Dresdale et al, 1956). Since then, it has been reported after minor violation of the pericardium, such as after percutaneous left ventricular puncture (Peter et al, 1966).

The precise etiology of this syndrome is still unknown. A common factor appears to be trauma and residual blood in the pericardial sac. Experimentally, it may be produced after an injection of autogenous blood or fat into the pericardial space (Ehrenhaft and Taber, 1952). Autoantibodies have been shown in rheumatic fever and in the postcommissurotomy syndrome (Kaplan, 1960). An antiheart antibody can be measured, and the serum concentration varies with the severity of the clinical symptoms (Engle et al, 1974). Whether this antibody is causative or simply registers the state of the disease is unknown.

Treatment is related directly to the severity of the syndrome. The course varies and is often self-limiting, requiring no therapy. In severe cases, accumulation of fluid in serous cavities may compromise cardiac or pulmonary function (Fig. 34–10). Salicylates and rest provide dramatic improvement in most cases. Salicylates should be given every 4 hours until improvement is noted. In severe cases, fluid balance and nutrition must be maintained, and complete bed rest is indicated. Corticosteroids usually produce improvement within 72 hours. After this short course of steroids, salicylates may be adequate to control symptoms. Prolonged use of steroids

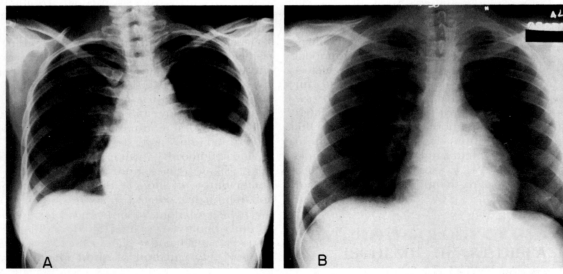

Figure 34–10. *A,* Chest film of a 40-year-old woman 10 days after open heart surgery. She had fever, pericardial friction rub, and a left pleural effusion. *B,* After 4 days' treatment with steroids and salicylates, the pleural effusion cleared, and the symptoms of postpericardiotomy syndrome did not return.

should be avoided, because rebound may occur with cessation of treatment. If this occurs, the patient should be maintained on the lowest dose of steroids that will control symptoms; the drug should be withdrawn gradually after 5 to 7 days. A low serum albumin, associated with poor nutrition as a factor in the development of clinical symptoms, has been described (Aronstam and Cox, 1966). Administration of albumin intravenously and reversal of the negative nitrogen balance resulted in clinical improvement. If collections of fluid persist, pericardiocentesis or thoracentesis may be necessary for precise diagnosis or for the relief of dyspnea.

Misdiagnosis with resultant failure to treat a specific infection, delay in recuperation with prolongation of hospitalization, and recurrences are always dangers in this syndrome. The recurrences are usually associated with withdrawal of therapy, commonly steroids, although recurrences may appear several years after the first episode. Postpericardiotomy syndrome usually does not have a role in the ultimate prognosis for the patient, even though the convalescent period can be prolonged. Persistent recurrent effusion is uncommon, but relief can be obtained with pericardiectomy.

Selected Bibliography

Engle, M. A., McCabe, J. C., Ebert, P. A., and Zabriskie, J.: The postpericardiotomy syndrome and antiheart antibodies. Circulation, 49:401, 1974.

This article describes the clinical course and possible etiologies of the postpericardiotomy syndrome. The immunologic significance of this rather common complication of cardiac surgery is emphasized. The findings of a heart reactive antibody that closely correlates with the clinical symptoms and the use of this as a diagnostic test in patients who have persistent pain and fever after thoracotomy are shown. The level of antibody is directly related to the clinical symptoms and could be used to predict recurrences.

Issacs, J. P., Carter, B. N., II, and Haller, J. A., Jr.: Experimental pericarditis: The pathologic physiology of constrictive pericarditis. Bull. Johns Hopkins Hosp., 90:259, 1952.

This represents one of the few well-detailed experimental studies in which constrictive pericarditis was produced. It emphasized the minimal effect of constriction about the atrium in raising venous pressure. The authors showed that all the systemic manifestations of constrictive pericarditis occurred when the constrictive component was present over the ventricles. In addition, the importance of removing the pericardium from the left ventricle before the right at operation was shown by the occurrence of pulmonary edema when left ventricular restriction was not relieved. The effect on the myocardium of constrictive pericarditis was emphasized by observing the marked change in the elasticity of the ventricle after removal of the constrictive scar. There is an excellent review of the hemodynamics associated with constrictive pericarditis and the effects on the systemic organs.

Kloster, F. E., Crislip, R. L., Bristow, J. D., et al: Hemodynamic studies following pericardiectomy for constrictive pericarditis. Circulation, 32:415, 1965.

This report very nicely shows the hemodynamic improvements in patients after relief of constrictive pericarditis. Improvements in

serum proteins and other blood components are emphasized. There are ventricular tracings in the article that show the effects of constrictive pericarditis on ventricular performance. The article gives a detailed discussion of pressure changes and hemodynamic patterns of patients with constrictive pericardial disease and emphasizes the diagnostic difficulty that is often encountered in distinguishing constrictive pericarditis from restrictive myocardial disease.

McCaughan, B. C., Schaff, H. V., Piehler, J. M., et al: Early and late results of pericardiectomy for constrictive pericarditis. J. Thorac. Cardiovasc. Surg., 89:340, 1985.

An excellent clinical review of 231 patients (10 months to 83 years of age) who had pericardiectomy for constrictive pericarditis at the Mayo Clinic between 1936 and 1982. The study was done to evaluate early and late results of this procedure. Four different incisions were used and included median sternotomy and left anterolateral thoracotomy. The authors prefer the latter incision. They refer to the depth and extent of resection and warn against the routine use of cardiopulmonary bypass.

Bibliography

Aronstam, E. M., and Cox, W. A.: A new concept of the pleuro-pericardial syndrome: Postpericardiotomy or postcardiotomy syndrome. J. Thorac. Cardiovasc. Surg., 51:341, 1966.

Barnard, H. L.: The functions of the pericardium. J. Physiol., 22:42, 1898.

Bates, J. C., and Leaver, F. Y.: Pericardial celomic cysts: Presentation of 5 new cases and 5 similar cases illustrating difficulty of diagnosis. Radiology, 57:330, 1951.

Beck, C. S.: Acute and chronic compression of the heart. Am. Heart J., 14:515, 1937.

Beck, C. S., and Griswold, R. A.: Pericardiectomy in the treatment of the Pick syndrome: Experimental and clinical observations. Arch. Surg., 21:1064, 1930.

Beck, C. S., and Moore, R. L.: The significance of the pericardium in relation to surgery of the heart. Arch. Surg., 11:550, 1925.

Bigelow, W. G., Dolan, F. G., Wilson, D. R., and Gunton, R. W.: The surgical treatment of chronic constrictive pericarditis. Can. Med. Assoc. J., 75:814, 1956.

Blakemore, W. S., Zinsser, H. F., Kirby, C. K., et al: Pericardiectomy for relapsing pericarditis and chronic constrictive pericarditis. J. Thorac. Cardiovasc. Surg., 39:26, 1960.

Blalock, A., and Levy, S. E.: Tuberculous pericarditis. J. Thorac. Surg., 7:132, 1937.

Bloomfield, R. A., Lauson, H. D., Cournand, A., et al: Recording of right heart pressures in normal subjects and in various types of cardio-circulatory disease. J. Clin. Invest., 25:639, 1946.

Borkon, A. M., Schaff, H. V., et al: Diagnosis and management of postoperative pericardial effusions and late cardiac tamponade following open-heart surgery. Ann. Thorac. Surg., 31:512, 1981.

Brawley, R. K., Vasko, J. S., and Morrow, A. G.: Cholesterol pericarditis. Am. J. Med., 41:235, 1966.

Bricheteau, I.: Observations d'hydropneumopéricarde. Arch. Gén. Méd., 4s, 4:334, 1844.

Burwell, C. S., and Blalock, A.: Chronic constrictive pericarditis: Physiologic and pathologic considerations. J.A.M.A., 110:265, 1938.

Bush, C. A., Stang, J. M., Wooley, C. F., et al: Occult constrictive pericardial disease. Circulation, 56:924, 1977.

Carroll, D.: Streptomycin in the treatment of tuberculous pericarditis. Bull. Johns Hopkins Hosp., 88:425, 1951.

Chester, M. H., and Tully, J. B.: Acute pericardial fat necrosis. J. Thorac. Surg., 38:62, 1959.

Cheevers, N.: Observations on the disease of the orifice and valves of the aorta. Guy's Hosp. Rep., 7:387, 1842.

Churchill, E. D.: Decortication of heart (Délorme) for adhesive pericarditis. Arch. Surg., 19:1457, 1929.

Churchill, E. D.: Pericardial resection in chronic constrictive pericarditis. Ann. Surg., *104*:516, 1936.

Cohnheim, J.: Lectures on general pathology. New Syndernham Soc., *1*:21, 1889.

Conti, C. R., and Friesinger, G. C.: Chronic constrictive pericarditis: Clinical and laboratory findings in 11 cases. Johns Hopkins Med. J., *120*:262, 1967.

Copeland, J. G., Stenson, E. G., Griepp, R. B., and Shumway, N. E.: Surgical treatment of chronic constrictive pericarditis using cardiopulmonary bypass. J. Thorac. Cardiovasc. Surg., *69*:236, 1975.

Cox, W. M.: Wounds of the heart. Arch. Surg., *17*:484, 1928.

Craddock, W. L.: Cysts of the pericardium. Am. Heart J., *40*:619, 1950.

Creech, O., Hicks, W. M., Snyder, H. B., and Erickson, E. E.: Cholesterol pericarditis: Successful treatment by pericardiectomy. Circulation, *12*:193, 1955.

Délorme, E.: Sur un traitement chirurgical de la symphyse cardopéricardique. Gaz. Hop., *71*:1150, 1898.

Doherty, J. E., and Jenkins, B. J.: Radiocarbon cholesterol turnover in cholesterol pericarditis. Am. J. Med., *41*:322, 1966.

Dresdale, D. T., Ropstein, C. B., Gusman, S. J., and Greene, M. A.: Postpericardiotomy syndrome in patients with rheumatic heart disease. Am. J. Med., *21*:57, 1956.

Effler, D. B., and Proudfit, W. L.: Pericardial biopsy: Role in diagnosis and treatment of chronic pericarditis. Am. Rev. Tuberc., *75*:469, 1957.

Ehrenhaft, J. L., and Taber, R. E.: Hemopericardium and constrictive pericarditis. J. Thorac. Surg., *24*:355, 1952.

Engle, M. A., McCabe, J. C., Ebert, P. A., and Zabriskie, J.: The postpericardiotomy syndrome and antiheart antibodies. Circulation, *49*:401, 1974.

Fitzpatrick, D. P., Wyso, E. M., Bosher, L. H., and Richardson, D. W.: Restoration of normal intracardiac pressures after extensive pericardiectomy for constrictive pericarditis. Circulation, *25*:484, 1962.

Fowler, N. O.: Physiology of cardiac tamponade and pulsus paradoxus. Mod. Concepts Cardiovasc. Dis., *47*:109, 1978.

Gillett, R. L.: Acute benign pericarditis and the Coxsackie viruses. N. Engl. J. Med., *261*:838, 1959.

Hitzig, W. M.: On mechanisms of inspiratory filling of the cervical veins and pulsus paradoxus in venous hypertension. J. Mt. Sinai Hosp., *8*:625, 1942.

Holman, C. W., and Steinberg, I.: The role of angiocardiography in the surgical treatment of massive pericardial effusions. Surg. Gynecol. Obstet., *107*:639, 1958.

Holman, E., and Beck, C. S.: The physiological response of the circulatory system to experimental alterations. II: The effect of variations in total blood volume. J. Exper. Med., *42*:681, 1925.

Holman, E., and Willett, F.: The surgical correction of constrictive pericarditis. Surg. Gynecol. Obstet., *89*:129, 1949.

Holman, E., and Willett, F.: Results of radical pericardiectomy for constrictive pericarditis. J.A.M.A., *157*:789, 1955.

Isaacs, J. P., Carter, B. N., II, and Haller, J. A., Jr.: Experimental pericarditis: The pathologic physiology of constrictive pericarditis. Bull. Johns Hopkins Hosp., *90*:259, 1952.

Jackson, R. C., Clagett, O. T., and McDonald, J. R.: Pericardial fat necrosis. J. Thorac. Surg., *33*:723, 1957.

Johnson, J., and Kirby, C. K.: A new incision for pericardiectomy. Ann. Surg., *133*:540, 1951.

Kaplan, M. H.: The conept of autoantibodies in rheumatic fever and in the postcommissurotomy state. Ann. N.Y. Acad. Sci., *86*:974, 1960.

Karanaeff: Paracentese des Brustkastens und des Pericardiums. Med. Z., *9*:251, 1840.

Klacsmann, P. G., Bulkley, B. H., and Hutchins, G. M.: The changed spectrum of purulent pericarditis. Am. J. Med., *63*:666, 1977.

Kloster, F. E., Crislip, R. L., Bristow, J. D., et al: Hemodynamic studies following pericardiectomy for constrictive pericarditis. Circulation, *32*:415, 1965.

Koucky, J. D., and Milles, G.: Stab wounds of the heart. Arch. Intern. Med., *56*:281, 1935.

Krook, H.: Acute non-specific pericarditis: Study in 24 cases including descriptions of 2 with later development into constrictive pericarditis. Acta Med. Scand., *148*:201, 1954.

Kussmaul, A.: Ueber schwielige Mediastino-Perikarditis und den paradoxen Puls. Berl. Klin. Wochenschr., *10*:433, 445, 461, 1873.

Laennec, R. T. H.: Traité d'Auscultation Médicale et des Maladies du Poumon et du Coeur. Paris, Brosson & J. S. Chaude, 1819.

Lam, C. R.: Pericardial celomic cyst. Radiology, *48*:239, 1947.

Lambert, A. V.: Etiology of thin-walled thoracic cysts. J. Thorac. Surg., *10*:1, 1940.

Lange, R. L.: Treatment of chronic constrictive pericarditis. Mod. Treat., *4*:162, 1967.

Lower, R.: Tractatus de Corde (London, 1669). In Major, R. H.: Classic Descriptions of Disease. Springfield, IL, Charles C Thomas, 1932, p. 630.

Mannix, E. P., Jr., and Dennis, C.: The surgical treatment of chronic pericardial effusion and cardiac tamponade. J. Thorac. Surg., *29*:381, 1955.

Martin, A.: Acute non-specific pericarditis: A description of nineteen cases. Br. Med. J., *2*:279, 1966.

Martin, J. W., and Schenk, W. G., Jr.: Pericardial tamponade: Newer dynamic concepts. Am. J. Surg., *99*:782, 1960.

McCaughan, B. C., Schaff, H. V., Piehler, J. M., et al: Early and late results of pericardiectomy for constrictive pericarditis. J. Thorac. Cardiovasc. Surg., *89*:340, 1985.

McKusick, V. A.: Chronic constrictive pericarditis: Some clinical and laboratory observations. Bull. Johns Hopkins Hosp., *90*:3, 1952.

McKusick, V. A., and Cochran, T. H.: Constrictive endocarditis. Bull. Johns Hopkins Hosp., *90*:90, 1952.

McKusick, V. A., Kay, J. H., and Isaacs, J. P.: Constrictive pericarditis following traumatic hemopericardium. Ann. Surg., *142*:97, 1955.

Morgagni, G. B.: De Sedibus et Causis Morborum per Anatomen Indagatis. Venetiis, typ. Remondiniana, 1761.

Mounsey, P.: The early diastolic sound of constrictive pericarditis. Br. Heart J., *17*:143, 1955.

Ofori-Krakye, S. K., Tyberg, T. L., et al: Late cardiac tamponade after open heart surgery: Incidence, role of anticoagulants in its pathogenesis and its relationship to the postpericardiotomy syndrome. Circulation, *63*:1323, 1981.

Parsons, H. G., and Holman, E.: Experimental Ascites. Surg. Forum (1950). Philadelphia, W. B. Saunders Company, 1951, p. 251.

Parsons, H. G., and Holman, E.: Experimental segmental pericarditis. Arch. Surg., *70*:479, 1955.

Peter, R. H., Whalen, R. E., Orgain, E. S., and McIntosh, H. D.: Postpericardiotomy syndrome as a complication of percutaneous left ventricular puncture. Am. J. Cardiol., *17*:718, 1966.

Pick, F.: Ueber chronische, unter dem Bilde der Lebercirrhose verlaufende Pericarditis (pericarditische Pseudolebercirrhose) nebst Bemerkungen ueber Zuckergussleber (Curshmann). Z. Klin. Med., *29*:385, 1896.

Potain, P. C.: Adhérence général du péricarde. Bull. Soc. Anat. Paris, Aug. 29, 1856.

Powers, P. P., Read, J. L., and Porter, R. R.: Acute idiopathic pericarditis simulating acute abdominal disease. J.A.M.A. *157*:224, 1955.

Rehn, I.: Zur experimentellen Pathologie des Herzbeutels. Verh. Dtsch. Ges. Chir., *42*:339, 1913.

Riolan, J.: Encheiridium Anatomicum et Pathologicum Lugduni Batavorum. Ex Officina Adriani Wyngaerden, 1649, p. 206.

Romero, cited by Baizeau: Mémoire sur le fonction du péricarde au point de vue chirurgical. Gaz. Med. Chir., 1868, p. 565.

Ronka, E. K. F., and Tessmer, C. F.: Congenital absence of pericardium: Report of case. Am. J. Pathol., *20*:137, 1944.

Rose, E.: Herz Tamponade (Ein Beitrag zur Herzchirurgie). Dtsch. Z. Chir., *20*:329, 1884.

Roshe, J., and Shumacker, H. B., Jr.: Pericardiectomy for chronic cardiac tamponade in children. Surgery, *46*:1152, 1959.

Sauerbruch, F.: Die Chirurgie der Brustorgane, Vol. II (Berlin, 1925).

Schmieden, V., and Fischer, H.: Die Herzbeutelentzundung und ihre Folgezustande. Ergeb. Chir. Orthop., *19*:98, 1926.

Schneider, S., and Rivier, J. L.: Hemopéricarde traumatique et péricarde calleux. Rev. Méd. Suisse Romande, *80*:171, 1960.

Schumacker, H. B., Jr., and Harris, J.: Pericardiectomy for chronic idiopathic pericarditis with massive effusion and cardiac tamponade. Surg. Gynecol. Obstet., 103:535, 1956.

Schumacker, H. B., Jr., and Roshe, J.: Pericardiectomy. J. Cardiovasc. Surg., 1:65, 1960.

Sellors, T. H.: Constrictive pericarditis. (Hunterian lecture abridged). Br. J. Surg., 33:215, 1946.

Sellors, T. H.: General observations on constrictive pericarditis with special reference to results of surgery: Minerva Cardioangiol. Europea, 4:489, 1956.

Senac, J. B.: Traité de la Structure du Coeur, de son Action, et de ses Maladies. Vol. 1. Paris, chez Briasson, 1749, p. 2.

Shackelford, R. T.: Hydropneumopericardium: Report of case with summary of the literature. J.A.M.A., 96:187, 1931.

Shidler, F. P., and Holman, E.: Mediastinal tumors: Presentation of 34 cases. Stanford Med. Bull., 10:217, 1952.

Soulen, R. L., Lapayowker, M. S., and Gimenz, J. L.: Echocardiography in the diagnosis of pericardial effusion. Radiology, 86:1047, 1966.

Turner, A. F., Meyers, H. I., Jacobson, G., and Lo, W.: Carbon dioxide cineangiocardiography in the diagnosis of pericardial disease. Am. J. Roentgenol., 97:342, 1966.

Vieussens, R.: Traité Nouveau de la Structure et des Causes du Mouvement Naturel de Coeur. Toulouse, J. Guillemette, 1715.

Weill, E.: Traité Clinique des Maladies du Coeur chez les Enfants. Paris, O. Doin Co., 1895.

Weir, E. K., and Joffe, H. S.: Purulent pericarditis in children: An analysis of 28 cases. Thorax, 32:438, 1977.

White, P.: Chronic constrictive pericarditis (Pick's disease) treated by pericardial resection. Lancet, 2:597, 1935.

White, P. D.: Heart Disease. 4th ed. New York, The Macmillan Co., 1951.

Wilkinson, P., Pinto, B., and Senior, J. R.: Reversible protein-losing enteropathy with intestinal lymphangiectasia secondary to chronic constrictive pericarditis. N. Engl. J. Med., 273:1178, 1965.

Wood, P.: Diagnosis of pericardial effusion by means of cardiac catheterization. Br. Heart J., 13:574, 1951.

Wood, P.: Diseases of the Heart and Circulation, 2nd ed. Philadelphia, J. B. Lippincott Company, 1956.

CHAPTER 35

ATRIAL SEPTAL DEFECT, ANOMALOUS PULMONARY VEINS, AND ATRIOVENTRICULAR SEPTAL DEFECTS (AV CANAL)

Frank C. Spencer

Defects in the atrial septum range from the simple, uncomplicated ostium secundum defect to the more complex ostium primum and atrioventricular (AV) canal, representing different degrees of severity of embryologic malformation of the atrial and ventricular septa. Partial anomalous drainage of the pulmonary veins is present in 10 to 15% of secundum defects and is almost always present with the sinus venosus defect. Because the physiologic burden with a secundum defect and partial anomalous drainage of pulmonary veins is identical, consisting of a left-to-right shunt, these two abnormalities are considered together in the following section. In later sections, the more severe abnormalities—total anomalous drainage of the pulmonary veins, ostium primum defect, and AV canal—are considered. In the last two malformations, insufficiency of the mitral and tricuspid valves is usually present in addition to the left-to-right shunt.

ATRIAL SEPTAL DEFECT AND PARTIAL ANOMALOUS DRAINAGE OF PULMONARY VEINS

Historical Considerations

The modern era of extracorporeal circulation (ECC) began in 1953, when the first successful intracardiac operation in man was done by Gibbon to close an atrial septal defect (Gibbon, 1954). Also in 1953, Lewis successfully closed a defect under direct vision by using hypothermia and inflow occlusion. These two pioneering achievements soon launched the modern era of ECC. Several ingenious techniques that did not require ECC were developed in earlier years but quickly became of historical interest only. The technique of hypothermia and inflow occlusion

was effective and safe, because temporary occlusion of the vena cava for 10 to 12 minutes at 28 to 30° C was well tolerated. This technique was used for several years until ECC became safer (Spencer and Bahnson, 1959). By 1960, ECC had developed to such an extent that other techniques were abandoned.

Pathologic Features

Secundum-type atrial defects are among the most common cardiac malformations and occur in 10 to 15% of all patients with congenital heart disease. Women are affected about twice as frequently as are men. No etiologic factors are known.

Atrial defects vary widely in size and location (Fig. 35–1). Most are 2 to 3 cm in diameter and range from as small as 1 cm to virtual absence of the atrial septum. Occasionally, the atrial septum is fenestrated with multiple defects. A foramen ovale is a normal opening, not an abnormality because it occurs in 15 to 25% of adult hearts. With its slit-like construction, it is normally sealed, unless there is a sharp rise in right atrial pressure.

Most secundum defects are in the midportion of the septum. *Low* defects may involve the orifice of the inferior vena cava, and caution is required at operation to avoid constriction of the caval orifice. In 5 to 10% of patients, a *high* defect occurs at the junction of the superior vena cava and the right atrium and is called a sinus venosus defect because of its embryologic origin. Anomalous drainage of the pulmonary veins from the right upper lobe into the superior vena cava occurs in almost all of these patients. Rarely, anomalous pulmonary veins enter the superior cava, but the atrial septal defect is small or absent. This requires the creation of an atrial septal defect at the time of operative correction. This is the

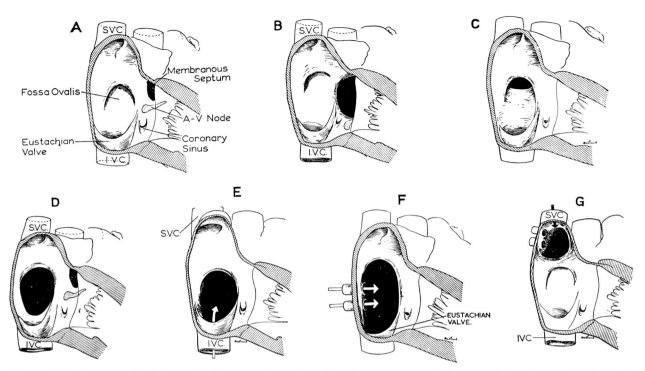

Figure 35–1. Anatomy of atrial septal defects, seen from the right atrium, as accurately shown and described in 1957 by Bedford and associates. The terminology is theirs. *A,* Normal atrial septum. *B,* AV type of defect. *C,* Widely patent foramen ovale. *D,* Fossa ovalis defect with complete septal rim. *E,* Low fossa ovalis defect astride inferior caval orifice with large eustachian valve. *F,* Large fossa ovalis defect without any posterior septal rim; pseudoanomalous right pulmonary veins. *G,* Superior caval type of defect, showing entrance of right upper pulmonary veins. (From Bedford, D. E., Sellors, T. H., Somerville, W., et al: Atrial septal defect and its surgical treatment. Lancet, *272:*1255, 1957.)

most common variety of atrial septal defect associated with anomalous pulmonary veins.

Less frequently, anomalous pulmonary veins enter directly into the posterior wall of the right atrium, anterior to the margin of the atrial septal defect. The rarest abnormality is entry of the pulmonary veins into the inferior vena cava. A variation of this unusual anomaly, associated with other malformations, has been called the "scimitar" syndrome, because of the radiologic appearance produced by the shadow of the anomalous pulmonary vein parallel to the right border of the heart. There are usually associated hypoplasia of the right lung and anomalous origin of the pulmonary arteries from the aorta. Because the amount of blood shunted through the hypoplastic lung is small, the physiologic disturbance is not severe.

Partial anomalous drainage of pulmonary veins usually involves the veins of only one lung, but a few examples of partial drainage of pulmonary veins from both lungs have been reported. One of the most detailed reports of the variety of pathologic patterns that occurs with anomalous pulmonary veins was published by Blake and associates (1965), an analysis of 113 patients from the Armed Forces Institute of Pathology. Twenty-seven patterns were found. This fact emphasizes the importance of routinely identifying the location of all pulmonary veins at the time of operation.

In a small percentage of patients with a secun-

dum defect, mitral stenosis is also present, a combination called Lutembacher's syndrome. With restriction of flow of blood into the left ventricle because of the mitral stenosis, an enormous left-to-right shunt develops, with massive dilatation of the pulmonary arteries. Craig and Selzer (1968) emphasized that the combination of lesions represented a true susceptibility of patients with secundum defects to rheumatic fever, because the frequency of the syndrome was greater than would occur from random association. Mitral stenosis, usually from prolapse of the mitral valve, is almost never found with other congenital lesions, such as ventricular septal defect.

Mitral insufficiency occasionally occurs in association with a secundum defect. It may be overlooked, unless specifically excluded by echocardiography or angiocardiography. Closure of the atrial defect without correcting the mitral insufficiency can result in serious, even fatal pulmonary congestion. Significant data are not yet available, but probably Carpentier's technique of mitral valve reconstruction could be used in most of these patients (Chapter 50).

Pathophysiology

An atrial septal defect results in a shunt of oxygenated blood from the left atrium to the right atrium because the left ventricle is a thicker muscle than the right ventricle. The difference in thickness

(10 to 12 mm versus 4 to 5 mm) is reflected by a difference in distensibility of the two ventricles, as a result of which, with an intact atrial septum, normal mean left atrial pressure is almost 8 to 10 mm Hg, whereas normal mean right atrial pressure is seldom more than 4 to 5 mm Hg. During the first 2 years of life, the right ventricle is similar to the left. Thus, only a small shunt may exist across an atrial septal defect but may increase in magnitude with growth of the child. Thus, an atrial septal defect may not be clinically evident in the first 2 years of life.

Rudolph (1974) offered an alternative explanation for infants in whom catheterization a few hours after birth detects a large shunt at the atrial level. Rudolph suggested that differences in the vascular resistance in the pulmonary and systemic circulations may be as important as the difference in distensibility of the two ventricles.

Depending on the size of the defect and the difference in distensibility between the two ventricles, the size of the shunt varies from as little as 1 l/min to as much as 20 l/min. Usually, the pulmonary blood flow is two to three times greater than the systemic blood flow. There is a reciprocal decrease in pulmonary vascular resistance with the increased pulmonary blood flow, so pulmonary hypertension is rare. In adults, pulmonary hypertension eventually develops in 15 to 20% of patients. An enigma of the pathophysiology of congenital heart disease is the frequency of development of a progressive increase in pulmonary vascular resistance, ultimately to a lethal degree, with an untreated ventricular septal defect or aortopulmonary window, whereas with an atrial septal defect, even with a large shunt, such an increase in pulmonary vascular resistance almost never develops in the first several years of life.

Because the intracardiac shunt causes a reduction in systemic blood flow, there may be retardation of growth and development, producing a gracile habitus. In adults, the cardiac index is usually near the lower limits of normal (2.5 l/m²/min). In a group of 128 adult patients studied by Craig and Selzer (1968), only 9 had a cardiac index of less than 2.0. A slight decrease in arterial oxygen saturation is frequent and probably results from mixing of oxygenated and unoxygenated blood in the atria. In the group studied by Craig and Selzer, 51 had an arterial oxygen saturation of 90 to 94%, and 17 had saturations of less than 90%. Severe hypoxia appears only when there is a marked increase in pulmonary vascular resistance.

The handicap from a pulmonary blood flow two to three times greater than normal is surprisingly well tolerated in most children. Most are asymptomatic; a few have dyspnea on extreme exertion. There may be some increase in susceptibility to pneumonia, as well as an increased susceptibility to rheumatic fever. Bacterial endocarditis is almost unknown. With the benign course of atrial defects in childhood in many patients, a natural question was whether such a course would continue in adult life.

In the 1968 Craig and Selzer report (128 patients over 18 years of age), most patients were limited only by dyspnea on exertion. Cardiac failure, with or without atrial fibrillation, was unusual before 40 years of age. The most alarming finding was an increase in pulmonary vascular resistance above the upper limits of normal (400 dyne-sec/cm⁻⁵) in 13% of patients. This finding represented a catastrophe, because the development of a major increase in pulmonary vascular resistance changed an atrial septal defect from an easily curable lesion to an inevitably lethal one. The pattern of development of the increase in pulmonary vascular resistance was studied in some detail in the 18 patients in whom it occurred and could not be correlated with age or with the degree of increase in pulmonary blood flow. Thus, it was not a "wear and tear" phenomenon. Apparently, an individual susceptibility of unknown type was the basic factor. The increased resistance occurred in approximately one-third of patients before 20 years of age, in another one-third in the third and fourth decades, and in the remainder after 40 years of age. In a few patients studied with serial catheterizations, the rise in pulmonary vascular resistance, once it began, continued rapidly. In two patients, it continued despite surgical closure of the defect.

The unpredictability of the development of an increase in pulmonary vascular resistance, although it never occurs in most patients, is sufficient reason in itself to close atrial septal defects routinely in all patients whenever they are diagnosed, even though most are asymptomatic.

Also in 1968, Gault and associates reported studies of 62 patients over 40 years of age. Compared with the younger group reported by Craig and Selzer, most were symptomatic, with 45% classified as Class III or Class IV cardiac patients. An increase in pulmonary vascular resistance was seen in 70%, a frequency identical to that found by Craig and Selzer.

Craig and Selzer commented on the rarity of a patient over 50 years of age with an atrial septal defect. Statistical analyses indicated that this low frequency was less than would occur in the normal population, which implied that most patients succumbed to cardiac failure or pulmonary hypertension before the sixth decade. The average life expectancy of all patients with atrial septal defects has been estimated to be near 40 years. Fifteen to 20% of patients die of pulmonary hypertension. The others die of cardiac failure 15 to 20 years earlier than the normal population.

Clinical Features

When symptoms are present, the most common are exertional dyspnea, fatigue, and palpitations. In a 1966 study of 275 patients who were operated on, Sellers and colleagues found that 113 were asymptomatic. As mentioned earlier, dyspnea is more frequent in adults and results from either pulmonary hypertension or cardiac failure. Atrial arrhythmias become more frequent in the fourth decade, probably from hypertrophy of the right atrium, and may precipitate or intensify symptoms of congestive failure. As with atrial fibrillation that develops with chronic mitral stenosis, these arrhythmias may be permanent and may remain even after closure of the septal defect. Cyanosis is rare except in the small percentage of patients in whom pulmonary vascular resistance has increased sufficiently to produce a large right-to-left shunt.

On physical examination, a soft, systolic murmur in the left second or third intercostal space near the sternum is the most common finding. The murmur arises from the increased flow of blood through the pulmonic valve. Wide, fixed splitting of the second sound is another important auscultatory finding.

On the chest film, slight to moderate cardiac enlargement from dilatation of the right ventricle may be evident. Enlargement of the pulmonary artery is frequent. The electrocardiogram usually shows typical abnormalities that include right ventricular hypertrophy with a right axis deviation and conduction abnormalities (Fig. 35–2). Two-dimensional echocardiography can usually confirm the diagnosis, thus some cardiac centers no longer do routine catheterization. Lack of catheterization has the hazard of overlooking associated anomalies, especially anomalous pulmonary veins.

The diagnosis can be confirmed by cardiac catheterization, which shows that blood in the right atrium has a greater degree of oxygen saturation than does blood in the venae cavae. The presence of anomalous pulmonary veins can be recognized if the cardiac catheter enters a pulmonary vein directly from the superior vena cava. If the pulmonary vein is entered from the right atrium, the diagnosis is uncertain, because the catheter may have traversed an atrial septal defect. Precise delineation of the pulmonary veins may be done with selective angiography. In most patients, the systolic right ventricular pressure is between 30 and 40 mm Hg. With large shunts, a gradient of 20 to 40 mm Hg may be found across a normal pulmonic valve because of the increased flow of blood.

Surgical Treatment

Indications and Contraindications. Operation is usually recommended if cardiac catheterization shows an increase in pulmonary blood flow more than one and one-half times greater than systemic blood flow. Because children with a shunt of this size are almost always asymptomatic, the decision for operation is based entirely on the findings at catheterization. The ideal time for operation is near the age of 5 or 6 years, before the child enters school, in order to avoid the psychologic school handicap of having a "heart problem."

The only contraindication to operation is a sharp increase in pulmonary vascular resistance, fortunately almost unknown in children. If the pulmonary vascular resistance has increased to more than 50%

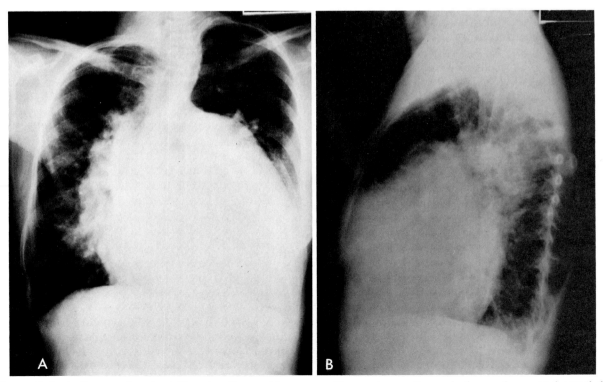

Figure 35–2. *A,* Preoperative chest film of a 45-year-old woman with massive cardiomegaly from a large atrial septal defect, operated on with blood cardioplegia. Recovery was uneventful. *B,* Preoperative lateral chest film of the patient described in *A.*

of systemic resistance, the risk of operation is high (30 to 40%), and surviving patients may show little benefit. As the progressive nature of the increasing pulmonary vascular resistance is well documented, these patients should be operated on, because operation is their only chance for long-term survival.

Age per se is not a contraindication, though mortality is increased and benefits are less with age. Several reports before 1970 described significant experiences with patients over 40 to 60 years of age.

Technique of Operation. All patients are operated on with extracorporeal circulation. The technique for ECC currently used at New York University is described in Chapter 50. A median sternotomy incision is used, unless cosmetic reasons are significant. A right thoracotomy in the fourth intercostal space gives satisfactory exposure if the patient is positioned properly in an anterolateral position, turned about 60 degrees from the horizontal plane. If there is any uncertainty about the diagnosis, a median sternotomy should be used, because the ability to treat previously unrecognized cardiac pathology is significantly hampered if operation is done through a right anterolateral incision. A submammary incision that had been used for more than a decade with satisfactory results was described in 1980 by Brom in Holland.

Once the pericardial cavity has been opened, the atrium is explored with a finger introduced through the atrial appendage. Seven or eight anatomic features should be routinely identified: the size and location of the atrial septal defect and its relation to the orifices of the superior and inferior venae cavae; the point of entry of the right and left pulmonary veins; the size and location of the coronary sinus ostium (a large ostium indicates a left superior vena cava); the presence of any mitral or tricuspid insufficiency; and the ventricular septum, which normally bulges in systole, unless a septal defect is present.

The superior vena cava is inspected for anomalous pulmonary veins that enter the cava directly. Absence of the left innominate vein usually indicates the presence of a left superior vena cava. This anomaly should be recognized and managed at operation with proper technique; otherwise the operative field is flooded with blood. A left superior vena cava can be detected by any of three methods: noting an enlarged coronary sinus on palpation, noting the absence of a left innominate vein, or elevating the heart and noting the left superior vena cava entering the coronary sinus just above the left atrial appendage.

When cardiopulmonary bypass has been established, the temperature is lowered to 25° C and the heart is arrested by infusion of cold blood with potassium as described under open mitral commissurotomy in Chapter 50. Topical hypothermia is routinely used and produces a myocardial temperature of 15 to 20° C. With the aorta clamped and the heart arrested and cooled, the right atrium is opened widely, the intracardiac structures are identified, and

the location of the structures previously palpated is confirmed. Ventilation of the lungs is stopped. A crucial point is to *avoid* aspirating intracardiac blood from the left of the septal defect, which will introduce air into the left atrium. If for any reason this is done because of uncertainty of pathology in the left side of the heart, the danger of air embolism is significant. Maneuvers for the removal of air similar to those used after replacement of the mitral valve should then be used. If the left atrium remains filled with blood during the procedure, the hazard of air embolism is much less.

Introduction of air into the left atrium is hazardous because blood in the aortic root, proximal to the occluding clamp, may drain into the left ventricle and be replaced by air arising from the left atrium into the aortic root, just as air enters a bottle filled with fluid when the bottle is turned upside down and the fluid is poured out.

The usual secundum defect can be readily identified as an opening of 2 to 4 cm located in the midportion of the atrial septum. Variations are numerous and range from a large defect that extends down to the inferior atrial wall to a superior defect near the point of entry of the superior vena cava. The location of the coronary sinus and the tricuspid valve should be noted. Normal entry of the right pulmonary veins into the left atrium can be confirmed by inserting a curved clamp through the defect and advancing it through the left atrium into the different pulmonary veins.

When the margins of the defect have been identified, closure can be done with a continuous suture (usually 3-0 Prolene) or a patch of pericardium or Dacron. Direct suture can be used in most patients (Fig. 35–3), especially children. The author's preference has shifted toward the use of an autologous patch of pericardium for most patients except for those with small defects. This choice is made primarily on a theoretical basis to minimize subsequent development of arrhythmias from distortion of the atrial septum by direct suture. In adult patients, the tissues in the atrial septum are less pliable, thus patch closure is usually done.

If the lower margin of the defect is near the inferior atrial wall or is missing, care must be taken during closure to avoid constriction of the orifice of the inferior vena cava. Care is also taken near the coronary sinus because of the proximity of the AV node near its medial border.

Complete heart block is rare and occurs more often in older patients, probably from traction or stretching in the region of the coronary sinus (Fig. 35–4), which is the reason why patch closure is preferable in older patients.

After all sutures have been placed but not tightened, the left atrium is filled with blood and the lungs are gently ventilated so that red blood visibly spurts from the left atrium through the defect, after which the sutures are tied while partly covered with blood. This method protects against trapping of air in the left atrium.

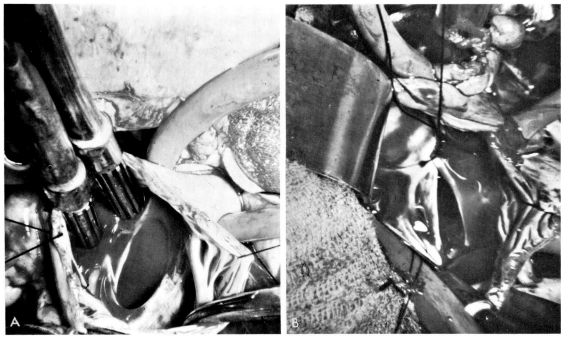

Figure 35–3. *A,* Atrial septal defect located in the midportion of the atrial septum. *B,* These defects can usually be closed by direct suture. A suture has been inserted at the top margin of the defect and will be continued caudad to approximate the two edges. Care is taken as the final sutures are inserted to avoid trapping air in the left atrial cavity.

Subsequently, ventricular fibrillation is induced, the aortic root is vented, and the aorta is unclamped. The right atriotomy incision is closed with the heart fibrillating, after which air is removed from the right atrium and the heart is defibrillated. The aortic root is routinely vented with gentle suction for a few minutes as a final precaution against air embolism, but usually none is seen.

After bypass, left atrial pressure should be meas-

ured to confirm the absence of mitral insufficiency. The correction of the left-to-right shunt can be confirmed by measuring and comparing oxygen saturation in blood aspirated from the superior and inferior cavae and the pulmonary artery.

Some patients are found at operation to have anomalous drainage of one or both pulmonary veins into the right atrium. This condition can be corrected with a patch closure of the atrial septal defect by

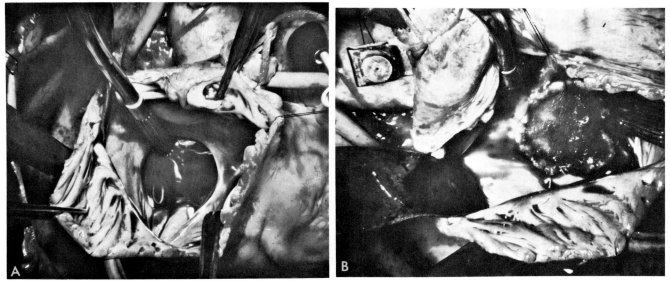

Figure 35–4. *A,* Large atrial septal defect in the lower portion of the atrial septum that extends to the orifice of the inferior vena cava. The patient, an adult, had gradually developed increasing congestive failure. *B,* Teflon felt patch attached with circumferential sutures to close the defect.

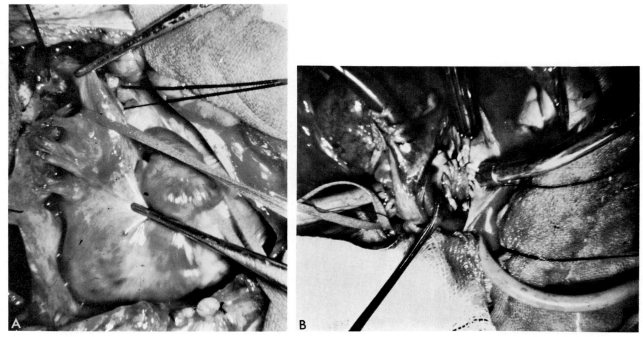

Figure 35–5. *A,* Three anomalous pulmonary veins entering the superior vena cava near its junction with the right atrium. This anomalous drainage is frequently encountered with the sinus venosus type of atrial septal defect. *B,* Pericardial patch applied to close the atrial septal defect in such a manner that the anomalous veins entering the superior vena cava are diverted into the left atrium. The cannula in the superior vena cava has been retracted upward, showing that insertion of the patch has not significantly narrowed the diameter of the superior vena cava.

simply suturing the patch to the right atrial wall in front of the point of entry of the anomalous veins.

In the presence of a sinus venosus defect—the combination of a high atrial septal defect and anomalous pulmonary veins entering the superior vena cava—certain guidelines are essential to prevent serious or lethal disasters such as thrombosis of the superior vena cava or the anomalous pulmonary veins.

The first principle is to dissect the extrapericardial superior cava superiorly above the point of entry of the azygos vein and encircle it at this point. Anomalous pulmonary veins that enter the superior vena cava above the point of entry of the azygos are almost unknown.

Second, the right pleural cavity should be opened to facilitate identification of the anomalous pulmonary vein when the cava is opened by simple introduction of a curved clamp into the ostium of the veins.

Third, the cardiac incision should begin in the right atrium and extend up the *right* anterolateral wall of the superior cava to remain well away from the area of the sinus node. The incision should be extended superiorly to expose the point of entry of the highest anomalous vein. If the superior vena cava has been snared above the azygos vein and occludes the azygos vein as well, exposure is usually excellent. If this has not been properly done, exposure can be difficult because of blood flowing from the orifice of the anomalous veins into the cava, especially when the caval cannula is retracted.

When adequate exposure has been obtained, a patch of pericardium can be inserted with a continuous suture of 4-0 Prolene; the patch is inserted superiorly around the point of entry of the pulmonary veins and inferiorly around the margins of the atrial defect so that a conduit is constructed to permit flow of blood from the anomalous veins into the left atrium (Fig. 35–5). The sutures are placed in the superficial portion of the posterior caval wall to avoid injury to the sinus node. Usually, the conduit can be constructed without significant stenosis of the superior cava, but if stenosis occurs, the superior cava can be widened by application of another patch of pericardium. After bypass, proper correction of the abnormality can be confirmed by measuring pressures in the superior vena cava, pulmonary veins, and right atrium.

More severe anomalies are unusual. Most of them are described in detail in the excellent textbook by Kirklin and Barratt-Boyes (1986). In the rare patient with absence of the atrial septum, and thus a single atrium, additional anomalies are common. The most frequent anomaly is a cleft in the mitral valve. Occasionally, a left superior vena cava enters the left atrium directly, rather than through the coronary sinus; this anomaly requires construction of an intracardiac tunnel to drain the left superior vena cava into the right atrium.

In most patients, convalescence after operation is uneventful. Atrial fibrillation is the most frequent postoperative arrhythmia but can be converted to sinus rhythm unless chronic atrial fibrillation is present. The risk of operation if pulmonary vascular resistance is normal is less than 1% and approaches zero per cent. Reports between 1966 and 1970 described experiences with more than 100 patients, with a mortality between 0 and 2% (Stansel et al, 1971). At New York University no deaths have occurred in children with uncomplicated secundum defect for the last 10 to 15 years, which supports the policy of routine closure of secundum defects of significant size.

Current data support a policy of routine closure of significant atrial septal defects, regardless of the age of the patient. The life expectancy of surgically untreated patients is shown in an actuarial curve in Figure 35–6. The 1988 report by Fiore and associates fully supports this policy. Fiore reported results for 51 patients over 50 years of age who were treated for 24 years, none of whom had a large increase in pulmonary vascular resistance. There were no operative deaths. Late results were excellent (mean follow-up was 9 years). No late systemic emboli occurred. Routine patch closure was recommended as primary repair and was associated with septal dehiscence in 2 of 15 patients.

Hawe and associates in 1969 analyzed late results for 546 patients at the Mayo Clinic. Atrial fibrillation was present in 30 to 40% of patients over 40 years of age. Late embolism occurred in 35 of 546 patients, which raised the question of long-term anticoagulation. In the 1988 report by Fiore, however, no late emboli were seen.

If pulmonary vascular resistance is elevated, the risk of operation is increased and long-term benefit is decreased. The question with regard to when operation should not be done because of increased vascular resistance has always been uncertain. The 1987 report from the Mayo Clinic by Steele and associates contains excellent data. During a period of 25 years, 40 patients with significant elevation of pulmonary vascular resistance (total resistance greater than 7 units/m^2) were treated, 26 surgically. In the surgically treated group, excellent results were obtained in 22 of the patients, whose total resistance was less than 15 units/m^2; 19 of the 22 were in good condition (follow-up averaged more than 10 years). Three of the four patients who had a resistance above 15 units/m^2 died. Of the 14 patients treated medically, 4 of 5 with a resistance of less than 15 died, and 6 of 9 with a resistance of above 15 died. Thus, in this series a total vascular resistance of 15 units/m^2 defined a group for whom neither medical nor surgical therapy was helpful.

PARTIAL ATRIOVENTRICULAR CANAL DEFECTS (OSTIUM PRIMUM)

The term AV septal defect, partial or complete, best describes this spectrum of malformations, which vary in severity with the extent of the deficiency in the AV septum. This concept is well discussed by Kirklin and Barratt-Boyes (1986, p. 543). The defects range from a simple atrial communication (ostium primum defect) to a severe defect with a common AV orifice and communications at both the atrial and ventricular levels (old term, atrioventricularis communis). The current terminology is based on the pathologic anatomy, rather than on the embryologic concepts that formed the basis for the previous terminology. These defects represent approximately 5% of all atrial septal defects and are found in 20 to 30% of children with Down's syndrome, but other than this association, no etiologic factors are known. AV septal defects with a common orifice (total defects) are discussed in a later section.

Anatomic studies over the past two decades have clarified the pathologic abnormality in these malformations. After the initial observations by Rastelli in 1966, further important observations were made by Piccoli, Carpentier, and Anderson. The 1985 paper by Penkoske and Anderson described observations of 130 AV septal defects from specimens in the pathologic collection of the Children's Hospital in Pittsburgh and summarized several important anatomic characteristics. First, the cardiac anatomy in both partial and complete AV septal defects is similar and varies only with the presence of the defect in the ventricular septum and the degree of malformation in the valve leaflets. Both the valve leaflets and the ventricular cavities are different from those found in normal hearts or other malformations. There are five leaflets at the two ventricular orifices, with various degrees of "bridging" across the ventricular septum. The left ventricular "mitral" valve is a trileaflet structure that comprises the left lateral, left superior, and left inferior leaflets (Fig. 35–7). The "cleft" dividing the left superior and left inferior leaflets (anterior leaflet of the mitral valve in old terminology) is actually a normal commissure. The extent of the cleft, which ranges from a small vertical opening to a triangular defect, is the principal determinant of the degree of mitral insufficiency. This subject is well discussed in the 1985 paper by Anderson. The conduction bundle, as originally described by Lev in 1958, is displaced posteriorly and inferiorly to lie between the inferior margin of the primum defect and the annulus of the tricuspid orifice.

The defect is readily recognized at operation by palpation or inspection. The superior border of the defect is a low crescent-shaped defect in the atrial septum, whereas the inferior border is the top of the ventricular septum with bridging of the leaflet tissue.

If the trileaflet mitral valve functions normally, there is no insufficiency. In at least 30 to 40% of patients there is moderate or severe insufficiency, either from the presence of the defect between the left superior and left inferior leaflets (the cleft) or from the absence of a varying extent of leaflet tissue that results in a triangular-shaped defect rather than in a simple cleft. Complete repair of incompetence may not be achieved in a few patients because of significant absence of leaflet tissue.

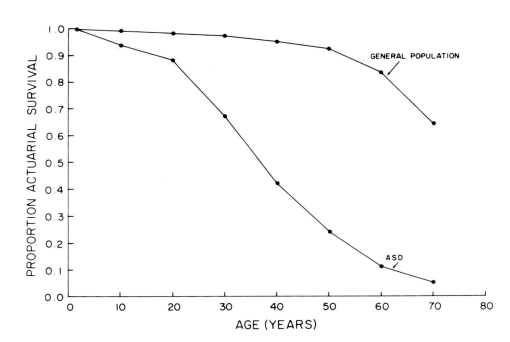

Figure 35–7. Diagrammatic representation of the AV valves seen from the atrial side (surgical orientation). *A,* Normal, with anterior and posterior mitral valve leaflets and septal, anterior, and posterior tricuspid valve leaflets. *B,* The leaflets in partial AV canal defects. The left superior, left inferior, and left lateral leaflets form the left AV valve; the right superior, right inferior, and right lateral leaflets form the right AV valve. *C,* The leaflets in complete AV canal defects are similar to those in *B.* However, the left superior and left inferior leaflets are not connected. The left inferior leaflet usually bridges a little (grade 1 or 2, on the basis of 1 to 5) across the crest of the ventricular septum. The left superior leaflet may bridge little or not at all (grade 0 or 1, Rastelli Type A) or moderately (grade 2 or 3, Rastelli Type B), or markedly (grade 4 or 5, Rastelli Type C). (AL = anterior leaflet; LIL = left inferior leaflet; LLL = left lateral leaflet; LSL = left superior leaflet; PL = posterior leaflet; RIL = right inferior leaflet; RLL = right lateral leaflet; RSL = right superior leaflet; SL = septal leaflet.) (From Kirklin, J. W., Pacifico, A. D., and Kirklin, J. K.: The surgical treatment of atrioventricular canal defects. *In* Arciniegas, E. [ed]: Pediatric Cardiac Surgery. Chicago, Year Book Medical Publishers. Copyright © 1985. Reproduced with permission.)

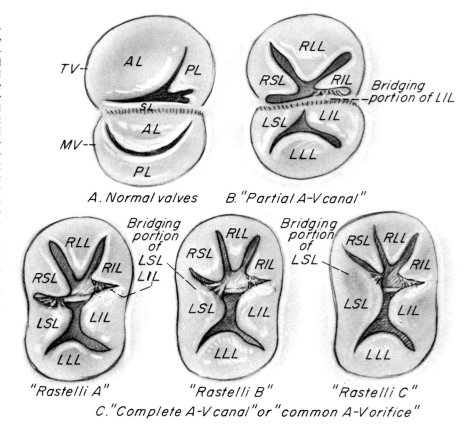

The chordae tendineae are usually normally attached along the margins of the two halves of the cleft leaflet (the commissure between the left superior and the left inferior leaflets) and are valuable guidelines during repair. There may be anomalous chordae that attach directly to the ventricular septum, because of the bridging of the leaflet tissue, and these may partly constrict the left ventricular outflow tract.

The anatomy of the different leaflets of the tricuspid valve varies. The septal leaflet is deficient or absent in almost 80% of patients, but significant tricuspid insufficiency is rare and does not require surgical treatment. Associated abnormalities are found in 10 to 15% (40 of 232 patients described by McMullan in 1973); the most common were secundum defect, pulmonary stenosis, and anomalous vena cava.

Pathophysiology

The two physiologic abnormalities are a left-to-right shunt at the atrial level and mitral insufficiency. When mitral insufficiency is small, the disability is identical to that of a secundum defect. When insufficiency is severe, cardiac failure and pulmonary hypertension often develop in the first 1 to 3 years of life. In the series by McMullan and associates (1973), catheterization data were described for 74 patients. The ratio of pulmonary flow to systemic flow was 2.7 and ranged from 1.3 to 5.6. Pulmonary resistance averaged 2.7 units/m² and ranged from 0.5 to 7.5. Systemic pulmonary artery pressure greater than 30 mm Hg was found in 36 patients.

With the range in degree of mitral insufficiency, there is a corresponding wide range in symptoms. With severe mitral insufficiency, exertional dyspnea is common, with other symptoms of pulmonary congestion if cardiac failure is more severe. In 30 patients described by Braunwald and Morrow (1966), 30 to 50% were asymptomatic.

On physical examination, the dominant finding is a loud systolic murmur along the left sternal border as well as at the cardiac apex, which indicates that an abnormality other than a simple secundum defect is present. The pulmonic second sound is increased in intensity and widely split. If cardiac failure is present, there may be signs of pulmonary and hepatic congestion.

Findings on the chest film vary. Enlargement of the pulmonary artery is the most frequent abnormality. With severe abnormalities, there is corresponding enlargement of the right ventricle. If mitral insufficiency is dominant, there is preponderant enlargement of the left ventricle.

The electrocardiogram almost always shows a left axis deviation and may provide the first clue to the correct diagnosis. There are various degrees of right and left ventricular hypertrophy. Conduction defects, with prolongation of the P-R interval, are frequent. The electrocardiographic abnormalities are due primarily to the conduction defect that results from displacement inferiorly of the conduction bundle.

A characteristic abnormality is usually present on the vector cardiogram; the frontal plane is inscribed in a counterclockwise loop, almost diagnostic of an ostium primum defect. The two-dimensional echocardiogram is virtually diagnostic; some physicians consider that cardiac catheterization is superfluous in uncomplicated defects. Cardiac catheterization and angiography are usually done; however, to determine the degree of mitral insufficiency, the presence of pulmonary hypertension, and any associated cardiac anomalies.

Surgical Treatment

In most patients, operation should be done between 1 and 4 years of age and before 2 years of age if there is significant cardiac failure or pulmonary hypertension. If mitral insufficiency is not present, the physiologic defect is the same as with a simple secundum defect. There is little urgency in operation, but correction before school is begun, near 5 years of age, is preferred.

The risk of operation is related to the degree of mitral insufficiency and pulmonary hypertension, and operative mortality averages 5 to 8%. Without these abnormalities, operative mortality is 1 to 2%.

Technique of Operation. The principal objectives are repair of the mitral insufficiency, avoidance of heart block, and closure of the atrial septal defect. A median sternotomy is preferable. A right anterior thoracotomy in the fourth intercostal space provides good exposure but is less satisfactory for prevention of air embolism. Palpation of the intracardiac chambers through the right atrial appendage readily confirms the diagnosis, with note being taken of the characteristic upper curved margin of the septal defect, as described earlier. The degree of mitral insufficiency can be estimated from the vigor of the regurgitant jet.

After palpation of the intracardiac structures, the heart is arrested with the cold blood potassium cardioplegia technique. The right atrium is then opened widely and appropriate retractors are inserted. The intracardiac anatomy is carefully examined, noting the size of the atrial septal defect, the extent and dimensions of the "cleft" in the mitral valve, the presence of abnormal chordae that might obstruct the aortic outflow tract, any abnormalities in the tricuspid valve, and the presence of any ventricular septal defect (Fig. 35–8).

The site and severity of mitral insufficiency are best evaluated at this time by injection of saline with a bulb syringe into the ventricular cavity to distend the valve leaflets.

The cleft in the mitral valve is repaired first, with figure-of-eight polyester sutures, usually Teflon (Fig. 35–9). As the edges of the cleft are rolled and thick-

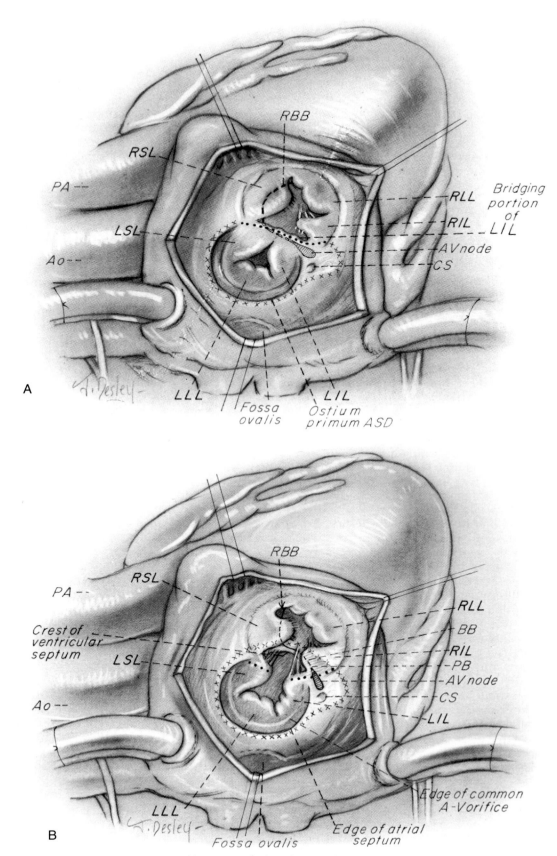

Figure 35–8 *See legend on opposite page*

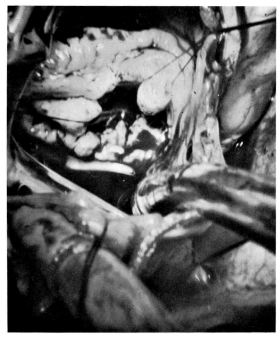

Figure 35–9. Operative photograph of cleft mitral valve through an incision in the atrial septum. Sutures have been placed in the margins of the cleft valve. The ventricular septum is visible in the midportion of the field, with the orifice of the tricuspid valve at the superior part of the field.

ened, the margins should be stretched to permit insertion of the sutures precisely in the free margin to prevent abnormal shortening of the reconstructed leaflet. The sutures are inserted from the ventricular septum medially out to near the insertion of the chordae tendineae on the valve leaflets centrally, depending on the degree of insufficiency. Care is taken with the sutures to avoid stretching the valve leaflets, which might create rather than correct insufficiency.

Good results have also been obtained by simply leaving the cleft alone, with a functioning trileaflet valve, if mitral insufficiency was not detected before operation. At New York University, routine suturing of the cleft as described has been consistently satisfactory. At least two patients at a second operation

(original operation was done elsewhere) had insufficiency that was corrected by suturing the cleft.

There has been a great deal of discussion with regard to whether the cleft should be sutured, because it is more properly recognized as a commissure and not as a cleft. The surgical significance of this debate seems to be minimal. The author has not recognized injury from routine suturing of the cleft. The extensive 1986 report from the Mayo Clinic by King and associates describes experiences with 199 patients during the previous 22 years. The cleft was routinely closed, regardless of the degree of preoperative valvular insufficiency. In two patients, who developed mitral insufficiency years after closure of the ostium primum defect in childhood without suture of the cleft, closure of the cleft at a second operation successfully eliminated regurgitation. In the 1987 report by Stewart and associates, which described experiences with 35 patients, the cleft was routinely closed. In the 1986 report by Pillai and associates, which described experiences with 84 patients at the Brompton Hospital in London during the previous 10 years, the cleft was sutured completely or partly in 72 of the group and was left alone in 11 patients.

Competency in the reconstructed leaflets is evaluated by injection of saline through a bulb syringe. In a few patients, a diffuse centrally located insufficiency can be shown and is probably due to a more severe absence of leaflet tissue. This is clearly not amenable to simple suturing of the cleft. Annuloplasty sutures at the commissure to narrow the mitral orifice have been used in a few of these patients, but significant data are not available (Kirklin and Barratt-Boyes, 1986).

After repair of the cleft in the mitral valve, the atrial defect is closed with a patch. The author's preference is for pericardium, although knitted Dacron appears to give equally good results. Avoidance of heart block caused by the sutures injuring the conduction bundle is crucial. The atrioventricular conduction bundle is at the inferior border of the defect and courses along the crest of the muscular ventricular septum. This bundle is displaced inferiorly from its usual course because of the absence of

---

Figure 35–8. The conduction system and suture siting in AV canal defects. The conduction system itself is in the same position in all types of AV canal defects, but the surgical problem is slightly different in defects without an interventricular communication than in those with one. (The stippled x's represent stitches for repair in the right ventricular aspect of the septum, beneath leaflet tissue. Stitches in the septal and atrial wall tissue are presented by the solid x's, and suture siting in leaflet tissue is represented by a *dotted line*.) *A,* Partial AV canal defect (AV canal defect without an interventricular communication). The AV node lies on the right side of the inferior (caudad) atrial septal remnant, at its junction with the floor of the right atrium over the crux cordis. The node pierces the abnormally formed central fibrous body to become the short penetrating portion of the His bundle. This structure immediately becomes the branching bundle, which gives off the left bundle branches earlier than normal as it courses along the crest of the ventricular septum. In its course, it is covered by the fibrous tissue that fuses the left inferior and left superior leaflets to the septal crest. At about the midportion of the crest of the septum, the branching bundle becomes the right bundle branch, which proceeds as shown. *B,* Complete AV canal defect (AV canal defect with common AV valve orifice and interventricular communication). The conduction system is in the same basic position as in the specimen in *A,* but the bundle of His is exposed as it passes along the crest of the septum. (Ao = aorta; ASD = atrial septal defect; AV = atrioventricular; BB = branching portion of bundle of His; CS = coronary sinus ostium; LIL = left inferior leaflet; LLL = left lateral leaflet; LSL = left superior leaflet; PA = pulmonary artery; PB = penetrating portion of bundle of His; RBB = right bundle branch; RIL = right inferior leaflet; RLL = right lateral leaflet; RSL = right superior leaflet.) (From Bharati, S., Lev, M., and Kirklin, J. W.: Cardiac Surgery and the Conduction System. New York, John Wiley & Sons. Copyright © 1983.)

the AV septum. With proper technique, heart block can be avoided in most patients, but the importance of technique is indicated by the variation in the frequency of heart block after operation, which ranges from 20% in operations done over 20 years ago to 1 to 2% in current reports. A series of interrupted sutures placed superficially to the left of the rim of the defect, directly in the annulus of the mitral valve, is preferred. This is done carefully, with traction on the mitral valve leaflet to stretch the tissue and define the annulus precisely. Excellent visualization is required, for the leaflet tissue bridges to merge with the leaflet tissue of the tricuspid orifice. Kirklin and Barratt-Boyes (1986) state that McGoon used this method for many years with excellent results. This method is used in the 199 patients described in King's report in 1986 and also in Stewart's report.

When the crucial sutures have been inserted through the patch and tied, the patch can be attached to the remaining margins of the defect with a continuous suture of 4-0 Prolene.

An alternative method places the sutures to the *right* of the conduction bundle and the coronary sinus and thus diverts the coronary sinus blood into the left atrium. This is well described by Kirklin and Barratt-Boyes (1986) and in the 1986 Pillai report. Either method appears to give excellent results.

After suturing of the different cardiac incisions, air should be carefully removed from the heart; air embolism was a frequent complication years ago and is now a rarity with appropriate techniques. After bypass, left atrial pressure should be measured as an index of residual mitral insufficiency. Intracardiac left atrial and right atrial catheters are left in place for postoperative monitoring. Pacemaker wires are also routinely left in the atrium and ventricle for a few days after operation, because transitory conduction defects are common, probably from edema near the conduction bundle.

Postoperative Considerations

Postoperative recovery is usually uneventful if the hazards described earlier are avoided. A permanent heart block is now uncommon with proper technique, but if it occurs, it should be treated by implantation of a pacemaker before the patient is discharged from the hospital. Most patients have a mild residual systolic murmur, usually of no hemodynamic significance. A loud systolic murmur warns of significant mitral insufficiency that may remain and should be evaluated by echocardiography and possibly ventriculography.

The risk of operation is small, in the range of 1 to 3%. The mortality was 5.5% in the 199 patients in King's report and has decreased to 3% since 1980. Mortality was 2% in Pillai's report and was almost 5% in Stewart's report. The principal factors that influence mortality are the degree of mitral insuffi-

ciency, presence of pulmonary vascular disease, and age of the patient. Several reports describe early and late results (Castenada et al, 1985; King et al, 1986; Pillai et al, 1986; Portman et al, 1985; Stewart et al, 1987). Generally, significant mitral insufficiency remains after operation in approximately 10% of patients. With severe insufficiency, patients often require another operation within a few years. Except for this group, long-term prognosis is excellent. In the Mayo Clinic series, 20 years after operation, survival was 96% and freedom from reoperation was 86%.

The unusual syndrome of severe hemolytic anemia after operation, described by Neill in 1964, has not been seen in the author's experience for more than 20 years. This syndrome has been avoided in almost all centers by an operative technique that prevents the development of localized mitral insufficiency.

COMPLETE ATRIOVENTRICULAR SEPTAL DEFECT (ATRIOVENTRICULARIS COMMUNIS)

As described earlier, this defect results from a more severe arrest in the development of the endocardial cushions than that which produces an ostium primum defect (partial AV canal). The basic defect is absence of the AV septum. Both the mitral and tricuspid valves are malformed and a combined septal defect that consists of an atrial and a ventricular septal defect is present. The atrial septal defect is similar to that with the ostium primum defect. The ventricular septal defect ranges from a small opening to a large one that extends into the muscular septum.

The classic pathologic studies by Rastelli and associates (1965, 1966, 1968) identified distinct anatomic types, called Types A, B, and C. These categories were based on the degree of bridging of the left superior leaflet of the mitral valve. In Type A the chordae extended to the rim of the ventricular septal defect. In Types B and C there was more extensive bridging with attachment of the chordae of the left superior leaflet to papillary muscles in the right ventricle. These concepts are well illustrated in Figure 35–7. The 1985 Penkoske-Anderson publication, based on a study of 130 specimens, clarifies and redefines the different Rastelli types.

The physiologic handicap with complete AV canals is far more severe than with an ostium primum defect. Cardiac failure occurs at an early age to the extent that 80% of untreated infants die within 2 years, and pulmonary vascular disease develops in almost all infants by 1 year of age. Diagnostic evaluation is identical to that described for the partial AV defect.

Surgical Treatment

The concepts of modern surgical treatment originated with Rastelli and associates at the Mayo Clinic,

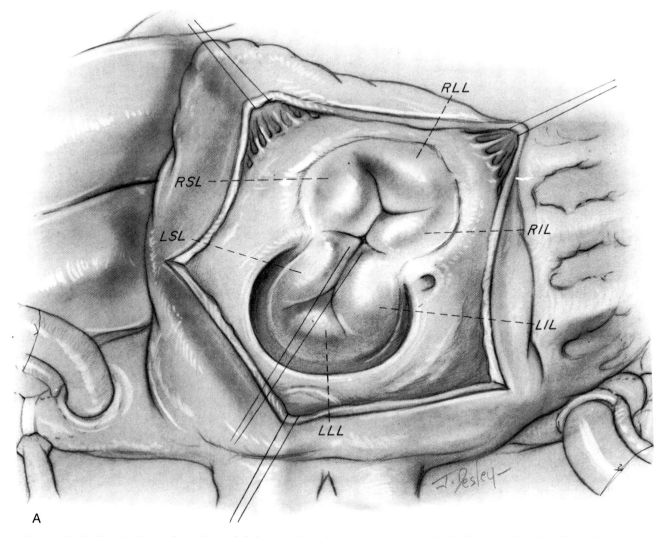

A

Figure 35–10. Repair of complete AV canal defect. *A,* After the atrium is opened, the leaflets are often closed exactly as they are in systole. If, instead, they are open, saline solution is injected into the ventricle to close them. At this point, the morphology of the leaflets, particularly their closure pattern, is studied, and the information obtained is used to plan the repair of any incompetence that may be present. A fine (6-0 polypropylene) suture is placed between the left superior leaflet (LSL) and left inferior leaflet (LIL) in the position shown, and left loose. (LLL = left lateral leaflet; RIL = right inferior leaflet; RLL = right lateral leaflet; RSL = right superior leaflet.)

Illustration continued on following page

who developed an operative technique based on their anatomic studies (1968). This procedure was described in detail in the 1972 report by McMullan and associates.

Most infants should be operated on in the first year of life, usually by 6 months of age, but earlier if severe symptoms are present. The techniques used for repair vary, depending on whether one or two patches are used, the method of treatment of a bridging left superior leaflet, and avoidance of the conduction bundle by staying on the left or right side. General principles are described here. Kirklin and Barratt-Boyes (1986) should be consulted for details.

In brief, the left superior and left inferior mitral leaflets are initially approximated and reconstructed (Fig. 35–10). A large prosthetic patch is then attached to the ventricular septum, with sutures placed to the right of the crest of the septum to avoid heart block.

The mitral and tricuspid valves are then attached at approximately the level where they would have attached to a normal intact ventricular septum. Finally, the atrial septal defect is closed by attaching the patch with a circumferential suture, and the conduction bundle is avoided by bringing the suture line to the right or the left.

Operative mortality varies with the degree of AV valve incompetence and ranges from almost 5% with mild incompetence to 10 to 15% with severe incompetence. Late results are excellent unless there is significant residual mitral incompetence or pulmonary vascular disease. Pulmonary vascular disease almost always subsides if a large pulmonary blood flow is present and operation is done in the first 2

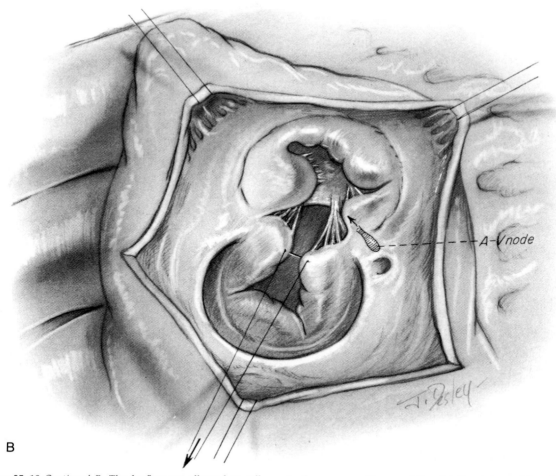

B

Figure 35–10 *Continued B,* The leaflets are allowed to collapse in the open position, and the details of the atrial and ventricular septal deficiencies and of the interatrial and interventricular communications are studied. The position of the coronary sinus is noted, and the positions of the unseen AV node and bundle of His are visualized by the surgeon from a knowledge of the anatomy.

years of life. With present techniques, significant residual incompetence is present in approximately 10% of patients.

TOTAL ANOMALOUS DRAINAGE OF PULMONARY VEINS

This severe anomaly is rare and occurs in 1 to 3% of patients with congenital heart disease. It is one of the most lethal congenital defects, because approximately 50% of infants die within 3 months without surgical treatment and another 30% die before 1 year of age. The 20% who survive beyond 1 year of age without surgical treatment are usually those with a large atrial septal defect as well.

There is now uniform agreement that operation should be done promptly after the diagnosis is made. In some infants operation is necessary in the first few days of life to prevent death.

The classification suggested by Darling and associates (1957), based on the point of emptying of the anomalous veins into the right side of the heart, is generally used. There are four basic types: supra-

cardiac (approximately 50% of patients), paracardiac (approximately 25%), infracardiac (15 to 20%), and mixed (3 to 5%). In the supracardiac type, the most common pattern of entry of the anomalous veins is through a left vertical vein, which, in turn, drains into the left innominate vein. A less frequent type is direct entry of the common venous sinus into the posterior aspect of the right superior cava.

With paracardiac drainage, the anomalous veins may enter the right atrium directly or, less often, drain into the coronary sinus, either directly or through a common venous sinus. With infracardiac drainage, the pulmonary veins enter a common sinus that travels caudad through the diaphragm to connect with the inferior vena cava through the portal vein in approximately two-thirds of the patients and through other veins in the remainder. This anomaly is rapidly fatal because the hepatic and portal venous channels progressively fibrose and obliterate.

Pathology and Pathophysiology

The anomalous veins usually enter a common venous sinus located behind the posterior pericar-

Figure 35–10 *Continued C,* A 5-0 silk stay suture is placed at point 2, the suture is then stretched toward the left leaflets, marked to the length between point 2 and the leaflets held with their chordae taut, removed, and used in cutting the interventricular Dacron patch to a proper width. The suture line of the interventricular patch to the ventricular septum and free wall is now visualized by the surgeon. As shown, this suture line lies on the right ventricular side of all of the chordae from the left-sided leaflets, including those from any bridging components of the LIL. The suture line goes beneath the right inferior leaflet (RIL), well away from the crest of the ventricular septum. The suture line begins at point 1. A stay suture is placed through the base of the RIL at point 3, where the suture line between interventricular patch and ventricle also ends by coming through the base of the RIL. Points 4 and 5 on the right atrium are on the suture line between the interatrial patch and the atrium. *D,* Point 6 is the area along which the base of the right inferior leaflet (RIL) is sandwiched between the interatrial and interventricular patches (the RIL has been removed here by the artist to facilitate visualization). Areas 7 and 8 are the portions of the LIL and LSL that are sandwiched between the interventricular and interatrial patches. Note that the suture lines completely avoid the AV node and bundle of His, the bundle lying in the muscle of the ventricular crest *beneath* valvar tissue. A 4-0 or 5-0 polypropylene suture is placed through the annulus at the base of any commissural tissue between the LSL and RSL at point 1. This suture will be used to begin suturing the Dacron patch to the ventricular septum. A marking suture of 5-0 polypropylene is placed through the base of the RIL leaflet at point 3. A fine silk stitch is placed and tied at point 4 and at point 5 to mark these locations. The position of the suture line between the Dacron patch and the ventricular septum, and the pericardial patch and the atrial wall and septum, can now be visualized, as well as that between the interventricular and interatrial patches. The latter suture line encloses the base of the LSL and LIL leaflets, as in a sandwich.

Illustration continued on following page

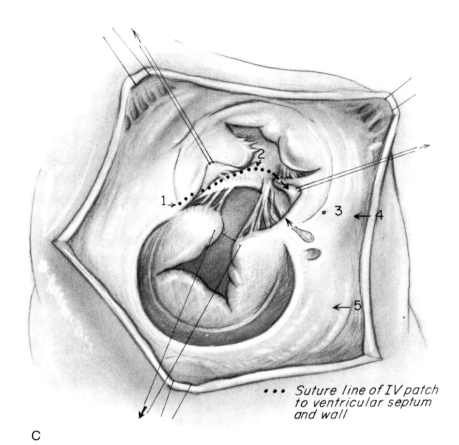

··· *Suture line of IV patch to ventricular septum and wall*

C

D

∘∘∘ *Suture line of IA patch to atrial septum and wall*
x x x *Suture line of IV to IA patch*

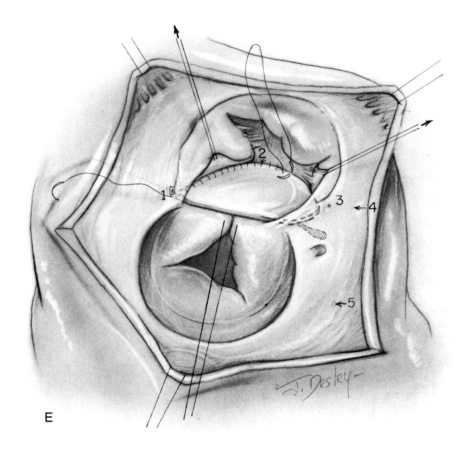

E

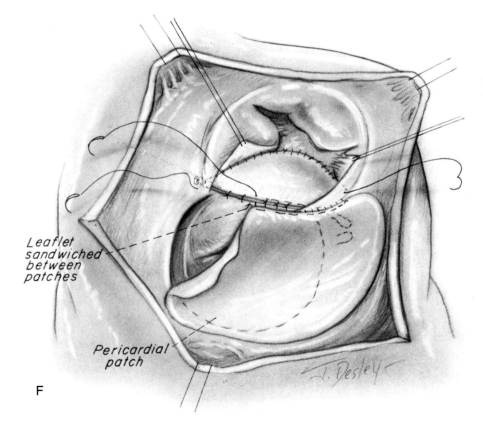

Leaflet
sandwiched
between
patches

Pericardial
patch

F

Figure 35–10 *Continued E,* After the Dacron patch has been trimmed according to measurements to fit precisely into position, it is sutured into place with the pledgetted mattress stitch previously placed at point 1. Note that the suture line is well on the right ventricular side of the crest of the ventricular septum, as shown in *D*. The suture line is approaching point 3, which previously was marked with a stay suture. *F,* The pericardial patch has now been cut according to measurements, and a new continuous mattress suture line is begun in the base of the RIL opposite point 3 (see *E*). This suture passes through the pericardial patch and base of the RIL, catches the Dacron patch, returns through the base of the leaflet to pass through the pericardial patch, and so on. After this suture line is completed, the pericardial patch is turned upward so that the left AV valve can be inspected. The stay suture previously placed between the anterior edge of the coapting surfaces of the LSL and LIL is passed through the edge of the Dacron patch at the appropriate point. A number of fine interrupted simple stitches are placed between the anterior aspect of these leaflets and the Dacron patch so as to perfectly align them. The previous suture used for the horizontal mattress stitches is now continued in the same manner through the pericardial patch, the base of the leaflets, and the Dacron patch, sandwiching the leaflet securely between the two patches in areas 7 and 8. (See text for currently preferred alternative suture technique.) After this suture line is completed, the pericardial patch is turned upward again, and the leaflets are closed by the injection of saline solution. If incompetence is present, the maneuvers described in the text are used to minimize or ablate the incompetence.

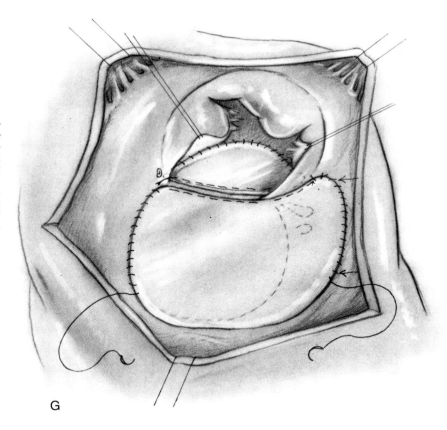

Figure 35–10 *Continued G,* With the previously held suture that has completed the attachment of the Dacron patch to the ventricular septum, shown in *F,* the pericardial patch is sutured to the atrial wall as shown, well away from the AV node and bundle of His. With the arm of the suture left after tying the two sutures at point 1, the pericardial patch is sutured to the superior aspect of the rim of the atrial septal defect. When this suture line is finished, the repair has been completed. (From Kirklin, J. W., Pacifico, A. D., and Kirklin, J. K.: The surgical treatment of atrioventricular canal defects. *In* Arciniegas, E. [ed]: Pediatric Cardiac Surgery. Chicago, Year Book Medical Publishers. Copyright © 1985. Reproduced with permission.)

G

dium, which, in turn, connects with the right side of the heart. An atrial septal defect must be present to maintain life, although the size varies considerably. A patent ductus arteriosus is present in most patients. In approximately one-third, other major cardiac anomalies are present.

As the oxygenated pulmonary venous blood and the systemic venous blood mix in the right atrium, there is always cyanosis, the degree of which depends on the pulmonary blood flow and the size of the atrial septal defect. As almost complete mixing of the systemic and pulmonary venous blood occurs in the right atrium, the findings at cardiac catheterization are unique and distinctive because oxygen saturations of blood drawn from the right atrium, right ventricle, pulmonary artery, and femoral artery are identical.

A severe physiologic handicap is pulmonary venous hypertension, which results from constriction at the point of entry of the anomalous pulmonary veins into the systemic venous system. This constriction apparently initiates the development of severe pulmonary hypertension. A predictable mathematical relationship exists between the degree of increased pulmonary vascular resistance, the pulmonary blood flow, and the severity of cyanosis. Because of the pulmonary venous obstruction, balloon septostomy to enlarge an atrial septal defect often has limited value.

In the fortunate few infants with adequate communication between the pulmonary veins and the systemic circulation, combined with a large atrial septal defect, the clinical course is like that of a large atrial septal defect except that there is a greater tendency to develop an increase in pulmonary vascular resistance.

The left atrium and left ventricle are small but are physiologically normal.

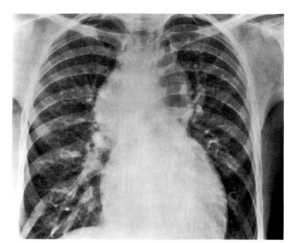

Figure 35–11. Chest film of a 24-year-old patient with total anomalous drainage of the pulmonary veins into a left vertical vein. The mediastinal shadow is composed of the dilated left vertical vein and the large superior vena cava. This roentgenographic appearance is frequently referred to as a "snowman" effect.

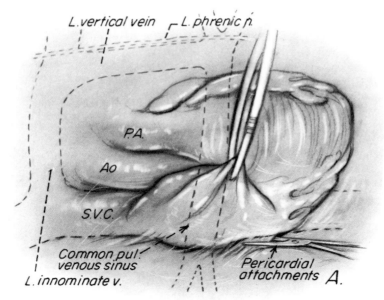

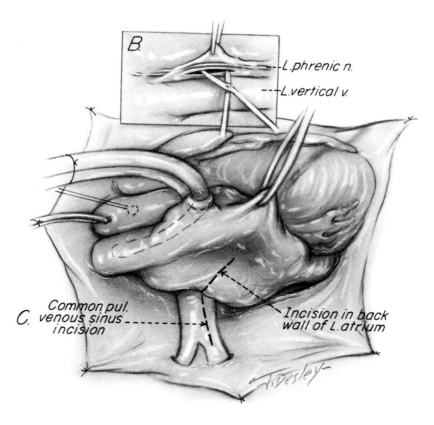

Figure 35–12. Technique of surgical correction of total anomalous drainage to left innominate vein. *A,* The posterior pericardial attachments are divided to mobilize the heart and expose the common pulmonary venous sinus located behind the pericardium. *B,* The left vertical vein is exposed and mobilized, with the phrenic nerve protected. *C,* The anterior wall of the pulmonary venous sinus is incised parallel to the long axis. The orifices of the left and right pulmonary veins are located and inspected. A corresponding incision is made in the back wall of the left atrium. The incision may have to be carried into the base of the left atrial appendage to the left and over to the atrial septum on the right.

Clinical Features

In the first few weeks of life *severe tachypnea* is the dominant symptom and is easily confused with aspiration pneumonia or primary pulmonary disease. After a few weeks, cyanosis, congestive failure, and progressive cardiac enlargement become more evident. Murmurs are not diagnostic.

The chest film may be diagnostic if there is drainage into a dilated left vertical vein, which creates a well-known double contour, called a "snowman" (Fig. 35–11). If pulmonary venous obstruction is severe, a diffuse ground glass-like type of pulmonary congestion is present.

If cyanosis is prominent, the differential diagnosis includes tetralogy of Fallot, transposition, and tricuspid atresia. The usual differential diagnosis is between anomalous drainage of pulmonary veins

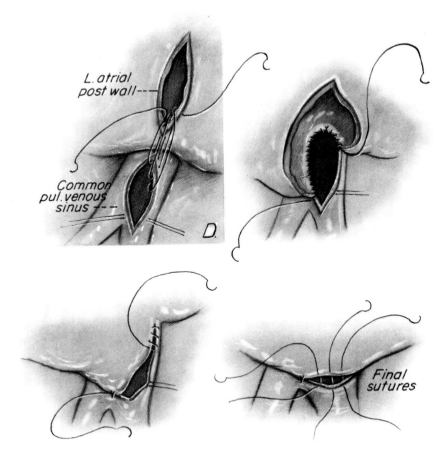

Figure 35–12 *Continued D,* A large anastomosis is constructed with continuous 4-0 or 5-0 polypropylene. (From Kirklin, J. W., and Barratt-Boyes, B. G.: Cardiac Surgery. New York, John Wiley & Sons. Copyright © 1986.)

and transposition, both of which produce cardiac enlargement and cardiac failure.

In the small group of patients with adequate pulmonary blood flow without pulmonary hypertension, the clinical findings are meager: a mild degree of cyanosis and some enlargement of the right side of the heart.

Two-dimensional echocardiography is virtually diagnostic, thus some centers no longer routinely do cardiac catheterization. In the 1988 report from London by Lincoln and associates, describing experiences with 83 patients, echocardiography was used without catheterization in 24 of the last 28 patients. Usually, cardiac catheterization and angiography are preferable to better define the abnormal venous anatomy, pulmonary blood flow, and associated anomalies. The similarity of oxygen saturation in all cardiac chambers is diagnostic.

Treatment

Operation should be done urgently as soon as the diagnosis is made, often within the first few days of life. Without operation, almost 50% of infants die within 3 months. For more than 10 years after the first successful correction with ECC by Kirklin in

1957, operative mortality in infants approached 50%. The outcome improved dramatically with the technique of hypothermia and circulatory arrest, which was developed near 1969 primarily by Barratt-Boyes and associates in New Zealand. This technique is the major reason for the low mortality when operation is necessary in the first month of life.

This low mortality is well illustrated in the 1980 report by Turley and associates, who described experiences with 22 infants operated on between 1975 and 1978. All six operated on within the first 4 days of life survived. Six others were operated on before 1 month of age and ten between 1 and 12 months. Of the total group of 22, 19 (87%) survived. There were two late deaths from progressive fibrosis of the pulmonary veins, an unsolved problem reported to occur in approximately 10% of infants within 1 year after operation.

The objective at operation is to make a large opening between the anomalous venous sinus and the left atrium, close the atrial septal defect, and ligate any abnormal communications. The operative technique is shown in Figure 35–12. The adequacy of the anastomosis constructed between the anomalous venous sinus and the left atrium should be confirmed at operation by showing the absence of any gradient between the two structures.

A staged operative procedure, with an anastomosis made but the atrial septal defect left for closure

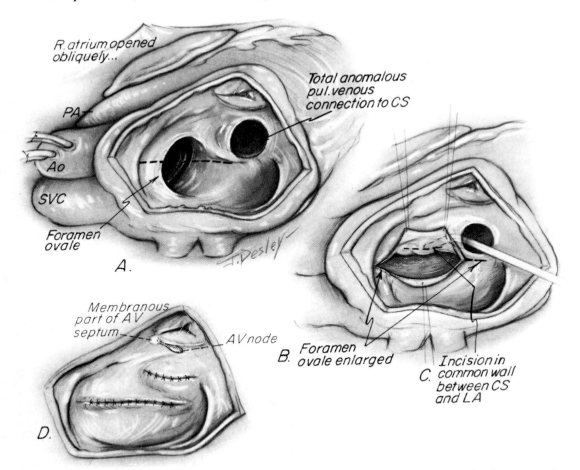

Figure 35–13. Repair of total anomalous pulmonary venous connection to coronary sinus. *A,* The foramen ovale is enlarged sufficiently to obtain adequate exposure within the left atrium. *B* and *C,* With a clamp placed in the coronary sinus, the coronary is "unroofed" with a long incision between the coronary sinus and the left atrium. *D,* The foramen ovale and the ostium of the coronary sinus are closed. (Ao = aorta; AV = atrioventricular; CS = coronary sinus; LA = left atrium; PA = pulmonary artery; SVC = superior vena cava.) (From Kirklin, J. W., and Barratt-Boyes, B. G.: Cardiac Surgery, New York, John Wiley & Sons. Copyright © 1986.)

at a later time, has not been beneficial. A palliative balloon septostomy to enlarge the atrial septal defect has also been disappointing because of the frequent presence of pulmonary venous obstruction. With the impressive results of operations in the first few days of life, immediate total correction appears to be the best approach.

When the anomalous veins drain through the coronary sinus, the technique suggested by Van Praagh in 1972 is commonly used. This is shown in Figure 35–13.

The original method of closure (Fig. 35–14) was to excise the common septum between the coronary sinus and the foramen ovale and then close the subsequent common opening. Although Van Praagh's approach is recommended by Kirklin and Barratt-Boyes (1986), and should decrease the frequency of atrial arrhythmias, the 1985 report by Castaneda and associates stated that they returned

to the original method after finding that the frequency of arrhythmias did not decrease with the more complex approach used by Van Praagh.

Surgical approaches for the more uncommon types of anomalous pulmonary veins, such as infracardiac or mixed types, are well described by Kirklin and Barratt-Boyes (1986).

Hospital mortality for operations done in the first year of life is between 15 and 20%. Kirklin and Barrett-Boyes reported 10 deaths in their experience with a total of 64 patients, a combination of the experiences of the two authors with those reported by Turley. The 1988 report by Lincoln and associates described a total of 12 deaths in 83 patients, with a 14% mortality.

After discharge from the hospital, infants should be monitored for the first year to determine whether a stricture of the pulmonary venous anastomosis occurs. This unusual but serious complication has

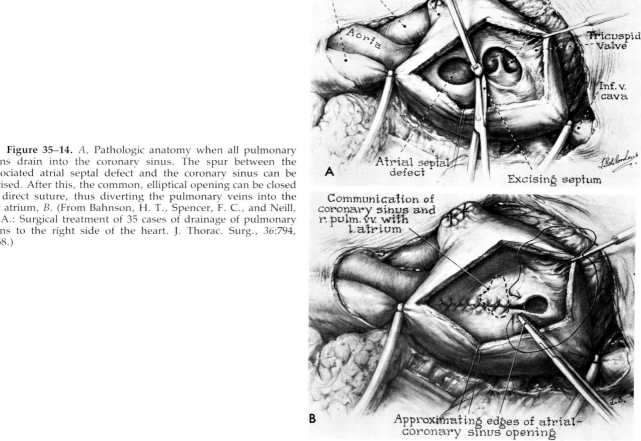

Figure 35–14. *A*, Pathologic anatomy when all pulmonary veins drain into the coronary sinus. The spur between the associated atrial septal defect and the coronary sinus can be excised. After this, the common, elliptical opening can be closed by direct suture, thus diverting the pulmonary veins into the left atrium, *B*. (From Bahnson, H. T., Spencer, F. C., and Neill, C. A.: Surgical treatment of 35 cases of drainage of pulmonary veins to the right side of the heart. J. Thorac. Surg., *36*:794, 1958.)

been reported in all series and has an incidence of almost 10%. Reoperation has often been necessary and has sometimes been unsuccessful.

In patients who survive the first year of life, operative mortality is low. Long-term results in both groups are excellent.

Selected Bibliography

Anderson, R. H., Zuberbuhler, J. R., Penkoske, P. A., et al: Of clefts, commissures, and things. J. Thorac. Cardiovasc. Surg., *90*:605, 1985.

Penkoske, P. A., Neches, W. H., Anderson, R. H., et al: Further observations on the morphology of atrioventricular septal defects. J. Thorac. Cardiovasc. Surg., *90*:611, 1985.

These two papers, published in a series, describe the anatomic findings in 130 hearts with atrioventricular septal defects, 50 hearts with ventricular septal defects, 7 hearts with isolated clefts, and 10 normal hearts. All specimens came from the cardiopathologic collection of the Children's Hospital of Pittsburgh.

The studies clearly show that the morphology of hearts with atrioventricular septal defects, partial or complete, is different from other hearts. The left atrioventricular valve is a three-leaflet valve that in no way resembles the normal mitral valve and differs in terms of its chordal support and its papillary muscle.

For more than two decades it has been debated whether the "cleft" in an ostium primum ("partial atrioventricular canal") defect should be sutured if there were no signs of mitral insufficiency. This reasoning was based on the anatomic fact that the cleft was actually a commissure and was not a true abnormality envisioned as an abnormal separation of the aortic leaflet of the normal mitral valve. Undoubtedly, in some patients without mitral insufficiency, repair has been satisfactory without placing any sutures in the cleft. However, most surgeons, including those at New York University, routinely suture the cleft regardless and take care not to distort the valvular anatomy. This is important because fibrosis and contraction in an unsutured cleft has later on caused recurrent insufficiency and a second operation.

Castaneda, A. R., Mayer, J. E., Jr., and Jonas, R. A.: Repair of complete atrioventricular canal in infancy. World J. Surg., *9*:590, 1985.

These data are from the Children's Hospital in Boston. Primary repair of complete atrioventricular canal in infancy is strongly recommended to prevent pulmonary vascular obstructive disease. Experiences with 48 patients treated for 5 years are presented (three early deaths and two late deaths). Three patients required reoperation for residual regurgitation; of 20 recatheterized patients, mitral regurgitation was severe in two patients.

King, R. M., Puga, F. J., Danielson, G. K., et al: Prognostic factors and surgical treatment of partial atrioventricular canal. Circulation, 74 (supp I):I-42, 1986.

Experiences at the Mayo Clinic with the surgical treatment of 199 patients with partial AV canal treated for 23 years are described. The 30-day operative mortality was almost 5%, less than 3% in the most recent 5 years. The average follow-up was 15 years, which makes this a valuable source of long-term data. Late survival was 91% at 1 year, 96% at 20 years. Reoperation was done on 18 patients, 15 for mitral insufficiency. No cases of complete heart block occurred after 1975.

This report is particularly significant because many of the modern techniques for closure of partial and complete atrioventricular canal defects were developed at the Mayo Clinic, especially by McGoon and Kirklin. The authors emphasize that their current practice is to close the cleft in the anterior mitral leaflet regardless of the degree of preoperative insufficiency.

Two patients have been treated in whom insufficiency developed months or years after the initial operation in which the cleft was not sutured. At a second operation in both patients, closure of the cleft successfully eliminated the regurgitation. Similar experiences have been observed at New York University.

Pillai, R., Ho, S. Y., Anderson, R. H., and Lincoln, C.: Ostium primum atrioventricular septal defects: An anatomical and surgical review. Ann. Thorac. Surg., 41:458, 1986.

Experiences with the treatment of 84 patients during a period of 10 years with the ostium primum type of defect at the Brompton Hospital in London are described. The patch that is used to close the atrial septal defect is inserted to avoid the displaced AV node, which diverts the coronary sinus into the left atrium. Only two patients had conduction problems.

The approach taken to the "cleft" mitral valve was selective. In most patients the cleft was completely sutured. In 11 patients, however, no sutures were inserted because of the complete absence of any preoperative insufficiency, whereas in 12 patients, only a few sutures were inserted. This approach is contrary to the approach taken at the Mayo Clinic that was discussed earlier.

Bibliography

Anderson, R. H., Zuberbuhler, J. D., Penkoske, P. A., and Neches, W. H.: Of clefts, commissures, and things. J. Thorac. Cardiovasc. Surg., 90:605, 1985.
Bahnson, H. T., Spencer, F. C., and Neill, C. A.: Surgical treatment of 35 cases of drainage of pulmonary veins to the right side of the heart. J. Thorac. Surg., 36:787, 1958.
Barratt-Boyes, B. G.: Primary definitive intracardiac operations in infants: Total anomalous pulmonary venous connection. In Kirklin, J. W. (ed): Advances in Cardiovascular Surgery. New York, Grune and Stratton, 1973, p. 127.
Bender, H. W., Jr.: Diagnosis and correction of anomalous pulmonary venous return. Ann. Thorac. Surg., 45:346, 1988.
Blake, H. A., Hall, R. C., and Manion, W. C.: Anomalous pulmonary venous return. Circulation, 32:406, 1965.
Braunwald, N. S., and Morrow, A. G.: Incomplete persistent atrioventricular canal. J. Thorac. Cardiovasc. Surg., 51:71, 1966.
Campbell, M.: Natural history of atrial septal defect. Br. Heart J., 32:820, 1970.
Castaneda, A. R., Mayer, J. E., Jr., and Jonas, R. A.: Repair of complete atrioventricular canal in infancy. World J. Surg., 9:590, 1985.
Craig, R. J., and Selzer, A.: Natural history and prognosis of atrial septal defect. Circulation, 37:805, 1968.
Darling, R. C., Rothney, W. B., and Craig, J. M.: Total pulmonary venous drainage into the right side of the heart: Report of 17 autopsied cases not associated with other major cardiovascular anomalies. Lab. Invest., 6:44, 1957.
de la Rivière, A. B., Brom, G. H. M., and Brom, A. G.: Horizontal submammary skin incision for median sternotomy. Ann. Thorac. Surg., 32:101, 1981.
Fiore, A. C., Naunheim, K. S., Kessler, K. A., et al: Surgical closure of atrial septal defect in patients older than 50 years of age. Arch. Surg., 123:965, 1988.
Gerbode, F., Sanchez, P. A., Arguero, R., et al: Endocardial cushion defects. Ann. Surg., 166:486, 1967.
Gibbon, J. H., Jr.: Application of a mechanical heart and lung apparatus to cardiac surgery. Minnesota Med., 37:171, 1954.
Hawe, A., Rastelli, G. C., Brandenburg, R. O., and McGoon, D. C.: Embolic complications following repair of atrial septal defects. Circulation, 39(Suppl 1):85, 1969.
Jonas, R. A., Smolinsky, A., Mayer, J. E., and Castaneda, A. R.: Obstructed pulmonary venous drainage with total anomalous pulmonary venous connection to the coronary sinus. Am. J. Cardiol., 59:431, 1987.
King, R. M., Puga, F. J., Danielson, G. K., et al: Prognostic factors and surgical treatment of partial atrioventricular canal. Circulation, 74(Suppl I):I-42, 1986.
Kirklin, J. W., and Barratt-Boyes, B. G.: Cardiac Surgery. New York, John Wiley & Sons, 1986.
Lewis, F. J., and Taufic, M.: Closure of atrial septal defects with the aid of hypothermia: Experimental accomplishments and the report of the one successful case. Surgery, 33:52, 1953.
Lincoln, C. R., Rigby, M. L., Mercanti, C., et al: Surgical risk factors in total anomalous pulmonary venous connection. Am. J. Cardiol., 61:608, 1988.
McGoon, D., and Puga, F.: Atrioventricular canal. Cardiovasc. Clin., 11:311, 1981.
McMullan, M. H., McGoon, D. C., Wallace, R. B., et al: Surgical treatment of partial atrioventricular canal. Arch. Surg., 107:705, 1973.
McMullan, M. H., Wallace, R. B., Weidman, W. H., and McGoon, D. C.: Surgical treatment of complete atrioventricular canal. Surgery, 6:905, 1972.
Neill, C. A.: Postoperative hemolytic anemia in endocardial cushion defects. Circulation, 30:801, 1964.
Penkoske, P. A., Neches, W. H., Anderson, R. H., and Zuberbuhler, J. R.: Further observations on the morphology of atrioventricular septal defects. J. Thorac. Cardiovasc. Surg., 90:614, 1985.
Paolillo, V., Dawkins, K. D., and Miller, G. A.: Atrial septal defect in patients over the age of 50. Int. J. Cardiol., 9:139, 1985.
Pillai, R., Ho, S. Y., Anderson, R. H., and Lincoln, C.: Ostium primum atrioventricular septal defect: An anatomical and surgical review. Ann. Thorac. Surg., 41:458, 1986.
Portman, M. A., Beder, S. D., Ankeney, J. L., et al: A 20-year review of ostium primum defect repair in children. Am. Heart J., 110:1064, 1985.
Rastelli, G. C., Kirklin, J. W., and Titus, J. L.: Anatomic observations on complete form of persistent common atrioventricular canal with special reference to atrioventricular valves. Mayo Clin. Proc., 41:296, 1966.
Rastelli, G. C., Weidman, W. H., and Kirklin, J. W.: Surgical repair of the partial form of persistent common atrioventricular canal, with special reference to mitral valve incompetence. Circulation, 31:31, 1965.
Rastelli, G. C., Rahimtoola, S. H., Ongley, P. A., and McGoon, D. C.: Common atrium: Anatomy, hemodynamics, and surgery. J. Thorac. Cardiovasc. Surg., 55:834, 1968.
Rudolph, A. M.: Congenital Diseases of the Heart. Chicago, Year Book Medical Publishers, Inc., 1974, p. 259.
Sellers, R. D., Ferlic, R. M., Sterns, L. P., and Lillehei, C. W.: Secundum type atrial septal defects: Results with 275 patients. Surgery, 59:155, 1966.
Spencer, F. C., and Bahnson, H. T.: Intracardiac surgery employing hypothermia and coronary perfusion performed on 100 patients. Surgery, 46:987, 1959.
Stansel, H. C., Jr., Talner, N. S., and Deran, M. M.: Surgical treatment of atrial septal defect: Analysis of 150 corrective operations. Am. J. Surg., 121:485, 1971.
Steele, P. M., Fuster, V., Cohen, M., et al: Isolated atrial septal defect with pulmonary vascular obstructive disease—long-term follow-up and prediction of outcome after surgical correction. Circulation, 76:1037, 1987.

Stewart, S., Alexson, C., and Manning, J.: Partial atrioventricular canal defect: The early and late results of operation. Ann. Thorac. Surg., 43:527, 1987.

Sutton, M., Tajik, A., and McGoon, D.: Atrial septal defect in patients 60 years or older: Operative results and longterm postoperative follow-up. Circulation, 64:402, 1981.

Trussler, G., Kazenelson, G., Freedom, R. M., et al: Late results following repair of partial anomalous pulmonary venous connections with sinus venosus atrial septal defect. J. Thorac. Cardiovasc. Surg., 79:776, 1980.

Turley, K., Tucker, W. Y., Uhyot, D. J., and Ebert, P. A.: Total anomalous pulmonary venous connection in infancy: Influence of age and type of lesion. Am. J. Cardiol., 45:92, 1980.

Turley, K., Wilson, J. M., and Ebert, P. A.: Atrial repairs of infant complex congenital heart lesions: Emphasis on the first three months of life. Arch. Surg., 115:1335, 1980.

Van Praagh, R., Harken, A. H., Delisle, G., et al: Total anomalous pulmonary venous drainage to the coronary sinus: A revised procedure for its correction. J. Thorac. Cardiovasc. Surg., 64:132, 1972.

CHAPTER 36

MAJOR ANOMALIES OF PULMONARY AND THORACIC SYSTEMIC VEINS

John W. Hammon, Jr.
Harvey W. Bender, Jr.

Major anomalies of pulmonary and systemic venous return represent one of the few forms of congenital heart disease in which the valves and ventricles are usually normal; thus, correction should offer excellent long-term results. Patients with total anomalous pulmonary venous connection (TAPVC) rarely survive beyond the first year of life without operative correction, and patients with anomalous systemic venous connections often become symptomatic in infancy and childhood. Operative correction of these conditions is usually successful, and knowledge of this relatively uncommon but important group of congenital anomalies is essential to ensure prompt, accurate diagnosis and therapy. Partial anomalous pulmonary venous connections are considered in Chapter 35.

EMBRYOLOGY

Pulmonary Venous System

At approximately 3½ weeks' gestation, the lung bud arises from the primitive foregut and becomes surrounded by a plexus of veins that has been called the pulmonary venous plexus (Fig. 36–1A) (Los, 1968). As differentiation proceeds, this venous system has no direct communication with the heart but instead shares the routes of drainage of the splanchnic plexus, that is, the cardinal and umbilicovitelline systems of veins (Fig. 36–1B). Normally, this pulmonary venous plexus eventually is connected to a vessel called the common pulmonary vein (Neill, 1956), a transient structure that arises from the undivided sinus venosus just to the left of the area in which the atrial septal primum develops (Fig. 36–1C). Eventually, connections to the systemic venous system terminate, and the common pulmonary vein is incorporated into the developing left atrium (Fig. 36–1D). Abnormal development of the common pulmonary vein is the embryologic basis for most of the congenital anomalies of the pulmonary veins (Lucas et al, 1962).

If atresia of the common pulmonary vein occurs when systemic communications are present to the cardinal and umbilicovitelline systems, one or several of these collateral channels can enlarge and provide total anomalous pulmonary venous connection to the systemic venous system (Fig. 36–2). If only the right or left portion of the common pulmonary vein is atretic, partial anomalous venous connection occurs.

Persisting segments of the cardinal veins eventually form the superior vena cava, the innominate vein, the coronary sinus, and the azygos vein. The umbilicovitelline system forms the inferior vena cava, the portal vein, and the ductus venosus. The anatomy of the anomalous venous connection is related to the early embryologic connection between the pulmonary venous plexus and the particular splanchnic component that persists. Direct anomalous connections to the right atrium are not explained by such an embryologic accident and are probably due to an abnormality of septation of the two atria, in which the atrial septum forms to the left of the pulmonary veins rather than to the right (Shaner, 1961). The systemic venous anatomy and the different systemic veins that can become the site of drainage of pulmonary venous blood in patients with TAPVC are shown in Figure 36–3.

When stenosis of the common pulmonary vein occurs, the result is *cor triatriatum* (Edwards, 1960). Usually, stenosis occurs late, after systemic venous connections have terminated (Fig. 36–4). Occasionally, cor triatriatum is associated with anomalous pulmonary venous connections to systemic veins, which suggests that significant stenosis of the common pulmonary vein is present at a time when systemic venous connections are still present.

Systemic Venous System

The first veins to appear in the embryo are the umbilical and vitelline veins (Fig. 36–5A). The cardinal veins are the next to develop (Streeter, 1942).

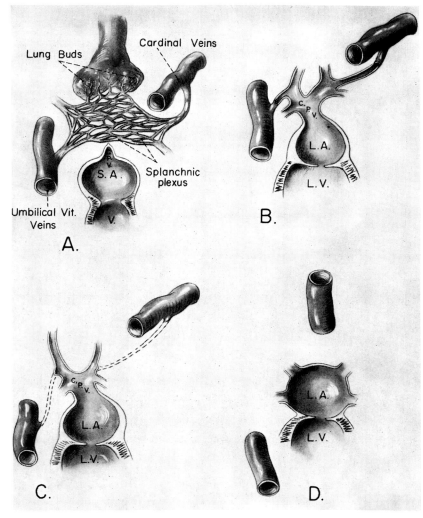

Figure 36–1. Normal development of the pulmonary venous system. *A,* The splanchnic plexus drains the lung buds and shares connections with the cardinal and umbilicovitelline systems. *B,* The common pulmonary vein (C.P.V.) has evaginated from the left atrium (L.A.) and has joined the splanchnic plexus. *C,* As pulmonary venous blood drains to the left side of the heart the primitive connections disappear. *D,* Finally, by differential growth the individual pulmonary veins are incorporated into the left atrium, and the common pulmonary vein disappears. (From Lucas, R. V., et al: Congenital causes of pulmonary venous obstruction. Pediatr. Clin. North Am., *10:*781, 1963.)

The anterior and posterior cardinal veins unite on each side to form a common cardinal vein. Eventually, the common cardinal, umbilical, and vitelline veins join the right and left horns of the sinus venosus (Fig. 36–5*B*). By the fourth week of fetal life, the sinus venosus has developed an invagination that separates its left horn from the left atrium and ultimately in which all systemic blood enters the right atrium (Fig. 36–5*C*) (Raghib et al, 1965).

At this stage, the cardinal systemic veins are symmetrical, except for their drainage into the right atrium. During the eighth week of fetal life, the left innominate vein develops and connects the two anterior cardinal veins. As flow through the left innominate vein increases, the left anterior cardinal vein decreases in size, and by the sixth fetal month it has been obliterated and the left common cardinal vein remains to drain only the coronary circulation to the right atrium as the coronary sinus (Fig. 36–5*C*). Occasionally, a small portion of the left anterior cardinal vein persists as the oblique ligament or vein of Marshall of the left atrium (Lucas and Schmidt, 1977).

Important abnormalities of the cardinal venous system result from two developmental aberrations: (1) Failure of obliteration of the left anterior cardinal vein results in persistence of the left superior vena cava. If invagination between the left horn of the sinus venosus has occurred, a coronary sinus is formed, which serves as an outlet for the left superior vena cava. (2) Failure of invagination between the left sinus horn and the left atrium and failure of obliteration of the left anterior cardinal vein result in the left superior vena cava draining directly into the left atrium.

The venous return of the caudal portion of the body drains via the posterior cardinal veins until the sixth week of fetal life. The inferior vena cava develops in the next 2 weeks (McClure and Butler, 1925).

Development of the inferior vena cava depends on the formation of two centrally located systems. The subcardinal system develops ventral and medial to the posterior cardinal veins. The supracardinal system forms dorsal and medial to the posterior cardinal veins, and anastomoses develop between the cardinal veins and both systems. The cardinal

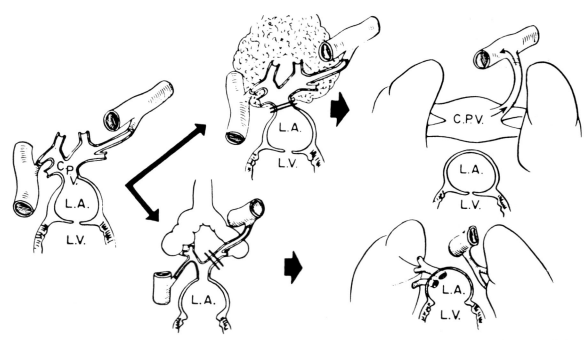

Figure 36–2. The embryologic explanation for anomalous pulmonary venous connections. *Upper,* If atresia of the common pulmonary vein occurs when systemic connections are still present, TAPVC results. *Lower,* Atresia of a branch of the common pulmonary veins results in partial anomalous pulmonary venous connection. (Adapted from Lucas, R. V., and Schmidt, R. E. *In* Moss, A. J., Adams, F. H., and Emmanouilides, G. C. [eds]: Heart Disease in Infants, Children and Adolescents, 2nd ed. Copyright 1977, The Williams & Wilkins Company, Baltimore. Reproduced by permission.)

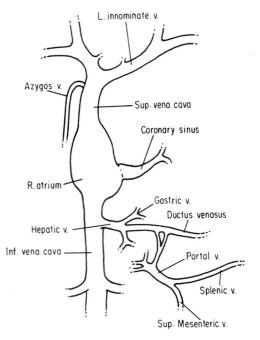

Figure 36–3. The systemic veins that can be the routes of drainage in TAPVC.

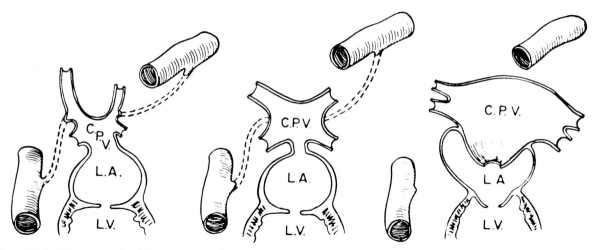

Figure 36–4. When stenosis of the common pulmonary vein occurs, the result is cor triatriatum. (Adapted from Lucas, R. V., and Schmidt, R. E. *In* Moss, A. J., Adams, F. H., and Emmanouilides, G. C. [eds]: Heart Disease in Infants, Children and Adolescents, 2nd ed. Copyright 1977, The Williams & Wilkins Company, Baltimore. Reproduced by permission.)

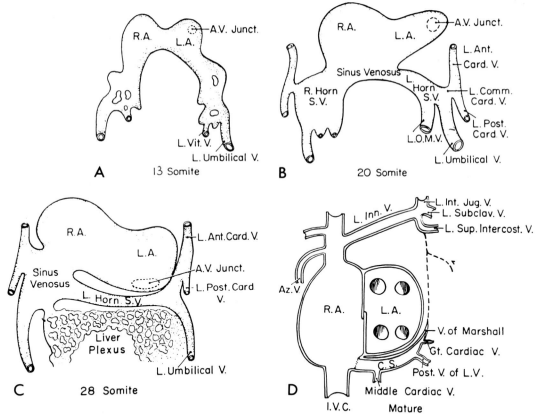

Figure 36–5. Normal embryology of the cardinal venous system. *A,* Bilaterally symmetrical umbilical and vitelline veins drain into the common atrium. Asymmetry begins with the atrioventricular junction to the left. *B,* The cardinal system develops with continuing asymmetrical development of the atrium. *C,* The left and right horns of the sinus venosus are completely separated, and all systemic blood drains to the right atrium. *D,* The left innominate vein (L. Inn. V.) develops, and the left anterior cardinal vein disappears. The left common cardinal vein becomes the coronary sinus (C.S.). (L. Ant. Card. V. = left anterior cardinal vein; L. Post. Card. V. = left posterior cardinal vein; L. Comm. Card. V. = left common cardinal vein; L. Umbilical V. = left umbilical vein; R.A. = right atrium; L.A. = left atrium; L. Int. Jug. V. = left internal jugular vein; L. Subclav. V. = left subclavian vein; L. Sup. Intercost. V. = left superior intercostal vein; V. of Marshall = vein of Marshall; Gt. Cardiac V. = great cardiac vein; Post. V. of L.V. = posterior vein of the left ventricle; Middle Cardiac V. = middle cardiac vein; I.V.C. = inferior vena cava; Az. V. = azygos vein; L. Vit. V. = left vitelline vein; R. Horn S.V. and L. Horn S.V. = right and left horns of the sinus venosus; A.V. Junct. = atrioventricular junction; L.O.M.V. = left omphalomesenteric vein.) (Adapted from Lucas, R. V., and Schmidt, R. E. *In* Moss, A. J., Adams, F. H., and Emmanouilides, G. C. [eds]: Heart Disease in Infants, Children and Adolescents, 2nd ed. Copyright 1977, The Williams & Wilkins Company, Baltimore. Reproduced by permission.)

system atrophies and no cardinal remnants persist between the iliac veins and the diaphragm. Anastomoses develop between the right and left supracardinal and subcardinal systems. Flow is preferentially directed to the right system, and the left system atrophies; the left supracardinal vein becomes the hemiazygos vein, which joins the right supracardinal (azygos) vein. The right subcardinal vein and hepatic veins join and form the inferior vena cava, which joins the right atrium at the junction of the right common cardinal vein and the atrium.

Failure of connection between the right subcardinal vein and the hepatic vein causes venous blood from the lower half of the body to be directed into the left subcardinal system and results in the common anomaly of interruption of the inferior vena cava with azygos continuation. The normal development of the inferior vena cava and the formation of interrupted inferior vena cava are detailed in Figure 36–6.

Direct *connection* of the inferior vena cava to the left atrium is not well defined embryologically (Meadows et al, 1961). The more common situation in which the inferior vena cava *drains* into the left atrium via an atrial septal defect is explained embryologically by persistence and overgrowth of the valves of the sinus venosus that usually form the eustachian and thebesian valves. Rarely, the right valve persists as a membrane that directs all systemic venous blood to the left atrium (Doucette and Knoblich, 1963).

TOTAL ANOMALOUS PULMONARY VENOUS CONNECTION

The term TAPVC defines the anomaly in which the pulmonary veins have no direct communication with the left atrium. Instead, they connect to the right atrium or to one of the systemic veins.

Historical Aspects

The first reported case of TAPVC was described in 1798, when Wilson reported a patient whose entire pulmonary venous return entered the coronary sinus. Additional reports were uncommon, until 1942, when Brody reviewed the subject with 37 autopsied cases from the literature. In 1957, Darling, Rothney, and Craig added 17 cases and classified the variants of this anomaly.

The first clinical diagnosis was made by Friedlich and associates in 1950 by using cardiac catheterization. In 1951, the first successful operation was reported by Muller, who provided palliation for the patient by anastomosing the left atrial appendage to anomalous veins from the left lung. In 1956, Lewis and associates reported the first successful open heart correction of the cardiac type of TAPVC in a 5-year-old patient by using hypothermia and inflow occlusion. Cooley and Ochsner (1957) reported the first

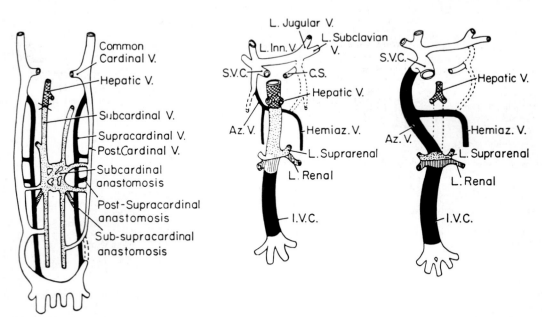

Figure 36–6. Embryology of the inferior vena cava (I.V.C.). *Left,* In early stages of development, blood can reach the heart by way of the posterior cardinal veins (Post. Cardinal V.), supracardinal veins, and the upper portion of the I.V.C. Multiple anastomotic sites exist in the renal area, as shown. *Center,* Normal development of the I.V.C. The I.V.C. is derived, from below upward, from the posterior cardinal system *(white),* the supracardinal system *(black),* the renal veins *(lined),* the subcardinal system *(stippled),* and the hepatic veins *(cross-hatched).* The supracardinal veins persist as the hemiazygos and azygos veins. *Right,* Interruption of the I.V.C. with azygos continuation. Absence of the I.V.C. above the renal veins occurs when the right subcardinal vein fails to join with the hepatic vein. The hepatic veins drain directly into the right atrium. All other blood from the lower body drains via the dilated azygos and hemiazygos systems. (From Lucas, R. V., and Schmidt, R. E. *In* Moss, A. J., Adams, F. H., and Emmanouilides, G. C. [eds]: Heart Disease in Infants, Children and Adolescents, 2nd ed. Copyright 1977, The Williams & Wilkins Company, Baltimore, Reproduced by permission.)

open heart correction by using cardiopulmonary bypass in a patient with a supracardiac anomaly. The first infracardiac anomaly was corrected in 1961 by Sloan, who used deep hypothermia, cardiopulmonary bypass, and a period of circulatory arrest (Sloan et al, 1962).

Anatomy

The anatomic prerequisite for TAPVC is an absence of connection between any pulmonary veins and the left atrium. The left atrium has no tributaries and receives all blood by an atrial septal defect. The term total anomalous pulmonary venous *connection* describes this anatomic abnormality and should not be confused with total anomalous pulmonary venous *drainage* in which the pulmonary veins terminate in the left atrium, but blood passes through an interatrial communication into the right atrium because of atresia of the mitral or aortic valves or a combination of both with total left-sided heart atresia. In 1957, Darling and associates described the most frequently used classification of TAPVC. They divided the anomaly into four subtypes that describe the anatomic connections of the pulmonary venous to the systemic venous circulation.

Type I—Supracardiac Connection. The anatomic site of anomalous venous connection in this type results in communications to the remnants of the right or left cardinal venous system. The most common form, in which pulmonary venous drainage is to a common pulmonary vein posterior to the left atrium, is shown in Figure 36–7. A left vertical vein connects this chamber with the innominate vein, and this vessel usually lies anterior to the left pulmonary artery. When the common pulmonary venous chamber connects with remnants of the right cardinal venous system, the connection may be to the superior vena cava or azygos vein or by an additional right vertical vein draining directly into the innominate vein. Occasionally, pulmonary veins separately enter the superior vena cava, azygos, or innominate vein; this type is associated with major cardiac anomalies (Ruttenberg et al, 1964).

Type II—Cardiac Connection. Cardiac connections are divided into two major subtypes. In the more common type, the left and right common pulmonary veins join to form a common venous sinus posterior to the left atrium, which connects to an enlarged coronary sinus in the atrioventricular groove (Fig. 36–8). In the second major group, the pulmonary veins drain individually or collectively into a sinus in the posterior right atrium (Fig. 36–9).

Type III—Infracardiac Connection. In this group, a common venous chamber posterior to the heart connects to an inferior vein that passes through the diaphragm anterior to the esophagus and then to the portal vein or one of its branches, or with the ductus venosus (Fig. 36–10). Occasionally, the anomalous descending vein passes through an accessory hiatus

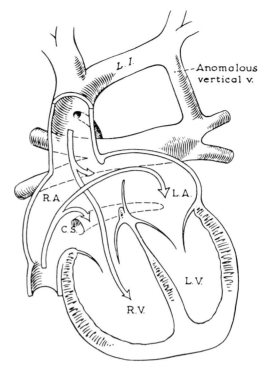

Figure 36–7. Representation of the most common type of supracardiac TAPVC (L.I. = left innominate vein; R.A. = right atrium; L.A. = left atrium; C.S. = coronary sinus; R.V. = right ventricle; L.V. = left ventricle).

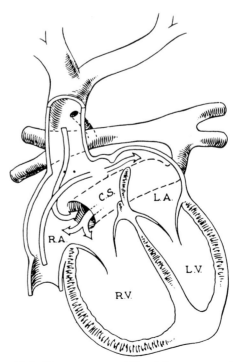

Figure 36–8. The anatomy and blood flow patterns in TAPVC when the pulmonary venous confluence connects to the coronary sinus (C.S.).

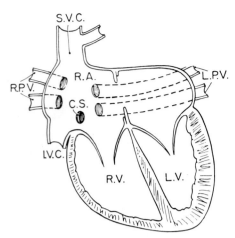

Figure 36–9. The type of TAPVC in which the pulmonary veins directly connect with the right atrium. (Redrawn from Lucas, R. V., and Schmidt, R. E. *In* Moss, A. J., Adams, F. H., and Emmanouilides, G. C. [eds]: Heart Disease in Infants, Children and Adolescents, 2nd ed. Copyright 1977, The Williams & Wilkins Company, Baltimore. Reproduced by permission.)

in the diaphragm and joins one of the systemic venous channels, usually the inferior vena cava or one of its branches.

Type IV—Mixed Connections. In this uncommon group, the pulmonary venous connections are divided so that one lung drains to one of the systemic veins, and pulmonary veins from the opposite side

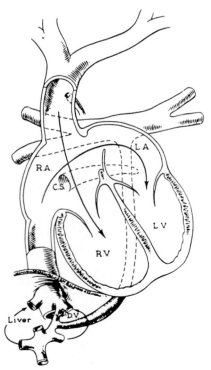

Figure 36–10. The most common type of infracardiac TAPVC in which the anomalous descending vein connects the pulmonary venous confluence with the ductus venosus (D.V.).

usually join one of the cardiac chambers, generally the coronary sinus.

Associated Cardiac Defects

An interatrial communication is required for persistence of life beyond the early neonatal period in patients with TAPVC and is present in almost all cases. The communication varies from a probe-patent foramen ovale to complete absence of the interatrial septum. Patent ductus arteriosus (PDA) is present in 25 to 50% of patients with this defect (Burroughs and Edwards, 1960). Infants with pulmonary venous obstruction have a high incidence of PDA, which is the physiologic means of decompressing obstructed pulmonary blood flow into the descending thoracic aorta. A very high incidence of TAPVC and severe congenital cardiac defects is associated with the asplenia syndrome (Ivemark, 1955).

Incidence

Approximately 1% of infants with congenital heart disease have TAPVC (Jensen and Blount, 1971). There is no known genetic predisposition to this lesion. Male infants are affected almost twice as often as female infants. The incidences of the various anatomic types of TAPVC are shown in Table 36–1. These data are taken from several collected series in the literature. The earlier series represent autopsy reports, and the later series are surgical. Supracardiac defects are the most common and affect 50% of the patients. The most common supracardiac anomaly is connection of the pulmonary venous chamber to a left anomalous vertical vein draining to the innominate vein. Type II defects are the second most common anomaly, with pulmonary venous connection to the coronary sinus most prevalent in this group.

Type III and Type IV defects are the least common, and Type III defects are reported more frequently in surgical series, as these infants survive to diagnosis and treatment. Patients with Type IV anomalies are not common in surgical series because most have major intracardiac defects that preclude correction.

Pathophysiology

Factors that influence the pathophysiology of TAPVC include obligatory mixing of pulmonary and systemic blood upstream of or at the right atrium, obstruction of the anomalous connection, the size of the atrial septal defect, and associated anomalies. The presence or absence of obstruction of the anomalous connection is the most significant factor in the patient's clinical condition.

In contrast to patients with atrial septal defects, the mixing of systemic and pulmonary venous blood

TABLE 36–1. COLLECTED CASES OF TAPVC CLASSIFIED BY TYPE

Types	Burroughs and Edwards (1960)	Bonham-Carter et al (1969)	Jensen and Blount (1971)	Snellen and Bruins (1968)	Cooley et al (1966)	Gathman and Nadas (1971)	Brecken-ridge et al (1973)	Applebaum et al (1975)	Turley et al (1980)	Hammon et al (1980)	Total	Incidence (%)
I												
Supracardiac												
Left anomalous vertical vein	56	34	12	12	28	26	11	21				
Right superior vena cava	31	9	2	1	7	8	3	2	9	12	284	51%
II												
Cardiac												
Coronary sinus	18	18	5	11	12	14	2	3	6	6		
Right atrium	30	3	6	7	8	3	1	3			156	28%
III												
Infracardiac	28	8	2	4	3	16	3	4	6	5	79	14%
IV												
Mixed	16	3	0	3	4	8	1	2	1	2	40	7%
Totals	179	75	27	38	62	75	21	35	22	25	559	100%

in TAPVC is obligatory and is not influenced by the compliance of the two ventricles and the end-diastolic pressure in both chambers. In theory, the oxygen saturation should be equal in all four cardiac chambers. The oxygen saturation may not be equal in patients with small atrial septal defects in which streaming of blood occurs, with most of the inferior vena caval blood directed through the patent foramen ovale or small atrial septal defect and with superior vena cava blood entering the right ventricle through the tricuspid valve. If the interatrial communication is large and the anomalous connection is not obstructed, there is adequate flow to the left atrium, and oxygen saturation is similar in the right and left heart chambers. In this condition, blood flow through the lungs is high, and systemic oxygen saturation is only slightly decreased.

In the patient with unobstructed TAPVC, the entire cardiac output is presented to the right ventricle, which accepts its maximal end-diastolic volume from the beginning of life. As the patient grows and exercises vigorously, cyanosis increases only when the pulmonary vascular resistance rises and a high pulmonary-systemic flow ratio cannot be maintained. Not all of these patients develop hyperkinetic pulmonary hypertension, but the incidence of this complication is higher in patients with TAPVC than in other high-flow–low-pressure lesions such as atrial septal defect (Gathman and Nadas, 1970; Newfield et al, 1980). Heart failure is more common in patients with hyperkinetic pulmonary hypertension but is not uncommon in patients with low pulmonary artery pressure and large left-to-right shunts.

The interatrial communication in patients with TAPVC is usually large, but in a very few patients this communication is small and obstructs flow to the left ventricle. In these patients, a gradient of 3 mm Hg or more between the right and left atrium

can indicate an obstructing atrial septal defect (Behrendt et al, 1972). The flow to the left side of the heart and thus the cardiac output is improved after a balloon atrial septostomy (Miller and Rashkind, 1968).

Anatomic obstruction of the anomalous connection is common in infants and can occur at several sites (Burroughs and Edwards, 1960). In patients with Type I anomalies, the left vertical vein can be constricted as it passes through the pericardial reflection or, rarely, between the left pulmonary artery and left mainstem bronchus. In Type III lesions, obstruction most commonly occurs when the PDA closes, if the connection attaches at this level. If the anomalous inferior vein communicates with the portal vein, obstruction is a prerequisite, because pulmonary venous blood must pass through the liver capillary bed before returning to the right side of the heart. Occasionally, anatomic obstruction occurs in infracardiac connections in which the vertical vein passes through the diaphragm and is constricted during tidal ventilation. In Type IV connections, obstruction usually occurs because of inadequate sites of communication between the pulmonary veins and the right side of the heart. Type II connections are rarely obstructed and present a more favorable situation for long-term survival.

The pathophysiologic consequences of an obstructed anomalous pulmonary venous connection are pulmonary edema and poor myocardial function. During the first few hours or days of extrauterine life, pulmonary blood flow increases. Pulmonary venous obstruction then causes elevation of pulmonary capillary hydrostatic pressure. When this pressure exceeds the net forces that retain fluid in the vascular space, interstitial pulmonary edema occurs. A vicious cycle ensues; interstitial edema causes decreased pulmonary compliance and increases in the work of breathing. Ventilation and perfusion are not balanced, and arterial oxygen desaturation results and further compromises the heart's ability to meet the body's oxygen demand. The result is alveolar flooding and perivascular hemorrhage, which ends in frank pulmonary collapse.

The combination of tachycardia, low coronary perfusion pressure, and cyanosis predisposes the myocardium to subendocardial ischemia. This is especially true in the right ventricle, which in this condition encounters an excessive afterload and in most cases has elevated end-diastolic pressure, which further increases oxygen demand and decreases subendocardial coronary blood flow. The low cardiac output that results promotes anaerobic metabolism, which creates a metabolic acidosis with an increase in plasma lactate. Because of these related events, infants with obstructed TAPVC rarely survive the first few weeks of life.

Infants born with obstructed connections often retain ductal patency, which serves to decompress the pulmonary artery and helps to unload the right ventricle. With ductal closure, severe right-sided heart failure and pulmonary and cardiovascular collapse can occur.

Diagnosis

Clinical Manifestations. The severity of the clinical manifestations of TAPVC is related to the presence of obstruction of the anomalous connection. With an obstructed connection, the infant usually becomes symptomatic in the first hours or days after birth. Mild to moderate cyanosis is evident, and the respiratory rate is rapid, with evidence of decreased pulmonary compliance, that is, intercostal retractions, nasal flaring, and sweating. Cardiac output is usually low, which is shown by decreased pulses and in some cases acidosis. In most of these infants, the obstruction accompanies infradiaphragmatic connections, but it can be seen with supracardiac or mixed connections. It is uncommon for these infants to present after 3 to 6 months of age, because most have expired from complications of pulmonary congestion and low cardiac output.

Children with partially obstructed connections or hyperkinetic pulmonary hypertension usually present in the first 1 to 2 years of life. These infants have all the hallmarks of pulmonary hypertension and right ventricular dysfunction with dyspnea on exertion, poor feeding, lack of weight gain, and cyanosis on crying or exercise. A history of frequent respiratory infections is often evident. On physical examination, the right ventricular impulse is prominent, and a left parasternal flow murmur is usually audible. The second heart sound is widely split and fixed and has a loud pulmonary component. Occasionally, there is a continuous murmur in the vicinity of the anomalous vertical vein.

Approximately 10 to 20% of infants with TAPVC

have no component of obstruction and do not develop pulmonary hypertension. These children can survive into adulthood, although with some restriction. These patients usually have Type I or II anomalous connections. Except for slight cyanosis, symptoms and signs are similar to those in patients with ostium secundum atrial septal defects but usually develop sooner. Dyspnea on exertion and fatigue at the end of the day with inability to keep up with their peers are hallmarks of this type of patient. Cyanosis is usually slight and not visible to the untrained eye. Respiratory infections may be more common than normal. The diagnosis in unobstructed connections may be delayed until the child is seen for a preschool examination. On physical examination, the right ventricle is prominent and hyperactive. The second cardiac sound is split and fixed, but the pulmonary component is not loud. The parasternal systolic flow murmur is present and is similar to that in patients with atrial septal defects.

Chest Film. In infants with obstructed TAPVC, the heart is often not enlarged or only mildly enlarged. Normally, after a day or two, the typical appearance of pulmonary venous congestion is seen on the plain chest film (Fig. 36–11). A fine reticular pattern with haziness of the entire area of the lung is often the hallmark of the diagnosis and should be considered to be pathognomonic of the condition when seen in the very sick infant. In patients with partially obstructed connections or when hyperkinetic pulmonary hypertension is present, the plain chest film shows increased pulmonary vascularity with cardiomegaly due to enlargement of the right

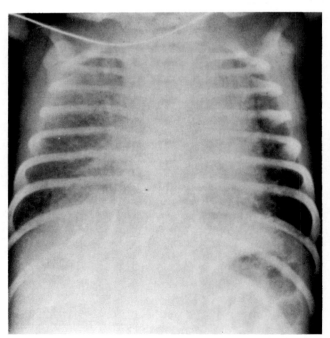

Figure 36–11. The plain chest film in an infant with obstructed TAPVC. Note the fine, reticular pulmonary markings and lack of cardiomegaly.

atrium and ventricle. In some older children, the mediastinal component of the anomalous connection, the dilated left vertical vein or coronary sinus, may be visualized on the chest film and can be diagnostic of the condition (Fig. 36–12). In patients with no pulmonary hypertension, the chest films show an increase in pulmonary vascularity and can show some right atrial and ventricular enlargement. Occasionally, pathognomonic mediastinal silhouettes are recognized.

Electrocardiogram. The electrocardiogram is least helpful in diagnosing TAPVC. Generally, all infants and children with TAPVC have deviation of the right axis and other electrocardiographic changes indicative of right ventricular hypertrophy. If the condition persists for more than 1 to 2 months, the signs of right atrial enlargement are present, and if the condition persists for some years, first-degree heart block may be evident, with prolongation of the PR interval.

Echocardiogram. Echocardiographic signs of right ventricular diastolic volume overload predominate in TAPVC. These signs are increased right ventricular dimension index and paradoxical ventricular septal movement. An echo-free space posterior to the left atrium represents the pulmonary venous confluence and is a reliable sign (Paquet and Gutgesell, 1975).

Cardiac Catheterization. As soon as the diagnosis of TAPVC is considered in an infant, cardiac catheterization should be done. In infants with obstructed connections, oxygen determinations may not be as helpful as anticipated because of the severe degree of pulmonary vascular obstruction and the degree of shunting, which may not be excessive. Severe pulmonary hypertension is present, usually with a right-to-left ductal shunt. Right ventricular cineangiocardiography may show such a large right-to-left ductal shunt that sluggish and insufficient pulmonary blood flow does not allow visualization of the pulmonary veins and their drainage. Visualization may be possible only with injection of contrast medium into individual pulmonary arteries or occlusion of the ductus arteriosus with a balloon catheter and injection of contrast material through a proximal port or separate catheter (Fig. 36–13). Left ventricular cineangiocardiography usually shows a small to normal-sized ventricle and a left atrium that is generally 50% of normal size (Graham and Bender, 1980).

Cardiac catheterization and cineangiocardiography in patients with TAPVC and only mild obstruction or hyperkinetic pulmonary hypertension show findings similar to those in infants with pulmonary venous obstruction, except that pulmonary blood flow is usually more than twice the systemic flow and pulmonary capillary wedge pressures and pulmonary vascular resistance are low. Cineangiocardiography shows a greatly dilated right ventricle, and the anomalous connection can easily be visualized with injection of contrast material into a pulmonary artery. In Type I connections, it is often

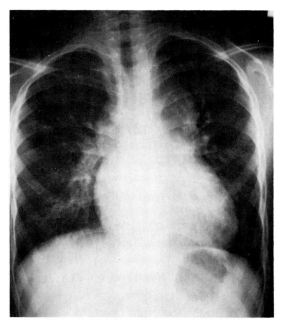

Figure 36–12. Typical chest film in an older child with nonobstructed supracardiac TAPVC. The prominent left upper mediastinal silhouette represents the dilated anomalous left vertical vein.

possible to delineate the connection by passing the catheter through the innominate vein to the anomalous connection with accurate delineation by injection of contrast material at this point.

In patients without pulmonary hypertension, the cardiac catheterization findings are similar to those of atrial septal defect, except that systemic oxygen saturations are slightly lower than normal and the anomalous connection is usually seen without difficulty after injection of contrast material into the pulmonary artery (Fig. 36–14).

Indications for Operation

More than 80% of infants born with TAPVC die before reaching 1 year of age (Burroughs and Edwards, 1980). The one variable that influences longevity is the presence or absence of significant pulmonary venous obstruction (Gathman and Nadas, 1970). Approximately 60 to 75% of infants with TAPVC have obstruction of the anomalous pulmonary venous pathway. Without operation, it is unusual for these children to survive after 1 year of age, and most die within 3 months after birth (Gathman and Nadas, 1970). Among the remaining 25 to 30% of children with unobstructed TAPVC, hyperkinetic pulmonary hypertension develops in a significant number more rapidly than in atrial septal defect (Jensen and Blount, 1971). Approximately 50% of these infants die within their first year, and few survive infancy, despite optimal medical management. Only 10 to 20% of all patients with TAPVC

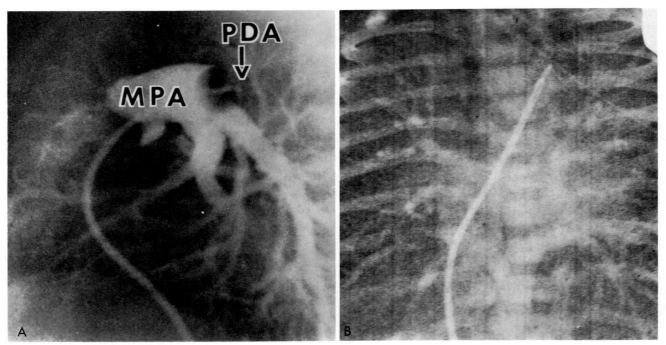

Figure 36–13. *A,* Cineangiocardiogram shows occlusion of the ductus arteriosus with a balloon catheter in an infant with infradiaphragmatic TAPVC. *B,* Subsequent contrast injection into the pulmonary artery reveals the pulmonary venous confluence and anomalous descending vertical vein.

have no pulmonary hypertension. Although heart failure often develops during infancy, most of these patients survive with proper medical management. The incidence of heart failure or other complications,

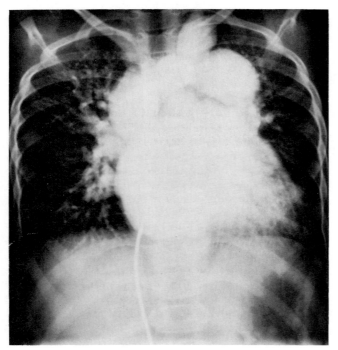

Figure 36–14. Pulmonary angiogram of a child with unobstructed TAPVC. During the venous phase of the study, the greatly dilated anomalous vertical vein that connects to a similarly large left innominate vein is shown.

such as hyperkinetic pulmonary hypertension, becomes obvious over the succeeding years, for very few reach adolescence and young adulthood without symptoms.

Because of the poor survival of patients with TAPVC, the diagnosis of TAPVC is in itself the indication for operation. In infants with pulmonary venous obstruction, operation should be done without delay because of progressive pulmonary insufficiency, low cardiac output, and acidosis that are refractory to conventional medical therapy. In infants with hyperkinetic pulmonary hypertension, operation can be scheduled at a convenient time but soon after cardiac catheterization. Children with unobstructed connections should have an operation within the first 5 years of life, and it is reasonable to repair these connections early to prevent damage to the distended right-sided cardiac chambers. In patients with small atrial septal defects and a large pressure gradient between the right and left atrium, balloon atrial septostomy is theoretically an effective method of increasing cardiac output while the infants are being prepared for operation. In one series, this procedure was not used and is rarely necessary (Hammon et al, 1980).

Operation is contraindicated only when irreversible changes of pulmonary vascular obstruction disease have developed. In these patients, intimal hyperplasia and muscular hypertrophy have increased pulmonary vascular resistance to more than 75% of the systemic level. This situation is rare in modern medical practice, and contraindication to operation in TAPVC is unusual.

Surgical Treatment

Cardiopulmonary bypass is used for all operations involving the correction of total anomalous pulmonary venous connection. The defect is best approached through a median sternotomy incision, and the type of perfusion support depends on the age of the patient. In children less than 1 year of age, either surface-induced hypothermia with cardiopulmonary bypass support (Barratt-Boyes, 1973) or cardiopulmonary bypass with profound hypothermia and low-flow perfusion (Turley et al, 1980) is the technique of choice. In small infants and children, prevention of intraoperative pulmonary venous distention and construction of an adequate anastomosis are facilitated by circulatory arrest or low-flow perfusion. Cardiopulmonary bypass assists with rapid cooling and rewarming and control of the circulation. The technique for surgical management of infants with profound hypothermia and circulatory arrest has been reported (Bender et al, 1979).

Infants are anesthetized with nitrous oxide and halothane, and cutdowns are done to permit monitoring of arterial and venous pressures. The infants are then transferred to a hypothermia chamber, where surface cooling to 30° C is established. Control of arterial oxygen concentration and acid base balance is essential during this period, because many infants with obstructive TAPVC have low cardiac output and require buffering to maintain the pH at normal levels. Acidosis that develops during the cooling period can predispose to serious arrhythmias, including ventricular fibrillation, and should be avoided at all cost. The infant is then transferred to the operating table, where a standard median sternotomy incision is made. After heparin is administered, the ascending aorta is cannulated, and the right atrium is cannulated through the right atrial appendage. Cardiopulmonary bypass is initiated, and the infant is further cooled to a nasopharyngeal temperature of 18° C. During this time, ventilation is continued, and the ductus is exposed by careful dissection and ligated. At 18° C, the ascending aorta is clamped and blood drained into the oxygenator. The venous cannula is removed, and the operative repair is made during a period of circulatory arrest. After repair, the venous cannula is reinserted, and the patient's blood volume is re-established. Air is vented from the left ventricular apex and ascending aorta, cardiopulmonary bypass is resumed, and the infant is rewarmed to an esophageal temperature of 35 to 37° C and cardiopulmonary bypass discontinued.

In infants weighing more than 10 kg or children more than 1 year of age, standard cardiopulmonary bypass techniques are used. A median sternotomy incision is made and the thymus is divided or one lobe is resected. After heparinization, the ascending aorta is cannulated, and venous cannulas are placed in the superior and inferior venae cavae after tapes are passed around these structures. Cardiopulmonary bypass is instituted, and moderate hypothermia to 25 to 28° C is established. The aorta is then cross-clamped, and hyperkalemic cardioplegic solution (10 ml/kg) is instilled through the aortic root. Topical hypothermic solution is poured over the heart to help reduce the intramyocardial temperature to 15° C. Cardiopulmonary bypass flows are reduced at this time to less than the calculated arterial flow. The repair is then made and the cardiac chambers are closed. The aortic cross-clamp is then removed, and before the heart is defibrillated, air is vented from the apex of the left ventricle and the aorta.

Supracardiac connections can be repaired by dissecting the right atrium and superior vena cava from their pericardial attachments (Fig. 36–15). With this method, the anastomosis between the left atrium and the posterior venous chamber can be constructed by a combination of lifting the heart upward and completing the anastomosis on the right side of the cavae. Pulmonary veins that have directly entered the right atrium or right superior vena cava are repaired through a right-sided atriotomy (Fig. 36–16). The atrial septal defect is enlarged, and a large pericardial patch is used to form a baffle that directs the pulmonary venous flow through the atrial septal defect. Intracardiac connections that drain into the right atrium by the coronary sinus are repaired similarly (Fig. 36–17).

In patients with Type II TAPVC draining to the coronary sinus, an oblique right atriotomy must be done so that the crista terminalis is not divided. The coronary sinus is then incised into the foramen ovale or atrial septal defect. The atrial septal defect or foramen ovale is then enlarged, and a pericardial patch is used to direct the coronary sinus blood into the left atrium. Incising the coronary sinus and removing a portion of the atrial septum may injure one or more of the internodal conduction tracts between the sinus and atrioventricular nodes. Preservation of the crista terminalis usually ensures sinus rhythm.

For Type III, or intracardiac, connections, the heart is elevated superiorly, and a large anastomosis is created between the posterior venous chamber and the left atrium (Fig. 36–18). In some patients, the posterior venous chamber is not a transverse structure but is an arborized, tree-like structure with the only large point of communication at the confluence of the descending anomalous vein (Kawashima et al, 1977). In these patients, it is necessary to make a Y-shaped incision in the anomalous venous chamber and connect this to a similarly shaped incision in the posterior left atrium. If ligating the descending anomalous vein compromises the size of the left atrium, this can be left open, as these connections are in all cases obstructed. Mixed (Type IV) TAPVC is repaired by using techniques described for this combination of lesions.

Enlargement of the usually small left atrium may be necessary (Bonham-Carter et al, 1969; Parr et al, 1974). On preoperative cineangiography (Graham and Bender, 1980), at operation (Goor et al, 1976),

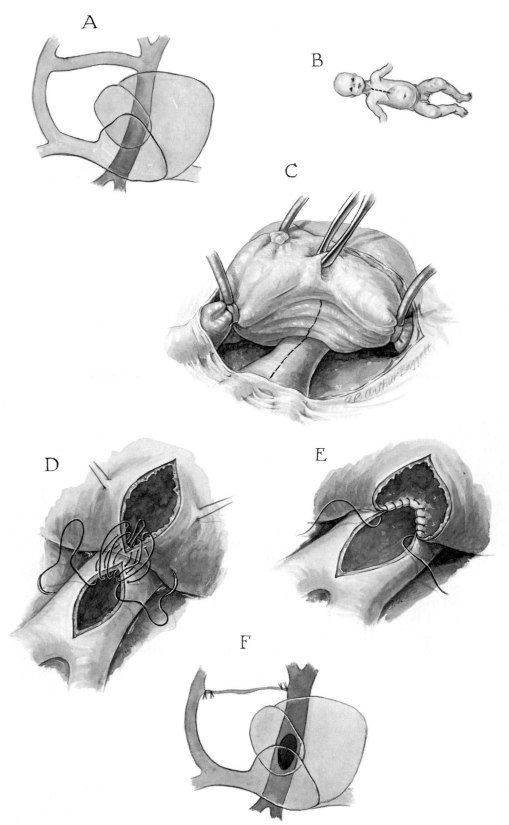

Figure 36–15. Steps in the repair of supracardiac TAPVC. *A,* Schematic anatomy as seen from the surgeon's view. *B,* Median sternotomy incision. *C,* After dissection of pericardial attachments, proposed incisions on the posterior left atrium and pulmonary venous confluence are shown. *D,* Generous incisions are made, and the first few stitches of a double-armed monofilament suture are shown. *E,* After the sutures are pulled tight, they should be interrupted in several places to avoid constricting the anastomosis. *F,* The final result. (From Kirklin, J. W.: Surgical treatment for total anomalous pulmonary venous connection in infancy. *In* Barratt-Boyes, B. G., Neutze, J. M., and Harris, E. A. [eds]: Heart Disease in Infancy: Diagnosis and Surgical Treatment. Edinburgh and London, Churchill Livingstone, 1973.)

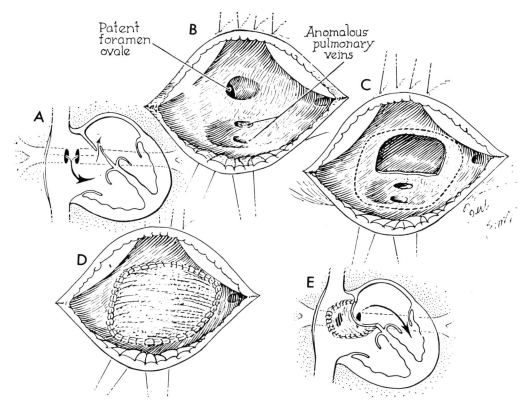

Figure 36–16. Repair of cardiac type of TAPVC in which the pulmonary veins drain directly to the right atrium. *A,* Anatomic representation. *B,* After right atriotomy. *C,* A generous portion of the atrial septum is excised. *D,* A large pericardial patch is used to direct pulmonary venous blood into the left atrium. (From Cooley, D. A., Hallman, G. L., and Leachman, R. D.: Total anomalous pulmonary venous drainage: Correction with the use of cardiopulmonary bypass in 62 cases. J. Thorac. Cardiovasc. Surg., *51*:88, 1966.)

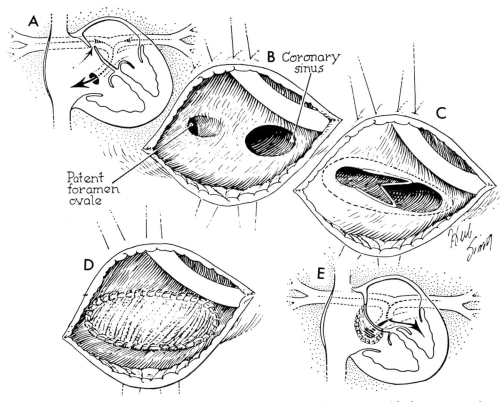

Figure 36–17. Repair of cardiac type of TAPVC in which the pulmonary veins connect with the coronary sinus. *A,* The surgical anatomy. *B,* A view of the dilated coronary sinus ostium after right atriotomy. *C,* The coronary sinus is incised into the left atrial wall and patent foramen ovale. *D,* A large pericardial patch is used to direct coronary sinus blood into the left atrium. *E,* The final result. (From Cooley, D. A., Hallman, G. L., and Leachman, R. D.: Total anomalous pulmonary venous drainage: Correction with the use of cardiopulmonary bypass in 62 cases. J. Thorac. Cardiovasc. Surg., *51:* 88, 1966.)

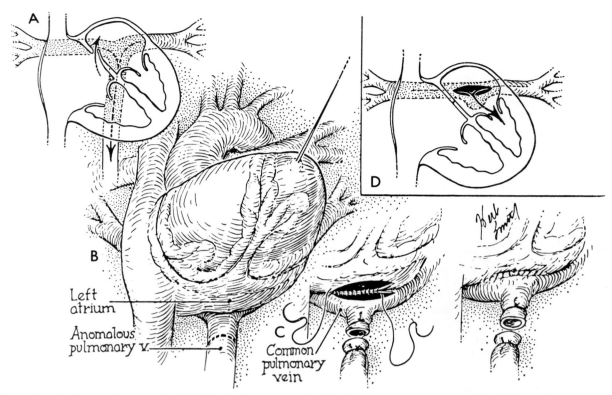

Figure 36–18. Repair of intracardiac TAPVC. *A*, The anatomy. *B*, The heart is deviated superiorly and the anomalous descending vein is ligated. *C*, Generous incisions are made in the venous confluence and the left atrium. These are anastomosed with a fine monofilament suture. *D*, The final result after closing the atrial septal defect or patent foramen ovale. (From Cooley, D. A., Hallman, G. L., and Leachman, R. D.: Total anomalous pulmonary venous drainage: Correction with the use of cardiopulmonary bypass in 62 cases. J. Thorac. Cardiovasc. Surg., *51*:88, 1966.)

and during the postoperative period (Parr et al, 1974), the left atrium is small, and reservoir function may be compromised because of poor compliance. Despite these reasons for using a pericardial patch to enlarge the left atrium, several authors have noted that these maneuvers do not appreciably increase survival (Hammon et al, 1980; Katz et al, 1978). There is no convincing evidence that the additional time and the construction of another suture line that may impair internodal conduction are necessary.

Postoperative care may be difficult in patients with TAPVC, especially infants. Stiff, wet lungs are difficult to ventilate, and excessive inspiratory pressure further decreases the function of a heart already compromised by preoperative and intraoperative ischemia. Positive end-expiratory pressure, used judiciously, can increase arterial oxygen concentration by better matching ventilation and perfusion and preventing atelectasis. Many infants require the infusion of catecholamines postoperatively. Isoproterenol in low to moderate doses (0.01 to 0.06 μg/kg/min) has a positive myocardial inotropic and chronotropic effect and serves to dilate both systemic and pulmonary arteries and thus decreases myocardial oxygen demands. Many infants are edematous, and administration of diuretics encourages the return to normal hydration. However, attention to blood and fluid replacement, arterial blood gases, and acid-base balance and maintenance of adequate cardiac output are essential to a successful result.

Results

The results of operations for TAPVC are related directly to the presence of obstruction and thus related indirectly to the type of connection present. Infants with obstructed connections usually present in extremis with very low cardiac output and are at great risk for the development of subendocardial necrosis. They are often difficult to ventilate because of poor pulmonary compliance and suffer the complications of mechanical ventilation that occur in infants with stiff lungs. Cardiac catheterization and operations in this group are usually done on an emergent basis, and mortality and the rate of complications have been high. The operative mortality in infants has decreased from nearly 50% in series reported in the 1960s to less than 30% in the modern era (Hammon et al, 1980; Turley et al, 1980). More of these infants survive to diagnosis and treatment, and these results represent a great improvement in the therapy of this condition. With more prompt diagnosis and therapy, the operative mortality can be expected to improve in these infants.

Operative mortality is even less in patients between 3 and 12 months of age (Behrendt et al, 1972). In older children and adults, operative mortality is probably less than 5% (Gomes et al, 1971). In most of these patients, the operative mortality is related to the presence of increased pulmonary vascular resistance from long-standing left-to-right intracardiac shunts.

Thus, it is the presence of obstruction in the anomalous connection that most affects the patient's survival both with and without operation. In a series of infants operated on at Vanderbilt University Hospital between 1970 and 1980, the age of the patient did not directly affect the operative mortality (Hammon et al, 1980). In all surgical series, there have been more deaths in Types I and III TAPVC; in these two groups the presence of anatomic obstruction to the anomalous connection is more prevalent, especially in Type III.

With successful operation, late complications and mortality are rare. In patients with severe pulmonary hypertension and impaired left ventricular function, normal pulmonary artery pressure (Fig. 36–19) and left ventricular function (Fig. 36–20) can be expected (Hammon et al, 1980; Mathew et al, 1977). Postoperative pulmonary venous obstructions due to a hypertrophic lesion in individual pulmonary veins after repair of various types of TAPVC in infancy have been reported (Behrendt et al, 1972; Breckenridge et al, 1973; Fleming et al, 1979; Turley et al, 1980; Whight et al, 1978). Although this complication is rare, it usually results in severe morbidity or death of the patient. The etiology of this problem is not clear; stenosis of individual pulmonary veins has a common embryologic etiology with TAPVC (Lucas et al, 1962), and these infants may have a combination of the two lesions. For older children and adults, late complication is rare and is usually due to an arrhythmia (Gomes et al, 1971).

Because repair of TAPVC involves a circumfer-

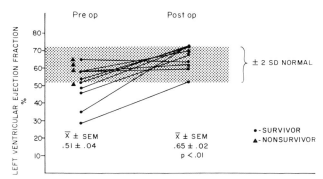

Figure 36–20. Preoperative and postoperative left ventricular ejection fraction calculated from left ventricular volume data obtained at cardiac catheterization. Note the return to normal function in postoperative patients. (From Hammon, J. W., Bender, H. W., Graham, T. P., et al: Total anomalous pulmonary venous connection in infancy. J. Thorac. Cardiovasc. Surg., *80*:544, 1980.)

ential suture line, late postoperative stenosis may result after significant growth occurs. In more than 50 patients operated on at Vanderbilt University Hospital, two cases of late postoperative pulmonary venous stenosis at the suture line occurred, both more than 10 years postoperatively. The stenotic suture line obstruction is shown in Figure 36–21, which also shows distended pulmonary veins. Operation is indicated when symptoms occur or when pulmonary artery pressure increases. Operation consists simply of enlarging the suture line by using a triangular pericardial or prosthetic patch. The risk is low and a good result can be expected.

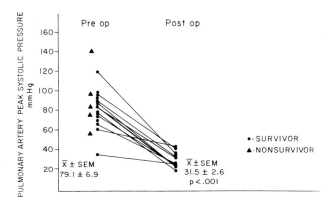

Figure 36–19. Preoperative and postoperative peak pulmonary artery pressures from a group of infants having repair of TAPVC in infancy. Note the marked reduction in postoperative patients. (From Hammon, J. W., Bender, H. W., Graham, T. P., et al: Total anomalous pulmonary venous connection in infancy. J. Thorac. Cardiovasc. Surg., *80*:544, 1980.)

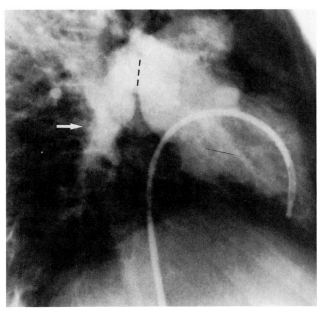

Figure 36–21. The venous phase of a pulmonary arteriogram in a patient with late postoperative suture line stenosis after repair of total anomalous pulmonary venous connection. The broken line shows the stenotic orifice between the pulmonary venous chamber and the left atrium. The *arrow* indicates an engorged pulmonary vein.

COR TRIATRIATUM

In *cor triatriatum*, the pulmonary veins enter a chamber superior to the left atrium that then joins the left atrium through a narrow opening. Alternatively, the accessory chamber is separate from the left atrium and has a direct communication with the right atrium or indirectly communicates with the right atrium by way of an anomalous channel.

Historical Aspects

The classic form of cor triatriatum was described in 1868 by Church. Anatomic classifications of cor triatriatum were given by Loeffler in 1949 and were further subdivided by Edwards in 1960. The first successful operation for total correction of cor triatriatum was reported by Vineberg and Gialloreto in 1956.

Incidence

Cor triatriatum is rare; the incidence of cor triatriatum in all patients with congenital heart disease has been reported to be 0.1 to 0.4% (Jegier et al, 1963; Niwayama, 1960). The male-female incidence is approximately equal in most series. Although the etiology is unknown, the accepted embryologic ex-

planation is that the accessory atrium is a common pulmonary vein that failed to become incorporated into the left atrium in a normal manner (Edwards, 1960).

Anatomy

The large number of subtypes of cor triatriatum requires a more inclusive classification than that proposed by Loeffler. The following classification is based on contributions of a number of individuals interested in this unusual anomaly (Edwards, 1960; Grondin et al, 1964; Loeffler, 1949; Niwayama, 1960).

Accessory Left Atrial Chamber Receives All Pulmonary Veins and Communicates with the Left Atrium. This type is the classic cor triatriatum in which a membranous partition with the shape of a windsock separates the more proximal chamber, which receives the pulmonary veins, from the more distal left atrium, which communicates with the mitral valve (Fig. 36–22A). The partition is usually directed toward the mitral valve and may have one or more orifices. This anomalous septum contains cardiac muscle fibers and is occasionally calcified. The true left atrium communicates with the left atrial appendage and contains a fossa ovalis. In most patients, there is no communication between the right and left atria, but, occasionally, a patent foramen ovale or secundum atrial septal defect allows

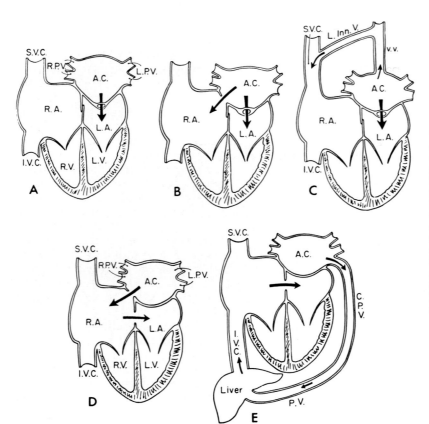

Figure 36–22. The various types of cor triatriatum. *A*, Classical cor triatriatum in which the accessory chamber receives the pulmonary veins and communicates with the left atrium. *B*, Classical cor triatriatum in which the accessory chamber communicates both with the left atrium and the right atrium or *C*, the systemic venous circulation via an anomalous venous connection. *D*, Cor triatriatum in which the accessory chamber communicates only with the right atrium or *E*, the systemic venous circulation via an anomalous vein. (Adapted from Lucas, R. V., and Schmidt, R. E. *In* Moss, A. J., Adams, F. H., and Emmanouilides, G. C. [eds]: Heart Disease in Infants, Children and Adolescents, 2nd ed. Copyright 1977, The Williams & Wilkins Company, Baltimore. Reproduced by permission.)

the lower left atrial chamber to communicate with the right atrium (Niwayama, 1960).

In a few patients, the accessory atrial chamber communicates directly with the left atrium through a stenotic opening and with the right atrium directly (Fig. 36–22*B*) or via an anomalous venous connection (Fig. 36–22*C*). The anatomy of complete cor triatriatum communicating with the left atrium was reported for 20 patients (Marin-Garcia et al, 1975). In 12 of the patients, a classic diaphragm divided the left atrium and contained one or more stenotic orifices. In 6 patients, the accessory venous chamber was obstructed by either an hourglass configuration or a tubular narrowing that obstructed flow into the normal left atrium. These obstructions were invariably associated with complex associated cardiac lesions. The remaining 2 patients had other anomalous connections to the right atrium.

Accessory Atrial Chamber Receives All Pulmonary Veins and Does Not Communicate with the Left Atrium. In this anomaly, the diaphragm separating the common venous chamber from the left atrium is complete and prevents direct flow of pulmonary venous blood to the left atrium. For the patient to survive, there is a direct communication from the common pulmonary venous chamber to the right atrium (Fig. 36–22*D*) or via an anomalous channel either to the innominate vein or to the portal vein, as in the supracardiac and infracardiac types of TAPVC (Fig. 36–22*E*).

Pathophysiology

In classic cor triatriatum in which there is no alternative pathway for pulmonary venous blood, the stenotic opening in the membranous partition between the accessory atrial chamber and the true left atrium results in supravalvular mitral stenosis with the features of elevated pulmonary venous pressure transmitted to the lungs that causes pulmonary edema. The clinical condition of the patient is determined by the size of the opening in the membrane. If the opening is 3 mm or less in diameter, the symptoms occur in infancy and are similar to those of TAPVC with obstruction. If the opening is larger, the symptoms occur later in infancy, in childhood, or occasionally later in life.

In other forms of cor triatriatum, the features of unobstructed TAPVC are found, with hyperkinetic pulmonary hypertension and communications of the pulmonary venous system with the right atrium either directly or through an anomalous channel.

Diagnosis

Clinical Manifestations. Most patients with cor triatriatum present with symptoms in the first few years of life (Niwayama, 1960). In these patients, signs of pulmonary venous obstruction are prevalent,

with bouts of pulmonary edema, extreme feeding difficulties, and poor weight gain. On physical examination, the predominant features are moist rales in the lower fields of the lung associated with a loud pulmonary second sound compatible with pulmonary hypertension. If there is a communication with the right atrium, there is a flow murmur at the left sternal border associated with the large left-to-right intracardiac shunt.

In the occasional patient who is discovered with this condition later in life, there is a history of breathlessness, frequent respiratory infections, and, in some cases, peripheral embolization. As with mitral stenosis, many patients are mistaken to have primary pulmonary disease. The physical examination in these patients reflects severe pulmonary hypertension: a loud pulmonary second sound, right ventricular lift, and pulmonary rales. In many patients, the signs of right-sided heart failure are prominent, with distended peripheral veins and an enlarged liver. The usual cardiac murmur is a soft, blowing, systolic murmur along the left sternal border. In some cases, a diastolic murmur is heard in the mitral area.

Chest Film. The plain chest film in cor triatriatum usually reflects pulmonary venous obstruction. Fine, diffuse, reticular pulmonary markings extend from the pulmonary hilus to involve the lower lung fields. In older patients, Kerley's B lines may be present, combined with prominent venous engorgement of the upper pulmonary vessels. There are also signs of left atrial enlargement produced by the dilated accessory chamber (Fig. 36–23).

Electrocardiogram. The electrocardiographic findings reflect right ventricular systolic overload. In many cases, there are tall peaked P waves, which suggest right atrial enlargement. Rarely, notched P waves are present, presumably because of the dilated accessory atrial chamber.

Echocardiogram. The echocardiographic features are variable in cor triatriatum. When the membrane that separates the accessory chamber from the true left atrium is thick and prominent, it is sometimes localized with the echocardiogram. In most cases, it is impossible to differentiate the large dilated accessory chamber from TAPVC draining to the coronary sinus or persistent left superior vena cava connecting to the coronary sinus.

Cardiac Catheterization. The hallmark of hemodynamic findings in cor triatriatum is a pressure gradient between the pulmonary capillary wedge pressure and the left atrial pressure. In most cases, oximetry excludes a left-to-right shunt, and significant pulmonary hypertension is the rule. Selective pulmonary arteriography usually shows cor triatriatum in the venous phase. Pulmonary transit time is prolonged. As the pulmonary veins are opacified, they drain into an accessory left atrial chamber. In most cases, there is a delay between the opacification of this chamber and the visualization of the true left atrium and left ventricle. With a high-quality study,

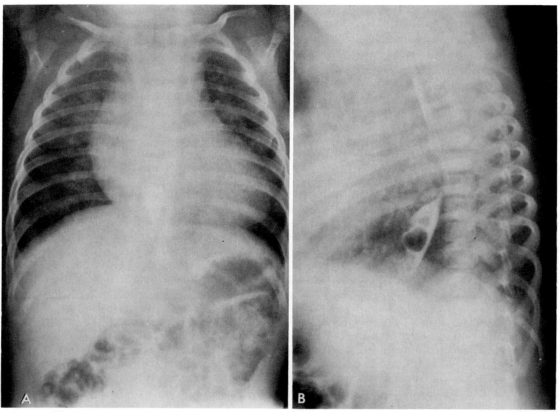

Figure 36–23. Plain chest film of a child with cor triatriatum. *A,* Posteroanterior view shows pulmonary venous engorgement and left atrial enlargement. *B,* Lateral view confirms left atrial enlargement produced by the dilated accessory chamber, which causes posterior displacement of the barium-filled esophagus.

the interatrial diaphragm can be identified as a linear or windsock-shaped filling defect between the accessory atrial chamber and the true left atrium (Fig. 36–24). The accessory atrial chamber usually remains opacified for some time and does not contract as does the normal left atrial chamber.

Surgical Treatment

The only successful therapy for cor triatriatum has been surgical. The indications for operation and preoperative preparation are similar to those for patients with TAPVC. Open correction is preferred in all patients. In infants, open correction is facilitated by hypothermia and circulatory arrest. In most cases, resection of the membrane between the accessory venous chamber and the left atrium can be done through the atrial septum in infants and in older children by an incision into the true left atrium by developing the interatrial groove. If the preoperative diagnosis suggests TAPVC, exploration of the heart exteriorly usually shows a dilated pulmonary venous chamber, which can be confused with the operative findings in congenital mitral stenosis. When anomalous connections between the accessory chamber and the systemic venous system are present, the

operative findings can be confusing, and only a careful and thorough intracardiac and extracardiac examination reveals the true cause of the anomaly, which can then easily be corrected. The number of cases reported in the literature is small, and thus it is difficult to estimate the operative mortality. Generally, the very sick infants with pulmonary venous obstruction have a higher mortality because of their preoperative condition. Mortality should be rare in older children and adults; however, late complications such as arrhythmias are more common.

MAJOR ANOMALIES OF THE THORACIC SYSTEMIC VENOUS SYSTEM

Developments in the diagnosis and treatment of cardiovascular disorders have brought anomalies of the thoracic systemic veins to the attention of the cardiologist and thoracic surgeon alike. Consideration of these diverse anomalies requires a simple and practical system classification. A classification based on anatomy tends to be cumbersome, whereas one based on physiology excludes conditions that result in hemodynamic derangement but may provide im-

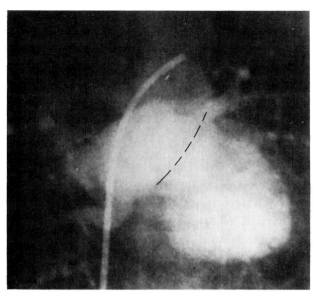

Figure 36–24. Venous phase of the pulmonary angiogram in a child with cor triatriatum. The position of the membrane that separates the dilated accessory chamber from the left atrium is shown *(broken line)*.

portant information about technical complications of cardiac catheterization and operation. A classification based on embryologic principles provides a more inclusive framework for discussion and practical consideration of the defects (Lucas and Schmidt, 1977). This system of classification includes anomalies of the cardinal venous system, anomalies of the inferior vena cava, and anomalies of the valves of the sinus venosus.

Anomalies of the Cardinal Venous System

Anomalies of the cardinal venous system involve aberrations in the development of the right and left superior vena cava and abnormalities of the coronary sinus. These anomalies present problems to the cardiac surgeon during repair of other defects or when the anomaly is associated with drainage of desaturated blood into the left atrium.

Persistent Left Superior Vena Cava. Persistent left superior vena cava is the most common anomaly of the superior vena cava system. In a series of 4,000 unselected autopsies, the prevalence was 0.3% (Geissler and Albert, 1956). The association in patients with additional cardiac defects ranges from 2.8 to 4.3% (Loogen and Rippert, 1958). Generally, persistent left superior vena cava is part of a bilateral superior vena caval system. Left superior vena cava is a normal stage in evolutionary development and in the growth of the human embryo. Its usual anatomic course begins where it arises from the junction of the left subclavian and the left internal jugular veins. It then descends vertically in front of the aortic arch. A short distance from its origin, it receives the superior left intercostal vein. It then passes in front of the left pulmonary artery and left pulmonary veins or in between these vessels (Winter, 1954). It usually receives a hemiazygos vein and then penetrates the pericardium and crosses the posterior wall of the left atrium obliquely to approach the posterior atrial ventricular groove. There it receives the great cardiac vein and becomes the coronary sinus (Fig. 36–25). Rarely, the right superior vena cava may be absent, and the entire venous return from the head and arms enters the coronary sinus (see Fig. 36–25). Associated anomalies are common with persistent left superior vena cava and include sinus venosus atrial septal defect or other congenital syndromes associated with cardiac malposition. The only clinical importance of persistent left superior vena cava is that cardiac catheterization is difficult when done from the left arm. In addition, at open cardiac operations, it is important to recognize the presence of the left superior vena cava and use appropriate cannulation techniques to eliminate the large amount of systemic venous blood that enters the heart through the coronary sinus. It is also important to recognize the absence of collateral vessels between the left and right superior vena cava or, rarely, the absence of the right superior vena cava, in which case ligation of the persistent left superior vena cava would result in venous engorgement in the head and arms.

Persistent Left Superior Vena Cava Associated with Failure of Coronary Sinus Development (Unroofed Coronary Sinus). In this defect, the left superior vena cava takes its usual course anterior to the aortic arch and the left pulmonary artery. Then, instead of crossing back to the left atrium to enter the coronary sinus, it directly connects to the upper portion of the left atrium between the atrial appendage and the left superior pulmonary veins (see Fig. 36–25C).

The physiologic consequences of this defect are almost always overshadowed by other major congenital cardiac malformations. The only contribution this defect makes to the overall hemodynamic findings at cardiac catheterization is a small right-to-left shunt at the atrial level.

This defect is almost invariably associated with other anomalies. In a series of eight surgical patients, a coronary sinus atrial septal defect was present in all patients (see Fig. 36–25D) (Quaegebeur et al, 1979). This anomaly is also associated with primitive-type cyanotic congenital heart defects, such as cor biloculare, anomalies of conotruncal development, and the syndrome of splenic agenesis (Campbell and Deuchar, 1954).

DIAGNOSIS. *Clinical Findings.* In most cases, features of a complex associated defect obscure the clinical effects of left superior vena cava directly connected to the left atrium. When a defect in the atrial septum is associated, the primary manifestations are those found in atrial septal defect. When drainage of the left superior vena cava to the left atrium is an isolated phenomenon, cyanosis is prev-

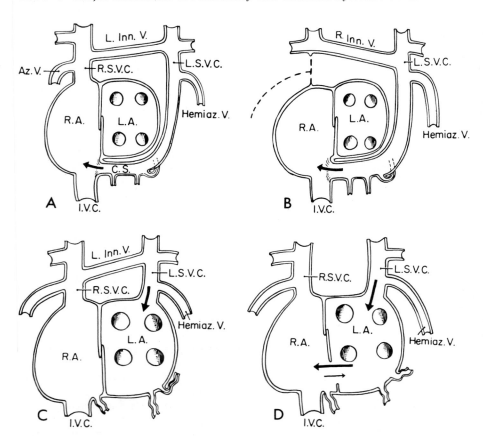

Figure 36–25. Variation of persistent left superior vena cava (L.S.V.C.). *A*, L.S.V.C. drains via the coronary sinus (C.S.) to the right atrium (R.A.). The sizes of the left innominate vein (L. Inn. V.) and L.S.V.C. vary inversely, and the former is often absent. *B*, Uncommonly, the right superior vena cava (R.S.V.C.) is atretic. *C*, The coronary sinus is absent, and the L.S.V.C. drains directly into the left atrium. Simple ligation of the L.S.V.C. provides a cure. *D*, The coronary sinus is absent, and there is no communication between the two superior venae cavae. A low-lying coronary sinus A.S.D. is present, and treatment requires baffling the L.S.V.C. into the right atrium and closing the A.S.D. (Adapted from Lucas, R. V., and Schmidt, R. E. *In* Moss, A. J., Adams, F. H., and Emmanouilides, G. C. [eds]: Heart Disease in Infants, Children and Adolescents, 2nd ed. Copyright 1977, The Williams & Wilkins Company, Baltimore. Reproduced by permission.)

alent in early infancy. Although the patient is asymptomatic, clubbing and polycythemia are usual. The heart is normal on auscultation and radiographic examination.

Cardiac Catheterization. Precise diagnosis of this defect is possible either by following the course of the cardiac catheter through the left superior vena cava or by dye injection in the left arm (Fig. 36–26). These findings in the presence of peripheral cyanosis suggest a systemic vein draining anomalously into the left atrium.

Surgical Treatment. The treatment in all cases is surgical. If there are competent bridging veins between the left and right superior vena cava, the treatment is simply ligation of the left superior vena cava and correction of the associated intracardiac defect. If, as in most cases, there are no bridging communications and the coronary sinus septum has not been formed, it is necessary to "roof" the coronary sinus with pericardium or a portion of the left atrium so that the left superior vena cava now drains into the right atrium (Fig. 36–27). Complications are usually related to the magnitude of operation for associated anomalies and not to the operative therapy for this uncommon situation.

Anomalies of the Inferior Vena Cava

Significant anomalies of the inferior vena cava are those that shunt unsaturated blood into the left atrium and that can complicate cardiac catheterization and cardiac operations for congenital heart disease. These anomalies are intrahepatic interruption of the inferior vena cava with azygos continuation

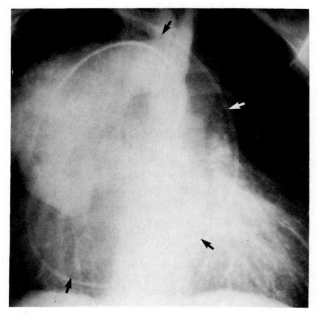

Figure 36–26. Cardiac catheter *(arrows)* passes from the right arm into a persistent left superior vena cava and into the right atrium in a child with complicated congenital heart disease.

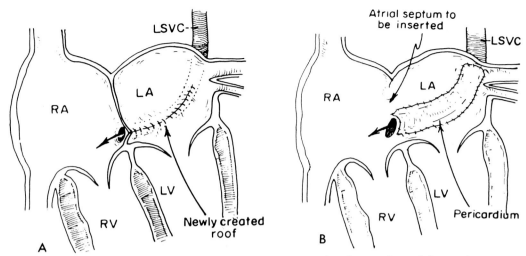

Figure 36-27. Repair (or roofing) of an unroofed coronary sinus associated with a persistent left superior vena cava (LSVC). *A,* The repair is made by bringing together the posterior left atrial wall to form a channel such that the LSVC communicates with the right atrium. *B,* The same repair is made in a patient with a common atrium by using pericardium. (Reprinted with permission from The Society of Thoracic Surgeons [The Annals of Thoracic Surgery, Vol. 27, 1979, p. 418–425].)

and anomalous drainage of the inferior vena cava into the left atrium.

Interrupted Inferior Vena Cava. Interruption of the inferior vena cava with azygos continuation is more prevalent in patients with congenital heart disease, particularly patients with polysplenia syndrome and with cardiac malpositions (Anderson and Varco, 1961). When interrupted inferior vena cava is an isolated anomaly, it is associated with normal longevity and no physiologic abnormalities. Problems arise when it occurs with other congenital anomalies that require surgical correction. During operations for congenital heart disease, ligation of the large azygos vein can result in a fatality and must be recognized (Effler et al, 1951). The anomaly also leads to difficulties in cannulation for cardiopulmonary bypass; details of this technical problem are given elsewhere (Bosher, 1959).

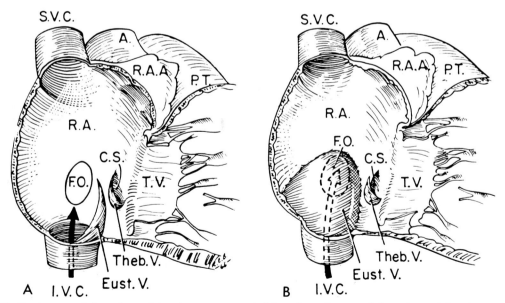

Figure 36-28. Persistence of the valves of the sinus venosus. *A,* Normal persistence of the valves of the sinus venosus results in the eustachian valve (Eust. V.) and the thebesian valve (Theb. V.). *B,* Abnormal persistence of the eustachian valve has resulted in a membrane that completely diverts inferior vena cava (I.V.C.) blood into the left atrium via the foramen ovale (F.O.). Similarly, the ostium of the coronary sinus (C.S.), the superior vena cava (S.V.C.) orifice, or all three may be isolated from the true right atrium by abnormal persistence of the valves of the sinus venosus. (R.A.A. = right atrial appendage; T.V. = tricuspid valve; P.T. = pulmonary trunk; A. = aorta.) (From Lucas, R. V., and Schmidt, R. E. *In* Moss, A. J., Adams, F. H., and Emmanouilides, G. C. [eds]: Heart Disease in Infants, Children and Adolescents, 2nd ed. Copyright 1977, The Williams & Wilkins Company, Baltimore, Reproduced by permission.)

Anomalous Drainage of the Inferior Vena Cava into the Left Atrium. When the inferior vena cava shunts blood directly into the left atrium, a distinction must be made between connection of the inferior vena cava to the left atrium with intact atrial septum and cases in which a low atrial septal defect allows drainage of inferior vena cava blood into the left atrium. Direct connection of the inferior vena cava to the left atrium is uncommon, and the embryology is obscure. The clinical features are comparable to those of left superior vena cava connections to the left atrium (Gardner and Cole, 1955). The risk of systemic embolization is present, and surgical therapy should be done. The placement of an interatrial baffle to provide normal systemic venous drainage is curative (Black et al, 1964). In some patients, persistence of the valves of the sinus venosus can direct inferior vena cava blood into the left atrium by an atrial septal defect or patent foramen ovale (Fig. 36–28) (Doucette and Knoblich, 1963). Treatment consists of incising the persistent valvular tissue and closing the interatrial communication. In some patients with an atrial septal defect, a large eustachian valve may be mistaken for the lower margin of the atrial septal defect. Care must be taken to close the atrial defect itself, because closure of the atrial septum onto the eustachian valve may then divert inferior vena cava blood into the left atrium (Mustard et al, 1964).

Selected Bibliography

Bender, H. W., Fisher, R. D., Walker, W. E., and Graham, T. P.: Reparative cardiac surgery in infants and small children: Five years experience with profound hypothermia and circulatory arrest. Ann. Surg., 190:437, 1979.

A summary of the results of operations in a large series (128) of infants and children by using hypothermia and circulatory arrest. The surgical techniques are detailed and the results are shown.

Darling, R. C., Rothney, W. B., and Craig, J. M.: Total pulmonary venous drainage into the right side of the heart. Lab. Invest., 6:44, 1957.

The first publication to characterize carefully the types of TAPVC. Beautifully illustrated description of the pathologic anatomy.

Hammon, J. W., Bender, H. W., Graham, T. P., et al: Total anomalous pulmonary venous connection in infancy. J. Thorac. Cardiovasc. Surg., 80:544, 1980.

This article on a series of patients with TAPVC emphasizes preoperative and postoperative hemodynamic and ventricular function studies and shows that operative survivors have normal hemodynamic and ventricular function.

Ivemark, B. I.: Implications of agenesis of the spleen on the pathogenesis of conotruncus anomalies in childhood: An analysis of the heart malformations in the splenic agenesis syndrome with fourteen new cases. Acta Paediatr. Scand. (Suppl.), 104:1, 1955.

One of the best descriptions of the pathologic anatomy, diagnosis, and surgical treatment of this uncommon anomaly.

Katz, N. M., Kirklin, J. W., and Pacifico, A. D.: Concepts and practices in surgery for total anomalous pulmonary venous connection. Ann. Thorac. Surg., 25:479, 1978.

An excellent review article that discusses many of the controversial features in the diagnosis and management of TAPVC.

Lucas, R. V., and Schmidt, R. E.: Anomalous venous connection, pulmonary and systemic. In Moss, A. J., Adams, F. H., and Emmanouilides, G. C. (eds): Heart Disease in Infants, Children and Adolescents. Baltimore, Williams & Wilkins, 1977, pp. 437–470.

A detailed explanation of the embryology of anomalies of pulmonary venous connection to the heart. Well illustrated and easily understandable.

Neill, C. A.: Development of the pulmonary veins: With reference to the embryology of anomalies of pulmonary venous return. Pediatrics, 18:880, 1956.

An important embryologic study that outlines the development of the pulmonary venous system and provides an embryologic explanation for anomalous pulmonary venous connections.

Sloan, H., MacKenzie, J., Morris, J. D., et al: Open-heart surgery in infancy. J. Thorac. Cardiovasc. Surg., 44:459, 1962.

A description of the first successful repair of Type III TAPVC in an infant. This work introduced the concept of deep hypothermia induced by surface cooling and cardiopulmonary bypass so that a period of circulatory arrest could be used for operative repair.

Bibliography

Anderson, R. C., and Varco, R. L.: Cor triatriatum: Successful diagnosis and surgical correction in a 3-year-old girl. Am. J. Cardiol., 7:436, 1961.

Appelbaum, A., Kirklin, J. W., Pacifico, A. D., et al: The surgical treatment of total anomalous pulmonary venous connection. Isr. J. Med. Sci., 11:89, 1975.

Barratt-Boyes, B. G.: Primary definitive intracardiac operations in infants; total anomalous pulmonary venous connection. In Kirklin, J. W. (ed): Advances in Cardiovascular Surgery. New York, Grune & Stratton, 1973, pp. 127–140.

Behrendt, D. M., Aberdeen, E., Waterson, D. J., and Bonham-Carter, R. E.: Total anomalous pulmonary venous drainage in infants. Circulation, 46:347, 1972.

Bender, H. W., Fisher, R. D., Walker, W. E., and Graham, T. P.: Reparative cardiac surgery in infants and small children: Five years experience with profound hypothermia and circulatory arrest. Ann. Surg., 190:437, 1979.

Black, H., Smith, G. T., and Goodale, W. T.: Anomalous inferior vena cava draining into the left atrium associated with intact interatrial septum and multiple pulmonary arteriovenous fistulae. Circulation, 29:258, 1964.

Bonham-Carter, R. E., Capriles, M., and Noe, Y.: Total anomalous pulmonary venous drainage: A clinical and anatomical study of 75 children. Br. Heart J., 31:45, 1969.

Bosher, L. H.: Problems in extracorporeal circulation relating to venous cannulation and drainage. Ann. Surg., 149:652, 1959.

Breckenridge, I. M., de Leval, M., Stark, J., and Waterston, D. J.: Correction of total anomalous pulmonary venous drainage in infancy. J. Thorac. Cardiovasc. Surg., 66:447, 1973.

Brody, H.: Drainage of the pulmonary veins into the right side of the heart. Arch. Pathol., 33:22, 1942.

Burroughs, J. T., and Edwards, J. E.: Total anomalous pulmonary venous connection. Am. Heart J., 59:913, 1960.

Campbell, M., and Deuchar, D. C.: The left-sided superior vena cava. Br. Heart J., 16:423, 1954.

Church, W. S.: Congenital malformation of the heart: Abnormal septum in left auricle. Trans. Pathol. Soc. (Lond.), 19:188, 1868.

Cooley, D. A., and Ochsner, A.: Correction of total anomalous pulmonary venous drainage. Surgery, 42:1014, 1957.

Cooley, D. A., Hallman, G. L., and Leachman, R. D.: Total anomalous pulmonary venous drainage: Correction with the use of cardiopulmonary bypass in 62 cases. J. Thorac. Cardiovasc. Surg., 51:88, 1966.

Darling, R. C., Rothney, W. B., and Craig, J. M.: Total pulmonary venous drainage into the right side of the heart. Lab. Invest., 6:44, 1957.

Doucette, J., and Knoblich, R.: Persistent right valve of the sinus venosus. Arch. Pathol., 75:105, 1963.

Edwards, J. E.: Malformations of the thoracic veins. In Gould, S. E. (ed): Pathology of the Heart, 2nd ed. Springfield, IL, Charles C Thomas, 1960, p. 484.

Effler, D. B., Greer, A. E., and Sifers, E. C.: Anomaly of the vena cava inferior. Report of fatality after ligation. J.A.M.A., 146:1321, 1951.

Eliot, R. S., and Edwards, J. E.: Congenital heart disease. In Hurst, J. W., and Logue, R. B. (eds): The Heart. New York, McGraw-Hill, 1966, pp. 587–620.

Fleming, W. H., Clark, E. B., Dooley, K. J., et al: Late complications following surgical repair of total anomalous pulmonary venous return below the diaphragm. Ann. Thorac. Surg., 27:435, 1979.

Friedlich, A., Bing, R. J., and Blount, S. G.: Physiological studies in congenital heart disease: IX: Circulatory dynamics in the anomalies of venous return to the heart, including pulmonary arteriovenous fistula. Am. Heart J., 86:20, 1950.

Gardner, D. L., and Cole, L.: Long survival with inferior vena cava draining into left atrium. Br. Heart J., 17:93, 1955.

Gathman, G. H., and Nadas, A. S.: Total anomalous pulmonary venous connection: Clinical and physiologic observations of 75 pediatric patients. Circulation, 42:143, 1970.

Geissler, W., and Albert, M.: Persistierende linke obere Hohlvene und Mitralstenose. A. Gesamte Inn. Med., 11:865, 1956.

Gomes, M. M. R., Feldt, R. H., McGoon, D. C., and Danielson, G. K.: Long-term results following correction of total anomalous pulmonary venous connection. J. Thorac. Cardiovasc. Surg., 61:253, 1971.

Goor, D. A., Yellin, A., Frand, M., et al: The operative problem of small left atrium in total anomalous pulmonary venous connection: Report of 5 patients. Ann. Thorac. Surg., 22:254, 1976.

Graham, T. P., and Bender, H. W.: Preoperative diagnosis and management of infants with critical congenital heart disease. Ann. Thorac. Surg., 29:272, 1980.

Grondin, C., Leonard, A. S., Anderson, R. C., et al: Cor triatriatum: A diagnostic surgical enigma. J. Thorac. Cardiovasc. Surg., 48:527, 1964.

Hammon, J. W., Bender, H. W., Graham, T. P., et al: Total anomalous pulmonary venous connection in infancy. J. Thorac. Cardiovasc. Surg., 80:544, 1980.

Ivemark, B. I.: Implications of agenesis of the spleen on the pathogenesis of conotruncus anomalies in childhood: An analysis of the heart malformations in the splenic agenesis syndrome with fourteen new cases. Acta Paediatr. Scand. (Suppl.), 104:1, 1955.

Jegier, W., Gibbons, J. E., and Wigglesworth, F. W.: Cor triatriatum: Clinical, hemodynamic, and pathologic studies: Surgical correction in early life. Pediatrics, 31:255, 1963.

Jensen, J. B., and Blount, S. G.: Total anomalous pulmonary venous return: A review and report of the oldest surviving patient. Am. Heart J., 82:387, 1971.

Katz, N. M., Kirklin, J. W., and Pacifico, A. D.: Concepts and practices in surgery for total anomalous pulmonary venous connection. Ann. Thorac. Surg., 25:479, 1978.

Kawashima, Y., Matsuda, H., Hakano, S., et al: Tree-shaped pulmonary veins in infracardiac total anomalous pulmonary venous drainage. Ann. Thorac. Surg., 23:436, 1977.

Kirklin, J. W.: Surgical treatment for total anomalous pulmonary venous connection in infancy. In Barratt-Boyes, B. G., Neutz, J. M., and Harris, E. A. (eds): Heart Disease in Infancy. Baltimore, Williams & Wilkins, 1973, pp. 89–100.

Lewis, J., Varco, R. L., Taufic, M., and Niazi, S. A.: Direct vision repair of triatrial heart and total anomalous pulmonary venous drainage. Surg. Gynecol. Obstet., 102:713, 1956.

Loeffler, E.: Unusual malformation of the left atrium: Pulmonary sinus. Arch. Pathol., 48:371, 1949.

Loogen, F., and Rippert, R.: Anomalien der grossen Korper und Lungenvenen. Z. Kreislaufforsch., 47:677, 1958.

Los, J. A.: Embryology. In Watson, H. (ed): Pediatric Cardiology. St. Louis, C. V. Mosby Co., 1968.

Lucas, R. V., and Schmidt, R. E.: Anomalous venous connection, pulmonary and systemic. In Moss, A. J., Adams, F. H., and Emmanouilides, G. C. (eds): Heart Disease in Infants, Children and Adolescents. Baltimore, Williams & Wilkins, 1977, pp. 437–470.

Lucas, R. V., Woolfrey, B. F., Anderson, R. C., et al: Atresia of the common pulmonary vein. Pediatrics, 29:729, 1962.

Marin-Garcia, J., Tandon, R., Lucas, R. V., Jr., and Edwards, J. E.: Cor triatriatum: Study of 20 cases. Am. J. Cardiol., 35:59, 1975.

Mathew, R., Thilenius, O. G., Replogle, R. L., and Arcilla, R. A.: Cardiac function in total anomalous pulmonary venous return before and after surgery. Circulation, 55:361, 1977.

McClure, C. F. W., and Butler, E. G.: The development of the vena cava inferior in man. Am. J. Anat., 35:331, 1925.

Meadows, W. R., Bergstrand, I., and Sharp, J. T.: Isolated anomalous connection of a great vein to the left atrium. Circulation, 24:669, 1961.

Miller, W. W., and Rashkind, W. J.: Palliative treatment of total anomalous pulmonary venous drainage by balloon atrial septostomy. Lancet, 2:387, 1968.

Muller, W. H.: The surgical treatment of transposition of the pulmonary veins. Ann. Surg., 134:683, 1951.

Mustard, W. T., Firor, W. B., and Kidd, L.: Diversion of the venae cavae into the left atrium during closure of atrial septal defects. J. Thorac. Cardiovasc. Surg., 47:317, 1964.

Neill, C. A.: Development of the pulmonary veins: With reference to the embryology of anomalies of pulmonary venous return. Pediatrics, 18:880, 1956.

Newfield, E. A., Wilson, A., Paul, M. H., and Reisch, J. S.: Pulmonary vascular disease in total anomalous venous drainage. Circulation, 61:103, 1980.

Niwayama, G.: Cor triatriatum. Am. Heart J., 59:291, 1960.

Paquet, M., and Gutgesell, H.: Echocardiographic features of total anomalous pulmonary venous connection. Circulation, 51:599, 1975.

Parr, G. V. S., Kirklin, J. W., Pacifico, A. D., et al: Cardiac performance in infants after repair of TAPVC. Ann. Thorac. Surg., 17:561, 1974.

Quaegebeur, J., Kirklin, J. W., Pacifico, A. D., and Bargeron, L. M.: Surgical experience with unroofed coronary sinus. Ann. Thorac. Surg., 27:418, 1979.

Raghib, G., Ruttenberg, H. D., Anderson, R. C., et al: Termination of left superior vena cava in left atrium, atrial septal defect, and absence of coronary sinus. Circulation, 31:906, 1965.

Ruttenberg, H. D., Neufeld, H. N., Lucas, R. V., et al: Syndrome of congenital cardiac disease with asplenia: Distinction from other forms of congenital cardiac disease. Am. J. Cardiol., 13:387, 1964.

Shaner, R. F.: The development of the bronchial veins with special reference to anomalies of the pulmonary veins. Anat. Rec., 140:159, 1961.

Sloan, H., MacKenzie, J., Morris, J. D., et al: Open-heart surgery in infancy. J. Thorac. Cardiovasc. Surg., 44:459, 1962.

Snellen, H. A., and Bruins, C.: Anomalies of venous return. In Watson, H. (ed): Pediatric Cardiology. St. Louis, C. V. Mosby Co., 1968.

Streeter, G. L.: Developmental horizons in human embryos. Description of age group XI, 13 to 20 somites, and age group XII, 21 to 20 somites. Carnegie Inst. Contrib. Embryol., 30(197):211, 1942.

Turley, K., Tucker, W. Y., Ullyot, D. J., and Ebert, P. A.: Total anomalous pulmonary venous connection in infancy: Influence of age and type of lesion. Am. J. Cardiol., 45:92, 1980.

Vineberg, A., and Gialloreto, O.: Report of a successful operation for stenosis of common pulmonary vein (cor triatriatum). Can. Med. Assoc. J., 74:719, 1956.

Whight, C. M., Barratt-Boyes, B. G., Calder, A. L., et al: Total anomalous pulmonary venous connection. J. Thorac. Cardiovasc. Surg., 75:52, 1978.

Wilson, J.: On a very unusual formation of the human heart. Phil. Trans. (Lond.), 88:332, 1798.

Winter, F. S.: Persistent left superior vena cava: Survey of world literature and report of thirty additional cases. Angiology, 5:90, 1954.

CHAPTER 37

ATRIOVENTRICULAR CANAL

Gordon K. Danielson
Francisco J. Puga
Dwight C. McGoon

The various congenital deformities of the atrioventricular canal are usually designated by the inclusive term "persistent common atrioventricular (AV) canal defect" (Feldt, 1976). The common AV canal is not seen in the normal, fully developed human heart but is encountered only in the embryo. It consists of the slightly narrowed zone between the one atrium and the one ventricle when the embryo is in its early tubular stage of development, and it serves as a broad area of connection and communication between the primitive atrium and the primitive ventricle.

During embryonic development, the ventricular septum ascends from the apex and the atrial septum descends from the cephalad atrial wall, and they thus divide the heart into right and left halves. As these septa converge at the AV junction or canal, "cushions" of endothelium form on the anterior and posterior margins of the canal. The progressive enlargement of these cushions contributes to separation of the common AV canal into right and left AV orifices and, together with delamination of ventricular myocardium, to development of their respective valves. Defective development in this area may result in incomplete septation of the AV canal and deformity of one or both AV valves. The underlying embryonic abnormality appears to be failure of normal fusion of the major AV endocardial cushions. The development of the central cardiac septum and the adjacent portions of the AV valves apparently depends on the normal development of the endocardial cushions.

CLASSIFICATION

When embryonic development of the area of the common AV canal is abnormal, the resultant malformation varies and depends on the extent of involvement of the atrial and ventricular septa as well as of the mitral and tricuspid valves. Concepts about classification of the various congenital cardiac defects have slowly evolved, and for the surgeon, a sur-

gically oriented classification is preferable. For the surgeon, the first distinction is whether an anomaly includes a fully displayed AV canal septal defect in the center of the heart that involves the ostium primum area of the atrial septum as well as the adjacent basal area of the ventricular septum, or whether the anomaly includes a lesser extent of septal defect or none at all and is therefore an incompletely displayed AV canal septal defect. The classification in Table 37–1 is based on this distinction. This table shows the 15 theoretically possible types of anomalies according to which combination of the four potential defects in embryogenesis of the AV canal has occurred. Note that both the ostium primum (O) and the basal ventricular (V) septal defects are present in each type of fully displayed form, whereas they are never associated in the same heart in any incompletely displayed form.

TABLE 37–1. THEORETICALLY POSSIBLE FORMS OF ATRIOVENTRICULAR CANAL DEFECT*

I. Fully displayed AV canal septal defect (both ostium primum [O] and ventricular [V] septal defects are present)
    1. OVMT
    2. OVM
    3. OVT
    4. OV

II. Incompletely displayed AV canal septal defect (O and V are not present together)
  A. Septal defect is present
    1. VMT
    2. OMT
    3. VM
    4. VT
    5. OM
    6. OT
    7. V
    8. O
  B. No septal defect is present
    1. MT
    2. M
    3. T

*Abbreviations: O = ostium primum atrial septal defect; V = basal (inlet) ventricular septal defect; M = typical mitral defect (cleft of anterior leaflet); T = typical tricuspid defect (cleft or partial absence of septal leaflet).

1298

Incompletely Displayed Forms

Incompletely displayed forms of the anomaly may result in isolated cleft formation in the anterior (aortic) leaflet of the mitral valve (M), isolated inlet ventricular septal defect (V), isolated atrial septal defect of the ostium primum type (O), or combined inlet ventricular septal defect and cleft mitral valve (VM), and so on. These forms of incompletely displayed AV canal septal defect are best classified with mitral valve deformities, atrial septal defects, or ventricular septal defects, whichever best pertains, and can be found in those respective chapters: therefore, they are not discussed further in this chapter. Emphasis is given to the tenet that to be classified as a fully displayed AV canal defect, an anomaly must include a central septal defect that involves both the ostium primum area of the atrial septum and the basal portion of the ventricular septum. This concept is important for clear appreciation of the anatomic and surgical aspects of this anomaly.

Fully Displayed Forms

It has been helpful from the surgical point of view to separate the fully displayed AV canal deformities into three types—partial, intermediate, and complete.

Partial AV Canal (Fig. 37–1A). In this type of deformity there is a centrally located septal defect with both involvement of the ostium primum area of the atrial septum and a deficiency ("scooping out") in the base of the ventricular septum. The distinctive feature of the partial AV canal is that the valvular leaflet tissue superadjacent to the ventricular septum has become fused continuously to the underlying crest of the ventricular septum. Although there is a deficiency, or "scooping out," of the base of the ventricular septum in partial AV canal, the fusion of the valvular leaflets to the crest of this deficient septum prevents a direct interventricular communication deep to the leaflets. This absence of direct interventricular communication is the hallmark of the partial AV canal anomaly. In addition, there is almost always a cleft in the anterior (aortic) leaflet of the mitral valve, and most hearts (85%) show incomplete development of the septal leaflet of the tricuspid valve, particularly in its anterior portion. Usually, the cleft in the anterior leaflet of the mitral valve does not extend across the crest of the ventricular septum; that is, the anterior and posterior portions of the anterior (aortic) mitral leaflet are fused to each other along the crest of the ventricular septum. This fusion in effect provides a complete circle to the mitral anulus and to the tricuspid anulus and thus divides the "complete" canal into separated mitral and tricuspid orifices.

The discerning reader of Table 37–1 might object that the theoretical OMT, OM, and O variations of AV canal defect should be dealt with in this chapter,

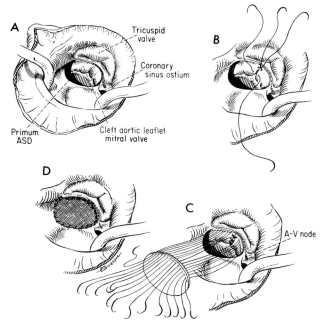

Figure 37–1. Partial AV canal. *A,* Surgical exposure, optimized by long atriotomy in the trabecular wall from the apex of the appendage to near the inferior caval orifice, and wide mobilization of venous cannulae. *B,* Beginning closure of the cleft in the anterior (aortic) mitral leaflet. *C,* Sutures placed between the patch and the junction of the mitral and tricuspid valves as initial stage of closure of the ostium primum atrial septal defect (see also Fig. 37–3A and B). *D,* Repair completed. (Reproduced with permission from Danielson, G. K.: Endocardial cushion defects. *In* Ravitch, M. M., et al (eds): Pediatric Surgery, 3rd ed., Vol. 1. Copyright © 1979 by Year Book Medical Publishers, Inc., Chicago.)

because they amount to an ostium primum atrial septal defect, with or without valvular involvement. However, a theoretically possible anomaly that consists of an isolated ostium primum defect (i.e., without an associated deficiency of the base of the ventricular septum) is *not* representative of a partial AV canal defect as typically encountered. Deficiency of the basal (inlet) portion of the ventricular septum is a constant component of the typical partial AV canal defect. In fact, the outflow tract of the left ventricle has the appearance of being elongated because of the ventricular septal deficiency into the "gooseneck" deformity typical of partial AV canal (Baron, 1968; Rastelli et al, 1967). The issue of deficiency at the base of the ventricular septum has relevance to the surgeon, particularly if valvular replacement is required, as discussed later.

Intermediate AV Canal. Intermediate AV canal is the rarest of the three types of fully displayed AV canal. Unfortunately, widely varying features are placed in this category by various authors (Bharati et al, 1980b). In the authors' usage, it is characterized by two features, one of which it has in common with the partial form of AV canal, and one it has in common with the complete form. In the intermediate form, distinct mitral and tricuspid valvular orifices have formed as a result of embryonic fusion between the anterior and posterior common leaflets of the common AV valve at their centers, just as in partial AV canal. Compared with partial AV canal, this centrally connected leaflet tissue does not fully fuse with the underlying crest of the ventricular septum. As a result, a space bordered superiorly by the leaflets and inferiorly by the crest of the ventricular septum allows a direct interventricular communication, as in the complete form of AV canal. This condition is truly intermediate between the partial and complete forms. Other authors have used a more liberal definition for the intermediate designation and include hearts that have any of various atypical features of the three basic types (partial, intermediate, and complete) of fully displayed AV canal.

Complete AV Canal (Fig. 37–2). This type of fully displayed AV canal is characterized by failure of the common AV valvular orifice to partition into separate mitral and tricuspid orifices; the anterior and posterior common leaflets of the common AV valvular orifice are not fused to each other centrally to form two separate orifices. The anterior and posterior common leaflets are also not fused with the crest of the underlying ventricular septum; thus, in complete AV canal, there *is* direct interventricular communication.

The three defined types of fully displayed AV canal septal defects may be correlated with the extent of involvement of the four possible components of the anomalies, which is shown in Table 37–1. All three types involve a central septal defect that consists of both an ostium primum atrial septal defect (O) and a deficiency or defect, or "scooping out," of the basilar ventricular septum (V). The complete AV canal defect always, by definition, has involvement of all four components, that is, OVMT. In the intermediate and partial types of AV canal, clefts or deformity of either the anterior leaflet of the mitral valve (M) or the septal leaflet of the tricuspid valve (T), or both, may be involved, or these leaflets may, rarely, be fully and normally developed. Thus, intermediate and partial types of AV canal can be of any one of the four patterns of fully displayed AV canal septal defect (OVMT, OVM, OVT, or OV) (see Table 37–1). (These abbreviations are used here only as symbols and not as a system of classification apart from the anatomic features for which the symbols stand.)

Subtypes of Complete AV Canal. Complete AV canal anomalies were subclassified into three types according to the configuration of the anterior common leaflet of the common AV valve by Rastelli and associates (1966). In Type A (see Fig. 37–2A), the anterior common leaflet has a natural division along the plane between its mitral and tricuspid components; there are also chordal attachments from the margins of this division to the crest of the underlying ventricular septum. Some 80% of patients with complete AV canal belong to this group. In Type B (see Fig. 37–2B), the anterior common leaflet is partially divided but is not attached by chordae directly to the crest of the underlying ventricular septum; instead, the edges of the division of the anterior common leaflet are attached by chordae to an abnormal papillary muscle that arises in the right ventricle near the apical portion of the ventricular septum. This form of complete AV canal is rare. In Type C (see Fig. 37–2C), the anterior common leaflet is undivided and appears as a single continuous leaflet that floats freely over the crest of the underlying ventricular septum, to which it is not attached. The chordal attachments of the leaflet at its right and left margins are to papillary muscles on the free wall of the right and left ventricles. Associated anomalies are common in this type of complete AV canal; for example, if pulmonary stenosis is associated with AV canal, it is almost always Type C.

No consistent relationship exists between the configurations of the anterior and posterior common leaflets. The attachment of the posterior common leaflet to the underlying ventricular septum can vary from sparse chordae to an imperforate "frenulum-like" membrane, and the division or notching between mitral and tricuspid portions also is variable. Although the structure of the posterior common leaflet does not enter into the scheme for subclassification of complete AV canal into Types A, B, and C, it is well, in describing individual hearts, to identify the characteristics of this leaflet, especially the extent of its fusion to the underlying crest of the ventricular septum.

Some workers have been persuaded by their studies to modify the aforementioned subtyping of complete AV canal in various ways (Carpentier, 1978; Piccoli et al, 1979). In the authors' surgical experience, the basic classification described earlier has correlated well with the selection of the best technique of repair, modified according to the individual variations that are common in congenital anomalies.

The location of the AV conduction system in AV canal defects is important to the surgeon. In all types, complete, intermediate, or partial, there is slight posterior displacement of the AV node compared with its normal relationship to the ostium of the coronary sinus (see Figs. 37–1, 37–3, and 37–6). There is also posterior displacement of the common bundle of His, the course of which is usually intimately related to the posterior rim of the "scooped out" basal portion of the ventricular septum.

ANATOMIC TERMINOLOGY

Anterior and Posterior. In these descriptions of the anatomic and surgical features of these anomalies, it may be helpful to be aware of the ambiguity of the terms "anterior" and "posterior" in relation to the common leaflets and to the respective portions of the ventricular and atrial septa. In the normal heart, the septa are not in a true sagittal plane but are obliquely oriented, with the anterior margins to the left and the posterior margins to the right. At

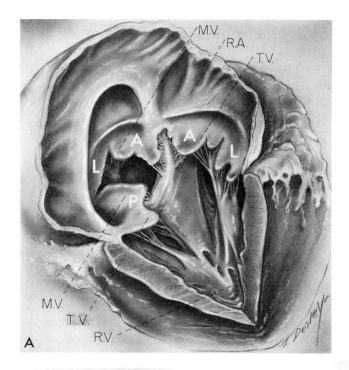

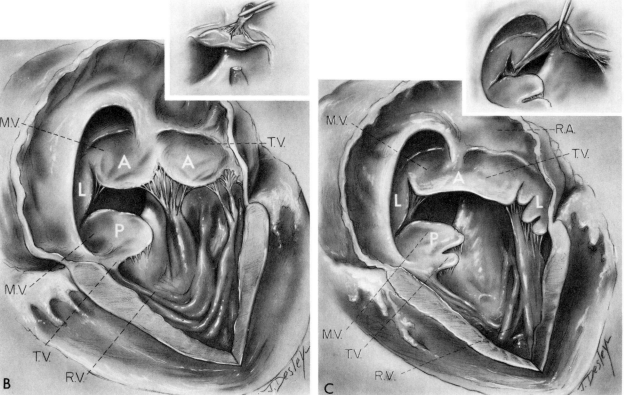

Figure 37–2. The three types of complete AV canal. *A,* Type A. Anterior common leaflet (A) divided and attached to the crest of the ventricular septum (M.V. = mitral valve; R.A. = right atrium; T.V. = tricuspid valve; P = posterior common leaflet; L = lateral leaflet; R.V. = right ventricle). *B,* Type B. Anterior common leaflet partially divided, with chordae from the central area of the leaflet attached to a single abnormal papillary muscle arising from the right ventricle. *C,* Type C. Anterior common leaflet is undivided and is not attached to the ventricular septum. The insets in *B* and *C* show the extent of the interventricular communication deep to the common anterior leaflet. Note that the ventricular septum below the valvular attachment approximates the position of the anterior rim of the atrial septal defect above the leaflet. Thus, the surgical incision to be made in the common anterior leaflet (see surgical technique) will be made to this area at the base of the common anterior leaflet. (From Rastelli, G. C., Kirklin, J. W., and Titus, J. L.: Anatomic observations on complete form of persistent common atrioventricular canal with special reference to atrioventricular valves. Mayo Clin. Proc., *41*:296, 1966.)

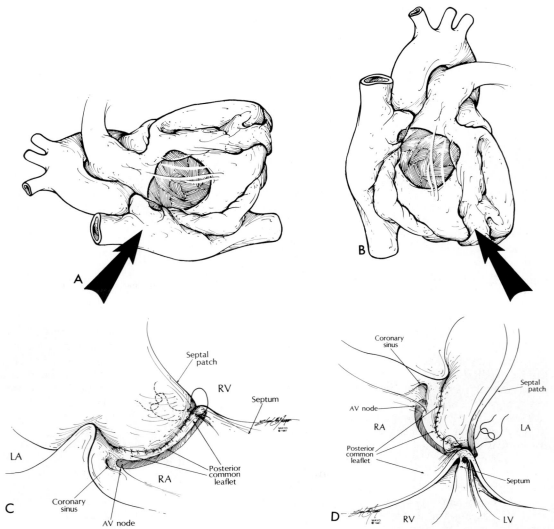

Figure 37–3. Detail of the positioning and suturing of the septal patch posteroinferiorly (posterocaudally) in partial AV canal. Drawings *A* and *B* provide orientation for the points of view for drawings *C* and *D*, respectively. The viewpoint shown in *A* and *C* is that of the surgeon at the operating table, whereas the viewpoint in *B* and *D* is, surgically speaking, a hypothetical one, as though the viewer were positioned anteroapically within the right ventricle. The central structure shown in *A* and *B* is for the purpose of designating the position within the heart of the septal defect typical of the AV canal anomaly. In *C* and *D*, the dark structure coursing along the crest of the ventricular septum, commencing at the AV node, is the bundle of His; its branches are not shown except in *D*, where part of the left bundle branch complex is seen in the cross-section of the ventricular septum. Views *C* and *D* show only the posterior aspect of the anomaly, the remainder of the heart having been "cut away" by the artist in (1) a transverse plane just superior to the level of the coronary sinus orifice, with the "cut" slicing through the posterior atrial wall and septum; and (2) in a coronal plane located toward the posterior part of the ventricular septum, with the "cut" slicing through the posterior common leaflet and through the septal patch.

To describe the principles for attachment of the patch in partial AV canal in this critical posteroinferior area, attention is first directed to the anterior aspect of the illustration (anterior is toward the right in both *C* and *D*). The patch is attached anteriorly to the line of junction of the mitral and tricuspid components of the posterior common leaflet, which is fused to the underlying crest of the ventricular septum. As the suturing progresses posteriorly, the line of attachment of the patch is deviated to the left, onto the base of the mitral component of the leaflet; still farther posteriorly after crossing the mitral annulus, the patch attachment remains to the left, away from the conduction tissue and to the left of the rim of the atrial septal defect. Thus, the widest possible separation is provided between the suture line and the AV node and penetrating portions of the conduction bundle. In the authors' experience with many operations in which suturing in this area was done with the heart beating, transient heart block was never encountered during suturing anterior to the middle *arrow* in the diagrams designating the posterior common leaflet, either in partial or in complete AV canal. All sutures shown were placed before lowering the patch into position, which allowed optimal exposure for suture placement.

operation, when the atrium is opened and the anterior lip of the atriotomy is retracted to the left, the heart becomes rotated counterclockwise on its longitudinal axis, as seen from above. Thus, the anterior margins of the septa become situated even more to the left. The crest of the ventricular septum, as seen by the surgeon, appears to be more in the coronal plane than in the sagittal plane so that which is called anterior becomes more strictly leftward, and vice versa.

Anterior or Posterior Common Leaflet. There is only one AV valve in complete AV canal. Anteriorly and posteriorly in such a valve are leaflets common to the left ventricular and right ventricular inlet orifices. These anterior and posterior common leaflets consist on the left side of tissue that would normally have been incorporated into the anterior leaflet (or aortic leaflet in some schemes of terminology) of the mitral valve, and on the right side of tissue that would have been incorporated into the septal leaflet of the tricuspid valve. In complete AV canal this normal differentiation into mitral and tricuspid valves does not occur, thus the leaflet tissue anteriorly and posteriorly remains part of the "common" AV valve and forms common leaflets. The terminology can be confusingly complex, especially when speaking of the anterior leaflet of the mitral valve. In Figure 37–2 the rudimentary components of the normal mitral valve are present; they consist of the lateral (L) leaflet (which would be called the posterior or mural leaflet of the normal mitral valve) and the left portion of the anterior common leaflet plus the left portion of the posterior common leaflet, which normally would have fused to form the anterior (aortic or septal) leaflet of the mitral valve.

Because the leaflet components that would have formed the mitral valve have failed to complete normal fusion, the valve does not have the usual appearance of a mitral valve. Some authors prefer to use the term "left atrioventricular valve." Similarly, the term "right atrioventricular valve" may be used synonymously with tricuspid valve in AV canal defects.

Cleft, Division, or Incision. A clear distinction should be made between the definitions of these three words. *Cleft* refers to the separation that partially persists between the two components of the anterior leaflet of the mitral valve, that is, a separation between the component originating from the anterior common leaflet and that originating from the posterior common leaflet; the term "cleft" is thus usually used in reference to the partial AV canal. A tricuspid counterpart of this cleft seldom exists. *Division* of the anterior common leaflet is found in Type A complete AV canal and refers to the naturally occurring separation, or division, between the mitral and tricuspid components of the common anterior leaflet. Some workers prefer to call this "division" a "commissure." As will be described under operative technique (see Figs. 37–5 and 37–6), it is often necessary for the surgeon to make an *incision* in the

anterior or posterior common leaflet to expose the underlying crest of the ventricular septum and to place a septal patch between the incised edges of the leaflet, especially in the Type C variety. Thus, "division" refers to a natural separation between the mitral and tricuspid components of the common leaflet, and "incision" refers to a surgically created separation between the components.

Ventricular Septal Defect and Interventricular Communication. Even the term "ventricular septal defect" is a potential source of confusion when speaking of AV canal defects, because *all* of the fully displayed forms of AV canal have a deficiency or defect in the base of the ventricular septum. It is not appropriate, strictly speaking, to state that a ventricular septal defect is not present in partial AV canal but is present in complete AV canal, because a defect is present in both forms. It is appropriate to state that a ventricular septal defect is present in both the partial and complete forms, but an *interventricular communication* is not present in the partial form but is present in the complete AV canal.

CLINICAL FEATURES

The partial form of AV canal was more commonly encountered than the complete form in earlier surgical experience, probably because of a greater mortality during infancy for babies born with a complete AV canal. Now that infants seriously ill with congenital heart disease are treated surgically, the complete form has become the more commonly encountered form at several centers.

The symptoms of AV canal defect are primarily related to increased pulmonary blood flow that results from the septal defect and to the presence of mitral regurgitation that results from mitral deformity. Approximately two-thirds of patients with partial AV canal are asymptomatic at the time of operation, and only one-sixth of patients who are operated on have had severe symptoms, which include dyspnea, fatigue, and frank congestive heart failure. Two-thirds of patients with complete AV canal have developed these symptoms of heart failure, most often during infancy. Patients with the partial form of AV canal are less likely to develop pulmonary hypertension or pulmonary vascular obstructive disease at any age, whereas in the complete form, pulmonary hypertension and progressive pulmonary vascular disease are common in infancy and childhood.

On physical examination, a systolic ejection murmur is noted at the pulmonary area due to increased flow across the pulmonary valve. A diastolic flow murmur across the tricuspid valve can be heard in many patients. A holosystolic apical murmur is often present, but the intensity depends on the degree of associated mitral regurgitation.

The vectorcardiogram helps to confirm the diagnosis, because a counterclockwise frontal loop is almost always present (Toscano-Barbosa et al, 1956); however, such a configuration may exist in other forms of congenital heart disease. Cardiac catheterization and angiography document the presence and magnitude of intracardiac shunting, help to define the degree of mitral regurgitation, and show the classic "gooseneck" configuration of the left ventricular outflow tract (Baron, 1968; Rastelli et al, 1967). The echocardiographic display of these lesions (Bloom et al, 1979; Hagler et al, 1979), particularly in the two-dimensional mode, is useful in distinguishing between the complete and partial forms as well as in defining the anatomic details of the subgroups that are not commonly shown by angiocardiography alone. Doppler echocardiography and color flow imaging allow excellent assessment of left-to-right shunt flow and of the site and degree of AV valve regurgitation (Reeder et al, 1986).

INDICATIONS FOR OPERATION

The guidelines for selecting patients for operation in AV canal anomaly are similar to those for patients who have any type of congenital anomaly that results in increased pulmonary blood flow (Berger et al, 1979). Operation is indicated at any age, including early infancy, when congestive heart failure or significant disability persists despite medical supportive measures or when there is evidence for development of pulmonary vascular disease.

For the asymptomatic infant with partial AV canal and absence of significant pulmonary hypertension, it has been customary to postpone correction until an age of 2 to 4 years. The current safety of operation in infancy makes it possible to operate at the time of diagnosis at any age. Operation is indicated on the basis of the relatively low anticipated hospital mortality for elective correction of partial AV canal (1 to 2%) and on the basis that progressive disability and cardiac failure are common during the second decade of life. For the patient with partial AV canal, the occurrence of progressive pulmonary vascular obstructive disease as a contraindication to operation is uncommon.

Most infants who have the complete form of AV canal have severe pulmonary hypertension and congestive heart failure that respond poorly to medical treatment. Surgical intervention is indicated for these infants. Some controversy remains with regard to whether palliative banding of the pulmonary artery or corrective operation is the better approach (Epstein et al, 1979; Studer et al, 1982). For surgical teams skilled in the repair of AV canal defects and in cardiac surgery for infants, corrective rather than palliative operation appears to be preferred. If the cumulative risks are the same, one operation is preferable to two, and banding of the pulmonary artery does not relieve the hemodynamic effects of mitral regurgitation, which may contribute to congestive heart failure. For the infant with complete AV canal who escapes significant disability and congestive heart failure in infancy, corrective operation is elective during the second year of life to prevent progressive pulmonary vascular obstructive disease (Newfeld et al, 1977).

OPERATIVE TECHNIQUE

Operation for both the partial and complete types of AV canal is done through a median sternotomy and with hypothermic total cardiopulmonary bypass. The ascending aorta is cannulated, and both caval lines are passed through the right atrial appendage so that they can be widely mobilized by the atriotomy to provide optimal intra-atrial exposure. Standard techniques of whole-body perfusion are maintained, including use of a slotted-needle air vent in the ascending aorta. Some surgeons have found that circulatory arrest during profound hypothermia is beneficial for very small infants, but the role of this modality is not firmly defined. Cardioplegic arrest is currently used for myocardial protection. The total time of extracorporeal circulation averages approximately 65 minutes for correction of the partial type of defect and 100 minutes for the complete type.

Partial Atrioventricular Canal

Repair of partial AV canal has two principal objectives: approximation and alignment of the edges of the cleft in the mitral valve and closure of the atrial septal defect with a patch (see Fig. 37–1). The aim is to close the cleft so that the competence of the mitral valve is optimized. Distortion of the leaflet is best avoided by suturing the cleft in an alignment that is the same as that during systolic closure of the valve. Saline is injected into the left ventricle to elevate the leaflets and show the line of closure. Thickened ridges are typically present along the edges of the cleft and are identical in length, as a result of closure of these edges against each other during systole throughout life. Accurate approximation of these ridges provides alignment of the valve, and the ridges themselves provide strength for the suture line. One or two simple sutures are first placed to approximate the cleft near the mitral ring. Then the thickened edges of the cleft at their farthest margin (closest to the free edge of the leaflet) are approximated; a pledgeted mattress suture may be used for additional security of closure. Finally, the intervening sutures are placed.

In the past, if incompetence was minimal or absent before operation, the cleft was often not closed. The authors have observed that mitral insufficiency has developed later in these patients, thus they now prefer to close the cleft. The authors have not found that mitral stenosis results from accurate repair of the mitral cleft. It is not the authors' practice to transect chordae of the mitral valve, including those attached to the ventricular septum, nor do the authors add tissue to the mitral leaflet in the form of a patch of pericardium or synthetic material. Preoperative mitral regurgitation is usually caused by incomplete closure of the cleft in the mitral valve during systole, especially at the base of the valve, and repair of the cleft is effective in reducing or obliterating the regurgitation. In some patients, regurgitation results from annular dilatation or, rarely, from a deficiency of leaflet length from base to free edge, which allows regurgitation through the central portion of the valve during systole. In these patients, insufficiency can often be controlled by a double purse-string annuloplasty around the free wall of the left ventricle, which reduces the circumference of the valve. Competence of the valve is tested by distending the ventricle with saline or blood so that refinements of the repair can be effected as indicated. Almost never is it so obvious that mitral repair will be unsuccessful that replacement of the mitral valve should be done at the time of the primary repair.

The interatrial communication is closed by a patch of pericardium or prosthetic material. The patch is attached to the mitral side of the junction of the mitral and tricuspid valves along the crest of the ventricular septum by using interrupted sutures, which are all placed before the patch is lowered into position (see Fig. 37–1). As this suturing continues toward the posterior (to the right) end of the crest of the ventricular septum, care must be taken to avoid injury to the bundle of His. Injury is avoided by carrying the suture line onto the base of the mitral valve leaflet (see Fig. 37–3). Delineation of the line of separation between the right and left atria along the posterior margin of the defect is facilitated by exerting traction on a suture placed for that purpose in the atrial septal rim of the ostium primum defect. The traction creates a small ridge that demarcates the right atrium from the left atrium. Sutures anchoring the patch should be placed on the left atrial side of that ridge until the suture line reaches the clearly defined septal rim of the ostium primum defect (see Fig. 37–3). The cephalad margin of the patch can then be attached to the rim of the atrial septal defect with continuous sutures.

Intermediate Atrioventricular Canal

So few intermediate types of AV canal have been encountered or reported that techniques for repair have not become standardized. The principles of repair are to leave the mitral and tricuspid valves intact, as for repair of the partial AV canal (with repair of the mitral cleft if appropriate), and to place two septal patches, one to close the interventricular communication and one for the interatrial communication. The two patches are separated from each other along their adjacent edges by the midline fused tricuspid and mitral leaflet tissue but are sutured to

each other by stitches that pass through this leaflet substance.

Complete Atrioventricular Canal

In the classic, one-patch technique, the first step in the repair of complete AV canal is to identify its anatomic characteristics. After the anatomy of the anterior and posterior common leaflets has been determined and the extent of the underlying interventricular communication has been defined, the next step in the repair is approximation of the mitral components of the anterior and posterior common leaflets so as to constitute an anterior (or aortic) leaflet of the mitral valve (Fig. 37–4A). As in partial AV canal, the objective is to avoid distortion of the mitral leaflet tissue as much as possible and to reconstruct the valve in the alignment it would assume during systole in the preoperative state. Again, this alignment is often determined best by floating the leaflets into their closed position by instillation of saline under pressure into the left ventricular cavity. Typically, there are no thickened ridges along the opposing edges of the anterior and posterior components of the anterior mitral leaflet that would correspond to the cleft of the anterior leaflet in the partial form of the defect; the absence of thickened ridges makes it difficult to obtain the appropriate alignment of the mitral valve in the complete form. Sufficient time must be devoted to this step in the reconstruction, even to placing and replacing reconstructing sutures in a trial-and-error manner. Commissural or central leaks found when the valve is tested are repaired by commissural annuloplasty sutures or double free wall purse-string sutures, respectively. As noted for repair of partial AV canal, valve replacement at the initial operation is rarely justified.

The second step in the one-patch repair is to expose the entire length of the crest of the ventricular septal rim of the interventricular communication. In Type A complete AV canal, the natural division in the anterior common leaflet has already resulted in such exposure of most of the underlying ventricular crest (see Fig. 37–4). Even when the division in the anterior common leaflet appears to deviate to the right near the anterior annulus, the underlying septum typically deviates similarly, which facilitates identification of the septal crest. In the Type C variant, it is necessary to incise the anterior common leaflet along a line estimated to demarcate the tricuspid from the mitral components of the anterior common leaflet (Fig. 37–5A, B). The proper site along the free edge for this incision is defined by the line of convergence of chordae from the papillary muscle of the left ventricle with those from the papillary muscle of the right ventricle. The location of the annular end of the incision in the common leaflet is established by the position of the underlying ventricular septum where it joins the annulus of the AV

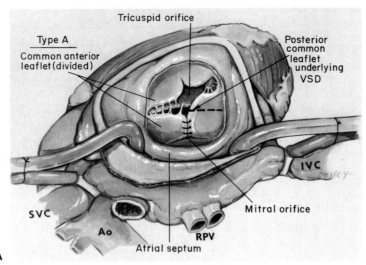

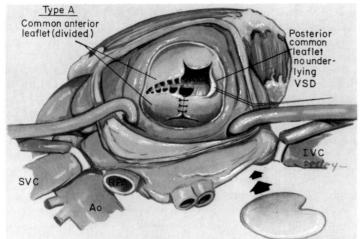

Figure 37–4. Repair of Type A complete AV canal. *A,* The anterior mitral leaflet has been constructed by approximating the edges of the mitral portions of the anterior and posterior common leaflets. The line for incision of the posterior common leaflet is identified by the *dashed* line. *B,* In this case, most of the posterior common leaflet is fused to the crest of the ventricular septum. Thus, there is no need to incise the posterior common leaflet, and the appropriately shaped patch (bottom right) can be attached to the atrial surface of the posterior common leaflet. *C,* The prosthetic patch is sewn to the right aspect of the ventricular septum with interrupted or pledgeted mattress sutures (see Fig. 37–6 for further detail).

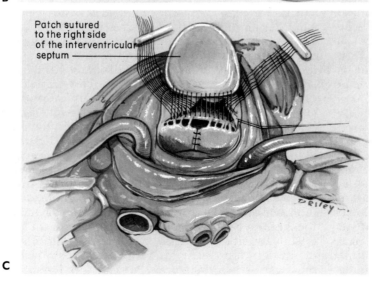

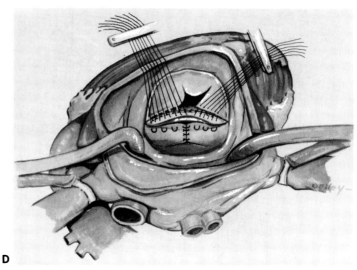

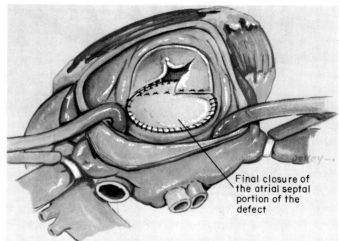

Final closure of the atrial septal portion of the defect

Figure 37–4 *Continued D,* The reconstructed anterior leaflet of the mitral valve is attached to the prosthetic patch with interrupted nonabsorbable mattress sutures in the same plane as the annulus of the AV valve. In this case, where the posterior common leaflet was incised, both edges of this incision (tricuspid and mitral) are attached to the respective surface of the patch. The authors usually prefer to use pledgets in these mattress sutures. *E,* The repair is completed by continuous suture approximation to the rim of the atrial septal defect. (SVC = superior vena cava; IVC = inferior vena cava; Ao = aorta; RPA = right pulmonary artery; VSD = ventricular septal defect; RPV = right pulmonary vein.) (From McMullan, M. H., Wallace, R. B., Weidman, W. H., and McGoon, D. C.: Surgical treatment of complete atrioventricular canal. Surgery, *72*:905, 1972.)

valve. When there is doubt, the authors prefer to err on the side of placing the incision more to the tricuspid aspect than to the mitral aspect of the anterior common leaflet, which is more likely to preserve adequate leaflet area for mitral function. The authors do not agree with the suggestion to incise the common leaflet far to the tricuspid side in a place remote from the underlying ventricular septum.

In the Type A deformity in which the division of the anterior leaflet is incomplete and in most cases of the Type B deformity (Pacifico and Kirklin, 1973), it is necessary to extend the division in the anterior common leaflet by incising the remaining intact bridging portion of the leaflet all the way to the annulus of the AV valve. A similar incision in the posterior common leaflet is almost always required but extends from the free margin of that leaflet only to the posterior limit of the underlying interventricular communication. Often, this interventricular communication does not reach the true annulus of the AV valve because there is a variable length of fibrous fusion of the base of the posterior common

leaflet to the crest of the ventricular septum (Figs. 37–4B and 37–6A, B). The latter is a favorable situation, because it provides a buffer area of intact fibrous septum that protects the conduction bundle from the suture line.

The next step is to close the cardiac septum with a patch of knitted synthetic material. The size of the patch is estimated by measuring the distance from the atrial septal rim to the ventricular septal rim of the defect with a segment of string and then by marking this distance on the patch. Similarly, the distance from the anterior to the posterior aspect of the annulus of the AV canal, that is, the anteroposterior dimension of the septal defect, is measured and marked off on the patch. It is important not to overestimate the anteroposterior dimension because that would enlarge the circumferences of the AV valve annuli and thus decrease the possibility of constructing competent valves. Usually, the two dimensions are approximately equal, and the patch assumes a circular configuration. The edge of the patch that will be approximated to the crest of the ventricular septum is then attached with a row of

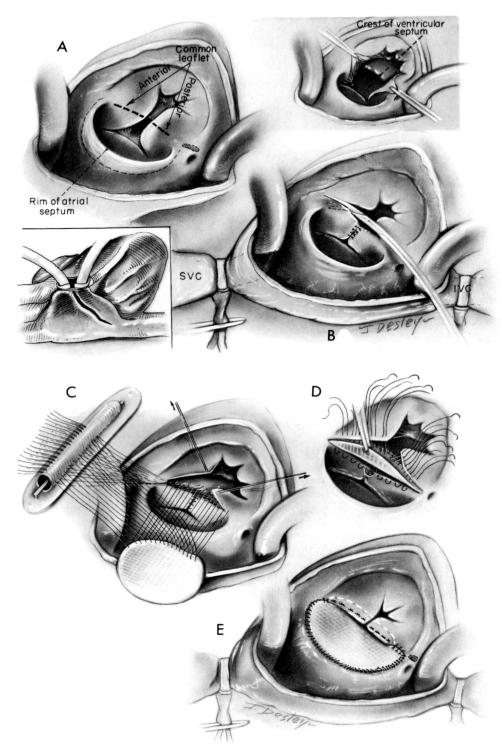

Figure 37–5. Surgical repair of Type C complete AV canal. *A, Heavy broken line* indicates line of incision of the common AV leaflets. *B,* Incisions are accomplished. *C–E,* The remainder of the repair is similar to that shown in Figure 37–4, except (as seen in *D* and *E*) both the tricuspid and the mitral edges of the incised anterior common leaflet are sutured to the respective sides of the patch. Currently, mattress sutures over felt pledgets are preferred to simple sutures. (From Rastelli, G. C., Ongley, P. A., and McGoon, D. C.: Surgical repair of complete atrioventricular canal with anterior common leaflet undivided and unattached to ventricular septum. Mayo Clin. Proc., *44*:335, 1969.)

interrupted sutures, which are placed before lowering the patch into position (see Figs. 37–4C and 37–5C). The authors prefer to use mattress sutures through felt pledgets that pass into the right aspect of the ventricular septum below its crest. Care is taken posteriorly to avoid encirclement of the nonbranching and penetrating portions of the conduction tissue.

In the situation in which the posterior limit of the interventricular communication is sealed off by a membrane between the ventricular septum and the overlying leaflet, the incision in the posterior common leaflet is extended posteriorly only to the limit of the interventricular communication (see Fig. 37–6A, B). From this point on, in a posterosuperior direction, the patch is sutured to the atrial surface of the posterior common leaflet, then to the posterior atrial wall as far to the left as possible, and finally to the atrial septum (see Fig. 37–6A, B) in the same manner as for repair of the partial AV canal described earlier (see Fig. 37–3C, D).

In hearts in which the interventricular communication (or perforating communication) extends all the way to the posterior valvular annulus (see Fig. 37–6C to F), there are two options for placement of the patch to achieve the least risk of heart block. Formerly, the incision was extended in the posterior common leaflet directly to the junction of ventricular septum and AV valvular annulus, with the intent of placing sutures for the patch superficially and close together in this area (see Fig. 37–6C, D). The authors now prefer to extend the incision in the posterior common leaflet along the annulus well to the right of the plane of the ventricular septum so that the patch crosses the anulus to the right of the junction of annulus and ventricular septum and thus to the right of the conduction tissue (see Fig. 37–6E,F). The atrial part of the patch, which is cut with an auricular extension, is attached around the coronary sinus so that it drains into the left atrium (Thiene et al, 1981).

The next step is to anchor the incised edges of the mitral and tricuspid components of the anterior and posterior common leaflets to their respective left and right sides of the prosthetic septal patch. This is done with a single row of interrupted mattress sutures (see Figs. 37–4D and 37–5D). These sutures may be buttressed by fine pledgets, especially in infants, when the valve tissues are thin and friable. This attachment of the mitral and tricuspid leaflets should be at a level on the patch that corresponds to the ideal plane of the orifice of the mitral and tricuspid valves. This level is considered to be along the line to which the leaflet would reach during systole when its retaining chordae were fully stretched and is also in the same plane as the annulus of the common AV valve. For the Type A deformity, the authors consider that it is appropriate to attach the mitral but not the corresponding tricuspid edge of the naturally divided anterior common leaflet to the patch (see Fig. 37–4D). This portion of the tricuspid valve corresponds to the anterior leaflet of the normally developed tricuspid valve, and the base of the anterior tricuspid leaflet does not normally attach to the septum. There is thus a complete deficiency of the anterior portion of the septal leaflet of the tricuspid valve in the Type A deformity (which corresponds to the usual situation in partial AV canal). Tricuspid regurgitation does not typically occur, despite this deficiency of the septal tricuspid leaflet. In Type C deformity, the incised edges of both the tricuspid and the mitral components of the anterior and posterior common leaflets are attached to the patch (see Fig. 37–5D). The tricuspid valve is tested by injecting saline into the right ventricle in a manner similar to testing of the mitral valve.

Interest has been rekindled in the use of two patches for the repair of complete AV canal defects (Carpentier, 1978). The authors have also used this technique successfully, and in infants it may minimize shortening of the reconstructed valve leaflets and decrease the chance for dehiscence of the valve from the prosthetic patch. The atrial patch is usually made from autologous pericardium.

A trifoliate repair of the mitral (left AV) valve has been proposed in which the anterior and posterior portions of the bridging leaflets are not approximated by sutures (Carpentier, 1978). The authors and others (Starr, 1982) found that this repair resulted in an increased incidence of reoperation for mitral insufficiency. Whether this problem represents lack of understanding of the procedure recommended or is inherent in the concept must still be determined. Late results of the trifoliate repair are awaited.

The final step of the repair is the attachment of the cephalad edge of the septal patch to the rim of the atrial septal defect with a continuous suture (see Figs. 37–4E and 37–5E).

After completion of the repair in both the partial and the complete forms, the right atriotomy is closed, air is evacuated from the heart, continuous aspiration is applied to a slotted-needle vent in the ascending aorta, and extracorporeal circulation is gradually discontinued.

The authors use double-sampling dye curves to assess competence of the mitral valve (Danielson, 1984). Intraoperative echocardiography, either with placement of the transducer directly on the heart or by the transesophageal route, can also be used to assess the accuracy of the repair.

The postoperative care of these patients is no different from that of other patients who have had repair of other forms of complex congenital cardiac defects. Right and left atrial and arterial pressures are monitored continuously throughout the first few days after operation. The postoperative course is typically uncomplicated. When a complication occurs, it is usually an arrhythmia of the supraventricular type or reduced cardiac output, which may be exacerbated by the presence of residual mitral regurgitation. The incidence of heart block has been negligible with utilization of the intraoperative precautions (King et al, 1986; McMullan et al, 1972, 1973).

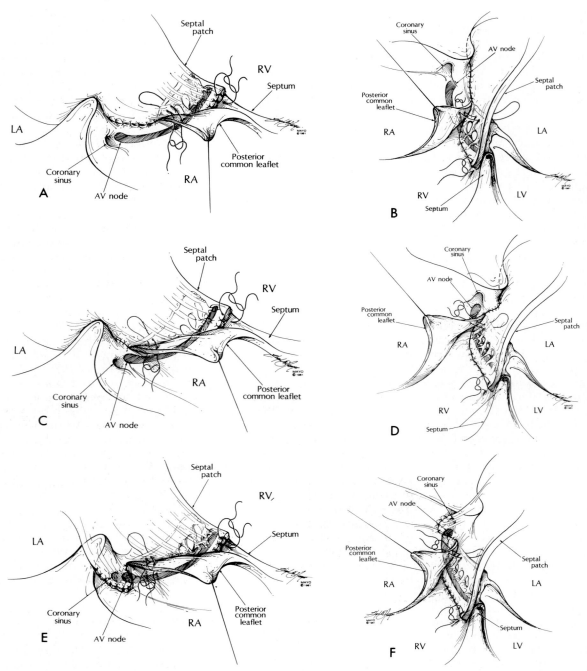

Figure 37–6. *See legend on opposite page*

The difficult surgical treatment of AV canal defect associated with anomalies such as tetralogy of Fallot and other conotruncal malformations has been increasingly successful (Bharati et al, 1980a; Pacifico et al, 1988; Sridaromont et al, 1975; Thiene et al, 1979; Uretzky et al, 1984; Vargas et al, 1986). Surgeons are also having increasing success with repair of AV canal anomalies combined with double-orifice mitral valve, common ventricle, atrial isomerism, AV discordance, and anomalies of cardiac situs and systemic and pulmonary venous return (Danielson, 1984; Lee et al, 1985; Pacifico et al, 1988).

Mitral Valve Replacement

When it is decided that mitral valve replacement is required, whether at the initial (rarely) or subsequent operation, an important anatomic feature bears re-emphasis: A deficiency of the basilar portion of the ventricular septum exists in both partial and complete AV canal lesions, and the patch that is placed to close the septal defect has a ventricular septal portion as well as an atrial septal portion. Stated differently, the plane of the mitral annulus lies at a level that does not follow the crest of the ventricular septum; rather it crosses the patch used to close the septal defect at a level centrally on the patch that is about 1 or 2 cm cephalad (or atrialward) from the crest of the scooped-out portion of the ventricular septum. The mitral valve prosthesis must be attached along the true plane of the mitral annulus. The prosthesis should be secured to the mural aspect of the mitral annulus as always, but on the septal aspect, the line of attachment leaves the edge of the resected natural valve and follows the left surface of the septal patch corresponding to the extended true plane of the mitral orifice.

Left-sided obstructive lesions are common in AV canal anomalies (Piccoli et al, 1982), and the left ventricular outflow tract is typically long and narrow in both the partial and complete forms. Thus, prosthetic valves can obstruct blood flow, produce ventricular arrhythmias by impingement on the ventricular septum, and produce poppet or disk malfunction. These risks are increased if the prosthesis is attached too high on the septal patch.

The principle for attachment of the mitral prosthesis avoids injury to the bundle of His, which courses along the ventricular septal crest. The only area in which the bundle of His is vulnerable in this technique is at the junction of the posterior annulus and the septal patch, thus suturing in this area should be done superficially.

RESULT OF OPERATION

In the entire experience with repair of partial AV canal, the mortality has been approximately 5% or less (King et al, 1986; McMullan et al, 1973). Mortality has not increased with the more frequent application of the operation for infants who are diagnosed or become symptomatic in the early months of life. Similarly, repair of partial AV canal in 52 adults up to 75 years of age (average age, 37 years) was done with a 6% risk (Hynes et al, 1981). The actuarial

freedom from reoperation is 86% at 20 years, and the incidence of late deaths, which are usually related to arrhythmias or the necessity for mitral valve replacement, is a small fraction of 1% per year (King et al, 1986). Most surviving patients with native valves are free of disability; approximately one-fourth show mild symptoms on strenuous exertion.

The results of operation for complete AV canal were unsatisfactory before the development of the current techniques of repair (McGoon et al, 1959). With the current techniques, the hospital mortality decreased from 60% to approximately 10% (McMullan et al, 1972). As more patients in the infant age group were operated on, the mortality initially increased, but more recently mortality for infants has decreased to 5 to 15% at the authors' institution and elsewhere (Bender et al, 1982; Mair and McGoon, 1977; Santos et al, 1986; Starr, 1982; Studer et al, 1982).

An important factor in the early and late results of repair of partial or complete AV canal deformities is the degree of residual mitral valve regurgitation. Intraoperative double-sampling dye dilution studies showed essentially complete absence of mitral regurgitation in approximately 50% of the operations; most of the remainder have mild to moderate regurgitation at the completion of operation. Although valve replacement at the initial operation might appear appropriate for the minority of patients who have persistence of moderate mitral regurgitation after repair, valve replacement is generally not elected because of its inherent limitations. These limitations include inability of the replacement valve to grow with the patient, the need for anticoagulant therapy if a mechanical valve is used, and uncertain durability, particularly of tissue valves. It appears preferable to accept moderate mitral regurgitation with the knowledge that reoperation will be required when mitral valve replacement can no longer be postponed. The overall incidence of reoperation for severe mitral regurgitation is less than 1% per year for older

---

Figure 37–6. Detail for anchoring septal patch posteroinferiorly in complete AV canal and for reconstructing posterior common leaflet. The view for A, C, and E corresponds to the orientation described for Figure 37–3A, and that for B, D, and F corresponds to the orientation described for Figure 37–3B. Illustrated in A and B is the repair used for hearts in which the basilar (or annular) portion of the posterior common leaflet is fused to the underlying ventricular septum by a sheet of fibrous tissue; C and D and E and F show alternatives for repair where no such fusion has occurred. In both situations, the posterior common leaflet has been incised beginning at its free margin (at the estimated point of junction of its tricuspid and mitral portions) to the posterior limit of any interventricular communication below the valve. In A and B, the incision extends only part way to the annulus, and in C, D, E, and F, it extends essentially to the annulus. In A and B, the septal patch is attached to the right surface of the ventricular septal crest where the leaflet has been incised, but continuing posteriorly the suture line then passes along the edge of the fibrous tissue fusing leaflet to septum until it reaches the apex of the incision in the leaflet. The suturing posteriorly from this point proceeds exactly as for partial AV canal, which is described in Figure 37–3. In reality, all the sutures shown were placed before lowering the patch into position, as in Figures 37–4C and 37–5C.

In C and D, which was the authors' usual technique, the incision in the posterior common leaflet extends posteriorly to the junction of atrium, ventricular septum, and annulus; the patch is again attached along the right surface of the ventricular septal crest, and the sutures become even more superficial and more closely spaced as work proceeds posteriorly. The suture at the apex of the leaflet incision (not shown) grasps only leaflet tissue near the annulus but does not penetrate the annulus; the suture line remains superficial as it crosses right to left to reach the left surface of the rim of the atrial septum, as in Figure 37–3.

The authors' currently preferred method is shown in E and F, in which the patch is placed entirely to the right of the conduction tissue; the incision in the posterior common leaflet is extended along the annulus to the right of the level of the coronary sinus ostium; the suture line for the patch passes even farther inferiorly on the right ventricular surface of the ventricular septum to reach the apex of the incision in the leaflet; the patch is then attached entirely to the right atrial side of the coronary-sinus ostium. An alternative would be to attach the patch along the inferior lip of the ostium, allowing the coronary sinus to drain to the right atrium.

patients but appears to be slightly higher for infants, probably because there is more severe valvular deformity in the infant group.

Selected Bibliography

Berger, T. J., Blackstone, E. H., Kirklin, J. W., et al: Survival and probability of cure without and with operation in complete atrioventricular canal. Ann. Thorac. Surg., 27:104, 1979.

This analysis of comparative data for nonsurgically and surgically treated patients with complete AV canal shows that only 54% of patients who did not have operation survived to 6 months of age and 15% survived to 24 months of age. The risk of correction was high in the early months of life but decreased to 1% by the age of 12 months. Among those surviving operation, the 5-year survival rate was excellent (91%).

Carpentier, A.: Surgical anatomy and management of the mitral component of atrioventricular canal defects. In Anderson, R. H., and Shinebourne, E. A. (eds): Paediatric Cardiology 1977. Edinburgh, Churchill Livingstone, 1978, p. 477.

This author has studied extensively and innovatively the surgical anatomy of AV canal defects. He espouses a three-leaflet functional concept for the mitral valve and describes techniques for the extensive mobilization of the leaflets and their support structures plus annular plication. For complete malformations, he recommends reconstruction of the septum with two separate patches, one ventricular and the other atrial.

Piccoli, G. P., Wilkinson, J. L., Macartney, F. J., et al: Morphology and classification of complete atrioventricular defects. Br. Heart J., 42:633, 1979.

This review of the anatomy and classification of the complete form of the anomaly was based on a study of 70 necropsied hearts in the hope of improving on Rastelli's classification. The subdivisions again depended on the morphology of the valve leaflets, but these authors identified five leaflets distinguished by their commissural pattern and support mechanisms. Some innovative surgical implications are discussed.

Thiene, G., Wenink, A. C. G., Frescura, C., et al: The surgical anatomy and pathology of the conduction tissues in atrioventricular defects. J. Thorac. Cardiovasc. Surg., 82:928, 1981.

These authors examined the hearts of 16 patients with AV defects in detail and described their findings from the surgeon's viewpoint. Ten hearts had complete defects and six had partial ones, and the disposition of the conduction tissue was the same in both groups. The anatomy of the triangle of Koch was found to be distorted, and the authors defined a "nodal triangle" lying between the coronary sinus ostium and the annulus that contained the AV node. Techniques for avoiding injury to the node and bundle were suggested.

Bibliography

Baron, M. G.: Endocardial cushion defects. Radiol. Clin. North Am., 6:343, 1968.
Bender, H. W., Jr., Hammon, J. W., Jr., Hubbard, S. G., et al: Repair of atrioventricular canal malformation in the first year of life. J. Thorac. Cardiovasc. Surg., 84:515, 1982.
Berger, T. J., Blackstone, E. H., Kirklin, J. W., et al: Survival and probability of cure without and with operation in complete atrioventricular canal. Ann. Thorac. Surg., 27:104, 1979.
Bharati, S., Kirklin, J. W., McAllister, H. A., Jr., and Lev, M.: The surgical anatomy of common atrioventricular orifice associated with tetralogy of Fallot, double outlet right ventricle and complete regular transposition. Circulation, 61:1142, 1980a.
Bharati, S., Lev, M., McAllister, H. A., Jr., and Kirklin, J. W.: Surgical anatomy of the atrioventricular valve in the intermediate type of common atrioventricular orifice. J. Thorac. Cardiovasc. Surg., 79:884, 1980b.
Bloom, K. R., Freedom, R. M., Williams, C. M., et al: Echocardiographic recognition of atrioventricular valve stenosis associated with endocardial cushion defect: Pathologic and surgical correlates. Am. J. Cardiol., 44:1326, 1979.
Carpentier, A.: Surgical anatomy and management of the mitral component of atrioventricular canal defects. In Anderson, R. H., and Shinebourne, E. A. (eds): Pediatric Cardiology 1977. Edinburgh, Churchill Livingstone, 1978, p. 477.
Danielson, G. K.: Repair of atrioventricular canal: The "classic" (one-patch) operative approach. In Moulton, A. L. (ed): Congenital Heart Surgery—Current Techniques and Controversies. Pasadena, CA, Appleton Davies, 1984, pp. 317–329.
Epstein, M. L., Moller, J. H., Amplatz, K., and Nicoloff, D. M.: Pulmonary banding in infants with complete atrioventricular canal. J. Thorac. Cardiovasc. Surg., 78:28, 1979.
Feldt, R. H.: Atrioventricular Canal Defects. Philadelphia, W. B. Saunders Company, 1976.
Hagler, D. J., Tajik, A. J., Seward, J. B., et al: Real-time wide-angle sector echocardiography: Atrioventricular canal defects. Circulation, 59:140, 1979.
Hynes, J. K., Tajik, A. J., Seward, J. B., et al: Partial atrioventricular canal defect in adults. Am. J. Cardiol., 47:466, 1981.
King, R. M., Puga, F. J., Danielson, G. K., et al: Prognostic factors and surgical treatment of partial atrioventricular canal. Circulation, 74:42, 1986.
Lee, C. N., Danielson, G. K., Schaff, H. V., et al: Surgical treatment of double-orifice mitral valve in atrioventricular canal defects: Experience in 25 patients. J. Thorac. Cardiovasc. Surg., 90:700, 1985.
Mair, D. D., and McGoon, D. C.: Surgical correction of atrioventricular canal during the first year of life. Am. J. Cardiol., 40:66, 1977.
McGoon, D. C., DuShane, J. W., and Kirklin, J. W.: The surgical treatment of endocardial cushion defects. Surgery, 46:185, 1959.
McMullan, M. H., McGoon, D. C., Wallace, R. B., et al: Surgical treatment of partial atrioventricular canal. Arch. Surg., 107:705, 1973.
McMullan, M. H., Wallace, R. B., Weidman, W. H., and McGoon, D. C.: Surgical treatment of complete atrioventricular canal. Surgery, 72:905, 1972.
Newfeld, E. A., Sher, M., and Paul, M. H.: Pulmonary vascular disease in complete atrioventricular canal defect. Am. J. Cardiol., 39:721, 1977.
Pacifico, A. D., and Kirklin, J. W.: Surgical repair of complete atrioventricular canal with anterior common leaflet attached to an anomalous right ventricular papillary muscle. J. Thorac. Cardiovasc. Surg., 65:727, 1973.
Pacifico, A. D., Kirklin, J. W., and Bargeron, L. M., Jr.: Repair of complete atrioventricular canal associated with tetralogy of Fallot or double outlet right ventricle: Report of 10 patients. Ann. Thorac. Surg., 29:351, 1980.
Pacifico, A. D., Ricchi, A., Bargeron, L. M., Jr., et al: Corrective repair of complete atrioventricular canal defects and major associated cardiac anomalies. Ann. Thorac. Surg., 46:645, 1988.
Piccoli, G. P., Ho, S. Y., Wilkinson, J. L., et al: Left-sided obstructive lesions in atrioventricular septal defects: An anatomical study. J. Thorac. Cardiovasc. Surg., 83:453, 1982.
Piccoli, G. P., Wilkinson, J. L., Macartney, F. J., et al: Morphology and classification of complete atrioventricular defects. Br. Heart J., 42:633, 1979.
Rastelli, G. C., Kirklin, J. W., and Kincaid, O. W.: Angiocardiography of persistent common atrioventricular canal. Mayo Clin. Proc., 42:200, 1967.
Rastelli, G. C., Kirklin, J. W., and Titus, J. L.: Anatomic observations on complete form of persistent common atrioventricular canal with special reference to atrioventricular valves. Mayo Clin. Proc., 41:296, 1966.

Reeder, G. S., Currie, P. J., Hagler, D. J., et al: Use of Doppler techniques (continuous-wave, pulsed wave, and color flow imaging) in the noninvasive hemodynamic assessment of congenital heart disease. Mayo Clin. Proc., 61:725, 1986.

Santos, A., Boucek, M., Ruttenberg, H., et al: Repair of atrioventricular septal defects in infancy. J. Thorac. Cardiovasc. Surg., 91:505, 1986.

Sridaromont, S., Feldt, R. H., Ritter, D. G., et al: Double-outlet right ventricle associated with persistent common atrioventricular canal. Circulation, 52:933, 1975.

Starr, A.: Discussion of Bender et al. J. Thorac. Cardiovasc. Surg., 84:515, 1982.

Studer, M., Blackstone, E. H., Kirklin, J. W., et al: Determinants of early and late results of repair of atrioventricular septal (canal) defects. J. Thorac. Cardiovasc. Surg., 84:523, 1982.

Thiene, G., Frescura, C., Di Donato, R., and Gallucci, R.: Complete atrioventricular canal associated with conotruncal malformations: Anatomical observations in 13 specimens. Eur. J. Cardiol., 9:199, 1979.

Thiene, G., Wenink, A. C. G., Frescura, C., et al: The surgical anatomy and pathology of the conduction tissues in atrioventricular defects. J. Thorac. Cardiovasc. Surg., 82:928, 1981.

Toscano-Barbosa, E., Brandenburg, R. O., and Burchell, H. B.: Electrocardiographic studies of cases with intracardiac malformations of the atrioventricular canal. Mayo Clin. Proc., 31:513, 1956.

Uretzky, G., Puga, F. J., Danielson, G. K., et al: Complete atrioventricular canal associated with tetralogy of Fallot: Morphologic and surgical considerations. J. Thorac. Cardiovasc. Surg., 87:756, 1984.

Vargas, F. J., Otero Coto, E., Mayer, J. E., Jr., et al: Complete atrioventricular canal and tetralogy of Fallot: Surgical considerations. Ann. Thorac. Surg., 42:258, 1986.

CHAPTER 38

SURGICAL TREATMENT OF VENTRICULAR SEPTAL DEFECT

A. D. Pacifico
John W. Kirklin
James K. Kirklin

A ventricular septal defect (VSD) is a hole in the interventricular septum that can occur as a primary anomaly with or without additional major associated cardiac defects. A VSD may occur as a single component of a wide variety of intracardiac anomalies that include the tetralogy of Fallot, complete atrioventricular canal defects, transposition of the great arteries, corrected transposition, and other anomalies. The defect in its isolated form is considered in this chapter.

HISTORICAL ASPECTS

A VSD was first repaired in 1954 by Lillehei and associates (1955) at the University of Minnesota. They described an experience with eight patients, five in their first year of life, who had VSD closure by using controlled cross-circulation with an adult as the pump oxygenator. Cardiac ischemia was avoided because the aorta was not cross-clamped, and six of the eight patients survived. This dramatic and spectacular experience was the beginning of the era of intracardiac surgery and is a great tribute to the skill and courage of these surgeons.

In 1956, an experience was reported from the Mayo Clinic with 20 patients who had intracardiac closure of large VSDs by using a mechanical pump oxygenator beginning in March 1955 (DuShane et al, 1956). The duration of cardiopulmonary bypass was from 10 to 45 minutes by using normothermic flow rates of 70 ml/kg/min or approximately 2.1 l/min/m². A pump sucker system was used to return intracardiac blood to the pump oxygenator. Four (20%) patients died in the hospital.

The feasibility of a transatrial approach to VSD closure was shown by Lillehei in 1957 (Stirling et al, 1957). Kirklin and associates (1961) reported an experience of primary repair of VSD in infants, as well as Sloan and associates (Sigmann et al, 1967). The

technique of profound hypothermia with surface cooling, total circulatory arrest, and rewarming by a pump oxygenator was applied successfully to infants with VSD by Okamoto and associates (1969). Barratt-Boyes reported an experience commencing in 1969 which showed that routine primary repair of VSD in six small infants was superior to pulmonary artery banding (Barratt-Boyes et al, 1976).

MORPHOLOGY

The interventricular septum can be considered as having three muscular components that are called the inlet septum, the apical trabecular septum, and the outlet (or infundibular) septum. In addition, there is a fourth component that is fibrous and is called the membranous septum (Fig. 38–1). In the normal heart, the tricuspid valve and mitral valves are attached to the ventricular septum at different levels so that the tricuspid valve attachment is apically

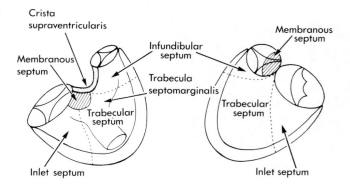

Figure 38–1. The components of the ventricular septum as seen from the right ventricle *(A)* and left ventricle *(B)*. (From Soto, B., et al: Classification of ventricular septal defects. Br. Heart J., 43:332, 1980.)

1314

displaced compared with that of the mitral valve. Thus, a portion of the ventricular septum is left and is placed between the right atrium and the left ventricle, which is called the atrioventricular muscular septum. It is usually present in most hearts with an isolated VSD. More anteriorly, the tricuspid valve attachment divides the area of the membranous septum into an interventricular component between the left and right ventricles and an atrioventricular component between the left ventricle and the right atrium. When an isolated VSD is present, the atrioventricular component of the membranous septum is usually intact.

Soto and associates (1980) proposed a classification of VSDs that is surgically useful (Fig. 38–2). Defects were classified as perimembranous when they were in the general area of the membranous septum, as muscular defects when they were completely surrounded by muscular tissue, and as subarterial defects when either the aortic or pulmonary valves formed part of the rim of the defect within the infundibular or outlet septum. Perimembranous defects can extend into the inlet, trabecular, or outlet septa and make them confluent with these areas (Fig. 38–3). The atrioventricular canal type of VSD is a perimembranous defect that extends into the inlet septum; the septal leaflet of the tricuspid valve forms its border on the right side. Perimembranous VSDs are related to the anteroseptal commissure of the tricuspid valve and also to the aortic valve. The annulus of these valves often forms part of the rim of the defect, but in some cases it is separated from the VSD by a thin rim of muscular tissue.

Approximately 10% of VSDs are located in the infundibulum or outlet septum. When the aortic and pulmonary valve annuli form part of the rim of the defect, they are called subarterial and form the majority of defects in this location. A few defects in the infundibular septum are surrounded completely by muscle and are called infundibular muscular defects. Most muscular defects are located in the trabecular portion of the ventricular septum where they may

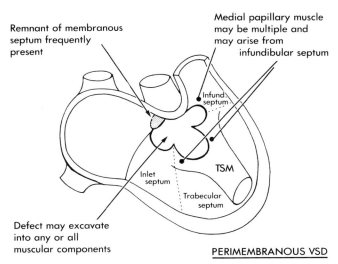

Figure 38–3. The types of perimembranous ventricular septal defects are shown with excavation into the inlet, trabecular and outlet septa. (TSM = trabecula septomarginalis; Infund = infundibular.) (From Soto, B., et al: Classification of ventricular septal defects. Br. Heart J., *43*:332, 1980.)

be single or multiple. When they are multiple, they are usually located in the anterior portion of the trabecular septum.

VSDs vary infinitely in size, and their division into groups is arbitrary. A large VSD is approximately the size of the aortic orifice or larger and results in systemic right ventricular pressure. Small VSDs have insufficient size to raise right ventricular systolic pressure, and the pulmonary-systemic flow ratio (Q_P/Q_S) does not increase above 1.75. Moderate-sized VSDs are "restrictive" but have sufficient size to raise the right ventricular systolic pressure to approximately half of the left ventricular pressure and may result in a Q_P/Q_S of 2 to 3.5. Several small defects may together behave as a large defect.

ASSOCIATED LESIONS IN "PRIMARY" VENTRICULAR SEPTAL DEFECT

Almost half of the patients having surgical treatment for "primary" VSD have an associated lesion (Barratt-Boyes et al, 1976; Blackstone et al, 1976). A *moderate- or large-sized patent ductus arteriosus* is present in approximately 6% of the patients of all ages, but in infants in heart failure, approximately 25% have an associated significant ductus (Barratt-Boyes et al, 1976). A VSD occurs in combination with *severe coarctation* in approximately 12% of patients. However, this combination is also more common among infants with large VSD coming to operation when less than 3 months old.

Congenital *valvar or subvalvar aortic stenosis* occurs in approximately 4% of patients requiring operation for VSD. Subvalvar stenosis is more common (Lauer et al, 1960) and may also occur in association with VSD and infundibular pulmonary stenosis. It may also develop after pulmonary artery banding (Freed

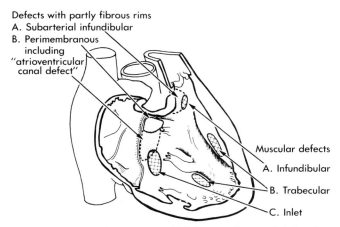

Defects with partly fibrous rims
A. Subarterial infundibular
B. Perimembranous including "atrioventricular canal defect"

Muscular defects
A. Infundibular
B. Trabecular
C. Inlet

Figure 38–2. Classification of VSDs according to their location within the septum. (From Soto, B., et al: Classification of ventricular septal defects. Br. Heart J., *43*:332, 1980.)

et al, 1973). This subvalvar stenosis is of two types. One type is in the form of a discrete fibromuscular bar that lies inferior (caudad or upstream) to the VSD. The other is distal (downstream) to the VSD and often consists of a displacement of infundibular septal muscle into the left ventricular outflow tract. This latter type is often associated with aortic arch anomalies (Dirksen et al, 1978; Moulaert et al, 1976; Van Praagh et al, 1971). Significant *congenital mitral valve disease* occurs in approximately 2% of patients. One or the other pulmonary artery may be absent or severely stenotic. Severe peripheral pulmonary artery stenoses rarely occur. Severe positional cardiac anomalies, such as isolated dextrocardia or situs inversus totalis, exist uncommonly in patients with simple VSD.

A number of minor anomalies may also be present in patients coming to operation for VSD (Table 38–1). In small infants, a large atrial septal defect coexisting with a large VSD may be a significant lesion (Barratt-Boyes et al, 1976).

PULMONARY VASCULAR DISEASE

The classic description of the pathology of hypertensive pulmonary vascular disease is that of Heath and Edwards (1958). They defined Grade 1 changes as being characterized by medial hypertrophy without intimal proliferation; Grade 2 by medial hypertrophy with cellular intimal reaction; Grade 3 by intimal fibrosis as well as medial hypertrophy, and possibly with early generalized vascular dilation; Grade 4 by generalized vascular dilation, an area of

TABLE 38–1. ASSOCIATED CONDITIONS OF MINOR ANATOMIC OR FUNCTIONAL SIGNIFICANCE IN 138 PATIENTS WITH LARGE "PRIMARY" VENTRICULAR SEPTAL DEFECTS AND WITHOUT ASSOCIATED CONDITIONS OF MAJOR ANATOMIC OR FUNCTIONAL SIGNIFICANCE AT UAB (1967–1976)*

Condition	No. and % of Patients†
None	73 (53%)
Mild or moderate pulmonary stenosis	27 (20%)
Atrial septal defect‡	24 (17%)
Persistent left superior vena cava	12 (9%)
Dextroposition of the aorta	7 (5%)
Aneurysm of membranous septum	2 (1%)
Mild or moderate coarctation of aorta	2 (1%)
Vascular ring	1 (0.7%)
Tricuspid incompetence, mild	2 (1%)
Mitral incompetence, mild	—
Pulmonary valve incompetence	1 (0.7%)
Hepatic veins entering right atrium directly	1 (0.7%)
Anomalous right ventricular muscle band without pulmonary stenosis	1 (0.7%)

*Modified from Blackstone, E. H., Kirklin, J. W., Bradley, E. L., et al: Optimal age and results in repair of large ventricular septal defects. J. Thorac. Cardiovasc. Surg., 72:661, 1976.

†Sum of percentages is > 100%, because some patients had more than one minor associated condition.

‡Exclusive of simple patent foramen ovale.

vascular occlusion by intimal fibrosis, and plexiform lesions; Grade 5 by other "dilation lesions" such as cavernous and angiomatoid lesions; and Grade 6 by, in addition, necrotizing arteritis.

The pulmonary resistance in patients with a large VSD (and those with a large patent ductus arteriosus) has been correlated positively with the histologic severity of the hypertensive pulmonary vascular disease by Heath and colleagues (1958). However, the authors have re-analyzed their data and find that the "confidence bands" are rather wide around the probability of severe pulmonary vascular disease as predicted from the pulmonary resistance. This is not unexpected, because the Heath-Edwards classification is based on the most severe lesion seen, regardless of its frequency. Furthermore, as emphasized by Wagenvoort (Wagenvoort et al, 1961; Wagenvoort and Wagenvoort, 1970) and by Yamaki and Tezuka (1976), the grading should include an assessment of the number of vessels affected. Moreover, the calculation of pulmonary vascular resistance is open to many errors.

A slightly different view of hypertensive pulmonary vascular disease in infants with large VSD has been provided by Reid and colleagues (Hislop et al, 1975). Other physicians had emphasized earlier that intimal proliferation (and thus Heath-Edwards changes of Grade 2 or more) rarely develops in infants with large VSD until 1 or 2 years of age (Wagenvoort et al, 1961), and yet, infants occasionally do have severely elevated pulmonary resistance. Reid and associates found that infants dying at 3 to 6 months of age with large VSD and high pulmonary vascular resistance (> 8 units/m²) with intermittent right-to-left shunting have marked medial hypertrophy affecting both large and small pulmonary arteries, including those less than 200 μ in diameter (Hislop et al, 1975). The usual number of intra-acinar vessels was present. However, they found that infants (3 to 10 months old) with large VSD, dying with a history of large pulmonary blood flow and congestive heart failure and normal or slightly raised pulmonary vascular resistance, have medial hypertrophy affecting mainly arteries with diameters larger than 200 μ. The intra-acinar vessels were less than usual.

The histologic reversibility of pulmonary vascular disease after closure of the VSD has not been documented. The favorable results in infants may be from an increased number of arterioles and capillaries as growth proceeds. Presumably, pulmonary vascular disease of Heath-Edwards Grade 3 or greater severity is not reversible.

PATHOPHYSIOLOGY

Determinants of Size and Direction of Shunt. The magnitude and direction of the shunt across a VSD depend on the size of the defect and the pressure gradient across it during the various phases of the cardiac cycle. The authors have observed these relations with biplane cineangiocardiograms in a large number of patients. Jarmakani and colleagues (1968) and Levin and associates (1966) have studied them with special techniques.

When the VSD is small, it offers considerable resistance to flow, and slight variations in the size of the defect are accompanied by large variations in the rate of flow (or shunting). Across small defects, only a large pressure difference, such as that which occurs during mid and late systole, results in significant flow. When the defect is large, it offers little resistance to flow, and small pressure differences between the left and right ventricle result in shunting. The pressure relations during the entire cardiac cycle must therefore be considered in patients with large defects.

The pressure relations late in systole appear mainly related to the output resistance to left and right ventricular ejection. The determinants of those during diastole and early systole are more complicated. They include the relative compliance of the two ventricles and the relative pressures in the two atria. Asynchronous systole of the two ventricles relates to the pressure relations in the early portion of systole and diastole.

The size of the VSD itself may vary during various phases of the cardiac cycle. Also, an apparently large VSD may be partially closed during ventricular systole by a flap of muscle or tissue. It is possible that defects in the muscular septum are considerably smaller during systole than during diastole or when seen at operation or autopsy.

Sequelae of Left-to-Right Shunting. When a left-to-right shunt is present at ventricular level, pulmonary blood flow is increased above normal and systemic blood flow. Thus, flow through the left atrium and the mitral valve orifice is similarly increased, and greater work is done by both the left and the right ventricles. The left atrium is enlarged to a degree corresponding to the magnitude of increase in pulmonary blood flow, and a diastolic murmur may be heard over the apex of the heart, reflecting the increase in the blood flow across the mitral valve. Left atrial pressure becomes raised relative both to normal and to right atrial pressure as the result of a natural adaptive process related to the Starling-Frank mechanism. The left ventricle is larger than normal, and the right ventricle is dilated.

The raised left atrial (and pulmonary venous) pressure causes many infants with VSD to have an increased amount of interstitial fluid in the lungs. As a result, they tend to have repeated pulmonary infections. The lungs are relatively noncompliant, and the work of breathing is increased. This increases energy expenditure, which, along with the relatively low systemic blood flow, causes these infants to have striking growth failure. These sequelae are well reflected in the physical findings, chest films, and electrocardiograms of patients with VSD and large pulmonary blood flow (DuShane and Kirklin, 1960).

When pulmonary resistance rises in patients with large VSD as a result of the development of pulmonary vascular disease, pulmonary blood flow is reduced, left atrial pressure lessens, and the sequelae of left-to-right shunting lessen. The infant or child appears to improve: as pulmonary infections subside, the work of breathing decreases, and growth improves. Unfortunately, further increases in pulmonary vascular resistance occur slowly, and the classic Eisenmenger complex results. In these patients with severe pulmonary hypertension and bidirectional shunting of equal magnitude in the two directions, the left ventricle is not enlarged and the right ventricle is hypertrophied, but its volume does not increase.

NATURAL HISTORY

Spontaneous Closure. VSDs have a tendency to close spontaneously, and this fact is relevant to decisions about operation (Collins et al, 1972). Spontaneous closure can be complete by 1 year of age, or the defect may have only narrowed by then. Complete closure takes considerably longer. The phenomenon of spontaneous closure or narrowing of VSDs explains the infrequency with which large VSDs are encountered in adults. An inverse relationship exists between the probability of eventual spontaneous closure and the age at which the patient is observed (Blackstone et al, 1976; Hoffman and Rudolph, 1965; Keith et al, 1971). (Fig. 38–4). This is highly relevant to clinical decisions about individual patients. According to these data, approximately 80% of individuals seen at 1 month of age with large VSDs have eventual spontaneous closure, as do approximately 60% of those seen at 3 months of age, approximately 50% of those seen at 6 months of age, and 25% of those seen at 12 months of age.

Pulmonary Vascular Disease. A large VSD predisposes the patient to the development of an increased pulmonary vascular resistance from hypertensive pulmonary vascular disease, which tends to grow worse as the individual gets older (Auld et al, 1963; Lucas et al, 1961). Thus, the proportion of patients with large VSD who have a severely raised pulmonary vascular resistance is related directly to the age of the patient. Patients with severe pulmonary vascular disease are usually dead by 40 years of age (Fig. 38–5).

The statement that some infants less than 2 years of age with large VSD have severely raised pulmonary vascular resistance is doubted by some physicians, but its occurrence is well documented (Barratt-Boyes et al, 1976). It is, however, uncommon. It occurs in some infants because they do not have the usual fall in pulmonary vascular resistance a few weeks to a few months after birth. Others do have this but later, in the first 2 years of life, develop a rapid increase in pulmonary vascular resistance (Hoffman and Rudolph, 1966). Some infants who

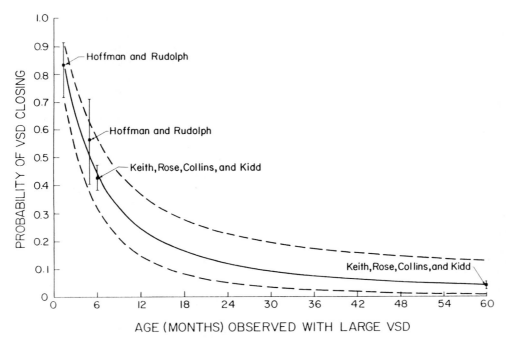

Figure 38–4. Probability of eventual spontaneous closure of a large VSD according to the age at which the patient is observed. The *broken lines* enclose the 70% CLs around the solid probability line. The specific ratios, with the 70% CLs reported by Hoffman and Rudolph (1966) and Keith and associates (1971), are shown centered on the mean or assumed ages of patients in their reports. ($p < 0.0001$.) (From Blackstone, E. H., Kirklin, J. W., Bradley, E. L., et al: Optimal age and results in repair of large ventricular septal defects. J. Thorac. Cardiovasc. Surg., 72:661, 1976.)

have a large VSD have normal or mildly raised resistance. They retain this through the first decade of life, and then, if their VSD is still large, later on develop more severe changes (Keith et al, 1971; Kirklin et al, 1963).

Bacterial Endocarditis. This is rare and occurs at a rate of approximately 0.3% per year in individuals with VSD (Campbell, 1971; Corone et al, 1977; Shah et al, 1966). Often, a pulmonary process is the presenting feature, presumably developing from emboli secondary to right-sided bacterial vegetations. Prognosis with treatment is excellent.

Premature Death. Previous experience and reports in the literature indicate that without surgical treatment some infants (approximately 9% of those with large VSD) die of their disease in the first year of life (Ash, 1964; Keith et al, 1971). Death may result from congestive heart failure, which may develop very early but usually occurs at approximately 2 to 3 months of age, presumably because at about this time the left-to-right shunt becomes larger as the medial hypertrophy present in the small pulmonary arteries at birth regresses. Death may also result from recurrent pulmonary infections secondary to pulmonary edema from the high pulmonary venous pressure. Death is most likely to occur in those infants with large VSD who have associated conditions of major anatomic or functional significance, such as patent ductus arteriosus, coarctation of the aorta, or a large atrial septal defect (Barratt-Boyes et al, 1976).

After the age of 1 year, few if any patients die because of their VSD until the second decade of life. By then, most patients whose VSDs have remained large have developed pulmonary vascular disease and in subsequent years die from complications of Eisenmenger complex (Clarkson et al, 1968) (see Fig. 38–5). These include hemoptysis, polycythemia, cerebral abscess or infarction, and right-sided heart failure.

Patients with *small* VSDs do not develop pulmonary vascular disease and are unlikely to die

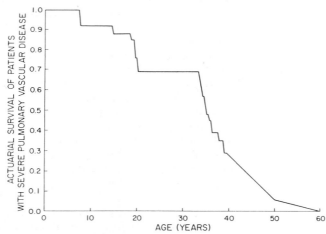

Figure 38–5. Actuarial survival of patients with large VSD who had proven elevation of pulmonary vascular resistance to a level that made them inoperable ($\geq$ 10 units/m²) demonstrated at cardiac catheterization done at various ages. Note that fatalities begin to occur in the second decade of life, that about one half of the patients are dead by 35 years of age, and that a few survive until 50 years of age. (Modified from Clarkson, P. M., Frye, R. L., DuShane, J. W., et al: Prognosis for patients with ventricular septal defect and severe pulmonary vascular obstructive disease. Circulation, *38*:129, 1968. By permission of the American Heart Association, Inc.)

prematurely. Their only real risk is bacterial endocarditis, the incidence of which is low (estimated to occur once in 500 patient years [Shah et al, 1966]). It is generally well treated by antibiotics.

Symptoms. Patients with small VSDs rarely have symptoms related to the defect. Patients with large VSDs may have symptoms of intractable heart failure in the first few months of life, with poor peripheral pulses, inability to feed, sweating, and chronic pulmonary edema. Approximately one-half of the patients coming to operation in the first 2 years of life do so because of this (Table 38–2) (Barratt-Boyes et al, 1976). During early life, rapid and labored respiration and recurrent pulmonary infections may occur secondary to high pulmonary venous pressure and chronic pulmonary edema. At any time in the first year of life, lobes of the lung may become chronically hyperinflated because of pressure of the large and tense pulmonary arteries on the bronchi, preventing complete escape of air during expiration (Oh et al, 1978). As a result of all this, many babies with large VSDs are small and physically underdeveloped. It is these symptomatic patients who fail to respond well to medical management who are at particular risk of dying in the first year of life. Some babies who survive through the first year of life with large VSD have controlled heart failure and failure to thrive in the second year of life as well.

Children and young adults with large VSDs are usually symptomatic and tend to be small both in height and weight. As pulmonary vascular disease develops, symptoms may regress.

Development of Aortic Incompetence. A small proportion of patients (probably approximately 5% in white and black races) develop aortic valve incompetence as a complication of VSD. The incompetence is not present at birth but develops during the first decade of life. It gradually worsens so that by the end of the second decade, it is usually severe. As the incompetence increases, the shunt often decreases, owing to occlusion of the VSD by the prolapsed aortic cusp.

Development of Infundibular Pulmonary Steno-

sis. A small proportion (perhaps 5 to 10%) of patients with large VSD and large left-to-right shunt in infancy develop infundibular pulmonary stenosis (Gasul et al, 1957; Hoffman and Rudolph, 1970; Keith et al, 1971). The mild and moderate infundibular pulmonary stenoses in patients operated on for "primary" VSD (see Table 38–1) as well as the more important stenoses probably develop in this way. The stenosis may become sufficiently severe to produce shunt reversal and cyanosis, and the condition can then properly be tetralogy of Fallot. Somerville's data (1970) indicate that this transformation occurs in approximately 6% of infants with isolated VSD. Those who have the transformation probably are born with some anterior displacement of the infundibular septum and its extensions.

DIAGNOSIS

Examination

The infant with a large VSD and increased pulmonary blood flow presents a particular and highly characteristic clinical picture. Tachypnea with marked subcostal retraction, severe growth failure, and lack of subcutaneous tissue are evident. A waxen complexion and evidence of profuse sweating such as hair that is damp or matted from recently dried perspiration may be noted. The external jugular venous pulses are usually prominent when the infant is supine and often even when he or she is held erect. A bulging precordium is a common finding. On palpation, a rapid, overactive heart is apparent. A thrill is maximal in the third to fifth intercostal spaces on the left. The loud pansystolic murmur is also maximal in the third to fifth intercostal spaces on the left. A short mid-diastolic murmur is usually appreciated at the apex and gives the entire cardiac cycle a gallop quality. The second sound at the base is usually loud and may be slightly split. The liver and spleen are usually enlarged, and the peripheral pulses are rapid and thready. These infants obviously have heart failure, and many are actually in shock.

In older patients with large VSDs, a protruding sternum, or so-called pigeon breast deformity, is found frequently. Presumably, this is due to the large right ventricle pushing the sternum anteriorly during the period of growth. A systolic thrill over the left precordium is often present. The characteristic murmur of VSD is a pansystolic harsh murmur heard in the second, third, and maximally in the fourth left interspace in the midclavicular line (Leatham and Segal, 1962). In patients with a large pulmonary blood flow, there may be a superimposed systolic ejection murmur originating in the area of the pulmonary valve. Characteristically, an early diastolic filling murmur is heard at the apex, indicating a large flow across the mitral valve. The first heart sound at the base is normal; the second sound at the base is abnormally split, owing both to shortened

TABLE 38–2. INDICATIONS FOR REPAIR OF VENTRICULAR SEPTAL DEFECT IN PATIENTS OPERATED ON IN THE FIRST 2 YEARS OF LIFE*

Indication for VSD Repair	No.	% of Total	Age in Months Average	Age in Months (Range)
Intractable congestive heart failure	30	53	2.9	(1 to 7)
Recurrent respiratory infections	3	5	8	(6 to 9)
Controlled congestive heart failure and failure to thrive	17	30	11.4	(4 to 21)
Increased pulmonary vascular resistance	7	12	14.6	(10 to 19)

*Modified from Barratt-Boyes, B. G., Neutze, J. M., Clarkson, P. M., et al: Repair of ventricular septal defect in the first two years of life using profound hypothermia-circulatory arrest techniques. Ann. Surg., *184*:376, 1976.

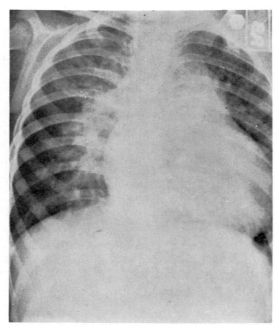

Figure 38–6. Chest film of a child with a large VSD, large pulmonary blood flow, and pulmonary hypertension, but only mild elevation of pulmonary vascular resistance. This is reflected in the evidence of left and right ventricular enlargement, enlargement of the main pulmonary artery, and sharp increase in pulmonary blood flow.

left ventricular ejection time and to prolonged right ventricular ejection time. The splitting is accentuated in inspiration.

These classic physical findings are altered by the size of the VSD and the magnitude of the pulmonary vascular resistance. Patients with small VSDs and small left-to-right shunts have only a systolic murmur. The heart is not hyperactive, and on palpation, there is no enlargement of the left ventricle and no right ventricular lift. Not only do patients with large VSD, mild elevation of pulmonary vascular resistance, and large pulmonary blood flow have the characteristic systolic murmur, but in addition, the heart is hyperactive, the left ventricle is enlarged on palpation, there is a right ventricular lift, there is an apical diastolic rumble, and the second sound at the base is moderately accentuated. In patients with a large VSD and high pulmonary vascular resistance, and consequently with a net left-to-right shunt that is small or with shunts that are bidirectional and of approximately equal magnitude in the two directions, the heart is quiet on examination. There is no evidence on palpation of left ventricular enlargement, but the right ventricular lift is prominent. The systolic murmur is soft and short, or may almost be absent. There is no apical diastolic rumble. The second sound at the base is greatly accentuated. Patients in whom the pulmonary vascular resistance has become higher than systemic resistance are, of course, cyanotic.

Chest Film

The chest film in a patient with a VSD reflects the pathophysiology. Patients with small VSDs and

small left-to-right shunts usually have normal chest films; those with large VSDs, mild elevation of pulmonary vascular resistance, and large left-to-right shunts have characteristic chest films (Fig. 38–6). In the latter, pulmonary arteries, both centrally and peripherally, are large, indicating large pulmonary blood flow. There may be evidence of some enlargement of the left atrium; the left ventricle is abnormally large; and the right ventricle appears dilated. When the physician sees *marked* enlargement of the left atrium in a patient suspected of having a VSD, the coexistence of significant mitral valvular incompetence should be suspected.

When the patient has a large VSD and severe rise in pulmonary vascular resistance, the appearance of the chest film is different. The peripheral pulmonary arteries are normal in size, and there is no evidence of increased pulmonary blood flow. The main pulmonary artery is often greatly enlarged. There is no evidence of left atrial or left ventricular enlargement. The right ventricle may appear slightly enlarged, but often the cardiac silhouette, other than the large pulmonary artery, is essentially normal (Fig. 38–7).

Electrocardiogram

If the defect is large and the pulmonary vascular resistance is only mildly raised, there is evidence of overload of both ventricles. The R wave from the right precordial leads is tall, and when right ventricular peak pressure is similar to left ventricular peak pressure it is notched on the upstroke. The left

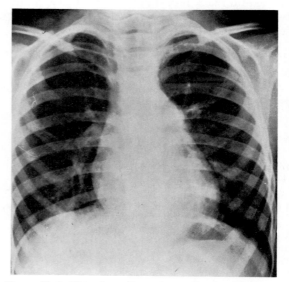

Figure 38–7. This chest film is in contrast to that shown in Figure 35–4. The heart is not enlarged overall. The main pulmonary artery is enlarged; there is no evidence of increased pulmonary blood flow. This patient has a large VSD, pulmonary hypertension, severe elevation of pulmonary vascular resistance, and pulmonary blood flow that is less than systemic blood flow. The condition is inoperable. (From DuShane, J. W., and Kirklin, J. W.: Selection for surgery of patients with ventricular septal defect and pulmonary hypertension. Circulation, 21:13, 1960. By permission of the American Heart Association, Inc.)

precordial leads in this situation have the pattern of ventricular overload previously described although here there may also be a deeper S wave. As long as evidence of left ventricular enlargement exists in these leads, the patient probably has a pulmonary-systemic flow more than approximately 1.8 and a pulmonary-systemic resistance less than approximately 0.6 and is operable. Absence of this pattern by itself is not clear evidence of a higher resistance ratio and inoperability.

Cardiac Catheterization and Cineangiography

Although clinical findings and the chest film usually allow estimation of the pulmonary blood flow and QP/QS, Doppler echocardiography with color flow mapping provides more precise information concerning the presence of a VSD. This noninvasive technique is useful in defining the status of the atrioventricular valves and left ventricular outflow tract. This technique, however, does not yet permit accurate identification of multiple VSDs and therefore the authors continue to advise cardiac catheterization studies and angled left ventriculography in projections designed to profile the ventricular septum (Bargeron et al, 1977). This technique also permits definition of the location of the defect and usually allows differentiation of perimembranous from muscular and subarterial defects.

INDICATIONS FOR OPERATION

When *infants* with *large VSDs* have severe intractable heart failure or intractable, severe respiratory symptoms at any time during the first 3 months of life, prompt primary repair is indicated. Operation is not advised *electively* in the first 3 months of life in the hope that spontaneous closure or narrowing of the defect may occur.

When severe symptoms, significant growth failure, or rising pulmonary vascular resistance is present in infants 3 months of age or older, prompt primary repair is advised.

When infants reach 6 months of age with a single large VSD, they are rarely thriving. The probability of cure by spontaneous closure of the VSD has decreased significantly (see Fig. 38–4). Operation generally should be advised at this time because the risk of repair is not demonstrably less at an older age. If the pulmonary vascular resistance is high (e.g., approximately 8 units/m² or more), repair is advisable without undue delay because further delay reduces the infant's chances of having a "surgical cure."

Patients with *large VSDs* who are first *seen after infancy* must be considered primarily on the basis of the *extent of their pulmonary vascular disease* (Kirklin and DuShane, 1963). When the pulmonary vascular

resistance is more than 10 units · m², in which circumstance the ratio of pulmonary to systemic blood flow (QP/QS) is usually less than 1.5 (with the patient at rest and breathing air), and when the clinical data are also consistent with this hemodynamic state (the systolic murmur is soft or absent; no apical diastolic flow murmur is present; the pulmonary fields on chest films are not plethoric; the left ventricle is normal or almost normal in size; and the electrocardiogram shows at least moderate right ventricular hypertrophy), operation is not advisable. Closure of the defect under these circumstances precludes right-to-left shunting during exercise; thus, exercise capacity and life expectancy are not as good with the defect closed as with it open. When pulmonary vascular resistance is elevated but within the "operable range" (5 to 10 units · m²), operation is generally advisable, with the knowledge that the long-term results may be compromised by persisting and possibly increasing pulmonary vascular disease. However, some patients with resistance values in this range at rest have rather fixed pulmonary vascular resistance, which does not fall during stress. Therefore, in patients with borderline operability who are old enough to cooperate, measurement of pulmonary and systemic blood flow and resistances during moderate exercise is helpful; even if QP/QS is 1.5 or 1.8 at rest, if it becomes 1.0 or less during moderate exercise (from systemic peripheral vasodilation and increased systemic blood flow, and a fixed and high pulmonary vascular resistance preventing increased pulmonary blood flow), operation is not indicated. The simple finding of a significant fall in arterial oxygen saturation during exercise (from right-to-left shunting across the VSD for the reasons described) is suggestive of inoperability. The response of the pulmonary vascular resistance to inhalation of high oxygen mixtures is not useful in determining operability in borderline situations.

A considerable number of children have a *moderate-sized VSD*, which is not sufficient to raise pulmonary artery pressure above 40 to 50 mm/Hg systolic and which will not result in later rise in pulmonary vascular resistance and yet produces a QP/QS of up to 3, moderate cardiomegaly, and significant pulmonary plethora. There are usually few if any symptoms. These patients should be kept under observation for about 5 years in the hope that there will be spontaneous reduction in the size of the VSD. If there is no change on subsequent recatheterization, closure is indicated.

It is not advised that young patients with *small VSDs* undergo repair, because they are suffering no significant ill effects and the defect will probably close.

Subpulmonary defects are a special situation. Even though apparently small, they should not be left untreated beyond 5 years of age, because aortic incompetence may develop, and they should be repaired promptly at an earlier age if an aortic diastolic murmur develops.

SURGICAL TECHNIQUE

The right atrial approach is preferred for most perimembranous and midmuscular VSDs and for some apical and subarterial defects. The right ventricular approach provides good exposure through a transverse infundibular incision for subarterial and infundibular defects, through an apical ventriculotomy for apical muscular defects, and through a longitudinal anterior right ventriculotomy for some multiple muscular defects. Rarely, a left ventriculotomy is used for multiple muscular VSDs in the trabecular septum.

Operations are done through a median sternotomy incision by using standard cardiopulmonary bypass methods with hypothermia to 24 to 28° C. During the procedure, periods of low flow (0.5 to 1 l/min/m²) or in rare circumstances, total circulatory arrest may be used. Ascending aortic cannulation is first accomplished by using a thin-walled, short-tip arterial cannula sized to result in a trans-cannula gradient ≤ 100 mm Hg at full flow (2.5 l/min/m²). Separate cannulation of each vena cava with appropriately sized thin-walled angled cannulas reduces the clutter in the surgical field and provides superb access for intracardiac exposure through the right atrium (Pacifico, 1988). The inferior vena cava (IVC) purse-string suture is placed directly on the IVC or at the caval-atrial junction and connected to a tourniquet. It is placed slightly to the right of the midline that reduces its interference with the right atriotomy. The superior vena cava (SVC) purse-string suture is placed directly on the SVC as an oval in its longitudinal axis and similarly connected to a tourniquet. The SVC snare is placed before establishing cardiopulmonary bypass (CPB) by mobilizing the SVC at the site of the right pulmonary artery, using a 0 silk ligature that is connected to a tourniquet. The IVC snare is placed after establishing CPB in an effort to avoid prebypass hypotension.

It is important to externally examine the cardiac chambers, making mental note of their size and position, and to determine the possible presence of anomalies of pulmonary or systemic venous return. The presence of a left SVC connecting to the coronary sinus in a small infant usually does not alter the cannulation regimen unless the right SVC is too small to cannulate. In this case, the left and right SVC return can be collected by an intracardiac sump sucker after opening the right atrium, and with periods of low flow or total circulatory arrest, the procedure is usually unhampered. Alternatively, CPB can be used with a single right atrial cannula for venous return, profound hypothermia induced and repair done during total circulatory arrest at 20° C (Barratt-Boyes et al, 1976; Rein et al, 1977). When a left SVC connects directly to the left atrium (unroofed coronary sinus syndrome), repair is more complicated and is best accomplished by using a period of total circulatory arrest in infants or by placing a third venous cannula into the anomalous left SVC in older subjects (Sand et al, 1986).

The patency of the ductus arteriosus should be known from preoperative studies. This detail is important because an open ductus combined with an open cardiotomy allows air to enter the aortic arch and later to go to the brain, if total circulatory arrest is used. Moreover, during CPB it results in increased intracardiac return and overdistends the pulmonary circulation resulting in potentially serious capillary damage to the lung. When a patent ductus arteriosus is present or suspected, it is ligated from the anterior approach.

CPB is established initially with only the IVC cannula in place, at a maximal flow rate of 1.6 l/min/m² at 25° C; the SVC cannula is inserted and "full flow" is established at 2 to 2.5 l/min/m². The water bath is then adjusted to "coldest temperature" to permit initial cooling of the myocardium by the perfusate. During this period, the IVC snare is placed, and a fine polyvinyl tube is passed into the left atrium through the right superior pulmonary vein for intraoperative and postoperative left atrial pressure monitoring. The action of the heart is usually ineffective by this time and the right atrium is opened obliquely (Fig. 38–8) and a disposable sump tip sucker is introduced into the left atrium through the foramen ovale or a small intra-atrial defect created in the fossa ovalis. Traction sutures are placed from the edges of the atriotomy to secure the atrial flaps to the subcutaneous tissue.

The aorta is cross-clamped and cold cardioplegic solution is injected into the aortic root. The temperature is now selected and is usually between 24 and 28° C. Colder temperatures are used for longer, more complex procedures and when the pulmonary venous return is large to provide "safe" periods of low flow. Generally, a flow rate of 0.5 l/min/m² or total circulatory arrest is "safe" for 45 minutes at a nasopharyngeal temperature of 22° C, 30 minutes at 26° C, and 20 minutes at 28° C. Usually, a flow rate of 1.6 l/min/m² is used during the intracardiac repair and until rewarming is commenced, when "full flow" is restored.

The heart is now soft and quiet from the cardioplegic solution infusion. Fine sutures are placed on the tricuspid valve leaflets, and traction is maintained by the weight of shodded clamps. This use and intermittent use of small eyelid or right-angled retractors provide excellent exposure for closure of most VSDs.

All VSDs are repaired with a patch. Although various methods of suturing are available, the authors prefer a continuous suturing technique with 4-0 polypropylene suture. The location of the specialized conduction tissue and its relation to the VSD must be understood.

The right atriotomy used for transatrial repair and the view of a perimembranous VSD through the tricuspid valve are shown in Figure 38–8. The sinus node is shown in the intact heart above and the AV

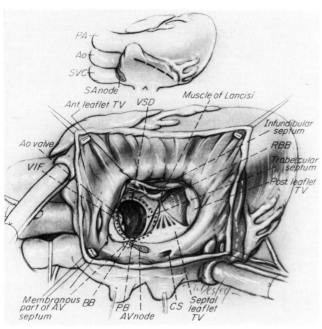

Figure 38–8. The sinus node and position of the right atriotomy is shown above. Transatrial exposure of a perimembranous VSD is shown below looking through the retracted tricuspid valve leaflets. The coronary sinus (CS) and the nearby atrioventricular (AV) node with the penetrating portion of the bundle of His (PB) and its branching portion (BB) as well as the right bundle branch (RBB) are shown in relation to the VSD. The pathway of the suture line that will secure the patch used to close the VSD is indicated by the x's along the muscular portion of the ventricular septum as well as the ventriculoinfundibular fold (VIF) and the dots shown in the base of the septal leaflet of the tricuspid valve (TV). The suture line remains well away from the inferior free edge of the VSD and on the tricuspid leaflet near its base to avoid the surgical creation of heart block. (Ao = aorta; PA = pulmonary artery; SVC = superior vena cava; SA = sinoatrial.) (By permission from Bharati, S., Lev, M., Kirklin, J. W.: Cardiac Surgery and the Conduction System. New York, John Wiley & Sons, 1983.)

node, penetrating portion of the bundle of His as well as its branching portion and right bundle in relation to the tricuspid valve and VSD below (see Fig. 38–8). The precise method of suturing the patch in place is shown in Figure 38–9.

In some cases, a perimembranous VSD is associated with an inlet muscular VSD leaving an intact muscle bar between them (Fig. 38–10). Usually, they can be nicely exposed by tricuspid valve leaflet retraction, but where the chordal pattern is particularly complicated, exposure is facilitated by incising the anterior and septal leaflets near their base and retracting the leaflets anteriorly (see Fig. 38–10). In this particular defect, the conduction tissue courses in the muscle bar and separates the two defects; its injury is avoided by using a single patch to cover both defects, leaving the muscle bar intact and placing the sutures in the path indicated.

The "atrioventricular canal type" of VSD and the course of the conduction tissue in relation to it are shown in Figure 38–11. No muscle tissue is present between the defect and the base of the septal tricuspid leaflet that is contiguous with the anterior

mitral leaflet and usually with part of the aortic valve annulus superiorly. The conduction tissue is related to the inferior border of the defect and the suture line used to attach the patch in this area is placed approximately 10 mm inferior to the free edge of the VSD.

The specialized conduction tissue is not related directly to a muscular VSD in the trabecular septum (Fig. 38–12). In this case, the patch suture line is placed circumferentially on the free edge of the defect.

Subarterial and muscular defects in the infundibular septum can sometimes be approached through the right atrium. They can always be nicely exposed through a transverse incision in the right ventricular infundibulum and sometimes through a pulmonary arteriotomy working through the retracted pulmonary valve and annulus.

Multiple anterior VSDs can be closed by mattress sutures placed over felt pledgets or strips working transatrially through the tricuspid valve or through a vertical right ventriculotomy incision made near the septum (Breckenridge et al, 1972). A left ventriculotomy also provides excellent exposure (Aaron and Lower, 1975; Singh et al, 1977), but the authors prefer not to use it routinely in infants because it has been associated with left ventricular dysfunction early and late postoperatively in some of the small patients. In older patients, avoidance of a left ventriculotomy appears to be less important.

The rare "Swiss-cheese" septum usually requires a left ventricular approach. An associated perimembranous defect should be repaired through the right atrium, because its repair from the left ventricular side increases the risk of heart block.

When VSD closure is completed, rewarming is commenced, the vent is removed, and the atrial septal defect is closed after inflating the lungs to expel air from the left atrium. Air is aspirated from the ascending aorta, the aortic cross-clamp released, and the right atriotomy is closed. De-airing is accomplished, and CPB is gradually discontinued. Decannulation is effected, and the incision is closed leaving temporary atrial and ventricular pacing electrodes.

POSTOPERATIVE CARE

Most infants convalesce normally after VSD repair, and special treatment is usually not required. Generally, the patients are extubated within 24 hours of operation and recover rapidly.

In the unusual case of low cardiac output after operation, in addition to the usual supportive treatment (Kirklin and Kirklin, 1981), consideration should be given to the possibility of an overlooked or incompletely closed VSD. This possibility must especially be considered if the left atrial pressure is considerably higher than the right atrial pressure. If recovery from the low output state does not occur within a few hours and in the absence of secure

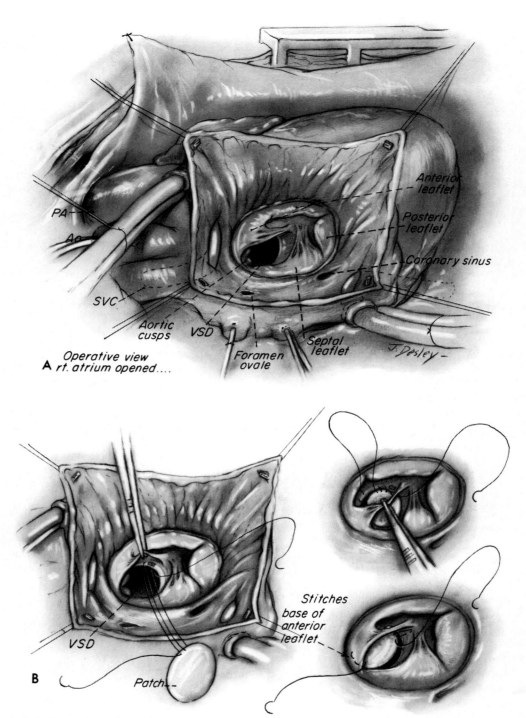

Figure 38–9. *A,* Right atrial incision and exposure of perimembranous VSD in the region of the tricuspid anteroseptal commissure. Stay sutures have been placed to slightly evert the atrial wall. Note that initially the superior edge of this typical perimembranous defect is not visible. The AV node is in the muscular portion of the AV septum, just on the atrial side of the commissure between the tricuspid septal and anterior leaflets. The bundle of His thus penetrates at the posterior angle of the VSD, where it is vulnerable to injury. *B,* The repair of the perimembranous VSD. This is begun by placing a mattress suture of 4-0 Prolene with a small pledget at the 12 o'clock position in the defect as seen by the surgeon through the tricuspid valve. A piece of knitted Dacron velour is trimmed to be slightly larger than the approximate size of the defect, and one arm of the suture is passed through the Dacron patch, back through the septum, and again through the patch. Either now or after placing several more stitches, the sutures are snugged up as the patch is lowered into place. The suture line between the cephalad rim of the defect and the patch is continued. The traction on the suture exposes the next areas to be stitched and provides good visibility. When the junction of the superior muscular rim (ventriculoinfundibular fold) and tricuspid annulus has been reached, the suture is passed through the base of the contiguous portion of the tricuspid valve (usually the anterior leaflet) from the ventricular to the atrial side, then back from the atrial to the ventricular side of the valve and through the patch. After passing the stitch back through the leaflet, the suture is tagged.

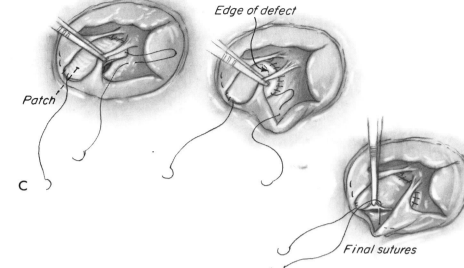

Figure 38–9 *Continued C,* Working now with the other limb of the suture, stitches are taken between the ventricular septum and the patch along the caudad side of the defect. These stitches are placed 3 to 5 mm away from the edge of the defect *to avoid the area most probably occupied by the bundle of His* and more posteriorly 5 to 7 mm back from the edge.

information from an indicator-dilution study or a Doppler examination with color flow mapping that a residual shunt is not present, urgent recatheterization and possible reoperation are indicated.

If complete atrioventricular dissociation was present for a time after CPB, but sinus rhythm reappeared, a demand pacemaker attached to ventricular wires should be in place for 1 week postoperatively, because, rarely, the atrioventricular dissociation recurs temporarily in the early postoperative period.

RESULTS OF SURGICAL TREATMENT

Early Results of Primary Repair

Hospital mortality for repair of VSD now approaches 0% in most centers properly prepared for this type of procedure, even in very small infants (Barratt-Boyes et al, 1976; Lincoln et al, 1977; Rein et al, 1977; Rizzoli et al, 1980). However, in earlier times, deaths did occur, and a number of incremental risk factors could be identified. The current very low hospital mortality is the result of the neutralization of most of these risk factors by scientific progress and by minimization of human error.

Type of VSD. The location of the *single large VSD* is not an incremental risk factor with regard to early or late results of repair. In the past, *multiple VSDs* have been an important incremental risk factor (Blackstone et al, 1976; Kirklin et al, 1980). The authors' more recent experience indicates that it is only a weak one (Rizzoli et al, 1980) (Table 38–3). This improvement is in part related to the general improvements in infant intracardiac operations, but is also related in a major way to a now higher proportion of patients with complete or almost com-

plete repair and little or no residual shunting. This improvement can be attributed primarily to better preoperative cineangiographic identification of the presence, size, and location of the multiple VSDs.

Age at Repair. There have been no deaths at the University of Alabama at Birmingham (UAB) among patients operated on at 24 months of age or older for repair of isolated large VSD in the last decade, and thus, for a long time, the risk of operation under these circumstances has approached 0%.

The incremental risk of young age was clearly apparent in the authors' early experience, as it was in many centers (Binet et al, 1970; Ching et al, 1971; Cooley et al, 1962; Johnson et al, 1974). However, a steady decrease in hospital mortality has occurred with time, and affects infants particularly. As a result, the previously apparent incremental risk of young age has been neutralized in more recent experiences (Barratt-Boyes et al, 1976; Rein et al, 1977; Rizzoli et al, 1980) (Table 38–4 and Fig. 38–13). This has resulted in part from scientific progress, with improved preoperative diagnostic accuracy, improved surgical and support techniques, and improved myocardial preservation. It has also resulted in part from a demonstrated decrease in the fatal human surgical and management errors as institutions have increased their experience and expertise with infant intracardiac surgery.

Pulmonary Artery Pressure and Pulmonary Vascular Resistance. At present, these are not determinants of hospital mortality, although they do affect late results (Blackstone et al, 1976). This is different from the earlier Mayo Clinic experiences (Cartmill et al, 1966), probably because the upper limit of acceptable ("operable") pulmonary vascular resistance is better understood and management has improved.

Major Associated Lesions. The frequency of ma-

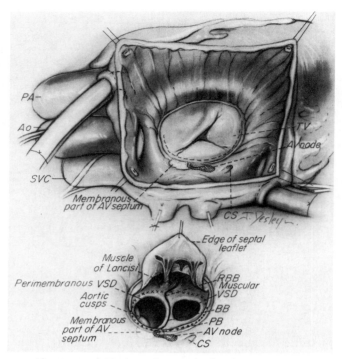

Figure 38–10. Transatrial exposure for closure of a perimembranous VSD associated with an inlet muscular VSD. The coronary sinus (CS) and atrioventricular (AV) node as well as an incision in the base of the anterior and septal tricuspid valve (TV) leaflets is shown above. The leaflets are retracted anteriorly in the lower part of the figure to expose the two VSDs. The penetrating portion of the bundle of His (PB), its branching portion (BB) and the right bundle branch (RBB) are shown in relation to the VSDs. The pathway of the suture line used to attach the Dacron patch along the muscular portion of the septum is indicated by x's and along the base of the tricuspid valve leaflet by dots. When repair is completed, the tricuspid leaflets are reattached to their basilar remnant by a continuous suture of fine polypropylene. (PA = pulmonary artery; Ao = aorta. SVC = superior vena cava.) (By permission from Bharati, S., Lev, M., Kirklin, J. W.: Cardiac Surgery and the Conduction System. New York, John Wiley & Sons, 1983.)

jor associated lesions, particularly in symptomatic infants with large VSDs, has already been emphasized. These do have, even currently, an incremental risk effect on hospital mortality. At the UAB, among 312 patients operated on for VSD from 1967 to 1979, 16 hospital deaths (6.3%; confidence limits (CL) 4.7 to 8.3%) occurred among 254 patients with single or multiple VSDs but no major associated lesion, whereas 14 (24%; CL 18 to 31%) occurred among 58 patients with major associated lesions (p < 0.0001) (Rizzoli et al, 1980). Additional technical and scientific progress will probably improve this situation.

Surgical Approach. The surgical approach for repair of the VSD (through the right atrium, through the right ventricle, or through both) has not been a determinant of hospital mortality after repair of single VSDs (Table 38–5). Neither has it been after the repair of muscular or multiple VSDs through a left ventriculotomy, an experience also reported by surgeons at the Boston Children's Hospital (Kirklin et al, 1980). However, concern continues about the

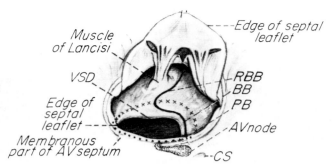

Figure 38–11. Transatrial exposure for repair of an "atrioventricular canal type" of VSD is shown after incision of the base of the tricuspid valve and anterior traction as in Figure 38–9. The coronary sinus (CS), atrioventricular (AV) node and its penetrating portion (PB), branching portion (BB) and the right bundle branch (RBB) are shown in relation to the VSD. The x's indicate the path of the suture line used to attach the patch to the muscular portion of the septum and the dots along the base of the tricuspid leaflet. Most defects of this type can be closed without incision of the tricuspid leaflets; however, when the chordal pattern is complex, this maneuver aids in exposure. (By permission from Bharati, S., Lev, M., Kirklin, J. W.: Cardiac Surgery and the Conduction System. New York, John Wiley & Sons, 1983.)

long-term functional results of left ventriculotomy in infants.

Late Results

Repair of VSD in the first year or two of life provides a cure for most patients and results in full functional activity and normal or almost normal life expectancy.

Improved Physical Development. This is a prom-

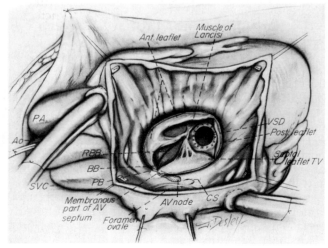

Figure 38–12. Transatrial exposure of a muscular defect in the trabecular portion of the septum is shown. The pathway of the suture line used to attach the patch to close the defect are along its free edge and indicated by the x's. (CS = coronary sinus; AV = atrioventricular; PB = penetrating portion of the bundle of His; BB = branching portion of the bundle of His; RBB = right bundle branch; Ao = aorta; SVC = superior vena cava; PA = pulmonary artery; Ant. = anterior; TV = tricuspid valve.) (By permission from Bharati, S., Lev, M., Kirklin, J. W.: Cardiac Surgery and the Conduction System. New York, John Wiley & Sons, 1983.)

TABLE 38–3. HOSPITAL MORTALITY* IN 29 PATIENTS HAVING PRIMARY REPAIR OF MULTIPLE VENTRICULAR SEPTAL DEFECTS WITHOUT MAJOR ASSOCIATED LESIONS AT UAB (1967–1979)†

Age (Months)	Total				1974–1979‡			
		Hospital Deaths				*Hospital Deaths*		
	No.	No.	%	70% CL (%)	No.	No.	%	70% CL (%)
<3	1	0	0	0–85	1	0	0	0–85
≥3 <6	4	2	50	18–82	2	0	0	0–61
≥6 <12	5	1	20	3–53	3	0	0	0–47
≥12 <24	7	3	43	20–68	4	1	25	3–63
≥24 <48	5	3	60	29–86	1	0	0	0–85
≥48	7	0	0	0–24	3	0	0	0–47
Total	29	9	31	21–42	14	1	7	1–22
	(15	8	53	37–69)§				

p = 0.22.

†From Rizzoli, G., Blackstone, E. H., Kirklin, J. W., et al: Incremental 131risk factors in hospital mortality after repair of ventricular septal defect. J. Thorac. Cardiovasc. Surg., *80*:494, 1980.

‡Note the greatly lowered mortality in this period.

§Numbers in parentheses are for the period from 1967 to 1974.

inent feature of the late postoperative course after repair of large VSDs in infants (Rein et al, 1977). Lillehei and colleagues first showed an impressive increase in weight after VSD repair in 1955. There is a less impressive increase in length and in head circumference (Clarkson et al, 1973). This improved physical development is usually associated with complete relief of symptoms. The authors have also reported increase in weight postoperatively in children in whom a large VSD had been repaired later in the first decade of life (Cartmill et al, 1966).

Permanent Heart Block (complete atrioventricular dissociation with independent atrial activity not conducted to the ventricles). This is uncommon with present techniques. For example, heart block was present at death or hospital dismissal in 1.5% (CL is 0.5 to 3%) of patients with large VSDs without associated lesions of major anatomic or functional significance in the UAB experience between 1967 and 1976 (Blackstone et al, 1976). The two patients were both unusual. One patient had multiple muscular defects and the other patient had Down's syndrome

and a large perimembranous defect. In the earlier report from the Mayo Clinic, no such case occurred among the 146 patients with large VSD operated on between 1962 and 1966.

Cardiac Function. Cardiac function late postoperatively is essentially normal when repair is done in the first 2 years of life by modern techniques through the right atrium or right ventricle. Graham and colleagues found that left ventricular end-diastolic volume, left ventricular systolic output, left ventricular mass, and left ventricular ejection fraction were all normal approximately 1 year after operation in a group of these patients (Cordell et al, 1976). Others have found persistent abnormalities of left ventricular size and function after repair of large VSDs at an older age, although all patients were asymptomatic (Jarmakani et al, 1971, 1972). This information lends support to the idea that, in general, patients with large VSDs should be operated on before they are 2 years old.

Residual Shunting. Postoperative left-to-right shunts of such magnitude as to indicate reoperation

TABLE 38–4. EFFECT OF AGE ON HOSPITAL MORTALITY* IN 166 PATIENTS HAVING PRIMARY REPAIR OF SINGLE LARGE VENTRICULAR SEPTAL DEFECT WITHOUT MAJOR ASSOCIATED LESIONS AT UAB (1967–1979)†

Age (Months)	Total					1974–1979				
			Hospital Deaths					*Hospital Deaths*		
	No.	%	No.	%	70% CL (%)	No.	%	No.	%	70% CL (%)
< 3	14	8.4	2	14	5–31	11	11.7	1‡	9	1–28
≥ 3 <6	12	7.2	0	0	0–15	10	10.6	0	0	0–17
≥ 6 <12	23	13.9	3	13	6–25	14	14.9	0	0	0–13
≥12 <24	21	12.7	1	5	1–15	11	11.7	0	0	0–16
≥24 <48	27	16.3	0	0	0–7	15	16.0	0	0	0–12
≥48	69	41.6	0	0	0–3	33	35.1	0	0	0–6
Total	166		6	3.6	2.1–5.8	94		1	1.1	0.1–3.6
	(72		5	6.9	3.9–11.5)§					

*The p value (*n* = 166) = 0.01.

†From Rizzoli, G., Blackstone, E. H., Kirklin, J. W., et al: Incremental risk factors in hospital mortality after repair of ventricular septal defect. J. Thorac. Cardiovasc. Surg., *80*:494, 1980.

‡A 1.2-month-old baby with preoperative seizures was admitted to surgery, intubated, and ventilated. Died on third postoperative day with acute cardiac failure.

§Numbers in parentheses are for the period from 1967 to 1974.

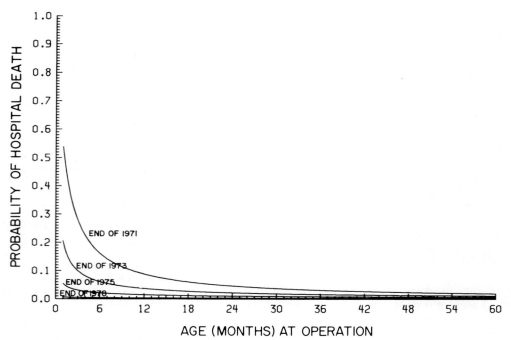

Figure 38–13. Probability of hospital death at UAB after repair of single large VSD in patients without major associated cardiac anomalies. Note that in 1971 and 1973 the risk was considerably increased in very young patients. By 1979, not only was the risk of hospital death less than 1%, but an incremental risk in patients of young age was no longer apparent. (From Rizzoli, G., Blackstone, E. H., Kirklin, J. W., et al: Incremental risk factors in hospital mortality after repair of ventricular septal defect. J. Thorac. Cardiovasc. Surg., *80:*494, 1980.)

are uncommon when proper techniques are used. One of 138 patients (0.7%; CL—0.1 to 2%) operated on at UAB for repair of large VSD has required reoperation (and this was for overlooked multiple muscular defects) (Blackstone et al, 1976). A report from Castaneda's group (Rein et al, 1977) stated that only 1 patient of 48 hospital survivors (2%; CL—0 to 7%) required reoperation for residual VSD.

Premature Late Deaths. Late death occurs rarely (<2.5% of patients) when pulmonary vascular resistance is low preoperatively. Presumably, these deaths are from arrhythmias, either ventricular fibrillation or the sudden late development of heart block.

Patients with a high pulmonary vascular resistance preoperatively have a tendency for this to progress and cause premature death; this becomes of some magnitude (±25% dying within 5 years of operation) when the resistance preoperatively is more than 10 units · m^2.

Pulmonary Hypertension. Generally, the younger the child is at the time of repair, the better his or her chances are of having an essentially normal pulmonary artery pressure 5 years later, and thus, presumably, for the rest of the child's life (Barratt-Boyes et al, 1976; Castaneda et al, 1971; DuShane and Kirklin, 1973; Hoffman and Rudolph, 1966; Lillehei et al, 1968; Maron et al, 1973; Sigmann et al, 1977; Yacoub et al, 1978). The lower the pulmonary vascular resistance or the pulmonary artery pressure

TABLE 38–5. EFFECT OF SURGICAL APPROACH ON HOSPITAL MORTALITY* IN 166 PATIENTS HAVING PRIMARY REPAIR OF SINGLE LARGE VENTRICULAR SEPTAL DEFECTS WITHOUT MAJOR ASSOCIATED LESIONS AT UAB (1967–1979)†

	Total				1974–1979			
		Hospital Deaths				Hospital Deaths		
Surgical Approach	*No.*	No.	%	70% CL (%)	*No.*	No.	%	70% CL (%)
RA‡	105	2	1.9	0.6–4.5	65	1	1.5	0.2–5.1
RA → RV§	4	0	0	0–38	2	0	0	0–61
RV	57	4	7	4–12	27	0	0	0–7
Total	166	6	3.6	2.1–5.8	94	1	1.1	0.1–3.6

*The p value (*n* = 166) = 0.23.

†From Rizzoli, G., Blackstone, E. H., Kirklin, J. W., et al: Incremental risk factors in hospital mortality after repair of ventricular septal defect. J. Thorac. Cardiovasc. Surg., *80:*494, 1980.

‡RA = right atrium.

§RV = right ventricle.

at the time of repair, the better are the patient's chances of having normal pulmonary artery pressure postoperatively.

Severe pulmonary hypertension postoperatively can increase with time (Friedli et al, 1974) and cause premature late death, usually within 3 to 10 years of operation (DuShane and Kirklin, 1973; Friedli et al, 1974; Hallidie-Smith et al, 1969). However, some patients with pulmonary hypertension and elevated pulmonary vascular resistance late postoperatively have neither progression nor regression of their disease for as long as 20 years, although with some limitation in exercise tolerance (DuShane and Kirklin, 1973; Hallidie-Smith et al, 1975). Their life expectancy, however, is probably not normal.

SPECIAL SITUATIONS

VSD Plus Coarctation of the Aorta. Although there has been controversy as to the management of young infants in congestive heart failure because of this combination, most centers, including the authors', now practice prompt repair of the coarctation (Bergdahl et al, 1982), *without* concomitant pulmonary artery banding. If the baby remains ventilator-dependent for 72 hours, the VSD is then closed. Usually, this is not the case, and prompt improvement occurs after repair of the coarctation. The VSD may then require repair 3 to 12 months later. Often, however, spontaneous reduction in size and eventual closure occur.

VSD Plus Patent Ductus Arteriosus. When a young infant with severe congestive heart failure has a large VSD and a patent ductus arteriosus of any size, operation is advisable, and both are repaired at operation, through a median sternotomy incision.

When the VSD is a moderate size or small and the patent ductus arteriosus is large and the infant is in the first few months of life, the ductus arteriosus is closed by way of a simple operation through a left thoracotomy incision. The VSD will usually become narrow and will close spontaneously.

Selected Bibliography

Barratt-Boyes, B. G., Neutze, J. M., Clarkson, P. M., et al: Repair of ventricular septal defect in the first two years of life using profound hypothermia—circulatory arrest techniques. Ann. Surg., *184*:376, 1976.

This classic paper describes the results of primary repair of VSD in 57 patients less than 2 years of age, with many of the patients being less than 6 months old. Hospital mortality was 4% in the patients without associated coarctation—a remarkable achievement. The late postoperative results are excellent. The method of profound hypothermia and total circulatory arrest and these superb results have had an important and worldwide impact on cardiac operations.

Hoffman, J. I. E., and Rudolph, A. M.: The natural history of ventricular septal defects in infancy. Am. J. Cardiol., *16*:634, 1965.

This classic paper reports data on 62 infants with VSD who were first catheterized under 1 year of age and were followed for 1 to 5 years after that. Forty were recatheterized. Fifty per cent of the infants had congestive heart failure. Spontaneous closure of the VSD occurred in 36% of the patients, and in an additional 28%, marked decrease in the size of the defect occurred. In this series, complete spontaneous closure occurred between 7 and 12 months of age. Sixteen per cent of the group studied did not do well. Five had severe and unrelenting congestive heart failure. One baby had a high pulmonary vascular resistance from birth that never regressed. Four babies had low pulmonary vascular resistance when first catheterized at less than 1 year of age, with significant rises of resistance to pathologic levels when recatheterized subsequently. These data form a rational basis for surgical patient management programs.

Lillehei, C. W., Cohen, M., Warden, H. E., et al: The results of direct vision closure of ventricular septal defects in eight patients by means of controlled cross-circulation. Surg. Gynecol. Obstet., *101*:446, 1955.

This classic article, reporting the first successful closures of VSDs, still makes superb and informative reading. Although cross-circulation is no longer used, it obviously was a superb support system for these small patients.

Rein, J. G., Freed, M. D., Norwood, W. I., and Castaneda, A. R.: Early and late results of closure of ventricular septal defect in infancy. Ann. Thorac. Surg., *24*:19, 1977.

The superb results obtained by Castaneda and colleagues in the operation of primary repair of VSD in the first year of life in 50 infants are reported here. The Kyoto-Barratt-Boyes technique of profound hypothermia and total circulatory arrest was used. Hospital mortality was 6%, no late death occurred, and the late functional status was excellent. This paper gave strong supportive evidence for the excellence of the results that can be obtained from primary repair of VSD, even in very young infants.

Rizzoli, G., Blackstone, E. H., Kirklin, J. W., et al: Incremental risk factors in hospital mortality after repair of ventricular septal defect. J. Thorac. Cardiovasc. Surg., *80*:494, 1980.

This paper describes the incremental risk (degree of difficulty, if you will) of numerous factors in 312 patients having repair of VSD from 1967 to 1979. More important, it describes how these incremental risk factors have gradually been neutralized by scientific advances and minimization of human errors. Thus, in the era beginning in 1978, the hospital mortality of repair of single large VSDs is less than 1%, no matter how young the patient (neutralization of the previous incremental risk of young age), and is approximately 5% for multiple VSDs, again without an incremental risk of young age. Major associated cardiac anomalies or procedures (large patent ductus arteriosus, simultaneous repair of coarctation or interrupted arch, and important mitral valve abnormalities) still increase risk.

Soto, B., Becker, A. E., Moulaert, A. J., et al: Classification of ventricular septal defects. Br. Heart J., *43*:332, 1980.

Many anatomic studies of VSD have been reported through the years, but this study by Anderson and colleagues has been particularly helpful to surgeons. Their work, described in this paper, forms the basis for the description of morphology used in this chapter. The ventricular septum is divided into a membranous and muscular portion, and the latter is divided into an inlet, trabecular, and infundibular (outlet) portion. This paper introduces the advisable phrase *perimembranous VSD* for those in the region of the membranous septum, right up against the tricuspid annulus. It also clarifies the fact that the so-called atrioventricular canal *type* of VSD is really a perimembranous one and extends particularly beneath the septal tricuspid leaflet. Beautiful anatomic and cineangiographic plates clarify the description.

Bibliography

Aaron, B. L., and Lower, R. R.: Muscular ventricular septal defect repair made easy. Ann. Thorac. Surg., 19:568, 1975.

Ash, R.: Natural history of ventricular septal defects in childhood lesions with predominant arteriovenous shunts. J. Pediatr., 64:45, 1964.

Auld, P. A. M., Johnson, A. L., Gibbons, J. E., and McGregor, M.: Changes in pulmonary vascular resistance in infants and children with intracardiac left-to-right shunts. Circulation, 27:257, 1963.

Bargeron, L. M., Jr., Elliott, L. P., Soto, B., et al: Axial angiocardiography in congenital heart disease. I: Concept, technical and anatomic considerations. Circulation, 56:1075, 1977.

Barratt-Boyes, B. G., Neutze, J. M., Clarkson, P. M., et al: Repair of ventricular septal defect in the first two years of life using profound hypothermia—circulatory arrest techniques. Ann. Surg., 184:376, 1976.

Bergdahl, L. A. L., Blackstone, E. H., Kirklin, J. W., et al: Determinants of early success in repair of aortic coarctation in infants. J. Thorac. Cardiovasc. Surg., 83:736, 1982.

Binet, J. P., Conso, J. F., Langlois, J., et al: Fermeture de certaines communications interventriculaires congénitales basses par le ventricule gauche. Arch. Mal. Coeur, 63:1345, 1970.

Blackstone, E. H., Kirklin, J. W., Bradley, E. L., et al: Optimal age and results in repair of large ventricular septal defects. J. Thorac. Cardiovasc. Surg., 72:661, 1976.

Breckenridge, I. M., Stark, J., Waterston, D. J., and Bonham-Carter, R. E.: Multiple ventricular septal defects. Ann. Thorac. Surg., 13:128, 1972.

Campbell, M.: Natural history of ventricular septal defect. Br. Heart J., 33:246, 1971.

Cartmill, T. B., DuShane, J. W., McGoon, D. C., and Kirklin, J. W.: Results of repair of ventricular septal defect. J. Thorac. Cardiovasc. Surg., 52:486, 1966.

Castaneda, A. R., Zamora, R., Nicoloff, D. M., et al: High-pressure, high-resistance ventricular septal defect. Surgical results of closure through right atrium. Ann. Thorac. Surg., 12:29, 1971.

Ching, E., DuShane, J. W., McGoon, D. C., and Danielson, G. K.: Total correction of ventricular septal defect in infancy using extracorporeal circulation: Surgical considerations and results of operation. Ann. Thorac. Surg., 12:1, 1971.

Clarkson, P. M.: Growth following corrective cardiac operation in early infancy. In Barratt-Boyes, B. G., Neutze, J. M., and Harris, E. A. (eds): Heart Disease in Infancy: Diagnosis and Surgical Treatment. London, Churchill Livingstone, 1973, p. 75.

Clarkson, P. M., Frye, R. L., DuShane, J. W., et al: Prognosis for patients with ventricular septal defect and severe pulmonary vascular obstructive disease. Circulation, 38:129, 1968.

Collins, G., Calder, L., Rose, V., Kidd, L., and Keith, J.: Ventricular septal defect: Clinical and hemodynamic changes in the first five years of life. Am. Heart J., 84:695, 1972.

Cooley, D. A., Garrett, H. E., and Howard, H. S.: The surgical treatment of ventricular septal defect: An analysis of 300 consecutive surgical cases. Prog. Cardiovasc. Dis., 4:312, 1962.

Cordell, D., Graham, T. P., Jr., Atwood, G. F., et al: Left heart volume characteristics following ventricular septal defect closure in infancy. Circulation, 54:294, 1976.

Corone, P., Doyan, F., Gaudeau, S., et al: Natural history of ventricular septal defect: A study involving 790 cases. Circulation, 55:908, 1977.

Dirksen, T., Moulaert, A. J., Buis-Liem, T. N., and Brom, A. G.: Ventricular septal defect associated with left ventricular outflow tract obstruction below the defect. J. Thorac. Cardiovasc. Surg., 75:688, 1978.

DuShane, J. W., and Kirklin, J. W.: Late results of the repair of ventricular septal defect on pulmonary vascular disease. In Kirklin, J. W. (ed): Advances in Cardiovascular Surgery. New York, Grune and Stratton, 1973, p. 9.

DuShane, J. W., and Kirklin, J. W.: Selection for surgery of patients with ventricular septal defect and pulmonary hypertension. Circulation, 21:13, 1960.

DuShane, J. W., Kirklin, J. W., Patrick, R. T., et al: Ventricular septal defects with pulmonary hypertension: Surgical treatment by means of a mechanical pump-oxygenator. J.A.M.A., 160:950, 1956.

Freed, M. D., Rosenthal, A., Plauth, W. H., Jr., and Nadas, A. S.: Development of subaortic stenosis after pulmonary artery banding. Circulation, 47, 48(Suppl. III):7, 1973.

Friedli, B., Kidd, B. S. L., Mustard, W. T., and Keith, J. D.: Ventricular septal defect with increased pulmonary vascular resistance. Late results of surgical closure. Am. J. Cardiol., 33:403, 1974.

Gasul, B. M., Dillon, R. F., Vrla, V., and Hait, G.: Ventricular septal defects. Their natural transformation into those with infundibular stenosis or into the cyanotic or non-cyanotic type of tetralogy of Fallot. J.A.M.A., 164:847, 1957.

Hallidie-Smith, K. A., Edwards, R. E., Wilson, R., and Zeidifard, E.: Long-term cardiorespiratory assessment after surgical closure of ventricular septal defect in childhood. (Abstract.) Proc. Br. Cardiac Soc., 37:553, 1975.

Hallidie-Smith, K. A., Hollman, A., Cleland, W. P., et al: Effects of surgical closure of ventricular septal defects upon pulmonary vascular disease. Br. Heart J., 31:246, 1969.

Heath, D., and Edwards, J. E.: The pathology of hypertensive pulmonary vascular disease: A description of six grades of structural changes in the pulmonary arteries with special reference to congenital cardiac septal defects. Circulation, 18:533, 1958.

Heath, D., Helmholtz, H. F., Jr., Burchell, H. B., et al: Relation between structural changes in the small pulmonary arteries and the immediate reversibility of pulmonary hypertension following closure of ventricular and atrial septal defects. Circulation, 18:1167, 1958.

Hislop, A., Haworth, S. G., Shinebourne, E. A., and Reid, L.: Quantitative structural analysis of pulmonary vessels in isolated ventricular septal defects in infancy. Br. Heart J., 37:1014, 1975.

Hoffman, J. I. E.: Diagnosis and treatment of pulmonary vascular disease. Birth Defects (original article series), 8:9, 1972.

Hoffman, J. I. E., and Rudolph, A. M.: Increasing pulmonary vascular resistance during infancy in association with ventricular septal defect. Pediatrics, 38:220, 1966.

Hoffman, J. I. E., and Rudolph, A. M.: The natural history of isolated ventricular septal defect, with special references to selection of patients for surgery. In Schulman, I. (ed): Advances in Pediatrics. Chicago: Year Book Medical Publishers, Inc., 1970, p. 57.

Hoffman, J. I. E., and Rudolph, A. M.: The natural history of ventricular septal defects in infancy. Am. J. Cardiol., 16:634, 1965.

Jarmakani, J. M., Edwards, S. B., Spach, M. S., et al: Left ventricular pressure volume characteristics in congenital heart disease. Circulation, 37:879, 1968.

Jarmakani, J. M., Graham, T. P., Jr., and Canent, R. V., Jr.: Left ventricular contractile state in children with successfully corrected ventricular septal defect. Circulation, 45, 46(Suppl. I):102, 1972.

Jarmakani, J. M., Graham, T. P., Jr., Canent, R. V., et al: The effect of corrective surgery on left heart volume and mass in children with ventricular septal defect. Am. J. Cardiol., 27:254, 1971.

Johnson, D. C., Cartmill, T. B., Celermajer, J. M., et al: Intracardiac repair of large ventricular septal defect in the first year of life. Med. J. Aust., 2:193, 1974.

Keith, J. D., Rose, V., Collins, G., and Kidd, B. S. L.: Ventricular septal defect: Incidence, morbidity, and mortality in various age groups. Br. Heart J., 33(Suppl.):81, 1971.

Kirklin, J. K., and Kirklin, J. W.: Management of the cardiovascular subsystem after cardiac surgery. Ann. Thorac. Surg., 32:311, 1981.

Kirklin, J. K., Castaneda, A. R., Keane, J. F., et al: Surgical management of multiple ventricular septal defects. J. Thorac. Cardiovasc. Surg., 80:485, 1980.

Kirklin, J. W., and DuShane, J. W.: Indications for repair of ventricular septal defects. Am. J. Cardiol., 12:79, 1963.

Kirklin, J. W., and DuShane, J. W.: Repair of ventricular septal defect in infancy. Pediatrics, 27:961, 1961.

Lauer, R. M., DuShane, J. W., and Edwards, J. E.: Obstruction of left ventricular outlet in association with ventricular septal defect. Circulation, 22:110, 1960.

Leatham, A., and Segal, B.: Auscultatory and phonocardiographic signs of ventricular septal defect with left-to-right shunt. Circulation, 25:318, 1962.

Levin, A. R., Boineau, J. P., Spach, M. S., et al: Ventricular pressure flow-dynamics in tetralogy of Fallot. Circulation, 34:4, 1966.

Lillehei, C. W., Anderson, R. C., Eliot, R. S., et al: Pre- and postoperative cardiac catheterization in 200 patients undergoing closure of ventricular septal defects. Surgery, 63:69, 1968.

Lillehei, C. W., Cohen, M., Warden, H. E., et al: The results of direct vision closure of ventricular septal defects in eight patients by means of controlled cross circulation. Surg. Gynecol. Obstet., 101:446, 1955.

Lincoln, C., Jamieson, S., Joseph, M., et al: Transatrial repair of ventricular septal defects with reference to their anatomic classification. J. Thorac. Cardiovasc. Surg., 74:183, 1977.

Lucas, R. V., Jr., Adams, P., Jr., Anderson, R. C., et al: The natural history of isolated ventricular septal defect: A serial physiologic study. Circulation, 24:1372, 1961.

Maron, B. J., Redwood, D. R., Hirschfeld, J. W., Jr., et al: Postoperative assessment of patients with ventricular septal defect and pulmonary hypertension: Response to intense upright exercise. Circulation, 48:864, 1973.

Moulaert, A. J., Bruins, C. G., and Oppenheimer-Dekker, A.: Anomalies of the aortic arch and ventricular septal defects. Circulation, 53:1011, 1976.

Oh, K. S., Park, S. C., Galvis, A. G., et al: Pulmonary hyperinflation in ventricular septal defect. J. Thorac. Cardiovasc. Surg., 76:706, 1978.

Okamoto, Y.: Clinical studies for open heart surgery in infants with profound hypothermia. Arch. Jpn. Chir., 38:188, 1969.

Pacifico, A. D.: Cardiopulmonary bypass and hypothermic circulatory arrest in congenital heart surgery. In Grillo, H. C., et al (eds): Current Therapy in Cardiothoracic Surgery. Toronto, B. C. Decker Inc., Publishers, 1988.

Rein, J. G., Freed, M. D., Norwood, W. I., and Castaneda, A. R.: Early and late results of closure of ventricular septal defect in infancy. Ann. Thorac. Surg., 24:19, 1977.

Rizzoli, G., Blackstone, E. H., Kirklin, J. W., et al: Incremental risk factors in hospital mortality after repair of ventricular septal defect. J. Thorac. Cardiovasc. Surg., 80:494, 1980.

Sand, M. E., McGrath, L. B., Pacifico, A. D., and Mandke, N. V.: Repair of left superior vena cava entering the left atrium. Ann. Thorac. Surg., 42:560, 1986.

Shah, P., Singh, W. S. A., Rose, V., and Keith, J. D.: Incidence of bacterial endocarditis in ventricular septal defects. Circulation, 34:127, 1966.

Sigmann, J. M., Perry, B. L., Behrendt, D. M., et al: Ventricular septal defect: Results after repair in infancy. Am. J. Cardiol., 39:66, 1977.

Sigmann, J. M., Stern, A. M., and Sloan, H. E.: Early surgical correction of large ventricular septal defects. Pediatrics, 39:4, 1967.

Singh, A. K., deLeval, M. R., and Stark, J.: Left ventriculotomy for closure of muscular ventricular septal defects. Ann. Surg., 186:577, 1977.

Somerville, J.: Personal communication, 1970.

Soto, B., Becker, A. E., Moulaert, A. J., et al: Classification of ventricular septal defects. Br. Heart J., 43:332, 1980.

Stirling, G. R., Stanley, P. H., and Lillehei, C. W.: Effect of cardiac bypass and ventriculotomy upon right ventricular function. Surg. Forum, 8:433, 1957.

Van Praagh, R., Bernhard, W. F., Rosenthal, A., et al: Interrupted aortic arch: Surgical treatment. Am. J. Cardiol., 27:200, 1971.

Wagenvoort, C. A., and Wagenvoort, N.: Primary pulmonary hypertension: A pathological study of the lung vessels in 156 clinically diagnosed cases. Circulation, 42:1163, 1970.

Wagenvoort, C. A., Neufeld, H. N., DuShane, J. W., and Edwards, J. E.: The pulmonary arterial tree in ventricular septal defect. A quantitative study of anatomic features in fetuses, infants, and children. Circulation, 23:740, 1961.

Yacoub, M. H., Radley-Smith, R., and deGasperis, C.: Primary repair of large ventricular septal defects in the first year of life. G. Ital. Cardiol., 8:827, 1978.

Yamaki, S., and Tezuka, F.: Quantitative analysis of pulmonary vascular disease in complete transposition of the great arteries. Circulation, 54:805, 1976.

CHAPTER 39

TETRALOGY OF FALLOT

Ross M. Ungerleider
David C. Sabiston, Jr.

Tetralogy of Fallot (TOF) is one of the most common congenital heart malformations. Depending on the criteria of definitions for this entity, it can occur in 3 to 6 infants per 10,000 births (Mitchell et al, 1971). It is appropriate to consider TOF within the spectrum of pulmonary stenosis (or atresia) with an accompanying ventricular septal defect (VSD). Affected infants usually present with cyanosis shortly after birth, and the diagnosis can be made with two-dimensional echocardiography or cardiac catheterization. Almost all patients are candidates for surgical correction, and there are several options that can provide excellent immediate and long-term results for most of these children.

HISTORICAL ASPECTS

Although Stensen deserves credit for the first description (1672) of what is now called the TOF, this congenital cardiac disorder was made known primarily by Fallot in 1888. Other physicians described the malformation earlier, including Sandifort (1777), John Hunter (1784), William Hunter (1784), Farre (1814), Gintrac (1824), Hope (1839), and Peacock (1866). Most of these descriptions were reports of pathologic curiosities. However, in his description of the disorder, Fallot was the first physician to describe accurately the clinical and complete pathologic manifestations. He emphasized that with a knowledge of the clinical manifestations the malformation could be diagnosed accurately during life.

In the original description, Fallot stated:

"This malformation consists of a true anatomopathological type represented by the following tetralogy: (1) stenosis of the pulmonary artery; (2) interventricular communication; (3) deviation of the origin of the aorta to the right; (4) hypertrophy, almost always concentric, of the right ventricle. Failure of obliteration of the foramen ovale may occasionally be added in a wholly accessory manner."

Fallot reported 55 patients with congenital heart disease, most of whom had the tetralogy malformation. Retrospectively, it is remarkable that such a large number of patients could have been reported by a single author at that time.

Despite the fact that an accurate clinical diagnosis could often be established after these contributions by Fallot, many years passed before definitive treatment of the condition became available. In 1944, Blalock operated on a severely ill infant with TOF who weighed only 4.5 kg. The child was severely cyanotic and had had multiple episodes of unconsciousness due to marked hypoxemia. A systemic-pulmonary anastomosis was created by joining the subclavian artery to the pulmonary artery, and the child benefited greatly. Several months later, Blalock and Taussig (1945) reported this patient and two others. With this epoch-making event, a new era opened in the field of cardiac surgery. The first successful open repair was done by Lillehei and Varco at the University of Minnesota in 1954 by using "controlled cross-circulation" with another patient serving as oxygenator and blood reservoir (Lillehei et al, 1955a, 1986). In the next year, Lillehei replaced this technique with the use of cardiopulmonary bypass and described the repair of TOF by using this technology (Lillehei et al, 1955b). Since then, several advances with life-support mechanisms as well as surgical techniques have made surgical treatment of pulmonary stenosis with a VSD one of the most interesting and often most satisfying procedures in cardiac surgery (Taussig, 1979).

ANATOMY

There is wide morphologic variation in the spectrum of pulmonary stenosis with VSD, which involves the size of the right ventricle, the size and distribution of the pulmonary arteries, the location of the pulmonary stenosis (i.e., subvalvular, valvular, or peripheral), and additional sources of pulmonary blood flow (i.e., systemic-pulmonary collaterals) (Figs. 39–1 to 39–7).

The lesion described by Fallot was considered to be four major defects: infundibular pulmonary stenosis, a VSD, dextroposition of the aorta, and hy-

1332

pertrophy of the right ventricle. Many experts now recognize that the two most important features of TOF are the right ventricular (RV) outflow tract obstruction, which almost always has an infundibular valvular location (Anderson et al, 1981; Arciniegas, 1980; Kirklin and Barratt-Boyes, 1986; Lev, 1964; Zerbini, 1965) and the VSD, which is usually large, subaortic, adjacent to the membranous septum (perimembranous), and associated with malalignment of

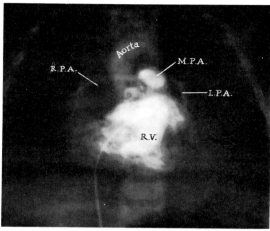

Figure 39–2. Angiocardiogram of an infant with TOF in whom the pulmonary arteries are very small. A palliative operation was done because of serious symptoms. The infant benefited greatly from the procedure. Evidence has been given that enlargement of the right and left pulmonary arteries is produced by a systemic-pulmonary anastomosis in these patients.

the conal septum (Kirklin and Barratt-Boyes, 1986; Lev, 1964). The conal septum is occasionally absent (TOF with subarterial VSD, or "acristal TOF") and the VSD is then subpulmonary as well (Vargas et al, 1986b). In 3 to 25% of patients with TOF, additional muscular VSDs may coexist with the typical subaortic VSD (Fellows et al, 1981) or the VSD may be surrounded by muscle (Anderson et al, 1981). This variation in anatomic presentation has led some physicians to urge discontinuation of the term "tetralogy of Fallot." Nevertheless, from both a diagnostic and therapeutic point of view, the term continues to be useful. A working definition of the tetralogy includes the basic principle that it is a

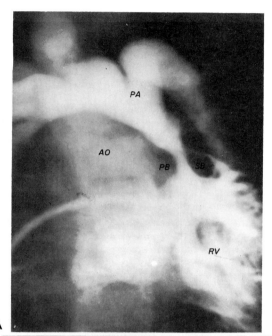

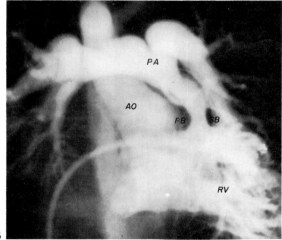

Figure 39–1. Obstruction in the region of the infundibulum. *A*, Frame made in systole. *B*, Frame made in diastole. The negative shadows of the hypertrophied parietal (PB) and septal (SB) bands are particularly well shown. The pulmonary valve appears to be domed, and was bicuspid, but not stenotic at operation. The aorta (AO) is opacified by this RV injection, and its diameter is three times that of the pulmonary artery. The underdevelopment of the infundibulum of the right ventricle, a basic characteristic of TOF, is apparent in this angiocardiogram. This patient has anatomy suitable for total correction. (RV = right ventricle; PA = pulmonary artery.) (From Kirklin, J. W., and Karp, R. B.: The Tetralogy of Fallot from a Surgical Viewpoint. Philadelphia, W. B. Saunders Company, 1970.)

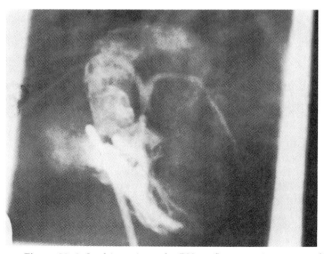

Figure 39–3. In this patient, the RV outflow tract is connected to a small main pulmonary artery with equally small branch pulmonary arteries. Because of the small size of these pulmonary arteries, total correction is not recommended and palliative systemic-pulmonary artery shunting should be done. (From Kirklin, J. W., and Barratt-Boyes, B. G.: Cardiac Surgery. Copyright © 1986 by John Wiley & Sons, New York.)

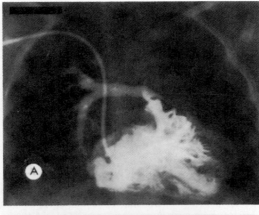

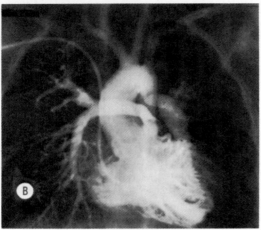

Figure 39–4. *A,* This patient seemingly has only a right main pulmonary artery with discrete valvular as well as subvalvular stenosis. *B,* Aortogram of the same patient shows that the left pulmonary artery arises as a continuation of the ductus arteriosus. (From Kirklin, J. W., and Barratt-Boyes, B. G.: Cardiac Surgery. Copyright © 1986 by John Wiley & Sons, New York.)

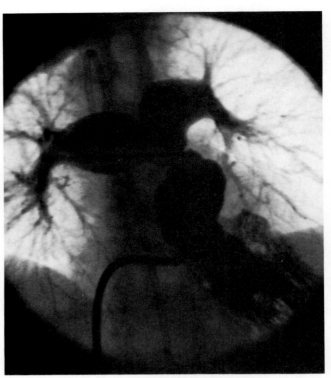

Figure 39–5. In absent pulmonary valve syndrome, there is no significant RV outflow tract stenosis and the pulmonary arteries are aneurysmally dilated.

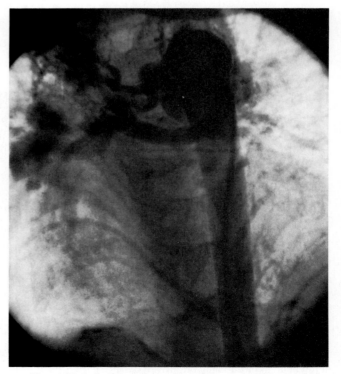

Figure 39–6. In this patient, the pulmonary arteries could be found only during aortography and are supplied entirely by collaterals off the descending aorta. This lesion has been called truncus arteriosus Type IV.

congenital cardiac malformation with a VSD, the size of which approximates the aortic orifice, and with pulmonary stenosis of such a degree that approximately equal pressures are present in both ventricles. There are various degrees of dextroposition of the aorta, and the degree and nature of the infundibular pulmonary stenosis vary. Several types of infundibular chambers have been described, depending primarily on the size of the chamber (Brock, 1952; Brock and Campbell, 1950). The infundibular chamber may be small when the outflow tract obstruction is near the pulmonary valve. At the opposite extreme, the muscular obstruction in the outflow tract may be situated proximally, resulting in a large infundibular chamber sometimes called a "third ventricle" (Fig. 39–8).

Physiologically, most patients with TOF have a high resistance to RV emptying owing to pulmonary stenosis. The predominant shunt is from right to left, with flow across the VSD into the aorta that produces cyanosis and a rise in hematocrit. When the pulmonary stenosis is less severe, bidirectional shunting may occur. In some patients, the infundibular ste-

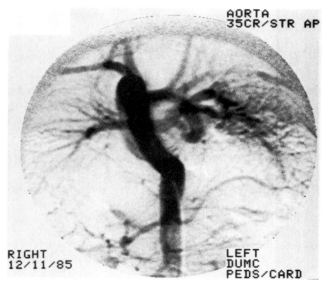

Figure 39–7. Digital subtraction angiography can show nicely the pulmonary artery anatomy as well as its source of flow in neonates. In this patient with pulmonary atresia, a VSD, and a right aortic arch, pulmonary flow depends on a large ductus arteriosus.

nosis is minimal and the predominant shunt is from left to right, which produces "the pink tetralogy." Although these patients may not appear to be cyanotic, they often have oxygen desaturation in the systemic arterial blood (Figs. 39–1 and 39–9). Three to 5% of these patients may present with small, vestigial pulmonary valve leaflets and are considered to have TOF with absent pulmonary valve syndrome (D'Cruz, 1964). In many patients, the infundibular stenosis is minimal and the child may have a net left-to-right shunt. The amount of pulmonary insuf-

ficiency is not trivial and the right and left pulmonary arteries are often enlarged aneurysmally and may compress on the mainstem bronchi causing respiratory distress (Lakier et al, 1974) (see Fig. 39–5). The severe pulmonary insufficiency may impair RV function (Hiraishi et al, 1983).

The pulmonary arteries can also vary in size and distribution. Occasionally, the left pulmonary artery may be absent (3%), although absence of the right pulmonary artery is rare. Some patients have a degree of stenosis of the peripheral pulmonary arteries that further restricts pulmonary blood flow. There may be no communication between the right ventricle and main pulmonary artery (pulmonary atresia), and in this situation pulmonary blood flow is maintained by a ductus arteriosus or some other form of bronchopulmonary collateral circulation. When both main pulmonary arteries are supplied by large bronchial collaterals, the condition is often classified as truncus arteriosus Type IV (see Fig. 39–6).

Overriding of the aorta is caused by true dextroposition and abnormal rotation of the aortic root causing an aorta that arises from the right ventricle to a varying degree. This feature often obscures the pulmonary artery from view on opening the chest—a situation that is made even more prominent when the main pulmonary artery is small and the left atrial appendage abuts the aortic root. Despite this dextroposition of the aorta, aortomitral fibrous continuity is usually maintained in TOF (compared with the subaortic conus that may be found in patients with double-outlet right ventricle).

The aortic arch may be on the *right* side in as many as 25 to 30% of patients with TOF, and the branching pattern of the arch vessels may be abnormal (Fig. 39–10). The ductus arteriosus occasionally

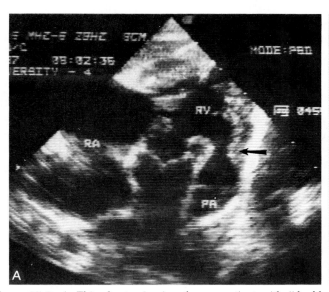 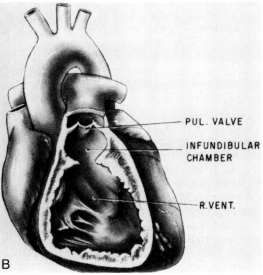

Figure 39–8. *A,* This short axis view from a patient with "double-chamber" right ventricle (RV) shows that the infundibular stenosis *(arrow)* divides the right ventricle into proximal and distal chambers. The distal chamber is proximal to the pulmonic valve. In this syndrome, the pulmonary valve annulus and pulmonary artery are normal and the pulmonary stenosis is entirely infundibular in location. *B,* The clarity of intraoperative echocardiography in delineating anatomy is emphasized when this diagram of "double-chamber" RV is compared with the echocardiogram in *A.*

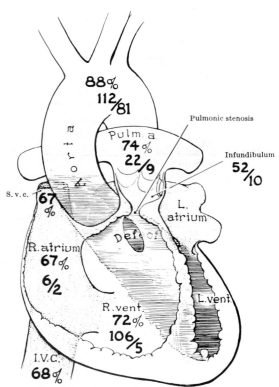

88%
112/81

Pulmonic stenosis

a
o
r
t
a

Pulm. a
74%
22/9

Infundibulum
52/10

s.v.c. **67%**

L. atrium

Defect

R. atrium
67%
6/2

L. vent.

R. vent.
72%
106/5

I.V.C.
68%

Figure 39–9. Results obtained at cardiac catheterization in a patient with TOF. This patient has a relatively high arterial oxygen saturation and represents one of the less severe anatomic types. Values of oxygen are expressed as percentage saturation. The pressures are given in millimeters of mercury (mm Hg). (From Sabiston, D. C., Jr., and Blalock, A.: *In* Derra, E. (ed): Encyclopedia of Thoracic Surgery. Heidelberg, Springer-Verlag, 1959.)

persists on the side opposite the arch (see Fig. 39–7), which could be called a systemic-pulmonary collateral, or it may be completely absent. An aberrant subclavian artery extending in a retroesophageal location may be present (5 to 10%) although it is rare for the retroesophageal subclavian vessels to cause dysphagia. A persistent superior vena cava occurs with almost the same incidence (Nagao et al, 1967).

Coronary arterial anomalies may also be present. Most notable is the origin of the left anterior descending coronary artery from the proximal right coronary artery causing the RV outflow tract to be crossed by this important coronary artery at various distances from the pulmonary valve annulus (Dabizzi et al, 1980; Fellows et al, 1975, 1981) (Fig. 39–11). Occasionally, all coronaries may arise from a single main coronary ostium (usually the left) or the left coronary artery may arise from the pulmonary artery (Akasaka et al, 1981).

Associated defects are not uncommon with TOF. The existence of an atrial septal defect (ASD) is sufficiently frequent to prompt its inclusion as "pentalogy" of Fallot. Other important defects include atrioventricular (AV) septal defects (Vargas, 1986a; Westerman, 1986), muscular VSDs (Fellows, 1981), anomalous pulmonary venous return (Kirklin and Barratt-Boyes, 1986), and aortic incompetence (Matsuda et al, 1980).

CLINICAL MANIFESTATIONS

The clinical presentation depends on the severity of the anatomic malformation. Infants with pulmonary atresia may become intensely cyanotic as the ductus arteriosus closes unless numerous bronchopulmonary collaterals are present, and heart failure is usually not a feature unless collaterals are extensive. Patients with RV to pulmonary continuity are cyanotic in relation to the degree of stenosis and consequent pulmonary blood flow. This balance is also affected by flow through a ductus arteriosus and symptoms usually increase when the ductus arteriosus begins to close shortly after birth. Occasionally, a child has sufficient pulmonary blood flow that cyanosis is not apparent and the lesion may be undetected until the child outgrows the pulmonary blood flow (Bonchek et al, 1973; Gotsman et al, 1966). A common method for these older children to increase pulmonary flow is to "squat," thus increasing peripheral vascular resistance and reducing the size of the right-to-left shunt across the VSD (see Fig. 39–12, color plate). This position has diagnostic significance and is highly characteristic of TOF. There is usually increasing effort with dyspnea as the child grows older (Kirklin and Karp, 1970).

Not all children require early surgical intervention although the natural history of the untreated lesion is unfavorable. This natural history is influenced greatly by the severity of the anatomic defect (McCord et al, 1957). Statistics show a 30% mortality by 6 months of age that increases to 50% by 2 years of age. Only 20% of patients can expect to reach 10 years of age and not more than 5 to 10% live to be 21 years of age (Bertranou et al, 1978; Garson et al, 1987; Kirklin and Barratt-Boyes, 1986) (Fig. 39–13). There are rare cases of patients whose shunts are so well balanced that they achieve a normal life span. One example of this is the American composer Gilbert, who had TOF and led a relatively productive life to the age of 60 without surgical therapy (White and Sprague, 1929).

The greatest risks include paradoxical emboli, leading to stroke or end-organ failure, cerebral or pulmonary thrombosis (from increasing polycythemia), and subacute bacterial endocarditis (Arciniegas, 1985). Heart failure is uncommon in untreated patients but poses a greater risk after the creation of a systemic to pulmonary artery shunt, especially if preexisting collaterals are not managed (Garson et al, 1987).

DIAGNOSTIC EVALUATIONS

Physical Examination

The patient may appear to be smaller than expected for age, and cyanosis of the lips and nail beds is usually apparent. The fingers and toes usually show clubbing (hypertrophic pulmonary osteoar-

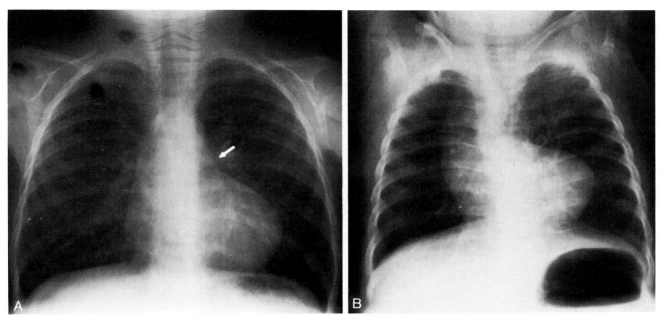

Figure 39–10. *A*, Chest film of a patient with TOF and a left aortic arch. The absence of the pulmonary artery shadow *(arrow)* gives the heart a characteristic "boot-shaped" appearance. *B*, In this patient, the boot-shaped appearance of the heart is made even more prominent due to the right aortic arch and accentuates the absence of pulmonary arterial shadow.

thropathy). On palpation of the chest, a thrill is usually present anteriorly. A harsh systolic murmur is audible over the pulmonary area and along the left sternal border. Absence of a murmur in a patient suspected of having TOF suggests pulmonary atresia. The second heart sound is usually single and rarely increases in intensity. During cyanotic episodes, murmurs may diminish, which suggests less RV outflow to the pulmonary arteries. A continuous murmur suggests a collateral source of pulmonary blood flow (either bronchopulmonary or a surgically created shunt).

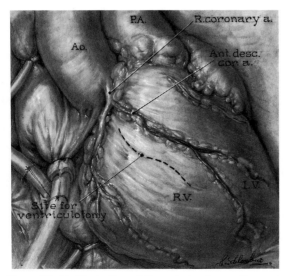

Figure 39–11. Illustration of the anterior descending coronary artery arising from the right coronary artery. Numerous options are available when this aberrancy is encountered.

Laboratory Studies

The hemoglobin, hematocrit, and erythrocyte count are usually raised. The magnitude of the increase is generally proportional to the degree of cyanosis, and hematocrit values vary from normal to as high as 90%; the majority are between 50 and 70%. Similarly, the oxygen saturation in the systemic arterial blood varies, usually between 65 and 70%. However, in severe forms of the malformation, the arterial oxygen saturation during exercise may fall to as low as 25%. A tendency to bleed is present in some patients with TOF, especially those in whom cyanosis is marked. The usual finding is a reduction in various factors responsible for blood coagulation, but none of the factors is reduced to critical levels. The platelet count and total blood fibrinogen are frequently slightly diminished, and clot retraction is sometimes poor and associated with prolonged prothrombin and coagulation times. Despite the defects in the clotting mechanism in some patients, the changes are usually insufficient to explain the hemorrhagic tendency seen at the time of operation (Hartmann, 1952; Porter and Silver, 1968). In infancy, the only significant alteration may be low arterial oxygen saturations.

Chest Films

In the early stages, the chest film may be normal, but in TOF the chest film usually shows diminished vascularity in the lungs and absence of prominence of the pulmonary artery. The shadow of the great vessels in the superior mediastinum is narrow owing

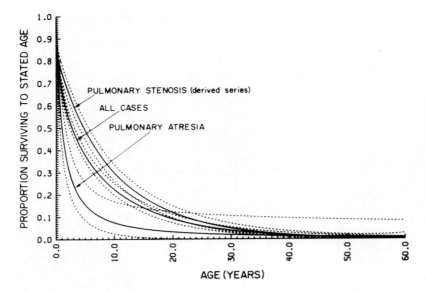

Figure 39–13. This nomogram shows the survival of operatively untreated patients with TOF. Patients with more severe RV outflow obstruction (i.e., pulmonary atresia) have a worse prognosis. *Smooth lines* indicate survival for each group and the *dashed lines* enclose the 70% CLs around each of these. (From Bertranou, E. G., Blackstone, E. H., Hazelrig, J. B., et al: Life expectancy without surgery in tetralogy of Fallot. Am. J. Cardiol., *42*:458, 1978.).

to the reduced caliber of the pulmonary artery. If cyanosis and dyspnea are prominent, the pulmonary vascular markings are usually greatly diminished. Later, the classic boot-shaped heart *(coeur en sabot)* may develop, and it is recognized as being characteristic of TOF (see Fig. 39–10). Diminution or absence of pulsations in the pulmonary arteries can be shown by fluoroscopy. RV enlargement is present and is best shown in the left anterior oblique position. The barium swallow provides evidence of the side on which the aortic arch descends. This is important because approximately one-fourth of the patients with TOF have a *right* aortic arch. The presence of a right aortic arch with cyanosis is strong evidence that the malformation is TOF. Occasionally there is asymmetric pulmonary vasculature with unilateral oligemia compared with the opposite lung. This finding suggests absent pulmonary valve syndrome with unilateral pulmonary artery agenesis or anomalous origin of one pulmonary artery from the aorta (see Fig. 39–4).

Electrocardiography

The electrocardiogram (ECG) usually shows RV hypertrophy, which is usually apparent in the standard leads and is found most consistently in the unipolar leads. The more commonly encountered findings include tall and peaked T waves, reversal of the RS ratio, and a normal PR interval and QRS duration. If RV hypertrophy is absent, a diagnosis of TOF should be questioned seriously and pulmonary or tricuspid atresia with hypoplastic right ventricle should be considered.

Echocardiography

Advances in two-dimensional echocardiography and color flow Doppler have increased the diagnostic

accuracy of this technique. It is not uncommon for infants and children to be accurately diagnosed by echocardiography before other laboratory tests, chest films, ECGs, or angiograms (Fig. 39–14). The addition of color flow mapping can detect quite sensitively the presence of a patent ductus arteriosus (PDA), additional muscular VSD, or small ASD. The physiology of a cyanotic episode with right-to-left shunting across a VSD that is reversed by a rise in peripheral vascular resistance has been nicely shown (Greeley, in press) (see Fig. 39–12, color plate). The coronary anatomy can be shown with remarkable accuracy, and abnormalities of valvular apparatus (i.e., straddling chords) may best be delineated with

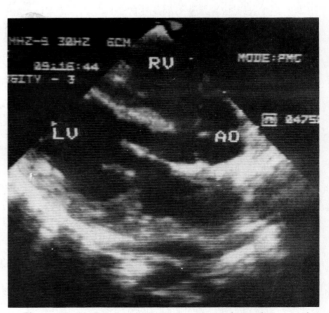

Figure 39–14. Long axis intraoperative echocardiogram that shows the typical features of TOF with a subaortic VSD and overriding of the aorta so that it appears to arise partially from the right ventricle.

this technology (Fig. 39–15). It is not uncommon to perform palliation or correction based on preoperative echocardiography data alone (Kisslo et al, 1988; Marino et al, 1987).

Angiocardiography and Cardiac Catheterization

Cardiac catheterization and angiography provide evidence of ventricular size, pulmonary arterial size, and with aortic root injection, sources of pulmonary blood flow as well as anomalies of coronary artery anatomy (see Figs. 39–1 to 39–7 and 39–9). Some authors base the prediction of the post-repair RV to left ventricular (LV) pressure ratio on data obtained from catheterization, thus assisting operative planning of the type of repair that should be done (Blackstone et al, 1979). Other pressure measurements should show equal pressures in both ventricles (distinguishing this condition from isolated pulmonary stenosis with intact ventricular septum in which the RV pressure may be considerably greater than that in the left ventricle). Angiograms are especially helpful after palliative shunt procedures before complete correction. They define the anatomy of the pulmonary arteries as well as any iatrogenic distortion caused by the shunt that might require attention. If pressure data (i.e., cardiac catheterization) are not needed, digital subtraction techniques can supply excellent views (see Fig. 39–7) with minimal invasion—a useful consideration because it is not unusual for cyanotic episodes and seizures to occur in these children during manipulation of a cardiac catheter.

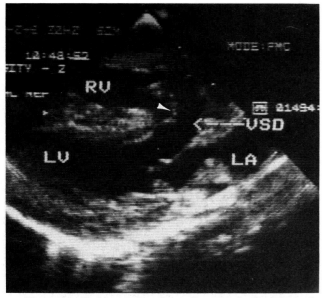

Figure 39–15. Long axis echocardiogram obtained from the epicardial surface at the time of operation shows an anterior papillary muscle giving rise to a chordal attachment on the ventricular septal crest of the VSD *(arrow)*. This information makes it possible to distinguish this anatomy from a straddling chord that would interfere with VSD closure.

INDICATIONS FOR OPERATION

As suggested by the natural history of this lesion, most patients require surgical intervention. Current trends are to do surgical correction as soon as possible, generally by 3 to 5 years of age. The urgency with which operation is done is affected by numerous variables including symptoms at presentation, age, and associated lesions. The use of prostaglandins (PGE_1) to stabilize patients with reduced pulmonary blood flow has greatly influenced the emergent care of these patients (Donahoo et al, 1981; Freed et al, 1981). Rather than doing systemic to pulmonary arterial shunts on critically ill, hypoxemic, and acidotic neonates, surgeons have the opportunity to more fully evaluate the patient's anatomy, while prostaglandins maintain ductal patency (and thus pulmonary blood flow), to arrive at the most appropriate decision for each individual patient. Although controversy continues concerning the preferred operation during infancy, there has been a general trend toward open correction (Calder et al, 1979; Tucker et al, 1979; Turley et al, 1980). The groups who urge early total correction at any time emphasize that it prevents the necessity for a second operation and that the current results are sufficiently encouraging to support this option. Some physicians believe that operation should be done in all patients with TOF irrespective of age or weight except for those with an anterior descending coronary artery arising from the right coronary artery or those with associated pulmonary atresia (Castaneda and Norwood, 1983; Castaneda et al, 1977; Gustafson et al, 1988). Opposition to this approach has been expressed by those who consider that palliation is preferable in infancy because the overall mortality is lower (Arciniegas et al, 1980a; Hammon et al, 1985; Kirklin et al, 1979; Rittenhouse et al, 1985). In addition, these observers are concerned whether the small heart in infancy will remain corrected as growth continues and that outflow tract obstruction of the right ventricle may occur (Kirklin et al, 1988). Various factors that increase the risk for early repair have been described (Table 39–1) and include pulmonary artery problems, major associated anomalies, small size (young age), more than one previous operation, and absent pulmonary valve syndrome (Kirklin et al, 1983). The type of palliation offered to infants, however, varies and is controversial (Figs. 39–16 and 39–17). Although the Blalock-Taussig shunt has been the most popular palliative procedure, many surgeons now use a modification of the Blalock-Taussig shunt by using polytetrafluoroethylene interposition between the subclavian artery and pulmonary artery (de Leval et al, 1981) or between the aorta and main pulmonary artery (central shunt) (Amato et al, 1988; Ebert, 1979). In selected patients, RV outflow patching to promote RV to pulmonary artery continuity and symmetric pulmonary artery growth has also been advocated (Ebert, 1980; Tucker et al, 1979). Irrespective of the type of palliation chosen, the goal

TABLE 39–1. RISKS OF PATIENTS HAVING CORRECTION OF TETRALOGY OF FALLOT*

Category	n	Hospital Deaths		
		No. of Patients	% of Patients	70% CL (%)†
Uncomplicated	89	2	2.2	0.7–5.3
Pulmonary arterial problems	22	3‡	14	6–26
Absent pulmonary valve	6	2§	33	12–62
Major associated cardiac anomalies	16	5‖	31	18–47
Multiple VSDs¶	4	2	50	18–82
Complete AV** canal defect	11	3	27	12–47
Others	1	0	0	0–85
More than one previous palliative operation	6	2††	33	12–62

*Patients with no risk factors have an overall operative mortality between 1 and 5% in most centers.
†CL = confidence limit.
‡One patient was 10 months old; two patients were 30 months old.
§Ages were 7 and 15 days old.
‖Ages were 8, 17, 17, 26, and 30 months old.
¶VSD = ventricular septal defect.
**AV = atrioventricular.
††Ages were 17 and 69 months old.

is to increase pulmonary blood flow, independent of ductal patency, to allow pulmonary artery growth and eventual total correction. Regardless of the approach chosen (one stage versus two stage), it appears that the early use of PGE₁ has saved more infants with TOF and has allowed them to be stabilized so that several surgical decisions can be considered.

SURGICAL TECHNIQUE

Palliative Procedures

The presence of pulmonary atresia or an anomalous left anterior descending coronary artery across the RV outflow tract may preclude the possibility of establishing transannular RV to pulmonary artery continuity and require eventual placement of a conduit. Although conduits can be used in infants (Ebert et al, 1976), patients with small pulmonary arteries may not tolerate total correction in infancy. Likewise, patients with small LV volumes (less than 60% of normal) may do better with initial palliation (Nomoto et al, 1984). Treatment for each patient must be individualized, but these considerations can provide adequate justification for doing a palliative rather than a corrective procedure when the patient is first diagnosed (Sabiston, 1976). Palliative procedures should be directed toward increasing pulmonary blood flow without dependence on the ductus arteriosus. A number of systemic to pulmonary artery shunts are done (see Fig. 39–16), but the most common shunts include (1) the classic Blalock-Taussig shunt, (2) the modified Blalock-Taussig shunt (de Leval et al, 1981), and (3) a central aortopulmonary shunt using prosthetic graft material. The shunts made popular by Potts (1946), Waterston (1962), and Glenn (1945) are no longer being widely used. The Waterston anastomosis (ascending aorta to right pulmonary artery) can cause kinking and stenosis at the

anastomotic site and may make subsequent open correction difficult (Gay and Ebert, 1973; Wilson et al, 1981), and the Potts' anastomosis (descending aorta to left pulmonary artery) can eventually enlarge and can produce an excessive shunt with pulmonary hypertension and often aneurysmal formation at the site of the anastomosis (Ross et al, 1958; Stephens, 1967). Moreover, a Potts' anastomosis is more difficult to close at the time of subsequent correction. Glenn's anastomosis, which is between the superior vena cava and right pulmonary artery, may be followed by good initial results, but more difficulty occurs after subsequent total correction.

Blalock-Taussig Operation

In performance of a subclavian-pulmonary anastomosis, the incision is generally made on the side opposite that on which the aorta descends (Fig. 39–18). Ideally, the subclavian branch of the innominate artery is used for the anastomosis because the angle produced at its origin from the parent vessel is better than that formed when the subclavian artery is used (Sabiston and Blalock, 1959). The latter arises directly from the aorta and is likely to kink at its origin when deflected inferiorly for an anastomosis to the pulmonary artery. If it is necessary to use the subclavian artery on the side of the arch, the modification introduced by Laks and Castaneda (1975) should be considered (see Fig. 39–17). Experimental studies have shown that approximately three-fourths of the blood that passes through a subclavian pulmonary shunt is directed to the lung on the side of the anastomosis (Fort et al, 1965). There is evidence that growth of the pulmonary arteries after shunting is influenced by their structural composition and proportion of elastin as well as by differential blood flow (Rosenberg et al, 1987). Close attention must be given to the performance of the Blalock-Taussig shunt, especially in the construction of the anastomosis.

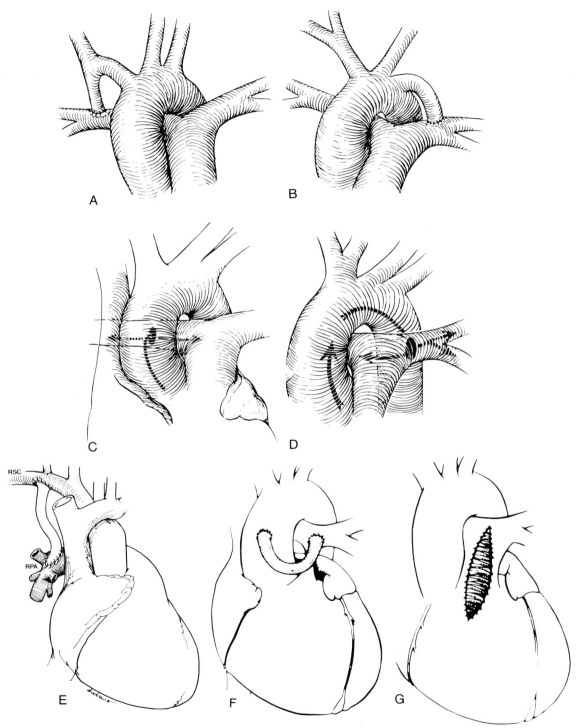

Figure 39–16. The most commonly encountered palliative shunts for increasing pulmonary blood flow in TOF. *A,* Classic Blalock-Taussig shunt. *B,* Blalock-Taussig shunt done on the side of the aortic arch. *C,* Waterston's shunt. *D,* Potts' shunt. *E,* Modified Blalock-Taussig shunt. (From Cooley, D. A.: Techniques in Cardiac Surgery, 2nd ed. Philadelphia, W. B. Saunders Company, 1984.) *F,* Central aortopulmonary shunt with prosthetic graft material. *G,* RV outflow tract patch with prosthetic material (or pericardium). (From Turley, K., Tucker, W. Y., and Ebert, P. A.: The changing role of palliative procedures in the treatment of infants with congenital heart disease. J. Thorac. Cardiovasc. Surg., *79:*194, 1980.)

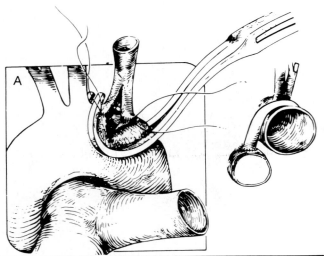

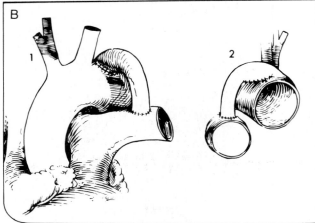

Figure 39–17. Subclavian arterioplasty. *A*, To avoid kinking of the ipsilateral subclavian artery when stretched over the prominence of the aorta *(inset)*, the aorta at the base of the subclavian artery is partially excluded with a C-type vascular clamp. A vertical incision is made approximately 1.5 cm in length, half on the aorta and half on the subclavian artery. The incision is closed transversely. *B*, This both enlarges the takeoff of the subclavian artery (1) and brings its orifice more anterior on the aorta arch (2). (Reprinted with permission from The Society of Thoracic Surgeons. The Annals of Thoracic Surgery, Vol. 19, 1975, p. 319.)

Constriction of the anastomosis must be prevented, and meticulous technique is essential. In infants it is preferable to use interrupted sutures to avoid constriction of the anastomosis. The advantages of the Blalock-Taussig shunt are that it produces a reliable shunt with excellent flow characteristics and shunt flow that is usually well matched to the size of the patient. Complications from transection of the subclavian artery are rare (Arciniegas et al, 1978). This shunt uses no prosthetic material and is easy to close at the time of total correction. The disadvantage is that the shunt requires meticulous and time-consuming dissection that may be difficult to justify in a severely ill infant. In addition, a Blalock shunt can cause distortion of the peripheral pulmonary artery, especially if technical difficulty is encountered during performance of the procedure. As the patient grows,

one pulmonary artery may develop more than the other due to flow characteristics, especially if there is anastomotic distortion. This pulmonary artery distortion may make subsequent total correction more hazardous (Kirklin et al, 1983). After creation of a Blalock-Taussig shunt, progression of the infundibular pulmonary stenosis has been encountered (Sabiston et al, 1964), which can also influence the future operative approach (i.e., transatrial versus transventricular). Despite these features, the classic Blalock-Taussig shunt is still an excellent and time-proven option for increasing pulmonary blood flow in these patients.

Modified Blalock-Taussig Shunt

With the advent of reliable prosthetic graft material, technically easier forms of systemic to pulmonary artery shunting as a method of palliation have become popular. In addition, because most patients return within 2 to 3 years for total correction, the temporary nature of "palliation" justifies the use of an artificial conduit that may not have optimal longevity but does allow for preservation of the subclavian arterial supply to the arm (Arciniegas et al, 1978; Lodge et al, 1983; Webb and Burford, 1952). The "Great Ormond Street" shunt (de Leval, 1981), or "modified" Blalock-Taussig shunt, requires interposition of a segment of polytetrafluoroethylene graft material (usually 4 or 5 mm in diameter) between the subclavian artery and the pulmonary artery (see Fig. 39–16E). Each anastomosis can be done with a partial occlusion clamp and continuous monofilament suture. The shunts can be constructed easily on either side because kinking of the subclavian artery is no longer a problem. Placement on the side of the aortic arch descent may be technically easier. They require limited dissection and are reasonably easy to construct. Although flow through this shunt is still controlled by the size of the subclavian artery, a long segment of prosthetic graft nevertheless supplies its own unique amount of resistance so that flow through these shunts can be more variable. Moreover, because the graft is fixed in size, distortion of the pulmonary artery by the shunt can be anticipated as the patient grows, although this has not been a universal experience (Lamberti et al, 1984; Ullom et al, 1987). These shunts can be slightly more difficult to close than is the Blalock-Taussig shunt and should probably be divided rather than ligated at the time of total correction. These have become the shunt of choice for some groups (Ilbawi et al, 1984) in infants less than 1 month of age.

Central Aortopulmonary Shunt

Several groups have been proponents of interposing a short segment of prosthetic graft material between the ascending aorta and main pulmonary

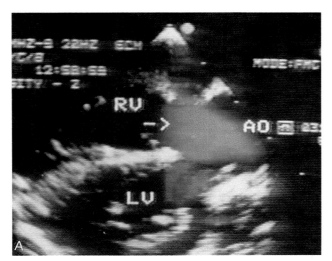 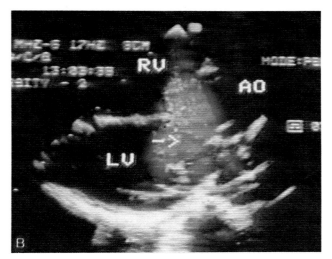

Figure 39–12 A & B

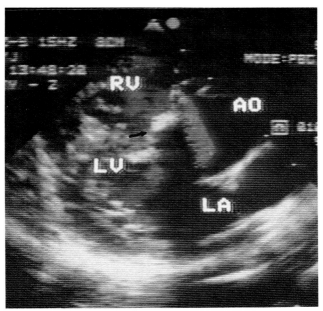

Figure 39–23

Figure 39–12. *A,* Intraoperative Doppler color flow image obtained during symptomatic tetralogy of Fallot. There is increased right-to-left shunting across the ventricular septal defect as demonstrated by "blue" blood flowing from the right ventricle into the aorta. *B,* With increase of systemic vascular resistance, this right-to-left shunt is reversed, thus improving systemic arterial oxygen saturation.

Figure 39–23. This intraoperative epicardial Doppler color flow image demonstrates the patch in place in the ventricular septum (*arrow*). There is no turbulence across the right ventricular outflow tract or across the aorta, nor is there any evidence of residual ventricular septal defect. This constitutes a complete repair.

PLATE 5

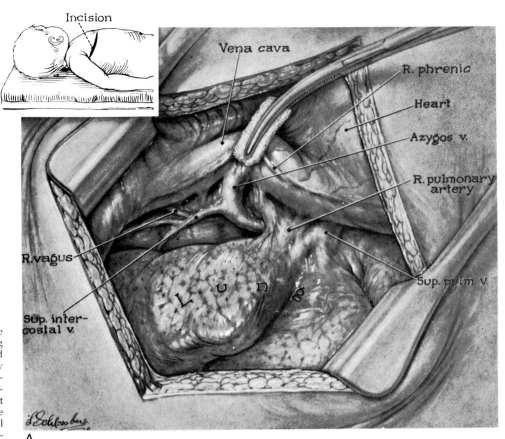

Incision

Vena cava

R. phrenic

Heart

Azygos v.

R. pulmonary artery

R. vagus

Sup. inter-costal v.

L u n g

Sup. pulm. v.

A

Figure 39–18. Performance of a classic Blalock-Taussig shunt. *A,* Initial dissection and exposure of the pulmonary artery for construction of a right subclavian-pulmonary artery anastomosis. The position of the patient is shown on the operating table *(inset).* The entry into the pleural cavity is through the second intercostal space. *B,* After the mediastinal pleura has been incised, the right pulmonary artery is easily identified and distinguished from the superior pulmonary vein. The vena cava is gently rolled anteriorly exposing the innominate artery with its termination in the subclavian and carotid arteries. The subclavian artery is dissected until its most prominent branch points are encountered. Care is taken to protect the recurrent laryngeal nerve that is located beneath the subclavian artery at this point. The subclavian artery is then divided and the distal end is oversewn. The subclavian artery is removed from the "sling" made by the recurrent laryngeal nerve.

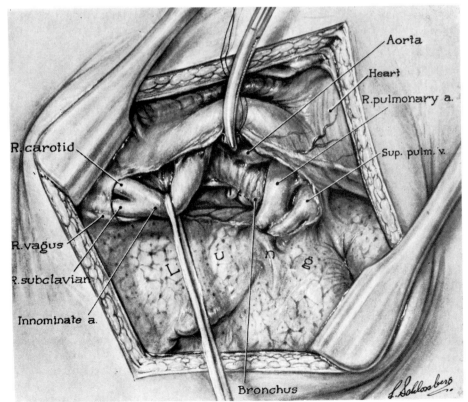

Aorta

Heart

R. pulmonary a.

R. carotid

Sup. pulm. v.

R. vagus

R. subclavian

L u n g

Innominate a.

Bronchus

B

Illustration continued on following page

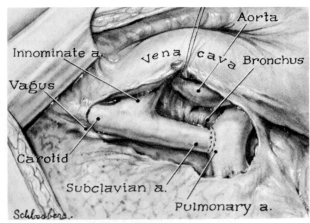

Figure 39–18 *Continued C,* The completed anastomosis. Note that the caliber of the subclavian artery at its origin from the innominate artery is circular. When the anastomosis is done between the subclavian branch of the aorta and the pulmonary artery, there is usually a kink (oval shape) of the subclavian artery at its origin, which thus diminishes the blood flow through the anastomosis. (From Blalock, A.: Surgical procedures employed and anatomical variations encountered in the treatment of congenital pulmonic stenosis. Surg. Gynecol. Obstet., 87:388, 390, 393, 1948.)

artery (Barragry et al, 1987; Ebert, 1979) (see Fig. 39–16*F*). This shunt is easily constructed and can usually be done without cardiopulmonary bypass (with partial occlusion clamps while pulmonary blood flow is maintained by the ductus arteriosus). Shunt flow is usually controlled by the size of the prosthetic material used and, although there have been numerous suggestions concerning the proper graft size, in most cases a 4-mm graft is appropriate for small infants (less than 3 kg) with a 5-mm preference for larger neonates. These grafts have the advantage of creating symmetric pulmonary blood flow and growth without distortion of peripheral pulmonary arteries. Although subsequent total correction requires a repeated sternotomy, this is usually not a problem and with their anterior location the shunts are easy to close. When constructing these shunts, it is important to prevent kinking of the prosthetic graft material because they have a tendency to thrombose if flow is impeded.

The goal of all of these palliative procedures is to increase pulmonary blood flow. The decision with regard to which procedure to use can be based on many factors including the experience of the surgeon. These procedures are generally temporary, and total correction will be needed later. Therefore, the shunt should be chosen which provides the best long-term preparation for repair. Individual problems with anatomy (e.g., proximal stenosis of the right or left pulmonary artery) should be considered, because in this case it may be more advantageous to do a central aortopulmonary shunt (even if cardiopulmonary bypass is necessary) to enable concomitant enlargement of the area of pulmonary artery stenosis. Creation of a peripheral subclavian to pulmonary shunt in such a situation might otherwise limit flow to the contra-

lateral pulmonary artery. A final palliative procedure that deserves mention is that of RV outflow tract patching (see Fig. 39–16*G*). This procedure must be done with cardiopulmonary bypass. Infundibular muscle is resected and the annular narrowing is incised so that there is no longer any obstruction between the right ventricle and pulmonary artery. The VSD is left unclosed and the incision is patched with pericardium or prosthetic material (in infants pericardium is preferred). This procedure is useful when the pulmonary arteries are small (less than one-third the size of the aorta) (see Fig. 39–3) because they will restrict the amount of shunt flow through the VSD. As the pulmonary arteries grow, over a few months, increased left-to-right shunting across the VSD occurs and enables complete repair to be made (Piehler et al, 1980; Tucker et al, 1979). Most patients return within 6 months of this procedure with enlarged pulmonary arteries and predominant left-to-right shunting and at such time require incision through the outflow patch, on cardiopulmonary bypass, for closure of the VSD that completes the repair. The authors' experience with this approach has been favorable in selected patients.

Total Correction

Total correction is the ideal operation for treatment of TOF and is accomplished with extracorporeal circulation. Through a median sternotomy, the pericardium is opened. The anatomy is inspected (if a previous sternotomy has been done for placement of a central aortopulmonary shunt or RV outflow tract patch, the anatomy should have been inspected and carefully commented on at that time). It is particularly important to assess the coronary artery anatomy as well as the size of the main and branch pulmonary arteries. Heparin is given intravenously, and the patient is cannulated for cardiopulmonary bypass. Arterial perfusion is usually accomplished through a cannula placed in the ascending aorta. The venous return can be obtained through bicaval cannulas, or (in patients under 8 kg) a single venous cannula into which holes have been cut. Before establishing cardiopulmonary bypass, previously placed systemic to pulmonary artery shunts should be identified for control. Cardiopulmonary bypass is initiated, and the patient is usually cooled to 25° C. During this time, previously placed shunts are divided or ligated. There are several methods for correcting TOF, and it is important for each surgeon to choose the procedure that yields the best results. The goal of operation, once cardiopulmonary bypass has been established, is closure of the VSD, resection of the area of infundibular stenosis, and relief of RV outflow obstruction (Figs. 39–19 to 39–22). The pulmonary valve should be sized and, if too small, the surgeon should not hesitate to do transannular incision with enlargement of the RV outflow tract out onto the pulmonary artery (Blackstone et al, 1979; Naito et al, 1980;

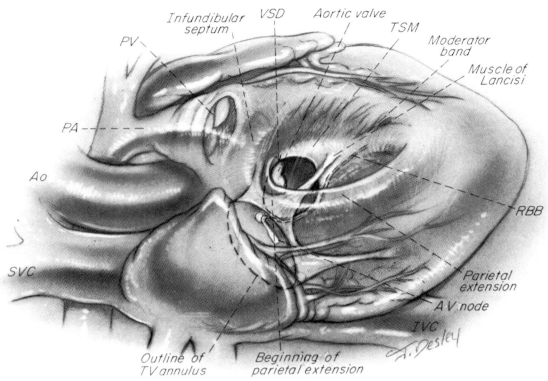

Figure 39–19. Knowledge of structural relationships necessary before correction of TOF. It is especially important to note the emergence of the conduction system in the membranous septum below the AV node. The conduction tissue is particularly at risk on the posterior portion of the VSD, and sutures in this region should be made well off the edge of the defect and kept on the RV side of the septum. The aortic valve should be visible through the defect, and care must be taken when placing sutures along the parietal infundibular fold to avoid the aortic leaflets. The parietal extension of the infundibular septum is usually the region of most severe stenosis and must be divided to enlarge the RV outflow tract. Clear understanding of these anatomic landmarks allows the surgeon to approach this lesion from either the ventricular or atrial approach. (From Kirklin, J. W., and Barratt-Boyes, B. G.: Cardiac Surgery. Copyright © 1986 by John Wiley & Sons, New York.)

Pacifico et al, 1977). Although transannular patches have been considered to be an incremental risk factor for later operative failure by leading to progressive RV dysfunction (Bove et al, 1983; Graham et al, 1976; Ilbawi et al, 1981), this association in the current era does not appear to be significant (Kirklin, 1988). Nevertheless, transannular patches should not be used unless necessary to provide adequate RV outflow, and when done should be constructed to limit the degree of pulmonary insufficiency to preserve long-term RV dynamics (He et al, 1986; Ilbawi et al, 1987; Kurosawa et al, 1986; Misbach et al, 1983). The VSD can be approached transatrially or transventricularly, although in patients with substantial infundibular stenosis the transventricular approach is probably preferable because a ventricular incision is usually necessary. The VSD should be closed with prosthetic material, because these defects are large and it is unwise to attempt primary closure. Knowledge of the location of the conduction tissue is important and, accordingly, sutures are placed along the posterior-inferior border (Bharati et al, 1983; Tamiya et al, 1985) (see Fig. 39–19). Several groups prefer to do this part of this procedure under conditions of moderate hypothermia (25° C) with cold potassium cardioplegic arrest, although the procedure can be accomplished on the cold, non-cross-

clamped, electrically fibrillating heart, or during a period of total circulatory arrest under profound hypothermic conditions (18° C). The optimal method of myocardial protection is still controversial and probably depends on numerous factors concerning the anatomy and physiology of each patient's lesion as well as on the age at the time of repair and the conduct of the operation (del Nido et al, 1988; Kirklin and Barratt-Boyes, 1986; Yamaguchi et al, 1986). After the defect has been adequately closed, attention must be given to relief of the RV outflow tract obstruction. Several groups have reported good results with relief of the subvalvular obstruction by means of transatrial exposure (thus avoiding ventriculotomy if the VSD was also closed by this approach), but a small incision in the infundibular portion of the ventricle can provide excellent results (Coles et al, 1988; Hudspeth et al, 1963; Kawashima et al, 1985; Pacifico et al, 1987). Because the conal septum is usually hypoplastic in these patients, it is important to transect the parietal and septal extensions of the conal septum to increase the size of the RV outflow tract. When all levels of obstruction have been relieved, the ventricular incision (if done) is patched (with pericardium or prosthetic material) and the patient is rewarmed and removed from cardiopulmonary bypass. Even if conduction problems do not occur, it is recommended

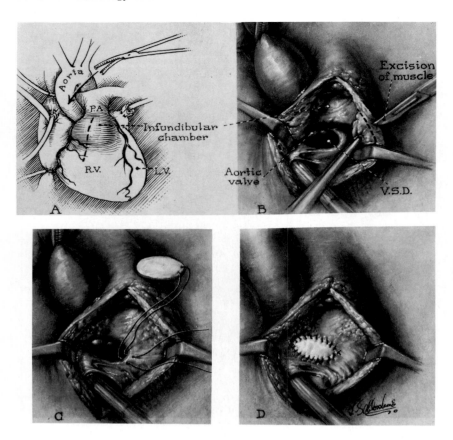

Figure 39–20. Transventricular approach for repair of TOF. *A* and *B*, The typical ventricular incision through the RV outflow tract below the pulmonary annulus. The VSD is identified and infundibular muscle on the parietal and septal side of the infundibular septum is excised. The valve annulus is sized and, if adequate, is preserved. Narrowing of the pulmonary artery can then be approached by a separate incision above the valve annulus if necessary. *C*, Initial suture for placement of the patch for closure of the VSD. *D*, The VSD patch is in place. The ventriculotomy incision is then closed with a patch of pericardium or prosthetic material.

that temporary atrial and ventricular pacing wires be left in place for the perioperative period. After the patient has been successfully removed from cardiopulmonary bypass and the cannulas have been removed, several methods can be used to assess residual ventricular septal shunting. These methods include selective atrial, ventricular, and pulmonary arterial oxygen saturations or pressure measurements. Dye curves have also been used. Experience with intraoperative color-flow Doppler, however, provides a more sensitive and accurate assessment of the adequacy of the intracardiac repair (see Fig. 39–23, color plate) (Hagler et al, 1988; Ungerleider et al, in press). When the surgeon is satisfied with the results of the repair, the chest is closed in the usual manner with mediastinal or pleural catheters and the patient is returned to the intensive care unit.

Special Situations

With the variation of anatomy in patients with TOF, numerous special situations should be mentioned. When the left anterior descending coronary artery crosses the RV outflow tract, a standard transannular enlargement is not feasible because this would cause transection of that coronary artery (see Fig. 39–11). In these cases (depending on the location of the stenosis) it may be possible to do a transverse incision on the infundibulum below the coronary artery for closure of the VSD and resection of the infundibular stenosis. If the pulmonary valve requires commissurotomy or the pulmonary artery requires additional enlarging, this can be done through a separate incision above the pulmonary annulus with patching of the pulmonary artery after

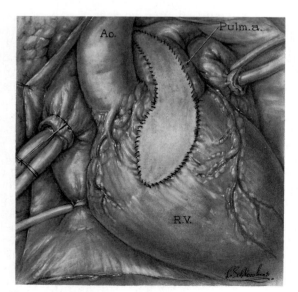

Figure 39–21. When a transannular incision is necessary, the patch should be continued out onto the main pulmonary artery to the level of pulmonary artery bifurcation. If there is stenosis of either branch of the pulmonary artery, the patch can be extended beyond that area of stenosis.

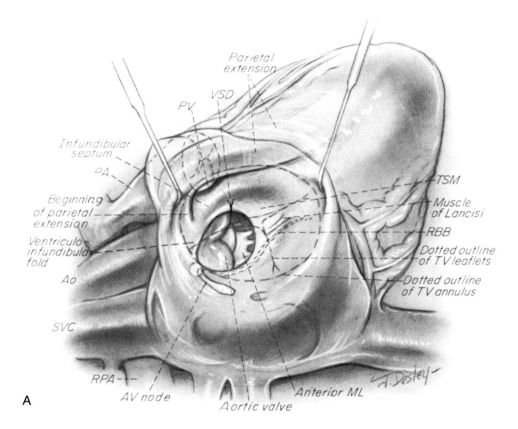

Figure 39–22. Transatrial approach to correction of TOF. *A,* The important landmarks are shown as seen through the tricuspid valve annulus. Note that the parietal extension of the infundibular septum, which must be resected, is now superior, as if it were on the ceiling of the ventricle. *B,* The parietal extension of the infundibular septum has been resected and the VSD is patched, which constitutes repair of the lesion. (From Kirklin, J. W., and Barratt-Boyes, B. G.: Cardiac Surgery. Copyright © 1986 by John Wiley & Sons, New York.)

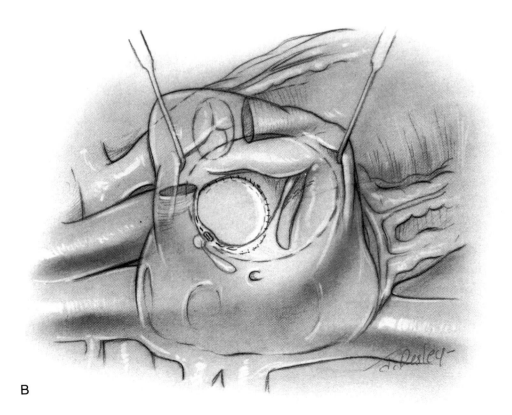

valvotomy has been done (Humes et al, 1987; Hurwitz et al, 1980). These two separate incisions may be preferable to dissecting the coronary artery off the outflow tract with placement of the patch beneath the coronary artery as described by Bonchek (1976), because RV distention, which is not uncommon in these patients, can cause coronary ischemia by stretching of the overlying coronary artery. Another alternative is the use of a systemic to pulmonary artery shunt that allows patients to grow until such time that they can accept an appropriately sized conduit between the right ventricle and pulmonary artery to allow correction by this method.

In patients with the absent pulmonary valve syndrome, the pulmonary arteries may be aneurysmally dilated (see Fig. 39–5). When this problem presents in infancy, it can be managed by plication of the dilated pulmonary arteries (with a running horizontal mattress suture) and closure of the VSD with relief of the subannular stenosis (McCaughan et al, 1985). It may be important to leave a small gradient between the right ventricle and pulmonary artery in these patients to curtail the degree of post repair pulmonary insufficiency (Ebert, personal communication). Some groups advocate a staged repair for severely symptomatic infants, with early systemic to pulmonary shunting together with interruption of right ventricle to pulmonary continuity followed by later correction with a valved conduit (Ilbawi et al, 1986). Regardless of the initial approach, it appears that with age these patients may require placement of a pulmonary valve that can be done with either a homograft or bioprosthesis (Ilbawi et al, 1981; Karl et al, 1986; Mavroudis et al, 1983).

Patients with pulmonary atresia who may need a conduit to re-establish continuity between the right ventricle and pulmonary arteries should be palliated with shunts until they are large enough to allow insertion of an adequate-sized conduit. Exploration by the authors through a median sternotomy has enabled placement of an RV outflow patch across the atretic area (on CPB) to establish RV to pulmonary artery continuity, thus potentially avoiding the necessity for future conduit reconstruction. The procedure for these children at the time of total correction is otherwise similar, with closure of the VSD through a transventricular approach. The ventricular incision can then be used for the proximal anastomosis of the conduit, with the distal anastomosis of the conduit being done to the bifurcation of the right and left main pulmonary arteries. Although these conduits do not require valves, increasing experience with homografts shows they serve quite well because the material is more manageable and more hemostatic than prosthetic conduits.

Occasionally, patients with previous Potts' shunts are encountered. Closure of these anastomoses can present more challenge than repair of the TOF lesion itself, and a useful technique is shown in Figure 39–24. Likewise, ligation of previously placed Blalock-Taussig shunts on the side of aortic arch descent can be difficult. A technique for this is also shown (Fig. 39–25).

RESULTS

The TOF is being corrected with an ever-diminishing mortality, and the results with open correction have been impressive. Nevertheless, it is important to realize that the spectrum of this lesion with respect to the age at presentation as well as the severity of the anatomical derangements can greatly affect the outcome. Overall, the mortality in most series is between 1 and 5% when the repair is done primarily or after a single systemic to pulmonary artery shunt. With improved techniques, excellent results with early one-stage repair in infants have been reported (Castaneda et al, 1977; Gustafson et al, 1988). Likewise, the mortality for infants treated with palliative shunts is low and can be expected to be between 0.5 and 3% depending on the severity of the lesion and the type of shunt chosen (Kirklin and Barratt-Boyes, 1986). Improved techniques of myocardial protection with hypothermia, cold cardioplegia, and even total circulatory arrest are enabling more precise anatomic repairs in younger infants with excellent results. Nevertheless, patients having total correction before 1 year of age have an increased risk compared with those over 1 year of age (Arciniegas, 1985; Arciniegas et al, 1980b; Kirklin et al, 1983), which may be a reflection of the severity of the anatomy.

Early postoperative risks include the creation of heart block, which should occur in less than 1%, and residual VSDs, which should occur in less than 4% (Arciniegas, 1985; Kirklin and Barratt-Boyes, 1986).

POSTOPERATIVE MANAGEMENT

Many variables must be monitored postoperatively. Pulmonary function is maintained by the use of an endotracheal tube and respirator until the patient's cardiac and respiratory status is stable, maintaining relatively normal values for the arterial PO_2, carbon dioxide, and pH. Maintenance of an adequate cardiac output is also important. Peripheral perfusion must be monitored as well as urine output and acid-base status. It is not uncommon for these patients to have elevated RV pressures postoperatively and some inotropic support may be necessary. Patients with this lesion have small RV volumes and can increase cardiac output more effectively by increasing heart rate rather than stroke volume. Therefore, atrial pacing to improve heart rate or the use of isoproterenol may be beneficial. The patients should be maintained on a ventilator until they are hemodynamically stable and show good evidence of no longer requiring ventilatory support. Poor peripheral perfusion, indicative of low cardiac output, should be treated aggressively. Mechanical causes such as cardiac tamponade should be excluded and, if nec-

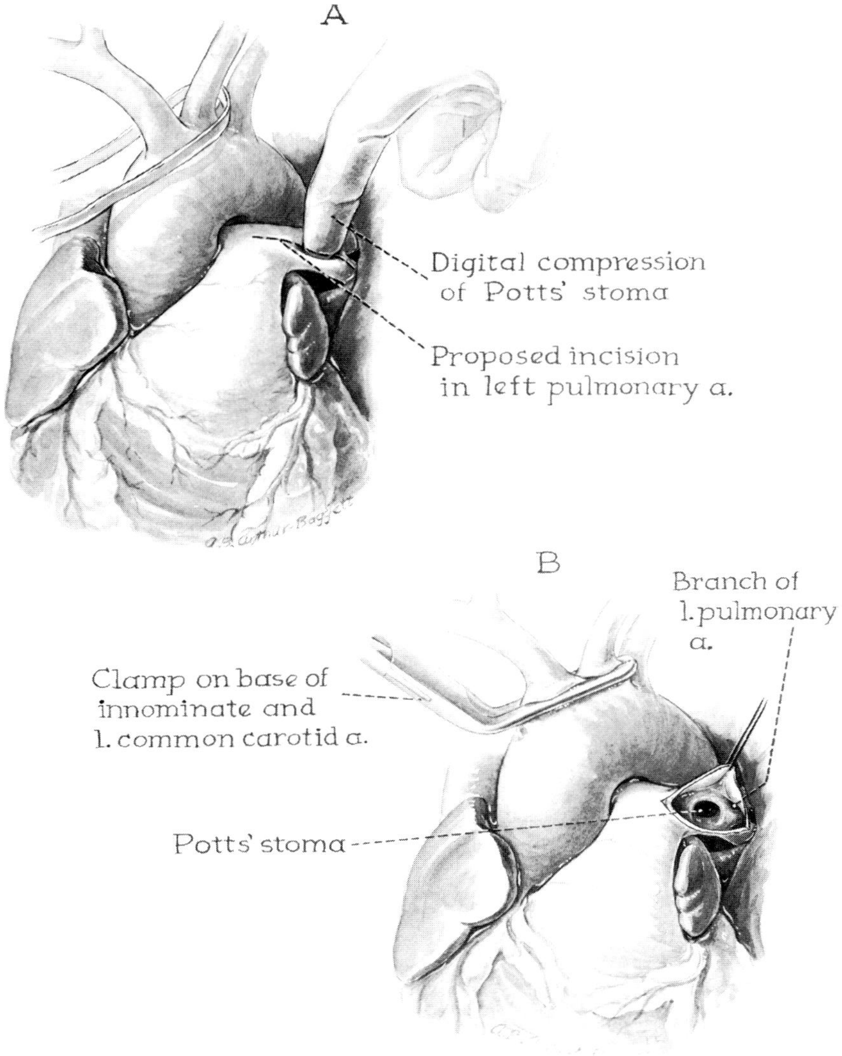

Figure 39–24. The technique for closing a Potts' anastomosis is shown. *A,* After the initiation of cardiopulmonary bypass, and during total body cooling, the Potts' stoma must be compressed to prevent excessive pulmonary blood flow. *B,* The pump is turned off, and the head vessels are clamped. Under total circulatory arrest the left pulmonary artery is opened and the Potts' anastomosis can be visualized and closed. (From Kirklin, J. W., and Karp, R. B.: Tetralogy of Fallot from a Surgical Viewpoint. Philadelphia, W. B. Saunders Company, 1970.)

essary, echocardiography done in the intensive care unit can immediately assess ventricular function or detect the presence of pericardial fluid. Central venous pressure should be adequate, and in these patients with poor RV compliance, central venous pressure may be maintained at slightly higher than normal values. In infants and small children, palpation of the liver edge can be a useful indicator of volume status. If the patient is adequately volume loaded, an inotropic agent such as dobutamine or dopamine to improve cardiac function should be administered. It is not uncommon for these patients to increase their need of inotropic support throughout the course of the first postoperative night. Daily weights should be obtained to follow volume status. These patients typically have a tendency toward fluid retention, and the use of diuretics may be helpful. Because prosthetic materials are used for palliation or correction of this lesion, perioperative broad-spectrum antibiotics should be given. Arrhythmias can often be diagnosed by the use of the temporary pacing wires to allow treatment directed specifically to each arrhythmia. Patients with heart block should be paced sequentially until conduction returns to normal through the AV node. If conduction has not returned in 5 to 6 days, the patient will probably require placement of a permanent pacemaker. The hemodynamic results after intracardiac repair of the TOF have been assessed in several series. Surgical repair of infants under deep hypothermia has been compared hemodynamically with correction by conventional cardiopulmonary bypass with the finding that the results are equal or better with deep hypothermia (Murphy et al, 1980). In a companion study, LV dysfunction as determined after an afterload stress was present postoperatively in patients who had open correction at an older age but not in patients who had repair during infancy. This raises the possibility that early definitive repair may help to preserve postoperative LV function (Borow et al, 1980). In another study, a group of patients with surgical correction of TOF who survived through adulthood were evaluated for their current state as adolescents and adults. Among 233 patients studied,

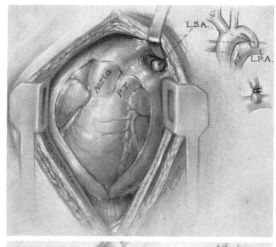
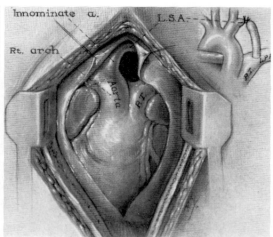
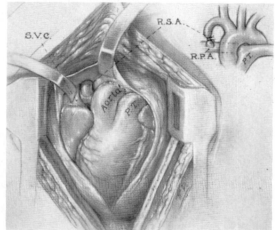

Figure 39–25. Techniques for controlling a previously placed shunt before initiating cardiopulmonary bypass. *A,* A classic Blalock-Taussig shunt can be located between the aorta and SVC where it is anastomosed to the right pulmonary artery. *B,* A classic Blalock-Taussig shunt off a right aortic arch can usually be ligated high in the neck at the origin of the subclavian artery. *C,* A Blalock-Taussig shunt on the left side in a patient with a left aortic arch (whether done in a classic fashion, with the Laks' modification, or as a modified Blalock-Taussig shunt) can be located by an extrapericardial approach. Care must be taken when using this approach to protect the phrenic nerve. (From Kirklin, J. W., and Payne, W. S.: Surgical treatment for tetralogy of Fallot after previous anastomosis of systemic to pulmonary artery. Surg. Gynecol. Obstet., *110:*711, 1960.)

it was concluded that clinical assessment alone did not predict the hemodynamic result and that cardiac catheterization should be done in all patients for objective assessment. The combination of persistent elevation of RV systolic pressure more than 60 mm Hg and ventricular premature depolarizations places the patient at risk of sudden death. However, 80% of the patients lived a normal life without impairment of intellect, exercise tolerance, or fertility (Garson et al, 1979).

With regard to the incidence of sudden death after correction of tetralogy, in a study of 243 patients evaluated with special emphasis on postoperative conduction disturbances, sudden death occurred in 7 patients; the average follow-up was 12 years (range of 6.5 to 16.5 years). Among these patients, four deaths occurred in those with right bundle branch block, and three of these four patients had premature ventricular contractions for more than 1 month postoperatively. Premature ventricular contractions were documented in 10 of 158 patients with right bundle branch block, and sudden death occurred in three patients. Three of the 10 patients with trifascicular block pattern died suddenly, but no deaths occurred

in 24 patients with bifascicular block pattern. The authors of this study concluded that the risk of sudden death in patients with right bundle branch block and premature ventricular contractions after repair of tetralogy is high and requires consideration of suppressive therapy (Quattlebaum et al, 1976). With the advances in detection and surgical treatment of recurrent sustained ventricular tachycardia, a new approach to the therapy of these problems has emerged. Ventricular tachyarrhythmias are estimated to occur in 0.3 to 3% of patients after complete repair and do not appear to be related to the hemodynamic success of the repair. A report on patients having 30 to 150 documented episodes of sustained ventricular tachycardia with failure of pharmacologic and pacing regimens indicated that the source of the arrhythmias was localized by electrophysiologic mapping to the right ventriculotomy scar (Harken et al, 1980). The scar was surgically excised, and ventricular tachycardia was not inducible after operation and has not recurred. These data support the enthusiasm for transatrial repair of tetralogy when possible although it must still be proved that this method will provide long-term protection from dysrhythmias.

Long-term success of repair appears to be based on many factors that mandate continued investigation (Zhao et al, 1985).

Of increasing significance are patients with TOF who also have additional major congenital cardiac anomalies. One of the more interesting associations is that with complete AV canal. Several studies have emphasized the fact that total correction of this combination consists of closure of the VSD as well as the ASD and reconstruction of the AV valve with relief of RV outflow tract obstruction (Arciniegas et al, 1981). A double-outlet right ventricle has also been reported with successful correction (Pacifico et al, 1980). In addition, patients with TOF and associated aortic insufficiency (Matsuda et al, 1980), with aorticopulmonary window (Castaneda and Kirklin, 1977), with anomalous origin of the left coronary artery from the pulmonary artery (Akasaka et al, 1981), and with diverticulum of the right ventricle (Magrassi et al, 1980) have been successfully repaired.

It is possible to correct the tetralogy with extracorporeal circulation in patients with sickle cell anemia, including those with glucose-6-phosphate dehydrogenase deficiency. Intracardiac procedures can be done safely on these patients if some guidelines are observed, especially the avoidance of hypoxia, hypothermia, acidosis, and dehydration. These patients should be prepared for operation with transfusion of normal red blood cells (Szentpetery et al, 1976).

PULMONARY STENOSIS WITH INTACT VENTRICULAR SEPTUM

Stenosis of the pulmonary valve with intact ventricular septum can be one of the congenital cardiac lesions most amenable to treatment. It can also be a highly lethal lesion with dismal prognosis. Much depends on the size of the RV chamber as well as on the age of the patient at presentation (Engle et al, 1964). For patients in whom a good outcome is likely, the symptoms are generally less pronounced than those seen with TOF, although there are numerous examples of infants with severe pulmonary stenosis that produces congestive heart failure. Some infants require immediate valvotomy as an emergency procedure, but in most infants the symptoms develop more slowly. In approximately three-fourths of this group, the foramen ovale is patent, and when increased pressure and decreased compliance develop in the right ventricle, blood is shunted to the left atrium and cyanosis is produced (Fig. 39–26). A jet of blood forced through the aperture under great pressure from the right ventricle into the pulmonary artery creates turbulence and a prominent thrill (Fig. 39–27). Poststenotic dilatation of the main pulmonary artery ensues (Fig. 39–28). In many cases, infundibular stenosis may be associated with valvular stenosis and an intact ventricular septum (Polansky et al,

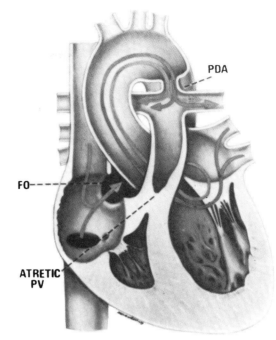

Figure 39–26. Pulmonary atresia with intact ventricular septum showing hypoplastic right ventricle, shunting via a patent foramen ovale, and ductus-dependent pulmonary blood flow. (PDA = patent ductus arteriosus; FO = foramen ovale; PV = pulmonary valve.) (From Moulton, A. M., Bowman, F. O., Jr., and Edie, R. N.: Pulmonary atresia with intact ventricular septum. J. Thorac. Cardiovasc. Surg., *78:*527, 1979.)

1984). Moreover, ASDs are also encountered, and the latter combination is called the *trilogy of Fallot.* The clinical findings depend on the severity of the valvar pulmonary stenosis and the patency of the foramen ovale (Engle and Taussig, 1950). In older children, exertional dyspnea is the most common complaint. Cyanosis is usually present in patients with a patent foramen ovale or an ASD. A harsh systolic murmur and thrill are present over the pul-

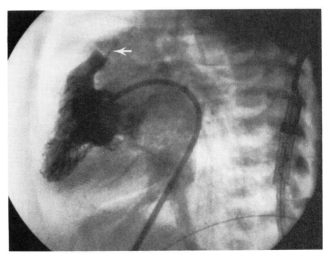

Figure 39–27. Angiocardiogram of a patient with critical pulmonary stenosis. Note the jet of blood *(arrow)* forced through the narrow pulmonary orifice. The main pulmonary artery shows poststenotic dilatation.

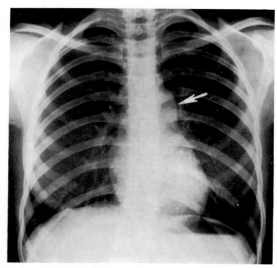

Figure 39–28. Chest film of a patient with isolated valvular pulmonary stenosis, showing typical appearance of poststenotic dilatation of the pulmonary artery *(arrow).*

monary area; the thrill can be palpated in the suprasternal notch. The pulmonary second sound is characteristically weak or absent, and the chest film is often typical, showing prominence of the pulmonary artery due to poststenotic dilatation (see Fig. 39–28). The angiocardiogram is also helpful in showing the classic dome-shaped pulmonary valve with small aperture and poststenotic dilation, or an ASD and infundibular stenosis combined with valvar stenosis. Cardiac catheterization shows a gradient between the right ventricle and the pulmonary artery without evidence of a shunt at the ventricular level. In severe forms, the pressure gradient between the pulmonary artery and the right ventricle may exceed 200 mm Hg.

Pulmonary atresia with an intact ventricular septum represents a serious condition in infancy. Although not a common lesion, it usually demands urgent therapy quite early in life. Infants with the combination of pulmonary atresia and an intact ventricular septum usually present within 24 to 48 hours of birth with dyspnea, tachypnea, and progressive cyanosis. A PDA is usually present as well as a RV heave and murmurs of tricuspid insufficiency. Ductal patency can be ensured by prostaglandin infusion while therapy is planned. Patients in whom symptoms are not as prominent until several weeks or several months later usually have a widely patent ductus arteriosus. Arrhythmias, probably the result of RV hypertension and right atrial dilatation, may be present. Cardiomegaly is shown on the chest film with diminished pulmonary vascular markings. The ECG usually shows a normal axis with LV predominance in the precordial leads. The size of the RV cavity can be assessed by echocardiography; the diagnosis together with details of anatomic and physiologic changes is best determined by cardiac catheterization and angiocardiography. Important factors in planning therapy in these infants include the size

of the main pulmonary artery and the right and left branches, the size and characteristics of the RV cavity, the presence of sinusoidal communications between the RV and coronary circulation, and the presence and relative size of a PDA (Joshi et al, 1986; Moulton et al, 1979; Weldon et al, 1984).

Treatment

Pulmonary valvotomy was introduced by Brock (1948) and consisted of transventricular valvotomy. A valvulotome was passed through the wall of the right ventricle into the pulmonary artery to open the stenotic valve. Later, an improved valvulotome was designed for transventricular use (Potts et al, 1950). Increased success is now being reported with the use of percutaneous balloon valvuloplasty in the cardiac catheterization laboratory (Kvelselis et al, 1985; Lababidi and Wu, 1983; Lock et al, 1987). Nevertheless, open repair of valvular stenosis under direct vision produces excellent results when balloon valvotomy fails. Although some groups recommend valvotomy under inflow occlusion (Coles et al, 1984), the use of extracorporeal circulation permits simultaneous correction of coexisting ASDs and of infundibular stenosis when indicated (McGoon and Kirklin, 1958; Polansky et al, 1985). Moreover, the use of cardiopulmonary bypass allows stabilization of critically ill neonates and affords the time necessary for appropriate surgical treatment, because patients in whom balloon valvuloplasty fails often have more complex anatomy (Fig. 39–29).

Most infants with the combination of pulmonary atresia and intact ventricular septum become critically ill quite early in life and require urgent therapy. In most, a PDA is responsible for maintenance of life, and the infusion of PGE_1 can be helpful in preventing ductal closure and the associated severe hypoxemia and acidosis that would otherwise follow. Although closed valvotomy, systemic-pulmonary shunt and combination procedures have been used, at present the preferred management appears to be combined open valvotomy and shunt (Joshi et al, 1986). Patients with normal-sized right ventricles may not need concomitant shunting (Cobanoglu et al, 1985), but most groups have found that placement of a systemic-pulmonary shunt at the time of open valvotomy ensures adequate pulmonary blood flow after the ductus is allowed to close and until RV compliance improves to provide substantial antegrade flow (Moulton et al, 1979). If there is satisfaction over the degree of right ventricle to pulmonary artery continuity established, then temporary postoperative continuation of prostaglandins may ameliorate the necessity of placement of a shunt at the time of valvotomy (Foker et al, 1986). Equal to the importance of ensuring pulmonary blood flow after valvotomy is the concept of establishing widely patent right ventricle–pulmonary artery continuity. Not only does this appear to prevent the development of

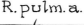
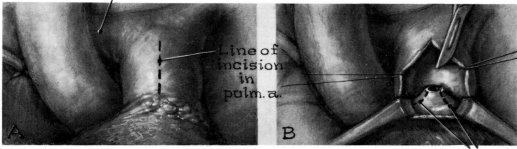

Figure 39–29. Pulmonary valvotomy can be done during inflow occlusion or, preferably, on cardiopulmonary bypass. *A,* The pulmonary artery is opened above the valve annulus. *B,* The valve is inspected. It can then be incised along the areas of commissural fusion. In addition, the RV chamber should be inspected and any areas of infundibular stenosis should be resected through the valvotomy. The pulmonary artery can be closed primarily or with a small patch of pericardium.

sinusoids between the right ventricle and coronary artery system, but it now seems fairly clear that it potentiates growth of the right ventricle to optimize its potential as a usable portion of the anatomy (Lewis et al, 1986; Weldon et al, 1984). Furthermore, with adequate relief of the RV outflow obstruction, infundibular hypertrophy appears to resolve with time and produces a more normal right ventricle (Griffith et al, 1982). These considerations are important because failure to encourage growth of the right ventricle may result in its ultimate inability to provide normal function and may require transformation of the circuit to a univentricular arrangement (Fontan's procedure).

Valvotomy by open correction of pulmonary valvular stenosis yields excellent results, and recurrence of the condition is rare. Moreover, the compensatory infundibular hypertrophy that frequently accompanies the valvular stenosis usually regresses with time. Although the gradient between the right ventricle and the pulmonary artery may not be totally abolished immediately after operation, regression of the secondary hypertrophy of the RV outflow tract occurs, and repeated catheterization later shows a sharp reduction in the gradient (Engle et al, 1958).

Isolated infundibular stenosis of the right ventricle may also occur as a congenital anomaly. The symptoms are similar to those of valvular stenosis, although the murmur may be located slightly lower in the precordium. The angiocardiogram shows the lesion with precision, and cardiac catheterization shows two gradients: one between the pulmonary artery and the other between the infundibulum and the right ventricle. Two-dimensional echocardiography shows this lesion well and shows why it is often referred to as a "double chamber" (see Fig. 39–8). Management of these patients consists of resection of the infundibular stenosis in the open heart by using extracorporeal circulation. The results are excellent.

Selected Bibliography

Arciniegas, E., Farooki, Z. Q., Hakimi, J., and Green, E. W.: Results of a two-stage surgical treatment of tetralogy of Fallot. J. Thorac. Cardiovasc. Surg., 79:876, 1980.

This group reports 109 consecutive patients having palliative shunt as the initial management for symptomatic TOF. The total early shunt mortality, including the Blalock-Taussig shunt as well as Waterston's shunt, was 2.7%. The mean patient age at the time of total repair was 4.8 years, and the second-stage corrective operation had a mortality of 1.6%. They consider the Blalock-Taussig shunt to be the shunt of choice in all symptomatic infants and small children with TOF and emphasize that the two-stage surgical approach compares favorably with primary total correction, particularly in infants under 1 year of age.

Bharati, S., Lev, M., and Kirklin, J. W.: Cardiac Surgery and the Conduction System. New York, Wiley Medical Publications, 1983.

This well illustrated monograph shows the location of cardiac conduction tissue through various standard surgical approaches. Increasing success with total repair of lesions such as TOF is related to greater understanding of the location of specialized conduction tissue so that injury to this tissue can be routinely and reliably prevented during open cardiac procedures. The contribution toward that understanding by these authors is extensive.

Blalock, A., and Taussig, H. B.: The surgical treatment of malformations of the heart in which there is pulmonary stenosis or pulmonary atresia. J.A.M.A., *128*:189, 1945.

In this paper, Blalock's first three operations for creation of a systemic-pulmonary anastomosis are reported. The first patient, a 15-month-old infant with severe cyanosis, had a history of multiple episodes of loss of consciousness. An anastomosis of the left subclavian artery to the left pulmonary artery was made, and the clinical improvement was striking. Two additional patients with successful results are also described. It is interesting that Blalock refers to earlier experimental work in which subclavian pulmonary anastomoses were done in the dog in an effort to produce pulmonary hypertension. Although these experiments did not succeed in producing an elevated pulmonary arterial pressure, the operation was later used for an entirely different purpose. This procedure was the first of many additional cardiac surgical advances.

Castaneda, A. R., Freed, M. D., Williams, R. G., and Norwood, W. I.: Repair of tetralogy of Fallot in infancy: Early and late results. J. Thorac. Cardiovasc. Surg., 74:372, 1977.

These authors report a series of 41 consecutive infants operated on for primary correction of the TOF with deep hypothermia and circulatory arrest. The infants ranged in age from 12 days to 1 year, with a mean age of 5 to 7 months. The authors conclude that the hospital mortality and early and late results justify continued evaluation of primary repair of TOF in symptomatic infants, regardless of weight or age. The contraindications they cite to reparative operation in symptomatic infants with the tetralogy are an anterior descending coronary artery arising from the right coronary artery or associated congenital pulmonary atresia.

Foker, J. E., Braunlin, E. A., St. Cyr, J. A., et al: Management of pulmonary atresia with intact ventricular septum. J. Thorac. Cardiovasc. Surg., 92:706, 1986.

These authors report clinical experiences with 50 neonates diagnosed with pulmonary atresia with an intact ventricular septum. The goal of therapeutic intervention was to re-establish the right ventricle to pulmonary artery continuity to encourage any potential RV growth. In addition, placement of a systemic to pulmonary artery shunt was avoided in all patients by utilizing continued PGE₁ infusion in the postoperative period. This study suggests that patients with pulmonary atresia can be managed adequately by attempts to salvage the right ventricle and that placement of an aortopulmonary shunt can often be avoided if re-establishment of antegrade flow from the right side of the heart can be achieved. With successful application of this technique, management of pulmonary atresia with an intact ventricular septum can be accomplished as a one-stage procedure.

Gustafson, R. A., Murray, G. F., Warden, H. E., et al: Early primary repair of tetralogy of Fallot. Ann. Thorac. Surg., 45:235, 1988.

These authors report an experience with total correction of TOF in 40 patients. Ten patients were less than 1 year of age and the mean age of the other 30 patients was 24 months. The operative mortality was zero. The results of the study suggest that early primary repair of TOF is justified in symptomatic children regardless of age or weight. In addition, no impact on operative mortality from the use of a transannular RV outflow tract (RVOT) patch was found.

Kirklin, J. W., and Barratt-Boyes, B. G.: Cardiac Surgery, New York, John Wiley and Sons, 1986, pp. 699–857.

This remarkable book includes the extraordinary experience of these two experts in the field of congenital heart surgery. The material included is among the most comprehensive and well-organized presentations available and should be read by anyone who desires in-depth reading in this field.

Kirklin, J. W., Blackstone, E. H., Kirklin, J. K., et al: Surgical results and protocols in the spectrum of tetralogy of Fallot. Ann. Surg., 198:251, 1983.

This study reports the results of this outstanding group with 1103 operations for TOF of all types between 1967 and 1982. Analysis of this large number of patients allows a description of the incremental risk factors for operative mortality as well as recommendations for patients who should have primary versus staged repair. Risks of correction were from 1.6 to 7.7% depending on the age of the patient and the nature of the lesion.

Kirklin, J. W., and Karp, R. B.: Tetralogy of Fallot from a Surgical Viewpoint. Philadelphia, W. B. Saunders Company, 1970.

This monograph is superb and has excellent presentations of the anatomy, natural history, hemodynamics, clinical features, and diagnosis of TOF. The techniques of palliative and open corrective procedures are well described and illustrated. A detailed account of the results is provided and ranks among the best in the world literature. The monograph is highly recommended for a complete analysis of the entire subject.

Lillehei, C. W., Varco, R. L., Cohen, M., et al: The first open heart repairs of ventricular septal defect, atrioventricular communis and tetralogy of Fallot using extracorporeal circulation by cross-circulation: A thirty year follow-up. Ann. Thorac. Surg., 414, 1986.

More than just a 30-year follow-up of the first patients to successfully have open cardiac correction of complex cardiac lesions, this reference provides a poignant recapitulation of early open heart surgery. Lillehei's historical account of the frustrations and ingenious attempts by the intrepid individuals who began the era of open heart surgery that is now so common should be read by everyone. Of equal impact are the thoughts offered by the discussants who include some of the more prominent experts in the field of cardiac surgery. After reading this book, the surgeon will have a better understanding of the historical debt that is owed these individuals who had the insight and creativity to attack the problems of open cardiac surgery.

Moulton, A. L., Bowman, F. O., Jr., Edie, R. N., et al: Pulmonary atresia with intact ventricular septum. Sixteen-year experience. J. Thorac. Cardiovasc. Surg., 78:527, 1979.

This is a review of 30 patients with pulmonary atresia and intact ventricular septum treated by various surgical approaches during a 16-year period. The authors conclude that in most patients the preferred operation is combined pulmonary valvotomy (or outflow patch) together with a systemic-pulmonary shunt. This approach has yielded the best long-term results so far.

Pacifico, A. D., Sand, M. E., Bargeron, L. M., Jr., and Colvin, E. C.: Transatrial-transpulmonary repair of tetralogy of Fallot. J. Thorac. Cardiovasc. Surg., 93:119, 1987.

These authors describe results with transatrial approach to total correction of TOF in 61 patients. There were no hospital or late deaths or reoperations among the entire group. This series indicates that successful repair of TOF can be accomplished in many patients by a transatrial approach, which may provide improved RV function over the long term.

Sabiston, D. C., Cornell, W. P., Criley, J. M., et al: The diagnosis and surgical correction of total obstruction of the right ventricle: An acquired condition developing after systemic artery-pulmonary artery anastomosis for tetralogy of Fallot. J. Thorac. Cardiovasc. Surg., 48:577, 1964.

In this report, the most severe forms of TOF, those with complete obliteration of the outflow tract of the right ventricle and its communication with the pulmonary artery, are described together with the details of operative corrections and results. In these patients who have no communication between the right ventricle and pulmonary artery and who, after correction, have total pulmonary insufficiency, the subsequent course is generally good (i.e., pulmonary valvular insufficiency can be well tolerated).

Taussig, H. B.: Tetralogy of Fallot: Early history and late results. Neuhauser Lecture. Am. J. Roentgenol., 133:423, 1979.

This classic and updated reference is written by a distinguished pediatric cardiologist. She summarizes the early and late results of the Blalock-Taussig operation in a large number of patients. An excellent historical review of the subject is also included.

Tucker, W. Y., Turley, K., Ullyot, D. J., and Ebert, P. A.: Management of symptomatic tetralogy of Fallot in the first year of life. J. Thorac. Cardiovasc. Surg., 78:494, 1979.

A series of patients is presented in whom correction of symptomatic TOF in the first year was recommended with excellent results. Criteria for early repair are given, and the concept of transannular outflow patching for patients with pulmonary arteries less than one-third the size of the aorta is suggested.

Turley, K., Tucker, W. Y., and Ebert, P. A.: The changing role of palliative procedures in the treatment of infants with congenital heart disease. J. Thorac. Cardiovasc. Surg., 79:194, 1980.

These authors question the need for palliation in some lesions, specifically transposition of the great arteries, TOF, VSD, and truncus arteriosus. Although previously palliated by many groups before the publication of this article, the feasibility and good results with early total correction are documented. In many ways, this important article encouraged many physicians to consider early total repair for complicated congenital heart defects.

Bibliography

Akasaka, T., Itoh, K., Ohkawa, Y., et al: Surgical treatment of anomalous origin of the left coronary artery from the pulmonary artery associated with tetralogy of Fallot. Ann. Thorac. Surg., 31:469, 1981.

Amato, J. J., Marbey, M. L., Bush, C., et al: Systemic-pulmonary polytetrafluoroethylene shunts in palliative operations for congenital heart disease: Revival of the central shunt. J. Thorac. Cardiovasc. Surg., 95:62, 1988.

Anderson, R. H., Path, M. R. C., Allwork, S. P., et al: Surgical anatomy of tetralogy of Fallot. J. Thorac. Cardiovasc. Surg., 81:887, 1981.

Arciniegas, E., Blackstone, E. H., Pacifico, A. D., and Kirklin, J. W.: Classic shunting operations as part of two-stage repair for tetralogy of Fallot. Ann. Thorac. Surg., 27:514, 1978.

Arciniegas, E., Farooki, Z. Q., Hakimi, M., et al: Early and late results of total correction of tetralogy of Fallot. J. Thorac. Cardiovasc. Surg., 80:770, 1980a.

Arciniegas, E., Farooki Z. Q., Hakimi, M., et al: Results of two-stage surgical treatment of tetralogy of Fallot. J. Thorac. Cardiovasc. Surg., 79:876, 1980b.

Arciniegas, E., Hakimi, M., Farooki, Z. Q., and Green, E. W.: Results of total correction of tetralogy of Fallot with complete atrioventricular canal. J. Thorac. Cardiovas. Surg., 81:768, 1981.

Arciniegas, E.: Tetralogy of Fallot. In Arciniegas, E. (ed): Pediatric Cardiac Surgery. Chicago, Year Book Medical Publishers, Inc., 1985.

Barragry, T. P., Ring, W. S., and Blatchford, J. W.: Central aorto-pulmonary artery shunts in neonates with complex cyanotic congenital heart disease. J. Thorac. Cardiovasc. Surg., 93:767, 1987.

Bertranou, E. G., Blackstone, E. H., Hazelrig, J. B., et al: Life expectancy without surgery in tetralogy of Fallot. Am. J. Cardiol., 42:458, 1978.

Bharati, S., Lev, M., and Kirklin, J. W.: Cardiac Surgery and the Conduction System. New York, Wiley Medical Publications, 1983.

Blackstone, E. H., Kirklin, J. W., Bertranou, E. G., et al: Preoperative prediction from cineangiograms of postrepair right ventricular pressure in tetralogy of Fallot. J. Thorac. Cardiovasc. Surg., 78:542, 1979.

Blackstone, E. H., Kirklin, J. W., and Pacifico, A. D.: Decision-making in repair of tetralogy of Fallot based on intraoperative measurements of pulmonary arterial outflow tract. J. Thorac. Cardiovasc. Surg., 77:526, 1979.

Blalock, A.: Surgical procedures employed and anatomical variations encountered in the treatment of congenital pulmonic stenosis. Surg. Gynecol. Obstet., 87:385, 1948.

Blalock, A., and Taussig, H. B.: The surgical treatment of malformations of the heart in which there is pulmonary stenosis or pulmonary atresia. J.A.M.A., 128:189, 1945.

Bonchek, L. I., Starr, A., Sunderland, C. O., et al: Natural history of tetralogy of Fallot. Circulation, 48:392, 1973.

Borow, K. M., Green, L. H., Castaneda, A. R., and Keane, J. F.: Left ventricular function after repair of tetralogy of Fallot and its relationship to age at surgery. Circulation, 61:1150, 1980.

Bove, E. L., Byrum, C. J., Thomas, F. D., et al: The influence of pulmonary insufficiency on ventricular function following repair of tetralogy of Fallot: Evaluation using radionuclide ventriculography. J. Thorac. Cardiovasc. Surg., 85:691, 1983.

Brock, R. C.: Pulmonary valvulotomy for the relief of congenital pulmonary stenosis: report of 3 cases. Br. Med. J., 1:1121, 1948.

Brock, R. C., and Campbell, M.: Infundibular resection or dilatation for infundibular stenosis. Br. Heart J., 12:403, 1950.

Brock, R. C.: Congenital pulmonary stenosis. Am. J. Med., 12:706, 1952.

Calder, A. L., Barratt-Boyes, B. G., Brandt, P. W. T., et al: Postoperative evaluation of patients with tetralogy of Fallot repaired in infancy. J. Thorac. Cardiovasc. Surg., 77:704, 1979.

Castaneda, A. R., Freed, M. D., Williams, R. G., and Norwood, W. I.: Repair of tetralogy of Fallot in infancy: Early and late results. J. Thorac. Cardiovasc. Surg., 74:372, 1977.

Castaneda, A. R., and Kirklin, J. W.: Tetralogy of Fallot with aorticopulmonary window: Report of two surgical cases. J. Thorac. Cardiovasc. Surg., 74:467, 1977.

Castaneda, A. R., and Norwood, W. I.: Fallot's tetralogy. In Stark, J., and de Leval, M. (eds): Surgery for Congenital Heart Defects. Orlando, FL, Grune & Stratton, 1983.

Cobanoglu, A., Metzdorff, M. T., Pinson, C. W., et al: Valvotomy for pulmonary atresia with intact ventricular septum. J. Thorac. Cardiovasc. Surg., 89:482, 1985.

Coles, J. G., Freedom, R. M., Olley, P. M., et al: Surgical management of critical pulmonary stenosis. Ann. Thorac. Surg., 38:458, 1984.

Coles, J. G., Kirklin, J. W., Pacifico, A. D., et al: The relief of pulmonary stenosis by a transatrial versus a transventricular approach to the repair of tetralogy of Fallot. Ann. Thorac. Surg., 45:7, 1988.

Cooley, D. A.: Techniques in Cardiac Surgery, 2nd ed. Philadelphia, W. B. Saunders Company, 1984.

Dabizzi, R. P., Caprioli, G., and Alazzi, L.: Distribution and anomalies of coronary arteries in tetralogy of Fallot. Circulation, 61:84, 1980.

D'Cruz, I., Lendrum, B. L., and Novak, G.: Congenital absence of the pulmonary valve. Am. Heart J., 68:728, 1964.

de Leval, M. R., McKay, R., Jones, M., et al: Modified Blalock-Taussig shunt: Use of subclavian artery orifice as flow regulator in prosthetic systemic-pulmonary artery shunts. J. Thorac. Cardiovasc. Surg., 81:112, 1981.

del Nido, P. J., Mickle, D. A., Wilson, G. J., et al: Inadequate myocardial protection with cold cardioplegic arrest during repair of tetralogy of Fallot. J. Thorac. Cardiovasc. Surg., 95:223, 1988.

Donahoo, J. S., Roland, J. M., Kan, J., et al: Prostaglandin E₁ as an adjunct to emergency cardiac operations in neonates. J. Thorac. Cardiovasc. Surg., 81:227, 1981.

Ebert, P. A., Robinson, S. J., Stanger, P., and Engle, M. A.: Pulmonary artery conduits in infants younger than six months of age. J. Thorac. Cardiovasc. Surg., 72:351, 1976.

Ebert, P. A.: Past, present, and future of palliative shunts. Adv. Cardiol., 26:127, 1979.

Ebert, P. A.: Discussion of Piehler, J. M., Danielson, G. K., McGoon, D. C., et al: Management of pulmonary atresia with ventricular septal defect and hypoplastic pulmonary arteries by right ventricular outflow construction. J. Thorac. Cardiovasc. Surg., 80:552, 1980.

Engle, M. A., Holswade, G. R., Goldberg, H. P., et al: Regression after open valvotomy of infundibular stenosis accompanying severe valvular pulmonic stenosis. Circulation, 17:862, 1958.

Engle, M. A., Tomiko, I., and Goldberg, H. P.: The fate of a patient with pulmonic stenosis. Circulation, 30:554, 1964.

Engle, M. A., and Taussig, H. B.: Valvular pulmonic stenosis with intact ventricular septum and patent foramen ovale: Report of illustrative cases and analysis of clinical syndrome. Circulation, 2:481, 1950.

Fallot, E. L. A.: Contribution à l'anatomic pathologique de la maladie bleue (cyanose cardiaque). Marseille Med., 25:77, 138, 207, 270, 341, 403, 1888.

Farre, J. R.: Pathological Researches. Essay I. On malformations of the human heart: Illustrated by numerous cases, and preceded by some observations on the method of improving the diagnostic part of medicine. London, Longmans, Green & Co., 1814.

Fellows, K. E., Freed, M. K., and Keane, J. R., et al: Results of routine preoperative coronary angiography in tetralogy of Fallot. Circulation, 51:561, 1975.

Fellows, K. E., Smith, J., and King, J. F.: Preoperative angiocardiography in infants with tetralogy of Fallot: Review of 36 cases. Am. J. Cardiol., 47:1279, 1981.

Foker, J. E., Braulin, E. A., St. Cyr, J. A., et al: Management of pulmonary atresia with intact ventricular septum. J. Thorac. Cardiovasc. Surg., 92:706, 1986.

Fort, L., III, Morrow, A. G., Pierce, G. E., et al: The distribution of pulmonary blood flow after subclavian-pulmonary anastomosis. An experimental study. J. Thorac. Cardiovasc. Surg., 50:671, 1965.

Freed, M. D., Heymann, M. A., Lewis, A. B., et al: Prostaglandin E₁ in infants with ductus arteriosus-dependent congenital heart disease. Circulation, 64:899, 1981.

Garson, A., Nihill, M. R., McNamara, D. G., and Cooley, D. A.: Status of the adult and adolescent after repair of tetralogy of Fallot. Circulation, 59:1232, 1979.

Garson, A., Jr., McNamara, D. G., and Cooley, D. A.: Tetralogy of Fallot in Adult Congenital Heart Disease. Philadelphia, F. A. Davis Company, 1987, pp. 493–519.

Gay, W. A., Jr., and Ebert, P. A.: Aorto-to-right pulmonary anastomosis causing obstruction to the right pulmonary artery. Ann. Thorac. Surg., 16:402, 1973.

Gintrac, E.: Observations et Recherches sur la Cyanose, ou Maladie Bleue. Paris, J. Pinard, 1924.

Glenn, W. W. L., and Patino, J. F.: Circulatory bypass of the right heart. I: Preliminary observation on direct delivery of vena caval blood into pulmonary arterial circulation: Azygos vein-pulmonary artery shunt. Yale J. Biol. Med., 27:147, 1954.

Gotsman, M. S.: Increasing obstruction to the outflow tract in Fallot's tetralogy. Br. Heart J., 28:615, 1966.

Graham, T. P., Jr., Cordell, D., Atwood, G. F., et al: Right ventricular volume characteristics before and after palliative and reparative operation in tetralogy of Fallot. Circulation, 54:417, 1976.

Greeley, W. J., Stanley, T. E., Ungerleider, R. M., and Kisslo, J. A.: Intraoperative hypoxemic spells in tetralogy of Fallot: An echocardiographic analysis of diagnosis and treatment. Anesth. Analg. (in press).

Griffith, B. P., Hardesty, R. L., Siewers, R. D., et al: Pulmonary valvulotomy alone for pulmonary stenosis: Results in children with and without muscular infundibular hypertrophy. J. Thorac. Cardiovasc. Surg., 83:577, 1982.

Gustafson, R. A., Murray, G. F., Warden, H. E., et al: Early primary repair of tetralogy of Fallot. Ann. Thorac. Surg., 45:235, 1988.

Hagler, D. J., Tajik, A. J., Seward, J. B., et al: Intraoperative two-dimensional Doppler echocardiography. Thorac. Cardiovasc. Surg., 95:516, 1988.

Hammon, J. W., Henry, C. L., Merrill, W. H., et al: Tetralogy of Fallot: Selective surgical management can minimize operative mortality. Ann. Thorac. Surg., 40:280, 1985.

Harken, A. H., Horowitz, L. N., and Josephson, M. E.: Surgical correction of recurrent sustained ventricular tachycardia following complete repair of tetralogy of Fallot. J. Thorac. Cardiovasc. Surg., 80:779, 1980.

Hartmann, R. C.: Hemorrhagic disorder occurring in patients with cyanotic congenital heart disease. Bull. Johns Hopkins Hosp., 91:49, 1952.

He, G. W., Kuo, C. C., and Mee, R. B.: Pulmonic regurgitation and reconstruction of right ventricular outflow tract with patch. J. Thorac. Cardiovasc. Surg., 92:128, 1986.

Hiraishi, S., Bargeron, L. M., Isabel-Jones, J. B., et al: Ventricular and pulmonary artery volumes in patients with absent pulmonary valve. Factors affecting the natural course. Circulation, 67:183, 1983.

Hope, J.: A treatise on the disease of the heart and great vessels, and on the affections which may be mistaken for them. London, J. Churchill & Sons, 1839.

Hudspeth, A. S., Cordell, A. R., and Johnston, F. R.: Transatrial approach to total correction of tetralogy of Fallot. Circulation, 27:796, 1963.

Humes, R. A., Driscoll, D. J., Danielson, G. K., et al: Tetralogy of Fallot with anomalous origin of left anterior descending coronary artery: Surgical options. J. Thorac. Cardiovasc. Surg., 94:784, 1987.

Hunter, J.: Medical Observations and Inquiries by a Society of Physicians in London. London, 1757–1784.

Hunter, W.: Three cases of malformation of the heart. II: Medical Observations and Inquiries by a Society of Physicians in London, 6:291, 1784.

Hurwitz, R. A., Smith, W., King, H., et al: Tetralogy of Fallot with abnormal coronary artery: 1967 to 1977. J. Thorac. Cardiovasc. Surg., 80:129, 1980.

Ilbawi, M. N., Fedorchik, J., Muster, A. J., et al: Surgical approach to severely symptomatic newborn infants with tetralogy of Fallot and absent pulmonary valve. J. Thorac. Cardiovasc. Surg., 91:584, 1986.

Ilbawi, M. N., Grieco, J., DeLeon, S. Y., et al: Modified Blalock-Taussig shunt in newborn infants. J. Thorac. Cardiovasc. Surg., 80:770, 1984.

Ilbawi, M. N., Idriss, F. S., DeLeon, S. Y., et al: Factors that exaggerate the deleterious effects of pulmonary insufficiency on the right ventricle after tetralogy repair: Surgical implications. J. Thorac. Cardiovasc. Surg., 93:36, 1987.

Ilbawi, M. N., Idriss, F. S., Muster, A. J., et al: Tetralogy of Fallot with absent pulmonary valve: Should valve insertion be part of the intracardiac repair? J. Thorac. Cardiovasc. Surg., 81:906, 1981.

Joshi, S. V., Brawn, W. J., and Mee, R. B. B.: Pulmonary atresia with intact ventricular septum. J. Thorac. Cardiovasc. Surg., 91:192, 1986.

Karl, T. R., Musumeci, F., de Leval, M., et al: Surgical treatment of absent pulmonary valve syndrome. J. Thorac. Cardiovasc. Surg., 91:590, 1986.

Kawashima, Y., Matsuda, H., Hirose, H., et al: Ninety consecutive corrective operations for tetralogy of Fallot with or without minimal right ventriculotomy. J. Thorac. Cardiovasc. Surg., 90:856, 1985.

Keagy, B. A., Wilcox, B. R., Lucus, C. L., et al: Constant postoperative monitoring of cardiac output after correction of congenital heart defects. J. Thorac. Cardiovasc. Surg., 93:658, 1987.

Kirklin, J. W., and Payne, W. S.: Surgical treatment for tetralogy of Fallot after previous anastomosis of systemic to pulmonary artery. Surg. Gynecol. Obstet., 110:707, 1960.

Kirklin, J. W., and Karp, R. B.: The Tetralogy of Fallot. Philadelphia, W. B. Saunders Company, 1970.

Kirklin, J. W., Blackstone, E. H., Pacifico, A. D., et al: Routine primary repair vs two-stage repair of tetralogy of Fallot. Circulation, 60:373, 1979.

Kirklin, J. W., Blackstone, E. H., Kirklin, J. K., et al: Surgical results and protocols in the spectrum of tetralogy of Fallot. Ann. Surg., 198:251, 1983.

Kirklin, J. W., and Barratt-Boyes, B. G.: Ventricular septal defect and pulmonary stenosis. In Cardiac Surgery. New York, John Wiley & Sons, 1986, pp. 699–857.

Kirklin, J. W., Blackstone, E. H., Colvin, E. V., and McConnell, M. E.: Early primary correction of tetralogy of Fallot. Ann. Thorac. Surg., 45:231, 1988.

Kisslo, J. A.: Doppler Color Flow Imaging. New York, Churchill Livingstone, 1988.

Kurosawa, H., Imai, Y., Nakazawa, M., et al: Standardized patch for infundibuloplasty for tetralogy of Fallot. J. Thorac. Cardiovasc. Surg., 92:396, 1986.

Kvelselis, D. A., Rocchini, A. P., Snider, A. R., et al: Results of balloon valvuloplasty in the treatment of congenital valvar pulmonary stenosis in children. Am. J. Cardiol., 56:527, 1985.

Lababidi, Z., and Wu, J. R.: Percutaneous balloon pulmonary valvuloplasty. Am. J. Cardiol., 52:560, 1983.

Lakier, J. B., Stanger, P., Heymann, M. A., et al: Tetralogy of Fallot with absent pulmonary valve: Natural history and hemodynamic considerations. Circulation, 50:167, 1974.

Laks, H., and Castaneda, A. R.: Subclavian arterioplasty for the ipsilateral Blalock-Taussig shunt. Ann. Thorac. Surg., 19:319, 1975.

Lamberti, J. J., Carlisle, J., Waldman, J. D., et al: Systemic-pulmonary shunts in infants and children. J. Thorac. Cardiovasc. Surg., 88:76, 1984.

Lev, M., and Eckner, F. A. Q.: The pathologic anatomy of tetralogy of Fallot and its variations. Dis. Chest, 45:251, 1964.

Lewis, A. B., Wells, W., and Lindesmith, G. G.: Right ventricular growth potential in neonates with pulmonary atresia and intact ventricular septum. J. Thorac. Cardiovasc. Surg., 91:835, 1986.

Lillehei, C. W., Cohen, M., Warden, H. E., and Varco, R. L.: The direct-vision intracardiac correction of congenital anomalies by controlled cross circulation: Results in 32 patients with ventricular septal defects, tetralogy of Fallot, and atrioventricular communis defects. Surgery, 38:11, 1955a.

Lillehei, C. W., Cohen, M., Warden, H. E., et al: Direct vision intracardiac surgical correction of the tetralogy of Fallot, pentalogy of Fallot, and pulmonary atresia defects: Report of first ten cases. Ann. Surg., 142:418, 1955b.

Lillehei, C. W., Varco, R. L., Cohen, M., et al: The first open-heart repairs of ventricular septal defect, atrio-ventricular communis, and tetralogy of Fallot using extracorporeal circulation by cross-circulation: A thirty-year follow-up. Ann. Thorac. Surg., 41:4, 1986.

Lock, J. E., Keane, J. F., and Fellows, K. E.: Diagnostic and Interventional Catheterization in Congenital Heart Disease. Boston, Martinus Nijhoff Publishing, 1987.

Lodge, F. A., Lamberti, J. J., Goodman, A. H., et al: Vascular consequences of subclavian artery transection for the treatment of congenital heart disease. J. Thorac. Cardiovas. Surg., 86:18, 1983.

Magrassi, P., Chartrand, C., Guerin, R., et al: True diverticulum of the right ventricle: Two cases associated with tetralogy of Fallot. Ann. Thorac. Surg., 29:357, 1980.

Marino, B., Corno, A., Pasquini, L., et al: Indication for systemic-pulmonary artery shunts guided by two-dimensional and Doppler echocardiography: Criteria for patient selection. Ann. Thorac. Surg., 44:495, 1987.

Matsuda, H., Ihara, K., Mori, T., et al: Tetralogy of Fallot associated with aortic insufficiency. Ann. Thorac. Surg., 29:529, 1980.

Mavroudis, C., Turley, K., Stanger, P., and Ebert, P. A.: Surgical management of tetralogy of Fallot with absent pulmonary valve. J. Cardiovasc. Surg., 24:603, 1983.

McCaughan, B. C., Danielson, G. K., and Driscoll, D. J.: Tetralogy of Fallot with absent pulmonary valve: Early and late results of surgical treatment. J. Thorac. Cardiovasc. Surg., 89:280, 1985.

McCord, M. C., van Elk, J., and Blount, G., Jr.: Tetralogy of Fallot clinical and hemodynamic spectrum of combined pulmonary stenosis and ventricular septal defects. Circulation, 16:736, 1957.

McGoon, D. C., and Kirkland, J. W.: Pulmonic stenosis with intact ventricular septum: Treatment utilizing extracorporeal circulation. Circulation, 17:180, 1958.

Misbach, G. A., Turley, K., and Ebert, P. A.: Pulmonary valve replacement for regurgitation after repair of tetralogy of Fallot. Ann. Thorac. Surg., 36:684, 1983.

Mitchell, S. C., Korones, S. B., and Berendes, H. W.: Congenital heart disease in 56,109 births: Incidence and natural history. Circulation, 43:323, 1971.

Moulton, A. L., Bowman, F. O., Jr., and Edie, R. N.: Pulmonary atresia with intact ventricular septum: Sixteen-year experience. J. Thorac. Cardiovasc. Surg., 78:527, 1979.

Murphy, J. D., Freed, M. D., Keane, J. F., et al: Hemodynamic results after intracardiac repair of tetralogy of Fallot by deep hypothermia and cardiopulmonary bypass. Circulation, 62(Suppl. I):168, 1980.

Nagao, G. I., Daoud, G. I., McAdams, A. J., et al: Cardiovascular anomalies associated with tetralogy of Fallot. Am. J. Cardiol., 20:206, 1967.

Naito, Y., Fujita, T., Manabe, H., and Kawashima, Y.: The criteria for reconstruction of right ventricular outflow tract in total correction of tetralogy of Fallot. J. Thorac. Cardiovasc. Surg., 80:574, 1980.

Nomoto, S., Muraoka, R., Yokota, M., et al: Left ventricular volume as a predictor of postoperative hemodynamics and a criterion for total correction of tetralogy of Fallot. J. Thorac. Cardiovasc. Surg., 88:389, 1984.

Pacifico, A. D., Kirkland, J. W., and Bargeron, L. M., Jr.: Repair of complete atrioventricular canal associated with tetralogy of Fallot or double-outlet right ventricle: Report of ten patients. Ann. Thorac. Surg., 29:351, 1980.

Pacifico, A. D., Kirkland, J. W., and Blackstone, E. H.: Surgical management of pulmonary stenosis in tetralogy of Fallot. J. Thorac. Cardiovasc. Surg., 74:382, 1977.

Pacifico, A. D., Sand, M. E., Bargeron, Jr., L. M., and Colvin, E. C.: Transatrial-transpulmonary repair of tetralogy of Fallot. J. Thorac. Cardiovasc. Surg., 93:919, 1987.

Peacock, T. B.: On Malformations of the Human Heart, etc. with Original Cases and Illustrations, 2nd ed. London, J. Churchill and Sons, 1866.

Piehler, J. M., Danielson, G. K., McGoon, D. C., et al: Management of pulmonary atresia with ventricular septal defect and hypoplastic pulmonary arteries by right ventricular outflow construction. J. Thorac. Cardiovasc. Surg., 80:552, 1980.

Polansky, D. B., Clark, E. B., and Doty, D. B.: Pulmonary stenosis in infants and young children. Ann. Thorac. Surg., 39:159, 1984.

Porter, J. M., and Silver, D.: Alterations in fibrinolysis and coagulation associated with cardiopulmonary bypass. J. Thorac. Cardiovasc. Surg., 56:869, 1968.

Potts, W. J., Gibson, S., Riker, W. L., and Leninger, C. R.: Congenital pulmonary stenosis with intact ventricular septum. J.A.M.A., 144:8, 1950.

Potts, W. J., Smith, S., and Gibson, S.: Anastomosis of the aorta to a pulmonary artery for certain types of congenital heart disease. J.A.M.A., 132:629, 1946.

Quattlebaum, T. G., Varghese, P. J., Neill, C. A., et al: Sudden death among postoperative patients with tetralogy of Fallot: A follow-up study of 243 patients for an average of twelve years. Circulation, 54:289, 1976.

Rittenhouse, E. A., Mansfield, P. B., Hall, D. G., et al: Tetralogy of Fallot: Selective staged management. J. Thorac. Cardiovasc. Surg., 89:772, 1985.

Rosenberg, H. G., Williams, W. G., Trusler, G. A., et al: Structural composition of central pulmonary arteries: Growth potential after surgical shunts. J. Thorac. Cardiovasc. Surg., 94:498, 1987.

Ross, R. S., Taussig, H. B., and Evans, M. H.: Late hemodynamic complications of anastomotic surgery for treatment of the tetralogy of Fallot. Circulation, 18L553, 1958.

Sabiston, D. C., Jr.: Role of the Blalock-Taussig operation in the hypoxic infant with tetralogy of Fallot. Ann. Thorac. Surg., 22:303, 1976.

Sabiston, D. C., Jr., and Blalock, A.: The tetralogy of Fallot, tricuspid atresia, transposition of the great vessels and associated disorders. In Derra, E. (ed): Encyclopedia of Thoracic Surgery, Vol. 2. Heidelberg, Springer-Verlag, 1959.

Sabiston, D. C., Jr., Cornell, W. P., Criley, J. M., et al: The diagnosis and surgical correction of total obstruction of the right ventricle: An acquired condition developing after systemic-pulmonary artery anastomosis for tetralogy of Fallot. J. Thorac. Cardiovasc. Surg., 48:577, 1964.

Sandifort, E.: Observationses Anatomico-Pathologicae. Lugdunum Batavorum, P.v.d. Eyk et D. Vygh, 1777, Chapter 1, Figure 1.

Stensen, H. (Nicholaus Steno). In Bartholin, T.: Acta Medica et Philosophica Hafnienca, 1671–72, Vol. 1, p. 302. Reprinted in Stenosis, N.: Opera Philosophica, Vol. 2. Copenhagen, Vilhelm Maar, 1910, pp. 49–53.

Stephens, H. B.: Aneurysm of the pulmonary artery following a Pott's shunt operation. J. Thorac. Cardiovasc. Surg., 53:642, 1967.

Szentpetery, S., Robertson, L., and Lower, R. R.: Complete repair of tetralogy associated with sickle cell anemia and G-6-PD deficiency. J. Thorac. Cardiovasc. Surg., 72:276, 1976.

Tamiya, T., Yamashiro, T., Matsumoto, T., et al: A histological study of surgical landmarks for the specialized atrioventricular conduction system, with particular reference to the papillary muscle. Ann. Thorac. Surg., 40:599, 1985.

Taussig, H. B.: Tetralogy of Fallot: Early history and late results: Neuhauser Lecture. Am. J. Roentgenol., *133:*423, 1979.

Tucker, W. Y., Turley, K., and Ullyot, D. J.: Management of symptomatic tetralogy of Fallot in the first year of life. J. Thorac. Cardiovasc. Surg., *78:*494, 1979.

Turley, K., Tucker, W. Y., and Ebert, P. A.: The changing role of palliative procedures in the treatment of infants with congenital heart disease. J. Thorac. Cardiovasc. Surg., *79:*194, 1980.

Ullom, R. L., Sade, R. M., and Crawford, F. A.: The Blalock-Taussig shunt in infants: Standard versus modified. Ann. Thorac. Surg., *44:*539, 1987.

Ungerleider, R. M., Greeley, W. J., Sheikh, K. H., et al: The use of intraoperative echo with Doppler color flow imaging to predict outcomes following repair of congenital cardiac defects. Ann. Surg., (in press, 1989).

Vargas, F. J., Coto, E. O., Mayer, J. E., Jr., et al: Complete atrioventricular canal and tetralogy of Fallot: Surgical considerations. Ann. Thorac. Surg., *42:*258, 1986a.

Vargas, F. J., Kreutzer, G. O., Pedrini, M., et al: Tetralogy of Fallot with subarterial ventricular septal defect. J. Thorac. Cardiovasc. Surg., *92:*908, 1986b.

Waterson, D. J.: Treatment of Fallot's tetralogy in children under 1 year of age. Rozhl. Chir., *41:*181, 1962.

Webb, W. R., and Burford, T. H.: Gangrene of the arm following use of the subclavian artery in a pulmonosystemic (Blalock) anastomosis. J. Thorac. Surg., *23:*199, 1952.

Weldon, C. S., Hartmann, A. F., Jr., and McKnight, R. C.: Surgical management of hypoplastic right ventricle with pulmonary atresia or critical pulmonary stenosis and intact ventricular septum. Ann. Thorac. Surg., *37:*12, 1984.

Westerman, G. R., Norton, J. V., and Van Devanter, S. H.: A double-outlet right atrium associated with tetralogy of Fallot and common atrioventricular valve. J. Thorac. Cardiovasc. Surg., *91:*205, 1986.

White, P. D., and Sprague, H. B.: The tetralogy of Fallot: Report of a case in a noted musician who lived to his sixtieth year. J.A.M.A., *92:*787, 1929.

Wilson, J. M., Mack, J. W., Turley, K., and Ebert, P. A.: Persistent stenosis and deformity of the right pulmonary artery after correction of the Waterston anastomosis. J. Thorac. Cardiovasc. Surg., *82:*169, 1981.

Yamaguchi, M., Imai, M., Ohashi, H., et al: Enhanced myocardial protection by systemic hypothermia in children undergoing total correction of tetralogy of Fallot. Ann. Thorac. Surg., *41:*639, 1986.

Zerbini, E. J., MacCruz, R., Bittencourt, D., et al: Total correction of complex of Fallot under extracorporeal circulation: Immediate results in a group of 221 patients. J. Thorac. Cardiovasc. Surg., *49:*430, 1965.

Zhao, H., Miller, D. C., and Reitz, B. A., et al: Surgical repair of tetralogy of Fallot. J. Thorac. Cardiovasc. Surg., *89:*204, 1985.

CHAPTER 40

TRUNCUS ARTERIOSUS

Gary K. Lofland

Truncus arteriosus (persistent truncus arteriosus, truncus arteriosus communis, common aorticopulmonary trunk) is a congenital heart malformation that involves the ventriculoarterial connection in which a single outlet is present and that is characterized by (1) the presence of a single semilunar valve annulus as the only exit from the heart, (2) a subarterial ventricular septal defect, and (3) absence or severe deficiency of the aortopulmonary septum. Two related but different malformations are aortopulmonary window and subarterial ventricular septal defect. The truncus thus provides the orifices of the coronary and pulmonary arteries before continuing as the aorta. This definition thus excludes hearts that have no true pulmonary arteries, in which case the lung is supplied by aortopulmonary collateral vessels (Type IV of Collett and Edwards, 1949).

Truncus arteriosus constitutes less than 3% of all congenital heart defects (de Leval, 1983).

HISTORICAL ASPECTS

The first well-documented case of truncus arteriosus was reported in 1798 (Wilson, 1798). In 1864 the entity was confirmed in a clinical and autopsy report on a 6-month-old infant (Buchanan, 1864). Taruffi (1875) reported a similar case, and other reports followed (Lev and Saphir, 1943; Shapiro, 1930; Victoria et al, 1969). In 1949, Collett and Edwards proposed a classification system after a review of all published cases (Fig. 40–1). An alternative system was proposed by Van Praagh and Van Praagh (1965).

The first successful correction of truncus arteriosus was done in 1962 but was not reported until 12 years later (Behrendt et al, 1974). The first successful repair was reported by McGoon and associates (1968) and an additional case was reported by Weldon and Cameron (1968). The first successful conduit repair in infancy was done by Barratt-Boyes in 1971 (Girinath, 1973). With some technical modifications, the technique described by McGoon (1983) for complete correction is used currently.

ANATOMY AND CLASSIFICATION

The classification system proposed by Collett and Edwards (1949) is based on the arrangement of the origins of the pulmonary arteries from the truncal artery (see Fig. 40–1). The classification system proposed by Van Praagh and Van Praagh (1965) also includes cases with a single pulmonary artery and various degrees of development of the ascending aorta and ductus arteriosus. In the Collett and Edwards Type I truncus, the pulmonary arteries arise from a common pulmonary trunk that originates from the truncus. In Type II, the right and left pulmonary arteries arise close together from the dorsal wall of the truncus arteriosus. In Type III, the pulmonary arteries arise separately from the lateral aspects of the truncus. In Type IV, the proximal pulmonary arteries are absent and pulmonary blood

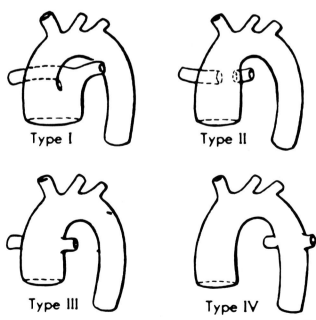

Figure 40–1. Anatomic types of truncus arteriosus. Collett and Edwards' classification. (From Heart Disease in Infancy and Childhood, by John D. Keith, Richard D. Rowe, and Peter Vlad. Copyright © 1958 The Macmillan Company; copyright renewed. Reprinted by permission of Macmillan Publishing Company, a div. of Macmillan, Inc.)

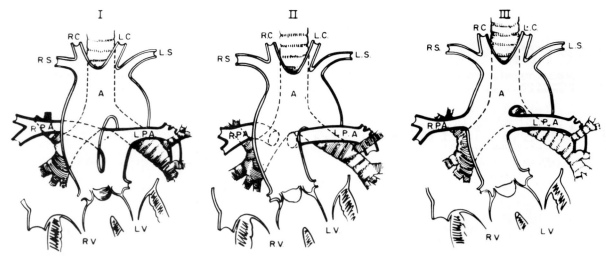

Figure 40-2. The three most common types of truncus arteriosus. The relationship of the truncal artery to the ventricular septal defect, coronary arteries, pulmonary arteries, and aortic arch is shown. The features have been exaggerated for purposes of illustration. The existence of Type III truncus, as shown here and in the Collett and Edwards' classification, is legitimately questioned.

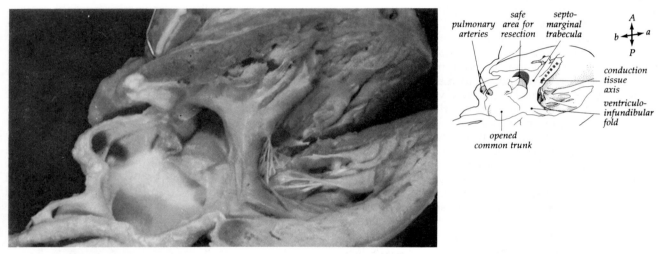

Figure 40-3. Opened anterior part of the right ventricle in surgical orientation shows the morphology of a subarterial defect with a muscular posterior inferior rim and a common trunk. The origin of both pulmonary arteries is from the left and posterior aspect of the trunk. (From Wilcox, B. R., and Anderson, R. H.: Surgical Anatomy of the Heart. New York, Raven Press, 1985, p. 7.20.)

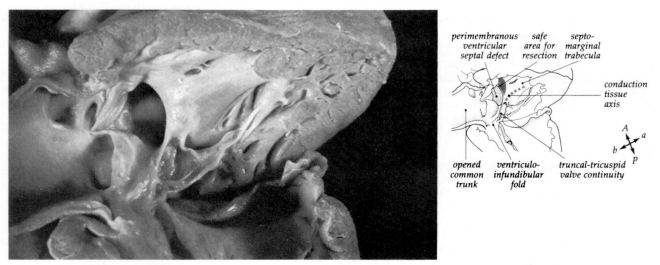

Figure 40-4. Common trunk with a perimembranous defect. The conduction axis is much closer to the posterior inferior rim than in Figure 40-3. The safe area for surgical resection or placement of sutures is in a similar position. (From Wilcox, B. R., and Anderson, R. H.: Surgical Anatomy of the Heart. New York, Raven Press, 1985, p. 7.20.)

flow originates from the multiple aorticopulmonary collateral vessels.

In practice, the distinction between Types I, II, and III truncus is imprecise, and the actual existence of Type III truncus with lateral origins of the pulmonary arteries is questioned (McGoon, 1983) (Fig. 40–2). The Type IV classification of Collett and Edwards should be replaced by the more precise designation, pulmonary atresia with ventricular septal defect. Also, the term "pseudotruncus" should be abandoned in favor of a more descriptive designation of a condition characterized by pulmonary atresia and patent ductus arteriosus (McGoon, 1983).

Morphologically, the arterial trunk or truncus is larger than a normal aorta and arises as a solitary vessel from the base of the heart. The truncus originates from both ventricles but usually overrides the septum to lie more over the right than over the left ventricle (Bharati et al, 1974; Crupi et al, 1977; Thiene et al, 1976). The coronary and pulmonary arteries arise from this truncus (Fig. 40–3).

Although coronary arteries usually arise from orifices in the truncal valve sinuses of Valsalva in a position close to the normal one (left arising posteriorly into the left and right arising anteriorly), variations in coronary anatomy have been reported (Anderson et al, 1978; Bharati et al, 1974; Crupi et al, 1977; Shrivastava and Edwards, 1977; Van Praagh and Van Praagh, 1965). The pulmonary arteries usually originate just downstream from the truncal valve, on the left posterolateral aspect of the truncus, although true lateral, true posterior, and true anterior origins have been described (Anderson et al, 1978). There is often a single orifice that soon divides into right and left pulmonary arteries (Type I of Collett and Edwards) (see Fig. 40–3). Less commonly, the pulmonary arteries have separate orifices (Type II of Collett and Edwards). These two types account for 86% of cases in the Barratt-Boyes series (Barratt-Boyes, 1986).

Rarely, only one pulmonary artery arises from the truncus, and a blood supply to the opposite lung arises from aorticopulmonary collaterals or a patent ductus arteriosus (Van der Horst and Gotsman, 1974).

Variations in great artery morphology are found in both the pulmonary and aortic pathways, and the pattern of the aortic arch has considerable surgical significance. Aortic arch interruption occurs (Calder et al, 1976) and is usually at the level of the isthmus, but it can be proximal to the origin of the left subclavian artery. In either case, the descending aorta is supplied by the ductus arteriosus. Truncus arteriosus with aortic arch interruptions is found in up to one-fifth of autopsy series (Bharati et al, 1974; Calder et al, 1976; Crupi et al, 1977; Van Praagh and Van Praagh, 1965).

The truncal valve is posterior and inferior in position but still points more anteriorly than the normal aortic valve (Calder et al, 1976). There is fibrous continuity between the posterior leaflet and the anterior mitral valve leaflet (Calder et al, 1976) (Fig. 40–4). The truncal valve usually has three cusps but may have two to six cusps. In one series, truncal valve incompetence was severe in 6%, moderate in 31%, and absent to minimal in 63% (Di Donato et al, 1985). Although dysplastic truncal valves have been seen with some frequency in autopsy series (Becker et al, 1971), they do not pose a major problem in surgical repair in infancy (Anderson, 1985).

The pathophysiology of truncus arteriosus is that of a large left-to-right shunt at a ventricular or great artery level, with a high ratio of pulmonary to systemic blood flow (Q_P/Q_S). Systemic pressures usually exist in the right ventricle and pulmonary arteries. There is an increased pulmonary vascular resistance (2 to 4 units/m^2) from birth. Rarely does truncal valve stenosis or a restrictive ventricular septal defect modify this hemodynamic pattern. Through infancy there is a progressive increase in pulmonary vascular resistance, with a gradual decrease in arterial oxygen saturation.

CLINICAL PRESENTATION AND DIAGNOSIS

The clinical symptoms of truncus arteriosus are those of severe congestive heart failure from infancy onward and they include tachypnea ("breathlessness"), tachycardia, irritability, poor feeding, respiratory infections, and ultimately failure to thrive. Cyanosis is not common in infants, but older children may be seen with cyanosis as Eisenmenger's physiology develops.

Physical examination reveals tachycardia and collapsing arterial pulses secondary to a runoff of systemic blood into the lower-pressure pulmonary circuit. The precordium is active, and a prominent systolic murmur is present. There may be an ejection click coincident with opening of the truncal valve. Truncal valve incompetence is associated with a coexistent diastolic murmur and is of concern, because an incompetent truncal valve is associated with a poorer prognosis than a competent valve.

The chest film shows pulmonary plethora and cardiomegaly and may demonstrate other abnormalities of the pulmonary arteries (Calder et al, 1976). Patients who survive into childhood have a gradual decrease in their pulmonary vascularity. Electrocardiographic findings are nonspecific but usually include left or biventricular hypertrophy and P-pulmonale. Echocardiography is diagnostic and shows a single great vessel, the subarterial ventricular septal defect, the origin of the pulmonary arteries, and the leaflets of the truncal valve (Marin-Garcia and Tonkin, 1982; Riggs and Paul, 1982). Echocardiography may even show the coronary artery distribution. Two-dimensional echocardiography combined with color flow Doppler is an excellent technique for evaluating truncal valve incompetence or stenosis and blood flow patterns and gradients across the ventricular septal defect.

Cardiac catheterization and angiocardiography are still used to define the pulmonary arteries, the aortic arch, and the hemodynamic state (Barratt-Boyes, 1986). Cineangiography with contrast injection shows the site of origin of both pulmonary arteries and, if a pulmonary artery is absent, enables the blood supply to the affected lung to be determined. Cardiac catheterization is also important in defining pulmonary vascular resistance.

SURGICAL CORRECTION

Total surgical correction involves closure of the ventricular septal defect and establishment of continuity between the right ventricle and pulmonary artery by using an extracardiac conduit. The basis of this repair was first described by two groups independently (McGoon et al, 1968; Weldon and Cameron, 1968). The complete procedure is shown in Figure 40–5.

The operation is done through a median sternotomy incision. After entry into the pericardium and creation of a pericardial cradle, dissection is done between the aorta and the pulmonary artery. The patient is cannulated for cardiopulmonary bypass, with the aortic cannula placed just proximal to the innominate origin. In infants in whom circulatory arrest is anticipated, a single atrial cannula is used. Otherwise, dual caval cannulation with maintenance of flow is preferred. Venting of the left ventricle is

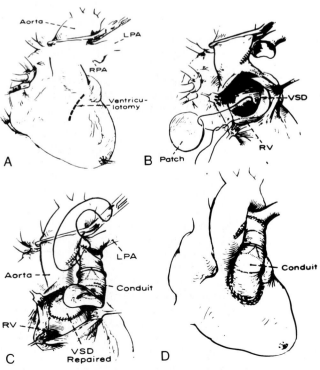

Figure 40–5. The complete procedure is shown.

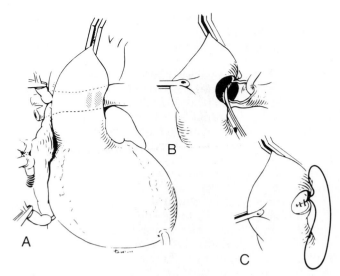

Figure 40–6. First step of surgical repair. *A,* Cardiopulmonary bypass is instituted and the ascending aorta is clamped. *B,* Excision of pulmonary arteries from the truncus. *C,* The defect in the truncus (aorta) is being repaired. (From Wallace, R. B., Rastelli, G. C., Ongley, P. A., et al: Complete repair of truncus arteriosus defects. J. Thorac. Cardiovasc. Surg., *57:*95, 1969.)

desirable to prevent overdistention as the patient is being cooled.

After bypass is begun, the patient is cooled to a rectal temperature of 20° C, which provides latitude for further cooling if circulatory arrest becomes necessary. During cooling, it is desirable to occlude blood flow to the pulmonary arteries partially or totally to prevent flooding of the lungs and overdistention of the left atrium and ventricle. It is also necessary to occlude flow to the pulmonary arteries during instillation of cardioplegic solution.

After cross-clamping the aorta, the pulmonary arteries are detached from the truncal artery, and the defect in the truncal artery is closed (Fig. 40–6). Closure must be done in such a way that no distortion of the truncal valve occurs. Placement of a patch rather than a primary closure may be necessary. It is desirable to leave intact as much proximal length of the truncal artery as possible to prevent distortion of the left coronary ostium.

When the coronary artery pattern over the right and left epicardium has been defined, a longitudinal or transverse incision is made in the right ventricular infundibulum. It is not necessary to excise any right ventricular free wall to accommodate the anastomosis between the right ventricle and the extracardiac conduit. After creation of the ventriculotomy, the ventricular septal defect is usually easily seen, because it involves the infundibular septum. The defect is closed with a synthetic patch by using either a continuous running or interrupted technique. A running 4-0 polypropylene suture is preferred. The cephalad margin of the suture line may be anchored to the epicardium and myocardium at the cephalad margin of the ventriculotomy (Fig. 40–7).

After closure of the ventricular septal defect, an

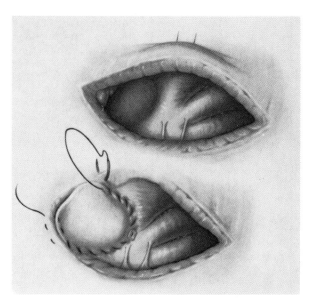

Figure 40–7. Longitudinal ventriculotomy shows the ventricular septal defect and closure of the ventricular septal defect by using a synthetic patch and continuous suture technique. (From de Leval, M.: Persistent truncus arteriosus. *In* Stark, J., and de Leval, M. [eds]: Surgery for Congenital Heart Defects. London, Grune & Stratton, 1983, p. 421.)

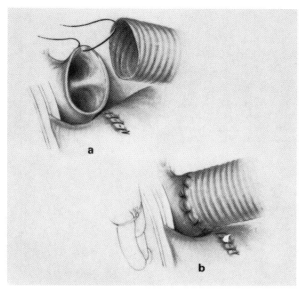

Figure 40–8. Anastomosis of the conduit to the pulmonary arteries. (From de Leval, M.: Persistent truncus arteriosus. *In* Stark, J., and de Leval, M. [eds]: Surgery for Congenital Heart Defects. London, Grune & Stratton, 1983, p. 421.)

extracardiac conduit is selected. Because of the increased pulmonary vascular resistance, a valved conduit is usually necessary, although correction of truncus arteriosus in neonates with nonvalved conduits has been reported (Peetz et al, 1982; Spicer et al, 1984). Valved conduits became commercially available in the 1970s and are supplied by several manufacturers in sizes ranging from 12 to 30 mm. These conduits usually give an excellent early result, but the valve component of the conduit tends to degenerate rapidly and must be replaced within 2 years in approximately 50% of patients (Ebert et al, 1984).

Aortic homografts preserved with various techniques have been used, even before the advent of commercially available conduits. With earlier preservation techniques, homografts tended to calcify, and their use was abandoned in most institutions (Moodie et al, 1976). Other groups who use fresh homografts have remained enthusiastic about their use (Shabbo et al, 1980).

Considering the disappointing results with synthetic valved conduits, cryopreservation techniques were improved, which resulted in improved viability of fibroblasts within a conduit. There has been a resurgence of interest in cryopreserved human aortic and pulmonary homografts, although the long-term durability of these conduits remains to be seen.

The conduit that is selected should be trimmed to an appropriate length by estimating the distance from the ventriculotomy to the transected pulmonary arteries. The length should be such that the conduit is not redundant and not subject to compression by the sternum. The anastomosis should also be under no tension and should not compress the left coronary artery.

The pulmonary anastomosis should be done first, and the author uses a continuous technique with fine polypropylene suture (Fig. 40–8). The origins of the pulmonary arteries may be enlarged with pericardial patches (Fig. 40–9) or by spatulating the pulmonary end of the valved conduit (Fig. 40–10).

The ventricular anastomosis is done by a similar technique. Care must be taken to avoid distortion of the conduit, and synthetic conduits may be beveled for this purpose (Fig. 40–11). If an aortic homograft

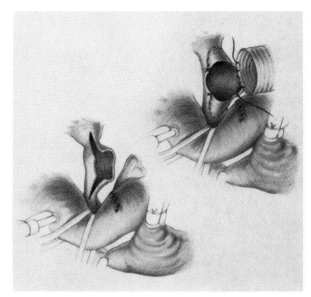

Figure 40–9. Enlargement of the origin of the pulmonary arteries with pericardium and anastomosis of the conduit to the enlarged pulmonary arteries. (From de Leval, M.: Persistent truncus arteriosus. *In* Stark, J., and de Leval, M. [eds]: Surgery for Congenital Heart Defects. London, Grune & Stratton, 1983, p. 423.)

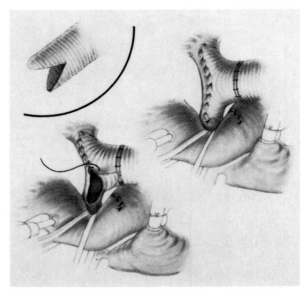

Figure 40–10. Enlargement of the pulmonary arteries by spatulating the pulmonary end of the conduit. (From de Leval, M.: Persistent truncus arteriosus. *In* Stark, J., and de Leval, M. [eds]: Surgery for Congenital Heart Defects. London, Grune & Stratton, 1983, p. 423.)

is used, the anterior mitral valve leaflet may be used as a gusset. The completed procedure is shown in Figure 40–12.

The ventricular anastomosis may be done with the aorta still cross-clamped or may be done during rewarming with the aorta unclamped and the heart beating. An aortic or pulmonary homograft may be tailored for a smaller patient (Fig. 40–13) if only larger homografts are available.

The presence of truncal valve insufficiency complicates the surgical procedure and should be assessed. Mild insufficiency may be tolerated, but the ventricle should be well vented and should not be allowed to overdistend. More severe truncal valve insufficiency may be amenable to valvuloplasty but usually requires extension of the operation and replacement of the valve (de Leval et al, 1974). Good results may be achieved with an aggressive approach. Pulmonary artery banding was previously attempted as a palliative procedure (Muller and Dammann,

1952). The mortality with this approach varied from 33 to 100% in a review by Poirier and associates (1975). Definitive correction in infancy has mainly replaced this approach.

RESULTS

Truncus arteriosus is relatively rare, so that few large series of patients have been described. One must be aware of the age of patients included in the series reports as well as the inclusion of patients who have coexistent anomalies or extracardiac valve conduits for other reasons.

A large review of results of surgical repair for truncus arteriosus as a discrete entity was provided by Marceletti and associates (1977) at the Mayo Clinic. The initial report of 92 patients was later expanded to 100 patients (McGoon et al, 1982) and then to 167 patients (Di Donato et al, 1985). Marceletti's report described 25% mortality within 30 days of operation and noted that mortality was correlated with the age of the patient at the time of repair; patients less than 2 years of age had a higher risk.

A more recent and encouraging experience was described by Ebert and associates (Ebert, 1981; Ebert et al, 1984; Stanger et al, 1977), who reported 11% mortality for repair of truncus arteriosus in 56 infants less than 6 months of age. They also reported that 50% of the conduits were replaced within 2 years after operation, but no mortality was associated with conduit replacement. This series provided support for early corrective operation. The results of several more recent series are shown in Table 40–1.

Incremental risk factors identified in the combined experience of the University of Alabama in Birmingham and Green Lane Hospital, Auckland, New Zealand, included the following (Barratt-Boyes, 1986):

1. Poor preoperative clinical status
2. Important truncal valve incompetence
3. A previously placed pulmonary artery band
4. Younger age
5. Pulmonary vascular disease
6. Earlier date of operation

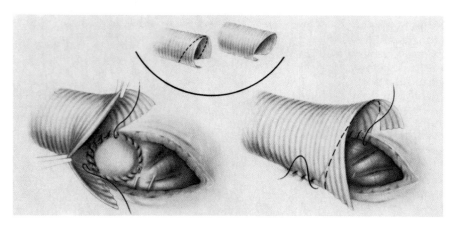

Figure 40–11. Completion of the ventricular septal defect closure; the ventricular end of the conduit is beveled to prevent distortion or kinking of the conduit. (From de Leval, M.: Persistent truncus arteriosus. *In* Stark, J., and de Leval, M. [eds]: Surgery for Congenital Heart Defects. London, Grune & Stratton, 1983, p. 422.)

TABLE 40–1. MORTALITY FOR SURGICAL REPAIR OF TRUNCUS ARTERIOSUS

Authors	Period	Total No. of Patients	Age at Correction	Early Mortality (%)	Late Mortality (%)
Ebert et al (1984)	1974–1981	106	<6 months	11	0
Di Donato et al (1985)	1965–1982	167	18 days to 33 years	28.7	15.6
Sharma et al (1985)	1979–1983	23	1 month to 2 years	13	0

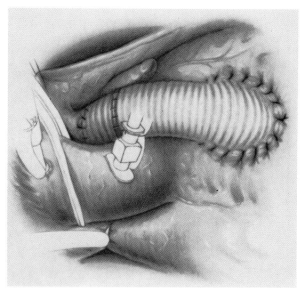

Figure 40–12. The completed repair. (From de Leval, M.: Persistent truncus arteriosus. *In* Stark, J., and de Leval, M. [eds]: Surgery for Congenital Heart Defects. London, Grune & Stratton, 1983, p. 422.)

7. Major coexisting cardiac anomalies (this is not supported by multivariate statistical analysis)

The pulmonary vascular structure in a large group of children with various congenital anomalies, including a large group with truncus arteriosus, was studied by Juaneda and Haworth (1984) by using quantitative morphometric techniques. These studies showed abnormal extension of muscle, increased pulmonary arterial medial thickness, and intimal proliferation even in infants less than 1 year of age with truncus arteriosus. Even in the presence of increased pulmonary vascular resistance (more than

or equal to 8 units/m²), the changes were potentially reversible in infants. These studies strongly support early intracardiac repair.

The natural history of truncus arteriosus is such that only approximately 10% of patients born with truncus survive to 1 year of age without operative intervention. Early definitive correction as described by Ebert and associates is clearly the approach of choice.

Selected Bibliography

Di Donato, R. M., Fyfe, D. A., Puga, F. J., et al: Fifteen-year experience with surgical repair of truncus arteriosus. J. Thorac. Cardiovasc. Surg., *89*:414, 1985.

This paper discusses 167 patients 18 days to 33 years of age with a mean age of 6 years. There were 48 hospital deaths (28.7%). The 119 hospital survivors had a 5-year survival of 84.4% and a 10-year survival of 68.8%. Reoperation was necessary for 36 patients (30%) during the follow-up period, primarily for right ventricular pulmonary arterial conduit replacement or for truncal valve replacement. This is the largest and most extensive experience in the literature.

Ebert, P. A., Turley, K., Stanger, P., et al: Surgical treatment of truncus arteriosus in the first 6 months of life. Ann. Surg., *200*:451, 1984.

One hundred infants had physiologic correction before 6 months of age. There were 11 operative deaths (a mortality of 11%). Of the 86 long-term survivors, 55 returned for conduit change within 2 years. This paper showed the feasibility of physiologic correction in the first 6 months of life, with low operative mortality and no mortality associated with conduit replacement. The low operative mortality indicated that corrective operation is the best method of intervention to control failure and reduce the likelihood of pulmonary vascular disease, even though reoperation for enlargement of the conduit will be required.

Juaneda, E., and Haworth, S. G.: Pulmonary vascular disease in children with truncus arteriosus. Am. J. Cardiol., *54*:1314, 1984.

Pulmonary vascular structure was analyzed by using quantitative morphometric techniques in lung biopsy specimens from 23 patients 18 days to 13 years of age with truncus arteriosus Type I or II. The paper showed that pulmonary vascular obstructive disease begins very early in this group of patients, but even in infants with increased pulmonary arteriolar resistance the changes were potentially reversible. The paper shows the type of in-depth morphometric analysis of pulmonary arteriolar structure that has increased our understanding of conditions involving large left-to-right shunts (increased QP/QS). The results strongly support early intracardiac repair to prevent development of permanent pulmonary vascular disease.

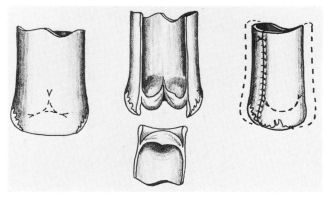

Figure 40–13. Illustration of a method for reducing the size of an aortic or pulmonary homograft.

Bibliography

Anderson, K. R., McGoon, D. C., and Lie, J. T.: Surgical significance of the coronary arterial anatomy in truncus arteriosus communis. Am. J. Cardiol., *41*:76, 1978.

Anderson, R. H.: Common arterial trunk. *In* Wilcox, B. R., and Anderson, R. H. (eds): Surgical Anatomy of the Heart. New York, Raven Press, 1985.

Angelini, P., Vrdugo, A. L., Illera, J. P., and Leachman, R. D.: Truncus arteriosus communis. Unusual case associated with transposition. Circulation, 56:1167, 1977.

Barratt-Boyes, B. G.: Truncus arteriosus. *In* Kirklin, J. W., and Barratt-Boyes, B. G. (eds): Cardiac Surgery. New York, John Wiley & Sons, 1986.

Becker, A. E., Becker, M. J., and Edwards, J. E.: Pathology of the semi-lunar valve in persistent truncus arteriosus. J. Thorac. Cardiovasc. Surg., 62:16, 1971.

Behrendt, D. M., Kirsch, M. M., Stern, A., et al: The surgical therapy for pulmonary artery–right ventricular discontinuity. Ann. Thorac. Surg., 18:122, 1974.

Bharati, S., McAllister, H. A., Rosenquist, G. C., et al: The surgical anatomy of truncus arteriosus communis. J. Thorac. Cardiovasc. Surg., 67:501, 1974.

Buchanan, A.: Malformation of the heart: Undivided truncus arteriosus. Heart otherwise double. Trans. Path. Soc. Lond., 15:89, 1864.

Calder, L., Van Praagh, R., Van Praagh, S., et al: Truncus arteriosus communis: Clinical, angiographic, and pathologic findings in 100 patients. Am. Heart J., 92:23, 1976.

Collett, R. W., and Edwards, J. E.: Persistent truncus arteriosus: A classification according to anatomic types. Surg. Clin. North Am., 29:1245, 1949.

Crupi, G., Macartney, F. J., and Anderson, R. H.: Persistent truncus arteriosus: A study of 66 autopsy cases with special reference to definition and morphogenesis. Am. J. Cardiol., 40:569, 1977.

de Leval, M. R., McGoon, D. C., Wallace, R. B., et al: Management of truncal valvular regurgitation. Ann. Surg., 180:427, 1974.

de Leval, M.: Persistent truncus arteriosus, *In* Stark, J., and de Leval, M. (eds): Surgery for Congenital Heart Defects. New York, Grune & Stratton, 1983.

Di Donato, R. M., Fyfe, D. A., Puga, F. J., et al: Fifteen-year experience with surgical repair of truncus arteriosus. J. Thorac. Cardiovasc. Surg. 89:414, 1985.

Ebert, P. A.: Truncus arteriosus. *In* Parenzan, L., Crupi, G., and Graham, G. (eds): Congenital Heart Disease in the First Three Months of Life, Medical and Surgical Aspects. Bologna, Patron Editore, 1981, p. 439.

Ebert, P. A., Turley, K., Stanger, P., et al: Surgical treatment of truncus arteriosus in the first 6 months of life. Ann. Surg., 200:451, 1984.

Girinath, M. R.: Case presentation: Truncus arteriosus: Repair with homograft reconstruction in infancy. *In* Barratt-Boyes, B.G., Neutze, J. M., and Harris, E. A. (eds.): Heart Disease in Infancy. Diagnosis and Surgical Treatment. Edinburgh, Churchill Livingstone, 1973, p. 234.

Juaneda, E., and Haworth, S. G.: Pulmonary vascular disease in children with truncus arteriosus. Am. J. Cardiol., 54:1314, 1984.

Kirklin, J. W., and Barratt-Boyes, B. G.: Truncus arteriosus. *In* Kirklin, J. W., and Barratt-Boyes, B. G. (eds): Cardiac Surgery. New York, John Wiley & Sons, 1986.

Lev, M., and Saphir, O.: Truncus arteriosus communis persistens. J. Pediatr., 20:74, 1943.

Marceletti, C., McGoon, D. C., Danielson, G. K., et al: Early and late results of surgical repair of truncus arteriosus. Circulation, 55:636, 1977.

Marin-Garcia, J., and Tonkin, L. D.: Two-dimensional echocardio-graphic evaluation of persistent truncus arteriosus. Am. J. Cardiol., 50:1376, 1982.

McGoon, D. C.: Truncus arteriosus. *In* Sabiston, D. C., Jr., and Spencer, F. C. (eds): Gibbons's Surgery of the Chest. Philadelphia, W. B. Saunders Company, 1983.

McGoon, D. C., Danielson, G. K., Puga, F. J., et al: Late results after extracardiac conduit repair for congenital cardiac defects. Am. J. Cardiol., 49:1741, 1982.

McGoon, D. C., Rastelli, G. C., and Ongley, P. A.: An operation for the correction of truncus arteriosus. J.A.M.A., 205:59, 1968.

Moodie, D. S., Mair, D. D., Fulton, R. E., et al: Aortic homograft obstruction. J. Thorac. Cardiovasc. Surg., 72:553, 1976.

Muller, W. H., Jr., and Dammann, J. F., Jr.: The treatment of certain congenital malformations of the heart by the creation of pulmonic stenosis to reduce pulmonary hypertension and excessive pulmonary blood flow: A preliminary report. Surg. Gynecol. Obstet., 95:213, 1952.

Peetz, D. J., Jr., Spicer, R. L., Crowley, D. C., et al: Correction of truncus arteriosus in the neonate using a nonvalved conduit. J. Thorac. Cardiovasc. Surg., 83:743, 1982.

Poirier, R. A., Berman, M. A., and Stansel, H. C., Jr.: Current status of the surgical treatment of truncus arteriosus. J. Thorac. Cardiovasc. Surg., 69:169, 1975.

Riggs, T. W., and Paul, M. H.: Two-dimensional echocardio-graphic prospective diagnosis of common truncus arteriosus in infants. Am. J. Cardiol., 50:1380, 1982.

Shabbo, F. P., Wain, W. H., and Ross, D. N.: Right ventricular outflow reconstruction with aortic homograft conduit: Analysis of the long-term results. Thorac. Cardiovasc. Surg., 28:21, 1980.

Shapiro, P. F.: Truncus solitarus pulmonalis: A rare type of congenital cardiac anomaly. Arch. Pathol., 10:671, 1930.

Sharma, A. K., Brawn, W. J., and Mee, R. B. B.: Truncus arteriosus: Surgical approach. J. Thorac. Cardiovasc. Surg., 90:45, 1985.

Shrivastava, S., and Edwards, J. E.: Coronary arterial origin in persistent truncus arteriosus. Circulation, 55:551, 1977.

Spicer, R. L., Behrendt, D. M., Crowley, D. C., et al: Repair of truncus arteriosus in neonates with the use of a valveless conduit. Circulation, 70:1, 1984.

Stanger, P., Robinson, S. J., Engle, M. A., and Ebert, P. A.: "Corrective" surgery for truncus arteriosus in the first year of life (Abstract). Am. J. Cardiol., 39:293, 1977.

Taruffi, C.: Sulle malattie congenite e sulle anomalie del cuore. Mem. Soc. Med. Chir. Bologna, 8:215, 1875.

Thiene, G., Bortolotti, A., Gallucci, V., et al: Anatomical study of truncus arteriosus communis with embryological and surgical considerations. Br. Heart J., 38:1109, 1976.

Van der Horst, R. L., and Gotsman, M. S.: Type 3C truncus arteriosus: Case report with clinical and surgical implications. Br. Heart J., 36:1046, 1974.

Van Praagh, R., and Van Praagh, S.: The anatomy of common aorticopulmonary trunk (truncus arteriosus communis) and its embryonic implications: A study of 57 necropsy cases. Am. J. Cardiol., 16:406, 1965.

Victoria, B. E., Krovetz, L. J., Elliott, C. P., et al: Persistent truncus arteriosus in infancy. Am. Heart J., 77:13, 1969.

Weldon, C. S., and Cameron, J. L.: Correction of persistent truncus arteriosus. J. Cardiovasc. Surg., 9:463, 1968.

Wilson, J.: A description of a very unusual malformation of the human heart. Philos. Trans. Roy. Soc. London (Biol.), 18:346, 1798.

CHAPTER 41

CONGENITAL AORTIC STENOSIS

Ross M. Ungerleider

Congenital aortic stenosis may be caused by a spectrum of lesions that obstruct the flow of blood from the left ventricle into the aorta (Fig. 41–1). Aortic stenosis may be of congenital origin in 3 to 10% of cases (Nadas and Fyler, 1972; Olley et al, 1978; Trinkle et al, 1975) and is frequently associated (in 8 to 30% of patients) (Bernhard et al, 1973; Mulder et al, 1968) with other cardiovascular anomalies, such as coarctation of the aorta, patent ductus arteriosus, endocardial fibroelastosis (EFE), ventricular septal defects, pulmonary stenosis, and mitral stenosis (Trinkle et al, 1975). Some forms of congenital aortic stenosis are often associated with predictable anomalies (Shone et al, 1963). The site of obstruction is classified anatomically as valvular, subvalvular, or supravalvular. A fourth form caused by hypertrophy of the interventricular muscular septum presents a type of subvalvular obstruction that differs physiologically from other forms of stenotic lesions and is considered to be a separate entity. Although these lesions usually occur separately, patients can have combinations of the anatomic varieties (Kirklin and Barratt-Boyes, 1986), and left ventricular outflow tract obstruction (LVOTO) is a more descriptive term for this spectrum of congenital anomalies.

HISTORICAL ASPECTS

Stenosis of the aortic valve was described by Riverius in 1646 and by Bonetti in 1700 and Morgagni in 1769 (Hallman and Cooley, 1983). It was not until 1844 that the congenital etiology of this form of stenosis was appreciated from Paget's description of bicuspid aortic valves. The potential clinical significance of this anomaly was recognized 42 years later, when Osler described a patient with endocarditis that occurred on a bicuspid aortic valve. More devastating implications were documented by Thursfield and Scott in 1913 when they described the sudden death of a 14-year-old boy with subaortic stenosis. Carrel (1910) and Jeger (1913) experimented independently with the use of conduits between the left ventricle and aorta to bypass aortic valvular obstruction. Tuffier (1914) first successfully dilated a calcific aortic valve and showed that it was possible to restore flow through the normal anatomic route. Initial therapeutic approaches involved aortic valvar dilatation, but in 1955 Swan and Kortz did the first open aortic valvotomy under direct vision by using systemic hypothermia with caval occlusion. Success with this technique was also reported by others (Lewis et al, 1956), but its popularity decreased after the advent of extracorporeal circulation, which allowed open

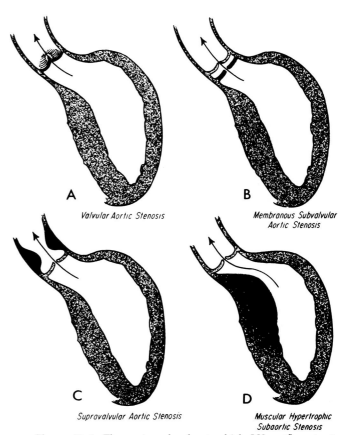

Figure 41–1. The various levels at which LV outflow tract obstruction can occur. (From Oldham, H. N., Jr.: Congenital aortic stenosis. *In* Sabiston, D. C., Jr. [ed]: Textbook of Surgery: The Biological Basis of Modern Surgical Practice, 13th ed. Philadelphia, W. B. Saunders Company, 1986.)

aortic valvotomy with cardiopulmonary bypass (Spencer, 1958). Since then, the treatment of the spectrum of lesions that cause LVOTO has expanded rapidly.

NATURAL HISTORY, CLINICAL PRESENTATION, AND DIAGNOSIS

Stenosis of the aortic valve may occur at any age. In most patients, it is a progressive problem that increases with growth (Ankeney et al, 1983; El-Said et al, 1972; Friedman et al, 1971). Few patients survive through the sixth decade without serious unfavorable signs or symptoms, and those who are initially asymptomatic should be monitored routinely because the untreated mortality can be 60% or more by the age of 40 (Campbell, 1968). Infants with symptoms have a 23% mortality if they are not treated in the first year of life, and the mean age of death for patients with untreated lesions is 35 years (Campbell, 1968). Congenital valvular aortic stenosis is three to four times more common in men than in women, and the natural history is influenced greatly by the age at presentation. When this lesion is seen in infancy the prognosis is worse than when it is seen later in life (Kirklin and Barratt-Boyes, 1986). Whereas infants with critical aortic stenosis may often present in New York Heart Association (NYHA) Class IV or V CHF with an urgent need for surgical relief, children who present after 1 year of age have few symptoms, and their greatest risk appears to be from the development of subacute bacterial endocarditis (SBE) or the ongoing risk of sudden death (Braverman and Gibson, 1957; Campbell, 1968; Glew et al, 1969). Although critically ill infants may need emergent aortic valvotomy, those who are found to have stenotic aortic valves later in life may live for many years with slowly progressive left ventricular (LV) outflow gradients before they require surgical intervention. The degree of stenosis present in children at the time of diagnosis predicts the likelihood of developing severe obstruction; only 20% of mild lesions progress to severe obstruction within 10 years, but 60% of moderate lesions become severe in that time frame (Friedman et al, 1971; Hossack et al, 1980; Mills et al, 1978).

Symptoms depend on the severity of the lesion and the age at presentation. Infants with critical aortic stenosis usually appear to be in fulminate congestive heart failure with poor peripheral perfusion, acidosis, tachypnea, pallor, perspiration, and inability to feed. If a patent ductus arteriosus is present, right-to-left shunting to support systemic perfusion may produce cyanosis. Physical examination shows a systolic ejection murmur with narrow pulse volume, but in severe lesions the diminished flow across the aortic valve combined with a depressed cardiac output may make the cardiac examination relatively unimpressive. The lungs may be congested and the liver may be engorged, and the infant shows signs of conges-

tive heart failure. Laboratory examination shows hypoxemia with acidosis due to congested pulmonary vasculature and poor peripheral perfusion. The chest film should reveal cardiomegaly and pulmonary edema. Electrocardiographic findings may show LV strain. Older children may be asymptomatic or may have fatigue, dyspnea, angina, or syncope with exercise. Laboratory parameters may be normal, and the chest film may show mild LV hypertrophy with prominence of the ascending aorta (Fig. 41–2).

The primary symptoms attributable to LV outflow tract obstruction are expected from increasing ventricular work. As the systolic pressure gradient across the outflow tract increases, flow can be maintained only by increasing LV pressure. In the neonate, it may not be possible to increase LV pressure and acute cardiac decompensation results. Peripheral perfusion can then be maintained by left-to-right shunting across a patent foramen ovale and right-to-left shunting across a patent ductus arteriosus. This mechanism explains the importance of maintaining ductal patency with prostaglandins in newborns with critical aortic stenosis (Jonas et al, 1985). In patients who survive infancy and have persistent aortic stenosis, the LV muscle undergoes concentric hypertrophy, which alters myocardial mechanics. The larger muscle mass creates greater systolic wall tension, which increases myocardial oxygen consumption—that is, increases the amount of oxygen necessary to meet the metabolic demands of the myocardium. The hypertrophied left ventricle is also

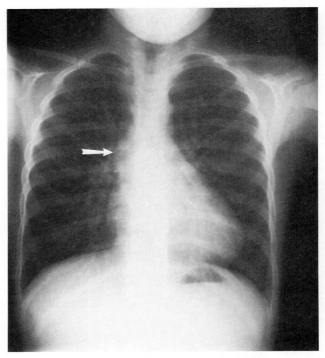

Figure 41–2. This chest film from an 8-year-old child with congenital valvular aortic stenosis shows the features characteristic of this lesion. Note the LV prominence and the enlargement of the ascending aorta *(arrow)* due to poststenotic dilatation.

slightly less compliant than the normal ventricle, and the end-diastolic pressure necessary for adequate volume loading of the ventricular chamber is increased. This higher end-diastolic pressure occurs when the myocardium receives its coronary blood flow and probably prevents an adequate supply to the subendocardial layer. Ischemia results because oxygen demand is increasing while the supply is decreasing, which leads to severe stenosis and eventually to heart failure (Spann et al, 1980). If the pressure gradient between the left ventricle and the aorta is less than 50 mm Hg and orifice size of the aortic valve is more than 0.7 cm²/m² body surface area, the heart usually adapts to increased demands without clinical evidence of failure (Oldham, 1986). Exercise necessitates an increase in cardiac output and therefore the flow per minute across the obstruction, which increases the severity of the lesion. Therefore, the measured gradient must be correlated with the cardiac index to provide an accurate estimate of its severity. The inability to increase forward flow to meet the metabolic demands of the body explains why most patients have initial symptoms with exercise. As the stenosis becomes more severe with growth, these symptoms may become more prominent, and they are thought to reflect hemodynamically severe obstruction that requires appropriate treatment to prevent death.

The proper time for therapeutic intervention must be determined, and periodic re-evaluation of children with suspicious murmurs is advised. These children may show little more than a harsh systolic ejection murmur most prominent over the second right intercostal space that radiates to the neck and is often associated with a thrill. As many as 22% of patients may have a diastolic murmur of aortic insufficiency, and there may also be a precordial lift (Braunwald et al, 1963). A number of criteria have been evaluated as indicators of more severe obstruction, because these children would be at greater risk. Symptoms rarely occur except with severe stenosis. A systolic precordial thrill usually suggests a gradient greater than 30 mm Hg. Narrowing of the peripheral pulse pressure (indicative of obstructed forward flow) suggests a severe stenosis. The chest film may be normal despite significant stenosis (see Fig. 41–2). Aortic valves rarely calcify until the fourth decade, but the presence of calcification in this location is evidence of an abnormal aortic valve. Although an electrocardiographic pattern of LV strain (ST segment and T wave abnormalities) often suggests an advanced form of disease, this correlation is not absolute, and children with a normal electrocardiogram have died suddenly with aortic stenosis (Glew et al, 1969; Hossack et al, 1980).

When significant stenosis is suspected, the diagnosis can be established by cardiac ultrasound, radionuclide angiography, or cardiac catheterization. Cardiac ultrasound with Doppler color flow imaging provides a sensitive and specific indicator of the severity and the site of obstruction (Kisslo et al,

1988). Color flow imaging also enables detection of minimal aortic insufficiency as well as associated small ventricular septal defects and other lesions. Doppler shifts allow measurement of the velocity across areas of stenosis (in meters per second [m/sec]) and, by using a simplification of Bernoulli's equation, gradients can be predicted accurately ($P = 4V^2$, where P is the peak instantaneous pressure gradient across the area of stenosis and V is the measured Doppler shift obtained by echocardiography. For example, a velocity of 5 m/sec across a stenotic valve causes a peak instantaneous pressure gradient of 100 mm Hg). Although the peak instantaneous pressure may overestimate the peak-to-peak gradient, especially in severe aortic stenosis, this noninvasive technology is useful for following the progression of aortic stenosis before, during, and after operation (Kisslo et al, 1988). There have been some studies of infants in which only echocardiography was used before operation and good results were obtained (Sink et al, 1984). However, because echocardiography cannot reliably show the anatomy of the aortic arch (and thus exclude coarctation or interruption), cardiac catheterization should be used if the patient's condition permits. For older patients, cardiac catheterization is still the standard for measurement of gradients and demonstration of anatomic defects (Fig. 41–3). However, gradients are significantly altered by the hemodynamic state, which is not normal in the cardiac catheterization laboratory or in the operating room, especially after cardiopul-

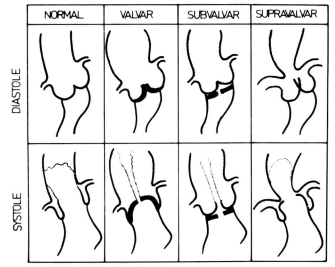

Figure 41–3. Diagrammatic representation of angiocardiographic signs of aortic stenosis. In valvular stenosis, there is systolic doming and a jet between the thickened leaflets. Poststenotic dilatation of the aorta is visible. In fibrous subvalvular stenosis, a jet may be seen and the leaflets may not open fully but doming is absent. The membrane should be visible, and there is often mild aortic incompetence. In supravalvular stenosis, the narrowing that starts above the aortic leaflets is visible. The sinuses of Valsalva are prominent, and the coronary arteries are often dilated. (From Kirklin, J. W., and Barratt-Boyes, B. G.: Cardiac Surgery. New York, John Wiley & Sons. Copyright © 1986.)

monary bypass, and the cardiac output at the time of measurement must be considered. Withdrawal of the catheter from the left ventricle into the ascending aorta provides critical pressure measurements that delineate the area of obstruction and quantitate the gradient across it at a particular cardiac index. Excellent examples of these are reproduced in the literature (Figs. 41–4 to 41–7) (Oldham, 1986). A gradient greater than 75 mm Hg or a valve area less than 0.5 cm^2/m^2 indicates severe stenosis. Increased LV end-diastolic pressure may indicate LV failure. By using various modalities, some quantification of the aortic valve gradient can be achieved. Mild stenosis is indicated by gradients less than 40 mm Hg at rest,

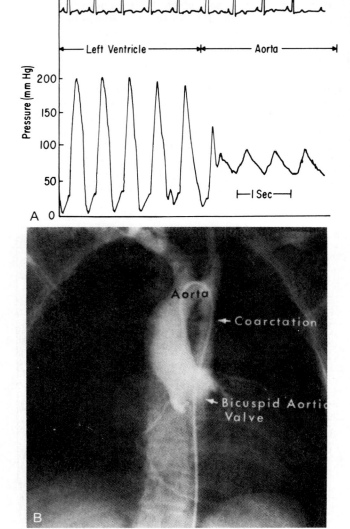

Figure 41–4. *A,* Pullback pressures from the left ventricle to the aorta in a patient with valvular aortic stenosis. *B,* The typical angiographic appearance of a bicuspid aortic valve. In this patient a coarctation of the aorta was also present, which is not an unusual combination. (From Oldham, H. N., Jr.: Congenital aortic stenosis. *In* Sabiston, D. C., Jr. [ed]: Textbook of Surgery: The Biological Basis of Modern Surgical Practice, 13th ed. Philadelphia, W. B. Saunders Company, 1986.)

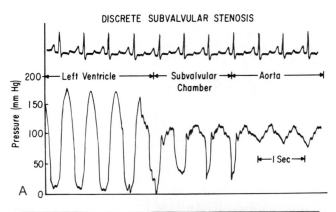

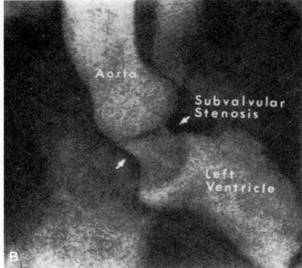

Figure 41–5. *A,* Pullback pressures in a patient with discrete subvalvular stenosis. *B,* The angiographic appearance of a subvalvular ring. (From Oldham, H. N., Jr.: Congenital aortic stenosis. *In* Sabiston, D. C., Jr. [ed]: Textbook of Surgery: The Biological Basis of Modern Surgical Practice, 13th ed. Philadelphia, W. B. Saunders Company, 1986.)

whereas patients who have gradients less than 75 mm Hg and usually with a mean of 50 mm Hg are considered to have moderate stenosis. Patients with severe stenosis have pressure gradients higher than 75 mm Hg and may have a mean calculated aortic valve area of 0.38 ± 0.15 cm^2/m^2 (Hossack et al, 1980).

INDICATIONS FOR OPERATION AND TREATMENT

Infants with congestive heart failure who respond poorly to medical management require operation (Hallman and Cooley, 1983; Kirklin and Barratt-Boyes, 1986). Older children and young adults with severe stenosis should also have surgical correction because they have a high risk of sudden death (de Leval, 1983; Hossack et al, 1980). A peak systolic gradient across the obstruction of 50 to 75 mm Hg during normal cardiac output and a valve surface

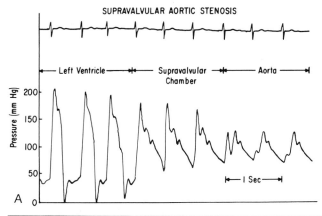

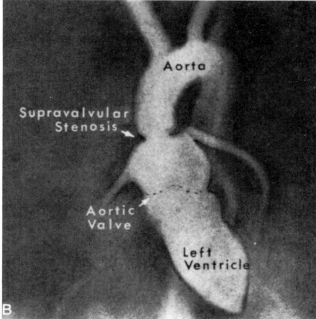

Figure 41-6. *A,* Pullback pressures in a patient with discrete supravalvular stenosis. *B,* The angiographic appearance of discrete supravalvular aortic stenosis. (From Oldham, H. N., Jr.: Congenital aortic stenosis. *In* Sabiston, D. C., Jr. [ed]: Textbook of Surgery: The Biological Basis of Modern Surgical Practice, 13th ed. Philadelphia, W. B. Saunders Company, 1986.)

area of less than 0.5 çm²/m² body surface area are generally accepted as parameters appropriate for operation. It is thought by some (Newfeld et al, 1976) that subvalvular stenosis requires early repair (i.e., a gradient of 40 mm Hg) to prevent progression of the lesion to a subaortic fibromuscular tunnel that can be more difficult to repair later (de Leval, 1983). Sudden death from arrhythmias (presumably due to progressive involvement of the bundle of His) has been reported to follow initially mild subaortic stenosis (James et al, 1988). The approach to aortic stenosis and the urgency with which the lesion is treated depend on the location of the obstruction and the age and condition of the patient. Critically ill infants in NYHA Class IV or V who are moribund and have metabolic acidosis may be treated initially with prostaglandin E_1 to maintain distal perfusion by

a patent ductus arteriosus and allow reversal of some of the metabolic defect before operation (Jonas et al, 1985).

Increasingly, some patients are treated nonoperatively by percutaneous balloon valvuloplasty. The use of this technique was first reported in 1983 (Lababidi), and the technique is now used by numerous pediatric cardiologists with various indications (Choy et al, 1987; Walls et al, 1984). Extensive experience with this approach has been described by Lock and associates (1987). Short-term results of balloon aortic valvotomy for congenital aortic stenosis appear to be comparable to results of surgical valvotomy. Neonates, who are the most difficult to treat with this technique, may obtain the greatest benefit as smaller catheters and low-profile balloons are

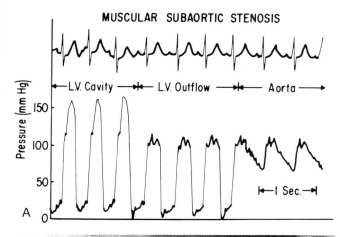

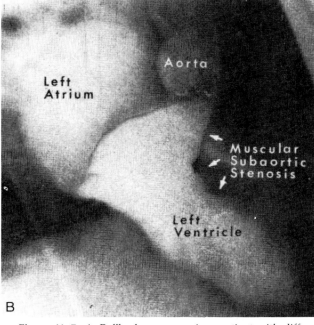

Figure 41-7. *A,* Pullback pressures in a patient with diffuse muscular subaortic stenosis. *B,* The angiographic appearance of muscular subaortic stenosis; narrowing of the LV outflow tract is shown. (From Oldham, H. N., Jr.: Congenital aortic stenosis. *In* Sabiston, D. C., Jr. [ed]: Textbook of Surgery: The Biological Basis of Modern Surgical Practice, 13th ed. Philadelphia, W. B. Saunders Company, 1986.)

developed. Aortic insufficiency contraindicates this option. Patients with aortic stenosis with severe aortic coarctation or interruption of the aortic arch are also not candidates for balloon valvuloplasty. The use of percutaneously introduced balloons for dilatation of valvar aortic stenosis may be appropriate in older children, because it appears that the balloon can open valves along the areas of commissural fusion and, when the technique is used properly, minimal if any regurgitation occurs.

Aortic valvotomy has also been attempted through a closed transventricular approach with dilators introduced through the LV apex (Duncan et al, 1987; Pelech et al, 1987). This approach has been useful in children with coexisting aortic coarctation because it can be used during left-sided thoracotomy for repair of the coarctation (Trinkle et al, 1975). Other surgeons described combined repair of coarctation with aortic valvotomy through a median sternotomy with cardiopulmonary bypass (Ungerleider and Ebert, 1987). Although closed transventricular valvotomy may be useful occasionally, most centers use an open transaortic valvotomy for this malformation.

Transaortic valvotomy done open and under direct vision has various technical alternatives. Repair of valvular aortic stenosis in infants with caval occlusion with various degrees of hypothermia has been reported (Castaneda and Norwood, 1985; Sink et al, 1984). With this technique, both cavae are occluded so that the heart is emptied and cardiac output is obliterated, which allows opening of the aorta proximal to a cross-clamp and quick repair of the lesion. During this time, neither the body nor the heart receives blood flow and the repair must be made in less than 2 to 3 minutes. This technique has been criticized by other surgeons experienced in this procedure (Messina et al, 1984), because these critically ill infants often cannot tolerate the additional hemodynamic insult of the technique. The long-term adequacy of valvotomy done in this manner is also questionable (Stewart et al, 1978). Overall, the usual procedures are best done with cardiopulmonary bypass. The introduction of an asanguineous prime by Cooley and associates (1965) increased the safety of repairing these lesions with cardiopulmonary bypass. Cardioplegia with moderate hypothermia can be added to provide a myocardium that is flaccid and protected, which allows the surgeon time to do the best possible procedure while the rest of the body is still perfused with oxygenated blood. Techniques for cardiopulmonary bypass vary between institutions. The author uses a median sternotomy, and for critically ill infants the pump prime is cooled to 7° C to achieve moderate hypothermia as soon as cardiopulmonary bypass is begun. This cooling produces a flaccid myocardium without the use of cardioplegia. The ascending aorta is cannulated near the innominate artery and a single venous cannula is used with extra perforations cut into it to improve venous return. Two venous cannulas can be used and are

especially useful for larger patients and patients who require more extensive procedures than simple aortic valvotomy. After cardiopulmonary bypass is started, the ascending aorta is cross-clamped. In infants, if only aortic valvotomy is planned, no cardioplegia is administered. Cardioplegic solution may be used for resections of subaortic membranes or for more extensive procedures to repair aortic stenosis. A standard transverse aortotomy is usually done unless it is thought that an aortoventriculoplasty may be required, in which case the aortotomy is done in a vertical manner. The aortic valve is inspected to permit the most direct and specific procedure to be used (Figs. 41–8 and 41–9). Before cardiopulmonary bypass is established, intraoperative Doppler colorflow imaging can be done with a hand-held epicardial probe. Placement of the probe directly on the epicardial surface eliminates chest wall attenuation and provides superb anatomic delineation of the LV outflow tract obstruction. In this manner, before cross-clamping the aorta, the anatomy of the aortic valve (number of cusps and areas of fusion) and any subvalvular lesions can be identified (Ungerleider et al, 1989). The aortotomy is closed after completion of the procedure with removal of air before release of the cross-clamp. When the patients are adequately warmed they are weaned from cardiopulmonary bypass. Temporary atrial and ventricular pacing wires can be left, which may be advisable if extensive subvalvular resection is done. The chest is usually closed over a single mediastinal tube and the patients are placed in an intensive care unit postoperatively. Details of the procedures vary with the types of lesions present.

VALVULAR STENOSIS

In 70 to 80% of patients LVOTO is caused by valvular lesions (Nadas and Fyler, 1972; Van Praagh, personal communication) and usually involves thickening of the valve leaflets and some degree of fusion of the commissures. The valves appear bicuspid, unicuspid, or rarely quadricuspid (see Fig. 41–9) (Peretz et al, 1969; Robicsek et al, 1969). Of hearts with unicuspid valves, 76% have associated EFE, whereas only 14% of hearts with bicuspid valves have EFE (Van Praagh, personal communication). In critically ill infants, the precise features of valve abnormality may be difficult to discern. Bicuspid valves occur in 0.7 to 2% of human hearts and in 70% of hearts with valvular aortic stenosis (Friedman and Johnson, 1987; Roberts, 1970). Although these valves may function normally, many calcify and become stenotic in later life. These valves are abnormal because of commissural fusion while the valve annulus and coronary arteries are normal. No surgical procedure can restore a stenotic valve to a completely normal one, and the goal of operation is to relieve stenosis. Operation is usually done with an incision separating the fused commissures (see

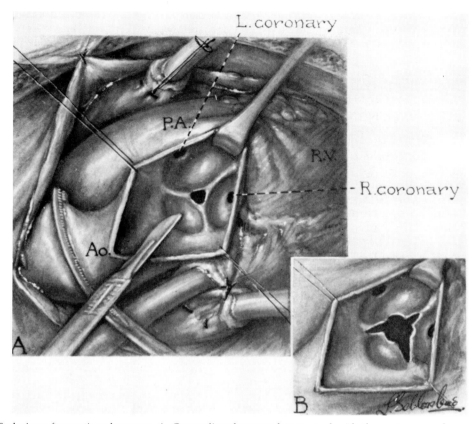

Figure 41–8. Technique for aortic valvotomy. *A,* On cardiopulmonary bypass and with the aorta cross-clamped, an aortotomy is done and the aortic valve is inspected. *B,* The valve can then be incised along the lines of commissural fusion. (From Spencer, F. C., Neill, C. A., Sank, L., and Bahnson, H. T.: Anatomical variations in 46 patients with congenital aortic stenosis. Am. Surg., *26:*204, 1960.)

Figure 41–9. Two lesions typical of valvular aortic stenosis. The uppermost valve is unicuspid. The commissure may be in any of the three possible normal locations for the valve commissure. Abortive commissures or raphes may be present. Repair is usually done by incision of the commissure toward the aortic annulus. Incision in the opposite direction, into the leaflet, can result in overwhelming aortic regurgitation. The lower valve is shown as bicuspid. The coronary arteries may arise on the same or opposite side of the commissure. A raphe may be present between the coronary arteries when they are on the same side of the commissure. When a bicuspid valve is stenotic, there is usually a small eccentric opening on one side of the commissure and correction involves incision in the fused portion of the commissure to enlarge this opening. Incision should not be made in the rudimentary raphes. (From de Leval, M.: Left ventricular outflow tract obstruction. *In* Stark, J., and de Leval, M. [eds]: Surgery for Congenital Heart Defects. New York, Grune & Stratton, 1983.)

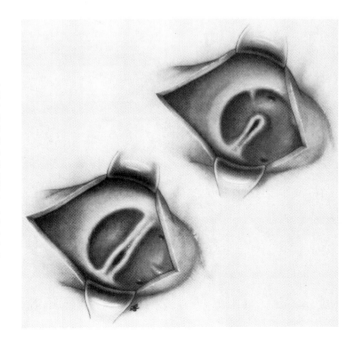

Fig. 41–8). This incision must not extend to the annulus, which could destroy the support mechanism of the leaflet and result in severe aortic insufficiency. Relief of stenosis is more easily accomplished in some anomalies than in others (see Fig. 41–9) (Dobell et al, 1981). In addition to relief of obstruction, some aortic insufficiency may be created. Infants may tolerate some aortic regurgitation better than they did the previous stenosis (Hallman and Cooley, 1983). Because these valves are still abnormal after relief of the stenosis, valvotomy is a palliative procedure. The goal of valvotomy should be to increase the size of the orifice as much as possible within the limitation of each individual valve.

Pressure gradients can be measured after valvotomy by various methods, including pressure catheter withdrawal across the repaired valve or comparison of direct trans-septal LV pressure and aortic pressure (Mavroudis et al, 1984). Intraoperative Doppler color-flow imaging can be used to predict the gradient of the repaired valve. Each method is helpful, but gradients must be related to the patient's cardiac output at the time of pressure measurement. Intraoperative color flow imaging can show the degree of aortic insufficiency that remains after valvotomy. Because of the association of EFE with aortic valve stenosis in neonates, the success of even the best procedures has been limited and mortality in infants has been between 9 and 33% (Gundry and Behrendt, 1986; Kugler et al, 1979; Messina et al, 1984; Pelech et al, 1987). Mortality is strongly affected by associated lesions and preoperative condition. Young age appears to be a risk factor only because it correlates with poorer preoperative functional status and associated lesions that lead to early presentation (Kirklin and Barratt-Boyes, 1986). Older children respond better and the mortality for valvotomy in children over 1 year of age should be almost zero (Kirklin and Barratt-Boyes, 1986).

AORTIC VALVE REPLACEMENT

Valvotomy is intended to reduce the aortic valve gradient and enable children to grow until they can accommodate placement of an adult-sized prosthetic valve if their LV outflow obstruction persists. Within 10 to 20 years after valvotomy, 35% of children require a second aortic valve operation. Reasons for reoperation range from recurrent stenosis to progressive aortic insufficiency and cannot always be managed by a repeated valvotomy. The need for reoperation does not appear to be related to age at initial valvotomy, although the second operation is more likely to be limited to repeat valvotomy if the initial valvotomy was done in infancy (Fulton et al, 1983). The usual interval until reoperation in patients who require one is 7 years (Johnson et al, 1985). If a second valvotomy can be done, it usually maintains the patient for 3 to 4 years before further aortic valve replacement is required. Only 70% of patients who survive an initial valvotomy are able to retain their

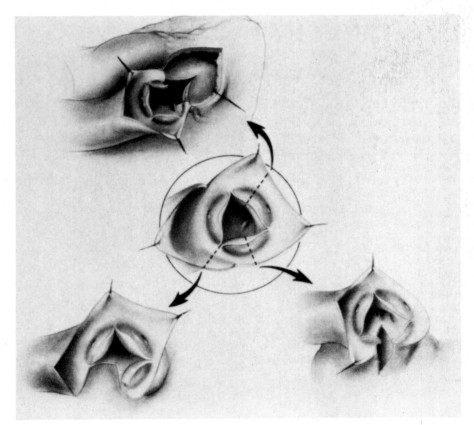

Figure 41–10. The various options available for enlarging the aortic annulus. Counterclockwise from the lower left are shown (1) the Rittenhouse-Manouguian procedure, (2) Nicks' (or Nunez') procedure, and (3) Konno-Rastan procedure. Manouguian's procedure (through the left coronary-noncoronary commissure) can be extended onto the anterior leaflet of the mitral valve, as shown. This area is then patched and can enlarge the aortic annulus by approximately 3 to 5 mm. Nicks' procedure extends through the noncoronary sinus and may or may not enter the roof of the left atrium. The Konno-Rastan aortoventriculoplasty provides the largest increase in aortic annular size and is the method of choice when there is associated subaortic fibromuscular stenosis. (From Doty, D. B.: Replacement of the aortic valve with cryopreserved aortic valve allograft: Considerations and techniques in children. J. Cardiovasc. Surg., 2:129, 1987.)

valve for more than 10 years (Kirklin and Barratt-Boyes, 1986). The smallest available prosthesis (17 mm) may be smaller than desirable, and in many cases of aortic valve replacement in children, annular enlarging procedures should be considered. Placement of an aortic valve that is too small to accommodate the patient's predicted growth can produce short-term success but eventual disappointment (Pugliese et al, 1984).

Several annular enlarging procedures are available (Fig. 41–10). The simplest method is to secure the prosthetic valve in a supra-annular position along the region of the noncoronary sinus (David and Uden, 1983; Olin et al, 1983). This sinus can be enlarged with graft material to allow placement of a larger valve (Najafi et al, 1969; Piehler et al, 1983). The aortic annulus can also be enlarged by incising through the annulus in various locations (Manouguian and Seybold-Epting, 1979; Nicks et al, 1970; Rittenhouse et al, 1979). Most of these procedures allow placement of a valve that is at most 3 to 5 mm larger than what could be accepted by the native annulus. For small children who require more radical enlargement of the aortic annulus, or for children who require relief of subaortic obstruction, the technique of aortoventriculoplasty can be used and has low mortality (Fig. 41–11) (Konno et al, 1975; Misbach et al, 1982; Rastan and Koncz, 1975). For the safe conduct of these procedures, the surgeon must appreciate the complex anatomic relationships of the aortic root to important cardiac morphologic and conduction structure (Sud et al, 1984).

The type of valve selected for children is important. After initial enthusiasm for the use of bioprosthetic valves (Sade et al, 1979), it was found that these valves often degenerate early in children and young adults (Thandroyen et al, 1980; Williams et al, 1982). For this reason, mechanical valves are preferred. Concerns about long-term anticoagulation in children have been raised. Although several groups report excellent results of the use of antiplatelet therapy for children with mechanical aortic prostheses (Hartz et al, 1986; Verrier et al, 1986), carefully monitored long-term anticoagulation with sodium warfarin (Coumadin) is standard therapy (Jaklitsch and Leyland, 1988; McGrath et al, 1987; Stewart et al, 1987). More recently, cryopreserved homografts placed in the aortic position have been used for valve replacement in children (Angell et al, 1987). Homografts may provide viable donor cells that may allow growth of the implanted valve (O'Brien et al, 1987). Only long-term follow-up will support the validity of this concept; cryopreserved homograft valves may be the best alternative in many cases for children and young adults. These valves can be placed in the normal annular position (Doty, 1987) or can be used during aortoventriculoplasty, although this procedure also requires reimplantation of the coronary arteries (Fig. 41–12) (McKowen et al, 1987; Somerville and Ross, 1982).

SUBVALVULAR STENOSIS

Discrete subvalvular stenosis was first described by Chevers in 1842. In 1956, Brock and Fleming described five patients with subvalvular aortic stenosis diagnosed during life. Initial treatment was by transventricular dilatation (Brock, 1959), but in 1960 Spencer and associates described surgical therapy of this lesion with cardiopulmonary bypass. A more severe form of muscular obstruction of the LV outflow tract was described by Spencer and associates (1960) and Reis and associates (1971). Attempts to resect this form of subaortic stenosis via the left atrium (Lillehei and Levy, 1963), left ventricle (Kirklin and Ellis, 1961), right side of the ventricular septum (Harken, 1961; Cooley et al, 1967), or aorta (Morrow, 1978) have been reported. Currently, the preferred approach for resection of most forms of subaortic stenosis is through the aorta.

Subvalvular aortic stenosis occurs in 8 to 20% of patients with LVOTO. It may be seen as a thin discrete membrane located anteriorly, immediately below the aortic valve, or less commonly as a diffuse fibromuscular "tunnel" beneath the aortic leaflets. Unusual variations caused by accessory endocardial cushion tissue (Nanton et al, 1979) and by tethering of the anterior leaflet of the mitral valve to the interventricular septum (Wright and Wittner, 1983) have been described. Correction of the membranous form necessitates an incision in the aorta, retraction of the usually normal aortic valve leaflets, and resection of the membrane with care being taken not to injure the conduction system or the anterior leaflet of the mitral valve, which is usually subjacent to the lesion (Fig. 41–13) (de Leval, 1983; Spencer et al, 1960; Sud et al, 1984). Early resection may prevent progression to the more severe fibromuscular variety (Oldham, 1986). The LVOTO caused by the more diffuse fibromuscular lesions may be amenable to resection of enough of the obstructing tissue to relieve the stenosis, although there is an increased danger of damaging the interventricular septum, the mitral valve, or the conduction system (Fig. 41–14). Some obstructions cannot be relieved safely by transaortic resection and require more complicated procedures such as aortoventriculoplasty (see Figs. 41–11 and 41–12) (Konno et al, 1975; Misbach et al, 1982; Rastan and Koncz, 1975; Schaffer et al, 1986) or implantation of a valved conduit between the left ventricle and the aorta that bypasses the normal outflow tract (Behrendt and Rocchini, 1987; Brown et al, 1984; Norwood et al, 1983). The indications for this procedure are debatable (Kirklin and Barratt-Boyes, 1986). In patients in whom the aortic valve and annulus are normal and there is elongated subaortic fibrous obstruction, a modified septoplasty to enlarge the subaortic area has been described (Fig. 41–15) (Cooley and Garrett, 1986).

A variation of subaortic stenosis is created by asymmetric septal hypertrophy. It has been described

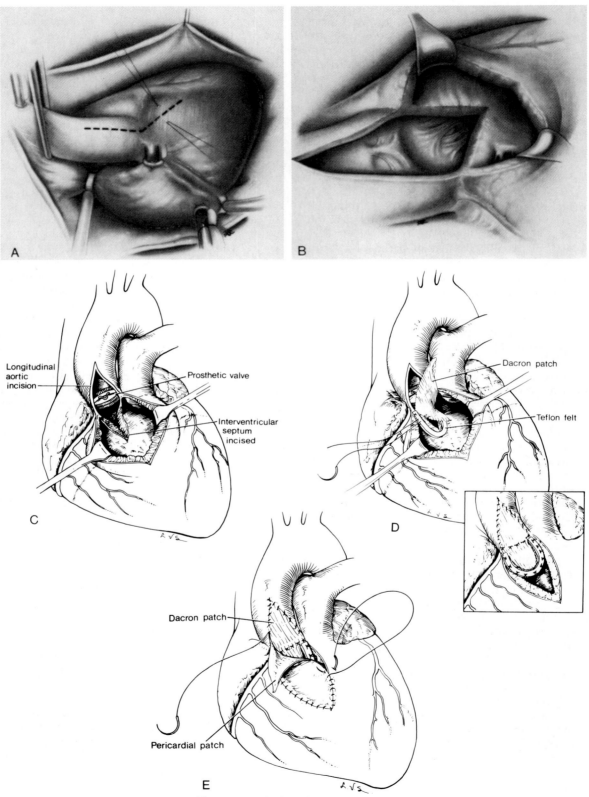

Figure 41–11 *See legend on opposite page*

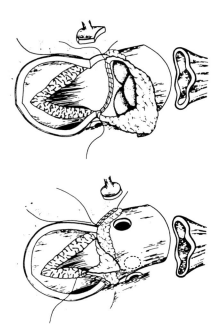

Figure 41–12. Technique for aortoventriculoplasty with a homograft valve. Incisions are the same as for a standard aortoventriculoplasty except that the coronary arteries are excised from the native aorta with substantial cuffs of tissue. The homograft is then sewn into place, and the mitral leaflet is used to patch the defect in the interventricular septum. The coronary arteries are implanted on the homograft above the valve leaflet in corresponding sinuses. The distal anastomosis between homograft and recipient aorta is then made. (From Clarke, D. R.: Extended aortic root replacement for the treatment of left ventricular outflow obstruction. J. Cardiac Surg., 2:121,1987.)

by Braunwald and associates (1964) and Morrow and associates (1975) and is called idiopathic hypertrophic subaortic stenosis. Unlike the other forms of fixed LVOTO, this condition appears to be a dynamic obstruction in which the hypertrophied septum interferes with outflow to an extent that depends on the contractile state of the heart and the LV systolic volume. This obstruction is increased by inotropic agents, by diminished blood volume, by Valsalva's maneuver, or by nitroglycerin (Braunwald et al, 1964). The gradient is reduced by propranolol or adrenergic blockage, by increased blood volume, or by general anesthesia (Oldham, 1986). These patients

can be treated medically with propranolol or managed surgically by myectomy with excision of part of the hypertrophied septum (through the aortic valve) (see Fig. 41–14) (Morrow, 1978). A surgical approach is indicated when the patient remains symptomatic despite appropriate medical management.

The surgeon who undertakes resection of muscle or fibrous membrane below the aortic valve must have clear knowledge of the anatomy of the conduction system, because this area is vulnerable during these procedures (Sud et al, 1984). In the discrete form of this lesion, in addition to resecting the fibrous membrane, a trough of muscle should be resected from the ventricular septum anteriorly centered beneath the commissure between the right and left aortic cusps (see Fig. 41–14), because the ventricular septum is always hypertrophied and may result in residual obstruction (Gallotti et al, 1981).

Discrete subvalvular aortic stenosis is rare in infancy and is more often seen in young children or young adults (Kirklin and Barratt-Boyes, 1986). The lesion may be associated with a ventricular septal defect and can occur after spontaneous closure of a ventricular septal defect. The lesion can progress rapidly and frequent follow-up is advised (Mody and Mody, 1975) with serial two-dimensional echocardiography with Doppler flow analysis. Indications for operative intervention are similar to those for valvular aortic stenosis, but the options for procedures appropriate for patients of various sizes makes the decision more complex. Depending on the extent of the lesion and the age of the patient, results for this form of LVOTO can be good; more than 80% of patients with correction of discrete obstructions live for more than 15 years. The rate of recurrent stenosis varies and continued follow-up is probably warranted, although recurrence may reflect inadequate initial resection, especially if no muscle is resected from the interventricular septum below the right or left coronary commissure (Katz et al, 1977; Kirklin and Barratt-Boyes, 1986). The results are not as good for patients with more severe forms of tunnel stenosis (Moses et al, 1984), especially if simple resection is done. More extensive procedures such as aortoventriculoplasty should be included in the plan for these patients. Aortoventriculoplasty in a 5-day-old infant has been reported (Guyton et al, 1986), but the

Figure 41–11. Aortoventriculoplasty can provide optimal enlargement of the aortic root as well as relief of subaortic stenosis. *A*, A vertical aortotomy is made and extended between the right and left coronary cusps into the right ventricular outflow tract. Care is taken to protect the right coronary artery ostium because the incision should remain well to the left of this region. The incision onto the right ventricular outflow tract must be below the pulmonary valve. *B*, When the right ventricular outflow tract is open, the aortic valve leaflets are excised and an incision is extended through the interventricular septum as far as necessary to relieve any area of subvalvular narrowing. (*A* and *B*, From de Leval, M.: Left ventricular outflow tract obstruction. *In* Stark, J., and de Leval, M. [eds]: Surgery for Congenital Heart Defects. New York, Grune & Stratton, 1983.) *C*, A prosthetic valve is then sewn in the normal annular position posteriorly with interrupted sutures. *D*, A patch of Dacron is used to enlarge the subvalvular interventricular septum and is continued onto the aorta. The anterior portion of the valve is anchored to this patch with interrupted sutures. *E*, Finally, the right ventricular outflow tract is reconstructed with pericardium and this patch extends onto the aortotomy to provide hemostasis. (*C*, *D*, and *E*, From Misbach, G. A., Turley, K., Ullyot, D. J., and Ebert, P. A.: Left ventricular outflow enlargement by the Konno procedure. J. Thorac. Cardiovasc. Surg., *84*:696, 1982.)

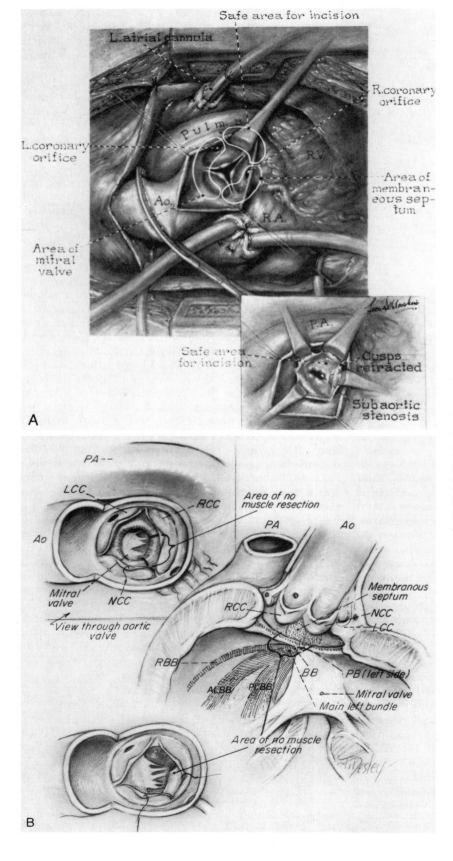

Figure 41–13. *A,* The areas that must be understood before resection of discrete subaortic stenosis. With the valve cusps retracted, the area of subaortic stenosis can be visualized *(lower panel).* It is important to preserve tissue in the area of the membranous septum. The mitral valve must be protected from damage during resection of the membrane in this region. (From Spencer, F. C., Neill, C. A., Sank, L., and Bahnson, H. T.: Anatomical variations in 46 patients with congenital aortic stenosis. *Am. Surg., 26:*204, 1960.) *B,* Appearance of the subvalvular area after resection of the membrane. Note that muscle along the region of the membranous septum is preserved to protect the conduction system. (From Bharati, S., Lev, M., and Kirklin, J. W.: Cardiac Surgery and the Conduction System. New York, John Wiley & Sons. Copyright © 1983.)

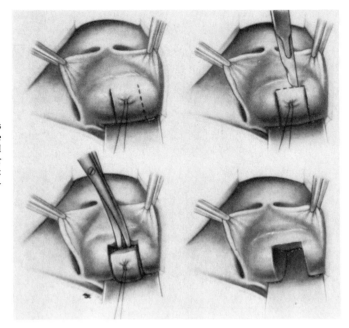

Figure 41–14. For patients with muscular subaortic stenosis (as in idiopathic hypertrophic subaortic stenosis), wedge of muscle in the outflow septum can be safely excised between the right and left aortic cusps as shown. (From de Leval, M.: Left ventricular outflow tract obstruction. *In* Stark, J., and de Leval, M. [eds]: Surgery for Congenital Heart Defects. New York, Grune & Stratton, 1983.)

procedure is usually delayed until patients are 4 years of age.

SUPRAVALVULAR STENOSIS

The first description of supravalvular aortic stenosis was by Mencarelli in 1930. In 1958, Denie and Verheugt showed how this form of LVOTO could be recognized by retrograde arterial catheterization with pullback pressures at various locations. In 1961, Williams and associates described the association of supravalvular aortic stenosis, mental retardation, and "elfin" facies (Fig. 41–16), a syndrome that now bears his name and that has been substantiated by others (Cornell et al, 1966). The presence of severe infantile hypercalcemia (Garcia et al, 1964; Hooft et al, 1963) or peripheral pulmonary stenosis (Beuren et al, 1964) has been associated with this syndrome. A form of supravalvular aortic stenosis occurs without the characteristic facies (Sissman et al, 1959). The first successful surgical correction of supravalvular aortic

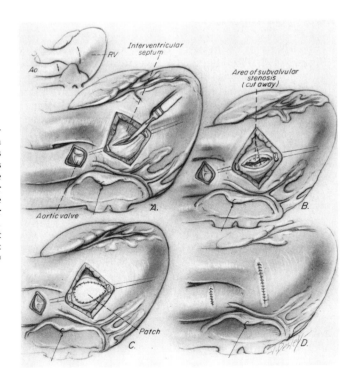

Figure 41–15. Modification of the aortoventriculoplasty procedure for patients with a normal aortic valve annulus but with significant subvalvular stenosis. *A,* A right ventricular incision is made through the right ventricular outflow tract to permit access to the interventricular septum below the aortic valve. *B,* The interventricular septum is incised and the area of subvalvular stenosis is removed. Careful placement of a clamp through the aortic valve helps direct this incision. *C,* The interventricular septum is then patched as is done for any ventricular septal defect. *D,* The incisions in the aorta and right ventricular outflow tract are repaired. (From Kirklin, J. W., and Barratt-Boyes, B. G.: Cardiac Surgery, New York, John Wiley & Sons. Copyright © 1986.)

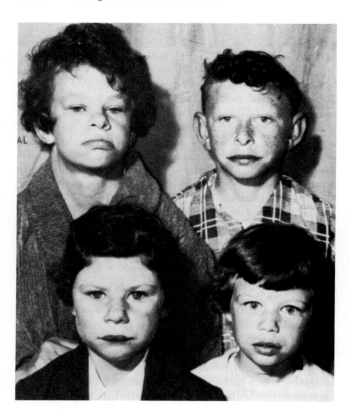

Figure 41–16. The "elfin" facies prominent in patients with supravalvular stenosis. Note the features of the ears, nose, and lips in these patients. (From Williams, J. C. P., Barratt-Boyes, B. G., and Lowe, J. B.: Supravalvular aortic stenosis. Circulation, 24:1311, 1961. By permission of the American Heart Association.)

stenosis by patch graft enlargement was reported by McGoon and associates at the Mayo Clinic in 1961. The first patient in this series was operated on in 1956. Reports of treatment for this lesion with resection and end-to-end anastomosis (Hara et al, 1962) and by excision of the intimal ridge without patch enlargement (Hancock, 1961) also appeared. Currently, patch aortoplasty is the recommended treatment.

This form of stenosis can be localized or diffuse (Fig. 41–17). The lesion is a coarctation or hypoplasia of the ascending aorta with various degrees of intimal hyperplasia. The disease is uncommon in adults, and it is speculated that untreated patients with supravalvular stenosis die before they become adults (Pasengrau et al, 1973). Presentation is similar to that in other forms of LVOTO, but associated anomalies such as peripheral pulmonary stenosis may complicate the clinical course.

Surgical treatment for this lesion includes cardiopulmonary bypass with moderate hypothermia, which was described earlier. The aorta is opened through the area of stenosis with an incision that extends into both the right and noncoronary sinus of Valsalva (Fig. 41–18). A Y-shaped patch of prosthetic material is used to enlarge the ascending aorta (Doty et al, 1977). Data suggest that resection of an intimal ridge opposite prosthetic patch aortoplasty increases the risk of aneurysm formation and indicate that this part of the procedure should be omitted (DeSanto et al, 1987; Hehrlein et al, 1986).

When the stenosis is of the more diffuse type with generalized hypoplasia of the ascending aorta, arterial cannulation may have to be done by the femoral route. The patient is then rapidly cooled to 18° C and the repair is made under total circulatory arrest. A longitudinal incision is made through the area of stenosis, which can be patched with prosthetic material or with a piece of homograft. During this procedure, the head vessels should be clamped and the incision should be extended onto the proximal portion of these vessels if stenosis exists at this level. Some groups suggest treating this form of stenosis with an LV apical to aortic bypass shunt (Keane et al, 1976).

Repair of the localized form of congenital supravalvular aortic stenosis has a lower hospital mortality and better long-term prognosis than repair of its diffuse counterpart. Operative mortality in the localized form should be almost 0%, whereas it can be as high as 40% in the diffuse form. Similarly, late survival is good and the reoperation rate should be low (Kirklin and Barratt-Boyes, 1986). Because this form of stenosis is a type of LV outflow tract obstruction, indications for operation are similar to those for valvular or subvalvular stenosis.

OVERALL RESULTS

In the evaluation of any procedure used for congenital lesions in young patients, the long-term benefits of surgical intervention must be assessed. The complications of LVOTO include sudden death,

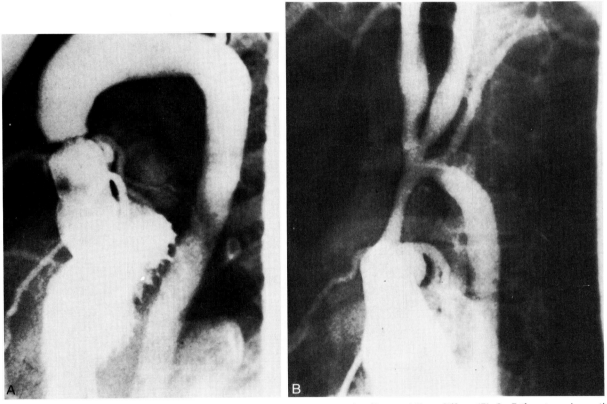

Figure 41–17. The angiographic appearance of supravalvular stenosis can be discrete (*A*) or diffuse (*B*). In *B* the stenosis continues onto the innominate, carotid, and subclavian arteries. (From Kirklin, J. W., and Barratt-Boyes, B. G.: Cardiac Surgery. New York, John Wiley & Sons. Copyright © 1986.)

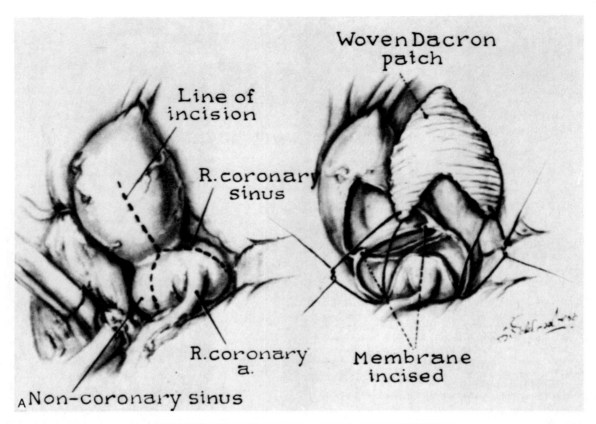

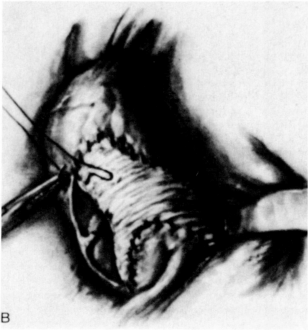

Figure 41–18. Technique of surgical correction for discrete supravalvular aortic stenosis. *A,* An incision is made in the ascending aorta and into the right coronary and noncoronary sinus. Care is taken to protect the right coronary artery. The intimal ridge can be excised, although recent data suggest that it should be left intact to protect the integrity of the aorta. A Y-shaped patch of Dacron is made to enlarge the aorta. *B,* The patch is sewn into place and provides enlargement of the aorta in the area of previous stenosis. (From Oldham, H. N, Jr.: Congenital aortic stenosis. *In* Sabiston, D. C., Jr. [ed]: Textbook of Surgery: The Biological Basis of Modern Surgical Practice, 13th ed. Philadelphia, W.B. Saunders Company, 1986.)

SBE, and heart failure (from chronic LV systolic overload or aortic insufficiency). Most procedures used for infants or young children are palliative; the intention is to relieve the stenosis and reduce the chance of early death. Many of these patients (with valvular lesions) eventually require valve replacement, and it is hoped that this can be done after they have become larger. The incidence of sudden death among patients with congenital aortic stenosis varies between 1 and 19% and in untreated patients the risk is estimated to be 0.9% each year (Campbell, 1968; Glew et al, 1969; Kirklin and Barratt-Boyes, 1986). Patients with more severe lesions, as proved by symptoms, pertinent physical findings, or objective pressure data, appear to be at greatest risk for sudden death (Braunwald et al, 1963; Glew et al, 1969; Hossack et al, 1980). Valvotomy does not eliminate this risk, but it reduces it to an estimated 0.29% each year (Stewart et al, 1978). SBE is always a risk in the presence of turbulence across abnormal anatomy. Without operation, approximately 3.1 episodes of SBE occur for every 1,000 patient-years with aortic stenosis; that is, there is a 1.4% chance of endocarditis in the first 30 years of life. The incidence of SBE increases after operation to 7.4% in the first 30 years of life (Stewart et al, 1978). Although the risk of heart failure from systolic overload is reduced by an adequate procedure, the incidence of aortic insufficiency probably triples in patients with primary valvular lesions from 11% preoperatively to 30 to 40% postoperatively (Stewart et al, 1978). Of these patients, 20% may be symptomatic.

Despite these figures, the survival of patients with significant stenotic lesions is improved by surgical therapy, but because the procedures for valvular aortic stenosis are palliative and result in increased risk of SBE and aortic regurgitation, they should probably be used only for children with severe lesions who have the higher risk of sudden death (Olley et al, 1978). Correction of subvalvular and supravalvular forms of LVOTO can lead to a better long-term result, depending on the nature of the lesion. The palliative nature of these procedures necessitates proper timing in selection of patients so that the current clinical condition is not replaced by new problems of equal or greater concern.

Selected Bibliography

Campbell, M.: The natural history of congenital aortic stenosis. Br. Heart J., 30:514, 1968.

For proper therapeutic decisions, it is essential to have an understanding of the natural history of a disease. This paper describes the expectations for various forms of aortic stenosis. Based on these data, current surgical decisions can be made.

Doty, D. B.: Replacement of the aortic valve with cryopreserved aortic valve allograft: Considerations and techniques in children. J. Cardiac Surg., 2:121, 1987.

A major contributor to this field, the author shares his perceptions on the proper approach to reconstruction of the aortic valve in patients with congenital aortic stenosis. He describes and illustrates his technique of homograft insertion in the aortic position in children and discusses the features that must be considered by the surgeon when attempting to re-establish "normal" aortic outflow.

Kirklin, J. W., and Barratt-Boyes, B. G.: Congenital aortic stenosis. In Kirklin, J. W., and Barratt-Boyes, B. G. (eds.): Cardiac Surgery. New York, John Wiley and Sons, 1986.

These authors share an extraordinary experience in the field of congenital heart surgery and provide a comprehensive and well-organized document that discusses all aspects of the presentation and treatment of the various forms of congenital aortic stenosis. This chapter is essential for anyone who wants in-depth knowledge of this field.

McKowen, R. L., Campbell, D. N., Woelfel, F., et al: Extended aortic root replacement with aortic allografts. J. Thorac. Cardiovasc. Surg., 93:366, 1987.

The authors describe a unique approach to aortoventriculoplasty with cryopreserved aortic homografts. The results in three patients are discussed and the technical features of the operation are described. With the current enthusiasm for aortic homografts, the operation may have wide application in the future.

Messina, L. M., Turley, K., Stanger, P., et al: Successful aortic valvotomy for severe congenital valvular aortic stenosis in the newborn infant. J. Thorac. Cardiovasc. Surg., 88:92, 1984.

The authors maintain that aortic valvotomy can be more safely performed in critically ill newborns by using the technique of cardiopulmonary bypass rather than inflow occlusion. They report 9% operative mortality (1 in 11 patients) with a mean cardiopulmonary bypass time of 21 minutes. Their technique is well described, and although some groups suggest that the use of prostaglandin E₁ to stabilize patients before operation may be more important than the technique of valvotomy (Jonas et al, 1985), this article nevertheless establishes the safety and efficacy of aortic valvotomy on cardiopulmonary bypass for critically ill newborns.

Misbach, G. A., Turley, K., Ullyot, D. J., and Ebert, P. A.: Left ventricular outflow enlargement by the Konno procedure. J. Thorac. Cardiovasc. Surg., 84:696, 1982.

The authors describe modifications of aortoventriculoplasty in which pericardium is used to reconstruct the right ventricular outflow tract and to provide additional hemostasis over the aortotomy. This approach makes aortoventriculoplasty a safe procedure for children who require enlargement of the subaortic region. Because of the safety of the procedure with their modifications, the authors suggest that an aortoventriculoplasty should be preferred over LV apical-aortic conduits.

Morrow, A. G.: Hypertrophic subaortic stenosis: Operative methods utilized to relieve left ventricular outflow obstruction. J. Thorac. Cardiovasc. Surg., 76:423, 1978.

This reference should be read in its entirety before any operation for hypertrophic subaortic stenosis. The report is a technical description of the operative methods developed by Morrow based on his extensive personal experience at the National Heart Institute. Each step of the procedure is precisely described and clearly shown by Schlossberg's lucid illustrations. The author's style is most apparent in the informative section entitled "Details considered to be of special importance." The article is a summary of experience with 217 patients and the results obtained.

O'Brien, M. F., Stafford, E. G., Gardner, M. A. H., et al: A comparison of aortic valve replacement with viable cryopreserved and fresh allograft valves, with a note on chromosomal studies. J. Thorac. Cardiovasc. Surg., 94:812, 1987.

This author, who has repopularized the use of aortic allografts by cryopreserving them in liquid nitrogen at −196° C, presents his results with 316 aortic valve replacements and compares cryopreserved allografts to fresh allografts stored at 4° C. He finds a marked difference in valve degeneration that favors the cryopreserved allografts. Freedom from reoperation for valve degeneration at 10 years was achieved in 89% of patients with fresh allografts compared with 100% of patients with cryopreserved implants. The author shows evidence of chromosomal studies which suggests that donor cells remain viable in the cryopreserved allografts, which may be a key to their durability.

Oldham, H. N., Jr.: Congenital aortic stenosis. In Sabiston, D. C., Jr. (ed): Textbook of Surgery: The Biological Basis of Modern Surgical Practice, 13th ed. Philadelphia, W. B. Saunders Company, 1986, pp. 2261–2279.

This well written chapter describes the spectrum of this disease. The author has had extensive experience with this disease entity, having worked with Dr. Morrow and colleagues at the National Heart Institute.

Sud, A., Parker, F., and Magilligan, D. J., Jr.: Anatomy of the aortic root. Ann. Thorac. Surg., 38:76, 1984.

These authors provide precise illustrations of the anatomy of the aortic root. A clear understanding of this anatomy is essential for safe surgical therapy for the various forms of congenital aortic stenosis.

Bibliography

Angell, W. W., Angell, J. D., Oury, J. H., et al: Long-term follow-up of viable frozen aortic homografts: A viable homograft valve bank. J. Thorac. Cardiovasc. Surg., 93:815, 1987.

Ankeney, J. L., Tzena, T. S., and Liebman, J.: Surgical therapy for congenital aortic valvular stenosis. J. Thorac. Cardiovasc. Surg., 85:41, 1983.

Behrendt, D. M., and Rocchini, A.: Relief of the left ventricular outflow tract obstruction in infants and small children with valved extracardiac conduits. Ann. Thorac. Surg., 43:82, 1987.

Bernhard, W. F., Keane, J. F., Fellows, K. E., et al: Progress and problems in the surgical management of congenital aortic stenosis. J. Thorac. Cardiovasc. Surg., 66:404, 1973.

Beuren, A. J., Schulze, C., Eberle, P., et al: The syndrome of supravalvular aortic stenosis, peripheral pulmonary stenosis, mental retardation and similar facial appearance. Am. J. Cardiol., 13:471, 1964.

Braunwald, E., Goldblatt, A., Aygen, M. M., et al: Congenital aortic stenosis. I: Clinical and hemodynamic findings in 100 patients. Morrow, A. G., Goldblatt, A., and Braunwald, E.: II: Surgical treatment and results of operations. Circulation, 27:426, 1963.

Braunwald, E., Oldham, H. N., Ross, J., et al: The circulatory response of patients with idiopathic hypertrophic subaortic stenosis to nitroglycerin and to the Valsalva maneuver. Circulation, 29:422, 1964.

Braverman, I. B., and Gibson, S.: The outlook for children with congenital aortic stenosis. Am. Heart J., 53:487, 1957.

Brock, R.: Aortic subvalvular stenosis with surgical treatment. Guy's Hosp. Rep., 108:144, 1959.

Brock, R., and Fleming, P. R.: Aortic subvalvular stenosis. A report of 5 cases diagnosed during life. Guy's Hosp. Rep., 105:391, 1956.

Brock, R. C.: Valvotomy for aortic stenosis. Br. Heart J., 16:471, 1954.

Brown, J. W., Girod, D. A., Hurwitz, R. A., et al: Apicoaortic valved conduits for complex left ventricular outflow obstruction: Technical considerations and current status. Ann. Thorac. Surg., 38:162, 1984.

Campbell, M.: The natural history of congenital aortic stenosis. Br. Heart J., 30:514, 1968.

Carrel, A.: On the experimental surgery of the thoracic aorta and the heart. Ann. Surg., 52:83, 1910.

Castaneda, A. R., and Norwood, W.: Left ventricular outflow tract obstruction. In Arciniegas, E. (ed): Pediatric Cardiac Surgery. Chicago, Year Book Medical Publishers, 1985.

Chevers, N.: Observations on the diseases of the orifice and valves of the aorta. Guy's Hosp. Rep., 7:387, 1842.

Choy, M., Beekman, R. H., Rocchini, A. P., et al: Percutaneous balloon valvuloplasty for valvar aortic stenosis in infants and children. Am. J. Cardiol., 59:1010, 1987.

Clarke, D. R.: Extended aortic root replacement for the treatment of left ventricular outflow obstruction. J. Cardiac Surg., 2:121, 1987.

Cooley, D. A., Beall, A. C., Jr., Grady, L., et al: Obstructive lesions of the left ventricular outflow tract: Surgical treatment. Circulation, 31:612, 1965.

Cooley, D. A., Bloodwell, R. D., Hallman, G. L., et al: Surgical treatment of muscular subaortic stenosis: Results from septectomy in twenty-six patients. Circulation, 35(Suppl. I):124, 1967.

Cooley, D. A., and Garrett, J. R.: Septoplasty for left ventricular outflow obstruction without aortic valve replacement: A new technique. Ann. Thorac. Surg., 42:445, 1986.

Cornell, W. P., Elkins, R. C., Criley, J. M., and Sabiston, D. C., Jr.: Supravalvular aortic stenosis. J. Thorac. Cardiovasc. Surg., 51:484, 1966.

David, T. E., and Uden, D. E.: Aortic valve replacement in adult patients with small aortic annuli. Ann. Thorc. Surg., 36:577, 1983.

de Leval, M.: Left ventricular outflow tract obstruction. In Stark, J., and de Leval, M. (eds): Surgery for Congenital Heart Defects. New York, Grune & Stratton, 1983.

Denie J. J., and Verheugt, A. P.: Supravalvular aortic stenosis. Circulation, 18:902, 1958.

DeSanto, A., Bills, R. G., King, H., et al: Pathogenesis of aneurysm formation opposite prosthetic patches used for coarctation repair: An experimental study. J. Thorac. Cardiovasc. Surg., 94:720, 1987.

Dobell, A. R. C., Bloss, R. S., Gibbons, J. E., and Collins, G. F.: Congenital valvular aortic stenosis. J. Thorac. Cardiovasc. Surg., 81:916, 1981.

Doty, D. B.: Replacement of the aortic valve with cryopreserved aortic valve allograft: Considerations and techniques in children. J. Cardiac Surg., 2:129, 1987.

Doty, D. B., Polansky, D. B., and Jenson, C. B.: Supravalvular aortic stenosis: Repair by external aortoplasty. J. Thorac. Cardiovasc. Surg., 74:362, 1977.

Duncan K., Sullivan, I., Robinson, P., et al: Transventricular aortic valvotomy for critical aortic stenosis in infants. J. Thorac. Cardiovasc. Surg., 93:546, 1987.

El-Said, G., Galioto, F. M., Mullins, C. E., et al: Natural hemodynamic history of congenital aortic stenosis in childhood. Am. J. Cardiol., 30:6, 1972.

Friedman, W. F., and Johnson, A. D.: Congenital aortic stenosis. In Roberts, W. C. (ed): Adult Congenital Heart Disease. Philadelphia, F. A. Davis Company, 1987.

Friedman, W. F., Modlinger, J., and Morgan, J. R.: Serial hemodynamic observations in asymptomatic children with valvar aortic stenosis. Circulation, 43:91, 1971.

Fulton, D. R., Hougen, T. J., Keane, J. F., et al: Repeat aortic valvotomy in children. Am. Heart J., 1067:60, 1983.

Gallotti, R., Wain, W. H., and Ross, D. N.: Surgical enucleation of discrete sub-aortic stenosis. Thorac. Cardiovasc. Surg., 29:312, 1981.

Garcia, R. E., Friedman, W. F., Kaback, M. M., and Rowe, R. D.: Idiopathic hypercalcaemia and supravalvular aortic stenosis: Documentation of a new syndrome. N. Engl. J. Med., 271:117, 1964.

Glew, R. H., Varghese, P. J., Krovetz, L. J., et al: Sudden death in congenital aortic stenosis: A review of eight cases with an evaluation of premonitory clinical features. Am. Heart J., 78:615, 1969.

Gundry, S. R., and Behrendt, D. M.: Prognostic factors in valvotomy for critical aortic stenosis in infancy. J. Thorac. Cardiovasc. Surg., 92:747, 1986.

Guyton, R. A., Michalik, R. E., McIntyre, A. B., et al: Aortic atresia and aortico-left ventricular tunnel: Successful surgical management by Konno aortoventriculoplasty in a neonate. J. Thorac. Cardiovasc. Surg., 92:1099, 1986.

Hallman, G. L., and Cooley, D. A.: Congenital aortic stenosis. In Sabiston, D. C., Jr., and Spencer, F. C. (eds): Gibbon's Surgery of the Chest. Philadelphia, W. B. Saunders Company, 1983.

Hancock, E.: Differentiation of valvular, subvalvular and supravalvular aortic stenosis. Guy's Hosp. Rep., 110:1, 1961.

Hara, M., Duncan, T., and Lincoln, B.: Supravalvular aortic stenosis. Report of successful excision and aortic re-anastomosis. J. Thorac. Cardiovasc. Surg., 43:212, 1962.

Harken, D. E.: Cited by Morrow, A. G., and Brockenbrough, E. C.: Surgical treatment of idiopathic hypertrophic subaortic stenosis: Technic and hemodynamic results of subaortic ventriculomyotomy. Ann. Surg., 154:181, 1961.

Hehrlein, F. W., Mulch, J., Rautenburg, H. W., et al: Incidence and pathogenesis of late aneurysms after patch graft aortoplasty for coarctation. J. Thorac. Cardiovasc. Surg., 92:226, 1986.

Hooft, C., Vermassen, A., and Blancquaert, A.: Observation concerning the evolution of the chronic form of idiopathic hypercalcaemia in children. Helv. Paediatr. Acta, 18:138, 1963.

Hossack, K. F., Neutze, J. M., Lowe, J. B., et al: Congenital valvar aortic stenosis: Natural history and assessment for operation. Br. Heart J., 43:561, 1980.

Jaklitsch, M., and Leyland, S.: Aspirin anticoagulation for mechanical heart valves and Reye's syndrome. J. Thorac. Cardiovasc. Surg., 95:246, 1988.

James, T. N., Jordan, J. D., Ridick, L., and Bargeron, L. M.: Subaortic stenosis and sudden death. J. Thorac. Cardiovasc. Surg., 95:247, 1988.

Jeger, E.: Die Chirurgie der Blutgefäss und des Herzens. Berlin, A. Hirschwald, 1913.

Johnson, R. G., Williams, G. R., Razook, J. D., et al: Reoperation in congenital aortic stenosis. Ann. Thorac. Surg., 40:156, 1985.

Jonas, R. A., Lang, P., Mayer, J. E., and Castaneda, A. R.: The importance of prostaglandin E₁ in resuscitation of the neonate with critical aortic stenosis. J. Thorac. Cardiovasc. Surg., 89:314, 1985.

Katz, N. M., Mortimer, J. B., and Liberthson, R. R.: Discrete membranous subaortic stenosis. Report of 31 patients, review of the literature, and delineation of management. Circulation, 56:1034, 1977.

Keane, J. F., Fellows, K. E., LaFarge, C. G., et al: The surgical management of discrete and diffuse supravalvular aortic stenosis. Circulation, 54:112, 1976.

Kirklin, J. W., and Barratt-Boyes, B. G.: Congenital aortic stenosis. In Kirklin, J. W., and Barratt-Boyes, B. E. (eds.): Cardiac Surgery. New York, John Wiley and Sons, 1986.

Kirklin, J. W., and Ellis, F. H.: Surgical relief of diffuse subvalvular aortic stenosis. Circulation, 24:739, 1961.

Kisslo, J. A., Adams, D. B., and Belkin, R. N. (eds.): Doppler Color Flow Imaging. New York, Churchill Livingstone, 1988.

Konno, S., Yasuharu, I., Yoshinau, I., et al: A new method for prosthetic valve replacement in congenital aortic stenosis associated with hypoplasia of the aortic valve ring. J. Thorac. Cardiovasc. Surg., 70:909, 1975.

Kugler, J. D., Campbell, E., Vargo, T. A., et al: Results of aortic valvotomy in infants with isolated aortic valvular stenosis. J. Thorac. Cardiovasc. Surg., 78:553, 1979.

Lababidi, A.: Aortic balloon valvuloplasty. Am. Heart. J., 106:751, 1983.

Lewis, F. J., Shumway, N. E., and Niazi, S. A.: Aortic valvulotomy under direct vision during hypothermia. J. Thorac. Cardiovasc. Surg., 32:481, 1956.

Lillehei, C. W., and Levy, M. J.: Transatrial exposure for correction of subaortic stenosis. J.A.M.A., 186:8, 1963.

Lock, J. E., Keane, J. F., and Fellows, K. E.: Diagnostic and Interventional Catheterization in Congenital Heart Disease. Boston, Martinus Nijhoff, 1987.

Manouguian, S., and Seybold-Epting, W.: Patch enlargement of the aortic valve ring by extending the aortic incision into the anterior mitral leaflet: New operative technique. J. Thorac. Cardiovasc. Surg., 78:402, 1979.

Mavroudis, C., Rees, A., Solinger, R., and Elbl, F.: The prognostic value of intraoperative pressure gradients with congenital aortic stenosis. Ann. Thorac. Surg., 38:237, 1984.

McGoon, D. C., Mankin, H. T., Vlad, P., and Kirklin, J. W.: The surgical treatment of supravalvular aortic stenosis. J. Thorac. Cardiovasc. Surg., 41:125, 1961.

McGrath, L. B., Gonzalez-Lavin, L., Eldredge, W. J., et al: Thromboembolic and other events following valve replacement in a pediatric population treated with antiplatelet agents. Ann. Thorac. Surg., 43:285, 1987.

McKowen, R.L., Campbell, D.N., and Woelfel, G.F.: Extended aortic root replacement with aortic allografts. J. Thorac. Cardiovasc. Surg., 93:366, 1987.

Mencarelli, L.: Stenosi sopravalvolare aortica and anello. Arch. Ital. Anat. Istol. Pat., 1:829, 1930.

Messina, L. M., Turley, K., Stanger P., et al: Successful aortic valvotomy for severe congenital valvular aortic stenosis in the newborn infant. J. Thorac. Cardiovasc. Surg., 88:92, 1984.

Mills, P., Leech, G., Davies, M., and Leatham, A.: The natural history of a non-stenotic bicuspid aortic valve. Br. Heart J., 40:951, 1978.

Misbach, G. A. Turley, K., Ullyot, D. J., and Ebert, P. A.: Left ventricular outflow enlargement by the Konno procedure. J. Thorac. Cardiovasc. Surg., 84:696, 1982.

Mody, M. R., and Mody, G. T.: Serial hemodynamic observations in congenital valvular and subvalvular aortic stenosis. Am. Heart J., 89:137, 1975.

Morrow, A. G.: Hypertrophic subaortic stenosis: Operative methods utilized to relieve left ventricular outflow obstruction. J. Thorac. Cardiovasc. Surg., 76:423, 1978.

Morrow, A. G., and Brockenbrough, E. C.: Surgical treatment of idiopathic hypertrophic subaortic stenosis: Technic and hemodynamic results of subaortic ventriculomyotomy. Ann. Surg., 154:181, 1961.

Morrow, A. G., Reitz, B. A., Epstein, S. E., et al: Operative treatment in hypertrophic subaortic stenosis: Techniques and the results of pre- and postoperative assessments in 83 patients. Circulation, 52:88, 1975.

Moses, R. D., Barnhart, G. R., and Jones, M.: The late prognosis after localized resection for fixed (discrete and tunnel) left ventricular outflow tract obstruction. J. Thorac. Cardiovasc. Surg., 87:410, 1984.

Mulder, D. G., Katz, R. D., Moss, A. J., et al: The surgical treatment of congenital aortic stenosis. J. Thorac. Cardiovasc. Surg., 88:786, 1968.

Nadas, A. S., and Fyler, D.: Pediatric Cardiology. Philadelphia, W. B. Saunders Company, 1972.

Najafi, H., Ostermiller, W. E., and Husang, J.: Narrow aortic root complicating aortic valve replacement. Arch. Surg., 99:690, 1969.

Nanton, M. A., Belcourt, C. L., and Gillis, D. A.: Left ventricular outflow tract obstruction owing to accessory endocardial cushion tissue. J. Thorac. Cardiovasc. Surg., 78:537, 1979.

Newfeld, E. A., Muster, A. J., Paul, M. H., et al: Discrete subvalvular aortic stenosis in childhood: Study of 51 patients. Am. J. Cardiol., 38:53, 1976.

Nicks, R., Cartmill, T., and Bernstein, L.: Hypoplasia of the aortic root. Thorax, 25:339, 1970.

Norwood, W. I., Lang, P., Castaneda, A. R., and Murphy, J. D.: Management of infants with left ventricular outflow obstruction by conduit interposition between the ventricular apex and thoracic aorta. J. Thorac. Cardiovasc. Surg., 86:771, 1983.

O'Brien, M. F., Stafford, E. G., Gardner, M. A., et al: A comparison of aortic valve replacement with viable cryopreserved and fresh allograft valves, with a note on chromosomal studies. J. Thorac. Cardiovasc. Surg., 94:812, 1987.

Oldham, H. N., Jr.: Congenital aortic stenosis. In Sabiston, D. C., Jr. (ed): Textbook of Surgery: The Biological Basis of Modern Surgical Practice, 13th ed. Philadelphia, W. B. Saunders Company, 1986, pp. 2261–2279.

Olin, C. L., Bomfim, V., Halvazulis, V., et al: Optimal insertion technique for the Bjork-Shiley valve in the narrow aortic ostium. Ann. Thorac. Surg., 36:567, 1983.

Olley, P. M., Bloom, K. R., and Rowe, R. D.: Aortic stenosis:

Valvular, subaortic, and supravalvular. *In* Keith, J. D., Rowe, R. D., and Vlad, P. (eds): Heart Disease in Infancy and Childhood, 3rd ed. New York, Macmillan Publishing Company, 1978, pp. 698–727.

Osler, W.: The bicuspid condition of the aortic valves. Trans. Assoc. Am. Physicians, 2:185, 1886.

Paget, J.: On obstructions of the branches of the pulmonary artery. Med. Chir. Trans., 27:162, 1844.

Pasengrau, D. G., Kioshos, J. M., Durnin, R. E., and Kroetz, F. W.: Supravalvular aortic stenosis in adults. Am. J. Cardiol., 31:635, 1973.

Pelech, A. N., Trusler, G. A., Olley, P. M., et al: Critical aortic stenosis. J. Thorac. Cardiovasc. Surg., 94:510, 1987.

Peretz, D. I., Changfoot, G. H., and Gourlay, R. H.: Four-cusped aortic valve with significant hemodynamic abnormality. Am. J. Cardiol., 23:291, 1969.

Piehler, J. M., Danielson, G. K., Pluth, J. R., et al: Enlargement of the aortic root or anulus with autogenous pericardial patch during aortic valve replacement. J. Thorac. Cardiovasc. Surg., 86:350, 1983.

Pugliese, P., Bernabei, M., Santi, C., et al: Posterior enlargement of the small annulus during aortic valve replacement versus implantation of a small prosthesis. Ann. Thorac. Surg., 38:31, 1984.

Rastan, H., and Koncz, J.: Plastische Erweiterung der linken Ausflussbahn: Eine neue Operationsmethode. Thorax-chirurgie, 23:169, 1975.

Reis, R. L., Peterson, L. M., Mason, D. T., et al: Congenital fixed subvalvular aortic stenosis: An anatomical classification and correlations with operative results. Circulation, 43(Suppl. I):I-II, 1971.

Rittenhouse, E. A., Sauvage, L. R., Stamm, S. J., et al: Radical enlargement of the aortic root and outflow tract to allow valve replacement. Ann. Thorac. Surg., 27:367, 1979.

Riverius, L.: Observations medical et curatives insignes, quebus accesserunt observations an Alles Communicatae. London, M. Flesher, 1646.

Roberts, W. C.: The congenitally bicuspid aortic valve: A study of 85 autopsy cases. Am. J. Cardiol., 26:72, 1970.

Robicsek, F., Sanger, P. W., Daugherty, H. K., and Montgomery, C. C.: Congenital quadricuspid aortic valve with displacement of the left coronary orifice. Am. J. Cardiol., 23:288, 1969.

Sade, R. M., Ballenger, J. F., Hohn, A. R., et al: Cardiac valve replacement in children: Comparison of tissue with mechanical prostheses. J. Thorac. Cardiovasc. Surg., 78:123, 1979.

Schaffer, M. S., Campbell, D. N., Clarke, D. R., et al: Aortoventriculoplasty in children. J. Thorac. Cardiovasc. Surg., 92:391, 1986.

Shone, J. D., Sellars, R. D., Anderson, R. C., et al: The developmental complex of "parachute mitral valve," supravalvular ring of left atrium, subaortic stenosis, and coarctation of aorta. Am. J. Cardiol., 11:715, 1963.

Sink, J. D., Smallhorn, J. F., Macartney, F. J., et al: Management of critical aortic stenosis in infancy. J. Thorac. Cardiovasc. Surg., 87:82, 1984.

Sissman, N. J., Neill, C. A., Spencer, F. C., and Taussig, H. B.: Congenital aortic stenosis. Circulation, 19:458, 1959.

Somerville, J., and Ross, D.: Homograft replacement of aortic root with reimplantation of coronary arteries: Results after 1–5 years. Br. Heart J., 47:473, 1982.

Spann, J. F., Bove, A. A., Natarajan G., et al: Ventricular performance, pump function and compensatory mechanisms in patients with aortic stenosis. Circulation, 62:576, 1980.

Spencer, F. C., Neill, C. A., and Bahnson, H. T.: The treatment of congenital aortic stenosis with valvotomy during cardiopulmonary bypass. Surgery, 44:109, 1958.

Spencer, F. C., Neill, C. A., Sank, L., and Bahnson, H. T.: Anatomical variations in 46 patients with congenital aortic stenosis. Am. Surg., 26:204, 1960.

Stewart, J. R., Paton, B. C., Blount, S. G., et al: Congenital aortic stenosis: Ten to 22 years after valvulotomy. Arch. Surg., 113:1248, 1978.

Stewart, S., Cianciotta, D., Alexson, C., and Manning, J.: The long-term risk of warfarin sodium therapy and the incidence of thromboembolism in children after prosthetic cardiac valve replacement. J. Thorac. Cardiovasc. Surg., 93:551, 1987.

Sud, A., Parker, F., and Magilligan, D. J., Jr.: Anatomy of the aortic root. Ann. Thorac. Surg., 38:76, 1984.

Swan, H., and Kortz, A. B.: Direct vision trans-aortic approach to the aortic valve during hypothermia: Experimental observations and report of successful clinical case. Ann. Surg., 144:205, 1956.

Thandroyen, F. T., Witthon, I. N., Pirie, D., et al: Severe calcification of glutaraldehyde preserved porcine xenografts in children. Am. J. Cardiol., 45:690, 1980.

Thursfield, H., and Scott, H. W.: Sub-aortic stenosis. Br. J. Child. Dis., 10:104, 1913.

Trinkle, J. K., Norton, J. B., Richardson, J. D., et al: Closed aortic valvotomy and simultaneous correction of associated anomalies in infants. J. Thorac. Cardiovasc. Surg., 69:758, 1975.

Tuffier, T.: État actuel de la chirurgie intrathoracique. Trans. Int. Cong. Med., London, 1914.

Ungerleider, R. M., and Ebert, P. A.: Indications and techniques for midline approach to aortic coarctation in infants and children. Ann. Thorac. Surg., 44:517, 1987.

Ungerleider, R. M., Greeley, W. J., Sheikh, K. H., et al: The use of intraoperative echo with Doppler color flow imaging to predict outcomes following repair of congenital cardiac defects. Ann. Surg., (in press).

Verrier, E. D., Tranbaugh, R. F., Soifer, S. J., et al: Aspirin anticoagulation in children with mechanical aortic valves. J. Thorac. Cardiovasc. Surg., 92:1013, 1986.

Walls, J. T., Lababidi, Z., Curtis, J. J., and Silver, D.: Assessment of percutaneous balloon pulmonary and aortic valvuloplasty. J. Thorac. Cardiovasc. Surg., 88:352, 1984.

Williams, D. B., Danielson, G. K., McGoon, D. C., et al: Porcine heterograft valve replacement in children. J. Thorac. Cardiovasc. Surg., 84:446, 1982.

Williams, J. C. P., Barratt-Boyes, B. G., and Lowe, J. B.: Supravalvular aortic stenosis. Circulation, 24:1311, 1961.

Wright, P. W., and Wittner, R. S.: Obstruction of the left ventricular outflow tract by the mitral valve due to a muscle band. J. Thorac. Cardiovasc. Surg., 85:938, 1983.

CHAPTER 42

CONGENITAL MALFORMATIONS OF THE MITRAL VALVE

Eli Milgalter
Hillel Laks

Congenital anomalies of the mitral valve are rare, occurring in 0.6% of autopsied patients with congenital heart disease and in 0.21 to 0.42% of clinical series (Baker et al, 1962; Collins-Nakai et al, 1977). They can occur as part of other more complex congenital cardiac malformations such as atrioventricular (AV) canal, univentricular heart, hypoplastic left heart syndrome, coronary artery anomalies, endocardial fibroelastosis, or corrected (L) transposition (Bharati and Lev, 1973). In these situations, the clinical course is usually determined by the major associated cardiac malformation, which is discussed in other chapters of this book. In this chapter congenital mitral deformities that are either *isolated* or associated with *discrete* congenital lesions, such as *coarctation of the aorta, aortic stenosis, patent ductus arteriosus, ventricular septal defect,* or *tetralogy of Fallot,* are reviewed (Bharati and Lev, 1973). The developmental malformation can affect each component of the valve and its supporting structures. The result may be mitral stenosis, incompetence, or a combined lesion. The severity of the clinical presentation depends on the degree of the mitral deformity as well as on the presence of associated anomalies.

HISTORICAL ASPECTS

Early descriptions of congenital mitral valve malformations are recorded as early as 1846 (Smith, 1846). In 1963, Shone described the "Shone heart" (Shone et al, 1963), which included supramitral ring, parachute mitral valve, left ventricular outflow tract obstruction, and coarctation of the aorta. Vlad (1954) and others (Carpentier et al, 1976; Devachi et al, 1971; Ruchman and Van Praagh, 1978) contributed to our understanding of the morphologic spectrum of congenital mitral valve disease.

Reports describing surgical treatment have appeared only in the last three decades. The first successful closed mitral commissurotomy in a child aged 5½ years was reported by Bower in 1952 (Bower and Gerrard, 1953). Starkey, in 1958, described the

treatment of congenital mitral regurgitation by both closed and open methods (Starkey, 1959). Young (1964) reported the first prosthetic mitral valve replacement in a 10-month-old infant. Initially, long-term results of both medical and surgical treatment were poor, as shown by an 18% late survival reported by Collins-Nakai in 1977 (Collins-Nakai et al, 1977). Improved results with surgical treatment were reported by Carpentier and associates who used innovative methods for reconstruction of the mitral valve (Carpentier et al, 1976).

EMBRYOLOGY

The mitral valve is formed from the endocardial cushions and from trabeculations of the primitive left ventricle (Van Mierap, et al, 1962). During the fourth week of embryonic life, the dorsal and ventral endocardial cushions, along with lateral infolds from the adjacent canal wall, partition the AV canal into atria and ventricles. After completion of ventricular and atrial septation during the fifth and sixth weeks, the future mitral and tricuspid valves are separated.

During the sixth and seventh weeks, the mitral leaflets are formed from the endocardial cushions and lateral projection tissue, while at the same time the papillary muscles and chordae are shaped from primitive muscular trabeculations of the left ventricle. Until the 24th week there is a slow process in which the ventricular trabeculations fuse into two distinct papillary muscles. The leaflets and chordae of the valve gradually change their muscular character into a thin delicate collagenous tissue.

SURGICAL ANATOMY

The normal mitral valve is composed of an annulus, two leaflets, two commissures, multiple chordae, and two papillary muscles.

The fibrous annulus separates the left atrium and the left ventricle. Anteriorly, it merges with the

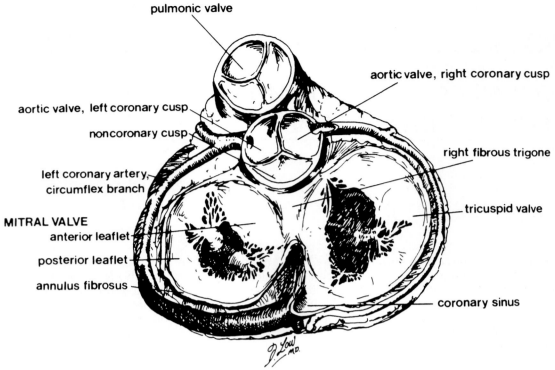

Figure 42–1. Cross-section of the heart showing the anatomic relations of the normal mitral valve. (From Edmunds, L. H., and Wagner, H. R.: Congenital anomalies of the mitral valve. *In* Arciniegas, E. [ed]: Pediatric Cardiac Surgery. Chicago, Year Book Medical Publishers, 1985.)

aortic valve annulus beneath the left and noncoronary aortic valve cusps. Laterally and posteriorly it lies deep in the AV groove, beneath the coronary sinus and the circumflex coronary artery. Medially, it joins the tricuspid valve annulus and the membranous interventricular septum (Fig. 42–1).

The two leaflets are separated by anterolateral and posteromedial commissures (see Fig. 42–1). The anterior leaflet is attached to about 150 degrees of the annulus and is wider than the posterior leaflet that is attached to 210 degrees of the circumference of the annulus and is significantly narrower. The posterior leaflet is often subdivided into a large central scallop and two or more smaller lateral scallops. The leaflets are usually thin and flexible; they have smooth surfaces and a line of coaptation that parallels the posterior part of the annulus and is a few millimeters proximal to the free margin of the leaflets on their left atrial surfaces.

There are three generations of chordae tendineae. The first-order chordae fuse with the free margins of the leaflets. Four to six chordae connect adjacent halves of the two leaflets to a papillary muscle. The second generation of chordae are attached to the undersurface of the leaflets, a few millimeters away from the free margin. The third-order chordae are attached to the leaflets close to the annulus and take their insertion either from the papillary muscle or the left ventricular free wall close to the annulus.

The two papillary muscles are separate structures and are attached at their bases to the ventricular wall. The anterolateral papillary muscle is attached to the lateral wall of the left ventricular wall and supports the anterolateral commissure. Its blood supply originates usually from the left circumflex coronary artery. The posteromedial papillary muscle is attached between the interventricular septum and posterior wall. It supports the posteromedial commissure and is supplied by branches of the posterior descending coronary artery. Each papillary muscle holds chordae connected to the appropriate half of both anterior and posterior leaflets.

During systole, this subvalvular apparatus arrests the upward tension on the leaflets so that the line of coaptation of the two leaflets is parallel to the level of the valve annulus. During diastole the leaflets collapse into the ventricle. The gap between the two leaflets is called the *primary orifice*. In congenital malformations of the mitral valve it is important to recognize the secondary mitral valve orifice that is the sum of the multiple gaps between the chordal network and between the papillary muscles and left ventricular wall.

CLASSIFICATION AND MORPHOLOGY

Early classifications were based on autopsy specimens of congenital mitral stenosis and described four discrete morphologic subtypes (Carpentier et al, 1976; Devachi et al, 1971; Ruckman and Van Praagh, 1978). These studies also reported a high incidence of associated congenital malformations (50 to 96%) that mainly obstructed lesions of the left ventricular outflow tract and the aorta.

Carpentier and colleagues (1976) suggested a more surgically oriented pathophysiologic classification, which was based on a series of 107 autopsy specimens and 70 open heart operations involving congenital mitral valve disease in children. According to this classification, the malformation can involve one or more levels of the mitral valve apparatus: adjacent left atrium (supramitral valve ring), valve annulus, leaflets, commissures, chordae tendineae, papillary muscles, and adjacent left ventricle (fibroelastosis, dilated left ventricle). According to Carpentier, the malformations are first classified with regard to whether there is *mitral valve stenosis* or *incompetence.* Second, the *leaflet motion* may be normal, prolapsed, or restricted. Third, the *papillary muscles* are either normal or abnormal. When there is more than one malformation along the mitral apparatus, the classification should be based on the most severe lesion. This pathophysiologic classification has proved to be an important guideline in the application of techniques of mitral valve reconstruction, the major aim of which is to restore *normal valve function* rather than *normal valve anatomy.* This basic classification and the breakdown of the subtypes in Carpentier's series are summarized in Table 42–1.

Morphology of Congenital Mitral Stenosis

Mitral valve stenosis is divided into two main groups according to the anatomy of the papillary muscles.

Mitral Stenosis with Normal Papillary Muscles

In this group there are four subtypes: commissural fusion, excess valvular tissue, annulus hypoplasia, and supravalvular ring.

Commissural Fusion. The two papillary muscles are fused directly with the leaflets without any chordae, or via thick deformed chordae (Carpentier et al, 1976). There is also fusion of the commissures that leaves a stenotic central orifice between the leaflets. This stenosis is increased further by obstruction of the secondary orifice of the valve by the thick papillary muscles (Fig. 42–2).

Excessive Mitral Valvular Tissue. The major malformation is excessive tissue that bridges and obliterates the interchordal spaces (Carpentier et al, 1976). The leaflets, papillary muscles, and valve motion are normal. A large bridge of valvular tissue sometimes joins the two leaflets, which thus creates a *double-orifice mitral valve* (Fig. 42–3).

TABLE 42–1. PATHOPHYSIOLOGIC CLASSIFICATION OF CONGENITAL MALFORMATIONS OF THE MITRAL VALVE AND BREAKDOWN OF THE DIFFERENT SUBTYPES IN 107 AUTOPSY SPECIMENS AND 70 SURGICAL CASES*

Malformation	Clinical	Autopsy
Mitral Valve Incompetence		
TYPE I: NORMAL LEAFLET MOTION	15	16
1. Isolated annulus dilatation	8	7
2. Cleft leaflet	6	4
a. True cleft leaflet		3
b. Three-leaflet valve		1
3. Leaflet defect	1	1
TYPE II: PROLAPSED LEAFLET	27	17
1. Absent chordae	5	6
2. Elongated chordae	14	11
3. Elongated papillary muscle	8	0
TYPE III: RESTRICTED LEAFLET MOTION	10	51
A. Normal Papillary Muscles		
1. Commissure fusion	2	4
2. Short chordae	1	18
3. Ebstein type mitral valve	0	0
B. Abnormal Papillary Muscles		
1. Parachute valve	2	5
2. Hammock valve	2	5
3. Papillary hypoplasia	3	19
Mitral Stenosis		
TYPE A: NORMAL PAPILLARY MUSCLES	10	18
1. Commissure fusion	7	11
2. Excess valvular tissue	1	2
3. Annulus hypoplasia	0	4
4. Supravalvular ring	2	1
TYPE B: ABNORMAL PAPILLARY MUSCLES	8	5
1. Parachute valve	3	1
2. Hammock valve	5	3
3. Absent papillary muscles	0	1

*From Carpentier, A., Branchini, B., Cour, J. C., et al: Congenital malformations of the mitral valve in children. J. Thorac. Cardiovasc. Surg., 72:854, 1976.

Annulus Hypoplasia. The "normal" size of the mitral valve annulus at different ages was reported by Rowlatt, Rimoldi, and Lev (1963) and is shown in Table 42–2. Hypoplasia of the mitral valve annulus is usually associated with the spectrum of hypoplastic left heart syndrome (Ruckman and Van Praagh, 1978). Rarely, isolated annular hypoplasia occurs (Carpentier et al, 1976). The degree of hypoplasia varies, and the remainder of the mitral valve apparatus and the left ventricle may develop normally.

Supravalvular Ring. In this condition there is a fibrous ring located on the left atrial side of the mitral valve annulus (Fig. 42–4). The size and the degree of obstruction can vary from a mild to a severe form causing pulmonary edema in the first days of life (Shone et al, 1963). It is a different entity from cor triatriatum, where the fibrous diaphragm is closer to the pulmonary veins and lies proximal to the left atrial appendage, and the mitral valve is normal. Although supravalvular ring can occur as an isolated anomaly, more often it coexists with other cardiac anomalies, especially the Shone syndrome, which

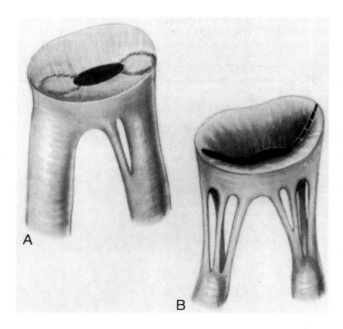

Figure 42–2. Congenital mitral stenosis. *A,* Papillary commissural fusion. Note the insertion of papillary muscles directly onto the fused commissures. *B,* After repair by commissurotomy and papillary splitting. (Reproduced with permission from Stark, J., and de Leval, M. (eds): Surgery for Congenital Heart Defects. Copyright 1983. Reproduced with permission from Grune & Stratton, Orlando, FL.)

includes supramitral ring, parachute mitral valve, left ventricular outflow tract obstructions, and coarctation of the aorta (Shone et al, 1963) (Fig. 42–5).

Mitral Valve Stenosis with Abnormal Papillary Muscles

This group contains three malformations: parachute mitral valve, hammock valve, and absent papillary muscles.

Parachute Mitral Valve. In this condition, all chordae are attached to a single papillary muscle, which is formed either from fusion of the two papillary muscles or from the presence of only one

papillary muscle, with the other being hypoplastic and without chordal connections (Fig. 42–5). The stenosis can be at the leaflet level, but more commonly it is at the secondary orifice of the valve due to obliteration of the interchordal spaces by excessive valve tissue (Shone et al, 1963). The parachute valve can appear as an isolated deformity or as part of the more complex *Shone heart.*

Hammock Mitral Valve. In this malformation the two normal papillary muscles are absent. They are replaced by numerous papillary muscles as well as muscular and fibrous bands, which are inserted high on the posterior wall of the ventricle, just below the mitral valve leaflets. As a result, the secondary orifice

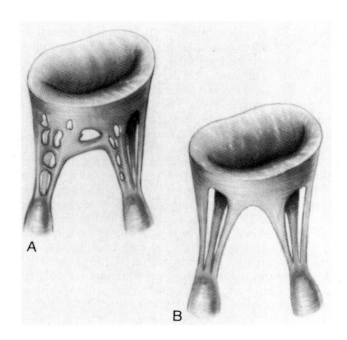

Figure 42–3. Congenital mitral stenosis. *A,* Excess mitral valve tissue. Note the obstruction of secondary orifice. *B,* After repair. (Reproduced with permission from Stark, J., and de Leval, M. (eds): Surgery for Congenital Heart Defects. Copyright 1983. Reproduced with permission from Grune & Stratton, Orlando, FL.)

TABLE 42–2. MEAN NORMAL VALVE DIAMETERS IN CHILDREN*

Body Surface Area (m²)	Mitral (mm)	Tricuspid (mm)	Aortic (mm)	Pulmonary (mm)
0.25	11.2	13.4	7.4	8.4
0.3	12.6	14.9	8.1	9.3
0.35	13.6	16.2	8.9	10.1
0.4	14.4	17.3	9.5	10.7
0.45	15.2	18.2	10.1	11.3
0.5	15.8	19.2	10.7	11.9
0.6	16.9	20.7	11.5	12.8
0.7	17.9	21.9	12.3	13.5
0.8	18.8	23.0	13.0	14.2
0.9	19.7	24.0	13.4	14.8
1.0	20.2	24.9	14.0	15.3
1.2	21.4	26.2	14.8	16.2
1.4	22.3	27.7	15.5	17.0
1.6	23.1	28.9	16.1	17.6
1.8	23.8	29.1	16.5	18.2
2.0	24.2	30.0	17.2	18.0

*Modified from Rowlatt, U. F., Rimoldi, H. J. A., and Lev, M.: The quantitative anatomy of the normal child's heart. Pediatr. Clin. North Am., 10:499, 1963.

The approximate standard deviations (±) are: mitral <0.3 m² = 1.9 mm, >0.3 m² = 1.6 mm; tricuspid <1 m² = 1.7 mm, >1 m² = 1.5 mm.

of the mitral valve is obstructed by the abnormal network of cords. The term *hammock valve* was coined by Carpentier (1976), whereas other physicians have used different terms: mitral arcade, obstructive papillary muscles, and hypertrophied papillary muscles (Castaneda et al, 1969).

Absent Papillary Muscle. In this condition there are no papillary muscles, and the chordae attach to the ventricular wall. There are variable imperforated interchordal spaces.

Morphology of Congenital Mitral Incompetence

Congenital lesions that cause mitral incompetence are divided into three groups according to the valve leaflet motion: normal, prolapsed, or restricted (Carpentier et al, 1976).

Regurgitation with Normal Leaflet Motion

The primary lesion may be dilatation of the annulus, cleft leaflet, or a leaflet defect.

Annulus Dilatation. Congenital primary dilatation of the mitral valve annulus is rare (Carpentier et al, 1976) and is often secondary to left ventricular dilatation. The annulus along most of the anterior leaflet is continuous with the aortic valve annulus and the fibrous trigone, and this protects this part of the mitral annulus from dilatation. The dilatation, therefore, mainly affects the posterior leaflet. An ostium secundum atrial septal defect is associated

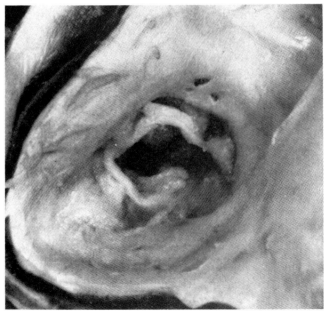

Figure 42–4. Left atrial view of an obstructing supramitral ring. (From Shone, J. D., Sellers, R. D., Anderson, R. C., et al: The developmental complex of "parachute mitral valve," supravalvular ring of left atrium, subaortic stenosis and coarctation of the aorta. Am. J. Cardiol., *11*:714, 1963.)

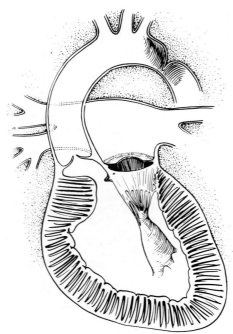

Figure 42–5. Description of the Shone complex: supramitral ring, parachute mitral valve, subaortic stenosis, and coarctation of the aorta. (From Shone, J. D. Sellers, R. D, Anderson, R. C., et al: The developmental complex of "parachute mitral valve," supravalvular ring of left atrium, subaortic stenosis and coarctation of the aorta. Am. J. Cardiol., 11:714, 1963.)

with 50% of the cases of primary annular dilatation of the mitral valve.

Cleft Leaflet. According to Carpentier (1976) two entities may be identified: true cleft versus a three-leaflet mitral valve. With a *true cleft,* the mitral valve is normal except for the cleft that vertically separates the two portions of the anterior leaflet. The two commissures and two papillary muscles are normal. A *three-leaflet mitral valve* is similar to the left-sided AV valve seen in AV canal defects, but there are no septal defects. In this subtype the papillary muscles are displaced laterally, and there is a separate, distinct, third triangular lateral mitral leaflet. The incompetence can start from poor coaptation, as well as from deformation of the annulus.

On rare occasions there are true posterior leaflet clefts, which should not be mistaken for the normal deep indentations that are common between the scallops of the posterior leaflet.

Leaflet Defects. Leaflet defects are holes due to localized agenesis of leaflet tissue, which are seen particularly in the posterior leaflet. In the absence of previous surgical therapy or infections, they are presumed to be congenital malformations.

Congenital Mitral Regurgitation with Prolapsed Leaflets

Prolapse of a leaflet is the condition in which the free margin of a leaflet reaches above the plane of the valve annulus in systole (Carpentier et al,

1976). Therefore, most cases of Barlow's syndrome are excluded.

Lesions that cause prolapse of mitral leaflets include *absent chordae,* where several chordae are missing from a segment of the free margin of a leaflet; *elongated chordae;* or *elongated papillary muscles.* Elongated papillary muscle was described as being a primary condition (Carpentier et al, 1976), which can also be caused by infarction of the papillary muscle in the context of anomalous origin of the left coronary artery from the pulmonary artery.

Congenital Mitral Regurgitation with Restricted Leaflet Motion

Restriction of leaflet motion can prevent coaptation and cause regurgitation. This group is divided further into two subtypes based on the papillary muscles.

Restricted Leaflet Motion with Normal Papillary Muscles. In this group the authors include *commissural fusion* where the commissures are obliterated and the papillary muscles are adherent to the commissures, which together cause central failure of coaptation and therefore regurgitation. In a second entity of *short chordae,* short thick chordae limit leaflet motion and cause regurgitation. There is usually also some stenosis at the secondary orifice of the valve. A third entity in this group is *Ebstein's anomaly* of the mitral valve, which is described by Ruschaupt (Ruschaupt et al, 1976). The major downward displacement is of the posterior leaflet.

Restricted Leaflet Motion with Abnormal Papillary Muscles. Regurgitation through the mitral valve can also be caused by malformations of the papillary muscles, which usually cause stenosis such as occurs in the parachute valve, hammock valve, or agenesis of papillary muscles.

COEXISTING CARDIAC ANOMALIES

Patients with congenital mitral valve disease also have a high incidence of coexisting cardiac anomalies. In the combined Greenlane Hospital and University of Alabama series (Kirklin and Barratt-Boyes, 1986), only 25% of cases had isolated congenital mitral stenosis. In 30% there was also a ventricular septal defect and in 40% there was some form of left ventricular outflow tract obstruction. Carpentier (1976) noted a 60% incidence, and Ruckman and Van Praagh (1978) found a 96% incidence of associated lesions.

These associated malformations are important because they may grow worse, mask, or be masked by the mitral valve anomaly. Therefore, they should be searched for and diagnosed before operation and should be treated at the time of mitral valve repair. In the very young, however, an associated patent ductus arteriosus or coarctation of the aorta may be better treated as a first stage before mitral valve repair (Carpentier et al, 1976).

CLINICAL COURSE

In general, the symptoms and signs are similar to those present in acquired mitral valve disease in older children and adults. The age at presentation and the severity of the disease vary greatly, depending mainly on the severity of the mitral deformity as well as on the severity and nature of coexisting lesions.

Both mitral stenosis and incompetence cause an increase in left artrial pressure and pulmonary arterial pressure. Pulmonary vascular resistance increases, and right ventricular hypertrophy develops. Pulmonary congestion and decreased pulmonary compliance increase the susceptibility to pulmonary infections.

In isolated mitral stenosis, the left ventricle has a normal size, unless other lesions are present, that can cause left ventricular failure and further increase pulmonary congestion. Isolated mitral regurgitation causes left ventricular dilatation as well as pulmonary venous hypertension. Associated obstructive lesions to the left ventricular outflow tract increase the amount of regurgitation.

The symptoms at presentation are usually those of pulmonary venous hypertension, including dyspnea, cough, and orthopnea. Feeding difficulties, failure to thrive, and recurrent pulmonary infection result. Frank pulmonary edema can develop in severe cases. The children usually have sinus tachycardia. In mitral stenosis, the pulmonary second sound increases, and there is a late diastolic murmur with presystolic accentuation at the apex. Compared with acquired mitral stenosis, an opening snap is usually not present in congenital mitral stenosis, which is probably due to the different morphologic features.

Mitral incompetence presents with an overactive precordium due to the left ventricular volume overload, an apical pansystolic murmur, and a third heart sound. If left untreated, right ventricular failure and congestive heart failure develop.

The age at presentation depends on the severity of the mitral valve lesions and coexistent deformities. Generally, mitral incompetence is better tolerated than stenosis and presents at a later age (Carpentier et al, 1976). The age of presentation also varies in medical and surgical series: Van der Horst and Hartreister (1967) reported the onset of symptoms during the first month of life in 33% of their patients and in 75% by 1 year of age. Once symptoms appeared, rapid deterioration followed: The mortality was 50% within 6 months. In the surgical series from Boston Children's Hospital (Collins-Nakai et al, 1977), the mean age at onset of symptoms was 1.6 years. In the University of Alabama series of mitral valve anomalies (Kirklin and Barratt-Boyes, 1986) by 4 years of age, 39% of patients with mitral incompetence,

62% of patients with mitral stenosis, and 86% of patients with coexisting anomalies have had surgical therapy for their anomaly. The mean age at operation in Carpentier's series was 3 years 1 month for mitral stenosis and 6 years 4 months for mitral incompetence (Carpentier et al, 1976).

Electrocardiographically, left atrial enlargement and right ventricular hypertrophy are usually present. In mitral regurgitation or with coexisting left ventricular outflow tract obstruction, signs of left ventricular hypertrophy and dilatation are also present. Compared with acquired mitral valve disease, atrial fibrillation is rare.

The chest film usually shows cardiomegaly that is more pronounced with mitral incompetence. Signs of left atrial enlargement and pulmonary venous hypertension are usually present. Massive enlargement of the left atrium may cause the left lung to collapse. Coexistent cardiac anomalies usually increase the severity of radiographic findings (Fig. 42–6).

Echocardiography has evolved as a most valuable diagnostic technique in the evaluation of congenital mitral valve disease (Celano et al, 1984; Grunadier et al, 1983). It is highly accurate in the delineation of supramitral ring, annulus size, leaflet size and motion, morphology of the papillary muscles, and ventricular function (Fig. 42–7). The severity of mitral regurgitation can be quantified particularly with color flow Doppler. Coexisting lesions can also be identified. Echocardiography has not eliminated the need for cardiac catheterization, which is essential to assess the severity of pulmonary hypertension, valve gradients, and also for the evaluation of coexisting cardiac lesions. Information from both echocardiography and cardiac catheterization is necessary for the accurate diagnosis and treatment of children with congenital mitral valve disease. Although helpful, these studies cannot definitely predict whether a valve can be repaired and this decision must be made intraoperatively.

TREATMENT

Because the repair of a valve is not always possible and replacement may be required, the timing of operation is important. Due to the poor prognosis once severe symptoms develop and the danger of developing irreversible pulmonary hypertension, these patients should be followed closely.

Medical management is based on controlling heart failure and preventing and treating pulmonary infection. Salt restriction, digitalis, and diuretics are effective initially, but once episodes of pulmonary edema occur or signs of severe pulmonary hypertension develop, surgical intervention is usually indicated. Chest films, echocardiography, and repeated cardiac catheterization are necessary to assess the progression of mitral regurgitation and pulmonary hypertension.

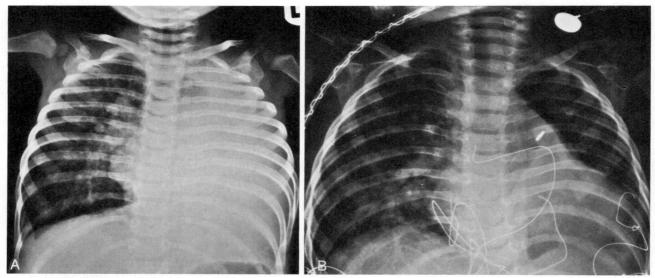

Figure 42–6. *A,* Chest film in a child with mitral incompetence. Left ventricular and left atrial enlargement and pulmonary venous congestion are evident, with atelectasis of the left lung. *B,* After mitral repair and plication of left atrium. Note the re-expansion of the left lung.

Most patients with congenital mitral valve lesions require an operation in infancy or early childhood. It is sometimes advisable to correct an associated extracardiac lesion first, such as patent ductus arteriosus or coarctation of the aorta, in the hope that the child will improve and mitral valve surgical therapy can be delayed. If operation on the mitral valve or associated intracardiac anomalies is indicated, every effort should be made to repair the mitral valve rather than replace it. Repair may result in better left ventricular function due to preservation of the chordal attachments (Carpentier et al, 1976; Kirklin and Barratt-Boyes, 1986). Insertion of a mitral prosthesis in an infant or small child requires reoperation as the child outgrows the prosthesis. Anticoagulation, which is required for a mechanical valve, is difficult to control in children. The porcine bioprostheses, which do not require anticoagulation, have an accelerated rate of calcification and early failure in children. Thus, even a functionally imper-

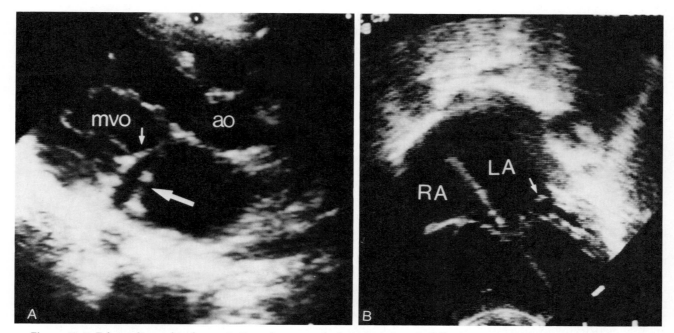

Figure 42–7. Echocardiographic demonstration of a supravalvular mitral ring. *A,* Off-axis parasternal left ventricular long axis. *B,* Apical four-chamber view. (Courtesy of Dr. Tom Santulli, UCLA Medical Center.)

fect mitral valve repair is superior to a prosthesis, as long as the child can grow and does not have severe signs of congestive heart failure or pulmonary hypertension.

SURGICAL TECHNIQUES

Carpentier (1976) has made major contributions to the techniques of mitral valve reconstruction. His pathophysiologic classification has proved to be an important guideline in the application of techniques of valve reconstruction. The main aim is to *restore a functional valve rather than normal mitral valve anatomy.*

Four techniques depend on the mitral abnormality: annuloplasty; leaflet resection and repair; chordal or papillary shortening; and chordal or papillary fenestration or splitting.

Operation is done through a median sternotomy with ascending aorta and bicaval venous cannulation. Carpentier (1976) recommended an evaluation of the valve in a cold, perfused, fibrillating heart, whereas Yacoub and associates (1981) preferred an evaluation of the beating perfused heart with the aorta clamped. The authors prefer the use of cold cardioplegia for both assessment and repair of the valve, which was reported by Kirklin (Kirklin and Barratt-Boyes, 1986).

The morphologic abnormalities of the mitral valve should be assessed in an orderly manner: First, the *left atrium* should be searched for clots, septal defects, or the presence of a supramitral ring. Valve function is then tested by injecting cold saline into the left ventricle and determining whether the valve is stenotic or incompetent, and whether the annulus is dilated, normal, or narrow. Next, assessment of the leaflets and commissures should be made. Leaflet motion should be classified as normal, prolapsed, or restricted, and commissural fusion, clefts, or leaflet defects should be sought. An evaluation of the chordal and papillary muscle anatomy completes the process of valve assessment.

REPAIR OF CONGENITAL MITRAL STENOSIS

As described earlier, there are two major groups according to the papillary muscle pathology.

Normal Papillary Muscles

The condition of *papillary muscle commissural fusion* is treated by commissurotomy, fenestration, and splitting of papillary muscle and resection of secondary chordae (see Figs. 42–2 and 42–3). Good results can often be achieved. With *excessive valve tissue* usually the secondary orifice is affected, and this is treated by chordal fenestration and papillary muscle splitting (see Fig. 42–3). *Isolated annular hypoplasia* is rare. In infancy, there are severe forms of tight isolated annular hypoplasia associated with an adequate sized left ventricle for which valve replacement is difficult. An extra cardiac valved conduit between left atrium and left ventricle has been used in this case (Laks et al, 1980; Mazzer et al, 1988). A supraannular ring is treated by resection and care is taken to avoid injury to the mitral valve and to exclude additional mitral deformities.

Abnormal Papillary Muscles

Mitral stenosis may be due to *parachute* or *hammock valves,* or *absent papillary muscles.* In *parachute valve,* the main obstruction is at the secondary orifice, which is treated by splitting of the papillary muscles and fenestration of the interchordal spaces. Again, a thorough search for additional anomalies of the mitral valve and left ventricular outflow tract should be made. In *hammock valve* severe obstruction of the secondary mitral valve orifice is the main lesion, which is caused by the numerous abnormal papillary muscles and bands, some of which cross from the anterior leaflet to insert onto the posterior wall of the left ventricle, immediately below the posterior mitral leaflet. Repair is difficult and is based on resection of all the chordae, papillary muscles, and bands that are not attached to the free leaflet margins. Valve replacement is frequently necessary. An incomplete repair and the frequent need for valve replacement also pertains to the rare condition of *absent papillary muscle.*

SURGICAL THERAPY FOR CONGENITAL MITRAL INCOMPETENCE

Severe heart failure and cardiomegaly, recurrent pulmonary infection, pulmonary edema, or signs of pulmonary hypertension are indications for surgical intervention. As classified earlier, mitral incompetence is subdivided into three groups according to leaflet motion.

Normal Leaflet Motion

Annular dilatation affects primarily the posterior leaflet annulus and can usually be repaired. These children usually come to operation after 5 to 6 years of age and have severe cardiomegaly. In children under 10 years of age or in those with a small annulus, it is preferable to avoid a mitral valve prosthetic ring because its insertion at an early age might lead to stenosis later in life. Other techniques of mitral annuloplasty may be used, such as the *DeVega's annuloplasty* (1977). Resection of part of the posterior leaflet with *annulus and leaflet plication* may be done. Up to one-half of the mural leaflet can be resected. Wooler's annuloplasty uses one or more heavy sutures anchored by pledgets at each commissure to plicate the adjacent annulus of the posterior leaflet (Wooler et al, 1962).

True cleft anterior leaflet is repaired by resection of abnormal chordal attachments to the free margins of the cleft, followed by closure of the cleft by several interrupted sutures. If the edges at the cleft are severely rolled and retracted, a pericardial patch reconstruction has been described to fill the gap between the leaflets and to achieve good coaptation (Carpentier et al, 1976). A Carpentier ring is often added to support the annulus.

A three-leaflet mitral valve (AV canal type in the absence of septal defects) is more difficult to repair. Compared with the true cleft where the basic mitral anatomy is normal, in a three-leaflet mitral valve the papillary muscles are displaced and there is a third, triangular lateral mitral leaflet and three commissures. If the third leaflet is large, suture of the cleft may be possible without causing mitral stenosis. An annuloplasty at the commissures may also be required to achieve a competent mitral valve. *True cleft posterior cleft* can usually be treated by suture of the cleft and plication of the annulus. *Leaflet defects* are more common in the posterior leaflet where they are treated by quadrangular resection and plication of the annulus. Anterior leaflet defects are repaired by direct sutures or pericardial patch repair.

Prolapsed Leaflet

Absent or ruptured chordae to the free margin of the posterior leaflet can be treated by one or more quadrangular resections of segments of the posterior leaflet and plication of the annulus. Resection cannot always be done on the anterior leaflet. Carpentier (1976) has suggested innovative techniques of reattaching secondary chordae or transferring posterior leaflet chordae to the anterior leaflet to achieve repair. Attempts to replace the missing chordae by pericardial strips failed (Carpentier et al, 1976). *Anterior leaflet chordal elongation* causing leaflet prolapse is treated by chordal shortening achieved by anchoring the proximal edge of the chordae to the depth of a groove made at the base of the corresponding papillary muscle (Carpentier et al, 1976). Elongation of posterior leaflet chordae is treated by either shortening or leaflet resection and plication of the annulus. The same principle is applied to *papillary muscle elongation,* which causes leaflet prolapse. The papillary muscle is buried in a trench created in the adjacent left ventricular wall (Carpentier et al, 1976).

Restricted Leaflet Motion

The papillary muscles are first evaluated. *With normal papillary muscles* the restricted motion results from *commissure fusion, short chordae* or, rarely, *Ebstein's anomaly* of the mitral valve. Repair can be achieved by combination of commissurotomy, papillary muscle splitting and fenestration, resection of secondary chordae, and remodeling of the annulus. Ebstein's anomaly of the mitral valve is rare and almost always requires mitral valve replacement.

When restricted leaflet motion is caused by *abnormal papillary muscles* (parachute, hammock, or papillary muscle agenesis), the lesions are usually complex, involving all levels of the mitral apparatus, and are often associated with stenosis of the valve, and additional lesions. Thus, repair is difficult, and often only some degree of palliation can be achieved initially to be followed by repair or usually replacement of the valve later in life (Carpentier et al, 1976). Slightly better results can be obtained with the parachute variety.

After completion of the valve repair, valve function is assessed by injecting cold saline into the cavity of the left ventricle by using a bulb syringe while applying suction on the aortic root vent to prevent air emboli. The repair is considered to be acceptable when the line of coaptation of the two leaflets is parallel to the annulus supporting the posterior leaflet and when there is a good line of coaptation of the two leaflets. Small leaks are acceptable and a mild degree of stenosis at the completion of the repair is also a common result that should still be accepted and is to be preferred over valve replacement in the very young (Carpentier et al, 1976).

After discontinuing cardiopulmonary bypass and before closing the chest, intraoperative echocardiography, preferably with color flow Doppler, is helpful in assessing mitral valve function.

Mitral valve replacement is done only when repair is impossible or has failed and the child is either symptomatic or has evidence of increased ventricular dysfunction or pulmonary hypertension. The largest possible low-profile prosthetic valve should be inserted; the authors prefer the St. Jude's valve (Kirklin and Barratt-Boyes, 1986), with its favorable annulus-to-orifice ratio and its low profile. Other valves with a higher profile may have their excursion affected by a small left ventricle or may cause obstruction of the left ventricular outflow tract (Kirklin and Barratt-Boyes, 1986). Placement of the prosthesis in the supra-annular position may be necessary in the presence of a small annulus. Although there are reports of the use of mechanical valves without anticoagulation (Pass et al, 1984), extended follow-up has shown significant thromboembolism. Coumadin anticoagulation is recommended for all mechanical valves in the mitral position in children (Edmunds and Wagner, 1985). Currently available bioprostheses should not be used in children because of the early accelerated fibrocalcification necessitating valve re-replacement in 50% of the children within 3 to 5 years.

In addition to either repair or replacement, there are few other therapeutic measures that can be added to the treatment of congenital mitral valve disease in infancy. Alday and Juaneda (1987) and Kveselis and associates (1986) reported successful percutaneous balloon dilatation for congenital mitral stenosis in infants. The valve area could be doubled in some patients. This modality is suitable only for isolated cases of commissural stenosis and cannot be used for most other lesions. Laks and associates (1980) and others (Lansing et al, 1983; Mazzer et al, 1988; Midgley et al, 1985) described left atrial to left ventricle external bypass by using a valved conduit, which might be the only surgical option in infants with a hypoplastic mitral valve and an adequate-sized left ventricle. Late follow-up on these case reports is *not* available.

It is worthwhile to reduce the size of the left atrium by free wall excision anterior to the right pulmonary veins along with longitudinal plication or excision of the posterior atrial wall midway between the right and left pulmonary veins (Kawazoe et al, 1983). Reduction in size of a giant left atrium helps to reduce bronchial compression and prevents pulmonary problems in the early postoperative period (see Fig. 42–6).

POSTOPERATIVE COURSE AND RESULTS

Early postoperative complications include low cardiac output, neurologic sequelae from intraoperative air emboli, bleeding, arrhythmias, pulmonary failure, and infection. Low cardiac output is frequent. Contributing factors are long-standing preoperative left ventricular dysfunction, high pulmonary resistance, and an incomplete valve repair. Therefore left and right atrial pressure monitoring and frequent echocardiographic assessment of ventricular function and adequacy of the repair or prosthesis function are necessary. These children usually need careful vol-

ume replacement and inotropic support in the first several days postoperatively, and often afterload reducing agents are beneficial.

The overall hospital mortality was higher than 50% in the early era of open heart procedures and is still high. Kirklin reported a 21% early mortality (Kirklin and Barratt-Boyes, 1986). Collins-Nakai reported 38% mortality (Collins-Nakai et al, 1977), whereas Carpentier reported 13% (Carpentier et al, 1976). Almost all deaths occur from sequelae of low cardiac output and pulmonary hypertension.

According to Kirklin, (Kirklin and Barratt-Boyes, 1986), incremental risk factors for hospital deaths were *young age at operation, functional status* of the child before operation, and the presence of *major associated cardiac anomalies.* The nature of the lesion (stenosis versus incompetence) or whether repair or replacement were done *did not* influence the results. Edmunds (Edmunds and Wagner, 1985) found better results in operations for mitral regurgitation than for mitral stenosis.

Long-term results are better for mitral valve repair. Kirklin and Barratt-Boyes (1986) reported a 63% 10-year survival for mitral repairs compared with a 30% 10-year survival for patients having replacement. Most survivors enjoy improved functional capacity; the majority were functional status I of II (Edmunds and Wagner, 1985). However, residual mitral stenosis or regurgitation is present in most patients and can progress. Therefore, patients should be followed closely late after operation. Collins-Nakai and associates (1977) showed that reduction of pulmonary hypertension was a critical factor in the long-term prognosis of these children and that late deaths occurred primarily in those with unsatisfactory repair and persistent or recurrent pulmonary hypertension. Active follow-up and reoperation when indicated might improve the long-term prognosis of this group

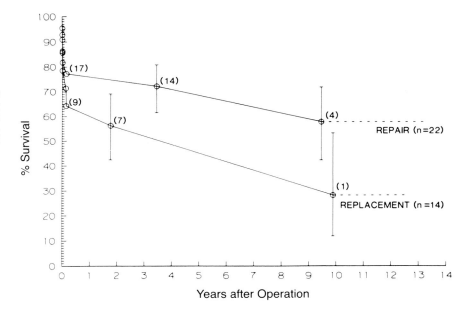

Figure 42–8. Actuarial survival after initial valve repair versus replacement for congenital mitral valve disease. (From Kirklin, J. W., Barratt-Boyes, B. G.: Cardiac Surgery. New York, John Wiley and Sons, Copyright 1986, pp. 1091–1106.)

(Kirkland and Barratt-Boyes, 1986). Of patients having repair 75% are *free* of reoperation at 10 years postoperatively, which indicates good overall results with repair despite the fact that in most patients some degree of stenosis or incompetence can be found (Fig. 42–8).

Reoperation after prosthetic mitral valve replacement is almost the rule, except for older children with cardiomegaly in whom an adult's size of prosthesis may be inserted initially. Sade and associates (1979) estimated that in children who had mitral valve replacement before 4 years of age, a second operation would be needed as they increased their weight by two-and-a-half to three times. The risk for late complications from the prosthesis is similar to that for adults (e.g., sudden death, thromboemboli, bleeding from anticoagulation, prosthetic endocarditis).

With improved understanding of the pathologic anatomy and with further experience, it is hoped that mitral valve repair will replace valve replacement in an increasing number of patients. This would justify operation at an earlier age to avoid the pulmonary hypertension and left ventricular dysfunction that may occur when surgical therapy is excessively delayed.

Bibliography

Alday, L. E., and Juaneda, E.: Percutaneous balloon dilatation in congenital mitral stenosis. Br. Heart J., *57*:479, 1987.

Baker, C. G., Benson, P. F., Joseph, M. C., et al: Congenital mitral stenosis. Br. Heart J., *24*:498, 1962.

Bharati, S., and Lev, M.: Congenital polyvalvar disease. Circulation, *49*:575, 1973.

Bower, B. D., and Gerrard, J. W.: Two cases of congenital mitral stenosis treated by valvotomy. Arch. Dis. Child., *28*:91, 1953.

Carpentier, A., Branchini, B., Cour, J. C., et al: Congenital malformations of the mitral valve in children. J. Thorac. Cardiovasc. Surg., *72*:854, 1976.

Castaneda, A. R., Anderson, R. C., and Edwards, J. E.: Congenital mitral stenosis resulting from anomalous arcade and obstructing papillary muscles. Am. J. Cardiol., *24*:237, 1969.

Celano, V., Pieroni, D. R., Morera, J. A., et al: 2D echocardiographic examination of mitral valve abnormalities associated with coarctation of the aorta. Circulation, *69*:924, 1984.

Collins-Nakai, R. L., Rosenthal, A., Castaneda, A. R., et al: Congenital mitral stenosis—a review of 20 years' experience. Circulation, *56*:1039, 1977.

Devachi, F., Moller, J. H., and Edwards, J. E.: Diseases of the mitral valve in infancy. Circulation, *43*:565, 1971.

DeVega, N. G.: La annuloplastica selectiva. Rev. Esp. Cardiol., *25*:555, 1977.

Edmunds, L. H., and Wagner, H. R.: Congenital anomalies of the mitral valve. *In* Arciniegas, E. (ed): Pediatric Cardiac Surgery. Chicago, Year Book Medical Publishers, 1985.

Grunadier, E., Sahn, D. J., Valdes-Crus, L. M., et al: Two-dimensional echo Doppler study of congenital disorders of the mitral valve. J. Am. Coll. Cardiol., *1*:873, 1983.

Kawazoe, K., Beppu, S., Takahara, Y., et al: Surgical treatment of giant left atrium combined with mitral valve disease. J. Thorac. Cardiovasc. Surg., *85*:885, 1983.

Kirklin, J. W., and Barratt-Boyes, B. G.: Cardiac Surgery, New York, John Wiley and Sons, 1986, pp. 1091–1106.

Kveselis, D. A., Rocchini, A. P., Beekman, R., et al: Balloon dilatation for congenital and rheumatic mitral stenosis. Am. J. Cardiol., *57*:348, 1986.

Laks, H., Hellenbrand, W. E., Kleinman, C., and Talner, N. S.: Left atrial to left ventricular conduit for relief of congenital mitral stenosis in infancy. J. Thorac. Cardiovasc. Surg., *80*:782, 1980.

Lansing, A. M., Elbe, F., and Solinger, R. E.: Left atrial to left ventricular bypass for congenital mitral stenosis. Ann. Thorac. Surg., *35*:667, 1983.

Mazzer, E., Corno, A., Didonato, J., et al: Surgical bypass of the systemic A-V valve in children by means of a valved conduit. J. Thorac. Cardiovasc. Surg., *96*:321, 1988.

Midgley, F. M., Perry, L. W., and Potter, B. M.: Conduit bypass of the mitral valve. Am. J. Cardiol., *56*:493, 1985.

Pass, H. I., Sade, R. M., Crawford, F. A., and Holm, A. R.: Cardiac valve prosthesis in children without anticoagulation. J. Thorac. Cardiovasc. Surg., *87*:832, 1984.

Rowlatt, U. F., Rimoldi, H. J. A., and Lev, M.: The quantitative anatomy of the normal child's heart. Pediatr. Clin. North Am., *10*:499, 1963.

Ruckman, R. N., and Van Praagh, R.: Anatomic types of congenital mitral stenosis; report on 49 autopsy cases. Am. J. Cardiol., *42*:592, 1978.

Ruschaupt, D. G., Bharati, S., and Lev, M.: Mitral valve malformations of Ebstein's type in the absence of corrected transposition. Am. J. Cardiol., *38*:109, 1976.

Sade, R. M., Ballenger, J. F., Hohn, A. R., et al: Cardiac valve replacement in children. J. Thorac. Cardiovasc. Surg., *78*:123, 1979.

Shone, J. D., Sellers, R. D., Anderson, R. D., et al: The developmental complex of "parachute mitral valve," supravalvular ring of left atrium, subaortic stenosis and coarctation of the aorta. Am. J. Cardiol., *11*:714, 1963.

Smith, E.: Premature occlusion of the foramen ovale, large pulmonary artery, and contracted left heart. Trans. Pathol. Soc. London, *1*:52, 1846. (Cited by Ferencz, C., et al: Congenital mitral stenosis. Circulation, *9*:161, 1954.)

Starkey, G. W. B.: Surgical experience in the treatment of congenital mitral stenosis and insufficiency. J. Thorac. Cardiovasc. Surg., *38*:336, 1959.

Van der Horst, R. L., and Hartreister, A. R.: Congenital mitral stenosis. Am. J. Cardiol., *20*:773, 1967.

Van Mierap, L. H. S., Alley, R. D., Kaasel, H. W., et al: The anatomy and embryology of endocardial cushion defects. J. Thorac. Cardiovasc. Surg., *43*:71, 1962.

Vlad, P.: Mitral valve anomalies in children. Circulation, *9*:161, 1954.

Wooler, G. H., Nixon, P. G. F., and Grimshaw, V. A.: Experience with the repair of the mitral valve in mitral incompetence. Thorax, *17*:49, 1962.

Yacoub, M., Halin, M., Radley Smith, R., et al: Surgical treatment of mitral regurgitation. Circulation, *64*:II-210, 1981.

Young, D., and Robinson, G.: Successful valve replacement in an infant with congenital mitral stenosis. N. Engl. J. Med., *270*:660, 1964.

CHAPTER 43

TRANSPOSITION OF THE GREAT ARTERIES

I THE MUSTARD PROCEDURE

George A. Trusler
Robert M. Freedom

Transposition of the great arteries (TGA) is a severe cardiac malformation in which the aorta arises from the right ventricle and the pulmonary artery arises from the left ventricle. The physiologic effects are acute, and cyanosis and distress are usually obvious soon after birth. Survival depends on the mixing of blood between pulmonary and systemic circulations, mainly through a patent foramen ovale, and with the assistance of a patent ductus arteriosus (PDA) and sometimes a coexistent ventricular septal defect (VSD). If left untreated, many infants die in the first week of life, and most die by 1 year of age. Survival is extended by procedures that increase mixing, mainly by enlarging the atrioseptal communication.

Although TGA was considered for many years to be lethal and uncorrectable, methods of repair were developed gradually. Once these techniques were widely available, there was a great upsurge in interest, study, and knowledge of TGA in both its simple and complex forms.

HISTORICAL ASPECTS

In 1797, Matthew Baillie first described the pathologic anatomy of TGA. The first palliative operation, an ingenious closed technique for creating an atrial septal defect (ASD), was done by Blalock and Hanlon in 1948. Lillehei and Varco (1953) tried to transfer the inferior vena cava to the left atrium and the right pulmonary veins to the right atrium. In 1956, Baffes described a palliative procedure, which was a partial repair, that consisted of suturing the right pulmonary veins to the right atrium and connecting the inferior vena cava to the left atrium with a graft. For some years, this procedure provided effective palliation for many children.

The first attempts at repair of TGA were directed toward the great arteries. In 1954, Mustard and associates described a technique for switching the arteries plus one coronary artery. They were unsuccessful, as were Bailey and co-workers (1954), Bjork and Bouckaert (1954), Kay and Cross (1955), Senning (1959), Idriss and colleagues (1961), and Baffes and associates (1961). It was not until 1975 that the first successful arterial repair was reported by Jatene and co-workers (1975, 1976). This encouraged other surgeons to attempt this operation, but the mortality was high. It is only in the last few years that the risk of arterial repair has improved, owing to better selection and management of patients.

A technique for complete repair by rearranging venous inflow at the atrial level was first suggested by Albert (1955), who later attempted an intra-arterial repair with a patch of plastic material. Later trials by Merendino and colleagues (1957), Kay and Cross (1955, 1957), Creech and associates (1958), and Wilson and associates (1962) using various materials were all unsuccessful. The first successful intra-atrial repair was done by Senning in 1959 with a clever but complicated procedure involving flaps of atrial wall and septum. Kirklin and colleagues (1961) used Senning's technique with success, but the mortality was high. In 1961, Barnard and co-workers did a successful intra-atrial repair by using a large crimped tube made of Teflon to connect the pulmonary veins to the tricuspid valve. In 1963 Mustard applied Albert's principle by using a patch or baffle of pericardium to partition the atria and redirect venous inflow to match the transposed arteries. This operation was not only relatively simple but could be reproduced safely; its success stimulated an immediate and widespread awakening of interest in the repair of TGA.

Other historical highlights include the development of Rastelli's procedure in 1969 for TGA with VSD and pulmonary stenosis and of intraventricular repair by McGoon in 1972 for patients with large and suitably positioned VSDs.

PATHOLOGIC ANATOMY

TGA refers to that condition in which the aorta originates from the morphologic right ventricle and the pulmonary artery is supported by the morphologic left ventricle. When complete TGA is present, the atrioventricular connections are concordant; that is, the morphologic right atrium connects with the morphologic right ventricle and the left atrium connects with the morphologic left ventricle. This definition of "transposition" excludes the concept of spatial relationships between the two great arteries because they vary so much and, by using a "connections" approach, is independent of infundibular anatomy.

Complete TGA can occur in hearts with dextrocardia or mesocardia, but the authors' experience indicates that levocardia is evident in more than 95% of patients. Similarly, more than 95% of patients with complete transposition show visceroatrial situs solitus, and only a few patients show visceroatrial situs inversus. A few patients with isomeric left atria, but with the right-sided atrium receiving the entire systemic venous return and the left-sided atrium receiving the pulmonary venous connections, have been identified. In this situation, the presence of normal or noninverted ventricles and discordant ventriculoarterial connections will result in the physiology of complete TGA. Among most patients with complete TGA and visceroatrial situs solitus, the ventricular relationship is that of a noninverted pattern—the so-called d-loop or "right-hand" pattern. In this pattern, the inlet-apical trabecular-outlet axis of the morphologic right ventricle is from right to left, and the outlet or infundibular component of the right ventricle is to the left of the inlet zone. With rare exceptions, the presence of concordant atrioventricular connections implies a d-ventricular loop. Hearts with superoinferior ventricles or cross-atrioventricular connections can have discordant ventriculoarterial connections (Freedom et al, 1978). Approximately 70% of patients with complete TGA have an intact ventricular septum, absence of left ventricular outflow tract obstruction (LVOTO), a small and inadequate interatrial communication, and a small PDA.

The morphology of the ventricular mass in hearts with TGA differs considerably from the normal heart (Smith et al, 1986). In hearts with transposition, the ventricular septum is a straight structure, and thus the ventricles have a side-by-side relationship. The entire atrioventricular septal area is reduced in size, and there is less wedging of the pulmonary outflow tract between the atrioventricular valves than in the deeply wedged aortic valve in the normal heart. Significant anomalies of the tricuspid valve and in the structure of the trabecula septomarginalis were observed in hearts with simple TGA. In addition, the inlet-outlet dimensions of the right ventricle in hearts with transposition are abnormal when compared with the normal heart, and the outlet-inlet ratio is increased.

Major Anomalies Associated with Transposition

The most common associated anomalies among patients with complete TGA include VSD or LVOTO (Rowe et al, 1981). VSDs can occur in any portion of the ventricular septum and may occur as a single defect or may be multiple defects. By using a tripartite schema of the ventricular septum, which was advocated by Soto and associates (1980), the septum can be seen as having an inlet component, an apical trabecular component, and an infundibular or subarterial component. In most patients, the VSD involves either the infundibular septum or the perimembranous septum (Oppenheimer-Dekker, 1978). As might be anticipated, a defect of one zone may be confluent with that of another zone. The infundibular (or subarterial) VSD can result from an isolated defect or deficiency of the infundibular septum (analogous to the isolated supracristal VSD in the otherwise normal heart), or it can result from a malalignment between the infundibular septum (the portion of interventricular septum that separates the aorta from the pulmonary artery) and the trabecula septomarginalis. When a malalignment defect is present, the infundibular septum is almost always deviated posteriorly, encroaching on the left ventricular outflow tract and resulting in a muscular subpulmonary stenosis. Anterosuperior deviation of the infundibular septum is infrequently identified in these patients. This deviation encroaches on the right ventricular subaortic outflow tract and may be seen in the patient with complete TGA, VSD, and an obstructive anomaly of the aortic arch. The complete form of atrioventricular defect rarely occurs in the patient with complete TGA, but it is identified more frequently in the patient with isomeric right or left atria and thus an ambiguous atrioventricular connection. The isolated defect of the inlet component of the ventricular septum is also uncommon. This defect can be accompanied by straddling of the tricuspid valve.

Moene and colleagues (1985, 1986) have characterized the VSD in 50 hearts with TGA and have compared these findings with 105 hearts with VSD and normally connected great arteries. The most common forms of VSD found in the normally connected group, the central muscular VSD, the perimembranous VSD with left-sided malalignment of the outlet septum, and perimembranous VSD with overriding posterior artery, were not found in hearts with VSD and transposition.

Chiu and colleagues (1984) have reviewed morphologic features of an intact ventricular septum that are susceptible to subpulmonary obstruction in complete transposition. This autopsy study focused on the "bulging" or "nonbulging" of the ventricular septum. A fibrous ridge was observed on the ventricular septum in 82% of those with the bulging ventricular septum, but no fibrous ridge was noted in those without a bulging ventricular septum. These authors suggest that the subpulmonary outflow tract is more susceptible to obstruction if the aorta lies more anterior and to the left of the pulmonary trunk rather than side-by-side and to the left.

It is difficult to consider the morphologic basis of LVOTO without first considering the basic pattern of infundibular anatomy among patients with complete TGA. Approximately 95% of patients have a subaortic infundibulum; thus, the aortic valve is separated from the tricuspid valve, whereas the pulmonary and mitral valves are in fibrous continuity. Approximately 4% of patients have bilateral muscular infundibula with neither semilunar valve in fibrous continuity with the atrioventricular valve. A rare patient will have bilaterally deficient infundibula, with both semilunar valves in continuity with the atrioventricular valves (Van Praagh et al, 1980).

LVOTO can result from one or more pathologic mechanisms (Aziz et al, 1979; Idriss et al, 1977; Jiminez and Martinez, 1974; Sansa et al, 1979; Shrivastave et al, 1976; Van Gils, 1978; Van Gils et al, 1978). These mechanisms include (1) posterior malalignment of the infundibular septum; (2) fibrous subpulmonary membrane; (3) accessory tissue tags, often pendunculated and mobile, originating from an atrioventricular valve and contiguous structures; (4) a muscular or tunnel form of subpulmonary obstruction; (5) aneurysm of the membranous or perimembranous interventricular septum; (6) straddling atrioventricular valve tissue; (7) pulmonary valve stenosis; (8) maladherent anterior leaflet of the mitral valve; (9) dynamic subvalvular obstruction due to posterior systolic bulging of the ventricular septum; or (10) combinations of these mechanisms. The most common mechanism results from the left-sided and posterior deviation of a malaligned infundibular septum (Van Gils et al, 1978), which is consistent with the observation that most of the patients with LVOTO complicating complete TGA have an associated VSD.

The spatial relationships between the great arteries at semilunar level in hearts with atrioventricular concordance and ventriculoarterial discordance vary, and, at least in part, the relative positions of the great arteries are predicated on the infundibular anatomy. The most common relationship is the location of the aorta to the right of and anterior to the pulmonary valve, but side-by-side, left-anterior, right-anterior, and left-posterior relationships have all been described. Thus, "transposition" should *not* be defined in terms of the relative position of the great arteries, but should be seen instead in terms of the ventriculoarterial connection.

Less Common Anomalies Associated with Transposition

Left juxtaposition of the right atrial appendage (Rosenquist et al, 1974) has been identified in approximately 1 to 2% of the authors' patients with complete transposition. These patients have had dextrocardia or mesocardia and often have an unusual spatial ventricular relationship. Almost any anomaly of the atrioventricular valve can complicate complete transposition (Layman and Edwards, 1967). Straddling of the tricuspid valve can be identified in some patients. It is particularly important to exclude an abnormality of the right atrioventricular junction in the patient with right ventricular hypoplasia (Riemenschneider et al, 1968). Structural anomalies of the mitral valve are not uncommon in patients with complete transposition (Rosenquist et al, 1975), but, fortunately, functional disturbances appear to be less frequent. Thus, although mitral stenosis or straddling of the anterior leaflet of the mitral valve has been recorded, these cases are uncommon. Tricuspid atresia may be more common than mitral atresia.

Huhta and colleagues from the Mayo clinic (1982) addressed structural anomalies of the tricuspid valve and identified these anomalies in 38 of 121 autopsied specimens. In addition to straddling and overriding of the tricuspid valve, abnormal chordal insertions were found in many cases. These abnormal chordal insertions to the infundibular septum could compromise the potential for the Rastelli operation and others.

Obstructive anomalies of the aortic arch, including coarctation, atresia, and complete interruption of the aortic arch, have been identified in approximately 6% of the authors' patients. Although severe coarctation can be found when the ventricular septum is intact and when the right ventricle is of normal size, these aortic arch anomalies are more frequently identified when a VSD is present or when the morphologic right ventricle is underdeveloped. Finally, aortic valve atresia can rarely complicate the condition of the patient with complete TGA and an intact ventricular septum (McGarry et al, 1980).

Thirty-two patients with complete TGA and coarctation of the aorta have been identified at this institution between 1963 and 1983 (Vogel et al, 1984 a and b). More than two-thirds of the patients had an associated VSD. Less than 20% had significant hypoplasia of the morphologic right ventricle. Subaortic stenosis resulting from a malaligned infundibular septum, or anomalous right ventricular muscle bundles, or a prominent right-sided ventriculoinfundibular fold, or combinations of these were identified in several of these 32 patients.

Moene and colleagues (1983) in a post-mortem study addressed the morphologic substrates responsible for anatomic obstruction of the right ventricular outflow tract in TGA. Seventy-one hearts of the 126 patients in this study had an intact ventricular septum, and only two of 71 patients had right ventricular outflow tract obstruction (RVOTO). However, of the 55 specimens with VSD, 15 (27%) had distinct RVOTO, and in 75% of those with obstruction, it resulted from wedging of the subaortic outflow tract between an anteriorly malaligned infundibular septum and a prominent right-sided ventriculoinfundibular fold.

Laterality of the Aortic Arch

A left-sided aortic arch is found in approximately 90 to 92% of patients with complete TGA; the aortic arch is right-sided in 8 to 10%. The lowest frequency of right-sided aortic arch (approximately 4%) is found in patients with an intact ventricular septum, and the highest incidence (approximately 16%) is seen among those with VSD and left ventricular outflow tract stenosis (Mathew et al, 1974).

Coronary Arteries

Knowledge of the aortic origin of the coronary arteries and their epicardial distribution is necessary for the operative management of some forms of transposition. The epicardial distribution must be defined before interposition of a right-ventricular pulmonary artery conduit. Because the anterior descending coronary artery can cross the right ventricular outflow tract, this distribution may prevent or make difficult interposition of a right ventricular conduit in the young or small patient. Since 1975, when Jatene and colleagues successfully did an anatomic repair with coronary artery reimplantation, there has been a resurgence of interest in the anatomy and variations of the origin of the coronary artery in these patients.

Kurosawa and colleagues (1986) did a morphometric study of the coronary arterioles in newborns, infants, and children and compared findings from normal hearts with those observed from patients with aortic atresia and TGA. Among patients with TGA the number of arterioles per surface area from birth to 1 year of age is below that anticipated from normal hearts. This difference was even more pronounced in the morphologic right ventricle than in the left ventricle. Moreover, the average medial thickness of the arterioles seems to be less than anticipated from the normal. The functional implications of these observations are unclear.

Wall Thickness of Ventricular Chambers in Transposition

Bano-Rodrigo and colleagues (1980) examined the wall thickness of ventricular chambers in TGA. The surgical implications of these findings with regard to the arterial switch are obvious. Among their patients with TGA and an intact ventricular septum, a significant decrease in the left ventricular-right ventricular ratio was found after the neonatal period, and after 8 months of age the thickness of the left ventricular wall in this group was under 95% confidence limits for normality. The same was true for patients with an associated large VSD after 18 months of age. Because of their findings, these authors could not recommend anatomic correction after 8 months of age for the patients with an intact ventricular septum or after 18 months of age for the patient with a large VSD.

Pulmonary Arteries

Among patients with complete TGA and an intact ventricular septum, the main and branch pulmonary arteries are usually dilated, especially after the newborn period. In addition, after the newborn period, the surgeon can recognize asymmetric distribution of the pulmonary blood flow between the right and left lungs (Muster et al, 1976). The inclination or geometry of the left ventricular outflow tract favors blood flow from the main pulmonary artery to the right pulmonary artery. This maldistribution of flow may increase when there is LVOTO or when there are anatomic stenoses in the left pulmonary artery. The disparity in perfusion between the two lungs may be progressive.

Patients with associated VSD and left ventricular outflow tract stenosis can have all of the anomalies of pulmonary arteries anticipated in patients with tetralogy of Fallot. Among patients with pulmonary atresia and VSD (but posterior pulmonary artery), it is necessary to define the site(s) or origin of the pulmonary arteries (e.g., single ductus; ascending aorta; aortopulmonary collaterals; and bilateral homologous ducts when the right and left pulmonary arteries are not confluent).

Left Pulmonary Vein Stenosis

Pulmonary vein stenosis has been described both as a sequela or complication of Mustard's operation, but unilateral left-sided pulmonary vein stenosis may also be a congenital anomaly that complicates complete TGA. Moreover, the degree of obstruction may become progressive as a result of the topography of the left ventricular outflow tract in hearts with transposition, which, postnatally, mandates preferential blood flow to the right lung (Vogel et al, 1984).

PATHOPHYSIOLOGY

The neonate with complete TGA, an intact ventricular septum, a small ASD, and a closing PDA can be seen to have two parallel circulations: a systemic circulation and a pulmonary circulation. Survival in this group of patients for even a short time is predicated on affording adequate mixing between the two parallel circulations. The presence of a large VSD or a large PDA affords some mixing between the two circulations. Thus, intense cyanosis is less common, and, frequently, these patients are only mildly to moderately cyanotic. However, in this group, congestive heart failure may be conspicuous and may not respond to anticongestive therapy.

The patient with associated VSD and LVOTO has a natural history similar to that of the patient with tetralogy of Fallot. An increased severity of LVOTO results in inadequate pulmonary blood flow, and thus hypoxia and polycythemia may become progressive. When the pulmonary arteries are not in continuity with the heart, pulmonary blood flow may be duct-dependent, or, depending on the site or origin of the pulmonary arteries, the patient may have reasonable saturation in the aorta.

CLINICAL MANIFESTATIONS

Data from the New England Regional Infant Cardiac Program reveal an incidence of 0.218 per 1,000 live births (Fyler, 1980). This study showed that of those infants with simple transposition 59% were hospitalized before the third day of life, compared with 34% of those with large associated VSD.

Two-thirds of patients with complete transposition are males (Fyler, 1980). Although 9% of patients with complete transposition included in the New England Regional Infant Cardiac Program had extracardiac congenital anomalies, the majority of these anomalies were minor. In reviewing 140 clinical and autopsy cases of complete transposition, Landtman and colleagues (1975) found extracardiac malformations in 39 patients, which were thought to be responsible for the death of 22 of these patients. Low birth weight was not a consistent feature.

The clinical manifestation depends on the presence or absence of associated cardiovascular anomalies. Because most patients with complete transposition have inadequate circulatory mixing, these patients inevitably present in the newborn period. The most striking physical sign of TGA is persistent cyanosis that does not respond to an increased oxygen concentration (Goldman et al, 1973; Jones et al, 1976; Shannon et al, 1972; Tooley and Stanger, 1972). Cyanosis, which is usually progressive, may be intense, especially when the neonate is also relatively polycythemic. It may be less intense, or even equivocal, in the patient with good circulatory mixing. When ductal patency is responsible for only equivocal cyanosis, the reprieve may be transient, and ductal closure may lead to rapid clinical deterioration (Rowe et al, 1981). Differential cyanosis with relatively pink lower extremities and deeper cyanosis of the upper extremities may be found in the patient with associated severe thoracic coarctation or interruption of the aortic arch. After cyanosis, the next most conspicuous finding in these patients is congestive heart failure, with tachycardia, tachypnea, dyspnea, and an enlarged liver. It would be distinctly uncommon for the patient with severe LVOTO to have signs of heart failure. Conversely, the patient with a large VSD or ductus arteriosus or severe obstructive anomaly of the aortic arch may present in severe cardiorespiratory distress and may have relatively mild to moderate hypoxia and cyanosis.

The profoundly acidotic infant may present in extremis.

The heart is usually overactive and has a prominent left parasternal lift. The heart sounds are usually loud and crisp; the second sound is single. When the ventricular septum is intact, there may be no murmur, or a soft systolic ejection murmur may be audible along the left sternal border. A soft pansystolic murmur may indicate the presence of a small or moderate VSD. It is uncommon to appreciate a typical "machinery" murmur of a PDA in the immediate newborn period. The caliber and timing of the femoral pulses may indicate an obstructive anomaly of the aortic arch.

LABORATORY FINDINGS

Radiologic Features. The typical radiographic appearance of TGA is that of an enlarged heart with the appearance of an egg on its side (Fig. 43–1). Pulmonary plethora may be conspicuous; beyond the first 1 or 2 months of life, a disparity in the pulmonary perfusion may be apparent and the right lung may be more plethoric than the left lung. Characteristically, the cardiac pedicle is narrow (Guerin et al, 1970; Kurlander et al, 1968; Moes, 1975; Nogrady and Dunbar, 1969; Tonkin et al, 1980). Although these features can be seen in the first few days of life, there are numerous exceptions to the classic appearance. Counahan and colleagues (1973) suggested that 10% of plain chest films obtained from infants less than 1 month of age with complete TGA were interpreted as being normal.

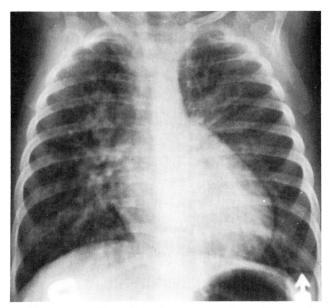

Figure 43–1. Chest film of a young patient with complete transposition of the great arteries. The cardiac pedicle is narrow, and the configuration is "egg-shaped." Pulmonary plethora is conspicuous. (Courtesy of C. A. F. Moes, M.D., Department of Radiology, The Hospital for Sick Children, Toronto.)

Electrocardiography. Most patients have normal sinus rhythm or a sinus tachycardia. Approximately 2% have the so-called coronary sinus rhythm with a negative P wave in leads 2, 3, and aVF, and a normal PR interval. The mean QRS axis congregates around 100 degrees to more than 120 degrees, although some patients have profound right-axis deviation of 150 degrees to more than 240 degrees. It is distinctly uncommon to identify left-axis deviation in patients with uncomplicated TGA.

There is not a clear-cut relationship between the pattern of ventricular hypertrophy and the presence or absence of a VSD or LVOTO. Most patients, especially hypoxic neonates, show a pattern of right ventricular hypertrophy of dominance, and the authors' data indicate that left ventricular hypertrophy or combined ventricular hypertrophy is uncommonly observed in the neonate. Even in the patient with severe LVOTO with or without a VSD, it is unusual for the electrocardiogram to show severe left ventricular hypertrophy.

ST-T wave changes are not uncommon and may reflect some degree of myocardial ischemia, especially in the severely hypoxic and acidotic neonate.

Echocardiography. Both M-mode and two-dimensional echocardiographic examinations have had a major impact on the noninvasive diagnosis of complete TGA. By using the two-dimensional technique, the demonstration of the abnormal spatial relationship between the aorta and the pulmonary artery (when compared with the normal relationship) and their respective origins from the discordant ventricle can be done in only a few minutes (Bierman

and Williams, 1979b; Houston et al, 1978). But what is the relevance of the echocardiographic examination to the surgeon?

When the diagnosis of complete transposition has been unequivocally confirmed, two-dimensional echocardiographic techniques should allow (1) visualization of the atrial septum and the adequacy of balloon atrial septostomy; (2) longitudinal assessment of ventricular contractility and wall motion; (3) assessment of the atrioventricular junction in the patient with complex transposition; (4) the recognition of the type of LVOTO when left ventricular angiography is unsatisfactory (Aziz et al, 1978, 1979); (5) imaging of the ventricular septum and quantitation of the number and type of VSD; and (6) imaging of the aortic isthmus and juxtaductal or juxtaligamental level with regard to the question of coarctation.

After the Mustard operation, echocardiographic techniques allow visualization of the baffle and serial assessment of right ventricular function. The use of microcavitation facilitates recognition of baffle leaks in the postoperative period or residual shunting at the ventricular level.

Angiocardiography. There is an extensive literature devoted to the angiocardiography of patients with complete TGA (Barcia et al, 1967; Deutsch et al, 1970; Fisher et al, 1970; Freedom et al, 1974; Paul, 1977; Sansa et al, 1979; Silove and Taylor, 1973).

Selective right ventriculography is usually done in frontal and lateral projections, and most institutions do selective angiocardiograms in the biplane mode. Frontal and lateral ventriculograms are most frequently done and show the discordant ventricu-

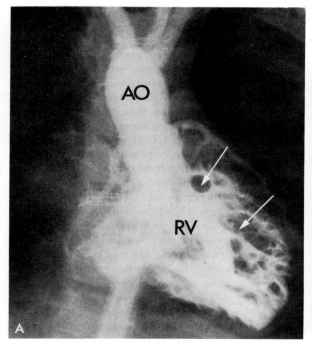
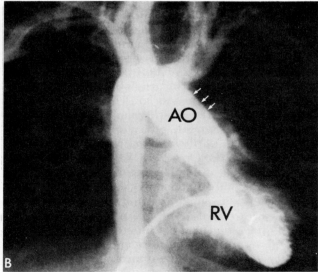

Figure 43–2. Complete TGA. *A,* Frontal right ventriculogram with opacification of aorta (AO). The right ventricle (RV) is heavily trabeculated *(white arrows).* The ascending aorta is in the usual position. *B,* In this patient with complete transposition, the aorta is relatively levopositioned and the ascending aorta *(white arrows)* forms the left border of the cardiac silhouette.

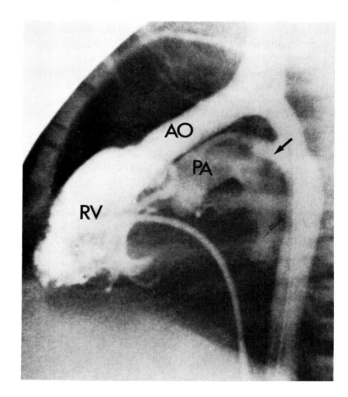

Figure 43–3. Complete transposition with PDA. Lateral right ventriculogram shows an anteriorly positioned, discordantly connected aorta (AO). The larger and posteriorly positioned pulmonary artery (PA) is opacified via a moderate-sized PDA *(arrow)*. (RV = right ventricle.)

loarterial connection, the subaortic infundibulum, the size and function (when using cine technique) of the right ventricle, and the presence or absence of tricuspid regurgitation, and when the ventricular septum is intact (or when only a small VSD is present), the status of the aortic isthmus, ductus arteriosus, and the presence or absence of a juxtaductal coarctation or other obstructive anomaly of the aortic arch (Figs. 43–2 and 43–3). When a significant VSD is

present, opacification of the main and left pulmonary arteries may obscure the aortic isthmus. Thus, selective aortography may be necessary to more completely define the caliber of the aortic isthmus and to exclude obstructive anomalies of the aortic arch (Fig. 43–4). In addition, the origin of the coronary arteries is best seen by aortography filmed in the biplane mode.

Selective biplane left ventriculography is best

Figure 43–4. Coarctation of the aorta *(arrow on right)* complicating complete TGA. This aortogram shows a relatively small ascending aorta (ao), a small aortic isthmus, and a discrete coarctation of aorta with a posterior shelf. The small patent ductus arteriosus (pda) opacifies the pulmonary artery (PA).

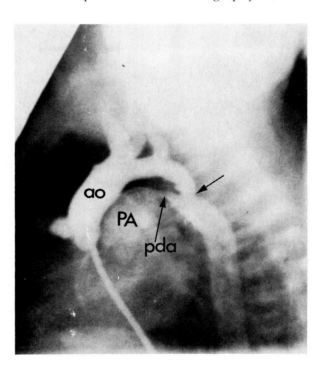

filmed by using axial cineangiography. These projections, which were advocated initially by Bargeron and colleagues (1977) and Elliott and associates (1977), elongate the left ventricular outflow tract and give two immediate advantages. First, it allows precise definition of the left ventricular outflow tract without the "shoulder" of the left ventricle compromising the immediate subpulmonary area (Fig. 43–5). Second, the left long axial oblique projection should profile the majority of the VSD involving the infundibular or perimembranous septum. When a more posteriorly positioned VSD is suspected, it would be advantageous to use the hepatoclavicular four-chamber projection. This profiles more adequately the inlet and posterior aspects of the ventricular septum.

As mentioned earlier, there is considerable heterogeneity among these anatomic causes of LVOTO. The left long axial oblique projection is ideal to show posterior malalignment of the infundibular septum and the resultant VSD. The presence of associated pulmonary valve stenosis, fibrous diaphragm, fibromuscular tunnel form of subpulmonary stenosis, and accessory tissue tags is also usually best profiled by using this projection, but the exact degree of obliquity must be individualized for every patient (Figs. 43–6 to 43–8).

Selective atrial angiography (right or left) may be necessary to define the presence or absence of a straddling atrioventricular connection. The authors advocate atrial angiography in patients with the superoinferior ventricular relationship or the appear-

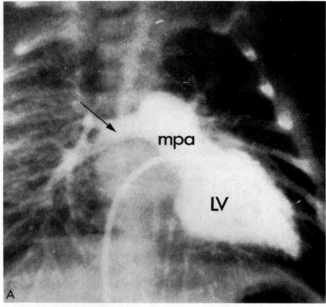

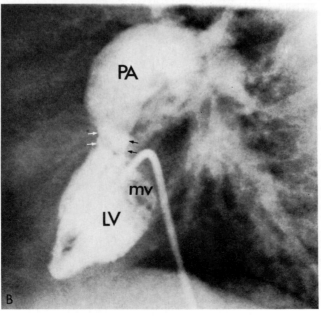

Figure 43–5. Left ventriculogram in a patient with complete TGA and an intact ventricular septum. *A*, Frontal left ventriculogram opacifies the discordantly connected pulmonary artery (mpa). There is preferential flow into the right pulmonary artery *(arrow)* because of the inclination of the left ventricular outflow tract. (LV = left ventricle.) *B*, An intact ventricular septum and absence of LVOTO (between *white* and *black arrows*). (mv = mitral valve.)

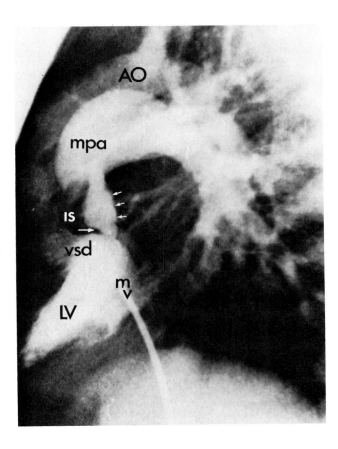

Figure 43–6. LVOTO at several sites in a child with complete TGA and malalignment type of ventricular septal defect. This long axial oblique left ventriculogram shows that the pulmonary artery (mpa) is supported by the left ventricle (LV). The infundibular septum (IS) is deviated posteriorly *(solitary white arrow)* and is seen superior to the large ventricular septal defect (vsd). The subpulmonary infundibulum is an elongated muscular structure *(small white arrows)*, and because it is well developed but poorly expanded, there is discontinuity between the pulmonary valve and the anterior leaflet of the mitral valve (mv). (AO = aorta.)

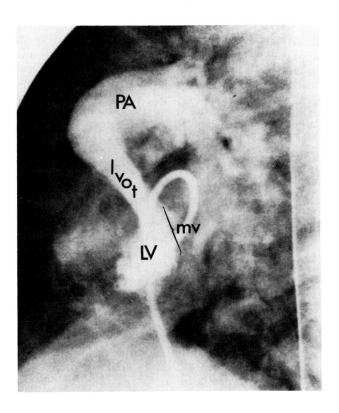

Figure 43–7. Muscular tunnel form of subpulmonary stenosis in a patient with complete TGA and multiple small VSDs. This lateral left ventriculogram shows the greatly elongated left ventricular outflow tract (lvot). The main pulmonary trunk (PA) has good caliber. Clearly, the mitral valve (mv) is not in continuity with the pulmonary valve. (LV = left ventricle.)

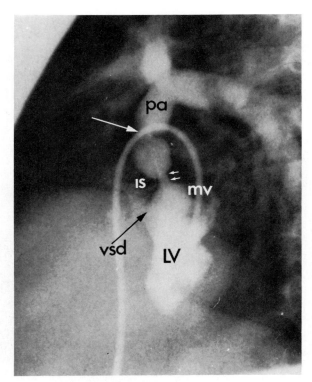

Figure 43–8. A relatively small ventricular septal defect (VSD) and severe subpulmonary obstruction are shown by this long axial oblique left ventriculogram done via the mitral valve (mv). The ventricular septal defect is inferior to the posteriorly malaligned infundibular septum (IS). There is concentric stenosis *(two small white arrows)* of the left ventricular outflow tract. The severely stenotic pulmonary valve *(long white arrow)* is partially obscured by the catheter. The muscular subpulmonary infundibulum prevents pulmonary valve-mitral valve fibrous continuity. (LV = left ventricle.)

ance of crossed atrioventricular connections, both conditions in which a straddling atrioventricular valve might be encountered. Atrial angiography may be useful in evaluating the atrioventricular junction when the concordant ventricle is underdeveloped. In addition, when mesocardia or dextrocardia is present, a selective right atrial angiogram excludes left juxtaposition of the right atrial appendage, a condition that makes Blalock-Hanlon's atrial septectomy or intra-atrial repair more difficult, especially in the very young and small patient (Rosenquist et al, 1975; Urban et al, 1976).

NATURAL HISTORY OF THE PATIENT WITH COMPLETE TRANSPOSITION OF THE GREAT ARTERIES

Before the introduction of balloon atrial septostomy by Rashkind and Miller in 1966, the natural history for these patients was clear: 90% of patients with TGA would not survive to their first birthday,

and almost half of all these patients would die by 1 month of age (Liebman et al, 1969). Although nonoperative atrial septostomy has irrevocably altered the natural history, a substantial number of patients with transposition still die before reaching 1 year of age. Data compiled from the New England Infant Cardiac Program (Fyler, 1980) show a crude first-year mortality of 39% for patients with complete transposition. In reviewing 112 consecutive neonates with complete transposition seen at the Texas Children's Hospital from 1967 to 1977, Gutgesell and colleagues (1979) found that the first month of life was the period of greatest risk and had an 8% mortality. Between the balloon atrial septostomy and baffle repair, 14 of 103 patients at risk either died or sustained a cerebrovascular accident. The mortality at baffle repair in their series was 14%, and there were three late postoperative deaths. Their actuarial analysis suggested that approximately 50% of newborns with TGA survive for 5 years with excellent function and that an additional 15 to 20% survive with one or more medical handicaps.

Plauth and associates (1968) reviewed serial hemodynamic studies among patients with complete TGA. Like the patient with a small VSD and an otherwise normal heart, the small VSD in the patient with complete TGA can decrease spontaneously in size or can close spontaneously. Reduction in size may be accompanied by aneurysmal transformation. Because the aneurysm protrudes into the left ventricular outflow tract, this may result in subpulmonary stenosis (Vidne et al, 1976). The spontaneous closure rate of a small VSD in the patient with complete transposition is assumed to be almost the same as that in the individual with an otherwise normal heart.

LVOTO can develop or may increase with time in the patient with an associated VSD or in the patient with an intact ventricular septum. The authors' data indicate that the development of LVOTO in the individual with an intact ventricular septum is in the range of 2 to 3% and is slightly higher in the patient with an associated VSD. Tonkin and coworkers (1980) provided excellent angiographic verification of developing LVOTO in patients with complete TGA and an intact ventricular septum.

Pulmonary vascular obstructive disease is uncommon within the first few years of life in the patient with complete TGA and an intact ventricular septum. However, Lakier and colleagues (1975) and Newfeld and associates (1974) described early onset of pulmonary vascular obstruction in a few patients. More common is the development of pulmonary vascular arteriopathy in patients with an associated large VSD or large PDA (Newfeld et al, 1974; Waldman et al, 1977). Although it is difficult and unwise to generalize, many patients with complete transposition and an unrestrictive VSD or ductus arteriosus may develop severe pulmonary vascular obstruction by 1 year of age (Yamaki and Tezuka, 1976).

MEDICAL TREATMENT

The initial medical therapy of the severely hypoxic neonate should be directed toward (1) correction of metabolic acidosis, (2) treatment of congestive heart failure with parenteral digoxin and diuretics, (3) maintenance of normothermia, (4) treatment of hypoglycemia, and (5) provision of adequate ventilation for the profoundly distressed infant. Echocardiographic examination should then be done as expeditiously as possible, and the neonate should be transferred to the cardiac catheterization laboratory. If the clinical and echocardiographic features of complete transposition are unequivocal in the critically ill neonate, the authors perform balloon atrial septostomy before hemodynamic and angiocardiographic investigations. Balloon atrial septostomy should be done with the largest balloon catheter that can be safely introduced. This can be done through a saphenofemoral venous cutdown, by the percutaneous approach, through the umbilical vein. The authors do the septostomy maneuver several times until no further resistance is met at the atrial septum. When hemodynamic recordings are obtained before balloon atrial septostomy, a withdrawal pressure tracing from the left to the right atrium after balloon septostomy is routinely recorded as well as obtaining arterial oxygen tension and saturation data before and after the procedure.

In some neonates, the clinical and echocardiographic features may not be entirely consistent with complete transposition. When this situation is encountered, complete hemodynamic data are obtained together with indicator dilution curves by injection of indocyanine green dye initially in the right atrium with withdrawal from the aorta and then by injection in the left atrium, again sampling in the aorta, which provides the correct diagnosis (Gingell et al, 1979). Dye dilution techniques to confirm the diagnosis in the acidotic infant are preferred because contrast material may hasten clinical deterioration. Today, with the routine application of cross-sectional echocardiography, the use of indicator dilution curves is rarely necessary. Again, when the unequivocal diagnosis of complete transposition is made, balloon atrial septostomy is indicated. Finally, complete hemodynamic and angiocardiographic investigations should be done. The use of flow-directed catheters facilitates entry into all the cardiac chambers, and usually both great arteries can be entered (Kelly et al, 1971). When possible, an umbilical artery catheter should be placed proximal to the origin of the ductus arteriosus. This allows efficient blood-gas analysis and may expedite the catheter study. Unless the left ventricular pressure is half systemic or less, the authors routinely attempt to record the pulmonary artery pressure.

There is not unanimity with regard to the definition of an adequate response to balloon atrial septostomy (the pertinent literature is summarized in Rowe et al, 1981). Some neonates remain hypoxic, despite an apparently adequate balloon atrial septostomy. The adequacy of the balloon atrial septostomy can be seen in terms of abolishing the interatrial pressure gradient and visualization of the atrial septum after septostomy to quantitate the adequacy of the tear (Bierman and Williams, 1979a; Clark et al, 1977; Korns et al, 1972).

The authors have tried two maneuvers to facilitate atrial mixing in neonates in whom a better response to balloon atrial septostomy would have been anticipated. If congestive heart failure is not a feature, hypertransfusion with 5 to 10 ml/kg of whole blood by increasing atrial filling may substantially improve arterial oxygen saturation. However, when an adequate tear of the atrial septum is obvious, the administration of an E type of prostaglandin may improve systemic oxygenation (Benson et al, 1979; Driscoll et al, 1979; Henry et al, 1981; Lang et al, 1979). The action of the E type of prostaglandin is to maintain patency of the ductus arteriosus (Coceani and Olley, 1973; Olley et al, 1978). The increase in pulmonary venous blood to the left atrium facilitated by the prostaglandin may alter the compliance of the left atrium; if an adequate interatrial communication is present, the result may be increased mixing. The authors urge care in the use of prostaglandin when the interatrial communication is marginal (Benson et al, 1979). When the interatrial defect is restrictive, the E type of prostaglandins, by increasing pulmonary blood flow, may actually precipitate or increase congestive heart failure. Despite an "adequate" balloon atrial septostomy, hypertransfusion, and the administration of an E type of prostaglandin, some infants, fortunately few, remain severely hypoxic. These infants may appear reasonably comfortable despite an arterial oxygen tension of 20 to 25 mm Hg, and the physician might become complacent. However, this type of patient tends to have a hypoxic cerebrovascular accident. Thus, if a neonate maintains an arterial oxygen tension consistently below 30 mm Hg, the authors advocate a Blalock-Hanlon atrial septectomy. In other institutions, a second balloon atrial septostomy might be done or an early intra-atrial baffle or Senning's repair may be done.

The medical management of the neonate with an associated small or moderate VSD is the same as that for the patient with an intact ventricular septum.

The patient with a large VSD or a large PDA poses a slightly different problem, and the authors' opinions about the surgical therapy of these groups of patients are changing. Congestive heart failure rather than hypoxia may be the more conspicuous sign, and, some of these infants have arterial oxygen saturations in the low to mid-80s. Nonetheless, the authors strongly urge that all patients with complete transposition (despite the associated lesion) have balloon atrial septostomy. Even a large ductus can close, and infants in whom this occurs can become acutely hypoxic. In addition, if a clinically "malignant" ductus requires surgical ligation, the magnitude of interatrial mixing becomes important. At present, the timing and type of surgical intervention reserved for the patient with TGA, a large VSD or a large PDA, and systemic levels of left ventricular hypertension are being reviewed. The surgical options for the infant with a large VSD and pulmonary artery hypertension include (1) intra-atrial repair and VSD closure; (2) pulmonary artery banding followed by the Mustard repair, VSD closure and debanding, or debanding with anatomic repair; or (3) primary anatomic repair. Because most patients with a nonrestrictive VSD develop pulmonary vascular obstruction, some type of surgical intervention is necessary within the first year of life. Other patients with intractable congestive heart failure and severe growth retardation may require surgical intervention within the first few weeks or months of life. Similarly, for the patient with transposition, an intact ventricular septum (IVS), and pulmonary artery (and left ventricular) hypertension secondary to a large ductus arteriosus, the surgical options include early duct ligation followed by a Mustard repair or operation within 3 months to 1 year of life with duct ligation and Mustard repair or duct ligation and anatomic repair.

TREATMENT

Palliative Procedures

The basic principle of palliation is to improve mixing between the pulmonary and systemic circulations by creating or enlarging an ASD. Enlargement of an ASD by balloon atrial septostomy (Rashkind and Miller, 1966) is done at initial cardiac catheterization in almost all infants with TGA.

In infants with TGA and intact ventricular septum (IVS) before balloon septostomy was done, some type of surgical atrial septectomy was an essential component of the management. Although closed techniques by using various ingenious instruments or open excision of the septum with inflow caval occlusion were often effective, the resultant ASD was relatively small and the palliation was sometimes barely adequate. The original operation by Blalock and Hanlon (1950) created a large ASD and remained the surgical procedure of choice for palliation (Fig. 43–9). The technique is demanding but, if done carefully, the results are excellent. Since 1968, at the Hospital for Sick Children, Toronto, there have been 9 (5.5%) deaths in 169 Blalock-Hanlon types of operations. Conduction disturbances may occur, and it is important to leave the superior margin of the atrial septum to preserve the artery to the sinoatrial (SA) node (Trusler et al, 1980).

During the last decade, improved techniques and management have reduced the mortality of TGA repair. The elective age for repair has decreased, and many surgeons now recommend primary repair at an early age whenever the protection given by balloon septostomy is no longer adequate (Bailey et al,

1982: Mahoney et al, 1982; Turley et al, 1982). Other surgeons recommend surgical septectomy for infants who require operation in the first 1 to 2 months of life and believe that repair at this age is associated with a slightly higher risk of operative death and postoperative complications. The choice rests with the surgeon who must consider the experience with both the Blalock-Hanlon type of operation and the repair.

Infants with TGA and large VSDs require treatment before the age of 6 months to prevent pulmonary vascular disease and often earlier to relieve congestive heart failure. Balloon atrial septostomy, soon after birth, helps by eliminating left atrial hypertension and improving oxygen saturation. Pulmonary artery banding, once the main type of palliation, is now seldom used and early atrial or arterial repair is preferred. Occasionally in very small ill infants or in the presence of some complicating feature, such as a large apical muscular VSD or hypoplastic ventricle, pulmonary artery banding rather than repair is advisable. In these patients, in order to apply an adequate band, there must be a satisfactory ASD. If not, a Blalock-Hanlon septectomy should be done with the banding. Both procedures can be done through a right anterolateral thoracotomy. Edwards described a modification of the Blalock-Hanlon operation (Edwards et al, 1964) in which the atrial septum is not resected but is sutured to the posterior wall of the left atrium medial to the right pulmonary venous orifices. This produces obligatory mixing of the right pulmonary venous return in the right atrium and, in infants with TGA and VSD, it appears to provide better palliation than the Blalock-Hanlon procedure when associated with pulmonary artery banding.

Infants with TGA plus VSD and LVOTO often require palliation before age permits repair. When the VSD is large and the LVOTO is a form that cannot be relieved directly, the best treatment is a Rastelli operation, but the risk is less if this is delayed until after the child's fifth birthday. If treatment is needed earlier, a shunt is done, preferably Blalock-Taussig anastomosis because it is the easiest shunt to close at repair and is associated with fewest complications. The modification using a prosthesis from the subclavian artery to the pulmonary artery, described by de Leval and associates (1981), is usually used. Other shunts (e.g., Potts' shunt, Waterston's shunt, Glenn's shunt) have been used, but most have serious disadvantages. At the Hospital for Sick Children, Toronto, from 1960 to 1987, 81 children with TGA had Blalock-Taussig shunts constructed with two (2.5%) deaths.

In infants with TGA and LVOTO without a VSD, creation of a large ASD usually provides adequate palliation until repair can be accomplished. If the LVOTO is severe and is in a form that cannot be relieved by a direct attack, it may be advisable to palliate the child for some years with a Blalock-Taussig shunt as well as with the Blalock-Hanlon

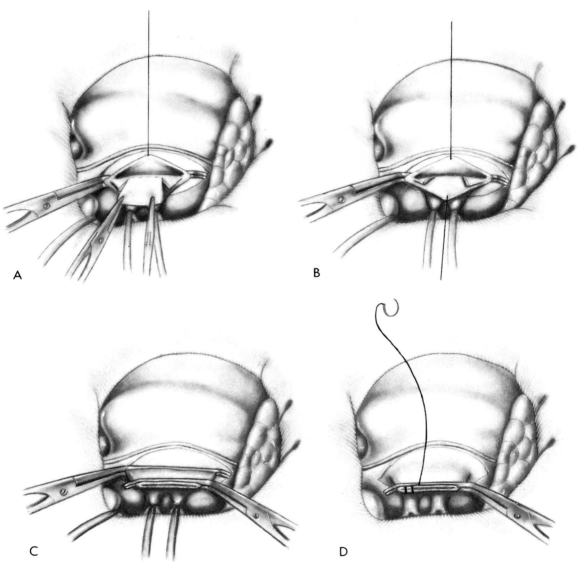

Figure 43–9. Approach by a right lateral thoracotomy through the fifth interspace with snares around the right pulmonary artery and the upper and lower right pulmonary veins, and a partial-occlusion clamp with one jaw posterior to the pulmonary veins and the other anterior so that a portion of the right and left atria has been included. The pericardium has been opened posterior to the right phrenic nerve, and the right and left atria have been opened by an incision parallel to the atrial septum. The atrial septum has been incised with scissors, the free edges have been grasped with hemostats, and an extra portion of atrial septum has been withdrawn from the heart while the partial-occlusion clamp was gently released *(A)*. The mobilized flap of atrial septum is then cut through its pedicle *(B)*, and a smaller partial-occlusion clamp is applied to the free edges of the incision in the left and right atria and lies anterior to the right pulmonary veins *(C)*. The larger occlusion clamp is then released, as are the snares on the pulmonary veins and the pulmonary artery. The incision in the atria can then be closed at leisure *(D)*. (From Aberdeen, E.: Blalock-Hanlon operation and Rashkind procedure. *In* Rob, C., and Smith, R.: Operative Surgery, 2nd ed., Vol. 2. London, Butterworth, 1968, pp. 193–199.)

septectomy. These palliated patients may be at risk for the early onset of pulmonary vascular obstructive disease and should be observed closely.

Surgical Repair

Various repair procedures are now available, and the choice is generally dictated by the anatomy. Arterial repair is used by some surgeons for TGA and IVS and by most surgeons for TGA with VSD. Rastelli's repair is used for TGA, VSD, and LVOTO and intraventricular repair for exceptional cases with large VSDs. There are two main operations for atrial repair: the Senning operation and the Mustard operation. The Senning operation is considered in a separate section. A description of the Mustard operation follows.

Technique of the Mustard Repair

Through a median sternotomy, the anterior aspect of the pericardial sac is cleared for a width of 5 to 6 cm and superiorly to the great arteries where the thymus is reflected. The pericardium is incised along the diaphragm and an approximately rectangular patch of pericardium is taken for use as the future atrial baffle (Fig. 43-10). The patch is hollowed or made concave on both sides to create a waist of 2.5 to 3 cm wide. Both ends are rounded for adequate caval channels. The inferior vena cava end (5 cm) is slightly larger than the superior vena cava (SVC) end (4 cm) and is more rounded to allow flexibility of choice in the position of the suture line. The long side of the patch is 7 cm long and is taken some distance from but almost parallel to the right phrenic nerve. It extends from the diaphragm below to the most prominent point on the ascending aorta above. The opposite side is 5 cm long. This size fits a child who weighs 10 kg body weight. In a 5-kg infant, the dimensions are 0.5 to 1 cm less on all sides. The size and shape of the pericardial baffle differs for each surgeon, and the trouser-shaped baffle advocated by Brom (1975) is preferred by some surgeons. Synthetic materials such as Dacron or Gore-Tex have also been used for the baffle.

At present, most patients with TGA have intracardiac repair in the first year of life by using deep hypothermia and circulatory arrest. Older children who weigh more than 10 kg are repaired with cardiopulmonary bypass and moderate hypothermia. Low-flow bypass and aortic cross-clamping are useful adjuncts to improve exposure for short periods.

Infants are allowed to cool moderately during the early part of the operation. After the pericardial baffle is prepared, cannulas are inserted into the ascending aorta and right atrial appendage, and bypass is begun with core-cooling to a rectal temperature of 16 to 18° C and esophageal temperature approximately 12° C. While cooling, tourniquets are placed around the cavae and the aorta; the thin

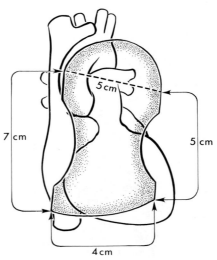

Figure 43-10. The pericardial patch (*stippled area*) for the intra-atrial baffle. Basic dimensions are 7 × 4 cm for a 10-kg child, 0.5 cm less for a 5-kg child. The slightly convex superior vena cava portion is taken along the diaphragm. The long border is on the right atrium and extends up to the ascending aorta. The other two borders are basically 5 cm long, but the superior border is fully rounded to allow flexibility in choosing the suture line position around the inferior vena cava.

cooling device pad is positioned surrounding the ventricles; and the cardioplegia line is filled and inserted into the ascending aorta.

During bypass cooling, the rectal temperature falls more slowly than the esophageal temperature and is thus likely to be a safer guide to the temperature of the brain. At 16 to 18° C (rectal), the pump is stopped and the aorta is cross-clamped. Cold (4° C) potassium blood cardioplegia is injected into the aortic root. The caval tourniquets are snugged; the venous cannula is removed; and the right atrium is opened with a longitudinal incision well away from the SA node (Fig. 43-11).

After cardioplegia is administered, the interior of the right atrium is examined as well as the pulmonary venous orifices, left atrial appendage, and mitral valve (Fig. 43-12). The remaining septum is partly excised. The first incision is made from the superior border of the ASD up to the middle of the SVC orifice. The ridge of septum to the left of this incision is preserved because it often contains the artery to the SA node and may also act as a conduction pathway between the SA node and atrioventricular node. The atrial septum to the right of this incision is excised completely. This excision is extended to include any septal remnant near the inferior vena cava (IVC). The coronary sinus is reflected back into the left atrium for approximately 1.5 cm, and any residual septum between IVC and coronary sinus is excised. The raw incised margins left by excising septum are oversewn with a 5-0 suture, and relatively small bites are taken to avoid a purse-string effect (Fig. 43-13).

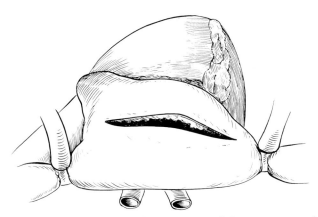

Figure 43–11. With circulatory arrest and the venous cannula removed, the caval tourniquets are tightened and a longitudinal incision is made in the right atrium.

The intra-atrial baffle is now sutured into the common atrium by using a double-armed continuous 3-0 braided synthetic suture (Fig. 43–14). The midpoint of the long side of the baffle is sutured and tied to the anterior margin of the internal orifice of the left pulmonary veins. The continuous suture line then passes around the orifice of the left superior pulmonary vein to reach the posterior wall of the left atrium, crosses that wall curving inferiorly for a short distance to create a larger SVC channel, and then passes between the right superior pulmonary vein and the SVC orifice. The first corner of the baffle, which is one end of the long border, should reach the lateral wall of the right atrium. The short SVC border of the baffle is now sutured around the internal orifice of the SVC, and the second corner of the baffle reaches partially across the roof of the right atrium between SVC and the residual ridge of atrial septum. Initially, on this border, relatively large bites of baffle and small bites of SVC orifice are taken to increase ballooning of the channel and to avoid flattening of the baffle across the SVC orifice. The SA node, approximately 1 cm away from this orifice, should be carefully avoided. This suture line contin-

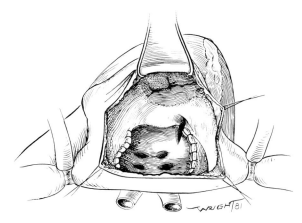

Figure 43–13. The first incision is made from the superior border of the ASD up to the middle of the SVC orifice. The ridge of septum to the left of this incision is preserved, because it often contains the artery to the SA node and may act as a conduction pathway between the SA node and the atrioventricular node. The atrial septum to the right of this incision is excised completely. This excision is extended to include any septal remnant near the IVC. The coronary sinus is incised back into the left atrium for a distance of approximately 1.5 cm, and any residual septum between the IVC and the coronary sinus is excised. The raw cut margins left by the excision of septum are oversewn with 5-0 suture material taking relatively small bites to avoid a purse-string effect.

ues onto the third border of the baffle, which, like the first, is made slightly concave. Part of this border is sutured to the roof of the right atrium and then to the residual atrial septum near the tricuspid valve; it stops at the middle of the septum.

The second end of the original 3-0 suture is now used to suture the remainder of the long border of the baffle around the internal orifice of the left inferior pulmonary vein and across the posterior wall of the left atrium to the right atrium. In crossing, the suture line curves up slightly to enlarge the IVC

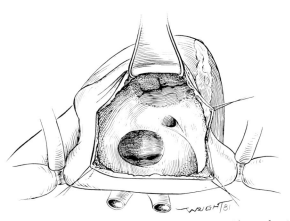

Figure 43–12. Interior of the right atrium with moderately large ASD.

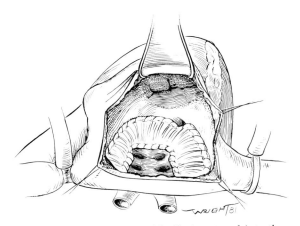

Figure 43–14. The intra-atrial baffle is sutured into the common atrial chamber with a double-armed continuous 3-0 braided synthetic suture. The IVC tourniquet is loosened to improve exposure for choice of suture line position. At the coronary sinus, which has been reduced, the suture line runs 5 to 8 mm to the left of the original coronary sinus orifice.

channel but should not be too close to the previous superior suture line because future baffle contraction may obstruct the left pulmonary veins. The corner of the baffle between the long border and the fully curved IVC border reaches the lateral wall of the right atrium between the right inferior pulmonary vein and the IVC, in a position that allows ample flow through both pulmonary and caval venous channels.

At this point, if there is circulatory arrest, it is expedient to remove the IVC tourniquet. With the IVC open, anatomic details can be distinguished easily and an appropriate path for the baffle suture line can be selected. If the eustachian valve is well formed and sturdy, the baffle may be sutured to it directly. If it is not, then either the base of the eustachian valve or some ridge nearby on the right atrial wall will serve. The last corner of baffle marking the end of the IVC border should reach a point approximately midway along the ridge that extends from the eustachian valve to the coronary sinus. The final border of the baffle is then sutured to this ridge. At the coronary sinus, the suture line extends down one cut edge of coronary sinus for 5 to 8 mm across the sinus 5 to 8 mm from its orifice and then back up the other cut edge and along the atrial septum a short distance to meet the first suture and complete the baffle. Before tying the suture, the left side of the heart is filled gently with saline to reduce the amount of trapped air. When completed, the baffle is inspected briefly and then the right atrial incision is closed.

The venous cannula is reinserted into the right atrium, and the infant is placed back on bypass to rewarm. The cardioplegia line is removed from the aortic root, but the suture is left loose to allow bleeding and evacuation of air. The tip of the venous cannula is inserted gently through the tricuspid valve for a few seconds to remove any major amount of air in the right ventricle. Reinsertion of the venous cannula into the right atrial appendage is simple and convenient. Because this is now the pulmonary venous atrium, there is some reduction in venous return to the pump for 2 to 3 minutes. Gentle cardiac massage and ventilation of the lungs move blood from the systemic venous side through the lungs to the cannula. The venous return becomes stable once the heart starts to beat spontaneously. While rewarming, two atrial and two ventricular temporary pacemaker wires are inserted for postoperative support and monitoring. When the infant's rectal temperature has returned to 34° C, bypass is terminated. The venous cannula is removed from the right atrial appendage, and a small plastic tube is inserted for postoperative monitoring of pulmonary venous pressure.

Variations in Surgical Repair

When there is left juxtaposition of the right atrial appendage, the right appendage is left as part of the systemic venous atrium by the repair. The new pulmonary venous atrium is smaller than usual and should be enlarged with a patch of pericardium. Mesocardia or dextrocardia with situs solitus makes access to the right atrium difficult from an anterior approach. A right lateral thoracotomy provides better exposure. Here, too, the right atrium may be small and may require enlargement with a pericardial patch.

Moderate to large VSDs are closed from the right atrium through the tricuspid valve. Very small VSDs are left untouched, not only to save time, but to avoid the danger of causing right bundle branch block. LVOTO is usually approached through the pulmonary artery and valve but alternatively is accessible through the mitral valve. When repair of one of the aforementioned is necessary in conjunction with a Mustard procedure, the time required may exceed the limits of safety for a single period of circulatory arrest. To avoid excessive ischemia, part of the repair is done on bypass by switching to two acutely curved cannulas that are inserted into the cavae through the open atriotomy.

When pulmonary vascular disease has become severe, patients can still be improved by a Mustard repair but leaving the VSD open (Lindesmith et al, 1972). Occasionally, severe pulmonary vascular disease develops in children with TGA and IVS. These children can be palliated with a Mustard operation and, in addition, creation of an apical VSD (Byrne et al, 1978).

A few infants with TGA and intact septum have a severe form of LVOTO that cannot be relieved directly. They should be treated palliatively with a Blalock-Taussig shunt with or without a Blalock-Hanlon atrial septectomy, and repair should be delayed until the child is older. When intra-atrial repair is done, the LVOTO should be relieved as completely as possible by direct means and, as necessary, the balance of the obstruction should be bypassed by using a valved conduit between the left ventricle and the pulmonary artery (Crupi et al, 1985).

If there is a large and high VSD, an option in some patients is the intraventricular repair described originally by McGoon (1972). The VSD is exposed through a right ventriculotomy. Excision of infundibular muscle and enlargement of the VSD are often necessary. A large patch directs blood from the left ventricle across the VSD to the aorta while leaving a channel for right ventricular blood to cross the VSD and reach the pulmonary artery (Fig. 43–15). Increased knowledge of this complex anatomy is leading to more aggressive resection and repair (Smolinsky et al, 1988).

Rastelli (1969) devised a repair for children with substantial VSD and LVOTO (Fig. 43–16). The VSD is closed with a patch that extends to include the aortic root, thus diverting flow from the left ventricle to the aorta. The pulmonary artery channel is closed, either within the ventricle through the VSD or by closing the pulmonary artery from outside of the artery. A valved conduit, either a homograft aorta

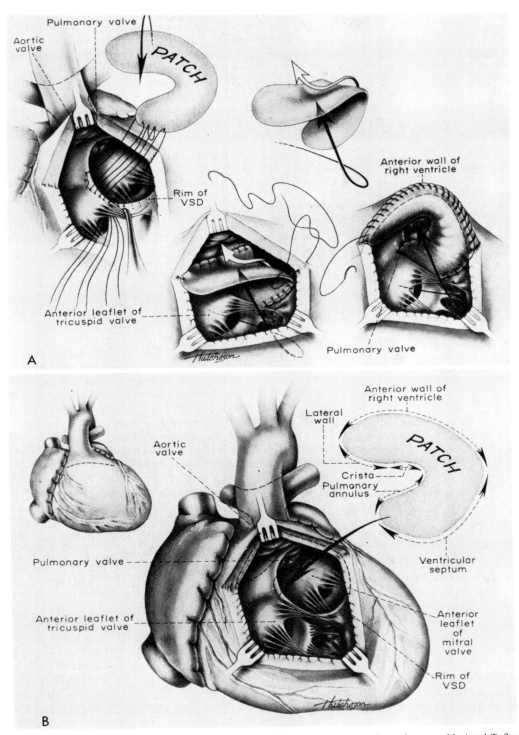

Figure 43–15. *A,* Anatomy of TGA associated with large basilar VSD. Line and sites of attachment of knitted Teflon patch, and its preferred contour, are shown. *B, Left,* Initial attachment of patch is the same as for any posterior high VSD. *Middle* and *right,* later steps in attachment of patch. (From McGoon, D. C.: Intraventricular repair of transposition of the great arteries. J. Thorac. Cardiovasc. Surg., *64*:430, 1972.)

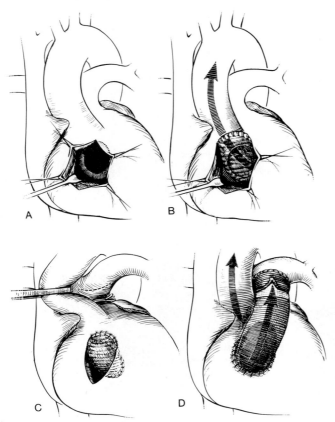

Figure 43–16. *A*, The right ventricle is incised with due regard for the position of the VSD, the distribution of the coronary arteries, and the desired placing of the conduit. *B*, The VSD is closed with a large patch that extends to cover the aortic root. *C*, The main pulmonary artery is securely ligated or divided and oversewn, and an incision is made near the bifurcation. *D*, The distal end of a valved conduit is sutured to the pulmonary artery bifurcation and the proximal end to the right ventricular incision. (From Trusler, G. A., and Freedom, R. M.: Complete transposition of the great arteries. *In* Arciniegas, E. [ed]: Pediatric Cardiac Surgery. Chicago, Year Book Medical Publishers, 1985.)

with aortic valve or one of the commercially available Dacron tubes with porcine valves is then interposed between the ventricular incision and the distal pulmonary artery. This repair is particularly appropriate in patients in whom the LVOTO cannot be relieved surgically. It requires a VSD that is the same size as the aortic root or at least one that can be enlarged to that size. LeCompte and associates (1982) proposed an alternative to the use of a valved conduit by transposing the distal pulmonary artery anterior to the aorta and with sufficient mobilization that it can be sutured directly to the right ventricle.

In arterial repair, the great arteries are divided and switched and the coronary arteries are transferred to the new aorta. After the first successful arterial repair by Jatene in 1975, this operation was attempted widely although originally with high mortality. Later on, mortality was reduced and continues to decline (Freedom et al, 1981; Yacoub et al, 1980).

It is best suited to patients with TGA with a normal left ventricular outflow tract, low pulmonary vascular resistance, and a left ventricle that is able to generate systemic pressures. Thus, the most appropriate children are those with TGA and VSD in the first 6 months of life before pulmonary vascular resistance increases. In this particular group of children, the results of atrial repair are poorest with relatively high early and late mortality and a high incidence of late problems. There has been increased application of the arterial switch procedure to infants with TGA, IVS, primarily in the newborn. As results improve, this operation is becoming increasingly competitive with atrial repair (Castaneda et al, 1984; Idriss et al, 1988; Quaegebeur et al, 1986). If there is diminished right ventricular function, arterial repair should be considered even in older infants who require preliminary pulmonary artery banding. Early arterial repair may prove the procedure of choice for newborn infants with TGA and a large ductus, a small group that can be difficult to manage by atrial repair.

RESULTS

Early Mortality

The overall early and late results with the Mustard operation at the Hospital for Sick Children, Toronto, are shown in Table 43–1 with this simple classification into four groups and comparing the first decade with the last 14 years. There was a total of 506 patients with 49 early hospital deaths. This early mortality (within 30 days of operation) has gradually decreased for all groups. The results of the Mustard procedure alone are evident in the 345 infants and children with TGA and intact ventricular septum (simple TGA) where the early mortality decreased from 11% in the first group to 0.8% in the last 239 patients (no deaths in 10 years, 170 operations). This finding is shown in Figure 43–17, which provides an actuarial comparison of two groups of patients with simple TGA, an early group repaired from 1963 to 1973, and a more recent group repaired from 1974 to 1985. In the recent group, there is a 5-year and 10-year survival rate of 93.7%. The overall results of the treatment protocol from the time that infants with simple TGA were first admitted to the hospital are shown in Figure 43–18 and include the effect of death related to cardiac catheterization and surgical septectomy as well as the atrial repair. Survival at 1 month, 1 year, 10 years, and 20 years is 95, 90, 83, and 80%, respectively. Mortality is higher in patients with complex TGA. Other surgeons have reported similar results (Arciniegas et al, 1981; Mahoney et al, 1982; Oelert et al, 1977; Piccoli et al, 1981; Stark et al, 1980).

The results reflect changing patterns of treatment. For example, in TGA with VSD, mortality was high initially because most children were operated on at an older age when they had pulmonary hyper-

TABLE 43–1. MUSTARD OPERATION FOR TRANSPOSITION OF THE GREAT ARTERIES

	May 1963—Dec. 1973			Jan. 1974—Dec. 1987		
	No. of Patients	Early Death	Late Death	No. of Patients	Early Death	Late Death
With intact ventricular septum (IVS)	106	11	22	239	2	10
With VSD	35	14	6	39	8	5
VSD + LVOTO	13	6	4	27	0	5
IVS + LVOTO	9	3	1	38	5	3
Total	163	34	33	343	15	23

tension. Mortality was later reduced by preliminary palliation with pulmonary artery banding and surgical septectomy and was decreased further when primary repair in the first 6 months of life became routine. Most infants in this group now have an arterial repair.

Similarly, the mortality for children with transposition with VSD and LVOTO changed when selected cases were treated by Rastelli's procedure. Atrial repair is now kept for those with relatively small VSDs and an obstruction that can be relieved surgically. In this particular subset, there has been no early mortality recently in the authors' series.

The most common causes of early mortality in the whole series were low output myocardial failure (26 patients), pulmonary vascular disease (10 patients), and dysrhythmias (4 patients). Pulmonary vascular disease is now avoided mainly by early repair, but myocardial failure is still the chief cause of death, particularly in infants with complex TGA. Other causes were bleeding (2 patients), other cardiac malformations (4 patients), and miscellaneous causes (3 patients).

Late Mortality

From May 1963 to December 31, 1987, in the authors' series, there were 304 early survivors among whom there were 47 late deaths, which occurred in all groups but more commonly in those with complex TGA. Five-year and 10-year actuarial survival after Mustard repair in patients with simple TGA since 1973 is 93.7% (see Fig. 43–17).

Cardiac failure was the most common cause of death (19 patients), which was likely related in part to the conduct of operation and has been reduced in recent years by improved myocardial protection by using lower temperatures, cardioplegia, shorter periods of myocardial ischemia, and local myocardial cooling. Inexplicable cases of failure still occur and continued refinement of methods of myocardial protection in infants is necessary. Perhaps myocardial

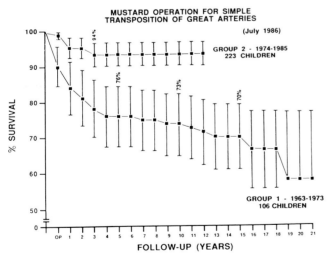

Figure 43–17. Graph comparing actuarial survivors in two groups of patients with simple transposition. Group I patients operated on from 1963 to 1973 had a 5-year and 10-year survival of 75.4 and 73.4%, respectively. However, Group II patients operated on from 1974 to 1985 had a 5-year and 10-year survival of 93.7%. (From Trusler, G. A., et al: Results with the Mustard operation in simple transposition of the great arteries 1963–1985. Ann. Surg., *206*:251, 1987.)

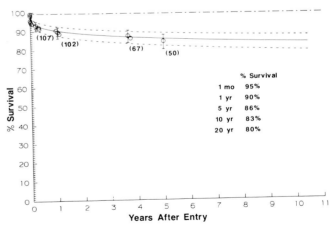

Figure 43–18. Survival after entry of 115 consecutive patients with simple TGA from 1976 to 1985. Each circle represents a death ($n = 16$) positioned along the horizontal axis according to the time of death and actuarially along the vertical axis. The *solid line* is the parametrically determined present survival, and the *dashed lines* are the 70% confidence intervals (limits). The *dashed and dotted line* shows the survival of an age-sex-race-matched general population. (From Williams, W. G., Trusler, G. A., Kirklin, J. W., et al: Early and late results of a protocol for simple transposition leading to an atrial switch [Mustard] repair. J. Thorac. Cardiovasc. Surg., *95*:717, 1988.)

damage can result from low output failure or even dysrhythmias postoperatively.

Dysrhythmia caused death in 11 patients and was the possible cause in another eight patients who died suddenly. Pulmonary venous obstruction was responsible in eight patients, but seldom occurs now. Pulmonary vascular disease was responsible for five late deaths early in the series. Other isolated causes were baffle detachment, congenital respiratory problems, pulmonary venous thrombosis, septicemia, and inferior vena cava obstruction.

Status of Survivors

The quality of life in the surviving children is good and most are asymptomatic. Infants and children grow at a more normal rate and regain their birth-weight percentile after TGA repair, which is considered to be an indication for early repair (Levy et al, 1978; Sholler et al, 1986; Takahashi et al, 1977). Stark and associates (1980) noted that many of their patients achieved a normal working capacity, but, as a group, there was a statistically significant reduction in exercise tolerance when compared with healthy children. They did not find a significant difference between the group of patients repaired in infancy and later. Newberger and associates (1984) found evidence to suggest that postponing repair to an older age was associated with progressive impairment of cognitive function; only 6 of 38 children studied had been repaired when less than 1 year of age.

COMPLICATIONS

Many of the complications of atrial repair for TGA are identical to those after any major cardiac repair. Postoperative bleeding, hemothorax, and cardiac tamponade may occur, particularly if there are pericardial adhesions from earlier palliative procedures, but can be prevented by meticulous hemostasis and maintenance of blood coagulability with appropriate blood clotting factors. Low output cardiac failure may occur after repair, especially in complicated cases, and cause early death or residual impairment of right ventricular contractility. This is likely due to inadequate myocardial protection and can be prevented mainly by the appropriate use of hypothermia and cardioplegia and avoiding prolonged myocardial ischemia. Air embolism is not a common problem if appropriate preventive measures are taken but is a constant danger, and the authors believe that transient and sometimes permanent neurologic problems are seen more often after repair of TGA than other heart malformations.

Phrenic nerve paralysis occurred in approximately 7% of operations, probably from dissection of the large pericardial patch. The incidence of paralysis rose to 10% in the presence of adhesions from pre-

vious palliative surgery (Watanabe et al, 1987). Nerve injury may be related to local mechanical trauma or cautery, particularly superiorly near the level of the great vessels, where the space between the two phrenic nerves is narrower; alternatively, perhaps strong traction on pericardial stay sutures near a phrenic nerve may cause injury.

Baffle Complications

Many complications are related to changes in the atrial partition and it is useful to consider what happens to it after operation. Mohri and associates (1970) found that the partition, regardless of the material used, was soon covered by a layer of fibrin that later fibrosed and formed a neoendocardium that with the underlying graft material, gradually contracted to approximately 50% of its original area. The neoendocardium that formed over Dacron was thicker than over pericardium. They concluded that adequate atrial volume would be maintained by growth of normal atrial wall.

The authors' observations at reoperation and necropsy indicate that baffle shrinkage is limited or restricted by tension, both from sutures and blood flow. Where the pericardium partially encircles a venous orifice, the appropriate channel is maintained if the sutures are secure. If several sutures withdraw, the pericardium contracts between the points of fixation partly obstructing the venous channel and creates a leak between the atrial chambers. When using pericardium, a relatively large patch can be used and the final shape is determined by the relative pressures and flow within the two atria as well as the security and position of the suture line. Soon after insertion, the mobile pericardium, covered by fibrin, may adhere to itself or other raw areas so that a redundant baffle should be avoided and raw areas of atrial wall should be oversewn.

Synthetic materials do not form as easily as pericardium and must be tailored precisely to avoid ridges or narrow channels. Excessive shrinkage or an error in the line of suture is more critical, especially in infants in whom all the venous orifices and channels are smaller, and there is less margin for error. This does not mean that synthetic materials should not be used, but pericardium appears to be safer for repair, particularly in infants.

Although baffle complications are identified fairly frequently, most are mild and have no consequence (Table 43–2). Thirty-three (7.2%) of the 457 children who were early survivors of the Mustard repair were considered to have major complications. A repair was attempted in 24 (5.3%) of the early survivors, and 10 (2.2%) patients died of the baffle complication.

Baffle Leaks. The most common late complication is a leak around the baffle. By December 31, 1987, 201 of 457 early survivors had one or more cardiac catheterizations after the Mustard repair.

TABLE 43–2. BAFFLE COMPLICATIONS*

Total No. of Complications	Total No.	No. of Major Complications	No. of Repairs	No. of Patients Who Died
Baffle leaks	47	7	6	1
SVC stenosis	35	11	5	0
IVC stenosis	6	2	2	1
PV stenosis	13	13	11	8
Total	101	33	24	10

*457 survivors of 201 catheterizations.

Forty-seven of these children had leaks. Fortunately, 39 were small leaks and only 8 were significant, 6 with left-to-right shunts over 1.5:1 and 2 with a right-to-left shunt. Leaks were easily repaired but, when associated with caval obstruction, it was necessary to patch the baffle to relieve the associated venous obstruction.

Superior Vena Cava Obstruction. This obstruction may cause symptoms and signs of increased SVC pressure soon after operation, although many patients are asymptomatic and are only identified at late cardiac catheterization. Occasionally there is persistent bilateral or right-sided pleural effusion or chylothorax, and communicating hydrocephalus has been described (Markowitz et al, 1984; Sweeney et al, 1982). The obstruction usually occurs where the new SVC channel crosses the plane of the atrial septum and may be due to a residual ridge of atrial septum or to flattening of the baffle (Figs. 43–19 and 43–20). If several sutures disengage, the baffle may contract across the caval orifice and cause obstruction. The incidence of SVC stenosis was increased by a change in the authors' technique of atrial septal excision with mild-to-moderate SVC narrowing resulting from the residual ridge of atrial septum between the SVC and the tricuspid valve. This was partly avoided by using a slightly larger and redundant baffle in this area. There have been 35 known cases of SVC stenosis among the 457 early survivors, which is an incidence of 8%. However, it is really not a major problem because only 5 (1% overall) required repair, two in association with baffle leaks. The incidence of SVC obstruction was increased when Dacron was used for the baffle material (Hagler et al, 1978; Kron et al, 1985; Stark et al, 1974).

Wyse and associates (1979) found that the echocardiographic jugular venous flow profile recording was an effective method of screening for SVC obstruction. Two-dimensional echocardiography with Doppler ultrasound or contrast is useful in assessing the status of the SVC pathway (Aziz et al, 1981; Silverman et al, 1981). Campbell and co-workers (1987) found echo-gated magnetic resonance imaging showing dilatation of the SVC and azygos complex were valuable adjuncts to echocardiography.

In most cases, the SVC stenosis has been relieved directly through a median sternotomy incision or a right-sided thoracotomy (Stark, 1983). Patching the narrow area of the baffle may be sufficient, but a more extensive revision may be necessary (e.g., revising the whole SVC end of the baffle and sometimes patching the adjacent wall of the atrium). A number of surgeons have relieved the SVC obstruction by anastomosing the innominate vein to the left atrial appendage either directly (Coulson et al, 1984) or with a graft (Abbruzzese et al, 1984; Danilowicz et al, 1981). Balloon dilatation has been used with some success, but Waldman (1983) found that the stenosis recurred within a few months.

Inferior Vena Cava Obstruction. This obstruction is uncommon. It may occur either at the plane of the atrial septum by the coronary sinus from a tight baffle or at the IVC orifice if several sutures dislodge. Severe obstruction is associated with increased IVC pressure and causes hepatomegaly and ascites or even a low output state. Protein-losing enteropathy has been reported (Kirk et al, 1988; Moodie et al, 1976).

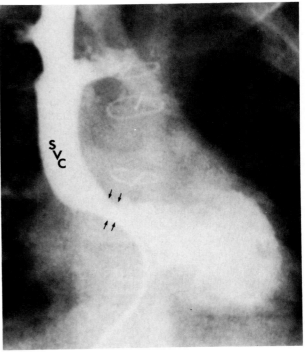

Figure 43–19. Mild narrowing *(arrows)* of the superior limb of the baffle after the Mustard operation. (SVC = superior vena cava.)

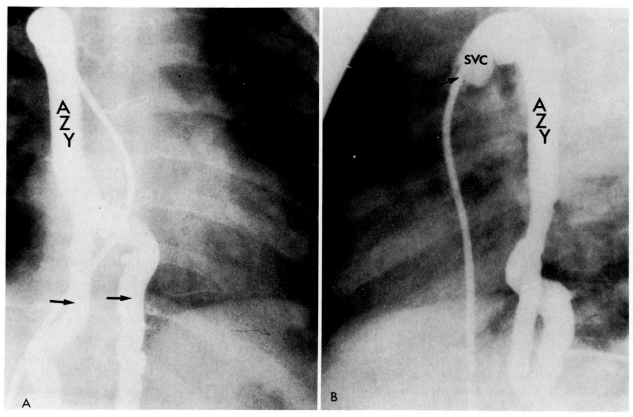

Figure 43–20. *A* and *B,* Severe stenosis of the superior limb of the baffle after the Mustard operation. This asymptomatic patient had paravertebral densities that proved to be venous in origin (Castellino et al, 1968; Polansky and Culham, 1980). Although the SVC could be probed from the venous route, most of the SVC blood passed via large azygos (AZY) and hemiazygos collaterals *(arrows)* and through the inferior limb of the baffle.

IVC obstruction was identified in 6 of the authors' 457 early survivors. In two children, it was associated with a baffle leak that required repair, and in one child the obstruction was identified at autopsy. The other three children are asymptomatic with partial obstruction that has not been repaired. Stark and associates (1974) described an increased incidence of IVC obstruction when Dacron was used as a baffle material in infants. Treatment is similar to SVC obstruction. Reducing the coronary sinus, if not done at the initial repair, may be an important part of the reoperation.

Pulmonary Venous Obstruction. This obstruction is the most serious baffle complication and has caused eight late deaths. There were 13 patients in the 457 early survivors, an incidence of 3%. Seven of the 13 patients had involvement of all four pulmonary veins. The obstruction occurred where the new pulmonary venous channel crossed the plane of the atrial septum, just anterior to the entrance of the right pulmonary veins, and appeared to be due to progressive adherence and fibrous stenosis between the baffle and adjacent margin of residual atrial septum by the right lateral atrial wall. This appears to occur more often if the raw cut margin of the atrial septum is not oversewn, and there is a large redun-

dant baffle that can make contact with the wall of the atrium. Routine patching of the right atrial wall extending down between the two right pulmonary veins or performance of a VY atrioplasty to accomplish this objective has been advocated for prevention of pulmonary venous obstruction (Barratt-Boyes, 1986). These children usually present within 3 to 6 months of operation with respiratory distress and pulmonary edema. Delayed presentation for 10 years after operation has been described (Campbell et al, 1986). Pulsed Doppler echocardiography has proved to be useful in the detection of pulmonary venous obstruction (Smallhorn et al, 1986). If diagnosed early, it can be treated successfully by patching both the baffle and the atrial wall between the two right pulmonary veins. Corno and associates (1987) suggested patching with pericardium in situ to allow for growth. With delayed diagnosis, there is rapid progression of severe pulmonary vascular disease and a high mortality. A high incidence of pulmonary venous obstruction has been found in several series and appears to be more common when repair is done in early infancy and where Dacron is used (Driscoll et al, 1977; Hagler et al, 1978). It has also been described as a result of using bovine pericardium for atrial augmentation (Cochrane et al, 1987).

An uncommon variation that the authors and others (Pappas, 1986) have encountered is isolated obstruction of the left pulmonary venous channel, which appears to result from excessive contraction of the baffle when the upper and lower suture lines between right and left pulmonary veins are brought too close together on the posterior wall of the left atrium. The orifices of the left pulmonary veins may also be involved in the stenosis, thus indicating that the suture line should not venture too close to these orifices. Affected children may present with chronic left pulmonary edema, pleural effusion, or with hemoptysis. Pulsed Doppler echocardiography is useful for diagnosis and, on angiocardiography, there is a sharp reduction in pulmonary blood flow to the left lung. Repair, which requires patching of both the posterior left atrial wall and the baffle itself at the site of obstruction, is often unsatisfactory because of the frequently associated stenosis of the left pulmonary venous orifices that is difficult to relieve.

Other Complications. Some degree of LVOTO appears to be common in children with TGA (Gomes et al, 1980; Idriss et al, 1977; Vidne et al, 1976). A pressure gradient of 10 mm Hg or more across the left ventricular outflow tract was identified in 54 children in the authors' series. Most stenoses were minor and due to bulging of the muscular septum into the outflow tract; only 20 had gradients over 25 mm Hg. Although some represented residual obstruction incompletely relieved by operation, the majority were children who were considered to have uncomplicated TGA. Fortunately, only one child has required operative intervention.

Other complications that have been identified include small persistent VSDs. Most of these are small defects that were recognized originally but were not treated because they had no physiologic significance. Pulmonary vascular disease of moderate or severe degree occurs in a few children after repair, some secondary to pulmonary problems and others without obvious cause. Mitral incompetence has developed in some children.

Dysrhythmias

Dysrhythmia is a relatively common and potentially serious complication that follows the Mustard operation due to the wide excision of the atrial septum and the long atrial suture line. It is generally accepted now that most dysrhythmias are due to interference with function of the SA node either directly or from injury to the SA node artery (El-Said et al, 1976; Gillette et al, 1980). Preservation of the node and its artery is an important principle of any operation (Rossi et al, 1986). The significance of obliterating or excising the pathways of impulse transmission from SA node to atrioventricular node is less clear, but it is possible that preservation of at least one pathway for internodal conduction is important.

There was a relatively high incidence of dysrhythmia in the early series, and some dysrhythmias were responsible for both early and late deaths, including a number of sudden unexpected deaths that were probably due to this cause. Temporary atrial and ventricular pacemaker wires were inserted routinely at operation and monitored carefully to maintain sinus rhythm and avoid serious dysrhythmias that are common for a few days after operation.

In recent years, with knowledge of the problem and attention to detail, the incidence of dysrhythmias is lower and most children remain in sinus rhythm (Lincoln and Southall, 1983). Since 1973, 92% of children with simple TGA who had a Mustard operation in Toronto were in sinus rhythm when discharged from the hospital. Of 180 patients available for review, 71.7% were still in sinus rhythm by last electrocardiogram whereas 18.3% showed junctional rhythm, 3.3% had sick sinus syndrome, 3.9% had a wandering pacemaker, 1.7% had atrial flutter, and 1.1% had SA-atrioventricular dysfunction (Trusler et al, 1987). Three children required pacemakers. These results were an improvement over the experience in the first 10 years.

The true incidence of abnormal rhythm, however, can be identified only by exercise studies and 24-hour monitoring. In the authors' experience with Holter recordings after Mustard repair in 126 patients, although sinus rhythm was observed in 90.5%, the predominant cardiac rhythm was a junctional bradycardia or atrial flutter. Multicatheter electrophysiologic studies an average of 52.5 months after operation showed frequent suppression of sinus node function and sometimes subtle abnormalities of AV node function.

In 23 children, electrophysiologic studies (EPS) were done preoperatively and on 1, 3 and 8 days postoperatively. Abnormal studies were frequent after the Mustard operation, and the incidence of abnormalities was similar to that of the patients studied for an average of 52.5 months after operation, which thus suggested that the conduction system abnormalities could be detected early after operation even if clinical manifestations appear later. This then differs slightly from the reports of several authors who suggest that the incidence of dysrhythmia increases with time (Duster et al, 1985; Flinn et al, 1984; Hayes and Gersony, 1986).

Bierman and associates (1983) in a series that included complex TGA reported only 30% of patients free of arrhythmias 9 years after repair, but symptoms from rhythm or conduction disturbances were rare. In the authors' experience only about one-quarter of children with abnormal rhythms are symptomatic.

Right Ventricular Dysfunction

Of greater significance is the recognition of some diminution of right ventricular contractility. In the authors' patients, this is a subjective assessment by the radiologist or the cardiologist, mainly from the angiocardiogram but also by echocardiography, and was recognized in 66 (33%) children at follow-up cardiac catheterization. Although most are mild changes, 11% of children with simple TGA show a definite decrease in function. Some children also have a degree, usually mild, of tricuspid incompetence and occasionally the incompetence occurs alone. A few of these children died later from cardiac failure usually within 4 years of operation and have been discussed as late deaths. Progressive right ventricular failure beyond 4 years postoperatively is uncommon. The incidence of right ventricular dysfunction is higher in the complicated forms of transposition where there is repair of a VSD. A reduction of right ventricular contractility at cardiac catheterization was found in 43 (29%) of 147 children with simple transposition and 17 (68%) of 25 children who also had a VSD repair. The incidence of accompanying tricuspid incompetence was higher in the latter group and suggests that the VSD repair may lead to tricuspid incompetence in some patients. In other patients, the incompetence may be related to pre-existing valve abnormalities, arrhythmia, or more commonly right ventricular dysfunction itself (Deal et al, 1985; Huhta et al, 1982; Smith et al, 1986).

There have been many studies of right ventricular function after atrial repair of TGA, and the ultimate significance is still not clear. Abnormal size and ejection fraction of the right ventricle after atrial repair were noted (Graham et al, 1975; Hagler et al, 1979; Jarmakani et al, 1974). By using gated equilibrium nuclear angiography, Benson and associates (1982) evaluated the right ventricular function response to the stress of supine bicycle exercise an average of 6.4 years after the Mustard operation. Although clinically well, 11 of 19 children had an abnormal response with a decrease or at least no increase in right ventricular ejection fraction. Similar results were obtained by others (Baker et al, 1986; Borow et al, 1981; Murphy et al, 1986). Parrish and associates (1983) also noted an abnormal left ventricular response to exercise in 10 of 11 children tested after a Mustard repair and concluded that biventricular dysfunction was frequently present. In each study, some children had normal right ventricular function at rest and during exercise, which suggests that the right ventricular problem may not be inevitable. Benson and associates (1986) reported normal systemic ventricular function in patients with congenitally corrected TGA. Ramsay and associates (1984) found an abnormal response to exercise by both right ventricle and left ventricle after Mustard repair but found no predictable correlation with clinical or hemodynamic criteria. Graham and co-workers (1985), comparing groups of patients after atrial repair of simple TGA, found an improvement in the postoperative right ventricular ejection fraction in patients operated on after 1974, whether by Mustard or Senning technique, compared with patients op-

erated on earlier. They suggest that this improvement may be due to a younger age at operation or changes in operative technique, particularly myocardial protection. Smith and associates (1986), however, warn that the general architecture of the ventricular mass and the atrioventricular valves is different from normal and the function of the normal heart may not always be an appropriate yardstick for comparison.

Likely, some of the right ventricular problems originate at operation, and the right ventricle in transposition is more susceptible to ischemic damage than the left ventricle in a normal heart. Every effort should be made to protect the myocardium during repair. Low output failure postoperatively and dysrhythmias may harm the myocardium and should be avoided if possible. Some cases of poor right ventricular function, however, occur in children who appear to have had a good operation and postoperative course, thus causing concern about the long-term fate of the right ventricle in transposition.

In the presence of severe right ventricular failure, Mee (1986) converted the Mustard atrial repair to an arterial switch repair. The pulmonary artery is banded as an initial first stage to prepare the left ventricle for systemic arterial pressures. Of four patients banded, two have had successful switches with promising improvement.

Clinical Status

Despite the threat of serious late problems, such as dysrhythmias and right ventricular dysfunction, most children are well. In the infants and children with simple TGA operated on from May 1963 to December 1985, late follow-up indicated that 76% were in NYHA Class I and 24% in NYHA Class II. No children were in Classes III or IV. Only 21% were taking medication, which was almost all for management of dysrhythmias. Most of the children were unrestricted in their activities and some children participated in athletic events. Stark and associates (1980) found that exercise performance of asymptomatic patients who appeared to be living normal lives 6 to 13 years after the Mustard operation were slightly diminished compared with a group of normal children, and this finding has also been shown by cardiopulmonary exercise testing (Mathews et al, 1983).

Senning Operation

In an attempt to reduce the incidence of complications, many surgeons have changed from the Mustard repair to the Senning repair. The Senning operation uses flaps of atrial wall to divert venous return, and because there is no pericardial baffle, there is less nonliving tissue and the new atrial walls have a greater potential for contraction and growth (Bjornstad et al, 1984). Where growth is most important, such as in infants less than 2 months old, there is likely to be an advantage to the Senning procedure with less chance of caval obstruction. When a high incidence of obstruction occurred, it was often related to the use of Dacron for the baffle (Cobanoglu et al, 1984). However, most complications that may occur after the Mustard operation have occurred after the Senning procedure, and the incidence in most series of Senning procedures is similar to the authors' experience with the Mustard repair (Bender et al, 1980). In addition, there is some suggestion that early and late actuarial survival is better with the Mustard operation (Castaneda et al, 1988).

In complex TGA, other procedures are preferred in many patients, the Rastelli operation for children with a large VSD and severe LVOTO, and arterial repair for infants with associated large VSDs. In simple TGA, the largest group of patients, however, the current decision is between some form of atrial repair and the arterial switch repair. Although this question must still be resolved, the authors, like many other surgical groups, have for the time being adopted a protocol involving arterial repair for neonates with simple TGA. As a result, whereas 10 years ago approximately 25 Mustard operations were done each year, in 1987 only 5 operations were done. This emphasizes that there are still patients who require atrial repair. The early mortality for the Mustard repair is now almost zero; however, there are some complications, such as a definite incidence of dysrhythmia and a danger of late right ventricular dysfunction. The mortality for arterial repair is higher although it is gradually decreasing. Complications requiring reoperation are more frequent than with the atrial repair, but the late results at this time show promise of being better with normal rhythm and ventricular function. Continuous appraisal is necessary, and continued improvement is expected.

mine the effect on cardiac rhythm. Mean resting heart rates were consistently lower than in age-matched normal children. Normal sinus rhythm was present in 76% at 1 year and 57% by the end of the eighth postoperative year. Twenty-five patients died during the follow-up period, 9 of whom died suddenly.

Although survival was good, 91% for 11 years and 71% for 15 years, over time there was a decreased prevalence of normal sinus rhythm as well as a small risk of sudden death.

Graham, T. P., Burger, J., Bender, H. W., et al: Improved right ventricular function after intra-atrial repair of transposition of the great arteries. Circulation, *72*:II-45, 1985.

This report is an extension of Graham's earlier studies evaluating right ventricular function after atrial repair and compares 32 patients after a Senning operation with 26 patients after a Mustard procedure. The authors documented a decrease in right ventricular ejection fraction after both procedures. Of particular interest was the observation that right ventricular performance was significantly better in both the Senning group and the later Mustard group (1975 to 1978) than in the earlier Mustard patients (1971 to 1974). They speculated that this resulted from a younger age at operation, better preoperative function, and, possibly, improved intraoperative myocardial protection. They also suggested that the earlier evidence indicating severe right ventricular dysfunction may not be a valid reason for the use of the arterial switch operation in patients with simple transposition.

Trusler, G. A., Williams, W. G., Duncan, K. F., et al: Results with the Mustard operation in simple transposition of the great arteries. Ann. Surg., *206*:251, 1987.

This is a review of the Toronto experience with the Mustard operation for simple TGA. For comparison, patients were divided into two groups—those operated on in the first decade (Group I, 1963 to 1973) and those repaired later (Group II, 1974 to 1985). Both early and late mortality were reduced significantly in the later group of patients with a 10-year actuarial survival rate of 93.7%. Major baffle complications, similar in both groups, occurred in 5.8%. Poor right ventricular function was identified in only 11% of survivors. By latest electrocardiogram, sinus rhythm appeared to be more prevalent in the second group but late ambulatory electrocardiography revealed that most patients had sinus node dysfunction or other dysrhythmias. Despite this, most patients were clinically well, and only 21% required cardiac medication. Both early and late results are encouraging and it must still be seen whether the overall results with arterial repair are better.

Selected Bibliography

Castaneda, A. R., Trusler, G. A., Paul, M. H., et al: The early results of treatment of simple transposition in the current era. J. Thorac. Cardiovasc. Surg., *95*:14, 1988.

This report is of a 20-institution study of 187 neonates with simple TGA, all of whom initially enter the study when they are less than 15 days old. Results with the Mustard, Senning, and arterial switch procedures are compared. The age at operation varied. The arterial switch was done earlier than either atrial repair. Overall survival rate was 81% at 1 year. The only risk factors for death were birth weight, date of entry in the study, and an arterial switch protocol in the group of institutions at high risk for arterial switch repair. The preliminary data suggested that the early (1-year) survival after the Mustard operation was better than either the Senning or arterial switch procedures.

Flinn, C. J., Wolff, G. S., Dick, M. II, et al: Cardiac rhythm after the Mustard operation for complete transposition of the great arteries. N. Engl. J. Med., *310*:1635, 1984.

In this multi-institutional review from eight pediatric cardiac centers, 372 patients, who survived a Mustard operation for repair of TGA, were followed for 0.4 to 15.9 (mean-4.5) years to deter-

Bibliography

Abbruzzese, P. S., Issenberg, H., Cobanoglu, A., et al: Superior vena cava obstruction after Mustard repair of d-transposition of the great arteries. Scan. J. Thorac. Cardiovasc. Surg., *18*:5, 1984.

Albert, H. M.: Surgical correction of transposition of the great vessels. Surg. Forum, *5*:74, 1955.

Arciniegas, E., Farooki, A. Q., Hakimi, M., et al: Results of the Mustard operation for dextro-transposition of the great arteries. J. Thorac. Cardiovasc. Surg., *81*:580, 1981.

Aziz, K. U., Paul, M. H., Bharati, S., et al: Two dimensional echocardiographic evaluation of Mustard operation for d-transposition of the great arteries. Am. J. Cardiol., *47*:654, 1981.

Aziz, R. U., Paul, M. H., Idriss, F. S., et al: Clinical manifestations of dynamic left ventricular outflow tract stenosis in infants with d-transposition of the great arteries with intact ventricular septum. Am. J. Cardiol., *44*:290, 1979.

Aziz, R. U., Paul, M. H., and Muster, A. J.: Echocardiographic assessment of left ventricular outflow tract in d-transposition of the great arteries. Am. J. Cardiol., *41*:543, 1978.

Baffes, T. G.: A new method for surgical correction of transposition of the aorta and pulmonary artery. Surg. Gynecol. Obstet., *102*:227, 1956.

Baffes, T. G., Ketola, F. H., and Tatooles, C. J.: Transfer of coronary ostia by "triangulation" in transposition of the great vessels and anomalous coronary arteries: A preliminary report. Dis. Chest, 39:648, 1961.

Bailey, C. P., Cookson, B. A., Downing, D. F., and Neptune, W. B.: Cardiac surgery under hypothermia. J. Thorac. Surg., 27:73, 1954.

Bailey, L. L., Jacobson, J. G., Merritt, M. H., et al: Mustard operation in the first month of life. Am. J. Cardiol., 49:766, 1982.

Baillie, M.: The Morbid Anatomy of Some of the Important Parts of the Human Body. London, Johnson and Nicol, 1797, p. 38.

Baker, E. J., Shubao, C., Clarke, S. E., et al: Radionuclide measurement of right ventricular function in atrial septal defect, ventricular septal defect and complete transposition of the great arteries. Am. J. Cardiol., 57:1142, 1986.

Bano-Rodrigo, A., Quero-Jiminez, M., Moreno-Granado, F., and Gamallo-Amat, C.: Wall thickness of ventricular chamber in transposition of the great arteries: Surgical implications. J. Thorac. Cardiovasc. Surg., 79:592, 1980.

Barcia, A., Kincaid, O. W., Davis, G. D., et al: Transposition of the great arteries: An angiocardiographic study. Am. J. Roentgenol., 100:249, 1967.

Bargeron, L. M., Jr., Elliott, L. P., Soto, B., et al: Axial cineangiography in congenital heart disease. I: Concept, technical and anatomical considerations. Circulation, 56:1075, 1977.

Barnard, C. N., Schrire, V., and Beck, W.: Complete transposition of the great vessels: A successful complete correction. J. Thorac. Cardiovasc. Surg., 43:768, 1962.

Barratt-Boyes, B. G.: Complete transposition of the great arteries. In Kirklin, J. W., and Barratt-Boyes, B. G. (eds): Cardiac Surgery. New York, John Wiley & Sons Inc., 1986, p. 1129.

Bender, H. W., Jr., Graham, T. P., Jr., Boucek, R. J., Jr., et al: Comparative operative results of the Senning and Mustard procedures for transposition of the great arteries. Circulation, 62:1197, 1980.

Benson, L. N., Bonet, J., McLaughlin, P., et al: Assessment of right ventricular function during supine bicycle exercise after Mustard's operation. Circulation, 65:1052, 1982.

Benson, L. N., Burns, R., Schwaiger, M., et al: Radionuclide angiographic evaluation of ventricular function in isolated congenitally corrected transposition of the great arteries. Am. J. Cardiol., 58:319, 1986.

Benson, L. N., Olley, P. M., Patel, R. G., et al: Role of prostaglandin E1 infusion in the management of transposition of the great arteries. Am. J. Cardiol., 44:691, 1979.

Bierman, F. Z., and Williams, R. G.: Prospective diagnosis of d-transposition of the great arteries in neonates by subxiphoid two-dimensional echocardiography. Circulation, 60:1496, 1979b.

Bierman, F. Z., and Williams, R. G.: Subxiphoid two-dimensional imaging of the interatrial septum in infants and neonates with congenital heart disease. Circulation, 60:80, 1979a.

Bierman, L. B., Neches, W. H., Fricker, F. J., et al: Arrhythmias in transposition of the great arteries after the operation. Am. J. Cardiol., 51:1530, 1983.

Bjork, V. O., and Bouckaert, L.: Complete transposition of the aorta and the pulmonary artery: An experimental study of the surgical possibilities for its treatment. J. Thorac. Surg., 28:632, 1954.

Bjornstad, P. G., Tjonnedland, S., and Semb, B. K. H.: Echocardiographic evaluation of atrial function after Senning and Mustard correction for transposition of the great arteries. Thorax, 39:114, 1984.

Blalock, A., and Hanlon, C. R.: The surgical treatment of complete transposition of the aorta and the pulmonary artery. Surg. Gynecol. Obstet., 90:1, 1950.

Borow, K. M., Keane, J. F., Castaneda, A. R., and Freed, M. D.: Systemic ventricular function in patients with tetralogy of Fallot, ventricular septal defect and transposition of the great arteries repaired during infancy. Circulation, 64:878, 1981.

Brom, G. A.: Technique of Mustard operation. In Hahn, C. (ed): Thorax Chirurgie, Leiden 1950–75. Leiden, Netherlands Drukkerij Bedrijf BC, 1975.

Byrne, J., Clarke, D., Taylor, J. F. N., et al: Treatment of patients with transposition of the great arteries and pulmonary vascular obstructive disease. Br. Heart J., 40:221, 1978.

Campbell, R. M., Moreau, G. A., Graham, T. P., Jr., and Bender, H. W.: Symptomatic pulmonary venous obstruction in adolescence after Mustard's repair of transposition in infancy. Am. J. Cardiol., 59:1218, 1987.

Campbell, R. M., Moreau, G. A., Johns, J. A., et al: Detection of caval obstruction by magnetic resonance imaging after intra-atrial repair of transposition of the great arteries. Am. J. Cardiol., 60:688, 1987.

Castaneda, A. R., Norwood, W. I., Jonas, R. A., et al: Transposition of the great arteries and intact ventricular septum: Anatomical repair in the neonate. Ann. Thorac. Surg., 38:438, 1984.

Castaneda, A. R., Trusler, G. A., Paul, M. H., et al: The early results of treatment of simple transposition in the current era. J. Thorac. Cardiovasc. Surg., 95:14, 1988.

Castellino, R. A., Blank, N., and Adams, D. F.: Dilated azygos and hemiazygos veins presenting as paravertebral intrathoracic masses. N. Engl. J. Med., 278:1087, 1968.

Chiu, I. S., Anderson, R. H., Macartney, F. J., et al: Morphologic features of an intact ventricular septum susceptible to subpulmonary obstruction in complete transposition of the great arteries. Am. J. Cardiol., 53:1633, 1984.

Clark, E. B., Sweeny, L. J., and Rosenquist, G. C.: Atrial defect size after Blalock-Hanlon atrioseptectomy. Am. J. Cardiol., 40:405, 1977.

Cobanoglu, A., Abbruzzese, P. A., Freimanis, I., et al: Pericardial baffle complications following the Mustard operation. J. Thorac. Cardiovasc. Surg., 87:371, 1984.

Coceani, F., and Olley, P. M.: The response of the ductus arteriosus in prostaglandins. Can. J. Physiol. Pharmacol., 51:220, 1973.

Cochrane, R. P., and McGough, E. C.: Bovine pericardium: A source of pulmonary venous obstruction in the Mustard procedure. Ann. Thorac. Surg., 44:552, 1987.

Corno, A. F., Laks, H., George, B., and Williams, R. G.: Use of in-situ pericardium for surgical relief of pulmonary venous obstruction following Mustard's operation. Ann. Thorac. Surg., 43:443, 1987.

Coulson, J. D., Pitlick, P. T., Miller, C., et al: Severe superior vena caval syndrome and hydrocephalus after the Mustard procedure: Findings and a new surgical approach. Circulation, 70:I-47, 1984.

Counahan, R., Simon, G., and Joseph, M.: The plain chest radiograph in d-transposition of the great arteries in the first month of life. Pediatr. Radiol., 1:217, 1973.

Creech, O., Jr., Mahaffey, D. E., Sayegh, S. F., and Sailors, E. L.: Complete transposition of the great vessels: A technique for intracardiac correction. Surgery, 43:349, 1958.

Crupi, G., Pillai, R., Parenzan, L., and Lincoln, C.: Surgical treatment of subpulmonary obstruction in transposition of the great arteries by means of a left ventricular-pulmonary arterial conduit. J. Thorac. Cardiovasc. Surg., 89:907, 1985.

Danilowicz, D., Isom, A. W., and Whiddon, L.: Superior vena caval syndrome after Mustard repair: Surgical decompression using a saphenous vein homograft. Am. Heart J., 101:862, 1981.

Deal, B. J., Chin, A. J., Sanders, S. P., et al: Subxiphoid two-dimensional echocardiographic identification of tricuspid valve abnormalities in transposition of the great arteries with ventricular septal defect. Am. J. Cardiol., 55:1146, 1985.

de Leval, M. R., McKay, R., Jones, M., et al: Modified Blalock-Taussig shunt. J. Thorac. Cardiovasc. Surg., 81:112, 1981.

Deutsch, V., Shem-Tov, A., Yahini, J. H., and Neufeld, H. N.: Cardioangiographic evaluation of the relationship between atrioventricular and semilunar valves: Its diagnostic importance in congenital heart disease. Am. J. Roentgenol., 110:474, 1970.

Driscoll, D. J., Kugler, J. D., Nihill, M. R., and McNanara, D. G.: The use of prostaglandin E1 in a critically ill infant with transposition of the great arteries. J. Pediatr., 95:259, 1979.

Driscoll, D. J., Nihill, M. R., Vargo, T. A., et al: Late development of pulmonary venous obstruction following Mustard's operation using a Dacron baffle. Circulation, 55:484, 1977.

Duster, M. C., Bink-Boelkens, M. T. E., Wampler, D., et al: Long term followup of dysrhythmias following the Mustard procedure. Am. Heart J., *109*:1323, 1985.

Edwards, W. S., Bargeron, L. M., Jr., and Lyons, C.: Reposition of right pulmonary veins in transposition of the great vessels. J.A.M.A., *188*:522, 1964.

Elliott, L. P., Bargeron, L. M., Jr., Bream, P. R., et al: Axial cineangiography in congenital heart disease. II: Specific lesions. Circulation, *56*:1084, 1977.

El-Said, G. M., Gillette, P. C., Cooley, D. A., et al: Protection of the sinus node in Mustard's operation. Circulation, *53*:788, 1976.

Fisher, E. H. R., Muster, A. J., Lev, M., and Paul, M. H.: Angiocardiographic and anatomic findings in transposition of the great arteries with left ventricular outflow tract gradients. Am. J. Cardiol., *25*:95, 1970.

Flinn, C. J., Wolff, G. S., Dick, M. II, et al: Cardiac rhythm after Mustard operation for complete transposition of the great arteries. N. Engl. J. Med., *310*:1635, 1984.

Freedom, R. M., Culham, J. A. G., Olley, P. M., et al: Anatomic correction of transposition of the great arteries: Preoperative and postoperative cardiac catheterization with angiocardiography in 5 patients. Circulation, *63*:905, 1981.

Freedom, R. M., Culham, G., and Rowe, R. D.: The criss-cross and supero-inferior ventricular heart: An angiocardiographic study. Am. J. Cardiol., *42*:620, 1978.

Freedom, R. M., Harrington, D. P., and White, R. I., Jr.: The differential diagnosis of levo-transposed or malposed aorta: An angiocardiographic study. Circulation, *50*:1040, 1974.

Fyler, D. C.: Report of the New England Regional Infant Cardiac Program. Pediatrics, *65*(Suppl):422, 1980.

Gillette, P. C., Kugler, J. D., Garson, A., Jr., et al: Mechanisms of cardiac arrhythmias after the Mustard operation for transposition of the great arteries. Am. J. Cardiol., *45*:1225, 1980.

Gingell, R. L., Freedom, R. M., Hawker, R. E., et al: Indicator dilution curves in the diagnosis of d-transposition of the great arteries in infancy. Cathet. Cardiovasc. Diagn., *5*:119, 1979.

Goldman, H. E., Maralit, A., Sun, S., and Lanzkowsky, P.: Neonatal cyanosis and arterial oxygen saturation. J. Pediatr., *82*:319, 1973.

Gomes, A. S., Nath, P. H., Singh, A., et al: Accessory flaplike tissue causing ventricular outflow obstruction. J. Thorac. Cardiovasc. Surg., *80*:211, 1980.

Graham, T. P., Jr., Atwood, G. F., Boucek, R. J., Jr., et al: Abnormalities of right ventricular function following Mustard's operation for transposition of the great arteries. Circulation, *52*:678, 1975.

Graham, T. P., Jr., Burger, J., Bender, H. W., et al: Improved right ventricular function after intra-atrial repair of transposition of the great arteries. Circulation, *72*:II–45, 1985.

Guerin, R., Soto, B., Karp, R. B., et al: Transposition of the great arteries: Determination of the position of the great arteries in conventional chest roentgenograms. Am. J. Roentgenol., *110*:747, 1970.

Gutgesell, H. P., Garson, A., and McNamara, D. G.: Prognosis for the newborn with transposition of the great arteries. Am. J. Cardiol., *44*:96, 1979.

Hagler, D. J., Ritter, D. G., Mair, D. D., et al: Clinical angiographic and hemodynamic assessment of late results after Mustard operation. Circulation, *57*:1214, 1978.

Hagler, D. J., Ritter, D. G., Mair, D. D., et al: Right and left ventricular function after the Mustard procedure in transposition of the great arteries. Am. J. Cardiol., *44*:276, 1979.

Hayes, C. J., and Gersony, W. M.: Arrhythmias after the Mustard operation for transposition of the great arteries: A long-term study. J. Am. Coll. Cardiol., *7*:133, 1986.

Henry, C. G., Goldring, D., Hartman, A. F., et al: Treatment of d-transposition of the great arteries: Management of hypoxemia after balloon atrial septostomy. Am. J. Cardiol., *47*:299, 1981.

Houston, A. B., Gregory, N. L., and Coleman, E. N.: Echocardiographic identification of aorta and main pulmonary artery in complete transposition. Br. Heart J., *40*:377, 1978.

Huhta, J. C., Edwards, W. D., Danielson, G. K., and Feldt, R. H.: Abnormalities of the tricuspid valve in complete trans-position of the great arteries with ventricular septal defect. J. Thorac. Cardiovasc. Surg., *83*:569, 1982.

Idriss, F. S., DeLeon, S. Y., Nikaidoh, H., et al: Resection of left ventricular outflow obstruction in d-transposition of the great arteries. J. Thorac. Cardiovasc. Surg., *74*:343, 1977.

Idriss, F. S., Goldstein, I. R., Grana, L., et al: A new technique for complete correction of transposition of the great vessels: An experimental study with a preliminary clinical report. Circulation, *24*:5, 1961.

Idriss, F. S., Ilbawi, M. N., DeLeon, S. Y., et al: Arterial switch in simple and complex transposition of the great arteries. J. Thorac. Cardiovasc. Surg., *95*:29, 1988.

Jarmakani, J. M. M., and Canent, R. V., Jr.: Preoperative and postoperative right ventricular function in children with transposition of the great vessels. Circulation, *49,50*:II–39, 1974.

Jatene, A. D., Fontes, V. F., Paulista, P. P., et al: Anatomic correction of transposition of the great vessels. J. Thorac. Cardiovasc. Surg., *72*:364, 1976.

Jatene, A. D., Fontes, V. F., Paulista, P. P., et al: Successful anatomic correction of transposition of the great vessels: A preliminary report. Arq. Bras. Cardiol., *28*:461, 1975.

Jiminez, M. Q., and Martinez, V. P.: Uncommon conal pathology in complete dextro-transposition of the great arteries with ventricular septal defect. Chest, *66*:411, 1974.

Jones, R. W. A., Baumer, J. H., Joseph, M. C., and Shinebourne, E. A.: Arterial oxygen tension and response to oxygen breathing in differential diagnosis of congenital heart disease in infancy. Arch. Dis. Child., *51*:667, 1976.

Kay, E. B., and Cross, F. S.: Surgical treatment of transposition of the great vessels. Surgery, *38*:712, 1955.

Kay, E. B., and Cross, F. S.: Transposition of the great vessels corrected by means of atrial transposition. Surgery, *41*:938, 1957.

Kelly, D. T., Krovetz, L. J., and Rowe, R. D.: Double-lumen flotation catheter for use in complex congenital cardiac anomalies. Circulation, *44*:910, 1971.

Kirk, C. R., Gibbs, J. L., Wilkinson, J. L., et al: Protein losing enteropathy caused by baffle obstruction after Mustard's operation. Br. Heart J., *59*:69, 1988.

Kirklin, J. W., Devloo, R. A., and Weidman, W. H.: Open intracardiac repair for transposition of the great vessels: 11 cases. Surgery, *50*:58, 1961.

Korns, M. E., Garabedian, H. A., and Lauer, R. M.: Anatomic limitation of balloon atrial septostomy. Hum. Pathol., *3*:345, 1972.

Kron, I. L., Rheuban, K. S., Joob, A. W., et al: Baffle obstruction following the Mustard operation: Cause and treatment. Ann. Thorac. Surg., *39*:112, 1985.

Kurlander, G. J., Petry, E. L., and Girod, D. A.: Plain film diagnosis of congenital heart disease in the newborn period. Am. J. Roentgenol., *103*:66, 1968.

Kurosawa, S., Kurosawa, H., and Becker, A. E.: The coronary arterioles in newborns, infants and children: A morphometric study of normal hearts and heart with aortic atresia and complete transposition. Int. J. Cardiol., *10*:43, 1986.

Lakier, J. B., Stanger, P., Heymann, M. A., et al: Early onset of pulmonary vascular obstruction in patients with aortopulmonary transposition and intact ventricular septum. Circulation, *51*:875, 1975.

Landtman, B., Louhimo, I., Rapola, J., and Tuuteri, L.: Causes of death in transposition of the great arteries: A clinical and autopsy study of 140 cases. Acta Paediatr. Scand., *64*:785, 1975.

Lang, P., Freed, M. D., Bierman, F. Z., et al: Use of prostaglandin E1 in infants with d-transposition of the great arteries and intact ventricular septum. Am. J. Cardiol., *44*:76, 1979.

Layman, T. E., and Edwards, J. E.: Anomalies of the cardiac valves associated with complete transposition of the great vessels. Am. J. Cardiol. *19*:247, 1967.

LeCompte, Y., Neveau, J. Y., Leca, F., et al: Reconstruction of the pulmonary outflow tract without prosthetic conduit. J. Thorac. Cardiovasc. Surg., *84*:727, 1982.

Levy, R. J., Rosenthal, A., Castaneda, A. R., and Nadas, N. S.: Growth after surgical repair of simple d-transposition of the great arteries. Ann. Thorac. Surg., *25*:225, 1978.

Liebman, J., Cullum, L., and Belloc, N. B.: Natural history of transposition of the great arteries: Anatomy and birth and death characteristics. Circulation, 40:237, 1969.

Lillehei, C. W., and Varco, R. L.: Certain physiologic, pathologic and surgical features of complete transposition of the great vessels. Surgery, 34:376, 1953.

Lincoln, C. R., and Southall, D.: Cardiac rhythm and conduction before and after Mustard's operation for complete transposition of the great arteries. Pediatr. Cardiol., 4:165, 1983.

Lindesmith, G. G., Stiles, Q. R., Tucker, B. L., et al: The Mustard operation as a palliative procedure. J. Thorac. Cardiovasc. Surg., 64:75, 1972.

Mahoney, J., Turley, K., Ebert, P., and Heymann, M. A.: Long term results after atrial repair of transposition of the great arteries in early infancy. Circulation, 66:253, 1982.

Markowitz, R. I., Kleinman, C. S., Hellenbrand, W. E., et al: Communicating hydrocephalus secondary to superior vena caval obstruction. Am. J. Dis. Child, 138:638, 1984.

Mathew, R., Rosenthal, A., and Fellows, K.: The significance of the right aortic arch in d-transposition of the great arteries. Am. Heart J., 87:314, 1974.

Mathews, R. A., Fricker, F. J., Beerman, L. B., et al: Exercise studies after the Mustard operation in transposition of the great arteries. Am. J. Cardiol., 51:1526, 1983.

McGarry, K. M., Taylor, J. F. N., and Macartney, F. J.: Aortic atresia occurring with complete transposition of the great arteries. Br. Heart J., 44:711, 1980.

McGoon, D. C.: Intraventricular repair of transposition of the great arteries. J. Thorac. Cardiovasc. Surg., 64:430, 1972.

Mee, R. B. B.: Severe right ventricular failure after Mustard or Senning operation. J. Thorac. Cardiovasc. Surg., 92:385, 1986.

Merendino, K. A., Jesseph, J. E., Herron, P. W., et al: Interatrial venous transposition—a one stage intracardiac operation for the conversion of complete transposition of the aorta and pulmonary artery to corrected transposition: Theory and clinical experience. Surgery, 42:898, 1957.

Moene, R. J., Oppenheimer-Dekker, A., and Bartelings, M. M.: Anatomic obstruction of the right ventricular outflow tract in transposition of the great arteries. Am. J. Cardiol., 51:1701, 1983.

Moene, R. J., Oppenheimer-Dekker, A., Bartelings, M. M., et al: Morphology of ventricular septal defect in complete transposition of the great arteries. Am. J. Cardiol., 55:1566, 1985.

Moene, R. J., Oppenheimer-Dekker, A., Bartelings, M. M., et al: Ventricular septal defect with normally connected great arteries and with transposed great arteries. Am. J. Cardiol., 58:627, 1986.

Moes, C. A. F.: Analysis of the chest in the neonate with congenital heart disease. Radiol. Clin. North Am., 13:251, 1975.

Mohri, H., Barnes, R. W., Rittenhouse, E. A., et al: Fate of autologous pericardium and Dacron fabric used as substitutes for total atrial septum in growing animals. J. Thorac. Cardiovasc. Surg., 59:501, 1970.

Moodie, D. S., Feldt, R. H., and Wallace, R. B.: Transient protein-losing enteropathy secondary to elevated caval pressures and caval obstruction after the Mustard procedure. J. Thorac. Cardiovasc. Surg., 72:379, 1976.

Murphy, J. H., Barlai-Kovach, M. M., Mathews, R. A., et al: Rest and exercise right and left ventricular function late after the Mustard operation: Assessment by radionuclide ventriculography. Am. J. Cardiol., 57:1142, 1986.

Mustard, W. T.: Successful two-stage correction of transposition of the great vessels. Surgery, 55:469, 1964.

Mustard, W. T. M., Chute, A. L., Keith, J. D., et al: A surgical approach to transposition of the great vessels with extracorporeal circuit. Surgery, 36:39, 1954.

Muster, A. J., Paul, M. H., Van Grondelle, A., and Conway, J. J.: Asymmetric distribution of the pulmonary blood flow between the right and left lungs in d-transposition of the great arteries. Am. J. Cardiol., 38:352, 1976.

Newberger, J. W., Silvert, A. R., Buckley, L. P., and Fyler, D. C.: Cognitive function and age at repair of transposition of the great arteries in children. N. Engl. J. Med., 310:1495, 1984.

Newfeld, E. A., Paul, M. H., Muster, A. J., and Idriss, F. S.: Pulmonary vascular disease in complete transposition of the

great arteries: A study of 200 patients. Am. J. Cardiol., 34:75, 1974.

Nogrady, M. B., and Dunbar, J. S.: Complete transposition of the great vessels: Re-evaluation of the so-called "typical configuration" on plain films of the chest. J. Can. Assoc. Radiol., 20:124, 1969.

Oelert, H., Laprell, H., Piepenbrock, S., et al: Emergency and non-emergency intra-atrial correction for transposition of the great arteries in 43 infants: Indications, details for the operative technique and results. Thoraxchirurgie, 25:305, 1977.

Olley, P. M., Coceani, F., and Rowe, R. D.: Role of prostaglandin E1 and E2 in the management of neonatal heart disease. Adv. Prostaglandin Thromboxane Res., 4:345, 1978.

Oppenheimer-Dekker, A.: Interventricular communications in transposition of the great arteries. In Van Mierop, L. H. S., Oppenheimer-Dekker, A., and Bruins, C. L. D. (eds): Embryology and Teratology of the Heart. Leiden, Leiden University Press, 1978, p. 136.

Pappas, G.: Left pulmonary vein stenosis associated with transposition of the great arteries. Ann. Thorac. Surg., 41:208, 1986.

Parrish, M. D., Graham, T. P., Jr., Bender, H. W., et al: Radionuclide angiographic evaluation of right and left ventricular function during exercise after repair of transposition of the great arteries. Circulation, 67:178, 1983.

Paul, M. H.: D-transposition of the great arteries. In Moss, A. J., Adams, F. H., and Emmanoulides, G. S.(eds): Heart Disease in Infants, Children and Adolescents. Baltimore, Williams & Wilkins Co., 1977, p. 301.

Piccoli, G. P., Wilkinson, J. F., Arnold, R., et al: Appraisal of the Mustard procedure for the physiologic correction of 'simple' transposition of the great arteries. J. Thorac. Cardiovasc. Surg., 82:436, 1981.

Plauth, H. W., Jr., Nadas, A. S., Bernhard, W. F., and Gross, R. E.: Transposition of the great arteries: Clinical and physiological observations on 74 patients treated by palliative surgery. Circulation, 37:316, 1968.

Polansky, S. M., and Culham, J. A. G.: Paraspinal densities developing after repair of transposition of the great arteries. Am. J. Roentgenol., 134:394, 1980.

Quaegebeur, J. M., Rohmer, J., Ottenkamp, J., et al: The arterial switch operation: An 8 year experience. J. Thorac. Cardiovasc. Surg., 92:361, 1986.

Ramsay, J. M., Venables, A. W., Kelly, M. J., and Kalff, M.: Right and left ventricular function at rest and with exercise after the Mustard operation for transposition of the great arteries. Br. Heart J., 51:364, 1984.

Rashkind, W. J., and Miller, W. W.: Creation of an atrial septal defect without thoracotomy: A palliative approach to complete transposition of the great arteries. J.A.M.A., 196:991, 1966.

Rastelli, G. C., McGoon, D. C., and Wallace, R. B.: Anatomic correction of transposition of the great arteries with ventricular septal defect and subpulmonary stenosis. J. Thorac. Cardiovasc. Surg., 58:545, 1969.

Riemenschneider, T. A., Vincent, W. R., Ruttenberg, H. D., and Desilets, D. T.: Transposition of the great vessels with hypoplasia of the right ventricle. Circulation, 38:386, 1968.

Rosenquist, G. C., Stark, J., and Taylor, J. F. N.: Anatomical relationships in transposition of the great arteries: Juxtaposition of the atrial appendage. Ann. Thorac. Surg., 18:456, 1974.

Rosenquist, G. C., Stark, J., and Taylor, J. F. N.: Congenital mitral valve disease in transposition of the great arteries. Circulation, 51:731, 1975.

Rossi, M. B., Ho, S. Y., Anderson, R. H., et al: Coronary arteries in complete transposition: The significance of the sinus node artery. Ann. Thorac. Surg., 42:573, 1986.

Rowe, R. D., Freedom, R. M., Mehrizi, A., and Bloom, K. R.: The neonate with congenital heart disease. Major Probl. Clin. Pediatr., 5:3, 1981.

Sansa, M., Tonkin, I. L., Bargeron, L. M., Jr., and Elliott, L. P.: Left ventricular outflow tract obstruction in transposition of the great arteries: An angiographic study of 74 cases. Am. J. Cardiol., 44:88, 1979.

Senning, A.: Surgical correction of transposition of the great vessels. Surgery, 45:966, 1959.

Shannon, D. C., Lusser, M., Goldblatt, A., and Bunnell, J. B.: The cyanotic infant—heart disease or lung disease? N. Engl. J. Med., *287*:951, 1972.

Sholler, G. F., and Celermajer, J. M.: Cardiac surgery in the first year of life: The effect on weight gain of infants with congenital heart disease. Austr. Paediatr. J., *22*:305, 1986.

Shrivastave, S., Tadavarthy, S. M., Fukuda, T., and Edwards, J. E.: Anatomic causes of pulmonary stenosis in complete transposition. Circulation, *54*:154, 1976.

Silove, E. D., and Taylor, J. F. N.: Angiographic anatomical features of subvalvular left ventricular outflow obstruction in transposition of the great arteries: The possible role of the anterior mitral valve leaflet. Pediatr. Radiol., *1*:87, 1973.

Silverman, N. H., Snider, A. R., Colo, J., et al: Superior vena caval obstruction after Mustard's operation by two-dimensional contrast echocardiography. Circulation, *64*:392, 1981.

Smallhorn, J. F., Gow, R., Freedom, R. M., et al: Pulsed Doppler echocardiographic assessment of the pulmonary venous pathway after the Mustard or Senning procedure for transposition of the great arteries. Circulation, *73*:765, 1986.

Smith, A., Wilkinson, J. L., Anderson, R. H., et al: Architecture of the ventricular mass and atrioventricular valves in complete transposition with intact septum compared with the normal. I: The left ventricle, mitral valve and interventricular septum. Pediatr. Cardiol., *6*:253, 1986a.

Smith, A., Wilkinson, J. L., Anderson, R. H., et al: Architecture of the ventricular mass and atrioventricular valves in complete transposition with intact septum compared with the normal. II: The right ventricle and tricuspid valve. Pediatr. Cardiol., *6*:299, 1986b.

Smolinsky, A., Castaneda, A. R., and Van Praagh, R.: Infundibular septal resection: Surgical anatomy of the superior approach. J. Thorac. Cardiovasc. Surg., *95*:486, 1988.

Soto, B., Becker, A. E., Moulaert, A. J., et al: Classification of ventricular septal defects. Br. Heart J., *43*:332, 1980.

Stark, J.: Concordant transposition-Mustard operation. *In* Stark, J, and de Leval, M. (eds): Surgery for Congenital Heart Defects. Orlando, FL, Grune & Stratton, 1983.

Stark, J., Silove, E. D., Taylor, J. F. N., and Graham, G. R. L.: Obstruction to systemic venous return following the Mustard operation for transposition of the great arteries. J. Thorac. Cardiovasc. Surg., *68*:742, 1974.

Stark, J., Weller, P., Leanage, R., et al: Late results of surgical treatment of transposition of the great arteries. Adv. Cardiol., *27*:254, 1980.

Sweeney, M. F., Bell, W. E., Doty, D. B., and Schieken, R. M.: Communicating hydrocephalus secondary to venous complications following intra-atrial baffle operation (Mustard procedure) for d-transposition of the great arteries. Pediatr. Cardiol., *3*:237, 1982.

Takahashi, M., Lindesmith, G. G., Lewis, A. B., et al: Long term results of the Mustard procedure. Circulation, *56*:85, 1977.

Tonkin, I. L., Sansa, M., Elliott, L. P., and Bargeron, L. M., Jr.: Recognition of developing left ventricular outflow tract obstruction in complete transposition of the great arteries. Radiology, *134*:53, 1980.

Tooley, W. H., and Stanger, P.: The blue baby—circulation or ventilation or both? N. Engl. J. Med., *287*:983, 1972.

Trusler, G. A., Castaneda, A. R., Rosenthal, A., et al: Current results of management in transposition of the great arteries with special emphasis on patients with associated ventricular septal defect. J. Am. Coll. Cardiol., *10*:1061, 1987.

Trusler, G. A., Williams, W. G., Izukawa, T., and Olley, P. M.: Current results with the Mustard operation in isolated transposition of the great arteries. J. Thorac. Cardiovasc. Surg., *80*:381, 1980.

Turley, K., Mavroudis, C., and Ebert, P. A.: Repair of congenital cardiac lesions during the first week of life. Circulation, *66*:1, 1982.

Urban, A. E., Stark, J., and Waterston, D. J.: Mustard's operation for transposition of the great arteries complicated by juxtaposition of the atrial appendages. Ann. Thorac. Surg., *21*:304, 1976.

Van Gils, F. A. W.: Left ventricular outflow tract obstruction in transposition with interventricular communication: Anatomical aspects. *In* Van Mierop, L. H. S., Oppenheimer-Dekker, A., and Bruins, C. L. D. (eds): Embryology and Teratology of the Heart. Leiden, Leiden University Press, 1978, p. 160.

Van Gils, F. A. W., Moulaert, A. J., Oppenheimer-Dekker, A., and Wenink, A. C. G.: Transposition of the great arteries with ventricular septal defect and pulmonary stenosis. Br. Heart J., *40*:494, 1978.

Van Praagh, R., Layton, W. M., and Van Praagh, S.: The morphogenesis of normal and abnormal relationship between the great arteries and the ventricle: Pathologic and experimental data. *In* Van Praagh, R., and Takao, A.(eds): Etiology and Morphogenesis of Congenital Heart Disease. Mt. Kisco, N.Y., Futura Publishing Co., 1980, p. 271.

Vidne, B. A., Subramanian, S., and Wagner, H. R.: Aneurysm of the membranous ventricular septum in transposition of the great arteries. Circulation, *53*:157, 1976.

Vogel, M., Ash, J., Rowe, R. D., et al: Congenital unilateral pulmonary vein stenosis complicating transposition of the great arteries. Am. J. Cardiol., *54*:166, 1984a.

Vogel, M., Freedom, R. M., Smallhorn, J. F., et al: Complete transposition of the great arteries and coarctation of the aorta. Am. J. Cardiol., *53*:1627, 1984b.

Waldman, J. D., Paul, M. H., Newfeld, E. A., et al: Transposition of the great arteries with intact ventricular septum and patent ductus arteriosus. Am. J. Cardiol., *39*:232, 1977.

Waldman, J. D., Waldman, J., and Jones, M. C.: Failure of balloon dilatation in mid-cavity obstruction of the systemic venous atrium after Mustard operation. Pediatr. Cardiol., *4*:151, 1983.

Watanabe, T., Trusler, G. A., Williams, W. G., et al: Phrenic nerve paralysis after pediatric cardiac surgery. J. Thorac. Cardiovasc. Surg., *94*:383, 1987.

Williams, W. G., Trusler, G. A., Kirklin, J. W., et al: Early and late results of a protocol for simple transposition leading to an atrial switch (Mustard) repair. J. Thorac. Cardiovasc. Surg., *95*:717, 1986.

Wilson, H. E., Nafrawi, A. G., Cardozo, R. H., and Aguillon, A.: Rational approach to surgery for complete transposition of the great vessels. Ann. Surg., *155*:258, 1962.

Wyse, R. K. H., Hawroth, S. G., Taylor, J. F. N., and Macartney, F. J.: Obstruction of superior vena caval pathway after Mustard's repair: Reliable diagnosis by transcutaneous Doppler ultrasound. Br. Heart J., *42*:162, 1979.

Yacoub, M., Bernhard, A., Lange, P., et al: Clinical and hemodynamic results of the two-stage anatomic correction of simple transposition of the great arteries. Circulation, *62*(Suppl. 1):190, 1980.

Yamaki, S., and Tezuka, F. L.: Quantitative analysis of pulmonary vascular disease in complete transposition of the great arteries. Circulation, *54*:805, 1976.

II THE SENNING PROCEDURE FOR TRANSPOSITION OF THE GREAT VESSELS

A. D. Pacifico

The operation described by Senning in 1959 and that by Mustard in 1964 are the most common types of procedures used to accomplish venous switching. The resurgence of the arterial switch operation, first successfully accomplished by Jatene in 1975, has reduced the role of venous switching for patients with transposition of the great arteries and similar malformations in many medical centers (Castaneda et al. 1988). Nevertheless, venous switching continues to be used uniformly in some centers and selectively in others.

Although the Senning operation was described 5 years earlier than the Mustard operation, the latter became the procedure of choice soon after it was introduced for patients with transposition of the great arteries. The probable reasons for this included the reported high early mortality for the Senning operation done as a single-stage procedure (Kirklin et al, 1961), which actually was related more to the selection of patients than to the operative procedure itself, and the belief that the Mustard procedure was simpler to do. The Mustard operation was done after a preliminary Blalock-Hanlon atrial septectomy and, therefore, the patients were older and larger and were often in the second to fourth year of life. As time passed, balloon atrial septostomy done at the time of neonatal catheterization was described (Rashkind and Miller, 1966) and supplanted the initial Blalock-Hanlon operation in many centers. The improvement resulting from balloon septostomy was not maintained as long as that from surgical septectomy, and this led to earlier performance of the Mustard operation with many groups advising it electively during the first year of life (Stark et al, 1974). Earlier performance of the Mustard procedure led to increased reports of pulmonary and systemic venous pathway obstructive complications that were reduced by various technical modifications.

In an attempt to reduce the obstructive complications after the Mustard procedure, Brom reintroduced the Senning operation (Quaegebeur et al, 1977), and it soon became the venous switching procedure of choice.

The Senning and Mustard operations both accomplish intra-atrial transposition of venous return by using living autologous atrial tissue in the former and a baffle tailored from autologous pericardium or synthetic material in the latter. At least theroretically, the intra-atrial venous pathways after the Senning procedure have greater potential for future growth because they are composed entirely of living atrial tissue. However, only part of the venous pathways of the Mustard operation consists of living tissue. A possible additional advantage of the Senning operation is that of atrial function that may be better preserved than after the Mustard procedure (Parenzan et al, 1978), although the incidence of atrial dysrhythmias is still similar.

TECHNIQUE

The technique that follows represents the one fundamentally described by Senning in 1959 and modified by the author (Pacifico, 1983). It can be applied in infants and older children, and the use of nonviable material is usually avoided.

The standard incision is a median sternotomy to expose the heart and great vessels. Purse-string sutures are placed in the ascending aorta for arterial cannulation and directly on each vena cava for venous cannulation. The purse string on the superior vena cava (SVC) is made oval to minimize narrowing of this structure when it is later tied. If the SVC is particularly small, the purse string is used solely to secure the cannula in place, and later the defect in the SVC is closed directly with a continuous fine monofilament suture. Separate caval cannulation, with thin-walled angled metal cannulas, provides excellent intracardiac exposure for this procedure and others and avoids the need for long periods of total circulatory arrest (Pacifico, 1988).

Before establishing cardipulmonary bypass, the circumference of the SVC and inferior vena cava (IVC) are each measured and recorded. Marking sutures are placed on the interatrial groove to define the cephalic (C) and caudal (D) extent of the left atriotomy (Fig. 43–21). Care is taken to place these marking sutures on the lateral margin of each vena cava and not posterior to them. A marking suture (A) may be placed 1 cm anterior to the crista terminalis at the superior extent of the right atrium. An additional marking suture (B) is placed a few millimeters cephalad from the junction of the IVC and right atrium, at a point measured from the caudal marking suture (D) on the interatrial groove, equal to two-thirds of the circumference of the IVC or a minimal distance of 15 mm (see Fig. 43–21). Points A and B define the superior and inferior extent of the longitudinal right atrial incision.

Cardiopulmonary bypass is established initially with the arterial and IVC cannulas in place, and later on the SVC cannula is inserted. The temperature of the perfusate is progressively reduced to cool the

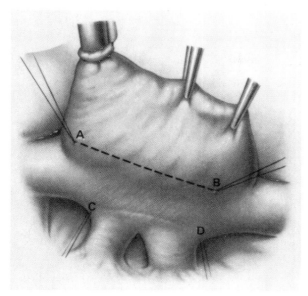

Figure 43–21. A marking suture (A) is placed 1 cm anterior to the crista terminalis at the superior extent of the right atriotomy incision. Marking suture (B) is placed a few millimeters cephalad from the junction of the inferior vena cava (IVC) and right atrium, at a measured point from the caudal marking suture (D) on the interatrial groove, equal to two-thirds the circumference of the IVC or a minimal distance of 15 mm. The *dashed line* shows the extent of the longitudinal right atrial incision. Points (C) and (D) are placed on the interatrial groove to define the cephalic and caudal extent of the left atrial incision. (From Pacifico, A. D.: Concordant transposition—Senning operation. *In* Stark, J., and DeLeval, M. [eds]: Surgery for Congenital Heart Defects. London, Grune & Stratton, 1983.)

patient to 24° C. Ligatures are placed about each vena cava for later occlusion around each caval cannula and the midportion of the interatrial groove is dissected about 1 cm to the left (Fig. 43–22). This dissection is limited by the previously placed marking sutures and must not extend beneath either vena cava, or it may later contribute to caval obstruction and distortion by the suture line used to construct the anterior wall of the pulmonary venous pathway. When cardiac ejections cease, a small incision is made into the left atrium at the right interatrial groove between points C and D, and a disposable sump tip vent is inserted. The aorta is cross-clamped, and cold cardioplegic solution is infused into the aortic root.

The right atrium is opened between points A and B (see Fig. 43–21) and the left margin of the atriotomy is sutured to the subcutaneous tissue for traction. The right margin is retracted by two sutures placed over the right chest wall and is held by the weight of a curved clamp. The atrial septum is inspected, and a flap is developed from the limbic tissue anteriorly toward the superior and inferior aspects of each respective right pulmonary vein. This flap remains attached at the right interatrial groove (Fig. 43–23). The flap has a trapezoid shape with a defect created by the existing interatrial communication. Formerly, a small patch of Dacron or pericar-

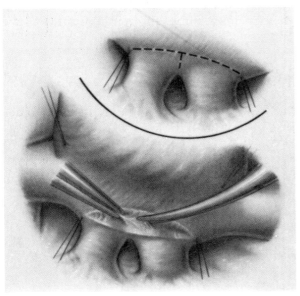

Figure 43–22. The midportion of the interatrial groove is dissected approximately 1 cm to the left. The dissection is limited by the previously placed marking sutures and must not extend beneath either vena cava. The *dashed line* above indicates the extent of the left atrial incision. (From Pacifico, A. D.: Concordant transposition—Senning operation. *In* Stark, J., and DeLeval, M. [eds]: Surgery for Congenital Heart Defects. London, Grune & Stratton, 1983.)

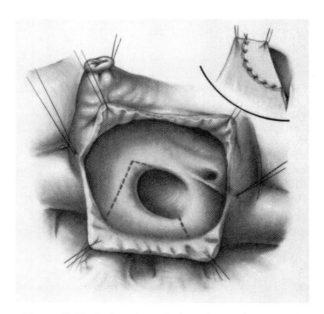

Figure 43–23. A view through the right atrial incision shows the atrial septum and its fossa ovalis defect. The coronary sinus can be seen to the right and anteriorly as well as the edge of the tricuspid valve annulus. The *dashed line* indicates the extent of the atrial septal incision to develop the septal flap. The incision is directed toward the superior aspect of the right superior pulmonary vein as well as the inferior aspect of the right inferior pulmonary vein. Formerly, a small patch of Dacron or pericardium *(inset)* was used to create a trapezoid configuration of the septal flap (see Fig. 43–24). (From Pacifico, A. D.: Concordant transposition—Senning operation. *In* Stark, J., and DeLeval, M. [eds]: Surgery for Congenital Heart Defects. London, Grune & Stratton, 1983.)

dium was sutured to the septal flap to accommodate this deficiency, leaving a trapezoid configuration (see Fig. 43–23). Currently, however, the coronary sinus is incised on its anterior margin, which is shown in Figure 43–24, to create a triangular-shaped coronary sinus flap. The tissue at the left apex of the coronary sinus flap and the left wall of the left atrium just above the left pulmonary veins is imbricated with a mattress suture to create a small roof above the left pulmonary veins. The coronary sinus flap is then combined with the atrial septal flap to form the roof of the left pulmonary venous pathway (Fig. 43–25). If the atrial septal defect (ASD) is small and centrally positioned, it is closed primarily before creating the septal flap, and the coronary sinus flap is not used. If a surgical atrial septectomy has been done earlier, a synthetic or pericardial patch may be required to reconstruct the atrial septum, although in some cases the coronary sinus flap and remaining atrial septal tissue suffice. The roof of the left pulmonary venous pathway is constructed as shown in Figures 43–25 and 43–26 by using continuous 4-0 polypropylene suture. The superior portion of the suture line lies above the left pulmonary veins and courses within the left atrium to the origin of the septal flap near the SVC junction. Similarly, the inferior border of the flap courses back to its origin near the IVC junction. These divergent suture lines are shown in Figure 43–26.

All of these maneuvers have been accomplished during standard cardiopulmonary bypass methods with core cooling. In some patients, suturing of the atrial septal flap above the left pulmonary veins is facilitated by the use of circulatory arrest. When this is used, the arrest time is usually between 5 and 10 minutes. If temporary total circulatory arrest had been established, cardiopulmonary bypass is reinstituted at 24° C when the septal flap suture lines have been completed.

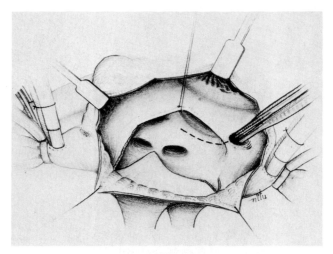

Figure 43–24. The coronary sinus is incised on its anterior margin to create a triangular-shaped coronary sinus flap. The tissue at the left apex of the coronary sinus flap and the left wall of the left atrium just above the left pulmonary veins is imbricated with a mattress suture to create a small roof above the left pulmonary veins.

The roof of the vena cava pathway is constructed with continuous 4-0 polypropylene suture. The inferior aspect of the right side of the free right atrial wall is sutured to the atrial tissue about the IVC orifice that continues superiorly to the coronary sinus (Fig. 43–27). If the coronary sinus has not been incised, it is left to drain with the pulmonary venous blood. When a coronary sinus flap has been used, care is taken to place this suture line slightly posterior to the remaining rim of the coronary sinus to avoid the area of the specialized conduction tissue. A second suture is used to complete the superior attachment of the right side of the free right atrial wall, attaching this about the SVC and along the limbic

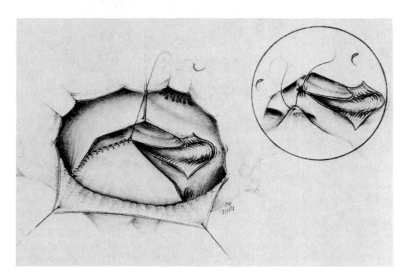

Figure 43–25. The coronary sinus flap is combined with the atrial septal flap to form the roof of the left pulmonary venous pathway.

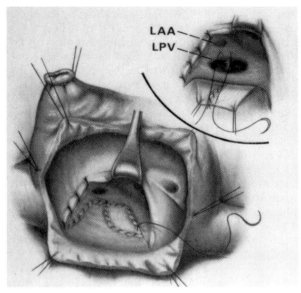

Figure 43–26. The roof of the left pulmonary venous pathway has been constructed with a continuous suture of 4-0 polypropylene. The superior portion of the suture line is above the left pulmonary veins (LPV, see *inset*) and posterior to the origin of the left atrial appendage (LAA). (From Pacifico, A. D.: Concordant transposition—Senning operation. *In* Stark, J., and DeLeval, M. [eds]: Surgery for Congenital Heart Defects. London, Grune & Stratton, 1983.)

tissue. The completed suture line is shown in Figure 43–28.

The incision in the left atrium that is used initially for the left atrial vent is extended between the marking sutures (C and D) on the interatrial groove (see Fig. 43–21), and the perimeter of the left atriotomy is lengthened by incising onto the right superior pulmonary vein for a distance of about 1 cm which is shown in Figure 43–29. When the right superior and inferior pulmonary veins are oriented more horizontally, the incision is made between them (Fig. 43–30). The original right atrial incision is extended anteriorly at each end, from A to A' and from B to B', which is shown in Figure 43–30. The length of each extension is almost one-quarter of the circumference of SVC and IVC, respectively, which will increase the perimeter of this flap by half the circumference of each vena cava, and leave additional length for attachment above the right pulmonary veins. These incisions permit the development of an advancement flap similar to that used in plastic surgical procedures. When properly made, they allow point A″ to reach point C without constricting or use of a purse string to the circumference of the superior vena cava pathway (see Fig. 43–30). Similarly, point B″ is brought to point D without compromising the IVC circumference. Initially, a 6-0 polypropylene suture attaches point A″ to point C and this suture is tied. A second suture is placed at point A, and is tied and retracted. The perimeter of the right atrial flap from A to A″ is then sutured superficially along the SVC pathway by using interrupted 6-0 polypropylene sutures (Fig. 43–31). Traction in opposite directions from points A through C permits the placement of accurate and superficial sutures, which

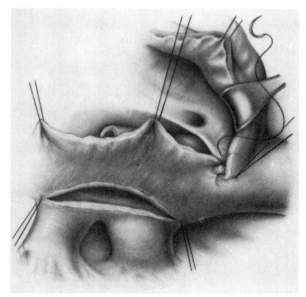

Figure 43–27. The roof of the caval pathway is formed by using the right side of the free right atrial wall beginning the suture line near the inferior vena cava and continuing beyond the area cephalad of the coronary sinus. A second suture is used to form this pathway near the superior vena cava. (From Pacifico, A. D.: Concordant transposition—Senning operation. *In* Stark, J., and DeLeval, M. [eds]: Surgery for Congenital Heart Defects. London, Grune & Stratton, 1983.)

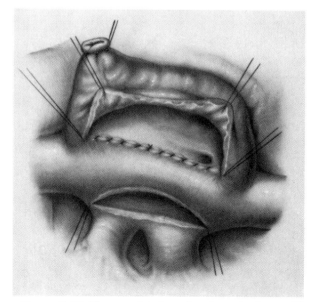

Figure 43–28. The completed caval pathway is shown. (From Pacifico, A. D.: Concordant transposition—Senning operation. *In* Stark, J., and DeLeval, M. [eds]: Surgery for Congenital Heart Defects. London, Grune & Stratton, 1983.)

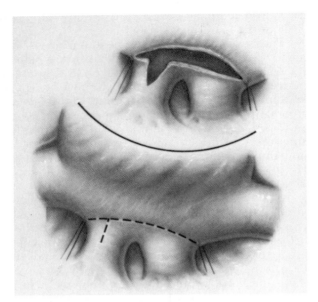

Figure 43–29. The extent of the left atrial incision is defined by the *dashed line*. The perimeter is enlarged by incising the right superior pulmonary vein, and the resultant atriotomy is shown above. When the right superior and inferior pulmonary veins are oriented horizontally, it is sometimes advantageous to enlarge the perimeter by incising between the right superior and inferior veins, which is shown in Figures 43–30 and 43–31. (From Pacifico, A. D.: Concordant transposition—Senning operation. *In* Stark, J., and DeLeval, M. [eds]: Surgery for Congenital Heart Defects. London, Grune & Stratton, 1983.)

avoids the area of the sinus node. Similarly, interrupted sutures placed at points B and D are tensed in opposite directions, and multiple interrupted 6-0 polypropylene sutures are used to attach this portion of the right atrial wall to the IVC pathway (Fig. 43–32). The use of interrupted sutures (compared with the continuous suture shown in Figure 43–31) obviates the potential purse-string effect of a continuous suture line that would reduce the circumference of each vena cava. Point E is then attached to point F with an interrupted 6-0 polypropylene suture, which is shown in Figure 43–32. Multiple interrupted sutures are placed to complete the attachment of the remaining segment of this flap to the right edge of the left atriotomy to complete the pulmonary venous pathway (Fig. 43–33). Rewarming is accomplished, air is removed from the heart and aorta, and the crossclamp is removed.

The technique described differs from that reported by Quaegebeur and associates (1977) primarily by the method of venous cannulation and also by not using the eustachian valve in construction of the inferior vena cava pathway. The eustachian valve may be well developed in some patients and essentially nonexistent in others, and therefore the author prefers not to rely on it. In addition, direct inferior vena cava cannulation sometimes results in injury of the eustachian valve. Avoiding the use of the eustachian valve, however, requires that the caudal aspect of the right atriotomy incision be directed more anteriorly (i.e., farther to the left or anterior from the

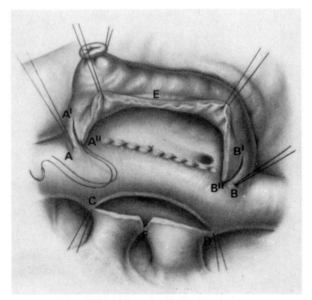

Figure 43–30. The original right atrial incision is extended anteriorly at each end, from A to A′ and from B to B′. The length of each extension is almost one-quarter the circumference of the superior and inferior vena cava respectively. An advancement flap has been created permitting point A″ to reach point C, and point B″ to reach point D. (From Pacifico, A. D.: Concordant transposition—Senning operation. *In* Stark, J., and DeLeval, M. [eds]: Surgery for Congenital Heart Defects. London, Grune & Stratton, 1983.)

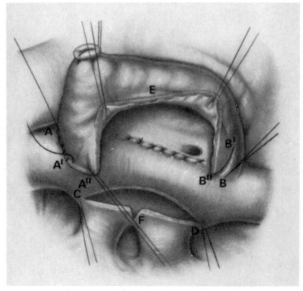

Figure 43–31. The perimeter of the right atrial flap from A to A″ is sutured superficially along the SVC pathway to point C. Interrupted 6-0 polypropylene sutures are preferred to avoid the purse-string effect of a continuous suture. (From Pacifico, A. D.: Concordant transposition—Senning operation. *In* Stark, J., and DeLeval, M. [eds]: Surgery for Congenital Heart Defect. London, Grune & Stratton, 1983.)

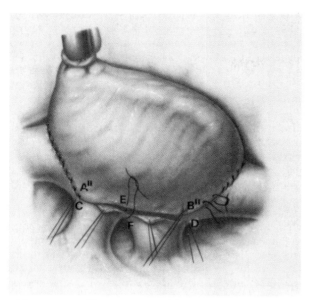

Figure 43–32. The perimeter of the right atrial flap from B to B″ is sutured along the inferior vena cava-right atrial junction. Interrupted sutures of 6-0 polypropylene are preferred. (From Pacifico, A. D.: Concordant transposition—Senning operation. *In* Stark, J., and DeLeval, M. [eds]: Surgery for Congenital Heart Defects. London, Grune & Stratton, 1983.)

interatrial groove) to leave sufficient right atrial tissue for construction of this segment of the caval pathway. The atriotomy incision presented here is similar to that used originally by Senning in 1959 but does require a greater perimeter of the remaining free right atrial wall for proper construction of the roof of the pulmonary venous pathway, which is achieved by using the advancement flap technique (see Fig. 43–30).

The use of the coronary sinus flap combined with the atrial septal flap avoids the use of a nonviable patch to fill in the atrial septal defect.

RESULTS

Hospital mortality after the Senning procedure in 146 patients with various forms of transposition of the great arteries, collected from three institutions was 2.7% (Pacifico, 1983). This procedure included 58 patients operated on in Leiden, Holland (Brom, 1982); 53 patients operated on at the Hospital for Sick Children at Great Ormond Street, London, England (Stark et al, 1984); and 35 patients operated on in Bergamo, Italy (Locatelli et al, 1979). This reflected the early experience with the Senning operation after its revival in 1977 by Quaegebeur and associates from Leiden, Holland.

The results of the Mustard and Senning operations were reviewed in 123 consecutive patients with transposition of the great arteries and intact ventricular septum who had atrial switching between 1972 and 1980 at the Children's Hospital Medical Center, Boston, Massachusetts (Marx et al, 1983). A Mustard

operation was done in 66 patients at a mean age of 15.5 months between 1972 and 1978. There were 7 (11%) deaths within 30 days of operation and 5 (8%) deaths during the follow-up period that extended to 43.5 months. However, a Senning operation was done in 57 patients between 1978 and 1980 at a mean age of 6.6 months. There were 3 (5%) deaths within 30 days of operation and 2 (4%) late deaths during the follow-up period that extended to 13.6 months.

In a more recent experience with 35 patients with transposition of the great arteries and intact ventricular septum, operated on between 1982 and 1985, there was 1 (2.9%) hospital death and no late mortality among 29 of 33 patients who were followed between 2 and 36 months postoperatively (mean = 14 ± 10) (George et al, 1987).

Some neonates with transposition of the great arteries and intact ventricular septum continue to be hypoxic despite an adequate balloon atrial septostomy. It was formerly believed that the performance of an atrial switch operation in the neonatal period was associated with high hospital mortality. DeLeon and associates (1984) reviewed their experience with the Senning operation in 19 patients who were operated on between 2 and 24 days of age (mean = 12 days). There were 2 (10%) early deaths and 1 (5%) late death during the follow-up interval that ranged between 7 and 40 months. The three deaths occurred in the first three infants operated on in the series, and the subsequent 16 patients were all alive and well at follow-up. This experience and others support the conclusion that the Senning operation can be done at low risk even in the sick hypoxemic neonate

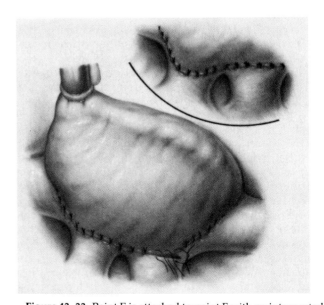

Figure 43–33. Point E is attached to point F with an interrupted 6-0 polypropylene suture and multiple similar interrupted sutures are used to complete the pulmonary venous pathway. (From Pacifico, A. D.: Concordant transposition—Senning operation. *In* Stark, J., and DeLeval, M. [eds]: Surgery for Congenital Heart Defects. London, Grune & Stratton, 1983.)

(Fortune et al, 1983; Matherne et al, 1985; Rubay et al, 1987; Turley et al, 1985).

In general, the early and late results of the Senning operation combined with closure of a large ventricular septal defect in infants with transposition are less good than for the group with intact ventricular septum. In one series of 46 infants ranging from 12 days to 12 months at operation (median = 5.1 ± 3.2 months) hospital mortality was 15.2% and late mortality was 5.1% (Penkoske et al, 1983). In another experience, there were no early (<30 days) deaths but 3 late deaths among 10 patients with various forms of complex transposition whose repair included a Senning operation (George et al, 1987).

Various complications can occur after the Senning operation that include systemic or pulmonary venous obstruction, baffle suture line leaks, tricuspid valve incompetence, residual or recurrent ventricular septal defect, or left ventricular outflow tract obstruction, arrhythmias, and reduction of systemic (right) ventricular function.

The incidence of superior vena caval obstruction ranges from 0 to 13% after the Senning operation (George et al, 1987; Marx et al, 1983). This obstruction has been implicated as a cause of early mortality, but its incidence appears to be no higher when the operation is done in younger and smaller subjects (DeLeon et al, 1984). This complication can result from a technical error during the initial construction of the systemic venous pathways and can also be related to narrowing of the perimeter of the superior vena cava by the suture line for the roof of the pulmonary venous pathway. Reoperation to repair systemic venous obstruction is uncommonly required, and in some patients it may be managed effectively by percutaneous catheter balloon dilatation. The living autologous tissue used in the Senning procedure may result in a lesser incidence of late baffle obstructive complications than that observed in patients after the Mustard type of repair.

Pulmonary venous obstruction in most series is rare after the Senning operation. It developed in 6 (11%) of 57 patients who had the Senning operation at a mean age of 6.6 months (Marx et al, 1983). This obstruction has not occurred in most series reported in the literature.

Baffle leaks can occur after the Senning operation but are uncommon. It was present in 1 (1.9%) of 54 survivors of the Senning operation in one series (Marx et al, 1983).

Tricuspid valve incompetence and systemic ventricular dysfunction can occur after atrial switch operations. In the Boston experience, mild and severe tricuspid valve incompetence was reported in three patients among 39 survivors of the Senning operation and VSD closure (Penkoske et al, 1983). Tricuspid valve replacement was required in the three patients with severe incompetence. Graham and associates (1985) studied right ventricular function after intraatrial repair of transposition of the great arteries. Postoperative right ventricular ejection fraction was

below normal (<0.49) in 16 of 32 patients who had the Senning procedure. Mean postoperative right ventricular ejection fraction was lower for patients operated on between 1971 and 1974 (0.39 ± 0.11) than for patients in either the Mustard group from 1975 to 1978 (0.47 ± 0.13, p < 0.03) or the Senning group (0.48 ± 0.09). Improved postoperative right ventricular performance was shown in patients who had a more recent intra-atrial repair, which leads to the speculation that younger age at operation, better preoperative function, and improved methods of myocardial protection may be responsible for improved postoperative ventricular performance.

The incidence of rhythm disturbances after the Mustard and Senning operation is similar. The incidence of sinus rhythm after the Senning operation varies between 88 and 100% with follow-ups ranging from 10 to 25 months. Rhythm disturbances are likely to be similar to those occurring after the Mustard procedure, and the incidence will probably increase progressively with time.

Although the quality of life and overall results after the Senning operation are very good, it is likely that the current trend to advise the arterial switch operation as the procedure of choice for patients with transposition of the great arteries will continue. Careful early and late follow-up after each type of procedure is necessary to provide a proper comparison of results.

Selected Bibliography

Castaneda, A. R., Trusler, G. A., Paul, M. H., et al: The early results of treatment of simple transposition in the current era. J. Thorac. Cardiovasc. Surg., 95:14, 1988.

This paper reports the early results in the modern era from 20 institutions in North America consisting of the Congenital Heart Surgeon's Society. A total of 187 neonates within the first 2 weeks of life were admitted into this cooperative study between January 1, 1985 and June 1, 1986. Seventy-six patients were initially entered into a protocol leading to an arterial switch repair, 45 into one leading to a Mustard type of repair and 49 into one leading to a Senning repair. The risk factors for death were low birth weight, earlier date of entry into the study, and an arterial switch protocol in the group of institutions at high risk for arterial switch repair. A detailed analysis of these patients is given and leads to the conclusion that the arterial and atrial switch repairs can have similar early results.

Quaegebeur, J. M., Rohmer, J., Brom, A. G., and Tinkelenberg, J.: Revival of the Senning operation in the treatment of transposition of the great arteries. Thorax, 32:517, 1977.

Although the Senning operation was used in a few institutions soon after it was introduced in 1959, it was abandoned in favor of the Mustard operation for many years. This paper was responsible for the revival of the Senning operation as a commonly performed procedure for transposition of the great arteries. The technique, which is used by the authors, is clearly detailed and the results are nicely analyzed.

Senning, A.: Surgical correction of transposition of the great vessels. Surgery, 45:966, 1959.

This paper describes the original surgical procedures done by

Senning for patients with transposition of the great arteries and forms the basis of the current Senning procedure.

Bibliography

Bender, H. W., Jr., Graham, T. P., Jr., Boucek, R. J., Jr., et al: Comparative operative results of the Senning and Mustard procedures for transposition of the great arteries. Circulation, 62(Suppl. I):197, 1980.

Brom, G.: The Senning procedure. In Moulton, A. (ed): Current Controversies and Techniques in Congenital Heart Disease. Pasadena, CA, Appleton Davis, Inc., 1982.

Castaneda, A. R., Trusler, G. A., Paul, M. H., et al: The early results of treatment of simple transposition in the current era. J. Thorac. Cardiovasc. Surg., 95:14, 1988.

DeLeon, V. H., Hougen, T. J., Norwood, W. I., et al: Results of the Senning operation for transposition of the great arteries with intact ventricular septum in neonates. Circulation, 70(Suppl. I):I–21, 1984.

Fortune, R. L., Pacquet, M., Collins-Nakai, R. L., and Duncan, N. F.: Intracardiac repair of dextro-transposition of the great arteries in the newborn period. J. Thorac. Cardiovasc. Surg., 85:371, 1983.

George, B. L., Laks, H., Klitzner, T. S., et al: Results of the Senning procedure in infants with simple and complex transposition of the great arteries. Am. J. Cardiol., 59:426, 1987.

Graham, T. P., Burger, J., Bender, H. W., et al: Improved right ventricular function after intraatrial repair of transposition of the great arteries. Circulation, 72(Suppl. II):II–45, 1985.

Jatene, A. D., Fontes, V. F., Paulista, P. P., et al: Successful anatomic correction of transposition of the great vessels: A preliminary report. Arg. Braz. Cardiol., 28:461, 1975.

Kirklin, J. W., Devloo, R. A., and Weidman, W. H.: Open intracardiac repair for transposition of the great vessels: 11 cases. Surgery, 50:68, 1961.

Locatelli, G., DiBenedetto, G., Villani, M., et al: Transposition of the great arteries: Successful Senning's operation in 35 consecutive patients. Thorac. Cardiovasc. Surg., 27:120, 1979.

Marx, G. R., Hougen, T. J., Norwood, W. I., et al: Transposition of the great arteries with intact ventricular septum: Results of Mustard and Senning operations in 123 consecutive patients. J. Am. Coll. Cardiol., 1:476, 1983.

Matherne, G. P., Razook, J. D., Thompson, W. M., Jr., et al: Senning repair for transposition of the great arteries in the first week of life. Circulation, 72:840, 1985.

Mustard, W. T.: Successful two-stage correction of transposition of the great vessels. Surgery, 55:469, 1964.

Pacifico, A. D.: Cardiopulmonary bypass and hypothermic circulatory arrest in congenital heart surgery. In Grillo, H. C., Austen, W. G., Wilkins, E. W., Jr., et al (eds): Current Therapy in Cardiothoracic Surgery. Toronto, B. C. Decker Inc., Publishers, 1988.

Pacifico, A. D.: Concordant transposition—Senning operation. In Stark, J., and DeLeval, M. (eds): Surgery for Congenital Heart Defects. London, Grune & Stratton, 1983, p. 345.

Parenzan, L., Locatelli, G., Alfieri, O., et al: The Senning operation for transposition of the great arteries. J. Thorac. Cardiovasc. Surg., 76:305, 1978.

Penkoske, P. A., Westerman, G. R., Marx, G. R., et al: Transposition of the great arteries and ventricular septal defect: Results with the Senning operation and closure of the ventricular septal defect in infants. Ann. Thorac. Surg., 36:281, 1983.

Quaegebeur, J. M., and Brom, A. G.: The trousers-shaped baffle for use in the Mustard operation. Ann. Thorac. Surg., 25:240, 1978.

Quaegebeur, J. M., Rohmer, J., Brom, A. G., and Tinkelenberg, J.: Revival of the Senning operation in the treatment of transposition of the great arteries. Thorax, 32:517, 1977.

Rashkind, W. J., and Miller, W. W.: Creation of an atrial septal defect without thoracotomy: A palliative approach to complete transposition of the great arteries. J.A.M.A., 196:173, 1966.

Rubay, J. E., de Halleux, C., Moulin, D., et al: Long-term follow-up of the Senning operation for transposition of the great arteries in children under 3 months of age. J. Thorac. Cardiovasc. Surg., 94:75, 1987.

Senning, A.: Surgical correction of transposition of the great vessels. Surgery, 45:966, 1959.

Stark, J.: Current operative approach to transposition of the great arteries with left ventricular outflow tract obstruction. In Moulton, A. L. (ed): Congenital Heart Surgery: Current Techniques and Controversies. Pasadena, Appleton Davies, Inc., 1984, p. 47.

Stark, J., de Leval, M. R., Waterston, D. J., et al: Corrective surgery of transposition of the great arteries in the first year of life: Results in 63 infants. J. Thorac. Cardiovasc. Surg., 67:673, 1974.

Turley, K., and Ebert, P. A.: Transposition of the great arteries in the neonate: Failed balloon atrial septostomy. J. Cardiovasc. Surg., 26:564, 1985.

III ANATOMIC CORRECTION OF TRANSPOSITION OF THE GREAT ARTERIES AT THE ARTERIAL LEVEL

Roberto M. Di Donato
Aldo R. Castaneda

Anatomic correction of transposition of the great arteries (TGA) includes any type of repair that connects the left ventricle (LV) with the aorta and the right ventricle (RV) with the pulmonary artery. This can be accomplished at the ventricular level (McGoon, 1972; Rastelli et al, 1969) or at the arterial level, either with (Jatene et al, 1975) or without coronary transfer (Aubert et al, 1978; Damus, 1975; Kaye, 1975; Stansel, 1975). This section describes primary repair of TGA at the arterial level with coronary transfer, the so-called *arterial switch operation* (ASO).

HISTORICAL ASPECTS

Mustard and colleagues (1954) were the first to attempt ASO and they used monkey lungs as an oxygenator in seven patients. This technique included transfer of only the left coronary artery, and none of the patients survived. Before the widespread use of cardiopulmonary bypass, attempts to switch the great arteries without coronary transfer experimentally (Bjork and Boukaert, 1954) and clinically (Bailey et al, 1954; Kay and Cross, 1955) also failed.

Despite the impressive results with the atrial inversion operation ("physiologic repair," that is, Mustard or Senning procedure), a few investigators continued to explore the possibility of switching the great arteries together with the coronary arteries. Senning (1959) reported three patients with TGA treated by a technique involving en-bloc transfer of the pulmonary valve and artery and diversion of the LV to the aorta through a ventricular septal defect (VSD). Idriss and associates (1961) translocated a segment of ascending aorta, including both coronary arteries, into the proximal pulmonary artery. None of these patients survived. Other experimental techniques were reported by Baffes and colleagues (1961) and by Anagnostopoulos (1973).

Jatene and colleagues (1975), in an epic report, described the first successful ASO in a patient with TGA and a large VSD. Many of the technical advances learned from coronary artery bypass and, more important, a clearer understanding of the need for a LV capable of supporting the systemic circulation contributed to the success of this first operation. Patients with TGA and VSD, or large patent ductus arteriosus (PDA), or left ventricular outflow tract obstruction (LVOTO) retain a LV pressure at or close to systemic levels after birth; therefore, Jatene and co-workers initially limited their operation to this subset of patients.

Because the early high operative mortality of the ASO was in part attributed to technical difficulties related to the transfer of the coronary arteries, alternative techniques, avoiding mobilization of the coronary arteries, were developed. These techniques included (1) baffling of the coronary arteries to a surgically created aortic-pulmonary window (Aubert et al, 1978); (2) translocation of the entire aortic root including the proximal coronary arteries (Bex et al, 1980); and (3) end-to-side proximal pulmonary artery to ascending aorta anastomosis with placement of a right ventricular to distal pulmonary artery conduit (Damus, 1975; Kaye, 1975; Stansel, 1975).

However, the ASO with coronary artery transfer (Jatene et al, 1982) retained its original appeal. Lecompte and colleagues (1981) added an important technical modification by transferring the distal pulmonary artery anterior to the ascending aorta, thus facilitating direct anastomosis of the neopulmonary artery without the need for conduit interposition.

Because approximately 75% of the patients with TGA have an intact ventricular septum (TGA-IVS), the application of the ASO principle to this largest subset of patients with TGA became of interest to several investigators. In addition to sporadic reports of successful primary ASO in infants (Abe et al, 1978; Mauck et al, 1977), most of the earlier attempts to use this approach failed, primarily because of LV

dysfunction. To prepare the LV for systemic pressure work, Yacoub and colleagues (1977) introduced a two-stage approach for TGA-IVS, by first banding the main pulmonary artery (with or without a systemic-pulmonary artery shunt) to stimulate the development of LV muscle mass, followed by an ASO several months later. The principle of doing the ASO as a primary repair in neonates with TGA-IVS, while the LV is still capable of systemic pressure work, was introduced successfully at the Boston Children's Hospital and at the University of Leyden in 1983 (Castaneda et al, 1984; Quaegebeur et al, 1986). Primary ASO for TGA-IVS in neonates has now become the operation of choice in many centers.

REASONS FOR THE ARTERIAL SWITCH OPERATION

The fate of the atrial or "physiologic" type of repairs is of increasing concern. Although the hospital mortality of both the Mustard and the Senning operations is extremely low, the long-term outcome of these procedures is affected by several complications, the most important being a high incidence of atrial dysrhythmias (more than 50% by 10 years) (Byrum et al, 1987; Duster et al, 1985; Hayes and Gersony, 1986; Vetter et al, 1987), and a less clearly established incidence of late RV (systemic ventricle) dysfunction (approximately 10%) (Benson et al, 1982; Borow et al, 1981; Graham et al, 1975; Trowitzsch et al, 1985).

Various theoretical considerations support the assumption that the LV is more suitable than the RV to serve the systemic circulation. The LV, because of its cylindrical shape, its concentric contraction pattern, and the location of both the inlet and the outlet orifices within its base, appears to be ideally adapted to work as a pressure pump. The RV, by comparison, because of its crescent-shaped cavity, its large internal surface area to volume ratio, its bellows-like contraction pattern, and its more separated inlet and outlet segments, appears to serve better as a volume pumping chamber.

The ASO recruits the LV as the systemic pump, and because atrial manipulation is essentially limited to closure of an atrial communication, it is also anticipated that atrial dysrhythmias will be significantly reduced after the ASO.

SURGICAL IMPLICATIONS

Suitability of the Left Ventricle for an Arterial Switch Operation

Most anatomic and functional features of a ventricle depend on the hemodynamic load to which the ventricle is subjected before and after birth (Hood et al, 1968; Van Doesburg et al, 1983). Ventricular wall stress is an index of the anatomic and functional responses to any specific pressure or volume load. Ventricular wall stress (WS) is directly proportional to intracavitary pressure (P), and diameter (D) and is inversely proportional to wall thickness (WT): WS = P × D/WT (Gaasch, 1979). In TGA, the LV works under different hemodynamic conditions depending on the presence of a VSD or an LVOTO, and its anatomic and functional features vary accordingly. In TGA-IVS, the pathophysiology is primarily that of a volume overload placed on the LV; in TGA with VSD or large PDA, both LV volume and pressure overload exist, and in TGA-LVOTO with or without a VSD, LV pressure overload is predominant. Generally, thickening of the LV free wall depends on a pressure load to levels more than 50% of the systemic pressure, but it is only minimally influenced by a pure volume load (Danford et al, 1985) (Fig. 43–34).

In TGA-IVS, the LV wall thickness is normal at birth. However, the rapidly decreasing pulmonary vascular resistance results in a drop of peak LV pressure and thus decreased development of LV muscle mass (Bano-Rodrigo et al, 1980; Danford et al, 1985; Huhta et al, 1982b; Maroto et al, 1983). By 1 month of age, many patients with TGA-IVS have a peak LV-RV pressure ratio equal to or less than 65%. Displacement of the ventricular septum to the left, secondary to the trans-septal pressure difference, causes a crescent-shaped transverse configuration of the LV cavity and may also cause dynamic LVOTO (Chiu et al, 1984; Van Doesburg et al, 1983). Furthermore, increased LV volume load due to augmented pulmonary blood flow leads to progressive LV dilatation (Smith et al, 1982). Therefore, in patients with TGA-IVS, performance of the ASO during the neonatal period when the LV is still prepared to support the systemic circulation by the intrauterine physiology is preferred. Ideally, the repair should be done within the first week of life. Because this is not always practical, empiric criteria for predicting postoperative LV performance have been developed. Before 2 weeks of age, all patients with TGA-IVS have repair regardless of preoperative LV pressure measurements. After this age, an LV-RV pressure ratio of 0.6 as the lowest limit of acceptable LV pressure is arbitrarily chosen. Helpful, but not yet clearly defined, two-dimensional echocardiographic indices of a LV suitable for ASO include ventricular septal position (Fig. 43–35), degree of LV wall thickness, LV volume, and LV muscle mass.

The authors' current indication for pulmonary artery banding in preparation for an ASO is limited to cases of TGA-IVS usually presenting beyond the

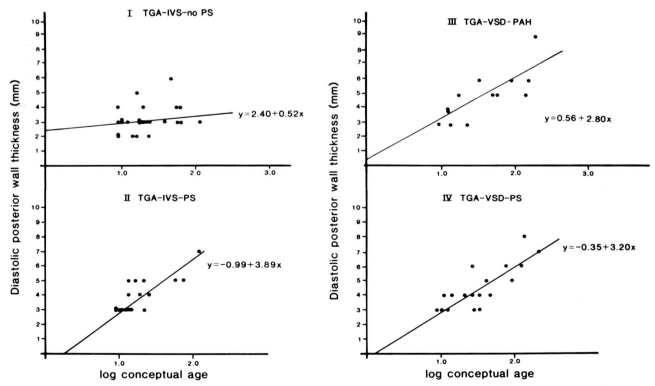

Figure 43–34. LV diastolic posterior wall thickness plotted against log conceptual age for each of four patient groups. Regression lines indicate, by their slope, the rate of increase of wall thickness in each group. Slope in Group I is significantly less than slopes in the other three groups (p < 0.05). Other slopes are not significantly different from each other. (PS = pulmonary stenosis; PAH = pulmonary artery hypertension.) (From Danford, D. A., Huhta, J. C., and Gutgesell, H. P.: Left ventricular wall stress and thickness in complete transposition of the great arteries: Implications for surgical intervention. J. Thorac. Cardiovasc. Surg., *89*:610, 1985.)

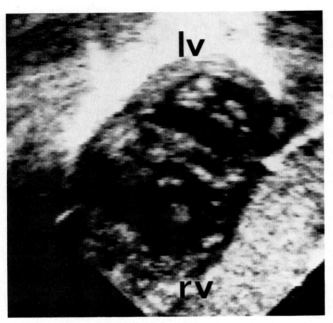

Figure 43–35. Two-dimensional echocardiogram of a newborn with TGA-IVS. This end-systolic subxiphoid short-axis view of the ventricular septum is at the level of the coapted mitral valve leaflets. Note the straight position of the septum, indicating balanced ventricular pressures.

first months of age with an LV-RV pressure ratio of less than 0.6 and to cases of RV failure late after an atrial inversion operation.

Laboratory studies have shown surprisingly rapid induction (within 48 hours) of the genes responsible for the isoenzyme adaptation response of rat myocardial myosin, actin, and tropomyosin to an acute pressure load. Furthermore, various proto-oncogenes involved in cell growth regulation accumulate in rat cardiac cells within 1 hour of an acute pressure load. Stress protein (HSP-70) also rises within 2 to 3 hours of an acute pressure load (Izumo et al, 1988). Consistent with these laboratory findings, in five patients ASO has been done 10 to 14 days after pulmonary artery banding.

Pulmonary Vascular Obstructive Disease

Patients with TGA typically develop early and rapidly progressive pulmonary vascular obstructive disease (Haworth et al, 1987; Newfeld et al, 1979). Although the precise cause of these lesions in TGA is unknown, contributing factors are increased pulmonary blood flow, elevated pulmonary artery pressure, high pulmonary arterial oxygen tension, low systemic arterial oxygen tension and oxygen saturation (with reduced oxygen supply to the pulmonary arterial wall by the bronchial arterial circulation), increased blood viscosity, and development of microthrombi. Also, pulmonary arterial vasospasm is believed to aggravate endothelial shear stress, thus

favoring the rapid progression of medial and intimal changes.

In the group of infants with TGA-VSD, Heath-Edwards Grade III lesions were found in 19% of patients less than 3 months of age, 24% of those 3 to 11 months of age, and in nearly 80% of those older than 1 year. In infants with TGA-IVS, Grade III lesions occur in less than 1% of those younger than 3 months and remain below 17% within the first year of life (Clarkson et al, 1976). Awareness of the accelerated development of pulmonary vascular obstructive disease in TGA is particularly important because of the unreliability of calculations of pulmonary blood flow and pulmonary vascular resistance in this disease. Therefore, in patients with TGA-VSD or TGA and a large PDA, closure of the VSD or PDA and an ASO within the first 2 months of life are recommended.

Coronary Arterial Anatomy

Several classifications of coronary anatomy have been proposed in TGA. A descriptive terminology (originated by Gittenberger-DeGroot et al, 1983), which includes the names of the three aortic sinuses, is preferred: left, right, and nonfacing sinus. The coronary arteries almost invariably originate from the facing sinuses and can generally be subdivided into three main coronary branches—that is, left anterior descending, left circumflex, and right coronary artery (Smith et al, 1986). The six most common types of coronary anatomy in TGA are shown in Figure 43–36.

Preoperative visualization of the coronary arteries in neonates with TGA is obtained by aortic root angiography and, more recently, by two-dimensional echocardiography (Pasquini et al, 1987) (Fig. 43–37).

Although most coronary arterial patterns in TGA lend themselves to the ASO, there are a few cases, particularly when the great arteries are side by side, in which the coronary transfer may be at risk for tension, torsion, or kinking. However, at this time, the coronary artery with an intramural course is probably the only absolute contraindication for an ASO (Gittenberg-DeGroot et al, 1986) (Fig. 43–38). Increased experience with the ASO tends to reduce the number of aborted arterial switches due to unusual coronary anatomy.

Associated Cardiac Defects

Ventricular Septal Defect. A VSD is present in approximately 25% of patients with TGA. All of the possible different locations of VSD have been encountered in TGA: perimembranous with or without malalignment, muscular, subaortic, subarterial, atrioventricular canal type, and multiple locations.

Atrioventricular Valve Abnormalities. Significant abnormalities of the tricuspid or mitral valve are

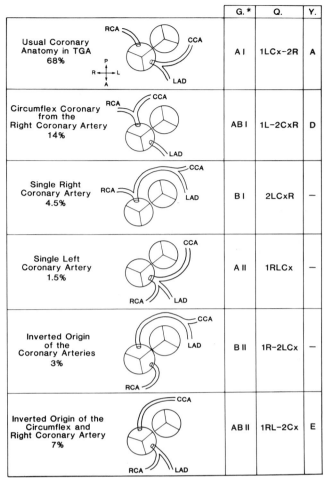

	G.*	Q.	Y.
Usual Coronary Anatomy in TGA 68%	A I	1LCx-2R	A
Circumflex Coronary from the Right Coronary Artery 14%	AB I	1L-2CxR	D
Single Right Coronary Artery 4.5%	B I	2LCxR	—
Single Left Coronary Artery 1.5%	A II	1RLCx	—
Inverted Origin of the Coronary Arteries 3%	B II	1R-2LCx	—
Inverted Origin of the Circumflex and Right Coronary Artery 7%	AB II	1RL-2Cx	E

* G.–Gittenberger–de–Groot, Q.–Quaegebeur, Y.–Yacoub

Figure 43–36. The six most common types of coronary artery anatomy in TGA. Descriptive terminology is on the left, and three classifications of TGA are on the right.

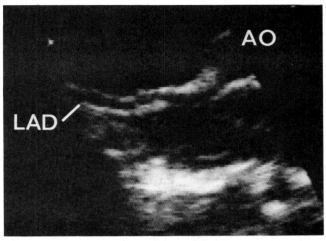

Figure 43–37. Two-dimensional echocardiogram of a newborn with TGA. The parasternal view, angled toward the left, shows the origin of the left descending coronary artery from the left facing aortic sinus and its course along the anterior interventricular groove.

by a localized fibrous ring, a long obstructing muscular tunnel, a protrusion of the ventricular septum, an anomalous attachment of the anterior mitral leaflet to the infundibular septum, other anomalies of the mitral valve (parachute mitral valve or accessory mitral valve), an aneurysm of the membranous ven-

rare and include anomalous chordal attachments, overriding annulus, and straddling tensor apparatus (Deal et al, 1985; Huhta et al, 1982a; Moene and Oppenheimer-Dekker, 1982). Significant straddling of an atrioventricular valve is commonly associated with hypoplasia of the respective ventricle, which may contraindicate the ASO. Preoperative tricuspid regurgitation is a strong indication for an ASO rather than for a physiologic repair.

Left Ventricular Outflow Tract Obstruction. LVOTO is present in approximately 20% of patients with TGA-IVS and in 30 to 35% of those with TGA-VSD. In TGA-IVS, the LVOTO is usually dynamic as a result of a left-sided displacement of the ventricular septum often accompanied by abnormal systolic motion of the anterior mitral leaflet (Chiu et al, 1984). More rarely, the obstruction is caused by a fibrous ring or by excrescences of endocardial cushion tissue in the subvalvular tract or, also, by pure valvular stenosis.

In cases of TGA-VSD, the LVOTO may be caused

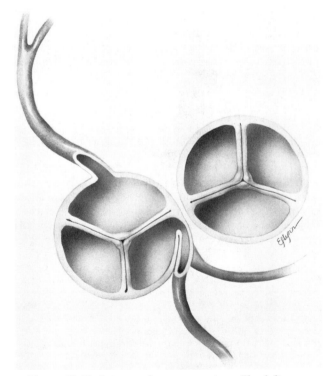

Figure 43–38. Intramural coronary artery. The left coronary artery (LCA) originates at an acute angle off the aorta and remains, for a short distance, partially embedded in the aortic wall. Note the normal angle of origin on the right coronary artery (RCA).

tricular septum, and, more rarely, valvular stenosis (Chin et al, 1985; Sansa et al, 1979).

Functional LVOTO is not a contraindication for an ASO; in fact, the gradients tend to disappear after the re-establishment of a normal LV-RV pressure ratio. However, long tunnel obstruction or any significant degree of organic pulmonary valve pathology is a contraindication for ASO.

Aortic Coarctation. Aortic coarctation coexists in approximately 5% of patients with TGA-VSD. In these cases, subaortic obstruction must be suspected (Moene et al, 1985; Schneeweiss et al, 1981).

Patent Ductus Arteriosus. Ductal patency is essential to maintain adequate oxygenation in the first few days of life. A large PDA may occasionally cause a low cardiac output syndrome and pulmonary edema. In these patients, the ASO should be accomplished as soon as possible unless the infant is significantly premature, in which case an emergency PDA ligation may prove to be the safest course of action.

Preoperative Management

All patients are evaluated preoperatively by two-dimensional echocardiography, cardiac catheterization, and angiography including aortic root injection. A balloon atrial septostomy during cardiac catheterization is generally recommended unless the ASO can be done immediately. In critically ill neonates, the balloon atrial septostomy can be accomplished at the patient's bedside under two-dimensional echocardiographic guidance.

When severe hypoxia or metabolic acidosis is present, prostaglandin E_1 may be added to maintain ductal patency and improve oxygenation (Lang et al, 1979).

Operative Technique

The operation is done through a midline sternotomy. A segment of pericardium is harvested and prepared with 0.6% glutaraldehyde solution. The ascending aorta and main pulmonary artery are then dissected free. After heparinization (2 mg/kg body weight), the aorta is cannulated as far distally as possible to allow adequate length for the aortic anastomosis. A single venous cannula is inserted through the right atrial appendage, and core cooling to profound hypothermia is initiated. During the

cooling period, the ductus arteriosus is divided. Both pulmonary arteries are dissected peripherally until the first pulmonary artery branches become visible. This maneuver allows eventual anastomosis of the pulmonary artery under no or minimal tension (Fig. 43–39A). At 20° C rectal temperature, the distal ascending aorta is clamped and cold cardioplegic solution (20 ml/kg body weight of St. Thomas' solution) is instilled into the proximal ascending aorta. Circulatory arrest can then be started. Alternatively, continuous deep hypothermic perfusion at low flows (20 to 50 ml/kg/min) can also be used, limiting the period of circulatory arrest to the closure of the atrial communication and of the VSD, if present.

The aorta is transected approximately 1 cm distal to the origin of the coronary arteries. The coronary ostia are inspected from within and are probed gently to identify anomalies of origin and branching. The pulmonary artery is then divided proximal to its bifurcation, and the native pulmonary valve is carefully explored (see Fig. 43–39B).

The left and right coronary ostia are then explanted, along with a generous flap of surrounding aortic wall. Only minimal dissection of the proximal segment of the coronary arteries is necessary. Small conal branches encountered during this dissection may occasionally have to be sacrificed (see Fig. 43–39C).

An equivalent V-shaped excision of the pulmonary arterial wall is excised from both the left and right anterior sinuses of the neoaorta. The coronary flaps are then sewn into these incisions with continuous 7-0 absorbable monofilament sutures (PDS) (see Fig. 43–39D). When the circumflex coronary artery arises from the right coronary artery, the site of implantation must be kept slightly higher to avoid kinking of the circumflex coronary artery. If two coronary arteries come from the same sinus, they can be included in the same aortic flap.

The distal pulmonary artery is then brought anterior to the aorta (Lecompte's maneuver), which can also be accomplished in most cases of a side-by-side relationship of the great arteries, although in isolated cases the pulmonary artery is better left in situ, anastomosing instead the neopulmonary artery to the main and right pulmonary arteries. The distal aorta is anastomosed to the proximal neoaorta with 6-0 continuous absorbable monofilament suture (PDS). Portions of the aortic flaps are incorporated into this anastomosis to compensate for discrepancies in size (see Fig. 43–39E). At this point, the right atrial

Figure 43–39. *A*, Surgical technique of ASO. After instituting cardiopulmonary bypass, the ductus arteriosus is divided between suture ligatures and the branch pulmonary arteries are thoroughly dissected. The *broken lines* represent the levels of transection of the aorta and the main pulmonary artery. Marking sutures are placed in the predicted sites of the coronary anastomoses. The *insert* shows the details of ductal division. *B*, Transection of the great arteries. Retraction sutures are placed at the level of the pulmonary valve commissures. *C*, The coronary arterial flaps are excised from the free edge of the aorta to the base of the sinus of Valsalva. In the inserts, details of the coronary flap excision in the tangential *(above)* and frontal *(below)* views are shown. *D*, The coronary arterial flaps are anastomosed to V-shaped excisions made in the pulmonary (neoaortic) wall. *E*, The pulmonary artery is brought anterior to the aorta (Lecompte's maneuver). Anastomosis of the proximal neoaorta to the distal aorta is shown. *F*, Filling of the coronary donor sites with pericardial patches. *G*, Anastomosis of the proximal neopulmonary artery and the distal pulmonary artery.

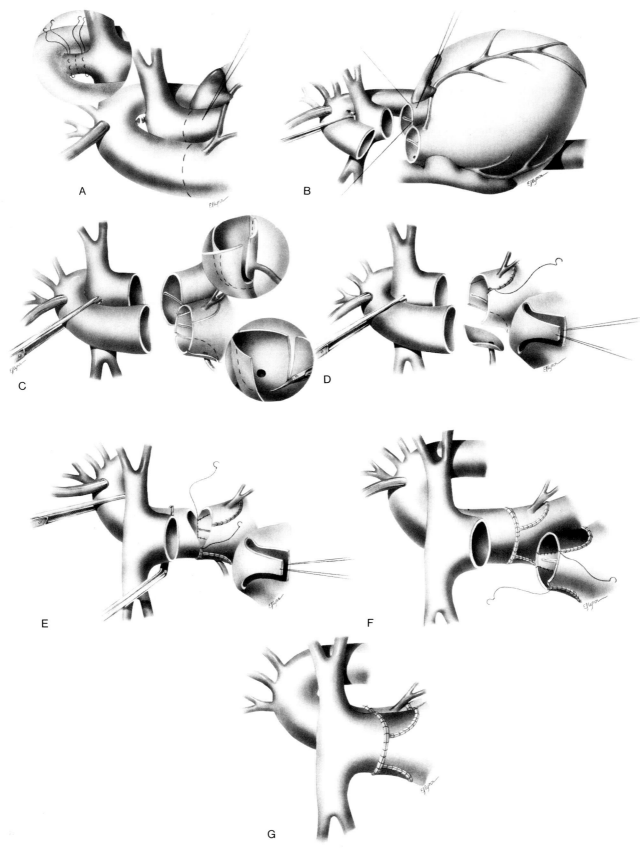

Figure 43–39 *See legend on opposite page*

communication is closed through a right atriotomy. If a VSD is present, it is also closed through the right atrium whenever possible. Alternatively, the VSD can be closed through a right ventriculotomy or atriotomy.

After closure of the right atriotomy, the venous cannula is reinserted, and cardiopulmonary bypass is reinitiated. The aortic cross-clamp can be removed at this point, provided that the left side of the heart is fully vented through a stab incision in the ascending aorta.

The coronary donor sites in the neopulmonary artery are then filled with segments of pretreated autologous pericardium (see Fig. 43–39E). Finally, the distal pulmonary artery is sewn to the proximal neopulmonary artery. Discrepancies in caliber of the two ends of the neopulmonary artery are reconciled with pericardial flaps derived from the distal redundant portions of the pericardial patches used to fill the coronary donor sites (see Fig. 43–39G).

Rewarming, usually started when the aortic clamp is released, is completed on bypass to a rectal temperature of 35° C. Weaning from cardiopulmonary bypass relies on close monitoring of heart rate and left atrial pressure. The systemic blood pressure is maintained at approximately 60 mm Hg, adding calcium and inotropic agents, usually dopamine, if necessary. Abnormalities of cardiac rhythm or of myocardial performance are considered to be suggestive of a coronary perfusion problem. If this is the case, the cause must be identified at this point and aggressively treated. After removal of the venous and arterial cannulas, a right atrial line is placed through the right atrial appendage.

Postoperative Management

Postoperative management is similar to that of neonates having repair of other complex cardiac lesions. Mechanical ventilation, sedation, and moderate inotropic support are provided during the first 24 to 48 hours or until hemodynamic stability is achieved.

RESULTS

From January, 1983, through December, 1987, 168 patients at the Children's Hospital in Boston had an ASO, 106 for TGA-IVS (Group I) and 62 for TGA-VSD or double-outlet right ventricle with subpulmonary VSD (Group II). Six patients with TGA-IVS had a two-stage approach: Four had pulmonary artery banding and right Blalock-Taussig shunt, one had only a pulmonary artery banding, and one only a right Blalock-Taussig shunt.

Hospital Outcome

The overall hospital mortality for ASO was 9.5% (16 of 168), 12.3% (13 of 106) in Group I and 4.8% (3

of 62) in Group II. In the last 2½ years (since July, 1984), the overall mortality has decreased to 4.8% (6 of 124), being only 3.7% (2 of 53) in patients with TGA-IVS operated on within the first week of life. Early results of ASO reported by other institutions are summarized in Tables 43–3 and 43–4.

Follow-up Data

Among 152 hospital survivors, three late deaths occurred. Most survivors presented with no cardiac symptoms. None of the patients were on cardiac medications, and all had a normal growth pattern.

Arterial Anastomotic Obstruction. Supravalvular pulmonary stenosis with RV to pulmonary artery gradients of more than 50 mm Hg was found in

TABLE 43–3. REVIEW OF THE RECENT LITERATURE ON THE EARLY RESULTS AFTER ASO FOR TGA-IVS

Institution	Period	No. of Patients	No. (%) of Deaths
Harefield Hospital (London, U.K.)	May 1982– Dec. 1983	11	1 (9.1%)
Brompton Hospital (London, U.K.)	Feb. 1981– Dec. 1984	8	1 (12.5%)
The Heart Institute (Tokyo, Japan)	Aug. 1982– May 1985	16	3 (18.7%)
Hospital des Enfantes Malades (Paris, France)	Apr. 1984– Jan. 1986	50	8 (16%)
University of Leiden (The Netherlands)	Jan. 1983– Apr. 1986	47	3 (6.4%)
Royal Children's Hospital (Melbourne, Australia)	May 1983– May 1986	51	0 (0%)
Multi-Institutional (North America)	Jan. 1985– June 1986	72	14 (19.4%)
University of Louisville (Kentucky, U.S.A.)	Jan. 1985– Oct. 1986	16	2 (12.5%)
Children's Memorial Hospital (Chicago, Illinois, U.S.A.)	Oct. 1983– Apr. 1987	38	3 (7.9%)
Boston Children's Hospital Massachusetts, U.S.A.	Jan. 1983– Dec. 1987	106	13 (12.3%)

TABLE 43–4. REVIEW OF THE RECENT LITERATURE ON THE EARLY RESULTS AFTER ASO FOR TGA-VSD OR DOUBLE-OUTLET RV WITH SUBPULMONARY VSD

Institution	Period	No. of Patients	No. (%) of Deaths
Brompton Hospital (London, U.K.)	Feb. 1981– Dec. 1984	22	7 (31.8%)
The Heart Institute (Tokyo, Japan)	Aug. 1982– May 1985	24	2 (8.3%)
University of Leiden (The Netherlands)	Jan. 1977– Apr. 1986	62	8 (12.9%)
Royal Children's Hospital (Melbourne, Australia)	May, 1983– May 1986	41	4 (9.8%)
Multi-Institutional (North America)	Jan. 1985– June 1986	14	3 (21.4%)
Children's Memorial Hospital (Chicago, Illinois, U.S.A.)	Oct. 1983– Apr. 1987	15	2 (13.3%)
Boston Children's Hospital (Massachusetts, U.S.A.)	Jan. 1983– Dec. 1987	62	3 (4.8%)

seven patients, all in Group I; five had reoperations. Two mechanisms for supravalvular pulmonary stenosis were identified: (1) tension on the anastomosis with anteroposterior flattening of the pulmonary artery and (2) circumferential narrowing of the anastomosis. These complications occurred early in the authors' experience and prompted some modifications of the technique, including more extensive dissection of the distal pulmonary arteries and enlargement of the expanded coronary donor areas with abundant patches of autologous pericardium to facilitate enlargement of the pulmonary artery anastomosis. Supravalvular aortic stenosis was uncommon. Only two patients had a transaortic gradient of more than 25 mm Hg.

Semilunar Valve Regurgitation. Mild pulmonary regurgitation was present in two patients, whereas trivial or mild aortic regurgitation was noted in 10% of the cases (15 of 152). These data compare favorably with the incidence of aortic regurgitation reported after the two-stage approach (31%) (Lange et al, 1986), which is most likely related to distortion of the native pulmonary valve by the pulmonary artery band.

Late Occlusion of Coronary Arteries. Occlusion of the left coronary artery occurred in three patients. One of these patients had the usual pattern of coronary anatomy, and two had a circumflex coronary artery arising from the right coronary artery, with only a small anterior descending coronary artery arising from the left facing sinus. All three patients had adequate retrograde perfusion through collaterals and showed no left ventricular dysfunction at two-dimensional echocardiography or cardiac catheterization. Late myocardial infarction with sudden death has been reported by Sidi and colleagues (1987) and may have been responsible for the single late death in the authors' series.

Pulmonary Vascular Obstructive Disease. Five patients in the group with TGA-VSD had persistent pulmonary hypertension and progression to pulmonary vascular obstructive disease. Their age at operation ranged from 6 to 28 months (mean = 16 months). Three of these patients had no previous pulmonary artery banding to protect the pulmonary arteries, whereas in the other two patients the pulmonary artery bands proved to be ineffective at preoperative cardiac catheterization. One patient with TGA-IVS and large PDA developed pulmonary vascular obstructive disease despite repair at 7 weeks of age.

Left Ventricular Dysfunction. LV dysfunction has not been observed in any of the authors' patients after primary ASO for TGA-IVS. In fact, both LV systolic and diastolic functions were normal, both on two-dimensional echocardiography and according to hemodynamic criteria.

Electrophysiology Data. Normal sinus rhythm was present for as long as 55 months after operation in 98% of the patients who had an ASO for TGA-IVS and in 88% of those who had an ASO for TGA-VSD. Only one patient had late sinus node dysfunc-

tion. Five patients in Group II had postoperative complete heart block (8%).

SUMMARY

It is still premature to assert that the ASO is superior to the atrial switch operation for the treatment of TGA. Although the different lengths of the respective follow-up studies do not allow adequate comparison, it appears that the hazard of death in the long run is less with the ASO. Although the ASO presents a single phase of rapidly declining risk, the atrial repair, in addition to an early phase of declining risk, shows a constant hazard phase that extends indefinitely. This difference becomes even more striking if one compares the hazard function per death in a protocol of routine early ASO versus a protocol of initial balloon atrial septostomy and atrial switch operation at 2 months (Quaegebeur, 1986) (Fig. 43–40).

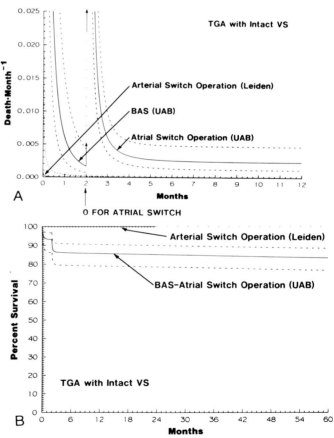

Figure 43–40. A comparison between a current protocol of routine ASO for patients with TGA-IVS (Leiden) with one of balloon atrial septostomy (BAS) followed by the atrial switch operation (Senning) at age of 2 months (UAB = University of Alabama) in a patient with a birth weight of 3.25 kg. *A,* Hazard function for death derived from multivariate equations. *B,* Parametric survivorship after repair by the two protocols. (From Quaegebeur, J. M., Rohmer, J., Ottenkamp, J., et al: The arterial switch operation: An eight-year experience. J. Thorac. Cardiovasc. Surg., *92:*361, 1986.)

Two differentiated preliminary reports derived from the same multi-institutional study on the current status of the treatment of TGA with both arterial and atrial repair have shown that surgical risk factors are low birth weight, early date of entry in the study, and the presence of major cardiac and noncardiac anomalies (more common in patients with TGA-VSD). According to this multicenter analysis, the 12-month predicted survival of a patient with TGA and with a weight of 3.4 kg currently entered into an atrial or arterial switch protocol is 92% (Castaneda et al, 1988; Trusler et al, 1987).

The early and intermediate results of the ASO have been progressively improving, and an optimal outcome can be currently achieved in the short term. The favorable intermediate echocardiographic and hemodynamic results of LV function and the electro-cardiographic and electrophysiologic data showing a 98% incidence of regular sinus mechanism 55 months after the ASO in patients with TGA-IVS are encouraging. However, the potential danger of late coronary insufficiency and aortic valve (anatomic pulmonary valve) dysfunction demand continued monitoring of these patients.

month). Pressure loading to levels above half of the RV pressure was associated with thickening (2.8 to 3.89 mm/log month).

Quaegebeur, J. M., Rohmer, J., Ottenkamp, J., et al: The arterial switch operation: An eight year experience. J. Thorac. Cardiovasc. Surg., *92*:361, 1986.

In this series, 66 patients (23 neonates with TGA-IVS, 33 infants and children with TGA-VSD and 10 with double-outlet RV with subpulmonary VSD) received an ASO between 1977 and 1985. There were eight hospital deaths (12.7%). Eleven-month actuarial survival rate for the entire group was 81%. Incremental risk factors for death included low birth weight, TGA-VSD, double-outlet RV with subpulmonary VSD, the presence of a PDA, and early date of operation. A formal comparison with the results of the atrial switch repair indicated that the ASO is superior.

Wernovsky, G., Hougen, T. J., Walsh, E. P., et al: Midterm results after the arterial switch operation for transposition of the great arteries with intact ventricular septum: Clinical, hemodynamic, echocardiographic, and electrophysiologic data. Circulation, *77*:1333, 1988.

This is a prospective study of 49 consecutive survivors of ASO for TGA-IVS by clinical examination, echocardiography, cardiac catheterization, ambulatory electrocardiographic, and invasive electrophysiologic evaluation. The mean length of follow-up was 29 ± 14 (SD) months after operation. This study has provided most of the follow-up data reported in this chapter.

Selected Bibliography

Castaneda, A. R., Norwood, W. I., Jonas, R. A., et al: Transposition of the great arteries and intact ventricular septum: Anatomical repair in the neonate. Ann. Thorac. Surg., *38*:438, 1984.

This is the first report of elective primary anatomic repair of TGA-IVS in newborns. Fourteen patients between 18 hours and 32 days of age with TGA-IVS had ASO, under deep hypothermic arrest. Preoperative LV-RV peak systolic pressure ratio ranged from 0.7 to 1.0 (mean = 0.92). The one hospital death was related to right coronary artery obstruction. The capacity of the left ventricle in a neonate to effectively assume the systemic circulation was clearly shown.

Castaneda, A. R., Trusler, G. A., Paul, M. H., et al: The early results of treatment of simple transposition in the current era. J. Thorac. Cardiovasc. Surg., *95*:14, 1988.

This prospective multi-institutional study compares the results of various treatment protocols for neonates with TGA-IVS. Of the 187 patients (less than 15 days of age) admitted to 20 North American participating institutions between January 1, 1985, and June 1, 1986, 76 were entered into a treatment protocol leading to an ASO, 45 to a Mustard's atrial repair, and 49 to a Senning's operation. Overall survival rate among the 187 patients was 18% at 1 year. The major risk factors for death were low birth weight and early date of entry into the study. Neither the arterial nor the atrial switch protocol was a risk factor in most institutions.

Danford, D. A., Huhta, J. C., and Gutgesell, H. P.: Left ventricular wall stress and thickness in complete transposition of the great arteries: Implications for surgical intervention. J. Thorac. Cardiovasc. Surg., *89*:610, 1985.

This is a combined echocardiographic and hemodynamic study of the effects of volume and pressure loading of the LV on posterior wall thickness and LV wall stress in TGA. Seventy-four patients with TGA were divided into four groups on the basis of hemodynamic data. Pure volume loading with low LV pressure resulted in little or no thickening of the LV posterior wall (0.52 mm/log

Bibliography

Abe, T., Kuribayashi, R., Sato, M., et al: Successful Jatene operation for transposition of the great arteries with intact ventricular septum—a case report. J. Thorac. Cardiovasc. Surg., *75*:64, 1978.

Anagnostopoulos, C. E.: A proposed new technique for correction of transposition of the great arteries. Ann. Thorac. Surg., *15*:565, 1973.

Aubert, J., Pannetier, A., Couvelly, J. P., et al: Transposition of the great arteries: New technique for anatomical correction. Br. Heart J., *40*:204, 1978.

Baffes, T. G., Ketola, H. K., and Tatooles, C. J.: Transfer of coronary ostia by "triangulation" in transposition of the great vessels and anomalous coronary arteries. Dis. Chest, *39*:648, 1961.

Bailey, C. P., Cookson, B. A., Downing, D. F., and Neptune, W. B.: Cardiac surgery under hypothermia. J. Thorac. Cardiovasc. Surg., *27*:73, 1954.

Bano-Rodrigo, A., Quero-Jimenez, M., Moreno-Granado, F., and Gamallo-Amat, C.: Wall thickness of ventricular chambers in transposition of the great arteries: Surgical implications. J. Thorac. Cardiovasc. Surg., *79*:592, 1980.

Benson, L. N., Bonet, J., McLaughlin, P., et al: Assessment of right ventricular function during supine bicycle exercise after Mustard's operation. Circulation, *65*:1052, 1982.

Bex, J. P., Lecompte, Y., Baillot, F., and Hazan, E.: Anatomical correction of transposition of the great arteries. Ann. Thorac. Surg., *29*:86, 1980.

Bjork, V. O., and Bouckaert, L.: Complete transposition of the aorta and the pulmonary artery. J. Thorac. Cardiovasc. Surg., *28*:632, 1954.

Borow, K. M., Arensman, F. W., Webb, C., et al: Assessment of left ventricular contractile state after anatomic correction of transposition of the great arteries. Circulation, *69*:106, 1984.

Borow, K. M., Keane, J. F., Castaneda, A. R., and Freed, M. D.: Systemic ventricular function in patients with tetralogy of Fallot, ventricular septal defect, and transposition of the great arteries repaired during infancy. Circulation, *64*:878, 1981.

Brawn, W. J., and Mee, R. B. B.: Early results for anatomic correction of transposition of the great arteries and for double-outlet right ventricle with subpulmonary ventricular septal defect. J. Thorac. Cardiovasc. Surg., *95*:230, 1988.

Byrum, C. J., Bove, E. L., Sondheimer, H. M., et al: Sinus node shift after the Senning procedure compared with the Mustard procedure for transposition of the great arteries. Am. J. Cardiol., 60:346, 1987.

Castaneda, A. R., Norwood, W. J., Lang, P., and Sanders, S. P.: Transposition of the great arteries and intact ventricular septum: Anatomical repair in the neonate. Ann. Thorac. Surg., 38:438, 1984.

Castaneda, A. R., Trusler, G. A., Paul, M. H., et al: The early results of treatment of simple transposition in the current era. J. Thorac. Cardiovasc. Surg., 95:14, 1988.

Chin, A. J., Yeager, S. B., Sanders, S. P., et al: Accuracy of two-dimensional endocardiographic evaluation of left ventricular outflow tract in complete transposition of the great arteries. Am. J. Cardiol., 55:759, 1985.

Chiu, I., Anderson, R. H., Macartney, F. J., et al: Morphologic features of an intact ventricular septum susceptible to sub-pulmonary obstruction in complete transposition. Am. J. Cardiol., 53:1633, 1984.

Clarkson, P. M., Neutze, J. M., Wardill, J. C., and Barratt-Boyes, B. G.: The pulmonary vascular bed in patients with complete transposition of the great arteries. Circulation, 53:539, 1976.

Damus, P. S.: Letter to the editor. Ann. Thorac. Surg., 20:724, 1975.

Danford, D. A., Huhta, J. C., and Gutgesell, H. P.: Left ventricular wall stress and thickness in complete transposition of the great arteries. J. Thorac. Cardiovasc. Surg., 89:610, 1985.

Deal, B. J., Chin, A. J., Sanders, S. P., et al: Subxiphoid two-dimensional echocardiographic identification of tricuspid valve abnormalities in transposition of the great arteries with ventricular septal defect. Am. J. Cardiol., 55:1146, 1985.

Duster, M. C., Bink-Boelkens, M. T. E., Wampler, D., et al: Long-term follow-up of dysrhythmias following the Mustard procedure. Am. Heart J., 109:1323, 1985.

Gaasch, W. H.: Left ventricular radius to wall thickness ratio. Am. J. Cardiol., 43:1189, 1979.

Gittenberger-DeGroot, A. C., Sauer, U., Oppenheimer-Dekker, A., and Quaegebeur, J.: Coronary arterial anatomy in transposition of the great arteries: A morphologic study. Pediatr. Cardiol., 4(Suppl. I):15, 1983.

Gittenberger-DeGroot, A. C., Sauer, U., and Quaegebeur, J.: Aortic intramural coronary artery in three hearts with transposition of the great arteries. J. Thorac. Cardiovasc. Surg., 91:566, 1986.

Graham, T. P., Atwood, G. F., Boucek, R. J., et al: Abnormalities of right ventricular function following Mustard's operation for transposition of the great arteries. Circulation, 52:678, 1975.

Haworth, S. G., Radley-Smith, R., and Yacoub, M.: Lung biopsy in transposition of the great arteries with ventricular septal defect: Potentially reversible pulmonary vascular disease is not always synonymous with operability. J. Am. Coll. Cardiol., 9:327, 1987.

Hayes, C. J., and Gersony, W. M.: Arrhythmias after the Mustard operation for transposition of the great arteries: A long-term study. J. Am. Coll. Cardiol., 7:133, 1986.

Hood, W. P., Rackley, C. E., and Rolett, E. L.: Wall stress in the normal and hypertrophied human left ventricle. Am. J. Cardiol., 22:550, 1968.

Huhta, J. C., Edwards, W. D., Danielson, G. K., and Feldt, R. H.: Abnormalities of the tricuspid valve in complete transposition of the great arteries with ventricular septal defect. J. Thorac. Cardiovasc. Surg., 83:569, 1982a.

Huhta, J. C., Edwards, W. D., Feldt, R. G., and Puga, F. J.: Left ventricular wall thickness in complete transposition of the great arteries. J. Thorac. Cardiovasc. Surg., 84:97, 1982b.

Idriss, F. S., Goldstein, I. R., Grana, L., et al: A new technique for complete correction of transposition of the great vessels. Circulation, 24:5, 1961.

Idriss, F. S., Ilbawi, M. N., DeLeon, S. Y., et al: Arterial switch in simple and complex transposition of the great arteries. J. Thorac. Cardiovasc. Surg., 95:29, 1988b.

Idriss, F. S., Ilbawi, M. N., DeLeon, S. Y., et al: Transposition of the great arteries with intact ventricular septum. Arterial switch in the first month of life. J. Thorac. Cardiovasc. Surg., 95:255, 1988a.

Izumo, S., Nadal-Ginard, B., and Mahdavi, V.: Protooncogene induction and reprogramming of cardiac gene expression produced by pressure overload. Proc. Natl. Acad. Sci., 85:339, 1988.

Jatene, A. D., Fontes, V. F., Paulista, P. P., et al: Successful anatomic correction of transposition of the great vessels: A preliminary report. Arq. Bras. Cardiol., 28:461, 1975.

Jatene, A. D., Fontes, V. F., Souza, L. C. B., et al: Anatomic correction of transposition of the great vessels. J. Thorac. Cardiovasc. Surg., 83:20, 1982.

Kanter, K. R., Anderson, R. H., Lincoln, C., et al: Anatomic correction for complete transposition and double-outlet right ventricle. J. Thorac. Cardiovasc. Surg., 90:690, 1985.

Kay, E. B., and Cross, F. S.: Surgical treatment of transposition of the great vessels. Surgery, 39:712, 1955.

Kaye, M. P.: Anatomic correction of transposition of the great arteries. Mayo Clin. Proc., 50:638, 1975.

Kurosawa, H., Imai, Y., Takanashi, Y., et al: Infundibular septum and coronary anatomy in Jatene operation. J. Thorac. Cardiovasc. Surg., 91:572, 1986.

Lang, P., Freed, M. D., Bierman, F. Z., et al: Use of prostaglandin E₁ in infants with D-transposition of the great arteries and intact ventricular septum. Am. J. Cardiol., 44:76, 1979.

Lange, P. E., Sievers, H. H., Onnasch, D. G. W., et al: Up to 7 years of follow-up after two-stage correction of simple transposition of the great arteries. Circulation, 74(Suppl. I):47, 1986.

Lecompte, Y., Zannini, L., Hazan, E., et al: Anatomic correction of transposition of the great arteries. A new technique without use of prosthetic conduit. J. Thorac. Cardiovasc. Surg., 82:629, 1981.

Maroto, E., Fouron, J. C., Douste-Blazy, M. Y., et al: Influence of age on wall thickness, cavity dimensions and myocardial contractility of the left ventricle in simple transposition of the great arteries. Circulation, 67:1311, 1983.

Mauck, H. P., Jr., Robertson, L. W., Parr, E. L., and Lower, R. R.: Anatomic correction of transposition of the great arteries without significant ventricular septal defect or patent ductus arteriosus. J. Thorac. Cardiovasc. Surg., 74:631, 1977.

Mavroudis, C.: Anatomical repair of transposition of the great arteries with intact ventricular septum in the neonate: Guidelines to avoid complications. Ann. Thorac. Surg., 43:495, 1987.

Mayer, J. E., Jonas, R. A., and Castaneda, A. R.: Arterial switch operation for transposition of the great arteries with intact ventricular septum. J. Cardiac Surg., 1:97, 1986.

McGoon, D. C.: Intraventricular repair of transposition of the great arteries. J. Thorac. Cardiovasc. Surg., 64:430, 1972.

Moene, R. J., and Oppenheimer-Dekker, A.: Congenital mitral valve anomalies in transposition of the great arteries. Am. J. Cardiol., 49:1972, 1982.

Moene, R. J., Ottenkamp, J., Oppenheimer-Dekker, A., and Bartelings, M. M.: Transposition of the great arteries and narrowing of the aortic arch: Emphasis on right ventricular characteristics. Br. Heart J., 53:58, 1985.

Mustard, W. T.: Successful two-stage correction of transposition of the great vessels. Surgery, 55:469, 1964.

Mustard, W. T., Chute, A. L., Keith, J. D., et al: A surgical approach to transposition of the great vessels with extracorporeal circuit. Surgery, 36:39, 1954.

Newfeld, E. A., Paul, M. H., Muster, A. J., and Idriss, F. S.: Pulmonary vascular disease in transposition of the great arteries and intact ventricular septum. Circulation, 59:525, 1979.

Pasquini, L., Sanders, S. P., Parness, I. A., and Colan, S. D.: Diagnosis of coronary artery anatomy by two-dimensional echocardiography in patients with transposition of the great arteries. Circulation, 75:557, 1987.

Quaegebeur, J. M.: The arterial switch operation—rationale, results, perspectives (Thesis). University of Leiden, Chapter 2, p. 45, 1986.

Radley-Smith, R., and Yacoub, M. H.: One-stage anatomic correction of simple complete transposition of the great arteries in neonates. Br. Heart J., 51:685, 1984.

Rastelli, G. C., Wallace, R. B., and Ongley, P. A.: Complete repair of transposition of the great arteries with pulmonary stenosis: A review and report of a case corrected by using a new surgical technique. Circulation, 39:83, 1969.

Sansa, J., Tonkin, I. L., Bargeron, L. M., Jr., and Elliott, L. P.: Left ventricular outflow tract obstruction in transposition of the great arteries: An angiographic study of 74 cases. Am. J. Cardiol., 44:88, 1979.

Schneeweiss, A., Motro, M., Shem-Tov, A., and Neufeld, H. N.: Subaortic stenosis: An unrecognized problem in transposition of the great arteries. Am. J. Cardiol., 48:336, 1981.

Senning, A.: Surgical correction of transposition of the great vessels. Surgery, 45:966, 1959.

Sidi, D., Planche, C., Karchaner, J., et al: Anatomic correction of simple transposition of the great arteries in 50 neonates. Circulation, 75:429, 1987.

Smith, A., Arnold, R., Wilkinson, J. L., et al: An anatomical study of the patterns of the coronary arteries and sinus nodal artery in complete transposition. Int. J. Cardiol., 12:295, 1986.

Smith, A., Wilkinson, J. L., Arnold, R., et al: Growth and development of ventricular walls in complete transposition of the great arteries with intact septum (simple transposition). Am. J. Cardiol., 49:362, 1982.

Stansel, H. C., Jr.: A new operation for D-loop transposition of the great vessels. Ann. Thorac. Surg., 19:565, 1975.

Trowitzsch, E., Colan, S. D., and Sanders, S. P.: Global and regional right ventricular function in normal infants and infants with transposition of the great arteries after Senning operation. Circulation, 72:1008, 1985.

Trusler, G. A., Castaneda, A. R., Rosenthal, A., et al: Current results of management in transposition of the great arteries, with special emphasis on patients with associated ventricular septal defects. J. Am. Coll. Cardiol., 10:1061, 1987.

Van Doesburg, N. H., Bierman, F. Z., and Williams, R. G.: Left ventricular geometry in infants with D-transposition of the great arteries and intact interventricular septum. Circulation, 68:733, 1983.

Vetter, V. L., Tanner, C. S., and Horowitz, L. N.: Electrophysiologic consequences of the Mustard repair of D-transposition of the great arteries. J. Am. Coll. Cardiol., 10:1265, 1987.

Yacoub, M. H., and Radley-Smith, R.: Anatomy of the coronary arteries in transposition of the great arteries and methods for their transfer in anatomical correction. Thorax, 33:418, 1978.

Yacoub, M. H., Radley-Smith, R., and MacLaurin, R.: Two-stage operation for anatomical correction of transposition of the great arteries with intact interventricular septum. Lancet, 1:1275, 1977.

PULMONARY ATRESIA WITH INTACT VENTRICULAR SEPTUM

James R. Malm

Pulmonary atresia with intact ventricular septum is an uncommon congenital cardiac anomaly associated with high infant mortality. One-third of the patients with this lesion are dead by the second week of life, and 50% die within 1 month unless they have surgical intervention. Longer survival depends on patency of the ductus arteriosus, and only rarely has survival been reported beyond childhood (Keith et al, 1978). This lesion was first described by Hunter, in 1783 (Hunter, 1869), but the clinical significance was not appreciated until 1951 (Edwards et al, 1965; Novelo et al, 1951). Pulmonary atresia with intact ventricular septum occurs in less than 1% of the total group of congenital malformations. This anomaly was described by Edwards and co-workers (1965) as complete obstruction of the pulmonary valve associated with a patent tricuspid valve and two distinct ventricles. The pulmonary valve is most frequently a diaphragm composed of three thick, fused leaflets and an annulus that is occasionally hypoplastic. The pulmonary arteries are confluent and normal in size as a result of flow through the patent ductus arteriosus. The main pulmonary artery is usually present to the level of the atretic pulmonary valve, and only a small segment of this atretic valve is in contact with the right ventricular cavity (Fig. 44–1).

ANATOMY

Anatomic variations of the right ventricle and tricuspid valve influence the extent and results of initial treatment and long-term management. The first variation is in the size of the right ventricular mass and its diastolic volume. A spectrum of dimensions do not fit conveniently into Greenwold's classification of a small or minuscule right ventricle (Group I) and a larger or normal right ventricle (Group II). Bull and associates (1982) proposed a more useful classification based on the presence of a sinus inlet portion, a trabecular part, and a conus or infundibular portion of the right ventricle. Right ventricular wall thickness was maximal when there

was no trabecular portion of the right ventricle and the conus was absent. Endocardial fibroelastosis is often present, decreasing diastolic compliance.

The second important anatomic feature of the anomaly is the size of the tricuspid orifice and anatomy of leaflets. Bull reported that the diameter of the tricuspid valve correlated with the size of the right ventricle and was smallest when the infundibular and trabecular portions of the ventricle were

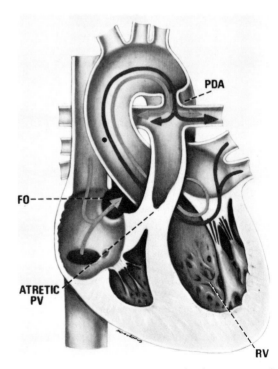

Figure 44–1. Schematic illustration of pulmonary atresia with intact ventricular septum showing the following anatomic features: a thick-walled right ventricle (RV) with a small cavity; pulmonary valve atresia (PV) with a normal-sized pulmonary artery; a patent foramen ovale (FO); and patent ductus arteriosus (PDA). (From Moulton, A. L., Bowman, F. O., Jr., Edie, R. N., et al: Pulmonary atresia with intact ventricular septum: A sixteen year experience. J. Thorac. Cardiovasc. Surg., 78:527, 1979.)

absent. Various degrees of tricuspid valve abnormalities and insufficiency are often present.

The third anatomic feature that influences management is the presence of sinusoidal communications between the right ventricular cavity and the coronary arteries. These fistulous pathways or sinusoids allow unsaturated blood to flow into the coronary circulation (Calder et al, 1987), and Hausdorf and colleagues (1987) reported apical left ventricular ischemia in these cases, presumably a result of blood flow steal from the coronary arteries. Fyfe and associates (1986) reported that these fistulas had an incidence of 35% and were associated with a high mortality after right ventricular decompression.

CLINICAL FINDINGS

Infants with pulmonary atresia with intact ventricular septum present characteristically with extreme cyanosis shortly after birth, often with arterial oxygen tension as low as 19 to 24 mm Hg. This condition is secondary to a large obligatory right-to-left shunt at the atrial level and inadequate pulmonary blood flow. Tricuspid regurgitation with signs of right-sided congestive heart failure may be present. No murmur is audible, or a soft systolic murmur of tricuspid regurgitation may be heard. The electrocardiogram is either normal or shows right-axis deviation in the frontal plane. Progressive changes occur with degrees of right-axis deviation, signs of right atrial overload, and right ventricular hypertrophy.

DIAGNOSIS

The chest film of an infant with pulmonary atresia varies and depends primarily on the degree of tricuspid regurgitation and right atrial enlargement (Ellis et al, 1971). The heart is often huge if there is significant tricuspid regurgitation secondary to the large right atrium. The preoperative evaluation of pulmonary atresia with intact ventricular septum is expedited by a detailed cardiac ultrasonographic assessment of the right ventricle and pulmonary artery morphology and size. The fundamental anatomy of the pulmonary valves, ventricular size, pulmonary artery size, and tricuspid valve morphology including annulus size and leaflet configuration are readily assessed with noninvasive imaging. Competency or stenosis of the tricuspid valve is shown with gated pulsed and continuous-wave Doppler ultrasound. Membranous atresia of the pulmonary valve with ventriculoatrial continuity and a satisfactory annulus size are readily displayed and also the less frequent hypoplasia of the infundibulum with a cord-like atresia of the proximal main pulmonary artery. The only feature not shown by ultrasound but revealed on the angiogram is the fistulous communications between the right ventricular chamber and the cor-

onary artery system. It is therefore possible to evaluate the patient and accomplish definitive therapy without catheterization based on a detailed cardiac ultrasonographic assessment. This modality is also helpful in the follow-up period for monitoring gradients across the right ventricular outflow tract, evaluating the relative growth of the right ventricular chamber, and identifying adaptations in the tricuspid valve.

Although initial emergent treatment has been done after echocardiographic studies alone, cardiac catheterization is usually done. A right atrial angiogram shows an obligatory right-to-left shunt, but it does not reliably define right ventricular anatomy or the source of pulmonary blood flow. Selective right ventricular angiography (Fig. 44–2) shows the size of the right ventricular chamber and allows measurement of right ventricular pressure and an estimation of the degree of tricuspid regurgitation. Left ventricular angiography (Fig. 44–3) shows the pulmonary artery filling retrograde through a patent ductus arteriosus and shows the level of atresia. Right ven-

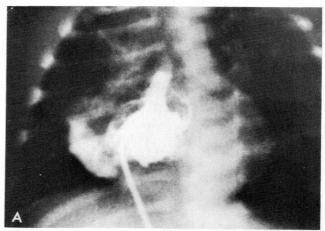
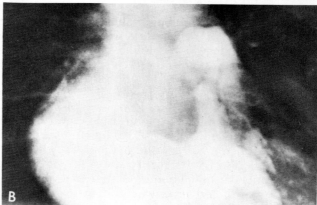

Figure 44–2. *A,* Anteroposterior right ventricular angiogram shows a small trabeculated right ventricular chamber with complete obstruction at the level of the pulmonary valve. *B,* This right ventricular angiogram shows tricuspid regurgitation resulting in marked right atrial enlargement. (From Bowman, F. O., Jr., Malm, J. R., Hayes, C. J., et al: Pulmonary atresia with intact ventricular septum. J. Thorac. Cardiovasc. Surg., *61:*85, 1971.)

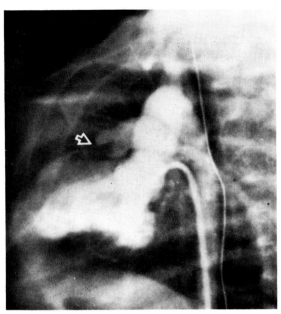

Figure 44–3. A lateral left ventricular angiogram shows a normal-sized left ventricle with intact ventricular septum and a normal-sized main pulmonary artery filling from a patent ductus arteriosus to the level of the atretic pulmonary valve *(arrow)*. (From Ellis, K., Cassarella, W. J., Hayes, C. J., et al: Pulmonary atresia with intact ventricular septum: New developments in diagnosis and treatment. Am. J. Roentgenol., *116*:501–513. Copyright © 1972 by Williams & Wilkins Company.)

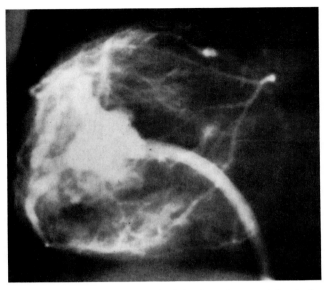

Figure 44–4. Right ventricular injection of contrast dye in the lateral projection shows filling of the entire left coronary artery through right ventricle-coronary artery communications.

tricular-coronary artery communications filling the left coronary system are shown in Figure 44–4.

SURGICAL MANAGEMENT

Most infants with pulmonary atresia and an intact ventricular septum are critically ill and have extreme cyanosis in the first hours of life when the ductus arteriosus constricts. These patients need urgent operative intervention. The introduction of prostaglandin E$_1$ infusion (Elliot et al, 1975; Heymann and Rudolph, 1977) has been valuable in maintaining duct patency and in delaying the onset of severe hypoxemia and resultant acidosis. Catheterization and operation may then be done under more stable conditions.

Definitive correction in newborns has not been recommended, but some type of pulmonary valvotomy or forward decompression of the right ventricle is necessary. Although this approach may provide adequate pulmonary blood flow in the presence of a right ventricle with a large chamber, it is usually inadequate. An initial rise in oxygen tension is followed by a decline in arterial saturation as prostaglandin influence on the duct patency is lost and pulmonary blood flow decreases. Foker and associates (1986), by using a right ventricular outflow patch for decompression, continue prostaglandin E until right ventricular function becomes adequate. This treatment provided long-term adequate forward flow into the pulmonary artery in 9 of 15 infants reported.

Decompression, regardless of how it is accomplished, is essential for preparation of the right ventricle for definitive repair. The authors' original report (Bowman et al, 1971; Moulton et al, 1979) clearly showed

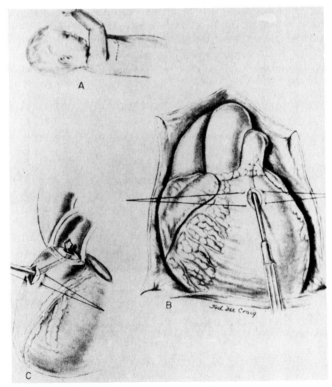

Figure 44–5. Through a right anterolateral incision, a transventricular pulmonic valvotomy is done, followed by a modified right Blalock shunt. (From Bowman, F. O., Jr., Malm, J. R., Hayes, C. J., et al: Pulmonary atresia with intact ventricular septum. J. Thorac. Cardiovasc. Surg., *61*:85, 1971. Published with the permission of the C. V. Mosby Company.)

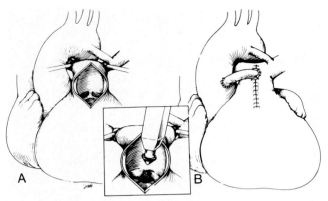

Figure 44–6. *A*, Pulmonary arteriotomy with hemostatic control of the origin of the branches. The insert shows a 4-mm punch used for valvotomy. *B*, Completed procedure with a 4-mm aortopulmonary shunt. (From Zollinger, R. W., Culpepper, W. S., III, and Ochsner, J: Simplified technique for the surgical palliation of pulmonary atresia with right ventricular hypoplasia and intact septum. Ann. Thorac. Surg., 41:222, 1986.)

TABLE 44–1. LATE RECONSTRUCTIVE PROCEDURES FOR REPAIR OF PULMONARY ATRESIA WITH INTACT VENTRICULAR SEPTUM

Anatomy	Procedure
Tripartite ventricle or trabecular cavity, adequate tricuspid valve	Valvotomy on bypass, closure of atrial septal defect Right ventricular outflow patch reconstruction
No trabecular cavity and small tricuspid valve	Right atrium to right ventricle valved conduit or repair II plus Glenn's shunt
No trabecular cavity or infundibular portion	Fontan procedure

right ventricular cavity growth after valvotomy over time, and this finding has been confirmed quantitatively by Lewis and co-workers (1986).

A concomitant shunt is usually required to provide reliable pulmonary blood flow. At the Columbia-Presbyterian Medical Center, a modified Gore-Tex right-sided Blalock shunt is preferred after a pulmonic valvotomy (Fig. 44–5). Several modifications of this combined approach have been reported (Joshi et al, 1986; Zollinger et al, 1986) (Figs. 44–6 and 44–7).

Of 42 infants treated under emergency conditions at the Columbia-Presbyterian Medical Center, 16 of 20 survived this combined management,

whereas only 8 of 22 infants survived valvotomy or shunt early in this series. The ductus is allowed to close and is re-evaluated at 6 to 9 months of age. If the right ventricular decompression is minimal, a second valvotomy or right ventricular outflow patch reconstruction is done. A more definitive open repair is deferred until 4 to 6 years of age, and the choice of procedure depends on the anatomy (Table 44–1). Of 14 patients who had repair, 11 had procedure I or II, one had a right atrial-right ventricular conduit (Bowman et al, 1973), one had a conduit and a Glenn operation, and one had a Fontan procedure. Three operative deaths and two late deaths occurred, indicating the continuing challenge in managing this defect. Alboliras and colleagues (1987) reported repair of the defect in 20 patients, with a 15% operative mortality. They selected right ventricular outflow repair or a modified Fontan procedure based on the size of the tricuspid valve, which was less than 55% of normal in 9 of the 20 patients. The high incidence

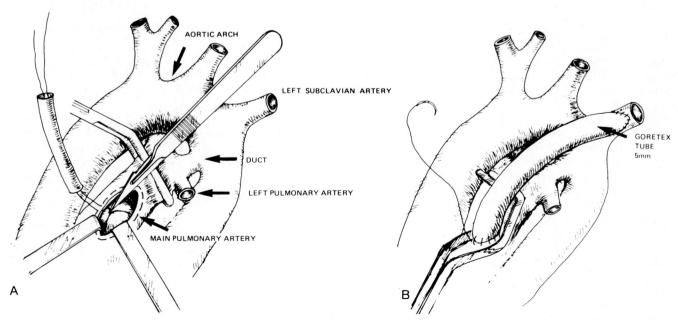

Figure 44–7. *A*, A direct pulmonary valvotomy is done by isolating the main pulmonary artery through the left side of the chest. *B*, A main pulmonary left subclavian shunt is done by using the incision in the pulmonary artery. The ductus is ligated. (From Joshi, S. V., Brawn, W. J., and Mee, R. B. B.: Pulmonary atresia with intact ventricular septum. J. Thorac. Cardiovasc. Surg., 91:192, 1986.)

PULMONARY ATRESIA AND INTACT VENTRICULAR SEPTUM TREATMENT PROTOCOL

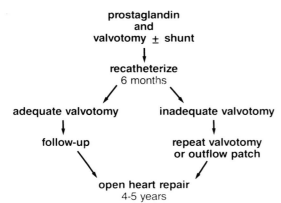

Figure 44–8. Treatment protocol is shown for pulmonary atresia with intact ventricular septum.

of Fontan's procedures suggests inadequate right ventricular preparation in early management, emphasizing the need for early right ventricular decompression to allow growth and development.

The initial surgical management must provide adequate pulmonary blood flow and allow development of the right ventricle without compromising future reconstructive surgery. The treatment protocol shown in Figure 44–8 is an overall management plan.

Selected Bibliography

Alboliras, E. T., Julsrud, P. R., Danielson, G. K., et al: Definitive operation for pulmonary atresia with intact ventricular septum: Results in twenty patients. J. Thorac. Cardiovasc. Surg., 93:454, 1987.

This article describes in detail the results of various types of definitive repair. The choice of the type of operation, repair versus a Fontan's procedure, is related primarily to the tricuspid annular circumference.

Bull, C., de Leval, M. R., Mercanti, C., et al: Pulmonary atresia and intact ventricular septum: A revised classification. Circulation, 66:266, 1982.

This excellent study of the anatomy of this anomaly clearly defines the important variations.

Waldman, J. D., Lamberti, J. J., Mathewson, J. W., and George, L.: Surgical closure of the tricuspid valve for pulmonary atresia, intact ventricular septum, and right ventricular to coronary artery communications. Pediatr. Cardiol., 5:221, 1984.

This interesting report describes closure of the tricuspid valve and plication of the right ventricle in a 5-month-old infant with right ventricle-coronary communications through sinusoids. One year later the sinusoid and right ventricle were not seen on angiogram. This unique and innovative approach should be further evaluated for this special problem.

Bibliography

Alboliras, E. T., Julsrud, P. R., Danielson, G. K., et al: Definitive operation for pulmonary atresia with intact ventricular septum: Results in twenty patients. J. Thorac. Cardiovasc. Surg., 93:454, 1987.

Bowman, F. O., Jr., Hancock, W. D., and Malm, J. R.: A valve-containing Dacron prosthesis. Arch. Surg., 107:724, 1973.

Bowman, F. O., Jr., Malm, J. R., Hayes, C. J., et al: Pulmonary atresia with intact ventricular septum. J. Thorac. Cardiovasc. Surg., 61:85, 1971.

Bull, C., de Leval, M. R., Mercanti, C., et al: Pulmonary atresia and intact ventricular septum: A revised classification. Circulation, 66:266, 1982.

Calder, A. L., Co, E. E., and Sage, M. D.: Coronary arterial abnormalities in pulmonary atresia with intact ventricular septum. Am. J. Cardiol., 59:436, 1987.

de Leval, M. R., Bull, C., Stark, J., et al: Pulmonary atresia and intact ventricular septum: Surgical management based on a revised classification. Circulation, 66:272, 1982.

Edwards, J. E., Carey, L. S., Neufeld, H. N., and Lester, R. G.: Congenital Heart Disease, Vol. II. Philadelphia, W. B. Saunders Company, 1965, pp. 575–578.

Elliot, R. B., Starling, M. P., and Neutze, J. M.: Medical manipulation of the ductus arteriosus. Lancet, 1:140, 1975.

Ellis, K., Casarella, W. J., Hayes, C. J., et al: Pulmonary atresia with intact ventricular septum: Report of 50 cases. Pediatrics, 47:370, 1971.

Ellis, K., Casarella, W. J., Hayes, C. J., et al: Pulmonary atresia with intact ventricular septum: New developments in diagnosis and treatment. Am. J. Roentgenol., 116:501, 1972.

Foker, J. E., Braulin, E. A., St. Cyr, J. A., et al: Management of pulmonary atresia with intact ventricular septum. J. Thorac. Cardiovasc. Surg., 92:706, 1986.

Fyfe, D. A., Edwards, W. D., and Driscoll, D. J.: Myocardial ischemia in patients with pulmonary atresia and intact ventricular septum. J. Am. Coll. Cardiol., 8:402, 1986.

Grant, R. T.: Unusual anomaly of coronary vessels in malformed heart of a child. Heart, 13:273, 1926.

Hausdorf, G., Gravinghoff, L., and Keck, E. W.: Effects of persisting myocardial sinusoids on left ventricular performance in pulmonary atresia with intact ventricular septum. Eur. Heart J., 8:291, 1987.

Heymann, M. A., and Rudolph, A. M.: Ductus arteriosus dilatation by prostaglandin E_1 in infants with pulmonary atresia. Pediatrics, 59:325, 1977.

Hunter, J.: Observations and Enquiries, 6:291, 1783. Cited in Peacock, T. B.: Malformations of the heart; atresia of the orifice of the pulmonary artery; aorta communicating with both ventricles. Trans. Pathol. Soc. Lond., 20:61, 1869.

Joshi, S. V., Brawn, W. J., and Mee, R. B. B.: Pulmonary atresia with intact ventricular septum. J. Thorac. Cardiovasc. Surg., 91:192, 1986.

Keith, J. D., Rowe, R. D., and Vlad, P.: Heart Disease in Infancy and Childhood, 3rd ed. New York, Macmillan, 1978.

Lewis, A. B., Wells, W., and Lindesmith, G. G.: Right ventricular growth potential in neonates with pulmonary atresia and intact ventricular septum. J. Thorac. Cardiovasc. Surg., 91:835, 1986.

Moulton, A. L., Bowman, F. O., Jr., Edie, R. N., et al: Pulmonary atresia with intact ventricular septum: A sixteen year experience. J. Thorac. Cardiovasc. Surg., 78:527, 1979.

Novelo, S., Chait, L. O., Zapata-Diaz, J., and Valasquez, T.: Atresia pulmonary estenosis tricuspidea sin co minicaciones interventricular. Arch. Inst. Cardiol. Mex., 21:325, 1951.

Zollinger, R. W., Culpepper, W. S., and Ochsner, J.: Simplified technique for the surgical palliation of pulmonary atresia with right ventricular hypoplasia and intact septum. Ann. Thorac. Surg., 41:222, 1986.

CHAPTER 45

UNIVENTRICULAR HEART

James R. Malm

In 1824, Holmes described a heart with one ventricle, and in 1936, Abbott reported 27 cases of single ventricle and with associated defects among 1,000 congenital heart malformations. Since then, the pathologic anatomy of hearts with one ventricle has been studied by many authors, causing various opinions of the entity itself as well as its embryology and classification. Van Praagh and associates (1964, 1965, 1972), Lev and co-workers (1969), and Anderson's group (1974, 1976, 1978) made major contributions to the understanding of the anatomy of single ventricle. A clinical diagnosis has become possible with the use of biplane cineangiocardiography and two-dimensional echocardiography. In selected cases, palliation or surgical correction has been done.

Anderson's terminology is practical for surgeons and has, therefore, been used throughout this chapter.* A univentricular heart (UVH) is defined by the commitment of the atrioventricular (AV) valves to only one chamber in the ventricular mass. A rudimentary chamber, which is either an outlet chamber or a trabecular pouch, is usually present. If this chamber gives rise to (more than half) a great artery, it is called an outlet chamber; otherwise, it is called a trabecular pouch. Common ventricle is defined by the absence or rudimentary presence (as a posterior rim) of the interventricular septum, with both right and left ventricular sinus myocardium present, and this form may be considered to be a large ventricular septal defect (VSD).

EMBRYOLOGY, ANATOMY, AND CLASSIFICATION

Three variations of UVH exist (Fig. 45–1). The most common form is UVH of left ventricular (LV) type in which the ventricle has a trabecular component of left ventricular morphology, which is associated with a rudimentary chamber of right ventricular (RV) type. The RV type of UVH is less common and is associated with a rudimentary chamber of the LV type. A UVH of indeterminate morphology, with-out a rudimentary chamber, has also been defined. The incidence of UVH of LV type has been reported to be approximately 63 to 80% of all cases of single ventricle, whereas UVH of RV type was present in approximately 5%. Ventricular arterial discordance (transposition of the great arteries [TGA]) was found in 76 to 90% of the hearts, with rather equal distribution of cases in which the aorta was anterior and to the right of the pulmonary artery and anterior and to the left of the pulmonary artery. Common ventricle (i.e., the absence of the ventricular septum in an otherwise "normal" heart) is now considered to be a large VSD.

Single ventricle and L-TGA may be associated with several types of intestinal malrotation, most commonly with the asplenia syndrome. Asplenia includes abdominal situs ambiguus and bilateral right bronchi, which facilitates the diagnosis on routine chest film. (Details of the embryology and anatomy of these defects are noted in the selected bibliography.)

Several aspects of the surgical anatomy of UVH deserve special attention: (1) the conduction tissue, (2) subarterial stenosis, (3) AV valves, and (4) coronary arteries.

Conduction Tissue. In a UVH of the LV type with an outlet chamber and discordant ventriculoarterial connection (i.e., transposed great arteries), the regular posterior AV node is rudimentary (Fig. 45–2). An anterolateral (right-sided) accessory AV node adjacent to the AV ring is present, from which the penetrating bundle descends onto the right rim of the trabecular septum at the outlet foramen. The relationship of the bundle and the posterior great artery (originating from the main chamber) depends on the position of the rudimentary chamber. A left-sided rudimentary chamber (again, in situs solitus of the atria) is associated with a long bundle in proximity to the ostium of the posterior great artery (the pulmonary artery) (see Fig. 45–2); whereas, with a right-sided rudimentary chamber, the bundle stays remote from the posteriorly located pulmonary artery and remains on the trabecula septomarginalis and is therefore not related to the pulmonary artery.

In common ventricle, the conduction tissue has an anatomy analogous to that of the conduction

---

*Exclusive of tricuspid and mitral atresia.

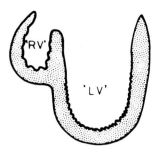 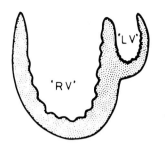 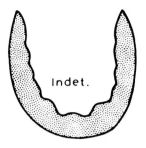

a) UVH of Left Ventricular Type with Rud. Chamber of RV Type

b) UVH of Right Ventricular Type with Rud. Chamber of LV Type

c) UVH of Indeterminate Type without Rudimentary Chamber

Figure 45–1. The ventricular morphologies of UVH. *Note:* Rudimentary chambers may be right-sided or left-sided in either LV or RV varieties of UVH. (LV = chamber of left ventricular morphology; RV = chamber of right ventricular morphology; Indet. = chamber of indeterminate morphology.)

tissue in VSD (i.e., the AV node is situated posteriorly and medially at the right AV valve orifice near the posterior ridge). The penetrating bundle extends to the posterior rim (i.e., at the rim of the rudimentary interventricular septum) (Fig. 45–3).

Detailed descriptions of the localization of the conduction tissue in other types of UVH have been reported: UVH of the LV type without an outlet chamber (Wilkinson et al, 1976), UVH of the RV type with a right-sided outlet chamber (Essed et al, 1980), and UVH of the RV type with a left-sided outlet chamber (Wilkinson et al, 1979).

Subarterial Stenosis (Fig. 45–4). Obstruction at the arterial outlet, either from the main chamber or from the rudimentary chamber, may be valvular or subvalvular. The obstruction can be present at birth or may be acquired during life. The obstruction can also form at the site of the bulboventricular foramen. Some evidence suggests that banding of the pulmonary artery may accelerate the development of subaortic stenosis if the anatomy is favorable to its formation.

The presence of a restrictive bulboventricular foramen has proved to be an incremental risk factor

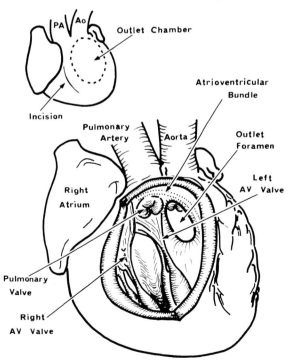

Figure 45–2. The surgeon's view of the conducting tissue in UVH of LV type with double inlet and left-sided rudimentary chamber. (From Anderson, R. H., Arnold, R., Thapar, M. K., et al: Cardiac specialized tissues in hearts with an apparently single ventricular chamber [double-inlet left ventricle]. Am. J. Cardiol., 33:95, 1975.)

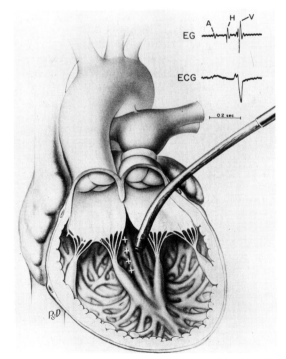

Figure 45–3. The intraventricular location of the bundle of His (+ +) in one patient with common ventricle. The electrical probe used for recording the operative electrogram (EG) is seen. Note on the EG the characteristic His (H) spike between the atrial (A) and ventricular (V) recordings. (From Edie, R. N., Ellis, K., Gersony, W. M., et al: Surgical repair of single ventricle. J. Thorac. Cardiovasc. Surg., 66:350, 1973.)

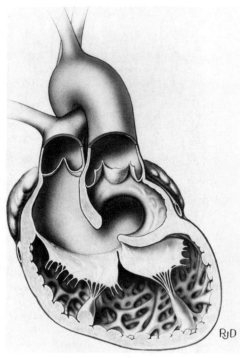

Figure 45–4. The UVH with LV morphology and left-sided subaortic outflow chamber with TGA. A single anatomic left ventricle is seen into which enter two separate AV valves. The rudimentary right ventricular infundibulum is in an inverted position and leads to a narrow aortic outflow tract. (From Edie, R. N., Ellis, K., Gersony, W. M., et al: Surgical repair of single ventricle. J. Thorac. Cardiovasc. Surg., *66*:350, 1973.)

in open repair of UVH. In UVH of the LV type with rudimentary chamber, the outlet foramen was restrictive in 33% of cases with ventriculoarterial discordance and resulted in an obstruction to the aortic flow. In 70% of cases with ventriculoarterial concordance, the outlet foramen resulted in obstruction to pulmonary flow. In one series, pulmonic stenosis was found in 83 of 145 cases of common ventricle. Occasionally, there is obstruction to both pulmonary and aortic flow.

Atrioventricular Valves. AV valve anomalies such as parachute deformities, clefts, valve stenoses, common papillary attachments, and common AV valves occur with a relatively high incidence. They have surgical significance; therefore, not only should preoperative analysis with echocardiography (especially two-dimensional and contrast M-mode) and cineangiocardiography be done to establish valve anatomy and function, but also sufficient time should be taken at operation for a complete evaluation of both AV valve apparatuses.

A special problem is presented by straddling of AV valves. In UVH, an overriding annulus is present when one AV valve ring is committed to both the ventricle and the rudimentary chamber; this is also called annular straddling. A straddling valve is defined as that condition in which either AV valve tensor apparatus enters both the ventricle and the rudimentary chamber with papillary and chordal attachments in both; this is also called peripheral straddling. Peripheral straddling precludes the insertion of a new interventricular septum, unless an AV valve prosthesis is used. Detachment of the straddling papillary muscles or chordae usually results in severe AV valve insufficiency. Therefore, in patients with straddling AV valve, a septation procedure is undesirable and a modified Fontan procedure is indicated.

AV valve regurgitation may develop, primarily after the first decade. This development may be due to congenital abnormal valve leaflets or tensor apparatus, but, more commonly, it is due to ventricular dilatation. This may be particularly prominent if an effective systemic-to-pulmonary artery shunt has been created and results in volume overloading of the ventricle. More likely, AV valve dysfunction is, apart from pulmonary vascular disease, the major precipitating cause of heart failure in adult life in the natural history of the disease.

Coronary Arteries. In the absence of an interventricular septum, the presence of a proper anterior descending coronary artery is unlikely. The terms right and left delimiting coronary arteries have been introduced and refer to vessels that demarcate the outlet chamber in UVH of the LV type. Keeton and associates (1979a) studied the coronary anatomy in 26 UVHs, 24 of which were of LV type with outlet chamber. Right and left delimiting coronary arteries outlined the outlet chamber in 16 (76%). In 95% of the hearts, large delimiting parallel branches of the right coronary artery crossed over the anterior wall of the heart. Especially because all hearts studied had marked hypertrophy with a poorly developed collateral circulation and little cross-circulation between the main coronary arterial systems, ischemic injury to the myocardium at the time of operation occurred frequently. Apparently normal coronary anatomy has also been described in UVH of the LV type. Therefore, during repair, the coronary anatomy should be determined intraoperatively.

NATURAL HISTORY

The incidence of single ventricle is approximately 3% in all congenital cardiac malformations, with a male predominance of 2.5:1. In the first year of life, single ventricle constitutes up to 10% of symptomatic cyanotic heart disease. Until recently, all diagnoses were made at autopsy, and in Abbott's series (1936), death occurred in a range from infancy to 37 years, with a mean of 7¾ years. Since that time, one-fifth of all reported patients have survived to adult life, and the mortality in the first year of life has been 47%.

The Mayo Clinic reported 122 patients with the diagnosis of common (single) ventricle followed from 6 months to 15 years (mean of 9 years), after diagnosis at the age of 7 days to 38 years (mean of 9.4 years). It was found that 44 patients died of congestive heart failure, dysrhythmias, or sudden unexplained death. Seventy-eight patients were alive (age 9 months to 40 years), of whom 62 patients were cyanotic and had diminished exercise tolerance. A positive or negative correlation with the presence or absence of an outlet chamber or obstruction to pulmonary blood flow could not be established. The oldest patient reported with one ventricle was 69 years old and died from congestive heart failure and atrial fibrillation with mild pulmonary stenosis. The author's experience suggests that survival depends on adequate resistance to pulmonary blood flow proximal to the pulmonary vascular bed. Longevity is most often associated with a flow-limiting degree of pulmonary stenosis.

PATHOPHYSIOLOGY, CLINICAL PRESENTATION, AND DIAGNOSIS

UVH and common ventricle are admixture types of lesions with clinical features dependent on the relative amount of systemic and pulmonary blood flow. Although preferential streaming in the ventricle may contribute to favorable blood flow (i.e., physiologic), the major determinant of the hemodynamic presentation is the degree of obstruction to pulmonary blood flow. Patients who do not have obstruction to pulmonary blood flow show clinical features typical of a large left-to-right shunt with congestive heart failure. The natural clinical course is determined by the development of pulmonary vascular disease.

If severe obstruction to pulmonary blood flow exists, patients are very cyanotic; lesser degrees of pulmonary stenosis are associated with arterial desaturation compatible with normal life.

Additional lesions (e.g., patent ductus arteriosus) contribute to the pathophysiology and clinical presentation according to their nature. Physical findings are not pathognomonic and depend mainly on the associated anomalies (e.g., pulmonic stenosis). The chest film appearance is not specific, and pulmonary vascular markings depend on pulmonary blood flow—oligemic pulmonary fields and a small heart in patients with severe obstruction to pulmonary blood flow and plethoric pulmonary fields with cardiomegaly in patients with pulmonary overcirculation. The determination of the cardiac position (e.g., dextrocardia) is important, and the atrial situs can be predicted. The electrocardiogram (ECG) is not diagnostic in UVH because of wide variations in the precordial lead patterns.

Echocardiography is valuable in establishing the diagnosis. Special criteria have been described with reference to the AV valves, the absence of the interventricular septum with apposition of the "septal" leaflets of the AV valves, the presence (or absence) of an outlet chamber, and echocardiographic continuity between the posterior great artery and the AV valves. Echocardiographic contrast studies have

proved to be most useful, particularly to show a common AV valve. Two-dimensional echocardiography has proved to be superior for an accurate diagnosis of UVH. The most diagnostic view in this technique is the apical four-chamber view. Echocardiography gives an indication of ventricular performance, provides cardiac dimensions, and allows the diagnosis of straddling AV valve. Although some echocardiographic studies have shown normal ventricular performance, Gibson and colleagues (1979) provided abnormal ventricular contraction patterns in UVH by using cineangiographic data.

Cardiac catheterization and cineangiocardiography provide the definitive diagnosis. Pressure tracings reveal outflow tract obstruction and its degree, and oximetry data show shunting. Flows as well as resistances should be calculated in order to make proper decisions regarding operation. Cineangiocardiography shows the anatomic and functional state of the major cardiac segments (Fig. 45–5).

To classify and manage UVH, the following features should be identified: AV valve anatomy and function, ventricular morphology, and the presence of a rudimentary chamber, and the ventriculoarterial connection.

The ejection fraction, independent from pulmonary stenosis, is depressed in single ventricle. Ventricular function and ventricular volume can be measured. Finally, the presence and nature of additional congenital cardiac malformation can be determined. The differentiation between UVH and common ventricle is important because of operative treatment. The most reliable sign to differentiate the UVH and common ventricle is the presence of a posterior rim between morphologic LV and RV trabecular portions.

TREATMENT

Surgical intervention is required for most patients with UVH. Patients with a naturally occurring obstruction to pulmonary blood flow require treatment when pulmonary blood flow is limited. When a severe, marked decrease in arterial desaturation occurs, a systemic-to-pulmonary artery shunt is indicated. The shunt procedure of choice is the Blalock-Taussig anastomosis by using either the native subclavian artery or a Gore-Tex prosthetic graft (connecting the subclavian artery to the pulmonary artery). It is possible to increase pulmonary blood flow by a transvalvular pulmonary valvotomy (Brock's procedure) in selected cases. A purely infundibular obstruction can be relieved by the insertion of a palliative outflow tract patch (with or without the aid of cardiopulmonary bypass). In older patients, a Glenn shunt (connecting the superior vena cava to the right pulmonary artery) can be done; its advantage over a Blalock-Taussig or Waterston shunt is the absence of volume loading (overloading) of the ventricle with subsequent ventricular dilatation and AV valve dysfunction. A Glenn shunt conditions the

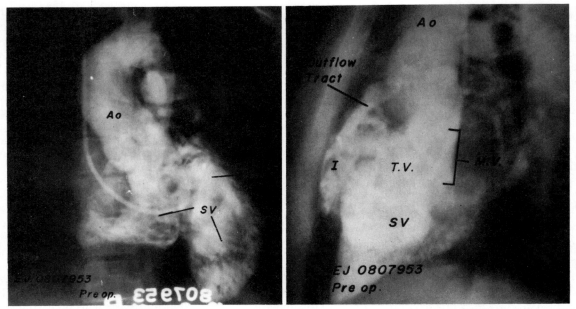

Figure 45–5. Preoperative anteroposterior and lateral angiocardiograms in a single ventricle of RV morphology with normal relationships of the great vessels. The catheter is through the tricuspid valve (T.V.) with the injection into a large, poorly defined single left ventricle (SV), which gives origin to both the aorta (Ao) and the narrow pulmonary outflow tract. The lateral view shows both the mitral (MV) and tricuspid (T.V.) valves entering the single ventricle with an anterior infundibulum (I) leading to the pulmonary outflow tract. (From Edie, R. N., Ellis, K., Gersony, W. M., et al: Surgical repair of single ventricle. J. Thorac. Cardiovasc. Surg., 66:350, 1973.)

heart favorably for a Fontan type of procedure. If pulmonary blood flow is adequate with normal pressure in the pulmonary artery, no treatment is necessary.

Patients with systemic pressure in the pulmonary artery will develop pulmonary vascular obstructive disease without surgical intervention. Banding of the pulmonary artery should be done at an early age, preferably during the first 6 months of life. The banding should be sufficient to reduce systolic pressure in the pulmonary artery distal to the band to 30 to 35% of the systemic arterial pressure.

If proper palliation or an adequate degree of pulmonary stenosis has allowed the patient to grow to the age of 4 to 8 years, two options exist for definitive repair of UVH: ventricular septation, which consists of the insertion of a prosthetic interventricular septum to divide the ventricle and thus make it into a physiologic biventricular pump, or a modified Fontan procedure, by which a univentricular pumping heart is established. Raised resistance in the pulmonary vascular bed contraindicates both types of repair.

VENTRICULAR SEPTATION

Construction of the ventricular septum by a prosthetic patch has been used to repair common ventricle (Fig. 45–6). The results obtained have been used to advocate septation for UVH, attention being focused on UVH of LV type with ventriculoarterial discordance (L-TGA).

A median sternotomy, or in young women, a horizontal submammary skin incision, is done before the median sternal split. Cardiopulmonary bypass by using hemodilution with hypothermia (18 to 24° C, which allows short periods of total circulatory arrest

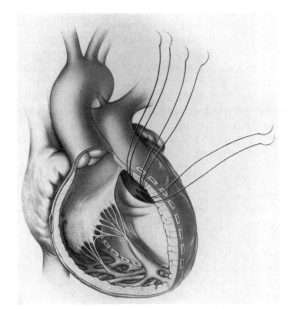

Figure 45–6. The operative technique used for reconstruction of the ventricular septum shows the large prosthesis separating the two AV valve mechanisms. The anterior sutures have been inserted from the outside of the heart through the entire wall thickness. (From Edie, R. N., Ellis, K., Gersony, W. M., et al: Surgical repair of single ventricle. J. Thorac. Cardiovasc. Surg., 66:350, 1973.)

if needed) is used, combined with low arterial flow, one period of aortic cross-clamping, and myocardial preservation by using cold potassium cardioplegia. Ventricular decompression via the right superior pulmonary vein or foramen ovale is established. Septation can be done through the atrium or via a ventriculotomy. The main advantage of the former is preservation of myocardial muscle; its disadvantage is the poor exposure for mapping the conduction tissue, as well as frequent inadequate exposure in general.

A longitudinal ventriculotomy is made in the plane of the anticipated attachment of the prosthetic patch, carefully avoiding the coronary arteries, or as a left-sided apical incision between the papillary muscles. The bundle of His can be localized by using a probe in 50% of patients, and its course can be anticipated by published anatomic studies. Mapping should be done before cardioplegia has been induced because the cessation of all electrical activity after administration of the cardioplegic solution prevents electrophysiologic studies.

A restrictive bulboventricular outlet foramen should be enlarged before septation, carefully avoiding the conduction tissue. The septal patch, for which a rather heavy noncompliant material is used, is shaped according to the anatomy. Insertion starts at the posterior aspect of the ventricle between the AV valves. Obviously, a common AV valve precludes the insertion of an interventricular septum unless a right-sided AV valve prosthesis is also inserted. Common atrium, which accompanies common AV valve, requires atrial septation.

Interrupted mattress sutures are used in the heavily trabecular areas taken from outside of the heart to prevent leaking. Papillary muscles are assigned to the appropriate ventricles because the patch is carefully sutured between them.

At the level of the semilunar valves, two options exist: The patch can be inserted between the semilunar valves, or both arterial outlets can be allowed to remain to the left side of the patch, which creates a double-outlet left ventricle. The former, especially in patients with L-TGA, implies suturing in the danger area between the semilunar valves with a high risk of inducing complete heart block. In the latter, re-establishment of RV pulmonary arterial continuity is necessary by using an external conduit. The use of a conduit is required when pulmonary stenosis is present, because reconstruction of the pulmonary outflow tract is hazardous, if at all possible, owing to its posterior localization.

Ventricle chambers are made of equal size. A patch that is too large or redundant tends to cause obstruction to the new RV outflow tract, whereas a patch that is too narrow impairs diastolic filling of both ventricles and places tension on the new septum predisposing to dehiscence.

Except for septation of the ventricle, additional abnormalities should be corrected and palliative shunts should be closed. Permanent pacing wires on the right atrium and the right ventricle are left in place because complete heart block occurs in approximately 50% of the patients.

MODIFIED FONTAN'S PROCEDURE

The modified Fontan procedure requires special venous cannulation techniques. To minimize surgical trauma to the right atrium, both venae cavae are directly cannulated by using right-angled Rygg cannulas. The right atrium is opened at the level of the right atrial appendage by a limited incision, which is later used to attach the valved conduit between the right side of the heart and the pulmonary artery. After the intracardiac anatomy has been determined, the right AV valve orifice is closed by using a pericardial patch. The patch is sutured so that the conduction tissue is avoided; therefore, it is attached to the atrial wall at least 5 mm from the AV valve ring. The coronary sinus is left draining into the ventricle beneath the patch. When mitral atresia is present, the patch should be semirigid, and the coronary sinus should be opened into the left atrium to avoid compression of pulmonary vein drainage by the elevated systemic venous pressure on the patch. A right atrial pulmonary artery connection is made after closing the pulmonic outflow. Obviously, again, all other anomalies should be corrected and palliative shunts should be closed. Special problems, such as arterial stenosis, are managed by more specific techniques (Doty et al, 1981).

If, coming off bypass, the patient's right atrial pressure is greater than 35 mm Hg, a superior vena cava-to-right pulmonary artery anastomosis (Glenn's shunt) can be done to unload the right atrium. A chest tube is left in place to drain pleural effusions that usually accompany Fontan's procedures. Postoperatively, early extubation promotes pulmonary blood flow, as will optimal positioning of the patient (semi-Fowler's position). Maintenance of an adequate cardiac output usually requires high systemic venous filling pressure and inotropic support. The use of drugs that lower pulmonary and systemic vascular resistance, such as sodium nitroprusside, is often helpful.

Treatment of common ventricle follows a course analogous to surgical therapy for VSD, although primary repair in infancy carries a higher risk. Palliation is usually accomplished by banding or partial closure of the defect with apical and septal patches, which were described by Ebert (1984). Because AV valve anatomy and arterial outflow are normal and the conduction tissue has a location similar to that in VSD, ventricular septation is the procedure of choice. Patch closure of the defect can be done, carefully avoiding the bundle at the posterior ridge of the rudimentary interventricular septum. If normal (ventriculoarterial concordance) relationship of the great arteries is present (in atrioventricular concordance), physiologic blood flow is obtained by septating the ventricle, leaving the arterial outlets to their respective ventricles. However, if ventriculoarterial discordance (i.e., transposition) is present, various options exist: a venous rerouting procedure at the atrial level (Mustard's or Senning's operation) can be done. When pulmonary stenosis is present a valved external conduit can be used by closing the pulmonary valve. A spiral interventricular patch can be inserted, which results in adequate interventricular rerouting, or an arterial switch procedure could be added to septation in order to achieve physiologic blood flow.

RESULTS

Palliative surgical treatment in UVH carries a substantial hospital mortality, primarily related to the age of the patient and the complexity of the lesion. The hospital mortality in patients with UVH and elevated pressure in the pulmonary artery who require banding has been 10%, whereas the hospital mortality in patients with decreased pulmonary blood flow requiring shunting procedures has been reported to be from 5 to 33%. The Blalock-Taussig anastomosis or the Gore-Tex graft modification is preferred. Although the Waterston shunt should be avoided, some patients may require multiple palliative procedures.

Late mortality is limited, and actuarial survival curves show an almost horizontally shaped curve after a few years' follow-up, the first part of the curve being greatly influenced by hospital mortality (Fig. 45–7). In 84 patients with common (single) ventricle, 70% were alive 10 years after diagnosis followed by palliative treatment. A survey has been published concerning palliative treatment of single ventricle during the first year of life. The overall mortality was 47%; it was 41% for the surgically treated patients and 58% for the medically treated patients as reported in the New England Regional Infant Cardiac Program.

Ventricular septation for double-inlet ventricle

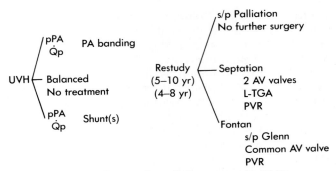

Figure 45–8. Proposed surgical treatment for UVH.

was reported by Pacifico (1986) among 36 patients. Thirteen (36%) patients died in the hospital, and 28 patients developed complete heart block. Five survivors required reoperation for patch dehiscence, AV valve replacement, or prosthetic replacement. Late functional status was described as being good. The author's experience with 12 patients confirms these results and must be compared with results of the Fontan procedure.

The immediate results of the Fontan procedure among a small reported series are now known. At the Columbia-Presbyterian Hospital, among 32 patients there were 6 hospital deaths (17%) and 6 late deaths (27%). The risk factors identified included complex systemic venous return, a hypertrophied noncompliant ventricle, AV valve incompetence, and pulmonary artery distortion by previous shunts. It is difficult to separate the tricuspid atresia patient from those with the more complex single ventricle in most reports, but the Fontan operation is technically more reproducible than septation for single ventricle. There is a trend toward the use of Fontan's procedure and at a younger age (4 to 8 years) before ventricular hypertrophy and AV incompetence occur in single ventricle. The late results published by Fontan report an actuarial survival rate of 90% exclusive of hospital mortality. The complications of chronic elevated systemic venous pressure can be avoided with strict criteria for selection.

PROPOSED SURGICAL TREATMENT

Patients with UVH usually require surgical treatment, most often in the first months of life. The indications for palliative correction are clearly defined: Elevated pressure in the pulmonary artery necessitates banding of that vessel, whereas decreased pulmonary blood flow causing hypoxic symptoms requires the creation of a systemic-to-pulmonary artery shunt.

When the patient has reached the age of 4 to 8 years, two options exist for total surgical correction: ventricular septation and a modified Fontan procedure (Fig. 45–8). In selected cases (UVH of LV type with two AV valves; L-TGA and no major additional abnormalities, such as subaortic obstruction), ventricular septation because of the good hospital results

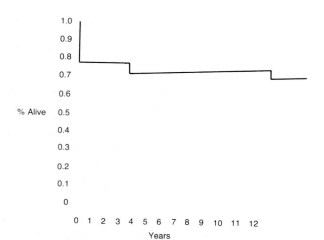

Figure 45–7. Actuarial survival after palliation of UVH.

and good long-term survival reported with this type of repair is favored. Adequate ventricular size seems to be very important so that the newly created right and left ventricles are of normal or greater than normal size (both naturally occurring and after previous pulmonary artery banding). A modified Fontan procedure is the correction of choice when a single AV valve is present. A management protocol is shown in Figure 45–8. The surgical management of UVH is still evolving.

Selected Bibliography

Anderson, R. H., Macartney, F. J., Tynan, M., et al: Univentricular-atrioventricular connection trap unsprung. Pediatr. Cardiol., 4:273, 1983.

The most recent and useful definition of this group of congenital cardiac lesions is the presence of an atrioventricular connection to one ventricle. This article provides a useful classification of these anomalies and should be a required reading for students.

Corno, A., Becker, A. E., Bulterijs, A. H., et al: Univentricular heart: Can we alter the natural history? Ann. Thorac. Surg., 34:716, 1982.

A thought-stimulating article that takes a reflective view of the efforts to correct and palliate the patients with UVH.

Pacifico, A. D.: Surgical treatment of double inlet ventricle ("single ventricle"). J. Cardiac Surg., 1:105, 1986.

This is the most current article on septation in a single ventricle. The anatomic features are reviewed and the surgical procedures are well illustrated.

Bibliography

Abbott, M. E.: Atlas of Congenital Heart Disease. New York, American Heart Association, 1936.

Anderson, R. H., Arnold, R., Thapar, M. K., et al: Cardiac specialized tissues in hearts with an apparently single ventricular chamber (double inlet left ventricle). Am. J. Cardiol., 33:95, 1975.

Anderson, R. H., and Shinebourne, E. A. (eds): Paediatric Cardiology, 1977. Edinburgh, Churchill Livingstone, 1978, pp. 305–406.

Anderson, R. H., Becker, A. E., Wilkinson, J. L., and Gerlis, L. M.: Morphogenesis of univentricular hearts. Br. Heart J., 38:558, 1976.

Anderson, R. H., Macartney, F. J., Tynon, M., et al: Univentricular-atrioventricular connection trap unsprung. Pediatric Cardiol., 4:273, 1983.

Anderson, R. H., Shinebourne, E. A., Becker, A. E., et al: Tricuspid atresia. J. Thorac. Cardiovasc. Surg., 74:325, 1977 (with reply by Bharati, S., and Lev, M., p. 328).

Beardshaw, J. A., Gibson, D. G., Pearson, M. C., et al: Echocardiographic diagrams of primitive ventricle with two AV valves. Br. Heart J., 39:266, 1977.

Bharati, S., and Lev, M.: Course of conductive tissue in single ventricle with L-loop and transposition of the great arteries. Circulation, 57:723, 1975.

Corno, A., Becker, A. E., Bulterijs, A. H., et al: Univentricular heart: Can we alter the natural history? Ann. Thorac. Surg., 34:716, 1982.

Doty, D. B., Marin, W. J., and Lauer, R. M.: Single ventricle with outflow obstruction. J. Thorac. Cardiovasc. Surg., 81:636, 1981.

Doty, D. B., Schrieken, R. M., and Lauer, R. M.: Septation of univentricular heart: Transatrial approach. J. Thorac. Cardiovasc. Surg., 78:423, 1979.

Ebert, P. A.: Staged positioning of single ventricle. J. Thorac. Cardiovasc. Surg., 88:908, 1984.

Edie, R. N., Ellis, K., Gersony, W. M., et al: Surgical repair of single ventricle. J. Thorac. Cardiovasc. Surg., 66:350, 1973.

Elliott, L. P., Bargeron, L. M., Soto, B., and Bream, P. R.: Axial cineangiography in congenital heart disease. Radiol. Clin. North Am., 18:515, 1980.

Elliott, L. P., Bream, P. R., and Gessner, I. H.: Single and common ventricle. In Moss, A. J., Adams, F. H., and Emmanouilides, C. (eds): Heart Disease in Infants, Children, and Adolescents, 2nd ed. Baltimore, Williams & Wilkins Co., 1977, p. 387.

Essed, C. E., Ho, S. Y., Hunter, S., and Anderson, R. H.: Atrioventricular conducting system in univentricular heart of right ventricular type with right-sided rudimentary chamber. Thorax, 35:123, 1980.

Feldt, R. H., Mair, D. D., Danielson, G. K., et al: Current status of the septation procedure for univentricular heart. J. Thorac. Cardiovasc. Surg., 82:93, 1981.

Fontan, F., Deville, C., Quaegebeur, J., et al: Repair of tricuspid atresia in 100 patients. J. Thorac. Cardiovasc. Surg., 85:647, 1983.

Freedom, R. M., Sondheimer, H., Dische, R., and Rowe, R. D.: Development of "subaortic" stenosis after pulmonary artery banding for common ventricle. Am. J. Cardiol., 39:78, 1977.

Gale, A. G., Danielson, G. K., McGoon, D. C., and Mair, D. D.: Modified Fontan operation for univentricular heart and complicated congenital anomalies. J. Thorac. Cardiovasc. Surg., 78:831, 1979.

Gibson, D. G., Traill, T. A., and Brow, D. J.: Abnormal ventricular function in patients with univentricular heart. Herz, 4:226, 1979.

Hallerman, F. J., Davis, G. D., Ritter, D. G., and Kincaid, O. K.: Roentgenographic patterns of common ventricle. Radiology, 87:409, 1966.

Holmes, W. F.: Case of malformation of the heart. Trans. Med. Clin. Soc. Edinburgh, 4:252, 1824 (Reprinted in Abbott, M. E.: Montreal Med. J., 30:522, 1901).

Kaiser, G. A., Waldo, A. L., Beach, P. M., et al: Specialized cardiac conductive system: Improved electrophysiologic identification techniques at surgery. Arch. Surg., 101:673, 1970.

Keeton, B. R., Lie, J. L., McGoon, D. C., et al: Anatomy of coronary arteries in univentricular hearts and its surgical implications. Am. J. Cardiol., 43:569, 1979a.

Keeton, B. R., Macartney, F. J., Hunter, S., et al: Univentricular heart of RV type with double or common inlet. Circulation, 59:403, 1979b.

Kitamura, S., Kawashima, Y., Shimazaki, Y., et al: Characteristics of ventricular function in single ventricle. Circulation, 60:849, 1979.

Lev, M., Liberthson, R. R., Kirckpatrick, J. K., et al: Simple (primitive) ventricle. Circulation, 39:577, 1969.

Liberthson, R. R., Paul, M. H., Muster, A. J., et al: Straddling and displaced AV orifices and valves with primitive ventricle. Circulation, 53:213, 1976.

Macartney, F. J., Partridge, J. B., Scott, O., and Deverall, P. B.: Common or single ventricle. Circulation, 53:543, 1976.

McGoon, D. C., Danielson, G. K., Ritter, D. G., et al: Correction of univentricular hearts having two AV valves. J. Thorac. Cardiovasc. Surg., 74:148, 1977.

McKay, R., Pacifico, A. D., Blackstone, E. H., et al: Septation of univentricular heart with left anterior subaortic outlet chamber. J. Thorac. Cardiovasc. Surg., 84:77, 1982.

Milo, S., Ho, S. Y., Macartney, F. J., et al: Straddling and overriding atrioventricular valves: Morphology and classification. Am. J. Cardiol., 44:1122, 1979.

Moodie, D. S., Tajik, A. J., and Ritter, D. G.: The natural history of common (single) ventricle (Abstract). Am. J. Cardiol., 39:311, 1977.

Moodie, D. S., Tajik, A. J., Ritter, D. G., and O'Falla, W. M.: Longterm follow-up of patients with common (single) ventricle after palliative surgery (Abstract). Am. J. Cardiol., *41*:390, 1978.

Pacifico, A. D.: Surgical treatment of double inlet ventricle ("single ventricle"). J. Cardiac Surg., *1*:105, 1986.

Quero-Jimenez, M., Perez-Martinez, V., Sarrion-Guzman, M., et al: Alterations des valves auriculoventricularies dans les ventricules uniques et anomalies similaires. Arch. Mal. Coeur, *68*:323, 1975.

Report of the New England Regional Infant Cardiac Program. Pediatrics, *65*:377, 1980.

Sakakibara, S., Tominaga, S., Imai, Y., et al: Successful total correction of common ventricle. Chest, *61*:192, 1972.

Schatz, J., Fenoglio, J., and Krongrad, E.: Electrophysiologic histologic correlation of the cardiac specialized conduction system in two cases of single ventricle and levo transposition of the great arteries. Am. Heart J., *96*:235, 1978.

Seki, S., and McGoon, D. C.: Surgical technique for replacement of the interventricular septum. J. Thorac. Cardiovasc. Surg., *62*:919, 1971.

Seward, J. B., Tajik, A. J., and Hagler, D. J.: 2D echocardiographic features of univentricular heart. *In* Lundstrom, N. R. (ed): Pediatric Echocardiography—Cross-Sectional, M Mode and Doppler. Amsterdam, Elsevier North Holland Biomedical Press, 1981, p. 129.

Seward, J. B., Tajik, A. J., Hagler, D. J., and Ritter, D. G.: Contrast echocardiography in single or common ventricle. Circulation, *55*:513, 1977.

Shimazaki, Y., Kawashima, Y., Mori, T., et al: Ventricular function of single ventricle after ventricular septation. Circulation, *61*:653, 1980a.

Shimazaki, Y., Kawashima, Y., Mori, T., et al: Ventricular volume characteristics of single ventricle before corrective surgery. Am. J. Cardiol., *45*:806, 1980b.

Shinebourne, E. A., Lau, K. C., Calcaterra, G., and Anderson, R. H.: UVH of RV type: Clinical, angiographic and electrocardiographic features. Am. J. Cardiol., *46*:439, 1980.

Somerville, J., Becu, L., and Ross, D. N.: Common ventricle with acquired subaortic obstruction. Am. J. Cardiol., *34*:206, 1974.

Van Praagh, R., Ongley, P. A., and Swan, H. J. C.: Anatomic types of single ventricle or common ventricle in man. Am. J. Cardiol., *13*:307, 1964.

Van Praagh, R., Plett, J. A., and Van Praagh, S.: Single ventricle. Herz, *4*:113, 1972.

Van Praagh, R., Van Praagh, S., Vlad, P., and Keith, J. D.: Diagnosis of the anatomic types of single or common ventricle. Am. J. Cardiol., *15*:345, 1965.

Wenink, A. G. C.: Conducting tissue in primitive ventricle with outlet chamber. J. Thorac. Cardiovasc. Surg., *75*:747, 1978.

Wilkinson, J. L., Anderson, R. H., Arnold, R., et al: The conducting tissues in primitive ventricular hearts without an outlet chamber. Circulation, *53*:930, 1976.

Wilkinson, J. L., Dickinson, D., Smith, A., and Anderson, R. H.: Conducting tissue in univentricular heart of right ventricular type with double or common inlet. J. Thorac. Cardiovasc. Surg., *77*:691, 1979.

CHAPTER 46

TRICUSPID ATRESIA

Robert M. Sade
Derek A. Fyfe

The hallmark of tricuspid atresia is the absence of direct communication between the right atrium and the right ventricle. Tricuspid atresia is the third most common congenital heart malformation causing cyanosis, after tetralogy of Fallot and transposition of the great arteries.

Tricuspid atresia served as the stimulus for the development of a corrective operation for children with only one functional ventricle: the Fontan operation. The concept underlying this procedure—that a pump is not needed for the pulmonary circuit—was startling when introduced in 1971 (Fontan and Baudet, 1971), but operative treatment is now considered to be safe and effective.

HISTORICAL ASPECTS

The first clear description of a heart with the anatomic features of tricuspid atresia is credited to Kreysig, in 1817 (Rashkind, 1982). A patient described earlier in the London Medical Review (1812) probably had tricuspid atresia, but absence of the tricuspid valve itself was not mentioned. Schuberg (1861) first called this malformation atresia. Although several patients with this malformation were described in the 19th century English language literature, the first use of the term *atresia* did not appear in that literature until 1917 (Hess). Kuhne (1906) recognized that patients with tricuspid atresia may have either normally related or transposed great arteries.

Surgical treatment for tricuspid atresia began in 1945 when Blalock performed a subclavian-to-pulmonary artery anastomosis in a patient with tricuspid atresia only a few months after he first used the operation in tetralogy of Fallot (Taussig et al, 1973). Other types of aortopulmonary anastomoses were introduced by Potts and colleagues (1946) and by Waterston (1962). A different type of palliative shunt, connecting a systemic vein directly to a pulmonary artery, was investigated experimentally by Carlon and co-workers (1951) and was clinically applied by Glenn (1958) and by Bakulev and Kolesnikov (1959).

Surgical palliation of tricuspid atresia may include enlargement of a restrictive atrial septal defect. A surgical method was first described by Blalock and Hanlon (1950), and a cardiac catheterization technique, balloon atrioseptostomy, was introduced by Rashkind and Miller (1966). A patient with tricuspid atresia with excessive pulmonary blood flow has occasionally benefited from the technique of pulmonary artery banding, first described by Muller and Dammann (1952).

Surgical correction of tricuspid atresia was first done by Fontan in 1968 and reported in 1971. His revolutionary procedure was based on the observation first made by Carlon and colleagues (1951) that pulmonary vascular resistance is so low that a pumping chamber is not needed for the pulmonary circuit. A wide variety of techniques to connect the systemic venous return to the pulmonary artery in various malformations have been developed and are referred to as modified Fontan operations.

CLASSIFICATION AND ANATOMY

The term *tricuspid atresia* is likely to remain in widespread use, although its embryologic, morphologic, and anatomic accuracy has been debated (Anderson and Rigby, 1987). Definitions of terms related to this malformation are shown in Table 46–1. Tricuspid atresia is the largest subgroup of a collection of anomalies referred to as univentricular atrioventricular connection (Anderson et al, 1984), which includes double-inlet left ventricle, mitral atresia, and other lesions. The logic of this grouping is reinforced by the fact that coronary artery distribution and ventricular morphology of hearts with tricuspid atresia and those with double-inlet left ventricle are almost identical (Deanfield et al, 1982).

The term *tricuspid atresia* is used in this discussion to describe hearts in which there is no direct communication between the right atrium (the atrial chamber receiving the systemic venous return) and a ventricular chamber. To describe a particular heart with tricuspid atresia, descriptions of ventriculoar-

TABLE 46–1. DEFINITIONS OF TERMS RELATED TO
TRICUSPID ATRESIA

Atrioventricular concordance: The morphologic right atrium is
connected to the right ventricle, and the left atrium is
connected to the left ventricle.
Atrioventricular discordance: The morphologic right atrium is
connected to the left ventricle, and the left atrium is connected
to the right ventricle.
Fontan's operation: Any operation on a heart with univentricular
atrioventricular connection in which the systemic and
pulmonary circuits are separated, the functional ventricle is
committed to the systemic circuit, and there is no ventricular
pump for the pulmonary circuit.
Outlet foramen: The opening between the dominant ventricular
chamber and the hypoplastic chamber in univentricular
atrioventricular connection; also called ventricular septal defect
or bulboventricular foramen.
Tricuspid atresia: A type of univentricular atrioventricular
connection in which no direct communication exists between
the systemic venous atrium and a ventricular cavity.
Univentricular atrioventricular connection: A group of
malformations (including tricuspid atresia) in which the
atrioventricular valves connect with only one functional
ventricle.
Ventriculoarterial concordance: Normally related great arteries.
Ventriculoarterial discordance: Transposition of the great
arteries.

terial relations and any subarterial obstruction are included. When appropriate, abnormalities of atrial situs or ventricular looping may be cited.

Edwards and Burchell's (1949) classification by associated malformations is still widely used in a modified form (Fig. 46–1), although it does not accommodate some examples of tricuspid atresia by the given definition (Anderson and Rigby, 1987). In the most common type of tricuspid atresia, Edwards and Burchell's type Ib, the atria are normally related and the tricuspid valve is represented by a dimple in the muscular floor of the right atrium. Systemic venous return cannot reach the ventricular cavity directly, thus it must cross an atrial septal communication from the right atrium to the left atrium, where it mixes with the pulmonary venous return. The mixed blood reaches the ventricular cavity by traversing the mitral valve, which is larger than normal, and enters a hyperplastic left ventricle. The mixed blood leaves the left ventricle through a normally connected aortic valve and aorta. Blood reaches the lungs from the left ventricle through an outlet foramen, into the hypoplastic right ventricle, which connects normally to a pulmonary valve and pulmonary artery. Additional pulmonary blood flow may come from a patent ductus arteriosus.

An atrial septal communication is always present. It is a patent foramen ovale in 60% of patients, and in the remainder it is an atrial septal defect that is usually an ostium secundum but may be of the ostium primum or sinus venosus type. The communication is usually widely patent but may be restrictive, especially when the ventriculoarterial connection is discordant (Weinberg, 1980).

The atresia of the right atrioventricular connection may assume many forms (Van Praagh et al, 1971). Most commonly, a dimple is located in the

floor of the right atrium directly overlying the left ventricle (Rosenquist et al, 1970), suggesting total absence of any relation between the right atrium and right ventricle. In those patients, the inlet portion of the right ventricle usually is completely absent. Rarely, a normally formed right atrium and right ventricle are separated by an imperforate membrane in the tricuspid orifice (Crupi et al, 1984). Three rare variations of tricuspid atresia have been described: Ebstein's malformation with imperforate tricuspid valve (Rao et al, 1973); total atrioventricular canal in which the connection of the common atrioventricular orifice to the right ventricle is absent; and a variation in which the right atrioventricular junction is open but is unguarded by a valve, and a partition, either membranous or muscular, completely separates the inlet from the outlet portion of the ventricle (Scalia et al, 1984).

The relationship of the right atrium to the ventricles is not constant. In cases of imperforate valve, the valve membrane is usually committed entirely to the right ventricle, but it may override an intact ventricular septum, relating to both the right ventricle and left ventricle (Ottenkamp et al, 1984). A similar spectrum in cases of absent valve was postulated by Wenink and Ottenkamp (1987) when they found that the dimple in the right atrial floor may connect by way of a fibrous strand with the right ventricle rather than the left ventricle. Thus, the relationship of the right atrium to the right ventricle may be concordant, discordant, or biventricular (Anderson and Rigby, 1987).

In patients with ventriculoarterial concordance, the morphology of the right ventricle is different from that in patients with discordance (Ottenkamp et al, 1985). In both situations, the inlet portion of the right ventricle is usually absent. In *ventriculoarterial concordance*, the outlet foramen (ventricular septal defect) separates the inferior trabeculated portion of the right ventricle from the superior infundibular portion. Obstruction to pulmonary blood flow is common (80% of patients) and is usually due to a small outlet foramen, often accompanied by infundibular stenosis and occasionally by valvular stenosis. However, in *ventriculoarterial discordance*, the right ventricle lacks not only an inlet portion but also an infundibular outlet so that the outlet foramen is immediately subjacent to the aortic valve and the outlet chamber (right ventricle) is completely trabeculated. Malalignment of the outlet septum lying between the pulmonary artery and aorta reciprocally affects the size of the subpulmonary and subaortic regions. Restricted pulmonary blood flow is encountered in 40% of patients with ventriculoarterial discordance, and subaortic stenosis rarely occurs; in patients with unrestricted pulmonary blood flow, subaortic stenosis is common and may be associated with aortic anomalies such as coarctation, isthmic hypoplasia or atresia, interruption of the aortic arch, or aortic valve atresia.

Other lesions of the heart and great vessels that

TRICUSPID ATRESIA WITH NORMALLY RELATED GREAT ARTERIES

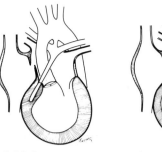 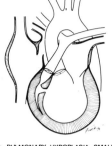 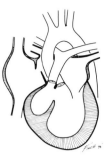

Ia PULMONARY ATRESIA   Ib PULMONARY HYPOPLASIA, SMALL   Ic NO PULMONARY HYPOPLASIA, LARGE
                                  VENTRICULAR SEPTAL DEFECT   VENTRICULAR SEPTAL DEFECT

TRICUSPID ATRESIA WITH *d*-TRANSPOSITION

Figure 46–1. Classification of tricuspid atresia according to associated lesions. Type I refers to normally related great arteries, II to *d*-transposition, and III to *l*-transposition. Subtype a refers to pulmonary atresia, b to pulmonary stenosis, and c to unobstructed pulmonary outflow tract. (From Keith, J. D., Rowe, R. D., and Vlad, P.: Heart Disease in Infancy and Childhood. New York, Macmillan Company, 1967.)

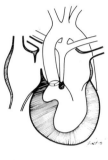 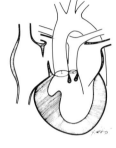 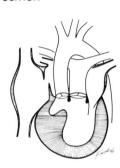

IIa PULMONARY ATRESIA   IIb PULMONARY STENOSIS   IIc LARGE PULMONARY ARTERY

TRICUSPID ATRESIA WITH *l*-TRANSPOSITION

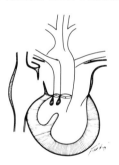

III SUBPULMONARY OR SUBAORTIC STENOSIS

may be associated with tricuspid atresia have important implications for surgical management. A left superior vena cava is present in 22% of patients (Weinberg, 1980); it usually drains to the coronary sinus but sometimes directly to the left atrium (Vargas et al, 1987b). Unusual interatrial communications may confound complete separation of the right from the left atrium. Coronary sinus septal defect (Lee and Sade, 1979) occurs in as many as 2.5% of patients with tricuspid atresia and, if not recognized, leaves a residual right-to-left shunt after the Fontan procedure (Coles et al, 1987; Rumisek et al, 1986). The same event may occur if cardiac veins connect the coronary sinus to the left atrium (Westerman et al, 1985). Anomalous pulmonary venous return (Scalia

et al, 1984) and coronary artery anomalies (Voci et al, 1987) occur rarely.

Congenital absence of the pulmonary valve (pulmonary orifice unguarded by a valve) may be associated with tricuspid atresia of the imperforate membrane type, usually with ventriculoarterial concordance, aortic dilatation, and intact ventricular septum (Marin-Garcia et al, 1973). Unlike the absence of the pulmonary valve in tetralogy of Fallot, in tricuspid atresia the pulmonary arteries are not large and bronchial compression does not occur (Forrest et al, 1987).

Juxtaposition of the atrial appendages occurs in tricuspid atresia in as many as 20% of patients with ventriculoarterial discordance (Scalia et al, 1984;

Weinberg, 1980). The smallness and inaccessibility of the right atrial appendage may affect the options for atriopulmonary anastomosis, and in addition, the volume of the right atrium itself is reduced (Scalia et al, 1984).

PATHOPHYSIOLOGY

Certain hemodynamic characteristics are common to all subtypes of tricuspid atresia. The entire systemic venous return must cross the atrial septum. The atrial septal communication is usually large and unobstructive, but in some patients with ventriculoarterial discordance it is obstructively small. The systemic and pulmonary venous returns are totally mixed in the pulmonary venous atrium. The oxygen saturations in the chambers and vessels downstream from the mitral valve are the same.

Patients with a restrictive subpulmonary pathway have reduced pulmonary blood flow and decreased pulmonary venous return so they are moderately to severely hypoxemic (71% of patients) (Keith et al, 1978). The small additional volume load on the left ventricle usually does not cause congestive heart failure.

Patients without subpulmonary obstruction have excessive pulmonary blood flow. The increased pulmonary venous return results in a highly oxygenated mixture of blood in the left atrium and systemic circulation, so these patients are frequently acyanotic. The left ventricle must do the work of pumping a large pulmonary blood flow, and this overload often leads to congestive heart failure. Severe congestive heart failure is common in patients with ventriculoarterial discordance. They may develop pulmonary vascular obstructive disease as a result of increased pulmonary blood flow and may continue to have a significant increase in pulmonary arterial smooth muscle despite banding of the pulmonary artery (Juaneda and Haworth, 1984).

Patients with ventriculoarterial concordance and unrestricted pulmonary blood flow usually have mild or moderate congestive heart failure that responds well to anticongestive medications. The outlet foramen, however, often decreases in size over time and leads to progressively increasing pulmonary outflow obstruction, increasing cyanosis, and the eventual need for a systemic-to-pulmonary artery shunt (Gallaher and Fyler, 1967).

CLINICAL FEATURES AND NATURAL HISTORY

Tricuspid atresia afflicts males and females almost equally, although there is a slight male predominance among the patients with ventriculoarterial discordance (Dick et al, 1975). The incidence is from 1% of all children with heart malformations in clinical series (Nadas and Fyler, 1972) to 3% in autopsy series (Keith et al, 1978). Of all infants who had a heart malformation and who were hospitalized or died in the first year of life, 2.5% had tricuspid atresia (Rosenthal, 1980).

Cyanosis or a heart murmur is present in 50% of patients on the first day of life, and 85% are recognized within the first 2 months. Cyanosis is the most constant clinical finding (Nadas and Fyler, 1972). Squatting is not common, and clubbing is usually present in cyanotic patients older than 2 years. Hypoxic episodes consisting of hyperpnea, increased cyanosis, and occasionally loss of consciousness occur in half of the patients.

Congestive heart failure occurs in 12% of patients (Dick et al, 1975), frequently during infancy. Mild congestive heart failure may remain stable for many years but, if severe, results in high mortality (Dick et al, 1975). Right-sided heart failure is manifested by systemic venous congestion, hepatomegaly, liver and jugular pulsation, and peripheral edema. It may be secondary to left-sided heart failure or may occur because of obstruction to emptying of the right side of the heart by a small atrial septal communication. Cerebral vascular accidents and brain abscess occur but are relatively uncommon (less than 5%). Infective endocarditis occurs in less than 5% of patients without previous operations.

The electrocardiogram demonstrates left-axis deviation in almost 90% of patients. Its presence in a cyanotic child should raise a strong suspicion of tricuspid atresia. Right-axis deviation occurs in patients with ventriculoarterial discordance and unrestricted pulmonary blood flow. Left ventricular hypertrophy is almost always present and may progress over time. The P wave may indicate right, left, or combined atrial hypertrophy. P-tricuspidale (notched P wave with a taller initial peak) is sometimes seen.

The appearance of the chest film varies greatly (Wittenborg et al, 1951). The size of the heart is usually normal or only slightly increased. Cardiomegaly may become quite marked, however, when pulmonary blood flow is large. The cardiac silhouette is not characteristic and may resemble the coeur en sabot that is seen in tetralogy of Fallot or the egg-shaped heart with a narrow vascular pedicle that is said to be typical of transposition of the great arteries. A right aortic arch is seen in 8% of patients.

Pulmonary vascular markings are usually reduced in patients with decreased pulmonary blood flow. Pulmonary plethora is seen in patients with increased pulmonary blood flow associated with a large outlet foramen, a large patent ductus arteriosus, or a large systemic-to-pulmonary artery shunt (Keith et al, 1978).

The natural history of tricuspid atresia is one of early death for most patients (Keith et al, 1978). Fifty per cent of patients die within the first 6 months of life, and two-thirds die within 1 year; by 10 years, 90% of patients have succumbed.

Patients with extremes of pulmonary blood flow usually die before the age of 3 months. Survival for several decades is associated with adequate but not excessive pulmonary blood flow, low pulmonary vascular resistance, and the absence of associated congenital heart malformations (Patterson et al, 1982). In one large series, 6 of 18 patients between the ages of 15 and 45 years had no previous operative procedures (Patterson et al, 1982). The longest survival without surgical intervention was 57 years (Patel et al, 1987): The patient had a large atrial septal defect, a small outlet foramen, and no pulmonary stenosis. The longest survival with associated pulmonary atresia (pulmonary circulation sustained by a patent ductus arteriosus) was 21 years (Breisch et al, 1983).

Certain anatomic and physiologic changes accompany increasing age. Progressive cyanosis occurs in association with decreasing size of the outlet foramen (Gallaher and Fyler, 1967; Rao, 1983a), which may progress to complete closure (Dick et al, 1975). In cases of greatly increased pulmonary blood flow, initial lack of cyanosis may give way to progressive cyanosis with the development and progression of pulmonary vascular obstructive disease (Patterson et al, 1982). Declining left ventricular function occurs with increasing age in unoperated patients and in patients with aortopulmonary shunts (LaCorte et al, 1975).

The grim prognosis of tricuspid atresia is reflected in life insurance practices in the United States (Talner et al, 1980). Although patients with many types of congenital heart disease are considered to be insurable at standard or increased rates, patients diagnosed as having tricuspid atresia are considered to be completely uninsurable by 89% of insurance companies (Truesdell et al, 1986).

DIAGNOSIS

Echocardiography

Two-dimensional, M-mode, and Doppler echocardiography are now the primary noninvasive imaging modalities for the diagnosis and classification of tricuspid atresia (Beppu et al, 1978; Rigby et al, 1981; Sahn et al, 1982; Seward et al, 1978) (Fig. 46–2). Segmental analysis clarifies details of anatomy and allows differentiation from other types of complex univentricular hearts: the size and location of cardiac chambers, valves, great arteries, and flow pathways, as well as atrial septal anatomy and communications and patency of the ductus arteriosus. Echocardiography also detects and defines associated malformations such as subaortic stenosis, coarctation of the aorta, left superior vena cava, and juxtaposition of the atrial appendages. It clarifies the relationship of the right atrium to the ventricular mass and distinguishes among the several types of tricuspid atresia.

Pulsed and continuous-wave Doppler echocardiography and color-flow mapping (two-dimensional

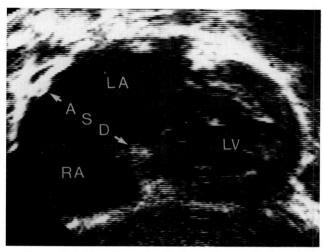

Figure 46–2. Two-dimensional echocardiogram in the subcostal view showing features of tricuspid atresia. A large atrial septal defect (ASD) is noted. The right atrium (RA) does not communicate with a ventricle. The left atrium (LA) and left ventricle (LV) appear to be normal.

Doppler echocardiography) show blood flow characteristics in patients with tricuspid atresia. Color-flow mapping allows a semiquantitative assessment of valvular regurgitation and shows spatial features of flow pathways through ventricular septal defects or obstructive outflow regions. Pressure gradients across stenotic orifices such as ventricular septal defect and subaortic or pulmonary outflow tracts are quantitated by Doppler detection with a high degree of accuracy and have correlated well with simultaneous catheterization pressures (Currie et al, 1986). Gradients across pulmonary artery bands (Fyfe et al, 1984) and systemic-to-pulmonary shunts give estimates of pulmonary artery pressure that are particularly useful when the pulmonary artery cannot be entered at catheterization. Interatrial pressure gradients can also be assessed by Doppler echocardiography and indicate the need for atrial septostomy or septectomy (Fyfe et al, 1987). Although central pulmonary arteries are usually easily demonstrable by echocardiography before palliative shunting, distortions occurring after shunting procedures may be difficult to visualize, although continuous-wave Doppler echocardiography may be able to show stenoses.

Magnetic Resonance Imaging and Radionuclide Scanning

The role of magnetic resonance (MR) imaging in the evaluation of tricuspid atresia is not established. In general, it provides anatomic information similar to that provided by echocardiography but is less useful in providing physiologic data. MR imaging has been successful in documenting the size of cardiac chambers, the anatomy of the great arteries, visceroatrial situs, the type of ventricular loop, and the relationships of the great arteries (Didier et al,

1986). MR imaging is helpful in distinguishing the types of tricuspid atresia: The right atrioventricular sulcus in typical tricuspid atresia is very deep and is filled with fat (Fletcher et al, 1987), appearing as a bright linear or triangular structure replacing the tricuspid valve. In patients with tricuspid atresia due to imperforate valve or Ebstein's anomaly, the right atrioventricular sulcus is shallow, as it is in a normal heart. Rarely, in a patient with an imperforate tricuspid valve, this information is important in planning operative intervention (Crupi et al, 1984).

Radionuclide studies are useful in tricuspid atresia, particularly for evaluation after corrective procedures. These techniques allow recognition of residual left-to-right shunts, right atrial outflow obstruction and stasis, left ventricular dysfunction, and pulmonary arteriovenous fistulas (Brendel et al, 1984; Covitz et al, 1982).

Cardiac Catheterization

The role of cardiac catheterization in the management and diagnosis of patients with tricuspid atresia has changed in recent years since echocardiography has become the primary diagnostic modality.

In infancy, catheterization is most useful in two circumstances. In patients with inadequate atrial communication, balloon septostomy may be done, and in patients with hypoplasia of the pulmonary arteries, the size and relationships of pulmonary blood vessels and brachiocephalic arteries may be clearly defined. Hemodynamic measurements during catheterization have limited value because of the special physiology of the neonate, such as pulmonary hypertension and patent ductus arteriosus, which may change later in infancy.

The greatest application of cardiac catheterization is in later childhood, especially for the assessment of the adverse impact of previous palliative procedures and for analysis of anatomic and physiologic risk factors before performance of a Fontan operation. Palliative shunts may cause distortion of pulmonary artery morphology that is best defined by angiocardiography. In patients with pulmonary stenosis after systemic-to-pulmonary shunts or pulmonary artery banding, it may not be possible to enter the pulmonary artery at catheterization despite special effort. In these cases, assessment of pressure gradients by Doppler echocardiography simultaneously with catheter measurements of ventricular or systemic arterial pressure enables accurate assessment of pulmonary artery pressure (Currie et al, 1986). Angiocardiography may allow inferences about pulmonary flow and resistance that cannot be obtained directly.

Several years after cavopulmonary anastomosis, arteriovenous fistulas may develop in the base of the shunted lung. These important communications may be shown by comparing arterial oxygen saturation in each of the pulmonary veins while the patient is breathing 100% oxygen. Arteriovenous fistulas adversely affect the outcome of the Fontan operation because residual right-to-left shunting causes systemic arterial oxygen desaturation (McFaul et al, 1977).

Other important factors that may affect suitability for Fontan operations, such as left ventricular outflow obstruction in patients with ventriculoarterial discordance, may be assessed by angiography and by measurement of pressure gradients. Even when subaortic stenosis is demonstrable by echocardiography or angiographic techniques, a pressure gradient at catheterization may not be present until provoked by isoproterenol infusion (Freedom et al, 1986).

Left ventricular end-diastolic pressure, size, and contractility may be quantitated at catheterization. Assessment of mitral regurgitation is often possible but may be hampered by the development of extrasystoles during contrast injection. Left ventricular angiocardiography may anatomically define the pulmonary outflow tract size (Fig. 46–3A). Right atrial angiocardiography shows the size and location of the atrial septal defect and confirms the absence of a connection with the ventricles (Fig. 46–3B).

Pressure data are characteristic for tricuspid atresia. The right ventricle cannot be entered through the tricuspid valve. There is a prominent a wave in the right atrium and a right-to-left shunt at the atrial level. In a substantial number of patients, left-to-right shunting occurs, usually as a result of instantaneous pressure differences between the two atria (Rao, 1983b) but occasionally as a result of an associated malformation such as anomalous pulmonary venous connection, coronary arteriovenous fistula to the right atrium, or sinus of Valsalva fistula to the right atrium. A large pressure gradient across the atrial septum may be associated with a small atrial septal defect. Almost identical oxygen saturation levels are found in the left atrium, left ventricle, right ventricle, and great arteries. If the right atrial appendage is not seen during selective right atrial injection in a patient with otherwise typical tricuspid atresia, an associated abnormality such as cor triatriatum dexter or anomalous systemic venous connection may be present (Hausdorf et al, 1985).

PALLIATIVE TREATMENT

The corrective operation for tricuspid atresia, the Fontan operation, cannot be done safely in infants, so palliative operations are needed in infants with insufficient pulmonary blood flow, excessive pulmonary blood flow, or an inadequate interatrial communication.

Systemic-to-Pulmonary Artery Shunt

The first palliative operation for congenital heart disease was a subclavian-to-pulmonary artery anas-

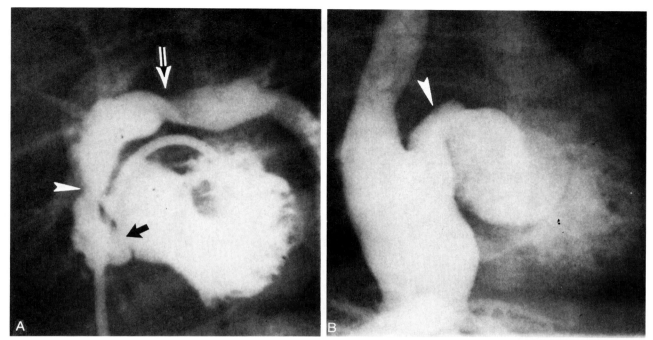

Figure 46–3. Angiocardiography in tricuspid atresia. *A,* Left anterior oblique view of left ventricular injection demonstrates three levels of obstruction to pulmonary blood flow: small ventricular septal defect *(black arrow),* obstructive infundibulum *(arrowhead),* and pulmonary annular stenosis *(white arrow). B,* Left anterior oblique view of right atrial injection shows the flow of contrast material directly into left atrium through an atrial septal communication *(arrowhead)* and no flow into right ventricle.

tomosis done by Blalock on November 19, 1944, in a patient with tetralogy of Fallot (Blalock and Taussig, 1945). A few months later, Blalock did a similar shunt in a patient with tricuspid atresia, the first palliation of that disease (Taussig et al, 1973). Later, Potts (1946) performed a descending aorta-to-left pulmonary artery anastomosis; Davidson (1955) anastomosed the main pulmonary artery to the aorta; and Waterston (1962) connected the ascending aorta to the right pulmonary artery.

Neonates who become severely cyanotic can be resuscitated by continuous infusion of prostaglandin E_1 to restore patency of the ductus arteriosus (Elliott et al, 1975; Hatem et al, 1980; Olley et al, 1976). Use of this agent has dramatically improved the results of a shunt operation in cyanotic neonates. Ductal patency maintains pulmonary blood flow and allows an elective operation on a stable patient. Infusion of prostaglandin E_1 may be continued for 1 week or longer if necessary (Teixeira et al, 1984).

The Blalock-Taussig shunt, either in its classic (direct anastomosis of the subclavian artery to a pulmonary artery) or modified form (interposition of a polytetrafluoroethylene [PTFE] graft between a subclavian artery and a pulmonary artery) (McKay et al, 1980) is now the most widely used systemic-to-pulmonary artery anastomosis. The current mortality risk of doing such a shunt in patients with tricuspid atresia is less than 10% (Cleveland et al, 1984). The advantage of the Blalock-Taussig shunt, both classic and modified, is that the lumen of the subclavian artery limits pulmonary blood flow; thus, congestive heart failure due to excessive pulmonary blood flow

and left ventricular volume overload is infrequent (Deverall et al, 1969), but systemic oxygen saturation is adequate. Disadvantages of this shunt include decreased growth of the ipsilateral arm (Currarino and Engle, 1965), tissue loss due to gangrene (Geiss et al, 1980), and phrenic nerve injury (Smith et al, 1986), which is often a lethal complication.

Two series in which the classic was compared with the modified Blalock-Taussig shunt (Moulton et al, 1985; Ullom et al, 1987) found the modified shunt to be superior to the classic shunt, especially in neonates, because it provides better immediate patency and arterial oxygen saturation, greater longevity of the shunt, better growth of the pulmonary arteries, and less distortion of the pulmonary arteries. Approximately 80% of patients with tricuspid atresia who have a systemic-to-pulmonary artery shunt are alive after 10 years (Kirklin and Barratt-Boyes, 1986; Trusler and Williams, 1980) (Fig. 46–4).

Several adverse anatomic and physiologic sequelae of systemic-to-pulmonary artery anastomoses militate against a successful future Fontan operation. These shunts may lead to distortion of the pulmonary arterial tree or to pulmonary artery hypertension with increased pulmonary arterial resistance and high left ventricular end-diastolic volume and pressure due to high pulmonary blood flow. These effects are most likely to occur after Potts' or Waterston's anastomoses because of difficulty in achieving accurate shunt size (Arciniegas et al, 1980). In addition, distortion of the pulmonary arteries after these shunts may require reconstruction at the time of corrective operation (Ashcraft, 1973; Gay and Ebert, 1973).

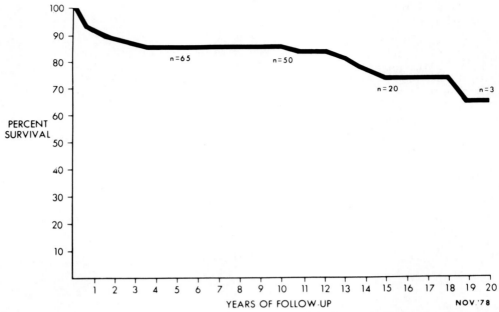

Figure 46–4. Actuarial survival of 104 patients who had tricuspid atresia and who survived an initial shunt operation. (Reprinted with permission from The Society of Thoracic Surgeons [The Annals of Thoracic Surgery, 29:312, 1980]).

Almost 25% of patients who have tricuspid atresia and who have an aortopulmonary shunt after the age of 1 year may develop a contraindication to a Fontan operation as a result of adverse anatomic and physiologic effects of the shunt (Mietus-Snyder et al, 1987); therefore, systemic-to-pulmonary artery anastomosis should probably be reserved for children who cannot safely have a Fontan operation (those under 1 year of age or older children with substantial contraindications to this operation).

Cavopulmonary Anastomosis

Direct connection of the superior vena cava to the pulmonary artery was proved to be feasible by Carlon and colleagues (1951), and this anastomosis was first done in a patient with congenital heart disease by Glenn (1958) and by Bakulev and Kolesnikov (1959). Cavopulmonary anastomosis has certain theoretical advantages over systemic-to-pulmonary artery anastomosis: The lung is supplied with pure systemic venous blood, the systemic venous pressure rises only slightly and remains in the physiologic range, and there is no volume load on the ventricles. Pulmonary artery hypertension seldom occurs, and endocarditis is rare (Robicsek et al, 1966).

Two important problems have been associated with the cavopulmonary anastomosis: The superior vena cava syndrome may occur early postoperatively, and failure of palliation due to increasing cyanosis and rising hematocrit may occur later. The superior vena cava syndrome results from too high a pressure in the superior vena cava and can be anatomically related to inadequate size of the pulmonary artery, so cavopulmonary anastomosis should not be done

unless the right pulmonary artery is at least the same diameter as the superior vena cava (Trusler and Williams, 1980). Proper selection of patients based on adequate size of right pulmonary artery and normal pulmonary vascular resistance in patients no younger than 18 months is associated with an operative mortality of less than 2% (DiCarlo et al, 1982).

Late clinical deterioration after cavopulmonary anastomosis may be related to progressive subvalvular obstruction to pulmonary blood flow into the left lung, ventilation-perfusion imbalance as bronchiolar collaterals displace caval flow from the upper and middle lobes to the lower lobe (Mathur and Glenn, 1973), development of pulmonary arteriovenous fistulas (Cloutier et al, 1985; McFaul et al; 1977) decreased right pulmonary artery flow due to development of collaterals from the superior vena cava to the inferior vena cava (Laks et al, 1977), or increased pulmonary vascular resistance because of the high viscosity associated with rising hematocrit (Mathur and Glenn, 1973). When clinical deterioration occurs, the treatment may be a Fontan operation if that operation is not contraindicated, or a contralateral aortopulmonary shunt (DiCarlo et al, 1982; Pennington et al, 1981).

The role of cavopulmonary anastomosis is not certain in tricuspid atresia. It is a safe operation and provides good long-term palliation, especially in children older than 5 years: Palliation is still adequate in 90% of patients at 5 years and in 60 to 70% at 10 years (DeBrux et al, 1983; DiCarlo et al, 1982). After Fontan's procedures, patients who have had an earlier cavopulmonary anastomosis may have fewer pericardial and pleural effusions and a shorter stay in the hospital (Pennington et al, 1981) and may be protected from sudden death and unusual catastrophic post-Fontan's events, such as acute occlusion of an atriopulmonary conduit (Covitz et al, 1982; DeLeon et al, 1983).

A variation of cavopulmonary anastomosis that may be useful as the first stage of an ultimate Fontan repair is the bidirectional cavopulmonary shunt in which the proximal end of the divided superior vena cava is connected to the side of the right pulmonary artery, permitting superior vena cava flow into both lungs. The physiologic benefits of this procedure are the same as for the classic shunt, but in addition, disproportionate commitment of 33% of the systemic venous return (superior vena cava) to 55% of the pulmonary capillary bed (right lung) is avoided, and the pulmonary arteries remain in continuity. In 12 of these operations before a Fontan procedure, cyanosis was relieved and no deaths, shunt failures, pulmonary artery deformities, or arteriovenous fistulas occurred (Hopkins et al, 1985).

Current Management of Decreased Pulmonary Blood Flow

Neonates with tricuspid atresia associated with decreased pulmonary blood flow are administered prostaglandin E_1 to stabilize them and to permit resuscitation if necessary. A day or two later, a modified Blalock-Taussig shunt is done using a 5-mm PTFE graft on the side of the aortic arch, usually the left (Fig. 46–5). Patients beyond the early newborn period also undergo a modified Blalock-Taussig shunt. If the shunt fails before the patient is 1 year old, a standard or modified Blalock-Taussig shunt is done on the opposite side. Patients who are older than 1 year and who require surgical intervention have a Fontan operation. If correction is contraindicated, then a cavopulmonary anastomosis or a contralateral modified Blalock-Taussig shunt is done.

Enlargement of Atrial Septal Communication

If the obligatory interatrial communication is obstructively small, peripheral edema, pulsatile and distended neck veins, and hepatomegaly denote right-sided heart failure. The electrocardiogram may have features of right atrial enlargement, and a large right atrium may be seen on the chest film. Echocardiography usually defines the diameter of the atrial septal defect, and Doppler echocardiography estimates the interatrial pressure gradient (Fyfe et al, 1987). Cardiac catheterization may show a pressure difference of 3 mm Hg or more between the atria.

If the atrial septal communication is inadequate, a balloon septostomy can be done at cardiac catheterization if the patient is less than 1 month old (Rashkind and Miller, 1966). In older children, increased septal thickness may require blade septos-tomy at cardiac catheterization (Park et al, 1982). If these measures fail, an atrial septal defect can be surgically created by the closed technique of Blalock and Hanlon (1950) by using open atrial septectomy under either inflow occlusion (Hallman et al, 1968) or cardiopulmonary bypass.

Reduction of Excessively Increased Pulmonary Blood Flow

Fortunately, less than 20% of all patients with tricuspid atresia (Keith et al, 1978) have unrestricted pulmonary blood flow, and only some of them have congestive heart failure of sufficient severity to require surgical treatment. Patients with tricuspid atresia and congestive heart failure due to increased pulmonary blood flow usually have ventriculoarterial discordance and little or no pulmonary stenosis. Pulmonary artery banding, which was originally suggested by Muller and Dammann (1952), increases resistance to flow from the right ventricle to the pulmonary artery and decreases pulmonary blood flow. The consequent decreased volume overload of the left ventricle alleviates congestive heart failure. Reduced pulmonary blood flow and pulmonary artery pressure decrease the possibility of later pulmonary vascular obstructive disease. The mortality of pulmonary artery banding for patients with tricuspid atresia is approximately 30%, but survivors usually have good resolution of congestive heart failure (Sade, 1983).

Although pulmonary artery banding provides successful palliation by decreasing pulmonary blood flow and congestive heart failure, it does not completely protect against the development of pulmonary vascular obstructive disease. Even when the pulmonary vascular resistance after banding is less than 4 units · m^2, significant pulmonary vascular abnormalities may remain: increased pulmonary vascular smooth muscle and occlusive organized pulmonary arterial thrombi (Juaneda and Haworth, 1984). The pulmonary artery band also frequently produces branch pulmonary arterial stenosis, more often on the right than on the left, and increases the risk in a later Fontan procedure.

In tricuspid atresia with ventriculoarterial discordance, as in other types of univentricular atrioventricular connection, a reciprocal relationship exists between the size of the systemic and the pulmonary ventricular outlet flow pathways; thus, patients with considerable pulmonary blood flow are likely to have some degree of subaortic obstruction (Ottenkamp et al, 1985). Subaortic obstruction may be present in patients with angiographic and two-dimensional echocardiographic evidence of a moderate or large outlet foramen, because the defect orifice may be oval and obstructively small in these patients (Freedom, 1987). In addition, when subaortic stenosis is clearly demonstrable anatomically, no pressure gradient may exist at rest, but a gradient

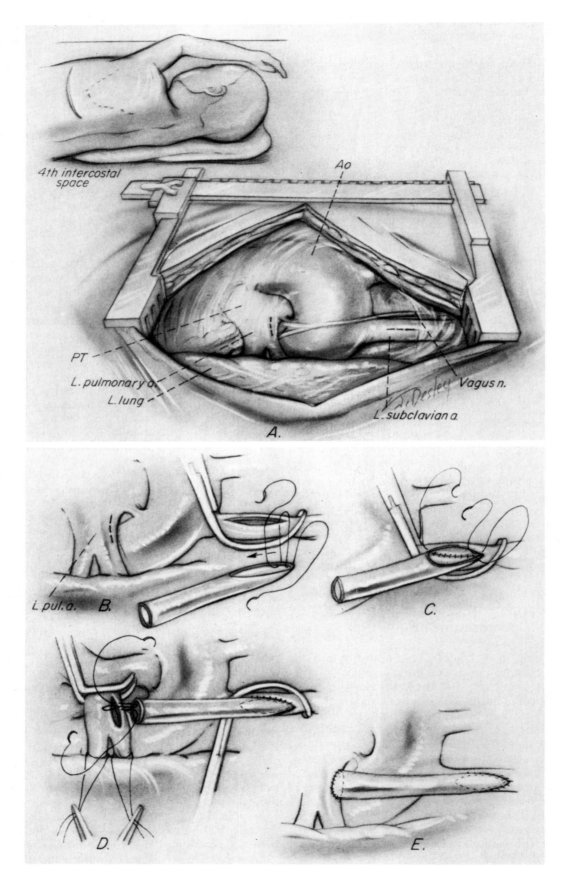

Figure 46–5 *See legend on opposite page*

can often be elicited with isoprenaline infusion at cardiac catheterization (Freedom et al, 1986). The outlet foramen in as many as 40% of patients with tricuspid atresia with ventriculoarterial discordance may decrease in size over time (Rao, 1983a), and this process may be accelerated by the presence of a pulmonary artery band (Freed et al, 1973). Because the outlet chamber is subaortic, decreasing size of the outlet foramen produces subaortic stenosis, ventricular hypertrophy, and a consequent decrease in ventricular diastolic compliance. There is increasing evidence that poor diastolic ventricular compliance and excessive left ventricular hypertrophy are important mortality risk factors after the Fontan operation (Freedom et al, 1986; Jonas et al, 1985; Kirklin et al, 1986; Penkoske et al, 1984).

For these reasons, the role of pulmonary artery banding in the surgical management of tricuspid atresia (and other types of univentricular atrioventricular connection) with increased pulmonary blood flow may be diminishing (Freedom, 1987). Subaortic stenosis may be resected or bypassed with a valve-bearing conduit from the left ventricular apex to the descending aorta (Penkoske et al, 1984; Rothman et al, 1987a), but neither procedure has had noteworthy success. Reasonable results have been achieved by creating an aortopulmonary window proximal to a pulmonary artery band (Park, 1982; Penkoske et al, 1984). The disadvantages of the pulmonary artery band itself, however, are not avoided with this procedure.

Several groups have used with success an alternative operation that employs the principle of the Norwood operation (Pigott et al, 1988) in this clinical situation and completely avoids the use of a pulmonary artery band. The main pulmonary artery is divided, and its proximal end is sutured to the side of the ascending aorta, thus bypassing the subaortic obstruction. The procedure is completed with a palliative shunt to the pulmonary artery or a corrective Fontan operation (Freedom, 1987; Jonas et al, 1985; Lin et al, 1986). Although the numbers of patients in these series are small, the approach appears to be promising.

Many uncertainties remain, but considering all the currently available information, certain recommendations can be made for patients with tricuspid atresia with unrestricted pulmonary blood flow. Anatomic and physiologic evaluation for subaortic obstruction should be done with two-dimensional and Doppler echocardiography and by cardiac catheterization by using exercise or pressors if no gradient can be shown at rest. If there is no evidence of subaortic stenosis in young infants, the pulmonary artery may be banded. In all infants with evidence of subaortic stenosis and in children beyond early infancy, a Norwood-type operation may be done: The pulmonary artery is divided, its proximal end is anastomosed to the ascending aorta, and the distal pulmonary artery is connected to the ascending aorta with an aortopulmonary shunt (4- to 5-mm PTFE graft, depending on the size of the patient). All patients with a pulmonary artery band need surveillance for the development of subaortic obstruction. At the first appearance of any gradient or anatomic evidence of subaortic stenosis with or without a gradient, the Norwood variant described earlier should be done in patients less than 1 year of age, or enlargement of the outlet foramen in patients older than 1 year, preceding or simultaneously with a Fontan operation.

FONTAN'S OPERATION

Surgical correction of tricuspid atresia was made possible by a radical conceptual shift: the recognition that a ventricle is not needed for the pulmonary circulation (Fontan and Baudet, 1971; Sade and Castaneda, 1975) because pulmonary vascular resistance is normally so low that a minor rise in caval pressure is needed to create a transpulmonary vascular pressure gradient sufficient to move the systemic venous return across the pulmonary capillary bed. Although the Fontan procedure has been done for many malformations associated with only one functional ventricle, operative mortality is lowest in patients with tricuspid atresia (Stefanelli et al, 1984).

Selection of Candidates

On the basis of their early experience, Fontan and colleagues developed a list of specific anatomic and physiologic criteria that would permit a Fontan procedure to be done safely by optimizing postoperative pulmonary blood flow and ensuring low caval pressures (Choussat et al, 1978); their criteria are summarized in Table 46–2. Most of these risk factors have now been found to be relative rather than absolute contraindications to correction.

Age. Age greater than 15 years is not a risk factor

Figure 46–5. Technique of modified Blalock-Taussig shunt. *A,* With the patient in the right lateral position, a left fourth intercostal space incision is made, the left pulmonary artery is dissected onto its branches, and the left subclavian artery is dissected from its bed. *B,* A vascular clamp is applied to the left subclavian artery, an incision is made, and the beveled end of a 5-mm Gore-Tex graft is sewn to this incision. *C,* The posterior wall is sewn from the inside of the graft and vessel, and the opposite side is completed with an external suture line. *D,* A vascular clamp or a vascular clamp with snares around the branch pulmonary arteries is used to occlude that vessel, which is incised, and, after the Gore-Tex shunt is cut to an appropriate length, its end is sewn to the pulmonary artery in the same manner as the subclavian anastomosis. *E,* The completed shunt is shown. Shunt patency is maintained intraoperatively and postoperatively by administering heparin, 100 units/kg, intravenously immediately after bleeding ceases from the anastomoses and every 4 hours for 24 hours after the operation. Phenylephrine hydrochloride (Neo-Synephrine) may be infused continuously at a rate that maintains the systolic blood pressure at 80 mm Hg or higher.

TABLE 46–2. SELECTION CRITERIA
FOR FONTAN'S PROCEDURE

Age more than 4 years or less than 15 years
Sinus rhythm
Normal drainage of the venae cavae
Normal volume of the right atrium
Mean pulmonary artery pressure no higher than 15 mm Hg
Pulmonary arterial resistance index less than 4 units/m²
Pulmonary artery-aortic diameter ratio at least 0.75
Normal function of dominant ventricle (ejection fraction at least 0.6)
No mitral incompetence
No impairing effects of a previous shunt

for operative survival (Mair et al, 1985; Mayer et al, 1986), although late survival may be adversely affected by deteriorating left ventricular function in some patients (Mair et al, 1985), and good operative survival in older patients may require more rigid adherence to selection criteria (Warnes and Somerville, 1987). Age less than 4 years was a risk factor in earlier series (Cleveland et al, 1984; Fontan et al, 1983; Mair et al, 1985), but this no longer appears to be true (Kirklin et al, 1986; Mayer et al, 1986). The lower age limit for safe operation is not established, but operation is known to be dangerous during infancy. It is likely that at very young ages the influence of other risk factors becomes more critical, particularly pulmonary vascular resistance more than 2 units · m² and pulmonary artery distortion due to pre-existing shunts (Mayer et al, 1986). Age-related decreases in exercise performance (Driscoll et al, 1986) and increases in ventricular hypertrophy (Kirklin et al, 1986) have suggested that the best age for a Fontan operation is before 6 years and may be as early as 1 to 2 years (Mayer et al, 1986).

Rhythm. Normal sinus rhythm is not required before operation. Pre-existing atrial flutter-fibrillation may be easier to control after Fontan's repair than before (Alboliras et al, 1985). Preoperative heart block can be treated with a pacemaker after corrective operation, and some patients clearly do not need atrioventricular synchrony to survive a Fontan operation.

Venous Drainage Pathways. Abnormal systemic and pulmonary venous connections can usually be accommodated during corrective operation (King et al, 1985; Mair et al, 1985; Mayer et al, 1986; Vargas et al, 1987b) and do not contraindicate Fontan's operations.

Pulmonary Artery Pressure. The mean pulmonary artery pressure need not be less than 15 mm Hg (Mair et al, 1985; Mayer et al, 1986) and may be acceptable up to 25 mm Hg if associated with increased pulmonary blood flow and a low calculated pulmonary vascular resistance.

Pulmonary Vascular Resistance. Pulmonary vascular obstruction is still an absolute contraindication to Fontan's repair: This may be indicated by a pulmonary vascular resistance more than 4 units · m² (Mair et al, 1985) or by incomplete arborization of the peripheral pulmonary arteries (Kirklin et al,

1986). There is an almost linear relationship between pulmonary vascular resistance and survival after corrective operation (Mair et al, 1985). Operative survival is likely to be good if the resistance is less than 2 units · m² (Mayer et al, 1986), but in selected patients may still be satisfactory when it is 2 to 4 units · m² (Mair et al, 1985).

Pulmonary Artery Anatomy. Very small pulmonary arteries contraindicate a Fontan repair. The pulmonary artery index (cross-sectional area of the branch pulmonary arteries normalized for body surface area) predicts survival if greater than 250 mm/m² (Nakata et al, 1984) but has been associated with survival when it is as low as 188 mm/m² (Girod et al, 1985). Local stenoses of the branch pulmonary arteries may be amenable to balloon dilatation at preoperative cardiac catheterization (Lock et al, 1983; Ring et al, 1985), but if this cannot be done, a corrective procedure may still be possible if the pulmonary artery deformity can be repaired at the time of corrective operation (Mair et al, 1985, Mayer et al, 1986). Pulmonary artery deformities produced by pulmonary artery banding may be correctable at Fontan operation (Kirklin et al, 1986; Mair et al, 1985), but these deformities contribute to a high operative mortality (Mayer et al, 1986). Pulmonary artery deformities associated with systemic-to-pulmonary artery shunts can be particularly difficult to manage (Mietus-Snyder et al, 1987; Ring et al, 1985). Patients with only a single pulmonary artery may safely have a Fontan operation, particularly if the opposite lung is hypoplastic (Sade et al, 1980).

Left Ventricular Function. Left ventricular end-diastolic pressure appears not to be a risk factor unless greater than 25 mm Hg (Mair et al, 1985), especially if associated with ventricular volume overload due to correctable causes such as increased pulmonary blood flow or atrioventricular valve insufficiency (Graham et al, 1986). Relief of volume overload and of myocardial hypoxia leads to improved left ventricular function postoperatively.

Ventricular hypertrophy is a significant risk factor, both early and late (Freedom, 1987; Kirklin et al, 1986). It may be associated with increased pulmonary blood flow with or without a pulmonary artery band; subaortic obstruction, especially in transposition of the great arteries (Freedom et al, 1986; Rothman et al, 1987a); and increasing age of the patient (Kirklin et al, 1986; Mair et al, 1985). Subaortic obstruction is associated with high mortality at corrective operation (Stark, 1986) and may require a preliminary operation to relieve the obstruction (Lin et al, 1986; Penkoske et al, 1984; Rothman et al, 1987a).

TECHNIQUE OF CORRECTIVE OPERATION

The goal of corrective procedures for tricuspid atresia is to separate the systemic and pulmonary circuits by connecting the systemic venous return directly to the pulmonary artery without obstruction and closing all communications between the right and left sides of the heart. Success depends primarily on a widely patent connection of the systemic venous return to the pulmonary circuit, sufficient cross-sectional area of pulmonary arteries, and low pulmonary venous and left atrial pressures. The operation requires the correction of all anatomic abnormalities that deter these requirements.

Fontan and Baudet's (1971) successful application of these principles in three patients was achieved against a background of considerable experimental and clinical work (Sade, 1982), including several unsuccessful clinical attempts to bypass the right ventricle (Harrison, 1962; Hurwitt et al, 1955; Shumacker, 1955). Fontan's approach included a cavopulmonary anastomosis and homograft valves in the inferior vena cava and in the atriopulmonary anastomosis (see Fig. 46–5E). Subsequent techniques simplified the operation by omitting the cavopulmonary shunt while connecting the right atrium to the main pulmonary artery with a homograft (Ross and Somerville, 1973) and, in addition, deleting the inferior vena cava valve (Kreutzer et al, 1973). Later modifications used the right ventricle by connecting it to the right atrium with a conduit with or without a valve or by directly anastomosing the right atrial appendage to the right ventricle (Bjork et al, 1979; Bowman et al, 1978; Fontan et al, 1978; Gago et al, 1976; Henry et al, 1974; Murray et al, 1977). Arterial switch with atriopulmonary anastomosis has been done in the setting of tricuspid atresia with ventriculoarterial discordance, pulmonary artery banding, and subaortic obstruction (Freedom et al, 1980). Orthotopic implantation of a tricuspid valve prosthesis is a theoretical possibility in patients with tricuspid atresia with an imperforate tricuspid valve and a normal-sized right ventricle (Crupi et al, 1984).

The most critical technical factor in determining the outcome of Fontan's procedure is the size of the atriopulmonary connection. Even minor degrees of obstruction are not well tolerated. Because Dacron grafts tend to become obstructed in the late postoperative period, they have largely been abandoned (DeLeon et al, 1984; Girod et al, 1987; Kreutzer et al, 1982). When a conduit is needed, homografts serve well for periods that now are as long as 16 years (Fontan et al, 1984; Girod et al, 1987). Externally supported PTFE grafts may also work well as conduits (Nawa et al, 1987). Anastomotic narrowing is perhaps best avoided by doing the aortopulmonary anastomosis behind the aorta (Doty et al, 1981; Kreutzer et al, 1982; Oelert and Borst, 1984). The posterior anastomosis can be done in patients with ventriculoarterial concordance or discordance (Kreutzer et al, 1982).

Early in the postoperative period, no functional pump exists in the pulmonary circuit with any atrial connection; therefore, connecting the right atrium to the right ventricle rather than to the pulmonary artery is not advantageous (DiSessa et al, 1984;

Kreutzer et al, 1982; Lee et al, 1986), although agreement on this is not universal (Coles et al, 1987). In the late postoperative period, however, differences have appeared.

There is now little doubt that connecting the right atrium to the right ventricle with a valve-bearing conduit leads to growth and function of the right ventricle as a pump, producing normally low right atrial pressures and a normal pulmonary artery pressure curve and pulmonary blood flow (Bowman et al, 1978; Bull et al, 1983; Fontan et al, 1983; Gussenhoven et al, 1986; Laks et al, 1984). One child had an excellent clinical result with pulmonary vascular obstructive disease, a pulmonary artery pressure of 50 mm Hg, and normal right atrial pressure (Williams, 1984).

Atrioventricular connection with a nonvalved conduit has been found by most authors to confer no long-term advantage over atriopulmonary connection, but one report showed better long-term survival in atrioventricular connection (Coles et al, 1987) and another showed better left ventricular function (Del Torso et al, 1985). Although no clear disadvantage of atrioventricular connection has been found, regurgitation from the right ventricle to the right atrium may rarely increase with time, leading to the need for valve interposition (Fontan et al, 1983; Laks et al, 1984). There appears to be little advantage to interposing a valve between the right atrium and pulmonary artery (Bull et al, 1983; Ishikawa et al, 1984; Laks et al, 1984; Sharratt et al, 1979), although Fontan (1983) has shown a slightly lower right atrial pressure when a valve is present.

Simple ligation of the pulmonary artery has been used during atriopulmonary anastomosis (Humes et al, 1987). A residual left-to-right shunt may occur through the ligature; therefore, division of the main pulmonary artery with oversewing of the proximal stump has been advocated (Girod et al, 1987).

A technique of total cavopulmonary connection has been described (de Leval et al, 1988; Matsuda et al, 1987; Puga et al, 1987). The superior vena cava is divided; the upstream end is anastomosed to the side of the right pulmonary artery, and the downstream end is anastomosed either to the other side of the right pulmonary artery or to the open end of the divided main pulmonary artery. In an effort to reduce turbulence and stasis, the inferior vena cava has been connected to the superior vena cava anastomosis with an intracardiac baffle, creating a nearly straight conduit. This procedure may result in fewer arrhythmias because most of the right atrial chamber is at low pressure, and reduced turbulence may prevent energy loss as blood flows from the cava to the pulmonary artery. The likelihood of right atrial thrombosis may be decreased because of reduced stasis (de Leval et al, 1988). More data are needed to evaluate these hypotheses.

Although associated anomalies are not as common with tricuspid atresia as with other forms of univentricular atrioventricular connection, they must

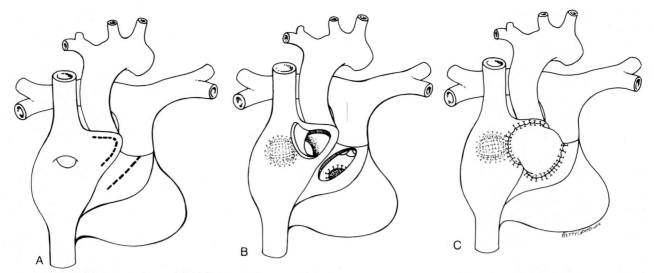

Figure 46–6. Right atrium to right ventricle connection with homograft. *A,* An incision is made in the right atrial appendage, and underlying muscular bands are divided. An incision is made in the hypoplastic right ventricle from the pulmonary annulus to the right ventricular sinus. *B,* The atrial septal communication is closed with a patch by using a continuous monofilament suture. All potentially obstructive muscle bands in the sinus of the right ventricle and the infundibulum are divided. The ventricular septal defect is closed with a patch by using either continuous or interrupted sutures. Care must be taken not to mistake the infundibular os for the ventricular septal defect. *C,* A homograft, either pulmonary or aortic, is appropriately trimmed and its proximal end sewn to the right atrium with a continuous nonabsorbable monofilament suture. The same is done at the pulmonary end.

be managed at the time of correction. A moderately or severely insufficient mitral valve may be repaired or replaced (Mair et al, 1985; Vargas et al, 1987a). Deformities of the pulmonary artery may be repaired directly by patch reconstruction or, in some cases, may be dilated intraoperatively by balloon angioplasty (Ring et al, 1985). A right-sided pulmonary artery deformed by a pre-existing Waterston shunt can be divided distal to the deformity and anastomosed to the side of the superior vena cava (Uretzky et al, 1983). Anomalies of the venous drainage can

usually be managed by intra-atrial baffles, but a left superior vena cava is best handled by division and anastomosis to the left pulmonary artery (Vargas et al, 1987b).

The patch closing the atrial septal communication should encircle the coronary sinus and leave it to drain into the left atrium. When the right atrial pressure exceeds 15 mm Hg, coronary sinus drainage and left ventricular function may be impaired (Ilbawi et al, 1986), although there is evidence that this impairment may not be significant (Ward et al, 1988).

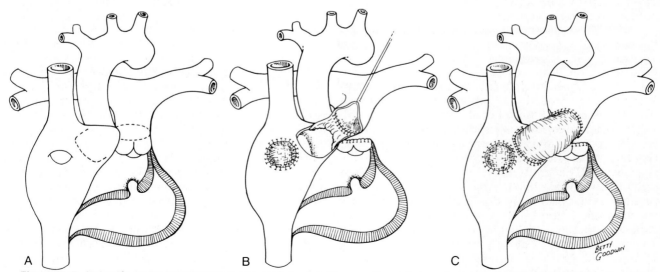

Figure 46–7. Atriopulmonary anastomosis in tricuspid atresia with normally related great arteries. *A,* A flap incision based medially on the right atrial appendage is made, and the main pulmonary artery is divided. *B,* The atrial septal defect is closed with a patch secured with a continuous nonabsorbable monofilament suture. The proximal stump of the main pulmonary artery is oversewn with a continuous suture, and the free edge of the atrial flap is sewn to the posterior edge of the pulmonary artery with a continuous absorbable monofilament suture. *C,* The anterior wall of the atriopulmonary conduit is completed with a patch of pericardium or prosthetic material by using a continuous nonabsorbable monofilament suture along the free edges of the atrial opening, the flap, and the pulmonary artery. (From Sade, R. M.: Tricuspid atresia. *In* Grillo, H., Austen, W. G., Wilkins, E. W., Jr., Mathisen, D. J., Vlahakes, G. J., [eds]: Current Therapy in Cardiothoracic Surgery. Toronto, B. C. Decker, 1989, p. 507.)

Leaving the coronary sinus in the left atrium has the additional advantage of obviating the possibility of a residual right-to-left shunt in the 2% of patients with tricuspid atresia who have a coronary sinus septal defect (Coles et al, 1987; Girod et al, 1987; Rumisek et al, 1986).

All pre-existing palliative shunts should be closed at the time of corrective operation, except for cavopulmonary anastomoses, which are usually left intact. To prevent commitment of a third of the systemic venous return to more than half of the pulmonary capillary bed, the authors have reconstructed the cavoatrial junction with a patch at Fontan's repair in patients with a previous cavopulmonary shunt to make the entire pulmonary capillary bed available to all of the systemic venous return.

Many of the uncertainties of the early experience with the Fontan operation have been clarified, and specific recommendations for operative management of patients with tricuspid atresia are possible. Patients with ventriculoarterial concordance, a normal pulmonary artery and valve, mild to moderate hypoplasia of the right ventricle, and adequate retrosternal space should have patch repair of both the outlet foramen and the atrial septal communication at the time a valved allograft is placed from the right atrium to the right ventricle (Fig. 46–6). Patients with ventriculoarterial concordance and severe right ventricular hypoplasia should have patch repair of the atrial septal communication, division of the main pulmonary artery with oversewing of the proximal stump, and anastomosis of the distal vessel to the right atrial appendage with a flap technique anterior to the aorta, if retrosternal space permits (Fig. 46–7), or posterior to the aorta (Fig. 46–8). Patients with ventriculoarterial discordance should have patch repair of the atrial septal communication and division of the main pulmonary artery with anastomosis to

the right atrial appendage posterior to the aorta (Fig. 46–9). Correction of associated anatomic abnormalities should accompany the repair.

POSTOPERATIVE MANAGEMENT

The immediate postoperative period is a time of dramatic hemodynamic adjustment to new circulatory physiology. No pump exists in the pulmonary circuit, and already impaired left ventricular function has been further compromised by recent operation. Because the two circulations are now separated and in series, cardiac output is limited by the pulmonary blood flow, which in turn varies directly with the transpulmonary pressure gradient. Cardiac output may be increased by increasing right atrial pressure, decreasing pulmonary vascular resistance, and decreasing left atrial pressure (Sade, 1982). Right atrial pressure can be increased by colloid transfusion. Pulmonary vascular resistance can be decreased by hyperventilation to achieve hypocarbia as low as 20 mm Hg and respiratory alkalosis to a pH of 7.45 to 7.50 or higher. Maintenance of a relatively low hematocrit (30 to 35%) decreases resistance by decreasing blood viscosity. Left atrial pressure can be reduced by improving left ventricular function with the use of inotropic agents and systemic arteriolar dilators (Matsuda et al, 1981; Sade et al, 1981; Sade and Dearing, 1981; Shemin et al, 1979).

In the immediate postoperative period, the requirement of a right atrial pressure of 17 mm Hg or greater predicts high morbidity and mortality (Sanders et al, 1982). When the cardiac output remains low despite a high right atrial pressure, low arterial carbon dioxide tension, high pH, inotropic agents, and vasodilators, intermittent abdominal compression may be used to good advantage (Guyton et al,

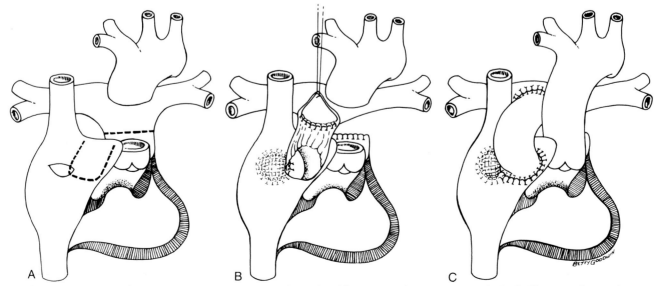

Figure 46–8. Atriopulmonary anastomosis in tricuspid atresia with transposed great arteries. *A, B, C,* The procedure is the same as in Figure 46–7, except that the atrial flap is based superiorly, and the anastomosis is posterolateral to the aorta.

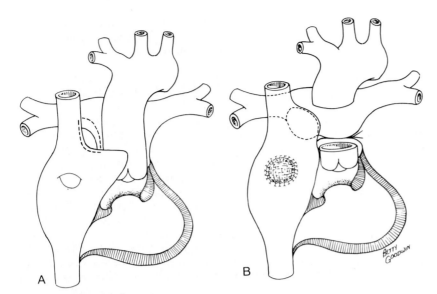

Figure 46–9. Atriopulmonary anastomosis in transposition of the great arteries. *A,* An incision is made in the right atrial appendage and extended into the superior vena cava immediately adjacent to the right pulmonary artery. A corresponding incision is made in the right atrial appendage into the superior vena cava to the level of the pulmonary arteriotomy. *B,* The atrial septal defect is closed with a patch secured with a continuous nonabsorbable monofilament suture. The proximal main pulmonary artery is ligated, and the opening in the right atrium and superior vena cava is sewn to the opening in the main and right pulmonary arteries with a continuous absorbable monofilament suture. If desired, the anterior aspect of the connection can be closed with a patch rather than by direct suture. (From Sade, R. M.: Tricuspid atresia. *In* Grillo, H. C., Austen, W. G., Wilkins, E. W., Jr., Mathisen, D. J., Vlahakes, G. J. [eds]: Current Therapy in Cardiothoracic Surgery. Toronto, B. C. Decker, 1989, p. 507.)

1985; Heck and Doty, 1981; Heilberg et al, 1977; Milliken et al, 1986). Several techniques of compression have been described. An adult arm or thigh blood pressure cuff may be wrapped loosely around the abdomen and connected to a ventilator or a pneumatic pressure-cycled extremity pump (Jobst Institute). The cuff is inflated to a pressure sufficient (usually 30 to 45 mm Hg) to maintain the left atrial pressure at 20 to 25 mm Hg. The cuff is inflated for 30 to 40 seconds and deflated for 15 to 30 seconds. The device is usually needed for 12 to 36 hours.

If cardiac output is still low despite all these measures, a specific cause should be sought, such as atriopulmonary obstruction, pulmonary hypertension, or left ventricular failure. If no correctable cause is found, the patient may require reoperation: The atriopulmonary anastomosis is disconnected, the atrial septum is opened, and a systemic-to-pulmonary artery shunt is done (DeLeon et al, 1986a).

Extracorporeal membrane oxygenation has been used with some success in children after open heart procedures, with a 38% long-term survival (Kanter et al, 1987); unfortunately, the only patient with tricuspid atresia in that series did not survive. Two experimental balloon pumps have been specifically designed for use in the right atrium (Jacobs et al, 1987) or pulmonary artery (de la Riviere, 1983) after a Fontan operation.

Arterial hypoxemia in the immediate postoperative period may be caused by intrapulmonary shunting due to atelectasis or interstitial edema and may respond to pulmonary toilet or addition of positive end-expiratory pressure. The latter should be used with caution because pressure greater than 6 mm Hg may be associated with substantial decreases in cardiac output (Williams et al, 1984). Persistent hypoxemia despite adequate ventilation may be related to pulmonary venous collaterals or arteriovenous fistula, especially in patients with a previous cavopulmonary anastomosis (Cloutier et al, 1985). Other anatomic causes of hypoxemia are dehiscence of the atrial septal closure, small atrial septal defects undetected at operation, unusual coronary vein connections between the right atrium and left atrium, or coronary sinus septal defect (Girod et al, 1987; Rumisek et al, 1986; Westerman et al, 1985). In these cases, early reoperation may be needed.

Atrioventricular sequential pacing in the early postoperative period is often helpful when rhythm is not sinus and cardiac output is marginal.

Almost all patients retain fluid after a Fontan operation for reasons that are not entirely clear. A general inflammatory response to cardiopulmonary bypass results in elevated complement levels (Kirklin et al, 1983), and atrial natriuretic peptide is abnormally elevated in patients after the Fontan operation (Stewart et al, 1987). Fluid retention is associated with pleural effusions, usually bilateral, requiring chest tube drainage for 1 to 3 weeks after operation. Chest tubes placed laterally may be required in addition to routine mediastinal tubes. Pleural effusion may be of shorter duration and lower volume in patients who have had a pre-existing Glenn shunt (DeLeon et al, 1983; Pennington et al, 1981).

RESULTS OF CORRECTIVE OPERATION

Results of Fontan's operations are often reported without differentiation between anatomic types of univentricular atrioventricular connection. This is reasonable, because there are few differences in morbidity and mortality among hospital survivors with tricuspid atresia or other types of univentricular atrioventricular connection (Coles et al, 1987; Humes et al, 1987). Some aspects of the results of Fontan's operation, however, are anatomic type-specific, such as hospital mortality (patients with tricuspid atresia do better than others). For these reasons, the following discussions of results do not distinguish between Fontan's operations done for tricuspid atresia and for other malformations, unless specifically stated.

Early Mortality

The hospital mortality for the Fontan operation in tricuspid atresia is 10 to 20% (Cleveland et al, 1984; Coles et al, 1987; DeBrux et al, 1983; de Vivie et al, 1986; Fontan et al, 1983; Humes et al, 1987; Mair et al, 1985; Mayer et al, 1986). Mortality is clearly related to preoperative risk factors. When Fontan's criteria are strictly observed, operative risk is very low, approximately 0 to 7% (Fontan et al, 1983; Humes et al, 1987; Laks et al, 1984). Most of the criteria, however, are relative risk factors. In the Mayo Clinic series, the operative mortality for all patients with tricuspid atresia was only 10%, yet 76% of the patients violated one to eight of the criteria (Humes et al, 1987). The mortality increases when more than two (Mayer et al, 1986) or three (Mair et al, 1985) risk factors are present, but these rates may still be acceptable in view of the long-term poor outcome of palliative surgery (Dick et al, 1975).

In the immediate postoperative period, a high right atrial pressure is associated with increased morbidity and mortality (Coles et al, 1987; Kirklin et al, 1986; Mayer et al, 1986) (Fig. 46–10).

Functional Results

Exercise capacity improves substantially from preoperative levels after a Fontan operation (Driscoll et al, 1986) and ranges from 50 to 100% of normal (Fontan et al, 1983; Kreutzer et al, 1982). The venti-

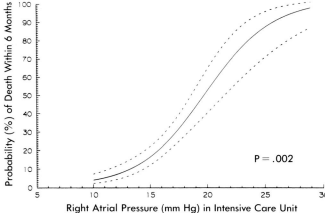

Figure 46–10. Right atrial pressure in the intensive care unit is an important predictor of mortality. The probability of death within 6 months of a Fontan operation, according to right atrial pressure about 2 hours after the operation, rises sharply when the pressure is greater than 16 to 17 mm Hg. The *broken lines* enclose the 70% confidence limits. (From Kirklin, J. K., Kirklin, J. W., Pacifico, A. D., and Bargeron, L. M., Jr.: The Fontan operation: Ventricular hypertrophy, age, and date of operation as risk factors. J. Thorac. Cardiovasc. Surg., *92*:1049, 1986.)

latory response to exercise also decreases toward normal after operation, compared with the preoperative response (Driscoll et al, 1986).

At postoperative cardiac catheterization, the cardiac index is usually in the low normal range (2.2 to 3.2 l/min/m²), the right atrial pressure is almost the same as the pulmonary artery pressure, approximately 15 mm Hg, the oxygen saturation is normal to low normal (91 to 98%), and the left ventricular end-diastolic pressure is normal (average of 8 mm Hg) (Driscoll et al, 1986; Kreutzer et al, 1982; Laks et al, 1984; Mair et al, 1985; Nakazawa et al, 1984).

The hemodynamic response to exercise is not normal. The cardiac index increases only 50 to 100% during exercise (Laks et al, 1984; Shachar et al, 1982), although in one study an almost normal response to exercise was found (Peterson et al, 1984). The left ventricular ejection fraction during exercise is abnormally low in most clinically well patients and correlates poorly both with resting ejection fraction measurements and with exercise capacity (Del Torso et al, 1985). Stroke volume may rise or fall slightly during exercise (Driscoll et al, 1986; Shachar et al, 1982). Much of the increase in cardiac index with exercise in post-Fontan patients is due to an increased heart rate that falls short of normal (Driscoll et al, 1986; Laks et al, 1984). During exercise, there is a sharp rise in right atrial pressure, which may (Shachar et al, 1982) or may not (Laks et al, 1984) be associated with atriopulmonary obstruction. When atriopulmonary flow is obstructed, a pressure gradient not demonstrable at rest may appear with exercise (Shachar et al, 1982).

Left ventricular ejection fraction is low to low normal and changes little from preoperative to postoperative determinations (Fontan et al, 1983; Sanders et al, 1982). Serial studies have shown that low ejection fraction early after Fontan operation does not deteriorate, but either remains stable or improves during 1 to 3 years (Hurwitz et al, 1986). There is a substantial (approximately two-thirds) decrease in left ventricular end-diastolic volume from preoperative to postoperative measurements, primarily because of closing of shunts and improvement in oxygen saturation (Graham et al, 1986; Mair et al, 1985; Sanders et al, 1982), as well as a concomitant decrease in left ventricular end-diastolic pressure by as much as 50% (Mair et al, 1985).

After a Fontan procedure, forward flow in the pulmonary artery is biphasic and occurs during early left ventricular diastole and atrial systole and again while the left atrium is filling during ventricular systole. Vena cava flow varies: It is often forward during ventricular systole and often reverses during atrial systole. Reversal of pulmonary blood flow occurs variably (DiSessa et al, 1984; Laks et al, 1984; Nakazawa et al, 1984). Flow patterns are independent of the type of connection: atriopulmonary or atrioventricular, with or without a valve in atriopulmonary connection (flow patterns have rarely been studied in atrioventricular valve connections). In atriopulmonary connections, the pulmonary valve remains open throughout the cardiac cycle (Bull et al, 1983; Ishikawa et al, 1984). The contribution of right atrial contraction to forward flow is minimal but may become important in patients with small pulmonary arteries (Nakazawa et al, 1987). Flow patterns in the right side of the heart are disorganized in patients with poor ventricular function or a residual shunt (Hagler et al, 1984).

Late Results

The following analysis combines the late follow-up of all patients having Fontan operations from the cited reports. Among 410 patients who had a Fontan operation, 25 (6%) died after leaving the hospital (Fontan et al, 1983; Humes et al, 1987; Laks et al, 1984; Stefanelli et al, 1984). Among the 25 deaths, 9 were related to failure of the dominant ventricle (36%), 6 were sudden deaths or were due to arrhythmias (24%), 5 were due to right heart failure (20%), and 5 were due to other causes (20%). Actuarial survival data (Fig. 46–11) suggest that most of the late mortality occurs within the first 6 months (Fig. 46–12) after a Fontan operation (Coles et al, 1987; Fontan et al, 1983; Humes et al, 1987; Kirklin et al, 1986; Stefanelli et al, 1984); annual mortality up to 16 years after operation may be 1% (Girod et al, 1987).

Among 321 patients for whom information is available, 29 (9%) had reoperation: residual shunt at the atrial or ventricular level (7 patients), obstructed

atriopulmonary connection (13 patients) including three clotting episodes, and other operations (9 patients) (Coles et al, 1987; Fontan et al, 1983; Kirklin et al, 1986; Laks et al, 1984). The need for reoperation is most frequent in the first 5 years after operation (Fig. 46–13).

Protein-losing enteropathy was a contributing factor in 8 of 23 late deaths in one large series (Humes et al, 1987) and may be associated with a high diastolic right atrial pressure (Hess et al, 1984), leading to *increased lymph production* because of high inferior vena cava and portal pressure, and leading to *obstruction of lymph drainage* due to high pressure in the superior vena cava. Loss of protein into the gut may lead to hypoalbuminemia with generalized edema and immunologic abnormalities. Treatment is a low-fat, medium-chain triglyceride diet, which may not become effective for several weeks or months. If diet fails, inflow valves in the vena cava may dramatically reverse this condition (Crupi et al, 1980).

Chronic pleural and pericardial effusions occur rarely, may be associated with high right atrial pressure, and are difficult to treat (Britton et al, 1986). Treatment with prednisone followed by slow tapering has been successful (Rothman et al, 1987b). High right atrial pressure may also lead to cardiac cirrhosis (Lemmer et al, 1983), but this complication remains rare, although many patients may have mild abnormalities of liver function (Girod et al, 1987).

Arrhythmias may require a pacemaker in as many as 5% of patients (Taliercio et al, 1985). Pacemakers in patients with a Fontan operation pose

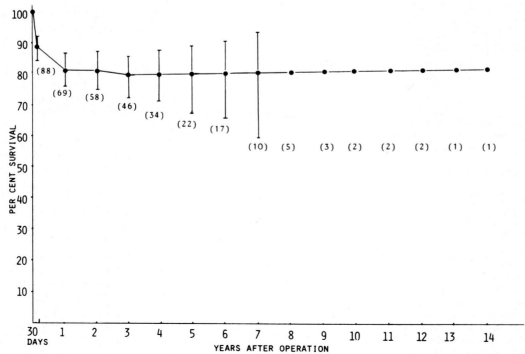

Figure 46–11. The actuarial survival rate of Fontan's first 100 patients. Note that most of the mortality occurs in the first year after operation. (From Fontan, F., Deville, C., Quaegebeur, J., et al: Repair of tricuspid atresia in 100 patients. J. Thorac. Cardiovasc. Surg., 85:647, 1983.)

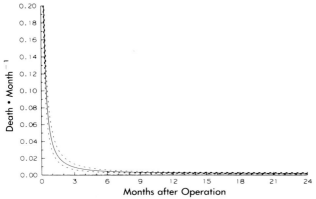

Figure 46–12. The hazard function (instantaneous risk of death in patients still living) after a Fontan operation (102 patients: 32 deaths). The *broken lines* enclose the 70% confidence limits. The greatest danger is within the first 2 to 3 months after operation. (From Kirklin, J. K., Kirklin, J. W., Pacifico, A. D., and Bargeron, L. M., Jr.: The Fontan operation: Ventricular hypertrophy, age, and date of operation as risk factors. J. Thorac. Cardiovasc. Surg., 92:1049, 1986.)

special anatomic problems but can be managed safely (Case et al, 1988). The incidence of supraventricular tachycardia increases linearly with time postoperatively, reaching 25% of patients followed 5 years postoperatively and 37% at 7.5 years (Porter et al, 1986). Appearance or reappearance of arrhythmias, including supraventricular, may be fatal in the late postoperative period, especially in the presence of atriopulmonary obstruction (Girod et al, 1987).

Thrombus formation in the right side of the heart is an uncommon event, but is usually fatal when it occurs. Twelve patients have been reported (Alboliras et al, 1985; Coles et al, 1987; Dajee et al, 1984; DiSessa et al, 1985; Dobell et al, 1986; Fontan et al, 1983; Putnam et al, 1988; Shannon et al, 1986). When recognized during life, thrombus may be surgically excised or may be treated successfully with streptokinase (Dajee et al, 1984; DiSessa et al, 1985). Some surgeons treat patients with warfarin for a few months after a Fontan operation in an effort to prevent this problem.

Cerebral infarction has been reported to be a late

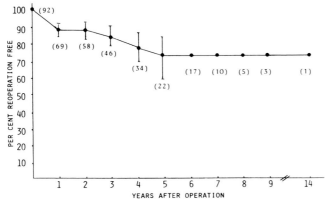

Figure 46–13. Reoperation-free actuarial curve in Fontan's first 100 patients shows a reoperation-free rate of 75% at 5 years after operation that persists.

complication. Risk factors for this event may include congestive heart failure, thrombocytosis, and arrhythmias (Mathews et al, 1986).

Late functional status is excellent in long-term survivors of a Fontan operation. In a combined group of 411 reported patients (Coles et al, 1987; Fontan et al, 1983; Humes et al, 1987; Kirklin et al, 1986; Laks et al, 1984), 380 (92%) were in Class I or II, 30 (7%) were in Class III, and only 1 was in Class IV. Almost all (97%) patients are able to work or attend school, and the majority (55%) require no medications (Humes et al, 1987).

The longest follow-up available is that of Fontan's earliest patients, 32 of whom survived at least 1 year and were monitored for 7 to 16 years (mean of 9 years). There were five late deaths (16%), three at reoperation and two sudden unexplained or due to arrhythmias. The most frequent problem in this group has been conduit obstruction, both of synthetic grafts and homografts, but 26 of the 27 survivors remain in Class I or II (Girod et al, 1987). Fontan's first patient, operated in 1968, is still alive, is married, and engages in the normal activities of a housewife (Fontan, 1986).

Selected Bibliography

Cleveland, D. C., Kirklin, J. K., Naftel, D. C., et al: Surgical treatment of tricuspid atresia. Ann. Thorac. Surg., 38:447, 1984.

This review of all surgical procedures for tricuspid atresia done at the University of Alabama since 1967 showed 9% mortality for the initial palliative operation, with a survival of 78% at 5 years. After Fontan's procedure, the mortality was 14%, and incremental risk factors were young age and complex associated procedures. Actuarial survival was 71% at 5 years, and 9% required subsequent reoperation.

Coles, J. G., Kielmanowizc, S., Freedom, R. M., et al: Surgical experience with the modified Fontan procedure. Circulation, 76(Suppl. 3):61, 1987.

This report summarizes the experience of the staff at the Hospital for Sick Children in Toronto with the modified Fontan operation. The hospital mortality was 14%, and risk factors included previous pulmonary artery banding and the use of a direct atriopulmonary connection. The researchers showed a survival advantage when the hypoplastic right ventricle was included as part of the repair, a conclusion that differs from that of other groups. Early Fontan's operation was recommended, particularly in patients requiring a palliative pulmonary artery band.

Fontan, F., Deville, C., Quaegebeur, J., et al: Repair of tricuspid atresia in 100 patients. J. Thorac. Cardiovasc. Surg., 85:647, 1983.

Fontan's first 100 consecutive patients with tricuspid atresia had a mortality of 12%, but by restrictive selection, this hospital mortality declined to 4% late in the series. Late mortality was 7%. Better results were obtained when a homograft valve was incorporated in the repair, regardless of the type of ventriculoarterial connection. Late results were excellent, and 94% of the surviving patients were in functional Class I or II.

Girod, D. A., Fontan, F., Deville, C., et al: Long-term results after the Fontan operation for tricuspid atresia. Circulation, 75:605, 1987.

Fontan has the longest follow-up available for patients who have had corrective operation for tricuspid atresia. In this study, 32 patients are evaluated 7 to 16 years after operation. Sixteen per cent died subsequently, and 25% had reoperation. All except 1 of the 27 survivors are in functional Class I or II. Conduit obstruction was associated with mortality, reoperation, and poor hemodynamic tolerance of arrhythmias.

Humes, R. A., Porter, C. J., Mair, D. D., et al: Intermediate follow-up and predicted survival after the modified Fontan procedure for tricuspid atresia and double-inlet ventricle. Circulation, 76(Suppl. 3, part 2):67, 1987.

The staff at the Mayo Clinic have reported the largest experience with the Fontan operation. This article is a summary of their work. Among 135 patients with tricuspid atresia, 10% died in the hospital, and 11% of the survivors succumbed later. Among patients leaving the hospital alive, actuarial survival in 5 years was 87%. Among survivors, 92% were in functional Class I or II, and 97% were able to work or attend school. Fifty-two per cent of the patients required no medications. A small number of patients, 16%, continued to have a problem with fluid retention.

Bibliography

Alboliras, E. T., Porter, C. J., Danielson, G. K., et al: Results of the modified Fontan operation for congenital heart lesions in patients without preoperative sinus rhythm. J. Am. Coll. Cardiol., 6:228, 1985.

Anderson, R. H., Becker, A. E., Tynan, M., et al: The univentricular atrioventricular connection: Getting to the root of a thorny problem. Am. J. Cardiol., 54:822, 1984.

Anderson, R. H., and Rigby, M. L.: The morphologic heterogeneity of "tricuspid atresia." Int. J. Cardiol., 16:67, 1987.

Arciniegas, E., Farooki, Z. Q., Hakimi, M., and Green, E. W.: Results of two-stage surgical treatment of tetralogy of Fallot. J. Thorac. Cardiovasc. Surg., 79:876, 1980.

Ashcraft, K. W.: Discussion of Gay W. A., Jr., and Ebert, P. A.: Aorta-to-right pulmonary artery anastomosis causing obstruction of the right pulmonary artery: Management during correction of tetralogy of Fallot. Ann. Thorac. Surg., 16:402, 1973.

Bakulev, A. N., and Kolesnikov, S. A.: Anastomosis of superior vena cava and pulmonary artery in the surgical treatment of certain congenital defects of the heart. J. Thorac. Surg., 37:693, 1959.

Beppu, S., Nimura, Y., Tamai, M., et al: Two-dimensional echocardiography in diagnosing tricuspid atresia: Differentiation from other hypoplastic right heart syndromes and common atrioventricular canal. Br. Heart J., 40:1174, 1978.

Bjork, V. O., Olin, C. L., Bjarke, B. B., and Thoren, C. A.: Right atrial-right ventricular anastomosis for correction of tricuspid atresia. J. Thorac. Cardiovasc. Surg., 77:452, 1979.

Blalock, A., and Hanlon, C. R.: The surgical treatment of transposition of the aorta and the pulmonary artery. Surg. Gynecol. Obstet., 90:1, 1950.

Blalock, A., and Taussig, H. B.: The surgical treatment of malformations of the heart in which there is pulmonary stenosis or pulmonary atresia. J.A.M.A., 128:189, 1945.

Bowman, F. O., Jr., Malm, J. R., Hayes, C. J., and Gersony, W. M.: Physiological approach to surgery for tricuspid atresia. Circulation, 58(Suppl. 1):83, 1978.

Breisch, E. A., Wilson, D. B., Laurenson, R. D., et al: Tricuspid atresia (type Ia): Survival to 21 years of age. Am. Heart J., 106:149, 1983.

Brendel, A. J., Wynchank, S., Choussat, A., et al: Radionuclide studies in postoperative evaluation of the Fontan procedure. A.J.R., 143:737, 1984.

Britton, L. W., Mayer, J. E., Galinanes, M., et al: Effusive complications of Fontan procedures. Circulation, 74(Suppl. 2):49, 1986.

Bull, C., de Leval, M. R., Stark, J., et al: Use of a subpulmonary ventricular chamber in the Fontan circulation. J. Thorac. Cardiovasc. Surg., 85:21, 1983.

Carlon, C. A., Mondini, P. G., and DeMarchi, R.: Surgical treatment of some cardiovascular diseases (a new vascular anastomosis). J. Int. Coll. Surg., 16:1, 1951.

Case, C., Gillette, P., Zeigler, V., and Sade, R. M.: Problems with permanent atrial pacing in the post Fontan patient. Pace, 11:484, 1988.

Choussat, A., Fontan, F., Besse, P., et al: Selection criteria for Fontan's procedure. In Anderson, R. H., and Shinebourne, E. A. (eds): Pediatric Cardiology, 1978. Edinburgh, Churchill Livingstone, 1978, pp. 559–566.

Cleveland, D. C., Kirklin, J. K., Naftel, D. C., et al: Surgical treatment of tricuspid atresia. Ann. Thorac. Surg., 38:447, 1984.

Cloutier, A., Ash, J. M., Smallhorn, J. F., et al: Abnormal distribution of pulmonary blood flow after the Glenn shunt or Fontan procedure: Risk of development of arteriovenous fistulae. Circulation, 72:471, 1985.

Coles, J. G., Kielmanowizc, S., Freedom, R. M., et al: Surgical experience with the modified Fontan procedure. Circulation, 76(Suppl. 3):61, 1987.

Covitz, W., Moore, H. V., Gray, B., et al: Assessment of Fontan graft patency by radionuclide perfusion pulmonary scan in tricuspid atresia with previous Glenn shunt. Am. Heart J., 103:1072, 1982.

Crupi, G., Locatelli, R., Tiraboschi, M., et al: Protein-losing enteropathy after Fontan operation for tricuspid atresia (imperforate tricuspid valve). Thorac. Cardiovasc. Surg., 28:359, 1980.

Crupi, G., Villani, M., Di Benedetto, G., et al: Tricuspid atresia with imperforate valve: Angiographic findings and surgical implications in two cases with AV concordance and normally related great arteries. Pediatr. Cardiol., 5:49, 1984.

Currarino, G., and Engle, M. A.: The effects of ligation of the subclavian artery on the bones and soft tissues of the arms. J. Pediatr., 67:808, 1965.

Currie, P. J., Hagler, D. J., Seward, J. B., et al: Instantaneous pressure gradient: A simultaneous Doppler and dual catheter correlative study. J. Am. Coll. Cardiol. 7:800, 1986.

Dajee, H., Deutsch, L. S., Benson, L. N., et al: Thrombolytic therapy for superior vena caval thrombosis following superior vena cava-pulmonary artery anastomosis. Ann. Thorac. Surg., 38:637, 1984.

Davidson, J. S.: Anastomosis between the ascending aorta and the main pulmonary artery in the tetralogy of Fallot. Thorax, 10:348, 1955.

Deanfield, J. E., Tommasini, G., Anderson, R. H., and Macartney, F. J.: Tricuspid atresia: Analysis of coronary artery distribution and ventricular morphology. Br. Heart J., 48:485, 1982.

DeBrux, J. L., Zannini, L., Binet, J. P., et al: Tricuspid atresia: Results of treatment in 115 children. J. Thorac. Cardiovasc. Surg., 85:440, 1983.

de la Riviere, A. B., Haasler, G., Malm, J. R., and Bregman, D.: Mechanical assistance of the pulmonary circulation after right ventricular exclusion. J. Thorac. Cardiovasc. Surg., 85:809, 1983.

DeLeon, S. Y., Idriss, F. S., Ilbawi, M. N., et al: The role of the Glenn shunt in patients undergoing the Fontan operation. J. Thorac. Cardiovasc. Surg., 85:669, 1983.

DeLeon, S. Y., Ilbawi, M. N., Idriss, F. S., et al: Persistent low cardiac output after the Fontan operation: Should takedown be considered? J. Thorac. Cardiovasc. Surg., 92:402, 1986a.

DeLeon, S. Y., Ilbawi, M. N., Idriss, F. S., et al: Fontan type operation for complex lesions: Surgical considerations to improve survival. J. Thorac. Cardiovasc. Surg., 92:1029, 1986b.

DeLeon, S. Y., Koopot, R., Mair, D. D., et al: Surgical management of occluded conduits after the Fontan operation in patients with Glenn shunts. J. Thorac. Cardiovasc. Surg., 88:601, 1984.

de Leval, M. R., Bull, C., and Kilner, P.: Total cavopulmonary connection: A logical alternative to atriopulmonary connection for complex Fontan operations—experimental studies and early clinical experience. J. Thorac. Cardiovasc. Surg., 96:682, 1988.

Del Torso, S., Kelly, M. J., Kalff, V., and Venables, A. W.: Radionuclide assessment of ventricular contraction at rest and during exercise following the Fontan procedure for either tricuspid atresia or single ventricle. Am. J. Cardiol., 55:1127, 1985.

Deverall, P. B., Lincoln, J. C., Aberdeen, E., et al: Surgical management of tricuspid atresia. Thorax, 24:239, 1969.

de Vivie, E. R., and Rupprath, G.: Long-term results after Fontan procedure and its modifications. J. Thorac. Cardiovasc. Surg., 91:690, 1986.

DiCarlo, D., Williams, W. G., Freedom, R.M., et al: The role of cava-pulmonary (Glenn) anastomosis in the palliative treatment of congenital heart disease. J. Thorac. Cardiovasc. Surg., 83:437, 1982.

Dick, M., Fyler, D. C., and Nadas, A. S.: Tricuspid atresia: Clinical course in 101 patients. Am. J. Cardiol., 36:327, 1975.

Didier, D., Higgins, C. B., Fisher, M. R., et al: Congenital heart disease: Gated MR imaging in 72 patients. Radiology, 158:227, 1986.

DiSessa, T. G., Child, J. S., Perloff, J. K., et al: Systemic venous and pulmonary arterial flow patterns after Fontan's procedure for tricuspid atresia or single ventricle. Circulation, 70:898, 1984.

DiSessa, T. G., Yeatman, L. A., Jr., Williams, R. G., et al: Thrombosis complicating balloon angioplasty of left pulmonary artery stenosis after Fontan's procedure: Successful treatment with intravenous streptokinase. Am. J. Cardiol., 55:610, 1985.

Dobell, A. R. C., Trusler, G. A., Smallhorn, J. F., and Williams, W. G.: Atrial thrombi after the Fontan operation. Ann. Thorac. Surg., 42:664, 1986.

Doty, D. B., Marvin, W. J., Jr., and Lauer, R. M.: Modified Fontan procedure: Methods to achieve direct anastomosis of right atrium to pulmonary artery. J. Thorac. Cardiovasc. Surg., 81:470, 1981.

Driscoll, D. J., Danielson, G. K., Puga, F. J., et al: Exercise tolerance and cardiorespiratory response to exercise after the Fontan operation for tricuspid atresia or functional single ventricle. J. Am. Coll. Cardiol., 7:1087, 1986.

Edwards, J. E., and Burchell, H. B.: Congenital tricuspid atresia: A classification. Med. Clin. North Am., 33:1177, 1949.

Elliott, R. B., Starling, M. B., and Neutze, J. M.: Medical manipulation of ductus arteriosus. Lancet, 1:140, 1975.

Fletcher, B. D., Jacobstein, M. D., Abramowsky, C. R., and Anderson, R. H.: Right atrioventricular valve atresia: Anatomic evaluation with MR imaging. A.J.R., 148:671, 1987.

Fontan, F.: Discussion of Lee, C. N., Schaff, H. V., Danielson, G. K., et al: Comparison of atriopulmonary versus atrioventricular corrections for modified Fontan/Kreutzer repair of tricuspid valve atresia. J. Thorac. Cardiovasc. Surg., 92:1038, 1986.

Fontan, F., and Baudet, E.: Surgical repair of tricuspid atresia. Thorax, 26:240, 1971.

Fontan, F., Choussat, A., Brown, A. G., et al: Repair of tricuspid atresia—surgical considerations and results. In Anderson, R. H., and Shinebourne, E. A., (eds): Pediatric Cardiology, 1977. Edinburgh, Churchill Livingstone, 1978, pp. 567–580.

Fontan, F., Choussat, A., Deville, C., et al: Aortic valve homografts in the surgical treatment of complex cardiac malformations. J. Thorac. Cardiovasc. Surg., 87:649, 1984.

Fontan, F., Deville, C., Quaegebeur, J., et al: Repair of tricuspid atresia in 100 patients. J. Thorac. Cardiovasc. Surg., 85:647, 1983.

Forrest, P., Bini, R. M., Wilkinson, J. L., et al: Congenital absence of the pulmonic valve and tricuspid valve atresia with intact ventricular septum. Am. J. Cardiol., 59:482, 1987.

Freed, M., Rosenthal, A., Planth, W. H., Jr., and Nadas, A. S.: Development of subaortic stenosis after pulmonary artery banding. Circulation, 47(Suppl. 3):7, 1973.

Freedom, R. M.: The dinosaur and banding of the main pulmonary trunk in the heart with functionally one ventricle and transposition of the great arteries: A saga of evolution and caution. J. Am. Coll. Cardiol., 10:427, 1987.

Freedom, R. M., Lee, N. B., Smallhorn, J. F., et al: Subaortic stenosis, the univentricular heart, and banding of the pulmonary artery: An analysis of the courses of 43 patients with univentricular heart palliated by pulmonary artery banding. Circulation, 73:758, 1986.

Freedom, R. M., Williams, W. G., Fowler, R. S., et al: Tricuspid

atresia, transposition of the great arteries, and banded pulmonary artery: Repair by arterial switch, coronary artery reimplantation, and right atrioventricular valved conduit. J. Thorac. Cardiovasc. Surg., 80:621, 1980.

Fyfe, D. A., Currie, P. J., Seward, J. B., et al: Continuous-wave Doppler determination of the pressure gradient across pulmonary artery bands: Hemodynamic correlation in 20 patients. Mayo Clin. Proc., 59:744, 1984.

Fyfe, D. A., Taylor, A. B., Gillette, P. C., et al: Doppler echocardiographic confirmation of recurrent atrial septal defect stenosis in infants with mitral valve atresia. Am. J. Cardiol., 60:410, 1987.

Gago, O., Salles, C. A., Stern, A. M., et al: A different approach for the total correction of tricuspid atresia. J. Thorac. Cardiovasc. Surg., 72:209, 1976.

Gallaher, M. E., and Fyler, D. C.: Observations on changing hemodynamics in tricuspid atresia without associated transposition of the great vessels. Circulation, 35:381, 1967.

Gay, W. A., Jr., and Ebert, P. A.: Aorta-to-right pulmonary artery anastomosis causing obstruction of the right pulmonary artery: Management during correction of tetralogy of Fallot. Ann. Thorac. Surg., 16:402, 1973.

Geiss, D., Williams, W. G., Lindsay, W. K., and Rowe, R. D.: Upper extremity gangrene: A complication of subclavian artery division. Ann. Thorac. Surg., 30:487, 1980.

Girod, D. A., Fontan, F., Deville, C., et al: Long-term results after the Fontan operation for tricuspid atresia. Circulation, 75:605, 1987.

Girod, D. A., Rice, M. J., Mair, D. D., et al: Relationship of pulmonary artery size to mortality in patients undergoing the Fontan operation. Circulation, 72(Suppl. 2):93, 1985.

Glenn, W. W. L.: Circulatory bypass of the right side of the heart. IV. Shunt between superior vena cava and distal right pulmonary artery—report of a clinical application. N. Engl. J. Med., 259:117, 1958.

Graham, T. P., Jr., Franklin, R. C. G., Wyse, R. K. H., et al: Left ventricular wall stress and contractile function in childhood: Normal values and comparison of Fontan repair versus palliation only in patients with tricuspid atresia. Circulation, 74(Suppl. 1):61, 1986.

Gussenhoven, W. J., The, H. K., Schippers, L., et al: Growth and function of the right ventricular outflow tract after Fontan's procedure for tricuspid atresia: A two-dimensional echocardiographic study. Thorac. Cardiovasc. Surg., 34:236, 1986.

Guyton, R. A., Davis, S. C., Michalik, R. E., et al: Right heart assist by intermittent abdominal compression after surgery for congenital heart disease. Circulation, 72(Suppl. 2):97, 1985.

Hagler, D. J., Seward, J. B., Tajik, A. J., and Ritter, D. G.: Functional assessment of the Fontan operation: Combined M-mode, two-dimensional and Doppler echocardiographic studies. J. Am. Coll. Cardiol., 4:756, 1984.

Hallman, G. L., Stasney, C. R., and Cooley, D. A.: Surgical treatment of tricuspid atresia. J. Cardiovasc. Surg., 9:154, 1968.

Harrison, R.: Discussion of Bopp, R. K., Larsen, P. B., Caddell, J. L., et al: Surgical considerations for treatment of congenital tricuspid atresia and stenosis: With particular reference to vena cava-pulmonary artery anastomosis. J. Thorac. Cardiovasc. Surg., 43:97, 1962.

Hatem, J., Sade, R. M., Upshur, J. K., and Hohn, A. R.: Maintaining patency of the ductus arteriosus for palliation of cyanotic congenital cardiac malformations. Ann. Surg., 192:124, 1980.

Hausdorf, G., Grävinghoff, L., Sieg, K., and Keck, E. W.: Pitfalls in the diagnosis of tricuspid atresia: Report of a new angiocardiographic sign. Clin. Cardiol., 8:189, 1985.

Heck, H. A., Jr., and Doty, D. B.: Assisted circulation by phasic external lower body compression. Circulation, 64(Suppl. 2):118, 1981.

Hellberg, K., Kirchoff, P. G., Orellano, L. E., et al: Supporting the pump function of the right atrium: A new therapeutic concept after physiological repair of tricuspid atresia. Thoraxchir. Vask. Chir., 25:400, 1977.

Henry, J. N., Devloo, R. A. E., Ritter, D. G., et al: Tricuspid atresia: Successful surgical "correction" in two patients using porcine xenograft valves. Mayo Clin. Proc., 49:803, 1974.

Hess, J. H.: Congenital atresia of the right auriculoventricular orifice with complete absence of tricuspid valves. Am. J. Dis. Child, 13:167, 1917.

Hess, J., Kruizinga, K., Bijleveld, C. M. A., et al: Protein-losing enteropathy after Fontan operation. J. Thorac. Cardiovasc. Surg., 88:606, 1984.

Hopkins, R. A., Armstrong, B. E., Serwer, G. A., et al: Physiological rationale for a bidirectional cavopulmonary shunt: A versatile complement to the Fontan principle. J. Thorac. Cardiovasc. Surg., 90:391, 1985.

Humes, R. A., Porter, C. J., Mair, D. D., et al: Intermediate follow-up and predicted survival after the modified Fontan procedure for tricuspid atresia and double-inlet ventricle. Circulation, 76(Suppl. 3, part 2):67, 1987.

Hurwitt, E. S., Young, D., and Escher, D. J. W.: The rationale of anastomosis of the right auricular appendage to the pulmonary artery in the treatment of tricuspid atresia. J. Thorac. Surg., 30:503, 1955.

Hurwitz, R. A., Caldwell, R. L., Girod, D. A., and Wellman, H.: Left ventricular function in tricuspid atresia: A radionuclide study. J. Am. Coll. Cardiol., 8:916, 1986.

Ilbawi, M. N., Idriss, F. S., Muster, A. J., et al: Effects of elevated coronary sinus pressure on left ventricular function after the Fontan operation: An experimental and clinical correlation. J. Thorac. Cardiovasc. Surg., 92:231, 1986.

Ishikawa, T., Neutze, J. M., Brandt, P. W. T., and Barratt-Boyes, B. G.: Hemodynamics following the Kreutzer procedure for tricuspid atresia in patients under two years of age. J. Thorac. Cardiovasc. Surg., 88:373, 1984.

Jacobs, M. L., Vlahakes, G. J., D'Ambra, M. N., et al: Augmentation of pulmonary blood flow by a right atrial balloon pump after the Fontan operation. Circulation, 76(Suppl. 3, part 2):72, 1987.

Jonas, R. A., Castaneda, A. R., and Lang, P.: Single ventricle (single- or double-inlet) complicated by subaortic stenosis: Surgical options in infancy. Ann. Thorac. Surg., 39:361, 1985.

Juaneda, E., and Haworth, S. G.: Pulmonary vascular structure in patients dying after a Fontan procedure: The lung as a risk factor. Br. Heart J., 52:575, 1984.

Kanter, K. R., Pennington, D. G., Weber, T. R., et al: Extracorporeal membrane oxygenation for postoperative cardiac support in children. J. Thorac. Cardiovasc. Surg., 93:27, 1987.

Keith, J. D., Rowe, R. D., and Vlad, P.: Heart Disease in Infancy and Childhood, 3rd ed. New York, Macmillan Company, 1978.

King, R. M., Puga, F. J., Danielson, G. K., and Julsrud, P. R.: Extended indications for the modified Fontan procedure in patients with anomalous systemic and pulmonary venous return. Pediatric Cardiology: Proceedings of the Second World Congress, New York, 1985, Springer-Verlag, p. 523.

Kirklin, J. K., Blackstone, E. H., Kirklin, J. W., et al: The Fontan operation: Ventricular hypertrophy, age, and date of operation as risk factors. J. Thorac. Cardiovasc. Surg., 92:1049, 1986.

Kirklin, J. K., Westaby, S., Blackstone, E. H., et al: Complement and the damaging effects of cardiopulmonary bypass. J. Thorac. Cardiovasc. Surg., 86:845, 1983.

Kirklin, J. W., and Barratt-Boyes, B. G.: Tricuspid atresia. In Kirklin and Barratt-Boyes: Cardiac Surgery. New York, John Wiley & Sons, 1986, pp. 857–888.

Kreutzer, G., Galindez, E., Bono, H., et al: An operation for the correction of tricuspid atresia. J. Thorac. Cardiovasc. Surg., 66:613, 1973.

Kreutzer, G. O., Vargas, F. J., Schlichter, A. J., et al: Atriopulmonary anastomosis. J. Thorac. Cardiovasc. Surg., 83:427, 1982.

Kreysig, F. L.: Krankenheiten des herzens, Vol. 3. Berlin, Maurer, 1817.

Kuhne, M.: Ueber zwei Faelle kongenitaler Atresie des Ostium venosum dextrum. Jahresber. Kinderh., 63:225, 1906.

LaCorte, M. A., Dick, M., Scheer, G., et al: Left ventricular function in tricuspid atresia: Angiographic analysis in 28 patients. Circulation, 52:996, 1975.

Laks, H., Milliken, J. C., Perloff, J. K., et al: Experience with the Fontan procedure. J. Thorac. Cardiovasc. Surg., 88:939, 1984.

Laks, H., Mudd, J. G., Standeven, J. W., et al: Long-term effect of the superior vena cava-pulmonary artery anastomosis on pulmonary blood flow. J. Thorac. Cardiovasc. Surg., 74:253, 1977.

Lee, C. N., Schaff, H. V., Danielson, G. K., et al: Comparison of atriopulmonary versus atrioventricular connections for modified Fontan/Kreutzer repair of tricuspid valve atresia. J. Thorac. Cardiovasc. Surg., 92:1038, 1986.

Lee, M. E., and Sade, R. M.: Coronary sinus septal defect: Surgical considerations. J. Thorac. Cardiovasc. Surg., 78:563, 1979.

Lemmer, J. H., Coran, A. G., Behrendt, D. M., et al: Liver fibrosis (cardiac cirrhosis) five years after modified Fontan operation for tricuspid atresia. J. Thorac. Cardiovasc. Surg., 86:757, 1983.

Lin, A. E., Laks, H., Barber, G., et al: Subaortic obstruction in complex congenital heart disease: Management by proximal pulmonary artery to ascending aorta end to side anastomosis. J. Am. Coll. Cardiol., 7:617, 1986.

Lock, J. E., Castaneda-Zuniga, W. R., Fuhrman, B. P., and Bass, J. L.: Balloon dilation angioplasty of hypoplastic and stenotic pulmonary arteries. Circulation, 67:962, 1983.

London Med. Rev., 5:252, 1812.

Mair, D. D., Rice, M. J., Hagler, D. J., et al: Outcome of the Fontan procedure in patients with tricuspid atresia. Circulation, 72(Suppl. 2):88, 1985.

Marin-Garcia, J., Roca, J., Blieden, L. C., et al: Congenital absence of the pulmonary valve associated with tricuspid atresia and intact ventricular septum. Chest, 64:658, 1973.

Mathews, K., Bale, J. F., Jr., Clark, E. B., et al: Cerebral infarction complicating Fontan surgery for cyanotic congenital heart disease. Pediatr. Cardiol., 7:161, 1986.

Mathur, M., and Glenn, W. W. L.: Long-term evaluation of cavapulmonary artery anastomosis. Surgery, 74:899, 1973.

Matsuda, H., Kawashima, Y., Hirose, H., et al: Modified Fontan operation for single ventricle with common atrium and abnormal systemic venous drainage: Usefulness of an additional superior vena cava to pulmonary artery anastomosis. Pediatr. Cardiol., 8:43, 1987.

Matsuda, H., Kawashima, Y., Takano, H., et al: Experimental evaluation of atrial function in right atrium-pulmonary artery conduit operation for tricuspid atresia. J. Thorac. Cardiovasc. Surg., 81:762, 1981.

Mayer, J. E., Jr., Helgason, H., Jonas, R. A., et al: Extending the limits for modified Fontan procedures. J. Thorac. Cardiovasc. Surg., 92:1021, 1986.

McFaul, R. C., Tajik, A. J., Mair, D. D., et al: Development of pulmonary arteriovenous shunt after superior vena cava-right pulmonary artery (Glenn) anastomosis: Report of four cases. Circulation, 55:212, 1977.

McKay, R., de Leval, M. R., Rees, P., et al: Postoperative angiographic assessment of modified Blalock-Taussig shunts using expanded polytetrafluoroethylene (Gore-Tex). Ann. Thorac. Surg., 30:137, 1980.

Mietus-Snyder, M., Lang, P., Mayer, J. E., et al: Childhood systemic-pulmonary shunts: Subsequent suitability for Fontan operation. Circulation, 76(Suppl. 3, part 2):39, 1987.

Milliken, J. C., Laks, H., and George, B.: Use of a venous assist device after repair of complex lesions of the right heart. J. Am. Coll. Cardiol., 8:922, 1986.

Moulton, A. L., Brenner, J. I., Ringel, R., et al: Classic versus modified Blalock-Taussig shunts in neonates and infants. Circulation, 72(Suppl. 2):35, 1985.

Muller, W. H., Jr., and Dammann, J. F., Jr.: The treatment of certain congenital malformations of the heart by the creation of pulmonary stenosis to reduce pulmonary hypertension and excessive pulmonary blood flow. Surg. Gynecol. Obstet., 95:213, 1952.

Murray, G. F., Herrington, R. T., and Delany, D. J.: Tricuspid atresia: Corrective operation without a bioprosthetic valve. Ann. Thorac. Surg., 23:209, 1977.

Nadas, A. S., and Fyler, D. C.: Pediatric Cardiology, 3rd ed. Philadelphia, W. B. Saunders Company, 1972.

Nakata, S., Imai, Y., Takanashi, Y., et al: A new method for the quantitative standardization of cross-sectional areas of the pulmonary arteries in congenital heart diseases with decreased pulmonary blood flow. J. Thorac. Cardiovasc. Surg., 88:610, 1984.

Nakazawa, M., Nakanishi, T., Okuda, H., et al: Dynamics of right heart flow in patients after Fontan procedure. Circulation, 69:306, 1984.

Nakazawa, M., Nojima, K., Okuda, H., et al: Flow dynamics in the main pulmonary artery after the Fontan procedure in patients with tricuspid atresia or single ventricle. Circulation, 75:1117, 1987.

Nawa, S., Matsuki, T., Shimizu, A., et al: Pulmonary artery connection in the Fontan procedure: Flexible polytetrafluoro- ethylene conduit for expansion. Chest, 91:552, 1987.

Oelert, H., and Borst, H. G.: Modified Fontan procedure using a retroaortic atriopulmonary anastomosis. Thorac. Cardiovasc. Surg., 32:392, 1984.

Olley, P. M., Coreani, F., and Badoch, E.: E-type prostaglandins: A new emergency therapy for certain cyanotic congenital heart malformations. Circulation, 53:728, 1976.

Ottenkamp, J., Wenink, A. C. G., Quaegebeur, J. M., et al: Tricuspid atresia: Morphology of the outlet chamber with special emphasis on surgical implications. J. Thorac. Cardio- vasc. Surg., 89:597, 1985.

Ottenkamp, J., Wenink, A. C. G., Rohmer, J., and Gittenberger- de Groot, A.: Tricuspid atresia with overriding imperforate tricuspid membrane: An anatomic variant. Int. J. Cardiol., 6:599, 1984.

Park, S. C., Neches, W. H., Mullins, C. E., et al: Blade atrial septostomy: Collaborative study. Circulation, 66:258, 1982.

Patel, M. M., Overy, D. C., Kozonis, M. C., and Hadley-Fowlkes, L. L.: Long-term survival in tricuspid atresia. J. Am. Coll. Cardiol., 9:338, 1987.

Patterson, W., Baxley, W. A., Karp, R. B., et al: Tricuspid atresia in adults. Am. J. Cardiol., 49:141, 1982.

Penkoske, P. A., Freedom, R. M., Williams, W. G., et al: Surgical palliation of subaortic stenosis in the univentricular heart. J. Thorac. Cardiovasc. Surg., 87:767, 1984.

Pennington, D. G., Nouri, S., Ho, J., et al: Glenn shunt: Long- term results and current role in congenital heart operations. Ann. Thorac. Surg., 31:532, 1981.

Peterson, R. J., Franch, R. H., Fajman, W. A., et al: Noninvasive determination of exercise cardiac function following Fontan operation. J. Thorac. Cardiovasc. Surg., 88:263, 1984.

Pigott, J. D., Murphy, J. D., Barber, G., and Norwood, W. I.: Palliative reconstructive surgery for hypoplastic left heart syndrome. Ann. Thorac. Surg., 45:122, 1988.

Porter, C. J., Battiste, C. E., Humes, R. A., et al: Risk factors for supraventricular tachyarrhythmias after Fontan procedure for tricuspid atresia. Am. Heart J., 112:645, 1986.

Potts, W. J., Smith, S., and Gibson, S.: Anastomosis of the aorta to a pulmonary artery. J.A.M.A., 132:627, 1946.

Puga, F. J., Chiavarelli, M., and Hagler, D. J.: Modifications of the Fontan operation applicable to patients with left atrioven- tricular valve atresia or single atrioventricular valve. Circula- tion, 76(Suppl. III):53, 1987.

Puga, F. J., Chiavarelli, M., and Hagler, D. J.: The Fontan operation for patients with left atrioventricular valve atresia. Circulation, 74(Suppl. 2):49, 1986.

Putnam, J. B., Lemmer, J. H., Jr., Rocchini, A. P., and Bove, E. L.: Embolectomy for acute pulmonary artery occlusion follow- ing Fontan procedure. Ann. Thorac. Surg., 45:335, 1988.

Rao, P. S.: Further observations on the spontaneous closure of physiologically advantageous ventricular septal defects in tricuspid atresia: Surgical implications. Ann. Thorac. Surg., 35:121, 1983a.

Rao, P. S.: Left to right atrial shunting in tricuspid atresia. Br. Heart J., 49:345, 1983b.

Rao, P. S., Jue, K. L., Isabel-Jones, J., and Ruttenberg, H. D.: Ebstein's malformation of the tricuspid valve with atresia. Am. J. Cardiol., 32:1004, 1973.

Rashkind, W. J.: Tricuspid atresia: A historical review. Pediatr. Cardiol., 2:85, 1982.

Rashkind, W. J., and Miller, W. W.: Creation of an atrial septal defect without thoracotomy: A palliative approach to complete transposition of the great arteries. J.A.M.A., 196:991, 1966.

Rigby, M. L., Anderson, R. H., Gibson, D., et al: Two-dimensional

echocardiographic categorisation of the univentricular heart: Ventricular morphology, type, and mode of atrioventricular connection. Br. Heart J., 46:603, 1981.

Ring, J. C., Bass, J. L., Marvin, W., et al: Management of congenital stenosis of a branch pulmonary artery with balloon dilation angioplasty. J. Thorac. Cardiovasc. Surg., 90:35, 1985.

Robicsek, F., Sanger, P. W., Gollucci, V., and Daugherty, H. K.: Long-term circulatory exclusion of the right heart. Surgery, 59:431, 1966.

Rosenquist, G. C., Levy, R. J., and Rowe, R. D.: Right atrial-left ventricular relationships in tricuspid atresia: Position of the presumed site of the atretic valve as determined by transillu- mination. Am. Heart J., 80:493, 1970.

Rosenthal, A.: Current status of treatment for tricuspid atresia: Introduction to symposium. Ann. Thorac. Surg., 29:304, 1980.

Ross, D. N., and Somerville, J.: Surgical correction of tricuspid atresia. Lancet, 1:845, 1973.

Rothman, A., Lang, P., Lock, J. E., et al: Surgical management of subaortic obstruction in single left ventricle and tricuspid atresia. J. Am. Coll. Cardiol., 10:421, 1987a.

Rothman, A., Mayer, J. E., and Freed, M. D.: Treatment of chronic pleural effusions after the Fontan procedure with prednisone. Am. J. Cardiol., 60:408, 1987b.

Rumisek, J. D., Pigott, J. D., Weinberg, P. M., and Norwood, W. I.: Coronary sinus septal defect associated with tricuspid atresia. J. Thorac. Cardiovasc. Surg., 92:142, 1986.

Sade, R. M.: Experimental observations on the physiology of the pulmonary circulation after right heart bypass. In Rao, P. S. (ed): Tricuspid Atresia. Mt. Kisco, NY, Futura Publishing Company, 1982, pp. 255–274.

Sade, R. M.: Tricuspid atresia. In Sabiston, D.C., Jr., and Spencer, F. C. (eds): Surgery of the Chest. Philadelphia, W. B. Saunders Company, 1983, pp. 1186–1203.

Sade, R. M., and Castaneda, A. R.: The dispensable right ventricle. Surgery, 77:624, 1975.

Sade, R. M., and Dearing, J. P.: Augmentation of pulmonary blood flow after right ventricular bypass. J. Thorac. Cardio- vasc. Surg., 81:928, 1981.

Sade, R. M., DeWet Lubbe, J. J., Simpser, M. D., and Strieder, D. J. S.: Mechanical ventilation as a pump for the pulmonary circulation. Eur. Surg. Res., 13:414, 1981.

Sade, R. M., Riopel, D. A., and Taylor, A. B.: Orthoterminally corrective operation in the presence of severe hypoplasia of a pulmonary artery. J. Thorac. Cardiovasc. Surg., 80:424, 1980.

Sahn, D. J., Harder, J. R., Freedom, R. M., et al: Cross sectional echocardiographic diagnosis and subclassification of univen- tricular hearts: Imaging studies of atrioventricular valves, septal structures and rudimentary outflow chambers. Circu- lation, 66:1070, 1982.

Sanders, S. P., Wright, G. B., Keane, J. F., et al: Clinical and hemodynamic results of the Fontan operation for tricuspid atresia. Am. J. Cardiol., 49:1733, 1982.

Scalia, D., Russo, P., Anderson, R. H., et al: The surgical anatomy of hearts with no direct communication between the right atrium and the ventricular mass—so-called tricuspid atresia. J. Thorac. Cardiovasc. Surg., 87:743, 1984.

Schuberg, W.: Beobachtung von Verkummerung des rechten Herzventrikels in Folge von Atresie des Ost. venos. dextr.; Perforation des Herzscheidewand und dadurch Bildung eines Canales, der durch den rudimentaren rechtaen Ventrikel in die Art. pulmon. fuhrt. Virchows Arch. [A] 20:294, 1861.

Seward, J. B., Tajik, A. J., Hagler, D. J., and Ritter, D. G.: Echocardiographic spectrum of tricuspid atresia. Mayo Clin. Proc., 53:100, 1978.

Shachar, G. B., Fuhrman, B. P., Wang, Y., et al: Rest and exercise hemodynamics after the Fontan procedure. Circulation, 65:1043, 1982.

Shannon, F. L., Campbell, D. N., and Clarke, D. R.: Right atrial thrombosis: Rare complication of the modified Fontan proce- dure. Pediatr. Cardiol., 7:209, 1986.

Sharratt, G. P., Johnson, A. M., and Monro, J. L.: Persistence and effects of sinus rhythm after Fontan procedure for tricuspid atresia. Br. Heart J., 42:74, 1979.

Shemin, R. J., Merrill, W. H., Pfeifer, J. S., et al: Evaluation of right atrial-pulmonary artery conduits for tricuspid atresia:

Experimental study. J. Thorac. Cardiovasc. Surg., 77:685, 1979.

Shumacker, H. B.: Discussion of Hurwitt, E. S., Young, D., and Escher, D. J. W.: The rationale of anastomosis of the right auricular appendage to the pulmonary artery in the treatment of tricuspid atresia. J. Thorac. Surg., 30:503, 1955.

Smith, C. D., Sade, R. M., Crawford, F. A., Jr., and Othersen, H. B.: Diaphragmatic eventration in infants. J. Thorac. Cardiovasc. Surg., 91:490, 1986.

Stark, J.: Discussion of Lee, C. N., Schaff, H. V., Danielson, G. K., et al: Comparison of atriopulmonary versus atrioventricular connections for modified Fontan/Kreutzer repair of tricuspid valve atresia. J. Thorac. Cardiovasc. Surg., 92:1038, 1986.

Stefanelli, G., Kirklin, J. W., Naftel, D. C., et al: Early and intermediate-term (10-year) results of surgery for univentricular atrioventricular connection ("single ventricle"). Am. J. Cardiol., 54:811, 1984.

Stewart, J. M., Seligman, K. P., Zeballos, G., et al: Elevated atrial natriuretic peptide after the Fontan procedure. Circulation, 76(Suppl. 3, part 2):77, 1987.

Taliercio, C. P., Vlietstra, R. E., McGoon, M. D., et al: Permanent cardiac pacing after the Fontan procedure. J. Thorac. Cardiovasc. Surg., 90:414, 1985.

Talner, N. S., McCue, H. M., Jr., Graham, T. P., et al: Guidelines for insurability of patient with congenital heart disease. Circulation, 62:1419A, 1980.

Taussig, H. B., Keinonen, R., Momberger, H., and Kirk, H.: Long-time observations on the Blalock-Taussig operation. IV: Tricuspid atresia. Johns Hopkins Med. J., 132:135, 1973.

Teixeira, O. H., Carpenter, B., MacMurray, S. B., and Vlad, P.: Long-term prostaglandin E$_1$ therapy in congenital heart defects. J. Am. Coll. Cardiol., 3:838, 1984.

Truesdell, S. C., Skorton, D. J., and Lauer, R. M.: Life insurance for children with cardiovascular disease. Pediatrics, 77:687, 1986.

Trusler, G. A., and Williams, W. G.: Long-term results of shunt procedures for tricuspid atresia. Ann. Thorac. Surg., 29:312, 1980.

Ullom, R. L., Sade, R. M., Crawford, F. A., Jr., et al: The Blalock-Taussig shunt in infants: Standard versus modified. Ann. Thorac. Surg., 44:539, 1987.

Uretzky, G., Puga, F. J., and Danielson, G. K.: Modified Fontan procedure in patients with previous ascending aorta-pulmonary artery anastomosis. J. Thorac. Cardiovasc. Surg., 85:447, 1983.

Van Praagh, R., Ando, M., and Dungan, W. T.: Anatomic types of tricuspid atresia: Clinical and developmental implications. Circulation, 44(Suppl. 2):115, 1971.

Vargas, F. J., Mayer, J. E., Jr., Jonas, R. A., and Castaneda, A. R.: Anomalous systemic and pulmonary venous connections in conjunction with atriopulmonary anastomosis (Fontan-Kreutzer): Technical considerations. J. Thorac. Cardiovasc. Surg., 93:523, 1987b.

Vargas, F. J., Mayer, J. E., Jr., Jonas, R. A., and Castaneda, A. R.: Atrioventricular valve repair or replacement in atriopulmonary anastomosis: Surgical considerations. Ann. Thorac. Surg., 43:403, 1987a.

Voci, G., Diego, J. N., Shafia, H., et al: Type Ia tricuspid atresia with extensive coronary artery abnormalities in a living 22 year old woman. J. Am. Coll. Cardiol., 10:1100, 1987.

Ward, K. E., Fisher, D. J., and Michael, L.: Elevated coronary sinus pressure does not alter myocardial blood flow or left ventricular contractile function in mature sheep. J. Thorac. Cardiovasc. Surg., 95:511, 1988.

Warnes, C. A., and Somerville, J.: Tricuspid atresia with transposition of the great arteries in adolescents and adults: Current state and late complications. Br. Heart J., 57:543, 1987.

Waterston, D. J.: The treatment of Fallot's tetralogy in children under one year of age (in Czech). Rozhl. Chir., 41:181, 1962.

Weinberg, P. M.: Anatomy of tricuspid atresia and its relevance to current forms of surgical therapy. Ann. Thorac. Surg., 29:306, 1980.

Wenink, A. C. G., and Ottenkamp, J.: Tricuspid atresia: Microscopic findings in relation to "absence" of the atrioventricular connection. Int. J. Cardiol., 16:57, 1987.

Westerman, G. R., Readinger, R. I., and Van Devanter, S. H.: Unusual interatrial communication after the Fontan procedure. J. Thorac. Cardiovasc. Surg., 90:627, 1985.

Williams, D. B., Kiernan, P. D., Metke, M. P., et al: Hemodynamic response to positive end-expiratory pressure following right atrium-pulmonary artery bypass (Fontan procedure). J. Thorac. Cardiovasc. Surg., 87:856, 1984.

Williams, W. G.: Discussion of Cleveland, D. C., Kirklin, J. K., Naftel, D. C., et al: Surgical treatment of tricuspid atresia. Ann. Thorac. Surg., 38:447, 1984.

Wittenborg, M. H., Neuhauser, E. B. D., and Sprunt, W. H.: Roentgenographic findings in congenital tricuspid atresia with hypoplasia of the right ventricle. Am. J. Roentgenol., 66:712, 1951.

CHAPTER 47

EBSTEIN'S ANOMALY

Gordon K. Danielson

PATHOLOGIC ANATOMY

The anomalous development of the tricuspid valve described by Wilhelm Ebstein in 1866 (Mann and Lie, 1979) is characterized by a deformity of the valve in which the posterior and septal leaflets are displaced downward in a spiral fashion below the true annulus (Fig. 47–1) (Anderson et al, 1979; Zuberbuhler et al, 1979). The displaced leaflets are hypoplastic, thickened, and often adherent to the wall of the right ventricle. Their displacement leaves a portion of the ventricle above the valve as an integral part of the right atrium; this is referred to as the "atrialized ventricle."

The anterior leaflet of the tricuspid valve in Ebstein's anomaly is typically larger than normal and has been described as sail-like. It may be fenestrated, and various portions of the leading edge may be attached to the right ventricular endocardium. The chordae tendineae and papillary muscles of the tricuspid valve are anomalous and abnormally positioned. The malformed tricuspid valve is usually incompetent, but it may occasionally be stenotic or, rarely, imperforate.

The atrialized ventricle is characteristically thinned and dilated, but careful observation shows that the entire wall of the right ventricle, both proximal and distal to the abnormal insertion of the tricuspid leaflets, including the infundibulum, is also dilated. Dilatation of the right ventricular wall is associated not only with thinning of the wall, but also with an absolute decrease in the number of myocardial fibers (Anderson and Lie, 1979). The atrioventricular node is located at the apex of the triangle of Koch, and the conduction system is normally situated. Atrial septal defect and other associated anomalies are common (Watson, 1974).

In those congenital cardiac anomalies in which there is atrioventricular discordance with ventriculoarterial discordance (corrected transposition), Ebstein's anomaly of the left atrioventricular valve is a common finding. The nature of the displacement of the septal and posterior leaflets in left-sided Ebstein's anomaly is similar to that in the right-sided form, but the anterior leaflet is smaller and anatomically different (Anderson et al, 1978). Other differences relate to the functional portion of the morphologically right ventricle, which is rarely dilated, and the atrialized portion of the ventricle, which has less thinning of the wall. The morphologically right ventricle is on the left side of the heart in this condition. The atrioventricular conduction tissue in corrected transposition is right-sided and anterior, at a distance from the left-sided tricuspid valve (Anderson et al, 1974). Thus, insertion of a prosthetic valve in the anatomic position has less risk of producing complete heart block in left-sided Ebstein's anomaly than in the right-sided form.

PATHOLOGIC PHYSIOLOGY

The functional impairment of the right ventricle and the incompetence of the deformed tricuspid valve retard forward flow of blood through the right side of the heart. Moreover, during contraction of the atrium, the atrialized portion of the right ventricle is in diastole and balloons out (if very thin) or acts

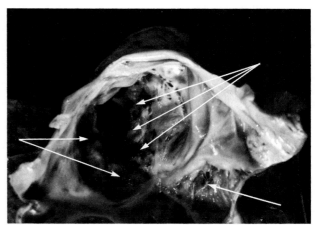

Figure 47–1. Ebstein's malformation in a 9-day-old infant. View from the right atrium. The *single arrow* indicates a patent foramen ovale. The anterior leaflet is enlarged and hooded *(double arrow)*. The posterior and septal leaflets are dysplastic and displaced in a spiral fashion toward the apex of the right ventricle *(triple arrow)*.

as a passive reservoir, decreasing the volume to be ejected; during ventricular systole it contracts, creating a pressure wave that impedes venous filling of the right atrium, which is in the diastolic phase. In most cases, the atrial septum is deficient owing to patency of the foramen ovale or fenestration of the fossa ovalis; a distinct secundum atrial septal defect is sometimes present. The movement of blood through the septal opening is generally from right to left but may be from left to right in some patients. The overall effect of these structural abnormalities on the right atrium is to produce gross dilatation, which may reach enormous proportions, even in infancy. This dilatation leads to further incompetence of the tricuspid valve and further widening of the interatrial communication.

CLINICAL FEATURES

Ebstein's anomaly is a rare cardiac anomaly that accounts for less than 1% of all congenital heart disease. It involves both sexes equally. Although a few patients reach advanced age, life expectancy for most is limited. The most common causes of death are congestive heart failure, hypoxia, and cardiac arrhythmias. When the diagnosis of Ebstein's anomaly is made in infancy, the prognosis is worse; one-third to one-half of these patients will die before 2 years of age (Giuliani et al, 1979; Kumar et al, 1971).

Because a broad spectrum of pathologic changes occur in Ebstein's anomaly, the hemodynamic alterations vary. Symptoms are related to the severity of the incompetence of the tricuspid valve, the presence or absence of an associated atrial septal defect, the impairment of right ventricular function, and the presence of associated cardiac anomalies.

In the early neonatal period, any tricuspid incompetence is accentuated by the normally occurring elevated pulmonary arteriolar resistance, and infants with Ebstein's anomaly may develop severe congestive heart failure. Because the foramen ovale is patent in early infancy, severe tricuspid incompetence, with its resultant elevation of right atrial pressure, will produce a right-to-left atrial-level shunt, and afflicted infants may be deeply cyanotic. If the infant survives this critical period, the degree of cyanosis and the symptoms often diminish as the fetal pulmonary hypertension regresses.

In older patients, the predominant symptoms are fatigability, dyspnea on exertion, and cyanosis. Less frequently, peripheral edema and palpitations in the form of paroxysmal atrial arrhythmias and premature ventricular beats are encountered.

In an experience with 67 patients who had a mean follow-up of 12 years, Giuliani and associates (1979) found that 39% remained in functional Class I or II and 61% progressed at some time into Class III or IV. Death occurred in 21% of the patients, who were characterized by one or more of the following features: (1) They were in functional Class III or IV;

(2) the cardiothoracic ratio was greater than 0.65; (3) they had cyanosis or an arterial oxygen saturation of less than 90%; or (4) they were infants when the diagnosis was made.

The physical signs vary. Heart sounds are usually soft, and a multiplicity of sounds and murmurs are often heard, all originating from the right side of the heart. A systolic murmur of tricuspid regurgitation is heard along the left sternal border. Low-intensity diastolic and presystolic murmurs may be heard. These murmurs result from anatomic or functional tricuspid stenosis. They characteristically become louder with inspiration. There is wide splitting of both the first and the second heart sounds. Atrial and ventricular filling sounds are relatively common and contribute to the cadence quality that is so often found in patients with Ebstein's anomaly. Summation of these gallop sounds may result from prolongation of atrioventricular conduction.

The arterial and jugular venous pulse forms are usually normal. A large v wave can sometimes be seen in the jugular venous pulse, but this is not usually prominent. The liver may be palpably enlarged, but it is almost never pulsatile.

DIAGNOSTIC CRITERIA

Electrocardiography. The electrocardiogram is usually abnormal, but it is not diagnostic. Complete or incomplete right bundle branch block and right-axis deviation are typically present. The P waves are large, and the R waves in leads V_1 to V_4 are small. The PR interval is often prolonged, and the QRS complex is slurred. Arrhythmias are common. Ventricular pre-excitation (Wolff-Parkinson-White syndrome) is encountered in approximately 13% of cases and is almost always of the right ventricular free-wall type, sometimes combined with a second pathway in the posterior septum.

Roentgenography. The cardiac silhouette may vary from almost normal to the typical configuration, which consists of a globular-shaped heart with a narrow waist similar to that seen with pericardial effusion. This appearance is produced by enlargement of the right atrium and displacement of the right ventricular outflow tract outward and upward. Vascularity of the pulmonary fields is either normal or decreased.

Cardiac Catheterization. The right atrial pressure is usually moderately elevated, and the pulse contour most often shows a dominant v wave with a steep y descent. However, in patients with a greatly dilated right atrium, the atrial pressure pulse may be normal despite the presence of severe tricuspid incompetence. Right ventricular pressure is most often normal, although the end-diastolic pressure may be elevated. One method of establishing the diagnosis is by intracardiac electrocardiography: When the catheter is pulled back from the right ventricle, the intracardiac electrocardiogram shows continued right ventricular electrical potentials after the pressure pulse has changed from a ventricular to an atrial contour. In some patients with severe tricuspid incompetence, however, the pressure pulses in the right atrium and right ventricle may have a similar contour, thus making interpretation of the intracardiac electrocardiogram difficult. Pulmonary artery pressure is normal or decreased. In patients with an associated atrial septal defect and right-to-left shunt, oximetry shows systemic arterial desaturation, and intracardiac dye-dilution curves from the venae cavae confirm the shunt. In the minority of cases having a left-to-right shunt through an atrial septal defect, this anomaly is also shown by oximetry and dye-dilution curves.

Angiography. Injection of contrast medium into the right atrium shows enlargement of this chamber and normal position of the tricuspid annulus. An indentation on the inferior wall of the right ventricle some distance to the left of the tricuspid annulus represents the site of origin of the displaced leaflets of the tricuspid valve. The leaflets sometimes appear as radiolucent lines laterally and superiorly within the body of the right ventricle. Contrast medium often moves back and forth between the right atrium and the right ventricle, and right-to-left shunting at the atrial level may be found in the presence of an atrial septal defect or a patent foramen ovale. Flow through the right side of the heart and lungs is slow.

Echocardiography. The M-mode echocardiogram is abnormal; the most reliable single criterion is the relationship of mitral valve closure to tricuspid valve closure (Giuliani et al, 1979). Two-dimensional echocardiography has become the definitive method for diagnosing Ebstein's anomaly. Cardiac catheterization is now rarely done unless associated lesions are present or a previous shunt has been done. Two-dimensional echocardiography allows an accurate evaluation of the anatomic relationships of the tricuspid leaflets to the right side of the heart, the size of the right atrium including the atrialized portion of the right ventricle, and the size and function of the right ventricle. It also provides the best method for assessing which patients are amenable to a valve reconstruction procedure and which require tricuspid valve replacement (Shiina et al, 1983).

When two-dimensional echocardiography is combined with the use of peripheral venous injections of indocyanine dye, the presence of a right-to-left shunt at the atrial level can be detected and semiquantitations of tricuspid regurgitation can be made by viewing reflux of dye into the inferior vena cava and the hepatic veins during systole.

New advances in Doppler echocardiography and color-flow imaging have essentially replaced the need for indocyanine dye curves to detect an atrial septal defect and the direction of shunt flow. In addition, color-flow imaging allows precise assessment of the site and degree of tricuspid valve regurgitation (Reeder et al, 1986).

SURGICAL CONSIDERATIONS

Medical management has little to offer patients with Ebstein's anomaly, except for management of fluid retention and treatment of some arrhythmias. The prognosis is poorest in those who have congestive heart failure, marked cyanosis, associated cardiac anomalies, extreme cardiomegaly (cardiothoracic ratio > 0.65), and diagnosis in infancy (Giuliani et al, 1979; Kumar et al, 1971). Serious cardiac arrhythmias may develop without associated congestive failure or hypoxemia. Patients who have survived infancy generally do well for a number of years; as long as they are only mildly symptomatic, continued observation is advised. Operative correction is generally postponed until deterioration is evident. Experience indicates that all patients with Ebstein's anomaly sooner or later show progressive deterioration, and all ultimately become potential candidates for surgical correction.

Patients who are in New York Heart Association Class III or IV are definitely surgical candidates. In view of the current low operative mortality, the fact that a plastic repair is feasible in the majority of cases and the encouraging follow-up results lead one to believe that surgical treatment is now advisable for patients who are less symptomatic but who show progressive, significant cardiomegaly, hypoxemia, or polycythemia or who have had a paradoxic embolus. The use of two-dimensional echocardiography to predict patients who are candidates for valvuloplasty and those who probably need valve replacement assists in the decision-making in borderline situations (Mair and Danielson, 1986).

Surgical attempts to treat Ebstein's anomaly began in the 1950s with the use of systemic-to-pulmonary artery shunts for relief of cyanosis. For the minority of patients who had obstruction of blood flow through the right side of the heart caused by pulmonary valvular or subvalvular stenosis or a stenotic or imperforate tricuspid valve, a shunt could be lifesaving. In the absence of obstructing lesions, results were uniformly poor.

A superior vena cava-to-pulmonary artery shunt was then proposed as a more physiologic method of improving oxygenation, but this approach has had limited use. In a collected series of 36 cases of cava-pulmonary artery shunts done for Ebstein's anomaly, 17 patients survived operation and 14 benefited from the procedure (Glenn et al, 1966). In 1954, Wright and co-workers effected surgical closure of a patent foramen ovale that was associated with Ebstein's anomaly; although the patient survived and improved, a residual shunt was shown at atrial level.

An operation for total correction of the hemodynamic abnormalities of Ebstein's anomaly was reported in 1958 by Hunter and Lillehei (Lillehei et al, 1967). Their method included repositioning the displaced posterior and septal leaflets, excluding the atrialized ventricular chamber, and closing the atrial septal defect when one was present. Both their

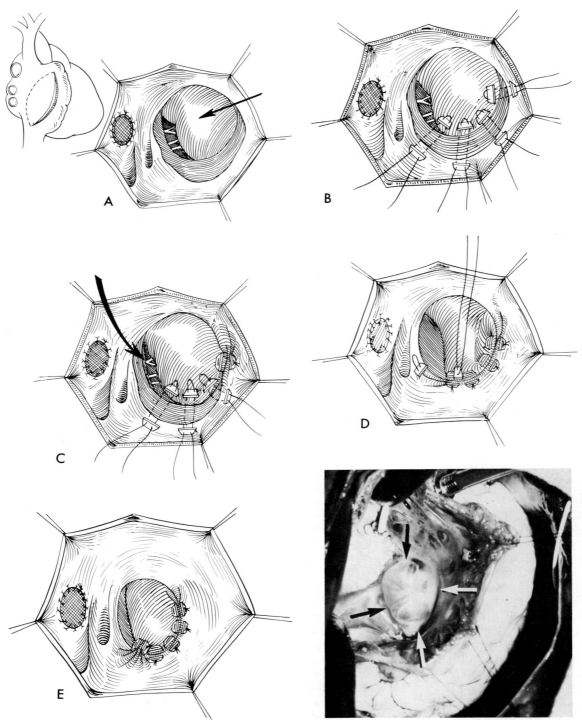

Figure 47–2. Diagram of repair. *A, Left,* The right atrium is incised from the atrial appendage to the inferior vena cava. Redundant portion of the right atrium is excised *(broken line)* so that the final size of the right atrium is normal. *Right,* Atrial septal defect is closed with a patch. The large anterior leaflet is indicated by the arrow. The posterior leaflet is displaced down from the annulus. The septal leaflet is hypoplastic and is not seen in this view. *B,* Mattress sutures passed through pledgets of Teflon felt are used to pull the tricuspid annulus and tricuspid valve together. Sutures are placed in the atrialized portion of the right ventricle (as shown) so that when they are subsequently tied, the atrialized ventricle is plicated and the aneurysmal cavity is obliterated. *C,* Sutures are tied down sequentially. Hypoplastic, markedly displaced septal leaflet is now visible *(arrow). D,* Posterior annuloplasty is done to narrow the diameter of the tricuspid annulus. Coronary sinus marks the posterior-left-sided extent of the annuloplasty, which is terminated there to avoid injury to the conduction bundle. Occasionally, one or two additional mattress sutures are required to obliterate the posterior aspect of the annuloplasty repair to render the valve totally competent. At this time, the tricuspid annulus will admit two or more fingers in adult patients. *E,* Completed repair, which allows the anterior leaflet to function as a monocuspid valve. *F,* Operative photograph of completed repair. Large anterior leaflet forms competent monocuspid valve *(arrows).* (From Danielson, G. K., Maloney, J. D., and Devloo, R. A. E.: Surgical repair of Ebstein's anomaly. Mayo Clin. Proc., *54:*185, 1979.)

TABLE 47–1. REPAIR OF EBSTEIN'S ANOMALY—
APRIL 1972–JANUARY 1988

Operation	No. of Patients	Operative Mortality	
		No.	%
Plastic repair	97	6	6.2
Valve replacement	33	1	3
Modified Fontan procedure*	4	0	0
Total	134	7	5.2

*Two patients previously had Glenn anastomoses.

patients sustained complete heart block, and neither survived.

Hardy and co-workers revived and modified the Hunter-Lillehei operation in 1964. They placed interrupted sutures close together on the spiral line of the displaced posterior and septal cusp bases and wider apart at the annulus. Tying the sutures created multiple tucks in the leaflets, narrowed the tricuspid orifice, and pulled the displaced leaflets back toward the tricuspid annulus. The technique was used in six patients; four were late survivors, and one of these had complete heart block (Hardy and Roe, 1969). Although some good results have later been reported with this procedure, it has not been generally effective in establishing a competent valve in the moderate and severe forms of Ebstein's anomaly. With suture placement in the septum as originally shown, heart block may occur. Moreover, it is not possible to transpose the septal leaflet and medial portions of the posterior leaflet to the tricuspid annulus, because the ventricular septum cannot be plicated in the same way as the free wall of the right ventricle. Finally, direct approximation of the displaced leaflet to the tricuspid annulus along the free wall does not obliterate the atrialized ventricle, which protrudes below the heart as an aneurysmal sac and, despite efforts to the contrary, usually remains in communication with the right ventricle.

In 1972, the author developed a new method of valve repair, which is described later. More recently, other types of valve reconstruction have been proposed (Carpentier et al, 1988; Schmidt-Habelmann et al, 1981), but the number of patients reported is small and late results are not available.

Prosthetic replacement of the deformed tricuspid valve was successfully accomplished by Barnard and

TABLE 47–2. REPAIR OF EBSTEIN'S ANOMALY—
ASSOCIATED PROCEDURES

Procedures	No. of Patients
Repair of atrial septal defect	116
Division of accessory pathway	17
Repair of pulmonary stenosis	12
Closure of shunt	6
Repair of ventricular septal defect	4
Repair of partial anomalous pulmonary venous connection	2
Closure of right atrial-left atrial fistula	1
Pericardiectomy	1
Implantation of automatic defibrillator leads	1

Schrire in 1963. In their technique, the sutures for anchoring the prosthesis were deviated cephalad to the coronary sinus and atrioventricular node to avoid injuring the node and the conduction bundle. With the sutures thus placed, blood from the coronary sinus drained directly into the right ventricle. The atrialized portion of the ventricle was not obliterated.

In 1967, Lillehei and colleagues reported tricuspid valve replacement with a Starr-Edwards ball valve in five patients with Ebstein's anomaly. In two patients, the prosthetic valve was sutured to the true annulus, thus causing complete atrioventricular dissociation; one of the two died. In the remaining three patients, attachment of the prosthesis according to the Barnard-Schrire technique avoided heart block.

Other operations include atrioventricular plication combined with tricuspid valve replacement (Timmis et al, 1967) and replacement of the tricuspid valve with a tissue valve combined with obliteration of the atrialized portion of the right ventricle and closure of the atrial septal defect (Ross and Somerville, 1970).

Prosthetic valve replacement, although it is still the most popular method for repair of Ebstein's anomaly, has produced less than ideal results for some patients. Valve replacement in the tricuspid area is associated with a higher frequency of valve malfunction and thrombotic complications than is replacement of the other cardiac valves. Tissue valves do not have the thromboembolic complications of mechanical valves, but they do have a limited life expectancy, particularly in infants and children. In the author's experience, the failure-free rate of porcine heterograft valves in children is only 58.5% at 5 years (Williams et al, 1982).

Since 1972, the author has used a repair that consists of plication of the free wall of the atrialized portion of the right ventricle, posterior tricuspid annuloplasty, and right reduction atrioplasty (Danielson et al, 1979). The repair is based on the construction of a monocuspid valve by the use of the anterior leaflet of the tricuspid valve, which, as noted earlier, is usually enlarged in this anomaly (Fig. 47–2). Repair is preferred to valve replacement whenever it is feasible because it avoids the problems of prosthetic valve dysfunction, anticoagulation, and, in children, the need for replacement of the prosthesis because of growth.

The author's operative management of patients with Ebstein's malformation consists of (1) electrophysiologic mapping for localization of accessory conduction pathways in patients having ventricular pre-excitation; (2) patch closure of the atrial septal defect or patent foramen ovale; (3) plication of the atrialized portion of the right ventricle; (4) plastic repair of the tricuspid valve, when feasible, or valve replacement with a prosthetic valve; (5) correction of associated anomalies, such as relief of pulmonary stenosis or division of accessory conduction pathways; and (6) excision of redundant right atrial wall.

The ventricular plication sutures are placed so

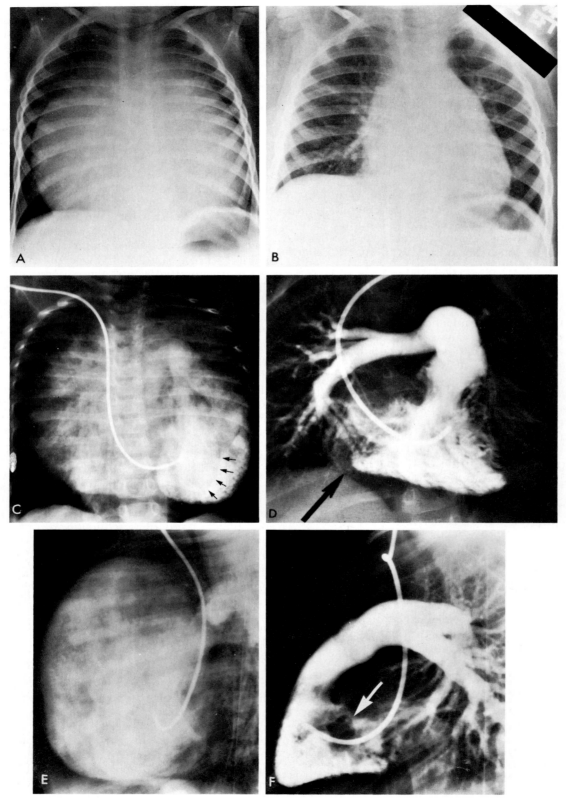

Figure 47–3 *See legend on opposite page*

that they avoid the posterior descending coronary artery and obvious large branches of the right coronary artery. When all plication sutures have been tied, the anterior and posterior aspects of the right ventricle are inspected to be certain that the major coronary arteries have not been injured.

At the completion of the procedure, the tricuspid valve is tested by injecting saline under pressure into the right ventricle with a bulb syringe and large catheter. Finally, after venous decannulation, an exploring finger is introduced into the right atrium for direct palpation of the tricuspid valve in the beating heart. Intraoperative echocardiography (transthoracic or transesophageal) is also useful for assessing tricuspid valve competency. Temporary pacemaker wires are attached to the right atrium and the right ventricle for postoperative monitoring of rhythm and for pacing in selected patients.

Modification of the procedure is necessary in a few patients. In those cases in which the tricuspid valve is only moderately displaced from the annulus but in which the leaflets adhere to the ventricular endocardium, the plicating sutures are extended across the leaflet down toward the apex of the right ventricle to the same level that would be appropriate if the leaflets had been displaced to the level of their adherence to the ventricular wall. This modification has produced results that are as good as those in cases in which there is no adherence of the displaced leaflet to the right ventricle.

Because repair is based on the presence of an enlarged anterior leaflet, significant abnormalities of the leaflet may compromise the result. For most patients with fenestrations or perforations of the anterior leaflet, the defects can be repaired satisfactorily with fine continuous sutures. If more significant abnormalities are present, such as linear attachment of the leading edge of the leaflet to the ventricular wall, this repair does not apply, and prosthetic valve replacement is required.

SURGICAL RESULTS

Between April 1972 and January 1988, 134 consecutive patients had operation for Ebstein's anomaly. The patients' ages were between 11 months and 64 years. Twenty-seven previous cardiac operations had been done, including nine systemic-pulmonary shunts, six Glenn procedures, four closures of atrial

septal defect, four pacemaker insertions, three attempted repairs elsewhere, and one pericardiectomy.

In 97 patients (72%), the repair described earlier could be done (Table 47–1). Associated procedures are shown in Table 47–2. In 17 patients with Wolff-Parkinson-White's syndrome, the accessory conduction pathways were successfully interrupted. No cases of permanent complete heart block resulted in the entire series.

Seven hospital deaths occurred, either suddenly in patients who were otherwise doing well but who had massive cardiomegaly (five patients, three with documented ventricular fibrillation), from low cardiac output (one patient), or from hemorrhage (one patient).

During follow-up, four late deaths occurred. Two patients who developed recurrent tricuspid insufficiency 1 and 7 years after repair, respectively, had successful tricuspid valve replacement. Most patients were in New York Heart Association functional Classes III and IV preoperatively; all but five patients were in functional Class I or II postoperatively. Six women have had successful pregnancy and delivery. Objective evaluation by exercise testing showed striking improvement in exercise tolerance and in the ventilatory response to exercise (Driscoll et al, 1988). An unexpected benefit was improved control of atrial arrhythmias; less than one-third of patients with preoperative paroxysmal supraventricular tachycardia and paroxysmal atrial fibrillation or flutter continued to have symptomatic tachycardia postoperatively (Oh et al, 1985).

Postoperative reduction in heart size was often dramatic (Fig. 47–3). The cardiothoracic ratio decreased in all patients who had a preoperative ratio greater than 0.5. Postoperative cardiac catheterization has shown satisfactory tricuspid valve function in most patients (see Fig. 47–3). Analysis by two-dimensional echocardiography showed significant reduction in the atrialized portion of the ventricle, reduced right atrial size, and good to excellent function of the reconstructed tricuspid valve. No perivalvular leaks were identified in patients who had tricuspid valve replacement, and no recurrent atrial septal defects were visible by indocyanine green dye injections or by echocardiographic Doppler and color-flow imaging techniques. These results are very favorable when compared with the natural history of patients who have Ebstein's anomaly and who are in functional Classes III or IV (Giuliani et al, 1979).

Figure 47–3. Two-year-old girl with Ebstein's anomaly and history of pneumonia, cardiorespiratory arrest, and failure to thrive. Chest films: A, Preoperative (cardiothoracic ratio—0.9). B, Thirteen days postoperatively (cardiothoracic ratio—0.55). Right ventricular angiogram, anteroposterior view: C, Preoperative. The contrast medium refluxes through the tricuspid valve to fill the entire cardiac silhouette. A radiolucent line within the cavity of the ventricle shows the location of the displaced tricuspid leaflets (arrows). D, Postoperative. There is rapid transit of contrast medium from the right ventricle to the pulmonary arteries with only a trace of tricuspid insufficiency. The arrow indicates the new plane of the tricuspid valve. Right ventricular angiogram, lateral view: E, Preoperative. F, Postoperative. The tricuspid valve is competent. The arrow points to filling defect created by the anterior leaflet. This patient is now 16 years old. She is asymptomatic, is taking no cardiac medications, and is an "A" student. (From Danielson, G. K., Maloney, J. D., and Devloo, R. A. E.: Surgical repair of Ebstein's anomaly. Mayo Clin. Proc., 54:185, 1979.)

Selected Bibliography

Kumar, A. E., Fyler, D. C., Miettinen, O. S., and Nadas, A. S.: Ebstein's anomaly: Clinical profile and natural history. Am. J. Cardiol., 28:84, 1971.

The clinical features, cardiac catheterization data, and natural history of 55 patients with Ebstein's anomaly are described. This review gives a good perspective of the clinical aspects of this anomaly, but current indications for operation and techniques for repair are not discussed.

Special Review of Ebstein's anomaly. Mayo Clin. Proc., 54:163, 1979.

This monograph describes the historical, clinical, morphologic, and surgical aspects of Ebstein's anomaly. The clinical features and natural history of 67 consecutive patients with Ebstein's anomaly who were monitored for a mean of 12 years are described. This monograph gives a good overview of the current knowledge of Ebstein's anomaly.

Bibliography

Anderson, K. R., Danielson, G. K., McGoon, D. C., and Lie, J. T.: Ebstein's anomaly of the left-sided tricuspid valve: Pathological anatomy of the valvular malformation. Circulation, 58:87, 1978.

Anderson, K. R., and Lie, J. T.: The right ventricular myocardium in Ebstein's anomaly: A morphometric histopathologic study. Mayo Clin. Proc., 54:181, 1979.

Anderson, K. R., Zuberbuhler, J. R., Anderson, R. H., et al: Morphologic spectrum of Ebstein's anomaly of the heart: A review. Mayo Clin. Proc., 54:174, 1979.

Anderson, R. H., Becker, A. E., Arnold, R., and Wilkinson, J. L.: The conducting tissues in congenitally corrected transposition. Circulation, 50:911, 1974.

Barnard, C. N., and Schrire, V.: Surgical correction of Ebstein's malformation with prosthetic tricuspid valve. Surgery, 54:302, 1963.

Carpentier, A., Chauvaud, S., Mace, L., et al: A new reconstructive operation for Ebstein's anomaly of the tricuspid valve. J. Thorac. Cardiovasc. Surg., 96:92, 1988.

Danielson, G. K., Maloney, J. D., and Devloo, R. A. E.: Surgical repair of Ebstein's anomaly. Mayo Clin. Proc., 54:185, 1979.

Driscoll, D. J., Mottram, C. D., and Danielson, G. K.: Spectrum of exercise intolerance in 45 patients with Ebstein's anomaly and observations on exercise tolerance in 11 patients after surgical repair. J. Am. Coll. Cardiol., 11:831, 1988.

Ebstein, W.: Über einen sehr seltenen Fall von Insufficienz der Valvula Tricuspidalis, Bedingt durch eine angeborene hochgradige Missbildung derselben. Arch. Anat. Physiol., 1866, pp. 238–254.

Giuliani, E. R., Fuster, V., Brandenburg, R. O., and Mair, D. D.: The clinical features and natural history of Ebstein's anomaly of the tricuspid valve. Mayo Clin. Proc., 54:163, 1979.

Glenn, W. W. L., Browne, M., and Whittemore, R.: Circulatory bypass of the right side of the heart: Cava-pulmonary artery shunt—indications and results (report of a collected series of 537 cases). In Cassels, D. E. (ed): The Heart and Circulation in the Newborn and Infant. New York, Grune & Stratton, 1966, pp. 345–357.

Hardy, K. L., May, I. A., Webster, C. A., et al: Ebstein's anomaly: A functional concept and successful definitive repair. J. Thorac. Cardiovasc. Surg., 48:927, 1964.

Hardy, K. L., and Roe, B. B.: Ebstein's anomaly: Further experience with definitive repair. J. Thorac. Cardiovasc. Surg., 58:553, 1969.

Hunter, S. W., and Lillehei, C. W.: Ebstein's malformation of the tricuspid valve: Study of a case, together with suggestions of a new form of surgical therapy. Dis. Chest., 33:297, 1958.

Lillehei, C. W., Kalke, B. R., and Carlson, R. G.: Evolution of corrective surgery for Ebstein's anomaly. Circulation, 35, 36(Suppl. 1):111, 1967.

Mair, D. D., and Danielson, G. K.: Ebstein's malformation. In Fortuin, N. J. (ed): Current Therapy in Cardiovascular Disease–2. Philadelphia, B. C. Decker, 1986, pp. 131–134.

Mann, R. J., and Lie, J. T.: The life story of Wilhelm Ebstein (1836–1912) and his almost overlooked description of a congenital heart disease. Mayo Clin. Proc., 54:197, 1979.

Oh, J. K., Holmes, D. R., Jr., Hayes, D. L., et al: Cardiac arrhythmias in patients with surgical repair of Ebstein's anomaly. J. Am. Coll. Cardiol., 6:1351, 1985.

Reeder, G. S., Currie, P. J., Hagler, D. J., et al: Use of Doppler techniques (continuous-wave, pulsed-wave, and color flow imaging) in the noninvasive hemodynamic assessment of congenital heart disease. Mayo Clin. Proc., 61:725, 1986.

Ross, D., and Somerville, J.: Surgical correction of Ebstein's anomaly. Lancet, 2:280, 1970.

Schmidt-Habelmann, P., Meisner, H., Struck, E., and Sebening, F.: Results of valvuloplasty for Ebstein's anomaly. Thorac. Cardiovasc. Surg., 29:155, 1981.

Shiina, A., Seward, J. B., Tajik, A. J., et al: Two-dimensional echocardiographic-surgical correlation in Ebstein's anomaly: Preoperative determination of patients requiring tricuspid valve plication vs. replacement. Circulation, 68:534, 1983.

Timmis, H. H., Hardy, J. D., and Watson, D. G.: The surgical management of Ebstein's anomaly: The combined use of tricuspid valve replacement, atrioventricular plication and atrioplasty. J. Thorac. Cardiovasc. Surg., 53:385, 1967.

Watson, H.: Natural history of Ebstein's anomaly of tricuspid valve in childhood and adolescence: An international co-operative study of 505 cases. Br. Heart J., 36:417, 1974.

Williams, D. B., Danielson, G. K., McGoon, D. C., et al: Porcine heterograft valve replacement in children. J. Thorac. Cardiovasc. Surg., 84:446, 1982.

Wright, J. L., Burchell, H. B., Kirklin, J. W., et al: Symposium on physiologic, clinical and surgical interdependence in study and treatment of congenital heart disease; congenital displacement of tricuspid valve (Ebstein's malformation); report of case with closure of associated foramen ovale for correction of right-to-left shunt. Proc. Staff Meet. Mayo Clin., 29:278, 1954.

Zuberbuhler, J. R., Allwork, S. P., and Anderson, R. H.: The spectrum of Ebstein's anomaly of the tricuspid valve. J. Thorac. Cardiovasc. Surg., 77:202, 1979.

CHAPTER *48*

HYPOPLASTIC LEFT HEART SYNDROME

William I. Norwood
John D. Murphy

Hypoplastic left heart syndrome is the fourth most common congenital cardiac anomaly presenting in the first year of life. It is the most common malformation in which there is only one ventricle, and as such is amenable to application of Fontan's procedure. However, the development of operative therapy for hypoplasia of left heart structures during the first 2 decades of open heart procedures appeared to be remote. Lev (1952) first described the pathology of "hypoplasia of the aortic tract complexes." This category included (1) isolated hypoplasia of the aorta, (2) hypoplasia of the aorta with ventricular septal defect, and (3) hypoplasia of the aorta with aortic stenosis or atresia with or without mitral stenosis or atresia. Noonan and Nadas (1958) referred to these lesions as hypoplastic left heart syndrome. Although the anatomic factors that result in the hypoplastic left heart syndrome are varied, the physiologic similarities among this collection of lesions have resulted in acceptance of this term. With the advent of surgical management for patients with hypoplastic left heart syndrome (Bailey et al, 1985; 1986a; 1986b; Doty and Knott, 1977; Jonas et al, 1986; Norwood et al, 1980; 1981, 1983; Sade et al, 1987), interest in a more precise anatomic definition has increased.

DEFINITION AND ANATOMY

Hypoplastic left heart syndrome consists of a group of cardiac malformations in which there is aortic valve hypoplasia, stenosis, or atresia with either hypoplasia or absence of the left ventricle and, as a consequence, hypoplasia of the ascending aorta (Fig. 48–1). This syndrome coexists most frequently with severe mitral hypoplasia or mitral atresia. A less common variation includes malalignment of the common atrioventricular canal with regard to the muscular ventricular septum over the right ventricle. Although 10% of patients have a double-outlet right ventricle rather than the usual normally related great arteries, cases involving transposition of the great arteries with hypoplasia of the left ventricle and pulmonary artery or hypoplasia of the right ventricle

and aorta are not considered to be hypoplastic left heart syndrome.

The anatomy of patients with aortic stenosis or atresia has been thoroughly described (Bharati and Lev, 1984; Bjerregaard and Laursen, 1980; Bulkley et al, 1983; Eliot et al, 1965; Elzenga and Gittenberger-de Groot, 1985; Hawkins and Doty, 1984; Jonas et al, 1986; Kanjuh et al, 1965; Lev, 1952; Moodie et al, 1986; Noonan and Nadas, 1958; O'Connor et al, 1982; Roberts et al, 1976; Sinha et al, 1968; van der Horst et al, 1983; Von Reuden et al, 1975; Watson and Rowe, 1962; Weinberg et al, 1985, 1986). The inferior vena cava and right superior vena cava enter the right atrium normally. In 2.5 to 4.3% of patients, a persistent left superior vena cava is found (Bharati et al, 1984; Roberts et al, 1976). The right atrium is dilated, and the tricuspid valve orifice is enlarged (Barber et al, 1986; Bharati and Lev, 1984; Hawkins and Doty, 1984; van der Horst et al, 1983). The right ventricle is enlarged (Bharati and Lev, 1984; Eliot et al, 1965; Kanjuh et al, 1965; van der Horst et al, 1983; Von Reuden et al, 1975), as well as the pulmonary orifice and main pulmonary artery. Bharati and Lev (1984) reported three patients with aortic atresia with pulmonary valve abnormalities (thickened nodular leaflets). Two of 198 patients with hypoplastic left heart syndrome presenting to Children's Hospital of Philadelphia since 1984 have had concurrent pulmonic stenosis. The left and right pulmonary arteries arise from the underside of the main pulmonary artery with the right branch orifice proximal to the left branch orifice. Patients dying before 2 weeks of age show no significant difference in the size and character of the small and medium-sized pulmonary artery branches (Sinha et al, 1968). Pulmonary venous connection is usually normal, but patients occasionally have anomalous or accessory pulmonary venous connection, usually through a persistent left vertical vein to left innominate vein (Watson and Rowe, 1962). The left atrium is small and frequently hypertrophied (Bharati and Lev, 1984; Eliot et al, 1965; Kanjuh et al, 1965; Roberts et al, 1976; van der Horst et al, 1983; Watson and Rowe, 1962). An interatrial communication is common, although a

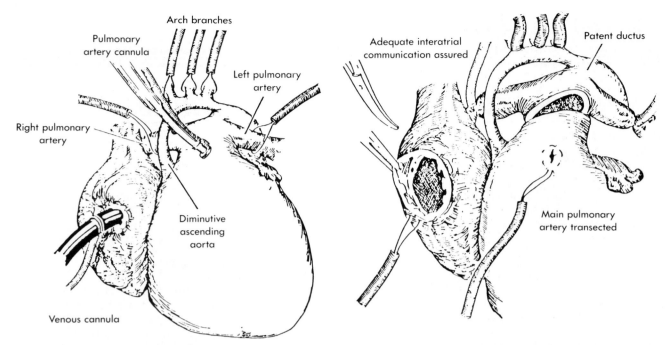

Figure 48–1. Cardiopulmonary bypass is established by arterial infusion in the ascending aorta. The branch pulmonary arteries are occluded with 2-0 Tevdek tourniquets. Through the atrial appendage the septum primum is excised. The main pulmonary artery is transected.

congenitally small foramen ovale may be present (Bharati and Lev, 1984; Eliot et al, 1965; Watson and Rowe, 1962; Weinberg et al, 1986). In an autopsy series, 65% of patients had a posterior and leftward displacement of the superior attachment of the septum primum relative to septum secundum (Fig. 48–2) (Weinberg et al, 1986).

Mitral stenosis or hypoplasia is present in approximately 60% of the patients, and the remaining 40% have mitral atresia (Bharati and Lev, 1984; Roberts et al, 1976). When there is mitral stenosis, the mitral valve leaflets are thickened and have short thick chordae attached to short papillary muscles (Bharati and Lev, 1984). Patients with mitral atresia may have either a blind dimple on the floor of the left atrium at the usual site of the mitral valve with no grossly recognizable mitral valve tissue (Elliot et al, 1965; Kanjuh et al, 1965) or may have atretic mitral valve tissue (Weinberg et al, 1985). The left ventricle does not form the apex of the heart. Patients with mitral hypoplasia or stenosis (patent left ventricular inflow) frequently have prominent endocardial fibroelastosis (Bharati and Lev, 1984; Lev, 1952; O'Connor et al, 1982; Roberts et al, 1976; Sinha et al, 1968) with myofibril disarray (Bulkley et al, 1983).

In a study by Bharati and Lev (1984), 87% of the patients had aortic atresia and 13% had aortic stenosis. The coronary arteries originate normally from the aortic root and have a normal distribution. The ascending and transverse portions of the aorta are hypoplastic. With aortic atresia, the size of the ascending aorta is usually 1 to 3 mm. In rare cases with aortic stenosis, the mean size of the ascending aorta

has been reported to be as large as 5 to 6 mm. True coarctation of the aorta is not a common finding. There is, however, a posterolateral intimal ridge at the junction of the aortic isthmus, ductus arteriosus, and thoracic aorta in most patients.

Malaligned Atrioventricular Canal. The anatomic features of malaligned atrioventricular canal are similar to those of any atrioventricular canal defect. Atrial communication is by an ostium primum atrial septal defect. An inlet ventricular septal defect may or may not be present. The development of the left ventricle depends on the degree of malalignment of the common atrioventricular valve. When there is no or almost no inlet into the left ventricle, left ventricular size is similar to that in patients with mitral atresia or stenosis. When part of the common atrioventricular valve enters the left ventricle, a left ventricle of intermediate size is present. This ventricle, however, still does not form the apex of the heart. Similarly, the size of the ascending and transverse aorta may be larger than in patients with aortic atresia but smaller than in patients with isolated aortic stenosis.

EMBRYOLOGY

The embryologic cause of hypoplastic left heart syndrome is not completely understood. Because this syndrome is a collection of lesions, multiple developmental anomalies probably can lead to the syndrome. The most likely embryologic cause of hypo-

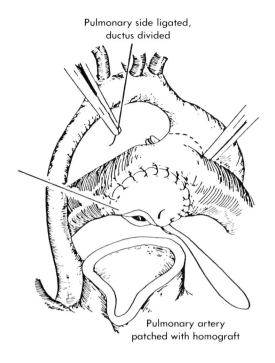

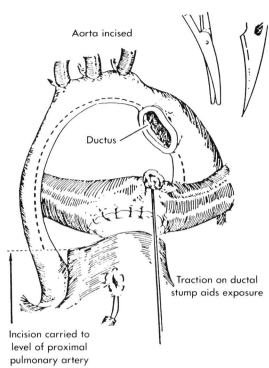

Figure 48–2. The distal main pulmonary artery is closed with a patch. The ductus arteriosus is ligated and divided after patch closure of the distal main pulmonary artery.

plastic left heart syndrome is either a limitation of left ventricular inflow or left ventricular outflow.

EPIDEMIOLOGY

Hypoplastic left heart syndrome has been reported to occur in at least 0.016 to 0.036% of live births, making it the most common defect in which there is only one ventricle (Brownell and Shokeir, 1976; Fyler, 1980). In pathologic series, it represents 1.4 to 3.8% of congenital heart disease (Abbott, 1936; Edwards, 1953) and has been reported to cause 23% of the deaths due to congenital heart disease in the newborn period (Watson and Rowe, 1962).

Males are affected slightly more often than females. Of the patients with hypoplastic left heart syndrome seen at The Children's Hospital of Philadelphia, 57% are male. The recurrence risk of siblings of patients with this syndrome has been reported to be 0.5%, with a 2.2% risk for other forms of congenital heart disease (Brownell and Shokeir, 1976; Holmes et al, 1972; Nora and Nora, 1978).

ETIOLOGY

The abnormal development of the left-sided cardiac structures results primarily from atresia or marked hypoplasia of the aortic valve. When left ventricular outflow obstruction accompanies an intact ventricular septum, the left ventricle is hypoplastic.

In the rare case of left ventricular outflow obstruction with an unrestrictive ventricular septal defect, normal left ventricular development can occur. Thus, a primary myocardial abnormality is unlikely to be the cause of hypoplastic left heart syndrome. The resultant elevation in left ventricular pressure that occurs with patent left ventricular inflow and obstructed left ventricular outflow in the absence of a ventricular septal defect probably causes the endocardial fibroelastosis encountered in some patients. Although a congenitally small or absent foramen ovale has been suggested as a possible cause of hypoplastic left heart syndrome (Bharati and Lev, 1984; Benner, 1939; Lehman, 1927; Lev et al, 1963), it is more likely to be the result of increased left atrial pressure secondary to the left ventricular outflow obstruction.

PHYSIOLOGY

The physiology of hypoplastic left heart syndrome is complex. The left ventricle is essentially a nonfunctional structure. Pulmonary venous return must therefore be to the right atrium through an atrial septal defect, a stretched foramen ovale, or, rarely, by an anomalous pulmonary venous connection. In the right atrium, systemic and pulmonary venous return mix. The right ventricle must maintain both the pulmonary and systemic output, and the ductus arteriosus must remain patent for systemic perfusion.

In utero, oxygenation occurs via the placenta.

Because the right ventricle is able to maintain systemic output by the ductus arteriosus, the fetus develops normally in utero. After birth, oxygenation occurs in the lungs. Systemic blood flow is maintained as long as the ductus arteriosus remains patent. Perfusion is retrograde through the transverse arch and ascending aorta to the carotid and coronary arteries. With the left and right pulmonary arteries connected parallel with the ductus arteriosus and descending aorta, the relative ratio of pulmonary to systemic blood flow depends on a delicate balance between pulmonary and systemic vascular resistances. In most patients, balanced systemic and pulmonary perfusion can be maintained. In some, however, a low ratio of pulmonary to systemic resistance results in excessive pulmonary blood flow. Although arterial oxygen saturation is elevated secondary to the high pulmonary blood flow, systemic perfusion is marginal in this circumstance and the child develops metabolic acidosis. In rare cases, a high ratio of pulmonary to systemic resistance is secondary to a severely restrictive interatrial communication. These patients appear to be very cyanotic because of inadequate pulmonary blood flow and can become acidotic because of hypoxemia. Arterial oxygen tension (PO_2) may be less than 20 mm Hg.

CLINICAL FEATURES

When hypoplastic left heart syndrome presents within 24 hours of birth, it is usually secondary to severe obstruction to blood flow at the interatrial level (congenitally small or absent foramen ovale). More typically, however, Apgar scores are normal. Within 24 to 48 hours of birth, most patients with this syndrome develop a dusky cyanosis with evidence of tachypnea and respiratory distress (Elliot et al, 1965; Noonan and Nadas, 1958; Roberts et al, 1976; Sinha et al, 1968; Watson and Rowe, 1962). Watson and Rowe (1967), however, reported that the onset of cyanosis and respiratory distress could be delayed for as long as 3 weeks. When the ductus arteriosus begins to close, the patient develops metabolic acidosis. Among 103 patients at The Children's Hospital of Philadelphia, the mean lowest preoperative pH was 7.22 ± 0.16, with a mean lowest preoperative bicarbonate concentration of 14 ± 5.5. Prostaglandin must be administered at this stage to ensure patency of the ductus arteriosus and allow palliative operative intervention. Both intravenous prostaglandin E_1 and oral E_2 have proved effective (Fujiseki et al, 1983; Lewis et al, 1981; Schlemmer et al, 1982; Yabek et al, 1979).

Physical examination typically shows a mildly cyanotic infant with tachypnea and tachycardia. Depending on the degree of ductal patency at the time of evaluation, peripheral pulses may be normal, diminished, or absent. Rales may be heard, although generally the fields of the lung are clear. Cardiac examination shows a dominant right ventricular impulse on palpation (Watson and Rowe, 1962), with a decreased left ventricular (apical) impulse. S1 is normal, and S2 is usually single and increased in intensity (Watson and Rowe, 1962). One-third of patients may have a gallop rhythm at the apex (Watson and Rowe, 1962). Fifty-eight to 67% of patients have a nonspecific soft grade 1 to 3/6 systolic murmur at the left sternal border (Roberts et al, 1976; Sinha et al, 1968; Watson and Rowe, 1962). An apical mid-diastolic flow rumble is heard in 20% of the patients (Eliot et al, 1965; Noonan and Nadas, 1958). The liver is frequently slightly enlarged.

The electrocardiogram often reflects the underlying pathology. Right atrial enlargement is encountered in 30 to 41%, and right ventricular hypertrophy is found in 78 to 92% of patients (Eliot et al, 1965; Noonan and Nadas, 1958; Sinha et al, 1968). Approximately 56% of patients have a QR pattern in lead V_1 (Sinha et al, 1968; Watson and Rowe, 1962). In patients with malaligned common atrioventricular canal, the QRS axis is to the left and superior.

The findings on the chest film in hypoplastic left heart syndrome are nonspecific. Cardiomegaly is reported in 75 to 85% of the patients, and pulmonary vascular markings are increased in 68 to 82% (Roberts et al, 1976; Sinha et al, 1968). In the occasional patient with a severely restrictive atrial septal defect, a reticular pattern may resemble that seen in total anomalous pulmonary venous connection with pulmonary venous obstruction.

Two-dimensional echocardiography is diagnostic in this lesion (Bash et al, 1986; Bass et al, 1980; Bierman, 1984; Farooki et al, 1976; Helton et al, 1986; Jonas et al, 1986; Mandorla et al, 1984; Mortera and Leon, 1980; Sahn et al, 1975 and 1982; Skovranek et al, 1981; Suzuki et al, 1982). The intracardiac anatomy should be examined with subcostal frontal, sagittal, left oblique, and right oblique views (Chin et al, 1985; Isaaz et al, 1985; Marino et al, 1985). Consistent with some obstruction at the interatrial level and an obligate atrial-level left-to-right shunt, the atrial septum is usually bowed from left to right. When the atrial septum is bowed from right to left, either severe tricuspid regurgitation or anomalous pulmonary venous connection should be suspected. When the atrial septum is thickened and severely bowed from left to right, a congenitally small or absent foramen ovale should be suspected. Septum primum should be examined for evidence of posterior and left-sided deviation of its superior attachment (Helton et al, 1986).

From suprasternal imaging, the anatomy of the ascending aorta, aortic arch, and upper descending aorta should be assessed by using frontal, sagittal, and left oblique views. A diminutive ascending aorta is characteristic of this malformation.

After the anatomic details are determined, color-flow imaging, pulsed Doppler, and continuous-wave Doppler are used to evaluate physiology. Of primary concern is the assessment of tricuspid or common atrioventricular valve for regurgitation (Barber et al,

1988). Fifty-six per cent of patients with hypoplastic left heart syndrome have tricuspid regurgitation preoperatively (35% mild, 16% moderate, and 5% severe) (Barber et al, 1988).

Because accurate diagnosis is possible by two-dimensional and Doppler echocardiography, cardiac catheterization is no longer routinely necessary in hypoplastic left heart syndrome. Moreover, because some obstruction to pulmonary venous return limits pulmonary overcirculation in patients with this syndrome, performance of a balloon atrial septostomy during cardiac catheterization may result in hemodynamic deterioration and should be avoided.

NATURAL HISTORY

Untreated, more than 95% of infants with hypoplastic left heart syndrome die within the first month of life (Fyler et al, 1981). This syndrome accounts for approximately 25% of cardiac deaths during the first week and 15% of cardiac deaths during the first month of life (Noonan and Nadas, 1958). Rarely, the ductus arteriosus remains patent. If pulmonary and systemic resistances are balanced, survival for 4 to 6 years has been reported sporadically (Ehrlich et al, 1986; Moodie et al, 1972). These patients expire secondary to pulmonary vascular obstructive disease.

PREOPERATIVE CARE

The preoperative care of the child with hypoplastic left heart syndrome is the same regardless of the surgical approach chosen. When the diagnosis is made, a continuous infusion of prostaglandin E_1 intravenously at a dose of 0.05 to 0.1 μg/kg/min should be administered. If available, orally administered prostaglandin E_2 may be used (Fujiseki et al, 1983; Schlemmer et al, 1982). An arterial line should be inserted for monitoring arterial oxygen saturation and acid-base balance. The umbilical artery should be used if possible, to preserve the peripheral arteries for future use.

The major goal in the preoperative period is to ensure adequate systemic perfusion for the metabolic needs of the child. Systemic perfusion depends on a delicate balance between pulmonary and systemic vascular resistances. The pulmonary resistance is usually less than systemic, and care must be taken not to decrease pulmonary resistance further. The main metabolic factor that appears to influence pulmonary resistance in this group of patients is carbon dioxide tension (PCO_2). Thus, care must be taken not to hyperventilate these patients, and hyperoxic ventilation should be avoided. Patients with hypoplastic left heart syndrome often have no abnormality of oxygen transport across the alveolar membrane. The effect of supplemental oxygen is to decrease pulmonary resistance and increase systemic resistance, re-

sulting in increased pulmonary blood flow and decreased systemic perfusion. In this case, the oxygen saturation of peripheral blood may be increased but oxygen delivery decreases, and metabolic acidosis can ensue. Similarly, inotropic agents often result in an unfavorable ratio of pulmonary to systemic resistance. Although overall cardiac output may increase, peripheral perfusion often decreases. Inotropic agents, although they may be necessary in cases of hypoplastic left heart syndrome with underlying abnormalities such as sepsis, are usually unnecessary and harmful in uncomplicated cases of hypoplastic left heart syndrome. Once the pulmonary vascular resistance has become very low, it is often difficult to stabilize the systemic perfusion. One method of increasing pulmonary resistance, and thus systemic perfusion in these patients, is elective endotracheal intubation. The PCO_2 can then be adjusted to 45 to 50 mm Hg. Pulmonary resistance is thus elevated, and peripheral perfusion is increased. Some degree of pulmonary venous obstruction, usually at the level of a patent foramen ovale or atrial septal defect, is a frequent component of pulmonary resistance in this lesion. Mild to moderate interatrial obstruction is beneficial to preoperative hemodynamics. In the absence of Pa_{O_2} less than 25 mm Hg, atrial septostomy should not be performed before surgical palliation.

In the rare patient with hypoplastic left heart syndrome and a congenitally small or absent foramen ovale, obstruction to pulmonary venous drainage may be sufficient to cause inadequate pulmonary blood flow. Compared with other patients with hypoplastic left heart syndrome, these patients have a low peripheral oxygen saturation. There is no diastolic reversal in the ductus arteriosus on Doppler echocardiogram, and they may require emergency surgical therapy because it may be impossible to stabilize them medically.

Two approaches to the surgical management of hypoplastic left heart syndrome have been advanced: reconstructive procedures and cardiac replacement. The reason for reconstructive procedures is based on the fact that the lungs, coronary anatomy, and myocardial biochemistry are inherently normal in this condition. Thus, if one considers hypoplastic left heart syndrome to be one of several cardiac malformations in which only one ventricle is effective, a surgical approach may be devised, leading to a modification of a Fontan procedure. A good functional result after a Fontan procedure can be expected when the pulmonary artery architecture is almost normal, the pulmonary vascular resistance is that of the normal mature lung, and ventricular function has been preserved (low end-diastolic pressure). However, because the systemic circulation in neonates with hypoplastic left heart syndrome depends on the patency of the ductus arteriosus, which characteristically closes in the first days of life, an urgent operative procedure is necessary. The pulmonary vascular resistance of the neonate is prohibitively high for a Fontan procedure; therefore, staged surgical therapy is necessary. The general goals of the initial stage are to establish unobstructed systemic output from the right ventricle, to ensure normal maturation of the pulmonary vasculature by regulating pulmonary arterial blood flow and pressure, and to ensure a widely patent interatrial communication, thus avoiding pulmonary venous hypertension. Although several approaches to these goals have been conceived, the surgical techniques outlined here are designed additionally to incorporate as much as possible the patient's own tissues and to avoid conduits or circumferential suture lines, thus minimizing the number of surgical interventions.

PALLIATION FOR HYPOPLASTIC LEFT HEART SYNDROME (STAGE I)

The operating room is maintained at 20° C to promote surface cooling of the patient. Induction of general anesthesia with pancuronium 0.2 mg/kg (Pavulon) (0.2 mg/kg) and fentanyl (10 μg/kg) is achieved. An additional dose of fentanyl (30 mg/kg) is administered once cardiopulmonary bypass has been established. Arterial and venous access is secured, and a urinary bladder drainage tube, a nasogastric tube, and nasopharyngeal, esophageal, and rectal temperature probes are placed. During this preparatory time, the rectal temperature typically decreases to 32 to 34° C.

A conventional midline sternotomy incision is made, and the thymus is partially excised to facilitate exposure of the diminutive aortic arch and its branch vessels. Cannulation for arterial infusion is most conveniently achieved in the proximal main pulmonary artery just above the sinuses of Valsalva by placing a single diamond-shaped purse-string suture through a small rubber tourniquet. A No. 10 French aortic cannula is fitted with a rubber bumper approximately 3 or 4 mm from the tip. After heparinization, a side-biting C clamp is placed to exclude the purse-string suture, the pulmonary artery is incised, and the cannula is introduced. Threading of the cannula through the ductus arteriosus should be avoided because it is unnecessary and requires excessive manipulation of the cardiovascular structures. Distortion, manipulation, and trauma of the delicate neonatal cardiovascular structures must be minimized to preserve anatomy and function.

A No. 16 French venous cannula is placed through the right atrial appendage, and cardiopulmonary bypass is instituted. The right and left pulmonary artery branches are rapidly exposed and occluded with 2-0 Tevdek tourniquets to ensure systemic perfusion through the ductus arteriosus. The infant is cooled to 20° C while esophageal, nasopharyngeal, and rectal temperatures are monitored. During this time, the branch vessels of the aortic arch are exposed and looped with 2-0 Tevdek tourniquets in preparation for circulatory arrest. Dissection is

extended around the aortic arch onto the thoracic aorta in the posterior mediastinum.

At this point, the branch vessels of the aortic arch are occluded, the circulation is discontinued, and the blood is drained into the venous reservoir. The arterial and venous cannulas are removed, and cardioplegic solution is infused through the pulmonary arterial cannulation site while the descending thoracic aorta is temporarily occluded with forceps. Through the right atrial cannulation site, the septum primum is identified and excised. Attention is then turned to the main pulmonary artery, which has been separated from the diminutive ascending aorta during the cooling phase of cardiopulmonary bypass. Adjacent to the takeoff of the right pulmonary artery, the main pulmonary artery is transected and the distal stump of the main pulmonary artery is oversewn with a patch by using a running monofilament suture technique. Patch closure is recommended to maintain better continuity between the right and left pulmonary artery branches.

The ductus arteriosus is then exposed, ligated, and transected at its entrance into the thoracic aorta. An incision in the aorta is extended distally 1 to 2 cm into the thoracic aorta and also proximally into the aortic arch and ascending aorta to the level of the rim of the transected proximal main pulmonary artery. Because the isthmus of the aorta and the aortic arch actually function as a branch of the main pulmonary artery-ductus-thoracic aorta continuum, the junction of the isthmus and thoracic aorta should be gusseted with a patch and the intimal ridge excised to minimize the development of distal aortic arch obstruction. A pulmonary homograft can be used for this patch and has the advantage of being thin, pliable, and hemostatic. Again, a monofilament running suture technique is used.

At this point, the authors favor the construction of a short central shunt of 4-mm polytetrafluoroethylene (PTFE) tube graft between the inferior aspect of the augmented aortic arch and the confluence of branch pulmonary arteries (Fig. 48–3). The reason for a central shunt is to obtain more even distribution of flow and thus growth of the right and left pulmonary arteries. The remaining pulmonary homograft gusset is then extended to approximately 5 mm above the end of the most proximal incision in the ascending aorta. The proximal anastomosis of the main pulmonary artery to the ascending aorta is begun with multiple interrupted fine monofilament sutures to avoid purse-stringing of the inlet into the diminutive aortic root (Fig. 48–4). The reconstruction is completed by anastomosis of the ascending aorta, main pulmonary artery, and pulmonary homograft, thus creating outflow from the right ventricle to the augmented aorta through the pulmonary valve. Cardiopulmonary bypass is reinstituted, and the patient is rewarmed to 37° C. The tourniquets on the branch vessels of the aortic arch are removed, but those on the branch pulmonary arteries remain until weaning from cardiopulmonary bypass.

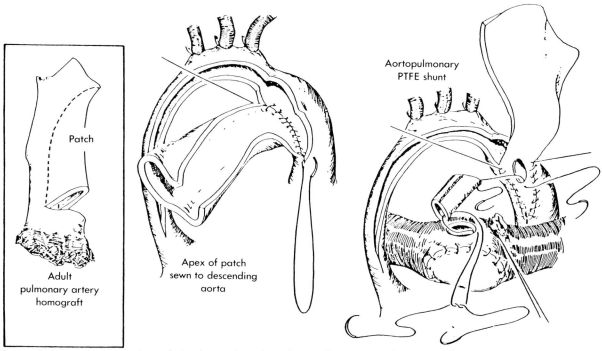

Figure 48–3. An aortotomy is made in the aortic arch and ascending aorta and is gusseted with a patch of pulmonary artery homograft. A 4-mm tube graft is interposed between the aortic arch and the branch pulmonary arteries.

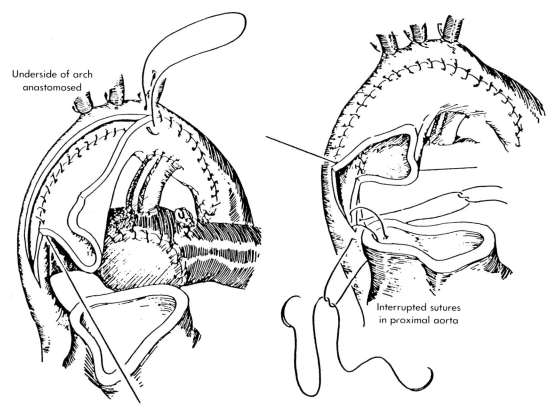

Figure 48–4. Reconstruction is completed by anastomosis of the main pulmonary artery to the ascending aorta and gusset.

After the patient is weaned from cardiopulmonary bypass, the cannulas are removed and a pressure monitoring line is placed through the right atrial appendage cannulation site. Using the lowest possible mean airway pressure, ventilation is adjusted to maintain the P_{CO_2} between 20 and 30 mm Hg to minimize pulmonary vascular resistance. Generally, the P_{O_2} will be between 40 and 45 mm Hg. An arterial P_{O_2} of 50 mm Hg or greater suggests a large pulmonary-to-systemic flow ratio, which may result in inadequate systemic perfusion. The ventilator may be used to adjust the pulmonary-to-systemic flow ratio when this occurs by rapidly decreasing the fraction of inspired oxygen ($F_{I_{O_2}}$) to 30 mm Hg and allowing P_{CO_2} to increase to 40 mm Hg. Pharmacologic support of any type is rarely necessary in the postoperative period.

FONTAN'S PROCEDURE (STAGE II)

After the previously described palliative operation, the right ventricle is subjected to both a volume and pressure load. With a goal of long-term preservation of ventricular function, assessment of suitability for Fontan's procedure is done at 12 to 18 months of age. At this age, the pulmonary resistance is likely to be low (<2.5 Wood's units) and ventricular end-diastolic pressure normal (<7 to 8 mm Hg), and the following surgical procedure may then be planned.

The heart is exposed through a midline sternotomy, and cannulation for cardiopulmonary bypass is achieved by placing an arterial cannula in the ascending aorta and a single venous cannula through the right atrial appendage. The systemic-to-pulmonary artery shunt is exposed and occluded as cardiopulmonary bypass is instituted, and the patient's core temperature is reduced to 20° C. During this cooling phase on cardiopulmonary bypass, the right and left pulmonary artery branches are exposed from pericardial reflection to pericardial reflection. This exposure is in preparation for widely augmenting the pulmonary arteries to avoid proximal pulmonary arterial obstruction from unrecognized irregularities in size.

The aorta is then cross-clamped, and cardioplegia solution is infused as the circulation is arrested and blood is drained into the venous reservoir. The pulmonary arteries are opened by a single incision extending from behind the right superior vena cava across the midline to the left lower lobe branch. An incision in the right atrium is made from the sulcus terminalis superiorly to the right lateral insertion of the eustachian valve inferiorly. The interatrial communication is inspected and enlarged if possible. A final incision is then made in the dome of the right atrium adjacent to the right pulmonary artery, and this incision is extended into the posterior aspect of the right superior vena cava immediately adjacent to the most right-sided aspect of the incision in the

right pulmonary artery. A suture line is begun between the inferior lip of the incised right pulmonary artery and the posterior lip of the right superior vena cava-right atrial incision with a running 5-0 monofilament suture, which provides the floor for the anastomosis of the systemic venous return to the pulmonary arterial tree.

A piece of PFTE tubing 10 mm in diameter and of sufficient length to extend from the inferior vena cava-right atrial junction to the right superior vena cava-right atrial junction is cut in half lengthwise for use as a baffle to channel inferior vena caval flow along the right lateral aspect of the right atrium to the superior anastomosis between the right atrium and the pulmonary arterial tree. The baffle is sutured with running 5-0 monofilament suture around the orifice of the inferior vena cava along the right lateral floor and free wall of the right atrium and around the patulous orifice in the superior dome of the right atrium. This particular baffling technique was introduced to minimize complications associated with tricuspid prolapse or regurgitation, or obstruction of pulmonary venous return to the right ventricle experienced early in this series with an alternate baffling technique. The construction of the systemic venous pulmonary arterial system is completed by gusseting the pulmonary arterial incision with an elongated triangular patch of pulmonary homograft material beginning on the left pulmonary artery with a running 5-0 monofilament suture (Fig. 48-5). As the right pulmonary artery and adjacent right superior vena cava are approached, the base of the triangular pulmonary homograft patch is sutured onto the superior lip of the right superior vena cava-right atrial incision, providing a roof for the anastomosis. The patient is placed back on cardiopulmonary bypass after closure of the initial right atriotomy with a running monofilament suture technique and is rewarmed to 37° C. Placement of 18-gauge pressure monitoring catheters in the right pulmonary artery and through the right atrial appendage (now receiving exclusively pulmonary venous return) allows postoperative assessment of right and left atrial pressures.

CONCLUSION

From October, 1984, through June, 1988, at the Children's Hospital of Philadelphia, 198 newborns had palliative operative procedures similar to those described for hypoplastic left heart syndrome. The hospital mortality among these patients was 28%. The 18-month actuarial survival was 61%. To date, 52 patients have undergone application of Fontan's procedure for the treatment of hypoplastic left heart syndrome. Of these 52 patients, there were 16 early and 2 late deaths, with 2 deaths in the last 15 patients. The results continue to improve for both initial palliation and later reconstructive procedures, as an increasing knowledge of the anatomy and physiology

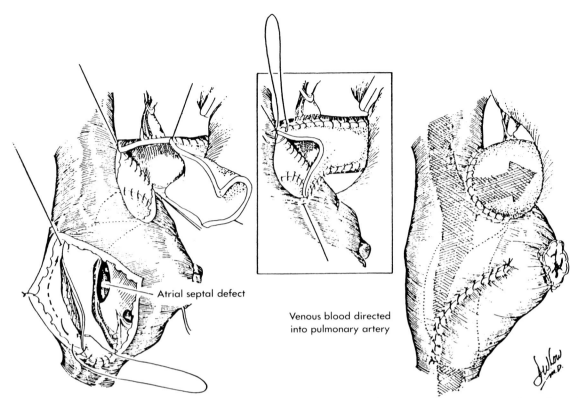

Atrial septal defect

Venous blood directed
into pulmonary artery

Figure 48–5. The modified Fontan procedure is structured to baffle the return from the inferior vena cava along the right lateral aspect of the right atrium to an anastomosis between the right superior vena cava, right atrium, and right pulmonary artery. A gusset of pulmonary artery homograft is used to augment the pulmonary artery atrial anastomosis.

of this complex group of patients is gained. The approach outlined here for reconstructive therapy for this malformation will continue to evolve. The challenge for the future is to characterize better this group of lesions so that the preoperative, operative, and postoperative management may be further improved.

Selected Bibliography

Bailey, L., Concepcion, W., Shattuk, H., and Huang, L.: Method of heart transplantation for treatment of hypoplastic left heart syndrome. J. Thorac. Cardiovasc. Surg., *92*:1, 1986.

Technical details of the investigational orthotopic cardiac transplantation for management of hypoplastic left heart syndrome in the neonate are given. A technique of extracorporeal perfusion and the need for extensive aortic arch reconstruction are emphasized. The source of donor graft in this case report was a subhuman primate, but it is emphasized that the donor graft makes little difference with regard to the unique technical aspects of cardiac transplantation in a ductus-dependent newborn infant with a diminutive aortic arch.

Bailey, L. L., Nehlsen-Cannarella, S. L., et al: Cardiac allotransplantation in newborns as therapy for hypoplastic left heart syndrome. N. Engl. J. Med., *351*:949, 1986.

These authors present the initial Loma Linda experience with heart replacement therapy for hypoplastic left heart syndrome. This report not only shows the feasibility of heart replacement in patients with the aortic arch anatomy of hypoplastic left heart syndrome but also illustrates the complex circumstances involved

in the procurement, within a limited time, of a heart sufficiently small to fit into the mediastinum of a neonate. Short-term results suggest that immunosuppressive management of neonates and small infants is no more complicated than that of adults.

Jonas, R. A., Lang, P., Hansen, D., et al: First stage palliation of hypoplastic left heart syndrome: The importance of coarctation and shunt size. J. Thorac. Cardiovasc. Surg., *92*:6, 1986.

This report describes the experience with palliative surgery for 25 neonates between January of 1984 and July of 1985. Six of the neonates died during this time. The authors emphasize the significance of a posterior shelf at the junction of the isthmus of the aorta with the thoracic aorta, because this anatomy can contribute to late coarctation of the aorta. Moreover, they point out the fact that careful ventilatory and pharmacologic management of the ratio of pulmonary to systemic vascular resistance is an essential part of the perioperative management of these neonates with two parallel competing circulations.

Noonan, J. A., and Nadas, A. S.: The hypoplastic left heart syndrome. Pediatr. Clin. North Am., *5*:1029, 1958.

This sentinel article coins the term *hypoplastic left heart syndrome* and outlines the anatomic-physiologic and natural historical features of this constellation of anatomic abnormalities in the development of the structures of the left heart. Although the modern concepts of hypoplastic left heart syndrome are slightly more focused today, this report represents the first time that this specific categorization is made.

Norwood, W. I., Lang, P., and Hansen, D.: Physiologic repair of aortic atresia—hypoplastic left heart syndrome. N. Engl. J. Med., *308*:23, 1983.

This report outlines early experience with reconstructive surgical management of hypoplastic left heart syndrome beginning in 1979.

This case report is of one patient in that series who had physiologic correction by modification of Fontan's operative procedure, showing the feasibility of reconstructive surgical management of hypoplastic left heart syndrome. The patient had physiologic correction at 16 months of age, at which time the pulmonary vascular resistance was calculated to be 2 Wood's units. The child was reported to be clinically well during 6 months of follow-up after physiologically corrective therapy. The boy is still clinically very well and has a right atrial pressure of 11 mm Hg determined by cardiac catheterization at 7 years of age.

Pigott, J. D., Murphy, J. D., Barber, G., and Norwood, W. I.: Palliative reconstructive surgery for hypoplastic left heart syndrome. Ann. Thorac. Surg., 45:122, 1988.

This report constitutes the experience from August of 1985 through August of 1987 with 104 consecutive nonselected neonates who had palliative procedures for hypoplastic left heart syndrome at the Children's Hospital of Philadelphia. It presents an evolution in technique to optimize pulmonary vascular development, minimize late aortic arch obstruction, and achieve a balanced pulmonary and systemic flow ratio. Such techniques were developed to achieve the best possible preparation for application of Fontan's procedure for the treatment of hypoplastic left heart syndrome.

Bibliography

Abbott, M. E.: Atlas of Congenital Cardiac Diseases. New York, American Heart Association, 1936, pp. 48 and 61.

Anderson, R. H., Ho, S. Y., Zuberbuhler, J. R., et al: Surgery for hypoplastic left heart syndrome: A fiction? Surgical anatomy and definition. In Marcelletti, C., Anderson, R. H., Becker, A. E., et al (eds): Paediatric Cardiology. New York, Churchill Livingstone, 1986, pp. 111–121.

Bailey, L., Concepcion, W., Shattuck, H., and Huang, L.: Method of heart transplantation for treatment of hypoplastic left heart syndrome. J. Thorac. Cardiovasc. Surg., 92:1, 1986a.

Bailey, L. L., Nehlsen-Cannarella, S. L., et al: Cardiac allotransplantation in newborns as therapy for hypoplastic left heart syndrome. N. Engl. J. Med., 315:949, 1986b.

Bailey, L. L., Nehlsen-Cannarella, S. L., Concepcion, W., and Jolley, W. B.: Baboon-to-human cardiac xenotransplantation in a neonate. J.A.M.A., 254:3321, 1985.

Barber, G., Helton, J. G., Aglira, B. A., et al: The significance of tricuspid regurgitation in hypoplastic left-heart syndrome. Am. Heart J., 116:1563, 1988.

Barber, G., Murphy, J. D., Pigott, J. D. and Norwood, W. I.: The evolving pattern of survival following palliative surgery for hypoplastic left heart syndrome. J. Am. Coll. Cardiol., 2:139A, 1988.

Bash, S. E., Huhta, J. C., Vick, G. W. III, et al: Hypoplastic left heart syndrome: Is echocardiography accurate enough to guide surgical palliation. J. Am. Coll. Cardiol., 7:610, 1986.

Bass, J. L., Ben-Shachar, G., and Edwards, J. E.: Comparison of M-mode echocardiography and pathologic findings in the hypoplastic left heart syndrome. Am. J. Cardiol., 45:79, 1980.

Benner, M. C.: Premature closure of the foramen ovale. Am. Heart J., 17:437, 1939.

Bharati, S., and Lev, M.: The spectrum of common atrioventricular orifice (canal). Am. Heart J., 86:553, 1973.

Bharati, S., and Lev, M.: The surgical anatomy of hypoplasia of aortic tract complex. J. Thorac. Cardiovasc. Surg., 88:97, 1984.

Bharati, S., Nordenberg, A., Brock, R. R., and Lev, M.: Hypoplastic left heart syndrome with dysplastic pulmonary valve with stenosis. Pediatr. Cardiol., 5:127, 1984.

Bidot-López, P., Matisoff, D., Talner, N. S., et al: Hypoplastic left heart in a patient with 45,X/46,XX/47,XXX mosaicism. Am. J. Med. Genet., 2:341, 1978.

Bierman, F. Z.: Two-dimensional echocardiography and its influence on cardiac catheterization. Cardiovasc. Intervent. Radiol., 7:140, 1984.

Bjerregaard, P., and Laursen, H. B.: Persistent left superior vena cava. Acta Paediatr. Scand., 69:105, 1980.

Brownell, L. G., and Shokeir, M. H.: Inheritance of hypoplastic left heart syndrome. Clin. Genet., 9:245, 1976.

Bulkley, B. H., D'Amico, B., and Taylor, A. L.: Extensive myocardial fiber disarray in aortic and pulmonary atresia. Circulation, 67:191, 1983.

Chin, A. J., Sanders, S. P., Sherman, F., et al: Accuracy of subcostal 2-dimensional echocardiography in prospective diagnosis of total anomalous pulmonary venous connection. Am. Heart J., 113:1153, 1987.

Chin, A. J., Yeager, S. B., Sanders, S. P., et al: Accuracy of prospective two-dimensional echocardiographic evaluation of left ventricular outflow tract in complete transposition of the great arteries. Am. J. Cardiol., 55:759, 1985.

Cloez, J. L., Isaaz, K., and Pernot, C.: Pulsed Doppler flow characteristics of ductus arteriosus in infants with associated congenital anomalies of the heart or great arteries. Am. J. Cardiol., 57:845, 1986.

Cobanoglu, A., Metzdorff, M. T., Pinson, C. W., et al: Valvotomy for pulmonary atresia with intact ventricular septum. J. Thorac. Cardiovasc. Surg., 89:482, 1985.

DiDonato, R. M., Fyfe, D. A., Puga, F. J., et al: Fifteen-year experience with surgical repair of truncus arteriosus. J. Thorac. Cardiovasc. Surg., 89:414, 1985.

Doty, D. B., and Knott, H. W.: Hypoplastic left heart syndrome: Experience with an operation to establish functionally normal circulation. J. Thorac. Cardiovasc. Surg., 74:624, 1977.

Edwards, J. E.: Congenital malformation of the heart and great vessels. In Gould, S. E. (ed): Pathology of the Heart. Springfield, IL, Charles C Thomas, 1953, p. 407.

Ehrlich, M., Bierman, F. Z., Ellis, K., and Gersony, W. M.: Hypoplastic left heart syndrome: Report of a unique survivor. J. Am. Coll. Cardiol., 7:361, 1986.

Eliot, R. S., Shone, J. D., Kanjuk, V. I., et al: Mitral atresia: A study of 32 cases. Am. Heart J., 71:6, 1965.

Elzenga, N. J., and Gittenberger-de Groot, A. C.: Coarctation and related aortic arch anomalies in hypoplastic left heart syndrome. Int. J. Cardiol., 8:379, 1985.

Farooki, Z. Q., Henry, J. G., and Green, E. W.: Echocardiographic spectrum of the hypoplastic left heart syndrome: A clinicopathologic correlation in 19 newborns. Am. J. Cardiol., 38:337, 1976.

Fontan, F., and Baudet, E.: Surgical repair of tricuspid atresia. Thorax, 26:240, 1971.

Friedman, S., Murphy, L., and Ash, R.: Congenital mitral atresia with hypoplastic nonfunctioning left heart. J. Dis. Child., 90:176, 1955.

Fujiseki, Y., Yamamoto, H., Hattori, M., et al: Oral administration of prostaglandin E_2 in hypoplastic left heart syndrome. Jpn. Heart J., 24:481, 1983.

Fyler, D. C.: Report of the New England Regional Infant Cardiac Program. Pediatrics., 65(Suppl.):463, 1980.

Fyler, D. C., Rothman, K. J., Buckley, L. P., et al: The determinants of five year survival of infants with critical congenital heart disease. In Engle, M. A. (ed): Pediatric Cardiovascular Disease, Cardiovascular Clinics. Philadelphia, F. A. Davis Company, 1981, pp. 393–405.

Harh, J. Y., Paul, M. H., Gallen, W. J., et al: Experimental production of hypoplastic left heart syndrome in the chick embryo. Am. J. Cardiol., 31:51, 1973.

Hastreiter, A. R., van der Horst, R. L., Dubrow, I. W., and Eckner, F. O.: Quantitative angiographic and morphologic aspects of aortic valve atresia. Am. J. Cardiol., 51:1705, 1983.

Hawkins, J. A., and Doty, D. B.: Aortic atresia: Morphologic characteristics affecting survival and operative palliation. J. Thorac. Cardiovasc. Surg., 88:620, 1984.

Helton, J. G., Aglira, B. A., Chin, A. J., et al: Analysis of potential anatomic or physiologic determinants of outcome of palliative surgery for hypoplastic left heart syndrome. Circulation, 74(Suppl. I):70, 1986.

Helton, J. G., Aglira, B. A., Chin, A. J., et al: Improvements in non-invasive evaluations of the aortic reconstruction for hypoplastic left heart syndrome. Am. Heart J., 7:48A, 1986.

Holmes, L. B., Rose, V., and Child, A. H.: Comment on hypoplastic left heart syndrome. *In* Birth Defects Original Article Series. Bergsma, D. (ed): Clinical Delineation of Birth Defects. XVI: Urinary System and Others. Baltimore, Williams & Wilkins, 1976, pp. 228–30.

Hutchins, G. M.: Coarctation of the aorta explained as a branch point of the ductus arteriosus. Am. J. Pathol., 63:203, 1971.

Isaaz, K., Cloez, J. L., Danchin, N., et al: Assessment of right ventricular outflow tract in children by two-dimensional echocardiography using a new subcostal view. Am. J. Cardiol., 56:539, 1985.

Jonas, R. A., Lang, P., Hansen, D., et al: First-stage palliation of hypoplastic left heart syndrome: The importance of coarctation and shunt size. J. Thorac. Cardiovasc. Surg., 92:6, 1986.

Kanjuh, V. I., Elliot, R. S., and Edwards, J. E.: Coexistent mitral and aortic valvular atresia: A pathologic study of 14 cases. Am. J. Cardiol., 15:611, 1965.

Kirklin, J. W., and Barnatt-Boyes, B. G.: Cardiac Surgery, Morphology, Diagnostic Criteria, Natural History, Techniques, Results, and Indications. New York, John Wiley & Sons, 1986, pp. 843–856.

Lehman, E.: Congenital atresia of the foramen ovale. Am. J. Dis. Child., 33:585, 1927.

Lev, M.: Pathologic anatomy and interrelationship of hypoplasia of the aortic tract complexes. Lab. Invest., 1:61, 1952.

Lev, M., Arcilla, R., Remoldi, H. J. A., et al: Premature narrowing or closure of the foramen ovale. Am. Heart J., 65:638, 1963.

Lewis, A. B., Freed, M., Heymann, M. A., et al: Side effects of therapy with prostaglandin E₁ in infants with critical congenital heart disease. Circulation, 64:893, 1981.

Lumb, G., and Dawkins, W. A.: Congenital atresia of mitral and aortic valves with vestigial left ventricle (three cases). Am. Heart J., 3:378, 1960.

Mandorla, S., Narducci, P. L., Migliozzi, L., et al: Fetal echocardiography: Prenatal diagnosis of hypoplastic left heart syndrome. G. Ital. Cardiol., 14:517, 1984.

Marino, B., Ballerini, L., Marcelletti, C., et al: Complete transposition of the great arteries: Visualization of left and right outflow tract obstruction by oblique subcostal two-dimensional echocardiography. Am. J. Cardiol., 55:1140, 1985.

Milo, S., Ho, S. Y., and Anderson, R. H.: Hypoplastic left heart syndrome: Can this malformation be treated surgically? Thorax, 35:351, 1980.

Moodie, D. S., Gill, C. C., Sterba, R., et al: The hypoplastic left heart syndrome: Evidence of preoperative myocardial and hepatic infarction in spite of prostaglandin therapy. Ann. Thorac. Surg., 42:307, 1986.

Moodie, D. S., Gallen, W. J., and Friedberg, D. Z.: Congenital aortic atresia: Report of long survival and some speculation about surgical approaches. J. Thorac. Cardiovasc. Surg., 63:726, 1972.

Mortera, C., and Leon, G.: Detection of persistent ductus in hypoplastic left heart syndrome by contrast echocardiography. Br. Heart J., 44:596, 1980.

Natowicz, M., and Kelley, R. I.: Association of Turner syndrome with hypoplastic left-heart syndrome. Am. J. Dis. Child., 141:218, 1987.

Noonan, J. A., and Nadas, A. S.: The hypoplastic left heart syndrome. Pediatr. Clin. North Am., 5:1029, 1958.

Nora, J. J., and Nora, A. H.: Genetics and counseling in cardiovascular diseases. Springfield, IL, Charles C Thomas, 1978, p. 181.

Norwood, W. I., Kirklin, J. K., and Sanders, S. P.: Hypoplastic left heart syndrome: Experience with palliative surgery. Am. J. Cardiol., 45:87, 1980.

Norwood, W. I., Lang, P., Castaneda, A. R., and Campbell, D. N.: Experience with operations for hypoplastic left heart syndrome. J. Thorac. Cardiovasc. Surg., 82:511, 1981.

Norwood, W. I., Lang, P., and Hansen, D.: Physiologic repair of aortic atresia—hypoplastic left heart syndrome. N. Engl. J. Med., 308:23, 1983.

O'Connor, W. N., Cash, J. B., Cottrill, C. M., et al: Ventriculocoronary connections in hypoplastic left hearts: An autopsy microscopic study. Circulation, 66:1078, 1982.

Oazi, Q. H., Kanchanapoomi, R., Cooper, R., et al: Brief clinical report: dup(12p) and hypoplastic left heart. Am. J. Med. Genet., 9:195, 1981.

Roberts, W. C., Perry, L. W., Chandra, R. S., et al: Aortic valve atresia: A new classification based on necropsy study of 73 cases. Am. J. Cardiol., 37:753, 1976.

Sade, R. M., Fyfe, D., and Alpert, C. C.: Hypoplastic left heart syndrome: A simplified palliative operation. Ann. Thorac. Surg., 43:309, 1987.

Sahn, D. J., Allen, H. D., Goldberg, S. J., et al: Pediatric echocardiography: A review of its clinical utility. J. Pediatr., 87:335, 1975.

Sahn, D. J., Shenker, L., Reed, K. L., et al: Prenatal ultrasound diagnosis of hypoplastic left heart syndrome in utero associated with hydrops fetalis. Am. Heart J., 104:1368, 1982.

Schall, S. A., and Dalldorf, F. G.: Premature closure of the foramen ovale and hypoplasia of the left heart. Int. J. Cardiol., 5:103, 1984.

Schlemmer, M., Khoss, A., Salzer, H. R., and Wimmer, M.: Prostaglandin E₂ in newborns with congenital heart disease. Z. Kardiol., 71:452, 1982.

Silverberg, B.: Coexistent aortic and mitral atresia associated with persistent common atrioventricular canal. Am. J. Cardiol., 16:754, 1965.

Sinha, S. N., Rusnak, S. L., Sommers, H. M., et al: Hypoplastic left ventricle syndrome: Analysis of thirty autopsy cases in infants with surgical consideration. Am. J. Cardiol., 21:166, 1968.

Skovranek, J., First, T., and Samanek, M.: Contribution of pulsed Doppler echocardiography to ultrasound diagnosis of congenital heart disease. Cor Vasa, 23:34, 1981.

Snider, A. R., and Silverman, N. H.: Suprasternal notch echocardiography: A two-dimensional technique for evaluating congenital heart disease. Circulation, 63:165, 1981.

Suzuki, K., Hitata, K., Eto, Y., et al: Echocardiographic assessment of anatomical detail in patients with hypoplastic left heart syndrome. J. Cardiogr., 12:991, 1982.

Tuma, S., Samanek, M., Benesova, D., and Voriskova, M.: Premature closure of the foramen ovale with levoatriocardinal vein. Eur. J. Pediatr., 129:205, 1978.

van der Horst, R. L., Hastreiter, A. R., DuBrow, I. W., and Eckner, F. A. O.: Pathologic measurements in aortic atresia. Am. Heart J., 106:1411, 1983.

Von Reuden, T. J., Knight, L., Moller, J. H., and Edwards, J. E.: Coarctation of the aorta associated with aortic valve atresia. Circulation, 52:951, 1975.

Watson, D. G., and Rowe, R. D.: Aortic-valve atresia report of 43 cases. J.A.M.A., 179:14, 1962.

Weinberg, P. M., Chin, A. J., Murphy, J. D., et al: Postmortem echocardiography and tomographic anatomy of hypoplastic left heart syndrome after palliative surgery. Am. J. Cardiol., 58:1228, 1986.

Weinberg, P. M., Peyser, K., and Hackney, J. R.: Fetal hydrops in a newborn with hypoplastic left heart syndrome: Tricuspid valve stopper. J. Am. Coll. Cardiol., 6:1365, 1985.

Weldon, C. S., Hartman, A. F., and McKnight, R. C.: Surgical management of hypoplastic right ventricle with pulmonary atresia or critical pulmonic stenosis and intact ventricular septum. Ann. Thorac. Surg., 37:12, 1984.

Yabek, S. M., and Mann, J. S.: Prostaglandin E₁ infusion in the hypoplastic left heart syndrome. Chest, 76:330, 1979.

CHAPTER 49

ACQUIRED DISEASE OF THE TRICUSPID VALVE

Robert B. Karp

Acquired tricuspid valve disease is classified surgically as either functional or organic. The physiology of the circulation and the surgical results are each related to the situation on the left side of the heart. Thus, functional tricuspid insufficiency results from left-sided mitral stenosis or regurgitation much less frequently than from isolated aortic valve disease. The degree of functional impairment is related to the severity of the left-sided lesion, the duration of aortic or mitral valve dysfunction and the resultant severity of the pulmonary vascular resistance, the degree of pulmonary artery hypertension, and the degree of right ventricular dilatation.

The causative factor most often associated with organic disease of the tricuspid valve is *rheumatic fever*. Organic disease of the tricuspid valve is also related to the left-sided disease, because rheumatic involvement rarely occurs on the tricuspid valve without also affecting the mitral or aortic valve.

Infrequent causes of organic tricuspid valve disease include trauma (penetrating or blunt) leading to incompetence, carcinoid syndrome, and nonbacterial endocarditis such as Libman-Sacks, eosinophilic leukemia, and diffuse collagen disorders. An increasingly frequent cause of organic tricuspid valve disease is infective endocarditis.

ANATOMY

The tricuspid orifice is the largest of the four cardiac valves, and in normal adults the valve area is approximately 10.5 cm² and the diameter is 36 ± 4.5 mm. In congestive heart failure, the tricuspid annulus may be 40 to 45 mm in diameter. The three tricuspid leaflets are supported by a tensor apparatus composed of chordae tendineae (primary, secondary, and tertiary) and papillary muscles (usually a single major anterior papillary muscle and several accessory papillary muscles). There is no tricuspid annulus, but the bases of the three leaflets are attached to the heart at the atrioventricular junction. In normal situs and connection, this "ring" is related to the base of

the aortic valve, the membranous septum, the central fibrous body, the right coronary artery, the lateral atrioventricular junction, the coronary sinus, and the bundle of His (clockwise from medially). With its tensor apparatus, the tricuspid valve in part defines the morphologic right ventricle. Of the three more or less well-defined tricuspid leaflets, the anterior is the largest, and the chordae are attached to the dominant papillary muscle. It is separated from the septal leaflet by the anterior septal commissure and from the small posterior leaflet by the posterior commissure. The base of the septal leaflet harbors the penetrating portion of the conducting system. Both the septal and posterior leaflets have chordae attaching directly to the right ventricular myocardium in the septal and parietal walls (Figs. 49–1 and 49–2).

The anterior commissure lies adjacent to the atrioventricular septum, and the tricuspid valve lies in a plane caudad to the mitral valve. Thus, a needle passed horizontally from the atrial side of the septal leaflet will exit into the left ventricle.

With right ventricular dilatation, the tricuspid annulus enlarges along the major portion of the attachment of the anterior leaflet, the posterior leaflet, and the lateral third of the septal leaflet.

PHYSIOLOGY

Disease of the tricuspid valve causes circulatory depression in several ways. Organic stenosis may limit flow into the pulmonary circulation and into the left side of the heart. With decreased preload to the left side of the heart, left ventricular stroke volume decreases, resulting in salt and water retention via the renin-aldosterone-angiotensin mechanism (forward heart failure). Tricuspid stenosis also may cause "backward heart failure," with hepatic congestion, ascites, and peripheral edema.

Tricuspid incompetence, organic or functional, also may limit preload to the left side of the heart. In addition, tricuspid incompetence leads to right

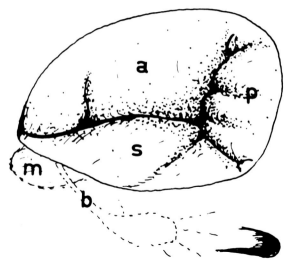

Figure 49–1. Normal tricuspid orifice. (a = anterior leaflet; p = posterior leaflet; s = septal leaflet; b = bundle of His; m = membranous septum.) (From Carpentier, A., Deloche, A., Hanania, G., et al: Surgical management of acquired tricuspid valve disease. J. Thorac. Cardiovasc. Surg., 67:53, 1974.)

ventricular dilatation. Right ventricular enlargement may also result from tricuspid regurgitation secondary to lesions in the left side of the heart.

The clinical signs of tricuspid valve disease are shown in Figure 49–3. Hepatojugular reflux is encountered in tricuspid regurgitation only, and increased intensity of murmurs with inspiration aids in distinguishing tricuspid murmurs from mitral murmurs.

Hepatic dysfunction often accompanies tricuspid valve disease and must be defined before surgical intervention.

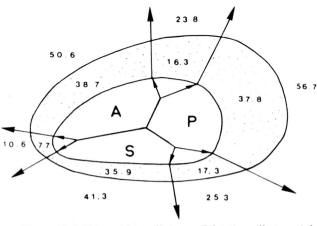

Figure 49–2. Tricuspid insufficiency. Dilatation affects mainly the posterior (P) and the anterior (A) leaflets. Numbers indicate the average lengths (in millimeters) of the attachment of the leaflets in a normal (central numbers) and a dilated (peripheral numbers) orifice. Most annuloplasties shorten the annulus at the anterior and posterior leaflets. (From Carpentier, A., Deloche, A., Hanania, G., et al: Surgical management of acquired tricuspid valve disease. J. Thorac. Cardiovasc. Surg., 67:53, 1974.)

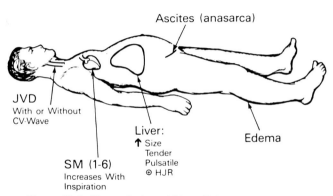

Figure 49–3. Signs of tricuspid insufficiency. (JVD = jugular venous distention; SM = systolic murmur; HJR = hepatojugular reflux.) (From Cohen, S. R., Sell, J. E., McIntosh, C. L., and Clark, R. E.: Tricuspid regurgitation in patients with acquired, chronic, pure mitral regurgitation. I: Prevalence, diagnosis, and comparison of preoperative clinical and hemodynamic features in patients with and without tricuspid regurgitation. J. Thorac. Cardiovasc. Surg., 94:481, 1987.)

INDICATIONS FOR OPERATION

Surgical indications in all but a few cases (of isolated tricuspid valve disease) are those related to the left-sided valvular dysfunction. Tricuspid valve dysfunction, both functional and organic, usually occurs in the late stages of left-sided valve problems. Thus, the results of tricuspid valve surgery must be interpreted with regard to early and late results of mitral and double-valve procedures. Also, it follows that tricuspid valve repair or replacement is almost always done in patients with New York Heart Association (NYHA) functional Classes III and IV.

RESULTS OF OPERATION

In 1974, Stephenson and colleagues (Stephenson et al, 1977) reported a 24% operative mortality (30-day) in 38 patients having triple-valve replacement (aortic, mitral, and tricuspid). The operative risk was influenced by NYHA functional class (18% for NYHA Class III and 40% for Class IV) (Fig. 49–4). Five-year survival for the entire group was 53%. Triple-valve replacement is seldom done now. Instead, tricuspid valve repair is used almost uniformly when tricuspid valve involvement is associated with important left-sided valve stenosis or incompetence. For example, Duran and colleagues (1980) reported 150 patients who had tricuspid valve involvement and in whom left-sided repair or replacement was done. Seventy-eight patients had organic disease, and 72 patients had functional tricuspid incompetence. One hundred nineteen patients had tricuspid valve repair (46 commissurotomies and 115 annuloplasties), and in 31 patients the tricuspid disease was surgically ignored. Postoperatively, 97% of patients with hemodynamically corrected left-sided lesions were NYHA functional Class I or II. In addition, appropriate repair of left-sided valve dysfunction determined the postop-

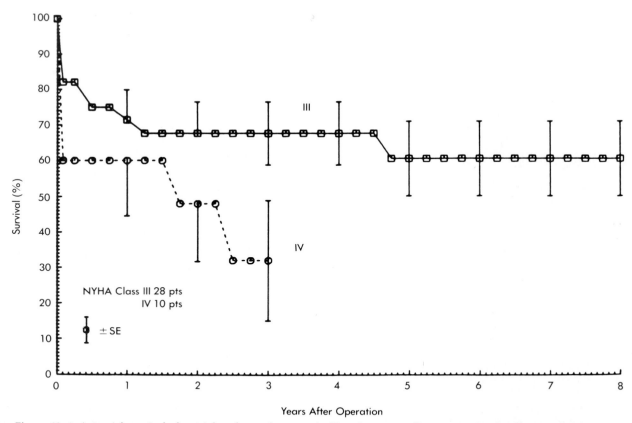

Figure 49–4. Actuarial survival after triple valve replacement in 38 patients according to preoperative functional class. (Reprinted with permission from The Society of Thoracic Surgeons [The Annals of Thoracic Surgery, Vol. 23, 1977, pp. 327–332].)

erative cardiac index. Operative mortality in that series was 8.4%. Residual tricuspid incompetence was present when pulmonary vascular resistance remained elevated. Eighty per cent of patients with preoperative tricuspid incompetence did not have postoperative regurgitation when pulmonary vascular resistance fell below 500 dyn-sec/cm^{-5}, compared with 47% of patients with pulmonary vascular resistance greater than 500 dyn postoperatively (i.e., 53% had residual tricuspid incompetence). Approximately 30% of patients have small or moderate postoperative tricuspid gradients after repair. Most residual gradients and incompetence are not clinically important if hemodynamic correction of the left-sided heart disease is adequate.

Baughman and colleagues (1984) at Massachusetts General Hospital reported 74 patients who had multiple valve surgery including procedures on the tricuspid valve. This report represents contemporary data—for example, congestive heart failure systems, Classes III and IV, were present preoperatively in 82%. Fifty-five of the 74 patients had had one or two previous cardiac operations. Thirty-day mortality was 22%, and the survival rate continued to decrease minimally to plateau at 70%. Male sex, NYHA functional Class IV, ascites or pulmonary edema, elevated preoperative bilirubin, mean pulmonary artery pres-

sure greater than 40 mm Hg, and pulmonary vascular resistance greater than 6 Wood's units all were associated with increased risk of death after operation. Multivariate risk analysis identified severity of peripheral edema and level of pulmonary artery pressure as the most predictive combination of those independent variables.

Indications for tricuspid valve surgery cannot be dissociated from operations on left-sided lesions. Results of tricuspid valve operations depend on the appropriate procedure for aortic or mitral valve lesions, the degree and reversibility of left ventricular dysfunction, the degree and reversibility of pulmonary vascular resistance, and the severity of right ventricular dysfunction. Therefore, better results occur if patients present for operation early in the course of congestive heart failure.

Although it cannot be documented, most surgeons believe that tricuspid valve repair is preferable to valve replacement. The hemodynamics are comparable: there is a higher incidence of mild incompetence with repair versus a higher gradient after replacement. The complications associated with replacement (e.g., thromboembolism, thrombosis, and anticoagulant-related problems) do not occur with operative procedures. These facts alone favor use of repair as often as possible.

TECHNIQUE OF OPERATION

Because most tricuspid valve operative procedures are associated with surgical therapy for aortic or mitral disease, the usual approach is through a median sternotomy. Infrequently, a right anterior thoracotomy approach can be used for isolated tricuspid valve operations or mitral and tricuspid valve procedures. Before cardiopulmonary bypass, the right atrial size is assessed and the thrill of tricuspid incompetence is palpated on the right atrial wall and, more definitively, by the index finger inserted through the right atrial appendage. At this time, organic changes in the tricuspid valve are determined. Scarring of the leaflets and thickening and adhesions or closure at the commissures, most frequently at the anterior commissure, are characteristic of organic valve disease. Shortening of the anterior leaflet and occasionally thickening of the chordae may also be present. Functional tricuspid incompetence exists in the absence of scarring and commissural changes. The annulus is dilated. The jet of tricuspid incompetence is graded I through VI. Generally, functional tricuspid incompetence, Grades I or II, is tolerated. Repair is done when there are organic changes or when tricuspid incompetence is Grade III to VI.

A single period of aortic cross-clamping is used, and myocardial protection is afforded by oxygenated crystalloid potassium cardioplegia and external myocardial cooling. The perfusate is stabilized at 26° C. The aortic or mitral valve or both are repaired or replaced.

TECHNIQUE OF TRICUSPID VALVE REPAIR

Commissurotomy for tricuspid stenosis is relatively straightforward. The anterior and occasionally posterior commissures are incised with a scapel. A suture or two is occasionally necessary to obliterate a cleft or to shorten the annulus posterolaterally.

Tricuspid annuloplasty can be accomplished by various techniques. The three basic methods are directed to narrowing the dilated tricuspid annulus while maintaining leaflet length and function and preserving the course of the conduction fibers as they penetrate from the right atrium to the membranous ventricular septum, posteromedially. The Kay or Wooler annuloplasty uses mattress or figure-of-eight sutures to obliterate the commissure and most of the annulus between the anterior and posterior leaflets (Fig. 49–5). The DeVega technique uses a double purse-string to narrow the annulus from the anterior commissure to the posterior septal commissure. A valve sizer is often inserted to gauge correctly the degree to which the annuloplasty suture is tightened (Fig. 49–6). A slightly more complex but perhaps more definitive procedure uses a Carpentier ring, which has actually evolved to an interrupted C-shaped configuration open at the area of the penetrating bundle of His. This ring is inserted at the level of the annulus to narrow and stabilize it. The tissue of the annulus is gathered by interrupted or continuous sutures to the slightly flexible Dacron-covered metal prosthetic annulus. A reproducible reduction in the circumference of the tricuspid an-

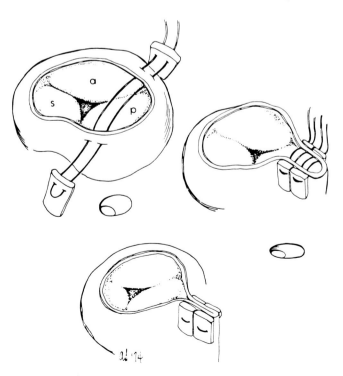

Figure 49–5. Basic commissural annuloplasty according to Kay or Wooler. (From Boyd, A. D., Engleman, R. M., Isom, O. W., et al: Tricuspid annuloplasty, five and one-half years' experience with 78 patients. J. Thorac. Cardiovasc. Surg., 68:344, 1974.)

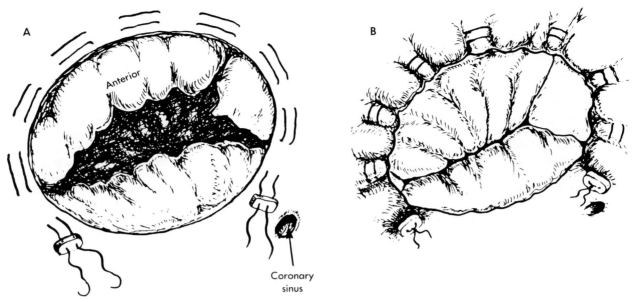

Figure 49–6. Double purse-string suture technique in DeVega's annuloplasty. (From Rabago, G., Fraile, J., Martinell, J., and Artiz, V.: Technique and results of tricuspid annuloplasty. J. Cardiovasc. Surg., *1*:247, 1986.)

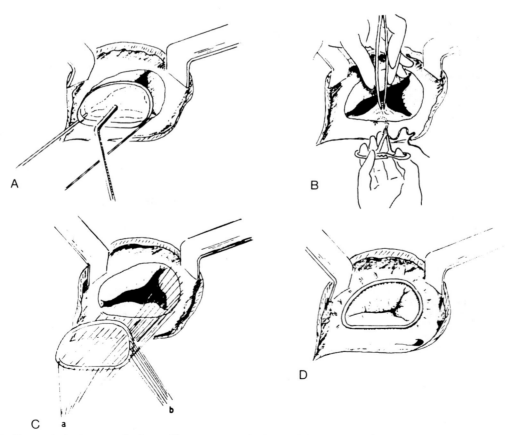

Figure 49–7. Carpentier's ring annuloplasty. The sutures at the base of the septal leaflet are passed through the corresponding segment of the prosthetic ring at the same intervals between them. The intervals are reduced to purse-string the anterior and septal annulus. (From Carpentier, A., Deloche, A., Hanania, G., et al: Surgical management of acquired tricuspid valve disease. J. Thorac. Cardiovasc. Surg., *67*:53, 1974.)

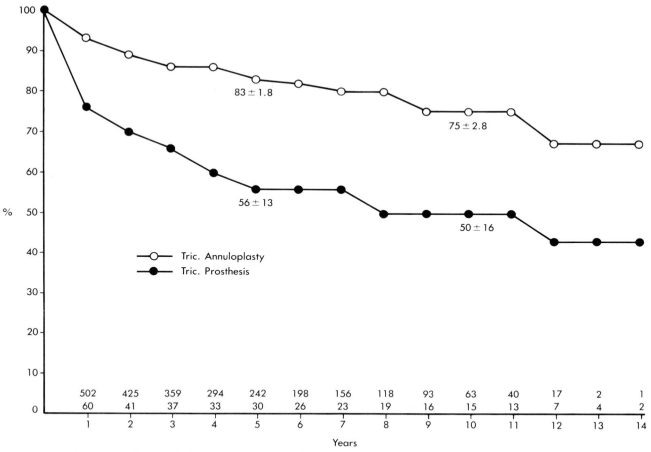

Figure 49–8. Comparative survival curves of patients with tricuspid prostheses or annuloplasty. (From Rabago, G., Fraile, J., Martinell, J., and Artiz, V.: Technique and results of tricuspid annuloplasty. J. Cardiovasc. Surg., 1:247, 1986.)

nulus is achieved. This repair may be more durable and more effective than either the Kay-Wooler or the DeVega technique (Fig. 49–7).

TRICUSPID VALVE REPLACEMENT

For severe organic tricuspid valve disease, valve replacement is occasionally necessary. In the tricuspid position, a tissue valve is used most often. Mechanical valves on the right side of the heart have a very high incidence of thromboembolism and thrombosis. Thus, a porcine xenograft or a pericardial valve is preferred. The bioprosthesis is inserted within the tricuspid annulus, where special care is taken in suturing near the bundle of His. The sutures are placed at the redundant septal leaflet and its base; otherwise, the needle bites pass through the annulus. A valve is occasionally placed supra-annularly—that is, on the atrial side of the tricuspid ring—with the coronary sinus draining into the right ventricle. This technique avoids the conduction system altogether.

In a nonconcurrent analysis, a study from the Mayo Clinic (Fig. 49–8) compares long-term survival in patients having tricuspid valve replacement versus those having repair. The groups are not strictly similar, but repair resulted in better survival.

INFECTIVE ENDOCARDITIS

An increasing indication for tricuspid valve surgical intervention is infective endocarditis, which has become more widespread because of the rising incidence of intravenous drug abuse. Some tricuspid endocarditis can be controlled effectively with specific antibiotic treatment. However, surgical intervention is necessary in the presence of continued sepsis, moderate or severe heart failure (secondary to tricuspid insufficiency), and multiple pulmonary emboli. Arbulu and Asfaw (1981) described tricuspid valvulectomy without replacement for this condition. The infected focus is removed, and sepsis is controlled. Valve replacement is not done because of the high incidence of recidivism. In most cases, congestive heart failure is present postoperatively but can be controlled. This valvulectomy approach is not favored. The incidence and severity of hepatic congestion are manifestly high, and reoperation for subsequent valve replacement is tedious, with considerable blood loss. For initial tricuspid valve endocarditis, intensive medical therapy is advocated. If operative intervention is necessary, valve replacement is done and aggressive counseling is offered to prevent further drug abuse.

Selected Bibliography

Boyd, A. D., Engelman, R. M., Isom, O. W., et al: Tricuspid annuloplasty: Five and one-half years' experience with 78 patients. J. Thorac. Cardiovasc. Surg., 68:344, 1974.

Boyd and colleagues at New York University Hospitals reported 78 tricuspid annuloplasties and 90 tricuspid valve replacements done in association with mitral or mitral and aortic valve procedures. Tricuspid insufficiency was not recognized preoperatively, either clinically or by cardiac catheterization, in 35% of these patients. This finding emphasizes the importance of routine digital palpation of the tricuspid valve. The hospital mortality was 14% in the group having annuloplasty and 34% in the group having replacement. Late survival of the patients having annuloplasty was perhaps slightly better than in those having tricuspid valve replacement.

Braunwald, N. S., Ross, J., and Morrow, A. G.: Conservative management of tricuspid regurgitation in patients undergoing mitral valve replacement. Circulation, 35 and 36(Suppl. I):63, 69, 1966.

Braunwald and colleagues at the National Institutes of Health were perhaps among the first to characterize functional tricuspid regurgitation. They reported 28 patients having mitral valve replacement. Twenty-five patients had no operative procedure on the tricuspid valve, and three had a tricuspid annuloplasty. Four patients died. Of the 24 survivors, 21 patients were asymptomatic and functional Class I or II. Mean right atrial pressures had an average of 5 mm Hg, and systolic pulmonary artery pressures had an average of 39 mm Hg, postoperatively. The authors concluded that in many patients who have a satisfactory left heart procedure, functional tricuspid regurgitation of mild, moderate, or even severe degree regresses postoperatively.

Bibliography

Arbulu, A., and Asfaw, I.: Tricuspid valvulectomy without prosthetic replacement: Ten years of clinical experience. J. Thorac. Cardiovasc. Surg., 82:684, 1981.
Baughman, K. L., Kallman, C. H., Yurchak, P. M., et al: Predictors of survival after tricuspid valve surgery. Am. J. Cardiol., 54:137, 1984.
Duran, C. M. G., Pomar, J. L., Colman, T., et al: Is tricuspid valve repair necessary? J. Thorac. Cardiovasc. Surg., 80:849, 1980.
Stephenson, L. W., Kouchoukos, N. T., and Kirklin, J. W.: Triple-valve replacement: An analysis of eight years' experience. Ann. Thorac. Surg., 23:327, 1977.

CHAPTER 50

ACQUIRED DISEASE OF THE MITRAL VALVE

Frank C. Spencer

HISTORICAL ASPECTS

In 1923, after detailed pathologic studies of diseased mitral valves, Cutler and Levine made a bold effort to perform mitral valvulotomy for mitral stenosis but, unfortunately, reasoned erroneously that resection of part of the stenosed valve was necessary. The first patient survived, but the next several died from insufficiency; thus the procedure was abandoned. In England, a digital commissurotomy was done in 1925 by Souttar on one patient, but for obscure reasons, no further commissurotomies were attempted. The field then remained static for more than 20 years, until Harken and associates (1948) and Bailey (1949) independently showed the feasibility and value of digital commissurotomy. This advance was dramatic because mitral stenosis was inevitably a fatal disease from either recurrent heart failure or cerebral emboli. Impressive results were quickly obtained in hundreds of patients and resulted in widespread adoption of the procedure throughout the world.

Because of the limitations of the extent to which the stenosed valve could be opened by digital commissurotomy, the stenosis recurred in as many as 50% of the patients within 4 to 5 years. In the following decade, a mitral valve dilator was developed in England by Tubbs (Logan and Turner, 1959). This permitted a more extensive commissurotomy, although mitral insufficiency resulted in a significant percentage of patients.

Open heart surgery had become feasible by this time, with the first successful operation by Gibbon in 1953, and the independent important achievements by Lillehei and Kirklin in 1955. Thus, there was increasing interest in the performance of commissurotomy by an open technique. Initially, the complications of cardiopulmonary bypass made the closed digital commissurotomy a safer procedure, but with improvements in cardiopulmonary bypass, an open valvulotomy with cardiopulmonary bypass was adopted in most centers by 1970 to 1972. Only in areas where a heart-lung machine is not available is digital commissurotomy still done with any frequency.

With mitral insufficiency, none of the ingenious closed techniques attempted before 1955 proved durable. With cardiopulmonary bypass (1955), different forms of annuloplasty were tried in many patients. Lillehei and Merendino independently described a selective form of annuloplasty in 1957. In 1960 McGoon described an effective technique for localized plication of a flail segment of mitral valve from ruptured chordae. However, nothing could be done for most patients. An intensive search in many cardiac laboratories was quickly initiated to develop a prosthetic mitral valve. The important accomplishment was the development of the ball valve prosthesis in 1961 by Starr and Edwards, who was a mechanical engineer. This finding launched the modern era of prosthetic valve replacement. They correctly reasoned from the earlier work of Hufnagel, who implanted a ball valve in the descending aorta of patients with aortic insufficiency without the use of a heart-lung machine, that a ball valve prosthesis could be successfully implanted. With the Starr-Edwards ball valve prosthesis, successful valve replacement became possible for the first time.

Since that time many types of ball valves and disk valves have been developed, but the ideal valve, durable but not requiring anticoagulants, still does not exist. The original ball valve initially had problems with the Silastic ball but these problems were corrected by 1966. The Silastic ball prosthesis developed near that time (Model No. 6120) is still one of the most durable and reliable prostheses used.

Disk prostheses, popularized by Björk in the 1960s, were later widely used. By 1979, Björk reported that more than 200,000 disk prostheses had been implanted. Because of problems with strut fracture in some patients in particular models of the Björk prostheses, combined with complex medicolegal concerns, the prosthesis has been temporarily withdrawn from the market but will, undoubtedly, be available soon. The most popular disk prosthesis is the St. Jude bileaflet prosthesis that was introduced in 1977. The results have been very good although little better than those of other types of disk prostheses. Unfortunately, all metallic prostheses require permanent anticoagulation to minimize the frequency of thromboembolism. Anticoagulant therapy has the associated hazard of hemorrhage. Even with ideal anticoagulant therapy, maintaining the prothrombin time one and one-half to two times normal, there is still a small but definite danger of thromboembolism or hemorrhage from anticoagulants. These two dangers clearly show the importance of permanent medical supervision of patients with prosthetic valves. A collective review by Edmunds in 1987 gave an excellent summary of the frequency of thrombotic and bleeding complications with different types of prosthetic valves.

Since the late 1960s, different types of tissue valves have been investigated, because it was quickly found that tissue valves have a lower frequency of thromboembolism and that they often do not require anticoagulants. Valves constructed from autogenous fascia lata or homologous dura mater were used for several years but have been discarded because of the high frequency of deterioration in less than 10 years. Homograft and heterograft valves have also been used widely but all ultimately failed because of fibrosis with stenosis or insufficiency until the glutaraldehyde-preserved porcine prosthesis was developed in the late 1960s, primarily by Carpentier in Paris and Hancock in the United States. Once the surprising 5-year durability, almost 95%, was established, this prosthesis was used widely because it usually did not require anticoagulant therapy. In 1986 experiences with 1,643 porcine prostheses implanted at New York University (NYU), between 1976 and 1983, were reported. Long-term durability, however, has been disappointing because 15 to 20% of prostheses failed within 10 years, and Magilligan reported in 1988 a 15-year failure rate exceeding 50%. Ionescu, in Leeds, England, developed glutaraldehyde-preserved valves constructed from bovine pericardium. Reul in 1985 reported experiences in which this prosthesis was implanted in 2,680 patients. Unfortunately, there was a high frequency of calcification and disruption within a few years; thus, the popularity of this prosthesis has greatly declined.

At NYU both metallic and porcine prostheses are widely used, and the patient is actively allowed to help to choose the prosthesis. If anticoagulant therapy can be safely taken, depending primarily on environmental and socioeconomic factors, a metallic prosthesis is recommended for most patients who are under 60 to 65 years of age. In older patients, with the attendant increased frequency of both stroke and hypertension, a porcine prosthesis is commonly recommended, but exceptions often occur. With porcine prostheses it is emphasized to all patients that there is at least a 20% probability that the prosthesis will require replacement within 10 years. Some young athletic patients insist on a porcine prosthesis and accept the probability of reoperation at some time during the next 10 to 15 years. Some older

patients, however, insist on a metallic prosthesis, rather than living with the possibility of the repeat operation at some time in the future.

After 1961, with a few exceptions, interest in mitral reconstruction sharply decreased for more than 20 years. Fortunately, at least three groups continued reconstruction with selected patients. The technique reported in 1960 by McGoon was used selectively at the Mayo Clinic; by 1985 Orzulak reported experiences with a total of 131 patients.

In 1963 Kay and Egerton described a technique of annuloplasty combined with repair of ruptured chordae. In 1986 Kay reported a repair in 101 of 141 patients treated for mitral regurgitation secondary to coronary disease.

Reed at NYU reported in 1965 an asymmetric exaggerated mitral annuloplasty that he has used since that time in selected patients with good results. A 17-year experience with 196 patients was reported in 1980 with a late mortality of 8.7% and only six arterial emboli. Reoperation was necessary in only 11 patients, six of whom were treated by a second repair. This technique has been useful primarily in children and young adults with pure mitral insufficiency.

In the 1970s, major contributions to the technique of mitral reconstruction were made by Carpentier in France and Duran in Spain. Initially, reconstruction consisted of a tailored annuloplasty ring; however, a most important step was the development of a method of quadrantic excision of diseased segments of mural leaflet as well as techniques of chordae shortening or leaflet transposition. These methods are well described in the report by Carpentier (1983) in his "Honored Guest Address" to the American Association for Thoracic Surgery.

Since 1980, under the leadership of Colvin at NYU, the Carpentier techniques of mitral reconstruction have been used with increasing frequency; current experiences include more than 300 patients. These experiences have been reported occasionally by this writer and by Galloway, and they are discussed in more detail in the section on mitral valve reconstruction.

MITRAL STENOSIS

Etiology and Pathology

Rheumatic fever is the only known cause of mitral stenosis, although a definite clinical history can be obtained in only about 50% of patients. For unknown reasons, women are affected more frequently than men. With the widespread effective prophylaxis of rheumatic fever in children for the previous decades, the frequency of mitral stenosis has decreased greatly in the United States, although in many areas of the world with limited health facilities, such as India and South Africa, mitral stenosis of advanced degree is commonly seen in childhood. Congenital mitral stenosis is rare. Less than 150 cases were found in the review by Tsuji and associates in 1967.

Although the rheumatic inflammatory process is a pancarditis involving the endocardium, myocardium, and pericardium, permanent injury is almost always limited to the cardiac valve. Rheumatic myocarditis is apparently seldom of permanent harm, although there is a puzzling, unexplained variation in cardiac reserve among patients after mitral replacement that could conceivably be caused by injury from a previous myocarditis.

Rheumatic valvulitis produces at least three distinct pathologic changes, with the degree varying widely among patients: fusion of the valve leaflets along the commissures; fibrosis of the leaflets with stiffening, retraction, and ultimate calcification; and fusion and shortening of the chordae tendineae. The more extensive changes are usually seen in patients with recurrent attacks of rheumatic fever.

Fusion of the valve leaflets is the most common result of rheumatic inflammation, because the endocardium ulcerates where the two leaflets normally oppose in systole. If commissural fusion alone is present, excellent results can be obtained by commissurotomy. However, if the valve leaflets have become fibrotic, contracted, and calcified, restoration of pliable valve leaflets is impossible and prosthetic replacement is necessary. An intermediate form of injury exists in which the underlying chordae tendineae are fibrotic and shortened. Often, by surgically separating these fused and divided chordae, perhaps combined with a form of annuloplasty if insufficiency is present, valve replacement can be avoided, although the long-term course of these diseased valves is uncertain. A large number, however, have functioned satisfactorily for more than 5 years.

After an initial attack of rheumatic fever, the pathologic changes often progress slowly, evolving over decades. Symptoms may not appear for 10 to 15 years. The process is apparently an initial fusion of the commissures followed by progressive fibrosis and stiffening of the commissures, underlying chordae, and valve leaflets. It is a remarkable biologic phenomenon to see patients in the fifth, sixth, or seventh decade of life with severe mitral stenosis, which apparently is the result of having rheumatic fever as a child. This late development, similar to that which occurs in some patients with mild congenital aortic stenosis, is probably the result of stiffening and fibrosis from turbulent flow of blood. This concept was proposed by Selzer and Cohen in 1972.

With recurrent episodes of untreated rheumatic fever, however, a totally different course evolves. Gross valvular destruction and calcification may develop by 10 to 12 years of age. This is rare with modern therapy in the United States but is commonly seen in Africa and India.

Pathophysiology

Although the cross-sectional area of the normal mitral valve is between 4 and 6 cm^2, varying with body size, significant hemodynamic changes do not appear until the cross-sectional area is reduced to less than 2 to 2.5 cm^2. Patients with this mild degree of mitral stenosis may have classic physical findings but become symptomatic only with extreme exertion (Class I). With more severe reduction in cross-sectional area to between 1 and 2 cm^2, symptoms appear more readily with lesser degrees of exertion (Class II). A patient with a mitral valve opening as small as 1 cm^2 is usually symptomatic at rest (Class III). An opening near 0.5 cm^2 is said to be about the smallest size compatible with life (Class IV).

The dominant physiologic change with mitral stenosis is a chronic increase in mean left atrial pressure above the normal limit of 10 to 12 mm Hg. Many of the symptoms of mitral stenosis can be interpreted as resulting from this chronic elevation in left atrial pressure. The restriction to flow of blood into the left ventricle from the mitral stenosis also causes a reduction in cardiac output and, in some patients (discussed later), an increase in pulmonary vascular resistance. In addition, the chronic elevation in left atrial pressure leads to the sequential changes of left atrial hypertrophy, atrial fibrillation, and, eventually, development of mural thrombi and systemic embolism.

The degree of increase in left atrial pressure above the normal limit of 10 to 12 mm Hg varies with three factors: the severity of the mitral stenosis, the cardiac output, and the cardiac rate, which determines the duration of diastolic filling of the left ventricle. Accordingly, any measurement of left atrial pressure must be related to the cardiac output. The most precise physiologic measurement is the cross-sectional area of the valve, calculated from the pressure gradient across the stenotic valve in combination with the cardiac output. Elevation in atrial pressure to levels of 15 to 20 mm Hg is commonly found at catheterization in patients with moderately severe stenosis. If mean left atrial pressure exceeds 30 mm Hg, above the oncotic pressure of plasma, transudation of fluid into the pulmonary interstitial tissues occurs. Pulmonary edema may or may not develop, depending on the transport capacity of the pulmonary lymphatic circulation.

Thus, the dominant symptoms of mitral stenosis are those of pulmonary congestion, such as cough, hemoptysis, orthopnea, paroxysmal nocturnal dyspnea, and pulmonary edema.

Because mitral stenosis restricts the flow of blood into the left ventricle, this chamber is often small and appears to be underdeveloped. Thus, patients with mitral stenosis may be treated medically for many years, using different measures to limit exercise activities and to avoid the accumulation of fluid in the lungs.

The decrease in cardiac output from restriction of flow through the stenotic orifice leads to fatigue, weakness, and the muscular wasting typically seen with cardiac cachexia. Any attempt by the patient to increase cardiac output with exercise results in severe dyspnea. The patient quickly learns to avoid such exertion. The widely recognized classic symptom of mitral stenosis, therefore, is "dyspnea on exertion." Patients with severe mitral stenosis may live for many years with a sedentary, semi-invalid type of existence.

The left atrial hypertension often produces pulmonary vasoconstriction and an increase in pulmonary vascular resistance. Hypertrophy of the intima and media of the pulmonary arterioles may be found on histologic studies of the lung, but permanent organic obstruction probably results principally from pulmonary emboli and thrombosis. There is great variation among individual patients in the degree of increase in pulmonary vascular resistance; probably more than 50% of patients never develop any significant increase, whereas others may develop an increase in resistance four to five times greater than normal, with pulmonary artery systolic pressures as great as 100 to 140 mm Hg. Fortunately, in the majority, the increase in vascular resistance subsides greatly after operation, in sharp contrast to the grim picture in congenital heart disease, in which elevated pulmonary vascular resistance is often an irreversible disease. A corollary to this fortunate fact is that pulmonary hypertension from mitral stenosis in adults, although it increases the operative risk, is never per se a contraindication to operation. Associated hypertrophy of the right ventricle, however, makes it necessary to protect the right ventricle as well as the left ventricle while the aorta is occluded at operation.

In 1988 Camara reported experiences with 88 patients with severe pulmonary hypertension treated for 10 years. Average systolic pulmonary artery pressure was 95 mm Hg, pressures ranging from 70 to 180 mm Hg. Operative mortality was 5%. On later follow-up, during an average of more than 4 years, excellent results were usually obtained. Only six late deaths were reported. With recatheterization in 14 patients there was an average decrease in systolic pressure from a mean preoperative value of almost 100 to approximately 40 mm Hg.

Eventually, as mentioned earlier, atrial fibrillation develops from hypertrophy of the smooth muscle of the left atrial wall. Cardiac output decreases 10 to 15% when this occurs, but the most serious complication is the development of thrombi from stasis in the left atrium. Rarely, huge thrombi, 5 to 10 cm in diameter, develop and almost fill the left atrial cavity. Systemic emboli, especially to the brain, are a constant threat and constitute a major indication for early operation, because the likelihood of systemic embolism can never be predicted. Emboli after successful commissurotomy, with closure of the atrial appendage, are rare, even though atrial fibrillation persists (Fig. 50–1).

Diagnostic Considerations

As mentioned earlier, the characteristic symptom of mitral stenosis is dyspnea on exertion. Often, this is the only symptom, except for general weakness and fatigue. The severity of mitral stenosis correlates to some degree with the degree of exertion required to produce dyspnea. As the symptoms of mitral stenosis primarily result from pulmonary congestion, the type of symptom varies with the effect of gravity on body fluids. Dyspnea that appears in a patient in the supine position is called orthopnea. At night, there may be paroxysmal nocturnal dyspnea or even pulmonary edema. Fortunately, hemoptysis, which is an alarming symptom, is rarely of great magnitude. Occasionally, it is severe enough to require urgent mitral commissurotomy to prevent death from asphyxia.

When right-sided heart failure develops, the familiar findings of chronic congestive failure with hepatomegaly, engorged veins, and peripheral edema gradually appear. With right-sided heart failure, pulmonary hypertension or tricuspid insufficiency is commonly present.

On physical examination, patients with chronic mitral stenosis are often thin and frail with diffuse muscular atrophy, which is a reflection of long-standing restriction of cardiac output. These chronic metabolic abnormalities, often reflected by anergy to skin tests and a negative nitrogen balance, decrease the overall tolerance to operation and increase the susceptibility to infection.

If right-sided heart failure has developed, engorged cervical veins, hepatomegaly, and peripheral edema are evident. Rubor or cyanosis of the lips, cheeks, and fingers is distinctive in some, a manifestation of increased oxygen extraction from the slow rate of blood flow through the peripheral capillaries because of the low cardiac output. The pulse is decreased in volume and is often irregular from atrial fibrillation. On examination of the chest, basilar inspiratory rales are frequently heard.

An important point to emphasize is that the size of the heart is usually normal and has an apical impulse of normal or decreased intensity. This occurs, of course, because the left ventricle is small. Finding a forceful apical impulse immediately suggests that additional valvular disease, such as mitral insufficiency or aortic valvular disease, has produced hypertrophy of the left ventricle. If pulmonary hypertension has produced hypertrophy of the right ventricle, a forceful systolic impulse may be palpable in the left parasternal area.

The three characteristic auscultatory findings of mitral stenosis, called "the auscultatory triad," include an apical diastolic rumble, an increased first sound, and an opening snap. These are sufficiently characteristic to establish the diagnosis with an accuracy of almost 100% on physical examination alone. The apical diastolic rumble, produced by blood flowing through the stenotic orifice, may be sharply localized to an area at the apex that is no larger than 1 inch in diameter. The intensity varies, usually Grade II or III, but in some patients, it is loud enough to produce a palpable thrill. However, the intensity

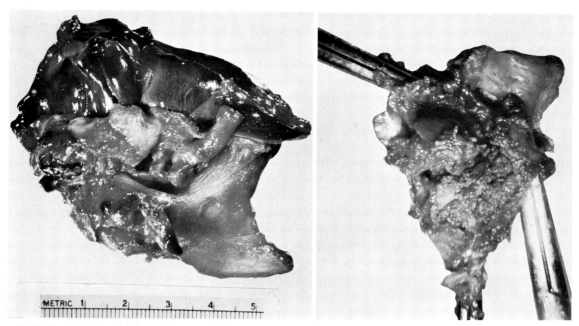

Figure 50–1. Massive left atrial thrombi removed from two patients during cardiopulmonary bypass. The thrombi almost filled the left atrial cavity and would obviously have led to catastrophic results if closed digital commissurotomy had been attempted.

of the murmur does not correlate with the severity of the stenosis. In some very advanced cases with a calcified immobile valve, so-called "silent" mitral stenosis is present, with no murmur detectable even by phonocardiography.

The increased first sound, probably resulting from thickening of the mitral leaflets, is one of the earliest findings. The opening snap can be identified on careful examination in most patients but is absent with rigid, immobile leaflets. A short apical systolic murmur occurs frequently and has little significance, but a loud pansystolic murmur, transmitted to the axilla, usually indicates mitral insufficiency. Associated tricuspid insufficiency may produce a systolic murmur near the apex, but usually, the murmur is loudest near the xiphoid process and characteristically varies with inspiration.

Several abnormalities are seen on the chest film. The earliest change is enlargement of the left atrium, typically seen on the posteroanterior film with a double contour visible behind the right atrial shadow (Fig. 50–2A). The earliest enlargement of the left atrium can be determined by the lateral film exposed during a barium swallow, showing concave indentation of the middle third of the esophagus (Fig. 50–2B). However, with the simplicity and precision of echocardiography, this test is now seldom done.

The overall cardiac size is often normal, but the enlargement of the left atrium and pulmonary artery obliterates the normal concavity between the aorta and the left ventricle, producing a "straight" left border of the heart. Calcification of the mitral valve, very extensive in an occasional patient, can be readily detected. In the pulmonary fields, several abnormalities result from pulmonary congestion. These include distention of the pulmonary arteries and veins,

engorgement of pulmonary lymphatics, and pleural effusion. Engorged pulmonary lymphatics, often termed "Kerley's lines," are seen with severe mitral stenosis and can be recognized as distinct horizontal linear opacities in the lower pulmonary fields.

The electrocardiogram is an inaccurate guide to assessment of the severity of the mitral stenosis and may be completely normal, even in patients with severe disease. An increased amplitude of the P wave from hypertrophy of the left atrium is the earliest change, but the changes are not consistent enough to have clinical value. Signs of right ventricular hypertrophy appear if there is an increase in pulmonary vascular resistance. If left ventricular hypertrophy is seen on the electrocardiogram, some disease other than isolated mitral stenosis, such as mitral insufficiency or aortic valvular disease, is probably present.

Echocardiography has become a valuable noninvasive technique for evaluating changes with mitral stenosis, measuring the cross-sectional area of the valve as well as the size of the left atrium and the left ventricle. This is discussed in detail in the section on mitral insufficiency later in the chapter.

Cardiac catheterization and angiography are unnecessary to establish the diagnosis of mitral stenosis but should be done routinely to evaluate associated diseases, such as pulmonary hypertension, mitral insufficiency, coronary disease, or aortic disease. This information, of course, has particular value in estimating the risk of operation, the likelihood of benefit, and the likelihood of prosthetic valve replacement being required. For example, if significant mitral insufficiency is present with severe calcification, prosthetic replacement is usually necessary. The significant points that can be determined from catheter-

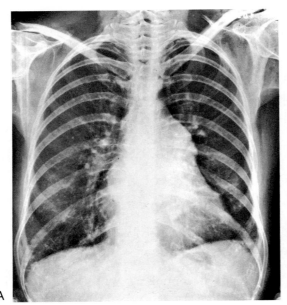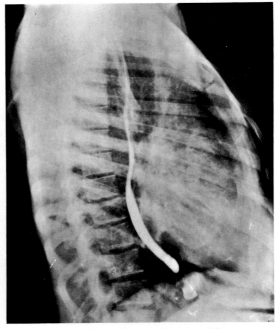

Figure 50–2. *A*, Chest film of a patient with mitral stenosis showing a heart of normal size. The prominent pulmonary artery along the left cardiac border is characteristic of this condition. The enlarged left atrium can be seen as a double density behind the shadow normally formed by the right atrium. *B*, Lateral roentgenogram of the same patient showing enlargement of the left atrium producing a concave displacement of the barium-filled esophagus.

ization include not only the presence of mitral stenosis and insufficiency, but also the presence of aortic stenosis and insufficiency; the nature of left ventricular function, reflected by left ventricular end-diastolic pressure, ejection fraction, and cardiac index; the presence of pulmonary hypertension; and the presence of coronary artery disease or calcification in the mitral valve or other areas.

Tricuspid stenosis or insufficiency may be difficult to detect on cardiac catheterization. Thus, an important routine is to always palpate the tricuspid valve at the time of operation by insertion of a finger through the right atrial appendage before the venous cannula is inserted.

OPERATIVE TREATMENT

Indications for Operation

In general, the author strongly believes that most patients with hemodynamically significant mitral stenosis (cross-sectional area less than 1.5 cm²) should be operated on, even though they are asymptomatic, unless concomitant disease creates a serious operative risk (Spencer, 1978). This opinion is in the minority and is not shared by many cardiologists because patients with few symptoms may be managed medically for years. However, during this time, there are two serious insidious dangers. The risk of cerebral embolism is always present, even though small as long as the patient is in sinus rhythm. Also, the turbulent flow of blood through the stenotic

orifice produces a relentless progressive deterioration of the valve from fibrosis and eventual calcification. These badly diseased valves must usually be replaced, but more than 90% of valves with less extensive injury can be treated effectively by commissurotomy.

The risk of early operation is very small, well under 1%, with a likelihood exceeding 90% that a commissurotomy can be done. Kirklin and Barratt-Boyes (1986) reported that only one death occurred after 259 operations done over a period of several years. Early commissurotomy, combined with obliteration of the atrial appendage, also provides marked protection from arterial embolism. Excellent long-term results in a group of 202 patients treated at NYU were reported by Gross and associates in 1981. Although uncommon, a grim clinical experience is seeing a patient who was asymptomatic until a massive cerebral embolus produced massive hemiplegia with aphasia and permanent neurologic deficit. Rarely such a patient is unaware of the presence of heart disease until the embolus occurs. Thus, this is one of the reasons why early operation is recommended for asymptomatic patients with hemodynamically significant mitral stenosis, similar to the policy followed for decades in children with atrial septal defects.

At the other extreme, it should be emphasized that patients rarely have such far advanced disease that operation cannot be done. Even in Class IV and Class V patients with mitral disease, with cardiac cachexia and massive ascites, operative risk with modern techniques is seldom more than 10%. Remarkable improvement can be obtained, although long-term results in these patients are inferior to those in patients operated on at an early stage. Five-year survival in Class IV patients is almost 60% compared with 90 to 95% in Class II patients.

The risk of operation in Class IV patients can be greatly reduced by intensive therapy with bedrest, nutritional support, and intensive diuresis for several days or even weeks before operation. The duration of effective preoperative therapy varies widely; thus, a fixed schedule cannot be planned. It should be continued for as long as the patient continues to improve, manifested by resolution of peripheral edema. Patients ultimately reach a plateau, at which time operation should be done. The most remarkable example seen in the author's medical center during the last two decades was a patient operated on several years ago. This patient lost *80 pounds* of edema fluid with intensive diuretic therapy over 2 months. Her later convalescence after mitral valve replacement was uneventful. She left the hospital in 2 weeks and later remained in good condition for the next few years.

Open Versus Closed Commissurotomy or Balloon Valvuloplasty

As stated earlier, since 1970 to 1972, an open approach for mitral commissurotomy has been used in most cardiac centers. There are several reasons why a closed commissurotomy is an inferior operation and should be done only in emergency cases such as severe cardiac failure with pregnancy or because of unavailability of a heart-lung machine. With open commissurotomy the operative risk is less than 1%, which is actually less than with closed commissurotomy. The risk of cerebral embolism is also less, almost 0%. Furthermore, a more effective commissurotomy can be done by separating fused chordae tendineae as well as fused commissures; mitral insufficiency, if present, can be precisely evaluated and treated. Results are described in a later section.

The goal with radical open valvuloplasty is not to simply open the valve enough to correct stenosis but to open it as widely as possible without producing insufficiency. The objective is not only to eliminate the diastolic gradient but also to minimize the turbulent flow of blood across the diseased mitral orifice. A mitral valve orifice enlarged to 2 cm^2 may have a good symptomatic result for a few years but is still much smaller than a normal mitral valve. The mediocre results that follow a limited mitral commissurotomy became abundantly clear in the 1950s. Despite widespread use of digital commissurotomy with excellent short-term results, as late as 1961 mitral stenosis recurred within 5 years in 20 to 50% of patients. It is now well known that this high frequency of "restenosis" was simply a progression of residual stenosis remaining after the initial limited

valvulotomy. Restenosis of a mitral valve after an extensive commissurotomy that eliminates the end-diastolic gradient is almost unknown.

These considerations are especially pertinent with the enthusiasm in several centers for balloon valvuloplasty, introduced in the last few years. This technique is valuable for a patient with associated diseases that create a serious operative risk, but the procedure has all of the limitations of the older closed commissurotomy and also does nothing to protect against future cerebral emboli from the fibrillating left atrial appendage. In all likelihood significant restenosis will occur within 5 years in a large number of patients; thus, in the good-risk patient, there would seem to be little justification to do a balloon valvuloplasty rather than an open commissurotomy.

The technique used at NYU for open mitral commissurotomy was first described by Mullin in 1974. In recent years, experiences gained with Carpentier's techniques of mitral reconstruction for mitral insufficiency have led to performance of an even more radical commissurotomy, including selective debridement of calcium and division of shortened secondary chordae that limit motion of the mural leaflet.

A median sternotomy incision is used. The tricuspid valve is palpated with a finger introduced through the right atrial appendage to detect insufficiency or stenosis. The thickness of the right atrial wall is a useful guide because an atrial wall of normal thickness indicates that any tricuspid insufficiency detected is probably of recent origin and will regress with correction of the mitral disease.

The bypass technique is a standard one with sufficient heparinization to produce an activated clotting time of more than 400 seconds, usually at least 4 mg/kg of heparin. Arterial cannulation is in the ascending aorta with separate cannulation of the venae cavae for venous return. The oxygenator is a membrane or a bubble oxygenator primed with a balanced crystalloid solution, almost 40 ml/kg of patient's body weight. Flow rate is almost 2.5 l/m^2/min at a temperature of almost 25° C. Blood is added to the perfusate if the hematocrit decreases below 20%. Once bypass is established, the aorta is clamped and cold potassium cardioplegia is induced by injecting 1,000 to 1,500 ml of cold blood (4 to 6° C) with potassium 30 to 35 mEq/l. The cold blood cardioplegia technique developed jointly at NYU and University of California at Los Angeles (UCLA) is used.

Once the heart has been arrested, sufficient blood is infused to confirm that all areas of the heart are cooled to at least 15° C. Temperatures are measured with a needle thermistor. After infusion of sufficient cold blood, the heart is wrapped in a laparotomy tape and cold electrolyte solution (4° C) infused onto the surface of the right ventricle, approximately 1 liter every 5 to 15 minutes, removing fluid from the operative field through a sump placed at the bottom of the pericardial cavity. This method of continuous topical hypothermia is particularly valuable for patients with hypertrophy of the right ventricle from pulmonary hypertension. Otherwise, this hypertrophied right ventricle is vulnerable to rewarming from lights in the operating room and other factors. With this technique the intramyocardial temperature usually remains well below 15° C. Six hundred to 800 ml of cold blood is reinfused every 30 minutes. Unless topical hypothermia is used, the myocardium may gradually rewarm because of the aorta lying posteriorly, the diaphragm inferiorly, and the operating room lights above. In all probability, this rewarming is the origin of right-sided heart failure reported by others in some patients after bypass; this is almost never seen at NYU.

Once the heart has been arrested and cooled, the left atrium is opened with a longitudinal incision in the interatrial groove, extending the atriotomy beneath and to the left of both the superior and inferior vena cava. The Carpentier mitral retractor (Fig. 50–3) is particularly valuable for providing adequate exposure, because its design permits multiple adjustments of the different blades. The crucial consideration is to adjust the tips of the retractor blades to apply traction to the atrial wall approximately 2 cm superior to the mitral annulus, usually well exposing the mitral ring.

Initially, the atrial cavity is examined for thrombi, especially inside the atrial appendage (see Fig. 50–1). Subsequently, for more than a decade, the atrial appendage has been excluded from the left atrium by closing the orifice with a continuous suture of 3-0 Prolene. This suture is placed carefully in a horizontal direction, not far beneath the endocardium, so that the shaft of the needle is faintly visible. This direction of needle insertion is parallel to the course of the circumflex coronary artery and has been uniformly safe. No problems have occurred in more than a decade, which refutes the myth that closure of the atrial appendage is inherently dangerous. Unless the appendage is closed, the patient naturally is still at risk after operation from emboli developing within the fibrillating appendage. The hazard of a fibrillating appendage has been seen at operation many times, and thrombi have been found only within the appendage. Usually, these are attached to the atrial endocardium but in some patients, for unknown reasons, thrombi 3 to 5 mm in diameter have been found lying "free" in the cavity of the appendage. The reason why these thrombi are not fused to the endocardium is unclear, but the frightful possibility is obvious that these emboli would be expelled quickly from the appendage if atrial contractions returned with a sinus rhythm.

After closure of the appendage, the mitral valve is exposed with a "triple right angle" technique. A suture is inserted in each leaflet, which, in turn, is grasped with a right angle clamp to apply "horizontal" traction to the leaflet, compared with simple vertical traction (Fig. 50–4). The application of horizontal traction stretches the leaflets and facilitates identification of the commissures. Several landmarks

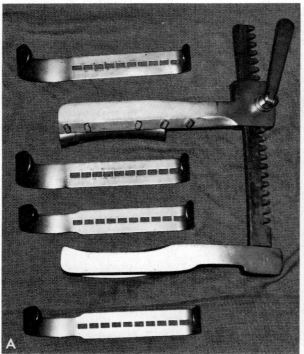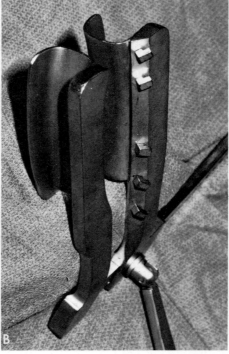

Figure 50–3. *A,* The sternal retractor developed by Carpentier in Paris with a variety of blades that can be attached to facilitate exposure of the mitral valve, greatly enhancing techniques of reconstruction. The instrument is very useful, with five different areas on the blades where the retractors can be attached with different degrees of tension. Adequate exposure is essential for complex techniques of reconstruction, even more so than for simple prosthetic replacement. *B,* Side view of the same instrument.

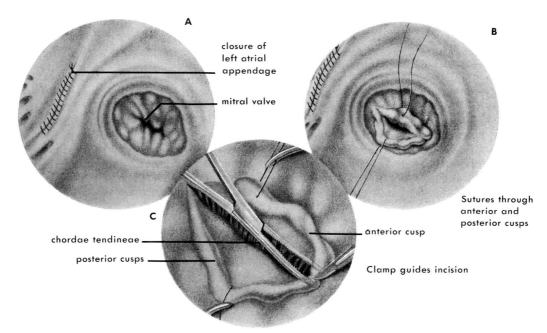

Figure 50–4. *A,* Closure of left atrial appendage. *B,* Exposure of mitral valve with horizontal traction on sutures. *C,* Third right-angle clamp guides incision.

identify a commissure, such as the "depressed trench" where the leaflets are fused, characterized by thickened tissue that is quite different in color and texture from the adjacent leaflets. A wide variation in visual appearance occurs, however. The fused commissures are immediately obvious in many patients. In other patients, the exact site of fusion must be determined carefully because landmarks have been obscured by the inflammatory process.

Once the commissure has been identified, the third right-angled clamp is introduced beneath the fused commissure between the chordae, and the blades are spread sufficiently to stretch the fused commissure. The commissure can then be carefully incised with a knife, 2 to 3 mm at a time, serially confirming that the separated margins of the commissure are attached to chordae tendineae. The usual commissurotomy curves anteriorly and does not go directly laterally.

Occasionally, landmarks are grossly distorted, and the leaflets fuse directly to underlying papillary muscles from shortening or obliteration of chordae tendineae. The suggestion made by Carpentier of starting the incision laterally, beyond the site of fusion with the papillary muscle, is followed. A stab wound is made in the commissure with a No. 15 small blade, after which the stab wound can be separated slightly with forceps and the incision can be carefully extended to the free margin of the mitral orifice, identifying and protecting the underlying chordae and subsequently incising the fused papillary muscle for 5 to 10 mm (Fig. 50–5).

The technique is a delicate one and requires a dry operative field with excellent exposure and careful identification of all structures before any incision is made. An incorrect incision, with division of chor-

dae tendineae, often results in insufficiency from a flail leaflet that may require prosthetic replacement. This precise technique is obviously inconsistent with the published reports from some institutions of doing an open commissurotomy in a few minutes.

In all operations, both commissures are opened as widely as possible, stopping a few millimeters from the valve annulus where the valve tissue becomes thin. This is the normal anatomic change and indicates the transition from the fused commissure to the normal commissural leaflet of the mitral valve.

Leaflet mobility is assessed after completion of commissurotomy and division of underlying chordae. Restricted motion may be improved by further separation of fused chordae or splitting the underlying papillary muscle. Shortened secondary chordae to the mural leaflet of the mitral valve may be divided and this was recommended by Carpentier. In a few patients, careful debridement of calcium from the leaflets with rongeurs and bone curette is feasible and obviously has the risk of perforation of the leaflet. The importance of doing more than a simple commissurotomy is evident from the operative records, which indicate that in more than 30% of patients more than a simple commissurotomy is needed and the procedure usually consists of separation of underlying fused chordae and splitting of papillary muscles. This observation was recorded by Roe in 1971.

After completion of the valvuloplasty, the presence of any mitral insufficiency can be visually assessed by inspection of the apposition of the valve leaflets when saline is injected forcefully into the ventricle to distend and coapt the leaflets. This is the standard technique used with the Carpentier reconstruction for mitral insufficiency and has been quite

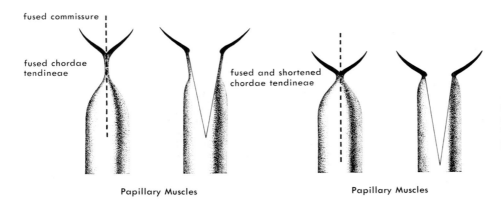

Figure 50–5. A, Separation of fused chordae tendineae with incision into papillary muscle. B, Deeper incision into papillary muscle when valve leaflets are fused to underlying papillary muscle.

reliable. The more cumbersome technique of retrograde insertion of a catheter with multiple perforations through a stab wound in the aorta across the aortic valve to distend the mitral leaflets is no longer used. If localized insufficiency exists, a selected annuloplasty can be done.

Thus, the absence of significant insufficiency is confirmed by digitally palpating the mitral valve with the heart beating and a systolic pressure near the preoperative level. This is done by introducing a finger through the untied suture line in the left atrium.

After commissurotomy, as the incision in the left atrium is sutured, a plastic catheter is placed across the mitral valve and is fixed into position to facilitate later removal of air. After the suture line is completed, fibrillation is induced and the aorta is unclamped. Air is then serially removed from different cardiac chambers by applying gentle suction to the catheter in the left atrium and ventricle. In addition, before the heart is defibrillated, a small catheter is placed in the aortic root, the head is lowered, and the aorta is partly clamped, after which the heart is defibrillated. Gentle suction is applied jointly to both the small aortic catheter and the left atrial catheter for 4 to 5 minutes, during which time the contracting heart is filled with blood, the lungs are ventilated, and the left ventricle is vigorously manipulated and shaken to dislodge any bubbles of air. Any signs of air embolism are almost unknown with this technique.

After bypass, when normal cardiac contractility and blood pressure have returned, correction of the mitral stenosis is confirmed by measuring left atrial and ventricular end-diastolic pressure, showing that no gradient remains. A residual gradient of 4 to 6 mm may have to be accepted in some patients with thickened stiff leaflets but warns that prosthetic replacement may be necessary within a few years.

Technique of Operation. The initial approach for mitral valve replacement is identical to that described earlier for open mitral commissurotomy. The tricuspid valve is routinely palpated at the time of insertion of the venous cannulas. Hypothermic potassium cardioplegia, described in detail in the section on mitral

commissurotomy, has considerably increased the safety of mitral valve replacement. In patients without coronary disease, periods of aortic occlusion as long as 2 to 3 hours are surprisingly well tolerated. The actual limit of safe occlusion is uncertain, probably between 3 and 4 hours, but much shorter periods of occlusion, almost 60 minutes, are adequate for most patients. The influence of aortic cross-clamp time on mortality is nicely shown in a group of 445 patients (Fig. 50–6). An ischemic time more than 60 minutes increased the operative risk only in seriously ill preoperative patients, New York Heart Association (NYHA) Classes IV and V.

As stated earlier, the Carpentier type of mitral retractor provides excellent exposure (see Fig. 50–3). After the orifice of the atrial appendage has been closed with sutures, the diseased mitral valve is removed, incising the leaflet tissue 3 to 4 mm from the annulus. A potentially hazardous problem exists with densely calcified valves. In these cases the calcium can be transected with heavy scissors or rongeurs, after carefully identifying and protecting the ventricular wall. In a few patients, massive calcification, extending from the annulus down into the left ventricle, exists. These are difficult technical problems, but with appropriate time and care, enough calcified tissue can be removed to permit insertion of the prosthetic valve without injuring the wall of the left ventricle or losing calcium fragments that could cause emboli.

The chordae tendineae are divided near their junction with the papillary muscles, usually carefully preserving a few chordae to the annulus of the mural leaflet.

Preservation of some chordae to the annulus of the mural leaflet has two theoretical advantages: protection from postoperative rupture of the left ventricle, discussed later on, and improvement in left ventricular function. The latter concept was first proposed by Lillehei and associates in 1964 and has been discussed many times since then but has never been proved. Available data were summarized by Kirklin and Barratt-Boyes (1986) with the statement that the question remained unsettled. Both Hetzer and Borst in 1983 and David (1983 to 1986) have had

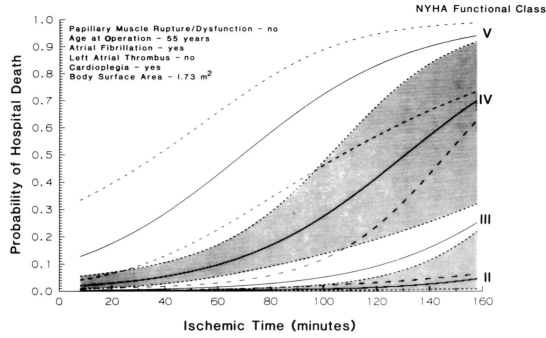

Figure 50–6. The interrelationship of the effect of aortic cross-clamp (ischemic) time and preoperative NYHA functional class on hospital mortality after isolated or combined primary mitral valve replacement using cold cardioplegic myocardial protection. The nomogram is based on the multivariate analysis shown in Table 11–8 of the source cited below (UAB; 1975—July 1979; $n = 445$; 20 events). The other values used in the equation are in the upper left corner of the figure. The mean value for age at operation among the 445 patients was 55 years, and that for body surface area was 1.73 m². The 70% confidence limits are indicated by the dashed lines, and those around NYHA Classes II and IV are crosshatched for ease of viewing. Note that with 60 minutes of ischemic time, the increased risk is evident only for NYHA Classes IV and V and that the increased risk of long cross-clamp (ischemic) time is only evident for functional Classes IV and V. (From Kirklin, J. W., and Barratt-Boyes, B. G.: Cardiac Surgery. New York, John Wiley & Sons, 1986.)

experiences encouraging preservation of chordae, but conclusive data do not exist.

After removal of the mitral valve, a prosthetic valve of appropriate size is selected with a plastic sizer. The type of prosthesis selected is discussed later. Except with small patients, a prosthetic valve with an orifice at least 29 mm in diameter or more is preferred. The position of the prosthesis in the ventricular cavity, as well as in the ventricular outflow tract, is carefully noted.

With porcine prostheses, a proper size is selected to confirm that the posterior post of the prosthesis lies freely in the ventricular cavity and does not impinge on the wall of the left ventricle. This impingement would create a serious hazard of rupture later when the left ventricle contracts. With ball valve prostheses, free motion of the ball within the cage of the prosthesis is confirmed after insertion. Similarly, with disk prostheses, free motion of the disk without contact with the ventricular wall or residual chordae is confirmed. This is rarely a problem with the St. Jude bileaflet prosthesis but can easily occur with the Björk disk prosthesis that was used earlier.

The prosthesis is then inserted with 12 to 16 mattress sutures of 2-0 Ticron, all buttressed with Dacron pledgets. The mattress suture pledget technique has been used since 1972 because it almost eliminates paravalvular leakage. Care is taken to insert the sutures precisely in the annulus of the mitral valve, usually readily confirmed both by inspection as well as by the tactile sense of resistance to insertion of the needle. Particular care is taken to avoid deeper insertion of the sutures that go beyond the annulus and may injure the circumflex coronary artery laterally and posteriorly, the atrioventricular node medially, and the aortic valve anteriorly.

After the prosthesis is lowered into position, great care is taken to tie the sutures gently, applying only enough tension to create a visible dimple on the surface of the cloth of the prosthesis. Greater force during tying of the sutures may inadvertently avulse the mitral annulus from the underlying ventricular muscle and result in rupture of the left ventricle.

After the prosthesis has been inserted, elevation of the ventricle is avoided to prevent to the risk of rupture of the left ventricle because the rigid prosthetic ring constitutes a fixed point that cannot bend if the apex of the left ventricle is raised. For similar reasons, a left ventricular vent is avoided in these patients.

Before the atriotomy incision is closed, a plastic catheter is placed across the prosthetic valve into the left ventricle to keep the prosthesis incompetent and to facilitate the removal of air. After closure of the atriotomy incision, fibrillation is induced and the aorta is unclamped. Air is then removed with the technique described in the preceding section for open mitral commissurotomy. After bypass, and neutralization of heparin with protamine, a small plastic catheter is left in the left atrium for monitoring left atrial pressure and a Swan-Ganz catheter is left in the pulmonary artery. Pacemaker wires are left in the atrium and ventricle. The mediastinal soft tissues are closed superiorly over the aorta, and the remaining pericardium is left open. One pleural cavity is routinely opened for drainage by this author, although other members of the NYU faculty leave both pleural cavities closed with equally good results. Chest tubes are inserted into the mediastinum, and in the pleural cavity, if opened, before the sternotomy incision is sutured.

Rupture of Left Ventricle After Mitral Valve Replacement. This rare but usually lethal complication can occur from at least three causes. The most frequent is partial avulsion of the mitral annulus from the underlying ventricular muscle from application of excessive traction during removal of the valve or insertion of the prosthesis (Zacharias, 1975). This can almost always be prevented by avoiding excessive traction during all parts of the operation and also by inserting sutures precisely into the annulus, rather than into the underlying ventricular muscle. The most common forms of traction injury are during excessive removal of calcium or fibrotic leaflet tissue, traction during insertion of sutures, traction while tying sutures, or later elevation of the apex of the left ventricle in the pericardial cavity.

A second type of left ventricular rupture results when a prosthesis that is too large for the ventricular cavity is inserted. The risk of this complication is greater with the use of potassium cardioplegia because the arrested heart is relaxed in diastole. This danger is primarily with porcine prostheses. In most patients the 29- or 31-mm prosthesis of the Carpentier-Edwards type can be inserted satisfactorily, but an important routine assessment is to examine the position of the posterior post of the prosthesis and the adjacent ventricular wall. The post should be at least 3 to 4 mm from the ventricular wall and should not lie against the ventricular endocardium. These two types of left ventricular rupture are well discussed in a 1974 report by Treasure.

The third type of rupture, the midventricular rupture, was designated as a "Type III" by Miller in 1978. This type of ventricular rupture is the most puzzling and occurs as a transverse rupture between the annulus of the mural leaflet and the papillary muscles. In an elegant report by Cobbs and associates from Emory University in 1980, seven fatal ruptures were described with the hypothesis that these ruptures evolve from strong contraction of the left ventricle after removal of chordae attached to the mural leaflet.

This "untethered loop" hypothesis proposed by Cobbs appears to be the most plausible explanation for this unusual complication. This subject was investigated in depth at NYU and was reported by this author in 1985. As the report describes, rupture of the left ventricle was recognized in 14 patients after mitral valve replacement during a period of 9 years. Until 1981 a traumatic injury was considered to be the most likely cause. In late 1981, however, during a period of 2 months, four fatal ruptures occurred after operations done by three different surgeons, in none of which was the application of undue traction recognized. This grim experience led to the prospective studies described in the 1985 report. In brief, in almost all operations since 1981 a few chordae have been preserved to the annulus of the mural leaflet. With this technique, left ventricular rupture almost never occurs. This writer has personally not encountered this complication since 1981. Whether this fortunate experience is due to preservation of chordae, or simply to a constant awareness of the hazard of the problem, is unknown. Similar experiences from Emory University were reported by Craver in 1985. The subject was also well analyzed in a collective review by Karlson in 1988.

ASSOCIATED PROCEDURES

Coronary Bypass

If significant coronary disease is present, concomitant coronary bypass grafting is almost always done. The frequency with which this was done at NYU from 1986 to 1988 is shown in Table 50–1.

As the ischemia time is longer, a precise sequence is used. After the aorta is clamped and the heart is arrested, a small incision is made in the left atrium and a coronary suction device is inserted to aspirate blood from the left atrium while the coronary bypasses are done. Otherwise, blood accumulates in the left atrium and rewarms the endocardial surface.

The distal anastomoses for the bypass grafts are then done, and cold blood is reinjected after each anastomosis is completed. The mitral valve is then replaced; fibrillation is induced; and the aorta is unclamped. After air is removed from the different cardiac chambers, the heart is defibrillated and allowed to beat while the proximal anastomoses are constructed. This technique minimizes the magnitude of myocardial ischemia during the procedure.

Treatment of Tricuspid Insufficiency

If significant tricuspid insufficiency is detected by digital palpation of the tricuspid valve, it is repaired routinely by a posterior annuloplasty, which was described by Boyd at NYU in 1974. It is a modification of the procedure described by Kay in 1965. As recommended by Reed, an 8-cm segment of tricuspid annulus underlying the septal and anterior leaflets is measured, after which the remaining annulus, principally beneath the posterior leaflet, is plicated between double-buttressed mattress sutures.

This produces an orifice almost 27 mm in diameter. Correction of insufficiency is confirmed by injection of saline with a bulb syringe into the ventricular cavity to distend and coapt the tricuspid leaflets.

This technique has been used for more than 15 years and excellent results have been obtained. Rarely has the leaflet disease been too extensive for correction by annuloplasty, requiring a prosthetic replacement. Significant recurrent insufficiency has rarely been found at a repeat operation years later, which became necessary because mitral valve disease with pulmonary hypertension recurred.

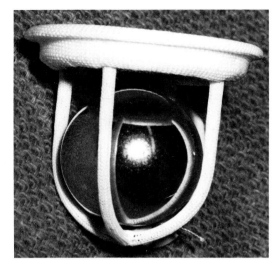

Figure 50–8. The Starr-Edwards cloth-covered steel ball prosthesis used at New York University for over a decade in more than 1,500 patients. The prosthesis was ultimately abandoned because of cloth wear, but it gave excellent results for many years.

In 1988 Nakano from Japan reported almost identical experiences with 133 patients treated by the Kay bicuspidalization procedure for 17 years. Only three tricuspid valve replacements were done. A reoperation was necessary in seven patients, six of whom had persistent mitral valve disease.

Kirklin and Barratt-Boyes prefer the Carpentier ring annuloplasty procedure (Fig. 50–7).

Selection of Prosthesis. A report from NYU by Galloway in 1988 summarized experiences with 1,424 mitral valve operations during the last 10 years. A porcine prosthesis was used in 975 patients; a mechanical prosthesis was used in 169 patients; and a Carpentier reconstruction was used in 280 patients. Selection of the type of mechanical prosthesis was primarily by preference of the surgeon. The Starr-Edwards ball valve prosthesis was used in 38% of patients (Fig. 50–8); the Björk disk prosthesis (no longer available) was used in 50% (Fig. 50–9) of patients; the St. Jude bileaflet prosthesis was used in 9% of patients; and other types of prostheses were used in 3% of patients (Figs. 50–10 and 50–11). Since the withdrawal of both the Björk disk prosthesis and the Duramedic bileaflet prosthesis from the market in early 1988, the St. Jude bileaflet prosthesis and the Starr-Edwards ball valve prosthesis have been uniformly used.

As discussed earlier, a selective policy with individual patients is followed. The patient actively participates in the choice of the prosthesis. If socioeconomic factors indicate that anticoagulant therapy can be done safely, a mechanical prosthesis is recommended for patients less than 65 years of age, whereas a porcine prosthesis is recommended for older patients because of the increased frequency of both hypertension and stroke. Many exceptions occur, however, primarily from the patient's preference. Currently, with the disappointing durability of porcine prostheses at 10 years and longer, mechanical

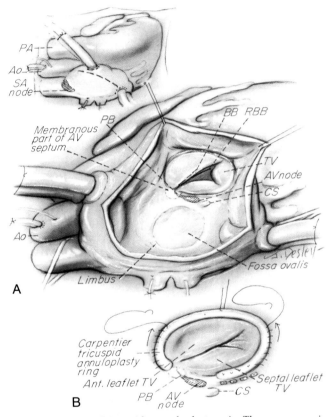

Figure 50–7. Tricuspid annuloplasty. *A,* The exposure is through the usual oblique right atriotomy. *B,* Stay sutures provide excellent exposure, and retractors are not needed. The surgeon identifies the anteroseptal tricuspid valve commissure, the membranous part of this atrioventricular septum, and the coronary sinus orifice. The surgeon can then mentally visualize the location of the atrioventricular node and the penetrating portion of the bundle of His. By using the appropriate sizers, notched at points corresponding to the anteroseptal and posteroseptal commissures at either end of the septal tricuspid leaflet, a proper-sized open, flexible Carpentier-Edwards tricuspid annuloplasty ring is selected. The ring is sewn into place with interrupted sutures (see text) or with interrupted pledgetted mattress sutures along the inferior aspect of the septal leaflet and continuous sutures elsewhere (see the figure), as described in the text. In either case, a stay suture is first placed through the annulus at the junction of the anterior and posterior leaflets and then through the marker on the annuloplasty ring, as shown. (Ao = aorta; AV node = atrioventricular node; BB = bundle branch; CS = coronary sinus; PB = penetrating bundle; RBB = right bundle branch; SA node = sinoatrial node; TV = tricuspid valve.) (From Bharati, S., Lev, M., and Kirklin, J. W.: Cardiac Surgery and the Conduction System. New York, John Wiley & Sons, 1983.)

TABLE 50–1. OPERATIVE MORTALITY: MITRAL VALVE REPLACEMENT WITH
AND WITHOUT CORONARY BYPASS (1986 TO 1988)

Procedure	No. of Deaths (%) in Hospital in 1986	No. of Deaths (%) in Hospital in 1987	No. of Deaths (%) in Hospital in 1988
Isolated MVR	71 (7.0%)	81 (2.5%)	50 (2.0%)
MVR + CAB	44 (9.1%)	34 (14.7%)	41 (9.8%)

prostheses are being used with increasing frequency. The relative frequency of the use of mechanical prostheses, porcine prostheses, and mitral reconstruction from 1986 to 1988 is shown in Table 50–2.

As stated earlier, the sobering report by Magilligan in 1988 found that more than 50% of porcine prostheses failed within 15 years after implantation. Unless recent technical modifications in the preparation of porcine prostheses yield considerably better results, it appears probable that most porcine prostheses will fail within 10 to 20 years after implantation.

Technique of Closed Commissurotomy

As stated earlier, this writer has not performed this operation for more than 15 years, because better and safer results are obtained with an open technique. Unless a heart-lung machine is not available for geographic reasons, almost the only indication for closed commissurotomy is during pregnancy because of the risks to the fetus from heparinization.

The technique of commissurotomy described in the last edition of this book is reproduced here.

The two main hazards with digital commissurotomy are hemorrhage from laceration of the left atrium and cerebral embolism from thrombi in the left atrium or calcific fragments dislodged from the mitral valve.

A left posterolateral thoracotomy in the fourth intercostal space, with the patient turned slightly beyond a true lateral position, approximately 110 degrees rather than 90 degrees, is best. The increased rotation facilitates exposure of the posterior aspect of the left atrium.

The pericardium is incised anterior to the phrenic nerve, and stay sutures are inserted for traction on the pericardial edges. The atrial appendage is then examined. An appendage containing an organized thrombus often has a rubbery consistency, which is very different from the soft, compressible feel of a normal appendage. A fibrotic, contracted appendage usually indicates chronic fibrotic organization of a thrombus over a long period of time.

A heavy purse-string suture is placed around the base of the appendage and secured with a snare that can be tightened around the finger to minimize the loss of blood. An important adjunct with the operation is to have the anesthesiologist identify both carotid pulses at the start of the operation so that intermittent digital occlusion for 30 to 60 seconds can be done during all intracardiac manipulations. Cerebral embolism is fortunately rare with this technique.

When the atrial appendage is incised, a jet of blood is allowed to flush from the opening momentarily to dislodge any free-floating thrombi. Rarely, a thrombus as large as 1 to 2 cm in diameter is expelled. Subsequently, the index finger is introduced, cautiously watching for undue resistance or laceration. If a tear begins, the finger should be withdrawn

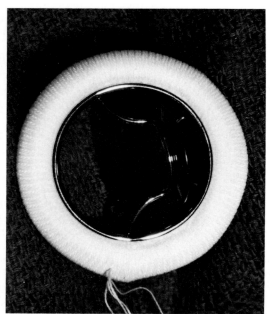

Figure 50–9. The Björk tilting-disk prosthesis, an excellent low-profile prosthetic valve. It was withdrawn from use for economic reasons early in 1988.

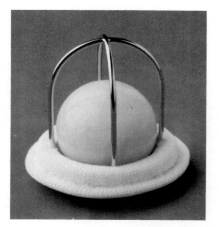

Figure 50–10. The mitral bare-strut Starr-Edwards Silastic ball valve currently in use. This was developed between 1965 and 1966 and is now the ball valve prosthesis of choice.

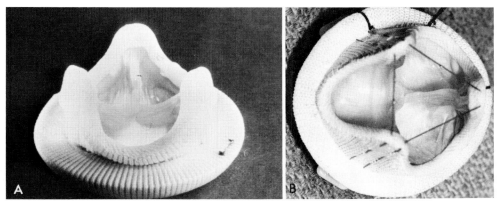

Figure 50–11. *A,* The Hancock porcine prosthesis. *B,* The Carpentier-Edwards porcine prosthesis. These are two of the most popular porcine prostheses currently in use. The Carpentier-Edwards prosthesis has been used almost exclusively at New York University for the last 4 to 5 years.

promptly and the atrial incision should be extended superiorly toward the left pulmonary vein. Lacerations in this area can be readily controlled, whereas those extending toward the circumflex coronary artery or beneath the pulmonary artery can produce lethal hemorrhage.

Once the index finger has been introduced into the atrium, the degree of stenosis, insufficiency, and valvular calcification is noted. If friable calcific granules are felt along the margins of the valve, there is a great risk of cerebral embolization. Thus, temporary occlusion of the carotid vessels is particularly important, if it is necessary to proceed with the procedure. If possible, the procedure should be terminated and an open commissurotomy should be done.

In the absence of a dangerous degree of calcification, commissurotomy is done by pressure with the index finger on the two commissures, opening each commissure gradually and noting any mitral insufficiency that results after each manipulation. A variety of digital maneuvers, varying with individual patients, is necessary to open a densely fused commissure.

Usually repeated efforts are necessary to open a fused commissure, gradually weakening and tearing the rigid scar tissue that initially may be quite resistant. A mechanical transverticular dilator can be used, which applies more mechanical force than is possible with the finger. However, insufficiency can readily result, and therefore, use of the dilator is no longer recommended. It is better to terminate the procedure and to do an open commissurotomy later.

Under ideal circumstances, unless mitral insufficiency is present, both commissures should be opened to within a few millimeters of the mitral annulus. Subsequently, after removal of the finger from the atrium, any gradient remaining across the mitral valve can be measured by needle puncture of the left atrium and left ventricle. It is hoped that the end-diastolic gradient will have been abolished.

With adequate precautions, the risk of operation is surprisingly small, 1 to 2%. As discussed earlier, the main objections are the inability to open the valve properly if fused chordae are present and the inability to correct any insufficiency produced at operation.

OPERATIVE MORTALITY

After Open Commissurotomy. The mortality is very low, almost 1%. A similar low mortality has been reported by several groups. In the Kirklin/Barratt-Boyes series, only one death occurred after 259 operations.

After Replacement or Reconstruction. In the 1988 report by Galloway of experiences at NYU with 1,424 mitral valve operations during the preceding decade, operative mortality for isolated valve replacement was almost 7% and rose to more than 11% for patients in whom additional procedures were done. By multivariate analysis the predictors of increased operative risk included age, NYHA Class IV status, earlier cardiac surgery, and the performance of concomitant cardiac surgical procedures. The type of valve procedure done did not predict operative risk. Kirklin and Barratt-Boyes (1986) described an operative mortality in the range of between 3 and 7% after a total of almost 661 operations. The major risk factors were the NYHA functional class and the age at

TABLE 50–2. FREQUENCY OF MITRAL VALVE PROCEDURES FROM 1986 TO 1988: PROSTHESES VERSUS RECONSTRUCTION

Procedure	No. (%) of Patients in 1986	No. (%) of Patients in 1987	No. (%) of Patients in 1988
Porcine MVR	70 (41.4%)	61 (35.3%)	50 (32.5%)
Mechanical MVR	38 (22.5%)	38 (22.0%)	47 (30.5%)
MV reconstruction	61 (36.1%)	74 (42.8%)	57 (37.0%)

operation. An excellent statistical analysis of their data found that addition of coronary bypass grafting was not, per se, an incremental risk factor. On superficial examination of the data, coronary bypass appeared to double the risk of replacement, but closer analysis found that the higher mortality was due to other factors.

Death was usually due to complications of a low cardiac output, either terminating as an arrhythmia or from organ failure, renal insufficiency, gastrointestinal bleeding or infection.

POSTOPERATIVE CARE

After Open Commissurotomy. The same treatment program, which is described later, is used for prosthetic valve replacement. However, in most patients after commissurotomy, the postoperative course is benign; thus patients are discharged within 7 to 8 days and gradually resume normal activities in the next 6 to 8 weeks. Postoperative echocardiography is normally done, estimating the orifice of the mitral valve as well as detecting any insufficiency.

After Prosthetic Replacement of the Mitral Valve. After operation, left atrial pressure, arterial pressure, and the electrocardiogram are monitored and visually displayed on an oscilloscopic screen in the recovery room. If pulmonary hypertension is present, the pulmonary artery systolic pressure is also monitored through the Swan-Ganz catheter. Cardiac output is measured periodically, and a cardiac index near 2.5 liters or higher is maintained by infusing sufficient fluid to maintain an appropriate left atrial pressure. Inotropic agents, usually small amounts of epinephrine or dobutamine (10 µg/kg/min), may be needed for short periods. If peripheral vascular resistance is elevated, an infusion of nitroprusside or nitroglycerin is given. The intracardiac catheters are removed in 24 to 48 hours. With the present techniques of myocardial preservation, significant depression of cardiac output is rarely seen.

Arrhythmias are common, especially atrial fibrillation; thus, monitoring of the cardiac rhythm is one of the most important aspects of postoperative care. Pacemaker wires are usually left in place for 5 to 7 days. Bradycardia is treated with electrical pacing, preferably atrioventricular pacing, and a rate of 80 to 85 beats per minute is best. Pacemaker wires are left routinely in place for several days.

The most frequently used antiarrhythmic drugs are lidocaine, procainamide (Procan), quinidine, and propranolol. If atrial fibrillation develops and persists despite appropriate drug therapy, cardioversion can be done, either during the postoperative course or a few weeks later.

A *pericardiotomy* syndrome frequently occurs, perhaps in 10 to 15% of patients after open heart operations. Although the syndrome has been recognized for more than two decades, the etiology is still obscure. The clinical manifestations vary but include fever, a white blood cell count of less than 10,000 cells per mm³, a pericardial or pleural effusion, and often a pericardial friction rub. Therapy with ibuprofen (Motrin) in appropriate doses for a few days is usually satisfactory.

Small *pericardial or pleural effusions* are common and usually require no specific treatment. Large pleural effusions are evacuated by aspiration. Large pericardial effusions, with the hazard of tamponade, usually respond to diuretic and anti-inflammatory drugs but rarely require subxiphoid drainage.

Prophylactic antibiotics are started before operation and given intravenously each 2 hours during the procedure. These drugs should be selected according to the prevailing bacterial flora found in wound infections in the hospital. Cefamandole (Mandol) has been used for the last several years, giving 2 g before operation and then 1 g every 2 hours during the procedure. It is continued after operation in a dosage of 2 g every 6 hours for 48 to 72 hours, usually until intracardiac catheters and central lines have been removed. Fortunately, infection of any type is uncommon. Infection in the sternotomy wound develops in approximately 1% of patients, usually responding to debridement and closed mediastinal irrigation with appropriate antibiotics; otherwise, a muscle flap procedure is used.

Postoperative endocarditis is rare. When it does occur, it often usually reflects bacterial contamination at operation and almost always requires prompt reoperation.

Anticoagulant therapy is started 2 to 3 days after operation with sodium warfarin (Coumadin), elevating the prothrombin time to above 20 seconds. A greater degree of anticoagulation, with the prothrombin time at almost twice normal levels, was found to be unnecessary several years ago. This higher degree of anticoagulation resulted in a greater frequency of hemorrhage but no greater protection from thromboembolism. With metallic prostheses warfarin is continued permanently, usually by adding dipyridamole (Persantine) as a platelet inhibitor.

With porcine prostheses, anticoagulation with warfarin is usually stopped after 3 months, subsequently using antiplatelet therapy with acetylsalicylic acid (Aspirin) and dipyridamole for at least 1 year. In a significant percentage of patients, especially those with atrial fibrillation, a large heart, or chronic congestive failure before operation, warfarin therapy is often continued indefinitely by the referring cardiologist unless problems with bleeding occur.

Patients are usually discharged from the hospital in 7 to 10 days and gradually resume normal activities during the next 2 to 3 months. Diuretic therapy is often necessary for a few months. This decision is made after taking daily measurements of body weight. Three to 6 months may be required to obtain full benefit from operation, especially in patients with previous advanced cardiac failure.

LONG-TERM MANAGEMENT AND RESULTS

After Open Commissurotomy. In 1981 Gross reported results in 202 patients having commissurotomy at NYU between 1967 and 1978, with a 98% complete follow-up. Late mortality was only 2.5%. Five years after operation, 87% of patients who had no residual valve dysfunction after commissurotomy were free of any complications. The frequency of thromboembolism was only 0.3% per year in the first 10 years after operation; ultimately 3% of the patients had an embolic episode.

Similar results were reported by Halseth (1980) who described experiences with 222 patients operated on during the previous decade. Operative mortality was 1.5%, and two of the three deaths occurred in patients operated on as an emergency. Only 7% of the 191 patients surviving commissurotomy later required mitral valve replacement; the 10-year survival was 81%.

Kirklin and Barratt-Boyes (1986) stated that 88% of patients were alive 8 years after commissurotomy, although 16% had required mitral valve replacement and 8% had had an embolic event.

Unfortunately, the rheumatic injury to cardiac valves appears to inflict permanent harm, because fibrosis and degeneration continue to appear even 15 to 20 years after successful commissurotomy, and usually produce mitral insufficiency. Thus, after commissurotomy patients should be periodically evaluated indefinitely because a high probability exists that eventually, perhaps after more than two decades, significant mitral disease will recur.

After Prosthetic Replacement of the Mitral Valve. An important principle to emphasize is that any patient with a prosthetic valve requires life-long periodic surveillance by a physician, similar to a patient with diabetes. Six common complications that occur are thromboembolism, anticoagulant hemorrhage, endocarditis, arrhythmias, malfunction of the prosthesis, and cardiac failure. These complications are discussed in the following paragraphs.

Data from eight large series of valve prostheses reported in recent years are summarized in the Selected Bibliography. See the entries under Arom (1987); Cobanoglu (1987); Czer (1987); Flemma (1988); Galloway (1988); Jamieson (1988); Lindblom (1988); and Murphy (1983).

THROMBOEMBOLISM. The 1988 report by Galloway from NYU described experiences with 975 porcine replacements and 169 mechanical replacements over 10 years (1976 to 1987). Average duration of follow-up (more than 96% complete) was almost 40 months. In the 169 patients selected for mechanical prostheses, there was a high freedom from thromboembolism at 5 years, 94%, much better than the 5-year freedom from thromboembolism of only 70 to 90% reported by most groups. This surprising finding probably indicates the importance of precise management of anticoagulant therapy by both the patient and the physician. Among the 975 porcine prostheses, freedom from thromboembolism was less, almost 87%, although many of these emboli were small without permanent injury. Freedom from anticoagulant hemorrhage was approximately 95% after mechanical or porcine prostheses. The significant frequency of hemorrhage with porcine prostheses reflected the continued use of warfarin in a significant percentage of patients with porcine prostheses.

In the series by Kirklin and Barratt-Boyes, approximately 90% of patients were free of thromboembolic complications 5 years after mitral valve replacement. Results were similar in patients with Björk disk prostheses who received anticoagulants and patients with porcine prostheses without anticoagulants. A report Tepley made from Starr's group in 1981 stated that since 1973 approximately 95% of patients were free of thromboemboli 5 years after insertion of a ball valve prosthesis, compared with approximately 70% in earlier years. A higher frequency with ball valve prostheses was reported by Miller, who found a frequency of thromboembolism of almost 45% 10 years after operation.

In the 1987 collective review of the frequency of thromboembolic complications by Edmunds, the percentage of patients free of thromboembolism at 5 years ranged from 65 to 89% with mechanical prostheses and between 90 and 97% with porcine prostheses.

HEMORRHAGE FROM ANTICOAGULANTS. Bleeding associated with anticoagulants is a significant danger in any patient with a metallic prosthesis. The importance of the selective use of prostheses is emphasized, because some patients may be unable to supervise anticoagulant therapy properly. The wide range in frequency of bleeding is well tabulated in the 1987 collective review by Edmunds, who reviewed data from more than 20 reports. The frequency in five large series reported in recent years is shown in Table 50–3, ranging from 1.2 per 100 patient years to 4.5. Fortunately, most of these are minor, but a fatal hemorrhage occasionally occurs in all series reported. Freedom from anticoagulant therapy is the main attraction of bioprostheses.

ENDOCARDITIS. Any patient with a prosthetic valve has a susceptibility to bacterial endocarditis during periods of transient bacteremia. The more common episodes occur after a dental extraction or cystoscopic procedures. Thus, it is important that appropriate antibiotic therapy be given for a short period before and after these elective procedures. This is effective in many patients, but unfortunately others develop endocarditis from unknown causes, similar to the well-known susceptibility of patients with valvular heart disease from rheumatic fever. Patients with porcine and metallic prostheses are equally susceptible. In the 1988 NYU report by Galloway, endocarditis occurred with a frequency of approximately 1% per year.

The frequency of endocarditis was almost 1%

TABLE 50–3. FREQUENCY OF ANTICOAGULANT-RELATED HEMORRHAGE IN RECENT REPORTS

Author (yr)	No. of Patients	Type of Prosthesis	Frequency in 100 Patient Years
Flemma (1988)	785	Björk disk	4.5
Lindblom (1988)	810	Björk disk	1.2
Arom (1987)	816	St. Jude	3.2
Czer (1987)	527	St. Jude	2.9
Murphy (1983)	958	Starr ball valve; Björk disk	~2.0

per year in the report of 809 prostheses by Murphy, almost 0.4% in the Flemma series (785 disk prostheses), and only 0.1% in the Lindblom series (810 disk prostheses). The reason for the very low frequency in the Lindblom series (in Sweden) is unknown.

Endocarditis is a serious complication. If appropriate antibiotic therapy does not promptly control signs of sepsis, surgical intervention is mandatory in most patients. Overall mortality from endocarditis was almost 25% in the NYU series and almost 50% in the patients in the series by Kirklin and Barratt-Boyes.

An important therapeutic principle that should be emphasized repeatedly is that delaying operation while ineffective antibiotic therapy is continued significantly increases overall mortality. The infection gradually spreads beyond the prosthesis into the annulus and adjacent tissues and creates a much more serious problem. When reoperation is done promptly, combined with the use of appropriate antibiotics, the risk is small and recurrent endocarditis is rare.

ARRHYTHMIAS. A high percentage of deaths that occur within 5 to 10 years after operation are "sudden," defined as developing within less than 1 hour after the onset of symptoms. These are apparently due to arrhythmias, because post-mortem examination usually reveals only various degrees of ventricular fibrosis. These events are more common in patients with serious impairment of ventricular function before operation, which probably explains the much higher frequency of death in the first 5 years after operation (30 to 40%) in NYHA Class IV patients compared with Class II patients (10%). Periodic monitoring of patients with known arrhythmias should be done, including 24-hour Holter monitoring, followed by use of appropriate antiarrhythmic drugs. Unfortunately, the effectiveness of these medications is limited; thus the best solution is probably operation before severe myocardial injury has developed. This possibility is one of the attractive features of mitral valve reconstructive procedures, rather than prosthetic replacement, because operation can be done at an earlier stage of the disease.

PROSTHESIS MALFUNCTION. Late deterioration is the serious handicap with porcine prostheses. In general, durability with porcine prostheses is almost 95% in the first 5 years after operation but after 7 to 8 years, failure increases at a more rapid rate, so that only about 80% are functioning 10 years after oper-

ation. The 15-year follow-up presented by Magilligan found that less than 50% of these prostheses were still functioning at that time. Thus, periodic evaluation of the patient, combined with echocardiography if murmurs develop, is important.

In the 1986 report of early results from NYU by this author of experiences with 1,643 porcine prostheses, over 7 years, with an average follow-up of 42 months, deterioration was recognized in only 42 patients, which was a frequency of less than 2%.

In 1988, Jamieson and associates reported experiences with 1,301 porcine prostheses implanted during 11 years, with an average follow-up of 5.6 years. Valve deterioration was identified in 104 prostheses; thus, the freedom from primary tissue failure at 10 years was almost 77%. Age had a major influence on the frequency of late deterioration. The worst results occurred in the younger patients. Patients less than 30 years of age had only 27% of valves functioning at 10 years; those between 30 and 60 years had only 77% of valves functioning; and those over 60 years had only 83% of valves functioning.

Mechanical failure with ball valve prostheses is almost unknown and was well documented in the report of 25 years' experience reported by Cobanoglu (1985). A similar high degree of reliability has been reported with the St. Jude bileaflet prostheses. The Björk disk prostheses, which are currently unavailable, had a small but serious frequency of thrombosis, primarily in the first few years after implantation.

LATE CARDIAC FAILURE. The degree of improvement after mitral valve replacement often cannot be determined for 3 to 4 months, depending on what degree of preoperative impairment of ventricular function was due to irreversible injury. When cardiac function initially improves but *late cardiac failure* appears months or years after mitral valve replacement, there are four common causes: paravalvular leakage, deterioration of the prosthesis, the development of additional cardiac disease, or left ventricular failure. A most important principle that should be emphasized is that *all* of these patients should be re-evaluated with cardiac catheterization. It is usually a serious mistake to treat these patients with increasing cardiac medications on the assumption that left ventricular failure is the primary cause.

At catheterization the diagnosis can be readily made. Primary left ventricular failure is manifested by an elevated end-diastolic pressure, which is often in the range of 20 to 25 mm Hg or higher. Other causes, which are surgically correctable, can be readily identified. Hopefully, the sad but familiar clinical picture of patients who improve for 2 to 3 years after operation, but who then return with advanced left ventricular failure, will decrease by operating on patients at an earlier stage of the disease.

LATE MORTALITY

As stated in the report by Cobanoglu from Starr's group, late survival is an insensitive indicator for comparing different valve prostheses because characteristics of patients are the most important factors. The dominant factors are age, degree of left ventricular failure, manifested by NHYA classification, and urgency of operation. In the series by Kirklin and Barratt-Boyes, approximately 80% of patients survived for 5 years; 60% survived for 10 years; and 45% survived for 15 years. Approximately 50% of late deaths were from heart failure and approximately 20% were from complications associated with the prosthetic valve such as thromboembolism, prosthesis degeneration, or infection. The dominant factors influencing late mortality were the severity of the preoperative symptoms (NYHA Class III or IV), reflecting left ventricular function, and older age at operation. The functional mitral lesion, an earlier valve replacement, or the type of prosthesis inserted did not affect late survival. The influence of age on late survival is shown in the report by Flemma of results after 10 years in 785 patients. Ten-year survival was 70% in the 20- to 49-year-old age group; 58% in the 50- to 59-year-old age group; and 48% in the 60- to 80-year-old age group.

In the 1988 report by Galloway of experiences at NYU during the previous decade, the overall 5-year survival rate was between 70 and 75%. This included the overall operative mortality of almost 12%. By multivariate analysis the strongest predictors of late death were age, a NYHA Class IV preoperative status, previous cardiac surgery, and performance of concomitant cardiac surgical procedures.

In 1983, Murphy reported a 7-year survival of almost 70% in a group of 447 mitral valve replacements done at the Massachusetts General Hospital. Operative mortality was excluded.

The 1985 report by Cobanoglu from Starr's group summarized experiences over 25 years. With the model 6120 ball valve prosthesis, 5-year survival was 73%; 10-year survival was 54%; and 15-year survival was 36%.

In the 1988 report by Flemma describing 268 mitral valve replacements with the Björk disk prosthesis, 5-year survival, excluding hospital deaths, was almost 85%.

MITRAL INSUFFICIENCY

Etiology and Pathology. Mitral stenosis is almost always due to rheumatic fever, but mitral insuffi-

ciency can result from several causes. Rheumatic fever was previously the most common cause but has decreased to where degenerative disease, (mitral prolapse and ruptured chordae), is now the most frequent cause. Other causes include endocarditis, coronary artery disease, and, rarely, congenital heart disease or myopathy. In the first 148 mitral reconstructions done at NYU, 43% were due to mitral prolapse, with or without ruptured chordae; 30% were due to rheumatic fever; approximately 12% resulted from coronary disease; and 12% resulted from endocarditis.

Four different structural components of the mitral valve may be injured. These components include the leaflets, chordae, annulus, and papillary muscle. All of these must be assessed at operation to determine the type of mitral reconstruction that should be done. The pathologic anatomy found in mitral insufficiency from different causes has been studied in detail by Carpentier.

With rheumatic valvular disease, the leaflets are often fibrotic and contracted and have focal areas of calcification. There is often fusion of the commissures. Valvular stenosis, insufficiency, or both, may be present (Fig. 50–12). The chordae tendineae are often thick, short, and fused, but are rarely elongated. Asymmetric dilatation of the annulus develops, primarily in the posteromedial portion, that changes the contour of the mitral valve from an ellipse with a long transverse axis between the commissures to an ellipse with a long axis in the anteroposterior direction. The annulus of the aortic leaflet is not dilated because it is fixed to the fibrous skeleton of the base of the heart, which is the important point in reconstruction.

Mitral valve prolapse (Barlow's syndrome) has been variously termed "floppy valve" or "myxomatous valve degeneration," emphasizing the leaflet and chordae abnormality. These abnormalities differ from those found in rheumatic valves. All chordae are thinned and elongated with thinning and increase in size of the mitral leaflets, the "billowing mitral valve." The posterior annular dilatation is symmetric and involves both commissures equally.

Rupture of chordae tendineae often occurs, supraimposed on the insufficiency initiated by the prolapsing valve. Alternately, rupture of isolated chordae may be the first sign of mitral valve disease, although this is probably a variation of prolapse.

Mild degrees of mitral valve prolapse are surprisingly common and are estimated to occur in almost 5% of the normal female population. In most of patients it has minor physiologic significance; however, in some patients it becomes more severe with age as turbulent flow of blood produces fibrosis and calcification of the leaflets. Before the widespread recognition of the frequency of mitral valve prolapse, these patients were erroneously considered to have had rheumatic fever in childhood, even though a clinical history could not be obtained.

With *coronary artery disease*, pathologic changes

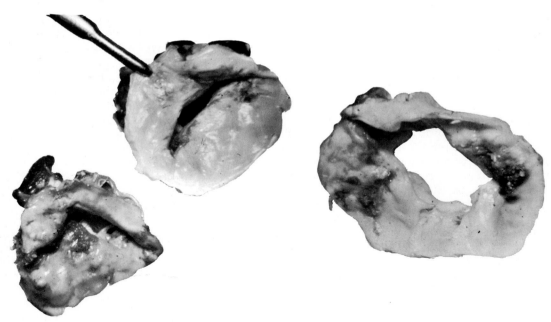

Figure 50–12. Mitral valves removed from three different patients, showing the fibrosis and calcification commonly encountered in patients with mitral insufficiency. An effort is made to remove the mitral valve intact to avoid fragmentation and possible displacement of calcium fragments into the left ventricle when the valve is removed.

are less precise and are not yet completely defined. Mitral insufficiency may be intermittent, apparently resulting from reversible ischemia in the papillary muscles. Few abnormalities may be found at operation in these patients. Severe ischemia may lead to diffuse scarring and contraction of a papillary muscle, or a localized infarction may significantly distort the wall of the myocardium from which the muscle originates. With advanced disease producing ventricular hypertrophy and dilatation there may be symmetric dilatation of the posterior annulus.

Dilatation of the mitral annulus is usually a secondary response to insufficiency from another cause. The primary cause is rarely dilatation alone, perhaps only in connective tissue disorders such as rheumatoid arthritis. This point is important and emphasizes why annuloplasty procedures alone have often given disappointing results because the pathology in the leaflets and chordae was not corrected.

Pathophysiology

The basic physiologic burden with mitral insufficiency is reflux of part of the stroke volume of the contracting left ventricle into the left atrium, reducing systemic blood flow and elevating left atrial pressure. Left atrial pressure tracings accordingly reveal a systolic spike as high as 30 to 40 mm Hg, rarely as high as 70 to 80 mm Hg, followed by an abrupt decline in diastole. At the end of diastole, pressure may remain slightly elevated, with a 5 to 10 mm Hg gradient across the mitral valve, even though no organic stenosis is present; this "flow gradient" results from the increased flow of blood during diastole. The

mean left atrial pressure is usually between 15 and 20 mm Hg; in some patients, it is normal.

Pulmonary vascular resistance is increased less often than in patients with mitral stenosis, probably because left atrial pressure is elevated only intermittently. Similarly, left atrial thrombi and systemic emboli occur less frequently than with mitral stenosis because of the absence of stasis in the left atrium. Left ventricular function may be adequate for surprisingly long periods, despite massive mitral regurgitation. This is indicated both by the absence of symptoms and by a left ventricular end-diastolic pressure less than 12 mm Hg. Initially the left ventricle compensates for the increased work load by dilatation and hypertrophy. Eventually, however, these compensatory mechanisms become inadequate as permanent injury of the ventricle evolves and progresses to cardiac failure. Once left ventricular failure occurs, the course progressively worsens, usually at a fairly rapid rate.

The blood regurgitating into the left atrium with each systolic contraction leads to progressive enlargement of the left atrium, often to gigantic proportions. A grotesque cardiac shadow may result in which the left atrial contour extends almost to the right chest wall, some of the largest degrees of left atrial enlargement encountered in clinical medicine. The degree of left atrial enlargement, however, does not correspond to the degree of mitral insufficiency. Why the degree of dilatation varies so much is unknown; it probably reflects an inherent variation in distensibility of left atrial muscle.

Diagnostic Considerations

In patients with mild mitral insufficiency, an apical systolic murmur is present without any disability. These patients may remain well for many years, with the left ventricle adapting adequately to the increased workload. An increased susceptibility to bacterial endocarditis is the only hazard. As stated earlier, the characteristic adaptation of the left ventricle is dilatation, increasing stroke volume by increasing the diastolic fiber length of the ventricular muscle. Thus, the principal question in evaluating the severity of mitral insufficiency is the degree of left ventricular enlargement.

As insufficiency progresses, the most common symptoms are weakness, fatigue, and palpitations, with some dyspnea on exertion. These symptoms reflect a decreased cardiac output as well as left atrial hypertension. Gradually, symptoms of pulmonary congestion become more prominent, as described in the section on mitral stenosis. Right-sided heart failure, with hepatic enlargement and peripheral edema, is a sign of far advanced disease, usually with a certain degree of permanent ventricular injury. Ideally, surgical therapy should be done well before this occurs.

On physical examination, the two characteristic findings are the apical systolic murmur and the forceful apical impulse with cardiac enlargement. The apical murmur is harsh and blowing in quality, transmitted to the axilla. Usually, it is Grade II or III in intensity, although there is wide variation. The severity of the insufficiency does not correlate with the intensity of the murmur, but the pansystolic characteristic does. With mild mitral insufficiency, the systolic murmur does not extend completely through systole, whereas with severe insufficiency, it occupies all of systole. A diastolic murmur may also be heard because of the increased volume of blood flowing across the mitral valve. However, compared with mitral stenosis, there is neither an opening snap nor an increased first sound.

The most important clinical finding on physical examination is the forceful apical impulse, reflecting the degree of enlargement of the left ventricle. This finding contrasts sharply with the normal or decreased apical impulse with mitral stenosis, in which the work requirements of the left ventricle are decreased rather than increased.

The characteristic change on the chest film is enlargement of the left atrium and the left ventricle (Fig. 50–13). Determining the degree of enlargement of the left ventricle is one of the most valuable measurements for deciding prognosis and therapy. As long as left ventricular size is normal, a nonoperative approach is satisfactory. With progressive degrees of enlargement of the left ventricle, however, operation should be done before irreversible injury occurs. A leading area of clinical investigation is to determine by echocardiography and other noninvasive techniques which abnormality of left ventricular function has the most accurate prognostic value for indicating when operation should be done. At present a fall in ejection fraction with exercise is one of the earliest indicators that serious ventricular dys-

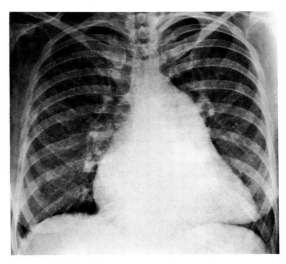

Figure 50–13. Chest film of a patient with mitral insufficiency. The distinctive features include an enlarged cardiac shadow with a prominent pulmonary artery. The shadow of the left atrium is visible in the right border of the cardiac shadow behind the shadow of the right atrium. The pulmonary vascular markings are prominent.

function is developing, and surgical therapy should be carefully considered. The goal is to select patients for operation on the basis of changes in left ventricular function, not symptoms, thus permitting operation before irreversible injury has occurred.

Changes in the pulmonary vasculature, similar to those described for mitral stenosis, may be present. Calcification of the mitral valve occurs less frequently but has considerable surgical importance. Extensive calcification often indicates that replacement, rather than reconstruction, will be necessary.

The electrocardiogram is not a precise guide. Signs of left ventricular hypertrophy are prominent in about half of the patients, whereas in other patients, right ventricular hypertrophy is more evident because of increased pulmonary vascular resistance. Atrial fibrillation is common. In some patients with extensive insufficiency, the electrocardiogram is nearly normal.

Echocardiography is one of the most valuable diagnostic techniques. Different abnormalities that cause mitral insufficiency can be recognized. Prolapse of the mitral valve can be readily detected. With coronary disease the impaired contraction of segments of ventricular wall from ischemia can be identified. With idiopathic hypertrophic subaortic stenosis (IHSS), the echocardiogram is highly sensitive and specific.

A separate important aspect of echocardiography is evaluating serial changes in left ventricular dysfunction. The size of the cardiac chambers in both systole and diastole can be measured as well as changes in thickness of the left ventricular wall during systole. The size of the left atrium indicates the chronicity and severity of the disease (a normal left atrium seldom has an internal diameter greater than 4 cm). Ejection fraction can be calculated from

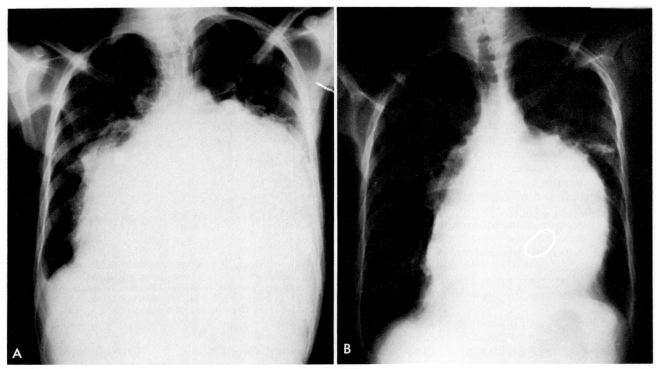

Figure 50–14. A and B, Chest films of a 42-year-old woman with long-standing mitral regurgitation who was operated on in August 1981. The preoperative film (A) shows the massive cardiac enlargement, found at operation to consist primarily of a gigantic left atrium with a tiny left ventricle. The postoperative film (B) was taken in September 1981, 6 weeks after operation. The Carpentier ring used for the annuloplasty can be faintly seen through the cardiac silhouette. Tricuspid annuloplasty was also done. At operation, the patient had rheumatic mitral insufficiency with fusion of the mural leaflet to the wall of the left ventricle. There were no ruptured chordae. The fused leaflets were mobilized, dividing secondary chordae, after which a Carpentier ring was inserted. The dramatic improvement well supports the role of annuloplasty in selected patients.

changes in left ventricular volume in systole and diastole. As stated earlier, a fall in ejection fraction with exercise, opposite to the normal response of an increase with exercise, is one of the earliest signs of serious ventricular dysfunction. A rise in left ventricular end-diastolic pressure above the normal value of 12 mm Hg to between 15 and 20 mm Hg indicates early, significant cardiac failure.

Cardiac catheterization and angiography constitute the ultimate invasive study, which is also the most important study performed. With angiography both the degree of regurgitation and ventricular contractility, expressed as ejection fraction, can be determined. Measurement of intracardiac pressures can detect the presence of cardiac failure as well as pulmonary hypertension.

OPERATIVE TREATMENT

Until 4 to 5 years ago, operation was usually considered for mitral insufficiency only when significant disability was present, manifested by symptoms, significant cardiac enlargement, and other signs of hemodynamic deterioration. This use of operation at a moderately advanced stage of the disease was based on the fact that most patients, more than 90%, required prosthetic valve replacement, which, in turn, has the well-known hazards from thromboembolism and anticoagulant therapy. This late use of operation, however, has the serious handicap that a significant degree of irreversible ventricular injury has already occurred; thus results 5 years after operation are considerably worse than those with patients operated on at an earlier stage of the disease. Currently, approximately 80% of hospital survivors of mitral valve replacement survive for 5 years, but approximately 50% of the late deaths are from heart failure. A major risk factor for death within 5 years after operation is a preoperative NYHA Class III or IV status. Five-year survival is 90 to 95% for patients preoperatively in Class I or II but only 60% for those in Class IV.

Thus, one of the most important developments in repair of the mitral valve is the increasing probability of successful repair, using Carpentier's techniques of reconstruction, in a high percentage of patients with nonrheumatic mitral disease. Because thromboembolism is rare after reconstruction, operation can be recommended at an earlier stage of the disease, which, in turn, should significantly lower the frequency of late death from left ventricular failure (Galloway, 1988). These concepts are elaborated in the following paragraphs.

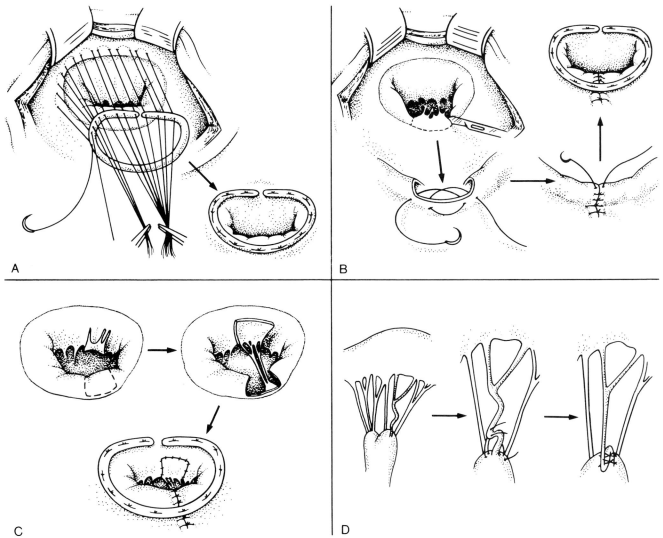

Figure 50–15. *A,* Insertion of annuloplasty ring. *B,* Posterior leaflet resection and leaflet repair followed by ring annuloplasty. *C,* Chordal transposition. *D,* Chordal shortening plasty. (From Galloway, A. C., Colvin, S. B., Baumann, F. G., et al: Current concepts of mitral valve reconstruction for mitral insufficiency. Circulation, *78:*1087, 1988. By permission of the American Heart Association, Inc.)

Prosthetic Replacement

Operative techniques for prosthetic replacement have been described in the earlier section under *mitral stenosis.*

Selected Annuloplasty Techniques

Some form of mitral annuloplasty for mitral insufficiency has been periodically evaluated for more than three decades. In 1957, before prosthetic valves were available, techniques were independently developed by Lillehei and Merendino, also by Wooler in England. After prosthetic valves became available in 1961 and 1962, however, most interest in annuloplasty ceased with the exception of three different groups described in the following paragraphs.

Unfortunately, these techniques have applied only to a small percentage of patients with mitral insufficiency.

In 1960 McGoon reported a method of treatment for isolated ruptured chordae of the mural leaflet. The flail segment was plicated, and the mitral annulus was narrowed by annuloplasty. Orzulak in 1985 reported later experiences with this technique at the Mayo Clinic and described experiences with 131 patients. Good results were obtained in most patients. Approximately 10% of surviving patients required a repeat operation within 5 years and approximately 25% in 10 years. The reason was usually due to progressive mitral insufficiency.

Kay and Egerton in Los Angeles in 1963 described techniques of selected annuloplasty of the mural leaflet, used for ruptured chordae, and subsequently applied posteromedial annuloplasty of the mural leaflet to patients with mitral insufficiency secondary to coronary disease. In 1986 Kay reported experiences with 141 patients with mitral insufficiency from coronary disease who had combined coronary revascularization and correction of mitral insufficiency. In 101 of these patients a mural leaflet annuloplasty was done, which reduced the mural annulus to about 30% of its original size.

Reed reported a technique of asymmetric annuloplasty, plicating part of the annulus of the aortic leaflet and the majority of the annulus of the mural leaflet, in 1973. This technique was particularly valuable in children with pure rheumatic mitral insufficiency and also applied to some adults. In a 1980 report, Reed summarized his experiences during 17 years with 196 patients. The frequency of thromboembolism was low; late mortality was only 9%; and only 8% of patients required a repeat operation.

CARPENTIER'S TECHNIQUES OF MITRAL VALVE RECONSTRUCTION

One of the most important developments in surgical therapy of the mitral valve in the last decade has been the increasing use of Carpentier's techniques of mitral valve reconstruction. During the 1970s, Carpentier, at the Hôpital Broussais in Paris, developed different techniques of mitral reconstruction, which were well summarized in his classic "Honored Guest Address" to the American Association for Thoracic Surgery in 1983. At that time, he described experiences with more than 1,400 patients, the majority of whom had mitral insufficiency from rheumatic fever. The techniques that had been developed included an annuloplasty ring, a technique of quadrantic segmental resection of diseased mural leaflet; shortening of elongated chordae; and transposition of mural leaflet chordae to the aortic leaflet. These techniques were based on the realization that the anatomic deformities that caused mitral insufficiency were usually multiple and often required more than one technique for correction. This important concept explains why a single form of annuloplasty has never been applicable for most patients with mitral insufficiency. As described in the preceding *pathology* section, the principal abnormalities are dilatation of the annulus of the mural leaflet, often with elongation or rupture of chordae, and segmental disease of the mural leaflet. Because the annulus of the aortic leaflet does not dilate, reconstruction is usually feasible as long as a functioning aortic leaflet is present.

Significant contributions were also made by Duran in Spain and later by Paneth and Yacoub in England.

The NYU experience began in 1980 after a visit by one of the faculty members, Stephen Colvin, to Paris.

A unique feature of the NYU series is that a decision was made initially to include one surgeon in almost all operations, permitting one person to gain a visual familiarity with the different types of valvular abnormalities encountered. Reconstruction was used carefully in a few patients initially until durability was determined because Carpentier's experience had been primarily with rheumatic patients, whereas degenerative disease with prolapse and insufficiency was more common in the United States (Fig. 50–14). As the significant durability became more certain, the frequency of mitral reconstruction rapidly increased. Initial experiences with 103 patients were reported by Spencer in 1985. At present, the NYU experience includes more than 300 patients. This experience was summarized by Galloway in a review article published in 1988.

In the first 148 patients operated on, an annuloplasty ring was used in 84%, mural leaflet resection in 65%, chordae shortening in 31%, and chordae transposition in 5%. In more than 90% of the patients two or more abnormalities were corrected. (Fig. 50–15A shows an annuloplasty ring.)

An important technical point is that 60 to 70% of the mural leaflet can be safely resected as a quadrangular resection (Fig. 50–15B). This astonishing fact is one of the important principles that make reconstruction usually feasible. Chordae shortening and chordae transposition were used less frequently (see Fig. 50–15C and D). All of these techniques were developed by Carpentier and were shown in his 1983 report.

In the NYU series, hospital mortality was 1% for isolated reconstruction. Five-year freedom from late cardiac death was 90%, and 5-year freedom from late valve replacement was 90%. A most significant point is the fact that among the late valve failures, only *one* failure occurred in a patient with degenerative disease; all others developed in patients with rheumatic disease (Fig. 50–16).

Anticoagulant therapy with warfarin and dipyr-

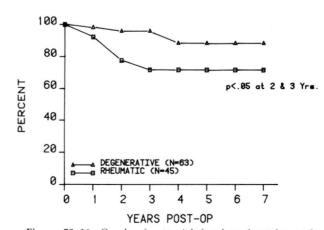

Figure 50–16. Graph of actuarial freedom from late valve failure after mitral reconstruction for patients with degenerative mitral disease compared with patients with rheumatic mitral disease. (From Galloway, A. C., Colvin, S. B., Baumann, F. G., et al: Current concepts of mitral valve reconstruction for mitral insufficiency. Circulation, *78*:1087, 1988. By permission of the American Heart Association, Inc.)

idamole was given for 3 months after operation, at which time warfarin was stopped but antiplatelet therapy continued for 1 year, using acetylsalicylic acid as well as dipyridamole. There has been a striking freedom from late thromboembolism, which is one of the major advantages of mitral valve reconstruction. Currently, 95% of patients are free of thromboemboli 7 years after operation (Fig. 50–17). Most emboli occur in the first few months after operation; beyond the first postoperative year, emboli are almost unknown. Endocarditis is rare and is almost zero in all reported series of mitral valve reconstruction. This constitutes another great advantage of the reconstructive techniques over insertion of prosthetic valves.

An unusual complication of Carpentier's reconstruction is left ventricular outflow tract obstruction associated with systolic anterior motion of the anterior mitral leaflet, which was reported by Kronzon and associates at NYU in 1983. This may develop with a frequency of approximately 10% of patients. In a subsequent 1986 report by Galler and associates 60 patients were studied with echocardiography more than 1 month after operation. Definite but insignificant narrowing of the outflow tract was found in most patients. Abnormal systolic anterior motion of the anterior mitral leaflet was found in six patients with gradients of 10 to 66 mm Hg measured by Doppler echocardiography. Fortunately, this degree of obstruction has not been associated with any symptoms.

Schiavone and associates in 1988 found an LVOT obstruction in 12 of 200 patients (6%) having reconstruction for degenerative mitral disease. Of the five obstructions detected intraoperatively with echocardiography, four were corrected by mitral valve replacement and one by removal of the ring. The

remaining seven were followed for more than 2 years. All had significant systolic anterior motion of the anterior leaflet but this remained clinically insignificant.

Cosgrove at the Cleveland Clinic similarly adopted Carpentier's methods and by 1986 reported good results with 117 patients. In a subsequent report in 1988, total experiences were stated to include approximately 300 patients. Kirklin in a review article in 1987 summarized available data and concluded that reconstruction rather than replacement should be used more frequently.

The 1988 Galloway report included a tabular summary of experiences with reconstruction in almost 3,000 patients reported from 13 different institutions. These data support the concept that reconstruction is widely applicable, safe, and durable.

Selected Bibliography

Arom, K. V., Nicoloff, D. M., Kersten, T. E., et al: St. Jude medical prosthesis: Valve-related deaths and complications. Ann. Thorac. Surg., 43:591, 1987.

Descriptions are given of experiences with 816 patients who were treated for 8 years. Of these patients 300 had mitral valve replacement. There was no malfunction of the valve, but thrombosis occurred in four patients (0.6%). Thromboembolism frequency was 1.78 per 100 patient years; anticoagulant hemorrhage frequency was 3.2.

Bjork, V. O., and Henze, A.: Ten years' experience with the Bjork-Shiley tilting disc valve. J. Thorac. Cardiovasc. Surg., 78:331, 1979.

A major development with prosthetic valves was the tilting disk valve, popularized by Bjork over 10 years ago. His decade of experience with more than 1,800 patients is summarized in this report.

Boyd, A. D., Engelman, R. H., Isom, O. W., et al: Tricuspid annuloplasty. J. Thorac. Cardiovasc. Surg., 68:344, 1974.

Many types of tricuspid valve reconstruction have been described in recent years. It remains a curiosity to the author why the technique of simple posterior leaflet annuloplasty has not been used more widely. As described initially in this report 9 years ago, it is simple and reliable and has been used at New York University for more than a decade with satisfactory results, unless advanced organic disease of the tricuspid valve requires valvular replacement.

Carpentier, A., Chauvaud, S., Fabiani, J. N., et al: Reconstructive surgery of mitral valve incompetence—Ten-year appraisal. J. Thorac. Cardiovasc. Surg., 79:338, 1980.

A major development of the recent years has been the elaboration of techniques of mitral valve reconstruction, compared with prosthetic valve replacement. Many contributions have been made by the group led by Carpentier in Paris. Experiences with 551 patients are summarized in this report. The prosthetic ring, developed by Carpentier, has been a major contribution.

Carpentier, A., Relland, J., Deloche, A., et al: Conservative management of the prolapsed mitral valve. Ann. Thorac. Surg., 26:294, 1978.

This remarkable paper describes the repair of prolapsed mitral

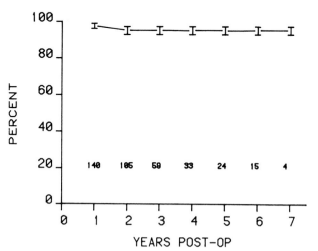

Figure 50–17. Actuarial freedom from late thromboemboli for 148 patients having mitral reconstruction. (Number over each end of interval mark on x axis indicates the number of patients who entered that interval.) (From Galloway, A. C., Colvin, S. B., Baumann, F. G., et al: Current concepts of mitral valve reconstruction for mitral insufficiency. Circulation, 78:1087, 1988. By permission of the American Heart Association, Inc.)

valves in 213 patients between 1969 and 1977, 109 of whom who had ruptured chordae as well. For uncertain reasons, Carpentier's methods of reconstruction have not become popular in the United States, although they have been enthusiastically adopted at New York University. Probably a simple lack of familiarity with this technique is the principal reason, although only time and meaningful data will provide the ultimate answer.

Cobanoglu, A., Grunkenmeier, G. L., Aru, G. M., et al: Mitral replacement: Clinical experience with the ball-valve prosthesis; 25 years later. Ann. Surg., 202:376, 1985.

This report from Albert Starr, whose classic report in 1961 launched the modern era of prosthetic valve replacements, summarizes his total experiences. Three different types of prostheses were evaluated but the Model 6120 has remained the standard for the last several years. A total of 318 prostheses were implanted.

The data showed a surprising decrease in frequency of thromboembolism after 1973, even though the prosthesis was the same. Since 1973, 93% of patients were free of thromboemboli 5 years after operation, compared with only 70% in the earlier group. There were no incidences of valve thrombosis or mechanical failure. The authors emphasize that survival is not a good measurement for valve evaluation because the dominant risk factors are age, NYHA class, left ventricular function, and urgency of operation. In this series, 5-year, 10-year, and 15-year survival was 73, 54, and 36%, respectively.

Cobbs, B. W., Jr., Hatcher, C. R., Jr., Craver, J. M., et al: Transverse midventricular disruption after mitral valve replacement. Am. Heart J., 99:33, 1980.

An infrequent but lethal complication of mitral valve replacement is rupture of the posterior wall of the left ventricle. This can occur in at least three areas, as described in detail in this chapter. The most bizarre is a transverse rupture of the muscle of the posterior ventricular wall, between the mitral annulus above and the stumps of the papillary muscles below. This paper is the most extensive report in the English literature of this unusual complication, which is perhaps a result of removal of the posterior papillary muscle in elderly people with small left ventricles.

Czer, L. S., Matloff, J. M., Chaux, A., et al: The St. Jude valve: Analysis of thromboembolism, warfarin-related hemorrhage and survival. Am. Heart J., 114:389, 1987.

Experiences with 527 patients treated for 8 years were analyzed. Five-year survival was 63%. No structural failures occurred. Valve thrombosis in six patients occurred without effective warfarin therapy. Most common complication was anticoagulant hemorrhage, 2.9% per patient year.

Edmunds, L. H.: Thrombotic and bleeding complications of prosthetic heart valves: Collective review. Ann. Thorac. Surg., 44:430, 1987.

This extensive report by Edmunds analyzes the reported frequency of thrombotic and bleeding complications with prosthetic valves in more than 20 different institutions. This is an excellent summary of the current magnitude of this serious problem.

Flemma, R. J., Mullen, D. C., Kleinman, L. H., et al: Survival and "event-free" analysis of 785 patients with Björk-Shiley spherical-disc valves at 10–16 years. Ann. Thorac. Surg., 45:258, 1988.

This large complete follow-up study included 268 mitral valve replacements. The mean follow-up was 12 years. Twelve-year survival was most closely related to age: less than 50 years, 70%; 50 to 59 years, 52%; over 60 years, 38%. The frequency of complications per 100 patient years was as follows: emboli: 1.8; thrombosis: 0.36; bleeding: 4.5; and endocarditis: 0.4.

Galloway, A. C., Colvin, S. B., Baumann, F. G., et al: Current

concepts of mitral valve reconstruction for mitral insufficiency. Circulation, 78:1087, 1988.

A detailed summary of late results with the first 148 patients operated on at NYU are presented. In addition current concepts regarding mitral reconstruction are summarized, and an analysis is made of the significant data published by others, totaling experiences with almost 3,000 patients from 13 different institutions.

Gross, R. I., Cunningham, J. N., Jr., Snively, S. L., et al: Long-term results of open radical mitral commissurotomy: Ten-year follow-up study of 202 patients. Am. J. Cardiol., 47:821, 1981.

With the increasingly good results with prosthetic valves, the value of mitral commissurotomy, compared with valve replacement, has been periodically questioned. This long-term follow-up conclusively shows that commissurotomy is superior to valve replacement if the gradient can be corrected without producing significant insufficiency.

Jamieson, W. R. E., Rosado, L. J., Munro, A. I., et al: Carpentier-Edwards standard porcine bioprosthesis: Primary tissue failure (structural valve deterioration) by age groups. Ann. Thorac. Surg., 46:155, 1988.

Experiences with 1,401 porcine prostheses for 11 years were analyzed, with a mean follow-up of 5.6 years. One hundred four prostheses failed. Freedom from primary tissue failure at 10 years was almost 80%. The freedom from deterioration increased by decades: 10 years after operation, only 27% of patients less than 30 years of age were all right; 30 to 59-year group, 77%; more than 60 years, 83%.

Lindblom, D.: Long-term clinical results after mitral valve replacement with the Björk-Shiley prosthesis. J. Thorac. Cardiovasc. Surg., 95:321, 1988.

This unique paper summarized long-term results with all Björk prostheses inserted at the Karolinska Hospital over 15 years, with a total of 810 prostheses. Follow-up was 100% complete with an average of 6 years. Actuarial survival at 5, 10, and 15 years was 78, 62, and 51%, respectively. Of late deaths 25% were related to the valve. The frequency of emboli was 1.6 per 100 patient years, and most occurred in the first year. Thrombosis also principally occurred in the first year, less commonly with the concave-convex model. Anticoagulant hemorrhage was at a constant rate of 1.2 per 100 patient years. Strut fracture occurred in seven patients with the concavo-convex. Endocarditis was rare, with only five patients (0.1 per 100 patient years).

Magilligan, D. J., Lewis, J. W., Allen, A. M., et al: The porcine valve prosthetic heart valve: Experiences over 15 years. Ann. Thorac. Surgery, (in press).

This report analyzed experiences with 1,015 patients operated on 1971 with a 100% follow-up. Fifteen years later, freedom from tissue degeneration after mitral replacement was only 41%, with 45% after aortic replacement. This report, which is the first report that provides a 15-year follow-up, clearly indicates that valve failure rapidly increases between 10 to 15 years after operation.

Miller, D. W., Jr., Johnson, D. D., and Ivey, T. D.: Does preservation of the posterior chordae tendineae enhance survival during mitral valve replacement? Ann. Thorac. Surg., 28:22, 1979.

The transverse ventricular rupture after the mitral valve replacement, described in the earlier cited report by Cobbs and associates, may be avoided by preservation of the chordae to the annulus of the mural leaflet of the mitral valve. This report, although certainly not conclusive, describes preliminary experiences with this technique, a concept suggested by Lillehei in the early 1960s for a different reason.

Murphy, D. A., Levine, F. H., Buckley, M. J., et al: Mechanical valves: A comparative analysis of the Starr-Edwards and Björk-Shiley prostheses. J. Thorac. Cardiovasc. Surg., 86:746, 1983.

This report from the Massachusetts General Hospital compared 105 disk valves with 342 ball valves inserted over 5 years. At 5-year follow-up the survival was the same, 78%. More patients were free from emboli at 5 years with the disk prosthesis than with the ball valve (89% versus 83%). However, the thrombosis rate with the disk valve was 8%. The frequency of endocarditis was similar, approximately 1% per year; anticoagulant hemorrhage was also similar at approximately 2% per year.

Spencer, F. C., Galloway, A. G., and Colvin, S. B.: A clinical evaluation of the hypothesis that rupture of the left ventricle following mitral valve replacement can be prevented by preservation of the chordae of the mural leaflet. Ann. Surg., 202:673, 1985.

Results with a prospective study at NYU concerning rupture of the left ventricle are described. Fourteen patients ruptured the left ventricle after mitral valve replacement over 9 years, ending in 1981. A prospective study, begun at that time, concentrated on preservation of some chordae to the annulus of the mural leaflet at operation. No further patients have been seen with rupture of the ventricle since this technique has been adopted.

Bibliography

Arom, K. V., Nicoloff, D. M., Kersten, T. E., et al: St. Jude medical prosthesis: Valve-related deaths and complications. Ann. Thorac. Surg., 43:591, 1987.
Bailey, C. P.: The surgical treatment of mitral stenosis (mitral commissurotomy). Dis. Chest, 15:377, 1949.
Bjork, V. O., and Henze, A.: Ten years experience with the Bjork-Shiley tilting disc valve. J. Thorac. Cardiovasc. Surg., 78:331, 1979.
Boyd, A. D., Tremblay, R. E., Spencer, F. C., and Bahnson, H. T.: Estimation of cardiac output soon after intracardiac surgery with cardiopulmonary bypass. Ann. Surg., 150:613, 1959.
Boyd, A. D., Engelman, R. H., Isom, O. W., et al: Tricuspid annuloplasty. J. Thorac. Cardiovasc. Surg., 68:344, 1974.
Camara, J. L., Aris, A., Padro, J. M., et al: Long-term results of mitral valve surgery in patients with severe pulmonary hypertension. Ann. Thorac. Surg., 45:133, 1988.
Carpentier, A.: Cardiac valve surgery—the "French correction." J. Thorac. Cardiovasc. Surg., 86:323, 1983.
Catinella, F. P., Cunningham, J. N., Jr., Srungaram, R. K., et al: Comparison of myocardial protection offered by three different techniques of blood potassium cardioplegia administration. Arch. Surg., 116:1509, 1981.
Cobanoglu, A., Grunkemeier, G. L., Aru, G. M., et al: Mitral replacement: Clinical experience with a ball-valve prosthesis. Ann. Surg., 202:376, 1985.
Cobb, L. A., Werner, J. A., and Trobaugh, G. B.: Sudden cardiac death. I: A decade's experience with out-of-hospital resuscitation. Mod. Concepts Cardiovasc. Dis., 49:31, 1980.
Cobbs, B. W., Jr., Hatcher, C. R., Jr., Craver, J. M., et al: Transverse midventricular disruption after mitral valve replacement. Am. Heart J., 99:33, 1980.
Cosgrove, D. M., Chavez, A. M., Lytle, B. W., et al: Results of mitral valve reconstruction. Circulation, 74:I-82, 1986.
Craver, J. M., Jones, E. L., Guyton, R. A., et al: Avoidance of transverse midventricular disruption following mitral valve replacement. Ann. Thorac. Surg., 40:163, 1985.
Cunningham, J. N., Jr., Adams, P. X., Knopp, E., et al: Preservation of ATP, ultrastructure, and ventricular function following aortic cross-clamping and reperfusion—clinical use of blood potassium cardioplegia. J. Thorac. Cardiovasc. Surg., 78:708, 1979.

Cutler, E. C., and Levine, S. A.: Cardiotomy and valvulotomy for mitral stenosis. Boston Med. Surg. J., 188:1023, 1923.
Czer, L. S., Matloff, J. M., C., Chaux, A., et al: The St. Jude valve: Analysis of thromboembolism, warfarin-related hemorrhage, and survival. Am. Heart J., 114:389, 1987.
David, T. E., and Ho, W. C.: The effect of preservation of chordae tendineae on mitral valve replacement for postinfarction mitral regurgitation. Circulation, 74:I-116, 1986.
Duran, C. G., Pomar, J. L., Revuelta, J. M., et al: Conservative operation for mitral insufficiency: Critical analysis supported by postoperative hemodynamic studies of 72 patients. J. Thorac. Cardiovasc. Surg., 79:326, 1980.
Edmunds, L. H., Jr.: Thrombotic and bleeding complications of prosthetic heart valves. Ann. Thorac. Surg., 44:430, 1987.
Flemma, R. J., Mullen, D. C., Kleinman, L. H., et al: Survival and "event-free" analysis of 785 patients with Björk-Shiley spherical-disc valves at 10 to 16 years. Ann. Thorac. Surg., 45:258, 1988.
Galler, M., Kronzon, I., Slater, J., et al: Long-term follow-up after mitral valve reconstruction: Incidence of post-operative left ventricular outflow obstruction. Circulation, 74:I-99, 1986.
Galloway, A. C., Colvin, S. B., Slater, J., et al: Long-term results of mitral valve reconstruction with Carpentier techniques in 148 patients with mitral insufficiency. Circulation, 78:I-97, 1988.
Galloway, A. C., Colvin, S. B., Baumann, F. G., et al: Current concepts of mitral valve reconstruction for mitral insufficiency. Circulation, 78:1087, 1988.
Galloway, A. C., Colvin, S. B., Baumann, F. G., et al: A comparison of mitral valve reconstruction with mitral valve replacement: Intermediate-term results. Ann. Thorac. Surg., 47:655, 1989.
Gross, R. I., Cunningham, J. N., Jr., Snively, S. L., et al: Long-term results of open radical mitral commissurotomy: Ten-year follow-up study of 202 patients. Am. J. Cardiol., 47:821, 1981.
Halseth, W. L., Elliott, D. P., Walker, E. L., and Smith, E. A.: Open mitral commissurotomy: A modern re-evaluation. J. Thorac. Cardiovasc. Surg., 80:842, 1980.
Harken, D. E., Ellis, L. B., Ware, P. F., and Norman, L. R.: The surgical treatment of mitral stenosis. N. Engl. J. Med., 239:801, 1948.
Hetzer, R., Bougioukas, G., Franz, M., and Borst, H. G.: Mitral valve replacement with preservation of papillary muscles and chordae tendineae—revival of a seemingly forgotten concept. Thorac. Cardiovasc. Surgeon, 31:291, 1983.
Isom, O. W., Spencer, F. C., Glassman, E., et al: Long-term results in 1375 patients undergoing valve replacement with the Starr-Edwards cloth-covered steel ball prosthesis. Ann. Surg., 186:310, 1977.
Jamieson, W. R., Rosado, L. J., Munro, A. I., et al: Carpentier-Edwards standard porcine bioprosthesis: Primary tissue failure (structural valve deterioration) by age groups. Ann. Thorac. Surg., 46:155, 1988.
Karlson, K. J., Ashraf, M. M., and Berger, R. L.: Rupture of left ventricle following mitral valve replacement. Ann. Thorac. Surg., 46:590, 1988.
Kay, G. L., Kay, J. H., Zubiate, P., et al: Mitral valve repair for mitral regurgitation secondary to coronary artery disease. Circulation, 74:I-88, 1986.
Kay, J. H., and Egerton, W. S.: The repair of mitral insufficiency associated with ruptured chordae tendineae. Ann. Surg., 157:351, 1963.
Kay, J. H., Maselli-Campagna, G., and Tsuji, H. K.: Surgical treatment of tricuspid insufficiency. Ann. Surg., 162:53, 1965.
Kirklin, J. W.: Mitral valve repair for mitral incompetence. Modern Concepts of Cardiovasc. Dis., 56:7, 1987.
Kirklin, J. W., and Barratt-Boyes, B. G.: Cardiac Surgery. New York, John Wiley & Sons, 1986.
Kronzon, I., Mercurio, P., et al: Echocardiographic evaluation of Carpentier mitral valvuloplasty. Am. Heart J., 106:362, 1983.
Lillehei, C. W., Gott, V. L., DeWall, R. A., and Varco, R. L.: Surgical correction of pure mitral insufficiency by annuloplasty under direct vision. Lancet, 77:446, 1957.
Lillehei, C. W., Levy, M. J., and Bonnabeau, R. C.: Mitral valve replacement with preservation of papillary muscles and chordae tendineae. J. Thorac. Cardiovasc. Surg., 47:532, 1964.

Lindblom, D.: Long-term clinical results after mitral valve replacement with the Björk-Shiley prosthesis. J. Thorac. Cardiovasc. Surg., *95*:321, 1988.

Logan, A., and Turner, R.: Surgical treatment of mitral stenosis with particular reference to the transventricular approach with a mechanical dilator. Lancet, 2:874, 1959.

Magilligan, D. J., Lewis, J. W., Allen, A. M., et al: The porcine valve prosthetic heart valve: Experiences in 15 years. Ann. Thorac. Surg., (in press.)

McGoon, D. C.: Repair of mitral insufficiency due to ruptured chordae tendineae. J. Thorac. Surg., *39*:357, 1960.

Miller, D. C., Oyer, P. E., Stinson, E. B., et al: Ten to 15 year reassessment of the performance characteristics of the Starr-Edwards model 6120 mitral valve prosthesis. J. Thorac. Cardiovasc. Surg., *85*:1, 1983.

Miller, D. W., Jr., Johnson, D. D., and Ivey, T. D.: Does preservation of the posterior chordae tendineae enhance survival during mitral valve replacement? Ann. Thorac. Surg., *28*:22, 1979.

Molajo, A. O., Bennett, D. H., Bray, C. L., et al: Actuarial Analysis of late results after closed mitral valvulotomy. Ann. Thorac. Surg., *45*:364, 1988.

Mullin, M. J., Engelman, R. M., Isom, O. W., et al: Experience with open mitral commissurotomy in 100 consecutive patients. Surgery, *76*:974, 1974.

Murphy, D. A., Levine, F. H., Buckley, M. J., et al: Mechanical valves: A comparative analysis of Starr-Edwards and Björk-Shiley prostheses. J. Thorac. Cardiovasc. Surg., *86*:746, 1983.

Nakano, S., Kawashima, Y., Nirose, H., et al: Evaluation of long-term results of bicuspidalization annuloplasty for functional tricuspid regurgitation. J. Thorac. Cardiovasc. Surg., *95*:340, 1988.

Orzulak, T. A., Schaff, H. V., and Danielson, G. K.: Mitral regurgitation due to ruptured chordae tendineae. Early and late results of valve repair. J. Thorac. Cardiovasc. Surg., *89*:491, 1985.

Penkoske, P. A., Ellis, F. H., Alexander, S., et al: Results of valve reconstruction for mitral regurgitation secondary to mitral valve prolapse. Am. J. Cardiol., *55*:735, 1985.

Qureshi, S. A., Halim, M. A., Campalani, G., et al: Late results of mitral valve replacement using unstented antibiotic sterilised aortic homografts. Br. Heart J., *50*:564, 1983.

Reed, G. E.: Repair of mitral regurgitation. Am. J. Cardiol., *31*:494, 1973.

Reed, G. E., Pooley, R. W., and Moggio, R. A.: Durability of measured mitral annuloplasty: Seventeen-year study. J. Thorac. Cardiovasc. Surg., *79*:321, 1980.

Reul, G. J., Jr., Cooley, D. A., Duncan, J. M., et al: Valve failure with the Ionescu-Shiley bovine pericardial bioprosthesis: Analysis of 2680 patients. J. Vasc. Surg., 2:192, 1985.

Roe, B. B., Edmunds, H., Jr., Fishman, N. H., and Hutchinson, J. C.: Open mitral commissurotomy. Ann. Thorac. Surg., *12*:483, 1971.

Schiavone, W. A., Cosgrove, D. M., Lever, H. M., et al: Long-term follow-up of patients with left ventricular outflow tract obstruction after Carpentier ring mitral valvuloplasty. Circulation, *78*:I-60, 1988.

Scott, W. C., Miller, D. C., Haverich, A., et al: Operative risk of mitral valve replacement: Discriminant analysis of 1329 procedures. Circulation, *72*:II-108, 1985.

Selzer, A., and Cohen, K. E.: Natural history of mitral stenosis: A review. Circulation, *45*:878, 1972.

Shore, D. F., Wong, P., Paneth, M., et al: Results of mitral valvuloplasty with a suture plication technique. J. Thorac. Cardiovasc. Surg., *79*:349, 1980.

Spencer, F. C.: A plea for early, open mitral commissurotomy. Am. Heart J., *95*:668, 1978.

Spencer, F. C., Colvin, S. B., Culliford, A. T., and Isom, O. N.: Experiences with the Carpentier techniques of mitral valve reconstruction in 103 patients (1980–1985). J. Thorac. Cardiovasc. Surg., *90*:341, 1985.

Spencer, F. C., Galloway, A. G., and Colvin, S. B.: A clinical evaluation of the hypothesis that rupture of the left ventricle following mitral valve replacement can be prevented by preservation of the chordae of the mural leaflet. Ann. Surg., *202*:673:1985.

Spencer, F. C., Grossi, E. A., Braumann, F. G., et al: Experiences with 1643 porcine prosthetic valves in 1492 patients. Ann. Surg., *203*:691, 1986.

Srungaram, R. K., Cunningham, J. N., Jr., Catinella, F. P., et al: Blood versus crystalloid cardioplegia. Which is superior for prolonged aortic cross-clamping? Surg. Forum, *32*:288, 1981.

Starr, A., and Edwards, M. L.: Mitral replacement: Clinical experience with a ball valve prosthesis. Ann. Surg., *154*:726, 1961.

Treasure, R. L., Rainer, W. G., Strevey, T. E., et al: Intraoperative left ventricular rupture associated with mitral valve replacement. Chest, *66*:511, 1974.

Yacoub, M., Halim, M., Radley-Smith, R., et al: Surgical treatment of mitral regurgitation caused by floppy valves: Repair versus replacement. Circulation, *64*:II-210, 1981.

Zacharias, A., Grones, L. K., Cheanvechai, C., et al: Rupture of the posterior wall of the left ventricle following mitral valve replacement. J. Thorac. Cardiovasc. Surg., *69*:259, 1975.

CHAPTER 51

COMPLICATIONS FROM CARDIAC PROSTHESES

I INFECTION, THROMBOSIS, AND EMBOLI ASSOCIATED WITH INTRACARDIAC PROSTHESES

Ellis L. Jones
Stephen W. Schwarzmann
William A. Check
Charles R. Hatcher, Jr.

INFECTION OF INTRACARDIAC DEVICES

Experience with infectious complications of prosthetic valve surgery shows that a useful purpose is served by classifying infective prosthetic valve endocarditis (PVE) according to the time at which infection occurs after surgical insertion of the valve. Infection that occurs within the first 60 days after operation is generally due to organisms acquired during or shortly after operation, whereas infection that occurs 2 months or longer after operation shares a pathogenesis with endocarditis on native heart valves. This classification also appears to be related to the relative morbidity and mortality of the infection and to the organism that causes the infection. The incidence of both early and late PVE is approximately 3.5%. Incremental risk factors for developing prosthetic endocarditis are a history of native valve endocarditis, black race, mechanical prosthesis, male sex, and prolonged cardiopulmonary bypass (Karp, 1987). The incidence of early PVE ranges between 0 and 7% with an average of 1% and the mortality ranges between 56 and 88%, with an average of 72%. The incidence of late PVE is related to the duration of follow-up of the patient. At 6 months the incidence of PVE averages 1.2%, but in at least one study (Clarkson and Barratt-Boyes, 1970), the incidence increased to 2.2% by 5 years after operation. The mortality from late PVE is between 31 and 66% with an average of 45%. In both the early and late groups, mortality appears to be lowest with streptococcal infection and highest with nonstreptococcal infec-

tions (staphylococci, gram-negative bacteria, and fungi). The fact that streptococcal infection is more common in late PVE may explain partly the lower mortality from late PVE. Other factors, such as a recent postoperative state with incomplete healing of the surgical field and tissue trauma, also affect the outcome of early PVE.

Early Prosthetic Valve Endocarditis

It is generally thought that the organisms responsible for early PVE are acquired during operation or in the early postoperative period. In a study designed to identify potential sources of contamination (Kluge et al, 1974), researchers found that the air in the operating room contained several organisms, mostly staphylococci and diphtheroids, and that the greatest microbial density occurred immediately above the operative field. Cultures from the operative site (i.e., the repaired area of myocardium or the prosthesis) were more often positive than not, especially when tested just before closure. Again, diphtheroids and staphylococci were the most commonly isolated organisms. Donor blood bags and the pump reservoir after bypass were less common sources of bacterial contamination; the blood bags were particularly likely to harbor gram-negative rods and yeasts and common skin contaminants. In the postoperative period, opportunities for infection of the freshly operated tissues include transient bacteremia as a complication of wound infections, pneumonia, emergency reoperation, urinary tract infec-

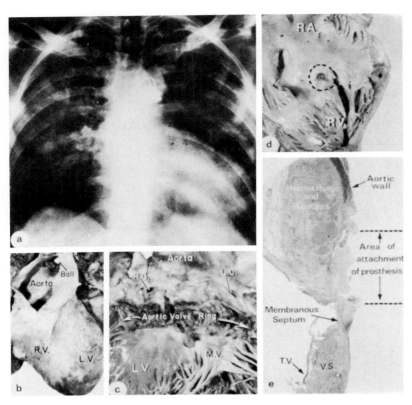

Figure 51–1. *Staphylococcus epidermidis* prosthetic aortic valve endocarditis in a 48-year-old man. He had been well for 11 months after insertion of the Starr-Edwards prosthesis when, 1 month before death and 6 weeks after dental extraction, shaking chills appeared and blood cultures were positive for *S. epidermidis*. Despite intensive antibiotic therapy, signs of aortic regurgitation appeared, and minutes before death he complained of "feeling funny." *a*, Chest film immediately postmortem showed that the prosthesis had dislodged and migrated to the aortic arch. *b*, Anterior view of the heart and opened ascending aorta. The detached prosthesis ball is visible, lodged in the transverse aorta. (L.V. = left ventricle; R.V. = right ventricle.) *c*, Opened aorta, aortic valve "ring," and left ventricle showing a totally necrotic aortic annulus. (M.V. = anterior mitral leaflet; R.C. = ostium of right coronary artery; L.C. = ostium of left coronary artery.) *d*, Opened right atrium (R.A.), tricuspid valve, and right ventricle (R.V.) showing a ring abscess *(circle)* that had extended from the aortic prosthetic annulus. *e*, Photomicrograph through the aortic valve "ring" showing a large ring abscess and the necrotic aortic annulus material, which extended through the membranous ventricular septum into the right atrium. (Hematoxylin and eosin stain; original magnification × 2.) (T.V. = tricuspid valve leaflet; V.S. = ventricular septum.) (From Arnett, E. N., and Roberts, W. C.: Active infective endocarditis: A clinicopathologic analysis of 137 necropsy patients. Curr. Probl. Cardiol., Vol. 1, p. 2. Copyright © 1976 by Year Book Medical Publishers. Reproduced with permission.)

tions, and especially contaminated intravascular catheters. In one study, 50% of intravascular catheter tips yielded various gram-positive and gram-negative organisms and fungi when routinely cultured immediately after removal. These infected catheters can become a source of bacteremia, with secondary seeding of micro-organisms on the newly inserted prosthetic heart valve. Measures such as removal of intravascular lines as soon as possible and frequent flushing of the lines appear to reduce the incidence of contamination, whereas manipulation without flushing appears to increase the likelihood of contamination.

The placement of a prosthetic valve in the setting of active native heart valve endocarditis could be considered to predispose the patient to early infection of the implanted prosthetic valve. However, this complication has not been a major factor; it occurs at a rate of approximately 4%, although the operative mortality when active infection is present is 20 to 30%. There appears to be no major difference in the risk of PVE between the use of a mechanical valve or heterograft tissue valve in this situation.

Late Prosthetic Valve Endocarditis

Late PVE may be acquired intraoperatively or postoperatively and simply has a long incubation period, perhaps because of the use of prophylactic antibiotics. Prophylactic antibiotics would then serve only to suppress growth of bacteria introduced intraoperatively or perioperatively and thus delay the clinical manifestations of the infection. This possibility is supported by data that showed a high incidence of valve infection due to staphylococci, diphtheroids, and gram-negative organisms in the first 18 months after operation, after which streptococci were responsible for 37% of all infections. This change in microbiologic etiology and the less acute clinical course in patients with delayed PVE suggest that the sources of the infection are much the same as in native heart valve infections (Santinga et al, 1984). These sources include transient bacteremias from genitourinary tract surgical therapy, dental manipulation or extraction, primary skin infection, or upper respiratory tract infections (Karchmer et al, 1978). Patients who have prosthetic heart valves require aggressive antibiotic prophylaxis when they undergo procedures that predispose them to endocarditis.

Epidemiology and Pathology

A study that included 51 patients who developed PVE in a group of 2,184 patients who received either heterograft tissue or mechanical heart valves showed several other features that characterize the epidemiology of PVE (Rossiter et al, 1978). There appeared to be no major difference in the risk of developing PVE between the use of heterograft tissue valves and mechanical valves (Cowgill et al, 1987). Compared with another study in which no early PVE was seen on heterograft tissue valves in the aortic position (Magilligan et al, 1977), the study by Rossiter and associates showed a significantly higher incidence of early PVE in heterograft tissue valves compared with mechanical valves in the aortic position. Concomitant aortocoronary bypass grafting was more common in the tissue valve group and resulted in increased operative time and additional risk of contamination by the saphenous vein graft. However, when infection was established, heterograft tissue valves appeared to be more easily sterilized. This impression was supported by the pathologic findings on recovered specimens; infection of heterograft valves was often limited to the valve leaflets, whereas ring infection was almost always present in mechanical valves. A ring abscess, whether associated with a heterograft valve or a mechanical valve, renders antibiotic sterilization almost impossible. A statistically significant finding that is universally reported is that there is a greater risk of developing PVE at the aortic site than at the mitral site, which is opposite to the situation in native valve endocarditis.

The pathologic focus of PVE is most often at the valve seat. Abscess formation and destruction of tissue are the hallmarks and often involve the entire circumference of the valve seat. With prosthetic aortic valves, the process may progress to dehiscence, with resultant paravalvular leaks and formation of mycotic aneurysms that border the prosthetic valve seat (Fig. 51–1). Extension of the ring infection to adjacent cardiac structures and the aorta is common and may produce fistula and disturbances of atrioventricular (AV) conduction (Fig. 51–2). Clinically, new regurgitant murmurs and various degrees of heart block may be observed. The appearance of left bundle branch block does not seem to indicate inflammatory invasion of the conduction system as reliably as does the presence of AV block.

Compared with the situation in aortic PVE, infection of a mitral prosthesis more commonly results in obstruction than regurgitation. Obstruction may result from immobilization of the disk or ball, in which case regurgitation may also occur, or fusion of the growths over the atrial surface of the valve may cause obstruction of the inflow site (Fig. 51–3). The development of obstruction by valve immobilization can often be recognized by changes in valve sounds and fluoroscopic evaluation of ball motion. Obstruction that occurs when infectious growth interferes with transmitral flow without interference with valve motion may appear simply as pulmonary congestion associated with evidence of pulmonary venous hypertension. This obstruction can be confirmed by measurement of a significant transmural gradient. Rapidly fatal disease due to significant obstruction of left ventricular flow with minimal evidence of valvular dysfunction has been reported, and these symptoms must always be investigated rapidly when there is a possibility of prosthetic mitral valve endocarditis (McAllister et al, 1974). In addition

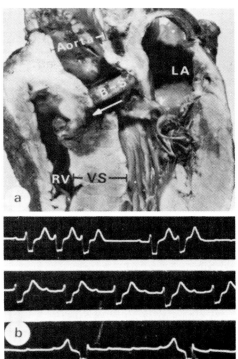

Figure 51–2. *Staphylococcus epidermidis* prosthetic aortic valve endocarditis in a 51-year-old man. His stenotic bicuspid aortic valve had been replaced with a Bjork-Shiley prosthesis 83 days before death. Fever was present in the early postoperative period, and shortly before death, complete heart block and signs of congestive heart failure appeared. *a,* Longitudinal section of the heart with the anterior portion removed. The Bjork-Shiley (B-S) prosthesis is partially detached, and the ring abscess *(arrow)* has burrowed through the ventricular septum (VS) into the right ventricle (RV). (LA = left atrium.) (From Arnett, E. N., and Roberts, W. C.: Active infective endocarditis: A clinicopathologic analysis of 137 necropsy patients. Curr. Probl. Cardiol., Vol. 1, p. 2. Copyright © 1976 by Year Book Medical Publishers. Reproduced with permission.)

to producing annular infection and abscess formation and its complications, endocarditis involving heterograft valves may be limited to the valve cusps (Fig. 51–4). This infection results in total destruction of the cusps or in vegetations that stiffen and obstruct the valve and make its replacement mandatory even if the infection has been eradicated.

Diagnosis and Microbiology

The diagnosis of PVE is generally accepted (1) if there are at least two positive blood cultures for the same organism in a patient with a compatible clinical syndrome and no other potential source of the bacteremia or (2) if histopathologic evidence of endocarditis is found in a surgical or autopsy specimen. A compatible clinical syndrome may include fever, development of a new regurgitant murmur, newly developed splenomegaly, or evidence of peripheral emboli. In most series, fever is the most common clinical finding and is observed in 95% of patients with early and late PVE. When fever occurs, a new

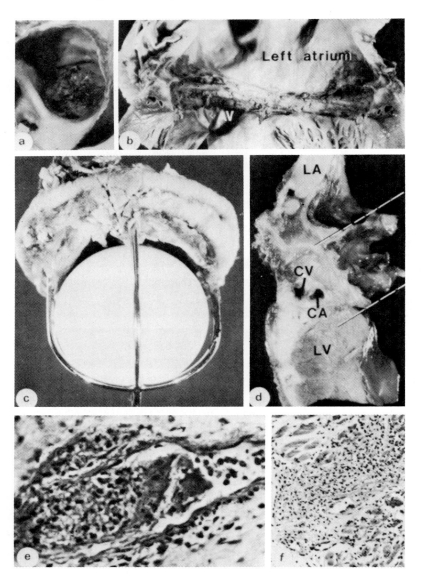

Figure 51–3. *Staphylococcus aureus* prosthetic mitral valve endocarditis in a 47-year-old man who had the onset of symptoms of infective endocarditis 4 months after valve replacement. He had done well during the first 3 months after operation but developed symptoms of infection after grafting of a cutaneous ulcer. Signs of prosthetic dysfunction were never detected clinically. *a*, Prosthetic mitral orifice obstructed by vegetative material, as seen from the left atrium. *b*, Opened left atrium, mitral annulus, and left ventricle after removal of the mitral prosthesis. The entire annulus is necrotic. (AV = aortic valve.) *c*, Mitral prosthesis showing infected thrombus at its base. *d*, Longitudinal section through left atrium (LA), mitral annulus, and left ventricle (LV). The former site of attachment of the prosthesis is designated by the dashed lines. The infective process burrowed through the wall of the heart and caused pericarditis. (CA = coronary artery; CV = coronary vein in the right atrioventricular sulcus.) (From Arnett, E. N., and Roberts, W. C.: Active infective endocarditis: A clinicopathologic analysis of 137 necropsy patients. Curr. Probl. Cardiol., Vol. 1, p. 2. Copyright © 1976 by Year Book Medical Publishers. Reproduced with permission.)

regurgitant murmur and septic shock are usually seen in early PVE; manifestations of peripheral emboli and splenomegaly are more commonly seen in late PVE. This difference is probably related to the duration of endocarditis before diagnosis.

The differential diagnosis of early PVE may be difficult in the early postoperative period when complications of sternal wound infection, pneumonia, septic phlebitis, or urinary tract infections have occurred. It may be difficult to discern whether positive blood cultures at this time indicate infection on the prosthetic heart valve. PVE was not usually the source of a sustained bacteremia due to gram-negative rods that occurred less than 25 days after operation and had obvious potential sites of origin in the absence of any changes in heart murmurs (Sande et al, 1972). However, multiple positive blood cultures that showed gram-positive organisms after the 25th postoperative day were likely to originate from the heart, especially if accompanied by new or changing heart murmurs. Exceptions to this clinical dictum

exist, particularly in relation to bacteremia with gram-negative rods in the early postoperative setting. Thus, the surgeon cannot confidently dismiss the diagnosis of PVE in this situation. Treatment for PVE is therefore often initiated in an effort to avoid its dismal prognosis.

The less acute course of late PVE may often be diagnosed as influenza or some other nonspecific cause of fever and weakness. In any event, the diagnosis must first be considered and then usually confirmed by blood culture. In one study, at least one of five blood samples was positive in 91% of patients, the first culture was positive in 87%, and all blood cultures were positive in 73% (Masur and Johnson, 1980). Antibiotic administration within a 2-week period before blood cultures are obtained reduces positive cultures only modestly and is therefore still very useful. In the case of fungal PVE, blood cultures are less reliable, and diagnosis is sometimes made by examination of peripheral emboli or histologic examination of the resected valve. When a

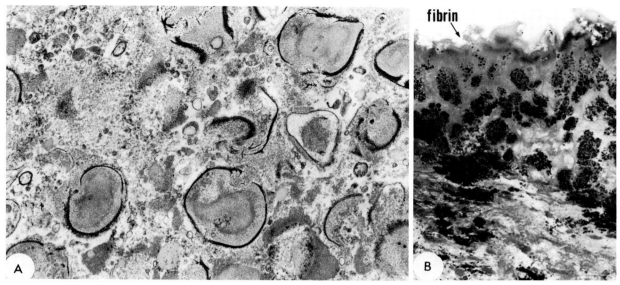

Figure 51–4. Infection of porcine bioprostheses. *A*, Electron micrograph showing lysed organisms in the substance of a porcine valve removed from a patient who developed signs of prosthetic stenosis and regurgitation and who had blood cultures positive for *Staphylococcus* (× 30,000). *B*, Clusters of gram-positive organisms in a fibrin meshwork on the surface of the valve leaflet shown in *A*, with invasion of the underlying valve tissue (toluidine blue stain, × 600). (Courtesy of Victor J. Ferrans, M.D., Ph.D.)

patient with strong clinical features of PVE has a negative blood culture, the physician should either initiate empiric antibiotic therapy or, preferably, do cardiac exploration. This procedure both confirms the diagnosis and allows replacement of the infected valve.

Other diagnostic aids include assessment of prosthetic valve stability by cinefluoroscopy and angiography. The former test generally requires an earlier study for comparison, although a single test that shows a valve that rocks more than 7 to 10 degrees is considered to be abnormal. Angiography may also be used to assess secure attachment of the valve to the valve seat or to identify the presence of a myocardial abscess or fistula.

The presence of growths on both native and prosthetic heart valves has been shown by two-dimensional echocardiography. Unlike M-mode echocardiography, which gives a relatively poor spatial impression of vegetations, the two-dimensional technique shows size, shape, attachment, and motion of vegetations. This diagnostic aid is most likely to be helpful in a more advanced infection, at which point salvageability is at its lowest.

The microbiology of PVE is reasonably consistent among several series of patients. Approximate proportions of the various organisms in early and late PVE are shown in Table 51–1. Staphylococcal species are the most common organisms in early PVE, and streptococcal species, including *Streptococcus viridans*, *Enterococcus*, and *Streptococcus pneumoniae*, are the largest group in late PVE. The fungal agents are most commonly *Candida* followed by *Aspergillus*. These agents appear more frequently in PVE. Organisms of the normal skin flora that are commonly considered nonpathogens (e.g., *Staphylococcus epidermidis*

and diphtheroids) are prominent in both early and late PVE, and antibiotic prophylaxis should be used for these organisms in addition to *Staphylococcus aureus*. No correlation between specific microorganisms and the type of prosthetic valve has been shown.

Diphtheroids may pose a difficult problem, both in their isolation from blood specimens and in in-vitro sensitivity testing. These organisms, which belong to the genus *Corynebacterium* and are part of the normal skin flora, are generally unclassified, except for *C. diphtheriae*. They often grow slowly and require 3 to 14 days of incubation to be recognized. Growth is best in brain-heart infusion (BHI) broth supplemented by 5% rabbit serum. Because of their slow growth, usual antibiotic sensitivity tests are often ineffective, and rabbit serum supplemented by BHI broth is useful for determination of broth dilution minimal inhibitory concentrations (MICs). Generally, diphtheroids are susceptible to gentamicin, amikacin, streptomycin, erythromycin, tetracycline, and vancomycin. A species of *Corynebacterium* designated by

TABLE 51–1. MICROBIOLOGY OF PROSTHETIC VALVE ENDOCARDITIS

Organism	Incidence in Early Endocarditis (%)	Incidence in Late Endocarditis (%)
Staphylococcus epidermidis	27.2	23.9
Staphylococcus aureus	18.6	12.7
Streptococci	6.2	38.5
Diphtheroids	8	4
Gram-negative (aerobic) organisms	21.5	12.8
Other bacteria	7.2	3.4
Fungi	11.3	4.7

the Special Bacteriology Section of the Centers for Disease Control as group JK has been recognized as a cause of serious and fatal diphtheroid infections in several clinical settings, including PVE. This organism is generally more resistant to antibiotics than other diphtheriod species, and only vancomycin had reliable activity against it (Murray et al, 1980).

Management

The therapeutic options for PVE include antibiotic therapy with or without replacement of the infected prosthetic valve. The approach to take in a particular situation can be determined by reviewing factors associated with mortality. Increased mortality is associated with early onset, nonstreptococcal etiology, paravalvular leak, heart failure, presence of multiple systemic emboli, and relapse of bacteremia after medical therapy. Generally, medical therapy alone is reserved for patients who have late onset of PVE due to a streptococcal organism and who show no evidence of a paravalvular leak, congestive heart failure, or multiple systemic emboli. Under these circumstances, the mortality is approximately 35%. When medical therapy alone is given to patients in other categories, the mortality increases greatly. In medically treated early-onset PVE, the mortality is 78%. When early or late PVE is complicated by a paravalvular leak or congestive heart failure, the mortality is 80 to 100%.

The success that has been achieved in the treatment of native valve bacterial and fungal endocarditis by means of prompt valve replacement suggested that this modality should be used for these high-risk PVE patients. Valve replacement plus antibiotic therapy was compared with antibiotic therapy alone for PVE at three medical centers and statistically significant benefits of replacement were shown in some patient categories. The overall mortalities in antibiotic-treated groups and valve replacement groups were 60 and 23%, respectively. The results were slightly different for early-onset and late-onset PVE. In early PVE, the mortality in the group who received antibiotic therapy only was 80%, compared with 60% in the group who had antibiotic therapy plus valve replacement. In late PVE, the corresponding mortalities were 42 and 12%, respectively. Valve replacement in addition to antibiotic therapy is recommended for all patients who have early PVE and for patients who have late PVE with any of the following conditions: infection by a nonstreptococcal organism, paravalvular leak, congestive heart failure, systemic emboli, or recurrence of medically treated infection. Early surgical intervention not only provides a better operative risk, but also prevents extension of the infection into vital or inaccessible myocardial tissue and reduces the risk of systemic embolism and congestive heart failure (Saffle et al, 1977). In more recent series the overall hospital mortality for valve replacement in the setting of PVE ranged from 23 to 32% (Baumgartner et al, 1983; Santinga et al, 1984). Early operation for endocarditis varied from 25% (Santinga et al, 1984) to 67% (Karp, 1987). Replacement of an infected prosthetic valve, however, may be technically difficult and in some situations may be impossible. The occurence of a grossly necrotic annulus at the time of reoperation poses major difficulties in the placement of a new valve, both in seating the prosthesis and in burrowing the sewing ring of the prosthesis into the necrotic annulus (Fig. 51–5). Despite these obstacles, valve replacement in this setting may be successful (Karp, 1987). Using logistic regression, Calderwood and associates (1986) identified two independent factors associated with development of "complicated" and morbid PVE infection of an aortic prosthesis and onset of infection within 12 months of valve implantation. According to Baumgartner and associates (1983), the primary predictors of operative mortality were peripheral emboli, renal dysfunction, active infection at the time of operation, and valve location.

The initial choice of an antibiotic regimen depends on identification of the organism and results of in vitro susceptibility tests modified by serum bactericidal assays. Bactericidal antibiotics are generally required because of barriers to host defense mechanisms presented by the prosthesis and infectious growth. Serum bactericidal levels of 1:8 or more are generally associated with a favorable outcome, although not in high-risk PVE.

Antibiotics are preferably administered intravenously on an intermittent schedule. Bactericidal levels should be obtained 2 to 3 days after antibiotics are started, and blood samples should be taken at a time estimated to represent the peak antibiotic blood level, that is, 30 to 60 minutes after administration. The selection and dose of antibiotics according to organism are shown in Table 51–2. Disk sensitivity testing for *Staphylococcus epidermidis* is often less reliable than more stringent methods of susceptibility testing, and serum bactericidal assays should always be done to ensure efficacy. Testing with inocula of 10^5 to 10^8 organisms in a broth assay has been recommended. When desired bactericidal antibiotic levels are achieved, they should be maintained for 6 to 8 weeks. Blood cultures should be obtained daily for the first few days to demonstrate efficacy and then weekly for the duration of antibiotic therapy and weekly for 1 month after antibiotics have been discontinued to confirm microbiologic cure. If relapse of infection occurs, the valve should be replaced and another course of bactericidal antibiotics should be given.

THROMBOEMBOLISM OF PROSTHETIC CARDIAC VALVES

When successful replacement of diseased aortic and mitral heart valves began in the early 1960s, it became clear that many recipients suffered compli-

Figure 51–5. *Staphylococcus epidermidis* endocarditis originally involving a Bjork-Shiley aortic valve prosthesis, which was excised and replaced with a Magovern prosthesis 28 days before death in a 69-year-old man. Fever and signs of aortic regurgitation appeared 7 months after aortic valve replacement with the Bjork-Shiley prosthesis. After replacement with the Magovern prosthesis, a murmur of aortic regurgitation reappeared. At necropsy, the sewing ring of the aortic wall, which probably produced prosthetic aortic stenosis. *a*, Longitudinal section of the heart through the aortic annulus with the Magovern prosthesis in place, and *b*, after removal of the prosthesis. The frame of the prosthesis has burrowed deeply into the necrotic annulus. (VS = ventricular septum; RV = right ventricular cavity; MV = mitral valve; LA = left atrium.) (From Arnett, E. N., and Roberts, W. C.: Active infective endocarditis: A clinicopathologic analysis of 137 necropsy patients. Curr. Probl. Cardiol., Vol. 1, p. 2. Copyright © 1976 by Year Book Medical Publishers. Reproduced with permission.)

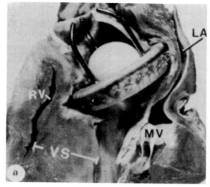
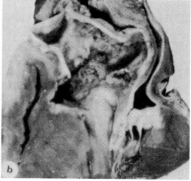

TABLE 51–2. RECOMMENDED ANTIBIOTIC THERAPY FOR PROSTHETIC VALVE ENDOCARDITIS IN AVERAGE-SIZED ADULTS WITH NORMAL RENAL FUNCTION

Organism	Antibiotic	Total Daily Dose	Frequency
Streptococci	Penicillin G	20 million units	q 4 h IV
	+		
	gentamicin	3–5 mg/kg	q 8 h IV
	or		
	vancomycin	2 g/day	q 12 h IV
	+		
	gentamicin	3–5 mg/kg	q 8 h IV
Staphylococcus aureus	Nafcillin	12 g	q 4 h IV
Staphylococcus epidermidis	± rifampin*	120 mg	q 12 h PO
Methicillin-resistant staphylococci	Vancomycin	2 g/day	q 12 h IV
	± rifampin*	1200 mg	q 12 h PO
Diphtheroids, penicillin-sensitive	Penicillin G	20 million units	q 4 h IV
	+		
	gentamicin	3–5 mg/kg	q 8 h IV
JK strain—penicillin-resistant (strain)	Vancomycin	2 g	q 12 h IV
Aerobic gram-negative bacilli†	Third-generation cephalosporin		
	Cefoperazone	4–8 g	q 12 h IV
	Ceftazidime	6 g	q 8 h IV
	Ceftizoxime	6 g	q 8 h IV
	Ceftriaxone	2–4 g	q 12–24 h IV
	Cefotaxime	8–12 g	q 4–6 h IV
	Ticarcillin	18 g	q 4 h IV
	+		
	gentamicin	3–5 mg/kg	q 8 h IV
Fastidious gram-negatives‡	Ceftriaxone	2–4 g	q 12–24 h IV
Fungi			
Candida	Amphotericin B	0.5–1.0 mg/kg	qd IV
	+		
	5-fluorocytosine	150 mg/kg	q 6 h PO
Aspergillus	Amphotericin B	0.5–1 mg/kg	qd IV
Etiologic agent unknown	Vancomycin	1 g/day	q 12 h IV
	+		
	gentamicin	3–5 mg/kg	q 8 h IV
	+		
	ampicillin	12 g	q 4 h IV

*May be added if serum bactericidal levels are inadequate on a single drug. Gentamicin can also be tested for presence of synergy when added to the beta-lactam antibiotic if these drugs are not effective.

†Aerobic gram-negative bacilli will show variable antibiotic sensitivity, and selection must be made appropriately.

‡Fastidious gram-negatives include *Hemophilus arphrophalus, H. paraphrophalus, H. parainfluenza, Cardiobacterium hominis, Actinobacillus actinomycetemcomitans, Kingella,* and *Capnocytophagia.*

cations from emboli that formed on the valve surfaces. Occasionally, the valve surfaces themselves were occluded by slowly developing thrombi. These problems appeared to be due to the inherent thrombogenicity of the materials used and to abnormalities in blood flow through the valves caused by the presence of a centrally occluding ball. The problem of thromboembolic complications has been approached by altering the materials used, changing the valve design, and using systemic anticoagulation. The most recent valves, made from porcine xenografts or bovine pericardium, give many patients improved cardiac function with a greatly reduced clotting risk and freedom from anticoagulant drugs. Not all surgeons are willing to use these valves in all patients. Several good reviews of the issues involved are available (Bonchek, 1981; Lefrak and Starr, 1979; Murphy and Kloster, 1979).

Incidence of Thromboembolic Complications with Mechanical Prosthetic Valves

The first type of valve used, the caged ball valve, was highly thrombogenic. Long-term systemic anticoagulation with warfarin or its derivatives greatly reduced the incidence of these complications. It was estimated that only 20% of patients who received the early Starr-Edwards caged ball valves would be free of emboli at 10 years without anticoagulation. Anticoagulant use reduced the incidence of these complications to approximately 5% in the aortic position and 7% in the mitral position per year. With recent changes in the selection of patients, the rates may now be even lower.

In 1967, the addition of a cloth covering over the cage struts and the inclusion of metal tracks for mobilization of the ball apparently reduced the thrombogenicity of this type of valve. The 10-year embolus-free survival without anticoagulants was increased to approximately 50%. With anticoagulants, thromboembolic incidents occurred in approximately 2% of replaced aortic valves per year and in 3 to 5% of mitral valves per year. Unfortunately, the cloth covering tends to wear, and the metal ball moving in a metal track creates a noise that is audible to most patients (Fig. 51–6).

The tilting disk valves, such as the Bjork-Shiley valve (introduced in 1969) and the Lillehei-Kaster valve, were designed to allow more central blood flow than the caged ball valves. It was hoped that reduced turbulence would decrease fibrin and thrombin deposition around the valve and decrease thromboembolic complications. Flow through tilting disk valves has been less than ideal, with such phenomena as eddy currents around the minor orifice creating the potential for platelet and thrombin accumulation. As a result, these valves appear to be no less thrombogenic than the caged ball valves, and pa-

tients who receive them still require lifelong anticoagulation. In a comparative study (Dale et al, 1980), deaths from thromboembolism occurred at a rate of 1.5 to 2% during a 5-year period with either the caged ball or tilting disk valves in the presence of continuous anticoagulation. With the tilting disk valves, nonfatal thromboembolic complications occur in various series at approximately 1 to 3% in the aortic position and 3 to 5% in the mitral position per year (Borst et al, 1979); these rates are similar to those found with caged ball prostheses. An additional problem with tilting disk valves is the occurrence of "sudden" thrombosis in which a thrombus forms on the valve itself (Fig. 51–7). Sudden thrombosis causes rapid loss of function and, in the absence of prompt reoperation, can result in high mortality. Bjork and Henze (1977) reported that sudden thrombosis in the absence of anticoagulation occurs at the rate of about 3% per year. Even with anticoagulation, 1% of patients with a tilting disk valve in the mitral position may have this complication.

In 1977, the St. Jude bileaflet valve was introduced. This device is designed to produce even more central flow. Early reports cited a low incidence of thromboembolism, but the incidence appears to be increasing with an increase in the number of valves inserted and the time of observation (Cohn, 1981). Two cases of valve thrombus have been reported. A review of the literature by Addonizio and Edmunds (1985) stated that the incidences of fatal and nonfatal thromboembolism for the ball valve in the aortic position varied between 0.2 and 1.2 per 100 patient years and 1.0 and 5.2 per 100 patient years, respectively. The incidences of fatal and nonfatal embolism for disk valves in the aortic position are also low (0 to 0.6 and 1.0 to 5.6 per 100 patient years, respectively). However, the occurrence of prosthetic thrombosis with disk valves is of greater concern than with ball valves.

The incidences of thromboembolic events in the mitral position were similar (0.7 to 1.7 fatal and 1.8 to 8.1 nonfatal), regardless of the type of mechanical valve used (Addonizio and Edmunds, 1985). In all reported series, the incidence of thromboembolic problems is higher for a prosthesis in the mitral position than in the aortic position. The St. Jude tilting disk valve may offer the lowest rate of thromboembolism of the mechanical prostheses (particularly in the mitral position), with incidences of 1.6 per 100 patient years for the aortic location and 1.2 per 100 patient years for the mitral location. Further observation is required to substantiate these findings.

Tissue Valves

Although anticoagulation was largely successful in reducing thromboembolic complications with mechanical prosthetic valves, the pharmacologic agents caused problems. "Serious" or "major" bleeding (bleeding that requires transfusion or hospitalization)

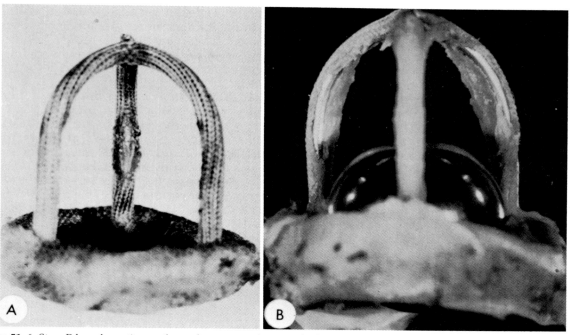

Figure 51–6. Starr-Edwards aortic prostheses from two patients; each shows cloth wear. *A,* Model 2300, size 8A prosthesis removed at operation 16 months after insertion. Focal wearing of the cloth was observed on the inner aspects of each of the three struts (the inner portion of only one strut is seen here). The cloth of the struts is nearly free of tissue ingrowth. *B,* Severe through-and-through wearing of the cloth exposing the metallic struts in this size 10A, Model 2310 prosthesis implanted for 25 months in a 47-year-old man who died suddenly and unexpectedly shortly after the onset of chest pain. Fibrin-platelet thrombus also is present on the struts. (From Winter, T. Q., Reis, R. L., Glancy, D. L., et al: Current status of the Starr-Edwards cloth-covered prosthetic cardiac valves. Circulation, *45, 46*(Suppl. 1):14, 1972. By permission of the American Heart Association, Inc.)

occurs at the rate of 1 to 3% each year with anticoagulation medication. Several investigators attempted to use valves made of cardiac tissue to avoid this problem.

One approach was to use human cadaver valves, rendered sterile with antibiotics and quick-frozen. Although these valves appear to be very effective, they are difficult to obtain and appropriate sizes are not always available.

In 1969, Carpentier and associates reported a more practical and effective prosthetic tissue valve, the porcine bioprosthesis, which is treated with glutaraldehyde to cross-link collagen fibers and is mounted on a support. The Carpentier-Edwards and Hancock porcine xenografts have been widely used, and this type of valve prosthesis is now the first choice of many surgeons for most patients. The device has very low thrombogenicity, perhaps because of its nearly central flow and decreased use of "unnatural" materials. Even without anticoagulation,

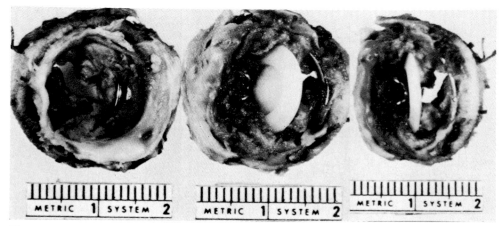

Figure 51–7. Three views of a thrombosed (noninfected) Bjork-Shiley aortic valve prosthesis. This prosthesis had been in place for 270 days, and the patient had not been receiving warfarin sodium. *A,* View from ventricular side. *B,* View from aortic side showing immobilization of the Delrin disk. *C,* View from aortic side showing orifice in its maximal dimension. Severe prosthetic obstruction was present. (From Roberts, W. C., and Hammer, W. J.: Cardiac pathology after valve replacement with a tilting disc prosthesis [Bjork-Shiley type]. Am. J. Cardiol., *37:*1024, 1976.)

porcine xenografts have a thromboembolic rate of only 1 to 3% per year in the aortic position and 2 to 4% per year in the mitral position (Jamieson et al, 1981). In one publication (Cohn et al, 1981), the actuarial embolus-free survival at 8 years with the Hancock valves was 97% for patients with aortic valve replacement, 82% for those with prosthetic mitral valves, and 72% with multiple valve replacement. Most patients were not taking anticoagulant medication.

Use of porcine heterograft tissue valves greatly decreases but does not eliminate the need for anticoagulants. Because of the high incidence of thrombi early after operation, anticoagulant drugs have been recommended for the first 6 to 8 weeks after insertion of the valve in the mitral position.

In addition, certain cardiac conditions predispose patients to clotting problems. These conditions include atrial fibrillation, enlarged left atrium, and low output syndrome (Fig. 51–8). (In these situations, it may be the disease itself, rather than the prosthetic valve, that induces the thromboembolic incidents.) In the series reported by Cohn and associates (1981), the 8-year embolus-free survival was approximately 95% for patients in sinus rhythm but only 70% for patients in atrial fibrillation. Recipients who have any of these three cardiac conditions (which frequently occur together) are given long-term systemic anticoagulation. Another indication for anticoagulation

cited by some authors is a history of emboli or the finding of thrombus during operation. Cohn and associates (1981) reported that 27% of recipients who had tissue valve replacement received anticoagulation for one or more of these indications.

Because many recipients of porcine xenograft tissue valves do not need anticoagulants, these valves appear to be ideal for the patients who have the grafts for the longest time—children and young adults. However, experience with bioprostheses in this population has shown that the failure rate with porcine tissue valves is much higher in younger patients. In a series of children who had the Hancock valves for reconstruction of the right ventricular outflow tract, it was projected that the failure rate would be 30% at 6 years (Bisset et al, 1981). In another group of patients between the ages of 1 and 20 years, 8 of the 25 Hancock valve recipients who survived for more than 20 months after operation required valve replacement (Sanders et al, 1980). Another group calculated a failure rate of almost 10% per year in a group of patients less than 15 years of age who had aortic or mitral valve replacement with porcine tissue valves (Oyer et al, 1980). Because removed xenograft valves have been heavily calcified and a high rate of xenograft failure is also seen in patients on renal dialysis, it was suggested that failure may be related to hyperactive calcium metabolism (Fig. 51–9).

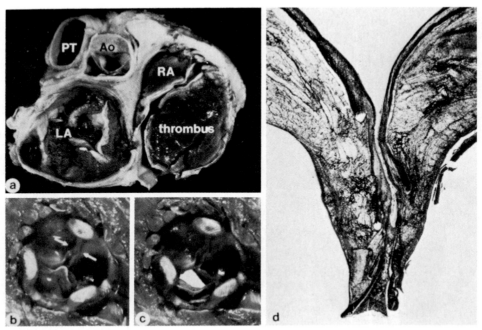

Figure 51–8. Stenosis of porcine bioprosthesis implanted 32 days earlier in a 61-year-old woman who had had rheumatic mitral stenosis and tricuspid regurgitation. The patient sustained an air embolus intraoperatively and remained comatose with severe low cardiac output after operation. *a,* At necropsy, both the right atrium (RA) and the left atrium (LA) were filled with organizing thrombi. (Ao = aortic root; PT = pulmonary trunk.) *b,* View of the 31-mm porcine bioprosthesis in the tricuspid position from the ventricular aspect as seen in systole. Thrombus is present in two of the three cusp sinuses, and there is fusion of the commissure between these leaflets *(arrows).* *c,* Bioprosthesis in simulated ventricular diastole. The fusion of two leaflets permits opening of only the one mobile leaflet, with resulting valve stenosis. *d,* Section through fused leaflets at level of arrows in *b* showing adherence of the leaflets by fibrin thrombus. (Phosphotungstic acid-hematoxylin stain, ×16, reduced by 24%.) (From Spray, T. L., and Roberts, W. C.: Structural changes in porcine xenografts used as substitute cardiac valves. Am. J. Cardiol., *40:*319, 1977.)

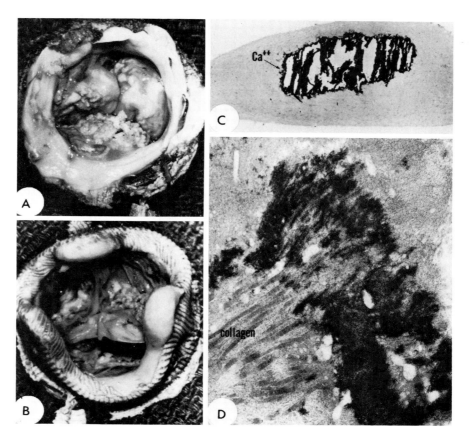

Figure 51–9. Calcification of porcine bioprostheses. *A* and *B,* Nodular calcific deposits in the leaflets of a mitral Hancock porcine valve implanted for 4 years in a 12-year-old male. Reoperation was required for prosthetic stenosis. *C,* Histologic section of one leaflet from a similar valve showing nodular calcific deposits (Ca^{2+}) in the substance of the valve leaflet. (VonKossa stain, ×40.) *D,* Electron micrograph showing calcium deposits associated with the collagen bundles in the valve leaflet (×47,000).

In older patients, the Hancock xenograft valve has an acceptably low rate of primary failure, approximately 1% per year. Studies of tissue valves recovered at autopsy suggest that the rate of failure may increase over the longer term (Ferrans et al, 1978) (Figs. 51–10 and 51–11), and a few investigators noticed acceleration of the failure rate between 5 and 6 years after insertion (Casarotto et al, 1979; Lakier et al, 1980; Oyer et al, 1980), but more extensive observation is necessary to resolve this question.

Anticoagulation

The basic agent for systemic long-term anticoagulation is warfarin or a derivative. In one study, the rate of emboli in patients receiving cloth-covered Starr-Edwards valves with no anticoagulation was 4% per year (Moggio et al, 1978). A similar group of patients treated concurrently with sodium warfarin (Coumadin) sustained only about one embolus per 100 patients per year. The same study showed that the embolic rate with aspirin used alone was 2.6% per year. However, generally both drugs are used in combination. In a group of high-risk patients who had caged ball valves for aortic replacement, emboli occurred at the rate of 9% per year when the patients were given warfarin (Dale et al, 1977). When these patients were subsequently treated with the addition of aspirin, the rate of emboli decreased to 2% per year. (Aspirin had to be discontinued in one-third of

these patients, primarily because of bleeding problems.) In a study in which the reverse order was used (Brott et al, 1981), 50 patients who received dipyridamole (Persantine) and aspirin had thromboembolic events at the rate of almost 9% per year. The addition of warfarin reduced this incidence to 1%.

Steele and associates (1979) showed that in-vitro measurements of platelet survival time strongly correlated with decreases in embolic events in patients who took aspirin. Patients who had decreased platelet survival times after valve replacement received antiplatelet drugs in addition to warfarin. During the next 4 years, there were no emboli among the 59 patients taking aspirin therapy whose platelet survival times increased, wheras one-third of the patients whose platelet survival times remained subnormal despite aspirin administration had emboli. These findings suggest that the effect of aspirin in reducing emboli is due to its antiplatelet action and show that antiplatelet therapy can be monitored by this in-vitro test.

Dipyridamole may be less effective than aspirin, although the evidence is not conclusive. Dipyridamole was given to a group of patients in Great Britain who received tilting disk valves (Thomsen and Alstrup, 1979). During the following years, these patients had a 22% incidence of thromboembolism. A similar group of patients who had valve replacement but received warfarin had only a 7% incidence of thromboembolism during the same period.

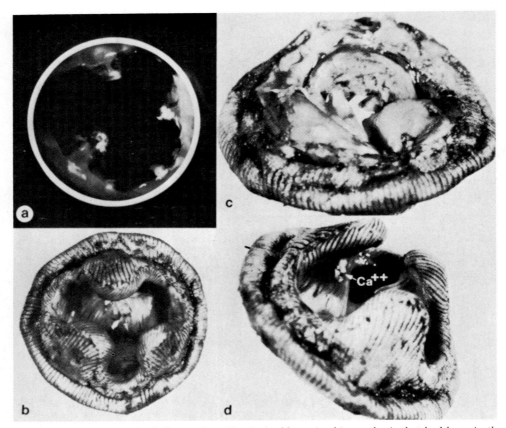

Figure 51–10. Tissue degeneration and calcification in a 75-month-old porcine bioprosthesis that had been in the mitral position. *a,* Roentgenogram of the removed bioprosthesis showing focal calcific deposits in the leaflets. *b,* View of the bioprosthesis from the ventricular aspect showing bowing-in of all three struts. *c,* View of the bioprosthesis from the atrial aspect showing tears and fraying of two of the three leaflets and prolapse of the leaflets toward the atrial side of the valve. The resulting regurgitation required reoperation and replacement of the bioprosthesis with a fresh prosthesis. *d,* Side view showing nodular calcific deposits (Ca^{2+}) at the commissural attachment of two leaflets. (From Spray, T. L., and Roberts, W. C.: Structural changes in porcine xenografts used as substitute cardiac valves. Am. J. Cardiol., *40*:319, 1977.)

Interruption of warfarin for short periods in patients who had noncardiac surgery resulted in a minimal risk of thromboembolic complications (Katholi et al, 1978; Tinker and Tarhan, 1978). Heparin may be given soon after operation to restore anticoagulation. Heparin can also be substituted for warfarin in women with prosthetic valves who become pregnant, but the need for valve replacement in a woman of childbearing age strongly indicates insertion of a tissue valve.

Diagnosis and Treatment of Valve Thrombosis

Clinically, the presence of thrombus formation on a valve can often be detected by the appearance of pulmonary edema associated with the disappearance of valve clicks, especially in cases of sudden valve thrombosis. Systolic murmurs may appear. Echocardiography may show an alteration in disk motion, especially if a baseline study is available. With tissue valves, serial echocardiography shows progressive thickening of the cusps. Magilligan and

associates (1980) reported that cusp thickening greater than 3 mm is correlated highly with tissue valve dysfunction. Phonocardiography can detect decreases in ejection time with aortic valves and a prolonged diastolic rumble with thrombosed mitral valves. Computer-assisted real-time sound spectrum analysis allowed detection of three of seven cerebral emboli and all four valve thrombi among 127 patients with disk valves (Kagawa et al, 1980). Two-dimensional echocardiography has been reported to be very accurate (Martin et al, 1980). Among 40 patients with suspected Hancock valve dysfunction, this technique correctly identified seven patients with normal valves, 18 of 19 patients with suspected endocarditis (12 positive, 6 negative), six patients with suspected recent cerebrovascular accident (3 with a valvular mass as a source of the embolus), and 8 patients with abnormal left ventricular function that caused congestive heart failure. The overall accuracy was 97%, compared with 67% with one-dimensional echocardiography in the same patients. The two-dimensional modality is more difficult to use, and the settings must be adjusted accurately because the sewing ring and stents produce stronger echoes than the valve leaflets.

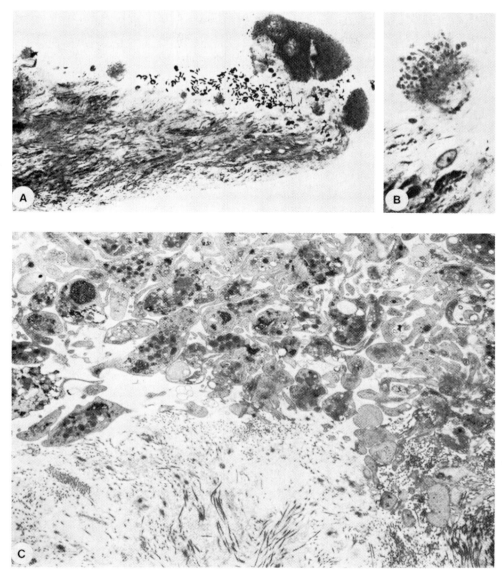

Figure 51–11. Light *(A* and *B)* and electron *(C)* micrographs of aggregates of platelets in a valve. *A,* Section through the area adjacent to a tear (the edge of which is seen at far right) in the leaflet. Collagen in this area is greatly disrupted, and layers of valve connective tissue are not recognizable. The outflow surface (top) is covered with red blood cells and with several aggregates of platelets. (Alkaline toluidine blue stain, ×250.) *B,* Aggregate of platelets (shown at upper left in *A)* is connected to the surface of the valve by a narrow pedicle (×750). *C,* Base of a platelet aggregate similar to that shown in *B.* The platelets are in direct contact with severely disrupted collagen in the valve surface; they are well preserved and contain abundant glycogen (×13,000). (From Ferrans, V. J., Spray, T. L., Billingham, M. E., and Roberts, W. C.: Structural changes in glutaraldehyde-treated porcine heterografts used as substitute cardiac valves. Am. J. Cardiol., *41:*1159, 1978.)

The most common treatment for thrombosed or failed valves is reoperation and replacement. Thromboembolic problems have been resolved by replacing mechanical valves with tissue valves. In one series, this strategy resulted in a 90% operative survival rate and 50% 10-year survival (Shemin et al, 1979).

An initial report from Europe on the use of fibrinolysis to treat valve thromboembolism was moderately encouraging (Witchitz et al, 1980). Of 13 episodes treated with intravenous streptokinase or urokinase for 1 to 4 days, complete regression resulted in 8 cases. Some of these patients had later thromboembolic episodes and required reoperation.

This technique may find a place in the treatment of an acute episode so that the patient can have reoperation in a nonemergency state.

Acknowledgment

Appreciation is expressed to Dr. Thomas L. Spray for preparing the illustrations for this chapter.

Selected Bibliography

Addonizio, V. P., Jr., and Edmunds, L. H., Jr.: Thromboembolic complications of prosthetic valves. Symposium on Cardiac Valve Surgery. Cardiol. Clin., 3:431–437, 1985.

Previous reports on patients with ball and pivoting disk valves are reviewed, and the follow-up in patient-years, incidence of late thromboembolism, and per cent free from thromboembolism during an adequate period of follow-up are given. The length of follow-up for each series is also shown. The risks of embolization of mechanical valves in both the aortic and mitral positions are given. This compilation of late follow-up series from the literature is well worth reading and offers an excellent basis for comparison with further data.

McGoon, D. C.: The risk of thromboembolism following valvular operations: How does one know? J. Thorac. Cardiovasc. Surg., *88*:782–786, 1984.

This review of the method of analysis for an important complication of valvular operations describes the adequacies and inadequacies of reporting in the literature. It summarizes the quality and value of available data on the thromboembolic risk of most valve prostheses. For future meaningful reporting of valve morbidity and mortality, criteria for analysis must be standardized and the appropriate questions posed before analysis of the data. The format used here should be extended to many other aspects of postoperative evaluation inquiries.

Bibliography

Addonizio, V. P., Jr., and Edmunds, L. H., Jr.: Thromboembolic complications of prosthetic valves. Cardiol. Clin., *3*:431, 1985.

Arnett, E. N., and Roberts, W. C.: Active infective endocarditis: A clinicopathologic analysis of 137 necropsy patients. Curr. Probl. Cardiol., *1*:2, 1976.

Baumgartner, W. A., Miller, D. C., Reitz, B. A., et al: Surgical treatment of prosthetic valve endocarditis. Ann. Thorac. Surg., *35*:87, 1983.

Bisset, G. S., III, Schwartz, S. C., Benzing, G., III, et al: Late results of reconstruction of the right ventricular outflow tract with porcine heterografts in children. Ann. Thorac. Surg., *31*:437, 1981.

Bjork, V. O., and Henze, A.: Isolated mitral valve replacement with the Bjork-Shiley tilting disc prothesis. Scand. J. Thorac. Cardiovasc. Surg., *11*:181, 1977.

Bonchek, L. I.: Current status of cardiac valve replacement: Selection of a prothesis and indications for operation. Am. Heart J., *101*:96, 1981.

Borst, H. G., Papagiannakis, N., Beddermann, C., and Oelert, H.: Cardiac valve replacement. Problems solved and unsolved. Thorac. Cardiovasc. Surg., *27*:76, 1979.

Brott, W. H., Zajchuck, R., Bowen, T. E., et al: Dipyridamole-aspirin as thromboembolic prophylaxis in patients with aortic valve prosthesis. J. Thorac. Cardiovasc. Surg., *81*:632, 1981.

Calderwood, S. B., Swinski, L. A., Karchmer, A. W., et al: Prosthetic valve endocarditis: Analysis of factors affecting outcome of therapy. J. Thorac. Cardiovasc. Surg., *92*:776, 1986.

Carpentier, A., Lemaigre, G., Robert, L., et al: Biological factors affecting long-term results of valvular heterografts. J. Thorac. Cardiovasc. Surg., *48*:467, 1969.

Casarotto, D., Bortolotti, U., Thiene, G., et al: Long-term results (from 5 to 7 years) with the Hancock S-G-P bioprosthesis. J. Cardiovasc. Surg., *20*:399, 1979.

Clarkson, P. M., and Barratt-Boyes, B. G.: Bacterial endocarditis following homograft replacement of the aortic valve. Circulation, *42*:987, 1970.

Cohn, L. H.: Valve replacement in children. Ann. Thorac. Surg., *31*:491, 1981.

Cohn, L. H., Mudge, G. H., Pratter, F., and Collins, J. J., Jr.: Five- to eight-year follow-up of patients undergoing porcine heart-valve replacement. N. Engl. J. Med., *304*:258, 1981.

Cowgill, L. D., Addonizio, V. P., Hopeman, A. R., and Harken, A. H.: A practical approach to prosthetic valve endocarditis. Ann. Thorac. Surg., *43*:450, 1987.

Dale, J., Levang, O., and Enge, I.: Long-term results after aortic valve replacement with four different prostheses. Am. Heart J., *99*:155, 1980.

Dale, J., Myhre, E., Storstein, O., et al: Prevention of arterial thromboembolism with acetylsalicylic acid: A controlled clinical trial in patients with aortic ball valves. Am. Heart J., *94*:101, 1977.

Ferrans, V. J., Spray, T. L., Billingham, M. E., and Roberts, W. C.: Structural changes in glutaraldehyde-treated porcine heterografts used as substitute cardiac valves. Am. J. Cardiol., *41*:1159, 1978.

Jamieson, W. R., Janusz, M. T., Miyagishima, R. T., et al: Embolic complications of porcine heterograft cardiac valves. J. Thorac. Cardiovasc. Surg., *81*:626, 1981.

Kagawa, Y., Sato, N., Nitta, S., et al: Real-time spectroanalysis for diagnosis of malfunctioning prosthetic valves. J. Thorac. Cardiovasc. Surg., *79*:671, 1980.

Karchmer, A. W., Dismukes, W. E., Buckley, M. J., and Austen, W. G.: Late prosthetic valve endocarditis. Am. J. Med., *64*:199, 1978.

Karp, R. B.: Role of surgery in infective endocarditis. *In* Brest, A. N. and McGoon, D. C. (eds): Cardiovascular Clinics, 17/3. Cardiac Surgery, 2nd ed. Philadelphia, F. A. Davis Company, 1987, pp. 141–162.

Katholi, R. E., Nolan, S. P., and McGuire, L. B.: The management of anticoagulation during noncardiac operations in patients with prosthetic heart valves: A prospective study. Am. Heart J., *96*:163, 1978.

Kluge, R. M., Calia, F. M., McLaughlin, J. S., and Hornick, R. B.: Source of contamination in open heart surgery. J.A.M.A., *230*:1415, 1974.

Lakier, J. B., Khaja, F., Magilligan, D. J., Jr., and Goldstein, S.: Porcine xenograft valves. Long-term (60–89 month) follow-up. Circulation, *62*:313, 1980.

Lefrak, E. A., and Starr, A.: Current heart valve prostheses. Am. Fam. Physician, *20*:93, 1979.

Magilligan, D. J., Jr., Lewis, J. W., Jr., Jara, F. M., et al: Spontaneous degeneration of porcine bioprosthetic valves. Ann. Thorac. Surg., *30*:259, 1980.

Magilligan, D. J., Jr., Quinn, E. L., and Davila, J. C.: Bacteremia, endocarditis and the Hancock valve. Ann. Thorac. Surg., *24*:508, 1977.

Martin, R. P., French, J. W., and Popp, R. L.: Clinical utility of two-dimensional echocardiography in patients with bioprosthetic valves. Adv. Cardiol., *27*:294, 1980.

Masur, H., and Johnson, W. D., Jr.: Prosthetic valve endocarditis. J. Thorac. Cardiovasc. Surg., *80*:31, 1980.

McAllister, R. G., Jr., Samet, J., Mazzoleni, A., and Dillon, M. L.: Endocarditis on prosthetic mitral valves. Chest, *66*:682, 1974.

Moggio, R. A., Hammond, G. L., Stansel, H. C., Jr., and Glenn, W. W.: Incidence of emboli with cloth-covered Starr-Edwards valve without anticoagulation and with varying forms of anticoagulation: Analysis of 183 patients followed for 3½ years. J. Thorac. Cardiovasc. Surg., *75*:296, 1978.

Murphy, E. S., and Kloster, F. E.: Late results of valve replacement surgery. II. Complications of prosthetic heart valves. Mod. Concepts Cardiovasc. Dis., *48*:59, 1979.

Murray, B. E., Karchmer, A. W., and Moellering, R. C., Jr.: Diphtheroid prosthetic valve endocarditis. Am. J. Med., *69*:838, 1980.

Oyer, P. E., Miller, D. C., Stinson, E. B., et al: Clinical durability of the (Hancock) porcine bioprosthesis valve. J. Thorac. Cardiovasc. Surg., *80*:824, 1980.

Roberts, W. C., and Hammer, W. J.: Cardiac pathology after valve replacement with a tilting disc prosthesis (Bjork-Shirley type). Am. J. Cardiol., *37*:1024, 1976.

Rossiter, S. J., Stinson, E. B., Oyer, P. E., et al: Prosthetic valve endocarditis. J. Thorac. Cardiovasc. Surg., *76*:795, 1978.

Saffle, J. R., Gardner, P., Schoenbaum, S. C., and Wild, W.: Prosthetic valve endocarditis: The case for prompt valve replacement. J. Thorac. Cardiovasc. Surg., *73*:416, 1977.

Sande, M. A., Johnson, W. D., Hook, E. W., et al: Sustained bacteremia in patients with prosthetic cardiac valves. N. Engl. J. Med., *286*:1067, 1972.

Sanders, S. P., Levy, R. J., Freed, M. D., et al: Use of Hancock porcine xenografts in children and adolescents. Am. J. Cardiol., *46*:429, 1980.

Santinga, J. T., Kirsh, M., and Fekety, R.: Factors affecting survival in prosthetic valve endocarditis: Review of the effectiveness of prophylaxis. Chest, *85*:471, 1984.

Shemin, R. J., Guadiana, V. A., Conkle, D. M., and Morrow, A. G.: Prosthetic aortic valves. Indications for and results of reoperation. Arch. Surg., *114*:63, 1979.

Spray, T. L., and Roberts, W. C.: Structural changes in porcine xenografts used as substitute cardiac valves. Am. J. Cardiol., *40*:319, 1977.

Steele, P., Rainwater, J., and Vogel, R.: Platelet suppressant therapy in patients with prosthetic cardiac valves: Relationship of clinical effectiveness to alteration of platelet survival time. Circulation, *60*:910, 1979.

Thomsen, P. B., and Alstrup, P.: Thromboembolism in patients without anticoagulants after aortic valve replacement with the Lillehei-Kaster disc valve. Thorac. Cardiovasc. Surg., *27*:313, 1979.

Tinker, J. H., and Tarhan, S.: Discontinuing anticoagulant therapy in surgical patients with cardiac valve prostheses. J.A.M.A., *239*:738, 1978.

Winter, T. Q., Reis, R. L., Glancy, D. L., et al: Current status of the Starr-Edwards cloth-covered prosthetic cardiac valves. Circulation, *45, 46*(Suppl. 1):14, 1972.

Witchitz, S., Veyrat, C., Moisson, P., et al: Fibrinolytic treatment of thrombus on prosthetic heart valves. Br. Heart J., *44*:545, 1980.

II THROMBOEMBOLIC COMPLICATIONS OF CARDIAC AND VASCULAR PROSTHESES

Edwin W. Salzman
J. Anthony Ware

Thromboembolism is a major cause of morbidity and mortality after implantation of prosthetic devices within the circulation or passage of blood through extracorporeal circuits, and it is a major deterrent to earlier operation for any procedure in which the blood comes in contact with artificial surfaces. Normally, platelets do not adhere to intact, functioning endothelium. Exposure of the blood to subendothelial connective tissue or to almost any artificial surface leads to deposition of a layer of adherent platelets, which can foster activation of the coagulation pathway and formation of a thrombus. Efforts have been made to understand the physical and chemical characteristics of surfaces that determine the nature of their interaction with blood. Detailed reviews of the subject are available (Leonard et al, 1987; Salzman and Merrill, 1987).

Plasma proteins also react with the subendothelium or with an artificial surface, which leads to activation of the intrinsic or extrinsic coagulation pathway (Fig. 51–12). Exposure to artificial surfaces typically leads to formation of enzymatically active Factors XIIa and XIa from their respective zymogens, which activates the intrinsic system and eventually results in thrombin generation and formation of a fibrin network. Activation of Factor XII also initiates the kininogen-kallikrein system, which leads to production of bradykinin and provides positive feedback for surface activation.

The reactions of the intrinsic system and the final common pathway are facilitated by initiation on a surface that concentrates the reactants. Alterations in the phospholipid plasma membrane of activated platelets provide such a surface, which binds calcium and clotting factors X and V and enhances formation of activated Factor X (Xa) and conversion of prothrombin to thrombin. In addition to converting fibrinogen to fibrin, thrombin is a powerful stimulant

for platelets, which can also be activated by contact with surfaces other than normal endothelium (Fig. 51–13). Several platelet- and plasma-associated proteins, including von Willebrand factor, fibrinogen, and probably thrombospondin and fibronectin, participate in platelet adhesion to artificial surfaces and to each other. After adhesion of individual platelets, additional platelets are recruited to form aggregates; this process depends on fibrinogen in solution and is aided by the secretion of platelet contents, including the platelet constituents serotonin and adenosine diphosphate (ADP), and the formation of thromboxane A_2 from platelet arachidonic acid. These substances and others released by adherent platelets, together with thrombin, influence other platelets to aggregate at the site of an endothelial defect or a foreign surface.

The relative composition of a thrombus, either plasma fibrin clot or cellular platelet aggregate, is dictated mainly by conditions of local blood flow. In areas of sluggish blood flow, where fluid shear stress is low or recirculating eddies permit prolonged exposure of blood elements to prosthetic surfaces, activation of clotting factors produces a local increase in concentration of procoagulants and leads ultimately to the formation of a plasma clot. The "red thrombus" or "stasis thrombus" is a clot composed of red blood cells entrapped in fibrin strands. This clot predominates in peripheral veins, behind stenotic cardiac valves, around the sewing rings of prosthetic heart valves, and in extracorporeal reservoirs. In regions in which blood flow is brisk and fluid shear stress is greater, such as in peripheral arteries, the "white thrombus" or "platelet thrombus" is more common. The white thrombus is found characteristically in arteries, in the tubing and cannulas of artificial circulatory systems, and on the

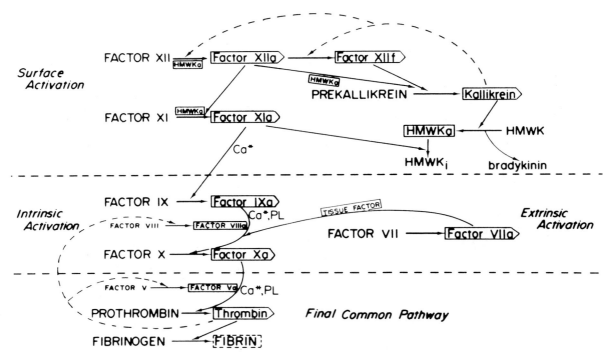

Figure 51–12. Schematic representation of the clotting cascade, divided arbitrarily into the sequences involved in surface (contact) activation, intrinsic and extrinsic activation, and the final common pathway. Interrupted lines show paths of positive feedback. HMWK$_g$ denotes high-molecular-weight kininogen. PL indicates phospholipid, which would be provided by platelet membranes in vivo. Factors XII, XI, IX, and X and prekallikrein and prothrombin are zymogens; Factors VIII and V are cofactors. (From Colman, R. W., Marder, V. J., Salzman, E. W., and Hirsh, J.: Overview of hemostasis. *In* Colman, R. W., Hirsh, J., Marder, V. J., and Salzman, E. W. [eds]: Hemostasis and Thrombosis, 2nd ed. Philadelphia, J. B. Lippincott, 1987.)

cages or struts of prosthetic heart valves that protrude into the bloodstream.

Exposure of the blood to an artificial surface can produce several pathologic responses. Thrombus for-

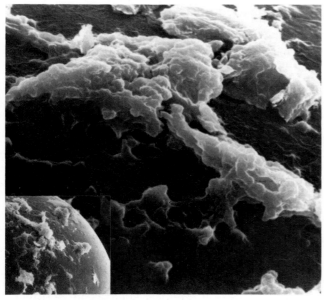

Figure 51–13. Scanning electron micrograph of clumps of washed platelets adherent to an artificial surface (a bead of polybutylmethacrylate). The platelets have become spiculated and have spread on the polymer surface. The same bead is shown at lower magnification *(inset)*. (Courtesy of Jack N. Lindon, Ph.D.)

mation can occur in an artificial intravascular device as a deposit on the surface facing the blood. Thrombosis on prosthetic heart valves can impair movement of the ball, disk, or leaflet. In conduits such as arterial grafts, obliteration of the lumen may result. Another potential result of thrombus formation is fragmentation and embolization downstream to distant organs, which sometimes leaves little trace behind. In patients with nontissue prosthetic mitral or aortic valves, thrombotic complications (together with bleeding caused by anticoagulants) account for 75% of the valve-related morbidity; with bioprosthetic valves, these events represent approximately 50% of the complications, and other problems such as degeneration, calcification, and infection represent the other half (Edmunds, 1987). Repeated generation of microscopic platelet aggregates and cellular debris may result from interaction of blood with artificial surfaces, such as prosthetic arterial graft segments or cardiac valvular prostheses, especially with extracorporeal circulation (Edmunds and Williams, 1983). Even when gross or microscopic thromboembolism is not demonstrable, accelerated destruction of hemostatic elements such as platelets and fibrinogen can be found (Harker and Slichter, 1972). Shortened platelet survival has been reported in patients with atrioventricular (AV) shunts for hemodialysis, vascular grafts, and artificial heart valves. In patients with artificial heart valves, Weily and Genton (1970) found a significant correlation between short platelet survival and earlier history of or later risk for thromboembolism. Davies and associates (1980) showed increased levels of fibrinopeptide A (an indicator of thrombin-fibrinogen interaction) and thromboxane B_2 (an indicator of platelet activation) in patients who had cardiopulmonary bypass for cardiac surgery; fibrinopeptide A was increased before cardiopulmonary bypass, which indicates stimulation of coagulation even before exposure of the blood to the extracorporeal circuit, probably caused by placement of intravascular cannulas. Activation of the hemostatic mechanism also induces remote systemic effects: contact activation of Factors XII and XI leads to production of kinins, which mediate blood vessel dilation, vascular permeability, white blood cell migration, and pain production. Platelet activation with release of platelet constituents (e.g., serotonin) is rarely responsible for phenomena such as bronchoconstriction with pulmonary embolism (Rosoff et al, 1971) and cerebral vasoconstriction with subarachnoid hemorrhage (Zervas et al, 1973). There may be decreased function of platelets and other hemostatic elements, especially during and after extracorporeal circulation (Mammen et al, 1985) when air bubbles cause denaturation of plasma proteins and lipids. Platelets are profoundly affected and show a qualitative defect that may be secondary to partial release of intracellular secretory granules (Harker et al, 1980).

PROSTHETIC HEART VALVES

The aspects of surface chemistry that govern interactions of blood with artificial materials are only partly understood (Salzman and Merrill, 1987). The usefulness of artificial circulatory devices depends less on the availability of bland thromboresistant surfaces than on skillful design to ensure favorable flow patterns and on the use of antithrombotic drugs to inhibit the response of the blood to contact with foreign surfaces.

In the early days of cardiac valve replacement, the frequency of thromboembolic complications was almost 50% if oral anticoagulants were not used (Duvoisin et al, 1967). Changes in design and materials and, in some cases, the use of bioprosthetic valves have reduced thromboembolic complications (Edmunds, 1987). Prosthetic valves are categorized according to flow type and materials in Table 51–3.

Thrombi that develop on prosthetic heart valves consist of many different hemostatic elements. Near the sewing ring at the base of a valve, where disturbed lines of blood flow with vortices and recirculating eddies allow prolonged contact for blood constituents, thrombi are primarily formed of fibrin. A white platelet thrombus is more typical on the cage or struts of the valve, which are in the regions of highest flow rates and are constantly exposed to rapidly moving blood. The composite nature of many thrombi might be responsible for the limited ability of long-term treatment with oral anticoagulants to prevent completely thromboembolic complications of prosthetic valves, although the occurrence of such events might reflect emboli from other sources (e.g., the left atrium in mitral valve disease) (Janusz et al, 1983). Thromboembolic rates are higher when more than one valve is implanted, which implies that the risk increases with each additional prosthetic valve, but the rates have improved with advances in valve design and the use of tissue valves (Braunwald, 1988). Prosthetic valves the fixed parts of which are covered by cloth may acquire an adherent layer of thrombus that, under ideal circumstances, is well tolerated by the blood and serves as a compatible coating. The thrombus layer is initially thin and delicate; its propagation into the orifice of the valve is limited by flow. Eventually, the thrombus is invaded by well-vascularized fibrous tissue that grows from the base of the valve. The development of an endothelial coat appears to decrease the frequency of embolic complications (Isom et al, 1973). In three different series, the Starr-Edwards valve had an embolus-free rate at 5 years of 65, 81, and 80% when placed in the mitral position in patients who were subsequently anticoagulated with warfarin (Cobanoglu et al, 1985; Miller et al, 1983; Sala et al, 1982). With aortic valve replacement, the 5-year embolus-free rate ranged from 85 to 92% with this valve (Farah et al, 1984; Miller et al, 1984; Perier et al, 1985).

The various tilting disk valves have slightly fewer thromboembolic complications than the caged ball valves with anticoagulation (Edmunds, 1987; Kinsley et al, 1986; Perier et al, 1985; Sethia et al, 1986). The previous incidence of gross valve thrombosis of 13% for the mitral position and 3% for the aortic position (Karp et al, 1981) in Bjork-Shiley tilting disk valves appears to be decreased, if not eliminated, by a design change in the tilting disk (Braunwald, 1988). Inadequate anticoagulation with warfarin increased the incidence of thrombotic obstruction (Edmunds, 1987), which was treated successfully with thrombolytic agents (Ledain et al, 1986). The St. Jude medical valve has a very low incidence of thromboembolism (0.7% per patient year) even with reduced dosages of warfarin (Kopf et al, 1987; Schaffer et al, 1987). One randomized trial compared the incidence of thromboembolism and death following implantation of three different tilting disk or bileaflet valves (Kuntze et al, 1989). In the first 6 postoperative months, the incidence of thromboembolism was approximately equal among the three valve types, and the death rate did not differ throughout the study. However, in the 6- to 37.5-month postoperative period, the incidence of thromboembolism for the Edwards-Duromedics valve and the Medtronic-Hall valve was 3.9 and 2.6 times higher, respectively, than that for the Bjork-Shiley valve.

TABLE 51–3. CHARACTERISTICS OF THE MAJOR TYPES OF PROSTHETIC CARDIAC VALVES IN CURRENT USE

Type of Valve	Trade Names of Valves	Flow	Material	Warfarin Required	Other Considerations
Caged ball valve	Starr-Edwards	Peripheral	Ball: metal or silicone; base and struts: metal; cloth covering: knitted Teflon, Dacron, polypropylene	Yes	
Tilting disk valves or bileaflet	Bjork-Shiley* Lillehei-Kaster St. Jude†	Central	Disk: pyrolate; base and struts: cobalt, titanium; cloth covering: Teflon	Yes	Sudden thrombosis has been reported to occur in both B-S and L-K, the latter only in the mitral position
Tissue valve	Hancock Carpentier-Edwards Ionescu-Shiley	Central	Valve: porcine (heterograft), bovine (xenograft); strut: polypropylene or metal; cloth covering of strut: Dacron, Teflon	Yes, for 3 postoperative months in all, and in mitral valves in patients at high risk for thromboembolism‡	Valve of choice for patients in whom anticoagulation is hazardous or in the elderly

*Related valves include the Omniscience, Omni Carbon, and Medtronic-Hall valves.
†Related valve is the Duromedics.
‡Those with atrial fibrillation, clot in the left atrium, and a history of thromboembolism.

Tissue valves such as the glutaraldehyde-preserved porcine valve are less thrombogenic and in many cases can be used without long-term anticoagulation (Edmunds, 1987). This relative thromboresistance probably derives more from their central flow, flexible leaflets, and favorable hemodynamics than from the material itself (Magilligan et al, 1984). Patients with bioprostheses in the aortic position were 94 to 99% free of emboli at 5 years and the comparable range for the mitral position was 90 to 97% (Brais et al, 1985; Gallucci et al, 1984; Oyer et al, 1984; Soots et al, 1984) with various anticoagulation regimens. In patients with atrial fibrillation, the incidence of emboli after implantation of a bioprosthesis into the mitral position is much higher than that in patients with sinus rhythm (Janusz et al, 1983). Use of anticoagulants after mitral valve replacement with a porcine valve in patients with atrial fibrillation is controversial. Because of the increased incidence of thromboembolism in the first 3 months after mitral valve replacement (Hetzer et al, 1982), with the low incidence of thromboembolic complications in patients treated with warfarin (Hill et al, 1982), and the success of a less intense warfarin therapy (Braunwald, 1988), it was recommended that all patients with bioprosthetic valves in the mitral position be treated for the first 3 months after valve insertion with this regimen, with long-term warfarin therapy reserved for patients at high risk for another thromboembolus (Stein et al, 1986). If warfarin cannot be given, aspirin may be efficacious in prevention of thromboemboli (Nunez et al, 1984).

Several groups have compared the thromboembolic rate of bioprosthetic valves with that of the Bjork-Shiley valve or the St. Jude valve. The rates appear similar, but bleeding complications are usually more frequent in the patients with mechanical prostheses who receive anticoagulants (Bloomfield et al, 1986; Douglas et al, 1985; Hammermeister et al, 1987).

EXTRACORPOREAL CIRCULATION

Extracorporeal circulation of the blood for cardiopulmonary bypass (CPB) or long-term respiratory assistance invariably results in damage to platelets and red blood cells, denaturation of plasma proteins, and activation of the coagulation mechanism. Bleeding after CPB necessitates reoperation in approximately 3% of patients who have operations on the heart, and 50% of all patients require transfusions of 2 to 4 units of packed red blood cells (Dodsworth and Dudley, 1985; Salzman et al, 1986). The enormous artificial surface of the heart-lung machine, combined with areas of stagnation and eddy currents, offers ample opportunity for blood-surface interaction. Blood also encounters other substances, including air bubbles, fibrin, tissue debris, platelet aggregates, and defoaming agents, which may be incorporated into microemboli; shear stresses and activation of complement may accelerate this process (Kirklin et al, 1983; Mammen et al, 1985).

Adequate anticoagulation before and during CPB is required to prevent thrombosis and fibrin deposition. Heparin is most commonly used for this purpose, and the degree of anticoagulation is usually measured by the activated clotting time, although more precise assays exist (Mammen et al, 1985). Heparin must be neutralized with protamine to ensure adequate surgical hemostasis before closure of the chest. Although the problems of inadequate heparinization, inadequate neutralization with protamine, protamine excess, and the heparin "rebound" phenomenon have received considerable attention as causes of bleeding after CPB, it is doubtful that, with currently accepted doses of heparin and protamine, they are important causes of hemorrhage (Bick, 1985).

Thrombocytopenia occurs within seconds of contact of the blood with the extracorporeal circuit (Gralnick and Fischer, 1971). This decrease in platelet numbers varies in different studies (Bick, 1985; Gluszko et al, 1987) and is rarely severe. The decrease is usually attributed to hemodilution (Mammen et al, 1985); adherence to foreign surfaces; sequestration in spleen, liver, and lungs; formation and filtration of microaggregates; and destruction in the cardiotomy suction system (Bick, 1985). Platelet consumption during CPB appears to be related to the exposure of platelet Gp IIB-IIIA fibrinogen receptors (Gluszko et al, 1987). The need to remove the circulating platelet aggregates and particulate matter that form during extracorporeal circulation has led to the development of micropore filters (Solis and Gibbs, 1972; Ware et al, 1982). These emboli and other systemic effects of bypass, such as hemolysis and complement activation, may be responsible for postoperative dysfunction of many viscera, including the brain, kidneys, and lungs. Extracorporeal circulation with membrane oxygenators appears to produce less hematologic derangement (e.g., hemolysis, platelet loss, protein denaturation) than the bubble type of oxygenators. Attempts to provide long-term respiratory support by using extracorporeal circulation have been frustrated by marked thrombocytopenia and serious bleeding complications (Zapol et al, 1979), but the apparatus has proved to be successful in the treatment of various respiratory distress syndromes in infants (Bartlett et al, 1982).

Extracorporeal circulation affects platelet function as well as number. Platelets may undergo partial "release" of intracellular granules, which results in an acquired storage pool deficiency (Harker et al, 1980). During bypass, circulating platelets become less responsive to soluble agonists (Edmunds and Williams, 1983; Ware et al, 1983). The etiology of this phenomenon is unknown. Evidence suggests that platelets may lose their surface receptors for epinephrine (Wachtvogel et al, 1985) and fibrinogen (Gluszko et al, 1987) by exposure to foreign surfaces. Other possible factors include changes in pH, anemia, altered oxygenation, circulating fibrin degradation products, and protamine, but platelet function has decreased even after these conditions have been corrected (Bick, 1985). A defect in platelet aggregation induced by ristocetin in patients on CPB (Mammen et al, 1985) suggests that an abnormality in von Willebrand's factor may be involved in altered platelet reactivity. This possibility is supported by the improvement in hemostasis after bypass produced by desmopressin acetate, an agent that increases levels of von Willebrand's factor (Salzman et al, 1986).

Fibrinolysis occurs in parallel with intravascular fibrin production, which is usually due to inadequate heparinization. When fibrinolysis occurs, fibrinogen-fibrin degradation products are formed, which are anticoagulants and prolong the thrombin time. With modern bypass equipment, fibrinolysis appears to be unusual (Brody et al, 1986). If fibrinolysis occurs, the patients might benefit from epsilon-aminocaproic acid (EACA), but there is no compelling evidence for its efficacy in these circumstances and, if disseminated intravascular coagulation (DIC) is present, EACA can lead to catastrophic thrombotic complications. Evidence that aprotinin, a serine proteinase inhibitor, reduces blood loss in patients having CPB was thought to reflect the favorable effect of the drug on platelet preservation rather than inhibition of fibrinolysis (Royston et al, 1987).

BLOOD PUMPS FOR CIRCULATORY SUPPORT

Blood pumps can be divided into two broad categories: (1) left ventricular assist devices, which bypass the diseased ventricle and are often referred to as heterotopic prosthetic ventricles or partial artificial hearts, and (2) the total artificial heart, also known as the biventricular replacement device, which usually replaces the diseased heart and thus is referred to as orthotopic. These means of circulatory support are considered for patients who cannot be sustained by pharmacologic therapy and intra-aortic balloon assistance and are increasingly used to provide complete circulatory support to patients awaiting cardiac transplantation (Farrar et al, 1988). With improvements in power supply and design, the indications for the use of these devices should increase. It is estimated that approximately 500 patients per year in the United States would benefit from permanent circulatory assistance; the current survival after temporary ventricular assistance is 25 to 50% (Clagett, 1987), and when a device of recent design was used as a bridge to cardiac transplantation, about two-thirds of the patients survived at long-term follow-up (Farrar et al, 1988).

The left ventricular assist devices consist of a flexible polyurethane blood sac and diaphragm with inlet and outlet prosthetic heart valves (porcine or Bjork-Shiley) that are connected to the great vessels by Dacron prosthetic grafts and to the left ventricular apex by a cannula. The device can be powered externally or internally by units that deliver pulses of compressed carbon dioxide (Hill et al, 1986; Pennock et al, 1986) or by an air-driven console (Schoen et al, 1986). Some recent devices have totally implantable pump units that are enclosed in titanium. Although the polyurethane surface appears to be less thrombogenic than the materials used earlier, embolic strokes and coagulopathies with clinically significant hemorrhage continue to be frequent complications (Farrar et al, 1988). To combat this problem, a recently developed device (Thermedics, Inc., Woburn, MA) has a polyurethane lining that is "flocked" with appendages so that a pseudoneointima can become anchored to the surface. It is not certain what anticoagulant therapy, if any, is optimal; low doses of intravenous heparin, low-molecular-weight dextran, and warfarin have all been used. In the patient who is bleeding or hemostatically incompetent because of prolonged CBP or for other reasons, anticoagulant therapy should be withheld at least temporarily.

The total artificial heart requires the use of two mechanical pumps that replace the native ventricles, and the inlet connectors are attached to the atria (rather than the ventricular apex) by Dacron felt sewing rings. This approach is most useful for a patient whose native heart is useless or is at risk for future hemodynamic or thrombotic problems; in particular, the function of the right ventricle with a left ventricular assist device in place has been difficult to predict. Also, with orthotopic replacement, the problems associated with implantation of a space-occupying mass are not seen. The most successful of these devices is the Jarvik heart, which has been used to support the circulation for long periods in several patients (DeVries, 1988, De Vries et al, 1984). Thromboembolism and hemorrhage from blood trauma and vigorous anticoagulation are still major hazards; the problem of thromboembolic strokes has been particularly persistent in these patients (Lawrie, 1988; Relman, 1984). Until more thromboresistant surfaces are developed, the most successful use of the total artificial heart is likely to be as a temporary measure before transplantation of a donor heart (Griffith et al, 1987).

INTRA-AORTIC BALLOON CARDIAC ASSISTANCE

Intra-aortic balloon pumping is a standard form of circulatory assistance for cardiogenic shock due to acute infarction or cardiac dysfunction after open heart surgery. It is also commonly used to support patients with unstable angina refractory to more conservative methods and for temporary support of preoperative patients with severe left ventricular failure. The primary benefits of balloon counterpulsation are those of stabilization before more definitive intervention, although patients can be maintained with these devices for several months (Freed et al, 1988).

High fluid shear rates in the thoracic aorta combined with streamlined design of the balloon and use of thromboresistant materials (i.e., polyurethane) have limited the rate of thromboembolic complications in the great vessels; the most common complication with this device is compromise of the circulation to the legs. Arterial insufficiency usually requires balloon removal (Alderman et al, 1987); if removal does not restore circulation, thrombectomy may be required. Anticoagulation with full-dose heparin is required to prevent this and other thromboembolic complications; administration of heparin and the trauma to the blood caused by the balloon result in a modest decrease in platelet count. Bleeding occurs

in about one-fifth of these patients (Freed et al, 1988) but is usually confined to the site of the arteriotomy. The incidence of other vascular complications is high; these complications include intimal injury, aortoiliac dissection, and perforation, and all of them are more common in women, diabetics, patients with pre-existing peripheral vascular disease (Alderman et al, 1987), and patients with percutaneous rather than open placement of the balloon (Goldberg et al, 1987).

VASCULAR PROSTHESES

Peripheral arteries and veins have been successfully replaced for four decades, despite the unavailability of truly nonthrombogenic materials for construction of vascular prostheses. Most prosthetic materials used today rely on deposition of a lining layer of adherent thrombus to create a relatively bland, thromboresistant surface. Large grafts, such as those to the aortoiliac vessels, have high patency rates because the neointimal thrombus does not significantly encroach on the lumen. High flow rates minimize layering of the thrombus, which would otherwise compromise the internal diameter of the graft. Because of thrombotic occlusion, prosthetic grafts to small (less than 4 mm in diameter) vessels such as the tibial and coronary arteries are not satisfactory in the long term, although glutaraldehyde-fixed bovine heterografts are being tested as possible coronary conduits. Larger grafts have a 5- to 10-year patency rate of 80 to 90%; this rate decreases to 15 to 50% with grafts to smaller vessels, especially grafts that cross a flexion crease such as femoral-popliteal bypasses or grafts placed in arteries with low flow rates (Clagett, 1987).

Several materials, which vary in thrombogenicity and mechanical properties, are used for fabrication of prosthetic vascular grafts (Table 51–4). Dacron grafts, either woven or knitted, rely on early deposition of plasma proteins, platelets, and fibrin to render their internal surfaces relatively thromboresistant. Within months, a neointimal lining of fibroblasts, smooth muscle cells, collagen, and elastin develops, although this lining is incomplete and leaves patches covered only by fibrin (Fig. 51–14). True endothelium grows from the ends of the graft for 1 to 2 cm, but endothelium in more central areas of the graft is rare in humans (Sauvage et al, 1975). In other species, endothelial recovering tends to be more nearly complete. Neointimal formation is facilitated by ingrowth of fibroblasts from the outside of the graft through its interstices. Factors such as wall thickness, porosity, and filamentous projection on the surface of the graft (i.e., velour) profoundly affect this ingrowth. Thrombotic occlusion of prostheses as a result of fracture of the neointima is a hazard long after implantation. Fibrous hyperplasia of the neointimal surface can occur and result in a stenosis at the anastomosis of the graft to the vessel; platelet pro-

TABLE 51–4. CHARACTERISTICS OF MATERIALS USED FOR FABRICATION OF
PROSTHETIC VASCULAR GRAFTS

Material	Construction	Porosity	Preclotting Required	Neointimal Formation	Platelet Adhesion to Graft
Dacron	Woven	Microporous	Optional	Yes	+
	Knitted (internal velour, external velour, or double velour)	Macroporous	Yes	Yes	+
Polytetrafluoroethylene (Teflon)	Expanded reinforced	Microporous	No	Yes	+
Human umbilical vein	Glutaraldehyde-stabilized (reinforced with Dacron mesh)	Nonporous	No	No	+
Autologous saphenous vein	Reversed because of valves or in situ	Nonporous	No	No (true endothelium preserved or regenerated)	−(+ if endothelium is injured)

duction of growth factors and mitogens is thought to be responsible for this phenomenon.

Autogenous saphenous vein is a better substitute for diseased medium-sized arteries, but its limited size restricts its use. Saphenous vein functions as a living tissue with considerable tensile strength and the inherent thromboresistance of its endothelial lining. Endothelial injury that results in platelet-fibrin thrombus occurs frequently on the intima of saphenous vein grafts, probably as a result of manipulation of the graft during its insertion (Shelton et al, 1988). Human umbilical vein grafts stabilized with glutar-

aldehyde and reinforced with Dacron mesh are promising when saphenous vein is unavailable. Processing makes the graft nonantigenic, and its nonporous structures prevent ingrowth of neointimal cells. After initial remodeling in vivo, the internal elastic membrane is retained, serves as the interface with the blood, and is apparently thromboresistant. Amorphous material is commonly found to line the graft when it is harvested after several months.

Grafts made of expanded microporous polytetrafluoroethylene (PTFE) have shown promise in various smaller vessel applications. Like Dacron, these

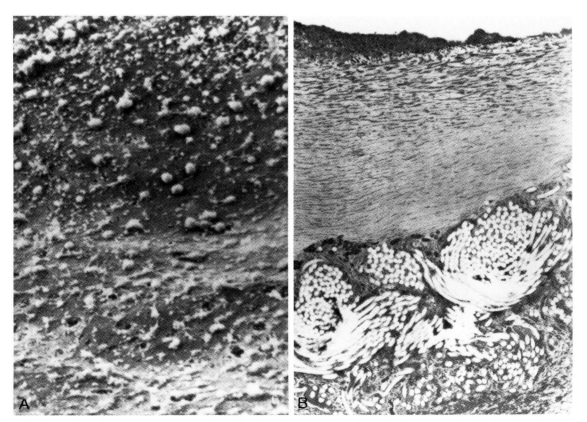

Figure 51–14. *A,* Scanning electron micrograph of the blood-contacting surface of a Dacron graft after implantation for 1 month; adherence of platelets and fibrin on a pseudoneointima is shown. *B,* Light micrograph of a similar graft 6 months after implantation. The surface is covered with a fibrin-platelet coagulum. (Reprinted by permission from Burkel, W. E., Graham, L. M., and Stanley, J. C.: Endothelial lining in prosthetic vascular grafts. Ann. N.Y. Acad. Sci., *516:*131, 1987.)

grafts rely on neointimal formation, but because of their low porosity, they do not require preclotting. Although there is evidence that porous grafts promote fibroblast ingrowth that stabilizes the intima, microporous and nonporous grafts have equivalent patency and compare well with saphenous vein grafts (Cranley and Hafner, 1981; LaSalle et al, 1982).

Heparin has been bonded to existing prosthetic materials to lessen thrombogenicity. There have been clinical successes with this approach (Donahoo et al, 1977), but its overall efficacy is not established. In an effort to provide a surface that inhibits platelet aggregation as well as fibrin formation, a prosthetic material coated with both prostaglandin E_1 and heparin is being tested (Kim et al, 1987).

Factors that contribute to occlusion of a vascular prosthesis are the early development of thrombosis and the later development of a proliferative fibrous stenosis, which is usually found at distal anastomoses (Clowes et al, 1985); the latter event can be complicated by thrombotic occlusion. There has been considerable attention to antithrombotic therapy in patients who receive artificial grafts. After implantation, a platelet-rich thrombus rapidly accumulates on the surface of vascular prostheses (Stratton et al, 1983); this deposit decreases in the next 6 months but can be detected during the following years. This acute process is associated with decreased platelet survival time after placement of aortic prostheses (Harker et al, 1977; Harker and Slichter, 1972) and with decreased levels of platelet dense granular contents, which suggests platelet activation (Savage et al, 1983). Administration of aspirin (325 mg three times daily) and dipyridamole (75 mg three times daily) reduces platelet uptake on both Dacron and PTFE arterial grafts (Goldman et al, 1983; Pumphrey et al, 1983); both platelet deposition and its reduction with antiplatelet agents are also seen on Dacron grafts even after months of implantation (Stratton and Ritchie, 1986). This effect of antiplatelet agents has been associated with improved short-term patency (Goldman et al, 1983), although clinical trials have not all been favorable (Kohler et al, 1984). Aspirin and dipyridamole therapy improves the patency of saphenous vein aortocoronary bypasses (Chesebro et al, 1982, 1984) at both early and late follow-up, but it has never been shown convincingly that dipyridamole contributes to this result (Fitzgerald, 1987; Lorenz et al, 1984). Aspirin improves the patency of clotted small-caliber prosthetic grafts after treatment with fibrinolytic agents (Curl et al, 1986). Thrombosis of these grafts responds to intravenous infusion of thrombolytic agents (Graor et al, 1986). Oral anticoagulants do not appear to protect prosthetic arterial reconstructions or aortocoronary bypass grafts from thrombosis (Genton et al, 1986).

Although both intraoperative heparin and dextran have been used in various protocols to prevent intraoperative arterial thrombosis and distal embolization, no trials support these approaches. Most vascular surgeons use heparin intraoperatively,

which has decreased thrombin generation in the ischemic limb (Sobel et al, 1987). That the saphenous vein bypass grafts do not have optimal antithrombotic surfaces has been shown by the superiority in long-term patency of internal mammary artery grafts compared with saphenous vein grafts (Loop et al, 1986). This improvement appears to derive from the lack of accelerated atherosclerosis in the internal mammary artery grafts (Shelton et al, 1988).

VASCULAR CATHETERS

Thrombotic occlusion of vessels that contain catheters for intravenous infusion is frequent and may occur even after removal of the catheter. Although material thrombogenicity is important, more significant factors are the length of time that the catheter is in place, the size of the artery or vein cannulated, the blood flow around the catheter, the nature and flow rate of the infused solution, and the coagulability of the patient's blood (Clagett, 1987). Arterial catheterization for angiography results in a low incidence of thromboembolism because of a favorable combination of these factors and because of the widespread use of anticoagulants and frequent flushing of the catheters with dilute heparin solutions. Thrombosis of the radial artery, which is often cannulated for longer periods for arterial monitoring and blood sampling, occurs in approximately one-third of the patients (Clagett, 1987). Significant hand ischemia is rare because of the presence of collateral circulation from the ulnar artery in more than 95% of patients.

With current standards of care, the most frequent serious thrombotic complication of vascular catheterization is associated with placement of central venous lines. These catheters are often left in place for several days and the frequently insidious thrombus formation can lead to axillary or subclavian venous thrombosis, superior vena caval syndrome, pulmonary embolization, and death. The incidence of asymptomatic thrombosis in the central veins approaches 50%; clinically evident thrombosis occurs in approximately 1 to 2% of cases, and pulmonary embolism occurs in less than 1% (Clagett, 1987). This thrombosis, even when asymptomatic, can be a nidus for infection. The incidence of venous thrombosis was decreased by the use of heparin-bonded catheters (Efsing et al, 1983; Hoar et al, 1981) and by the use of heparin in intermittently infused solutions (Brismar et al, 1982; Fabri et al, 1982).

ANTITHROMBOTIC DRUGS

Pharmacologic agents that interfere with hemostatic processes may reduce the thrombotic tendency of blood exposed to artificial surfaces. The drugs available include heparin and coumarin compounds, which interfere with fibrin formation, and numerous agents that alter platelet activity. Heparin is a strongly anionic sulfated polysaccharide that must be administered parenterally. Heparin binds to and activates antithrombin III, a natural inhibitor of several serine protease coagulation factors, including thrombin and Factors XIIa, XIa, IXa, and Xa. Cleavage by thrombin of fibrinopeptides A and B from fibrinogen is prevented, which stops fibrin production. An undesirable side effect is the induction of platelet clumping, which accounts in part for thrombocytopenia in patients who receive heparin. The heparin fractions that are most responsible for this phenomenon are the fractions that have the least anticoagulant activity, and there is hope that preparations of heparin subfractions of lower molecular weight will cause fewer bleeding complications without an increase in the incidence of thromboembolism (Salzman, 1986). These special heparin preparations might be indicated for patients with heparin-induced thrombocytopenia, which, when associated with thrombosis, has a high morbidity and mortality (Ware et al, 1988).

Cardiopulmonary bypass requires anticoagulation with heparin to prevent the formation of fibrin in the extracorporeal circuit. Heparin is frequently used by vascular surgeons during peripheral arterial reconstruction and graft placement (Genton et al, 1986). Low-dose heparin is commonly used in surgical patients to prevent venous thromboembolism; full-dose heparin is recommended in the treatment of established deep or central venous thrombi or pulmonary emboli, during arterial catheterization, and for selected patients in whom warfarin administration is impossible or hazardous. Because hemorrhagic complications are common when pre-existing coagulation defects are present, a simple assessment of hemostasis is made before heparin therapy and should include platelet count, prothrombin time, and partial thromboplastin time. The risk of major bleeding complications is greater within 48 hours of major surgical procedures or within 6 weeks of neurosurgery or intracranial bleeding. Hemorrhagic complications occur in 10 to 20% of patients who have normal hemostasis before heparinization and in up to 50% of patients with uremia or thrombocytopenia (Ware et al, 1988).

For long-term anticoagulation of patients with vascular or valvular prostheses, warfarin is preferred to heparin because of ease of administration, relatively simple regulation of dosage, and freedom from the side effects peculiar to heparin, such as thrombocytopenia, osteoporosis, and alopecia. Warfarin inhibits the synthesis of vitamin-K-dependent Factors VII, IX, and X and prothrombin. The clinical response depends on vitamin K stores, albumin binding, and hepatic degradation but is usually related to the degree of anticoagulation as shown by the prothrombin time. Warfarin is essential for patients with nontissue cardiac valvular prostheses and is used in bioprosthetic valve recipients for 3 to 6 months. Warfarin is continued in patients in the latter group

who have atrial fibrillation or enlargement or who have previously had a thromboembolic event; some surgeons recommend warfarin therapy for all patients with a bioprosthetic valve in the mitral position. The use of oral anticoagulants for patients who have had arterial reconstruction with implantation of vascular prostheses has not been beneficial. Late patency rates do not improve by anticoagulation, nor is the ultimate progression of arteriosclerosis affected.

Bleeding during warfarin administration is dose related. Patients should be monitored with a clotting test, such as the prothrombin time. The therapeutic goal for the prothrombin time is prolongation to 1.5 to 2 times the control level, although low-risk patients without mechanical prostheses can be anticoagulated adequately with prolongation of the prothrombin time to 1.2 to 1.5 times (Hull et al, 1982; Poller and Tabener, 1982). When a patient bleeds despite proper anticoagulation, an underlying lesion, such as an ulcer, neoplasm, or arteriovenous malformation, should be suspected. Another complication of warfarin therapy is skin necrosis, which reflects local capillary thrombosis and is due to an abrupt decrease in the level of protein C, a vitamin-K-dependent natural anticoagulant, that occurs on initiation of therapy with this agent. The use of warfarin in the first trimester of gestation (specifically the 6th through the 13th weeks) can cause serious congenital abnormalities and an increased incidence of fetal death. Heparin can be substituted for warfarin in the first trimester soon after conception and in the last 2 weeks of the third trimester (Iturbe-Alessio et al, 1986; Lee et al, 1986), but the incidence of thromboemboli and of fetal abortion is still high even with these precautions.

Some drugs that alter platelet function have a clinically important antithrombotic effect. These drugs function by various mechanisms (Fig. 51–15). Aspirin in small doses inhibits platelet synthesis of prostaglandins by irreversibly blocking the enzyme cyclooxygenase and thus impairs platelet secretion and aggregation for the life span of the platelet (10 days). Other nonsteroidal anti-inflammatory agents block the same synthetic pathway, but their effect is reversible and dose related. Dipyridamole increases platelet cyclic adenosine monophosphate (AMP) levels by inhibiting the enzyme phosphodiesterase, which normally degrades cyclic AMP, and thus dipyridamole might be expected to inhibit aggregation and adhesion; however, it is not certain that this action is clinically important (Fitzgerald, 1987). A combination of dipyridamole and warfarin is more effective than warfarin alone in patients with prosthetic valves who have an embolus despite adequate warfarin treatment (Sullivan et al, 1969). Warfarin was shown to protect patients with prosthetic heart valves from thromboembolism better than either a combination of pentoxifylline and aspirin or a combination of dipyridamole and aspirin (Mok et al, 1985).

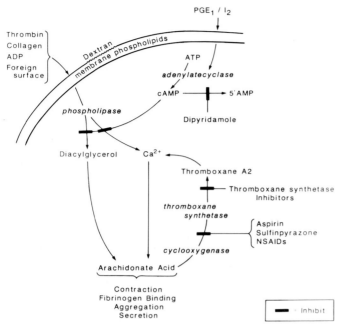

Figure 51–15. Site of action of antiplatelet drugs. Enzyme names appear in italics. (NSAIDs = nonsteroidal anti-inflammatory drugs.)

Sulfinpyrazone, a drug introduced as a uricosuric agent, inhibits platelet prostaglandin synthesis, but the precise mechanism of action is not understood. Sulfinpyrazone decreased the rate of thrombotic occlusion of arteriovenous shunts used for hemodialysis (Kaegi et al, 1974) and corrected shortened platelet survival in patients with prosthetic heart valves (Weily and Genton, 1970), but there are few generally accepted indications for its clinical use.

Low-molecular-weight dextran impairs platelet adhesion and aggregation by mechanisms that also are not well understood. Dextran is often used empirically for its antiplatelet and antithrombotic effect, but no well-designed studies support its efficacy and there are no generally accepted indications for its use. It may be used most effectively in prevention of thromboembolism in orthopedic and general surgical patients (Ware et al, 1988).

Generally, aspirin in combination with an anticoagulant such as heparin or warfarin is associated with increased bleeding and should be avoided (Chesebro et al, 1983; Torosian et al, 1978).

Prostaglandin E_1 (PGE$_1$) and prostacyclin (PGI$_2$) have reversible short-lived antiplatelet effects that derive from their ability to increase platelet cyclic AMP, which inhibits platelet adhesion and aggregation. These drugs are potent platelet inhibitors, but it has been difficult to administer them in effective doses because of their vasodilator properties (Harker and Fuster, 1986). Cardiopulmonary bypass with PGE$_1$ preserved platelet number and function without undue bleeding in monkeys (Addonizio et al, 1978). Both drugs have been infused during clinical CPB and have preserved platelet number and func-

tion, reduced platelet deposition on artificial surfaces, and reduced postoperative blood loss, but the resultant hypotension has led to questions about their safety (Edmunds, 1987). PGI$_2$ has been used instead of heparin in hemodialysis without adverse effects. Several studies evaluated the use of PGI$_2$ in peripheral arterial disease and showed mixed results (Ware et al, 1988). A clinical trial of PGI$_2$ in patients who had CPB showed that the postoperative blood loss was not significantly reduced (Fish et al, 1986).

NONTHROMBOGENIC MATERIALS

Many vascular mechanisms that protect against thrombosis require an intact endothelial surface. These mechanisms include the protein C, protein S, and thrombomodulin system; the heparin-antithrombin III system; and the generation of prostacyclin. Artificial surfaces must rely on inherent physiochemical properties that render them relatively compatible with blood. Prosthetic devices are less than perfect in this regard and owe much of their in-vivo success to the cleansing effects of blood flow, limited surface area, antithrombotic drugs, and deposition of neointimal thrombus (Clagett, 1987).

The properties of a surface that affect reactivity toward the blood are not entirely understood. Proteins are adsorbed by foreign surfaces within seconds after contact with blood. These proteins appear to mediate subsequent interaction with platelets and formation of thrombus. The importance of these early protein-surface interactions is illustrated by the fact that a material coated with albumin is relatively thromboresistant, whereas the same material coated with fibrinogen fosters platelet reactivity (Salzman and Merrill, 1987). Platelet adhesion to an artificial surface may increase with increased surface coverage by adsorbed fibrinogen molecules that retain their normal conformation (Lindon et al, 1986).

Surface charge was thought to be important in blood compatibility after early reports that electrodes placed across a blood vessel in an animal caused thrombosis at the positive pole. Efforts were made to produce materials with a fixed negative charge at their surface, which would electrostatically repel negatively charged blood elements such as plasma proteins and platelets. However, surface charge is an average value that results from summation of a mosaic of molecular charges arrayed at the surface, and it has had limited value for prediction of the behavior of an artificial material in contact with blood.

Surface-wetting ability as an expression of surface-free energy is also cited as an important characteristic of artificial surfaces. Wettable surfaces have been thought to promote thrombosis (Neubauer and Lampert, 1930). More recent evidence suggests that hydrophobic (nonwettable) surfaces may actually be more thrombogenic than more hydrophilic surfaces (Merrill et al, 1981). Other properties that may influence thrombogenicity are surface roughness, capacity for electrostatic (ionic) interaction, chain flexibility in polymers, and a host of contaminants such as waxes, plasticizers, and mold-release agents.

Blood compatibility has been improved by binding heparin to a polymer surface (Lindon et al, 1985). This approach might seem to be paradoxic, because heparin dissolved in blood does nothing to impede platelet adhesion or other platelet reactions, except those mediated by thrombin. In fact, heparin induces platelet aggregation in platelet-rich plasma and whole blood in vitro and "sensitizes" the platelets to subsequent stimulation with ADP, epinephrine, or collagen. Why does binding of heparin to various polymers render them less thrombogenic? First, heparin bonded to a surface electrostatically or ionically may leach from the material and create a thin layer of anticoagulated blood in contact with the surface. Second, heparin that remains bound to the material may participate in formation of heparin-antithrombin complexes, which "passivate" artificial surfaces in vitro (Salzman et al, 1981). Improved techniques for binding heparin to artificial surfaces and the use of heparin fractions selected for high antithrombin III affinity and low platelet reactivity may lead to materials with better blood compatibility.

Selected Bibliography

DeVries, W. C.: The permanent artificial heart. J.A.M.A., *259*:849, 1988.

A clinically oriented description and case presentations of patients who received the Jarvik heart. Also see editorials by Lawrie (1988) and Relman (1984) for critical assessments of the progress thus far and articles by Griffith and associates (1987) and Hill and associates (1986), who described the more successful trials in which prosthetic ventricles were used as a bridge to cardiac transplantation.

Edmunds, L. H.: Thrombotic and bleeding complications of prosthetic heart valves. Ann. Thorac. Surg., *44*:430, 1987.

A comprehensive review of the many clinical series of cardiac valve replacements, with emphasis on comparisons between caged ball, disk, and bioprosthetic valves. Also see Perier and associates (1985), who found that the lower incidences of thromboembolism and anticoagulant-related hemorrhage with the porcine bioprosthetic valve compared with either the Starr or Bjork valve led to marked decreases in morbidity and mortality at 8-year follow-up.

Leonard, E. F., Turitto, V. T., and Vroman, L. (eds): Blood in contact with natural and artificial surfaces. Ann. N.Y. Acad. Sci., *516*:1–686, 1987.

This book is a collection of reviews by a number of groups who are investigating the biochemical and physical aspects of artificial surfaces. Almost every major experimental approach to understanding blood-surface contact is described, and a good view of possible future developments in this field is given.

Bibliography

Addonizio, V. P., Strauss, J. F., Macarak, E. J., et al: Preservation of platelet number and function by prostaglandin E during total cardiopulmonary bypass in rhesus monkeys. Surgery, *83*:619, 1978.

Alderman, J. D., Gabliani, G. I., McCabe, C. H., et al: Incidence and management of limb ischemia with percutaneous wire-guided intraaortic balloon catheters. J. Am. Coll. Cardiol., *9*:524, 1987.

Bartlett, R. H., Andrews, A. F., Toomasian, J. M., et al: Extracorporeal membrane oxygenation (ECMO) for newborn respiratory failure: 45 cases. Surgery, *92*:425, 1982.

Bick, R. L.: Hemostasis defects associated with cardiac surgery, prosthetic devices and other extracorporeal circuits. Semin. Thromb. Hemost., *11*:249, 1985.

Bloomfield, P., Kitchin, A. H., Wheatley, D. J., et al: A prospective evaluation of the Bjork-Shiley, Hancock, and Carpentier-Edwards heart valve prostheses. Circulation, *73*:1213, 1986.

Brais, M. P., Bedard, J. P., Goldstein, W., et al: Ionescu-Shiley pericardial xenografts: Follow up of up to 6 years. Ann. Thorac. Surg., *39*:105, 1985.

Braunwald, E.: Valvular heart disease. *In* Braunwald, E. (ed): Heart Disease. Philadelphia, W. B. Saunders Company, 1988, p. 1023.

Brismar, B., Hardstedt, C., Jacobson, S., et al: Reduction of catheter-associated thrombosis in parenteral nutrition by intravenous heparin therapy. Arch. Surg., *117*:1196, 1982.

Brody, J. I., Pickering, N. J., and Fink, G. B.: Concentrations of factor VIII-related antigen and factor XIII during open-heart surgery. Transfusion, *26*:478, 1986.

Chesebro, J. H., Clements, I. P., Fuster, V., et al: A platelet-inhibitor-drug trial in coronary artery bypass operations. Benefit of perioperative dipyridamole and aspirin therapy on early postoperative vein-graft patency. N. Engl. J. Med., *307*:73, 1982.

Chesebro, J. H., Fuster, V., Elveback, L. R., et al: Effect of dipyridamole and aspirin on late vein-graft patency after coronary bypass operations. N. Engl. J. Med., *310*:209, 1984.

Chesebro, J. H., Fuster, V., Elveback, L. R., et al: Trial of combined warfarin plus dipyridamole or aspirin therapy in prosthetic heart valve replacement: Danger of aspirin compared with dipyridamole. Am. J. Cardiol., *51*:1537, 1983.

Clagett, G. P.: Artificial devices in clinical practice. *In* Colman, R. W., Hirsh, J., Marder, V. J., and Salzman, E. W. (eds): Hemostasis and Thrombosis, 2nd ed. Philadelphia, J. B. Lippincott, 1987, p. 1348.

Clowes, A. W., Gown, A. M., Hanson, S. R., and Reidy, M. A.: Mechanisms of arterial graft failure. 1. Role of cellular proliferation in early healing of PTFE prostheses. Am. J. Pathol., *118*:43, 1985.

Cobanoglu, A., Grunkemeier, G. L., Aru, G. M., et al: Mitral replacement: Clinical experience with the ball-valve prosthesis. Ann. Surg., *202*:376, 1985.

Cranley, J. J., and Hafner, C. D.: Newer prosthetic material compared with autogenous saphenous vein for occlusive arterial disease of the lower extremity. Surgery, *89*:2, 1981.

Curl, G. R., Jakubowski, J. A., Deykin, D., and Bush, H. L., Jr.: Beneficial effect of aspirin in maintaining the patency of small-caliber prosthetic grafts after thrombolysis with urokinase or tissue-type plasminogen activator. Circulation, *74*:I-21, 1986.

Davies, G. C., Sobel, M., and Salzman, E. W.: Elevated plasma fibrinopeptide A and thromboxane B_2 levels during cardiopulmonary bypass. Circulation, *61*:808, 1980.

DeVries, W. C.: The permanent artificial heart. J.A.M.A., *259*:849, 1988.

DeVries, W. C., Anderson, J. L., Joyce, L. D., et al: Clinical use of the total artificial heart. N. Engl. J. Med., *310*:273, 1984.

Dodsworth, H., and Dudley, H. A. F.: Increased efficiency of transfusion practice in routine surgery using preoperative antibody screening and selective ordering with an abbreviated crossmatch. Br. J. Surg., *72*:102, 1985.

Donahoo, J. S., Bawley, R. K., and Gott, V. L.: The heparin-coated vascular shunt for thoracic aortic and great vessel procedures: A ten-year experience. Ann. Thorac. Surg., *23*:509, 1977.

Douglas, P. S., Hirshfield, J. W., Jr., Edie, R. N., et al: Clinical comparison of St. Jude and porcine aortic valve prostheses. Circulation, *72*:II-135, 1985.

Duvoisin, G. E., Brandenburg, R. O., and McGoon, D. C.: Factors affecting thromboembolism associated with prosthetic heart valves. Circulation, 35(Suppl. 1):70, 1967.

Edmunds, L. H.: Thrombotic and bleeding complications of prosthetic heart valves. Ann. Thorac. Surg., 44:430, 1987.

Edmunds, L. H., and Williams, W.: Microemboli and the use of filters during cardiopulmonary bypass. In Utley, J. R. (ed): Pathophysiology and Techniques of Cardiopulmonary Bypass. Baltimore, Williams & Wilkins, 1983, p. 101.

Efsing, H. O., Lindblad, B., Mark, J., and Wolff, T.: Thromboembolic complications from central venous catheters: A comparison of three catheter materials. World J. Surg., 7:419, 1983.

Fabri, P. J., Mirtallo, J. M., Ruberg, R. L., et al: Incidence and prevention of thrombosis of the subclavian vein during total parenteral nutrition. Surg. Gynecol. Obstet., 155:238, 1982.

Farah, E., Enriques-Sarano, M., Vahanian, A., et al: Thromboembolic and haemorrhage risk in mechanical and biologic aortic prosthesis. Eur. Heart J., 5(Suppl. D):43, 1984.

Farrar, D. J., Hill, J. D., Gray, L. A., Jr., et al: Heterotopic prosthetic ventricles as a bridge to cardiac transplantation: A multicenter study in 29 patients. N. Engl. J. Med., 318:333, 1988.

Fish, K. J., Sarnquist, F. H., van Steennis, C., et al: A prospective, randomized study of the effects of prostacyclin on platelets and blood loss during coronary bypass operations. J. Thorac. Cardiovasc. Surg., 91:436, 1986.

Fitzgerald, G. A.: Dipyridamole. N. Engl. J. Med., 316:1247, 1987.

Freed, P. S., Wasfie, T., Zado, B., and Kantrowitz, A.: Intraaortic balloon pumping for prolonged circulatory support. Am. J. Cardiol., 61:554, 1988.

Gallucci, V., Bortolotti, U., Milano, A., et al: Isolated mitral valve replacement with the Hancock bioprosthesis: A 13 year appraisal. Ann. Thorac. Surg., 38:571, 1984.

Genton, E., Clagett, G. P., and Salzman, E. W.: Antithrombotic therapy in peripheral vascular disease. Chest, 89:75S, 1986.

Gluszko, P., Rucinski, B., Musial, J., et al: Fibrinogen receptors in platelet adhesion to surfaces of extracorporeal circuit. Am. J. Physiol., 252:H615, 1987.

Goldberg, M., Kantrowitz, A., Rubenfire, M., et al: Intraaortic balloon pump insertion: A randomized study comparing percutaneous and surgical techniques. J. Am. Coll. Cardiol., 9:515, 1987.

Goldman, M. D., Simpson, D., Hawker, R. J., et al: Aspirin and dipyridamole reduce platelet deposition on prosthetic femoropopliteal grafts in man. Ann. Surg., 198:713, 1983.

Gralnick, H. R., and Fischer, R. D.: The hemostatic response to open-heart operations. J. Thorac. Cardiovasc. Surg., 61:909, 1971.

Graor, R. A., Risius, B., Lucas, F. V., et al: Thrombolysis with recombinant human tissue-type plasminogen activator in patients with peripheral artery and bypass graft occlusions. Circulation, 74(Suppl. I):I, 1986.

Griffith, B. P., Hardesty, R. L., Kormos, R. L., et al: Temporary use of the Jarvik-7 total artificial heart before transplantation. N. Engl. J. Med., 316:130, 1987.

Hammermeister, K. E., Henderson, W. G., Burchfield, C. M., et al: Comparison of outcome after valve replacement with a bioprosthesis versus a mechanical prosthesis: Initial 5 year results of a randomized trial. J. Am. Coll. Cardiol., 10:719, 1987.

Harker, L. A., and Fuster, V.: Pharmacology of platelet inhibitors. J. Am. Coll. Cardiol., 8:21B, 1986.

Harker, L. A., Malpass, T. W., Branson, H. E., et al: Mechanism of abnormal bleeding in patients undergoing cardiopulmonary bypass: Acquired transient platelet dysfunction associated with selective a-granule release. Blood, 56:824, 1980.

Harker, L. A., and Slichter, S. J.: Platelet and fibrinogen consumption in man. N. Engl. J. Med., 287:999, 1972.

Harker, L. A., Slichter, S. J., and Sauvage, L. R.: Platelet consumption by arterial prostheses: The effects of endothelialization and pharmacologic inhibition of platelet function. Ann. Surg., 186:594, 1977.

Hetzer, R., Topalidis, T., and Borst, H. G.: Thromboembolism and anticoagulation after isolated mitral valve replacement with porcine heterografts. In Cohn, C. H., and Gallucci, V.

(eds): Proceedings, Second International Symposium on Cardiac Bioprostheses. New York, Yorke Medical Books, 1982, p. 170.

Hill, J. D., Farrar, D. J., Hershon, J. J., et al: Use of a prosthetic ventricle as a bridge to cardiac transplantation for postinfarction cardiogenic shock. N. Engl. J. Med., 314:626, 1986.

Hill, J. D., Lizellen, L. B. A., Szarnicki, R. J., et al: Risk-benefit analysis of warfarin therapy in Hancock mitral valve replacement. J. Thorac. Cardiovasc. Surg., 83:718, 1982.

Hoar, P. F., Wilson, R. M., Mangano, D. T., et al: Heparin bonding reduces thrombogenicity of pulmonary artery catheters. N. Engl. J. Med., 305:993, 1981.

Hull, R., Delmore, T., Gento, E., et al: Warfarin sodium versus low-dose heparin in the long term treatment of venous thrombosis. N. Engl. J. Med., 301:855, 1979.

Hull, R., Hirsh, J., Jay, R., et al: Different intensities of oral anticoagulant therapy in the treatment of proximal vein thrombosis. N. Engl. J. Med., 307:1676, 1982.

Isom, O. W., Williams, D., Falk, E. A., et al: Evaluation of anticoagulant therapy in cloth-covered prosthetic valves. Circulation, 48(Suppl 3):48, 1973.

Iturbe-Alessio, I., del Carmen Fonseca, M., Mutchinik, O., et al: Risks of anticoagulant therapy in pregnant women with artificial heart valves. N. Engl. J. Med., 315:1390, 1986.

Janusz, M. T., Jamieson, W. R. E., Burr, L. H., et al: Thromboembolic risks and the role of anticoagulants in patients in chronic atrial fibrillation following mitral valve replacement with porcine bioprostheses. J. Am. Coll. Cardiol., 1:587, 1983.

Kaegi, A., Pineo, G. F., Shimize, A., et al: Arteriovenous-shunt thrombosis: Prevention by sulfinpyrazone. N. Engl. J. Med., 290:304, 1974.

Karp, R. B., Cyrus, R. J., Blackstone, E. H., et al: The Bjork-Shiley valve: Intermediate-term follow-up. J. Thorac. Cardiovasc. Surg., 81:602, 1981.

Kim, S. W., Jacobs, H., Lin, J. Y., et al: Nonthrombogenic bioactive surfaces. In Leonard, E. F., Turitto, V. T., and Vroman, L. (eds): Blood in Contact with Natural and Artificial Surfaces. Ann. N.Y. Acad. Sci., 516:116, 1987.

Kinsley, R. H., Antunes, M. J., and Colsen, P. R.: St. Jude medical valve replacement: An evaluation of valve performance. J. Thorac. Cardiovasc. Surg., 92:349, 1986.

Kirklin, J. W., Westaby, S., Blackstone, E. H., et al: Complement and the damaging effects of cardiopulmonary bypass. J. Thorac. Cardiovasc. Surg., 86:845, 1983.

Kohler, T. R., Kaufman, J. L., Kacoyanis, G., et al: Effect of aspirin and dipyridamole on the patency of lower extremity bypass grafts. Surgery, 96:462, 1984.

Kuntze, C. E. E., Ebels, T., Eijgelaar, A., et al: Rates of thromboembolism with three different heart valve prostheses: Randomized study. Lancet, 1:514, 1989.

Kopf, G. S., Hammond, G. L., Geha, A. S., et al: Long-term performance of the St. Jude medical valve: Low incidence of thromboembolism and hemorrhagic complication with modest doses of warfarin. Circulation, 76:III-132, 1987.

LaSalle, A. J., Brewster, D. C., Corson, J. D., and Darling, R. C.: Femoropopliteal composite bypass grafts: Current status. Surgery, 92:36, 1982.

Lawrie, G. M.: Permanent implantation of the Jarvik-7 total artificial heart: A clinical perspective. J.A.M.A., 259:892, 1988.

Ledain, L. D., Ohayon, J. P., Colle, J. P., et al: Acute thrombotic obstruction with disc valve prostheses: Diagnostic considerations and fibrinolytic treatment. J. Am. Coll. Cardiol., 7:743, 1986.

Lee, P.-K., Wange, R. Y. C., Chow, J. S. F., et al: Combined use of warfarin and adjusted subcutaneous heparin during pregnancy in patients with an artificial heart valve. J. Am. Coll. Cardiol., 8:221, 1986.

Leonard, E. F., Turitto, V. T., and Vroman, L. (eds): Blood in contact with natural and artificial surfaces. Ann. N.Y. Acad. Sci., 516:1–686, 1987.

Lindon, J. N., McManama, G., Kushner, L., et al: Does the conformation of adsorbed fibrinogen dictate platelet interactions with artificial surfaces? Blood, 68:355, 1986.

Lindon, J. N., Salzman, E. W., Merrill, E. W., et al: Catalytic activity and platelet reactivity of heparin covalently bonded to surfaces. J. Lab. Clin. Med., 105:219, 1985.

Loop, F. D., Lytle, B. W., Cosgrove, D. M., et al: Influence of the internal mammary artery graft on 10 year survival and other cardiac events. N. Engl. J. Med., *314*:1, 1986.

Lorenz, R. L., Weber, M., Kotzur, J., et al: Improved aortocoronary bypass patency by low-dose aspirin (100 mg daily): Effects on platelet aggregation and thromboxane formation. Lancet, *1*:1261, 1984.

Magilligan, D. J., Jr., Oyama, C., Klein, S., et al: Platelet adherence to bioprosthetic cardiac valves. Am. J. Cardiol, *53*:945, 1984.

Mammen, E. F., Koets, M. H., Washington, B. C., et al: Hemostasis changes during cardiopulmonary bypass surgery. Semin. Thromb. Hemostasis, *11*:281, 1985.

Merrill, E. W., Salzman, E. W., Sa da Costa, V., et al: Molecular factors in blood polymer interaction: Hydrophobic, hydrophilic, hydrogen bonding and aromatic. AIChE Symposium, 1981.

Miller, D. C., Oyer, P. E., Mitchell, R. S., et al: Performance characteristics of the Starr-Edwards model 1260 aortic valve prosthesis beyond ten years. J. Thorac. Cardiovasc. Surg., *88*:193, 1984.

Miller, D. C., Oyer, P. E., Stinson, E. B., et al: Ten to fifteen year reassessment of the performance characteristics of the Starr-Edwards model 6120 mitral valve prosthesis. J. Thorac. Cardiovasc. Surg., *85*:1, 1983.

Mok, C. K., Boey, J., Wang, R., et al: Warfarin versus dipyridamole-aspirin and pentoxifylline-aspirin for the prevention of prosthetic heart valve thromboembolism: A prospective randomized clinical trial. Circulation, *72*:1059, 1985.

Neubauer, O., and Lampert, H. A.: A new blood transfusion apparatus. Munch. Med. Wochenschr., *77*:582, 1930.

Nunez, L., Gil Aguado, M., Larrea, J. L., et al: Prevention of thromboembolism using aspirin after mitral valve replacement with porcine bioprosthesis. Ann. Thorac. Surg., *37*:84, 1984.

Oyer, P. E., Stinson, E. B., Miller, D. C., et al: Thromboembolic risk and durability of the Hancock bioprosthetic cardiac valve. Eur. Heart J., *5*(Suppl. D):81, 1984.

Pennock, J. L., Pierce, W. S., Campbell, D. B., et al: Mechanical support of the circulation followed by cardiac transplantation. J. Thorac. Cardiovasc. Surg., *92*:944, 1986.

Perier, P., Bessou, J. P., Swanson, J. S., et al: Comparative evaluation of aortic valve replacement with Starr, Bjork and porcine valve prostheses. Circulation, *72*(Suppl. II):140, 1985.

Poller, L., and Tabener, D. A.: Dosage and control of oral anticoagulants: An international collaborative survey. Br. J. Haematol., *51*:479, 1982.

Pumphrey, C. W., Chesebro, J. H., Dewanjee, M. K., et al: In vivo quantitation of platelet deposition on human peripheral arterial bypass grafts using indium-111-labeled platelets. Am. J. Cardiol., *51*:796, 1983.

Relman, A. S.: Artificial hearts—permanent and temporary. N. Engl. J. Med., *314*:644, 1984.

Rosoff, C. B., Salzman, E. W., Gurewich, V., et al: Reduction of platelet serotonin and the response to pulmonary emboli. Surgery, *70*:12, 1971.

Royston, D., Taylor, K. M., Bidstrup, B. P., and Saphsford, R. N.: Effect of aprotinin on need for blood transfusion after repeat open-heart surgery. Lancet, *2*:1289, 1987.

Sala, A., Schoevaerdts, J. C., Jaumin, P., et al: Review of 387 isolated mitral valve replacements by the model 6120 Starr-Edwards prosthesis. J. Thorac. Cardiovasc. Surg., *84*:744, 1982.

Salzman, E.: Low molecular weight heparin: Is small beautiful? N. Engl. J. Med., *315*:957, 1986.

Salzman, E. W., and Merrill, E. W.: Interaction of blood with artificial surfaces. *In* Colman, R., Hirsh, J., Marder, V., and Salzman, E. (eds): Hemostasis and Thrombosis, 2nd ed. Philadelphia, J. B. Lippincott, 1987, p. 1335.

Salzman, E. W., Silane, M., Lindon, J., et al: Thromboresistance of heparin-coated surfaces. *In* Lundblad, R. L., Brown, W. V., Mann, K. G., and Roberts, H. R.: Chemistry and Biology of Heparin. New York, Elsevier North-Holland, 1981, p. 435.

Salzman, E. W., Weinstein, M. J., Weintraub, R. M., et al: Treatment with desmopressin acetate to reduce blood loss after cardiac surgery. N. Engl. J. Med., *314*:1402, 1986.

Sauvage, L. R., Berger, K., Beilin, L., et al: Presence of endothe-

lium in an axillary-femoral graft of knitted Dacron with an external velour surface. Ann. Surg., *182*:749, 1975.

Savage, B., Malpass, T. W., Stratton, J. R., and Harker, L. A.: Platelet adenine nucleotide levels in patients with Dacron vascular prostheses. Thromb. Res., *32*:365, 1983.

Schaffer, M. S., Clarke, D. R., Campbell, D. N., et al: The St. Jude medical cardiac valve in infants and children: Role of anticoagulant therapy. J. Am. Coll. Cardiol., *9*:235, 1987.

Schoen, F. J., Palmer, D. C., Bernhard, W. F., et al: Clinical temporary ventricular assist: Pathologic findings and their implications in a multi-institutional study of 41 patients. J. Thorac. Cardiovasc. Surg., *92*:1071, 1986.

Sethia, B., Turner, M. A., Lewis, S., et al: Fourteen years' experience with the Bjork-Shiley tilting disc prosthesis. J. Thorac. Cardiovasc. Surg., *91*:350, 1986.

Shelton, M. E., Forman, M. B., Virmani, R., et al: A comparison of morphologic and angiographic findings in long-term internal mammary artery and saphenous vein bypass grafts. J. Am. Coll. Cardiol., *11*:297, 1988.

Sobel, M., Gervin, C. A., Qureshi, D. G., and Greenfield, L. J.: Coagulation responses to heparin in the ischemic limb: Assessment of thrombin and platelet activation during vascular surgery. Circulation, *76*:III-8, 1987.

Solis, R. T., and Gibbs, M. B.: Filtration of the microaggregates in stored blood. Transfusion, *12*:245, 1972.

Soots, G., Pieronne, A., Roux, J. P., et al: Experience with 813 aortic or mitral valve replacements with a Carpentier-Edwards bioprosthesis: Five year results. Eur. Heart J., *5*(Suppl. D):87, 1984.

Stein, P. D., Collins, J. J., and Kantrowitz, A.: Antithrombotic therapy in mechanical and biological prosthetic heart valves and saphenous vein bypass grafts. Chest, *89*:46S, 1986.

Stratton, J. R., and Ritchie, J. L.: Reduction of indium-111 platelet deposition on Dacron vascular grafts in humans by aspirin plus dipyridamole. Circulation, *73*:325, 1986.

Stratton, J. R., Thiele, B. L., and Ritchie, J. L.: Natural history of platelet deposition on Dacron aortic bifurcation grafts in the first year after implantation in man. Am. J. Cardiol., *52*:371, 1983.

Sullivan, J. M., Harken, D. E., and Gorlin, R.: Effect of dipyridamole on the incidence of arterial emboli after cardiac valve replacement. Circulation, *39–40*:1–149, 1969.

Torosian, M., Michelson, E. L., Morganroth, J., et al: Aspirin and Coumadin-related bleeding after coronary artery bypass graft surgery. Ann. Intern. Med., *89*:325, 1978.

Turitto, V. T., and Baumgartner, H. R.: Platelet surface interactions. *In* Colman, R., Hirsh, J., Marder, V., and Salzman, E. (eds): Hemostasis and Thrombosis. Philadelphia, J. B. Lippincott, 1987, p. 555.

Wachtvogel, Y. T., Musial, J., Jenkin, B., et al: Platelet alpha-2 adrenergic receptors during simulated extracorporeal circulation. J. Lab. Clin. Med., *105*:601, 1985.

Ware, J. A., Lewis, J. L., and Salzman, E. W.: Antithrombotic therapy. *In* Rutherford, R. B. (ed): Vascular Surgery. Philadelphia, W. B. Saunders Company, 1988, (in press).

Ware, J. A., Reaves, W. H., Horak, J. K., and Solis, R. T.: Defective platelet aggregation in patients undergoing surgical correction of cyanotic congenital heart disease. Ann. Thorac. Surg., *36*:289, 1983.

Ware, J. A., Scott, M. A., Horak, J. K., and Solis, R. T.: Platelet aggregation during and after cardiopulmonary bypass: Effect of two different cardiotomy filters. Ann. Thorac. Surg., *34*:204, 1982.

Weily, H. S., and Genton, E.: Altered platelet function in patients with prosthetic mitral valves: Effects of sulfinpyrazone therapy. Circulation, *42*:967, 1970.

Weily, H. S., Steele, P. P., Davies, H., et al: Platelet survival in patients with substitute heart valves. N. Engl. J. Med., *290*:534, 1974.

Zapol, W. M., Snider, M. T., Hill, J. D., et al: Extracorporeal membrane oxygenation in severe acute respiratory failure: A randomized prospective study. J.A.M.A., *242*:2193, 1979.

Zervas, N. T., Kuwayama, A., Rosoff, C. B., et al: Cerebral arterial spasm. Arch. Neurol., *28*:400, 1973.

CHAPTER 52

ACQUIRED AORTIC VALVE DISEASE

Marshall L. Jacobs
W. Gerald Austen

HISTORICAL ASPECTS

In 1914, Tuffier in Paris reported the first attempt to relieve aortic stenosis in a patient by dilatation of the aortic valve with the surgeon's finger inserted through the wall of the aorta. In 1947, Smithy and Parker reported an experimental study of aortic valve surgery, and in 1952 Bailey and associates inserted a mechanical dilator into the left ventricle of patients; the dilator passed retrograde through the aortic valve to separate the fused valve commissures. Others reported digital dilatation of the aortic valve (Ellis and Kirklin, 1955) by using a sleeve sewn onto the ascending aorta. In 1953 Hufnagel and Harvey at Georgetown University inserted a prosthetic ball valve into the descending aorta to reduce the physiologic effects of aortic valve regurgitation. Because of the risks associated with proximal hypertension and distal hypoperfusion during clamping of the descending thoracic aorta, the prosthesis was designed for rapid insertion by using fixation rings placed outside the aorta around each end of the prosthesis (Fig. 52–1).

The era of effective surgical management of aortic valve disease began with the development of the pump oxygenator by Gibbon in 1954. Kirklin and Mankin (1960), Scannell and associates (1963), and others used cardiopulmonary bypass and performed aortic valvotomies or aortic valve incision and debridements with removal of calcific deposits to enhance leaflet mobility. Bahnson and associates (1960), Harken and associates (1960), Hufnagel and Conrad (1961), McGoon (1961), and others used single-leaflet prostheses for partial replacement of diseased aortic valves. Lillehei and associates (1961) and Muller and associates (1961) replaced the entire aortic valve with a prosthesis in the subcoronary position. The development independently by Harken and associates (1960) and by Starr of the ball valve prosthesis and its use for aortic valve replacement (Starr et al, 1963) began an era of conceptual and technologic advances in the design and manufacture of aortic valve prostheses.

Coincident with these efforts to design a practical mechanical prosthetic substitute for the aortic valve, others explored replacement of the diseased aortic valve with biologic tissues. Murray (1956) transplanted a homograft aortic valve into the descending thoracic aorta of a patient with aortic insufficiency. Ross (1962), Barratt-Boyes (1965), and Duran and Gunning (1962) achieved successful orthotopic insertion of homograft aortic valves. Various other biologic materials were used to create partial or complete aortic valve substitutes. Senning (1967) used the patient's own fascia lata to create individual leaflets for valve replacement. Ionescu and Ross (1969) used autologous fascia lata mounted on a frame as a complete bioprosthesis. Zerbini (1975) used allograft dura mater valves preserved in glycerol. These fascia lata and dura mater valves were abandoned eventually because of infectious complications and limited durability. The first stent-mounted porcine aortic valves were implanted by Binet and associates (1965). Formaldehyde fixation proved to be unsatisfactory because the valves degenerated rapidly, and Carpentier (1974) modified the fixation process and introduced the glutaraldehyde-preserved, stent-mounted porcine xenograft, which proved to be more durable. Ionescu (1972) introduced the glutaraldehyde-treated, stent-mounted bovine pericardium prosthesis.

FUNCTIONAL ANATOMY OF THE AORTIC VALVE

The aortic valve, located at the junction of the left ventricle and the outflow tract of the ascending aorta, is normally tricuspid and is composed of a fibrous skeleton, three cusps, and the sinuses of Valsalva. The fibrous skeleton consists of three U-shaped structures that adjoin one another as at the points of a crown. The skeleton is in fibrous continuity with the anterior leaflet of the mitral valve (subaortic curtain) and with the membranous septum. The cusps are delicate fibrous leaflets that insert

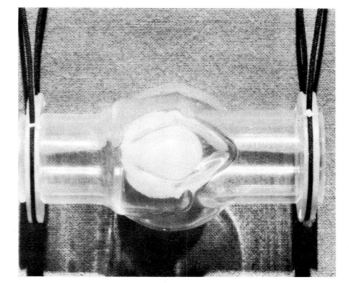

Figure 52–1. The prosthetic ball valve used by Hufnagel in the early 1950s. The prosthesis consists of a Lucite housing and a spherical silicon occluder. Fixation rings at each end facilitate rapid insertion into the descending thoracic aorta. (The original model of this prosthesis had a Lucite occluder, which combined with the Lucite housing had a noise level that was unacceptable to the recipients.)

into the outline of the valve skeleton. The free edge of each cusp is concave, is tougher and thicker than the rest of the leaflet, and has at its midpoint a fibrous nodule called the nodulus Arantius (Fig. 52–2). At the beginning of systole, the three cusps rapidly retract to form a triangular orifice (Fig. 52–3). Pulse duplicator studies show eddy currents within the sinuses of Valsalva that cause a slow wave-like motion of the free edge and billowing of the base of each cusp and thus prevent occlusion of the coronary ostia. During ventricular diastole, the cusps fall passively into the lumen of the aorta, support the ejected column of blood, and prevent regurgitation into the ventricle. In a healthy valve, approximation of the cusps during diastole is complete; the three noduli Arantii come together near the center of the aortic lumen. As much as 80% of coronary blood flow occurs during *diastole*.

The sinuses of Valsalva are slightly dilated pockets of the aortic root between the cusps and the aortic wall. The coronary arteries arise from two of the sinuses of Valsalva. These two sinuses and the corresponding valve cusps derive their names from the left and right coronary arteries that arise therein. The remaining sinus and cusp are termed noncoronary. Because the aortic valve lies in an oblique plane, the origin of the left coronary artery is slightly superior to that of the right coronary artery.

AORTIC VALVE DISEASE

Acquired diseases that affect the aortic valve cause valve lesions that may be classified functionally into the categories of aortic stenosis, aortic regurgitation, and mixed aortic valve disease. Hypertrophic cardiomyopathy, a disease of the myocardium that can produce obstruction to left ventricular outflow, is also considered in this chapter.

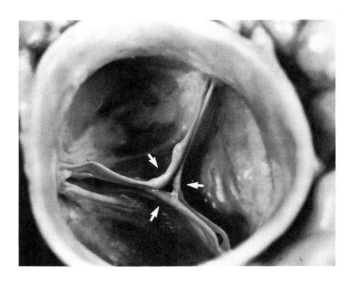

Figure 52–2. Post-mortem specimen of a normal aortic valve in the closed position. The free edge of each leaflet is slightly thicker than the remainder of the leaflet. There is a fibrous nodule, the nodulus Arantius, at the approximate midpoint of each free edge. The three noduli Arantii meet near the midpoint of the valve during closure *(arrows)*. (From Sutton, G. C., and Anderson, R. H. [eds]: Slide Atlas of Cardiology. London, England, Medi-Cine Productions, 1978.)

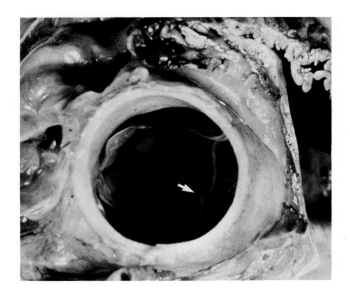

Figure 52–3. Post-mortem specimen of a normal aortic valve in the open position. The three cusps have retracted toward the aortic wall and form a roughly triangular orifice. Even in this fixed specimen, the wave-like pattern of motion of the free edges of the cusps can be appreciated *(arrow)*. (From Sutton, G. C., and Anderson, R. H. [eds]: Slide Atlas of Cardiology. London, England, Medi-Cine Productions, 1978.)

Aortic Stenosis

Pathophysiology. Aortic stenosis is a narrowing of the aortic valve orifice that obstructs left ventricular emptying. The degree of stenosis is expressed in terms of aortic valve area and the pressure gradient between the left ventricular chamber and the supravalvular aorta. In severe valvular obstruction, the left ventricular pressure during systole is increased and the systolic ejection period is prolonged (Fig. 52–4), which results in a delay in the upstroke and an increase in the duration of the systemic arterial pulse. These physiologic alterations are associated with an increase in myocardial oxygen consumption during the cardiac cycle. The relationship between the aortic valve area and the gradient across the aortic valve is expressed by the Gorlin formula (Gorlin and Gorlin, 1951).

$$\text{Aortic valve area (cm}^2) = \text{aortic valve flow} \div 44.5 \times \sqrt{\text{aortic valve mean systolic gradient}}$$

The number 44.5 is an acceleration constant. With clinically significant aortic valve stenosis, the systolic gradient across the valve is usually greater than 50 mm Hg. If there is severe depression of cardiac output and thus of flow across the aortic valve, a gradient of less than 50 mm Hg may be measured

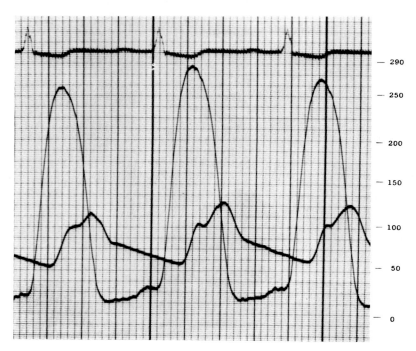

— 290

— 250

— 200

— 150

— 100

— 50

— 0

Figure 52–4. Hemodynamic tracing obtained during left-sided heart catheterization of a patient with severe aortic stenosis. Systolic pressure in the left ventricle is 270 to 285 mm Hg. Radial artery pressure is 110 to 120/60 mm Hg. The peak systolic gradient across the aortic valve is more than 150 mm Hg. The upstroke of the radial artery pressure tracing is delayed relative to the left ventricular pressure tracing. (From Thibault, G. E., DeSanctis, R. W., and Buckley, M. J.: Aortic stenosis, Chapter 18. *In* Johnson, R. A., Haber, E., and Austen, W. G. [eds]: The Practice of Cardiology. Boston, Little, Brown and Company, 1980, p. 478.)

across a critically narrowed valve with an area of less than 0.5 cm²/m² of body surface area. Inaccuracies of the Gorlin formula may be magnified in states of extremely low flow, but the relationship between aortic valve area, aortic valve flow, and systolic gradient generally holds true (Friedlich and Buckley, 1980). The increase in systolic left ventricular pressure caused by aortic valve obstruction generally leads to concentric hypertrophy of the left ventricle. Increased ventricular wall thickness is associated with diminished left ventricular compliance, which, if sufficiently severe, may be reflected by an increase in left ventricular end-diastolic pressure. Left ventricular cavity size is generally normal, but the chamber may become dilated in the advanced stages of aortic stenosis or in association with other lesions (including aortic regurgitation, coronary occlusive disease, and mitral regurgitation). Resting cardiac output is generally well maintained in severe aortic stenosis, but aortic valve obstruction results in inability to raise the cardiac output during exercise.

Etiology. Aortic stenosis in adults may be due to secondary changes that affect a congenitally abnormal aortic valve, to rheumatic heart disease, or to senile degenerative aortic valve disease.

One of the most common congenital cardiac anomalies is the congenitally bicuspid aortic valve (Fig. 52–5). As many as 1% of the general population may have this anomaly (Fenoglio et al, 1977). With advancing age, the abnormal aortic valve undergoes fibrocalcific degenerative changes. Most patients with a congenitally bicuspid aortic valve do not have significant aortic valve obstruction during childhood but do have abnormal valvular calcification by the age of 20, and nearly all show calcification by 30 years of age (Friedberg, 1966). Roberts (1970) showed by demographic and pathologic studies that most

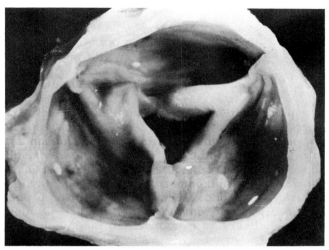

Figure 52–6. Post-mortem specimen of aortic valve with stenosis due to rheumatic valvulitis. The leaflets are thickened, and there is commissural fusion that results in a triangular central orifice. (From Sutton, G. C., and Anderson, R. H. [eds]: Slide Atlas of Cardiology. London, England, Medi-Cine Productions, 1978.)

cases of isolated aortic stenosis in young adults result from degenerative changes in a congenitally abnormal valve. Also, stenotic aortic valves that require valvotomy in infancy or childhood generally undergo degenerative changes including calcification (Friedberg, 1966), which may necessitate repeat valvotomy or valve replacement during adult life (Sandor et al, 1980).

Rheumatic fever was once thought to be the cause of most cases of valvular aortic stenosis in young adults. Studies by Roberts and associates (1970, 1973) showed that this is not the case, but it is clear that the pathologic changes of rheumatic valvulitis do progress to aortic stenosis. The inflammatory process results in edema, lymphocytic infiltration, and neovascularization of valve leaflets. Thickening of the valve leaflets progresses to commissural fusion between adjacent cusps. The leaflets eventually calcify, and an immobile ring of rigid valvular tissue with a fixed triangular central orifice forms (Fig. 52–6). While the reduced orifice significantly obstructs left ventricular emptying, the immobility of the leaflets generally also causes insufficiency of the valve. Rheumatic aortic stenosis is often also associated with disease of the mitral or tricuspid valves.

Senile degenerative calcific aortic stenosis is the most common cause of aortic stenosis in patients 65 years of age and older (Roberts et al, 1971). Histologic and histochemical studies of the aortic valve showed that clinically occult degenerative changes (collagen disruption and small calcific deposits) were present in nearly all aortic valve tissue from patients who died in mid-life of non-valve-related causes (Sell and Scully, 1965). Calcification begins in the sinuses of Valsalva and may not only progress to involve fusion

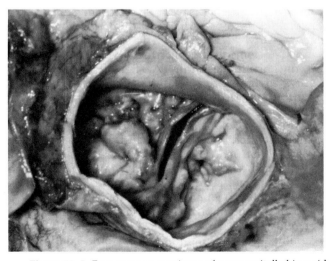

Figure 52–5. Post-mortem specimen of a congenitally bicuspid aortic valve shows secondary changes including significant calcification of both cusps, with valvular stenosis. (From Sutton, G. C., and Anderson, R. H. [eds]: Slide Atlas of Cardiology. London, England, Medi-Cine Productions, 1978.)

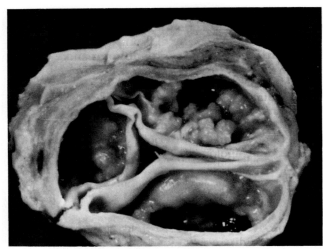

Figure 52–7. Post-mortem specimen that shows senile degenerative calcific aortic stenosis. The calcification not only involves the leaflets but also extends to the adjacent aortic wall. (From Sutton, G. C., and Anderson, R. H. [eds]: Slide Atlas of Cardiology. London, England, Medi-Cine Productions, 1978.)

at the commissures and extensive calcification of the leaflets but also extend into the adjacent aortic wall and onto the anterior leaflet of the mitral valve. Although calcification is characteristic of senile degenerative aortic stenosis (Fig. 52–7), some aortic valve calcification occurs in the advanced stages of aortic stenosis regardless of etiology. Complications may result from extension of calcification into the interventricular septum in the region of the bundle of His or into the region of the ostia of the coronary arteries with consequent obstruction.

Clinical Findings. Angina, syncope, and exertional dyspnea (left ventricular failure) are the principal symptoms of severe aortic stenosis. Typical exertional angina can be experienced by patients with aortic stenosis in the absence of coronary artery disease. The angina generally occurs after effort or excitement and is a manifestation of the relative inadequacy of coronary blood flow in a setting of hypertrophied myocardium and increased ventricular systolic pressure. The syncope occurs during increased cardiac work and may be due to an arrhythmia, to inability to increase cardiac output in response to exercise-induced vasodilatation in muscle beds, or to sudden inability of the left ventricle to eject against the stenotic valve (Schwartz et al, 1969). Occasionally, critical aortic stenosis may present as unheralded myocardial infarction or as sudden death due to ventricular arrhythmia.

Physical signs of aortic stenosis are evident long before the onset of symptoms. The contour of the arterial pulse is the physical finding that most accurately reflects the severity of aortic stenosis, and it is best evaluated by palpation of the carotid arteries. The carotid pulses of patients with significant aortic stenosis have a delayed upstroke and prolonged duration. An anacrotic notch or a thrill may be

present. In the very elderly, the rigidity of the carotid arteries due to loss of elasticity may mask these findings. Generally, the left ventricular impulse has the same delayed and sustained character as the arterial pulse. Auscultation reveals a diamond-shaped (crescendo-descrescendo) systolic ejection murmur that is loudest over the second right intercostal space and that may be transmitted to the left precordium, to the carotid arteries, and to the cardiac apex. The character of the murmur is not as useful an indication of the severity of obstruction as the character of the arterial pulse. In severe heart failure due to aortic stenosis, the murmur may almost be inaudible because of depressed cardiac output. Paradoxic splitting of the second heart sound (narrowing during inspiration, widening during expiration) is heard if the aortic valve leaflets are relatively mobile. As the valve becomes more rigid, the aortic component of the second heart sound becomes less prominent; when calcification causes the valve to be nearly immobile, the aortic component is generally not heard.

The electrocardiogram of a patient with isolated aortic stenosis generally shows normal sinus rhythm and the pattern of left ventricular hypertrophy with strain (Fig. 52–8). Intraventricular conduction defects such as fascicular block or right or left bundle-branch block may be present, especially when there is extensive calcification (Thompson et al, 1979a).

Evidence of aortic stenosis on the chest film includes calcification in the region of the aortic valve,

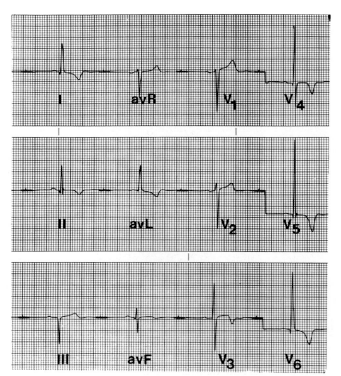

Figure 52–8. Electrocardiogram of a patient with aortic stenosis. The pattern of left ventricular hypertrophy with strain is present.

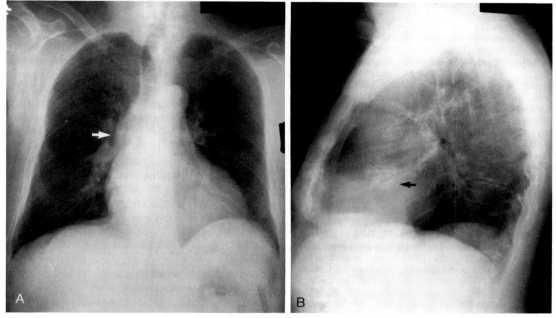

Figure 52–9. Chest film of a patient with critical calcific aortic stenosis and symptoms of congestive heart failure. *A,* The posteroanterior film shows a cardiac silhouette with left ventricular prominence and evidence of poststenotic dilatation of the ascending aorta *(arrow)*. *B,* The lateral film shows extensive calcification in the region of the aortic valve *(arrow)*.

poststenotic dilatation of the ascending aorta, and left ventricular configuration of the cardiac silhouette (Fig. 52–9). A significantly increased cardiothoracic ratio is generally a late finding and indicates left ventricular failure.

Echocardiography shows restricted movement of valve leaflets and calcification in the region of the aortic valve (Fig. 52–10). The degree of left ventricular hypertrophy and the quality of left ventricular systolic function may also be measured. Doppler echocardiography may be used to measure accurately the peak aortic valve gradient and to estimate the severity of aortic regurgitation (Takenaka et al, 1986) and is also useful in distinguishing valvular aortic stenosis from supravalvular or subvalvular obstruction.

Cardiac catheterization is not mandatory to establish the diagnosis of aortic stenosis but it should be done when the severity of the lesion or the site of the obstruction is not known with certainty. Cardiac catheterization is also done when there is suspicion of associated lesions of the mitral or tricuspid valves or of associated coronary artery disease. Selective coronary angiography should be done in patients over 40 years of age or patients with symptoms or electrocardiographic findings that suggest coronary artery disease. At catheterization, the aortic valve can usually be crossed, and the systolic gradient across the valve can be measured directly. In severe aortic stenosis, the gradient usually exceeds 55 mm Hg and may be as high as 125 mm Hg or more. When aortic stenosis is complicated by severe left ventricular failure, the cardiac output may be low and the gradient across the aortic valve may be small despite critical obstruction.

Indications for Operation. Asymptomatic patients with aortic stenosis may do well for many years, but the onset of symptoms (angina, syncope, or heart failure) is generally followed by rapid deterioration. Morrow and associates (1968) showed that

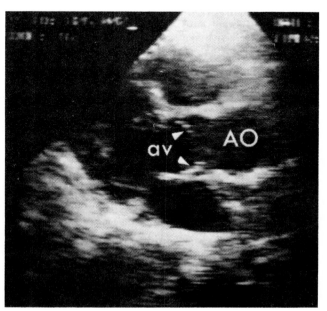

Figure 52–10. Two-dimensional echocardiogram of a patient with valvular aortic stenosis. This systolic frame shows the domed aortic valve (av) and mild poststenotic dilatation of the ascending aorta (AO). (From Feigenbaum, H.: Echocardiography. *In* Braunwald, E. [ed]: Heart Disease. Philadelphia, W. B. Saunders Company, 1988, p. 108.)

the average life expectancy was 5 years after the onset of angina, 3 years after syncope, and 2 years after heart failure. Operation is indicated for any symptomatic patient with significant aortic stenosis. Indications for operation in asymptomatic patients with significant aortic stenosis include progressive cardiac enlargement and objective findings of left ventricular dysfunction (such as elevation of left ventricular end-diastolic pressure at rest or with exercise during cardiac catheterization). Less clear answers are available for asymptomatic young adults with significant aortic stenosis and without any of the abnormalities indicated earlier who wish to be physically active.

Aortic Regurgitation

Pathophysiology. Failure of the aortic valve leaflets to coapt and thus obliterate the valve orifice at the end of ventricular systole results in failure of the valve to support the column of ejected blood. A fraction of the column of blood passes retrograde through the valve into the left ventricular chamber during diastole. The severity of aortic regurgitation is determined by the size of the regurgitant orifice and the pressure gradient during diastole between the systemic circulation and the left ventricle. The left ventricle is subjected to an increased work load. Both preload and afterload are increased. In the compensated state, the left ventricle responds to the increased burden in two ways: dilatation and hypertrophy. As the left ventricular chamber becomes dilated, ventricular end-diastolic volume increases and preload increases. The result is increased stroke volume (by Starling's principle), but at the cost of higher wall tension and increased myocardial oxygen consumption. With increased volume work and increased wall tension, gradual hypertrophy of the left ventricular myocardium takes place. For a time, sys-tolic function is maintained because of the increase in left ventricular mass. In advanced stages of aortic regurgitation, the compensatory changes of the left ventricle (dilatation and hypertrophy) are inadequate to meet circulatory demands (Boucher et al, 1989). Symptoms of congestive heart failure or coronary insufficiency become evident. In the chronically dilated and hypertrophied left ventricle, ultrastructural changes with fibrosis and fiber slippage are seen (Braunwald, 1988). Systolic function deteriorates and with it the capacity of the ventricle to respond to stress. Ventricular compliance decreases, which also compromises diastolic function.

Etiology. The cause of aortic regurgitation influences the progression of the disease and its symptoms (Rottman et al, 1971), and the outcome of surgical therapy (Shean et al, 1971). Although rheumatic valvulitis represents a significant percentage of cases of chronic aortic regurgitation, the percentage has probably been overestimated in the past. On the basis of post-mortem studies, Roberts (1970) maintained that pure aortic regurgitation is seldom due to rheumatic disease. However, in most large clinical series, such as that from the Massachusetts General Hospital (Samuels et al, 1979) and that of Barratt-Boyes and associates (1986), 30 to 50% of cases of chronic aortic regurgitation were estimated to be of rheumatic origin. The changes in rheumatic valvulitis that lead to pure aortic regurgitation differ from those that result in stenosis. Failure of the cusps to coapt at the end of systole is due primarily to scarring of the leaflets with shortening of the distance between the annulus and free edge (Fig. 52–11). The leaflets need not show marked thickening, and commissural fusion need not be present.

Annuloaortic ectasia due to cystic medial necrosis may also cause aortic regurgitation. Cystic medial necrosis is a disease of the aorta rather than of the valve itself, but it can produce both chronic aortic regurgitation from dilatation of the annulus and acute

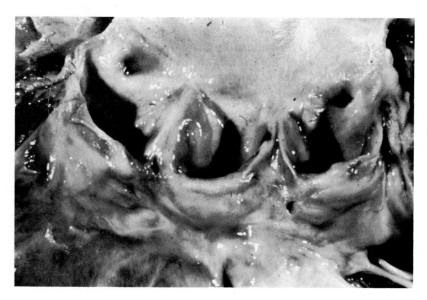

Figure 52–11. Opened post-mortem specimen of an aortic valve showing typical changes of rheumatic aortic incompetence. All three cusps are fibrotic and retracted, which results in shortening of the distance between annulus and free edge and thus in failure of the cusps to coapt at the end of systole. (From Sutton, G. C., and Anderson, R. H. [eds]: Slide Atlas of Cardiology. London, England, Medi-Cine Productions, 1978.)

aortic regurgitation from aortic dissection (DeSanctis et al, 1987). Cystic medial necrosis is a feature of Marfan's syndrome, a generalized disorder of connective tissue that is inherited as an autosomal dominant trait. At least 60% of adults with Marfan's syndrome have cardiovascular anomalies. The most common anomaly is dilatation of the aortic annulus, the sinuses of Valsalva, and the ascending thoracic aorta. Progressive enlargement of the aortic annulus leads to aortic regurgitation. The characteristic pathologic changes in the aorta (Roberts and Honig, 1982) include degeneration of elastic elements of the aortic wall with abnormal organization of smooth muscle bundles and increased amounts of collagen. Cystic vacuoles may be observed in the media, as may faults that contain a mucopolysaccharide-rich ground substance. It has been proposed that because similar degenerative changes in the aortic media are observed in patients with aortic disease but without Marfan's syndrome (Hirst and Gore, 1983), the term cystic medial necrosis should be replaced by a broader descriptive term, such as medial degeneration, that does not necessarily imply association with a particular biochemical or inherited disease. Estimates of the frequency of cystic medial necrosis as the etiology for aortic regurgitation vary widely; some series include only cases of documented Marfan's syndrome, whereas others include all cases that share the cardiovascular pathology and refer to the form without other stigmata of Marfan's syndrome as a forme fruste of the disease.

Atherosclerotic and syphilitic aneurysms of the ascending aorta may produce valvular incompetence by the same mechanism (annular dilatation) as cystic medial necrosis but are much less frequently complicated by dissection. In luetic aortitis, inflammatory changes and thickening of the valve leaflets themselves may result in decreased leaflet mobility and incomplete leaflet coaptation.

Arthritic inflammatory diseases such as rheumatoid arthritis, ankylosing spondylitis, and Reiter's syndrome may be associated with aortitis. The inflammatory process may involve the aortic valve leaflets, such as in typical rheumatic valvulitis, and may result in aortic valvular regurgitation (Bulkley and Roberts, 1973).

A congenitally bicuspid valve may have some incompetence, but in most cases aortic regurgitation with a congenitally bicuspid valve is due to surgical or balloon catheter valvotomy or to changes secondary to bacterial endocarditis. Endocarditis is an important cause of aortic regurgitation (26% in the series reported by Samuels and associates [1979]). Endocarditis may occur on a structurally normal valve but is more likely to occur on a congenitally malformed or rheumatically scarred valve. Acute aortic regurgitation may result from perforation through a leaflet (Fig. 52–12) or prolapse of a leaflet secondary to destruction of a commissure. Extensive infection of the aortic root may be associated with fistulas between the aorta and one or more contiguous cardiac chambers.

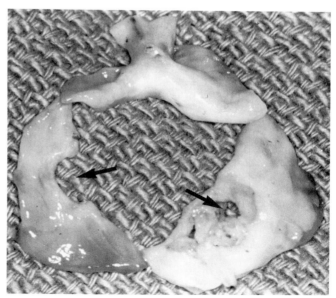

Figure 52–12. Surgical specimen of aortic valve leaflets from a 17-year-old Ethiopian girl with aortic insufficiency due to previous endocarditis. Leaflets are scarred and thickened and have perforations (*arrows*) that measure up to 7 mm in diameter.

Acute aortic regurgitation may also be produced by blunt chest injury with cusp rupture or by penetrating injury with perforation of one or more cusps.

In as many as 25% of patients, aortic regurgitation is attributed to unknown causes. Many of these patients have the pathologic features of myxoid degeneration of the valve (Lakier et al, 1985), including cystic degeneration, loss of cellularity, and increase in mucopolysaccharide ground substance. Patients with these degenerative changes of the aortic valve frequently have a history of chronic hypertension.

Clinical Features. Patients with chronic aortic regurgitation may be asymptomatic for years. Augmented force of the heartbeat may be the first sign of which the patient is cognizant. Effort intolerance, or more precisely exertional dyspnea, is generally the first symptom of aortic regurgitation. Effort intolerance is usually correlated with elevation of mean left atrial pressure during effort, which indicates one or more of the following: increased end-diastolic volume, decreased left ventricular contraction, or decreased left ventricular compliance. The other principal symptom of aortic regurgitation is angina pectoris. Myocardial ischemia results from increased left ventricular work (increased preload and afterload) and mass and from decreased coronary blood flow due to decreased coronary perfusion pressure (decreased diastolic blood pressure). Coronary atherosclerosis need not be present for a patient with aortic regurgitation to experience typical angina pectoris. Most patients with aortic regurgitation who have exertional angina due only to aortic regurgitation also have symptoms of congestive heart failure. In patients with aortic regurgitation and no heart failure, coronary atherosclerosis may be principally responsible for exertional angina. In very advanced aortic regurgitation, patients may have angina decubitus. Syncope and presyncopal lightheadedness are more often symptoms of aortic stenosis but may occur in patients with pure aortic regurgitation (Samuels et al, 1979).

The high-pitched decrescendo diastolic murmur of aortic incompetence is best heard at the upper left sternal border or in the second right interspace. The intensity of the murmur generally increases with the severity of regurgitation, but in patients with severe regurgitation and heart failure the murmur may almost be inaudible. The most reliable indication of the severity of aortic regurgitation is the character of the pulsation palpated over the carotid arteries or the cardiac apex. The sharpness of the upstroke, rapidity of the downstroke, and width of the pulse pressure are usually correlated with the severity of aortic regurgitation (Friedlich and Buckley, 1980). The auscultated diastolic blood pressure is usually less than 60 mm Hg in moderate regurgitation and lower in severe aortic regurgitation.

The chest film of patients with aortic regurgitation may show left ventricular enlargement and enlargement of the ascending aorta (Fig. 52–13). The evaluation of heart size on serial chest examinations is important.

In severe aortic regurgitation, the electrocardiogram generally shows voltage indications of left ventricular hypertrophy and may show left ventricular strain pattern (T-wave inversion in the lateral precordial leads).

Echocardiography has become important in the noninvasive assessment of aortic regurgitation. Left ventricular function can be assessed with two-dimensional echocardiography, and regurgitant flow can be estimated by using Doppler (Fig. 52–14) or color flow techniques. Echocardiography is a particularly valuable noninvasive method of serial evaluation of asymptomatic and minimally symptomatic patients (Stewart et al, 1985).

Cardiac catheterization with supravalvular aortography is the definitive diagnostic study for patients with aortic insufficiency (Fig. 52–15). In addition to the severity of regurgitation, this study shows associated pathology of the aortic root, the coronary arteries, and other valves and permits quantification of such prognostic features as ventricular function and pulmonary hypertension.

Indications for Operation. Patients with heart failure or angina should have definitive diagnostic testing, and if significant aortic regurgitation is present, operation should usually be done. There is little place for chronic medical therapy in symptomatic patients with significant aortic regurgitation, because delay of operation is associated with progression of left ventricular disease (Friedlich and Buckley, 1980). Hegglin and associates (1968) described the natural history of symptomatic patients with aortic regurgitation who were not treated surgically. They reported

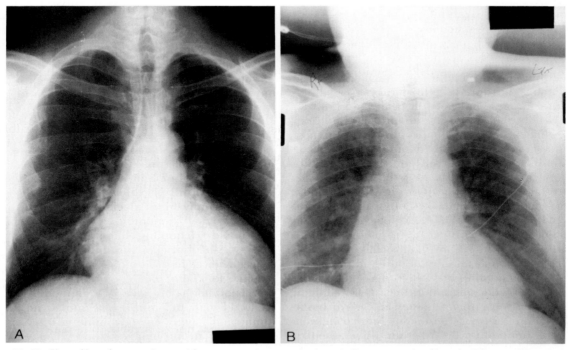

Figure 52–13. Chest film of two patients with severe aortic regurgitation. *A,* Posteroanterior film of a 37-year-old man with severe aortic insufficiency of unknown etiology. There is marked cardiomegaly. Pulmonary vascular markings are prominent. The patient later had isolated aortic valve replacement. *B,* Anteroposterior film of a 59-year-old man with annuloaortic ectasia, severe aortic insufficiency, and coronary artery disease. The heart and the ascending aorta are enlarged. The pulmonary fields show evidence of interstitial pulmonary edema. The patient had successful emergency aortic root replacement with a composite valved conduit and multiple saphenous vein coronary bypass grafts.

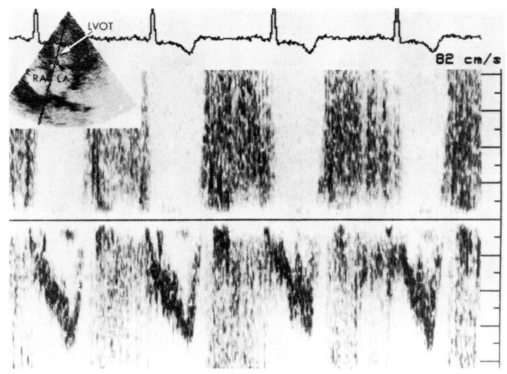

Figure 52–14. Pulsed Doppler echocardiogram of a patient with aortic regurgitation. The sample volume is in the left ventricular outflow tract *(arrow)*. High-velocity flow is recorded at this site during diastole and indicates aortic regurgitation. (LVOT = left ventricular outflow tract; RA = right atrium; LA = left atrium.) (From Feigenbaum, H.: Echocardiography, 4th ed. Philadelphia, Lea & Febiger, 1986, p. 291.)

50% mortality of patients with severe aortic regurgitation 5 years after the development of angina or 2 years after the development of heart failure. Patients with few or no symptoms pose a more difficult problem. One would like to be able to identify the point in a patient's course at which aortic valve

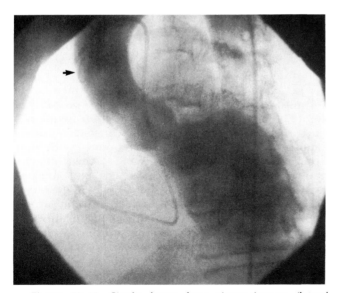

Figure 52–15. Single frame from cineangiogram (lateral oblique) of a supravalvular aortogram of a 59-year-old man with severe aortic regurgitation. The end of the pigtail catheter *(arrow)* is in the ascending aorta well above the level of the aortic valve. The regurgitant jet almost reaches to the apex of the left ventricle.

replacement would be expected to preserve or restore normal ventricular function. The preservation of ventricular function is the primary goal in surgical therapy for asymptomatic or minimally symptomatic patients but must be weighed against the risk of operation and the problems associated with even the best aortic valve substitutes. In evaluating the risk of aortic valve replacement for aortic insufficiency, Thompson and associates (1979b) and Bonow and associates (1984) found that patients with a resting left ventricular ejection fraction of more than 45% had a relatively low risk of operative mortality, compared with patients with resting left ventricular ejection fractions of less than 45%. Increased left ventricular end-systolic volume during exercise and increased cardiothoracic ratio ($\geq$ 0.55) were also predictors of poor outcome. No studies have clearly shown the levels of ejection fraction and end-systolic volume at which the changes in ventricular function become irreversible despite aortic valve replacement. With a goal of restoring aortic valve function to normal before significant irreversible changes in left ventricular function occur, the authors currently proceed with catheterization and operation in asymptomatic or minimally symptomatic patients who show (1) progressive increase in heart size or left ventricular size, (2) left ventricular ejection fraction at rest less than 0.5 or a progressive fall in ejection fraction over time, or (3) signs correlated with increased left ventricular end-diastolic pressure (Boucher et al, 1989).

Mixed Aortic Valve Disease

Patients with severe aortic stenosis often have mild to moderate aortic insufficiency, usually because of commissural fusion and leaflet immobility that result in incomplete leaflet coaptation during diastole. In many cases of severe calcific aortic valve stenosis there is a small valve orifice that is nearly fixed and through which regurgitation occurs during diastole. Occasionally, a patient with severe aortic insufficiency has some degree of stenosis as well. In patients with balanced aortic valve lesions (both stenosis and regurgitation that are significant), the symptoms are primarily those of aortic stenosis (Kirklin and Barratt-Boyes, 1986). Approximately half of the patients who require surgical therapy for balanced aortic stenosis and incompetence have congenitally abnormal aortic valves; most of the other cases are due to rheumatic disease, and a small percentage are due to other nonrheumatic inflammatory disease or are of unknown etiology (Kirklin and Barratt-Boyes, 1986).

HYPERTROPHIC CARDIOMYOPATHY

The obstructive form of hypertrophic cardiomyopathy (HCM), formerly referred to as idiopathic hypertrophic subaortic stenosis (IHSS), should be distinguished from other causes of left ventricular outflow tract obstruction, notably valvular aortic stenosis. First systematically described by Teare (1958), the disease has the morphologic hallmark of inappropriate myocardial hypertrophy, which generally involves the interventricular septum (Fig. 52–16).

Pathophysiology. In patients with obstructive HCM, the ratio of the thickness of the interventricular septum to the thickness of the left ventricular free wall generally exceeds 1.3 to 1, whereas in normal subjects and in patients with left ventricular hypertrophy not due to HCM the ratio is almost always less and is most often nearly 1 to 1 (Wynne and Braunwald, 1988). There are exceptions, and two-dimensional echocardiographic studies have shown that the distribution and extent of left ventricular hypertrophy vary greatly among patients with HCM (Maron et al, 1987a; 1987b). Patients with obstructive HCM commonly have pronounced hypertrophy of the basal portion of the interventricular septum, to which the descriptive term asymmetric septal hypertrophy (ASH) has been applied. Other features of the disease that contribute to the impedance to left ventricular emptying include abnormal anterior displacement of the mitral valve apparatus and systolic anterior motion (SAM) of the anterior mitral valve leaflet. The result of these abnormalities is a dynamic narrowing of the left ventricular outflow tract. The mechanism of SAM of the mitral valve is still debated, but there is a close relationship between the degree of SAM and the magnitude of the outflow gradient (Maron, 1985). The degree of mitral regurgitation is

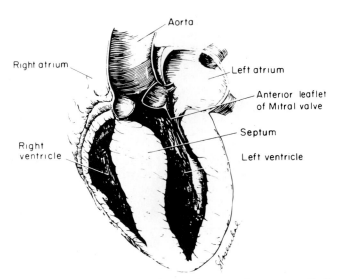

Figure 52–16. Hypertrophic cardiomyopathy. Longitudinal section through the heart shows generalized hypertrophy of the left ventricle and disproportionate thickening of the upper portion of the interventricular septum. (From Powell, W. J., Jr.: Hypertrophic nondilated cardiomyopathy: Idiopathic hypertrophic subaortic stenosis and its variants. *In* Johnson, R. A., Haber, E., and Austen, W. G. [eds]: The Practice of Cardiology. Boston, Little, Brown and Company, 1980, p. 648.)

thought by some surgeons to be related to the extent and timing of the anterior motion of the mitral valve during systole (Wigle et al., 1968). Mitral regurgitation of a mild degree is invariably present in patients with significant obstruction; severe mitral regurgitation usually implies intrinsic mitral valve disease. Patients with HCM with significant obstruction to left ventricular emptying (those previously considered to have IHSS) are a minority of all patients with HCM. Patients with the nonobstructive variant of the disease can be comparably symptomatic. Abnormalities of diastolic function due to increased myocardial stiffness, altered ventricular compliance, and, perhaps, myocardial ischemia are common to both types of HCM and contribute significantly to clinical symptoms.

Etiology. HCM, or more precisely the susceptibility to the development of HCM, is probably inherited (Ciro et al, 1983). The disorder is often familial and is transmitted in a pattern consistent with an autosomal dominant trait. The frequency with which sporadic (nonfamilial) cases of HCM occur suggests the possibility of other etiologies. The clinical expression of the disease in sporadic cases cannot be distinguished from that in familial cases (Maron et al, 1987a, 1987b). Histologically, the myocardium of patients with HCM shows disorganization of muscle bundles and a characteristic whorled pattern. Autopsy studies show myocardial fibrosis that ranges from a patchy interstitial process to transmural scars. Abnormal intramural coronary arteries that have markedly thickened walls and apparently narrowed lumens have been described (Maron et al, 1987a, 1987b).

Clinical Findings. Pathologic findings of HCM have been seen in almost all age groups, but symptomatic HCM is generally a disease of young adults. In an early report from the National Institutes of Health, the average age of presentation with symptoms was 26 years (Braunwald et al, 1964). The primary symptoms reported by patients with HCM include dyspnea, angina, fatigue, and episodes of near syncope or syncope. The pattern of symptoms in a patient represents the interactions of the components of the disease: left ventricular hypertrophy, subaortic obstruction, abnormal diastolic function, and myocardial ischemia (Maron et al, 1987a, 1987b). Sudden death is most common in young patients (less than 30 years of age), and it is most often attributable to arrhythmias, particularly to ventricular tachycardia (Maron et al, 1981). The symptoms and their severity are unreliable indicators of the likelihood of sudden death (Shah et al, 1974).

In patients with HCM, the first and second heart sounds are usually normal, although rarely paradoxic splitting of the second sound may be heard in the obstructive form. A fourth heart sound is usually present. The systolic murmur of obstructive HCM is typically a harsh crescendo-decrescendo murmur that is best heard between the cardiac apex and the left sternal border. The murmur increases in intensity after maneuvers that decrease left ventricular preload (Valsalva, standing), increase contractility (post-premature contraction), or decrease left ventricular afterload (vasodilators). The murmur decreases with maneuvers that increase preload (leg raising, squatting), decrease contractility (beta-blockade), or increase afterload (pressor agents). A more holosystolic murmur is often heard in the region of the cardiac apex and in the axilla and signifies coexisting mitral regurgitation. A systolic thrill may be felt over the cardiac apex or the lower left sternal border. Unlike patients with severe valvular aortic stenosis, patients with HCM have a rapid carotid upstroke. The arterial impulse or the cardiac apical impulse may have a palpable bifid contour, which is probably caused by

rapid ejection during early systole by the hyperdynamic ventricle and then a more prolonged impulse as the ventricle continues to eject in the presence of increased left ventricular outflow obstruction (Powell, 1980).

The principal finding on the electrocardiogram is left ventricular hypertrophy with strain, which is present in at least half the patients with HCM. Electrocardiographic signs of left atrial enlargement and a pattern of pseudoinfarction (resembling an old anterior or inferior myocardial infarction) may be present. The chest film may be unrevealing or may show enlargement of the heart (particularly with prominence of the left ventricle). Left atrial enlargement may be seen when significant mitral regurgitation is present.

The echocardiogram is most helpful in the diagnosis of HCM. M-mode echocardiography shows systolic anterior motion of the anterior mitral leaflet (Fig. 52–17) and the abnormal ratio of septal to left ventricular free wall thickness. Two-dimensional echocardiography provides additional critical information about the extent and distribution of hypertrophy and the presence or absence of associated abnormalities. Concomitant Doppler studies allow estimation of the magnitude of the outflow gradient in patients with obstruction and provide data on diastolic filling characteristics. Cardiac catheterization is usually reserved for patients with obstructive HCM who remain symptomatic after optimal medical therapy. Other indications for catheterization are the presence of a coexisting disorder (e.g., coronary artery disease) or continued uncertainty about the diagnosis of the disease after echocardiography.

Indications for Operation. Initial treatment of patients with HCM consists of medical therapy directed at symptomatic relief and control of arrhythmias, when present. Agents that may increase the forcefulness of ventricular contraction (including digitalis preparations) are generally excluded. The main type of medical therapy is beta-adrenergic blockade. Inhibition of the sympathetic stimulation of the heart

Figure 52–17. M-mode echocardiogram from a patient with hypertrophic cardiomyopathy. Abnormal systolic anterior motion of the mitral valve is clearly seen *(arrows)*. The septum is considerably thicker than the posterior wall of the left ventricle. (From Powell, W. J., Jr.: Hypertrophic nondilated cardiomyopathy: Idiopathic hypertrophic subaortic stenosis and its variants. *In* Johnson, R. A., Haber, E., and Austen, W. G. [eds]: The Practice of Cardiology. Boston, Little, Brown and Company, 1980, p. 657.)

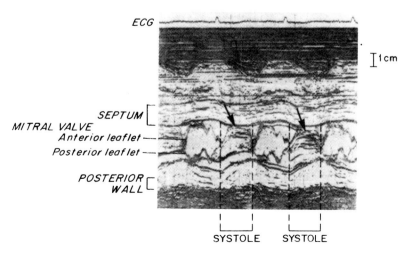

decreases the heart rate and the forcefulness of ventricular contraction. In patients with obstruction, this negative inotropic effect may decrease the magnitude of the outflow gradient. Whether beta-blockade directly improves left ventricular diastolic function or merely enhances left ventricular filling by decreasing the heart rate is controversial (Speiser and Krayenbuehl, 1981). Initially, almost half of symptomatic patients with HCM have significant relief of symptoms with the use of beta-blocking drugs. For patients whose symptoms continue despite maximal doses of beta-blocking agents, addition of calcium channel blockers, particularly verapamil, may be effective. In one study (Rosing et al, 1985), nearly 60% of patients with HCM who were given verapamil because of persistent symptoms despite beta-blockade had significant symptomatic improvement. The calcium channel blockers, beta-adrenergic blockers, and conventional antiarrhythmic agents do not appear to prevent sudden death in HCM (McKenna, 1983). Amiodarone may hold promise in the treatment of ventricular and supraventricular arrhythmias and in the prevention of sudden death in patients with HCM (McKenna et al, 1984). The effectiveness of amiodarone does not appear to be related to depression of left ventricular function. Surgical therapy of HCM is indicated for patients with a demonstrable left ventricular outflow gradient (generally 50 mm Hg or more) and persistence of significant symptoms despite medical therapy.

SURGICAL THERAPY FOR AORTIC VALVE DISEASE

Preoperative Preparation

Patients who have aortic valve surgery should receive the same systematic evaluation as all patients who have open heart surgery. Emphasis should be placed on certain features. Dentition should be evaluated and abscessed teeth or severe periodontal disease should be corrected, usually by operative treatment, before aortic valve surgery. (In some patients with critical aortic stenosis and heart failure, oral surgery must be postponed until after aortic valve replacement.) Infectious processes elsewhere, such as in the urinary tract or tracheobronchial tree, are also managed before aortic valve surgery. The risk of excessive bleeding associated with operation or long-term anticoagulation is assessed by evaluation of coagulation parameters, including the platelet count, prothrombin time, and partial thromboplastin time, and by assessment of liver function; it is also important to obtain a detailed patient history that includes previous surgical procedures, history of a bleeding tendency, and presence or absence of peptic ulcer disease. Aspirin and other anti-inflammatory agents that affect platelet function should be eliminated for several weeks before elective surgical procedures. Smoking is discontinued as early before

operation as possible. Patients are evaluated by a respiratory therapist before operation for assessment of respiratory function and are introduced to techniques of postoperative respiratory care. Digoxin is generally discontinued 24 to 48 hours before operation unless it is required for control of chronic atrial fibrillation.

Aortic Valve Replacement

Intraoperative monitoring of the patient includes the surface electrocardiogram (limb leads and a precordial lead), temperature measurements at the nasopharynx and the rectum, and continuous collection of urine with a Foley catheter. Anesthetic techniques for cardiac surgery include invasive monitoring that generally consists of peripheral arterial cannulation (radial artery is generally preferred) and placement of a Swan-Ganz catheter to permit continuous assessment of intracardiac pressures and periodic determination of cardiac output by the thermodilution technique.

Median sternotomy is done in a standard fashion (see Chapter 7) and the patient is then heparinized. The authors' technique of cannulation for bypass generally consists of an arterial perfusion cannula (Nos. 20 to 24 French) in the distal ascending aorta and separate venous drainage catheters in the superior and inferior venae cavae. Alternatively, venous drainage can be accomplished with a single large cannula in the right atrium. In some reoperations or when there is significant aneurysmal disease or severe calcification of the ascending aorta, the femoral artery may be used as the site of insertion of the arterial perfusion cannula. The authors use a crystalloid prime and establish bypass at an initial flow of 2 to 2.5 l/min/m² body surface area. The perfusate temperature is adjusted so that the patient is gradually cooled to 25° to 28° C (measured in the esophagus). At that temperature, a flow of approximately 1.6 to 2 l/min/m² body surface area is generally maintained. Left ventricular decompression is accomplished with a catheter introduced into the left atrium from the right side (often through the right superior pulmonary vein) and guided through the mitral valve into the left ventricular cavity or, alternatively, with a left ventricular vent catheter inserted directly through the apex of the ventricle. In patients with significant aortic insufficiency, myocardial cooling and consequent slowing of the heart may be associated with cardiac distention, at the first sign of which the left ventricular vent is promptly inserted.

The myocardium is protected during aortic cross-clamping by infusion of cardioplegic solution into the coronary arteries. The authors use a fully oxygenated crystalloid cardioplegic solution to which a small amount of autologous blood has been added (Daggett et al, 1987). The initial dose of cardioplegic solution infused to arrest and cool the myocardium is in the range of 12 to 20 ml/kg body weight. During cross-clamping, continuous topical irrigation of the heart with cold (4° C) lactated Ringer's solution is maintained. In the absence of significant aortic incompetence, an initial dose of cardioplegic solution is infused through a needle in the ascending aorta. If the valve is incompetent and the aortic root does not remain distended during infusion of the solution, aortotomy and direct infusion into the coronary ostia should be used instead. Care must be taken to avoid injury to the ostia of the coronary arteries and to ensure satisfactory flow of cardioplegic solution into each coronary artery system. The left main coronary artery may bifurcate early, and the catheter tip must be positioned so that it will not obstruct flow into either branch of the left coronary artery. At some centers, myocardial temperature is monitored with a needle thermistor inserted directly into the interventricular septum. With reinfusion of cardioplegic solution directly into the ostia of the coronary arteries at intervals of 20 to 30 minutes and with topical cold irrigation, it is routinely possible to maintain myocardial temperature at or below 15° C.

The aortotomy incision is begun anteriorly, 10 to 15 mm distal to the origin of the right coronary artery, with a transverse orientation (Fig. 52–18). After the initial incision, inspection of the interior of

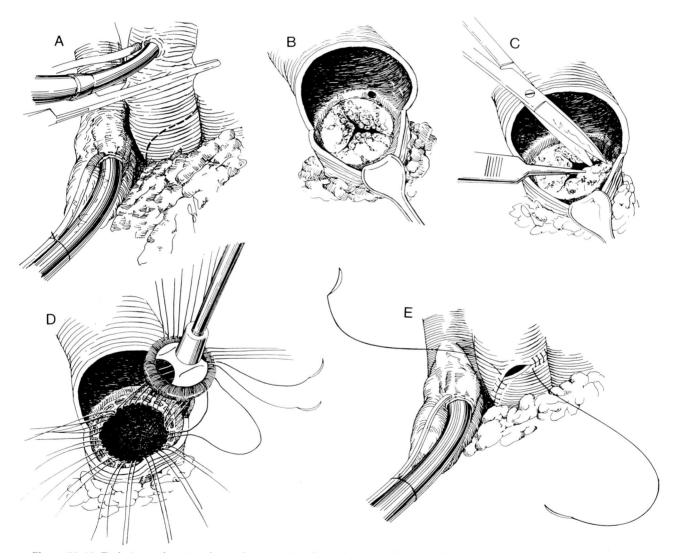

Figure 52–18. Technique of aortic valve replacement (mechanical or stented tissue valve prosthesis). *A,* The aortic cross-clamp has been placed proximal to the site of insertion of the aortic perfusion cannula. An oblique aortotomy incision is made, as indicated by the *broken line.* To the left, the incision is carried to a point on the medial wall of the aorta, in the sulcus between the aorta and the main pulmonary artery. To the right, the extension of the incision is angled obliquely toward the heart, into the center of the noncoronary sinus. *B,* The anterior edge of the proximal aortic wall is gently retracted, which gives excellent exposure of the aortic valve. *C,* Excision of the valve is begun at a point that lends itself most readily to incision. In this example, this point is at the commissure between the left and right coronary cusps. After the valve leaflets have been excised, the annulus is carefully debrided by using rongeurs to remove as much calcium as possible (not shown). *D,* Pledgeted mattress sutures are passed through the aortic annulus and then through the sewing ring of the prosthetic valve. In the example shown, the mattress sutures have been placed so that the felt pledgets are on the aortic side of the annulus. (See text for discussion of this method and alternatives of suture placement.) *E,* The aortotomy incision is closed with continuous monofilament sutures.

the aortic root affords better control during the extension of the aortotomy toward the right and left sides. The incision is extended toward the left to a point on the medial wall of the aorta, in the sulcus between the aorta and the main pulmonary artery; this extension may be done in transverse manner or at a slightly oblique angle so that it is located slightly more distally on the aorta than the level of the initial incision. The extension of the incision to the right side is most important; here the incision is angled obliquely toward the heart, into the center of the noncoronary sinus.

Some surgeons prefer to insert a gauze sponge in the left ventricular cavity at this point, although that is generally not the authors' practice. Excision of the valve is begun at the point that lends itself most readily to incision, often at the commissure between the right and noncoronary cusps. If the valve is not heavily calcified but must be replaced, the leaflets are excised precisely at the level of attachment of the cusps to the annulus. When the valve is very heavily calcified, it is often easiest and safest to begin at a point within the valve orifice, at the free edge of the most mobile leaflet, and cut toward the annulus and then continue the excision of the valve with scissors or scalpel blade at the junction of the cusps and the annulus. Too radical an initial excision of the valve can result in a cut that extends through the wall of the aorta at the level of the annulus. This problem can be avoided by beginning with a more conservative excision of the calcified valve, followed by thorough debridement of the annulus with rongeurs. After the valve has been excised, the gauze sponge (if used) is removed from the ventricular cavity and the aortic root, annulus, and ventricular cavity are irrigated vigorously with cold saline to remove residual particulate debris. The authors protect the ostium of the left coronary artery by gently occluding it with the tip of a suction device during this maneuver to prevent embolization of debris into the coronary circulation. Additional cardioplegic solution (to a total of approximately 7 to 10 ml/kg body weight) is infused at this time into the ostia of the coronary arteries. Similar amounts are given at intervals of 20 to 30 minutes during the remainder of the cross-clamp period, or at any time if there is evidence of electrical activity on the electrocardiographic monitor.

The choice of a prosthesis depends on many factors and is discussed later. At this point in the operation, the annulus is sized by using valve templates that correspond to the type of valve substitute that has been chosen. If a mechanical prosthesis or a stented bioprosthesis is to be implanted, interrupted valve sutures are placed through the annulus at the junction of annulus and aortic wall. Several suture techniques are acceptable. The authors' practice is to place 12 to 20 2-0 Dacron polyester sutures through the annulus either in figure-of-eight fashion or as horizontal mattress sutures that are buttressed with Teflon felt pledgets. Horizontal mattress sutures

are generally placed so that the felt pledgets are on the aortic side of the annulus, which results in a degree of eversion of the annulus about the edges of the sewing ring. Although this technique is useful if the annulus is soft or friable, it may necessitate the use of a prosthesis one size smaller than would otherwise fit and so may be undesirable if the aortic root is small. Alternatively, mattress sutures may be placed with pledgets on the ventricular side of the annulus, which results in implantation of the prosthesis at a slightly supra-annular level. Disadvantages of this technique are the potential problem of retrieving a pledget from the ventricular chamber if a suture breaks while being tied and the possibility of the sewing ring encroaching on and causing obstruction of a coronary ostium when the valve is implanted at the supra-annular level. Some surgeons prefer to use a series of simple nonpledgeted interrupted sutures. After all sutures have been placed through the annulus, they are passed through the sewing ring of the prosthesis. The valve is then lowered into position and all sutures are tied. If a mechanical prosthesis is used, unimpeded motion of the poppet, disk, or leaflets must be confirmed by using rubber-shod instruments before the aortotomy incision is closed.

If a nonstented aortic valve homograft is to be inserted (Fig. 52–19), the aortic diameter is measured at the level of the annulus and the commissures, and the banked homograft of appropriate size is thawed and rinsed. Generally, the diameter of the homograft should be 2 to 3 mm less than that of the recipient root and annulus. The trimmed homograft is inserted by using two layers of continuous 4-0 polypropylene monofilament sutures. Alternative suturing techniques have been associated with satisfactory results (Barratt-Boyes et al, 1965; Khanna et al, 1981; Ross, 1962).

Rewarming of the perfusate is initiated as the closure of the aortotomy is begun. The incision is closed with continuous 3-0 or 4-0 monofilament nonabsorbable sutures. One suture is placed as a pledgeted mattress suture at either end. Great care is taken when placing the sutures at the end of the incision in the noncoronary sinus, which may otherwise be the site of troublesome bleeding. The sutures are then each carried to the midpoint of the aortotomy. At this point the authors partially occlude the venous return and temporarily discontinue the left ventricular vent; the lungs are then ventilated and the heart is massaged gently to fill the heart with blood and displace air from the cardiac chambers and the aortic root. The patient is placed in moderate Trendelenburg position and the ascending aorta is vented (either at the site of the cardioplegia needle or at the midpoint of the as yet untied aortotomy suture line) while the aortic cross-clamp is released and the heart is reperfused. The lungs are ventilated again to displace any remaining air from the pulmonary veins and left atrium. The heart may be gently elevated, and an aspirating needle may be placed directly

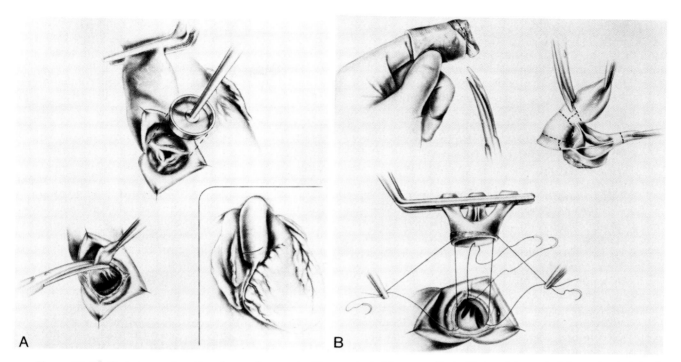

Figure 52–19. Technique of aortic valve replacement with nonstented homograft. *A,* The aortotomy incision extends into the noncoronary sinus of Valsalva. The annulus is measured and the valve is excised. *B,* Excessive ventricular septal muscle is trimmed from the aortic homograft. Aortic sinus tissue is excised, leaving a rim of 3 to 4 mm of aortic tissue for attachment to the recipient aorta. The valve is oriented within the recipient aortic root by placing three sutures, one beneath each of the commissures.

Illustration continued on following page

through the apex of the left ventricle during positive pressure ventilation. It is most important to select a series of maneuvers to remove air from the heart and ascending aorta with which the surgeon is comfortable. If the left ventricle begins to become distended, the vent suction is resumed at a low level appropriate to keep the heart decompressed. Excessive return from the left ventricular vent may indicate incompetence of the prosthesis, particularly if it persists after the cardiac rhythm has been restored. Defibrillation of the heart, if necessary, is accomplished by direct currect (DC) cardioversion. Temporary atrial and ventricular pacing wires are secured on the epicardium. These wires are useful in the postbypass and perioperative periods, as temporary atrioventricular dissociation and interventricular conduction defects are common. Permanent complete heart block is an occasional complication of aortic valve replacement, particularly if calcification extends into the region of the membranous septum and bundle of His. Before bypass is discontinued, the left ventricular vent is removed and a catheter may be inserted to monitor left atrial pressure. Bypass is discontinued when the cardiac rhythm is stable and hemodynamics are satisfactory.

Special Considerations

Aortic Valve Replacement and Coronary Bypass Grafting. The benefit of coronary bypass grafting in patients with both aortic valve disease and coronary occlusive disease is controversial. However, the combined operation can be done without significantly greater risk than aortic valve replacement alone (Jacobs et al, 1980; Wideman et al, 1981), and 5 to 20% of late deaths after aortic valve replacement in the era before direct coronary revascularization were related to coronary artery disease (Kirklin and Barratt-Boyes, 1986). Most cardiac surgeons routinely do coronary bypass grafting of all significantly stenotic arteries of appropriate size that supply viable myocardium at the time of aortic valve replacement. Many operative strategies for coronary revascularization and aortic valve replacement have given satisfactory results. The authors' preference is to construct the proximal anastomoses of the saphenous vein grafts to the ascending aorta before cardiopulmonary bypass, which minimizes total bypass time. After bypass is established, the aorta is cross-clamped and cardioplegic arrest is achieved (with delivery of cardioplegic solution into the aortic root if possible, or directly into the coronary ostia when necessary because of aortic incompetence). The distal vein grafts to coronary artery anastomoses are then done in the order dictated by the severity of the respective coronary occlusive lesions. Cardioplegic solution is reinfused after the completion of each graft. When all grafts have been completed, replacement of the aortic valve is done in the usual manner. It is helpful to make the vein grafts slightly longer than would otherwise be necessary so that they do not lie across

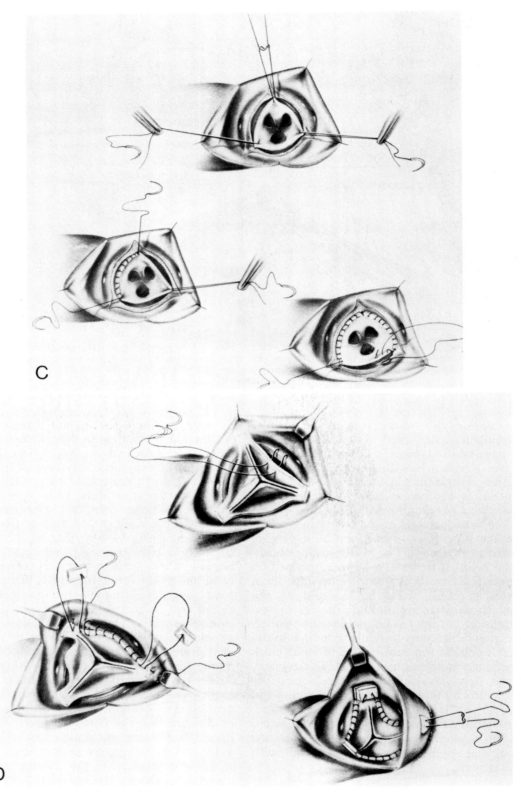

Figure 52–19 *Continued C*, The homograft is lowered into the recipient aortic root and the commissures are inverted. The edge of the graft is sutured to the outflow tract below the aortic annulus with continuous sutures. *D*, The inverted commissures are brought back up into the aortic root. The rim of sinus tissue of the homograft is sutured to the sinus of the recipient aorta with continuous sutures. The tops of the commissures are secured with Teflon pledgets. (*A* to *D*, From Doty, D. B.: Replacement of the aortic valve with cryopreserved aortic valve allograft: Considerations and techniques in children. J. Cardiac. Surg., 1(Suppl.):130, 1987.)

the proposed location of the aortotomy incision and obstruct access to the aortic valve.

Alternative operative strategies can be equally effective, as long as they include a satisfactory method of myocardial protection. One strategy involves the construction of distal vein grafts to coronary artery anastomoses first, with sequential delivery of cardioplegic solution into the proximal end of each vein graft. In general, the aortic valve is replaced after all distal coronary anastomoses have been constructed. The aortic cross-clamp can then be removed, and the proximal vein grafts to ascending aortic anastomoses are constructed during reperfusion and rewarming.

The internal mammary artery may be used as a conduit for revascularization of one or more coronary arteries, but its use does not allow delivery of cardioplegic solution via the internal mammary artery bypass to the myocardium beyond a critical coronary artery stenosis. Accordingly, the anastomosis of an internal mammary artery to a coronary artery may be done after the construction of saphenous vein grafts or after replacement of the aortic valve and just before removal of the aortic cross-clamp.

The Small Aortic Root. In adult patients with a smaller than normal aortic root, several techniques can be used to achieve aortic valve replacement with minimal gradient between the left ventricle and ascending aorta. Usually, a mechanical prosthesis is chosen that has satisfactory hemodynamics in small sizes (see Choice of Prosthesis). Occasionally, when the size of the annulus is satisfactory but the supraannular aortic root is small, the use of an oval gusset of Dacron or expanded polytetrafluoroethylene (PTFE) will permit closure of the aortotomy, which would not otherwise be possible with a stented xenograft or high-profile mechanical prosthesis. When the annulus itself is too small (e.g., smaller than 19 to 21 mm in an adult patient of average size), a prosthesis slightly larger than the size of the annulus can often be implanted at an oblique angle by positioning some of it (corresponding to the noncoronary cusp) in a supra-annular position. Alternatively, the annulus can be enlarged in a number of ways. Most commonly, the aortotomy incision, which has been extended to the midpoint of the noncoronary sinus, may be extended through the remnant of the noncoronary cusp and down into the anterior leaflet of the mitral valve (Manouguian and Seybold-Epting, 1979; Nicks et al, 1970). Valve sutures may be placed at the apex of the incision and a patch may be used in closure of the aorta, or alternatively (Fig. 52-20) an elliptical patch may first be sewn into the defect created in the subaortic (anterior) leaflet of the mitral valve and the valve sutures may be placed through the patch at the level of the annulus. The superior portion of the patch is used to close the aortotomy. These maneuvers are usually sufficient to enlarge the aortic root, but if they are not, more radical procedures that involve incision and patching of the roof of the left atrium and mitral valve (Rittenhouse et al, 1979) or incision

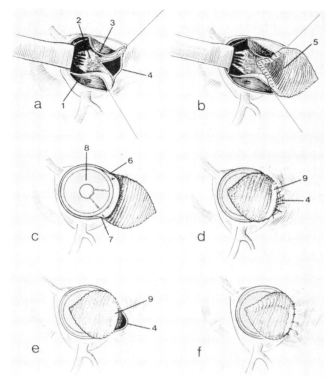

Figure 52-20. Technique for patch enlargement of the aortic annulus by extending the aortotomy incision into the anterior leaflet of the mitral valve. *A,* The aortic incision is extended toward the center of the anterior mitral leaflet. Extension of the incision 1 cm into the anterior mitral leaflet results in enlargement of the aortic valve ring by approximately 15 mm. An elliptical Dacron patch is sutured into the V-shaped defect in the anterior leaflet of the mitral valve. *C,* The resulting enlargement of the aortic annulus allows implantation of a prosthesis that is larger than the original aortic valve ring. *D,* A portion of the sewing ring of the prosthesis is sutured to the Dacron patch and the edge of the left atrium. *E,* Any residual defect between the left atrial wall and the patch is closed with continuous sutures or with mattress sutures that also pass through the sewing ring of the aortic prosthesis. *F,* The prosthesis is secured in place. The superior portion of the Dacron patch will be incorporated into the closure of the aortotomy. *1,* Left coronary cusps; *2,* anterior leaflet of mitral valve; *3,* noncoronary cusp; *4,* left atrial wall; *5,* prosthetic patch; *6, 7,* enlargement of aortic annulus; *8,* aortic valve prosthesis; *9,* sewing ring of aortic valve prosthesis. (From Manouguian, S., and Seybold-Epting, W.: Patch enlargement of the aortic valve ring by extending the aortic incision into the anterior mitral leaflet. J. Thorac. Cardiovasc. Surg., *78:*402, 1979.)

through the ventricular septum and patch enlargement of the left ventricular outflow tract (Konno et al, 1975) may be used. The latter procedure is often used for diffuse congenital hypoplasia of the left ventricular outflow tract and aortic valve ring (see Chapter 41). Even if the annulus is very small, it may be possible to replace the aortic valve with minimal or no gradient between the left ventricle and ascending aorta by using a nonstented aortic homograft valve and by inserting the valve freehand (Kirklin and Barratt-Boyes, 1986). Rarely, when the left ventricular outflow tract is considered to be unreconstructible, a valved conduit may be placed between the apex of the left ventricle and the descending thoracic or abdominal aorta (Norman et al, 1976).

Coexisting Mitral Valve Disease. When organic disease of the mitral valve coexists with significant aortic valve disease, a combined operation with definitive treatment of both valves should be done. Various operative strategies have been used for combined aortic and mitral valve operation. The authors prefer the following sequence: Bypass is established in the usual manner, and the left ventricle is vented with a catheter that is inserted into the left atrium just posterior to the interatrial groove and then passed through the mitral valve into the left ventricular cavity. The aorta is cross-clamped and cardioplegic solution is infused initially and at appropriate intervals such as for aortic valve replacement. The aortotomy incision is made, the aortic valve is excised, and the annulus is debrided. Valve sutures are placed through the aortic annulus and then through the sewing ring of an appropriate prosthesis. The aortic prosthesis is not seated in the annulus at this point but rather is put aside on the operating field and protected with a sterile towel. Next, the left atrium is opened at a level just posterior to the interatrial groove. Exposure of the mitral valve by retraction of the anterior portion of the left atrium is facilitated by the fact that the rigid aortic valve prosthesis has not yet been implanted, while the possibility of trauma to the aortic prosthesis is avoided. The mitral valve is then repaired or replaced with a suitable prosthesis (see Chapter 50). After the mitral procedure, the left atrial retractor is removed and attention is directed to the aortic valve. The aortic prosthesis is seated in the annulus and all sutures are tied. While the aortotomy incision is being closed, the patient is warmed in anticipation of removal of the aortic cross-clamp. The aortic root is de-aired, and the aortic cross-clamp is removed. The heart is reperfused, and the left atriotomy incision is closed during the completion of warming.

Moderately severe mitral incompetence may occur in the presence of severe aortic stenosis or regurgitation, although organic disease of the mitral valve and subvalvular apparatus is mild or absent. In such circumstances, mitral regurgitation should be reduced significantly or absent after aortic valve replacement (Austen et al, 1967). In addition to the catheterization and angiographic and echocardiographic findings, several maneuvers help to show the extent of mitral valve disease. These maneuvers include palpation of the mitral valve through the left atrium before aortic valve replacement and inspection of the mitral valve through the aortic root after excision of the aortic valve, which can sometimes help to indicate the presence of organic mitral disease. If the mitral valve is preserved, the phasic left atrial pressure trace should be monitored after separation from cardiopulmonary bypass to be certain that significant residual mitral regurgitation is not present.

Aortic Dissection with Aortic Insufficiency. When aortic insufficiency complicates dissection of the ascending aorta and the valve is morphologically normal, it may be possible after obliteration of the false channel to resuspend the aortic valve by placing mattress sutures at the level of the commissures and passing them through all layers of the aortic wall. Replacement of the ascending aorta at the supracoronary level with a sleeve graft completes the procedure. If there is any doubt that this maneuver will result in satisfactory competence of the aortic valve, the authors generally replace the aortic valve with a prosthesis to minimize the chance that aortic valve replacement will be needed later because of progressive aortic incompetence. In such cases, the aortic valve may be replaced in the usual manner and the ascending aorta then replaced at the supracoronary level with a sleeve graft (see Chapter 33, IV). When there is significant involvement of the proximal aorta, a composite graft replacement with a valved conduit (Bentall and DeBono, 1968) is the procedure of choice (see Chapter 33, IV). An aortic valve prosthesis is attached directly to the proximal end of a sleeve graft. The prosthesis is sewn to the aortic annulus, generally with pledgeted mattress sutures. The distal end of the sleeve graft is anastomosed to the transected distal aorta, after obliteration of the false lumen. The ostia of the coronary arteries are usually reimplanted directly onto the graft. When there is significant coronary occlusive disease or the dissection involves the proximal portions of one or both coronary arteries, coronary revascularization may be achieved with reversed saphenous vein grafts from the ascending aortic sleeve graft to the coronary arteries. If the dissection involves the transverse portion of the aortic arch, the replacement or reconstruction of this portion of the aorta is best done during a period of profound hypothermia and circulatory arrest and is generally accomplished without cross-clamping the distal aorta (Crawford et al, 1988).

Ascending Aortic Aneurysm with Aortic Insufficiency. When aortic insufficiency occurs in the setting of annuloaortic ectasia due to cystic medial necrosis, optimal therapy consists of composite replacement of the aortic valve and ascending aorta with reimplantation of the coronary arteries into the aortic graft (see Chapter 33, IV).

Aortic Valve Endocarditis. Operation may be indicated during antibiotic therapy for native valve bacterial endocarditis because of the occurrence of one or more of the following: resistance of the infection to antibiotic therapy (indicated by persistent fever more than 1 week after achieving therapeutic levels of appropriate antibiotics), presence of new conduction disturbances or arrhythmias that suggest extension of infection beyond the valve, recurrent peripheral emboli, or hemodynamic deterioration. These indications mandate prompt surgical intervention, because survival is considerably better with aortic valve replacement than with continued medical therapy (Ormiston et al, 1981). Active native valve endocarditis has been reported to be a significant risk factor for early prosthetic valve endocarditis (Ionescu and Tandon, 1978), although in a retrospective case-control study of 72 patients with early prosthetic valve endocarditis at the Massachusetts General Hospital, native valve endocarditis at the time of operation was not a significant determinant of risk (Jacobs et al, 1986b). Some surgeons consider that the risk of prosthetic valve endocarditis is minimized by insertion of a homograft or a porcine xenograft bioprosthesis (Magilligan et al, 1977; Ormiston et al, 1981).

When endocarditis is limited to the valve leaflets, aortic valve replacement is done in the usual manner. Extension of infection beyond the valve tissue is often associated with abscesses at the annular or subannular level, and it is important to debride these abscesses after excision of the valve and, when possible, to obliterate the abscess cavities. Occasionally, abscess formation is so extensive that it threatens to disrupt continuity of the ventricle and aortic root. Various techniques have been described to deal with this situation (Buckley et al, 1971). One technique consists of translocation of the prosthetic aortic valve to a supracoronary position with construction of vein bypass grafts to the coronary arteries and, in the Stanford experience, 75% operative survival was achieved with this method (Reitz et al, 1981). Composite replacement of the aortic valve and aortic root with either a prosthetic valve and conduit (Frantz et al, 1980) or a homograft valve and homograft ascending aorta (Donaldson and Ross, 1984) has been done successfully for patients with extensive endocarditis with left ventricular-aortic discontinuity.

Valve-Preserving Techniques. There has been a resurgence of interest in procedures to relieve aortic stenosis without replacement of the valve. These approaches may apply particularly to older patients for whom the risk of aortic valve replacement and chronic anticoagulant therapy is greater than for younger patients. Mindich and associates in 1985 reported a series of 15 elderly patients (mean age of 75.4 years) who had open aortic valvuloplasty procedures with cardiopulmonary bypass for relief of aortic stenosis. All the patients had small aortic roots and contraindications to anticoagulation. The procedures resulted in significant decreases in the mean gradients between left ventricle and aorta, with significant increases in calculated valve areas. Similar initial results with open aortic valvuloplasty were reported nearly 25 years earlier from this institution by Scannell and Austen (1964), who advocated valve-preserving techniques for the management of aortic stenosis in selected patients. Long-term follow-up of these patients indicated a high incidence of recurrence. Modern technology has contributed to the possibility of success with open valvuloplasty procedures. Several centers are experimenting with the use of the Cavitron ultrasonic surgical aspirator. This ultrasonic scalpel, which has been widely used in cataract surgery, neurosurgery, and hepatic surgery,

consists of a probe that vibrates longitudinally at more than 18,000 cycles per second, which results in precisely controlled fragmentation of tissue that comes in contact with the distal end of the probe. The system includes irrigation and suction to remove the debris (Hodgson, 1979). The Cavitron has been used successfully to debride slightly and moderately calcified aortic valves. Long-term follow-up is not yet available.

Other reconstructive techniques have been used for repair of rheumatic aortic valve disease in patients with concomitant mitral valve disease. Duran (1988) reported a series of 50 patients who had aortic valve reconstruction at the time of mitral valve reconstruction. All of the patients had severe mitral disease, and most patients had mixed aortic valve disease (stenosis and insufficiency). Aortic lesions were managed by a combination of four techniques: commissurotomy, cusp free edge unfolding, commissural annuloplasty, and supra-aortic crest enlargement. Only 4 of 50 patients had significant residual aortic regurgitation that required late reoperation (follow-up of 1 to 13 years; mean follow-up of 7.7 years). In these patients with combined mitral and aortic valve disease whose mitral disease was amenable to valve-preserving reconstructive procedures, it was often possible to improve aortic valve function and to avoid problems associated with a prosthesis.

Percutaneous Balloon Aortic Valvotomy. Encouraged by the initial results of percutaneous balloon mitral valvotomy, several centers are experimenting with techniques for balloon dilatation of stenotic aortic valves in adults (Block and Palacios, 1987; McKay et al, 1987). The procedure is done in the cardiac catheterization laboratory under local anesthesia and uses standard cardiac catheterization approaches and a large fluid-filled balloon similar to the balloon used in the treatment of congenital pulmonic valve stenosis. The aortic valve can be crossed by a retrograde approach from the femoral artery or by an antegrade approach from the femoral vein and across the atrial septum. Under fluoroscopic control and with continuous hemodynamic monitoring, the balloon is inflated with a mixture of contrast medium and saline. Inflations are repeated until the balloon expands fully at the level of the aortic valve. Several centers have reported favorable results with significant reduction of the peak transvalvular gradient (Cribier et al, 1986; McKay et al, 1987; Palacios and Block, 1987). Postdilatation aortic valve areas have been improved but usually by only a slight to moderate degree. The most frequent complications have been transient hypotension and bleeding or thrombosis at the site of catheter introduction. A slight increase in the amount of aortic regurgitation is common after balloon aortic valvotomy, but significant aortic regurgitation occurs in less than 3% of patients (Cribier et al, 1986). Hospital mortality is 3 to 5% and is related to the patient's functional class (Block and Palacios, 1987). Myocardial infarction, tamponade, and embolic complications occur with low frequency. No long-term follow-up data are available, but it appears that this technique may be suitable for short-term palliation of a selected group of patients at a prohibitively high risk for surgical therapy, such as elderly patients with severe multisystem disease.

OPERATIONS FOR HYPERTROPHIC CARDIOMYOPATHY

Septal myotomy-myectomy is the most widely used operative technique for HCM. The largest experience with this technique is that of Morrow and associates (1975). This procedure involves resection of the obstructing muscle through an aortotomy incision alone (Fig. 52–21). Approximately 70% of patients in the early series had significant symptomatic improvement for up to 25 years after operation (Maron et al, 1978). Kirklin and Ellis (1961) and Agnew and associates (1977) advocated a combined approach through the aorta and left ventricle for resection of the obstructing muscle. Most groups recommend mitral valve replacement only when myotomy-myectomy has not significantly decreased the dynamic left ventricular outflow gradient or when significant mitral regurgitation has not regressed. Cooley and associates (1973), however, advocated mitral valve replacement as the primary surgical therapy of obstructive HCM. McIntosh and associates (1989) at the National Institutes of Health reported excellent results with mitral valve replacement used selectively for patients with atypical septal morphology, thin septum (less than 18 mm) in the region of usual resection, or previous myomectomy with residual obstruction.

The authors use myotomy-myectomy for patients with significant gradients who have not had symptomatic relief with beta-blocking agents or calcium channel blockers. Potential complications of this operation include conduction disturbances (incidence of complete heart block was 5% in the series reported by Maron and associates, 1978), perioperative myocardial infarction, and, rarely, iatrogenic ventricular septal defect. Iatrogenic aortic and mitral incompetence is a rare complication and should be avoided with appropriate surgical technique. Adequate myotomy and myectomy routinely result in a decrease in the gradient between the left ventricle and the aorta; failure to relieve the obstruction is associated with the persistence of symptoms (Kelly et al, 1966). Surgical correction of the dynamic outflow obstruction relieves symptoms and improves the quality of life, but no conclusive studies have shown that life is prolonged.

CHOICE OF AORTIC VALVE PROSTHESES

The choice of a prosthesis for aortic valve replacement must be individualized and must take into consideration patient-related factors such as age, lifestyle, other medical problems, and ability to comply with a program of follow-up that may include chronic anticoagulation therapy. Valve-related factors including availability, durability, hemodynamic performance, thrombogenicity, patient acceptance, and potential modes of failure must also be considered in the choice of a valve substitute.

Since the early aortic valve replacements with biologic prostheses and mechanical caged-ball prostheses almost three decades ago, great progress has been made in prosthetic valve design and construction and in the handling, preparation, and preservation of biologic valve substitutes. At present, a number of excellent mechanical prostheses and bioprostheses, as well as human aortic valve homografts, are available. Valve substitutes are usually divided into two groups: mechanical valves and tissue valves. The two groups differ with regard to durability, hemodynamic performance, thrombogenicity, patient acceptance, and potential modes of failure. In addition, within each broad category, a specific prosthesis may be superior to the others in a particular area.

Mechanical valves all share the disadvantage of thrombogenicity and the potential for thromboembolic complications. Chronic anticoagulant therapy of some type is almost universally used after implantation of mechanical prostheses. The mechanical valves have durability as their principal advantage. Some types, such as the Starr-Edwards caged-ball model 1200 and 1260 aortic valves (Fig. 52–22), have been in continuous use for more than two decades. These Starr-Edwards valves are the most widely used caged-ball prostheses and have an excellent record of durability. Cobanoglu and associates (1988) reported the 20-year follow-up of patients operated on by Starr and associates. The overall valve-related mortality at 20 years was 13%. The linearized rate of a first thromboembolic event was 2.8% per patient year and of all thromboembolic events was 3.3% per patient year, which are comparable to rates for other mechanical prostheses currently in use. The linearized rate of hemorrhagic complications was 2.5% per patient year. Caged-ball prostheses, as compared with tilting disk and bileaflet mechanical valves, have the disadvantages of high-profile design (which may necessitate aortic root enlargement in some patients) and significant transvalvular gradients in small sizes.

The Wada-Cutter, standard spherical Bjork-Shiley, and Lillehei-Kaster tilting disk valves were developed during the 1960s, followed more recently by the Medtronic Hall (previously Hall Kaster) tilting disk valve. The principal design objective for this group of tilting disk valves has been to minimize transvalvular gradients. In the open position, the tilting disk occluder presents a thin cross-section to the column of flowing blood and thus more closely approximates the physiologic condition of central laminar flow. Counterbalancing the advantage of slightly better hemodynamics (particularly in small sizes) is the higher incidence of thrombosis of the

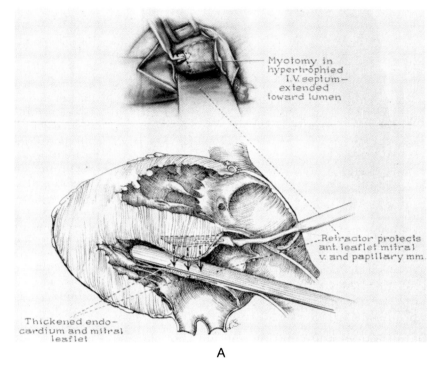

Figure 52–21. Technique of myotomy-myectomy for idiopathic hypertrophic subaortic stenosis as used by Morrow and associates at the National Institutes of Health. *A,* A flat ribbon retractor is used to displace and protect the anterior mitral leaflet and papillary muscles. A knife blade is passed into the muscular septum just below the base of the right coronary leaflet of the aortic valve at a point 2 to 3 mm to the right of the intercoronary commissure. After a second incision has been made parallel and approximately 1 cm to the right of the first incision, the bar of muscle between the two myotomies is excised. *B,* Resected area of the septum is shown with its relationship to the aortic valve, the area of the conduction system, and the anterior leaflet of the mitral valve. (From Morrow, A. G., Reitz, B. A., Epstein, S. E., et al: Operative treatment in hypertrophic subaortic stenosis: Techniques and results of pre- and post-operative assessment in 83 patients. Circulation, 52:88, 1975. By permission of the American Heart Association, Inc.)

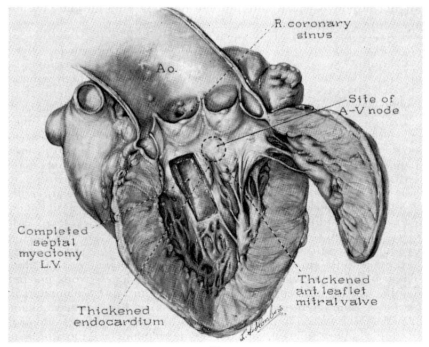

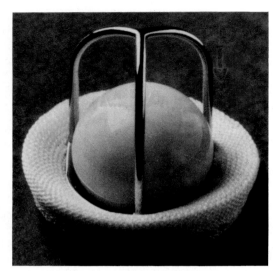

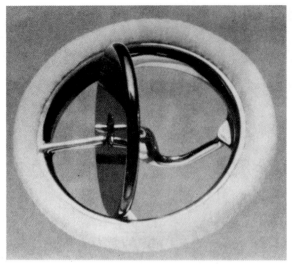

Figure 52–22. The model 1260 Starr-Edwards caged-ball aortic valve prosthesis. The cage is made of Stellite, the ball is made of Silastic, and the sewing ring is made of Teflon and polypropylene cloth. This prosthesis has been continuously used for more than two decades.

Figure 52–24. The Medtronic Hall aortic valve prosthesis. This valve (formerly the Hall-Kaster prosthesis) was introduced in 1977. The valve housing and S-shaped disk guide strut are titanium, and the disk is made of pyrolite-coated graphite. The sewing ring is Teflon. The disk opens to 75 degrees.

valve prosthesis itself. Bjork and Henze (1979) reported an incidence of valve thrombosis of 0.3 episodes per 100 patient years with the standard Bjork-Shiley aortic prosthesis (Fig. 52–23). In the authors' experience with 624 patients who were followed for 10 years after isolated aortic valve replacement, the rates of all thromboembolic complications (inclusive of valve thrombosis) did not differ significantly between the caged-ball (Starr-Edwards model 1260) and tilting disk (standard spherical disk Bjork-Shiley) groups (Jacobs et al, 1986). The standard spherical disk Bjork-Shiley prosthesis was modified in an attempt to improve hemodynamic performance (convexoconcave disk Bjork-Shiley prosthesis), but this

resulted in durability problems (strut fracture and disk escape) and the convexoconcave disk Bjork-Shiley prosthesis has been withdrawn from use. Sale of the standard spherical disk Bjork-Shiley prosthesis has also been discontinued in the United States; both of these valves may be replaced with the newer Bjork-Shiley monostrut tilting disk prosthesis when it receives FDA approval. The Medtronic Hall valve (Fig. 52–24) appears to have many of the advantages of tilting disk design with excellent durability (Beaudet et al, 1986). The Wada-Cutter valve is no longer used.

Bileaflet mechanical valves, such as the St. Jude medical prosthesis, have the design feature of central flow and consequently have excellent hemodynamics and small transvalvular gradients even in small sizes. Durability of the St. Jude Medical aortic valve prosthesis (Fig. 52–25), which was introduced for clinical evaluation in 1977, has been excellent at medium-term follow-up (Arom et al, 1985; Baudet et al, 1985; Kinsley et al., 1986). Linearized rates of thromboembolic events after St. Jude aortic valve replacement are 0.6 to 2.3% per patient year (Edmunds, 1987). There have been trials of aspirin alone or aspirin and dipyridamole without warfarin as anticoagulant therapy for children and adults with St. Jude prosthetic valves, but most of the data suggest the need for warfarin anticoagulation in all patients with mechanical valve prostheses (Edmunds, 1987).

Aortic bioprostheses (stented tissue valves) have been developed with the principal goals of achieving physiologic central flow with minimal gradients and minimizing the risk of thromboembolic complications without the need for chronic anticoagulation. To varying degrees, these needs have been met by various bioprostheses, but none has matched the durability of selected mechanical valves. Bio-

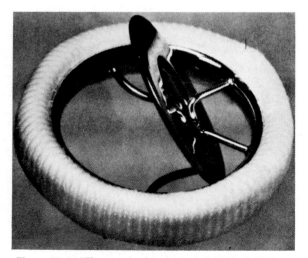

Figure 52–23. The standard (spherical disk) Bjork-Shiley aortic valve prosthesis. The valve consists of a Stellite cage, Teflon cloth sewing ring, and pyrolytic carbon disk that opens to 60 degrees.

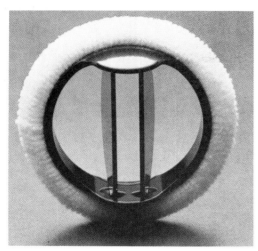

Figure 52–25. The St. Jude Medical aortic valve prosthesis. The bileaflet design results in central laminar flow with minimal obstruction. The leaflets and housing are made of pyrolytic carbon. The leaflets pivot open to 85 degrees. The sewing ring is made of Dacron.

prostheses include stented xenografts; stented valves made from other biologic tissues such as fascia lata, dura mater, and bovine pericardium; and stented aortic homograft valves (prepared and preserved in various ways).

The Carpentier-Edwards valve (Fig. 52–26) and the Hancock valve are representative of stented porcine xenograft bioprostheses. These glutaraldehyde-treated porcine aortic valves are stent-mounted with cushioned sewing rings. The central flow characteristics of these valves are associated with excellent hemodynamics in medium to large sizes. The use of small porcine xenograft bioprostheses in adults with normal cardiac outputs may be associated with significant gradients. The long-term durability of the glutaraldehyde-preserved porcine bioprostheses is affected by primary tissue degeneration and calcification. In patients who had isolated aortic valve replacement at Massachusetts General Hospital from

1975 to 1980, actuarial freedom from valve failure was 94% at 5 years and 88% at 8 years for those who received porcine xenografts, compared with 95% at 5 years and 93% at 8 years for patients who received Starr-Edwards model 1260 or standard spherical Bjork-Shiley mechanical aortic valve prostheses (Jacobs et al, 1986a). The higher incidence of valve failure of the bioprostheses compared with the mechanical prostheses at 8 years is due to the significant incidence of calcification and tissue degeneration in that time interval. Beyond approximately 7 years, failure of the porcine xenograft bioprostheses due to calcification and tissue degeneration appears to accelerate. Gallo and associates (1988) reported the follow-up of patients who received the Hancock porcine bioprostheses between 1974 and 1976. At 12.5 years' follow-up, the calculated actuarial probability of freedom from primary tissue valve failure was 58 ± 6% for the aortic prostheses. For the Carpentier-Edwards and Hancock porcine bioprostheses, design changes have been made to minimize transvalvular gradients in the smaller sizes, and changes in the methods of chemical fixation have been made to retard the processes of calcification and tissue degeneration that have been the principal modes of valve failure (Jones et al, 1986). Long-term anticoagulation is generally not required after implantation of porcine bioprostheses in the aortic position, because a very low incidence of thromboembolic complications is associated with these valves. A retrospective evaluation of patients who received Hancock or Carpentier-Edwards porcine xenograft prostheses in the aortic position from 1975 to 1980 showed a calculated actuarial probability of freedom from thromboembolic complications of 96 ± 1% at 5 years and 93 ± 2% at 8 years (Jacobs et al, 1986a). After early enthusiasm for the use of porcine bioprostheses (and avoidance of anticoagulation) in pediatric patients, the use of these valves in children has decreased greatly because of the accelerated xenograft calcification and higher rates of early valve failure in young patients than in adults (Williams et al, 1982).

Several of the earliest bioprostheses were constructed of nonvalvular tissue mounted on a supporting frame. Valves made of fascia lata and dura mater are no longer used because they tend to deteriorate rapidly, but several stent-mounted pericardial bioprostheses are currently available. The Ionescu-Shiley bovine pericardial prosthesis is one such valve. Glutaraldehyde-treated bovine pericardium is mounted in a trileaflet configuration on a rigid stent with a cushioned sewing ring. In small sizes the transvalvular gradients across this bioprosthesis are slightly less than gradients across the porcine xenografts in comparable sizes. The incidence of thromboembolism is comparable to that associated with the porcine xenografts (Revuelta et al, 1986), but the durability of pericardial aortic valve prostheses, particularly in small sizes, is reported by some surgeons to be less than that of porcine xenografts (Nistal et al, 1986; Reul et al, 1985).

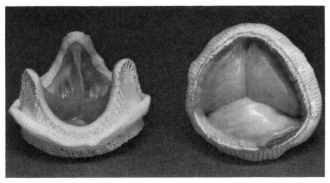

Figure 52–26. The Carpentier-Edwards porcine xenograft aortic bioprosthesis. The glutaraldehyde-preserved porcine aortic valve is mounted on a flexible frame made of Elgiloy (a corrosion-resistant alloy of cobalt and nickel) that is covered with Teflon cloth.

The homograft (allograft) aortic valve has been used for orthotopic (subcoronary) aortic valve replacement with and without a stent in various forms since 1962 (Ross, 1962). Irradiated and chemically sterilized valves had unacceptably high rates of early failure by cusp rupture. Techniques of preservation evolved in a number of centers in the latter half of the 1960s. Antibiotic sterilization and nutrient medium storage of fresh homografts produced more favorable medium- and long-term results (Barratt-Boyes et al, 1977; Verdi et al, 1986). More recently, experience with unstented homografts treated with antibiotics and then cryopreserved in liquid nitrogen at $-196°$ C has been compared with experience with fresh antibiotic-sterilized unstented homografts (O'Brien et al, 1987). Most of the fresh valves were implanted 3 to 4 days after procurement and were essentially nonviable as determined by tissue culture techniques, histologic demonstration of viable cells, and measurement of glucose utilization. (Viability of the aortic homograft was inferred from the results of testing of the pulmonary valve, which had been harvested at the same time and subjected to identical handling.) The cryopreserved valves were viable at the time of implantation. Freedom from thromboembolism (without anticoagulant therapy) for both groups was 97% at 10 years. The two groups differed in freedom from reoperation for valve degeneration at 10 years: 89% for the fresh homografts and 100% for the cryopreserved homografts. Also, explanted valves from the cryopreserved group (which were removed because of technical malalignment) consistently had evidence of persisting viability. Few follow-up data beyond 10 years are available for the cryopreserved valves, but it appears that preservation of long-term viability of valvular tissue is associated with greater freedom from degeneration. Because of the other advantages of nonstented aortic valve homografts (excellent hemodynamics even in small sizes and relative infrequency of thromboembolic complications without anticoagulant therapy), there has been renewed interest in homograft aortic valve replacement. Limited availability of normal homograft aortic valves and the cost and effort of procurement, handling, and preservation will continue to affect the choice of aortic valve substitutes. Freehand implantation of homograft aortic valves is considered by many to be technically more demanding than the implantation of a mechanical prosthesis or stented bioprosthesis. Use of a homograft valve of inappropriate size for the recipient's aortic root or a technical error in implantation can result in valvular incompetence of various degrees.

RESULTS OF AORTIC VALVE REPLACEMENT

Operative Mortality

The operative mortality in many of the earliest reports of sizable series of aortic valve replacements was moderately low, 3 to 8% (Barratt-Boyes et al, 1965; McGoon et al, 1965). The risk of hospital mortality has been reduced with improvements in patient management. These improvements include better preoperative evaluation, improved cardiac anesthetic management, better postoperative care, and, most important, refinements in operative technique and improvements in myocardial protection. At the same time, aortic valve replacement has been extended to a broader patient population.

Overall hospital mortality for aortic valve replacement with or without coronary revascularization currently is 2 to 5% (Jacobs et al, 1980; Kirklin and Barratt-Boyes, 1986). The preoperative functional status of the patient is the strongest predictor of operative mortality. For a consecutive group of 200 patients from the Massachusetts General Hospital, the operative mortality was 8.3% for patients in New York Heart Association functional Class IV, compared with 1.9% for all other patients ($p = 0.039$). Preoperative functional class was also a stong predictor of operative risk in the University of Alabama series (Kirklin and Barratt-Boyes, 1986) and the Stanford experience (Scott et al, 1985). In some series, hemodynamic parameters such as ventricular end-diastolic pressure, pulmonary capillary wedge pressure, and left ventricular ejection fraction showed some correlation with operative risk, but none of these is as strong a predictor of operative risk as the preoperative functional class. Age at operation is also correlated with risk of operative mortality (Craver et al, 1984). In the University of Alabama series, the risk of operative mortality at 40 years of age was approximately 1% and at 75 years of age was approximately 5% (Kirklin and Barratt-Boyes, 1986). In that series, age was also an incremental risk factor for significant postoperative hemorrhage. Type of aortic valve disease (stenosis, incompetence, or mixed) is a predictor of mortality in some series. In the Stanford experience (Scott et al, 1985), the subgroup with aortic regurgitation had the highest operative mortality (10%, compared with 6% for the subgroup with aortic stenosis and 5% for the subgroup with combined stenosis-regurgitation), but there was a sharp decrease over time in the operative mortality within the group with aortic regurgitation. Whether the decrease can be attributed to changing patterns of patient selection or to evolving techniques of myocardial protection cannot be determined conclusively. In a consecutive group of 200 patients, the mortality was the same for isolated aortic stenosis and incompetence (5.6% versus 5.9%), and there were no deaths among 22 patients in this group with mixed stenosis and incompetence (Jacobs et al, 1980). That operative mortality is not prosthesis related is generally conceded, but the Green Lane Hospital experience (Kirklin and Barratt-Boyes, 1986) suggests that operative mortality is less for patients who receive freehand homografts than for those who receive mechanical prostheses or xenografts. Whether this reflects superiority of the homografts or pattern of patient selection for the various types of valves or some other reason cannot be determined from their analysis.

One randomized study showed no difference in risk of operative mortality between groups who had aortic valve replacement with continuous coronary perfusion and those who had cold potassium cardioplegia (Sapsford et al, 1974), but most recent series report lower operative mortality with cardioplegia (Jacobs et al, 1980). In addition, the use of cold potassium cardioplegia has largely eliminated the importance of aortic cross-clamp time as an incremental risk factor. In the experience at the Cleveland Clinic, cold cardioplegia (compared with other methods of myocardial protection) was associated with decreased mortality in patients who had combined aortic valve replacement and coronary revascularization (Lytle et al, 1983). Coronary revascularization at the time of aortic valve replacement does not appear to be an incremental risk factor for operative mortality. Isolated aortic valve replacement without revascularization in patients with significant coronary disease has a higher risk than isolated aortic valve replacement in patients without coronary artery disease (Miller et al, 1979).

In general, the risk of operative mortality in elective re-replacement of the aortic valve does not differ significantly from that of primary aortic valve replacement (Parr et al, 1977). Re-replacement of aortic valves because of infection and urgent re-replacement of aortic valves because of severe hemodynamic deterioration have significantly higher risks (20 to 50%) (Syracuse et al, 1979).

Complications

Prosthesis-related complications such as thromboembolism, anticoagulation-related hemorrhage, and infection of the prosthesis are considered elsewhere (see Chapter 51). The principal perioperative complications of aortic valve replacement are hemorrhage, neurologic deficits, and myocardial infarction. Lytle and associates (1989) reported a series of 1,689 consecutive patients who had isolated aortic valve replacement from 1972 to 1986 at the Cleveland Clinic: 194 patients (11.5%) required reoperation for postoperative bleeding; 29 (1.7%) sustained a neurologic deficit that persisted to the time of discharge from the hospital; 19 (1.1%) had wound complications; 49 (2.9%) had respiratory failure that required prolonged ventilation; and 16 (1.0%) required tracheostomy. Renal failure that required dialysis occurred in 12 patients (0.7%). There was a 2% incidence of perioperative myocardial infarction. In all, 17% of the patients had one or more morbid perioperative event. The incidence of in-hospital death was 10.8% for patients who required reoperation for bleeding and 11.4% for those who had perioperative myocardial infarctions (compared with an overall in-hospital mortality of 3.4%). The incidence of bleeding complications varies from one center to another and is

generally in the range of 5 to 12% (5.8% in a series from Massachusetts General Hospital; Jacobs et al, 1980). The risk of hemorrhage is related to the patient's age and functional class (Kirklin and Barratt-Boyes, 1986) but can be decreased by meticulous surgical technique, particularly in closure of the aortotomy. Neurologic complications that result from particulate or air embolism should also be avoided. Some incidence of atherosclerotic embolization may be unavoidable in operations that involve cardiopulmonary bypass and aortic cross-clamping. The incidence of perioperative myocardial infarction has decreased (from 3.0% for the first 442 patients in the Cleveland Clinic series to 1.3% for the last 308 patients), at least partly because of improved methods of myocardial protection. Although temporary conduction defects are common in the early perioperative period after aortic valve replacement, permanent complete heart block is a rare complication that is related to the debridement of calcific deposits and the placement of sutures in the region of the membranous septum, with trauma to the bundle of His.

Late Results

Evaluation of 987 patients who had isolated aortic valve replacement at Massachusetts General Hospital between 1975 and 1980 showed 5-year survival rates of 83 ± 2% for those with Starr-Edwards model 1260 and Bjork-Shiley standard spherical disk mechanical prostheses, and 84 ± 2% for those with Hancock and Carpentier-Edwards bioprostheses. At 8 years, survival rates were 70 ± 3% and 74 ± 3%, respectively (Jacobs et al, 1986a). These medium-term survival rates are comparable with rates from other major centers (Barnhorst et al, 1975a, 1975b; Davila et al, 1978; Ionescu and Tandon, 1979). Lytle and associates (1989) reported survival of 85% at 5 years, 66% at 10 years, and 56% at 12 postoperative years, for 1,317 in-hospital survivors of isolated aortic valve replacement (with various mechanical prostheses and bioprostheses) from 1972 to 1983. The actuarial 5-year survival rate for patients with bioprostheses was slightly higher than for patients with mechanical prostheses, but at 10 years the actuarial survival rates for the two groups were essentially the same (Fig. 52–27). That aortic valve replacement does not give recipients the normal life expectancy of age-matched controls from the general population is not surprising (Barnhorst et al, 1975a, 1975b).

Results of aortic valve replacement must be evaluated not only in terms of survival but also in terms of patient rehabilitation. At medium-term follow-up (4.3 years), 87% of patients were in NYHA Class I or II, 79% had improved by one class or more over their preoperative status, and only 1% had a poorer NYHA classification than before operation (Jacobs et al, 1980). In the report by Copeland and associates (1977) of Stanford University's long-term follow-up after isolated aortic valve replacement, 90% of patients

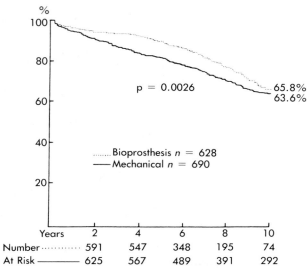

Figure 52–27. Actuarial survival curves of 1,318 patients who had isolated aortic valve replacement at the Cleveland Clinic from 1972 to 1983. (In-hospital deaths are not included in this analysis.) The patients have been divided into groups according to prosthesis type (628 patients with bioprostheses and 690 patients with mechanical prostheses). The percentage of patients who survived at 5 years was higher for the group with a bioprosthesis than for the group with a mechanical prosthesis. The percentage of patients who survived at 10 years was similar for the two groups. (From Lytle, E. W., Cosgrove, D. M., Taylor, P. C., et al: Primary isolated aortic valve replacement: Early and late results. J. Thorac. Cardiovasc. Surg., 97:675, 1989.)

followed for 8 years were in NYHA Class I or II. Perhaps most impressive are the University of Alabama data which indicated that 70% of patients who were preoperatively in NYHA Class IV became Class I or II after operation (Kirklin and Barratt-Boyes, 1986). As quality of life after aortic valve replacement is directly related to freedom from valve-related complications, improvement is primarily related to the development of mechanical prostheses with fewer thromboembolic complications and biologic valve substitutes of greater durability.

Selected Bibliography

Baudet, E. M., Oca, C. C., Roques, X. E., et al: A 5½ year experience with the St. Jude Medical cardiac valve prosthesis. J. Thorac. Cardiovasc. Surg., 90:137, 1985.

Baudet and associates from Bordeaux, France, report the results of their experience with the St. Jude medical valve prosthesis. Between June 1978 and June 1983, 671 patients had implantation of St. Jude Medical valve prostheses including 500 aortic valve replacements. Hospital mortality was 3.6% (18 of 500 patients) for aortic valve replacements. No hospital deaths after aortic valve replacement were valve-related. The actuarial survival rate at 5½ years was 91% for patients who had aortic valve replacement. The linearized rate of systemic embolic events was 0.34% per patient year for patients who received anticoagulants and 6.15% per patient year for patients who did not receive anticoagulants. There were no cases of aortic valve thrombosis among the patients who received anticoagulants. There were 4 cases of aortic valve throm-

bosis among the 65 patients who did not receive anticoagulants. On the basis of this 5½ years of experience, the authors concluded that the St. Jude Medical valve is an excellent mechanical prosthesis in terms of hemodynamic performance and low thrombogenicity in patients who receive anticoagulants.

Cobanoglu, A., Fessler, C. L., Guvendik, L., et al: Aortic valve replacement with the Starr-Edwards prosthesis: A comparison of the first and second decades of follow-up. Ann. Thorac. Surg., 45:248, 1988.

This review of the long-term follow-up of patients who had aortic valve replacement with the Starr-Edwards prosthesis by Starr and associates in Portland, Oregon, between January 1965 and December 1986, is unique in describing the course of patients who received an aortic valve prosthesis that is currently available and has been essentially unmodified during the last 20 years. Valve-related mortality at 20 years was 13%. The incidence of thromboembolic complications was 3.3% per year. There were no cases of structural deterioration of the prostheses and no evidence of an increased rate of valve-related complications during the second decade.

Gallo, I., Nistal, F., Blasquez, R., et al: Incidence of primary tissue valve failure in porcine bioprosthetic heart valves. Ann. Thorac. Surg., 45:66, 1988.

This report gives long-term follow-up data on 324 patients who received a Hancock porcine xenograft bioprosthesis in the aortic or mitral position or in both positions between 1974 and 1976. This series included 126 aortic bioprostheses. There were 41 cases of primary tissue valve failure among the aortic bioprostheses. The calculated actuarial probability of freedom from primary tissue valve failure was 58 ± 6% for the aortic prostheses at 12.5 years of follow-up. Follow-up was 99.7% complete. This carefully executed retrospective study clearly documents the increased rate of primary tissue failure of porcine aortic valve bioprostheses after approximately 7 years.

Lytle, B. W., Cosgrove, D. M., Loop, F. D., et al: Replacement of aortic valve combined with myocardial revascularization: Determinants of early and late risk for 500 patients, 1967–1981. Circulation, 68:1149, 1983.

These authors from the Cleveland Clinic review their experience with 500 consecutive patients who had aortic valve replacement and coronary revascularization in the years 1967 to 1981. Overall hospital mortality was 5.9%, with a reduced mortality of 3.4% in the final 3 years of the study. Determinants of early and late risk were identified by univariate and multivariate analyses. Female sex, aortic insufficiency, and advanced age were associated with increased in-hospital mortality. The use of cardioplegia for myocardial protection was associated with decreased in-hospital mortality. Patients who received bioprostheses and did not receive anticoagulants had higher long-term survival and event-free survival rates than patients with bioprostheses who received anticoagulants or patients with mechanical valves with or without anticoagulants.

Maron, B. J., Bonow, R. O., Cannon, R. O., et al: Hypertrophic cardiomyopathy: Interrelations of clinical manifestations, pathophysiology, and therapy. Part I. N. Engl. J. Med., 316:780, 1987.

Maron, B. J., Bonow, R. O., Cannon, R. O., et al: Hypertrophic cardiomyopathy: Interrelations of clinical manifestations, pathophysiology, and therapy. Part II. N. Engl. J. Med., 316:844, 1987.

This comprehensive review of the subject of hypertrophic cardiomyopathy by authors from the Cardiology Branch of the National Heart, Lung, and Blood Institute of the National Institutes of Health is a valuable updated resource by undisputed experts on the subject. It includes detailed reviews of the pathology, pathophysiology, diagnostic studies, and modes of therapy of this disease. The clinical experience with hypertrophic cardiomyopathy at the NIH has been more extensive than at any other center in the world. Current controversies are covered in detail and views other than those of the authors are clearly represented. Newer pharmacologic agents and their potential roles in the control of symptoms and arrhythmias associated with hypertrophic cardiomyopathy are covered in detail.

O'Brien, M. F., Stafford, E. G., Gardner, M. A., et al: A comparison of aortic valve replacement with viable cryopreserved and fresh allograft valves, with a note on chromosomal studies. J. Thorac. Cardiovasc. Surg., 94:812, 1987.

This report reviews the experience with allograft aortic valves at the Prince Charles Hospital in Brisbane, Australia, between December 1969 and December 1986. Two different methods were used consecutively for preservation of aortic valve allografts. In the earlier experience fresh allografts were refrigerated at 4° C. More recently allografts were cryopreserved in liquid nitrogen at −196° C. Freedom from thromboembolism was comparable for the two groups. Freedom from reoperation for valve degeneration was considerably better in the cryopreserved (and more recent) group. Valves from the cryopreserved group that were explanted because of technical malalignment consistently showed evidence of viability on tissue culture, metabolic studies, and histologic appearance. Chromosomal studies showed the donor origin of these cells. Although the comparison involved a consecutive (and not a randomized) series, this careful study suggests that persistence of cell viability within the cyropreserved valve is important in terms of functional durability.

Scott, W. C., Miller, D. C., Haverich, A., et al: Determinants of operative mortality for patients undergoing aortic valve replacement. J. Thorac. Cardiovasc. Surg., 89:400, 1985.

These authors present the Stanford University experience with 1,479 isolated aortic valve replacements (1967 to 1981). Overall operative mortality was 7%. In this series, the highest operative mortality (10%) was associated with the subgroup with aortic regurgitation. Discriminant analysis identified advanced New York Heart Association functional class, renal dysfunction, physiologic subgroup, atrial fibrillation, and older age as independent determinants of operative mortality.

Bibliography

Agnew, T. M., Barratt-Boyes, B. G., Brandt, P. W. T., et al: Surgical resection in idiopathic hypertrophic subaortic stenosis using a combined approach through aorta and left ventricle: A long-term follow-up study of 49 patients. J. Thorac. Cardiovasc. Surg., 74:307, 1977.

Arom, K. V., Nicoloff, D. M., Kersten, T. E., et al: Six years of experience with the St. Jude Medical valvular prosthesis. Circulation, 72:2-153, 1985.

Austen, W. G., Kastor, J. A., and Sanders, C. A.: Resolution of functional mitral regurgitation following surgical correction of aortic valvular disease. J. Thorac. Cardiovasc. Surg., 53:255, 1967.

Bahnson, H. T., Spencer, F. C., Busse, E. F. G., and Davis, F. W., Jr.: Cusp replacement in coronary artery perfusion in open operations on the aortic valve. Ann. Surg., 152:494, 1960.

Bailey, C. P., Ramirez, H. P., and Larselere, H. B.: Surgical treatment of aortic stenosis. J.A.M.A., 150:1647, 1952.

Barnhorst, D. A., Oxman, H. A., Connolly, D. C., et al: Isolated replacement of the aortic valve with the Starr-Edwards prosthesis: A 9 year review. J. Thorac. Cardiovasc. Surg., 70:113, 1975a.

Barnhorst, D. A., Oxman, H. A., Connolly, D. C., et al: Long-term follow-up of isolated replacement of the aortic or mitral valve with the Starr-Edwards prothesis. Am. J. Cardiol., 35:228, 1975b.

Barratt-Boyes, B. G.: A method for preparing and inserting a homograft aortic valve. Br. J. Surg., 52:847, 1965.

Barratt-Boyes, B. G.: Homograft replacement for aortic valve disease. Mod. Concepts Cardiovasc. Dis., 36:1, 1967.

Barratt-Boyes, B. G.: The timing of operation in valvular insufficiency. J. Cardiac Surg., 2:435, 1987.

Barratt-Boyes, B. G., Lowe, J. B., Cole, D. S., and Kelly, D. T.: Homograft valve replacement for aortic valve disease. Thorax, 20:495, 1965.

Barratt-Boyes, B. G., Roche, A. H. G., and Whitlock, R. M. L.: Six year review of the results of freehand aortic valve replacement using an antibiotic sterilised homograft valve. Circulation, 55:353, 1977.

Baudet, E. M., Oca, C. C., Roques, X. F., et al: A 5½ year experience with the St. Jude Medical cardiac valve prosthesis. J. Thorac. Cardiovasc. Surg., 90:137, 1985.

Beaudet, R. L., Poirier, N. L., Doyle, D., et al: The Medtronic-Hall cardiac valve: 7½ years' clinical experience. Ann. Thorac. Surg., 42:644, 1986.

Bentall, H. H., and DeBono, A.: A technique for complete replacement of the ascending aorta. Thorax, 23:338, 1968.

Binet, J. P., Duran, C. G., Carpentier, A., and Langlois, J.: Heterologous aortic valve transplantation. Lancet, 2:1275, 1965.

Bjork, V. O., and Henze, A.: Ten years' experience with the Bjork-Shiley tilting disc valve. J. Thorac. Cardiovasc. Surg., 78:331, 1979.

Bjork, V. O., Henze, A., and Holmgren, A.: Five years' experience with the Bjork-Shiley tilting-disc valve in isolated aortic valvular disease. J. Thorac. Cardiovasc. Surg., 7:1, 1973.

Block, P. C., and Palacios, I. F.: Comparison of hemodynamic results of anterograde versus retrograde percutaneous balloon aortic valvuloplasty. Am. J. Cardiol., 60:659, 1987.

Bonow, R. O., Picone, A. L., and McIntosh, C. L.: Survival and functional results after valve replacement for aortic regurgitation from 1976 to 1983. Impact of preoperative left ventricular dysfunction. Circulation, 70:4, 1984.

Boucher, C. A., Friedlich, A. L., and Buckley, M. J.: Aortic regurgitation. In Eagle, K. A., Haber, E., De Sanctis, R. W., and Austen, W. G. (eds): The Practice of Cardiology, 2nd ed. Boston, Little, Brown and Company, 1989.

Braunwald, E.: Valvular heart disease. In Braunwald, E. (ed): Heart Disease: A Textbook of Cardiovascular Medicine. Philadelphia, W. B. Saunders Company, 1988, pp. 1023–1092.

Braunwald, E., Lambrew, C. T., Rockoff, S. D., et al: Idiopathic hypertrophic subaortic stenosis. Circulation, 29/30(Suppl. 4):1, 1964.

Buckley, M. J., Mundth, E. D., Daggett, W. M., and Austen, W. G.: Surgical management of the complications of sepsis involving the aortic valve, aortic root, and ascending aorta. Ann. Thorac. Surg., 12:391, 1971.

Bulkley, B. H., and Roberts, W. C.: Ankylosing spondylitis and aortic regurgitation: Description of the characteristic cardiovascular lesion from study of eight necropsy patients. Circulation, 48:1014, 1973.

Carpentier, A., Deloche, A., Relland, J., et al: Six-year follow-up of glutaraldehyde-preserved heterografts. J. Thorac. Cardiovasc. Surg., 68:771, 1974.

Ciro, E., Nichols, P. F., III, and Maron, B. J.: Heterogeneous morphologic expression of genetically transmitted hypertrophic cardiomyopathy. Circulation, 67:1227, 1983.

Clark, C. E., Henry, W. L., and Epstein, S. E.: Familial prevalence and genetic transmission of idiopathic hypertrophic subaortic stenosis. N. Engl. J. Med., 189:709, 1973.

Cobanoglu, A., Fessler, C. L., Guvendik, L., et al: Aortic valve replacement with the Starr-Edwards prosthesis: A comparison of the first and second decades of follow-up. Ann. Thorac. Surg., 45:248, 1988.

Cooley, D. A., Leachman, R. D., and Wukasch, D. C.: Diffuse muscular subaortic stenosis: Surgical treatment. Am. J. Cardiol., 31:1, 1973.

Copeland, J. G., Griepp, R. B., Stinson, E. B., and Shumway, N. E.: Long-term follow-up after isolated aortic valve replacement. J. Thorac. Cardiovasc. Surg., 74:875, 1977.

Craver, J. M., Goldstein, J., Jones, E. L., et al: Clinical, hemodynamic, and operative descriptors affecting outcome of aortic valve replacement in elderly versus young patients. Ann. Surg., 199:733, 1984.

Crawford, E. S., Svensson, L. G., Coselli, J. S., et al: Aortic dissection and dissecting aortic aneurysms. Ann. Surg., 208:254, 1988.

Cribier, A., Savin, T., Saoudi, N., et al: Percutaneous transluminal valvuloplasty of acquired aortic stenosis in elderly patients: An alternative to valve replacement? Lancet, 1:63, 1986.

Daggett, W. M., Jacobs, M. L., Geffin, G. A., and O'Keefe, D. D.: The role of oxygenated solutions in cardioplegia. In Roberts, A. J. (ed): Myocardial Protection in Cardiac Surgery. New York, Marcel Dekker, 1987, pp. 295–302.

Davila, J. C., Magilligan, D. J., Jr., and Lewis, J. W., Jr.: Is the Hancock porcine valve the best cardiac valve substitute today? Ann. Thorac. Surg., 26:303, 1978.

DeSanctis, R. W., Doroghazi, R. M., Austen, W. G., and Buckley, M. J.: Aortic dissection. N. Engl. J. Med., 317:1060, 1987.

Donaldson, R. M., and Ross, D. M.: Homograft aortic root replacement for complicated prosthetic valve endocarditis. Circulation, 70: I-178, 1984.

Duran, C. G.: Reconstructive techniques for rheumatic aortic valve disease. J. Cardiac Surg., 3:23, 1988.

Duran, C. G., and Gunning, A. J.: A method for placing a total homologous aortic valve in the subcoronary position. Lancet, 2:488, 1962.

Edmunds, L. H., Jr.: Thrombotic and bleeding complications of prosthetic heart valves. Collective Review. Ann. Thorac. Surg., 44:430, 1987.

Ellis, F. H., Jr., and Kirklin, J. W.: Aortic stenosis. Surg. Clin. North Am., 35:1029, 1955.

Fenoglio, J. J., Jr., McAllister, H. A., Jr., DeCastro, C. M., et al: Congenital bicuspid aortic valve after age 20. Am. J. Cardiol., 39:164, 1977.

Frantz, P. T., Murray, G. F., and Wilcox, B. R.: Surgical management of left ventricular-aortic discontinuity complicating bacterial endocarditis. Ann. Thorac. Surg., 29:1, 1980.

Friedberg, C. K.: Diseases of the Heart, 3rd ed. Philadelphia, W. B. Saunders Company, 1966.

Friedlich, A. L., and Buckley, M. J.: Aortic regurgitation. In Johnson, R. A., Haber, E., and Austen, W. G. (eds): The Practice of Cardiology. Boston, Little, Brown and Company, 1980.

Gallo, I., Nistal, F., Blasquez, R., et al: Incidence of primary tissue valve failure in porcine bioprosthetic heart valves. Ann. Thorac. Surg., 45:66, 1988.

Gibbon, J. H.: Application of a mechanical heart and lung apparatus to cardiac surgery. Minn. Med., 37:171, 1954.

Golden, R. L., and Lakin, H.: The forme fruste in Marfan's syndrome. N. Engl. J. Med., 260:797, 1959.

Gorlin, R., and Gorlin, S. G.: Hydraulic formula for calculation of the area of the stenotic mitral valve, other cardiac valves, and central circulatory shunts. Am. Heart J., 41:1, 1951.

Harken, D. E., Soroff, H. S., Taylor, W. J., et al: Partial and complete prostheses in aortic insufficiency. J. Thorac. Cardiovasc. Surg., 40:744, 1960.

Hegglin, R, Scheu, H., and Rothlin, M.: Aortic insufficiency. Circulation, 37,38:V-77, 1968.

Hirst, A. E., and Gore, I.: The etiology and pathology of aortic dissection. In Doroghazi, R. M., and Slater, E. E. (eds): Aortic Dissection. New York, McGraw-Hill, 1983, pp. 13–54.

Hodgson, W. J. B.: The ultrasonic scalpel. Bull. N.Y. Acad. Med., 55:10, 1979.

Hufnagel, C. A., and Conrad, P. W.: The direct approach for the correction of aortic insufficiency. J.A.M.A., 178:275, 1961.

Hufnagel, C. A., and Harvey, W. P.: The surgical correction of aortic regurgitation: Preliminary report. Bull. Georgetown U. Med. Ctr., 6:60, 1953.

Hurley, P. J., Lowe, J. B., and Barratt-Boyes, B. G.: Debridement valvotomy for aortic stenosis in adults: A follow-up of 76 patients. Thorax, 22:314, 1967.

Ionescu, M. I., Pakrashi, B. C., Holden, M. P., et al: Results of aortic valve replacement with frame-supported fascia lata and pericardial grafts. J. Thorac. Cardiovasc. Surg., 64:340, 1972.

Ionescu, M. I., and Ross, D. N.: Heart-valve replacement with autologous fascia lata. Lancet, 2:1, 1969.

Ionescu, M. I., and Tandon, A. P.: Long-term clinical and hemodynamic evaluation of the Ionescu-Shiley pericardial xenograft valve. Thorax Chirurgie, 26:250, 1978.

Ionescu, M. I., and Tandon, A. P.: The Ionescu-Shiley pericardial xenograft heart valve. In Ionescu, M. I. (ed): Tissue Heart Valves. London, Butterworth, 1979.

Jacobs, M. L., Buckley, M. J., Austen, W. G., et al: A comparative evaluation of mechanical and bioprosthetic heart valves: Long-term results. In Bodnar, E., and Yacoub, M.: (eds): Biologic Bioprosthetic Valves. Proceedings of the Third International Symposium on Cardiac Bioprostheses, 1986a.

Jacobs, M. L., Buckley, M. J., Austen, W. G., et al: Mechanical valves: Ten year follow-up of Starr-Edwards and Bjork-Shiley prostheses (Abstract). Circ., 72:III-208, 1985.

Jacobs, M. L., Buckley, M. J., Austen, W. G., et al: Early prosthetic valve endocarditis (PVE): Analysis of risk factors. In Bodnar, E., and Yacoub, M. (eds): Biologic Bioprosthetic Valves: Proceedings of the Third International Symposium. New York, Yorke Medical Books, 1986b.

Jacobs, M. L., Fowler, B. N., Vezeridis, M. P., et al: Aortic valve replacement: A 9-year experience. Ann. Thorac. Surg., 30:439, 1980.

Jones, M., Eidbo, E. E., Walters, S. M., et al: Effects of 2 types of preimplantation processes on calcification of bioprosthetic valves. In Bodnar, E., and Yacoub, M. (eds): Biologic Bioprosthetic Valves. Proceedings of the Third International Symposium. New York, Yorke Medical Books, 1986, pp. 451–459.

Kelly, D. T., Barratt-Boyes, B. G., and Lowe, J. B.: Results of surgery and hemodynamic observations in muscular subaortic stenosis. J. Thorac. Cardiovasc. Surg., 51:353, 1966.

Khanna, S. K., Ross, J. K., and Monro, J. L.: Homograft aortic valve replacement: Seven years' experience with antibiotic-treated valves. Thorax, 36:330, 1981.

Kinsley, R. H., Antunes, M. J., and Colsen, P. R.: St. Jude Medical valve replacement: An evaluation of valve performance. J. Thorac. Cardiovasc. Surg., 92:349, 1986.

Kirklin, J. W., and Barratt-Boyes, B. G.: Aortic valve disease. In Cardiac Surgery. New York, John Wiley & Sons, 1986, pp. 373–429.

Kirklin, J. W., and Ellis, F. H.: Surgical relief of diffuse subvalvular aortic stenosis. Circulation, 25:739, 1961.

Kirklin, J. W., and Mankin, H. T.: Open operation in the treatment of calcific aortic stenosis. Circulation, 21:578, 1960.

Konno, S., Imai, Y., Iida, Y., et al: A new method for prosthetic valve replacement in congenital aortic stenosis associated with hypoplasia of the aortic valve ring. J. Thorac. Cardiovasc. Surg., 70:909, 1975.

Lakier, J. B., Copans, H., Rosman, H. S., et al: Idiopathic degeneration of the aortic valve: A common cause of isolated aortic regurgitation. J. Am. Coll. Cardiol., 5:347, 1985.

Lillehei, C. W., Barnard, C. N., Long, D. M., et al: Aortic valve reconstruction and replacement by total valve prostheses. In Merendino, K. A. (ed): Prosthetic Heart Valves for Cardiac Surgery. Springfield, IL, Charles C Thomas, 1961, pp. 527–575.

Lytle, B. W., Cosgrove, D. M., Loop, F. D., et al: Replacement of aortic valve combined with myocardial revascularization: Determinants of early and late risk for 500 patients, 1967–1981. Circulation, 68:1149, 1983.

Lytle, B. W., Cosgrove, D. M., Taylor, P. C., et al: Primary isolated aortic valve replacement: Early and late results. J. Thorac. Cardiovasc. Surg., 97:675, 1989.

Magilligan, D. J., Jr., Quinn, E. L., and Davila, J. C.: Bacteremia, endocarditis and the Hancock valve. Ann. Thorac. Surg., 24:508, 1977.

Manouguian, S., and Seybold-Epting, W.: Patch enlargement of the aortic valve ring by extending the aortic incision into the anterior mitral leaflet: New operative technique. J. Thorac. Cardiovasc. Surg., 78:402, 1979.

Maron, B. J.: Asymmetry in hypertrophic cardiomyopathy: The septal to free wall thickness ratio revisited. Am. J. Cardiol., 55:835, 1985.

Maron, B. J., and Roberts, W. C.: Hypertrophic cardiomyopathy and cardiac muscle cell disorganization revisited: Relation between the two and significance. Am. Heart J., 102:95, 1981.

Maron, B. J., Bonow, R. O., Cannon, R. O., et al: Hypertrophic cardiomyopathy: Interrelations of clinical manifestations, pathophysiology, and therapy. Part I. N. Engl. J. Med., 316:780, 1987a.

Maron, B. J., Bonow, R. O., Cannon, R. O., et al: Hypertrophic cardiomyopathy: Interrelations of clinical manifestations, pathophysiology, and therapy. Part II. N. Engl. J. Med., 316:844, 1987b.

Maron, B. J., Ferrans, V. J., and Roberts, W. C.: Myocardial ultrastructure in patients with chronic aortic valve disease. Am. J. Cardiol., 35:725, 1975.

Maron, B. J., Gottdiener, J. S., and Epstein, S. E.: Patterns and significance of distribution of left ventricular hypertrophy in hypertrophic cardiomyopathy: A wide-angle two-dimensional echocardiographic study of 125 patients. Am. J. Cardiol., 48:418, 1981.

Maron, B. J., Merrill, W. H., Freier, A. P., et al: Long-term clinical course and symptomatic status of patients after operation for hypertrophic subaortic stenosis. Circulation, 57:1205, 1978.

McGoon, D. C.: Prosthetic reconstruction of the aortic valve. Staff Meet. Mayo Clin., 36:88, 1961.

McGoon, D. C., Ellis, F. H., Jr., and Kirklin, J. W.: Late results of operation for acquired aortic valvular disease. Circulation, 31,32:I-108, 1965.

McIntosh, C. L., Greenberg, G. J., Maron, B. J., et al: Clinical and hemodynamic results after mitral valve replacement in patients with obstructive hypertrophic cardiomyopathy. Ann. Thorac. Surg., 47:236, 1989.

McKay, R. G., Safian, R. D., Lock, J. E., et al: Assessment of left ventricular and aortic valve function after aortic balloon valvuloplasty in adult patients with critical aortic stenosis. Circulation, 75:192, 1987.

McKenna, W. J.: Arrhythmia and prognosis in hypertrophic cardiomyopathy. Eur. Heart J., 4:225, 1983.

McKenna, W. J., Harris, L., Rowland, E., et al: Amiodarone for long-term management of patients with hypertrophic cardiomyopathy. Am. J. Cardiol., 54:802, 1984.

Miller, D. C., Stinson, E. B., Oyer, P. E., et al: Surgical implications and results of combined aortic valve replacement and myocardial revascularization. Am. J. Cardiol., 43:494, 1979.

Mindich, B. P., Guarino, T., and Goldman, M. E.: Aortic valvuloplasty for acquired aortic stenosis. Circulation, 72(Suppl. 3):209, 1985.

Morrow, A. G., Reitz, B. A., Epstein, S. E., et al: Operative treatment in hypertrophic subaortic stenosis: Techniques, and the results of pre- and post-operative assessment in 83 patients. Circulation, 52:88, 1975.

Morrow, A. G., Roberts, W. C., Ross, J., Jr., et al: Obstruction to left ventricular outflow. Ann. Intern. Med., 69:1255, 1968.

Muller, W. H., Jr., Littlefield, J. B., and Dammann, J. F.: Subcoronary prosthetic replacement of the aortic valve. In Merendino, K. A. (ed): Prosthetic Heart Valves for Cardiac Surgery. Springfield, IL, Charles C Thomas, 1961, pp. 493–526.

Murray, G.: Homologous aortic valve segment transplant as surgical treatment for aortic and mitral insufficiency. Angiology, 7:466, 1956.

Nicks, R., Cartmill, T., and Bernstein, L.: Hypoplasia of the aortic root. Thorax, 25:339, 1970.

Nistal, F., Garcia-Satue, E., Artinano, E., et al: Primary tissue failure in bioprosthetic glutaraldehyde-preserved heart valves: Bovine pericardial versus porcine tissue in the mid-term. In Bodnar, E., and Yacoub, M. (eds): Biologic Bioprosthetic Valves. Proceedings of the Third International Symposium. New York, Yorke Medical Books, 1986, pp. 233–244..

Norman, J. C., Cooley, D. A., Hallman, G. L., and Nihill, M. R.: Left ventricular apical-abdominal aortic conduits for left ventricular outflow tract obstructions: Clinical results in nine patients with a special composite prosthesis. Circulation, 54(Suppl.):100, 1976.

Norman, J. C., Nihill, M. R., and Cooley, D. A.: Valved apico-aortic composite conduits for left ventricular outflow tract obstructions. Am. J. Cardiol., 45:1265, 1980.

O'Brien, M. F., Stafford, E. G., Gardner, M. A., et al: A comparison of aortic valve replacement with viable cryopreserved and fresh allograft valves, with a note on chromosomal studies. J. Thorac. Cardiovasc. Surg., 94:812, 1987.

Ormiston, J. A., Neutze, J. M., Agnew, T. M., et al: Infective endocarditis: A lethal disease. Aust. N.Z. J. Med., 11:620, 1981.

Palacios, I., and Block, P. C.: Antegrade balloon valvotomy for aortic stenosis (Abstract). J. Am. Coll. Cardiol., 9:14A, 1987.

Parr, G. V. S., Kirklin, J. W., and Blackstone, E. H.: The early risks of replacement of aortic valves. Ann. Thorac. Surg., 23:319, 1977.

Powell, W. J., Jr.: Hypertrophic nondilated cardiomyopathy: Idiopathic hypertrophic subaortic stenosis and it variants. In Johnson, R. A., Haber, E., and Austen, W. G., (eds): The Practice of Cardiology. Boston, Little, Brown and Company, 1980, pp. 647–663.

Reitz, B. A., Stinson, E. B., Watson, D. C., et al: Translocation of the aortic valve for prosthetic valve endocarditis. J. Thorac. Cardiovasc. Surg., 81:212, 1981.

Reul, G. J., Cooley, D. A., Duncan, J., et al: Valve failure with the Ionescu-Shiley bovine pericardial bioprosthesis: Analysis of 2,680 patients. J. Vasc. Surg., 2:191, 1985.

Revuelta, J. M., Garcia-Rinaldi, R., Ubago, J. L., and Duran, C. G.: The Ionescu-Shiley pericardial valve in the small aortic anulus: A 7-year experience. In Bodnar, E., and Yacoub, M. (eds): Biologic and Bioprosthetic Valves. Proceedings of the Third International Symposium. New York, Yorke Medical Books, 1986, pp. 227–232.

Rittenhouse, E. A., Sauvage, L. R., Stamm, S. J., et al: Radical enlargement of the aortic root and outflow tract to allow valve replacement. Ann. Thorac. Surg., 27:367, 1979.

Roberts, W. C.: Anatomically isolated aortic valvular disease. The case against its being of rheumatic etiology. Am. J. Med., 49:151, 1970a.

Roberts, W. C.: The congenitally bicuspid aortic valve. A study of 85 autopsy cases. Am. J. Cardiol., 26:72, 1970b.

Roberts, W. C.: Valvular, subvalvular, and supravalvular aortic stenosis: Morphologic features. Cardiovasc. Clin., 5:97, 1973.

Roberts, W. C., and Honig, H. S.: The spectrum of cardiovascular disease in the Marfan syndrome: A clinico-morphologic study of 18 necropsy patients and comparison of 151 previously reported necropsy patients. Am. Heart J., 104:115, 1982.

Roberts, W. C., Kehoe, J. A., Carpenter, D. F., and Golden, A.: Cardiac valvular lesions in rheumatoid arthritis. Arch. Intern. Med., 122:141, 1980.

Roberts, W. C., Morrow, A. G., McIntosh, C. L., et al: Congenitally bicuspid aortic valve causing severe, pure aortic regurgitation without superimposed infective endocarditis. Am. J. Cardiol., 47:206, 1981.

Roberts, W. C., Perloff, J. K., and Costantino, T.: Severe valvular aortic stenosis in patients over 65 years of age. Am. J. Cardiol., 27:497, 1971.

Rosing, D. R., Idanpaan-Heikkila, U., Maron, B. J., et al: Use of calcium-channel blocking drugs in hypertrophic cardiomyopathy. Am. J. Cardiol., 55(Suppl):185B, 1985.

Ross, D. N.: Homograft replacement of the aortic valve. Lancet, 2:487, 1962.

Rottman, M., Morris, J. J., Behar, V. S., et al: Aortic valvular disease: Comparison of types and their medical and surgical management. Am. J. Med., 51:241, 1971.

Samuels, D. A., Curfman, G. D., Friedlich, A. L., et al: Valve replacement for aortic regurgitation: Long-term follow-up with factors influencing the results. Circulation, 60:647, 1979.

Sandor, G. G. S., Olley, P. M., Trusler, G. A., et al: Long-term follow-up of patients after valvotomy for congenital valvular aortic stenosis in children: A clinical and actuarial follow-up. J. Thorac. Cardiovasc. Surg., 80:171, 1980.

Sapsford, R. N., Blackstone, E. H., Kirklin, J. W., et al: Coronary perfusion versus cold ischemic arrest during aortic valve surgery: A randomized study. Circulation, 49:1190, 1974.

Scannell, J. G., and Austen, W. G.: Operative treatment of aortic stenosis in the elderly patient. N. Engl. J. Med., 270:96, 1964.

Scannell, J. G., Shaw, R. S., Burke, J. F., et al: Aortic valvuloplasty under direct vision. N. Engl. J. Med., 262:492, 1960.

Scannell, J. G., Shaw, R. S., Burke, J. F., et al: Operative treatment of aortic stenosis in the adult. Circulation, 27:772, 1963.

Schwartz, L. S., Goldfischer, J., Sprague, G. J., et al: Syncope and sudden death in aortic stenosis. Am. J. Cardiol., 23:647, 1969.

Scott, W. C., Miller, D. C., Haverich, A., et al: Determinants of operative mortality for patients undergoing aortic valve replacement. J. Thorac. Cardiovasc. Surg., 89:400, 1985.

Sell, S., and Scully, R. E.: Aging changes in the aortic and mitral valves. Histologic and histochemical studies, with observations on the pathogenesis of calcific aortic stenosis and calcification of the mitral annulus. Am. J. Pathol., 46:345, 1965.

Senning, A.: Fascia lata replacement of aortic valves. J. Thorac. Cardiovasc. Surg., 54:465, 1967.

Shah, P. M., Adelman, A. G., Wigle, E. D., et al: The natural (and unnatural) history of hypertrophic obstructive cardiomyopathy. Circ. Res., 34/35:179, 1974.

Shean, F. C., Austen, W. G., Buckley, M. J., et al: Survival after Starr-Edwards aortic valve replacement. Circulation, 44:1, 1971.

Smithy, H. G., and Parker, E. F.: Experimental aortic valvulotomy, preliminary report. Surg. Gynecol. Obstet., 34:625, 1947.

Speiser, K. W., and Krayenbuehl, H. P.: Reappraisal of the effect of acute beta-blockade on left ventricular filling dynamics in hypertrophic obstructive cardiomyopathy. Br. Heart J., 2:21, 1981.

Starr, A., Edwards, M. L., McCord, C. W., and Griswold, H. E.: Aortic replacement: Clinical experience with a semirigid ball-valve prosthesis. Circulation, 27:779, 1963.

Stewart, W. J., Galvin, K. A., Gillam, L. D., et al: Comparison of high pulse repetition frequency and continuous-wave Doppler echocardiography in the assessment of high flow velocity in patients with valvular stenosis and regurgitation. J. Am. Coll. Cardiol., 6:565, 1985.

Syracuse, D. C., Bowman, F. O., Jr., and Malm, J. R.: Prosthetic valve reoperations: Factors influencing early and late survival. J. Thorac. Cardiovasc. Surg., 77:346, 1979.

Takenaka, K., Dabestani, A., Gardin, J. M., et al: A simple Doppler echocardiographic method for estimating severity of aortic regurgitation. Am. J. Cardiol., 57:1340, 1986.

Teare, R. D.: Asymmetrical hypertrophy of the heart in young adults. Br. Heart J., 20:1, 1958.

Thibault, G. E., DeSanctis, R. W., and Buckley, M. J.: Aortic stenosis. In Johnson, R. A., Haber, E., and Austen, W. G. (eds): The Practice of Cardiology. Boston, Little, Brown and Company, 1980.

Thompson, R., Mitchell, A., Ahmed, M., et al: Conduction defects in aortic valve disease. Am. Heart J., 98:3, 1979a.

Thompson, R., Yacoub, M., Ahmed, M., et al: Influence of preoperative left ventricular function on results of homograft replacement of the aortic valve for aortic stenosis. Am. J. Cardiol., 43:929, 1979b.

Tuffier, T.: Étude expérimentale sur la chirurgie des valves de coeur. Bull. Acad. Med. Paris, 71:293, 1914.

Verdi, I. S., Monro, J. L., and Ross, J. K.: Aortic valve replacement with antibiotic-sterilized homograft valves: 11-year experience at Southampton. In Bodnar, E., and Yacoub, M. (eds): Biologic and Bioprosthetic Valves. Proceedings of the Third International Symposium. New York, Yorke Medical Books, 1986, p. 29.

Wideman, F. E., Blackstone, E. H., Kirklin, J. W., et al: The hospital mortality of re-replacement of the aortic valve: Incremental risk factors. J. Thorac. Cardiovasc. Surg., 82:870, 1981.

Wigle, E. D., Trimble, A. S., Adelman, G., and Bigelow, W. G.: Surgery in muscular subaortic stenosis. Prog. Cardiovasc. Dis., 11:83, 1968.

Williams, D. B., Danielson, G. K., McGoon, D. C., et al: Porcine heterograft valve replacement in children. J. Thorac. Cardiovasc. Surg., 84:446, 1982.

Wynne, J., and Braunwald, E.: The cardiomyopathies and myocarditides. In Braunwald, E. (ed): Heart Disease: A Textbook of Cardiovascular Medicine. Philadelphia, W. B. Saunders Company, 1988, pp. 1410–1469.

Zerbini, E. J.: Results of replacement of cardiac valves by homologous dura mater valves (Abstract). J.A.M.A., 233:1433, 1975.

CHAPTER 53

CARDIAC PACEMAKERS AND CARDIAC CONDUCTION SYSTEM ABNORMALITIES

James E. Lowe
Lawrence D. German

Although cardiac electrostimulation has a long and fascinating history beginning in the 18th century, the modern artificial cardiac pacemaker has followed technologic advances during the last 2 decades. The implantable pacemaker is one of modern medicine's greatest contributions to prolonging and improving human life. The exact number of persons now living with an artificial pacemaker is unknown. However, estimates are that approximately 500,000 persons now living in the United States have pacemakers, and each year 100,000 or more require permanent pacemaker implantation (Parsonnet et al, 1984). It is estimated that 1.5 to 2 million pacemakers have been implanted worldwide during the last 20 years (Chung, 1984).

Advances in pacemaker design are now occurring so rapidly that refinements that previously required years of research and development are now achieved within months. Recent technologic improvements resulting from aerospace research programs are mainly responsible for this progress. The development and application of future pacemakers and antiarrhythmic devices require an interdisiplinary interface between cardiovascular surgeons, cardiologists, basic electrophysiologists, and biomedical engineers in an era of continued cost containment and expense justification.

HISTORICAL ASPECTS

Cardiac electrostimulation began in the mid-18th century with the use of currents from the Leyden's jar or voltaic pile to stimulate cardiac nerves and cardiac muscle in animals and to attempt resuscitation of intact dead animals (Schechter, 1971). Electrostimulation was suggested for human resuscitation in a number of communications to the Royal Humane Society of London by Squires, Henley, and Fothergill between 1774 and 1784 (Registers of the Royal Humane Society of London, 1774–1784; Schechter, 1971). However, Aldini, in 1774, was the first to use intermittent precordial electrical stimulation to successfully revive a child who had fallen downstairs (Aldini, 1819). These reports may have led Hunter (1776) to recommend that electrostimulation be attempted as a last resort in the resuscitation of drowning victims. Nysten (1802), using the body of a recently executed convict, demonstrated that the heart lost its ability to be electrically reactivated, first in the left ventricle, then in the right ventricle, then in the left atrium, and then in the right atrium. Later in the 19th century, Walshe (1862) and Duchenne (1872) advocated electrostimulation for cardiac standstill. During this same period, Althaus (1864) and Steiner (1871) reported successful resuscitation of cardiac arrest victims by electrical currents applied through transthoracic needles.

Von Ziemssen (1882) reported a 42-year-old woman, Catharina Serafin, who had a huge defect of the anterior left chest wall after resection of an enchondroma. The heart was covered only by a thin layer of skin and was visible and palpable (Fig. 53–1). Von Ziemssen noted that application of electrodes to the heart produced rhythmic stimulation only if the rate of stimulation was greater than the spontaneous heart rate. Slower stimulation rates produced erratic and occasionally slower heart rates. He also noted while placing the electrodes that the most sensitive area for stimulation was in the region of the atrioventricular (AV) groove. This observation was made more than a decade before His (1893) and Kent (1893) described the location of the AV node and the bundle of His.

Prevost and Battelli (1899) showed that electrical currents could cause ventricular fibrillation that often could be reversed by another powerful discharge of alternating or direct current. Robinovitch (1907–1909), in a series of reports, confirmed this work and designed the first portable electrical resuscitative apparatus for ambulances. MacWilliam, in many publications beginning in 1899 and extending until World War I, further elucidated the pathophysiology of ventricular fibrillation and described deterioration of

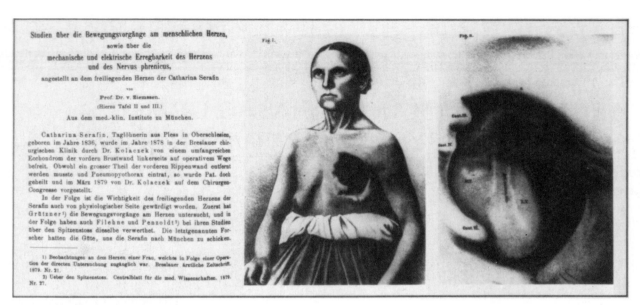

Figure 53–1. Hugo von Ziemssen's manuscript describing Catharina Serafin. Frau Serafin had a large defect in the left anterior chest wall after resection of an enchondroma. As shown in the second panel, the heart was covered only by skin, thus allowing von Ziemssen the opportunity to electrically stimulate various parts of the human heart. (From Schechter, D. C.: Exploring the origins of electrical cardiac stimulation, VII World Symposium on Cardiac Pacing, Vienna, Austria, May 1983. Minneapolis, Medtronic, Inc., 1983. Reprinted with permission of Medtronic, Inc.)

cardiac pump function by both tachyarrhythmias and bradyarrhythmias (Schechter, 1972).

These early experimental and clinical experiences did not lead to immediate clinical trials of cardiac pacing or electrical defibrillation. Schechter suggested that this initial apathy may have been due to the medical profession's interest in other techniques of cardiac reanimation, including pharmacologic injections, blood transfusions, electrolyte infusions, and cardiac massage (Schechter, 1971, 1972). The efforts of Kouwenhoven and colleagues (1932) and Beck and associates (1947) helped electrical defibrillation become widely applied clinically. Delayed communications and unnoticed publications were also an obstacle to progress in the development of cardiac pacing (Samet and El-Sherif, 1980). Studies in Europe by Marmorstein (1927) using both transvenous and transthoracic electrodes to pace the right atrium, right ventricle, and left ventricle in dogs were essentially unnoticed in the United States. This is evident from the reports of Bigelow and colleagues (1950), who independently described similar studies using transvenous electrodes to pace the right atrium of dogs. If these investigators had advanced electrodes into the right ventricle, which was done by Marmorstein, a clinical method to treat complete heart block might have been developed earlier. Similarly, the contributions of Gould, who designed a pulse generator and transthoracic pacing needle electrode and successfully resuscitated a patient, went unnoticed in the United States. This work was presented in Australia but was not published except for mention of it later by Hyman (1932). However, a report by Mond and associates (1982) suggests that Gould did not exist and that the Australians actually

responsible for the development of the first impulse generator were Lidwill and Booth.

Developments Leading to the Modern Pacemaker

Hyman (1932) developed a machine for controlled repetitive electrostimulation of the heart and called this device "the artificial cardiac pacemaker" (Fig. 53–2). This device was used successfully in a

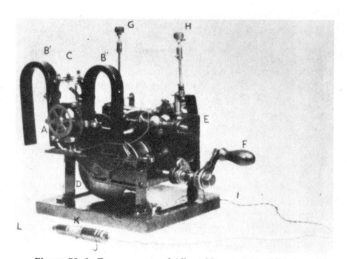

Figure 53–2. Components of Albert Hyman's "artificial cardiac pacemaker." Regular-spaced, repeated stimuli were delivered through a needle passed across the intact chest wall into the right atrium. (From Schechter, D. C.: Exploring the origins of electrical cardiac stimulation, VII World Symposium on Cardiac Pacing, Vienna, Austria, May 1983. Minneapolis, Medtronic, Inc., 1983. Reprinted with permission of Medtronic, Inc.)

number of animal experiments. By using a transthoracic needle electrode, the artificial cardiac pacemaker was subsequently used to resuscitate for brief intervals several patients with complete heart block and syncope. Unfortunately, these reports were never published because Hyman was subjected to abusive correspondence and even lawsuits from those who regarded his attempts at resuscitation by pacing as tampering with "Divine Providence" (Schechter, 1983).

Zoll (1952) first described successful pacing through external metal electrodes applied to the anterior chest wall in two patients (Fig. 53–3). The initial impulse generator was a Grass stimulator. This noninvasive technique was easy to apply and was much better accepted than the invasive techniques of Hyman or Bigelow and Callaghan. Zoll's continued work and many publications convinced the medical profession as well as the general public that cardiac pacing was both feasible and lifesaving. Disadvantages of the external pacing technique included skin burns when inadequate electrode jelly was applied, painful chest wall muscle contractions in some patients, and inability to pace in thick-chested or emphysematous patients.

The new field of cardiac operations provided a major impetus in pacemaker development, because complete heart block was sometimes created during operations such as pulmonic commissurotomy and closure of ventricular septal defect (VSD). Brockman and colleagues (1958) used a wire electrode to successfully pace the heart of an infant who developed complete heart block after closure of a VSD. Although this patient died, pacing was effective and uninterrupted for 10 hours. Intramyocardial electrodes placed at the time of operation or introduced percu-

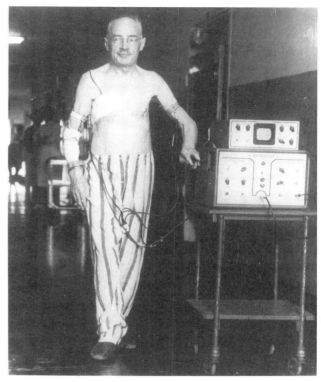

Figure 53–4. The feasibility of prolonged cardiac pacing using a right ventricular endocardial wire electrode connected to an external generator was demonstrated by Furman in 1958. Successful pacing was maintained for 96 days. The unipolar catheter attached to the external impulse generator allowed the patient to ambulate. (Courtesy of Dr. Seymour Furman.)

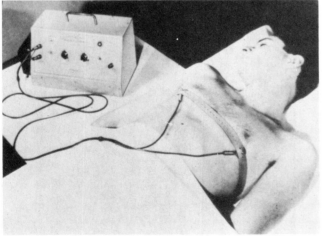

Figure 53–3. Zoll's successful pacing technique using external metal electrodes applied to the anterior chest wall. Zoll's contributions convinced the medical profession as well as the general public that cardiac pacing was both feasible and lifesaving. (From Schechter, D. C.: Exploring the origins of electrical cardiac stimulation, VII World Symposium on Cardiac Pacing, Vienna, Austria, May 1983. Minneapolis, Medtronic, Inc., 1983. Reprinted with permission of Medtronic, Inc.)

taneously through a needle were popularized in 1957 by the researchers at the University of Minneapolis (Allen and Lillehei, 1957; Gott et al, 1960; Lillehei et al, 1960, 1964; Thevenet et al, 1958; Weirich and Roe, 1961; Weirich et al, 1957, 1958a, 1958b). The electrodes were insulated silver-plated copper wires with exposed tips. These intramyocardial electrodes were connected to a self-contained external pacemaker containing transistors and a mercury battery. The disadvantages of this technique included lead dislodgment and steadily rising thresholds of the myocardial wire electrode.

In August of 1958, Furman and Schwedel used a right ventricular endocardial wire electrode connected to an external generator to successfully pace for 96 hours a 76-year-old patient with complete heart block (Furman and Robinson 1959; Furman et al, 1961; Schwedel et al, 1960) (Fig. 53–4). This experience showed that prolonged cardiac pacing with low voltages could be accomplished with an endocardial right ventricular electrode connected to an external pacemaker. Other important and independent developments in the field of cardiac electrostimulation also occurred during this period. Elmquist and Senning (1960) first implanted a rechargeable pacemaker in an epigastric pocket connected to electrodes that passed subcutaneously to the heart. Glenn and associates (1959) developed a method of cardiac pacing that used radiofrequency transmission. This method required an external pulse generator but had the advantage of leaving the skin intact.

Chardack and colleagues (1960) developed a transistorized, self-contained implantable pacemaker connected to modified Hunter-Roth epicardial electrodes (Hunter et al, 1959). This was the first implantable permanent pacemaker with the pacing lead attached to the heart by thoracotomy (Fig. 53–5). Other completely implantable units developed by Zoll and colleagues (1961) and by Kantrowitz and associates (1962) followed. The technique for inserting a permanent transvenous bipolar pacemaker was developed in the United States by Parsonnet and colleagues (1962) and in Sweden by Ekestrom and associates (1962). In the most common method of pacing, the permanent impulse generator is now implanted near the site where the lead enters the cephalic or subclavian vein.

These initial implantable permanent pacemakers were fixed-rate asynchronous devices that delivered the impulse independently of the underlying cardiac rate. Noncompetitive demand pacing of the ventricles was later introduced by Leatham and associates (1956) and by Nicks and co-workers (1962) using external pacemakers. A brief period of asystole (1 to 2 seconds) triggered the onset of pacing, but deactivation of pacing required manual intervention. The use of implantable demand pacemakers that initiated pacing automatically in response to a single R-R interval prolongation with suppression on return of rhythm to a baseline R-R rate was first reported by Lemberg and associates (1965). Extensive clinical trials showing the efficacy of demand pacing were later reported by Goetz and associates (1966), Parsonnet and colleagues (1966), and Furman and co-workers (1967).

During the late 1960s, increased numbers' of patients with sinus bradycardia and intact conduction were recognized. R wave inhibited and synchronous pulse generators began to be applied to the atrium, and eventually bifocal pacemakers were designed to provide AV sequential pacing in patients with sinus bradycardia and heart block (Berkovits et al, 1969; Smyth et al, 1971). During the 1960s, new and improved pacemaker power sources were developed. Mercury-zinc batteries were used initially and usually lasted for less than 2 years. The mass of these cells

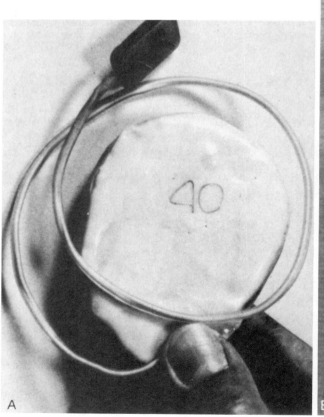
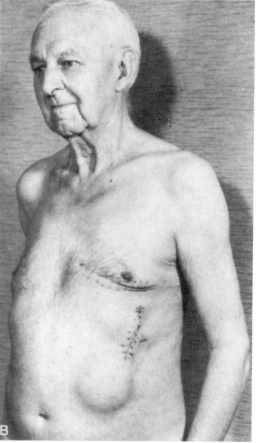

Figure 53–5. *A,* The first totally implantable pacemaker developed in 1960 by Chardack, Gage, and Greatbach. The pacemaker was connected to modified Hunter-Roth epicardial electrodes. *B,* The first patient to receive a Chardack, Gage, Greatbach totally implantable pacemaker. (From Schechter, D. C.: *In* Exploring the origins of electrical cardiac stimulation, VII World Symposium on Cardiac Pacing, Vienna, Austria, May, 1983, Medtronic, Inc., 1983. Reprinted with permission of Medtronic, Inc.)

represented two-thirds to three-quarters of the volume and even more of the weight of the pacemaker. Although various new power sources were tested, the lithium-iodine battery was soon recognized to be the best power source. In general, it is thought that the modern lithium-iodine battery may last for as long as 10 to 12 years. Nuclear-powered plutonium pacemakers are thought to last for a minimum of 10 to more than 20 years. However, cost and environmental restrictions have essentially eliminated their use in the United States.

NORMAL CARDIAC CONDUCTION SYSTEM

Impulse Formation

In the resting state, the myocardial cell maintains an electrical gradient or voltage potential across its cell membrane known as the *resting membrane potential*. The cell membrane is a semipermeable barrier through which ions can pass with various degrees of ease. In addition to the passive diffusion of ions along chemical or electrical gradients, active transport processes or "pumps" move ions against these gradients. The resting potential is the result of transmembrane differences in the concentrations of various ions, mainly sodium and potassium. The intracellular potassium concentration is much higher than that in the extracellular fluid. The opposite is true for sodium ions. The cell membrane is more permeable to potassium than to sodium, and potassium ions tend to pass outward through the cell membrane down the concentration gradient. This outward flow of positively charged ions causes a voltage gradient across the cell membrane. Because the flux of potassium ions is greater, potassium is the chief determinant of the voltage gradient at equilibrium. This equilibrium potential can be approximated by Nernst's equation, which relates the transmembrane potential to the ratio of extracellular and intracellular potassium concentrations:

$$V = \frac{RT}{F} \ln \frac{[K^+]_o}{[K^+]_i}$$

where R is the universal gas constant, T is the absolute temperature, and F is the Faraday constant. The cell membrane is a biologic system subject to variation, and the relationship between transmembrane potential and potassium levels becomes nonlinear at extremes of intra- or extracellular potassium concentrations. Changes in membrane permeability to other ions such as sodium at these extremes may also make their contribution to transmembrane potential more significant.

At equilibrium, when there is no net change in ion concentrations across the cell membrane, the equilibrium or resting potential is constant. For myocardial cells, the equilibrium potential is approxi-

mately -90 mV. *Depolarization* refers to a change in membrane potential to a less negative value (toward zero). When cell membranes are depolarized to a particular critical value, the threshold potential, a chain reaction of events is triggered, resulting in complete, rapid depolarization followed by repolarization. When these events are recorded from a microelectrode placed inside the cell, an action potential is obtained (Fig. 53–6A). The phases of the action potential are the result of various transmembrane ionic currents, and rapid inward flux of sodium is mainly responsible for the rapid upstroke (phase 0) of the action potential recorded from myocardial cells and Purkinje fibers.

Certain cells, notably those in the sinoatrial (SA) node, display the property of automaticity. Automaticity refers to the spontaneous phase IV depolarization noted in recordings from these cells (Fig. 53–6B). The resting membrane potential of these cells is considerably lower (less negative) than that in myo-

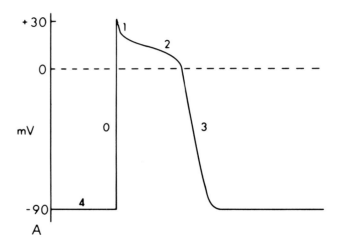

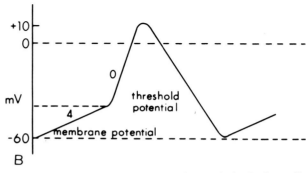

Figure 53–6. *A,* An action potential typical of a Purkinje fiber or ventricular myocardial cell. The resting membrane potential is -90 mV, and there is no spontaneous phase 4 depolarization. The upstroke (phase 0) is rapid. *B,* An action potential recorded from a cell displaying automaticity such as found in the SA and AV nodes. Spontaneous phase IV depolarization is present. The resting membrane potential is lower (-60 mV), and the upstroke is slower.

cardial cells and Purkinje fibers, and phase 0 is slower. The depolarization of these cells depends on slow channel currents, thought to be carried by calcium as well as sodium ions. The transmembrane potential in cells displaying automaticity does not remain constant in phase IV, but undergoes spontaneous depolarization until the threshold potential is reached and an action potential is generated. A wave of depolarizing current then passes from one cell to another throughout the myocardium. Automaticity is normally a property of cells in the SA node and, to a lesser extent, cells of the AV node. Under abnormal conditions, Purkinje fibers and myocardial cells may also develop automaticity.

Myocardial cells can also be depolarized by means of artificially applied electrical stimuli. The stimulus must have sufficient strength to bring a critical number of cells up to the threshold potential, which results in a propagated impulse. When an activation wavefront is initiated by an artificial stimulus, it propagates throughout the myocardium. This unique property of myocardial cells forms the basis for artificial cardiac pacing.

Functional Anatomy of the Conduction System

The SA node is a group of specialized cells located subepicardially at the lateral junction of the superior vena cava with the right atrium, although some anatomic variation may occur with extension of the node anteriorly across the caval-atrial junction. The SA node is especially vulnerable to surgical trauma because of its location. Three types of cells can be found in the human SA node, in addition to supporting elements of fibrocytes, nerves, and vessels (Lowe et al, 1988). Pacemaker or polygonal cells are polyhedral and contain prominent nuclei and sparse numbers of contractile elements. These cells are believed to be the site of impulse formation in the SA node, although electrophysiologic confirmation in humans is lacking. Transitional cells are found surrounding pacemaker cells and interposed between nodal cells and atrial myocardium. These cells have some features of both nodal cells and myocardial cells, with larger numbers of contractile elements. Atrial myocardial cells with prominent longitudinally oriented myofibrils may also be found in SA node tissue.

The AV node is located subendocardially in the triangle of Koch, an anatomic region on the medial wall of the right atrium formed by the tendon of Todaro, the eustachian valve of the coronary sinus, and the tricuspid annulus. The AV node is composed of a transitional zone and a compact zone. The cells of the compact zone are more distal and are arranged in fascicles that merge into the penetrating bundle of His (Anderson et al, 1981). The cells of the transitional zone are thought to provide distinct input pathways into the AV node from the atrium, and although the orientation of atrial muscle fibers appears to produce preferential pathways of conduction, evidence for functionally distinct conduction pathways across the atrium from the SA node (internodal tracts) is lacking.

Decremental conduction is a characteristic feature of conduction through the AV node. This refers to the normal slowing of conduction that occurs as impulses traverse the node from the atrium to the bundle of His. The AV node is the site of physiologic AV block (Wenckebach's or Mobitz Type I) that occurs when excessively rapid atrial rates (usually more than 150 to 160 beats per minute) are present. Conduction through the AV node depends heavily on autonomic tone. Withdrawal of vagal tone due to exercise or administration of atropine results in accelerated AV conduction, whereas increased vagal tone results in slower AV conduction or transient AV block.

The delay in conduction that occurs in the AV node is responsible for the majority of the P-R interval of the standard electrocardiogram (ECG) as well as the AH interval of the bundle of His recording. Normal conduction times across the AV node are between 60 and 120 msec, whereas conduction throughout the entire His-Purkinje system to the ventricles normally requires only 35 to 45 msec.

Conduction of impulses may proceed retrogradely from ventricle to atrium across the AV node. Retrograde conduction has been estimated to be intact in two-thirds of normal humans (Akhtar, 1981). Retrograde VA block often occurs in or below the bundle of His, compared with antegrade conduction block that normally occurs in the AV node.

When the cardiac impulse traverses the AV node, it rapidly courses down the bundle of His, which pierces the central fibrous body and divides into the left and right bundle branches. The bundle branches are composed of specialized cells oriented longitudinally with end-to-end connections. These conduction fibers traverse the subendocardium of the interventricular septum and carry the impulse to the distal ramifications of the Purkinje system, where activation of ventricular myocardium occurs. The right bundle branch is a single distinct strand of fibers, whereas the fibers to the left ventricle divide into numerous ramifications with multiple interconnections.

INDICATIONS FOR PACEMAKER THERAPY

Artificial cardiac pacing has clearly led to the prolongation and improvement of the lives of thousands of patients with conduction system disorders. However, pacing is a costly type of therapy. In 1976, the average cost of pacing was estimated to be $102 per month per patient for the lifetime of the individual (Stoney et al, 1976). Inflation and rising hospital costs combined with the additional expense of improved pacing technology have further increased the overall cost of cardiac pacing. However, each advance in cardiac pacing has proved to be cost-effective (Goldman and Parsonnet, 1979). Important advances containing the cost of permanent pacing have included improved electrodes and power sources, hermetic sealing of impulse generators, transtelephonic follow-up, and multiprogrammability of impulse generators. These advances have led to decreased rehospitalization and reoperation rates and lower follow-up costs. In fact, based on 1970 dollars, the current cost of pacing per patient year is approximately $40 per month (Goldman and Parsonnet, 1979). A major challenge facing pacemaker manufacturers is the continued development of new products that provide improved clinical results with lower overall medical costs. Recent advances indicate that this goal is possible and should be a major consideration in the design of future pacing systems. Physicians, however, must be responsible for choosing the appropriate pacing system, either permanent or temporary, for the specific cardiac conduction disorder being treated. In the early 1960s, symptomatic complete AV block was almost the sole indication for permanent pacing. Although complete heart block is still a major indication, symptomatic patients with the sick sinus syndrome now represent the most common indication for permanent pacing.

Although there is still some controversy regarding indications for temporary and permanent cardiac pacing as well as the type of pacing system chosen, most physicians would agree with the following guidelines.

Indications for Temporary Pacing

Three major factors that help to determine the indications for temporary pacing include (1) symptoms such as dizziness, near syncope, frank syncope, hypotension, and heart failure; (2) ventricular rate; and (3) clinical circumstances, which include the patient's underlying heart disease and the direct cause of the dysrhythmia being evaluated for temporary pacing. In general, ventricular rates less than 45 beats per minute produce symptoms and require temporary pacing. Acute dysrhythmias require temporary pacing more often than chronic arrhythmias. This appears to be particularly important in dealing with acute dysrhythmias associated with recent myocardial infarction. Indications for temporary pacing are shown in Table 53–1.

Symptomatic, Second Degree, and Complete AV Block. Wenckebach's (Mobitz Type I) AV block rarely requires temporary pacing unless the patient is symptomatic or the ventricular rate is slower than 45 beats per minute. Wenckebach's AV block is commonly due to enhanced vagal tone. In high-grade AV block, symptoms and the ventricular rate are the

TABLE 53–1. INDICATIONS FOR TEMPORARY PACING

Symptomatic second-degree and complete AV block

Symptomatic bradyarrhythmias after acute myocardial infarction

New bifascicular or trifascicular block after acute myocardial infarction

Sick sinus syndrome (selected patients before permanent pacemaker insertion)

Symptomatic drug-induced bradyarrhythmias

Drug-resistant tachyarrhythmias (selected patients)

Carotid sinus syncope (selected patients)

Before permanent pacemaker implantation in selected patients

Therapeutic trial in patients with medically refractory low cardiac output

After cardiac surgery

Ventricular tachycardia (torsades de pointes) associated with long Q-T interval or bradycardia

determining factors for insertion of a temporary pacemaker. Generally, temporary pacing is indicated in this group of patients who have symptoms that include dizziness, near syncope, frank syncope, hypotension, or congestive heart failure. Infranodal advanced or complete AV block frequently requires permanent pacing. Temporary pacing may be indicated before implantation of a permanent pacemaker, depending on the patient's ventricular rate and on the presence or absence of symptoms.

Symptomatic Bradyarrhythmias After Acute Myocardial Infarction. Acute diaphragmatic myocardial infarction often leads to bradyarrhythmias that are usually transient and seldom require artificial pacing. However, when the ventricular rate is significantly slow (less than 45 beats per minute), or when the bradyarrhythmia becomes refractory to pharmacologic agents such as atropine and isoproterenol, or if symptoms develop, temporary pacing is indicated. Although less common, AV block due to anterior myocardial infarction usually represents infranodal block, which usually requires permanent cardiac pacing. However, a temporary pacemaker may be necessary before permanent pacing when the patient is symptomatic or the ventricular rate is inadequate.

New Bifascicular or Trifascicular Block After Acute Myocardial Infarction. In general, prophylactic temporary pacing should be considered in patients with acute bifascicular block or trifascicular block after acute infarction. Although some cardiologists have recommended prophylactic pacing for isolated acute left bundle branch block or for isolated left posterior hemiblock and right bundle branch block after infarction, the role of pacing in these disorders is still uncertain. Most physicians would agree that temporary pacing is not indicated in patients with myocardial infarction who display only acute left anterior hemiblock or in those with pre-existing bifascicular block.

Sick Sinus Syndrome. Patients with advanced sick sinus syndrome often require permanent pacing. Many develop bradyarrhythmias as well as tachyarrhythmias and require a combination of pacemaker therapy and antiarrhythmic drug therapy. Temporary cardiac pacing is occasionally necessary before permanent pacemaker implantation in those patients who are symptomatic and have near syncope or syncope. In most of these patients, temporary pacing can be accomplished with conventional ventricular demand pacing. However, in those who require the atrial component to cardiac filling, temporary atrial pacing or dual-chamber pacing may be required.

Symptomatic Digitalis-Induced Bradyarrhythmias. Temporary cardiac pacing is indicated in symptomatic patients with marked bradyarrhythmia due to digitalis toxicity. Digitalis-induced bradyarrhythmias include sinus bradycardia, sinus arrest, second-degree AV block, and advanced or complete AV block.

Drug-Resistant Tachyarrhythmias. When tachyarrhythmias, particularly ventricular tachycardia, become refractory to antiarrhythmic drug therapy, artificial overdrive pacing (80 to 120 beats per minute) is occasionally effective. Various modes of temporary pacing can be attempted, but atrial or coronary sinus pacing is usually ideal, particularly in patients in whom the atrial contribution to cardiac output is essential.

Carotid Sinus Syncope. Permanent pacemaker implantation is indicated in patients with carotid sinus syncope or near syncope resulting from bradycardia. Syncope due to hypotension (vasodepressor syncope) do not respond to pacing. In some patients, hypersensitive carotid sinus reactions may be greatly exaggerated by drugs such as digitalis, methyldopa, guanethidine, and propranolol. Temporary pacing is occasionally indicated in this group while the offending drug is withdrawn.

Before Permanent Pacemaker Implantation. Most patients requiring permanent pacemaker implantation do not require a preoperative temporary pacemaker. However, temporary pacing is essential before permanent implantation in patients with acute arrhythmias, especially after acute myocardial infarction or in symptomatic patients with complete AV block.

Therapeutic Trial for Congestive Heart Failure, Cardiogenic Shock, and Cerebral or Renal Insufficiency. It is becoming increasingly apparent that some patients with intractable congestive heart failure, cardiogenic shock, and cerebral or renal hypoperfusion may be improved by an increased heart rate. Generally, atrial or coronary sinus pacing is chosen because the atrial contribution to cardiac output appears to be essential in patients with low perfusion states. Therefore, temporary pacing should be considered as a therapy in this difficult subgroup of patients. In patients who respond, permanent pacemaker implantation may be considered for long-term therapy.

After Cardiac Surgery. Temporary atrial or AV sequential pacing through temporary epicardial electrodes may decrease the need for inotropic support in the perioperative period. Transient conduction disturbances are often encountered in the immediate perioperative period, and temporary epicardial pacing is essential. An additional advantage is that atrial dysrhythmias that occur perioperatively can be diagnosed more accurately through recording of electrograms from these temporary wires, and overdrive pacing can often be used to convert perioperative atrial flutter and occasionally atrial fibrillation (Waldo and MacLean, 1980). Most cardiac surgeons routinely attach temporary atrial and ventricular pacing wires after major cardiac surgical procedures.

Indications For Permanent Pacing

Implantation of a permanent cardiac pacemaker commits the physician and patient to a lifetime of appropriate follow-up care and also exposes the patient to the possible complications of permanent pacing. In the early 1960s, after the introduction of the completely implantable pacing system, the major indication for permanent pacemaker therapy was complete AV block associated with presyncope or syncope. During the last several years, however, indications for implantation of permanent pacemakers have changed. Although complete AV block remains a definite indication for permanent pacing, most permanent pacemakers implanted are in patients with the sick sinus syndrome. Many patients with this syndrome have coexisting conduction disturbances, including AV block or fascicular block or both. When it has been decided that a patient is a candidate for a permanent pacemaker, the type and mode of the pacemaker most suitable for each patient must be determined. Factors involved in selecting an appropriate pacing system include the patient's age, general condition, underlying heart disease, and the characteristics of the dysrhythmia being treated. When sinus rhythm predominates, a simple ventricular inhibited-demand pacemaker is often adequate. However, in patients in whom frequent or constant pacing is anticipated, a pacemaker that allows a changing heart rate according to physiologic demands with exercise should be used. Dual-chamber pacing is indicated in those who have shown that the atrial component of cardiac filling is essential for adequate cardiac output. The general trend now is toward the use of more dual-chamber or single-chamber rate-modulated pacemakers with multiprogrammable capability so that various pacing parameters can be adjusted noninvasively as the patient's need for pacing changes.

As with temporary pacing, opinions about the indications for permanent cardiac pacing differ. Indications for permanent pacing have been outlined in detail by a joint task force of the American College of Cardiology, and the American Heart Association (1984) and are shown in Table 53–2.

Sick Sinus Syndrome and Bradycardia-Tachycardia Syndrome. Pharmacologic therapy alone is often ineffective in patients with the sick sinus syndrome, and permanent pacing is indicated in those who remain symptomatic because of bradycardia. The most common manifestation of the sick sinus syndrome is marked sinus bradycardia associated with intermittent sinus arrest or SA node block and episodes of AV junctional escape rhythm. In more advanced forms of the sick sinus syndrome, chronic atrial fibrillation may develop and may be associated with a slow ventricular rate secondary to advanced AV block. An additional group of patients develop various atrial tachyarrhythmias in association with the sick sinus syndrome. These components of the sick sinus syndrome are referred to as the bradyarrhythmia-tachyarrhythmia syndrome, which is a common result of advanced sick sinus syndrome.

In many patients, a ventricular inhibited-demand pacemaker is adequate therapy. However, in patients in whom the atrial contribution to cardiac output is essential, dual-chamber pacing should be used. Atrial arrhythmias can be suppressed occasionally by atrial pacing. In patients with the bradyarrhythmia-tachyarrhythmia syndrome, one or more antiarrhythmic agents are frequently required in addition to permanent pacemaker therapy.

Mobitz Type II AV Block. It is generally believed that permanent pacing is indicated for patients with Mobitz Type II AV block, associated with a wide QRS complex, regardless of whether the patient is symptomatic or not. It has been documented that Mobitz Type II AV block frequently leads to advanced AV block (Dhingra et al, 1974).

TABLE 53–2. INDICATIONS FOR PERMANENT PACING

Complete AV block with
  Syncope or presyncope
  Congestive heart failure
  Ventricular tachycardia
  Heart rate less than 40 or asystole greater than 3 seconds
  Cerebral hypoperfusion

Second-degree AV block with symptoms

Acute myocardial infarction with persistent second-degree AV block or complete AV block

Chronic bifascicular or trifascicular block with symptomatic intermittent complete or second-degree AV block

Sinus bradycardia or sinus pauses with symptoms

Hypersensitive carotid sinus syndrome with recurrent syncope

Atrial fibrillation with slow ventricular rate and symptoms

Complete AV Block. Before pacemaker therapy became clinically available, 50% of patients with complete heart block died within 1 year (Friedberg et al, 1964; Johansson, 1969). Complete heart block is frequently caused by sclerodegenerative disease of the cardiac skeleton or of the conduction system itself and is often preceded by the development of bifascicular blocks such as right bundle branch block with left- or right-axis deviation and left bundle branch block. Therefore, most surgeons would agree that complete AV block represents a definite indication for permanent cardiac pacing. In addition to sclerodegenerative diseases, other causes of acquired complete AV block include ischemic myocardial injury, infiltrative cardiomyopathies, Chagas' disease, traumatic injuries, and cardiac procedures. Permanent pacing is usually recommended for surgically induced complete heart block lasting more than 1 week after operation. Complete AV block associated with acute anterior wall myocardial infarction is often irreversible and requires permanent pacemaker implantation (Domenighetti and Perret, 1980; Hindman et al, 1978). Conversely, complete AV block after a diaphragmatic myocardial infarction can usually be reversed and may only require temporary pacing. Permanent pacing is generally recommended in all patients with myocardial infarction when complete AV block continues for more than 10 to 14 days.

Symptomatic Bifascicular and Trifascicular Block. Bifascicular or trifascicular block usually signifies extensive conduction system pathology. Symptoms in patients with bundle branch block may be due to intermittent episodes of advanced or complete AV block or to ventricular tachycardia. Permanent pacing should be considered in symptomatic patients with bifascicular or trifascicular block and prolonged HV intervals of 100 msec or longer. In patients with documented episodes of complete AV block associated with bundle branch block, implantation of a permanent pacemaker should be an urgent consideration. Dual-chamber pacing is generally perferred in patients in whom progression to permanent complete AV block is likely.

Bifascicular or Trifascicular Block with Intermittent Complete AV Block After Acute Myocardial Infarction. Clinical studies have shown that the potential risk of sudden death within 6 months after acute myocardial infarction increases in patients with bifascicular or incomplete trifascicular block associated with intermittent complete AV block during the peri-infarction period (Domenighetti and Perret, 1980; Hindman et al, 1978). Therefore, it is now recommended that this group of patients be considered to be candidates for permanent pacemaker implantation before discharge from the hospital after their infarction.

Carotid Sinus Syncope. As mentioned earlier, a permanent pacemaker may be indicated in patients with carotid sinus syncope or near syncope when a significant cardioinhibitory component can be implicated.

Recurrent Drug-Resistant Tachyarrhythmias Improved by Temporary Pacing. Some patients with tachyarrhythmias, particularly paroxysmal ventricular tachycardia, can be managed successfully by temporary pacing. In patients who respond, permanent pacing techniques can be considered to be part of their therapy. Because of the excellent surgical results obtained in patients with Wolff-Parkinson-White syndrome and ventricular tachycardia associated with left ventricular aneurysms and micro-reentry, operation should be considered to be primary therapy. However, in patients who are not surgical candidates, various antitachycardia pacing techniques are useful. Torsades de pointes due to a long Q-T interval as encountered with drug toxicity or electrolyte imbalance can be managed successfully with temporary overdrive pacing.

Intractable Congestive Heart Failure and Cerebral or Renal Insufficiency Benefited by Temporary Pacing. As described earlier, patients with refractory congestive heart failure and decreased perfusion causing cerebral or renal insufficiency may be improved occasionally by increasing heart rate with temporary pacing. If temporary pacing has proved to be effective under these conditions and long-term therapy is indicated, permanent pacing should be considered. Most of these patients require atrial contraction to improve cardiac output. Therefore, dual-chamber atrial synchronous pacing is usually indicated in this subgroup. In patients with sinus bradycardia or atrial arrhythmias, single-chamber rate-modulated pacing should be considered. These examples show that choice of the exact mode of pacing depends on a thorough knowledge of the underlying conduction disturbance.

IMPULSE GENERATOR

An implantable cardiac pacemaker consists of an impulse generator, lead wire, and electrode (Fig. 53–7). The impulse generator contains a power source or battery, hybrid circuits, and a lead connector (Fig. 53–8). All of these components are kept in a hermetically sealed metal container. The size and weight of the impulse generator depend on the size of the battery and the number of electronic components. Impulse generators are usually kept in rectangular or oval packages with rounded edges and weigh between 32 and 135 g.

Power Sources

The power source used in a totally implantable pacemaker may be biologic, rechargeable, nuclear, or chemical. Biologic power sources convert mechanical or chemical energy of the body into electrical energy using piezoelectric crystals, biogalvanic cells, or biofuel cells (Armour et al, 1966; Cywinski et al, 1978; Myers et al, 1964). Theoretically, these power

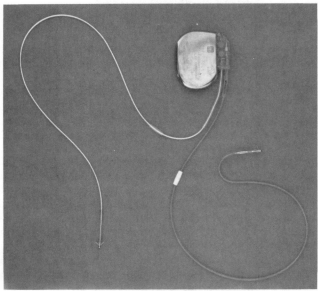

Figure 53–7. The modern implantable cardiac pacemaker consists of an impulse generator, lead wire, and electrode. A bipolar dual-chamber impulse generator (Symbios 7006, Medtronic, Inc.) is shown connected to an atrial J tined lead (Medtronic, Inc., model 4512) and a ventricular tined lead (Medtronic, Inc., model 4002). Devices such as the system shown here represent the current state of the art in pacemaker technology.

sources can be renewed potentially for the patient's lifetime, but they have not been developed to a point at which they are clinically practical. In 1973, a highly reliable, hermetically sealed, nickel-cadmium rechargeable pacemaker was developed at Johns Hopkins University and introduced commercially by Pacesetter, Inc. (Fischell et al, 1975). The useful battery life of such a rechargeable pacemaker has been calculated to be 70 to 80 years. Rechargeable pacemakers, although reliable, are not widely used, primarily because of the necessity for weekly recharging. Nuclear-powered impulse generators have been implanted in more than 3,000 patients worldwide. Their longevity is predicted to be longer than 20 years; however, nuclear generators are infrequently used because of cost, the improved longevity of newer chemical power sources, legislative restrictions, and concerns about the risk of chronic low-level radiation exposure. Chemical power sources continue to be the primary component of power cells in implantable pacemakers.

The modern power cell or battery is composed of an anode, a cathode, and an electrolyte. The power cell is generally named for the materials used in the anode and cathode—for example, lithium-iodine. Current solid-state cells have a dry, crystalline electrolyte between the anode and cathode. Electric current is produced by ionization of the anode, resulting in the migration of positively charged metallic ions through the electrolyte toward the cathode. Electrons are left behind on the anode, which becomes negatively charged relative to the cathode. When

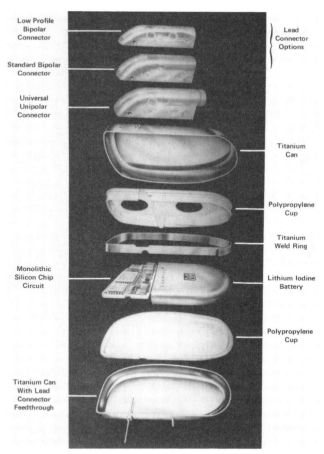

Figure 53–8. Exploded view of a modern multiprogrammable impulse generator. Various lead connectors are available to accept a variety of epicardial and transvenous leads. The battery and pacemaker electronics are enclosed in a titanium metal case. Hybrid circuit technology allows all components of the circuit including semiconductors, resistors, and capacitors to be diffused into a substrate to produce what is called a monolithic silicon chip. As shown, the major advantage of the silicon chip circuit is its extremely small size. This technology combined with the improved lithium power source has allowed modern multiprogrammable pacemakers to be much smaller, lighter, and more reliable than earlier pacemakers. (Courtesy of Paul Craven, Joe Hitselberger, and Gene Boone, Medtronic, Inc.)

the anode and cathode are connected by a conductive pathway, a flow of electrons passes from the anode to the cathode. The higher the resistance in the conductor, the slower the flow of electrons and the longer the power cell will last. In the modern lithium-iodine power cell, the migrating or positively charged ions are lithium, which combines with iodine from the cathode to form a lithium-iodide electrolyte barrier (Tyers and Brownlee, 1981). Most currently available lithium-powered pacemakers contain a single power cell, unlike the original mercury-zinc generators, which were powered by multiple-cell batteries.

Lithium power cells are available in five chemical types: (1) lithium-iodine (polyvinyl pyridine), (2) lithium-lead sulfide, (3) lithium-silver chromate, (4) lithium-copper sulfide, and (5) lithium-thionyl chloride

(Tyers and Brownlee, 1981). All of these lithium power sources have been extremely reliable and durable when compared with the earlier mercury-zinc systems. Most current pacemaker implants worldwide contain a solid-state lithium-iodine cell, which appears to be the power source of choice. Overall, pulse generator performance based on the type of power source is shown in Figure 53–9. The results with rechargeable impulse generators are essentially parallel to those of the nuclear power sources. The power source longevity of lithium pacemakers is estimated to be 10 to 12 years. However, because of wound, lead-electrode, and functional problems relating to pacing and sensing, it appears that approximately 20% of patients have required reoperation 4 to 5 years after implantation of a lithium-powered pacemaker (Tyers and Brownlee, 1981). Therefore, it is unwise to suggest to a patient that the life of the pacemaker is governed only by the predicted life expectancy of the power cell. Even modern lithium-powered pacemakers have been associated with a small incidence of random failure (Welti, 1981).

Pacemaker Electronics

The first implantable pacemakers contained individual or discrete components including resistors, capacitors, diodes, transistors, reed switches, and wire coils for induction. These individual components were mounted on or between printed circuit boards. A major advance in pacemaker electronics has been the development of "hybrid" circuits. Hybrid technology allows all components of the circuit

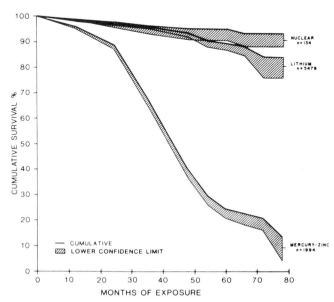

Figure 53–9. Impulse generator performance based on the type of power source. (From Bilitch, M., Hauser, R. G., Goldman, B. S., et al: Performance of cardiac pacemaker pulse generators. PACE, 4:254, 1981.)

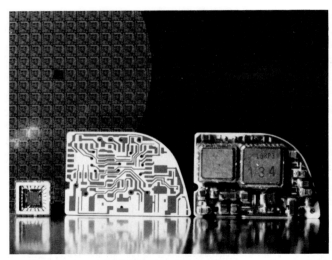

Figure 53–10. A highly magnified view of a modern hybrid circuit. Hybrid technology allows all components of the circuit including semiconductors, resistors, and capacitors to be diffused into a substrate to produce what is called a monolithic silicon chip. The obvious advantage of the single-chip circuit is its small size. Such hybrid circuits are used in almost all multiprogrammable pacemakers and may include as many as 40,000 transistors on 4-mm² wafer. Such a hybrid circuit is exceptionally reliable and capable of providing both multiprogrammable and physiologic pacing functions. However, its capacity for monitoring and data processing is limited, and it may be replaced in the future by single-chip microcomputers.

including semiconductors, resistors, and capacitors to be diffused into a substrate to produce a monolithic silicon chip (Fig. 53–10). The major advantage of the single-chip circuit is its small size. Customized digital, silicon, large-scale integrated circuits are used in almost all multiprogrammable pacemakers and may include as many as 40,000 transistors on a 4-mm² wafer (Tyers and Brownlee, 1981). This technology combined with the improved lithium power source has allowed modern multiprogrammable pacemakers to be much smaller, lighter, and more reliable than earlier simpler pacemakers. The lithium-powered pacemaker containing a custom integrated circuit design is exceptionally reliable and capable of providing both multiprogrammable and physiologic pacing functions. However, its capacity for monitoring and data processing is limited (Tyers and Brownlee, 1981). Single-chip microcomputers are now available, although high-current drain and software limitations have prevented their widespread use in pacemakers. Future pacemakers will most likely use low current drain, custom microcomputers consisting of a central processing unit, a memory unit, and an input-output circuit (Barold and Mugica, 1982). Pacemakers containing microcomputers are now capable of monitoring various physiologic changes to control in online manner pacemaker function. Physiologic changes that can be monitored include cardiac output requirements as determined by online measurement of temperature, Q-T interval, oxygen saturation, body motion, and respiratory rate. Moreover, microcom-

puter-based pacemakers can automatically select an appropriate pacing technique for the control of various dysrhythmias. Future pacemakers will be able to automatically detect loss of capture due to threshold changes and adjust their output accordingly.

Hermetic Seal

The electronics and power source of the first totally implantable pacemakers were protected by epoxy resins and silicone rubber (Tyers and Brownlee, 1981). Gradually, however, moisture gained access to the interior of the pacemaker, causing short circuits, sudden cessation of pacing, battery explosion, pacemaker runaway, and occasionally even ventricular fibrillation (Tyers and Brownlee, 1976). Fluid infiltration problems were responsible for the massive recalls that eventually terminated the use of mercury-zinc, epoxy-enclosed pacemakers (Tyers and Brownlee, 1976).

The modern pacemaker is hermetically enclosed, rendering it airtight and fluid tight. Pacemaker manufacturers determine the quality of the hermitic seal in terms of a leak rate for an inert gas under standard conditions (Tyers and Brownlee, 1981). For example, an acceptable helium leak rate of 10^{-8} ml/sec at one atmosphere involves the passage of less than 0.01 ml of helium per 24 hours. Permeability to fluid is many orders of magnitude lower. Hermitic seal is now achieved by encasing the power source and electronics in a sealed metal container, which usually requires laser welding. The materials chosen for enclosure have included stainless steel, Haynes' alloy, and titanium. Most modern pacemakers are enclosed in titanium.

Lead Connector

Impressive advances have been made in leads and electrodes and in pacemaker power sources and circuitry. As described by Tyers (1981), the ideal pacemaker connector should be tangential to reduce electrode stress, universal to accept all available leads without adapters, simple, and short-circuit proof. A standard coaxial bipolar connector that has been developed may represent an industry standard that will eliminate incompatibilities between various leads and pacemakers. This universal lead connector is referred to as the VS-1 (voluntary standard) and is a 3.2-mm-diameter connector designed to fit potentially all bipolar pacemakers (Calfee and Saulson, 1986) as well as to reduce the size of the connector itself (see Fig. 53–8).

LEAD-ELECTRODE

A pacemaker lead is an insulated wire used to connect the pacemaker impulse generator to the heart. The electrode is the uninsulated, electrically active metal tip that is in contact with the myocardium (see Fig. 53–7). The lead-electrode system in a demand pacemaker has two equally important functions: It conducts the electric stimulus from the impulse generator to the myocardium and transmits an endocardial electrogram from the heart to the pacemaker (Tyers and Brownlee, 1981). In unipolar systems, only the cathode is in the heart and the indifferent electrode, or anode, which is a part of the metallic pacemaker case, is in soft tissue. In a bipolar system, a double wire runs from the pacemaker to the heart and the two electrodes are separated by approximately 1 cm within the heart. The lead wire is most often a continuous helical coil or braided wire that is resistant to fracture caused by repeated flexion. Carbon leads as well as multistrand leads made of combinations of metals such as nickel alloy and silver are now under evaluation in Europe and in the United States. These new leads may offer improved flexibility and lower resistance, which will result in decreased energy consumption. In the past, the lead was most commonly insulated with silicone rubber. Polyurethane insulation has been introduced because of its greater elasticity and tensile strength, which allows lead diameter to be reduced with improved durability. Furthermore, polyurethane has a smoother surface, which improves handling characteristics during multilead placement and reduces the risk of venous thrombosis (Williams et al, 1978).

The uninsulated electrically active metal tip of the lead in contact with the myocardium is the electrode. This exposed tip is usually made of platinum, iridium, nickel alloys, or activated carbon. Platinum-iridium electrodes are now the most common and may be either porous or solid.

Two general types of lead-electrode systems exist. The most common are the systems passed transvenously to embed within the subendocardium of the right atrium or right ventricle or both. The second group are those placed transthoracically; they are directly attached to the myocardium of any chamber. These leads have been referred to as epicardial leads, but this term is a misnomer because they are actually embedded within the myocardium and not just within the epicardium. Transthoracic leads are used primarily in small infants and children, after repeated failure of the transvenous approach, and sometimes when the chest is already open, such as after cardiac surgical procedures. Generally, transvenous lead-electrode systems are preferred because of their improved chronic thresholds and decreased incidence of lead fracture.

Transvenous systems are referred to as active or passive. Passive leads have a small flanged expansion just proximal to the exposed distal electrode or have short, flexible tines (Fig. 53–11A). These tined leads are designed to catch beneath trabeculas and reduce the incidence of dislodgment, which should be less than 1% (Furman et al, 1981). Active fixation leads are designed for insertion into large, smooth-walled

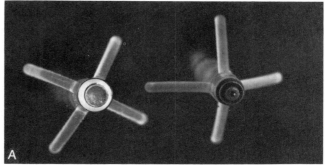

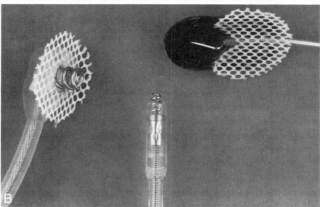

Figure 53–11. *A,* Examples of transvenous passive leads. These tined leads are designed to catch beneath trabeculae and reduce the incidence of dislodgment. They can be used in both the right atrium and right ventricle. Shown on the left is a tined lead with a polished platinum electrode tip (Medtronic, Inc., model 6971). Shown on the right is a platinum-iridium target tip electrode (Medtronic, Inc., model 4011). It appears that target tip electrodes have improved sensing function because the interstices increase the sensing area without increasing overall electrode size and subsequent energy stimulation requirements for pacing. *B,* Active leads contain either barbs, hooks, or screws. Shown on the left is a three-turn epicardial screw-in lead (Medtronic, Inc., model 6917). In the center, a transvenous endocardial screw-in lead is shown. The screw can be remotely activated or retracted. The lead is shown with the screw activated (Medtronic, Inc., model 6957). On the far right, an epicardial fishhook lead is shown (Medtronic, Inc., model 4951). The authors have found that the fishhook lead provides improved pacing and sensing thresholds in both the atrial and ventricular epicardial positions.

ventricular cavities, as well as for lead placement in the atrial appendage. Currently used active fixation leads contain sharpened screws that may be remotely activated and retractable (Tyers and Brownlee, 1981) (Fig. 53–11B). The authors prefer polyurethane-coated tined leads for routine transvenous ventricular pacing and sharp corkscrew-type screw-in electrodes for placement in the right atrium or the right ventricle under adverse circumstances when the rate of dislodgment is increased. Leads designed primarily for placement in the atrial appendage by the transvenous route differ from ventricular leads in that when the stylet is withdrawn they assume a J shape, which allows them to be positioned well up into the atrial appendage (see Fig. 53–7).

As mentioned earlier, pacemaker lead-electrode systems are referred to as being either bipolar or unipolar. Possible advantages of a unipolar system include a more simple connection, slightly decreased energy requirements, lower risk of pacemaker-induced fibrillation, and decreased risk of anodal corrosion (Tyers and Brownlee, 1981). Advantages of bipolar pacing include reduced risk of skeletal muscle stimulation, lower susceptibility to electromagnetic interference, elimination of pacemaker suppression by skeletal myopotentials, decreased risk of "crosstalk" between atrial and ventricular stimuli, and increased sensing selectivity (Tyers and Brownlee, 1981). The advantages and disadvantages of unipolar and bipolar pacing should be considered when selecting the most appropriate pacemaker for a particular patient.

To a certain extent, decreasing electrode tip size results in lower thresholds, both at the time of implant as well as chronically because of higher current density. However, better sensing function is directly related to electrode area and is adversely affected by small electrode size (Hughes et al, 1976). Therefore, a compromise between pacing and sensing efficiency is required. Typical electrode surface areas for pacing are between 8 and 10 mm². The effective surface area for sensing is increased many times through the use of microporous electrodes. These porous-tip electrodes improve sensing for a given electrode size because the interstices increase the sensing area without increasing overall electrode size and subsequent stimulation energy requirements (Lagergren and Johansson, 1963) (see Fig. 53–11A). Techniques such as platinization of the electrode or use of activated carbon result in lower stimulation thresholds by reducing polarizing currents at the electrode surface.

OPERATIVE TECHNIQUES AND EVALUATION OF PACEMAKER FUNCTION

Operative Techniques

Implantation of a permanent impulse generator and lead-electrode system should be done in a fluoroscopic unit or a cardiac catheterization laboratory under sterile conditions. Various impulse generators and lead electrodes as well as a pacing system analyzer should be readily available. Most commonly, the pacemaker lead-electrode is passed transvenously under local anesthesia to become embedded within the subendocardium of the right atrium or right ventricle. Transthoracic leads are used primarily in small infants and children, after repeated failure of the transvenous approach, and sometimes after cardiac procedures when a permanent pacemaker is indicated. In general, for elective permanent pacemakers, transvenous leads are preferred because of

their improved chronic thresholds and decreased incidence of lead fracture.

Preoperatively, patients receive a therapeutic dose of an antistaphylococcal antibiotic based on the proven beneficial effects of prophylactic antibiotic administration in general and thoracic surgical procedures. Antibiotics are discontinued 24 hours postoperatively. Regardless of the planned approach for implantation, the entire anterior chest from the chin to the umbilicus should be prepared and draped as a sterile field. This wide field of preparation allows conversion from one transvenous approach to another and permits a limited anterior thoracotomy without interruption of the procedure.

Based on the work of Lagergren and Johansson (1963) in Sweden and by Furman and Schwedel (1959) and Chardack and colleagues (1965) in the United States, the transvenous approach under local anesthesia is now used in more than 90% of patients requiring pacemakers. The venous anatomy of the anterior chest wall is particularly well suited for implantation of pacing leads (Fig. 53–12). Generally, the pacemaker pocket is placed over the anterior side of the chest beneath the junction of the inner and

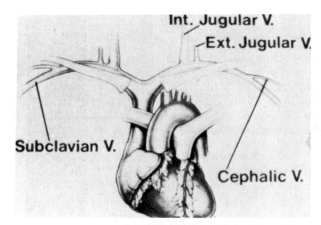

Figure 53–12. Anatomy for preferred venous approaches. Any vein in the neck, chest, or shoulder may be used for a permanent transvenous lead, but it is preferable to expose the vein through the same incision used for making the pocket. In order of preference, acceptable veins are as follows: (1) Cephalic vein, a tributary of the subclavian vein. It lies in the deltopectoral groove and is usually big enough to admit a lead up to No. 7 or 8 French. In 10% of patients, it is quite delicate and may not be usable. It is occasionally absent. (2) Subclavian vein or tributary. If the cephalic vein cannot be used, it is always possible to expose another tributary of the subclavian or the subclavian vein itself through the same incision by freeing the pectoralis major from its lateral origin from the inferior surface of the clavicle. The subclavian vein is now commonly used as the primary choice for lead insertion with introducer techniques. (3) External jugular vein. This is usually the most prominent visible vein in the neck, although it may be absent in 10% of patients. Because of the necessity of tunneling the electrode over or under the clavicle, with an increased incidence of fracture and erosion, this is a poor choice for permanent pacing. (4) Internal jugular vein. This is also a poor choice, unless purulent infections exist at every other potential site or an unusually large electrode is required as for an implantable defibrillator. (From Parsonnet, V.: Implantation of Transvenous Pacemakers. Tarpon Springs, FL, Tampa Tracings, 1972.)

middle thirds of the clavicle on the patient's nondominant side. The cephalic or subclavian veins are the preferred venous approaches for lead introduction. Implantation through the external or internal jugular veins requires a separate neck incision, and the lead must be tunneled over or under the clavicle to reach the pacemaker pocket and generator. Passing the lead over the clavicle predisposes to skin erosion and lead fracture; tunneling beneath the clavicle increases the risk of hemorrhage due to vascular injury.

An oblique incision on the anterior chest wall inferior to the deltopectoral groove provides excellent exposure to the cephalic vein and also allows introducer cannulation of the subclavian vein (Fig. 53–13). The pacemaker pocket should be as far medial as is comfortable for the patient to minimize pectoral stimulation. It should be made only slightly larger than the impulse generator so that migration laterally, which tends to follow the curvature of the chest wall, is minimized. Small arterial and venous bleeders are ligated or electrocoagulated to avoid postoperative hematoma formation. The pacemaker generator pocket should be just superficial to the pectoralis major in thick-chested individuals or beneath the premuscular fascia or muscle itself in thin-chested patients.

Techniques for cephalic and subclavian vein cannulation are shown in Figures 53–14 to 53–16). A gentle, twisting motion is used to introduce the lead-electrode system into the right atrium. The guide wire is then exchanged for one with a J tip, which allows the lead to be passed across the tricuspid valve. The lead is then advanced across the pulmonary valve to confirm that the right ventricle has been cannulated and not the coronary sinus. The

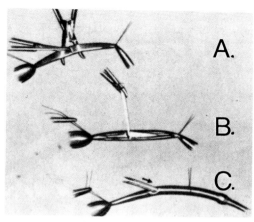

Figure 53–14. Small-vein introduction technique. If the vein is large, insertion of an electrode can be performed simply by any standard method. When the vein is small, gentle handling and care permit insertion of an electrode that at first may seem to be much larger than the vein. The vein is ligated distally, a loose, nonabsorbable suture is placed proximally, and a transverse incision is made one-third of the way across the anterior wall of the vessel (A). A plastic inserter (present in the lead packages from many manufacturers) is carefully slipped into the opening (B). With upward traction on the inserter, which is concave on its inferior surface, the electrode can be passed underneath the inserter, which is not withdrawn until the tip of the electrode has passed medially a centimeter or so. As the electrode is advanced, the proximal ligature is loosened and then tightened to prevent bleeding. Countertraction on the distal ligature is maintained to assist passage into the subclavian vein (C). Traction on the distal ligature is easily maintained by pulling it over the self-retaining retractor shown in Figure 53–13 and by placing a straight hemostat across it, with the tip of the hemostat underneath the ratchet of the retractor. (From Parsonnet, V.: Implantation of Transvenous Pacemakers. Tarpon Springs, FL, Tampa Tracings, 1972.)

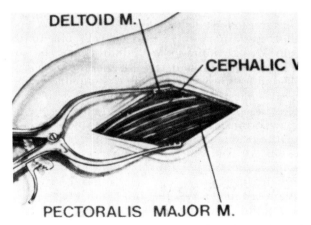

Figure 53–13. Cephalic vein approach. After making the incision below the clavicle, the deltopectoral groove is identified. The cephalic vein is usually found with ease in the fat pad that fills the groove. Division of a few fibers of the pectoralis major from the clavicle will allow dissection of the vein proximally, and if gentle traction is applied, the angle of entrance of the cephalic vein into the subclavian vein can be made more oblique. Passage of the electrode toward the heart rather than into the axilla is thus facilitated. (From Parsonnet, V.: Implantation of Transvenous Pacemaker. Tarpon Springs, FL, Tampa Tracings, 1972.)

lead is then withdrawn into the cavity of the right ventricle, and the curved guidewire is replaced with a straight wire. The lead is then gradually withdrawn until the electrode falls and points toward the apex of the right ventricle. The guidewire is then withdrawn a few millimeters and the lead is gently maneuvered to lodge the pacing and sensing electrode beneath right ventricular trabeculae (see Fig. 53–16). If a dual-chamber procedure is planned, ventricular lead placement is accomplished first, followed by placement of an atrial J lead, which is designed to lodge in the right atrial appendage. If stable positioning of an atrial J lead cannot be accomplished, an endocardial screw-in lead is placed into the wall of the right atrium. After transvenous positioning and testing of thresholds, the lead is anchored at the fascial or venous exit site to prevent dislodgment. After testing the impulse generator, the lead-electrode system is then connected to the impulse generator, which is then positioned in its pocket. Finally, the wound is irrigated with a dilute bacitracin-saline solution and closed in layers by using absorbable suture.

Permanent transthoracic leads can be placed through either a small left anterior thoracotomy or subxiphoid mediastinotomy. Generally, sutureless

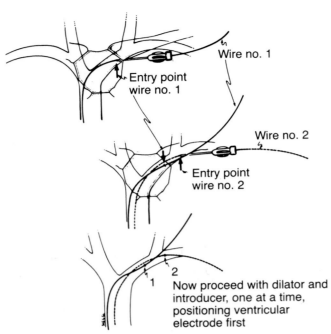

Figure 53–15. Two-entry point dual-lead introducer technique. Method for inserting separate guide wires, introducers, and sheaths with a small distance between the electrode entrance sites. (From Parsonnet V., Werres R., Atherley, T., et al: Transvenous insertion of double set of permanent electrodes: Atraumatic technique for atrial synchronous and atrial ventricular sequential pacemakers. J.A.M.A., 243:62–64, 1980. Copyright 1980, American Medical Association.)

screw-in or hook leads are used and tunneled beneath the costal margin to the pacemaker pocket, which is created over the left upper quadrant of the abdomen well above the belt line or occasionally placed retroperitoneally in either lower quadrant in small infants (Fig. 53–17). The electrode is placed by opening the pericardium and by identifying a fat-free area on the anterior or lateral aspect of the left ventricle. The electrode should not be placed too close to the apex of the heart because of its thinness and because increased motion in this area may cause electrode dislodgment or lead fracture. In addition, the electrode should not be placed in myocardium adjacent to the pericardial course of the phrenic nerve, which could cause diaphragmatic pacing.

Evaluation of Pacemaker Function

A thorough evaluation of pacing threshold energy requirements, atrial and ventricular endocardial electrograms, and impulse generator parameters should be done at the time of initial pacemaker implantation as well as at the time of replacement (Calvin, 1978; Kleinert et al, 1979; Parsonnet et al, 1980; Venkataraman and Bilitch, 1979). A pacing system analyzer simulates the function of the pacemaker's output and sensing circuits and is also capable of evaluating the integrity of the impulse gen-

erator itself (Fig. 53–18). The pacemakers' energy output and sensing circuits communicate with the myocardium through the implanted lead at the electrode-myocardial interface. The pacemaker impulse generator delivers an electrical discharge, which passes through its output circuit into the lead, to the electrode-myocardial interface, and back through body tissue to an indifferent electrode. This system is a simple series electrical circuit described by Ohm's law (resistance = voltage/current.) The factors determining resistance are summarized in Figure 53–19.

The electrical pulse discharged by the impulse generator's output circuit is designed to initiate cardiac depolarization. The pacing threshold of the electrode-myocardial interface can be expressed in terms of energy, current, or voltage. The electrical energy discharged by the impulse generator is defined as follows: energy = voltage × current × time. This electrical energy has both an amplitude (voltage or current) and a time component (pulse width or duration). The lowest voltage or current that is delivered to the heart at a given pulse width and that results in cardiac depolarization is referred to as the stimulation threshold. A strength-duration curve (Fig. 53–20) is a graphic plot that shows the stimulation threshold for each pulse width. Any amplitude pulse width combination on or above the strength-duration curve is sufficient to initiate cardiac depolarization. As shown in Figure 53–20, the amplitude component approaches an infinite value at very short pulse widths, such as less than 0.1 msec, and it approaches a minimal value at long pulse

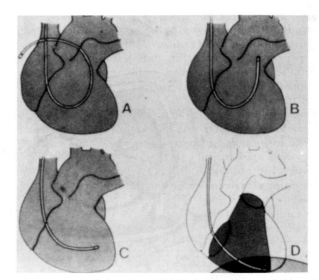

Figure 53–16. Right ventricular lead positioning technique. If the catheter is advanced into the pulmonary artery (A), which is easily confirmed by seeing the tip in the lung fields, there can be no question that on slow withdrawal of the electrode tip (B) it will fall into the ventricle (C), assuming the absence of ventricular septal defects. D, The shaded area reflects the approximate shape of the right ventricle. Note that the apex is far lateral and that the electrode usually lies below the dome of the left diaphragm as seen fluoroscopically. (From Parsonnet, V.: Implantation of Transvenous Pacemakers. Tarpon Springs, FL, Tampa Tracings, 1972.)

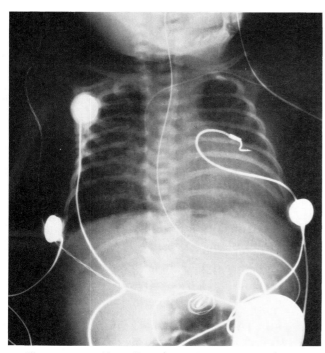

Figure 53–17. Chest film of a 36-hour-old infant born with congenital complete heart block. A fishhook lead electrode (Medtronic, Inc., model 4951) was embedded over the lateral aspect of the left ventricle. The lead was then tunneled beneath the musculature of the anterior abdominal wall down to the left lower quadrant. A left lower-quadrant incision was made, and the anterior abdominal wall musculature was split. The peritoneum was identified and swept down and medially to create a retroperitoneal pacemaker pocket. The lead was connected to a Pacesetter Programalith III unipolar impulse generator. Most children who require pacemakers do not require a retroperitoneal pocket because of the small size of current impulse generators. However, in an extremely small infant, it is occasionally necessary to place the impulse generator in a retroperitoneal position.

widths, such as greater than 1.5 msec. As can be seen from the strength-duration curve, at a short pulse width, the stimulation threshold may exceed the output of the pacemaker and result in loss of pacing. Conversely, excessively long pulse widths do not lower the pacing threshold and waste energy. In right ventricular implants using currently available transvenous electrodes, a pulse width of at least 0.5 msec is usually used acutely to obtain a voltage threshold of less than or equal to 0.5 volts. Generally, an acute threshold greater than 1 volt is unsatisfactory. Atrial pacing thresholds are usually comparable with ventricular thresholds but may be slightly higher. Atrial thresholds greater than 2 volts are unsatisfactory. In general, a low acute threshold provides a substantial safety margin because acute thresholds generally rise to higher values during the first several weeks and then decline slightly to their chronic levels secondary to maturation of the electrode-myocardial interface.

In addition to measuring pulse amplitude (voltage and current) and pulse width, resistance is also

determined. As described by Ohm's law, resistance is calculated by dividing voltage by current. Resistance calculations are made at a voltage near that of the pacemaker's output. The calculated resistance at 5 volts should range from 300 to 800 ohms. Low resistances result in higher currents and are unsatisfactory for pacing. An unsatisfactorily low resistance can develop secondary to location of the electrode in the ventricular chamber or because of a separate competing electrical pathway (parallel circuit) (Fig. 53–21). If a competing pathway exists, current flows through a stimulating and nonstimulating pathway. The current flow through the nonstimulating pathway lowers the resistance and represents wasted energy. This phenomenon can be seen with poorly positioned endocardial electrodes, as well as with epicardial electrodes. Very low acute resistances are unsatisfactory because current is wasted and battery life is shortened, which results in a potential for exit block or an increased incidence of muscle stimulation due to increased current. Conversely, excessively high resistances (> 800 ohms) increase battery life but decrease the current delivered to the heart for both constant-voltage and con-

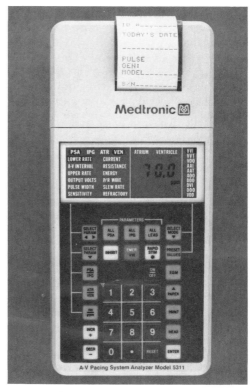

Figure 53–18. A pacing system analyzer (PSA) simulates the function of the pacemaker's output and sensing circuits and is also capable of evaluating the integrity of the impulse generator itself. A thorough evaluation of pacing threshold energy requirements, atrial and ventricular endocardial electrograms, and impulse generator parameters should be performed at the time of initial pacemaker implantation as well as at the time of generator or lead electrode replacement.

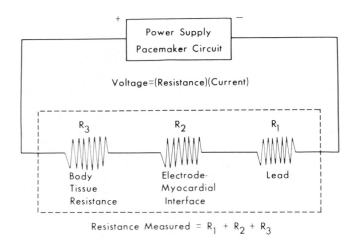

Voltage = (Resistance)(Current)

Resistance Measured = $R_1 + R_2 + R_3$

Figure 53–19. Simple series circuit. A simple series circuit is an accurate model for the standard pacemaker-body circuit. The electrical properties of this circuit are expressed by Ohm's law: V = R × I. The resistance of the lead (R_1), the electrode-myocardial interface (R_2), and the body tissue acting as the return pathway back to the pacemaker's indifferent electrode (R_3) are series resistances that add up to the total resistance of the circuit (i.e., total resistance of the circuit = $R_2 + R_2 + R_3$). This is the resistance measured across the circuit by a PSA device. (From Byrd, C.: *In* Samet, P., and El-Sherif, N. [eds]: Cardiac Pacing, 2nd ed. New York, Grune & Stratton, 1980, p. 229.)

Figure 53–20. Strength-duration curve. A strength-duration curve demonstrates the relationship between the pulse amplitude (volts and current) and the pulse width. Each point on the curve is the stimulation threshold for that respective pulse amplitude and pulse width. The area above the strength-duration curve represents the pulse amplitude and pulse width combinations that will stimulate an endocardial depolarization. The area below the curve represents the combinations of pulse amplitude and pulse width insufficient to stimulate a depolarization. (From Byrd, C.: *In* Samet, P., and El-Sherif, N. [eds]: Cardiac Pacing, 2nd ed. New York, Grune & Stratton, 1980).

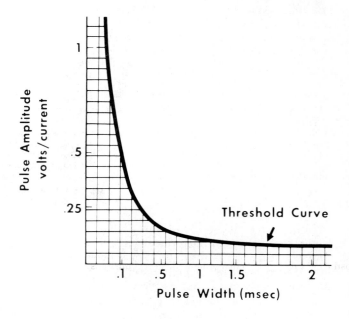

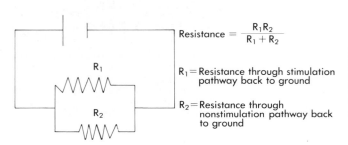

$$Resistance = \frac{R_1 R_2}{R_1 + R_2}$$

R_1 = Resistance through stimulation pathway back to ground

R_2 = Resistance through nonstimulation pathway back to ground

Figure 53–21. Parallel circuit. A stimulating and a nonstimulating circuit represent two separate pathways back through the body tissue to the indifferent electrode. Parallel circuits may occur in bipolar lead implants, epicardial lead implants, and with current leaks from a damaged lead system. (From Byrd, C.: *In* Samet, P., and El-Sherif, N. [eds]: Cardiac Pacing, 2nd ed. New York, Grune & Stratton, 1980, p. 229.)

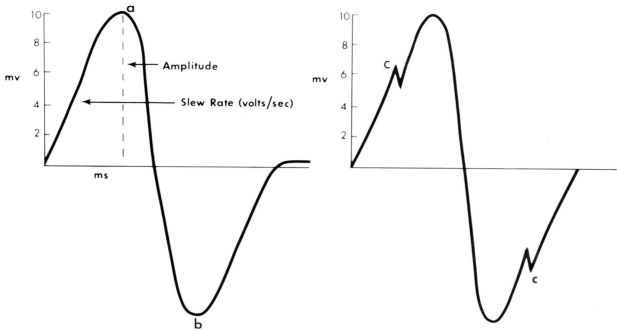

Figure 53–22. Endocardial waveform analysis. An endocardial waveform, as demonstrated on an electrogram, consists of deflections above and below the baseline. The pacemaker sensing circuit evaluates these deflections by rapidly determining the slew rate (rate of change of the amplitude with respect to time) and amplitude of that deflection. The amplitude is defined by a sensing circuit as the maximal uninterrupted excursion of the wave deflection at a constant slew rate (point a and point b). A change in the slew rate for a deflection such as a notch (point c) on the wave will be interpreted as a point of maximal excursion (the amplitude or peak for that deflection). Modern sensing circuits can determine not only the peak deflections (points a, b, and c) from the baseline but the peak-to-peak deflections across the baseline (point a to point b). The sensing circuit samples only a small portion of the waveform to determine the slew rate and amplitude. The slew rate obtained from a peak deflection above and below the baseline or a peak-to-peak analysis can be extrapolated into a frequency measurement, assuming the entire waveform has that slew rate. (From Byrd, C.: *In* Samet, P., and El-Sherif, N. [eds]: Cardiac Pacing, 2nd ed. New York, Grune & Stratton, 1980, p. 229.)

stant-current pacemakers. For example, current flow from a 5-volt battery through a resistance greater than 1,000 ohms is reduced below 5 mA, which is an inadequate safety margin to compensate for eventual chronic threshold elevation.

In addition to measuring stimulation thresholds and resistance, the sensing circuit of the pacemaker must be evaluated. The sensing circuit monitors spontaneous myocardial depolarizations. A cardiac depolarization waveform (P wave or R wave) passes from the myocardium into the electrode and is transmitted via the lead to the sensing circuit of the impulse generator. The sensing circuit is designed to detect electrical signals above a particular amplitude within the frequency range of endocardial electrograms. Measurements of amplitude and frequency are essential to ensure proper operation of the sensing circuit. As shown in Figure 53–22, an endocardial waveform has both an amplitude and a frequency component. The frequency component of the endocardial signal is approximated by the slew rate for the measured portion of the waveform. The slew rate is defined as millivolts per millisecond (mV/msec) and represents the rate of change of the amplitude with respect to time. As shown in Figure

53–22, the amplitude of the atrial or ventricular electrogram is measured in millivolts. As this waveform passes through the sensing circuit of the pacemaker, both the amplitude and the slew rate (rate of amplitude rise or frequency) must be acceptable for the signal to be detected. In general, ventricular endocardial electrograms greater than 4 mV and atrial endocardial electrograms greater than 1.5 mV in amplitude can be detected and provide a safety margin over time. A slew rate of 0.5 or greater is sufficient for detection of both types of signal.

A pacing system analyzer that is capable of simulating the function of a given pacemaker's output and sensing circuits is provided by each pacemaker manufacturer. In addition, the pacing system analyzer is used to evaluate the pacemaker's rate, interval, pulse width, voltage, current, sensitivity, refractory period, and AV interval in dual-chamber devices. After complete testing of threshold energy requirements, atrial and ventricular endocardial signals, and pacemaker parameters, high-voltage settings are used to detect diaphragmatic or phrenic nerve stimulation, which require lead repositioning. The patient is then asked to do deep-breathing and coughing exercises to attempt to produce electrode dislodgment before securing the pacemaker leads and implanting the generator.

PHYSIOLOGY OF PACING

Pacing Modes

Perhaps the most dramatic example of the advancement in pacemaker technology is the various ways in which the heart can be paced. The way in which an impulse generator functions is referred to as the pacing mode. An accurate description of pacing mode must convey not only the chamber of the heart that is being paced, but also the chamber sensed by the pacemaker and the manner in which the pacemaker responds to sensed activity. Simple descriptive terms such as *ventricular-demand pacemaker* sufficed well for single-chamber devices but have become more awkward as the complexity of pacemakers increases. Devices that pace and sense both atrial and ventricular activity are now frequently implanted. To meet the need for a uniform method of describing pacemaker function, the Intersociety Commission for Heart Disease Resources (ICHD) recommended a five-letter code that succinctly and accurately describes various pacing modes (Parsonnet et al, 1981). This code was updated in 1987 to accommodate newer pacemakers (Table 53–3) (Bernstein et al, 1987).

The ICHD code uses the letters A and V for atrium and ventricle. The letter D stands for "dual," indicating both chambers, or when indicating a mode of response, more than one mode. The two traditional response modes to sensed activity, either inhibition or triggering, are indicated by I and T. When no function or response is possible, the letter O is used. In the three-letter code system, the first letter designates the chamber(s) paced, the second letter

the chamber(s) sensed, and the third letter the mode of response of the pacemaker to sensed activity. Thus, a pacemaker that paces only the ventricle senses ventricular activity when intrinsic beats are present, and it responds to the sensed activity by inhibiting its output (the well-known ventricular-demand pacemaker is designated VVI in the ICHD code). An asynchronous ventricular pacemaker that does not sense but that paces at a constant rate regardless of intrinsic cardiac rhythm would be designated VOO (the ventricle is paced, neither chamber is sensed, and there is therefore no response mode to sensed events). In the case of the standard AV sequential pacemaker in which both the atrium and ventricle are paced but only ventricular activity is sensed, the designation is DVI.

The five-letter code has a tremendous advantage in describing not only a certain pacemaker, but also various possible modes of function incorporated into a single programmable pacemaker. The magnet mode of a pacemaker may also be described. This is the test mode in which a pacemaker functions when the internal reed switch is closed by the external application of a strong magnet. Thus, a VVI pacemaker generally functions in the VOO (asynchronous) mode when an external magnet is applied. Likewise, a sophisticated DDD pacemaker, discussed later, may be programmed to function in one of many modes, including DVI, VVI, AAI, AOO, VDD, and many more.

Fourth and fifth letters are used to denote programmability and antitachycardia capabilities, respectively (see Table 53–3). In this system, the letter P in the fourth position indicates the ability to program one or two parameters, and the letter M represents multiprogrammability. The letter R in the fourth position is used to designate a rate-modulated pacemaker (e.g., VVI-R); an O in the fourth position indicates a nonprogrammable pacemaker. In the fifth

TABLE 53–3. NBG (NASPE*/BPEG†) GENERIC PACEMAKER CODE‡

Position/Category	I Chamber(s) Paced	II Chamber(s) Sensed	III Response to Sensing	IV Programmability, Rate Modulation	V Antitachyarrhythmia Function(s)
	O = None	O = None	O = None	O = None	O = None
	V = Ventricle	V = Ventricle	T = Triggers pacing	P = Simple programmable	P = Pacing (antitachyarrhythmia)
Letter Codes	A = Atrium	A = Atrium	I = Inhibits pacing	M = Multiprogrammable	S = Shock
	D = Dual (A + V)	D = Dual (A + V)	D = Dual (T + I)	C = Communicating (telemetry)	D = Dual (P + S)
				R = Rate modulation	

NOTE: Positions I through III are used exclusively for antibradyarrhythmia pacing.
    Manufacturers may use "S" in positions I and II to indicate single chamber (A or V).
    A minimum of four positions is required to describe a pacemaker.

*NASPE = North American Society of Pacing and Electrophysiology.
†BPEG = British Pacing and Electrophysiology Groups.
‡Adapted from Bernstein, A. D., Camm, A. J., Fletcher, R. D., et al.: The NASPE/BPEG Generic Pacemaker Code for antibradyarrhythmia and adaptive-rate pacing and antitachyarrhythmia devices. PACE, 10:794, 1987.

position, various antitachycardia functions may be indicated, including P for pacing, S for shock, and D (for both pacing and shock). These modes are discussed later in detail.

Multiple pacing modes are potentially feasible, although only seven modes have real significance in clinical practice. Of these, two (VVI and DVI) have comprised the majority of pacing applications until recently (Table 53–4).

VVI Pacing. Single-chamber ventricular pacing has been the main type of cardiac pacing but is being replaced by more physiologic pacing modes. This mode, often referred to as ventricular-demand pacing, is the simplest of the pacing modes that is routinely used. As the ICHD code states, the pacemaker senses intrinsic ventricular activity and is inhibited when this activity exceeds the standby or escape rate of the pacemaker. When the intrinsic ventricular rate falls below the escape rate of the pulse generator, the pacemaker begins to function at its programmed rate. The escape rate and the automatic rate (pacing rate) may be identical or may be different if hysteresis is programmed into the pacemaker.

Potential disadvantages of VVI pacing are the lack of AV synchrony and the inability to increase heart rate with physiologic stress. Loss of coordinated contraction of the atria and ventricles may cause unpleasant symptoms due to atrial contraction against a closed tricuspid valve and may produce symptoms of low cardiac output referred to as the pacemaker syndrome. The magnet mode for VVI pacemakers (VOO) allows the function of the pacemaker to be observed even when an intrinsic rhythm is present that would otherwise inhibit pacemaker function.

Asynchronous ventricular pacing was used clinically before units capable of inhibition were available. Because of the potential dangers of asynchronous pacemaker function, with paced beats falling in the T wave of preceding spontaneous beats and inducing ventricular arrhythmias, VOO pacing is now relegated to the rare situation in which oversensing results in inappropriate inhibition that cannot be corrected by reprogramming.

AAI Pacing. Atrial pacing is potentially of great benefit in patients with intact AV conduction and sinus bradycardia, as in the sick sinus syndrome.

Until recently, atrial pacing was not used extensively because of technical problems related to stability of endocardial atrial leads. In addition to achieving stable pacing, the atrial electrode must be able to sense an adequate atrial electrogram to avoid asynchronous atrial pacing, although this is not frought with the potential hazards of asynchronous ventricular pacing. Advances in electrode technology have resulted in preformed J-shaped atrial tined leads that may be placed in position in the atrial appendage and active fixation leads that can be screwed into the atrial endocardium in other locations. These leads are capable of providing reliable atrial pacing in most patients.

Single-Chamber Rate-Modulated Pacing. Single-chamber rate-modulated pacing (VVI-R or AAI-R) has become an important and frequently used pacing mode with the commercial availability of pacemakers using various sensors to regulate the pacing rate. In rate-modulated pacing, the pacing rate is determined by a physiologic parameter, other than atrial rate, that is measured by a special sensor in the pacemaker or pacing lead. Examples of physiologic parameters that are currently used in rate-modulated pacing include body motion, venous blood temperature, the Q-T interval, and respiratory rate. Other parameters that are being developed include mixed venous oxygen saturation, contractility, and stroke volume. Although these pacing systems can theoretically respond to various physiologic stimuli with an increase in heart rate, their chief use is to provide an increase in cardiac output with exercise.

Patients who have chronic or intermittent atrial fibrillation and in whom atrial synchronous pacing is impossible may be able to maintain normal heart rate responses to exercise through the use of ventricular-rate–modulated pacing. In patients with normal AV conduction and sinus bradycardia that does not respond to exercise, rate-modulated atrial pacing may be indicated.

DVI Pacing. Dual-chamber pacing has provided an important improvement over simple ventricular pacing in approximately 40% of patients in whom optimal cardiac function depends on the atrial contribution to cardiac output. Before the development of atrial synchronous pacing, "bifocal" or AV sequential pacing was the only modality available.

In this mode, both the atrium and the ventricle are paced, with an artificial AV delay programmed between the atrial and ventricular impulses. In other respects, these devices function similarly to VVI pacemakers. Only ventricular activity is sensed, thus atrial stimulation is asynchronous if the spontaneous atrial rate exceeds the paced rate. DVI pacemakers may be of two varieties: committed or noncommitted. Committed systems are those in which the ventricular output must be delivered when the atrial pulse has occurred. In these systems, a QRS appearing in the AV interval will not inhibit ventricular output, and the ventricular pulse will fall in the QRS or ST segment (Fig. 53–23). The advantage of the commit-

TABLE 53–4. COMMONLY USED PACING MODES

ICHD* Code	Description
VVI	Ventricular demand
VOO	Ventricular asynchronous
AAI	Atrial demand
AOO	Atrial asynchronous
DVI	AV sequential fixed rate
VDD	Atrial synchronous
DDD	AV "universal"
VVI-R	Ventricular rate modulated

*ICHD = Inter-Society Commission for Heart Disease.

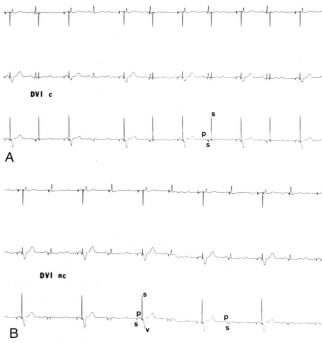

Figure 53–23. *A,* Simultaneous three-channel rhythm strip showing a normally functioning DVI pacemaker in the committed mode. Even though a normally conducted QRS occurs in the AV interval (second, sixth, eighth, and tenth complexes), a ventricular pacing output occurs after the QRS. Note that there is no atrial sensing in the DVI mode. The pacemaker is completely inhibited only when a QRS occurs sufficiently early to inhibit both atrial and ventricular outputs (fourth complex). *B,* A normally functioning noncommitted DVI pacemaker. P waves are not sensed in the DVI mode (second, fourth, sixth, eighth, and tenth complexes) and atrial pacing artifacts occur in the P-R interval. Conducted QRS complexes that follow these P waves inhibit the ventricular output.

systems have used a compromise between these two modes in which sensed ventricular activity after the atrial output results in a paced beat with a shortened AV interval, thus providing protection from failure to pace and diminishing the chance that the paced beat will fall in the vulnerable period, causing an arrhythmia.

VDD Pacing. One of the primary limitations of DVI pacing is its fixed rate and the need for pacing at a rate faster than the patient's intrinsic sinus rate if the benefits of AV synchrony are to be maintained. Atrial synchronous pacing allows the ventricle to be paced after sensed atrial activity (Fig. 53–24). This method has the advantage of preserving AV synchrony and allowing the ventricular rate to vary as the sinus rate varies. VDD pacing is differentiated from an earlier form of atrial synchronous pacing (VAT) in which the ventricle was paced synchronously with atrial activity, but without sensing in the ventricle.

Advanced forms of dual-chamber pacing (VDD or DDD) have no fixed rate, but rather are programmed to lower and upper rate limits. The way in which the pacemaker functions when the atrial rate exceeds the upper rate limits is also an important feature of these devices.

The upper rate limit is the rate beyond which the pacemaker does not continue to track atrial activity. This is a programmable function that can be set according to the patient's needs. When the atrial rate reaches the upper rate limit, the pacemaker continues to pace at a constant rate (the upper rate), and an apparent Wenckebach's sequence appears (Fig. 53–25).

When atrial activity decreases to the rate programmed as the lower rate limit of the pacemaker, the pacemaker responds in much the same manner as a VVI pacemaker at its escape interval. Because the VDD pacemaker cannot pace the atrium, VVI pacing occurs at the pacemaker's lower rate limit. Failure to sense in the atrium results in pacemaker function at lower rate limits despite the presence of faster atrial activity. A VDD pacemaker has no technologic advantage over present DDD units because both require atrial and ventricular leads, and devices capable only of VDD pacing are now obsolete.

ted system is that false inhibition of the ventricular output due to cross-talk from the atrial channel cannot result in inappropriate failure to pace. In noncommitted systems, ventricular activity occurring in the AV interval results in inhibition of the ventricular output. Cross-talk from the atrial channel is prevented by means of a blanking period of approximately 20 to 30 msec after atrial output during which the ventricular sensing circuits are closed. Some

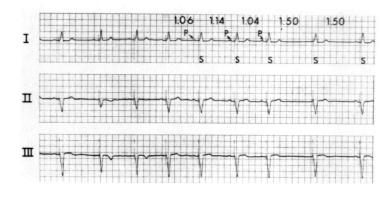

Figure 53–24. A normally functioning VDD pacemaker. Spontaneous atrial activity is sensed and followed by paced ventricular beats, resulting in slight variation in cycle length. When the atrial activity falls below the lower rate limit of the pacemaker, in this case a rate of 40 beats per minute (R-R interval of 1.5 second), ventricular pacing results. In the case of a DDD device, DVI pacing as seen in Figure 53–23 would be present at the lower rate.

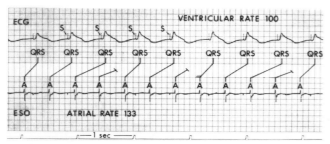

Figure 53–25. An atrial synchronous pacemaker functioning at the upper rate limit. The atrial rate is 133 beats per minute, and the upper rate limit of the pacemaker has been programmed to 100 beats per minute. The interval between sensed atrial activity recorded from an esophageal lead, and the pacing stimulus progressively lengthens until a P wave cannot be "tracked," which results in a dropped beat.

DDD Pacing. "Universal" or "automatic" pacing represents the height of pacing technology at the present time, although, as will be discussed in the section on physiologic pacing, not necessarily the optimal form of pacing for every patient. The primary difference between early DDD pacemakers and VDD pacemakers was the ability to pace the atrium at the lower rate limit. Thus, instead of VVI pacing at the low rate, AV synchrony was maintained by DVI pacing. Newer and more sophisticated DDD pacemakers can now be programmed to almost every pacing mode conceivable in addition to DDD, including AAI, VVI, DVI, VVT, and VOO.

With atrial rates above the lower rate limit of the pacemaker, the atrial output is inhibited and the pacemaker tracks atrial activity and responds with ventricular pacing after the programmed AV delay. This method provides a range of rate variation between the lower and the upper rate limits. An upper rate limit is programmed to avoid excessive paced rates in the event of rapid atrial rhythms. When the patient's atrial rate exceeds the upper rate limit of the pacemaker, the pacemaker maintains a fixed ventricular rate, resulting in an apparent Wenckebach's sequence with gradually lengthening AV intervals.

The fastest atrial rate the pacemaker can follow is also governed by the duration of total atrial refractoriness, composed of the AV interval and the postventricular atrial refractory period. If the atrial rate becomes so rapid that alternating P waves fall during the pacemaker's period of atrial refractoriness, they will not be sensed at all and the pacemaker will track only every other P wave. Injudicious programming of the atrial refractory period of the pacemaker may therefore result in abrupt reversion to 2:1 conduction by the pacemaker at or near the upper rate limit, and the patient has an abrupt decrease in heart rate.

Unipolar Versus Bipolar Pacing. The pacing configuration of any implanted system may be unipolar or bipolar. A unipolar system is one in which the cathode, or negative pole, of the pacemaker battery is connected to the stimulating electrode and the anode, or positive pole, is connected to an indifferent electrode remote from the actual site being paced. In practice, this indifferent electrode is usually the exterior of the pulse generator. To prevent stimulation of the adjacent skeletal muscle, most of the surface of the pulse generator is insulated and only a small area is left bare.

A bipolar system is one in which two electrodes in proximity are connected to the anode and cathode of the pulse generator. Because cathodal stimulation requires lower energy than anodal stimulation, the electrode in best contact with the myocardium is connected to the cathode in either unipolar or bipolar systems. In bipolar transvenous systems, the anode is usually the proximal electrode of the bipolar lead, and the cathode (negative pole) is connected to the distal or tip electrode.

In addition to pacing, sensing is also affected by the configuration of the pacing system. The bipolar system excludes remote electrical activity and is therefore less easily affected by extraneous electrical activity such as skeletal muscle potentials. When patients with unipolar systems are subjected to ambulatory monitoring, a significant incidence of sensing abnormalities is found, chiefly related to oversensing of myopotentials with inappropriate inhibition of the pacemaker (Breivik and Ohm, 1980; Secemsky et al, 1982).

Programmability

Programmability is defined as the ability to permanently and noninvasively change one or more of the operating characteristics of an implanted pacemaker. The advantages of modifying pacemaker function after implantation have been apparent for a long time. Early devices were made with the capability of changing rate by inserting a transcutaneous needle that turned a potentiometer in the pacemaker. Noninvasive programming was made possible originally through the use of an external magnet that activated a switch inside the pacemaker and changed its rate in incremental steps.

Almost all pacemakers implanted now have at least one programmable function. The use of programmability in terms of avoiding reoperation for pacing system malfunction and in improving the patient's tolerance of the pacemaker has been documented (Billhardt et al, 1982), and essentially no indications exist for the implantation of nonprogrammable pacemakers. Simple programmability usually includes the ability to change rate, pulse width, mode (usually from inhibited to asynchronous), and refractory period. The ability to change many parameters is called multiprogrammability (Table 53–5). The various programmable functions found on current devices are discussed in detail later in this section.

TABLE 53–5. COMMONLY PROGRAMMABLE FUNCTIONS OF A MULTIPROGRAMMABLE PULSE GENERATOR

Mode	Hysteresis
Rate	Polarity
Pulse width	AV interval*
Output	Upper rate limit*
Sensitivity	Lower rate limit*
Refractory period	

*Dual-chamber devices only.

To effect programming of an implanted pacemaker, a signal must be sent from a programmer to the pacemaker. In practical terms, a programmer must be placed relatively close to the pacemaker to transmit coded information to the pacemaker that is specific for the change desired. The pacemaker must be able to reject inappropriate signals from the environment or from other programmers that could potentially cause unwanted changes in pacemaker function. The pacemaker may respond by returning a signal to the programmer, indicating acceptance of the programming instructions (Fig. 53–26).

Programming features that are desirable include the ability of the programmer to interrogate the pacemaker and to retrieve two kinds of information: (1) the programmed settings of the pacemaker—that is, what the pacemaker is supposed to be doing; and (2) measured data from the pacemaker that indicate what the pacemaker is actually doing, what kind of sensed electrograms the pacemaker is receiving, and the state of the electrode and battery.

Most pacemakers now use radiofrequency signals to transmit coded information to and from the pacemaker. The functions that can be programmed in a given pacemaker vary considerably depending on the manufacturer and model. Obviously, the functions subject to programmability depend a great deal on the type of pacemaker (e.g., VVI, DVI, DDD). The most important functions for programmability are generally considered to be rate, pulse width, and sensitivity. Most of the potentially correctable problems encountered with implanted pacemakers can be managed by using these functions. Other functions that can be programmed in various models include refractory period, mode, and hysteresis. In dual-chamber pacemakers, the AV interval, upper and lower rate limits, and the mode of response to upper rate limit may be programmed. In sophisticated units, the pacemaker may actually be programmed off, blanking periods on atrial and ventricular channels can be changed, polarity can be programmed from bipolar to unipolar, and the pacemaker can even be programmed to respond or not respond to an external magnet.

Rate Programmability. The ability to change the rate of an implanted pacemaker is the single most useful programmable function. In patients with chronic cardiac disease, cardiac output may be highly rate dependent. The ability to increase rate allows the individual patient's heart rate to be changed to accommodate temporary changes in physical condition (e.g., cardiac procedures, heart failure, angina pectoris). Some patients develop an unpleasant sensation during pacemaker function or may actually have adverse hemodynamic effects from ventricular pacing. These situations may be remedied by lowering the pacing rate to allow more time in sinus rhythm. The ability to change rate also allows one pacemaker model to be used in all patient age groups, obviating the need for different models for use in pediatric patients who may require higher rates. In most pacemakers, rate can be programmed in steps from 40 to 130 pulses per minute.

Output Programmability. The output of the pacemaker in terms of total pacing energy is a function of both voltage and pulse width. Standard lithium-iodine batteries have an output of approximately 2.5 volts. The nominal voltage output of most pacemakers is 5 volts, achieved by the use of a voltage multiplier circuit. The ability to program the voltage output down to the lower value may help greatly in prolonging the battery life when chronic lead thresholds permit a lower stimulation energy. In addition, some models have the capability of increasing voltage output to the 7- to 10-volt range, thus accommodating unusually high pacing thresholds.

Pulse width programmability also allows the output of the pacemaker to be lowered to prolong battery life. Lowering pulse width below 0.3 msec is not generally recommended, because very high stimulation voltages may be required. Unfortunately, as evident from the strength-duration curve, increasing the pulse width beyond approximately 1 msec does little to lower the stimulation threshold; thus, raising pulse width in situations of high threshold has often little value (see Fig. 53–20).

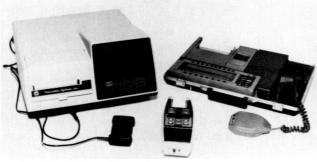

Figure 53–26. Three programmers currently in use, showing the range of complexity and size. *A,* The programmer for Pacesetter Systems, Inc., models 281, 283, and 285 pacemakers. The programming head is placed over the pacemaker for programming or interrogation. *B,* A portable hand-held programmer that is capable of performing many of the same functions as the larger unit on the left. The programming head is incorporated into the device itself. *C,* The Medtronic model 9710 programmer with printer and programming head. This device is compatible with all programmable Medtronic pulse generators.

Sensitivity Programmability. The sensitivity setting of the pacemaker determines the amplitude of the patient's intrinsic cardiac activity required for proper sensing to occur. A balance must be reached between settings that are oversensitive and may allow inhibition by extraneous signals such as myopotentials or T waves, and settings that are too insensitive and result in failure to sense intrinsic electrograms. Most pacemakers have a ventricular R wave sensitivity ranging from 1.25 to 5 mV (the lower value representing the highest sensitivity). In the atrium, sensitivity values of 1.5 to 2.5 mV are usual. Whether a given electrogram is sensed by a pacemaker depends not only on the actual amplitude of the electrogram, but also on the slew rate, or change in voltage per time (dV/dt). Thus, the programmed sensitivities do not necessarily guarantee adequate sensing of an electrogram based on its peak-to-peak amplitude. The ability to program sensitivity frequently corrects sensing problems that might otherwise require lead repositioning. Failure to sense premature ventricular contractions (PVCs) is a common example of a situation in which failure to sense may develop, despite proper sensing of sinus beats.

Refractory Period Programmability. The refractory period of the pacemaker is the interval after a sensed or paced event during which the pacemaker is incapable of sensing any electrical activity. This feature prevents inappropriate inhibition of the pacemaker due to artifacts from the stimulus and theoretically prevents sensing of other waveforms of the ECG such as the T wave. When electrodes are implanted in the atrium for AAI pacing, the refractory period should be extended to prevent sensing of far-field R waves. Occasionally, a pacemaker fails to sense closely coupled PVCs that fall in the refractory period of the pacemaker. This problem can be managed by shortening the refractory period.

Hysteresis. Hysteresis is a feature that has more theoretical appeal than practical applicability. Hysteresis is usually expressed in terms of the number of pulses per minute below the programmed rate required to initiate pacing. Thus, the escape interval is longer than the automatic or pacing interval. A pacemaker programmed to pace at a rate of 60 pulses per minute with 20 pulses per minute of hysteresis would remain inhibited until a sensed rate of 40 pulses per minute was present, at which time the pacemaker would begin to pace at a rate of 60 pulses per minute. The theoretical advantage of this function is that the patient is allowed to remain in sinus rhythm at intermediate rates between 40 and 60 beats per minute, but when pacing is required, the heart rate is maintained at the faster rate. A problem often encountered with hysteresis is that the patient's intrinsic rate must exceed the automatic rate to inhibit the pacemaker again. For patients who tend to maintain slow rates, hysteresis works well on the front end of the loop, but when pacing is initiated, patients may be unable to elevate their heart rate sufficiently to once again inhibit the pacemaker.

Physiologic Pacing

Physiologic pacing is a term used to describe pacing modes that attempt to duplicate normally conducted sinus rhythm (Sutton et al, 1980; Wirtzfield et al, 1987). This concept assumes an understanding of the physiologic relationships between the conduction of the cardiac impulse and the hemodynamic events it initiates and implies that duplication of this physiology can be achieved with an artificial pacemaker. At best, current artificial pacemakers are only crude substitutes for normal sinus rhythm; therefore, the term *physiologic pacing* must be considered to be an oversimplification. Physiologic pacing has also been recognized as synonymous with dual-chamber pacing, although this is not necessarily true.

It has been well established that AV synchrony—that is, the contraction of the atria and the ventricles with normal sequence and timing—provides some margin of improved cardiac output when compared with ventricular pacing alone at comparable rates (Kappenberger et al, 1982; Ogawa et al, 1978; Sutton et al, 1980, 1983; Wirtzfield et al, 1987). Appropriately timed atrial contraction has been shown to increase cardiac output by as much as 25% (Kappenberger et al, 1982; Reiter and Hindman, 1982; Samet et al, 1965). This difference may be even greater during exercise or in certain pathologic states (Narahara and Blettel, 1983; Rickards and Donaldson, 1983; Shapland et al, 1983). The deleterious effects of AV dissociation due to ventricular pacing vary greatly from one patient to another and depend on the heart's ability to compensate for a fixed rate, the presence of retrograde VA conduction, and the patient's overall level of activity.

The ability to increase heart rate to meet increased metabolic demand is also an important feature of normal cardiac conduction. Cardiac output is related directly to heart rate and stroke volume, and when cardiac disease impairs the ability to increase stroke volume, increased heart rate is the only mechanism remaining to increase cardiac output. Therefore, a physiologic pacing system has two aspects: the maintenance of AV synchrony and the preservation of rate variation. Obviously, these two features can be separated and may not be found in the same pacemaker. The familiar DVI pacemaker, for example, preserves AV synchrony without being able to vary rate in response to physiologic demands. Rate-modulated pacemakers can respond to physiologic stimuli including respiratory rate, Q-T interval, body motion during exercise, mixed venous oxygen saturation, and temperature (Rickards and Donaldson, 1983; Wirtzfield et al, 1987). These devices are particularly suited for patients with chronic atrial fibrillation. Thus, physiologic pacing should not be thought of as only dual-chamber pacing, but rather any pacing system that meets the physiologic needs of the patient.

The pacing modes that offer some preservation

of normal physiologic relationships include AAI-R, DVI, VVI-R, and DDD. AAI-R pacing has the advantages of maintaining normal AV conduction, requiring only one electrode, and offering rate variation and is used in patients with chronic sinus bradycardia with intact AV conduction. DVI pacing obviates the concern for AV conduction but has the limitation of fixed rate. DDD pacing offers both rate variation and AV synchrony and is the optimal pacing mode when normal sinus node function is present.

The acute benefits of AV sequential or atrial synchronous pacing compared with ventricular pacing have been well documented (Reiter and Hindman, 1982). Numerous studies have also substantiated a sustained hemodynamic benefit of physiologic pacing modalities compared with fixed-rate ventricular pacing. Improvement in acute and chronic exercise capacity, symptoms (dyspnea and fatigue), and even survival have been attributed to rate-modulated and dual-chamber atrial synchronous pacing when compared with simple ventricular pacing (Alpert et al, 1986; Faerestrand and Ohm, 1985; Kappenberger et al, 1982; Kristensson et al, 1985; Kruse and Ryder, 1981; Kruse et al, 1982; Levy et al, 1979; Perrins et al, 1983; Rickards and Donaldson, 1983; Sutton et al, 1983; Videen et al, 1986; Wirtzfield et al, 1987; Yee et al, 1984).

An often neglected aspect of dual-chamber pacing systems is the AV interval. This function is programmable on most current models, but little is known regarding the effects of changes in programmed AV interval. The optimal AV interval must be defined in relationship to the pacing rate, because physiologically AV conduction shortens with increasing heart rate. A shorter AV interval may be more appropriate for a patient with an atrial synchronous system in which optimal function during exercise is desired. The surgeon must also appreciate the differences in AV interval with atrial synchronous pacing compared with DVI pacing. The latency from the atrial stimulus to the onset of atrial systole results in a longer AV interval than occurs when ventricular pacing follows a sensed atrial event. The location of the atrial electrode also has an effect on the timing of ventricular systole in an atrial synchronous system.

It might be held that patients with normal cardiac function and potentially high levels of normal activity should benefit the most from physiologic pacing systems, whereas patients with limited exercise capacity should benefit the least. However, the former patients are probably best able to compensate for a fixed-rate ventricular pacing system through an increase in stroke volume, whereas patients with cardiac disease may depend completely on an increase in heart rate to increase their cardiac output.

An aspect of pacing that may also have significance in terms of physiologic pacing is the pacing site. Normal ventricular contraction is related to the sequence of myocardial depolarization. Ventricular dyssynergy is present during artificial ventricular pacing. This may cause an increase in myocardial oxygen consumption, inefficient ventricular emptying, and abnormal mitral valve function. The deleterious effects of artificial ventricular stimulation may depend on pacing site and are present even when AV synchrony is maintained with DVI pacing. Thus, in patients with intact AV conduction and sinus bradycardia, atrial pacing can be expected to be superior to both VVI and DVI pacing.

Indications for Pacing Modes

AAI Pacing. Atrial fixed-rate pacing may be indicated in patients with resting sinus bradycardia and intact AV conduction. Patients with the sick sinus syndrome may be included in this category; however, the potential effects of antiarrhythmic drugs on AV conduction must be considered before an atrial pacing system is implanted. Likewise, the intermittent occurrence of atrial fibrillation would render this pacing mode ineffective. AAI-R (rate-modulated) pacing is indicated when a normal increase in sinus rate with exercise is absent.

Technical problems with atrial lead stability have been mainly overcome with the use of tined J leads, as well as the availability of endocardial screw-in leads. These active fixation leads make atrial pacing possible in patients who have had cardiac procedures with cannulation of the right atrial appendage. Screw-in leads may also be useful in other patients in whom a stable pacing site cannot be found in the atrial appendage. Atrial pacing from the coronary sinus has also been an effective method (Moss and Rivers, 1978).

VVI Pacing. VVI pacing is indicated in patients who are receiving a pacemaker for the prevention of intermittent symptoms and who have normal sinus rhythm most of the time. VVI pacing systems should not be implanted in patients who would benefit from dual-chamber pacemakers because of unfamiliarity with these systems. The development and ready availability of more sophisticated pacing modalities compel the physician to implant a VVI unit in favor of a dual-chamber or rate-modulated system.

VVI-R pacing is indicated when dual-chamber pacing is not possible because of atrial arrhythmias and when a normal chronotropic response of heart rate to exercise is not present.

VVT Pacing. Ventricular-triggered pacing is rarely indicated. Inappropriate inhibition resulting in failure to pace may be managed by using the VVT mode when reprogramming the sensing threshold is not successful. Another potential application of VVT pacing is in the treatment of re-entrant tachycardias. An external stimulator is used to trigger the pacemaker, causing interruption of the arrhythmia. To prevent sensing of T waves and pacing in the vulnerable period, the sensing refractory period should be extended in pacemakers programmed to the VVT mode.

DVI Pacing. Fixed-rate AV sequential pacing devices are rapidly giving way to pulse generators capable of atrial synchronous pacing. The indications for the use of these systems now are essentially limited to patients with chronic stable sinus brady-cardia with unstable AV conduction. As a pacing mode within the capabilities of a DDD system, DVI may be useful when atrial sensing is unreliable or concomitant arrhythmic therapy results in sinus bradycardia.

DDD Pacing. Atrial synchronous pacing systems are indicated in patients with chronic AV block (second-degree or third-degree) with stable sinus rhythm. Patients with exercise-induced second-degree AV block are also good candidates for a DDD pacemaker.

The pacemaker syndrome is an unusual problem associated with ventricular pacing, although, if carefully sought, symptoms that suggest suboptimal cardiac output may be found more frequently. It may be difficult to prove a causal relationship between nonspecific symptoms such as fatigue and ventricular pacing in patients who often have coexisting cardiopulmonary disease, and care should be taken before replacing a normally functioning VVI system with a dual-chamber system in an attempt to relieve these symptoms. Patients who clearly have hypotension or diminished exercise capacity with a fixed-rate VVI system or who are troubled by symptomatic jugular venous pulsations due to asynchronous atrial contractions may, however, benefit greatly from a dual-chamber pacing system.

Whenever an atrial synchronous system is contemplated, the presence of retrograde VA conduction must be considered. Retrograde conduction may be a particular problem in patients with the pacemaker syndrome. In these patients, retrograde conduction resulting in a reversed sequence of AV synchrony during ventricular pacing appears to exacerbate the hemodynamic abnormality (Fig. 53–27). Most atrial synchronous devices have features designed to accommodate retrograde conduction and prevent the development of pacemaker-mediated tachycardia (PMT). Mechanisms built into atrial synchronous pacemakers to prevent sensing retrograde atrial activity and initiating PMT include programmable atrial refractory period, automatic extension of the atrial refractory period after premature ventricular beats, and temporary reversion to the DVI mode after a premature ventricular beat. If the atrial sensing refractory period of the pacemaker exceeds the VA interval of the retrograde P wave, the P wave is not sensed and PMT cannot develop. Extending the atrial refractory period may be useful in this regard but necessarily limits the upper tracking rate of the pacemaker. Because retrograde VA conduction is likely after a premature ventricular beat, some devices attempt to prevent PMT and at the same time preserve upper rate flexibility by keeping the atrial refractory period short normally, but automatically extending the atrial refractory period to a longer

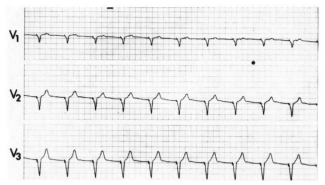

Figure 53–27. VVI pacing at a rate of 60 beats per minute with retrograde conduction. A retrograde P wave can be seen in the ST segment of each paced beat. This patient had symptoms of low cardiac output due to pacemaker syndrome.

value when the pacemaker senses a ventricular event not preceded by an atrial event. Even extending the atrial refractory period cannot guarantee that the retrograde P wave will always fall within that refractory period. A further extension of this principle is to totally disable the sensing function of the atrial circuit for one cycle after a premature ventricular beat. This causes the pacemaker to pace AV sequentially and hopefully will restore the normal atrial activation sequence.

The use of dual-chamber pacing systems in patients in whom pacemaker implantation is indicated for the prevention of syncope or presyncope due to carotid sinus hypersensitivity is controversial. In these patients, a VVI pacing system may not provide the required hemodynamic support during episodes of bradycardia and hypotension (Madigan et al, 1984; Morley et al, 1982; Stryjer et al, 1986).

An algorithm for choosing pacing modes based on the presence of atrial arrhythmias and AV conduction is shown in Figure 53–28.

ANTITACHYCARDIA PACING

Mechanisms of Arrhythmias

Tachycardias are traditionally considered to follow one of three mechanisms: re-entry, triggered activity, or abnormal automaticity. Arrhythmias due to triggered activity are rarely documented clinically. Sinus rhythm is the prototype automatic rhythm, and although other arrhythmias due to abnormal automaticity are encountered occasionally, they are not generally amenable to termination by pacing. Arrhythmias due to re-entry are potentially amenable to termination by pacing.

Re-entry may occur around an anatomic circuit such as that created by the presence of an accessory AV pathway in Wolff-Parkinson-White syndrome, or may be created by functionally abnormal tissue such as in coronary artery disease with myocardial infarction or ischemia. The conditions that favor the de-

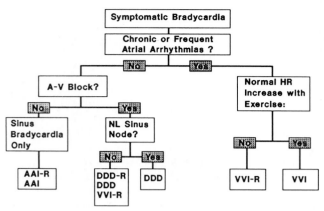

Figure 53–28. Algorithm for choosing pacing mode. Patients with frequent atrial arrhythmias are generally not considered to be candidates for dual-chamber systems, but may do well with a rate-modulated pacemaker if they do not increase their heart rate with exercise. Patients with an insufficient heart rate response to exercise and AV conduction abnormalities are candidates for the newer DDD-R pacemakers. Atrial pacing alone should be used only when AV conduction is known to be reliably intact.

velopment of re-entry are abnormally slow conduction in the re-entrant circuit and the presence of unidirectional block in one limb of the circuit. Re-entrant circuits that are large and anatomically defined are easily penetrated by pacing stimuli, whereas smaller re-entrant circuits that may exist within functionally abnormal regions of the heart may be relatively protected and difficult to interrupt.

Supraventricular re-entrant arrhythmias that may be terminated by pacing include reciprocating tachycardia due to the presence of an accessory AV pathway (Wolff-Parkinson-White syndrome), AV node re-entrant tachycardia, some cases of atrial flutter, and less commonly re-entrant tachycardias due to partial AV nodal bypass (Mahaim's) fibers. Ventricular tachycardia is also often amenable to termination by pacing, although the use of pacing techniques in treating ventricular tachycardia is limited by the frequent acceleration of the arrhythmia or the degeneration of the arrhythmia to ventricular fibrillation during attempts at termination.

Factors that determine the ease with which a re-entrant arrhythmia is terminated by pacing include the size of the re-entrant circuit, the location of the pacing site relative to the re-entrant circuit, and the rate of the tachycardia. The functional properties of the myocardium between the site of stimulation and the site of the arrhythmia are also important. Termination of re-entrant tachycardia by pacing stimuli depends on the ability of the paced activation wavefront to penetrate the re-entrant circuit and create an area of refractoriness ahead of the re-entrant wavefront. When the re-entrant wavefront collides with the area of refractoriness created by the paced impulse, the arrhythmia cannot propagate further and terminates. If the paced impulse fails to block the re-entrant circuit, it may instead penetrate the re-entrant

circuit and advance or accelerate the tachycardia. Pacing during an arrhythmia may also result in fibrillation. These complications are more serious when ventricular tachycardia is the arrhythmia being treated than in the case of supraventricular arrhythmias and may limit the use of pacing techniques in many patients. In addition, extensive electrophysiologic testing before implantation of the pacing device is mandatory to ensure safety and efficacy.

Some clinical considerations are important in the selection of an antitachycardia pacing device. The arrhythmia must be reliably terminated by the technique being considered. In addition, if the patient is to activate the device, the arrhythmia must be well tolerated hemodynamically, and the patient must be able to accurately sense the presence of the arrhythmia and distinguish between the arrhythmia and sinus tachycardia.

Modes of Pacing

Several pacing techniques have been used successfully to terminate arrhythmias. These techniques include competitive or underdrive pacing, burst pacing, overdrive pacing, and critically timed premature stimuli.

Underdrive pacing was one of the first modalities to be applied and is easily accomplished by applying an external magnet to the implanted pulse generator, resulting in asynchronous pacing. Termination of the arrhythmia depends on the chance occurrence of an appropriately timed stimulus. Underdrive pacing can also be accomplished by extending the sensing refractory period of a VVI-AAI pacemaker to exceed the cycle length of the tachycardia. Thus, when the heart rate exceeds the refractory period of the pulse generator (spontaneous R-R interval is less than the pulse generator's refractory period), the pulse generator can no longer sense spontaneous activity and begins to function asynchronously. This "reverse" mode of pacing, response to a rapid heart rate as well as a slow one, is often called dual-demand pacing. To make this mode of tachycardia reversion feasible, a pulse generator with a refractory period programmable to greater than 400 msec is necessary. Devices manufactured by Siemens-Elema and Telectronics have programmable refractory periods as long as 437 msec, resulting in dual-demand pacing when the heart rate exceeds 137 beats per minute.

Overdrive pacing (pacing at a rate less than 30 beats per minute faster than the tachycardia cycle length) is used frequently on a temporary basis to suppress both atrial and ventricular arrhythmias. Permanent overdrive pacing to suppress arrhythmias has been used most notably in patients with bradycardia-related ventricular tachycardia.

Burst pacing (defined as pacing at a rate greater than 30 beats per minute faster than the tachycardia) (Fisher et al, 1982) is often successful in terminating

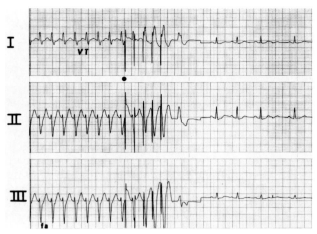

Figure 53–29. Termination of ventricular tachycardia (VT) with a manually activated radiofrequency pacemaker. A short burst of pacing stimuli results in interruption of the tachycardia. Extensive preimplantation testing was done to show safety and efficacy.

re-entrant tachycardias (Fig. 53–29). Burst pacing may be activated by the patient or may be done automatically by an implanted device that senses the onset of tachycardia and responds with a preprogrammed pacing sequence. A device that has been available for routine use for a number of years is the Medtronic model 5998. This device consists of an implantable radiofrequency receiver that is connected to the pacing lead and an external transmitter that can easily be set to the desired pacing rate. The pacing burst is delivered as long as the external device is activated by the patient. This device has the advantage of not requiring an implantable battery, thus eliminating reoperation for battery changes, simplicity of operation, and ease of adjustment. The disadvantages of this system are the need for patients to be able to reliably sense their tachycardia and distinguish arrhythmia from sinus tachycardia. In addition, the tachycardia must be hemodynamically well tolerated to allow the patient time to use the transmitter. Pacing can be done at only one rate without readjustment of the transmitter, although the tachycardia rate may change under various conditions, rendering the device less effective at particular times.

A variation on patient-activated pacing is provided by pulse generators that can be programmed to the triggered mode. An external stimulator applied to the chest wall causes the pacemaker to respond to the transthoracic stimuli and pace the heart at whatever rate or stimulation sequence the external device is set to function. An advantage of this system is the ability of the external device to transmit not only pacing bursts but also timed extrastimuli.

The introduction of critically timed premature stimuli is also an effective method of terminating re-entrant tachycardias (Fig. 53–30). Devices that function automatically to detect and terminate tachycardia are now commerically available. Stimuli may be de-

livered at preset coupling intervals after recognition of tachycardia. In addition, the pacemaker automatically cycles through combinations of coupling intervals if the first sequence fails to terminate the tachycardia. The successful sequence is "remembered" by the device, which automatically begins with these coupling intervals with the next episode of tachycardia, hopefully resulting in prompt arrhythmia conversion. Newer devices also have backup pacing capability to manage the bradycardia that follows tachycardia termination in some patients.

The major limitation of the widespread use of antitachycardia pacemakers in the treatment of serious ventricular arrhythmias has been the potential for arrhythmia acceleration or fibrillation. With ventricular arrhythmias, these adverse effects can be fatal. Extensive preimplant testing has therefore been important to document the efficacy and safety of pacing techniques, because even the development of atrial fibrillation, although not often life threatening, is usually undesirable.

AUTOMATIC IMPLANTABLE CARDIOVERTER DEFIBRILLATOR

Mortality in patients with recurrent malignant ventricular dysrhythmias refractory to antiarrhythmic therapy, electrophysiologically directed surgical procedures, and antitachycardia pacing is still a significant problem. After a decade of experimental work, the automatic implantable defibrillator was introduced in 1980 to treat patients at risk of sudden cardiac death. Since February of 1980, the automatic implantable cardioverter defibrillator (AICD) has been implanted in more than 1,500 patients (Fig. 53–31). Sudden death has been reduced to 2 to 4% annually (Watkins et al, 1988). The AICD system consists of a lithium-powered pulse generator that weighs 250 g and occupies a volume of 148 ml. The

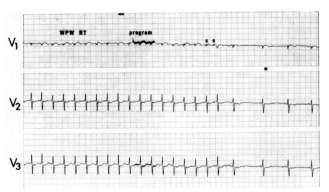

Figure 53–30. Terminating of reciprocating tachycardia (RT) in a patient with Wolff-Parkinson-White syndrome by an automatic device. During testing, the device is inhibited while tachycardia is induced and is then programmed on during tachycardia. After four sensed beats of tachycardia, the pacemaker responds with two premature stimuli, terminating the arrhythmia.

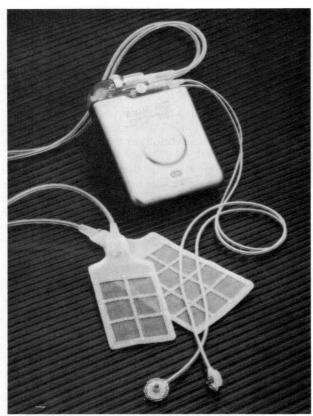

Figure 53–31. Automatic implantable cardioverter defibrillator. Through a median sternotomy, epicardial sensing electrodes are attached at the level of the anterior aspect of the interventricular septum. Plaque electrodes are sutured onto the right ventricle and lateral aspect of the left ventricle. The defibrillating shock is delivered from the smaller RV plaque, and the large LV plaque serves as a grounding electrode. After implantation of the sensing electrodes and defibrillating electrodes, all leads are tunneled beneath the xiphoid to a left upper-quadrant pocket, where they are attached to the AICD generator.

lead system consists of bipolar sensing electrodes for synchronized cardioversion via defibrillating plaques. The defibrillator continuously monitors the patient's heart rate and electrogram waveform. When a probability density function and heart rate exceed specified values, a truncated exponential pulse of 25 joules is delivered approximately 15 to 20 seconds after the onset of arrhythmia. The generator can be activated or inactivated noninvasively by using a doughnut-shaped magnet. Warranty lifetime is 50 pulses or 18 months (Watkins et al, 1988). An external analyzer (AID-check) is available to measure and digitally display battery charge time as well as the number of discharges. In addition to the standard AICD described earlier, a variation of the system referred to as a "rate only device" is available. A preset cutoff value for heart rate determines when the device will fire (Watkins et al, 1988).

Patients at high risk of sudden death from ventricular arrhythmias refractory to either pharmacologic therapy or electrophysiologically guided oper-

ative procedures are candidates for implantation of an AICD system. Excluded are patients with (1) recent myocardial infarction, (2) drug toxicity, (3) mental or psychological disorders that preclude informed consent, and (4) life expectancy of less than 6 months (Watkins et al, 1988).

The system can be implanted through a subxiphoid approach anterior thoracotomy, median sternotomy, or subcostal technique. In a recent report by Watkins and associates (1988), the operative mortality among 200 patients receiving the entire system was 4%; after implantation, the annual sudden death rate is approximately 2%. As summarized by Watkins and associates (1988), current clinical results indicate that the device can be safely implanted in a high-risk group of patients, and more important, improved long-term survival can be achieved in this exceptionally high-risk group. However, the cost of a complete AICD system is approximately $16,000, and the generator must be replaced at 18-month intervals (additional $14,000 per generator replacement).

COMPLICATIONS

As summarized in Table 53–6, pacemaker complications can be divided into four categories: immediate surgical complications, wound problems, delayed complications, and pacemaker malfunctions. Fortunately, all are relatively uncommon, making pacemaker insertion an exceptionally safe procedure when done by experienced surgeons.

Immediate Surgical Complications

As described earlier, perhaps the safest way of inserting a permanent transvenous lead-electrode system is via the cephalic vein. The risk of pneumothorax, vascular injury, air embolism, and air entrapment within the pacing pocket are increased when the subclavian vein access route is chosen. Air entrapment within the pacemaker pocket secondary to either pneumothorax with subcutaneous emphysema or secondary to air entrapped during pacemaker pocket closure can result in pacemaker failure in unipolar systems secondary to insulation of the unipolar anodal plate (indifferent electrode) from the subcutaneous tissues (Hearne and Maloney, 1982; Kreis et al, 1979; Lasala et al, 1979). Neural injury to both the phrenic and recurrent laryngeal nerves has been reported when the lead-electrode system is introduced through the internal jugular vein (Dieter et al, 1981). Regardless of the venous access route chosen, cardiac perforation can occur but fortunately rarely leads to hemopericardium and tamponade (Fig. 53–32) (Irwin et al, 1987). A final complication is immediate electrode dislodgment. The risk of this complication can be reduced by doing provocative maneuvers such as coughing and deep breathing at the time of initial implantation. Transvenous elec-

TABLE 53–6. PACEMAKER COMPLICATIONS

Immediate Surgical Complications	*Delayed Complications*
Pneumothorax	Venous thrombosis
Vascular injury	Pulmonary embolism
Air embolism	Twiddler's syndrome
Cardiac perforation	Constrictive pericarditis
Tamponade	Tricuspid insufficiency
Lead-electrode dislodgment	Pacemaker syndrome
Neural injury—phrenic, recurrent laryngeal	
Air entrapment in pocket	

Wound Problems	*Pacemaker Malfunctions*
Hematoma	Radiation damage
Infection	Runaway pacemaker
Skin erosion	Pacemaker-induced ventricular fibrillation
Migration of impulse generator	Irregular pacing
Skeletal muscle stimulation	Failure of sensing
	Failure of capture
	Electrode fracture
	Knotting of lead
	Inhibition of pacemaker by skeletal myopotentials
	Electromagnetic interference

trode dislodgment problems have not been significantly increased in patients with congenitally corrected transposition of the great vessels, although this would have been expected because of the decreased trabeculation of the embryologic left ventricle, which is where the pacing lead lies (Estes et al, 1983).

Wound Problems

Perhaps the most common wound problem associated with permanent pacemaker implantation is a hematoma. Obviously, this complication can be prevented by strict attention to hemostasis at the time of implantation. In patients who require impulse generator change, the pacemaker pocket should be debrided of excess pseudocapsule to prevent the formation of a sterile seroma. Fortunately, wound infection is a rare problem prevented by meticulous operative technique and the appropriate use of prophylactic antibiotics. In general, when

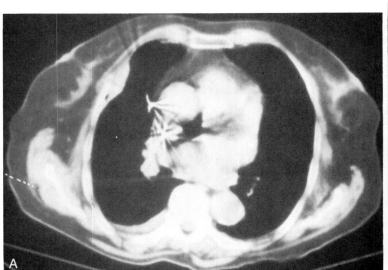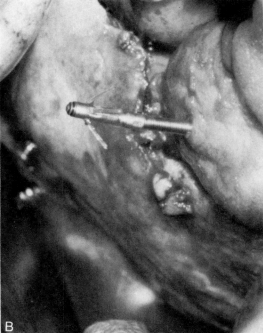

Figure 53–32. Transvenous atrial lead perforation. An 80-year-old woman was referred to Duke University Medical Center several months after implantation of a DDD pacemaker system. The patient initially had done well but was referred for evaluation of a recent syncopal episode. During evaluation, she was noted to have hiccups that coincided with atrial pacing. An ECG demonstrated atrial pacing without atrial capture. The admission chest film showed a new right pleural effusion and suggested displacement of the atrial lead outside of the cardiac silhouette. A repeat echocardiogram could not show the position of the atrial lead, but a chest computerized tomographic scan *(A)* clearly showed that the atrial lead perforated the atrium. A pneumomediastinum was also noted. The patient was taken to the operating room and had a right anterior thoracotomy *(B)* for removal of the lead and atrial repair under direct visualization. An atrial epicardial lead was placed and tunneled across the chest subcutaneously to the chronic left pectoral pacemaker pocket, where the ventricular endocardial lead was still attached. The patient recovered uneventfully. This case demonstrates that unlike ventricular perforations, which often seal with retraction of the pacing wire, the thin-walled atrium may not seal and indeed, as in this case, may require surgical repair. (From Irwin, J. M., Greer, G. S., Lowe, J. E., et al: Atrial lead perforation: A case report. PACE, *10*:1378, 1987.)

infection occurs, the entire pacing system including the impulse generator and lead-electrode system should be removed, the patient should be treated with appropriate intravenous antibiotics, and a temporary pacemaker should be used for an interim period. When infection has completely cleared, a new pacemaker system is implanted through another access site. Skin erosion by either the impulse generator or lead can be prevented by proper positioning of pacemaker hardware deep within the subcutaneous tissues or beneath the fascia of the pectoralis major muscle. Unipolar impulse generators can cause muscle stimulation if placed immediately adjacent to skeletal muscle. However, bipolar impulse generators can be placed either in the subcutaneous tissue or beneath muscle. Migration of the impulse generator most commonly occurs in infraclavicular pacemaker pockets. Migration tends to follow the curvature of the chest wall, and the impulse generator tends to migrate laterally. This can be prevented by creating an anteromedial pocket sufficiently large to contain the impulse generator and lead. In susceptible individuals, the impulse generator can be further secured to the chest wall to prevent migration.

Delayed Complications

Unusual delayed complications associated with transvenous pacemakers include thrombosis of the superior vena cava with resultant superior vena caval syndrome, axillary vein thrombosis with upper-extremity edema, cerebral venous sinus thrombosis, and right atrial and right ventricular thrombosis (Bradof et al, 1982; Branson, 1978; Cholankeril et al, 1982; Fritz et al, 1983; Girard et al, 1980; Gunderson et al, 1982; Kinney et al, 1979; Krug and Zerbe, 1980;

Mitrovic et al, 1983; Nicolosi et al, 1980; Pauletti et al, 1979; Youngson et al, 1980). Pulmonary thromboembolism has also been recognized as a rare but lethal complication that occurs most often in patients with low cardiac output and underlying right atrial or right ventricular thrombi (Kinney et al, 1979). Constrictive pericarditis has been reported in patients who have received both transvenous and transthoracic electrodes (Foster, 1982; Schwartz et al, 1979). Tricuspid insufficiency is rare, usually asymptomatic, and is secondary to either lead placement or lead removal (Gibson et al, 1980; Ong et al, 1981). Electrode dislodgment and lead fracture can be caused by unconscious or habitual "twiddling" of the impulse generator (Fig. 53–33). Twiddler's syndrome has been reported most commonly in patients with transvenous pacing systems but has also been reported in those with transmediastinal pacing systems (Rodan et al, 1978). Finally, several reports have suggested that permanent pacemaker implantation with the impulse generator lying over the infraclavicular area is associated with an increased risk of breast carcinoma in women. However, based on a careful review by Magilligan and Isshak (1980), the appearance of breast cancer in women with pacemakers is probably coincidental and is not related to materials, electrochemical stimulation, or chronic trauma.

Pacemaker Malfunctions

Biomedical engineering improvements have led to exceptionally durable and reliable permanent pacemakers. However, random failures still occur and emphasize the need for appropriate long-term follow-up. Pacemaker malfunctions are secondary to alter-

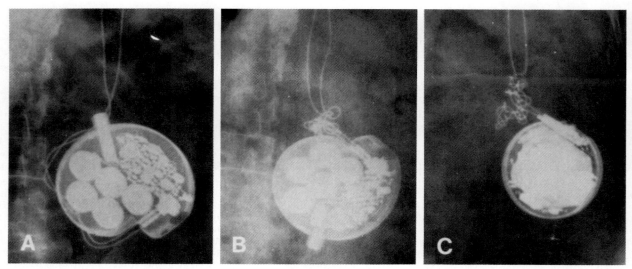

Figure 53–33. Abdominal films. *A*, Film 1 year after initial implant shows normal relationship between the wires and the impulse generator. *B*, Film 2 years later shows rotation of impulse generator 180 degrees and twisting of wires close to the generator. *C*, 6 months after implantation of a new impulse generator, additional twisting is evident. (From Rodan, B. A., Lowe, J. E., and Chen, J. T. T.: Abdominal twiddler's syndrome. Am. J. Roentgenol., *131*:1084, 1978. Copyright © 1978 by Williams & Wilkins Company.)

ations of the preset pacing rate (acceleration or slowing), irregular pacing, failure of sensing, failure of cardiac capture or depolarization, and various combinations of these events. Sudden acceleration of pacing rate, called "runaway pacemaker," results in pacemaker-induced ventricular tachycardia. This complication was most often a manifestation of malfunction of fixed-rate devices. Fortunately, the runaway pacemaker has been rarely encountered because demand ventricular pacemakers have gradually replaced fixed-rate models. In advanced runaway pacemaker syndrome, ventricular fibrillation may occur and lead to sudden death. The runaway pacemaker is a medical emergency and is treated immediately by placement of a new impulse generator.

Slowing of the pacing rate is a more common manifestation of pacemaker malfunction in modern demand impulse generators. Irregular pacing usually indicates an advanced form of malfunction and may be associated with acceleration or slowing of the pacing rate. Failure of sensing can occur as an isolated finding but is commonly associated with failure of cardiac capture. Failure of sensing results in a demand unit that functions as a fixed-rate pacemaker when its sensing circuit does not work properly. Failure of cardiac capture may be complete but is usually intermittent. The most common cause of failure of capture is malposition of the pacemaker electrode or lead fracture. Electrode displacement may be observed at any time but most often occurs within the first few days after implantation. Late causes of failure of capture are fibrosis around the pacemaker electrode, advancement of underlying heart disease, severe hyperkalemia or hypokalemia, and drug toxicity, especially with quinidine and procainamide. If none of these factors is present, the pacemaker impulse generator itself is most likely malfunctioning.

Ventricular fibrillation can occur during insertion, especially when ventricular fibrillation thresholds are low, such as in patients with acute myocardial infarction. Ventricular fibrillation is uncommon because the R on T phenomenon should not occur in a properly functioning demand pacemaker.

Inhibition of demand pacemakers by myopotentials is always a possibility when unipolar pacing systems are used. Inhibition of bipolar demand pacemakers by noncardiac muscle potentials, however, is a relatively uncommon phenomenon. Transient pacemaker inhibition of unipolar pacemakers may also result from active contraction of the diaphragm, such as that created by deep inspiration, straining, and coughing.

It was previously thought that ionizing radiation did not have any adverse affect on the function of impulse generators. However, reports have suggested that ionizing radiation can cause malfunction of new-generation programmable pacemakers. No deleterious effects can be attributed to diagnostic x-ray exposure, but radiation for therapeutic purposes can cause permanent malfunction of susceptible programmable devices (Adamec et al, 1982; Katzenberg et al, 1982). The mode of failure cannot be predicted.

The effect of magnetic resonance imaging (MRI) machines on pacemakers is unpredictable (Holmes et al, 1986). Pacemakers contain small amounts of ferrous metals and are therefore only slightly attracted to magnetic fields. The presence of a strong magnetic field such as is present in MRI scanners results in closure of the reed switch, which would be expected. This results in asynchronous operation of most pacemakers, except for those in which the magnet mode of operation can be programmed "off." The radiofrequency pulses used during MRI may also affect pacemaker function, and some devices have for unknown reasons paced at the rapid rate of the radiofrequency pulse. However, permanent reprogramming or damage to pacemakers from MRI equipment has not been encountered. Patients with pacemakers who require MRI should be able to have this procedure safely if they are monitored carefully for the possibility of rapid pacing during the procedure.

A syndrome that describes a complex of symptoms caused by pacemaker insertion has been recognized. This "pacemaker syndrome" is characterized by vertigo, light-headedness, syncope, and hypotension occurring after implantation of a ventricular pacemaker. The cause has been attributed to a decrease in cardiac output during ventricular pacing secondary to loss of atrial contribution to ventricular end-diastolic volume. As discussed earlier, the pacemaker syndrome is most likely to occur in patients who require the atrial contribution to cardiac output. The symptoms can usually be relieved by placement of a dual-chamber pacing system that allows more physiologic pacing if lowering the demand pacing rate is ineffectual.

PACEMAKER FOLLOW-UP

An organized follow-up program for pacemaker patients should be provided by every clinic engaged in implanting permanent pacemakers. An adequate follow-up program must do more than merely document normal or abnormal function of a pacemaker, and the purpose of pacemaker follow-up is not just to detect pacemaker failure. Instead, a comprehensive program should provide preimplant and postimplant teaching, continued reassurance for the patient and family, transtelephonic monitoring of both the pacemaker and the patient's spontaneous rhythm, office or clinic visits when necessary, and assistance when admission to the hospital is required for complications, for routine battery changes, or for reasons not related to the pacemaker directly.

A properly designed follow-up program should not only provide support for the patient with a pacemaker, but should also be capable of providing important information concerning the patient's pacemaker for the physicians who are involved in care.

The functions of the pacemaker follow-up program may be summarized as involving the education of both the patient and physician, documentation of normal and abnormal pacemaker function, detection of complications (surgical and related to pacemaker function), facilitation of efficient medical care for the patient with the pacemaker, and storage of critical data regarding the pacemaker and electrodes for each patient in an organized system so that it is available to any physician who takes care of the patient. Commercial services can provide transtelephonic ECG tracings and monitor pacemaker function, but these services cannot substitute for a program that involves the medical personnel involved in pacemaker implantation and patient follow-up.

Although commonly thought to involve primarily transtelephonic ECG recording, pacemaker follow-up should be an integrated system of postimplant teaching, clinic visits, and telephone transmissions. The purposes of teaching the patient when the pacemaker is implanted are to allay the patient's and family's concerns about the pacemaker, to inform the patient about the normal function of the pacemaker, and to teach the patient how to use the telephone transmission equipment. A schedule of call-in times should be arranged before discharge, and the use of the transmitter should be practiced with the personnel who will receive the calls. Baseline recordings should be made of the ECG with and without magnet and an overpenetrated chest film obtained to document lead position.

The patient should be observed as an outpatient at 6 weeks after implantation, at which time a noninvasive assessment of pacing threshold should be made. This assessment is done in different ways, depending on the model and manufacturer of the pacemaker. Pulse generator output can be decreased in a stepwise fashion by shortening pulse width in some generators and by lowering output voltage in others. By observing the point at which capture is lost, an estimation of the chronic pacing threshold can be obtained and the pacemaker's output programmed down to lower levels to prolong battery life. A margin of safety of at least 2:1 over the capture threshold should be maintained. Because pacing thresholds may rise during the first few weeks after implantation, decreasing pacing output, either by reprogramming pulse width or voltage, should not be done earlier than 4 to 6 weeks after implantation.

The return visit also provides an opportunity to carefully examine the surgical site for signs of excessive skin tension, inflammation, or improper wound healing.

Telephone transmissions should begin immediately after discharge and are done weekly for the first 4 weeks to document proper function. Subsequent telephone transmissions should be made regularly, but at longer intervals. In most patients, transmissions are probably not required more frequently than every 6 months in the absence of symptoms. At the time of the telephone transmission, recordings should be made of the spontaneous rhythm, and then with the application of the external magnet. Readings of pulse width and AV interval (for dual-chamber devices) can also be obtained. These data are recorded in the follow-up files so that proper pacemaker function can be documented and future malfunctions ascertained. Some pacemakers respond to magnet application with a change in rate and may also automatically begin a cycle of decreasing output to check pacing threshold. It should be borne in mind that the magnet response can be programmed off in some pacemakers.

As the pacemaker begins to approach its theoretical end of life, the frequency of telephone transmissions should be increased. In some models, the pulse width gradually extends before the pacemaker actually begins to change its rate. Thus, the approach of end of life can be monitored as pulse width extends, and the frequency of telephone transmissions can be increased when pulse width has doubled. When the pacemaker finally shows its end of life indicator, usually a drop in rate, elective admission can be arranged and the pacemaker can be replaced.

Finally, records of any reprogramming should be maintained in the follow-up files so that changes in pacemaker function that appear on routine tracings can be properly interpreted.

FUTURE TRENDS

Future trends in cardiac pacing will undoubtedly continue to follow the advances in technology that have characterized the field during the last 10 years. Improvements in lead-electrode technology can be expected to result in smaller leads and improved electrodes with lower chronic pacing thresholds resulting in lower energy requirements and longer battery life. The ability to pace with less energy output may permit the use of smaller batteries, and thus smaller pulse generators.

One of the predictable areas of continued progress is the field of antitachycardia pacing. Devices that can terminate supraventricular tachycardia are currently available and are being refined. Successful treatment of ventricular tachycardia requires the development of devices that incorporate both antitachycardia pacing and backup defibrillation.

The proliferation of programmable pacemakers has required pacemaker centers to stock an increasingly large number of different manufacturer's programmers. At present, there is no compatibility between the various programmers. Unfortunately, it is unlikely that a device will be devised to program all existing pacemakers. In the future, it would seem to be in the best interests of efficiency and cost reduction to work toward a universal system for pacemaker programmability.

Finally, continued advances in physiologic pacing devices can also be expected. Among these advances will be pacemakers that respond to various physiologic parameters and allow changes in heart rate that correspond with the patient's physiologic needs (Wirtzfield et al, 1987).

With further technologic advances in the field of physiologic pacing, improved ways of determining which patients will benefit from these devices will be necessary. This can be accomplished only through clinical databases located at centers that implant and closely monitor large numbers of patients with pacemakers.

Selected Bibliography

Bernstein, A. D., Camm, A. J., Fletcher, R. D., et al: The NASPE/BPEG generic pacemaker code for antibradyarrhythmia and adaptive-rate pacing and antitachyarrhythmia devices. PACE, *10*:794, 1987.

Because of the variety of complex modes of operation available in pacemakers, letter codes were established in 1974 to indicate pacing modes in a condensed form. Recent technical advances in pacemakers have increased the need for an expanded code to reflect these developments. A new pacemaker code proposed by the North American Society of Pacing and Electrophysiology (NASPE) and the British Pacing and Electrophysiology Groups (BPEG) is called the NBG Generic Pacemaker Code. The NBG code expands on the previous Inter-Society Commission for Heart Disease (ICHG) code and was designed to meet two major needs previously not met by other codes. As described in detail in this report, the NBG pacemaker code shows the use of a rate-modulation mechanism to respond adaptively to changes in a physiologic variable, and it indicates the presence of one or more antitachyarrhythmia functions without identifying them specifically. The new five-digit NBG pacemaker code is an expansion of the three-digit ICHG code so that either code can be used with clarity.

Furman, S., Hayes, D. L., and Holmes, D. R.: A Practice of Cardiac Pacing. Mt. Kisco, NY, Futura Publishing Co., 1986.

This well-written, concise, and complete text presents all aspects of permanent and temporary cardiac pacing including electrophysiologic and hemodynamic concepts, indications, implantation techniques, and troubleshooting. Much practical information is provided and also answers to frequently posed questions with regard to pacemakers.

Mond, H. G.: The Cardiac Pacemaker: Function and Malfunction. New York, Grune & Stratton, 1983.

This comprehensive monograph discusses pacemaker function and malfunction in detail and also provides a great deal of historical and fundamental technical information on pacing leads, electrodes, batteries, and circuitry. This source is highly recommended for readers who desire more in-depth information regarding technical considerations in pacemaker design and function.

Morse, D., Steiner, R. M., and Parsonnet, V.: A Guide to Cardiac Pacemakers. Supplement, 1986–1987. Philadelphia, F. A. Davis, 1986.

Almost every modern pacemaker in current use is described in detail in this atlas. Radiographs of each pacemaker are included, and identification codes are thoroughly explained. Available pacemaker lead electrode systems and pacing system analyzers are also covered in detail.

Schechter, D. C.: Exploring the Origins of Electrical Cardiac Stimulation. Medtronics, Inc., 1983.

This monograph contains selected works of Schechter on the history of electrotherapy. Areas covered in detail include the origins of electrotherapy, the background of clinical cardiac electrostimulation, and early observations on the pathophysiology of ventricular fibrillation. This special volume is exceptionally well illustrated and referenced and represents an outstanding source for those interested in the fascinating history of cardiac pacing.

Watkins, L., Jr., Guarnieri, T., Griffith, L. S. C., et al: Implantation of the automatic implantable cardioverter defibrillator. J. Cardiovasc. Surg., *3*:1, 1988.

This manuscript throughly describes the automatic implantable cardioverter defibrillator, indications for implantation, surgical techniques, and clinical results. Since February of 1980, the automatic implantable cardioverter defibrillator has been implanted in approximately 1,500 patients, and sudden death rates have been reduced to 2 to 4% annually. This report reviews the clinical experience in 200 patients evaluated by the authors.

Bibliography

Adamec, R., Haefliger, J. M., Killisch, J. P., et al: Damaging effect of therapeutic radiation on programmable pacemakers. PACE, *5*:146, 1982.
Akhtar, M.: Retrograde conduction in man. PACE, 4:548, 1981.
Aldini, G.: General Views on the Application of Galvanism to Medical Purposes. London, J. Callow, 1819.
Allen, P., and Lillehei, C. W.: Use of induced cardiac arrest in open heart surgery: Results in seventy patients. Minn. Med., *40*:672, 1957.
Alpert, M. A., Curtis, J. J., San Felippo, J. F., et al: Comparative survival after permanent ventricular and dual chamber pacing for patients with chronic high degree atrioventricular block with and without pre-existent congestive heart failure. J. Am. Coll. Cardiol., *7*:925, 1986.
Althaus, J.: Report of the committee appointed by the Royal Medical and Chirurgical Society to inquire into the uses and the physiological, therapeutical and toxic effects of chloroform. Med. Chir. Trans., *47*:416, 1864.
Anderson, R. H., Becker, A. E., Tranum-Jensen, J., and Janse, M. J.: Anatomico-electrophysiological correlations in the conduction system—a review. Br. Heart J., *45*:67, 1981.
Armour, J. A., Roy, O. Z., Firor, W. B., et al: A battery-less biological cardiovascular pacemaker. Surg. Forum, *17*:164, 1966.
Barold, S. S., and Mugica, J.: Advances in technology and clinical applications. *In* Barold, S. S. (ed): The Third Decade of Cardiac Pacing. Mt. Kisco, N.Y., Futura Publishing Co., 1982.
Beck, C. S., Pritchard, W. H., and Feil, H. S.: Ventricular fibrillation of long duration abolished by electric shock. J.A.M.A., *135*:985, 1947.
Berkovits, B. V., Castellanos, A., Jr., and Lemberg, L.: Bifocal demand pacing. Circulation, *39*:44, 1969.
Bernstein, A. D., Camm, A. J., Fletcher, R. D., et al: The NASPE/BPEG generic pacemaker code for antibradyarrhythmia and adaptive-rate pacing and antitachyarrhythmia devices. PACE, *10*:794, 1987.
Bigelow, W. G., Callaghan, J. C., and Hopps, J. A.: General hypotherma for experimental intracardiac surgery. The use of electrophrenic respirations, an artificial pacemaker for cardiac standstill, and radio-frequency rewarming in general hypothermia. Ann. Surg., *132*:531, 1950.
Billhardt, R. A., Rosenbush, S. W., and Hauser, R. G.: Successful management of pacing system malfunctions without surgery: The role of programmable pulse generators. PACE, *5*:675, 1982.

Bradof, J., Sands, M. J., and Lakin, P. C.: Symptomatic venous thrombosis of the upper extremity complicating permanent transvenous pacing: Reversal with streptokinase infusion. Am. Heart J., 104:1112, 1982.

Branson, J. A.: Radiology of cardiac pacemakers and their complications with three cases of superior vena caval obstruction. Australas. Radiol., 22:125, 1978.

Breivik, K., and Ohm, O.: Myopotential inhibition of unipolar QRS-inhibited (VVI) pacemakers, assessed by ambulatory Holter monitoring of the electrocardiogram. PACE, 3:470, 1980.

Brockman, S. K., Webb, R. C., Jr., and Bahnson, H. T.: Monopolar ventricular stimulation for the control of acute surgically produced heart block. Surgery, 44:910, 1958.

Calfee, R. V., and Saulson, S. H.: A voluntary standard for 3.2 mm unipolar and bipolar pacemaker leads and connectors. PACE, 9:1181, 1986.

Calvin, J. W.: Intraoperative pacemaker electrical testing. Ann. Thorac. Surg., 26:165, 1978.

Chardack, W. M., Gage, A. A., Federico, A. J., et al: Five years' clinical experience with an implantable pacemaker: An appraisal. Surgery, 58:915, 1965.

Chardack, W. M., Gage, A. A., and Greatbatch, W.: A transistorized self-contained, implantable pacemaker for the long-term correction of heart block. Surgery, 48:643, 1960.

Cholankeril, J. V., Joshi, R. R., and Ketyer, S.: Benign superior vena cava syndrome caused by transvenous cardiac pacemaker. Cardiovasc. Intervent. Radiol., 5:40, 1982.

Chung, E. K.: Artificial Cardiac Pacing: Practical Approach, 2nd ed. Baltimore, Williams & Wilkins, 1984.

Cywinski, J. K., Hahn, A. W., Nichols, M. F., et al: Performance of implanted biogalvanic pacemakers. PACE, 1:117, 1978.

Dhingra, R. C., Denes, P., Wu, D., et al: The significance of second degree atrioventricular block and bundle branch block: Observations regarding site and type of block. Circulation, 49:638, 1974.

Dieter, R. A., Jr., Asselmeier, G. H., Hamouda, F., et al: Neural complications of transvenous pacemaker implantation: Hoarseness and diaphragmatic paralysis: Case reports. Milit. Med., 146:647, 1981.

Domenighetti, G., and Perret, C.: Intraventricular conduction disturbances in acute myocardial infarction: Short- and long-term prognosis. Eur. J. Cardiol. 11:51, 1980.

Duchenne de Boulogne: De L'Electrisation Localisée et son Application à la Pathologie et à la Therapeutique. Paris, Baillière, 1872.

Ekestrom, S., Johansson, L., and Lagergren, H.: Behandling av Adams-Stokes syndrom med en intracardiell pacemaker elektrod. Opusc. Med., 7:1, 1962.

Elmquist, R., and Senning, A.: Implantable pacemaker for the heart. In Smyth, C. N. (ed): Medical Electronics. Proceedings of the Second International Conference on Medical Electronics. Paris, June, 1959; London, Iliffe & Sons, Ltd., 1960.

Estes, N. A. M., III, Salem, D. N., Isner, J. M., and Gamble, W. J.: Permanent pacemaker therapy in corrected transposition of the great arteries: Analysis of site of lead placement in 40 patients. Am. J. Cardiol., 52:1091, 1983.

Faerestrand, S., and Ohm, O-J.: A time-related study of the hemodynamic benefit of atrioventricular synchronous pacing evaluated by Doppler echocardiography. PACE, 8:838, 1985.

Fischell, R. E., Lewis, K. B., Schulman, J. H., et al: A long-lived, reliable, rechargeable cardiac pacemaker. In Schaldach, M. (ed): Advances in Pacemaker Technology, New York, Springer-Verlag, 1975, p. 357.

Fisher, J. D., Kim, S. G., Furman, S., and Matos, J. A.: Role of implantable pacemakers in control of recurrent ventricular tachycardia. Am. J. Cardiol., 49:194, 1982.

Foster, C. J.: Constrictive pericarditis complicating an endocardial pacemaker. Br. Heart J., 47:497, 1982.

Friedberg, C. K., Donoso, E., and Stein, W. G.: Nonsurgical acquired heart block. Ann. N.Y. Acad. Sci., 111:835, 1964.

Fritz, T., Richeson, J. F., Fitzpatrick, P., and Wilson, G.: Venous obstruction: A potential complication of transvenous pacemaker electrodes. Chest, 83:534, 1983.

Furman, S., Escher, D. J. W., Solomon, N., et al: Electrocardiographic manifestation of standby pacing. J. Thorac. Cardiovasc. Surg., 54:723, 1967.

Furman, S., Pannizzo, F., and Campo, I.: Comparison of active and passive leads for endocardial pacing. II. PACE, 4:78, 1981.

Furman, S., and Robinson, G.: Stimulation of the ventricular endocardial surface in control of complete heart block. Ann. Surg., 150:841, 1959.

Furman, S., and Schwedel, J. B.: An intracardiac pacemaker for Stokes-Adams seizures. N. Engl. J. Med., 261:943, 1959.

Furman, S., Schwedel, J. B., Robinson, G., and Hurwitt, E. S.: Use of an intracardiac pacemaker in the control of heart block. Surgery, 49:98, 1961.

Gibson, T. C., Davidson, R. C., and DeSilvey, D. L.: Presumptive tricuspid valve malfunction induced by a pacemaker lead: A case report and review of the literature. PACE, 3:88, 1980.

Girard, D. E., Reuler, J. B., Mayer, B. S., et al: Cerebral venous sinus thrombosis due to indwelling transvenous pacemaker catheter. Arch. Neurol., 37:113, 1980.

Glenn, W. W. L., Mauro, A., Longo, E., et al: Remote stimulation of the heart by radiofrequency transmission: Clinical application to a patient with Stokes-Adams syndrome. N. Engl. J. Med., 261:948, 1959.

Goetz, R. H., Dormandy, J. A., and Berkovits, B.: Pacing on demand in the treatment of atrioventricular conduction disturbances of the heart. Lancet, 2:599, 1966.

Goldman, B. S., and Parsonnet, V.: Cardiac pacing, data collection, and world surveys. PACE, 2:115, 1979.

Gott, V. L., Sellers, R., and Lillehei, C. W.: The development of an epicardial-endocardial electrode for permanent placement in Stokes-Adams disease. Surg. Forum, 11:250, 1960.

Guidelines for Permanent Cardiac Pacemaker Implantation, May 1984. Subcommittee on Pacemaker Implantation—Joint AC/AHA Taskforce on Assessment of Cardiovascular Procedures. J. Am. Coll. Cardiol., 4:434, 1984.

Gundersen, T., Abrahamsen, A. M., and Jorgensen, I.: Thrombosis of superior vena cava as a complication of transvenous pacemaker treatment. Acta Med. Scand., 212:85, 1982.

Hearne, S. F., and Maloney, J. D.: Pacemaker system failure secondary to air entrapment within the pulse generator pocket: A complication of subclavian venipuncture for lead placement. Chest, 82:651, 1982.

Hindman, M. C., Wagner, G. S., Jo Ro, M., et al: The clinical significance of bundle branch block complicating acute myocardial infarction. II: Indications for temporary and permanent pacemaker insertion. Circulation, 58:689, 1978.

His, W.: Die Thatigkeit des embryonalen Herzens und deren Bedeutung fur die tehre von der Herzbewegung beim Erwachsenen. In Curschmaun, H. (ed): Arbeiten aus der Medicinischen Klinik zu Leipzig. Leipzig, Vogel, 1893.

Holmes, D. R., Jr., Hayes, D. L., Gray, J. E., and Merideth, J.: The effects of magnetic resonance imaging on implantable pulse generators. PACE, 9:360, 1986.

Hughes, H. C., Jr., Brownlee, R. R., and Tyers, G. F.: Failure of demand pacing with small surface area electrodes. Circulation, 54:128, 1976.

Hunter, J.: Proposals for recovery of people apparently drowned. Philos. Trans. R. Soc. Lond., 66:412, 1776.

Hunter, S. W., Roth, N. A., Bernardez, D., et al: A bipolar myocardial electrode for complete heart block. Lancet, 70:506, 1959.

Hyman, A. S.: Resuscitation of the stopped heart by intracardial therapy. II: Experimental use of an artificial pacemaker. Arch. Intern. Med., 50:283, 1932.

Irwin, J. M., Greer, G. S., Lowe, J. E., et al: Atrial lead perforation: A case report. PACE, 10:1378, 1987.

Johansson, B. W.: Longevity in complete heart block. Ann. N.Y. Acad. Sci., 167:1031, 1969.

Kantrowitz, A., Cohen, R., Raillard, H., et al: The treatment of complete heart block with an implanted, controllable pacemaker. Surg. Gynecol. Obstet., 115:415, 1962.

Kappenberger, L., Gloor, H. O., Babotai, I., et al: Hemodynamic effects of atrial synchronization in acute and long-term ventricular pacing. PACE, 5:639, 1982.

Katzenberg, C. A., Marcus, F. I., Heusinkveld, R. S., et al: Pacemaker failure due to radiation therapy. PACE, 5:156, 1982.

Kent, A. F. S.: Researches on the structure and function of the mammalian heart. J. Physiol. (Lond.), 14:233, 1893.

Kinney, E. L., Allen, R. P., Weidner, W. A., et al: Recurrent pulmonary emboli secondary to right atrial thrombus around a permanent pacing catheter: A case report and review of the literature. PACE, 2:196, 1979.

Kleinert, M., Elmqvist, H., and Strandberg, H.: Spectral properties of atrial and ventricular endocardial signals. PACE, 2:11, 1979.

Kouwenhoven, W. G., Hooker, D. R., and Langworthy, O. R.: Current flowing through the heart under conditions of electric shock. Am. J. Physiol., 100:344, 1932.

Kreis, D. J., Jr., Licalzi, L., and Shaw, R. K.: Air entrapment as a cause of transient cardiac pacemaker malfunction. PACE, 2:641, 1979.

Kristensson, B. E., Arnmon, K., Smedgard, P., and Ryden, L.: Physiological versus single-rate ventricular pacing: A double-blind cross-over study. PACE, 8:73, 1985.

Krug, H., and Zerbe, F.: Major venous thrombosis: A complication of transvenous pacemaker electrodes. Br. Heart J., 44:158, 1980.

Kruse, I., Arnman, K., Conradson, T. B., and Ryden, L.: A comparison of the acute and long-term hemodynamic effects of ventricular inhibited and atrial synchronous ventricular inhibited pacing. Circulation, 65:846, 1982.

Kruse, I. B., and Ryder, L.: Comparison of physical work capacity and systolic time intervals with ventricular inhibited and atrial synchronous ventricular inhibited pacing. Br. Heart J., 46:129, 1981.

Lagergren, H., and Johansson, L.: Intracardiac stimulation for complete heart block. Acta Chir. Scand., 125:562, 1963.

Lasala, A. F., Fieldman, A., Diana, D. J., and Humphrey, C. B.: Gas pocket causing pacemaker malfunction. PACE, 2:183, 1979.

Leatham, A., Cook, P., and Davies, J. G.: External electric stimulator for treatment of ventricular standstill. Lancet, 2:1185, 1956.

Lemberg, L., Castellanos, A., Jr., and Berkovits, B.: Pacing on demand in AV block. J.A.M.A., 191:12, 1965.

Levy, S., Gerard, R., Jausseran, J. M., et al: Long-term results of permanent atrioventricular sequential demand pacing. PACE, 2:175, 1979.

Lillehei, C. W., Gott, V. L., Hodges, P. C., Jr., et al: Transistor pacemaker for treatment of complete atrioventricular dissociation. J.A.M.A., 172:2007, 1960.

Lillehei, C. W., Levy, M. J., Bonnabeau, M. D., Jr., et al: The use of a myocardial electrode and pacemaker in the management of acute postoperative and postinfarction complete heart block. Surgery, 56:463, 1964.

Lowe, J. E., Hartwich, T., Takla, M. W., and Schaper, J.: Ultrastructure of Electrophysiologically Identified Human Sinoatrial Nodes. Basic Research in Cardiology, 83:401, 1988.

MacGregor, D. C., Wilson, G. J., Lixfeld, W., et al: The porous-surfaced electrode: A new concept in pacemaker lead design. J. Thorac. Cardiovas. Surg., 78:281, 1979.

Madigan, N. P., Flaker, G. C., Curtis, J. J., et al: Carotid sinus hypersensitivity: Beneficial effects of dual-chamber pacing. Am. J. Cardiol., 53:1034, 1984.

Magilligan, D. J., Jr., and Isshak, G.: Carcinoma of the breast in a pacemaker pocket. Simple recurrence or oncotaxis? PACE, 3:220, 1980.

Marmorstein, M.: Contribution à l'étude des excitations électriques localisées sur le coeur en rapport avec la topographie de l'innervation du coeur chéz le chien. J. Physiol. (Paris), 25:617, 1927.

Mitrovic, V., Thormann, J., Schlepper, M., and Neuss, H.: Thrombotic complications with pacemakers. Int. J. Cardiol., 2:363, 1983.

Mond, H. G., Sloman, J. G., and Edwards, R. H.: The first pacemaker. PACE, 5:278, 1982.

Morley, C. A., Perrins, E. J., Grant, P., et al: Carotid sinus syncope treated by pacing: Analysis of persistent symptoms and role of atrioventricular sequential pacing. Br. Heart J., 47:411, 1982.

Moss, A. J., and Rivers, R. J., Jr.: Atrial pacing from the coronary vein: Ten-year experience in 50 patients with implanted pervenous pacemakers. Circulation, 57:103, 1978.

Myers, G. H., Parsonnet, V., Zucker, I. R., et al: Biologically-energized cardiac pacemakers. Am. J. Med. Electron., 3:233, 1964.

Narahara, K. A., and Blettel, M. L.: Effects of rate on left ventricular volumes and ejection fraction during chronic ventricular pacing. Circulation, 67:323, 1983.

Nicks, R., Stening, G. F., and Hulme, E. C.: Some observations on the surgical treatment of heart block in degenerative heart disease. Med. J. Aust., 49:857, 1962.

Nicolosi, G. L., Charmet, P. A., and Zanuttini, D.: Large right atrial thrombosis: Rare complication during permanent transvenous endocardial pacing. Br. Heart J., 43:199, 1980.

Nysten, P. H.: Experiences sur le Coeur et les Autres Parties d'un Homme Décapité le 14 Brumaire, Au XI. Paris, Levkault, 1802.

Ogawa, S., Dreifus, L. S., Shenoy, P. N., et al: Hemodynamic consequences of atrioventricular and ventriculoatrial pacing. PACE, 1:8, 1978.

Ong, L. S., Barold, S. S., Craver, W. L., et al: Partial avulsion of the tricuspid valve by tined pacing electrode. Am. Heart J., 102:798, 1981.

Parsonnet, V., Bernstein, A. D., and Norman, J. C.: Dual-chamber pacing for cardiac arrhythmias: Controversies in cloning the conduction system. Tex. Heart Inst. J., 11:208, 1984.

Parsonnet, V., Furman, S., and Smyth, N. P.: A revised code for pacemaker identification. PACE, 4:400, 1981.

Parsonnet, V., Myers, G. H., and Kresh, Y. M.: Characteristics of intracardiac electrograms. II: Atrial endocardial electrograms. PACE, 3:406, 1980.

Parsonnet, V., Zucker, I. R., Gilbert, L., et al: An intracardiac bipolar electrode for interim treatment of complete heart block. Am. J. Cardiol., 10:261, 1962.

Parsonnet, V., Zucker, I. R., Gilbert, L., et al: Clinical use of an implantable standby pacemaker. J.A.M.A., 196:784, 1966.

Pauletti, M., Pingitore, R., and Contini, C.: Superior vena cava stenosis at site of intersection of two pacing electrodes. Br. Heart J., 42:487, 1979.

Perrins, E. J., Morley, C. A., Chen, S. L., and Sutton, R.: Randomized controlled trial of physiological and ventricular pacing. Br. Heart J., 50:112, 1983.

Prevost, J. L., and Battelli, F.: La mort par les courant electriques. Courant alternatif a bas voltage. J. Physiol. (Paris), 1:399, 1899.

Registers of the Royal Humane Society of London. London, Nichols and Sons, 1774–1784.

Reiter, M. J., and Hindman, M. C.: Hemodynamic effects of acute atrioventricular sequential pacing in patients with left ventricular dysfunction. Am. J. Cardiol., 49:687, 1982.

Rickards, A. F., and Donaldson, R. M.: Rate responsive pacing. Clin. Prog. Pacing Electrophysiol., 1:12, 1983.

Robinovitch, L. G.: Triple interrupter of direct currents for resuscitation: Portable model for ambulance service. J. Ment. Path., 8:195, 1907–1909.

Rodan, B. A., Lowe, J. E., and Chen, J. T. T.: Abdominal twiddler's syndrome. Am. J. Roentgenol., 131:1084, 1978.

Samet, P., Bernstein, W. H., Nathan, D. A., and Lopez, A.: Atrial contribution to cardiac output in complete heart block. Am. J. Cardiol., 16:1, 1965.

Samet, P., and El-Sherif, N.: Cardiac Pacing, 2nd ed. New York, Grune & Stratton, 1980, pp. 631–643.

Schechter, D. C.: Background of clinical cardiac electrostimulation. I: Responsiveness of quiescent, bare heart to electricity. N.Y. State J. Med., 71:2575, 1971.

Schechter, D. C.: Background of clinical cardiac electrostimulation. IV: Early studies on the feasibility of accelerating heart rate by means of electricity. N.Y. State J. Med., 72:395, 1972.

Schechter, D. C.: Early experience with resuscitation by means of electricity. Surgery, 69:360, 1971.

Schechter, D. C.: Exploring the origins of electrical cardiac stimulation. Minneapolis, Medtronic, Inc., 1983, p. 91.

Schwartz, D. J., Thanavaro, S., Kleiger, R. E., et al: Epicardial pacemaker complicated by cardiac tamponade and constrictive pericarditis. Chest, 76:226, 1979.

Schwedel, J. B., Furman, S., and Escher, D. J. W.: Use of an intracardiac pacemaker in the treatment of Stokes-Adams seizures. Prog. Cardiovasc. Dis., 3:170, 1960.

Secemsky, S. I., Hauser, R. G., Denes, P., and Edwards, L. M.: Unipolar sensing abnormalities: Incidence and clinical significance of skeletal muscle interference and undersensing in 228 patients. PACE, 5:10, 1982.

Shapland, J. E., MacCarter, D., Tockman, B., and Knudson, M.: Physiologic benefits of rate responsiveness. PACE, 6:329, 1983.

Smyth, N. P. D., Basu, A. P., Bacos, J. M., et al: Permanent transvenous synchronous cardiac pacing. Chest, 59:493, 1971.

Steiner, F.: Ueber die Electropunctur des Herzens als Wiederbelebungsmittel in der Choroformsyncope zugleich eine Studie uber Stichwunden des Herzens. Arch. Klin. Chir., 12:741, 1871.

Stoney, W. S., Alford, W. C., Jr., Burrus, G. R., et al: Cost of cardiac pacing. Am. J. Cardiol., 37:23, 1976.

Stryjer, D., Friedensohn, A., and Schlesinger, Z.: Ventricular pacing as the preferable mode for long-term pacing in patients with carotid sinus syncope of the cardioinhibitory type. PACE, 9:705, 1986.

Sutton, R., Morley, C., Chan, S. L., and Perrins, J.: Physiological benefits of atrial syncrony in paced patients. PACE, 6:327, 1983.

Sutton, R., Perrins, J., and Citron, P.: Physiological cardiac pacing. PACE, 3:207, 1980.

Sutton, R., Perrins, E. J., Morley, C., and Chen, S. L.: Sustained improvement in exercise tolerance following physiological cardiac pacing. Eur. Heart J., 4:781, 1983.

Thevenet, A., Hodges, P. C., and Lillehei, C. W.: The use of a myocardial electrode inserted percutaneously for control of complete atrioventricular block by an artificial pacemaker. Dis. Chest, 34:621, 1958.

Tyers, G. F., and Brownlee, R. R.: The non-hermetically sealed pacemaker myth, or, Navy-Ribicoff 22,000—FDA-Weinberger. J. Thorac. Cardiovasc. Surg., 71:253, 1976.

Tyers, G. F. O., and Brownlee, R. R.: Power pulse generators, electrodes and longevity. Prog. Cardiovasc. Dis., 23:421, 1981.

Venkataraman, K., and Bilitch, M.: Intracardiac electrocardiography during permanent pacemaker implantation: Predictors of cardiac perforation. Am. J. Cardiol., 44:225, 1979.

Videen, J. S., Huang, S. K., Bazgan, I. D., et al: Hemodynamic comparison of ventricular pacing, atrioventricular sequential pacing, and atrial synchronous ventricular pacing using radionuclide ventriculography. Am. J. Cardiol., 57:1305, 1986.

Waldo, A. L., and MacLean, W. A. H.: Diagnosis and treatment of cardiac arrhythmias following open heart surgery: Emphasis on the use of atrial and ventricular epicardial wire electrodes. Mt. Kisco, N.Y., Futura Publishing Co., 1980, p. 115.

Walshe, W. H.: A Practical Treatise on the Diseases of the Heart and Great Vessels Including the Principles of Physical Diagnosis. Philadelphia, Blanchard & Lee, 1862.

Watkins, L., Jr., Guarnieri, T., Griffith, L. S. C., et al: Implantation of the automatic implantable cardioverter defibrillator. J. Cardiovasc. Surg., 3:1, 1988.

Weirich, W. L., Gott, V. L., and Lillehei, C. W.: The treatment of complete heart block by the combined use of myocardial electrode and an artificial pacemaker. Surg. Forum, 8:360, 1957.

Weirich, W. L., Paneth, M., Gott, V. L., and Lillehei, C. W.: Control of complete heart block by use of an artificial pacemaker a myocardial electrode. Circ. Res., 6:410, 1958a.

Weirich, W. L., Paneth, M., Gott, V. L., and Lillehei, C. W.: The treatment of complete heart block by the use of an artificial pacemaker and a myocardial electrode. Am. J. Cardiol., 2:250, 1958b.

Weirich, W. L., and Roe, B. B.: The role of pacemakers in the management of surgically induced complete heart block. Am. J. Surg., 102:293, 1961.

Welti, J. J.: Premature lithium batteries depletion. PACE, 4:349, 1981.

Williams, E. H., Tyers, G. F., and Shaffer, C. W.: Symptomatic deep venous thrombosis of the arm associated with permanent transvenous pacing electrodes. Chest, 73:613, 1978.

Wirtzfield, A., Schmidt, G., Himmler, F. C., and Stangl, K.: Physiologic pacing: Present status and future developments. PACE, 10:41, 1987.

Yee, R., Benditt, D. G., Kostuk, W. J., et al: Comparative functional effects of chronic ventricular demand and atrial synchronous ventricular inhibited pacing. PACE, 7:23, 1984.

Youngson, G. G., McKenzie, F. N., and Nichol, P. M.: Superior vena cava syndrome: Case report. A complication of permanent transvenous endocardial cardiac pacing requiring surgical correction. Am. Heart J., 99:503, 1980.

Ziemssen, H. von: Studien uber die Bewegungsvorgange am menschlichen Herzen, sowie uber die mechanische und elektrische Erregbarkeit des Herzens und des Nervus phrenicus, angestellt an dem freiliegenden Herzen der Catharina Serafin. Dtsch. Arch. Klin. Med., 30:270, 1882.

Zoll, P. M.: Resuscitation of the heart in ventricular standstill by external electric stimulation. N. Engl. J. Med., 247:768, 1952.

Zoll, P. M., Frank, H. A., Zarsky, L. R. N., et al: Long-term electric stimulation of the heart for Stokes-Adams disease. Ann. Surg., 154:330, 1961.

CHAPTER 54

THE CORONARY CIRCULATION
I PHYSIOLOGY OF CORONARY BLOOD FLOW, MYOCARDIAL FUNCTION, AND INTRAOPERATIVE MYOCARDIAL PROTECTION

J. Scott Rankin
David C. Sabiston, Jr.

A detailed knowledge of normal and pathologic physiology of the heart is of primary importance to the practice of cardiac surgery. Many patients are referred for surgical procedures with pre-existing myocardial ischemia or hypertrophy, and operations have the potential for superimposing further physiologic defects. Unlike other organs, the heart must resume adequate function immediately after the procedure, and prevention of intraoperative myocardial injury with restoration of optimal cardiac performance is critical for survival. In this section three topics are reviewed: the normal and pathologic physiology of the heart; basic aspects of intraoperative myocardial preservation; and practical techniques of myocardial protection found useful in surgical practice.

NORMAL PHYSIOLOGY

Coronary blood flow delivers oxygen and metabolic substrates to the myocardium and simultaneously removes carbon dioxide and metabolic byproducts by transcapillary exchange. The function of the heart is to transfer this metabolic energy into the mechanical energy of circulatory pressure and flow. Therefore, the cardiac ventricles and their fundamental units, the sarcomeres, can be considered physiologically to be chemomechanical energy transducers. Normal coronary blood flow approximates 0.7 to 0.9 ml per gram myocardium per minute and delivers 0.1 ml of oxygen per gram per minute to the heart, which is an extreme rate of energy utilization compared with the remainder of the body (Rowe et al, 1959). The extraction of oxygen in the coronary bed is very high, averaging 75% under normal conditions and increasing to almost 100% during stress.

Coronary artery blood flow occurs primarily during diastole (Sabiston and Gregg, 1957) because systolic myocardial contraction increases intramyocardial vascular resistance (Fig. 54–1). Normally, mean coronary resistance is three to six times greater than the total vasodilated value; and, because of the high baseline oxygen extraction, increased oxygen delivery during stress is provided primarily by vasodilatation (Gibbs, 1978). Assuming adequate perfusion pressure, total and regional myocardial blood flow under normal conditions is determined by autoregulation of regional arteriolar resistance that is modulated by local metabolic demand (Bache et al, 1974; Berne and Rubio, 1979).

According to the most accepted theory, the fundamental unit of myocardial contraction is the myosin crossbridge (Squire, 1981). With electrical depolarization of the myocardial cell membrane, ionized calcium fluxes into the cytoplasm and causes the myosin molecule to hydrolyze adenosine triphosphate (ATP) into adenosine diphosphate and inorganic phosphate. When ATP is split, a considerable amount of chemical energy is released from the ATP molecule and is transferred into a conformational change in the myosin crossbridge (Fig. 54–2). This chemomechanical alteration in the crossbridge* in some way produces sliding of myosin filaments relative to actin and shortening of the sarcomere. Over the physiologic range of sarcomere lengths (1.6 to 2 μ), the surface area of available crossbridge interactions and, therefore, the metabolic energy transferred into mechanical energy during sarcomere contraction are linearly proportional to end-diastolic sarcomere length (Fig. 54–3). This length dependency of crossbridge interaction at the

---

*Theories of crossbridge dynamics are beyond the scope of this work. For further reading see Squire, 1981.

1635

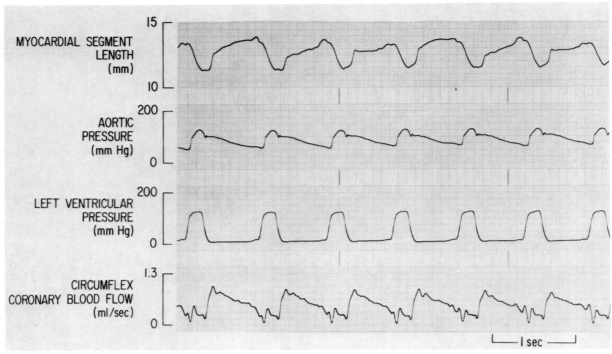

Figure 54–1. Coronary blood flow and myocardial functional characteristics are observed under normal conditions in the conscious dog. Myocardial segment length was measured with pulse transit ultrasonic dimension transducers; pressures were obtained with high-fidelity micromanometers; and coronary blood flow was assessed with an implanted electromagnetic flow transducer.

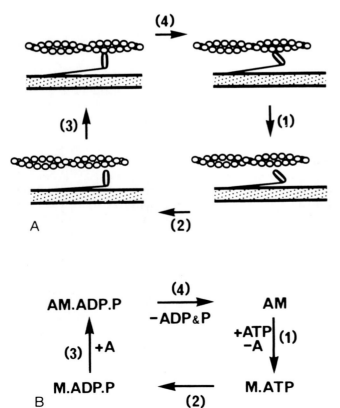

Figure 54–2. Comparison of the mechanical steps thought to be involved in the force generating crossbridge cycle in muscle (*A*) and the corresponding biochemical steps (*B*). In step 3, a crossbridge attaches to the adjacent actin filament; in step 4, it changes its angle of attachment and causes relative sliding of the actin and myosin filaments (ADP and P are released); in step 1, the crossbridge detaches after binding ATP; and in step 2, it reverts to the configuration in which it can reinitiate its attachment cycle. (From Offer, G. *In* Bull, A. T., Lagnado, J. R., Thomas, J. O., and Tipton, K. F. (eds): Companion to Biochemistry. London, Longmans, 1974, pp. 623–671. [After E. W. Taylor].)

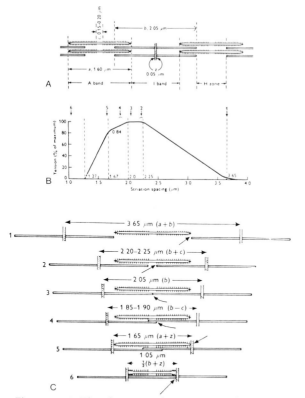

Figure 54–3. The alteration of tension actively generated by the contractile apparatus as a function of sarcomere length (*B*) and its interpretation in terms of the changing overlap of the thick and thin filaments (*A* and *C*). (From Gordon, A. M., Huxley, A. F., and Julian, F. J.: The variation in isometric tension with sarcomere length in vertebrate muscle fibres. J. Physiol. (London), *184*:170, 1966.)

sarcomere level constitutes the basis for the Frank-Starling relationship. As a final step in the process, calcium is removed from the cell by active transport of the cytoplasmic reticulum, and ATP is regenerated at the mitochondrial level by aerobic metabolism of oxygen and substrates (Braunwald, 1974).

In many ways, the intact cardiac ventricles function as an integrated total of their component sarcomeres. The production of mechanical energy, in the form of external stroke work, is a direct linear function of end-diastolic volume (Fig. 54–4) and is not influenced significantly by physiologic changes in afterload (Glower et al, 1985). Therefore, short-term alterations in myocardial inotropism (defined as load-independent intrinsic myocardial performance) can be assessed by the slope of the stroke work–end-diastolic volume relationship (Fig. 54–5). This fundamental Frank-Starling property of the heart probably directly reflects sarcomere and myosin crossbridge dynamics.

Energetically, cardiac metabolic activity over time can be assessed by myocardial oxygen consumption. Each milliliter of oxygen used by the heart provides 2.02 joules of energy to the contractile apparatus via aerobic metabolic pathways and ATP. Thus, oxygen consumption can be used to quantify

myocardial *energy utilization*. Myocardial *energy expenditure* has two components: external energy, which is stroke work or the integral of the ventricular pressure (P) volume (V) loop; and internal energy, which is the thermodynamic cost of maintaining systolic ventricular pressure at a particular volume (Feneley et al, 1987). Internal energy expenditure is estimated to be the product of ventricular mean ejection pressure (P_{ME}) and end-diastolic volume (V_{ED}) and constitutes the sole production of mechanical energy during isovolumic contraction. Thus, total mechanical energy expenditure (TME) for each cardiac cycle can be calculated as

$$TME = \int PdV + (P_{ME} \times V_{ED})$$

Because 1 mm Hg/ml is equivalent to 1.333×10^{-4} joule, total mechanical energy expenditure can be compared with metabolic energy use to obtain a measure of metabolic to mechanical energy transfer efficiency (Fig. 54–6). Oxygen consumption appears to be tightly coupled to mechanical energy expenditure (Maier et al, 1988), on both a steady state and a beat-to-beat basis (Elbeery et al, 1989).

ISCHEMIC PATHOPHYSIOLOGY

The pathophysiology of coronary blood flow is complicated. Reduction in myocardial oxygen supply

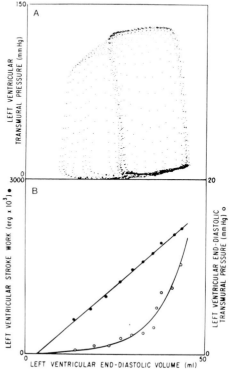

Figure 54–4. *A,* Dynamic left ventricular pressure-volume loops obtained in the conscious dog during vena caval occlusion with data digitized at 200 Hz. *B,* Stroke work–end-diastolic volume and diastolic pressure-volume curves are shown.

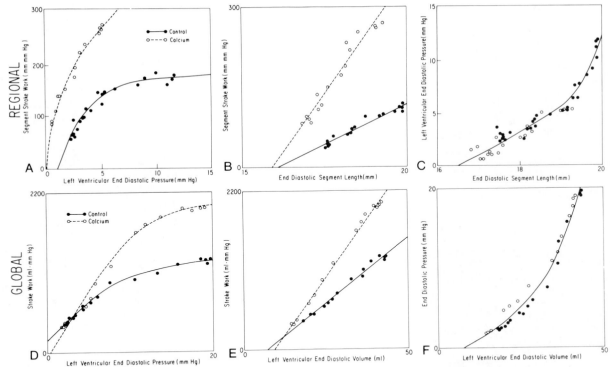

Figure 54–5. Typical effects of calcium infusion on stroke work versus end-diastolic pressure (*A, D*), stroke work versus end-diastolic dimension relationships (*B, E*), and end-diastolic pressure versus dimension relationships (*C, F*). *A, B,* and *C,* Typical data are shown from one regional study. *D, E,* and *F,* A representative global study is shown. (From Glower, D. D., Spratt, J. A., Snow, N. D., et al: Linearity of the Frank-Starling relationship in the intact heart: The concept of preload recruitable stroke work. Circulation, *71:*994, 1985. By permission of the American Heart Association, Inc.)

during ischemia or increased oxygen demand during hemodynamic stress produces regulatory coronary vasodilation. With decreased arteriolar resistance, impedance to coronary blood flow is shifted proximally in the coronary circuit, and diastolic intramyocardial pressure becomes a more important determinant of mean myocardial perfusion. In the presence of adequate arterial pressure and low diastolic cavitary pressure, the modest transmural gradient of diastolic intramyocardial force has little effect on regional myocardial perfusion through the dilated vascular bed. In this situation, however, transmural

flow becomes pressure dependent and, if perfusion pressure decreases or diastolic intracavitary pressure increases, coronary blood flow may be redistributed away from the subendocardium where intramural compressive forces are highest (Bache et al, 1974). This redistribution of flow can cause subendocardial ischemia, even in the presence of normal coronary arteries (Buckberg et al, 1972), and together with an inherent subendocardial metabolic vulnerability (Lowe et al, 1983) contributes to subendocardial myocardial infarction.

When an atherosclerotic plaque in a proximal

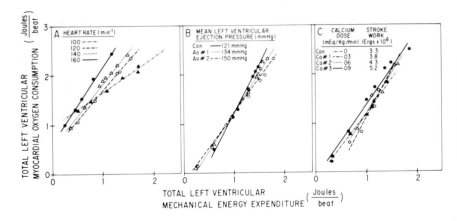

Figure 54–6. Metabolic to mechanical energy transfer characteristics of the left ventricle in the conscious dog as a function of variations in heart rate (*A*), afterload (*B*), and inotropic state (*C*). (From Maier, G. W., Owen, C. H., Feneley, M. P., et al: The mechanical determinants of myocardial oxygen consumption in the conscious dog. Circulation, *78*(suppl II): II-67, 1988. By permission of the American Heart Association, Inc.)

coronary artery decreases the cross-sectional area by 75% or more, the resistance to flow caused by the plaque becomes significant (Sabiston, 1974). The dominant point of coronary vascular impedance moves even more proximally, and the critical stenosis can restrict myocardial perfusion to a fixed value. Although flow may be adequate at rest, exercise or other factors that increase myocardial oxygen demand can induce relative ischemia, a fall in the coronary pressure distal to the stenosis, and redistribution of blood flow away from the subendocardium. This appears to be the mechanism of exercise-induced angina pectoris and associated transient regional myocardial dysfunction. Superimposed on this phenomenon, coronary vasospasm or unstable thrombotic plaques can compound the obstructive physiology.

Because of high metabolic demand and tight coupling between use and expenditure of energy, acute coronary hypoperfusion produces an immediate decrement in myocardial performance (Fig. 54–7). Work function of the ischemic segment ceases, and myocardial necrosis begins in the subendocardium after approximately 15 to 20 minutes. Reperfusion in the first hours after occlusion can produce partial functional recovery, but after approximately 4 to 6 hours, infarction becomes irreversible. Excep-

tions do exist, however, including infarctions with minor persistent antegrade flow and those with well-established collaterals (Gregg, 1974).

Even with a totally reversible injury produced by a 15-minute coronary occlusion, dysfunction can be prolonged, and a period of up to 24 to 48 hours can be required for full recovery (Fig. 54–8). Ischemic myocardial dysfunction in this setting is characterized by a diminished slope of the stroke work–end-diastolic segment length relationship, together with a shift to the right of the x-intercept (l_0) called *diastolic creep* (Glower et al, 1988). With reperfusion, the slope recovers rapidly, but l_0 remains overstretched, diminishing work capacity at any given preload (Fig. 54–9). Subsequent recovery of systolic function tends to occur slowly and is associated with a reversal of the ischemic-induced creep (Glower et al, 1988). Pressure afterloading or a second ischemic event during early reperfusion can produce prolonged dysfunction and delay ultimate recovery (Gall et al, 1988; Williams et al, 1985). Postischemic systolic dysfunction and diastolic creep can be correlated at an ultrastructural level with myofilament relaxation, increased Z-band separation, and widening of the I bands (Fig. 54–10). Thus, ischemic myocardial dysfunction appears to represent some degree of disengagement of actin-myosin filaments and possibly a fundamental abnor-

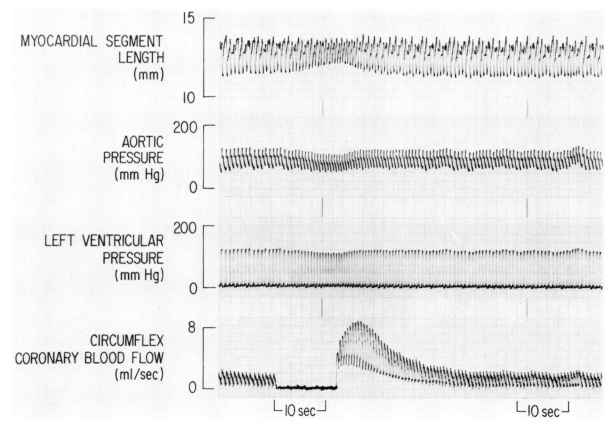

Figure 54–7. Myocardial dimension, pressure, and blood flow data obtained during a 12-second coronary occlusion in the conscious dog. Myocardial shortening begins to diminish rapidly after coronary occlusion, and vasodilation associated with postischemic reactive hyperemia increases coronary blood flow severalfold.

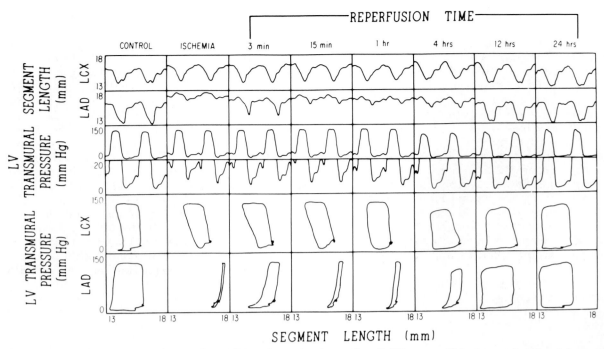

Figure 54–8. Raw data tracings of circumflex (LCX) and anterior descending (LAD) myocardial segment lengths, left ventricular transmural pressure, and pressure-length work loops in the control state, during 15 minutes of LAD occlusion, and after 3 minutes, 15 minutes, 1 hour, 4 hours, 12 hours, and 24 hours of LAD reperfusion. (From Glower, D. D., Spratt, J. A., Kabas, J. S., et al: Quantification of regional myocardial function after acute ischemic injury: Application of preload recruitable stroke work. Am. J. Physiol., *255*:H85, 1988.)

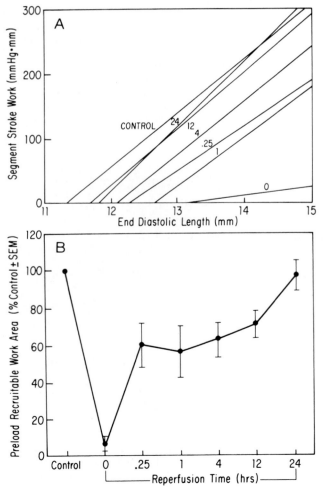

Figure 54–9. Segment stroke work–end-diastolic segment length relationships for a representative dog under control conditions, after 15 minutes of coronary occlusion (0), and after 0.25, 1, 4, 12, and 24 hours of coronary reperfusion (*A*). *B*, Mean values for the area beneath the curve are observed in eight studies during the same time intervals.

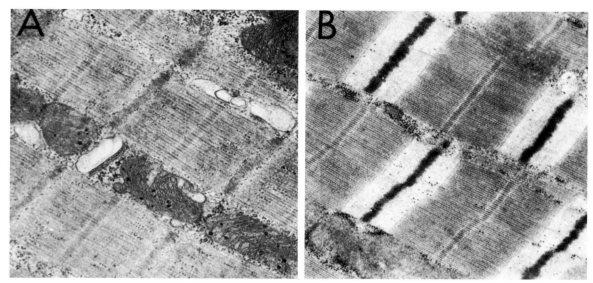

Figure 54–10. Typical electron micrographs of nonischemic (*A*) and ischemic (*B*) myocardium after 15 minutes of coronary occlusion. Ischemic tissue displays myofilament relaxation with increased Z-band separation and widening of I bands. (From Glower, D. D., Schaper, J., Kabas, J. S., et al: Relation between reversal of diastolic creep and recovery of systolic function after ischemic myocardial injury in conscious dogs. Circ. Res., *60*:850, 1987. By permission of the American Heart Association, Inc.)

mality in crossbridge registration (Glower et al, 1987). Accompanying the functional abnormalities of early reperfusion, metabolic to mechanical energy transfer is altered (Fig. 54–11) representing either excess repair energy or a metabolic transfer block.

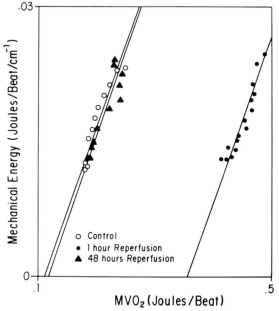

Figure 54–11. Regional mechanical to metabolic energy transfer characteristics in a conscious dog obtained during control conditions at 1 hour of reperfusion after a 15-minute coronary occlusion and after 48 hours of reperfusion. In the early reperfusion period, myocardial oxygen consumption (MVO_2) increased relative to mechanical energy expenditure, which suggests decreased efficiency of energy utilization. (Unpublished data, courtesy of Dr. J. Elbeery.)

Acute coronary thrombosis in an area of atherosclerotic narrowing is clearly the dominant mechanism of myocardial infarction. With persistent ischemia during infarction, ultrastructural changes become more prominent, and distinct irreversible alterations are evident by 30 to 40 minutes (Jennings and Ganote, 1974). The cell nucleus shows peripherally aggregated chromatin and numerous swollen perinuclear mitochondria (Fig. 54–12). Some mitochondria contain amorphous matrix densities, and the Z bands bisect the I bands of the myofibrils. After 60 minutes of ischemia, glycogen is almost absent, and the myofibrils are stretched to an even greater extent (Fig. 54–13). Mitochondrial and sarcolemmal abnormalities progress to total myofibrillar disruption and distortion of Z lines. When irreversibly injured myocardium is reperfused, explosive cellular swelling, deposition of calcium phosphate, and intense contracture are observed; these changes ultimately progress to cell rupture and death. Healing of infarcted myocardium is characterized by resorption of necrotic tissue, wall thinning, and replacement of infarcted myofibrils by fibrous tissue.

PRINCIPLES OF INTRAOPERATIVE MYOCARDIAL PROTECTION

Minimizing Operative Injury

Most cardiac operations require arrest of the heart along with interruption of coronary blood flow; thus a precise technical procedure can be done in a quiet bloodless field. The historical development of surgical cardioplegia has been reviewed earlier (Ran-

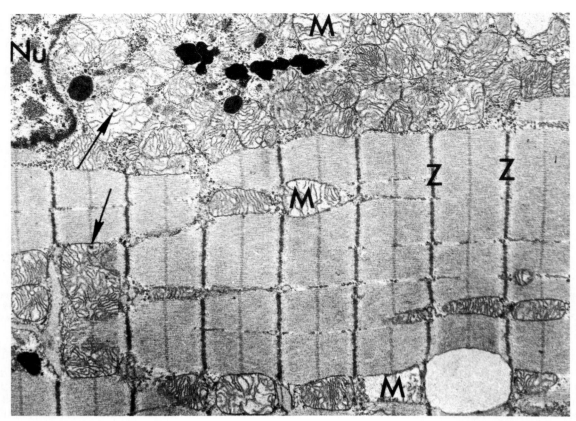

Figure 54–12. Electron micrograph of myocardial ultrastructure after 40 minutes of ischemia, which shows irreversible injury. This portion of a myocardial cell illustrates a nucleus (Nu) with peripherally aggregated chromatin and numerous swollen perinuclear mitochondria (M). Some mitochondria contain tiny amorphous matrix densities. The Z bands (Z) bisect the I bands of the myofibrils. The dark bodies in the perinuclear zone are pigment granules (lysomes, lipofuchsin) and are structurally intact. (Osmium fixation; magnification × 31,000.) (From Jennings, R. B., and Ganote, C. E.: Structural changes in myocardium during acute ischemia. Circ. Res., *34, 35* [Suppl. 3]:156, 1974. By permission of the American Heart Association, Inc.)

kin and Sabiston, 1983; Silverman and Levitsky, 1987). At present, general agreement exists that the period of induced operative ischemia should be kept as short as possible by appropriate planning of the procedure. Even with current methods of hypothermic cardioplegia, ischemic tissue injury progresses exponentially with time, which emphasizes the fact that there is no substitute for an expeditiously performed operation. With modern surgical techniques, however, even the most complicated cardiac operations can be accomplished within 150 minutes, a period of ischemia that is well tolerated with appropriate myocardial protection. Care should be taken during the operation to minimize retraction of cardiac structures because direct damage to the heart may negate even the best method of myocardial preservation.

When the heart is being perfused during cardiopulmonary bypass, close attention should be given to maintaining adequate coronary perfusion pressure (with a mean of at least 50 to 60 mm Hg) to ensure satisfactory transmural blood flow distribution. Ventricular distention can restrict subendocardial flow and should be prevented by appropriate perfusion

techniques. Ventricular fibrillation creates a continuous myocardial wall stress, which, combined with increased oxygen demand, predisposes the heart to subendocardial injury (Buckberg and Hottenrott, 1975). Periods of ventricular fibrillation should thus be avoided or minimized during the procedure. Finally, there is no substitute for a well-performed operation. Good myocardial protection combined with adequate correction of physiologic defects should optimize operative results.

Hypothermia

Hypothermia is still the most important component of myocardial preservation during induced ischemia. The protective effects of hypothermia are related to reduction in cardiac cellular metabolism (Buckberg et al, 1977). This metabolic effect diminishes energy and ATP consumption during ischemia and reduces the toxic products of metabolism such as carbon dioxide (Fig. 54–14) and hydrogen ions (Flaherty et al, 1979). Because tissue acidosis may produce ultrastructural damage (Gevers, 1977), in-

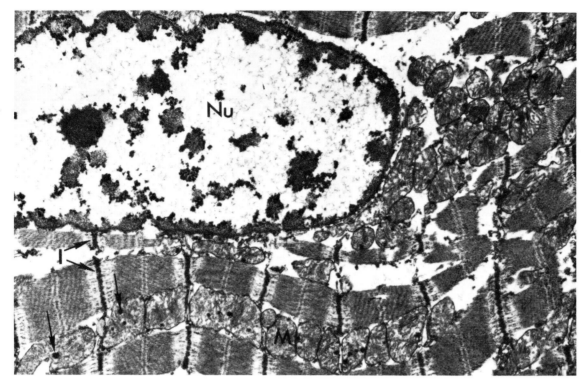

Figure 54–13. Myocardial ultrastructure after 60 minutes of ischemia, with irreversible injury. Note the margination of the chromatin in the nucleus (Nu). The myofibrils are relaxed and have prominent I bands (I); an N band is also present in the I bands. The mitochondria are swollen and contain amorphous matrix densities at the *arrows*. Little or no glycogen is expected to be present, but this tissue cannot be used to illustrate this fact because the fixative extracts glycogen during processing. (Osmium fixation with uranyl acetate in block; magnification × 16,628.) (From Jennings, R. B., and Ganote, C. E.: Structural changes in myocardium during acute ischemia. Circ. Res., *34, 35* [Suppl. 3]:156, 1974. By permission of the American Heart Association, Inc.)

Figure 54–14. Effect of hypothermia on myocardial carbon dioxide tension during ischemic arrest of the isolated cat heart. Myocardial P_{CO_2} was measured with mass spectrometry by a probe positioned at the midmyocardial level. (From Flaherty, J. T., Schaffy, H. V., Goldman, R. A., and Gott, V. L.: Metabolic and functional effects of progressive degrees of hypothermia during local ischemia. Am. J. Physiol., *236*:H839, 1979.)

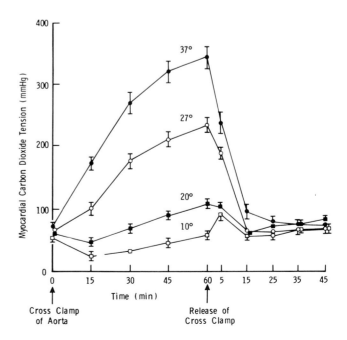

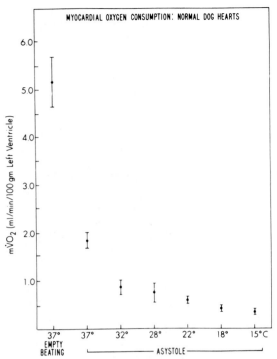

Figure 54–15. Effects of hypothermia on myocardial oxygen consumption in the potassium-arrested dog heart. (From Chitwood, W. R., Sink, J. D., Hill, R. C., et al: The effects of hypothermia on myocardial oxygen consumption and transmural coronary blood flow in the potassium-arrested heart. Ann. Surg., *190*:106, 1979.)

hibition of proton production is one of the most important considerations. As shown in Figure 54–15, oxygen consumption at 10 to 20° C in the chemically arrested nonworking heart is less than 5% of the normal value (Chitwood et al, 1979) and permits safe ischemic arrest for prolonged periods without permanent injury.

Initial rapid induction of myocardial hypothermia is best accomplished by infusion of *cold cardioplegia solution* into the aortic root after aortic clamping. In current practice, 1.2 liters of 4° C crystalloid solution is infused during a 3-minute to 5-minute interval to achieve a measured myocardial temperature below 10 to 12° C. Occasionally, with marked ventricular hypertrophy, critical coronary obstruction, or a highly developed noncoronary collateral circulation, more cardioplegia solution is required to produce the desired myocardial hypothermia. Recirculation of the cardioplegia solution between infusions with a commercially available cannula system* and a roller pump has been helpful in maintaining uniform temperature of the solution. The solution is periodically reinfused every 30 to 45 minutes as necessary to assist in maintenance of hypothermia.

Myocardial hypothermia is also accomplished by using combinations of other techniques. *External top-*

*DLP, Inc., Walker, Michigan.

ical cooling is one important method and is readily achieved by a continuous infusion of 4° C saline at 50 to 100 ml/min over the heart and into the pericardial cavity (Hurley et al, 1964; Shumway et al, 1959). Excess fluid is removed by a suction catheter in the inferior aspect of the incision. The effectiveness of myocardial cooling with the topical method appears to be related to the size of the heart. In large hypertrophied ventricles, cooling may be slow and reduction in endocardial temperature may be less uniform. Endocardial cooling can be facilitated by continuous or intermittent intracavitary infusion of cold saline either directly into the heart, such as in aortic or mitral valve replacement, or through an indwelling catheter (Hearse et al, 1981; Rosenfeldt and Watson, 1979; Schachner et al, 1976). The use of topical saline ice slush is also useful in maintaining a low myocardial temperature.

Along with bronchial blood flow and noncoronary collateral circulation, return of the systemic perfusate to the heart is the major source of rewarming during hypothermic arrest (Rosenfeldt and Watson, 1979). Therefore, an additional technique, *low-flow systemic hypothermia*, is important in minimizing myocardial rewarming during the period of aortic occlusion (Fig. 54–16) (Conti et al, 1978; Grover et al, 1981; Tyers et al, 1977a). In current practice, systemic perfusate temperature is lowered to 24° C, and systemic pump flow is lowered to between 1.0 and 1.5

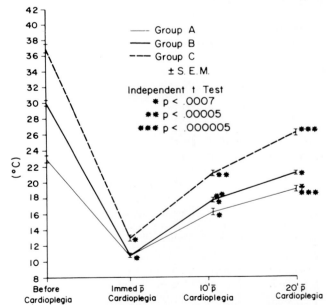

Figure 54–16. Effects of lowering systemic perfusate temperature on myocardial rewarming. Ventricular septal temperature (° C) was measured after infusion of 4° C potassium cardioplegia solution into the aortic root. In Group A, systemic perfusate temperature was maintained at 23° C, in Group B at 30° C, and in Group C at 37° C. Lowering systemic perfusate temperature reduced the rate of myocardial rewarming. (From Grover, F. L., Fewel, J. G., Ghidoni, J. J., and Trinkle, J. K.: Does lower systemic temperature enhance cardioplegic myocardial protection? J. Thorac. Cardiovasc. Surg., *81*:11, 1981.)

liters/min/m² of calculated values during the arrest period. Rewarming is begun 5 to 10 minutes before the aortic clamp is released. Lowering systemic blood flow not only reduces noncoronary collateral perfusion but also assists with right atrial decompression during atrial venous cannulation. The importance of systemic hypothermia should not be underestimated, and clinical experience suggests that it is a *major factor* in myocardial protection. In selected cases that require longer arrest times, individual vena cava cannulation with occluding tapes in combination with endocardial cold saline lavage can further reduce the rewarming associated with venous return (Daily et al, 1987).

In the presence of severe proximal coronary stenosis or occlusion, impairment in regional cooling during antegrade delivery of cardioplegia solution can occur because of the obstruction. In this situation, the first bypass graft is usually placed on the involved vessel, and then cardioplegia solution is delivered through the graft (Silverman et al, 1985). Reinfusion of cardioplegia solution every 30 to 45 minutes is generally done, and most studies would support periodic reinfusion to replenish the arresting agents, to maintain myocardial hypothermia, and to wash out metabolic wastes (Buckberg, 1979; Nelson et al, 1976). Retrograde delivery of cardioplegia solution via the coronary sinus or right atrium currently is being investigated in a number of centers. Although the rationale for improved hypothermia in regions with severe inflow obstruction is logical, results have been inconclusive, and the technique of retrograde cardioplegia has not been established clinically at present (Fabiani et al, 1986; Guiraudon et al, 1986; Menasché and Piwnica, 1987; Schaper et al, 1985).

Cardioplegic Additives

Rapid metabolic arrest of the heart can be achieved with a number of chemical components. Potassium arrest is probably the most widely used technique (Gay and Ebert, 1973). High extracellular potassium reduces the transmembrane potassium gradient, depolarizes the cell, and eliminates the energy cost of maintaining membrane ionic pumps. The concentration of potassium is critical. Optimal results are achieved in most studies with 15 to 20 mM/l (Hearse et al, 1975; Tyers, 1975). *High* concentrations of potassium, such as those present in the Melrose solution, can be associated with myocardial contracture and other forms of injury (Melrose, 1978). Conversely, lower concentrations of potassium are less effective in producing immediate arrest. Evidence exists that potassium levels in the range of 25 to 30 mM/l may be necessary with blood cardioplegia (Buckberg, 1979).

Magnesium is a major intracellular cation contained primarily within mitochondria and myofibrils. On the cell membrane, magnesium competes for calcium receptor sites and delays calcium influx into the cell. Magnesium is an important component of high-energy phosphate molecules and is a cofactor for cellular enzyme systems. When used to induce arrest, magnesium appears to inhibit excitation-contraction coupling, although it is not a very good arresting agent because of its slow onset of action. Absence of magnesium during ischemia or reperfusion can impair synthesis of ATP. Thus, magnesium can be useful in crystalloid cardioplegia solutions, and during the ischemic interval, magnesium concentrations in the range of 15 to 20 mM/l provide the best protection in experimental systems (Hearse et al, 1978b).

Calcium is an essential component of actin-myosin interaction and contributes importantly to the regulation of myocardial contraction (Katz, 1977). Calcium is also required for maintenance of membrane integrity and numerous intracellular functions. Because intracellular calcium deposition has a significant role in ischemic and reperfusion injury (Shen and Jennings, 1972), extracellular calcium should be regulated carefully during cardioplegic arrest. Reduction in calcium has been shown to diminish the cellular influx associated with ischemic injury and to improve functional recovery (Hearse et al, 1977). Minute quantities of calcium, however, are essential for maintenance of cellular integrity, and ischemic arrest of isolated myocardium with calcium-free solutions is associated with severe reperfusion injury when re-exposed to calcium (Zimmerman et al, 1967). The magnitude of this "calcium paradox" can be reduced by hypothermia and is influenced to some extent by the severity of the ischemic insult. In the in-vivo situation, calcium paradox may not be a major factor because small amounts of calcium are provided to the myocardium through the noncoronary collateral circulation. However, maintenance of a minimal concentration of calcium is probably useful for cardioplegia formulations (Jynge et al, 1977).

The availability of calcium during the ischemic period can be diminished in several ways. First, in crystalloid solutions, calcium can be reduced to a concentration of 0.5 to 1 mM/l, which has been beneficial in numerous studies (Hearse et al, 1981). When blood cardioplegia is used, calcium in the blood can be chelated with small amounts of citrate (Follette et al, 1978a). Cellular calcium influx can also be limited by cardioplegia additives such as magnesium and procaine (Hearse et al, 1981). Finally, slow channel calcium-blocking agents have been investigated in a number of centers (Clark et al, 1981; Lowe et al, 1977; Robb-Nicholson et al, 1978). These drugs selectively inhibit the sarcolemmal slow calcium channel and prevent cellular calcium accumulation and degradation of ATP. They can be used to induce and maintain cardiac arrest either primarily or in combination with other agents. Although effective in preventing ischemic and reperfusion injuries, the clinical application of slow channel blockers may be limited by myocardial depression and conduction disturbances that can occur after reperfusion (Barner et al, 1987; Christakis et al, 1986b; Clark, 1986; Flameng et al, 1986; Hicks and Deweese, 1985). It also is not clear how much additional protection is given by these agents beyond that provided by current cardioplegia techniques.

The optimal concentration of sodium to be used in cardioplegia solutions has been a subject of controversy. The formulations of Bretschneider and Kirsch are based on an *intracellular* composition that has little or no sodium in the solutions (Bretschneider et al, 1975; Kirsch et al, 1972). Sudden sodium depletion rapidly arrests the heart by eliminating transmembrane gradients and by producing cell depolarization. However, arrest by sodium depletion favors influx of calcium into the cell, and strict control or elimination of calcium with this technique is essential. Most American surgeons now prefer physiologic *extracellular* sodium concentration, based on the data from the group at St. Thomas' Hospital and others (Hearse et al, 1981; Tyers et al, 1977b). As with magnesium, one protective effect of sodium is exerted through its control of intracellular calcium movement. Sodium concentrations in the range of 100 to 130 mM/l provide the best protection of isolated myocardium when used in conjunction with hyperkalemic arrest. Extensive clinical experience with extracellular cardioplegic solutions has been very favorable (Craver et al, 1978; Hearse et al, 1981; Tyers et al, 1977b).

Local anesthetic agents have been used for cardioplegia for many years. Especially in Europe, procaine has been extensively evaluated and constitutes a major protective component of Bretschneider's solution (Bretschneider, 1964). These agents induce cardiac arrest by blocking the sodium channel of the sarcolemma and also provide protection by inhibiting the cellular influx of calcium. Inclusion of local anesthetics in cardioplegia solutions also diminishes the incidence of ventricular fibrillation in the early reperfusion period (Vercillo et al, 1987). When used with hyperkalemic extracellular solutions, procaine concentrations in the range of 0.05 to 1 mM/l have proved to be most effective in isolated studies on the heart (Hearse et al, 1981). Inclusion of vasodilators in cardioplegia solutions does not appear to be helpful (Hines et al, 1985; Slogoff et al, 1986).

Buffering

As discussed earlier, tissue acidosis during ischemia can produce direct myocardial injury. Therefore, maintenance of appropriate pH is important for repletion of ATP and for sustaining low levels of cellular function. Hydrogen ions are produced continuously during the ischemic period so that a stable source of buffering is required. In most cardioplegia formulations, pH is controlled by the addition of specific buffering systems. The choice of buffers varies, but most clinically tested solutions utilize bicarbonate, phosphate, or tris (hydroxymethyl) aminomethase (TRIS) as the major component. Lactate should be avoided because of its poor buffering

capacity and because lactate inhibits anaerobic metabolism independent of pH (Hearse et al, 1976; Tyers, 1975).

Available information suggests that cellular integrity during hypothermia is best maintained with a slightly alkaline pH (Becker et al, 1981; Rahn et al, 1975; White, 1981). Normally, when blood is cooled, pH increases approximately 0.15 per 10° C of hypothermia (Rosenthal, 1948). Thus, at temperatures below 20° C, cellular pH in excess of 7.7 may be necessary. This concept is further substantiated by the observation that the pH of poikilothermic animals increases to approximately 7.8 with hypothermia. Recovery of myocardial function is better when a pH of 7.6 to 7.8 is maintained (Follette et al, 1981), and most investigators recommend appropriate composition and buffering of cardioplegia solutions to maintain pH in the alkaline range of normal.

Osmolarity

Cellular swelling and myocardial edema consistently accompany ischemic injury (Leaf, 1970). The primary mechanisms responsible appear to be altered cellular energetics and permeability related to the ischemic state (Lee et al, 1980; MacKnight and Leaf, 1977). Thus, one important aspect of minimizing water gain is the efficacy of myocardial protection, and less edema occurs in well-protected hearts. The osmolarity of the perfusate also influences myocardial edema, and hearts perfused with hypotonic solutions rapidly gain water (Foglia et al, 1979). Conversely, hyperosmotic formulations in excess of 400 mOsm/kg of H_2O produce myocardial dehydration and impair functional recovery (Hearse et al, 1978a; Wildenthal et al, 1969). Although the direct influence of minor degrees of cellular edema on ultimate functional recovery is unclear, most surgeons would recommend slightly hyperosmolar cardioplegic solutions. Oncotic agents such as albumin or mannitol are also effective in preventing myocardial edema and contributing to functional preservation (Bodenhamer et al, 1983; Lucas et al, 1980; Powell et al, 1976), although clinical trials have been less positive (Bodenhamer et al, 1985).

Oxygen Delivery and Blood Cardioplegia

The concept of using blood as the vehicle for cardioplegic arrest was reintroduced by Buckberg and associates (Follette et al, 1978a, 1978b). Blood is diluted to a hematocrit of 20% with a cardioplegia solution so that the final potassium concentration is 25 to 30 mM/l. The solution is oxygenated, cooled, and delivered through standard cannulas. Initially, 500 to 750 ml is administered at 16 to 20° C, and then 250 ml is reinfused every 20 minutes. Before releasing the aortic clamp, 500 to 750 ml of 37° C blood cardioplegia solution is infused to warm and reoxygenate the heart while maintaining arrest (Follette et al, 1981).

When used in this manner, blood cardioplegia has several potential advantages. Blood is the most physiologic solution. The heart is arrested while being oxygenated, thus ATP is not depleted before asystole. Reinfusion of oxygenated blood provides a source of oxygen for continued metabolism and ATP repletion during the period of hypothermic arrest. Although little oxygen is released from hemoglobin during hypothermia, enough oxygen is probably dissolved in the plasma to sustain metabolism when reinfusion is done every 20 minutes. Reinfusion of the solution maintains myocardial hypothermia, washes out waste products, and provides metabolic substrate. Hyperkalemia maintains chemical arrest with its inherently lower metabolic requirements. Formulation of the blood from the oxygenator is simple, and hemodilution is usually not significant unlike certain asanguineous cardioplegia techniques. The buffering and oncotic characteristics of blood are excellent. Trace metals, cofactors, hormones, or other as yet undefined but important constituents are provided. Finally, reperfusion with alkalotic, hyperkalemic, hypocalcemic blood is facilitated with this system, minimizing fibrillation and reperfusion injury and providing a source of oxygen during the initial rewarming period (Follette et al, 1981).

Clinical experience with blood cardioplegia has been positive. Follette and associates (1978b) reduced the perioperative myocardial infarction rate from 6.4% with intermittent ischemia to 1.3% with blood cardioplegia, and operative mortality declined. Similar results have been reported by Culliford and associates (1980), who also noted good preservation of myocardial ultrastructure and ATP. These authors indicated that the "safe" aortic clamping time was extended beyond 2 hours with this technique. Barner and colleagues (1981) confirmed these findings, and many surgeons believe that blood cardioplegia offers distinct advantages. Oxygenation of crystalloid cardioplegia represents a variation on this concept and has been used extensively in recent years with favorable results (Daggett et al, 1987; Guyton et al, 1985; Heitmiller et al, 1985). Although oxygenated fluorocarbon compounds are still being investigated, they have shown promise in several studies (Magovern et al, 1982; Novick et al, 1985).

The relative merits of intermittent or regional hypothermic ischemic arrest, standard crystalloid cardioplegia, oxygenated crystalloid cardioplegia, and blood cardioplegia have been controversial, and experimental and clinical studies have yielded mixed results. Several authors have advocated continued use of hypothermic fibrillation or intermittent ischemic arrest for routine coronary bypass (Akins and Carroll, 1987; Baur et al, 1986; Bonchek and Burlingame, 1987). Although it may be difficult to define differences in clinical end-points between different techniques in low-risk patients who require short arrest times, current experimental and clinical expe-

riences suggest that cold potassium cardioplegia is superior to hypothermic ischemic arrest. Cold cardioplegia is certainly no worse, probably provides better protection (van der Vusse et al, 1986), has a greater margin of safety, and offers significant advantages of technical simplification.

Schaper and co-workers (1986) showed that the St. Thomas' and Hamburg crystalloid cardioplegia solutions provided excellent preservation of myocardial ultrastructure in humans, whereas Kirsch's solution was inadequate. Several studies have shown improved protection with blood cardioplegia, compared with crystalloid (Christakis et al, 1986a; Codd et al, 1985), whereas others yielded inconclusive results (Mullen et al, 1986a, 1986b). Results with variations on the theme of blood cardioplegia have also been inconclusive (Roberts et al, 1985; Teoh et al, 1986).

The authors' experience with crystalloid cardioplegia in low-risk and high-risk patients has been excellent (Rankin et al, 1985, 1986), suggesting that properly performed crystalloid techniques, paying strict attention to maximizing myocardial hypothermia, are adequate. In addition, Lovell and Rankin (unpublished data) recently completed a random survey of 714 centers in the United States performing cardiac surgery (Lovell et al, unpublished data). Although 90% of centers were satisfied with the quality of their myocardial protection, the relative utilization of blood (44%) versus crystalloid (45%) versus both (11%) suggests that large clinical differences between techniques may not be apparent.

To further address this issue, Maier and Rankin (unpublished data) evaluated blood versus St. Thomas' cardioplegia in the hearts of dogs undergoing 3 hours of ischemic arrest. Left ventricular cavitary volume and wall volume were measured with ultrasonic crystals, and micromanometers recorded left ventricular pressure. Systolic ventricular function was evaluated before and 1 hour after the arrest period by using the stroke work–end-diastolic volume model (Fig. 54–17). No significant differences in preservation of ventricular function could be appreciated between the two techniques (Table 54–1), which suggests that factors common to both, such as hypothermia and potassium arrest, may be the most relevant variables.

CLINICAL MYOCARDIAL PROTECTION WITH CRYSTALLOID CARDIOPLEGIA

Although numerous methods of myocardial protection exist and probably vary slightly between most centers, the crystalloid cardioplegia technique used by the authors during the last 5 years is described in this section as being a standardized and reliable method. The technique is a variation of that described by the St. Thomas' Hospital group (Braimbridge et al, 1977) and has produced excellent results in a wide range of clinical practice. The basic steps are first

TABLE 54–1. EFFICACY OF CRYSTALLOID VERSUS BLOOD CARDIOPLEGIA SOLUTIONS FOR PRESERVATION OF LEFT VENTRICULAR FUNCTION

Solution	n	Δ MV† (ml)	SW-EDV* Relationships		
			Δ X-intercepts (ml)	Δ Slope (10⁴ erg/ml)	A‡ (% control)
STS§	8	+12 ± 2	+5 ± 3	−1.9 ± 2.2	50 ± 10
BC‖	9	+ 20 ± 3	+5 ± 3	+1.3 + 1.8	60 ± 9
p value		<0.05	>0.2	>0.2	>0.1

Control slopes were 12.5 for STS and 10 for BC; data are expressed as mean ± SEM.
*SW − EDV = Stroke work–end-diastolic volume.
†MV = myocardial volume.
‡A = area beneath stroke work–end-diastolic volume curve.
§STS = St. Thomas' crystalloid cardioplegia.
‖BC = blood cardioplegia.

described and are followed by clinical data on the physiologic adequacy.

Aortic arch cannulation is almost uniformly employed by using the metal-tip Sarns cannula.* For most coronary bypass and aortic valve procedures, single venous cannulation is accomplished through the right atrial appendage, and direct cardiac venting is now omitted (Fig. 54–18). Cardiopulmonary bypass is initiated at 32° C, distal coronary grafting sites are visualized, and internal mammary artery flow is measured (Rankin and Smith, 1989; Rankin et al, 1986). As the cardioplegia cannula† is inserted into the distal ascending aorta, pump inflow temperature is reduced to 16° C to "precool" the myocardium. Myocardial precooling with the bypass circuit allows

*Sarns, Inc., Ann Arbor, Michigan.
†DLP Inc., Walker, Michigan.

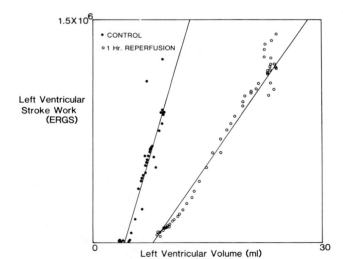

Figure 54–17. Changes in mechanical performance of the left ventricle observed after a 3-hour cardiac arrest using crystalloid cardioplegia. A standard functional response to ischemic injury is observed with an increase in the x-intercept, a diminished slope, and a decreased area under the stroke work–end-diastolic volume curve, which reflects a decrement in myocardial work capacity. (From Maier, G. W., and Rankin, J. S.: Unpublished data.)

better and more uniform myocardial hypothermia for a particular volume of cardioplegia infusion. A silicone rubber catheter is placed in the posterior pericardium via the transverse sinus and is connected to a cold saline lavage system. A metal coil submerged in a mixture of ice and alcohol acts as a heat exchanger to cool the pericardial saline, and infusion is begun at 100 ml/min. A suction catheter at the inferior aspect of the incision collects the pericardial lavage and returns it to a cell-saver device to scavenge shed blood. A myocardial temperature probe is placed into the interventricular septum. When myocardial temperature falls below 24° C, the aorta is occluded with a Fogarty clamp, and 1,200 ml of cold crystalloid cardioplegia solution (Table 54–2) is infused by the DLP cannula for 3 to 5 minutes. A commercial (Plegisol, Abbott Laboratories) St. Thomas' Hospital cardioplegia solution is preferred to reduce the risk of contamination from bacteria or of human error during formulation (Hughes et al, 1986). Reduction in myocardial temperature well below 15° C is usually achieved, and topical saline ice slush is applied as well to assist further in achieving low myocardial temperatures. If myocardial hypothermia is inadequate, additional volumes of cardioplegia solution are infused to attain the desired temperature. Coincident with aortic clamping, systemic perfusate temperature is returned to 24° C, and flow is reduced to 1 to 1.5 l/min/m². Systemic arterial pressure during the arrest period is adjusted to approximately 40 mm Hg. A side arm on the cardioplegia cannula is used for venting the aorta and left ventricle during aortic occlusion. The cardiac procedure is then done, and

TABLE 54–2. COMPOSITION OF MODIFIED ST. THOMAS' HOSPITAL CARDIOPLEGIC SOLUTION

Composition	Concentration
Sodium chloride	110.0 mmol/l
Potassium chloride	16.0 mmol/l
Magnesium chloride	16.0 mmol/l
Calcium chloride	1.2 mmol/l
Sodium bicarbonate	10.0 mmol/l
Procaine	0.05 mmol/l
Sodium heparin	1000 U/l
Human serum albumin	12.5 g/l

324 mOsm/kg of H_2O; pH 7.8.

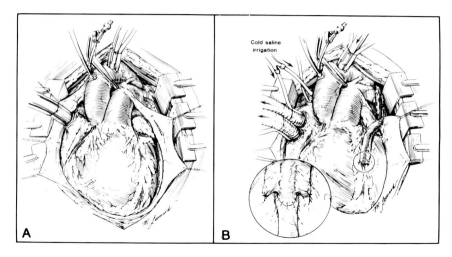

Figure 54–18. Simple perfusion technique (*A*) used for most coronary bypass procedures consisting of aortic cannulation for arterial flow, single right atrial cannulation for venous return, and aortic venting via the cardioplegia cannula. For more complex procedures including mitral value and multiple valve operations. (*B*), individual vena cava cannulation with occluding tapes and endocardial right atrial cold saline lavage are used to augment topical cardiac hypothermia.

additional 200 to 500 ml volumes of cardioplegia solution are infused every 30 to 45 minutes to maintain a myocardial temperature below 15° C. Full rewarming is begun 5 to 10 minutes before aortic unclamping, and a 200-mg dose of lidocaine is administered into the oxygenator to diminish reperfusion arrhythmias. After aortic unclamping, additional procedures such as proximal aorto-vein graft anastomoses are completed, and cardiopulmonary bypass is discontinued after adequate rewarming.

For mitral valve procedures, or for unusual cases in which long periods of arrest are required in the presence of preoperative ventricular impairment, individual vena cava cannulation is used with occluding tapes (see Fig. 54–18). A side arm from the pericardial lavage system is inserted into the right atrium adjacent to one of the venous cannulas, and the purse string is left loose to allow uninhibited egress of the endocardial saline lavage. Aortic venting is usually used, thus this method differs from the routine technique only by requiring one additional venous cannula and caval tapes. Experimental and clinical evidence suggests that the additional hypothermia provided by this method can significantly enhance myocardial protection for procedures requiring more than 90 minutes of cardiac arrest. In the authors' experience as well as that of others (Daily et al, 1987), this method has provided excellent cardiac protection for aortic occlusion times up to 150 minutes, extending the safe arrest period significantly. Thus, the more involved technique is used primarily in complex valve-coronary or aortic replacement valve-coronary operations; the simpler method is used almost uniformly for routine coronary bypass.

CLINICAL RESULTS

This method of crystalloid cardioplegia has been assessed clinically in several ways. First, functional adequacy of coronary bypass operations was evaluated by postoperative ventriculographic wall motion analysis in 149 patients (Rankin et al, 1985). Within this group, only one patient had a significant decrement in regional wall motion (at the site of an occluded vein graft), and 37% had significant postoperative improvement (Fig. 54–19). The perioperative myocardial infarction rate with this technique of

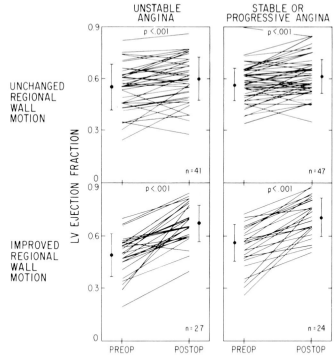

Figure 54–19. Perioperative ventriculographic ejection fraction data for 139 patients having coronary bypass with the myocardial protection technique described in this section. The categories are separated into unstable angina (*left panels*) and stable or progressive angina (*right panels*), and subdivided further according to the observed change in regional wall motion. Improvement in global ejection fraction was statistically significant in each category and in the entire group. (From Rankin, J. S., Newman, G. E., Muhlbaier, L. H., et al: The effects of coronary revascularization on left ventricular function in ischemic heart disease. J. Thorac. Cardiovasc. Surg., *90*:818, 1985.)

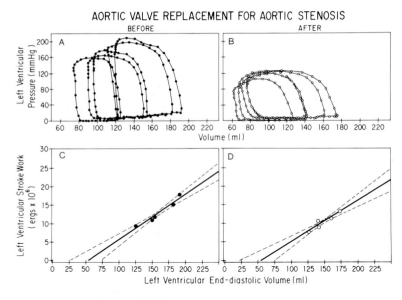

AORTIC VALVE REPLACEMENT FOR AORTIC STENOSIS

Figure 54–20. Representative left ventricular pressure-volume and stroke work–end-diastolic volume relationships obtained before (*closed circles*) and after (*open circles*) crystalloid cardioplegia in a patient having aortic valve replacement for aortic stenosis. Pressure-volume data were obtained with a 3F Millar micromanometer and a portable first-pass RNA camera. End-diastolic volume varied by blood infusion or by withdrawal via the aortic perfusion cannula. Note the reduction in systolic left ventricular pressure and improved ejection fraction associated with valve replacement (*A* versus *C*). The linear stroke work–end-diastolic volume relationships (±95% confidence limits) were well-preserved (*B* versus *D*) by crystalloid, cold potassium cardioplegia. (From Harpole, D. H., Wolfe, W. G., Rankin, J. S., et al: Assessment of left ventricular functional preservation during isolated cardiac valvular operations. Circulation, *80*:III, (in press). By permission of the American Heart Association, Inc.)

crystalloid cardioplegia was 1.6%. Left ventricular ejection fraction improved significantly in the group as a whole and also in those with improved wall motion, with an average of +0.18 in the latter. Thus, crystalloid cardioplegia, together with topical hypothermia and a physiologically adequate coronary revascularization, appears to provide excellent myocardial protection in patients with coronary bypass.

The physiologic adequacy of crystalloid cardioplegia has also been evaluated in patients with valvular heart disease with significant ventricular hypertrophy (Fig. 54–20). Stroke work–end-diastolic volume relationships were determined by radionuclide techniques and high-fidelity micromanometry immediately before and after cardiopulmonary bypass (Harpole et al, 1988). Sixteen patients had isolated aortic or mitral valve procedures, and significant ventricular hypertrophy was present in most patients. Left ventricular performance, which was assessed by the stroke work–end-diastolic volume method, was well preserved by crystalloid cardioplegia, and left ventricular performance characteristics were not significantly diminished postoperatively in either the entire group or any subgroup (Table 54–3). Thus, crystalloid cardioplegia provides excellent myocardial protection for isolated cardiac valve operations accompanied by cardiac hypertrophy.

Finally, the clinical results of 1,106 consecutive cardiac operations done by a single surgeon during the 4-year period ending on June 30, 1988, were evaluated (Rankin, unpublished data). Eighty-eight per cent were coronary bypass procedures with or without left ventricular aneurysm resections, and significant risk factors in this population included multivessel or left main disease, 94%; emergency bypass for refractory unstable or postinfarction angina or acute evolving myocardial infarction, 48%; age older than 65 years, 37%; ejection fraction less than 0.4, 24%. Within this group, there were *no* deaths in the operating room. There was a 2.1% overall hospital mortality and a 1.3% elective hospital mortality.

The remainder of the patients had cardiac valvular repair or replacement procedures (*n* = 122). Again, there were *no* deaths in the operating room, and the hospital mortality was 5.4% (5/91) for all nonischemic valve procedures. The hospital mortality for acute ischemic mitral regurgitation was 19.3% (6 of 31). Although adequate surgical repair is obviously an important factor in optimizing results, the elimination of operating room mortality and a low incidence of postoperative ventricular dysfunction support the adequacy of myocardial protection provided by the crystalloid technique described in this section.

TABLE 54–3. EFFICACY OF CRYSTALLOID CARDIOPLEGIA IN PRESERVING VENTRICULAR FUNCTION DURING CARDIAC VALVE OPERATIONS

| | *n* | LV* Mass (g/m²) | SW-EDV† Relationships | | |
			Slope (10⁴ erg/ml)	X-intercept (ml)	r
Prebypass	12	130 ± 56	11 ± 5	66 ± 38	0.95 ± 0.03
Postbypass	12	138 ± 53	9 ± 5	59 ± 38	0.94 ± 0.04
p value		0.1	>0.1	>0.1	

Data are presented as mean ±SD. LV mass was assessed with 2-D transesophageal echocardiography.
*LV = left ventricular.
†SW-EDV = stroke work–end-diastolic volume.

In conclusion, current cardioplegia techniques have been developed to the point that myocardial protection no longer constitutes a major problem in cardiac operations. Although methods undoubtedly will be refined further, the clinical results that can be achieved with current systems are quite good and contribute significantly to the management of cardiac surgical patients.

Selected Bibliography

Berne, R. M., and Rubio, R.: Coronary circulation. *In* Handbook of Physiology, Vol. I. Bethesda, MD, American Physiology Society, 1979, pp. 873–952.

A comprehensive review of the physiology of coronary blood flow by two outstanding experts.

Follette, D. M., Fey, K., Mulder, D., et al: Advantages of blood cardioplegia over intermittent ischemia during prolonged hypothermic aortic clamping. Circulation, *58* (Suppl. 1):200, 1978.

This is the original work on blood cardioplegia on which clinical application has been based.

Gay, W. A., and Ebert, P. A.: Functional, metabolic and morphologic effects of potassium-induced cardioplegia. Surgery, *74*:284, 1973.

This paper was responsible for reintroducing potassium cardioplegia into clinical practice. The work is not only a major contribution but is also a model of simplicity and innovation.

Hearse, D. J., Braimbridge, M. V., and Jynge, P.: Protection of the Ischemic Myocardium: Cardioplegia. New York, Raven Press, 1981.

This is a definitive work on myocardial preservation, and emphasis is placed on both basic scientific and practical surgical techniques. The world literature on this subject has been reviewed and analyzed by the investigators from St. Thomas' Hospital, London.

Sabiston, D. C., Jr.: The coronary circulation. The William F. Rienhoff, Jr. Lecture. Johns Hopkins Med. J., *134*:314, 1974.

This is a review of the anatomy, physiology, and pathologic aspects of the coronary circulation. The data are based on experimental and clinical findings in normal and pathologic conditions. The first saphenous vein bypass for the aorta in humans in 1962 is also described in this article.

Bibliography

Akins, C. W. and Carroll, D. L.: Event-free survival following nonemergency myocardial revascularization during hypothermic fibrillatory arrest. Ann. Thorac. Surg., *43*:628, 1987.

Bache, R. J., Cobb, R. F., and Greenfield, J. C., Jr.: Myocardial blood flow distribution during ischemia-induced coronary vasodilation in the unanesthetized dog. J. Clin. Invest., *54*:1462, 1974.

Barner, H. B., Kaiser, G. C., Codd, J. E., et al: Clinical experience with cold blood as the vehicle for hypothermic potassium cardioplegia. Ann. Thorac. Surg., *29*:224, 1981.

Barner, H. B., Swartz, M. T., Devine, J. E., et al: Diltiazem as an adjunct to cold blood potassium cardioplegia: A clinical assessment of dose and prospective randomization. Ann. Thorac. Surg., *43*:191, 1987.

Baur, H. R., Peterson, T. A., Yasmineh, W. G., and Gobel, F. L.: Cold potassium versus topical hypothermia and intermittent aortic occlusion for myocardial protection during coronary artery surgery: A randomized clinical study. Ann. Thorac. Surg., *41*:511, 1986.

Becker, H., Vinten-Johansen, J., Buckberg, G. D., et al: Myocardial damage caused by keeping pH 7.4 during systemic deep hypothermia. J. Thorac. Cardiovasc. Surg., *81*:810, 1981.

Berne, R. M., and Rubio, R.: Coronary circulation. *In* Handbook of Physiology. Bethesda, MD, American Physiological Society, 1979, pp. 873–952.

Bigelow, W. G., Mustard, W. T., and Evans, J. G.: Some physiologic concepts of hypothermia and their application to cardiac surgery. J. Thorac. Cardiovasc. Surg., *28*:463, 1954.

Bodenhamer, R. M., DeBoer, L. W. V., Geffin, G. A., et al: Enhanced myocardial protection during ischemic arrest: Oxygenation of a crystalloid cardioplegic solution. J. Thorac. Cardiovasc. Surg., *85*:769, 1983.

Bodenhamer, R. M., Johnson, R. G., Randolph, J. D., et al: The effect of adding mannitol or albumin to a crystalloid cardioplegic solution: A prospective, randomized clinical study. Ann. Thorac. Surg., *40*:374, 1985.

Boncheck, L., and Burlingame, M. W.: Coronary artery bypass without cardioplegia. J. Thorac. Cardiovasc. Surg., *93*:261, 1987.

Braimbridge, M. V., Chayen, J., Bitensky, L., et al: Cold cardioplegia or continuous coronary perfusion? Report on preliminary clinical experience as assessed cytochemically. J. Thorac. Cardiovasc. Surg., *74*:900, 1977.

Braunwald, E. (ed): Symposium on myocardial metabolism. Proceedings of a symposium held in Ponte Vedra, Florida, November 4 to 6, 1973. American Heart Association Monograph No. 44. Circ. Res., *34, 35* (Suppl. 3):1, 1974.

Bretschneider, H. J.: Überlebenszeit un Wiederbelebungszeit des Herzens bei Normo-und Hypothermie. Verh. Dtsch. Ges. Kreislaufforsch., *30*:11, 1964.

Bretschneider, H. J., Hubner, G., Knoll, D., et al: Myocardial resistance and tolerance to ischemia: Physiological and biochemical basis. J. Cardiovasc. Surg., *16*:241, 1975.

Buckberg, G. D.: A proposed "solution" to the cardioplegic controversy. J. Thorac. Cardiovasc. Surg., *77*:803, 1979.

Buckberg, G. D., and Hottenrott, C. E.: Ventricular fibrillation: Its effect on myocardial flow, distribution, and performance. Ann. Thorac. Surg., *20*:76, 1975.

Buckberg, G. D., Brazier, J. R., Nelson, R. H., et al: Studies on the effects of hypothermia on regional myocardial blood flow and metabolism during cardiopulmonary bypass. I: The adequately perfused beating, fibrillating, and arrested heart. J. Thorac. Cardiovasc. Surg., *73*:87, 1977.

Buckberg, G. D., Fixler, D. E., Archie, J. P., and Hoffman, J. I. E.: Experimental subendocardial ischemia in dogs with normal coronary arteries. Circ. Res., *30*:67, 1972.

Chitwood, W. R., Sink, J. D., Hill, R. C., et al: The effects of hypothermia on myocardial oxygen consumption and transmural coronary blood flow in the potassium-arrested heart. Ann. Surg., *190*:106, 1979.

Christakis, G. T., Fremes, S. E., Weisel, R. D., et al: Reducing the risk of urgent revascularization for unstable angina: A randomized clinical trial. J. Vasc. Surg., *3*:764, 1986a.

Christakis, G. T., Fremes, S. E., Weisel, R. D., et al: Diltiazem cardioplegia. J. Thorac. Cardiovasc. Surg., *91*:647, 1986b.

Clark, R. E.: Verapamil, cardioplegia, and coronary artery bypass grafting. Ann. Thorac. Surg., *41*:585, 1986.

Clark, R. E., Christlieb, I. Y., Ferguson, T. B., et al: The first American clinical trial of nifedipine in cardioplegia: A report of the first 12 months' experience. J. Thorac. Cardiovasc. Surg., *82*:848, 1981.

Codd, J. E., Barner, H. B., Pennington, D. G., et al: Intraoperative myocardial protection: A comparison of blood and asanguineous cardioplegia. Ann. Thorac. Surg., *39*:125, 1985.

Conti, V. R., Bertranou, E. G., Blackstone, E. H., et al: Cold cardioplegia versus hypothermia for myocardial protection: Randomized clinical study. J. Thorac. Cardiovasc. Surg., *76*:577, 1978.

Craver, J. M., Sams, A. B., and Hatcher, C. R.: Potassium-induced cardioplegia: Additive protection against ischemic myocardial injury during coronary revascularization. J. Thorac. Cardiovasc. Surg., 76:24, 1978.

Culliford, A. T., Cunningham, J. N., Jr., Adams, P. X., et al: Clinical experience with potassium cold blood cardioplegia at New York University Medical Center. In Moran, J. M., and Michaelis, L. L. (eds): Surgery for the Complications of Myocardial Infarction. New York, Grune & Stratton, 1980, pp. 119–134.

Cunningham, J. N., Jr., Adams, P. X., Knopp, E. A., et al: Preservation of ATP, ultrastructure, and ventricular function after aortic crossclamping and reperfusion: Clinical use of blood potassium cardioplegia. J. Thorac. Cardiovasc. Surg., 78:708, 1979.

Daggett, W. M., Randolph, J. D., Jacobs, M., et al: The superiority of cold oxygenated dilute blood cardioplegia. Ann. Thorac. Surg., 43:397, 1987.

Daily, P. O., Pfeiffer, T. A., Wisniewski, J. B., et al: Clinical comparisons of methods of myocardial protection. J. Thorac. Cardiovasc. Surg., 93:324, 1987.

Elbeery, J. R., Owen, C. H., Savitt, M. A., et al: Myocardial metabolic to mechanical energy transfer characteristics obtained from single vena caval occlusions. J. Am. Coll. Cardiol., 13:87A, 1989.

Fabiani, J., Deloche, A., Swanson, J., and Carpentier, A.: Retrograde cardioplegia through the right atrium. Ann. Thorac. Surg., 41:101, 1986.

Feneley, M. P., Maier, G. W., Gayor, J. W., et al: Comparison of elastic and non-elastic predictive models of myocardial oxygen consumption in conscious dogs. Circulation, 76:IV-543, 1987.

Flaherty, J. T., Schaffy, H. V., Goldman, R. A., and Gott, V. L.: Metabolic and functional effects of progressive degrees of hypothermia during global ischemia. Am. J. Physiol., 236:H839, 1979.

Flameng, W., De Meyere, R., Daenen, W., et al: Nifedipine as an adjunct to St. Thomas' Hospital cardioplegia. J. Thorac. Cardiovasc. Surg., 91:723, 1986.

Foglia, R. P., Steed, D. L., Follette, D. M., et al: Iatrogenic myocardial edema with potassium cardioplegia. J. Thorac. Cardiovasc. Surg., 78:217, 1979.

Follette, D. M., Fey, K., Mulder, D., et al: Advantages of blood cardioplegia over continuous coronary perfusion or intermittent ischemia: Experimental and clinical study. J. Thorac. Cardiovasc. Surg., 76:604, 1978a.

Follette, D. M., Steed, D. L., Foglia, R., et al: Advantages of intermittent blood cardioplegia over intermittent ischemia during prolonged hypothermic aortic clamping. Circulation, 58(Suppl.1):200, 1978b.

Follette, D. M., Fey, K., Buckberg, G. D., et al: Reducing postischemic damage by temporary modification of reperfusate calcium, potassium, pH, and osmolarity. J. Thorac. Cardiovasc. Surg., 82:221, 1981.

Gall, S. A., Maier, G. W., Gaynor, J. W., et al: Repetitive ischemia delays recovery of regional myocardial function in awake dogs. J. Am. Coll. Cardiol., 11:94A, 1988.

Gay, W. A., and Ebert, P. A.: Functional, metabolic and morphologic effects of potassium-induced cardioplegia. Surgery, 74:284, 1973.

Gevers, W.: Generation of protons by metabolic processes in heart cells. J. Mol. Cell. Cardiol., 9:867, 1977.

Gibbs, C. L.: Cardiac energetics. Physiol. Rev., 58:174, 1978.

Glower, D. D., Schaper, J., Kabas, J. S., et al: Relation between reversal of diastolic creep and recovery of systolic function after ischemic myocardial injury in conscious dogs. Circ. Res., 60:850, 1987.

Glower, D. D., Spratt, J. A., Kabas, J. S., et al: Quantification of regional myocardial function after acute ischemic injury: Application of preload recruitable stroke work. Am. J. Physiol, 255:H85, 1988.

Glower, D. D., Spratt, J. A., Snow, N. D., et al: Linearity of the Frank-Starling relationship in the intact heart: The concept of preload recruitable stroke work. Circulation, 71:994, 1985.

Gregg, D. E.: The natural history of coronary collateral development. Circ. Res., 35:335, 1974.

Grover, F. L., Fewel, J. G., Ghidoni, J. J., and Trinkle, J. K.: Does lower systemic temperature enhance cardioplegic myocardial protection? J. Thorac. Cardiovasc. Surg., 81:11, 1981.

Guiraudon, G. M., Campbell, C. S., McLellan, D. G., et al: Retrograde coronary sinus versus aortic root perfusion with cold cardioplegia: Randomized study of levels of cardiac enzymes in 40 patients. Circulation, 74:III-105, 1986.

Guyton, R. A., Dorsey, L. M. A., Craver, J. M., et al: Improved myocardial recovery after cardioplegic arrest with an oxygenated crystalloid solution. J. Thorac. Cardiovasc. Surg., 89:877, 1985.

Harpole, D. H., Wolfe, W. G., Rankin, J. S., et al: Assessment of left ventricular preservation during isolated cardiac valvular operations. Circulation, 80:III (in press).

Hearse, D. J., Braimbridge, M. V., and Jynge, P.: Protection of the Ischemic Myocardium: Cardioplegia. New York, Raven Press, 1981.

Hearse, D. J., Garlick, P. B., and Humphrey, S. M.: Ischemic contracture of the myocardium: Mechanisms and prevention. Am. J. Cardiol., 39:986, 1977.

Hearse, D. J., O'Brien, K., and Braimbridge, M. V.: Protection of the myocardium during ischemic arrest: Dose-response curves for procaine and lignocaine in cardioplegia solutions. J. Thorac. Cardiovasc. Surg., 81:873, 1981.

Hearse, D. J., Stewart, D. A., and Braimbridge, M. V.: Hypothermic arrest and potassium arrest, metabolic and myocardial protection during elective cardiac arrest. Circ. Res., 36:481, 1985.

Hearse, D. J., Stewart, D. A., and Braimbridge, M. V.: Myocardial protection during bypass and arrest: A possible hazard with lactate-containing infusates. J. Thorac. Cardiovasc. Surg., 72:880, 1976.

Hearse, D. J., Stewart, D. A., and Braimbridge, M. V.: Myocardial protection during ischemic cardiac arrest: Possible deleterious effects of glucose and mannitol in coronary infusates. J. Thorac. Cardiovasc. Surg., 76:16, 1978a.

Hearse, D. J., Stewart, D. A., and Braimbridge, M. V.: Myocardial protection during ischemic cardiac arrest: The importance of magnesium in cardioplegic infusates. J. Thorac. Cardiovasc. Surg., 75:877, 1978b.

Heitmiller, R. F., DeBoer, L. W. V., Geffin, G. A., et al: Myocardial recovery after hypothermic arrest: A comparison of oxygenated crystalloid to blood cardioplegia: The role of calcium. Circulation, 72 (Suppl. II):241, 1985.

Hicks, G. L., and DeWeese, J. A.: Verapamil potassium cardioplegia and cardiac conduction. Ann. Thorac. Surg., 39:324, 1985.

Hines, G. L., Wehbe, W., and Mele, V.: Papaverine hydrochloride as an adjunct to asanguinous cardioplegia: Is it beneficial? J. Cardiovasc. Surg., 26:196, 1985.

Hughes, C. F., Leckie, B. D., and Baird, D. K.: Cardioplegic solution: A contamination crises. J. Thorac. Cardiovasc. Surg., 91:296, 1986.

Hurley, E. J., Lower, R. R., Dong, E., Jr., et al: Clinical experience with local hypothermia in elective cardiac arrest. J. Thorac. Cardiovasc. Surg., 47:50, 1964.

Jennings, R. B., and Ganote, C. E.: Structural changes in myocardium during acute ischemia. Circ. Res., 34, 35 (Suppl. 3):156, 1974.

Jynge, P., Hearse, D. J., and Braimbridge, M. V.: Myocardial protection during ischemic cardiac arrest: A possible hazard with calcium-free cardioplegic infusates. J. Thorac. Cardiovasc. Surg., 73:848, 1977.

Katz, A. M.: Physiology of the Heart. New York, Raven Press, 1977.

Kirsch, U., Rodewald, G., and Kalmar, P.: Induced ischemic arrest. J. Thorac. Cardiovasc. Surg., 63:121, 1972.

Leaf, A.: Regulation of intracellular fluid volume and disease. Am. J. Med., 49:291, 1970.

Lee, B. Y., Wilson, G. J., Domnech, R. J., and MacGregor, D. C.: Relative roles of edema versus contracture in the myocardial "no-reflow" phenomenon. J. Surg. Res., 29:50, 1980.

Lowe, J. E., Cummings, R. G., Adams, D. H., and Hull-Ryde, E. A.: Evidence that ischemic cell death begins in the subendocardium independent of variations in collateral flow or wall tension. Circulation, 68:190, 1983.

Lowe, J. E., Kleinman, L. H., Reimer, K. A., et al: Effects of cardioplegia produced by calcium flux inhibition. Surg. Forum, 28:279, 1977.

Lucas, S. K., Gardner, J. J., Flaherty, J. T., et al: Beneficial effects of mannitol administration during reperfusion after ischemic arrest. Circulation, 62 (Suppl. I):34, 1980.

MacKnight, A. C., and Leaf, A.: Regulation of cellular volume. Physiol. Rev., 57:510, 1977.

Magovern, G. J., Flaherty, J. T., Gott, V. L., et al: Optimal myocardial protection with Fluosol cardioplegia. Ann. Thorac. Surg., 34:249, 1982.

Maier, G. W., Owen, C. H., Feneley, M. P., et al: The mechanical determinants of myocardial oxygen consumption in the conscious dog. Circulation, 78:II-67, 1988.

Melrose, D. G.: Elective cardiac arrest: Historical perspective. In Longmore, D. (ed): Modern Cardiac Surgery. Baltimore, MD, University Park Press, 1978, pp. 271–275.

Menasché, P. and Piwnica, A.: Retrograde cardioplegia through the coronary sinus. Ann. Thorac. Surg., 44:214, 1987.

Mullen, J. C., Cristakis, G. T., Weisel, R. D., et al: Late postoperative ventricular function after blood and crystalloid cardioplegia. Circulation, 74 (Suppl. III):89, 1986a.

Mullen, J. C., Fremes, S. E., Weisel, R. D., et al: Right ventricular function: A comparison between blood and crystalloid cardioplegia. Ann. Thorac. Surg., 43:17, 1986b.

Nelson, R., Fey, K., Follette, D. M., et al: The critical importance of intermittent infusion of cardioplegic solution during aortic cross clamping. Surg. Forum, 27:241, 1976.

Novick, R. J., Stefaniszyn, H. J., Michel, R. P., et al: Protection of the hypertrophied pig myocardium. A comparison of crystalloid, blood, and Fluosol. DA cardioplegia during prolonged aortic clamping. J. Thorac. Cardiovasc. Surg., 89:547, 1985.

Powell, W. J., DiBona, D. R., Flores, J., and Leaf, A.: The protective effect of hyperosmotic mannitol in reducing ischemic cell swelling and minimizing myocardial necrosis. Circulation, 53 (Suppl. I):45, 1976.

Rahn, H., Reeves, R. B., and Howell, B. J.: Hydrogen ion regulation, temperature and evolution. Am. Rev. Respir. Dis., 112:165, 1975.

Rankin, J. S., and Sabiston, D. C., Jr.: Physiology of the coronary circulation and intraoperative myocardial protection. In Sabiston, D. C., Jr., and Spencer, F. C. (eds): Gibbon's Surgery of the Chest, 4th ed. Philadelphia, W. B. Saunders Company, 1983.

Rankin, J. S., and Smith, L. R.: Utilization of the internal mammary arteries for coronary artery bypass. In Sabiston, D. C., Jr., and Spencer, F. C. (eds): Gibbon's Surgery of the Chest, 5th ed. Philadelphia, W. B. Saunders Company, 1989.

Rankin, J. S., Newman, G. E., Bashore, T. M., et al: Clinical and angiographic assessment of complex mammary artery bypass grafting. J. Thorac. Cardiovasc. Surg., 92:832, 1986.

Rankin, J. S., Newman, G. E., Muhlbaier, L. H., et al: The effects of coronary revascularization on left ventricular function in ischemic heart disease. J. Thorac. Cardiovasc. Surg., 90:818, 1985.

Robb-Nicholson, C., Currie, W. D., and Wechsler, A. S.: Effects of verapamil on myocardial tolerance to ischemic cardiac arrest. Circulation, 58 (Suppl. 1):119, 1978.

Roberts, A. J., Woodhall, D. D., Knauf, D. G., and Alexander, J. A.: Coronary artery bypass graft surgery: Clinical comparison of cold blood potassium cardioplegia, warm cardioplegic induction, and secondary cardioplegia. Ann. Thorac. Surg., 40:483, 1985.

Rosenfeldt, F. L., and Watson, D. A.: Interference with local myocardial cooling by heat gain during aortic cross-clamping. Ann. Thorac. Surg., 27:13, 1979.

Rosenthal, T. B.: The effect of temperature on the pH of blood and plasma in vitro. J. Biol. Chem., 173:25, 1948.

Rowe, G. G., Castillo, C. A., Maxwell, G. M., and Crumpton, C. W.: Comparison of systemic and coronary hemodynamics in the normal human male and female. Circ. Res., 7:728, 1959.

Sabiston, D. C., Jr.: The coronary circulation: The William F. Rienhoff, Jr. Lecture. Johns Hopkins Med. J., 134:314, 1974.

Sabiston, D. C., Jr., and Gregg, D. E.: Effect of cardiac contraction on coronary blood flow. Circulation, 15:14, 1957.

Schachner, A., Schmimert, G., Lajos, T. S., et al: Selective intracavitary and coronary hypothermic cardioplegia for myocardial preservation. Arch. Surg., 111:1197, 1976.

Schaper, J., Scheld, H. H., Schmidt, U., and Herlein, F.: Ultrastructural study comparing the efficacy of five different methods of intraoperative myocardial protection in the human heart. J. Thorac. Cardiovasc. Surg., 92:47, 1986.

Schaper, J., Walter, P., Scheld, H., and Hehrlein, F.: The effects of retrograde perfusion of cardioplegic solution in cardiac operations. J. Thorac. Cardiovasc. Surg., 90:882, 1985.

Shen, A. C., and Jennings, R. B.: Myocardial calcium and magnesium in acute ischemic injury. Am. J. Pathol., 67:417, 1972.

Shumway, N. E., Lower, R. R., and Stofer, R. C.: Selective hypothermia of the heart in anoxic cardiac arrest. Surg. Gynecol. Obstet., 109:750, 1959.

Silverman, N. A., and Levitsky, S.: Intraoperative myocardial protection in the context of coronary revascularization. Prog. Cardiovasc. Dis., 29:413, 1987.

Silverman, N. A., Wright, R., Levitsky, S., et al: Efficacy of infusion route and regional wall motion on preservation of adenine nucleotide stores. J. Thorac. Cardiovasc. Surg., 89:90, 1985.

Slogoff, S., Keats, A. S., Cooley, D. A., et al: Addition of papaverine to cardioplegia does not reduce myocardial necrosis. Ann. Thorac. Surg., 42:60, 1986.

Squire, J.: The Structural Basis of Muscular Contraction. New York, Plenum Press, 1981.

Teoh, K. H., Christakis, G. T., Weisel, R. D., et al: Accelerated myocardial metabolic recovery with terminal warm blood cardioplegia. J. Thorac. Cardiovasc. Surg., 91:888, 1986.

Tyers, G. F. O.: Metabolic arrest of the heart. Ann. Thorac. Surg., 20:91, 1975.

Tyers, G. F. O., Manley, J. J., Williams, G. H., et al: Preliminary clinical experience with isotonic hypothermic potassium induced arrest. J. Thorac. Cardiovasc. Surg., 74:674, 1977b.

Tyers, G. F. O., Williams, E. H., Hughes, H. C., and Todd, G. J.: Effect of perfusate temperature on myocardial protection from ischemia. J. Thorac. Cardiovasc. Surg., 73:766, 1977a.

van der Vusse, G. J., van der Veen, F. H., Flameng, W., et al: A biochemical and ultrastructural study on myocardial changes during aorto-coronary bypass surgery: St. Thomas' Hospital cardioplegia versus intermittent aortic cross-clamping at 34 and 25°. Eur. Surg. Res., 18:1, 1986.

Vercillo, A. P., Squier, R. C., Chawla, S., et al: Procaine versus magnesium in cardioplegia solution. Conn. Med., 51:74, 1987.

White, F. N.: A comparative physiological approach to hypothermia (Editorial). J. Thorac. Cardiovasc. Surg., 82:821, 1981.

Wildenthal, K., Mierzwiak, D. S., and Mitchell, J.: Acute effects of increased serum osmolarity on left ventricular performance. Am. J. Physiol., 216:898, 1969.

Williams, R. F., Maier, G. W., Davis, J. W., and Rankin, J. S.: The effects of systolic loading on myocardial recovery after ischemic injury. Circulation, 72 (Suppl. III):280, 1985.

Zimmerman, A. N. E., Daems, W., Hulsmann, W. C., et al: Morphological changes of heart muscle caused by successive perfusion with calcium-free and calcium-containing solutions (calcium paradox). Cardiovasc. Res., 1:201, 1967.

II PATHOLOGY OF CORONARY ATHEROSCLEROSIS

William C. Roberts

Atherosclerotic coronary artery disease (CAD) is the most common cause of death in the western world. One American dies every minute of atherosclerotic CAD. In the United States alone, 5.5 to 7.5 million individuals have symptomatic myocardial ischemia because of atherosclerotic CAD. Approximately 250,000 coronary artery bypass grafting operations, and similar numbers of coronary angioplasty procedures, are now done annually in the United States. The cause of atherosclerosis is now clear; the evidence is overwhelming that atherosclerosis is a cholesterol problem. The higher the blood total cholesterol level (especially the low-density lipoprotein level) the greater is the risk for developing symptomatic CAD, fatal CAD, and atherosclerotic plaques. Lowering the blood total cholesterol level decreases the chances of development of symptomatic or fatal CAD, and the possibility that some atherosclerotic plaques will actually regress increases.

Although the coronary arteries have been examined visually at necropsy for more than 100 years, only recently has the extent of the atherosclerotic process in the coronary arteries in patients with symptomatic or fatal CAD become appreciated. This chapter concerns the status of the major epicardial coronary arteries in various subsets of patients with fatal atherosclerotic CAD.

NUMBER OF MAJOR EPICARDIAL CORONARY ARTERIES SEVERELY NARROWED IN THE VARIOUS "CORONARY EVENTS"

The most common method for describing the severity of CAD in patients with clinical evidence of myocardial ischemia is by the number of major epicardial coronary arteries narrowed by more than 50% in luminal diameter by angiography. Thus, patients are divided into groups of one-vessel, two-vessel, three-vessel, and "left main" CAD. Because a 50% diameter reduction in general is equivalent to a 75% cross-sectional area narrowing, the cut-off point of "significant" compared with "insignificant" luminal narrowing at necropsy is the 75% cross-sectional area point. Physiologically, there is no obstruction to arterial flow until the lumen is narrowed by more than 75% in cross-sectional area (Fig. 54–21).

The numbers of major (right, left main, left anterior descending, and left circumflex) epicardial coronary arteries narrowed by more than 75% in cross-sectional area by atherosclerotic plaque alone

in patients with fatal CAD are summarized in Table 54–4. Among the 129 patients with fatal CAD studied at necropsy, 516 major epicardial coronary arteries were examined and of them 345 (67%) were narrowed at some point by 76 to 100% in cross-sectional area by atherosclerotic plaque. However, of 40 control subjects, mainly victims of acute leukemia, and without clinical evidence of myocardial ischemia during life, 160 major epicardial coronary arteries were examined and of them 60 (37%) were narrowed at some point by more than 75% in cross-sectional area by plaque. Among the 129 patients with coronary artery problems, only 11 (8%) had a single coronary artery severely narrowed (controls = 23%); 37 (29%) had two arteries so narrowed (controls = 13%); 64 (50%) had three arteries severely narrowed (controls = 5%) and 17 patients (13%) had all four major arteries so narrowed (controls = 0). Thus, of the four major coronary arteries in the coronary patients, an average of 2.7 were narrowed by more than 75% in cross-sectional area by plaque and among the control subjects 0.7 of the four major arteries.

The numbers of major coronary arteries severely narrowed by atherosclerotic plaque among the various subsets of coronary patients were relatively similar except for the patients with unstable angina (see Table 54–4). Among the 31 patients who died unexpectedly (*sudden coronary death*) (Roberts and Jones, 1979), all of whom died outside the hospital, usually within a few minutes of onset of symptoms of myocardial ischemia, an average of 2.8 of the four major arteries were severely narrowed, a number almost identical to that of the 27 patients with *transmural acute myocardial infarction* (Roberts and Jones, 1980), all of whom died in a coronary care unit. Only 2 of the 31 victims of sudden death and none of the 27 victims of acute myocardial infarction had only a single coronary artery ("one-vessel disease") severely narrowed.

The *healed myocardial infarction* group was divided into three subgroups. One group consisted of patients who had had an acute myocardial infarct in the past which had healed, and thereafter there was no evidence of myocardial ischemia clinically. These patients died from noncardiac causes, usually from cancer (Virmani and Roberts, 1981). Nevertheless, the average number of major coronary arteries severely narrowed at necropsy was 2.2 of four. Another subgroup consisted of patients who had chronic congestive heart failure after healing of an acute myocardial infarction but in the absence of a left ventricular aneurysm (Virmani and Roberts, 1980). The diagnosis in this group might be called *ischemic*

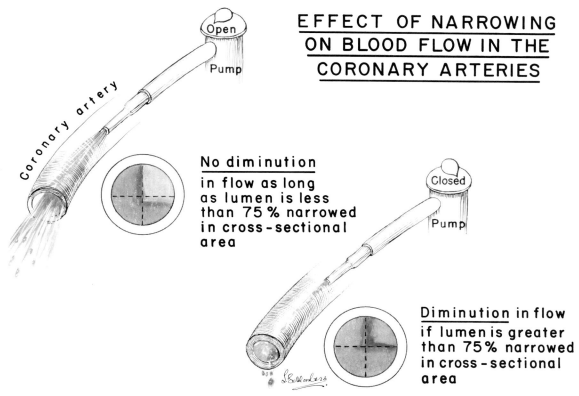

EFFECT OF NARROWING ON BLOOD FLOW IN THE CORONARY ARTERIES

No diminution in flow as long as lumen is less than 75% narrowed in cross-sectional area

Diminution in flow if lumen is greater than 75% narrowed in cross-sectional area

Figure 54–21. The amount of luminal narrowing necessary to reduce flow through a coronary artery.

cardiomyopathy. The average number of major coronary arteries severely narrowed in them was also 2.2 of four. The other subgroup of patients with healed myocardial infarction had a true left ventricular aneurysm (Cabin and Roberts, 1980). The average number of major coronary arteries severely narrowed in them was 2.5 of four.

The final subgroup consisted of 22 patients with *unstable angina pectoris,* and 19 of these patients had had coronary artery bypass grafting procedures

within 7 days of death (Roberts and Virmani, 1979). Preoperatively, all had normal left ventricular function and none had had a clinically apparent acute myocardial infarct or congestive heart failure at any time. The average number of major coronary arteries severely narrowed by plaque was 3.2 of four, and 10 of the 22 patients had severe narrowing of the left main coronary artery as well as severe narrowing of the other three major coronary arteries ("four-vessel disease"). (Another study by Bulkley and Roberts,

TABLE 54–4. NUMBER OF MAJOR (RIGHT, LEFT MAIN, LEFT ANTERIOR DESCENDING, LEFT CIRCUMFLEX) CORONARY ARTERIES NARROWED MORE THAN 75% IN CROSS-SECTIONAL AREA BY ATHEROSCLEROTIC PLAQUE IN FATAL CORONARY ARTERY DISEASE

Coronary Event	No. of Patients	Mean Age (Yrs)	No. of 4 Arteries Per Patient >75% CSA* by Plaque				
			4	3	2	1	Mean
Sudden coronary death	31	47	3	20	6	2	2.8
Acute myocardial infarction	27	59	3	14	10	0	2.7
Healed myocardial infarction							
A. Asymptomatic	18	66	0	7	7	4	2.2
B. Chronic CHF† without aneurysm	9	63	0	3	5	1	2.2
C. Left ventricular aneurysm	22	61	1	12	6	3	2.5
Angina pectoris/unstable	22	48	10	8	3	1	3.2
Totals	129	56	17	64	37	11	2.7
	(%)		(13)	(50)	(29)	(8)	
Controls	40	52	0	5	12	21	0.7
	(%)		(0)	(5)	(13)	(23)	

*CSA = cross-sectional area.
†CHF = congestive heart failure.

1976, suggested that severe narrowing of the left main coronary artery is usually an indication that the other three major arteries are also severely narrowed.) The group with unstable angina thus had the largest average number of major coronary arteries severely narrowed of the subgroups, but nevertheless these patients had excellent left ventricular function.

QUANTITATIVE APPROACH TO ATHEROSCLEROTIC CORONARY ARTERY DISEASE

Although the one-, two-, three-, and four-vessel disease approach has been useful clinically, this type of severity analysis might be thought of as a *qualitative* approach and differences in degrees of coronary narrowing in the various subsets of coronary patients are usually not discernible by this approach.

To obtain a better appreciation of the extent of the atherosclerotic process in patients with fatal CAD, several years ago the author and colleagues began examining each 5-mm segment of each of the four major coronary arteries. In adults, the average length of the right coronary artery is 10 cm; the left main coronary artery is 1 cm; the left anterior descending artery is 10 cm; and the left circumflex is 6 cm. Thus, 27 cm of major epicardial coronary arteries are available for examination in each adult. Because each 1 cm is divided into two 5-mm segments, an average of 54 5-mm segments is available to examine in each heart. This approach allows one to ask not only how many of the 5-mm segments are narrowed 76 to 100% in cross-sectional area, but also how many are narrowed by 51 to 75%, 26 to 50%, and 0 to 25%. This approach, compared with the one-, two-, three-, and four-vessel disease approach, might be considered to be *quantitative*.

The same patients described earlier by the qualitative approach also were examined at necropsy by the quantitative approach, and the findings are summarized in Table 54–5. A total of 6,461 5-mm segments were sectioned and were later examined histologically. The sections were stained by Movat's method to delineate the internal elastic membrane. The findings in the 129 coronary patients were compared with those in 1,849 5-mm segments in 40 control subjects. In each coronary subgroup, the 5-mm segments from each of the four major coronary arteries were pooled together so that by this approach the amount of narrowing in an individual patient could not be discerned. The percentage of 5-mm segments narrowed 76 to 100% in cross-sectional area by atherosclerotic plaque was 35% for the coronary patients and 3% for the control subjects; the percentage narrowed 51 to 75% was 36% for the coronary patients and 22% for the control subjects. Thus, 71% of the 5-mm segments in the coronary patients were narrowed more than 50% in cross-sectional area by atherosclerotic plaque and 25% in the control subjects. However, only 29% of the 5-mm segments in the coronary patients were narrowed less than 50%, and only 8% even approached normal (i.e., narrowed 25% or less in cross-sectional area). In contrast, 75% of the 5-mm segments in the control subjects were narrowed less than 50% and 31% of them were normal or almost normal. Thus, in the coronary patients 92% of the 6,461 5-mm segments of the four major epicardial coronary arteries were narrowed more than 25% in cross-sectional area by atherosclerotic plaque. Accordingly, the coronary atherosclerotic process is a diffuse one in patients with fatal CAD, and to believe that the atherosclerotic process is a focal one in patients with fatal CAD is to believe a myth.

Among the various subsets of coronary patients, those with *sudden coronary death* (Roberts, 1986; Roberts and Jones, 1979), and *acute myocardial infarction* (Roberts and Jones, 1979) (Fig. 54–22) had similar percentages of 5-mm segments narrowed 76 to 100%

TABLE 54–5. AMOUNTS OF CROSS-SECTIONAL AREA NARROWING OF EACH 5-MM SEGMENT OF THE FOUR MAJOR EPICARDIAL CORONARY ARTERIES* BY ATHEROSCLEROTIC PLAQUES IN SUBJECTS OF FATAL CORONARY ARTERY DISEASE

Subgroup	No. of Patients	Mean Age (Yrs)	No. of 5-mm Segments	Segments Narrowed (%) 0–25%	26–50%	51–75%	76–100%	Mean Score	Mean % Narrowing Per 5-mm Segments
Sudden coronary death	31	47	1,564	7	23	34	36	2.98	67
Acute myocardial infarction	27	59	1,403	5	23	38	34	3.01	68
Healed myocardial infarction									
A. Asymptomatic	18	66	924	11	23	35	31	2.87	64
B. Chronic CHF† without aneurysm	9	63	529	11	23	37	31	2.78	61
C. Left ventricular aneurysm	22	61	992	4	21	42	29 33	3.03	68
Angina pectoris/unstable	22	48	1,049	11	12	29	48	3.12	70
Totals	129	56	6,461	8	21	36	35	2.98	67
Controls	40	52	1,849	31	44	22	3	1.97	32

*Right, left main, left anterior descending, and left circumflex arteries.
†CHF = congestive heart failure.

ACUTE MYOCARDIAL INFARCTION

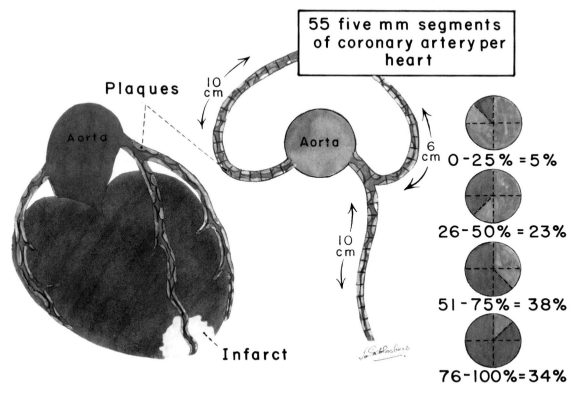

Figure 54–22. The percentage of 5-mm segments of the four major epicardial coronary arteries narrowed to four categories of cross-sectional area narrowing by atherosclerotic plaque in 27 patients with fatal transmural acute myocardial infarction.

in cross-sectional area by plaque (36 and 34%, respectively); patients with *healed myocardial infarction* (Cabin and Roberts, 1980; Virmani and Roberts, 1980, 1981) (Fig. 54–23) as a group had the least severe narrowing (31% of segments narrowed more than 75%), and the patients with *unstable angina pectoris* (Roberts and Virmani, 1979) had the most severe narrowing of all (48% of the 5-mm segments were narrowed more than 75% by plaque).

In an attempt to provide a single number for the amount of coronary arterial narrowing in each patient, a score system was used. A segment narrowed 0 to 25% was assigned a score of 1; a segment narrowed 26 to 50% had a score of 2; a segment narrowed 51 to 75% had a score of 3; and one narrowed 76 to 100% had a score of 4. The mean score for all 129 patients or for each of the 6,461 5-mm coronary segments was 3 and that for the 40 control subjects or 1,849 5-mm segments was 2. Again, the unstable patients with angina had the most extensive coronary narrowing by this approach.

A possible criticism of the 5-mm segment approach to quantifying coronary arterial narrowing is that the epicardial coronary arteries were fixed in an unphysiologic pressure state, namely a zero pressure state, rather than at a systemic arterial diastolic pressure. In an attempt to take into account the unphysiologic fixation state, the degrees of narrowing were conservatively judged; thus, if a segment was more or less in between two quadrants (51 to 75% and 76 to 100%), the lesser degree of narrowing was always chosen. Second, in any segment in which a portion of wall was collapsed by the fixation process, the degree of narrowing was determined as if the segment were expanded. Most important, the segments narrowed the most (i.e., more than 75% in cross-sectional area) were affected the least by the fixation process. Irrespective of whether the histologic technique used in this study was perfect or imperfect, the same technique was used in all subsets of coronary patients and also on all control subjects, and, therefore, the comparison data were highly reliable. Irrespective of whether the degrees of luminal narrowing should be slightly greater or slightly less than that determined by this technique, it is clear that the atherosclerotic process is a diffuse one in almost all patients with fatal CAD. The accuracy of the technique of determining degrees of cross-sectional area narrowing by estimating from stained histologic sections magnified about 40 times is similar ($\leq$5%) to that determined by planimetry (Isner et al, 1980).

HEALED MYOCARDIAL INFARCTION

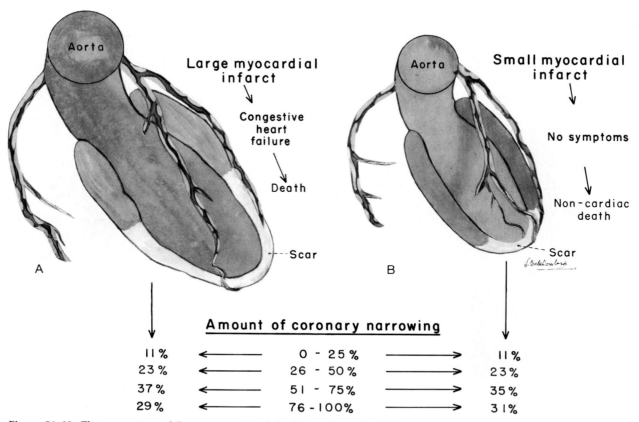

Figure 54–23. The percentage of 5-mm segments of the four major epicardial coronary arteries narrowed to four categories of cross-sectional area narrowing by atherosclerotic plaque in 18 patients with healed myocardial infarcts and chronic congestive heart failure (*A*) and in 18 patients with healed myocardial infarcts and noncardiac death (*B*). The percentage of 5-mm coronary segments narrowed to each of the four categories of narrowing were similar in each group. Thus, the size of a myocardial infarct that heals is not indicative of the degree of coronary arterial narrowing.

Another possible concern of the aforementioned quantitative data is applicability to living patients with symptomatic or other clinical evidence (e.g., positive exercise test) of myocardial ischemia. The author believes that the major difference in coronary arterial narrowing occurs at the stage of conversion from the asymptomatic to the symptomatic myocardial ischemia state and that there is relatively little difference in degrees of coronary narrowing between the symptomatic and the fatal states. Support for this belief can be obtained by the presence of severe and extensive coronary narrowing by angiography during life and by studying the coronary tree at necropsy in patients who, during life, had a coronary event and who died later from a noncardiac cause. Although data from the latter situation are minimal, the degrees of coronary narrowing at necropsy are similar to those in other patients with symptomatic myocardial ischemia that is fatal (Virmani and Roberts, 1980, 1981). Finally, among the subsets of coronary patients described earlier, those with unstable angina pectoris had the worst degrees of coronary narrowing, and the subjects in this group were the only ones in

whom their natural course was interrupted by an iatrogenic event, namely coronary artery bypass grafting (within 7 days of death).

DISTRIBUTION OF SEVERE NARROWING IN EACH OF THE THREE LONGEST EPICARDIAL CORONARY ARTERIES IN FATAL CORONARY ARTERY DISEASE

In all of the aforementioned quantitative coronary arterial studies, the amount of cross-sectional area luminal narrowing by atherosclerotic plaque in the right, left anterior descending, and left circumflex coronary arteries was similar if the 5-mm segments in each of the three longest coronary arteries were pooled together from a number of patients. This statement might be best understood by examining a single subset of coronary patients with fatal CAD. Among the 27 patients with fatal transmural acute myocardial infarction, a total of 1,358 5-mm segments were analyzed from the right, left anterior descending, and left circumflex coronary arteries, and the percentage of segments narrowed 0 to 25, 26 to 50, 51 to 75, and 76 to 100% was similar at each of these four categories of cross-sectional area narrowing in each of these three major epicardial coronary arteries (Fig. 54–24). The same findings were observed in the patients with sudden coronary death, healed myocardial infarction, and unstable angina pectoris.

In a single patient, however, the percentage of 5-mm coronary segments severely (more than 75% in cross-sectional area) narrowed by atherosclerotic plaque in one major epicardial coronary artery may be greater or less than that of another major coronary artery. If the segments from one coronary artery (e.g., right coronary artery), however, were pooled

together from several patients with fatal CAD and compared with pooled 5-mm segments from another coronary artery (e.g., left anterior descending coronary artery) from several patients with fatal CAD, the percentage of segments narrowed at each of the four categories of cross-sectional area narrowing in each artery are similar. The definition of "several" has not yet been established, but with few exceptions, this principle may apply to as few as three patients with pooled 5-mm segments from each of the three major coronary arteries. Thus, the quantity of atherosclerotic plaque is similar for similar lengths of the right, left anterior descending, and left circumflex coronary arteries. Furthermore, because the amount of atherosclerotic plaque is similar, the amount of resultant luminal narrowing is also similar. The cholesterol thesis might not be tenable if the amount of atherosclerotic plaque were highly different in the different major epicardial coronary arteries because the same serum cholesterol level is present presumably in each major coronary artery.

CLINICAL USE OF THE QUANTITATIVE APPROACH TO CORONARY ARTERY DISEASE

The information derived at necropsy quantitating the severity and extent of atherosclerosis in the four major epicardial coronary arteries in fatal CAD is potentially useful clinically in two areas: in interpreting degrees of coronary narrowing by angiography during life, and in deciding which of the major coronary arteries needs a conduit at the time of coronary artery bypass grafting.

Without coronary angiography, neither coronary bypass nor angioplasty would be done. The only way during life to obtain information on the status of the epicardial coronary arteries is angiography, and, therefore, this procedure revolutionized diagnosis of CAD just as aortocoronary bypass grafting revolutionized therapy of CAD. However, angiography—as good as it is—has certain deficiencies. An angiogram is a luminogram and a narrow segment is compared with a less narrowed segment that is assumed to be normal. The angiogram does not delineate the internal elastic membrane of the artery, and, therefore, the artery's true lumen is still uncertain.

The aforementioned coronary quantitative studies demonstrated in fatal CAD that 93% of the 5-mm segments of the four major epicardial coronary arteries were narrowed more than 25% in cross-sectional area by atherosclerotic plaque. Thus, only 7% of the 5-mm segments approached normal and almost none was normal. Thus, at least in fatal CAD, and probably also in live patients with symptomatic myocardial ischemia, it is infrequent that an angiographically severely narrowed segment of a coronary artery can be compared with a segment of coronary artery that is actually normal. In other words, in patients with

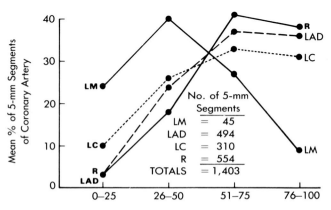

A

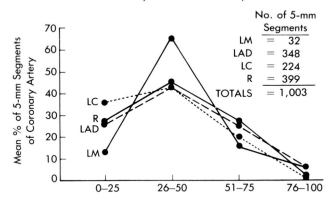

B

Figure 54–24. Mean percentage of 5-mm segments of each of the four major coronary arteries narrowed to various degrees in the 27 patients with acute myocardial infarction (A) and in the 22 control subjects (B). The amount of luminal narrowing of the left anterior descending (LAD), left circumflex (LC), and right (R) coronary arteries is similar. The degree of severe narrowing of the left main (LM) coronary artery is considerably less than that of the other three arteries in the patients in the study. (From Roberts, W. C. and Jones, A. A.: Quantification of coronary arterial narrowing at necropsy in acute transmural myocardial infarction: Analysis and comparison of findings in 27 patients and 22 controls. Circulation, 61:786, 1980. By permission of the American Heart Association, Inc.)

symptomatic myocardial ischemia, the coronary angiogram measures degrees of narrowing by comparing severely narrowed segments with segments that are less narrowed and by no means normal (Fig. 54–25). Accordingly, coronary angiograms in patients with symptomatic myocardial ischemia usually underestimate the degrees of luminal narrowing (Arnett et al, 1979; Isner et al, 1981). This fact is well appreciated by most cardiac surgeons, but is less well appreciated by cardiologists.

The unit of measuring degrees of narrowing by angiography differs from the unit of measurement at necropsy. In the anatomic quantitative studies presented here, the unit was *cross-sectional area* narrowing. The unit of angiography is *diameter* narrowing. Generally, a 75% cross-sectional area narrowing is equivalent to a 50% diameter reduction, and, there-fore, a 50% or more diameter reduction during life has generally been considered to be the cut-off point between clinically significant and clinically insignificant coronary narrowing (see Fig. 54–25).

The second potential use of the information derived from the quantitative CAD studies at necropsy is the appreciation that the atherosclerotic process in patients with symptomatic myocardial ischemia is usually diffuse and severe and, therefore, that more rather than fewer aortocoronary conduits provide a higher frequency of relief or improvement in symptoms of myocardial ischemia, in improvement in results of exercise testing, and in prolonging life. Among patients surviving for less than 30 days or at later periods after aortocoronary bypass operations, the amount of severe narrowing in the *nonby-passed native* coronary arteries is usually similar to

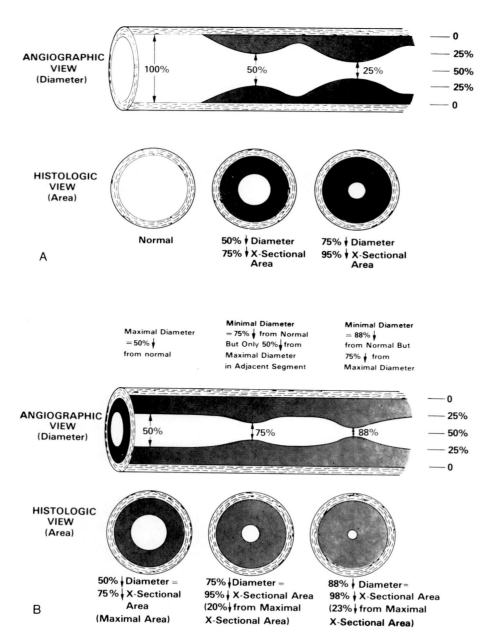

Figure 54–25. The relation between longitudinal narrowing (diameter reduction) as seen by coronary angiography and cross-sectional area narrowing as seen by histologic examination of a coronary artery. A coronary arterial segment with a 50% longitudinal width narrowing has a 75% reduction in cross-sectional area. A 75% reduction in longitudinal width corresponds to a 95% reduction in cross-sectional area. The theoretical situation by which a narrowing is compared with an adjacent perfectly normal segment of artery is shown (A) and the usual real situation is shown (B). The least-narrowed segment below has a 50% reduction in longitudinal width (75% loss of cross-sectional area) and a central, round residual lumen. Because the angiogram is a luminogram and the width of the original arterial lumen is unknown, the least narrowed segment is often presumed to be normal. The width of more narrowed segments is compared with that of the least narrowed segments, but, nevertheless, narrowed segment. If the least narrowed segment is 50% narrowed, what appears to be a 50% narrowing in an adjacent segment is really a 75% longitudinal narrowing (95% reduction in cross-sectional area); what appears to be a 75% narrowing in an adjacent segment is really an 88% longitudinal narrowing (98% reduction in cross-sectional area). (From Arnett, E. N., Isner, J. M., Redwood, D. R., et al: Coronary artery narrowing in coronary heart disease: Comparison of cineangiographic and necropsy findings. Ann. Intern. Med., 91:350, 1979.)

that in the *bypassed native* coronary arteries. From study at necropsy of 102 patients dying either early (≤60 days) or late (2.5 to 108 months [mean, 35]) after bypass operations (Waller and Roberts, 1980, 1981), it was found that the bypassed and nonbypassed native coronary arteries had similar degrees of severe luminal narrowing by atherosclerotic plaques. Specifically, in 213 (94%) of the 226 bypassed native arteries and in 73 (91%) of 80 nonbypassed native arteries the lumens were narrowed more than 75% in cross-sectional area by atherosclerotic plaque. The reason why the native arteries were not bypassed was not because they were too small or severely narrowed distally, but because by angiogram the lumens were judged not to be sufficiently narrowed to warrant the insertion of a conduit. Thus, if two of the major coronary arteries are severely narrowed by angiography and the third major artery is "insignificantly" narrowed and if a bypass operation is to be done, the insertion of a conduit in all three major coronary arteries could be reasonably considered. There is, of course, potential danger in insertion of a conduit in an artery that is insignificantly narrowed; nevertheless, it may be more advantageous to err on the side of too many conduits than too few. At necropsy, "three-vessel disease" is more frequent than "two-vessel disease," and when only two of the three major arteries at necropsy are narrowed more than 75% in cross-sectional area, the third one is usually narrowed 51 to 75% in cross-sectional area. Thus, an appreciation of the diffuse nature of coronary atherosclerosis in fatal CAD and probably also in symptomatic myocardial ischemia encourages the use of more rather than fewer conduits at coronary bypass operations.

Bibliography

Arnett, E. N., Isner, J. M., Redwood, D. R., et al: Coronary artery narrowing in coronary heart disease: Comparison of cineangiographic and necropsy findings. Ann. Intern. Med., *91*:350, 1979.

Bulkley, B. H., and Roberts, W. C.: Atherosclerotic narrowing of the left main coronary artery: A necropsy analysis of 152 patients with fatal coronary heart disease and varying degrees of left main narrowing. Circulation, *53*:823, 1976.

Cabin, H. S., and Roberts, W. C.: True left ventricular aneurysm and healed myocardial infarction: Clinical and necropsy observations including quantification of degrees of coronary arterial narrowing. Am. J. Cardiol., *46*:754, 1980.

Isner, J. M., Kishel, J., Kent, K. M., et al: Accuracy of angiographic determination of left main coronary arterial narrowing: Angiographic-histologic correlative analysis in 28 patients. Circulation, *63*:1056, 1981.

Isner, J. M., Wu, M., Virmani, R., et al: Comparison of coronary arterial luminal narrowing determined by visual inspection of histologic sections under magnification among three independent observers and comparison to that obtained by video planimetry: An analysis of 559 five-millimeter segments of 61 coronary arteries from eleven patients. Lab. Invest., *42*:566, 1980.

Roberts, W. C.: Sudden cardiac death: Definitions and causes. Am. J. Cardiol., *57*:1410, 1986.

Roberts, W. C., and Jones, A. A.: Quantitation of coronary arterial narrowing at necropsy in sudden coronary death: Analysis of 31 patients and comparison with 25 control subjects. Am. J. Cardiol., *44*:39, 1979.

Roberts, W. C., and Jones, A. A.: *Quantification* of coronary arterial narrowing at necropsy in *acute transmural myocardial infarction:* Analysis and comparison of findings in 27 patients and 22 controls. Circulation, *61*:786, 1980.

Roberts, W. C., and Virmani, R.: Quantification of coronary arterial narrowing in clinically-isolated unstable angina pectoris: An analysis of 22 necropsy patients. Am. J. Med., *67*:792, 1979.

Virmani, R., and Roberts, W. C.: Disappearance of symptomatic coronary heart disease and death from a noncardiac condition. Chest, *77*:91, 1980.

Virmani, R., and Roberts, W. C.: Non-fatal healed transmural myocardial infarction and fatal non-cardiac disease: Qualification and quantification of coronary arterial narrowing and of left ventricular scarring in 18 necropsy patients. Br. Heart J., *45*:434, 1981.

Virmani, R., and Roberts, W. C.: Quantification of coronary arterial narrowing and of left ventricular myocardial scarring in healed myocardial infarction with chronic eventually fatal, congestive cardiac failure. Am. J. Med., *68*:831, 1980.

Waller, B. F., and Roberts, W. C.: Amount of narrowing by atherosclerotic plaque in 44 nonbypassed and 52 bypassed major epicardial coronary arteries in 32 necropsy patients who died within 1 month of aortocoronary bypass grafting. Am. J. Cardiol., *46*:956, 1980.

Waller, B. F., and Roberts, W. C.: Amount of luminal narrowing in bypassed and non-bypassed native coronary arteries in necropsy patients dying early and late after aortocoronary bypass operations. In Mason, D. T., and Collins, J. J. Jr. (eds): Myocardial Revascularization, Medical and Surgical Advances in Coronary Disease. New York, Yorke Medical Books, 1981, pp. 503–510.

III CORONARY ARTERIOGRAPHY

Charles J. Davidson
Thomas M. Bashore

HISTORICAL ASPECTS

Forssmann (1929) is credited with having performed the first human cardiac catheterization. While receiving training as a surgeon in Eberswalde, Germany, he used fluoroscopic guidance to advance a catheter through his own left antecubital vein into the right atrium. In an attempt to develop a technique for direct delivery of drugs into the heart, he catheterized himself on several occasions. However, as a result of intense criticism, he eventually abandoned this pursuit and undertook a career as a urologist. Zimmerman and co-workers (1950) did the first left-sided heart catheterization. This technique was facilitated greatly by the development of the percutaneous technique for catheter introduction by Seldinger (1953). Early attempts to visualize the coronary arteries in humans were accomplished with nonselective injection of radiopaque contrast medium into the ascending aorta (Radner, 1945). In 1958, Sones did the first selective injection of contrast media into the coronary arteries (Sones et al, 1959). Several percutaneous transfemoral coronary arteriographic techniques were developed by Ricketts and Abrams (1962), Amplatz and colleagues (1967), and Judkins (1967). However, the femoral technique introduced by Judkins and the brachial technique pioneered by Sones are the most widely used today. Each method has its own set of disadvantages and advantages. For example, the brachial technique is useful particularly in patients with severe peripheral vascular disease involving the abdominal aorta and the iliac and femoral arteries, but is done usually via cutdown on the artery. The femoral approach offers the advantage of not requiring arteriotomy and arterial repair. It can therefore be done several times in the same patient, and less technical skill is required to do the procedure in its entirety.

Gruentzig and colleagues (1977, 1979) developed percutaneous transluminal coronary angioplasty (PTCA). While working in Zurich, and later at Emory University, Gruentzig introduced an intra-arterial therapeutic technique that has revolutionized the approach to patients with coronary artery disease. His innovation opened a new era in the interventional approach to coronary artery stenoses and has led to other potential modalities such as atherectomy and laser techniques.

ANATOMY

Physicians performing coronary arteriography as well as cardiac surgeons need to have a clear understanding of normal coronary artery anatomy and its common anomalies. In most patients, two separate ostia arise from the ascending aorta to supply the left and right main coronary arteries. Variations of the usual pattern are discussed later in the section on coronary artery anomalies.

Normal Arterial Anatomy (Fig. 54–26)

Left Coronary Artery

The left main coronary artery arises from the left posterior coronary sinus. It courses laterally between the posterior portion of the pulmonary artery and the anterior portion of the left atrial appendage. After a distance of less than 1 mm to as much as 30 mm, it bifurcates into two major branches, the left anterior descending and left circumflex arteries. A trifurcation

often occurs when the ramus intermedius or optional diagonal originates between the anterior descending and the circumflex arteries. It may be difficult angiographically to distinguish the third branch from a proximal branch of the left anterior descending or circumflex arteries. Infrequently, the left main coronary artery is absent, and the left anterior descending and circumflex arteries arise from common or separate ostia. In these cases, selective left coronary arteriography of each branch is done.

Left Anterior Descending Artery. The left anterior descending artery courses behind the pulmonary trunk into the anterior interventricular sulcus, extending to and often around the left ventricular apex. The left anterior descending artery provides major branches that penetrate the interventricular septum and LV free wall. A variable number of small right ventricular branches may also arise proximally and distally from the left anterior descending artery. A large proximal branch may course toward similar branches of the right conus artery to form the circle of Vieussens.

Many septal perforating branches provide arterial supply to the anterior two-thirds and apical portions of the interventricular septum and are the characteristic landmarks of the anterior descending artery. The first and usually largest septal perforator supplies the base of the septal myocardium. Septal perforators tend to become progressively smaller toward the left ventricular apex.

Diagonal Branches. As the left anterior descending artery courses along the interventricular sulcus, several branches arise diagonally over the left ventricular surface. The diagonal (anterolateral) branches arise, as their name implies, diagonally over the left ventricular surface. Two to six diagonal branches may be present, running parallel to each other. Generally, the largest diagonal arteries originate from the proximal portion of the left anterior descending coronary artery and become progressively smaller distally. If an intermediate artery is present, these diagonal branches may be less prominent, because the intermediate artery supplies this area of myocardium. Occasionally, diagonal branches may be the source of septal perforating arteries.

Left Circumflex Artery. The left circumflex artery originates from the left main coronary artery at an acute angle or occasionally from a separate ostium of the left coronary sinus. It courses posteriorly under the left atrial appendage along the left atrioventricular (AV) groove. Its termination is highly dependent on the length of the right coronary artery; in most cases, it terminates at the acute left margin of the heart. From the obtuse margin of the heart, one to four marginal branches of various dimensions emerge from the main circumflex artery. These obtuse marginal arteries course along the lateral aspect of the left ventricle and are named by the order of emergence from the main body of the circumflex artery. Branches arising most distally are often referred to as posterolateral branches from the circum-

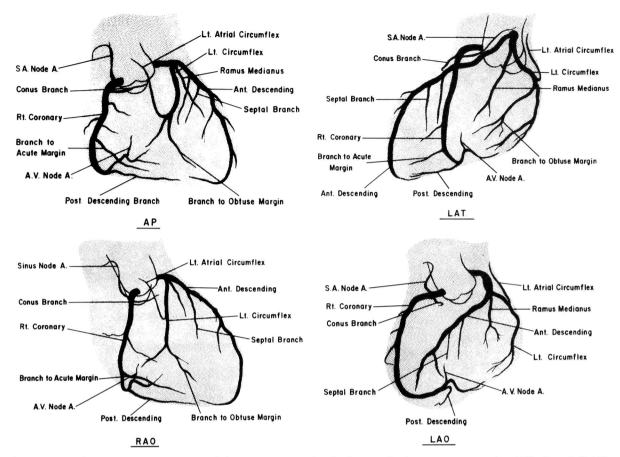

Figure 54–26. Anatomic representation of the coronary arteries in four projections: anteroposterior (AP), lateral (LAT), right anterior oblique (RAO), and left anterior oblique (LAO). (From Abrams, H. L., and Adams, D. F.: The coronary arteriogram: Structural and functional aspects. N. Engl. J. Med., *281*:1276, 1969.)

flex artery and course toward the apex perpendicular to the AV groove.

In approximately 10% of patients, the circumflex artery extends to the interventricular groove and beyond the crux of the heart. In these cases, it supplies the posterior descending and frequently AV nodal arteries as it courses along the posterior interventricular sulcus. This pattern of circulation is called *left dominant* or *predominant* (Fig. 54–27).

A large left atrial branch arises proximally from the left circumflex artery in 30 to 40% of patients. It courses superiorly along the left atrium, posterior to

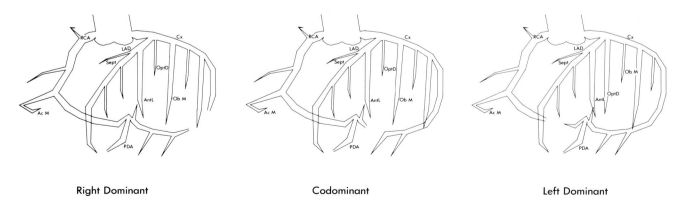

Figure 54–27. Diagrams of the coronary artery tree demonstrating right, left, and co-dominance based on the variation in blood supply to the posterior diaphragmatic surface. (RCA = right coronary artery; LAD = left anterior descending; Cx = circumflex artery; PDA = posterior descending artery; Ac M = acute marginal artery; AntL = anterolateral (*diagonal*) arteries; OptD = optional diagonal artery; Ob M = obtuse marginal arteries; Sept = septal perforator artery.)

the aorta, continuing to the anterior interatrial sulcus. In addition to being an important source of blood supply to the left atrium and providing collateral flow to the right coronary artery, it initiates the sinus node artery in slightly less than 50% of human hearts.

Right Coronary Artery

The right coronary artery emerges from its ostium in the right coronary sinus. Lying deep in epicardial fat, it courses anteriorly along the right AV sulcus between the right atrium and right ventricle. The extent of the right coronary artery is usually related inversely to the length of the circumflex artery. In approximately 90% of patients, it courses in the AV sulcus to the posterior interventricular sulcus and has a C shape in left anterior oblique projection. If any vessels arise after the posterior descending takeoff, the system is referred to as *right dominant*.

The conus artery may originate as a separate ostium anterior to the right coronary artery or as the most proximal branch of the right coronary artery. It is an important collateral artery source to the left anterior descending distribution. The conus artery courses across the anterior surface of the right ventricle near the pulmonic valve and terminates in the anterior interventricular sulcus.

The sinus node artery arises from the proximal right coronary artery in about half of patients studied. It takes a course posteriorly along the right atrium, traveling in an almost opposite direction as the conus artery. While supplying small branches to both atria and the interatrial septum, the sinus node artery terminates as it encircles the superior vena cava. Many small atrial branches arise from the right coronary artery, but they usually have little significance as sources for collateral circulation to the left ventricle (see the section on coronary collaterals).

Other prominent branches of the right coronary artery include the acute marginal artery and anterior ventricular branches. The acute marginal artery courses along the right aspect of the heart and may occasionally supply all or a portion of the posterior descending artery. In a left dominant circulation, the acute marginal artery may represent the last prominent branch of the right coronary artery.

In most cases, the right coronary artery bifurcates into the posterior descending artery and posterior left ventricular branches (posterolaterals to the left ventricle). The posterior descending artery courses toward the apex through the interventricular groove. The actual length of the posterior descending artery is related inversely to the extent of the left anterior descending artery. Several small anterior branches are usually present. These branches arise from the posterior descending artery and perforate the interventricular septum supplying the lower one-third of the septum. These septal perforating arteries may help angiographically to distinguish between the posterior descending artery and the larger left

ventricular branches. Posterolaterals to the left ventricular branches are a continuation of the right coronary artery beyond the takeoff of the posterior descending artery.

The AV node artery arises from the right coronary artery in approximately 90% of patients. The location of the AV node artery is related to whether the right coronary artery or left circumflex artery crosses the posterior interventricular groove (crux). In 90%, the right coronary artery extends beyond the crux and supplies the posterior descending and left ventricular branches (right dominant). In 10% of patients, the left circumflex crosses the crux and supplies branches to the right ventricle (left dominant). Occasionally, posterior descending arteries arise from both the right coronary and left circumflex arteries and produce a *balanced*, mixed, or codominant circulation (see Fig. 54–27). Angiographically, if the right coronary terminates in the posterior descending artery with no further branches to the left ventricle, the anatomy is considered to be *codominant*.

Anomalies

With widespread use of coronary arteriography, a knowledge of coronary artery anomalies is essential to avoid potential misdiagnosis or complications. Two reviews of 4,250 and 3,750 patients having diagnostic cardiac catheterization indicate that the incidence of anomalies is approximately 1% (Chaitman et al, 1976; Engel et al, 1975). These congenital abnormalities may or may not be clinically significant. Insignificant anomalies are due primarily to an abnormal origin from the aorta or unusual distribution of the coronary arteries. Hemodynamically significant anomalies such as coronary fistula or the origin of a coronary artery from the pulmonary artery cause abnormalities of coronary perfusion. A list of coronary artery anomalies is provided in Table 54–6.

TABLE 54–6. ANOMALIES OF THE CORONARY ARTERIES

Minor Anomalies
Circumflex artery from the right coronary artery or right sinus of Valsalva
Left anterior descending artery from the right coronary artery or right sinus of Valsalva
Left main coronary artery from the right sinus of Valsalva
Right coronary artery from the left sinus of Valsalva
Right coronary artery from the posterior (noncoronary) sinus of Valsalva
Single coronary artery
Multiple coronary ostia

Major Anomalies
Coronary artery fistulas
Anomalous origin of the left or right coronary artery from the pulmonary artery
Coronary artery atresia
Coronary artery hypoplasia
Congenital coronary artery aneurysms
Congenital coronary artery stenosis

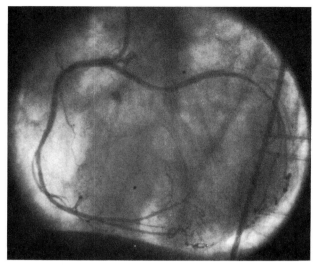 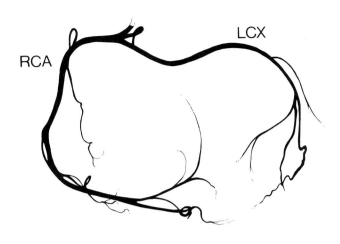

Figure 54–28. Coronary arteriogram and diagram of the most common anomaly, which is in the left circumflex coronary artery (LCX) arising from the right sinus of Valsalva and coursing between the aorta and main pulmonary artery. (RCA = right coronary artery.)

The most common congenital variation encountered by the angiographer is the origin of the circumflex artery from the right coronary artery or the right coronary sinus (Figs. 54–28 and 54–29). This malformation occurs in approximately 0.5% of patients (Chaitman et al, 1976, Engel et al, 1975). Typically, this anomalous circumflex artery takes a posterior course behind the great vessels to reach the left AV groove. This anomaly may be associated with transposition of the great vessels (Ogden, 1970) and is generally considered to be benign.

Anomalous origin of the anterior descending artery from the right sinus of Valsalva is similar in several respects to the origin of left main coronary

Figure 54–29. Schematic representation of aberrant coronary artery patterns. (A = aorta; R.V. Inf = right ventricular infundibulum; R = right sinus of Valsalva; L = left sinus of Valsalva; N = noncoronary sinus.) Numbers in parentheses indicate the frequency of the aberrant pattern in this series of 21 cases. (From Liberthson, R. R., Dinsmore, R. E., Bharati, S., et al: Aberrant coronary artery origin from the aorta. Circulation, 50:774, 1974. By permission of the American Heart Association, Inc.)

• ABERRANT ORIGIN OF THE LAD and LEFT CX (6 CASES)

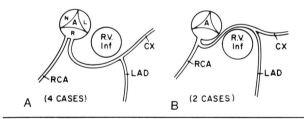

A (4 CASES)   B (2 CASES)

• ABERRANT ORIGIN OF THE LEFT CX (11 CASES)

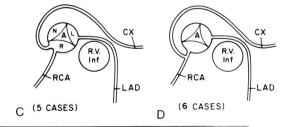

C (5 CASES)   D (6 CASES)

• ABERRANT RCA (4 CASES)

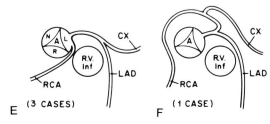

E (3 CASES)   F (1 CASE)

artery from the right sinus of Valsalva. The anterior descending artery may arise from a separate ostium in the right sinus of Valsalva or directly from the right coronary artery (see Fig. 54–29). It initially courses similarly to the conus artery. It then extends across the anterior aspect of the right ventricular infundibulum to reach the anterior interventricular sulcus. This is the most common coronary artery anomaly associated with tetralogy of Fallot and has been reported to occur in 2% of these patients (McManus et al, 1982; Meng et al, 1965). Because inadvertent transection of this anomalous anterior descending artery has been reported to occur during operative repair of tetralogy of Fallot, preoperative coronary arteriography has been recommended (McManus et al, 1982) in this population. Compared with left main coronary artery from the right sinus of Valsalva, origin of the anterior descending artery from the right coronary artery or right sinus of Valsalva is generally considered to be benign.

Origin of the left main coronary artery and the right coronary artery from the right sinus of Valsalva is a rare anomaly that has been associated with sudden death in young adults. The left main coronary artery may take one of three courses. Most commonly, it originates anterior to the right coronary artery and courses between the pulmonary artery and the aorta, then bifurcates into the anterior descending and circumflex arteries (see Fig. 54–29). More rarely, the left main coronary artery may pass either anterior to the right ventricular outflow tract or posterior to the aorta. Liberthson and co-workers (1974) postulated that sudden death may result from acute occlusion of this aberrant left main coronary artery. Because cardiac output rises during exercise, the left main coronary artery could become compressed between the dilated aorta and pulmonary artery or stretched between them with subsequent occlusion of the sharply angulated proximal segment of the vessel.

Anomalous origin of the right coronary artery from the left sinus of Valsalva has been reported to be present in 0.17% (Engel et al, 1975) and 0.16% (Chaitman et al, 1976) of patients having routine cardiac catheterization (Fig. 54–30). In this anatomic variation, the right coronary artery courses between the ascending aorta and the pulmonary artery to reach the right AV sulcus. Roberts and colleagues (1982) reported that in 10 patients with this anomaly, the ostium of the right coronary artery was slit-like. He postulated that coronary blood flow might be altered when the aorta dilated and further compressed the right coronary artery during exercise.

The origin of both coronary arteries from a single ostium has been reported to occur in from 0.04% (Sharbaugh and White, 1974) to 0.1% (Douglas et al, 1985) of the population. Single right and left coronary arteries are present in about equal numbers (Sharbaugh and White, 1974). An example of a single right coronary artery is shown in Figure 54–31. As described earlier for other coronary artery anomalies, the clinical features of this anomaly depend on the luminal diameter of the orifice and the degree of compression or angulation of the artery as it courses through or around the great vessels. Myocardial infarction, angina pectoris, congestive heart failure, or sudden death have been reported before the age of 40 in as many as 15% of patients with a single coronary artery (Douglas et al, 1985).

The most common hemodynamically significant coronary anomaly is a precapillary fistula that connects a major coronary artery directly with a cardiac chamber, coronary sinus, superior vena cava, or pulmonary artery (Levin et al, 1978). Although a physiologic left-to-right shunt is present, except in rare cases in which termination is in a left-sided heart

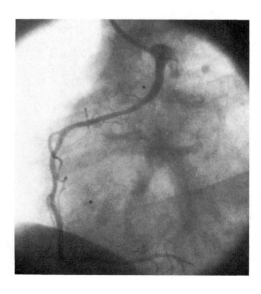

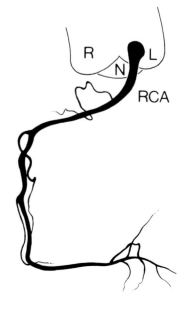

Figure 54–30. Anomalous origin of the right coronary artery from the left sinus of Valsalva (LAO view).

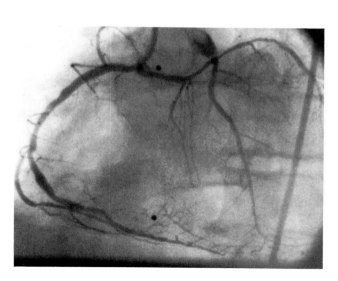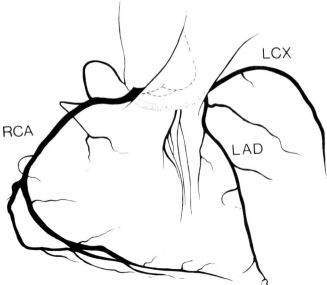

Figure 54–31. Coronary arteriogram and diagram in LAO view showing a single right coronary ostium initiative, right and left main coronary arteries. Note that the course of the left main coronary artery is between the pulmonary artery and the aorta (anteroposterior view). (LAD = left anterior descending coronary artery; LCX = left circumflex coronary artery; RCA = right coronary artery.)

chamber, approximately 50% of patients have catheterization for an asymptomatic continuous murmur (Oldham et al, 1971). Others may develop congestive heart failure, endocarditis (endarteritis), myocardial ischemia due to a steal phenomenon, or rupture of an aneurysmal fistula (Oldham et al, 1971). Levin and others (Levin et al, 1978) reviewed 363 reported cases of coronary artery fistulas and noted that 50% arose from the right coronary artery, 42% arose from the left coronary artery, and 5% arose from both coronary arteries. Drainage occurred most commonly into the right ventricle (41%), followed by the right atrium (26%), pulmonary artery (16%), coronary sinus (7%), left atrium (5%), left ventricle (3%), and superior vena cava (1%). An example of a right coronary artery to right atrial fistula is shown in Figure 54–32. Angiography provides the definitive diagnosis, although oximetry may help to estimate the size of the shunt (but the degree of the shunt is frequently too small for accurate assessment). The originating coronary artery is usually dilated and tortuous and often resembles saccular aneurysms. In approximately 3% of patients with coronary artery fistulas, the contralateral coronary artery is absent.

The four types of anomalous origin of the coronary arteries from the pulmonary trunk are the origin of the left coronary artery, the right coronary artery, both arteries, and an accessory coronary artery. In approximately 90% of patients with this anomaly, the left coronary artery arises from the pulmonary artery (Ogden, 1970). Angina-like symptoms of dyspnea, tachypnea, pallor, and restlessness often begin early after birth as pulmonary artery pressures decline, leading to coronary artery steal and inadequate perfusion of the myocardium. Myocardial infarction,

papillary muscle dysfunction with mitral insufficiency, and sudden death are common. Aortography reveals a large right coronary artery, an absent left coronary artery, and delayed appearance of collateral vessels from the right coronary artery that opacify the left anterior descending and circumflex arteries. When an extensive collateral circulation is present, contrast appears in the pulmonary artery and outlines the left-to-right shunt.

Congenital coronary artery stenosis occurs most commonly in conjunction with other congenital le-

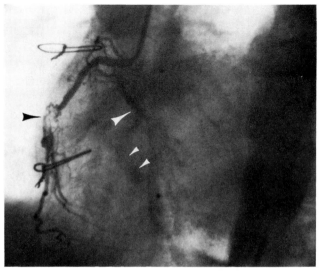

Figure 54–32. Right coronary artery to right atrial fistula (LAO view) (*single, large, white arrow*). Note the area of contrast dye pooling in the right atrium (*double white arrows*). Incidental severe stenosis of the right coronary artery (*black arrow*) is shown.

sions such as calcific coronary sclerosis, supravalvular aortic stenosis, homocystinuria, Friedreich's ataxia, Hurler's syndrome, and rubella syndrome (Levin et al, 1978). Congenital coronary artery aneurysm is a rare lesion, and most occur secondary to conditions such as atherosclerosis, inflammatory processes, or a coronary fistula. These aneurysms are caused presumably by structural weakness in the arterial wall and are often difficult to distinguish from acquired coronary artery aneurysms.

Coronary Venous Anatomy

Gensini and colleagues (1965) explored the anatomy of the coronary circulation with coronary venography in living humans. Specially designed bal-

loon-tip catheters were used. Satisfactory balloon inflation and occlusion were determined by a characteristic change from the atrial waveform of the unoccluded coronary sinus to ventricular complexes of occluded coronary venous pressure.

The normal anatomy of coronary veins can be represented diagramatically by two large triangles with apices on either side of the apex of the heart and hinged at their bases on the great cardiac vein and the coronary sinus (Fig. 54–33). The first triangle is larger and medially located. The sides of the triangle are formed by the anterior and posterior interventricular veins. The second triangle is smaller and is located on the free wall of the left ventricle; the sides are formed by the left diagonal and obtuse marginal veins.

This entire system drains approximately 85% of

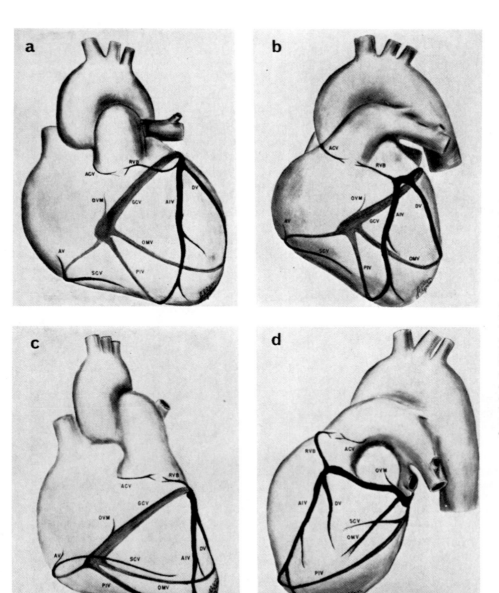

Figure 54–33. Four projections of the human coronary venous anatomy. *A,* anteroposterior view; *B,* left anterior oblique; *C,* right anterior oblique; *D,* left lateral. Black vessels are anteriorly located; gray are posteriorly located. (GCV = great cardiac vein; AIV = anterior interventricular vein; OMV = obtuse marginal vein; DV = diagonal vein; PIV = posterior interventricular vein [middle cardiac vein]; OVM = oblique vein of Marshall; SCV = small cardiac vein [right marginal vein]; ACV = anterior cardiac vein.) (From Gensini, G. G., DiGiorgi, S., Coskun, O., et al: Anatomy of the coronary circulation in living man: Coronary venography. Circulation, *31:*778, 1965. By permission of the American Heart Association, Inc.)

coronary blood flow, including the interventricular septum, left ventricular free wall, and part of the right ventricle. The remaining 15% is drained by the anterior cardiac veins and thebesian channels.

A small left atrial vein of great anatomic significance is the oblique vein of Marshall. It courses diagonally on the posterior surface of the left atrium and is directed medially and caudally. The great cardiac vein becomes the coronary sinus at the point at which the vein of Marshall drains into it.

Hutchins and co-workers (1986) investigated the interrelationships between the intramural arteries and veins by angiography, serial sectioning, and graphic microconstruction. They showed that epicardial vessels begin to divide within the epicardium and that muscle fibers are oriented in the same direction as the interstitial space. An unconventional pattern of branching exists; the vein begins as a large vessel that divides and then rejoins its branches, forming a large vessel. The arteriole intertwines between veins.

Penetrating arteries lie in the interstitial spaces and are related closely to accompanying veins. The interstitial veins partially surround and are indented by branch arteries. A second system of veins lies within the muscle fascicles between interstitial spaces and is not related to arteries. The isolated veins have collateral connections with interstitial veins and join them in the subepicardium. Therefore, there are twice as many veins as arteries. The auxillary venous system not adjacent to the artery could be an alternative route for increased blood flow, preventing rapid washout of metabolic end-products during ischemia (Hutchins et al, 1986).

PATHOANATOMIC CORRELATES

Interpretation of Coronary Artery Disease

In the angiographic evaluation of coronary artery disease, it is imperative to define the degree of stenosis that constitutes either prognostic or hemodynamic significance. Generally, the severity of stenosis is assessed by visually comparing the percentage diameter reduction relative to an adjacent "normal" segment. Although a 50% narrowing in diameter has been considered to be clinically significant, the American Heart Association (1975) has recommended that an 80% decrease in luminal diameter should be considered to be a significant lesion. This recommendation is based on data obtained at the time of operation indicating that this degree of stenosis was necessary to measure a pressure gradient. It has further been shown that a 50% decrease in diameter represents a small reduction in peak coronary artery flow, whereas a 70% stenosis results in a severe reduction in peak flow (McMahon et al, 1979; Peterson et al, 1983). Exercise-induced ischemia has been documented by first-pass radionuclide angiography in patients with 75% stenosis

determined by cardiac catheterization, and 40 mm Hg pressure gradients allowed discrimination of patients with and without exercise ischemia (American Heart Association Committee Report, 1975). Length of stenosis, although not generally measured, has been shown to limit coronary flow when greater than 10 mm (Feldman et al, 1978).

Studies of coronary flow reserve measured by Doppler flowmeters have shown the inadequacy of measurement of percentage diameter narrowing alone (Gould et al, 1986; Kirkeeide et al, 1986; White et al, 1984). Consideration of all dimensions may be necessary to adequately evaluate the physiologic significance of a lesion. These dimensions of a lesion include percentage diameter stenosis, absolute minimal cross-sectional area, absolute stenosis diameter, and minimal stenosis luminal area. The entry and exit angles entering and leaving the lesion also affect lesion resistance. Thus, consideration of all parameters of lesion length, absolute diameter, and percentage narrowing may be necessary to correctly predict the functional severity of stenosis, at least as defined by coronary flow reserve (Gould et al, 1986; Kirkeeide et al, 1986).

Despite the fact that prognostic information based on the number of diseased vessels can be obtained by qualitative interpretation, it must be appreciated that visual interpretation has multiple sources of error. Various studies have documented the wide interobserver and intraobserver variation that exists when cineangiograms are visually evaluated. DeRouen and colleagues (1977) reported that when 11 experienced angiographers interpreted ten angiograms, disagreement regarding the number of vessels with greater than 70% stenosis occurred in one-third of the cases. The Coronary Artery Surgery Study (CASS) (Kennedy et al, 1982) found that in the posterior descending artery one observer did not identify a lesion in 28.5% of patients, whereas another reader identified a lesion of greater than 50%. A second area in which interobserver variation was large was in the left main coronary artery; whereas one angiographer interpreted a lesion of more than 50%, a second reader failed to identify the same lesion 15.7% of the time. The scattergram results of the CASS study describing interobserver and intraobserver variation in the proximal left anterior descending artery are shown in Figure 54–34.

Similarly, a poor correlation exists between visually assessed coronary arteriograms and corresponding post-mortem coronary artery specimens. In general, coronary arteriography tends to underestimate the severity of most lesions. The presence of diffuse atherosclerosis in patients with clinically symptomatic disease (Blankenhorn and Curry, 1982) or dilatation of the nearby normal vessel as a result of aging or poststenotic enlargement may make definition of a "normal" segment difficult. The agreement between angiography and pathology is improved when either minimal lesions or severe lesions are present; variation increases when the stenosis is

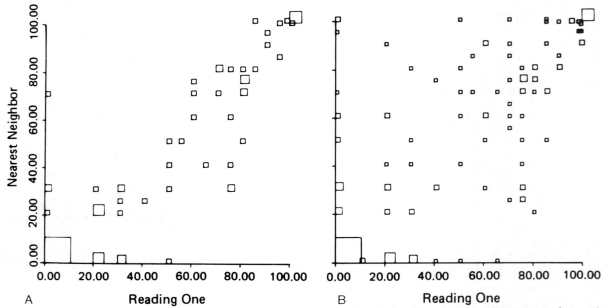

Figure 54–34. Scattergram showing intraobserver (A) and interobserver (B) variation. Data from visually interpreted stenosis of the proximal left anterior descending artery in the CASS registry. The size of each square represents the number of each observation. (From Kennedy, J. W., Fisher, L. D., and Killip, T.: In Bond, M. A., Insull, W., and Glagov, S. [eds]: Clinical Diagnosis of Atherosclerosis: Quantitative Methods of Evaluation. New York, Springer-Verlag 1982, pp. 475–491.)

from 51 to 75%. Minimal lumen area may be a better predictor of the physiologic significance of a coronary lesion than the calculated percentage of stenosis (Harrison et al, 1984).

Computerized edge-detection algorithms have been applied to digitally acquired image data or to standard cine film that has been digitized. Some of these techniques of analysis are labor intensive and time consuming and require two orthogonal views of the lesion. One version of quantitative coronary arteriography that uses a fully automated algorithm to determine the vessel centerline and the vessel borders has recently been validated (Le Free et al, 1986). By using the coronary artery catheter for calibration, this automated algorithm has been applied to detect the edges of digitized cineangiograms and digitally subtracted images (Fig. 54–35). Measurements done on digital subtraction angiograms have compared favorably with pathologic data of vessels fixed in barium gelatin and contrast injections into perfused hearts (Skelton et al, 1987).

Videodensitometry has been used to quantitate artery diameter and percentage stenosis. This method analyzes the optical density of selected cross-sections of the artery. Abrupt changes identify the borders of the arteriographic lumen. This concept forms the basis of the edge-detection algorithms used for quantitative coronary arteriography. By using videodensitometric techniques, the optical density of an arterial segment can be expressed as a function of the volume of contrast medium within the lumen of the artery and represents the volume of the segment. The optical density profile can thus provide an estimate of the cross-sectional area of the artery. Three-

dimensional information can therefore be derived from two-dimensional images. Normal segment optical density can then be compared with the area of greatest vessel narrowing and a percentage area reduction determined (Laufer and Buda, 1985).

The motivation for the development of videodensitometric techniques has been the desire to avoid the need for geometric assumptions characteristic of the previously described qualitative and quantitative coronary artery analysis methods. Generally, all single-plane methods of quantitative coronary arteriography assume circular lesions, and those that require orthogonal views to assess eccentric lesions assume an elliptical shape. In comparison, measurements of videodensitometry data of either cineangiograms or digital images theoretically yield measurements of cross-sectional area and vessel thickness for any shape of lesion. Nichols and co-workers (1984) have validated that relative cross-sectional area determinations from digitized cinefilm correlate well with phantoms and post-mortem specimens.

Mancini and associates (1987) have shown anatomic and physiologic validation in vivo of a fully automated edge-detection algorithm by doing digital coronary arteriograms and cine angiograms on dogs with intraluminal stenosis created by plastic cylinders. An excellent correlation was found between known and measured minimal diameter stenosis (r = 0.87 to 0.98). Interobserver and intraobserver analyses were highly reproducible (r = 0.9 to 0.97). Furthermore, measures of percentage diameter stenosis, percentage area stenosis (geometric and videodensitometric), and absolute minimal cross-sectional diameter (geometric and videodensitometric) all sig-

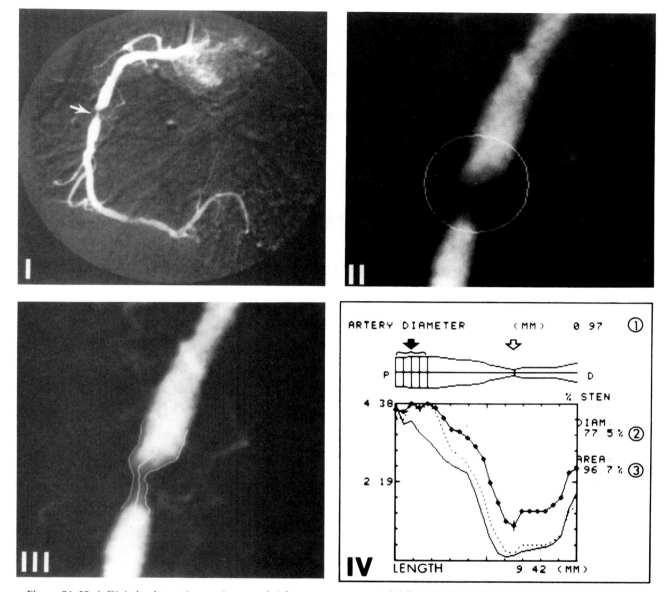

Figure 54–35. *I,* Digital substraction angiogram of right coronary artery in LAO projection with severe stenosis (*arrow*). *II,* Area of interest as defined by the surgeon is encircled and magnified four times. *III,* Automated algorithm of edge defection by centerline method traces normal and stenosed vessel margins. *IV,* Quantitative data display describing lesion characteristics of diameter and area reduction. (1 = minimal lesion diameter; 2 = percent diameter stenosis determined by geometric diameter change; 3 = percent area reduction by using videodensitometric changes.)

nificantly correlated with coronary blood flow measured by electromagnetic flow probes.

The widespread use of videodensitometric methods is still limited, however, because the linearity of the relationship between the video signal and the thickness of the contrast-filled vasculature often deviate from the ideal situation. Contrast streaming, variation in film processing, and fluctuations in light source during projection or variable digital acquisition are potential sources of error with this technique. Other limitations include x-ray scatter and veiling glare within the image intensifier. Some standard other than visual assessment of percentage stenosis will most likely emerge from continued studies to

develop accurate and reproducible quantitative lesion descriptors that can be used in routine clinical practice.

LESION MORPHOLOGY

Quantitation and imaging of coronary artery atherosclerosis should ideally be concerned with four related, yet distinguishable, anatomic manifestations of lesions: (1) extent, (2) severity, (3) lesion composition, and (4) complication (Glagov and Zarins, 1982) (Fig. 54–36). Extent of disease refers to the mass of

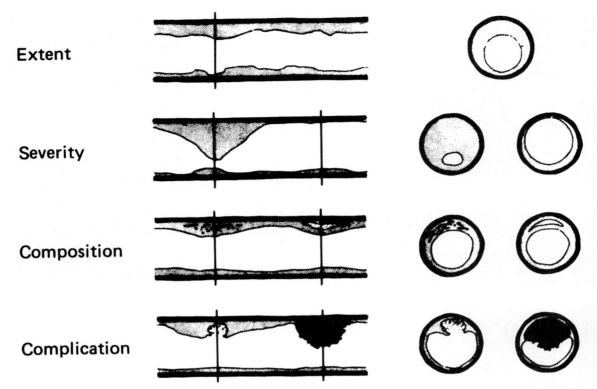

Figure 54–36. Schematic representation of atherosclerotic lesions demonstrating quantifiable aspects. Each feature is illustrated in longitudinal (*left*) and transverse (*right*) cross-section. *Vertical lines* indicate the level of transverse cross-section. Shaded areas are intimal lesions. See the text for a description of the extent, severity, composition, and complication. (From Glagov, S., and Zarins, C. K.: Quantitative atherosclerosis: Problems of definition. *In* Bond, M. G., Insull, W., and Glagov, S. [eds]: Clinical Diagnosis of Atherosclerosis: Quantitative Methods of Evaluation. New York, Springer-Verlag, 1982, pp. 11–35.)

atherosclerotic intimal tissue in an artery or arterial segment. The location of narrowing should be defined as precisely as possible, because diffuse disease may be distributed in various patterns. Severity of disease is a measure of the degree to which atherosclerosis has narrowed the lumen of the artery and compromised flow. This may be quantitated by measuring absolute diameter and length of each stenosis with respect to the number of stenoses in an artery. In most cases, severity is expressed as percentage stenosis by comparing nearby "normal" segments with diseased segments.

The composition of the lesion deals with the nature, consistency, and distribution of the stenosis. It evaluates the cellular and matrix constituents of lesions. Stenosis can be dense, hard, and calcific or soft and semisolid. A complicated lesion refers to fragmentation, ulceration, plaque hemorrhage, or thrombosis of the lesion.

Minor irregularities of the arterial wall are an early manifestation of atherosclerosis. This intimal plaque formation can be seen in many patients older than 45 years. These plaques occur irregularly along the vessel but are more evident on proximal segments.

Atheroma and vessel calcification are frequently associated. Calcification may be visible during fluoroscopy before injection of contrast and tends to be most extensive proximally. Calcium within the coronary arteries is associated with significant disease in 50 to 75% of patients, although the stenosis may not be at the site of calcification (Bartel et al, 1974; Hamby et al, 1974).

In reality, the actual extent of disease or the composition of lesions cannot be well defined by coronary arteriography. The irregularities and stenoses visualized may represent ulcerations or thrombi or alternatively complex lesions that override each other. Even detection of thrombus depends on the size and type of thrombus. Although small thrombi may be difficult to discern, organizing thrombi may conform to the atherosclerotic lesion and be difficult to distinguish from underlying plaque. Large and fresh thrombi extending from the wall into the lumen and those associated with disintegration of plaque can often be detected when multiple views are obtained.

CORONARY BLOOD FLOW DETERMINATIONS IN THE CARDIAC CATHETERIZATION LABORATORY

Four methods are generally used to measure human coronary blood flow in the cardiac catheterization laboratory: thermodilution, digital subtraction angiography, Doppler velocity probes, and electromagnetic flowmeters. Although most current methods measure relative changes in coronary blood flow, useful information regarding the physiologic significance of stenosis (Wilson et al, 1987), cardiac hypertrophy (Marcus, 1983), and pharmacologic interventions (Klocke et al, 1987) can be obtained from these measurements.

Ganz and colleagues (1971) introduced thermodilution methods for measuring coronary sinus flow in humans. This inexpensive, widely available technique is the most frequently applied method for measuring global coronary blood flow in humans (Marcus et al, 1987). By injecting iced saline in the distal end of the catheter placed in the coronary sinus and measuring the temperature change from a proximal thermistor, the rate of change in temperature can be used to define coronary flow. The frequency response of this system is sufficient to measure flow changes that occur in 2 to 3 seconds and are greater than 30% (Ganz et al, 1971). This technique suffers from several serious limitations, however (Marcus et al, 1987). Although the method has been validated in vitro with the thermodilution catheter attached to the coronary sinus (Ganz et al, 1971), weaker correlations have been shown when the thermodilution catheter is allowed to move within the coronary sinus (Mathey et al, 1978). Meanwhile, no studies have clearly demonstrated the accuracy of this method in patients with severe coronary artery disease or myocardial infarction. Other fundamental limitations include the fact that (1) rapid changes in flow cannot be assessed because of the slow time constant of the technique, (2) right atrial and ventricular perfusion cannot be evaluated because the venous drainage is not via the coronary sinus, and (3) regional function and specifically transmural coronary flow cannot be assessed.

By using digital subtraction angiography, contrast medium is power injected into a coronary artery at a rate and quantity sufficient to replace blood within the artery completely. It is assumed that the contrast bolus is undiluted until the peak concentration has been imaged distally in the arterial segment. Regional flow reserve can be calculated in a number of ways, including the use of downstream appearance time and maximal contrast concentration before and during reactive hyperemia (Klocke, 1987). The assumption is that transit time within a region is inversely proportional to coronary blood flow in that region. This is true if the volume of distribution is constant. The technique is limited by a slow time constant and the inability to measure absolute flow. This method of evaluation of coronary flow reserve has been validated in dogs by comparing digital flow ratio estimates with electromagnetic flow ratio measurements (Cusma et al, 1987; Hodgson et al, 1985). In humans, flow reserve has been shown to be abnormal in stenosed arteries and bypass grafts and after coronary angioplasty (Vogel, 1985). However, with only limited animal validation studies reported,

clinical application of digital angiographic techniques awaits further validation in humans.

The Doppler flowmeter is based on the principle of the Doppler effect. High-frequency sound waves are reflected from moving red blood cells and undergo a shift in sound frequency that is proportional to the velocity of the blood flow. In pulsed-wave Doppler methods, a single piezoelectric crystal can transmit and receive these high-frequency sound waves. These methods have been applied successfully in humans by using tiny crystals fixed to the tip of catheters. Validation studies have been performed that compare Doppler flow probes with labeled microspheres (Wangler et al, 1981) and electromagnetic flow probes (Marcus et al, 1981). The use of this technique in 200 patients in the cardiac catheterization laboratory has been reported (Wilson and White, 1987). It has the advantage of permitting repeated sampling and at high frequency, thus allowing measurements after physiologic or pharmacologic interventions. With the use of smaller Doppler catheters, selective coronary artery flow velocity can be measured. By noting the increase in flow velocity following a strong coronary vasodilator, such as papaverine, the coronary flow reserve can be defined. Coronary flow reserve may provide an index of the functional significance of coronary lesions that obviates some of the vagaries of anatomic description (Wilson et al, 1987). The limitation of the current Doppler probe method is that only changes in flow velocity rather than absolute velocity or flow are measurable. Furthermore, there is concern that changes in luminal diameter and arterial cross-sectional area during interventions are not reflected in measurements of flow velocity, thus potentially causing underestimation of the true volume flow (Klocke, 1987).

The electromagnetic flowmeter is based on Faraday's induction law, which states that a conductor moving in an electric field produces current. A major advantage of electromagnetic flowmeters is the high-frequency response (Marcus, 1983). Although these flowmeters have been used to measure aortic blood flow velocity in humans (Klinke et al, 1980), they have not developed to the point at which they are useful for measuring coronary blood flow at catheterization, in part because most methods require placement directly around the coronary artery. Electromagnetic flowmeters are occasionally still used intraoperatively to evaluate flow in aortocoronary bypass grafts.

COLLATERAL CIRCULATION

Coronary collaterals provide an alternative blood supply to a major artery that has become obstructed. In humans, the collaterals represent an initially unused pathway that can be recruited when the original vessel is unable to provide adequate flow. Collateral vessels may arise de novo or alternatively be pre-existing, with dilatation and expansion in response to severe obstruction. Collaterals are classified as being intercoronary if they connect branches of different arteries. Intercoronary collaterals are present in individuals with fixed coronary artery disease and have been visualized acutely during angiography when coronary artery spasm occurs (Maseri et al, 1978). Intracoronary collaterals have been divided into two subtypes, secondary and tertiary. Secondary connections link branches of the same coronary artery, are found in 50 to 60% of normal hearts, and form one-third of the normal heart's collateral network (Cohen, 1985). Tertiary collaterals join proximal and distal segments of the same branch and are observed only in patients with occlusive coronary artery disease (Cohen, 1985).

Levin (1974) examined 200 coronary arteriograms and left ventriculograms of patients with significant coronary disease and found that collateral circulation was usually visualized when the degree of stenosis exceeded 90% diameter narrowing. The major patterns of these collateral routes to the coronary arteries are shown in Figures 54–37 to 54–39. In patients with severe narrowing of the right coronary artery, the most common collateral source involves the left anterior descending artery via septal branches to the posterior descending branch of the right coronary artery or distal left circumflex to the distal right coronary artery (see Fig. 54–37). Individuals with severe or complete obstruction of the left anterior descending artery most commonly show intercoronary collaterals via the acute marginal branch of the right coronary artery and intracoronary collaterals via proximal septal branches (see Fig. 54–38). In circumflex artery occlusion, intracoronary collaterals are frequently observed. These collaterals include the left

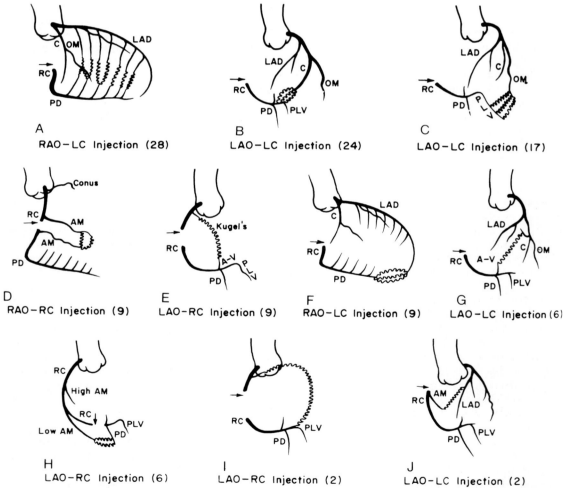

Figure 54–37. Coronary collateral pathways observed in patients with right coronary artery obstruction (*arrow*). (RAO = right anterior oblique projection; LAO = left anterior oblique projection; LC = left coronary artery; AM = acute marginal branch of the right coronary artery; PD = posterior descending branch of the right coronary artery; PLV = posterior left ventricular branch of the right coronary artery; A-V = atrioventricular node artery; LAD = left anterior descending artery; C = circumflex artery; OM = obtuse marginal branch of circumflex artery.) Numbers in parentheses signify the frequency of a particular collateral pathway in this series. (From Levin, D. C.: Pathways and functional significance of the coronary collateral circulation. Circulation, *50*:831, 1973. By permission of the American Heart Association, Inc.)

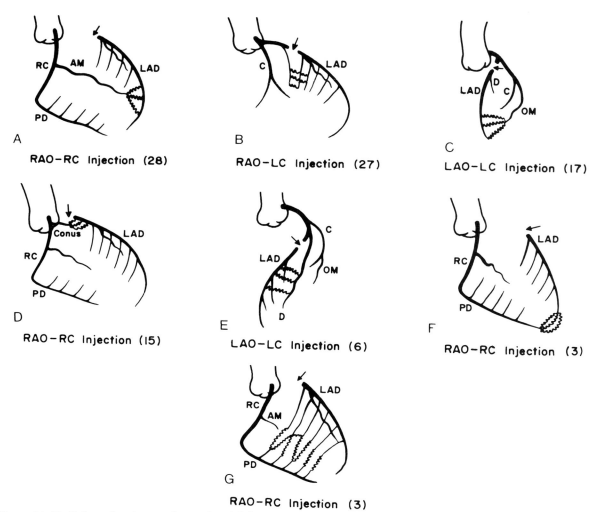

Figure 54–38. Collateral pathways observed with left anterior descending artery obstruction (*arrow*). (AM = acute marginal branch of the right coronary artery; C = circumflex artery; D = diagonal [anterolateral] branch of the left anterior descending artery; LAD = left anterior descending artery; OM = obtuse marginal branch of circumflex artery; PD = posterior descending branch of the right coronary artery.) (From Levin, D. C.: Pathways and functional significance of the coronary collateral circulation. Circulation, *50:*831, 1973. By permission of the American Heart Association, Inc.)

atrial circumflex branch to the distal circumflex and the proximal obtuse marginal branch to a more distal obtuse marginal artery (see Fig. 54–39). Finally, in patients with adequate collaterals manifested by good distal runoff, regional left ventricular function is often preserved.

CORONARY SPASM

Coronary artery spasm when detected by angiography can be clinically benign catheter-induced spasm, spontaneous spasm occurring in patients with variant (Prinzmetal's) angina, or provocatively induced spasm in patients with variant angina. When no vasodilating agents have been administered before catheterization, coronary artery spasm has occurred in up to 1 to 3% of patients (Chahine et al, 1975; Linhart, 1974). In most cases, spasm is me-

chanically induced by the catheter tip and is especially frequent when cannulating the right coronary artery. It is presumably due to local irritation, rarely produces symptoms, and usually responds to removal of the catheter and administration of nitroglycerin. A repeat arteriogram should be done after administration of nitroglycerin if associated coronary spasm is suspected.

Coronary artery spasm may also occur spontaneously in angiographically normal coronary arteries, producing transient ST segment elevation and angina. When it occurs, spasm is most frequently noted in a section of the coronary artery with atheromatous involvement (MacAlpin, 1980). It is often irregular and eccentric and may involve long segments of single or multiple arteries. Even in patients with known Prinzmetal's angina, spontaneous spasm occurs only in the minority of patients during coronary angiography (Maseri et al, 1978). Therefore, provoc-

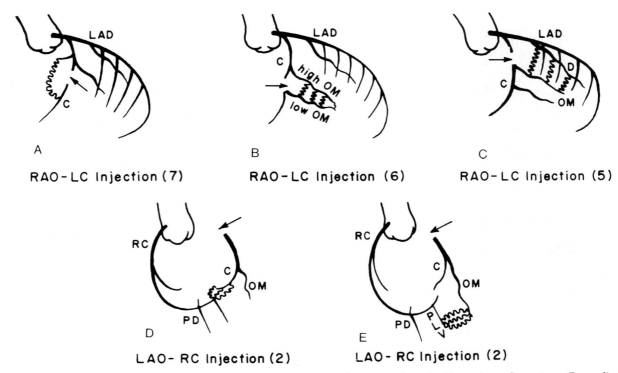

Figure 54–39. Collateral pathways observed in circumflex artery obstruction (*arrow*). (C = circumflex artery; D = diagonal [anterolateral] branch of the left anterior descending artery; LAD = left anterior descending artery; OM = obtuse marginal branch of circumflex artery; PD = posterior descending branch of the right coronary artery; PLV = posterior left ventricular branch of the right coronary artery.) (From Levin, D. C.: Pathways and functional significance of the coronary collateral circulation. Circulation, *50*:831, 1973. By permission of the American Heart Association, Inc.)

ative testing to precipitate spasm during arteriography can be used in patients who have symptoms that suggest variant angina and in whom insignificant stenosis of a major coronary artery is seen. Provocative testing should generally not be used if significant stenoses are evident on the initial coronary angiogram or if there is well-documented ECG evidence of transient transmural ischemia.

The most commonly used provocative test for coronary artery spasm is intravenous administration of ergonovine maleate (Heupler et al, 1978; Waters et al, 1983), which is an alpha-adrenergic and serotonin receptor agonist in epicardial coronary vessels. Spasm can often be induced in patients with known variant angina and has been reported to occur in approximately 5% of patients with atypical anginal symptoms (Bertrand et al, 1982). Other agents that have been used include intravenous methacholine, epinephrine, propranolol, tris-buffer, or the use of the cold pressor test (placing the hands in iced saline). Intracoronary injection of acetylcholine has been reported to be a useful, safe, and reliable method to document multivessel coronary spasm in patients with variant angina (Okumura et al, 1988). The patient should be withdrawn from nitrates and calcium antagonists before provocative testing.

For ergonovine testing, progressive incremental doses of 0.05 mg, 0.1 mg, and then 0.15 mg are administered intravenously at 3-minute to 5-minute intervals. Because severe spasm can occur instantly,

intracoronary nitroglycerin (usual dose 300 to 500 mg) should be made available for use. The patient should be asked about the presence of symptoms, and multilead electrocardiography should be done before and during the procedure. Even in the absence of symptoms or electrocardiographic changes, repeat arteriography of the left and right coronary arteries should be done. Traditionally, a positive response is identified if focal vasospasm exceeding 70% diameter narrowing is associated with typical anginal symptoms or electrocardiographic ST segment changes. Based on the previous discussion of the role of lesion length, diffuse spasm might also be considered to be flow limiting, however. An example of intense spasm of the right coronary artery after administration of ergonovine maleate in a patient with variant angina is shown in Figure 54–40.

MYOCARDIAL BRIDGES

The major coronary arteries pass primarily along the epicardial surface of the heart. Segments of the epicardial artery occasionally dip below the surface and into the myocardium. The myocardial fibers thus form a bridge over the involved arterial segment. Myocardial bridging is shown angiographically by systolic compression of the intramyocardial arterial segment that reverts to a normal caliber during diastole. It is most often observed in the middle

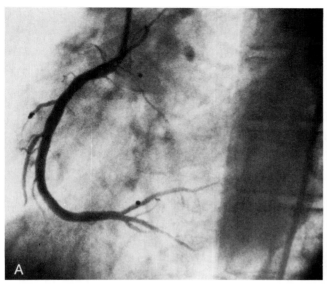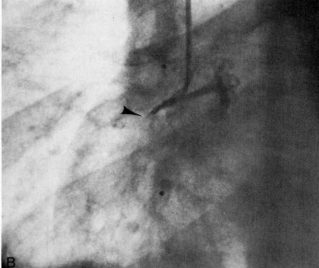

Figure 54–40. LAO projection of the right coronary artery before (*A*) and after (*B*) intravenous ergonovine injection. Note the severe spasm resulting in total occlusion of the coronary (*arrow*).

segment of the left anterior descending coronary artery. Systolic compression is angiographically apparent in 1.6 to 5% of patients studied (Bertrand et al, 1982; Huepler et al, 1978; MacAlpin, 1980; Waters et al, 1983). Myocardial bridges are more frequently discovered during autopsy than during cardiac catheterization. The incidence is higher in men and in patients with hypertrophic cardiomyopathy. In the latter disease, bridging of septal vessels is particularly prominent.

Rare reports have suggested that myocardial bridges cause ischemia and resultant angina (Ishimori et al, 1977; Kramer et al, 1982), myocardial infarction (Ross et al, 1980), and sudden death (Angelini et al, 1983; Morales et al, 1980). Although these data are inconclusive, it appears that in some patients bridging may alter coronary flow sufficiently to produce symptoms of ischemia. In one report (Hill et al, 1981), the persistence of luminal narrowing in early diastole appeared to blunt the normal early influx of coronary perfusion observed at this time; loss of early diastolic filling may therefore contribute to reduced coronary flow. There appears to be a decreased incidence of atherosclerotic changes at the level of intramural coronary arteries. In 1,100 consecutive patients with coronary artery disease studied with angiography, no luminal defects were noted in diastole at the level of systolic narrowing (Angelini et al, 1983). An example of myocardial bridging of the left anterior descending artery and otherwise normal coronaries is shown in Figure 54–41.

TECHNIQUES

Before cardiac catheterization, the procedure and potential complications should be explained to the patient and a written informed consent should be obtained from the patient. The patient is generally fasting and is often premedicated with antihistamines such as diphenhydramine, 25 to 50 mg intravenously. Sedatives including intravenous or oral benzodiazepam may help before the procedure. An intravenous line should be established before the catheterization. The patient is brought to the catheterization laboratory and prepared and draped in a sterile manner.

Electrocardiographic monitoring and recording should be visible to the angiographer and the catheterization team. Systemic blood pressure should be monitored through the intra-arterial catheter and displayed on the same screen as the electrocardiogram. A defibrillator should be located in each laboratory (for further details, see Chapter 31).

Percutaneous Femoral Technique—Judkins' Technique

Judkins' technique (1967), because of its relative ease, speed, reliability, and slightly lower complication rate (Davis et al, 1979), has become the most widely used method of coronary arteriography in the United States. The preformed catheters used for Judkins' technique are shown in Figure 54–42. These catheters are made of polyurethane and polyethylene and contain either steel braid or nylon in the wall of the shaft to allow better torque control. The catheters are designed with a single end hole for contrast injection and a tapered blunt tip to reduce intimal trauma. Although the original catheters were usually No. 8 French, Nos. 5, 6, and 7 French of a standard 100-cm length are currently available for use. The Nos. 6 and 7 French catheters are the most commonly used for adult coronary arteriography. All catheters have a primary, secondary, and tertiary curve. The Judkins' left and right coronary catheters are available

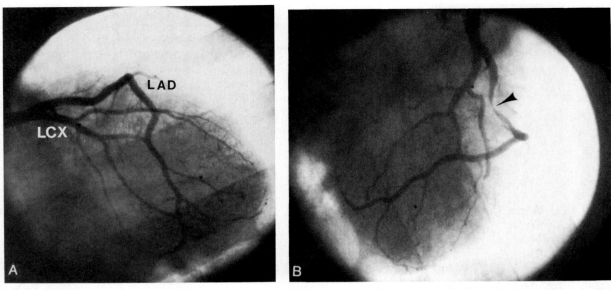

Figure 54–41. RAO caudal view of left coronary artery demonstrating muscle bridging. The left anterior descending artery (LAD) shows normal caliber during diastole (A), but shows profound systolic narrowing in B (*arrow*). (LCX = left circumflex coronary artery.)

in four sizes and are commonly referred to as JL3.5, JL4, JL5, JL6 (left) and JR3.5, JR4, JR5, JR6 (right). The numbers describe the length in centimeters of the secondary arm of the catheters. The JL4 catheter is most commonly used in patients with normal-sized aortic roots, whereas the Nos. 5 and 6 catheters are used in patients with progressively elongated or dilated aortic roots. The secondary bend constitutes the major difference in the left and right coronary catheters. The secondary bend of the left coronary catheter approaches 180 degrees, whereas the right coronary bend is approximately 30 degrees.

After local anesthesia with 1% lidocaine (Xylo-

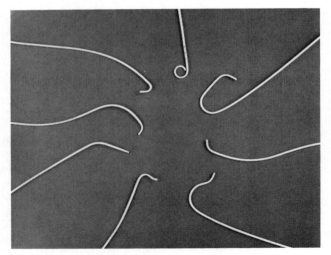

Figure 54–42. Various types of catheters used in cardiac catheterization with the percutaneous femoral technique. Beginning clockwise from 12 o'clock, the pigtail catheter, the left and right Judkins catheters, the left and right Amplatz catheters, a multipurpose catheter, a bypass graft catheter, and an internal mammary artery catheter.

caine), percutaneous entry of the femoral artery is achieved by puncturing the vessel 1 to 3 cm below the inguinal ligament. The ligament, which can be palpated as it courses from the anterior superior iliac spine to the superior pubic ramus, should be the landmark used rather than the inguinal crease, which is often misleading. A transverse skin incision is made over the femoral artery with a scapel. A No. 18-gauge thin-wall needle is inserted at a 30-degree to 45-degree angle into the femoral artery, and a 0.035-inch J-tip Teflon-coated guidewire is advanced into the needle. The wire should pass freely up the aorta. Fluoroscopy should be used to reveal the cause of any resistance to advancement. While pressure is firmly applied over the femoral artery, the needle is removed and a dilator equal in size to the catheters to be used is introduced. With the guidewire within the aorta, the coronary catheter is passed over the wire to the ascending aorta. After the guidewire is removed, 3 to 4 ml of blood is aspirated from the catheter, which is then flushed with heparinized saline. The catheter is attached to a catheter-syringe manifold assembly that allows pressure monitoring as well as contrast injection. It is generally recommended that patients should receive systemic heparinization after arterial access.

The left coronary catheter is initially advanced near but not into the orifice of the left main coronary artery. With the image intensifier in a shallow left anterior oblique (LAO) projection, a flush injection of contrast is made to visualize the left main ostium before entry of the catheter. After this and each subsequent injection, arterial pressure should be noted first before selective angiography. If damping (decrease in catheter tip pressure) or ventricularization (normal systolic pressure but low diastolic pressure) occurs, it may indicate a significant stenosis of the left main coronary artery and implies that the catheter tip has created total or almost total obstruction of the vessel. Alternatively, it suggests an adverse position of the catheter against the wall of the artery. In either situation, the catheter should be removed immediately from the ostium. The angiographer should re-evaluate the possibility of high-grade proximal coronary stenosis with further flush injections of the artery in multiple views. If ostial stenosis is present, additional injections must be made quickly and followed by immediate withdrawal of the catheter. Lengthy injections in this situation may result in prolonged ischemia or dissection of the artery.

After arteriography of the left coronary artery is done in multiple views with satisfactory visualization of any abnormalities (see later section on angiographic views), the left coronary catheter is withdrawn to the level of the diaphragm. The guidewire is reintroduced, and the left coronary catheter is replaced with Judkins right catheter. The catheter is advanced to the ascending aorta approximately 3 cm above the right sinus of Valsalva, and the patient is imaged in the LAO position. The Judkins left catheter almost automatically seeks out the ostium, but the right catheter may require considerable manipulation. The right coronary catheter tip is slowly rotated clockwise (anteriorly) and steadily withdrawn until it enters the orifice of the artery. The withdrawal is necessary because the catheter tends to descend within the aortic root as it is torqued clockwise.

Unlike the left coronary artery, damping and ventricularization of the right coronary artery are commonly due to catheter tip–induced spasm. Other potential causes include a small-caliber artery, superselective cannulation of the conus artery, or severe proximal stenosis. The cause can usually be determined by nonselective test injections or administration of nitroglycerin. Once again, cautious injections with rapid catheter withdrawal should be accomplished to avoid unnecessary ischemic complications.

Selective injection of aortocoronary bypass grafts via the percutaneous femoral approach can be accomplished with a right Judkins catheter, a right Amplatz catheter, or specifically designed graft catheters. To engage posterior or medial grafts, a specifically designed Judkins bypass catheter, which is similar to a right coronary catheter but modified so that the tip has a smooth downward terminal curve, may be used (see Fig. 54–42). Performing arteriography of aortocoronary bypass grafts is greatly facilitated if rings or metal clips are placed at the origin of the graft.

Arteriography of internal mammary artery grafts can be done with a Judkins right coronary catheter or a specifically designed internal mammary catheter (see Fig. 54–42). Injection of these grafts with contrast media often causes patients various degrees of pain in the extremities.

After coronary arteriography has been done, the catheters are removed and firm pressure is applied to the femoral area for 10 to 15 minutes, either by hand or by a mechanical clamp. The patient should be instructed to lie in bed for several hours with the leg remaining straight to prevent hematoma formation.

The main advantage of Judkins' technique is the speed and ease of selective catheterization. However, these attributes should not preclude gaining extensive operator experience to ensure quality studies with an acceptable degree of safety. The main disadvantage of this technique is that its use in patients with ileofemoral atherosclerotic disease may prevent retrograde passage of catheters through areas of extreme narrowing or tortuosity.

Brachial Artery Technique

Sones and colleagues (1959) introduced the first technique for coronary artery catheterization via a brachial artery cutdown. Sones' technique is still popular in many centers. The Sones catheter is available in a thin-walled woven Dacron or polyurethane design. It is 100 cm long and No. 7 or 8 French in diameter, tapering to No. 5.5 French at the tip. It has an end hole and two to four side holes near the catheter tip. After direct exposure of the brachial artery (usually the right brachial artery), an arteriotomy is made. The catheter is connected to a manifold and is advanced through the subclavian artery and innominate artery to the ascending aorta under fluoroscopic and pressure control. If a tortuous innominate or subclavian artery is encountered, a guidewire may be useful. The patient may attempt maneuvers such as shrugging the shoulders, turning the head to the left, or taking a deep breath in these situations. Pressure monitoring and safety precautions are the same as those with Judkins' techniques.

With the catheter in the central aorta, systemic heparinization is administered. In Sones' technique, the same catheter is used for both right and left coronary injections. After a flush injection of the left main coronary artery, selective left and right coronary arteriography may be done. With the patient in the LAO projection, the catheter is advanced to the left sinus of Valsalva and a J loop is made. The catheter is then advanced and withdrawn until the left ostium is engaged.

To cannulate the right coronary artery, the catheter is withdrawn from the left coronary artery while maintaining a gentle loop and applying clockwise rotation. Damping due to spasm, selective catheterization of the conus artery, or wedging within a stenosis may occur as well with Sones' technique.

When the catheter is removed from the brachial artery, proximal and distal bleeding are permitted to flush potential small thrombi. A small probe may be placed gently into the distal artery if distal flow is inadequate. A Fogarty thrombectomy catheter may be used for this purpose. The arteriotomy site is usually closed with a purse-string suture. After the skin is closed, a light pressure dressing is placed over the area.

Disadvantages of Sones' technique are that it is more difficult to master and the left coronary artery may be extremely difficult to cannulate. Furthermore, catheter seating may be less stable than using Judkins' technique, and biplane ventriculography or aortography may be difficult because the patient is being studied from the arm. Left internal mammary grafts may require the use of a left brachial approach. Advantages of Sones' technique are that the entire procedure including bypass grafts may be done with one catheter, and the technique is especially useful in patients with severe ileofemoral vascular disease. In addition, patients can ambulate soon after the procedure.

A modification of Sones' technique is the percutaneous brachial technique with preformed Judkins' catheters. This technique uses the Seldinger method of percutaneous brachial artery entry. A No. 6 French sheath is placed into the brachial artery, and 5,000 units of heparin are infused into the side port. A guidewire is then advanced to the ascending aorta under fluoroscopic control. No. 5 or 6 French left, right, and pigtail catheters are passed over the guidewire for routine arteriography and ventriculography. The guidewire may be necessary occasionally to direct the left coronary catheter into the left sinus of Valsalva and the ostium of the left main coronary artery. The main advantage of the percutaneous brachial technique is that it avoids a brachial artery cutdown and repair.

Angiographic Views

To visualize coronary arteries adequately, it is necessary to identify the left and right coronary arteries in multiple projections. Because of considerable overlap, tortuosity, and branching of vessels, additional views may be required to assess atherosclerotic lesions. As discussed in the section on pathoanatomic correlates, eccentric lesions necessitate orthogonal views of a lesion to quantify the severity of stenosis.

Early angiographic studies of the heart depended on transverse views. Therefore, only different degrees of LAO and right anterior oblique views (RAO) were done. As expected, these limited views were often inadequate to assess the severity of the lesion when eccentricity and branching obscured visualization.

Several reports in the 1970s documented the use of cranial and caudal angulation of the x-ray beam (Aldridge et al, 1975, 1984; Arani et al, 1975; Sos and Baltaxe, 1977). These sagittal plane views have allowed improved evaluation of foreshortened and partially obscured vessels (Fig. 54–43). In particular, it has been well documented that stenosis of the origin of the posterior descending artery and the distal left main coronary artery may be difficult to quantify reliably, even when multiple views are available (Kennedy et al, 1982).

X-ray systems now in routine use are capable of providing any combination of transverse angulation with cranial or caudal angulation. The proposed and generally accepted (Aldridge et al, 1975; Sos and Baltaxe, 1977) terminology for angiographic views is based on how one views the arteries from the image intensifier. Thus, in the LAO cranial view, one visualizes the coronary arteries as if looking over the patient's left shoulder. Likewise, in the RAO caudal view, coronary arteries are viewed as if looking from the inferior aspect of the left thorax.

The left coronary artery with its major branches may require as many as six views to assess the anatomy adequately. RAO, LAO, LAO cranial, RAO cranial, RAO caudal, and LAO caudal are the standard projections used. The left main coronary artery is typically best viewed in a shallow LAO and RAO projection, with the artery just off the spine. However, in many cases additional injections with cranial and caudal angulation are necessary.

The left anterior descending artery should be seen at minimum in the LAO and RAO projections.

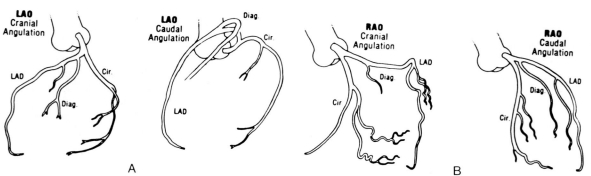

Figure 54–43. Diagrammatic representation of the left coronary artery when visualized with cranial and caudal angulation of the x-ray beam. (LAD = left anterior descending artery; Cir. = circumflex artery; Diagn. = diagonal artery.) (From Sos, T. A., and Baltaxe, H. A.: Cranial and caudal angulation for coronary angiography revisited. Circulation, 56:119, 1977. By permission of the American Heart Association, Inc.)

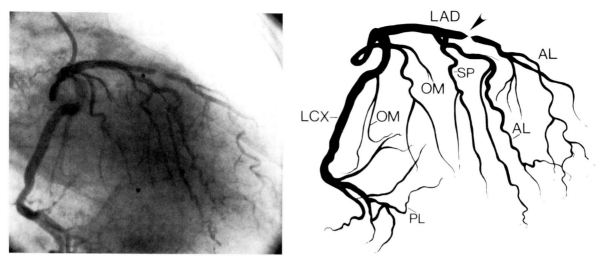

Figure 54–44. Coronary arteriogram and diagram in RAO projection of severe stenosis of the mid left anterior descending coronary artery (LAD). (AL = anterolateral (diagonal) artery; LCX = left circumflex coronary artery; OM = obtuse marginal branch of circumflex artery; SP = septal perforator; PL = posterolateral artery.)

The addition of cranial angulation to these views may facilitate identification of lesions, especially those in the proximal left anterior descending artery, the septal perforators, and the diagonal (anterolateral) branches (Figs. 54–43 to 54–45). The left circumflex coronary artery is best evaluated in the LAO caudal, RAO, and LAO projections (Figs. 54–43 and 54–46). In a left dominant circulation, the posterior descending artery from the circumflex artery is best visualized in the LAO and LAO cranial projections. A RAO caudal projection aids in separation and visualization of the marginal branches. Although it is appreciated that all views may not be necessary in all patients, the angiographer should individualize the examination to obtain the maximal amount of information with the least number of injections.

Occasionally, complex overlap of proximal left coronary artery vessels can be better defined by rolling the camera during the view.

The right coronary artery is usually viewed in shallow RAO and LAO projections (Figs. 54–47 and 54–48). However, when the posterior descending artery or the origin of the right coronary artery is obscured, an LAO cranial or a steep RAO view may be useful to overcome foreshortening. Cranial angulation of the LAO view helps to visualize the bifurcation of the right coronary artery into the posterior descending artery and left ventricular branches. The LAO caudal view (spider view) allows evaluation of the left main, proximal left anterior descending and proximal circumflex artery, including the optional diagonal artery.

Figure 54–45. Coronary arteriogram and diagram of LAO cranial view of left anterior descending artery (LAD) stenosis described in Figure 54–44. (AL = anterolateral (diagonal) artery; LCX = left circumflex coronary artery; LM = left main coronary artery; OM = obtuse marginal branch of circumflex artery; PL = posterolateral artery.)

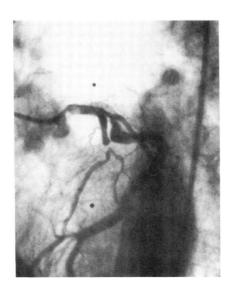
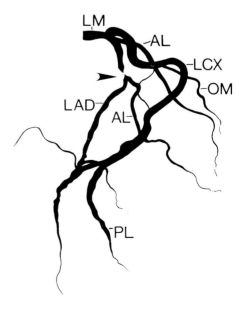

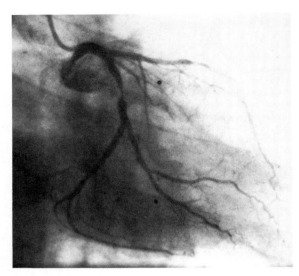
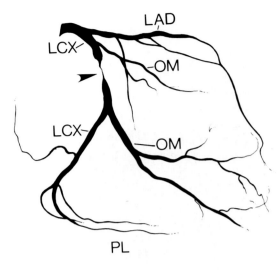

Figure 54–46. RAO caudal view of mid-left circumflex lesion. (LAD = left anterior descending coronary artery; LCX = left circumflex coronary artery; OM = obtuse marginal branch of circumflex artery; PL = posterolateral artery.)

UNUSUAL CORONARY ANATOMY

Coronary artery aneurysms and ectasia are usually caused by atherosclerotic infiltration of the media of the artery, although congenital aneurysms may also occur (Fujita et al, 1983). Other less common causes include periarteritis, syphilis, trauma, rheumatic fever, bacterial endocarditis, and Kawasaki's disease. Coronary aneurysms are present angiographically or at autopsy in as many as 1.5% of patients (Glickel et al, 1978). Aneurysms have been classified as being diffuse or localized (Kalke and Edwards, 1968). Diffuse aneurysms are generally considered to be congenital, whereas localized aneurysms can be due to atherosclerosis or inflammatory diseases. They are frequently encountered when arteriovenous fistulas are present. The diagnosis of

coronary artery aneurysms and ectasia can best be made by coronary arteriography (Figs. 54–49 and 54–50). Multiple views should be obtained to exclude the presence of coexisting atherosclerotic disease.

Angiographically, a fresh or organized coronary artery thrombus appears as an eccentric filling defect that usually extends from the arterial wall into the lumen. These may be difficult to distinguish in vivo from fixed atherosclerotic stenosis and, in many cases, are attached to an atherosclerotic plaque. Coronary artery thrombus appears to be a frequent observation in patients with acute myocardial infarction or unstable angina. However, coronary artery emboli are separate from the intima of the artery and may have a tail-like appearance. Coronary artery embolism may result from endocarditis, mural thrombi secondary to valvular disease or cardiomy-

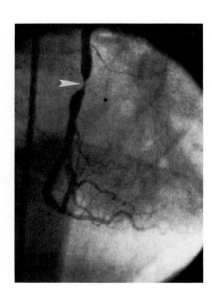
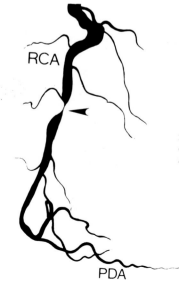

Figure 54–47. RAO view of mid-right coronary artery obstruction (*arrow*). (RCA = right coronary artery; PDA = posterior descending artery.)

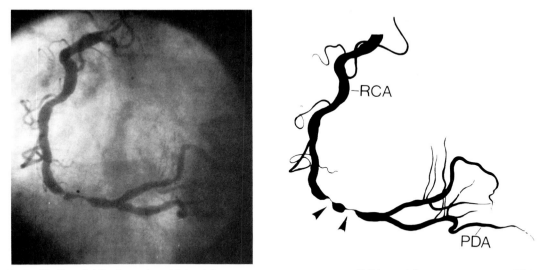

Figure 54–48. Shallow LAO view of multiple right coronary artery stenoses. (RCA = right coronary artery; PDA = posterior descending artery.)

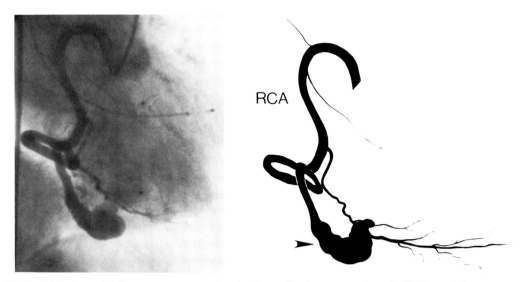

Figure 54–49. RAO view of right coronary artery showing large distal aneurysm (*arrow*). (RCA = right coronary artery.)

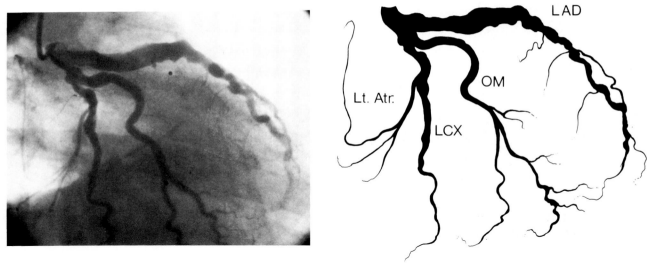

Figure 54–50. RAO projection of left coronary artery with multiple areas of ectasia within the left anterior descending (LAD) and left circumflex (LCX) arteries. (OM = obtuse marginal branch of circumflex artery; Lt. Atr. = left atrial branch.)

opathy, or intracardiac tumors (in particular myxoma). Iatrogenic coronary occlusion due to embolism is a well-recognized complication of coronary arteriography, especially during interventional procedures (Fig. 54–51).

CORONARY ARTERY BYPASS GRAFTS
(Figs. 54–52 and 54–53)

Coronary artery bypass grafts should appear smooth and equal or larger in size than the native coronary artery. Stenosis may occur at the proximal anastomosis, in the body of the graft, or at distal anastomosis. In aortocoronary bypass grafts, stenosis of the origin is best viewed in multiple orthogonal projections because of the potential eccentricity of the lesions. Total occlusion of the graft appears as a dimple or stump arising from the aortic root during selective angiography. If total stenosis occurs anywhere within the graft, the vessel may occlude back to the aortic anastomosis. Although aortography may assist in localizing unmarked grafts, an inability to visualize graft patency by this method should not be taken as conclusive evidence of graft occlusion. Selective angiography is necessary to fully evaluate the patency of a graft.

Midgraft or distal graft stenosis may appear as either smooth intimal proliferation or as a typical atherosclerotic plaque. To avoid confusion, the significance of a lesion within an aortocoronary bypass graft should probably be interpreted in relation to the diameter of the normal native artery rather than the "normal" part of the saphenous vein.

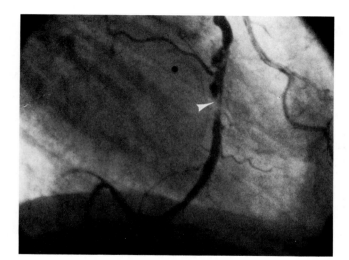

Figure 54–51. RAO projection of the right coronary with intracoronary thrombus present at the site of severe stenosis. Thrombus occurred as a complication of routine coronary arteriography.

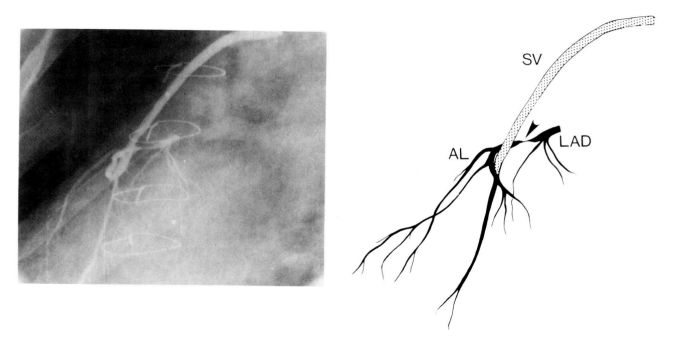

Figure 54–52. LAO view of saphenous vein graft to left anterior descending (LAD) artery. Note the stenosis of the LAD proximal to insertion of the graft. (AL = anterolateral artery; SV = saphenous vein graft.)

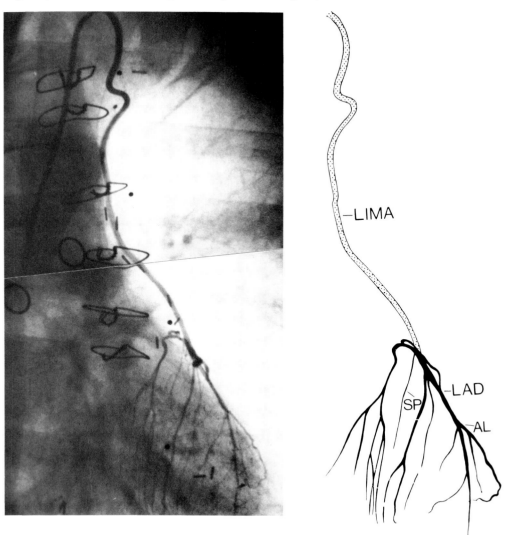

Figure 54–53. RAO view of left internal mammary artery (LIMA) graft to left anterior descending (LAD) artery. (AL = anterolateral artery; SP = septal perforator.)

Selected Bibliography

Angelini, P., Trivellato, M., Donis, J., and Leachman, R. D.: Myocardial bridges: A review. Prog. Cardiovasc. Dis., 26:75, 1983.

This article is a comprehensive review of myocardial bridging. Definitions, comparative anatomy, and human anatomic studies are described. Included is an extensive discussion of the angiographic features and an evaluation of systolic narrowing of the arteries. The role of coronary artery surgery in the setting of isolated myocardial bridges and bridges associated with fixed stenoses are reviewed. The article concludes with a discussion of the physiology of myocardial bridges.

The authors conclude that myocardial bridges are a frequent anatomic finding and are common among the general population. Patients with equal degrees of systolic narrowing do not show common clinical patterns. Finally, the pathophysiologic ways in which myocardial bridges cause ischemia have been poorly demonstrated, particularly because systolic narrowing can affect only 5 to 30% of total coronary blood flow.

Chaitman, B. R., Lesperance, J., Saltiel, J., and Bourassa, M. G.: Clinical, angiographic, and hemodynamic findings in patients with anomalous origin of the coronary arteries. Circulation, 53:122, 1976.

This study describes the clinical and angiographic features of 31 patients with an anomalous origin of the coronary arteries. The course of aberrant circumflex, left coronary artery, and right coronary artery are described. The relationship between each anomaly and its clinical significance is reviewed. In addition, coronary blood flow during exercise and myocardial metabolism during pacing are assessed in five patients with aberrant left coronary arteries. It is concluded that aberrant left coronary artery origin from the right sinus of Valsalva can result in significant myocardial ischemia and infarction.

Kennedy, J. W., Fisher, L. D., and Killip, T.: Coronary angiography quality control in CASS study. In Bond, M. G., Insull, W., Glagov, S., et al (eds): Clinical Diagnosis of Atherosclerosis: Quantitative Methods of Evaluation. New York, Springer-Verlag, 1982, pp. 475–491.

This report describes the quality control of the CASS registry. In particular, problems related to the performance and interpretation of coronary arteriograms are outlined. In 870 arteriograms read independently by readers at different centers, an absolute difference in percentage stenosis of between 5 and 10% was found, depending on the arterial segment analyzed. The proximal left main was a particularly difficult area to interpret reproducibly. If one angiographer read a stenosis of 50% or more, it was estimated that a second angiographer would find no stenosis 15.7% of the time. Although intrareader variation was one-half of interreader variation, a scattergram results when comparing reading one with reading two. The data presented clearly show the drawbacks of visual interpretation of lesion severity, and more routine use of quantitative methods of evaluation is recommended.

Levin, D. C.: Pathways and functional significance of the coronary collateral circulation. Circulation, 50:831, 1974.

This classic article reports the results of 200 coronary arteriograms and left ventriculograms in patients with significant coronary artery disease. The diagrams of collateral circulation outline the pathways observed in left anterior descending, left circumflex, and right coronary artery obstruction. These diagrams are reproduced in this chapter.

The author examines the role of collateral circulation in preserving myocardial function and concludes that regional wall motion is preserved in the presence of adequate collateral circulation.

Levin, D. C., Fellows, K. E., and Abrams, H. L.: Hemodynamically significant primary anomalies of the coronary arteries. Circulation, 58:25, 1978.

This study is a comprehensive review of the radiologic aspects of hemodynamically significant coronary artery anomalies that cause abnormalities of myocardial perfusion. The four major types described are coronary fistulas, origin of the left coronary artery from the pulmonary artery, congenital coronary stenosis or atresia, and origin of the left coronary artery from the right sinus of Valsalva with the artery coursing between the aorta and pulmonary artery. The relative incidence, angiographic appearance, associated abnormalities, and physiologic significance of the anomalies are discussed.

Mancini, G. B. J., Simon S. B., McGillem, M. J., et al: Automated quantitative coronary arteriography: Morphologic and physiologic validation in vivo of a rapid digital angiographic method. Circulation, 75:452, 1987.

This study assesses for the first time the performance in vivo of a fully automatic rapid coronary quantitation program. Dogs were instrumented with high-fidelity micromanometer catheters, electromagnetic flow, and plastic cylinders to create intraluminal stenoses of the left anterior descending and circumflex arteries. Interobserver and intraobserver variation was low, and the correlation between known and measured luminal diameter was high. The measures of percentage diameter stenosis, percentage area stenosis (geometric and videodensitometric), and absolute minimal cross-sectional area (geometric and videodensitometric) all were correlated with independent measures of coronary flow reserve. Therefore, this report provides direct anatomic and physiologic validation of a quantitative method of analysis for digital angiograms and cineangiograms.

Marcus, M. L., Wilson, R. F., and White, C. W.: Methods of measurement of myocardial blood flow in patients: A critical review. Circulation, 76:245, 1987.

This article critically reviews the currently available methods of studying coronary flow in humans and provides insight into newer methods under investigation and development. The methods discussed include thermodilution, gas clearance, densitometry, electromagnetic and Doppler flow probes, positron-emission tomography, ultrafast computed tomography, contrast echocardiography, and magnetic resonance imaging. The article discusses the relative merits and limitations of each technique and strongly recommends more widespread use of Doppler catheters. An extensive list of current references is provided.

Waters, D. D., Szlachic, J., and Bonan, R.: Comparative sensitivity of exercise, cold pressor and ergonovine testing in provoking attacks of variant angina in patients with active disease. Circulation, 67:310, 1983.

This study evaluates the sensitivity of ergonovine, exercise, and the cold pressor test in provoking attacks of variant angina in patients with well-documented active variant angina. The patients had recent cardiac catheterization. Anginal attacks and electrocardiography were monitored to evaluate effects of provocative testing. In patients with active variant angina, an attack can be provoked by ergonovine in more than 90% of cases, by exercise in approximately 30%, and by the cold pressor test in approximately 10%. Therefore, ergonovine provocation was recommended as the most sensitive test to detect variant angina.

Wilson, R. F., Marcus, M. L., and White, C. W.: Prediction of the physiologic significance of coronary artery lesions by quantitative lesion geometry in patients with limited coronary artery disease. Circulation, 75:723, 1987.

This study examines the relationship between coronary flow reserve measured by Doppler coronary catheter and luminal stenosis of individual lesions in patients with discrete coronary artery stenoses. They show that in patients with limited coronary atherosclerosis, precise angiographic measurements by quantitative angiography correlated closely with a physiologic measurement of coronary obstruction. Lesions in major coronary arteries with less than a 70% area stenosis or minimal cross-sectional area greater than 2.5 cm² did not functionally impair coronary blood flow or result in significant translesional pressure gradient.

The physiologic conclusions emerging from this study are as follows: (1) Coronary stenosis of more than 90% luminal area stenosis was associated with a wide range of coronary flow reserve. (2) Lesions of less than a 70% area stenosis or greater than 2.5 mm² cross-sectional area may also result in myocardial ischemia. (3) There is usually only modest reduction in coronary blood flow reserve in lesions with 70 to 80% area obstruction.

Bibliography

Aldridge, H. E.: A decade or more of cranial and caudal angled projections in coronary arteriography—another look. Cathet. Cardiovasc. Diagn., 10:539, 1984.

Aldridge, H. E., McLoughlin, M. J., and Taylor, L. W.: Improved diagnosis in coronary cinearteriography with routine use of 110 degree oblique views and cranial and caudal angulations: Comparison with standard oblique views in 100 patients. Am. J. Cardiol., 36:568, 1975.

American Heart Association Committee Report: A reporting system on patients evaluated for coronary artery disease. Circulation, 51:7, 1975.

Amplatz, K., Formonek G., Stranger, P., and Wilson, W.: Mechanics of selective coronary artery catheterization via the femoral approach. Radiology, 89:1040, 1967.

Angelini, P., Trivellato, M., Donis, J., and Leachman, R. D.: Myocardial bridges: A review. Prog. Cardiovasc. Dis., 26:75, 1983.

Arani, D. T., Bunnell, I. L., and Greene, D. G.: Lordotic right posterior oblique projection of the left coronary artery: A special view for special anatomy. Circulation, 52:504, 1975.

Bartel, A. G., Chen J. T., Peter, R. H., et al: The significance of coronary artery calcification detected by fluoroscopy. Circulation, 49:1247, 1974.

Bertrand, M. E., La Blanche, J. M., Tilmant P. Y., et al: Frequency of provoked coronary arterial spasm in 1089 consecutive patients undergoing coronary arteriography. Circulation, 65:1299, 1982.

Blankenhorn, D. H., and Curry, P. J.: The accuracy of arteriography and ultrasound imaging for atherosclerotic measurement. Arch. Pathol. Lab. Med., 106:483, 1982.

Chahine, R. A., Raizner, A. E., Ishimon, T., et al: The incidence and clinical implications of coronary artery spasm. Circulation, 52:972, 1975.

Chaitman, B. R., Lesperance, J., Saltiel, J., and Bourassa, M. G.: Clinical, angiographic, and hemodynamic findings in patients with anomalous origin of the coronary arteries. Circulation, 53:122, 1976.

Cohen, M. V.: Morphologic considerations of the coronary collateral circulation in man. In Cohen, M. V. (ed): Coronary Collaterals: Clinical and Experimental Observation. Mount Kisco, NY, Futura Publishing Co., 1985, pp. 1–91.

Cusma, J. T., Toggart, E. J., Folts, J. D., et al: Digital subtraction angiographic imaging of coronary flow reserve. Circulation, 75:461, 1987.

Davis, K., Kennedy, J. W., Kemp, H. G., et al: Complications of coronary arteriography. Circulation, 59:1105, 1979.

DeRouen, T. A., Murray, J. A., and Owen, W.: Variability in the analysis of coronary arteriograms. Circulation, 55:324, 1977.

Douglas, J. S., Franch, R. H., and King, S. B.: In King, S. B., and Douglas, J. S. (eds): Coronary Arteriography. New York, McGraw-Hill Book Company, 1985, pp. 33–85.

Engel, H. J., Torres, C., and Page, H. L.: Major variations in anatomical origin of the coronary arteries. Cath. Cardiovasc. Diagn., 1:157, 1975.

Feldman, R. L., Nichols, W. W., Pepine, C. J., and Conti, C. R.: Hemodynamic significance of the length of a coronary arterial narrowing. Am. J. Cardiol., 41:865, 1978.

Forssmann, W.: The catheterization of the right side of the heart. Klin. Wochenschr., 8:2085, 1929.

Fujita, S., Murakami, E., TakeKoshi, N., et al: Congenital coronary arterial aneurysm without arteriovenous fistula resulting in myocardial infarction. Jpn. Circ. J., 47:363, 1983.

Ganz, W., Tamura, K., Marcus, H. S., et al: Measurement of coronary sinus blood flow by continuous thermodilution in man. Circulation, 44:181, 1971.

Gensini, G. G., DiGiorgi, S., Coskun, O., et al: Anatomy of the coronary circulation in living man: Coronary venography. Circulation, 31:778, 1965.

Glagov, S., and Zarins, C. V.: Quantitative atherosclerosis: Problems of definition. In Bond, M. A., Insull, W., Glagov, S., et al (eds): Clinical Diagnosis of Atherosclerosis: Quantitative Methods of Evaluation. New York, Springer-Verlag, 1982.

Glickel, S. Z., Maggs, P. R., and Ellis, F. H.: Coronary artery aneurysm. Ann. Thorac. Surg., 25:372, 1978.

Gould, K. L., Goldstein, R. A., Mullani, N. A., et al: Noninvasive assessment of coronary stenoses by myocardial perfusion imaging during pharmacologic coronary vasodilation. VII: Clinical feasibility of position cardiac imaging without a cyclotron using generator-produced rubidium-82. J. Am. Coll. Cardiol., 7:775, 1986.

Gruentzig, A. R., Myler, R. K., Hanna, E. S., et al: Coronary transluminal angioplasty (Abstract). Circulation, 56:11, 1977.

Gruentzig, A. R., Senning, A., and Siegenthaler, W. E.: Nonoperative dilation of coronary artery stenoses: Percutaneous transluminal coronary angioplasty. N. Engl. J. Med., 301:61, 1979.

Hamby, R. I., Tabrah, R., Wisoff, B. G., and Hartenstein, M. L.: Coronary artery calcification: Clinical implications and angiographic correlates. Am. Heart J., 87:565, 1974.

Harrison, D. G., White, C. W., and Hiratzka, L. F.: The value of cross-sectional area determined by quantitative coronary arteriography in assessing the physiologic significance of proximal left anterior stenosis. Circulation, 69:1111, 1984.

Heupler, F. A., Proudfit, W. L., Razavi, M., et al: Ergonovine meleate: Provocative test for coronary artery spasm. Am. J. Cardiol., 41:631, 1978.

Hill, R., Chitwood, W. R., Bashore, T. M., et al: Coronary flow and regional function before and after supraarterial myotomy for myocardial bridging. Ann. Thorac. Surg., 31:176, 1981.

Hodgson, J. M., LeGrand, V., Bates, E. R., et al: Validation in dogs of a rapid digital angiographic technique to measure relative coronary blood flow during routine cardiac catheterization. Am. J. Cardiol., 55:188, 1985.

Hutchins, G. M., Moore, W., and Hatton, E. V.: Arterial-venous relationships in the human left ventricular myocardium: Anatomic basis for countercurrent regulation of blood flow. Circulation, 74:1195, 1986.

Ishimori, T., Raizner, A. E., Chahine, R. A., et al: Myocardial bridges in man: Clinical correlation and angiographic accentuations with nitroglycerin. Cathet. Cardiovasc. Diagn., 3:59, 1977.

Judkins, M. P.: Selective coronary arteriography. I: A percutaneous transfemoral technique. Radiology, 89:815, 1967.

Kalke, B., and Edwards, J. E.: Localized aneurysms of the coronary arteries. Angiology, 19:460, 1968.

Kennedy, J. W., Fisher, L. D., and Killip, T.: Coronary angiography quality control in CASS study. In Bond, M. G., Insull, W., Glagov, S., et al (eds): Clinical Diagnosis of Atherosclerosis: Quantitative Methods of Evaluation. New York, Springer-Verlag, 1982, pp. 475–491.

Kirkeeide, R. L., Gould, K. L., and Parsel, L.: Assessment of coronary stenoses by myocardial perfusion imaging during pharmacologic coronary vasodilation. VII: Validation of coronary flow reserve as a single integrated functional measure of stenosis severity reflecting all its geometric dimensions. J. Am. Coll. Cardiol., 7:103, 1986.

Klinke, W. P., Christie, L. G., Nichols, W. W., et al: Use of catheter-tip velocity-pressure transducer to evaluate left ventricular function in man: Effects of intravenous propranolol. Circulation, 61:946, 1980.

Klocke, F. J.: Measurement of coronary flow reserve: Defining pathophysiology versus making decisions about patient care. Circulation, 76:1183, 1987.

Klocke, F. J., Ellisa, K., and Canty, J. M., Jr.: Interpretation of changes in coronary flow that accompany pharmacologic interventions. Circulation, 75 (Suppl. V):34, 1987.

Kramer, J. R., Kitazume, H., Proudfitt, W. L., and Sones, F. M.: Clinical significance of isolated coronary bridges: Benign and frequent condition involving the left anterior descending artery. Am. Heart J., 103:283, 1982.

Laufer, N., and Buda, A.: Quantitative coronary arteriography. In Buda, A. J., and Delp, E. J. (eds): Digital Cardiac Imaging. Boston, Martinus Nijhoff, 1985, pp. 119–139.

LeFree, M. T., Simon, S. B., Mancini, G. B. J., and Vogel, R. A.: Digital radiographic assessment of coronary artery diameter and videodensitometric cross-sectional area. Proc. SPIE, 626:334, 1986.

Levin, D. C.: Pathways and functional significance of the coronary collateral circulation. Circulation, 50:831, 1974.

Levin, D. C., Fellows, K. E., and Abrams, H. L.: Hemodynamically significant primary anomalies of the coronary arteries. Circulation, 58:25, 1978.

Liberthson, R. R., Dinsmore, R. E., Bharak, S., et al: Aberrant coronary artery origin from the aorta: Diagnosis and clinical significance. Circulation, 50:774, 1974.

Linhart, J. W.: Prinzmetal variant of angina pectoris. J.A.M.A., 228:342, 1974.

MacAlpin, R. N.: Relation of coronary artery spasm to sites of organic stenosis. Am. J. Cardiol., 46:143, 1980.

Mancini, G. B. J., Simon, S. B., McGillem, M. J., et al: Automated quantitative coronary arteriography: Morphologic and physiologic validation in vivo of a rapid digital angiographic method. Circulation, 75:452, 1987.

Marcus, M. L.: Effects of cardiac hypertrophy on the coronary circulation. In Marcus, M. L. (ed): The Coronary Circulation in Health and Disease. New York, McGraw-Hill Book Company, 1983, p. 285.

Marcus, M. L., Wilson, R. F., and White, C. W.: Methods of measurement of myocardial blood flow in patients: A critical review. Circulation, 76:245, 1987.

Marcus, M., Wright, C., Doty, D., et al: Measurement of coronary velocity and reactive hyperemia in the coronary circulation in humans. Circ. Res., 49:877, 1981.

Maseri, A., Severi, S., deNes, M., et al: "Variant" angina: One aspect of a continuous spectrum of vasospastic myocardial ischemia: Pathogenetic mechanisms, estimated incidence, and clinical and coronary arteriographic findings in 138 patients. Am. J. Cardiol., 42:1019, 1978.

Mathey, D. G., Chatterjee, K., Tyberg, J. V., et al: Coronary sinus reflux: A source of error in the measurement of thermodilution coronary sinus flow. Circulation, 57:778, 1978.

McMahon, M. M., Brown, G. B., Cuckingnon, R., et al: Quantitative coronary angiography: Measurement of the critical stenosis in patients with unstable angina and single vessel disease without collaterals. Circulation, 60:106, 1979.

McManus, B. M., Waller, B. F., Jones, M., et al: The case for preoperative coronary angiography in patients with tetralogy of Fallot and the complex congenital heart disease. Am. Heart J., 103:451, 1982.

Meng, C. C., Eckner, F. A., and Lev, M.: Coronary artery distribution in tetralogy of Fallot. Arch. Surg., 90:363, 1965.

Morales, A. R., Romanell, R., and Boucek, R. J.: The mural left anterior descending coronary artery, strenuous exercise and sudden death. Circulation, 62:230, 1980.

Nichols, A. B., Gabrich, C. F. O., Fenoglio, J. J., and Esser, P. D.: Quantification of relative coronary arterial stenosis by cinevideodensitometric analysis of coronary arteriograms. Circulation, 69:512, 1984.

Ogden, J. A.: Congenital anomalies of the coronary arteries. Am. J. Cardiol., 25:474, 1970.

Okumura, K., Yasue, H., Horio, Y., et al: Multivessel coronary spasm in patients with variant angina: A study with intracoronary injection of acetylcholine. Circulation, 77:535, 1988.

Oldham, H. N., Ebert, P. A., Young, W. G., and Sabiston, D. C.: Surgical management of congenital coronary artery fistula. Ann. Thorac. Surg., 12:503, 1971.

Peterson, R. J., King, S. B., Farjam, W. A., et al: Relationship of coronary artery stenosis and gradient to exercise-induced ischemia. J. Am. Coll. Cardiol., 1:673, 1983.

Radner, S.: Attempt at roentgenologic visualization of coronary blood vessels in man. Acta Radiol., 26:492, 1945.

Ricketts, J. H., and Abrams, H. L.: Percutaneous selective coronary arteriography. J.A.M.A., 181:620, 1962.

Roberts, W. C., Siegel, R. J., and Zipes, D. P.: Origin of the right coronary artery from the left sinus of Valsalva and its functional consequences: Analysis of 10 necropsy patients. Am. J. Cardiol., 49:863, 1982.

Ross, L., Dander, B., Nidasio, G. P., et al: Myocardial bridges and ischemic heart disease. Eur. Heart J., 1:239, 1980.

Seldinger, S. I.: Catheter replacement of the needle in percutaneous arteriography: A new technique. Acta Radiol., 39:368, 1953.

Sharbaugh, A. H., and White, R. S.: Single coronary artery: Analysis of the anatomic variation, clinical importance, and report of five cases. J.A.M.A., 230:243, 1974.

Skelton, T. N., Kisslo, K. B., Mikat, E. M., and Bashore, T. M.: Accuracy of digital angiography for quantitation of normal coronary luminal segments in excised, perfused hearts. Am. J. Cardiol., 59:1261, 1987.

Sones, F. M., Jr., Shivey, E. K., Proudfit, W. L., and Westcott, R. N.: Cinecoronary arteriography (Abstract). Circulation, 20:773, 1959.

Sos, T. A., and Baltaxe, H. A.: Cranial and caudal angulation for coronary arteriography revisited. Circulation, 56:119, 1977.

Vogel, R. A.: Digital radiographic assessment of coronary flow reserve. In Buda, A. J., and Delp, E. J. (eds): Digital Cardiac Imaging. Boston, Martinus Nijhoff, 1985, pp. 106–118.

Wangler, R. D., Peters, K. G., Laughlin, D. E., et al: A method for continuously assessing coronary velocity in the rat. Am. J. Physiol., 10:H816, 1981.

Waters, D. D., Szlachic, J., and Bonan, R.: Comparative sensitivity of exercise, cold pressor, and ergonovine testing in provoking attacks of variant angina in patients with active disease. Circulation, 67:310, 1983.

White, C. W., Wright, C. B., Doty, D. B., et al: Does visual interpretation of the coronary arteriogram predict the physiologic importance of a coronary stenosis? N. Engl. J. Med., 310:819, 1984.

Wilson, R. F., Marcus, M. L., and White, C. W.: Prediction of the physiologic significance of coronary artery lesions by quantitative lesion geometry in patients with limited coronary artery disease. Circulation, 75:723, 1987.

Wilson, R. F., and White, C. W.: Measurement of maximal coronary flow reserve: A technique for assessing the physiologic significance of coronary arterial lesions in humans. Herz, 12:163, 1987.

Zimmerman, H. A., Scott, R. W., and Becker, N. O.: Catheterization of the left side of the heart in man. Circulation, 1:357, 1950.

IV CONGENITAL MALFORMATIONS OF THE CORONARY CIRCULATION

James E. Lowe
David C. Sabiston, Jr.

Congenital coronary arterial malformations have long been recognized, but the frequency of these reports in the literature has increased greatly since the introduction of selective coronary arteriography by Sones in 1959. In a review of 224 patients with coronary malformations, Ogden (1970) proposed three basic classifications: (1) *major anomalies*, in which there is an abnormal communication between an artery and a cardiac chamber or abnormal origin of a major coronary artery from the pulmonary artery; (2) *minor anomalies*, in which there is variation of the origin of the vessels from the aorta but the distal circulation is normal; and (3) *secondary anomalies*, in which the coronary arterial variation probably represents a circulatory response of the primary intracardiac pathologic defect. The distribution of coronary artery anomalies in these 224 patients is shown in Table 54–7.

Major anomalies that are amenable to surgical correction include congenital coronary fistulas, anomalous origin of either the left or right coronary artery from the pulmonary artery, congenital aneurysms of the coronary arteries, and congenital membranous obstruction of the ostium of the left main coronary artery. Minor anomalies, in which there is variation in the origin of the coronary arteries from the aorta with normal distal circulation, and secondary anomalies, associated with congenital heart defects, such as transposition of the great vessels, truncus arteriosus, and tetralogy of Fallot, seldom require surgical intervention. In this section, the clinical manifestations, evaluation, and surgical management of patients with major coronary anomalies, including congenital coronary artery fistulas, congenital origin of either the left or right coronary artery from the pulmonary artery, congenital coronary artery aneurysms, and membranous obstruction of the ostium of the left main coronary artery, are described.

Based on the authors' experience and supported by that of others, it is recommended that most patients with major congenital coronary arterial malformations be considered to be candidates for surgical correction. In most cases, the natural history of these lesions is not associated with a normal life expectancy, with the possible exception of patients with congenital origin of the right coronary artery from the pulmonary artery. Because these malformations can now be safely corrected and long-term results are gratifying, surgical intervention should be strongly recommended when a precise diagnosis has been established.

CORONARY ARTERY FISTULAS

Since Krause first described a coronary artery fistula in 1865, almost 400 additional patients with this malformation have been reported in the literature. Increasing numbers of patients with this anomaly are being recognized each year because of the widespread use of cardiac catheterization and selective coronary arteriography in the evaluation of various cardiac problems (Fig. 54–54).

Coronary artery fistulas are characterized by normal origin of the coronary artery from the aorta with a fistulous communication with the atria or ventricles or with the pulmonary artery, coronary sinus, or superior vena cava. These fistulas represent

TABLE 54–7. CONGENITAL VARIATIONS OF THE CORONARY ARTERIES IN 224 PATIENTS*

Congenital Variations	No. of Cases
Major coronary anomalies (75 cases)	
Coronary "arteriovenous" fistula†	31
Anomalous origin from the pulmonary artery	44
Left coronary artery	39
Right coronary artery	4
Both coronary arteries	1
Minor coronary variations (63 cases)	
High takeoff	2
Multiple ostia	6
Anomalous circumflex artery origin	14
Anomalous anterior descending artery origin	11
Absent proximal ostium/single ostium in other aortic sinus	10
Absent proximal ostium/multiple ostia in other aortic sinus	10
Hypoplastic proximal coronary artery	5
Congenital proximal stenosis	2
Congenital distal stenosis	1
Coronary artery from the posterior aortic sinus	1
Ventricular origin of an accessory coronary artery	1
Second coronary anomalies (86 cases)	
Secondary coronary "arteriovenous" fistula	3
Variations in transposition of the great vessels	65
Variations in truncus arteriosus	6
Variations in tetralogy of Fallot	4
Ectasia of coronary arteries in supravalvular aortic stenosis	5
Mural coronary artery	3

*Adapted from Ogden, J. A.: Congenital anomalies of the coronary arteries. Am. J. Cardiol., 25:474, 1970.
†This category does not include cases of adult anomalous origin of the right or left coronary artery from the pulmonary artery.

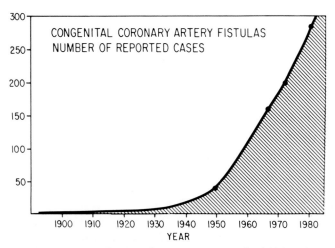

Figure 54–54. This graph represents a total of 286 patients with congenital coronary fistulas, including 28 in the present series from Duke University Medical Center. Increased numbers are being recognized each year because of the widespread use of cardiac catheterization and selective coronary arteriography in the evaluation of cardiac problems. (From Lowe, J. E., Oldham, H. N., Jr., and Sabiston, D. C., Jr.: Surgical management of congenital coronary artery fistulas. Ann. Surg., *194*:371, 1981.)

TABLE 54–8. MAJOR PRESENTING CLINICAL MANIFESTATIONS OF CORONARY ARTERY FISTULAS WHEN PRESENT AS SOLE CARDIAC ANOMALY*

	No. of Cases	Percentage of Total
Asymptomatic murmur	67	45
Dyspnea on exertion; fatigue	34	22
Congestive heart failure	21	14
Angina or nonspecific chest pain	10	7
Bacterial endocarditis	9	6
Frequent upper respiratory infections	9	6
Total	150	

*From Daniel, T. M., Graham, T. P., and Sabiston, D. C., Jr.: Coronary artery-right ventricular fistula with congestive heart failure: Surgical correction in the neonatal period. Surgery, *67*:985, 1970.

the most common of the congenital coronary malformations. Coronary artery fistulas are found in 1 of every 50,000 patients with congenital heart disease and in 1 of every 500 patients who have coronary arteriography (Wenger, 1978). The right coronary artery is involved most frequently, and the abnormal communication most often is to the right ventricle, followed in incidence by drainage into the right atrium and pulmonary artery. Left coronary artery fistulas are less common but may drain into the right ventricle, right atrium, or coronary sinus. On rare occasion, right or left coronary fistulas may communicate with the superior vena cava. The size of the fistulous communication may vary widely but generally becomes larger with time.

Clinical Manifestations

It is commonly believed that most patients with coronary artery fistulas are asymptomatic. However, based on the authors' experience with 30 patients and supported by a review of 258 others reported in the literature, 55% are symptomatic at the time of presentation (Lowe et al, 1981; Lowe and Sabiston, 1982). Because the underlying pathophysiology is essentially that of a left-to-right cardiac shunt, it follows that the most common manifestation is congestive heart failure. Other common symptoms are angina pectoris, secondary to a steal of coronary arterial flow through the fistulous communication, and subacute bacterial endocarditis. Bacterial endocarditis, anemia, and glomerulonephritis in the same patient have been reported (Sabiston et al, 1963). Infants and children with this lesion may demon-

strate a failure to thrive. Less commonly, patients present with acute myocardial infarction, aneurysm formation with subsequent rupture or embolization, or symptoms secondary to pulmonary hypertension.

The major presenting features of coronary artery fistulas are shown in Table 54–8 (Daniel et al, 1970). The age of onset of congestive heart failure in 21 patients who had this feature in a group of 150 studied is shown in Figure 54–55. In addition, the age of onset of dyspnea on exertion, the appearance of bacterial endocarditis, and the age of onset of angina pectoris in this series are shown in Figures 54–56 to 54–58.

Congestive heart failure may actually appear quite early; the chest films and arteriogram of a 1-month-old infant with this complication are shown

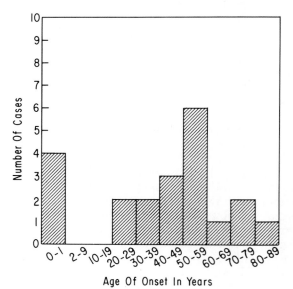

Figure 54–55. Age of onset of congestive heart failure in patients with an isolated coronary artery fistula. (From Daniel, T. M., Graham, T. P., and Sabiston, D. C., Jr.: Coronary artery-right ventricular fistula with congestive heart failure: Surgical correction in the neonatal period. Surgery, *67*:985, 1970.)

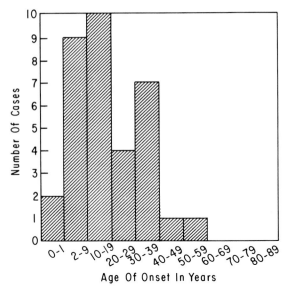

Figure 54–56. Age of onset of dyspnea on exertion or fatigue in patients with isolated coronary artery fistula. (From Daniel, T. M., Graham, T. P., and Sabiston, D. C., Jr.: Coronary artery-right ventricular fistula with congestive heart failure: Surgical correction in the neonatal period: Surgery, *67*:985, 1970.)

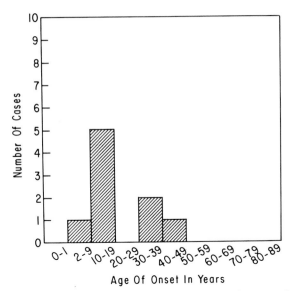

Figure 54–58. Age of onset of bacterial endocarditis in patients with an isolated coronary artery fistula. (From Daniel, T. M., Graham, T. P., and Sabiston, D. C., Jr.: Coronary artery-right ventricular fistula with congestive heart failure: Surgical correction in the neonatal period. Surgery, *67*:985, 1970.)

in Figures 54–59 and 54–60. The infant was managed by closure of the communication between the anterior descending coronary artery and the right ventricle, and clinical results were excellent. The postoperative aortogram is shown in Figure 54–61B (Daniel et al, 1970).

In patients who are asymptomatic, the diagnosis is usually made after coronary angiography is done

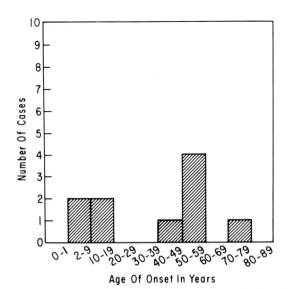

Figure 54–57. Age of onset of angina or chest pain in patients with an isolated coronary artery fistula. (From Daniel, T. M., Graham, T. P., and Sabiston, D. C., Jr.: Coronary artery-right ventricular fistula with congestive heart failure: Surgical correction in the neonatal period. Surgery, *67*:985, 1970.)

for evaluation of asymptomatic murmurs, mild cardiomegaly discovered on routine chest film, or persistent electrocardiographic abnormalities.

The main clinical manifestation of coronary artery fistulas is a continuous murmur over the site of the abnormal communication. This murmur may closely resemble that of a patent ductus arteriosus, and, in fact, the first patient on whom closure was performed was operated on by Bjork and Crafoord in 1947 for a presumed patent ductus. Because a patent ductus was not found, the pericardium was opened, and a coronary artery fistula draining into the pulmonary artery was identified and obliterated. The differential diagnosis of coronary artery fistulas, in addition to patent ductus arteriosus, includes congenital aortic-pulmonary fistulas, sinus of Valsalva fistulas, ventricular septal defect with aortic insufficiency, pulmonary arteriovenous malformations, and fistulas of systemic vessels such as the subclavian and internal mammary arteries connecting to veins of the chest wall or to the lung.

Involved Coronary Artery and Site of Fistulous Communication. The right coronary artery is most often involved in the development of a congenital coronary artery fistula (56%) (Table 54–9) and most commonly communicates with a chamber of the right side of the heart (Table 54–10). The fistula usually involves the right ventricle (39%), followed closely in incidence by drainage into the right atrium (33%), including the coronary sinus and superior vena cava, or the pulmonary artery (20%). Left coronary artery fistulas are less common but usually drain into the right ventricle or right atrium. Rarely, coronary artery fistulas may drain into the left atrium or left ventricle.

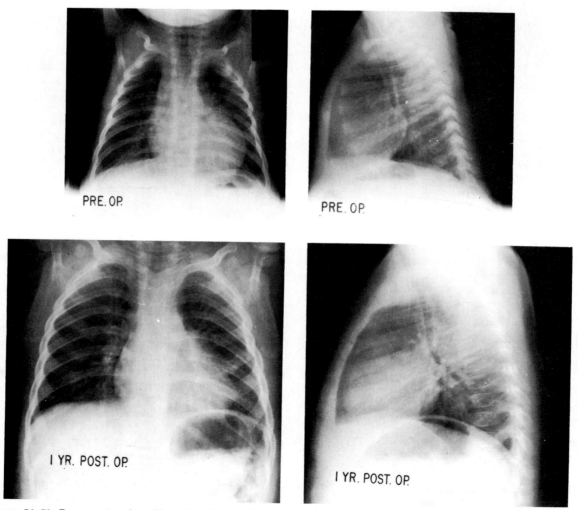

PRE. OP.

PRE. OP.

I YR. POST. OP.

I YR. POST. OP.

Figure 54–59. Preoperative chest films of an infant with a coronary artery fistula at 5 weeks of age. The interpretation included biventricular enlargement, left atrial enlargement, and increased pulmonary vasculature. Chest films 1 year after operation show decrease in cardiomegaly. (From Daniel, T. M., Graham, T. P., and Sabiston, D. C., Jr.: Coronary artery-right ventricular fistula with congestive heart failure: Surgical correction in the neonatal period. Surgery, *67*:985, 1970.)

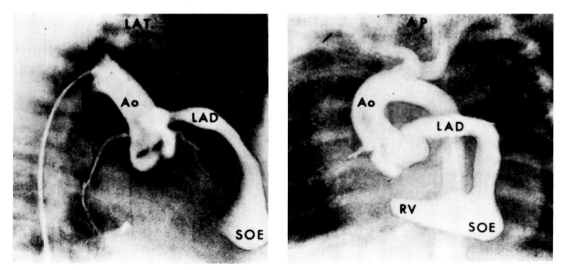

Figure 54–60. Ascending aortogram (lateral and anteroposterior views) in a 6-week-old infant who presented with severe congestive heart failure. The aortogram shows a left coronary artery-right ventricular fistula. (Ao = aorta; LAD = left anterior descending coronary; SOE = site of entry of the fistula into the right ventricle; RV = incompletely opacified right ventricle.) (From Daniel, T. M., Graham, T. P., and Sabiston, D. C., Jr.: Coronary artery-right ventricular fistula with congestive heart failure: Surgical correction in the neonatal period. Surgery, *67*:985, 1970.)

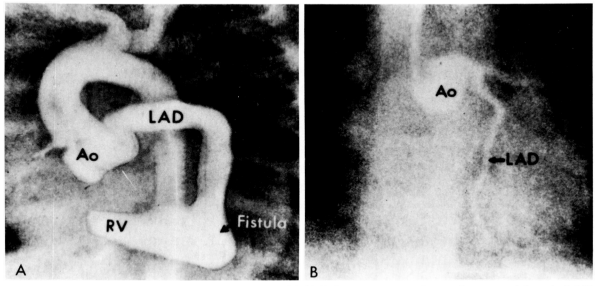

Figure 54–61. *A,* Preoperative aortogram of patient in Figure 54–60. *B,* Repeat aortogram 1 year after successful surgical obliteration of the fistula. The left anterior descending coronary artery has returned to normal size. (From Daniel, T. M., Graham, T. P., and Sabiston, D. C., Jr.: Coronary artery-right ventricular fistula with congestive heart failure: Surgical correction in the neonatal period. Surgery, *67*:985, 1970.)

TABLE 54–9. CONGENITAL CORONARY ARTERY FISTULAS—INVOLVED CORONARY ARTERY IN 286 PATIENTS*

	%
Right coronary artery	56
Left coronary artery	36
Both right and left coronary arteries	5
Single coronary artery	3

*From Lowe, J. E., Oldham, H. N., Jr., and Sabiston, D. C., Jr.: Surgical management of congenital coronary artery fistulas. Ann. Surg., 194:371, 1981.

Evaluation

The successful surgical management of patients with congenital coronary artery fistulas depends on a thorough preoperative evaluation that precisely defines the anatomy and pathophysiology of the anomaly. Although echocardiography (Barton et al, 1986; Pickoff et al, 1982; Reeder et al, 1980) and computed chest tomography (Slater et al, 1984) have been used to noninvasively identify coronary fistulas, the precise diagnosis requires arteriographic demonstration of the involved coronary artery, the recipient cardiac chamber, and the exact site of communication. It should be emphasized that the clinical manifestations and the radiographic and electrocardiographic findings do not exclude other lesions such as patent ductus arteriosus, sinus of Valsalva fistulas, or a ventricular septal defect with aortic insufficiency. In patients with a large fistula, injection of contrast medium into the aortic root may clearly delineate the lesion. In patients with a smaller fistula or fistulous communications from both coronary arteries, selective coronary arteriography is preferable and may be essential to establish the diagnosis.

Based on the authors' experience and supported by that of others in the literature, it is recommended that almost all patients with a major coronary artery fistula be considered to be candidates for surgical correction. In most cases, the natural history of these lesions is not associated with a normal life expectancy because of the eventual development of congestive heart failure, angina, myocardial infarction, subacute bacterial endocarditis, aneurysm formation with rupture or embolization, or the development of pulmo-

TABLE 54–10. CONGENITAL CORONARY ARTERY FISTULAS—SITE OF FISTULOUS COMMUNICATION IN 286 PATIENTS*

	%
Right ventricle	39
Right atrium (coronary sinus, superior vena cava)	33
Pulmonary artery	20
Left atrium	6
Left ventricle	2

*From Lowe, J. E., Oldham, H. N., Jr., and Sabiston, D. C., Jr.: Surgical management of congenital coronary artery fistulas. Ann. Surg., 194:371, 1981.

nary hypertension. Spontaneous closure of a coronary fistula is rare, and only two documented cases have been reported (Griffiths et al, 1983; Mahoney et al, 1982). It should be emphasized that the ideal time for elective surgical closure is before the development of symptoms and major pathologic changes in the heart, the coronary arteries, and the pulmonary circulation. As shown by Liberthson and associates (1979), most patients with congenital coronary artery fistulas develop both symptoms and fistula-related complications with increased age and are subject to increased morbidity and mortality when operation is done later in life.

Surgical Management

Because patients with coronary artery fistulas have had a precise and detailed angiographic examination showing the involved coronary artery, the recipient cardiac chamber, and the exact site of communication, it can often be anticipated preoperatively whether cardiopulmonary bypass is required. Patients with a single communication that is easily dissected usually do not require bypass for suture obliteration. However, in patients with multiple communications or large, tortuous, draining channels, the fistula is best obliterated by opening the recipient cardiac chamber with the patient on bypass in order to completely close all fistulous tracts. Finally, if fistula obliteration in any way jeopardizes distal coronary arterial flow, a saphenous vein or internal mammary bypass graft should be placed under hypothermic potassium cardioplegic arrest. In any event, these procedures are always planned with pump stand-by.

After a median sternotomy or anterior thoracotomy is done and a pericardial cradle is created, the fistulous communication is dissected and obliterated by using multiple transfixion sutures of nonabsorbable material. If a cardiac chamber or the main pulmonary artery must be opened to close larger or multiple fistulous tracts, the patient is placed on cardiopulmonary bypass (Figs. 54–62 to 54–64). An arterial perfusion cannula is placed in the ascending aorta or femoral artery, and venous return cannulas are placed in the superior and inferior venae cavae. Tapes are placed around both the inferior and superior venae cavae. If the right atrium, right ventricle, or pulmonary artery is opened, the tapes are drawn tightly around the venous cannulas to prevent venous return to the right side of the heart except for coronary sinus flow. The heart is then fibrillated, and the recipient cardiac chamber is opened. If the fistulous communication is with the left side of the heart and obliteration requires opening the left atrium or left ventricle or if saphenous vein bypass grafting is planned, the aorta is cross-clamped by using cold potassium cardioplegic arrest and topical hypothermia. After operative correction, intraoperative shunt curves are obtained to be certain that there is no residual left-to-right shunt.

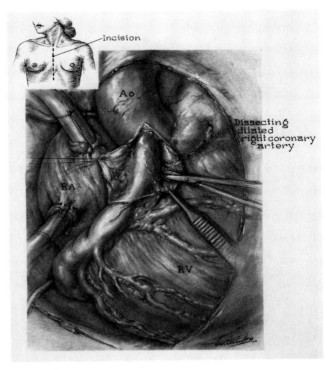

Figure 54–62. Right coronary-right atrial congenital coronary fistula as seen at operation in a 76-year-old woman who presented with severe congestive heart failure. Through a median sternotomy, the patient was placed on cardiopulmonary bypass with separate venous return cannulas placed in the superior and inferior venae cavae. (From Lowe, J. E., and Sabiston, D. C., Jr.: Congenital coronary malformations. *In* Cohn, L. [ed]: Modern Technics in Surgery, Cardiac-Thoracic Surgery. Mt. Kisco, NY, Futura Publishing Co., 1981.)

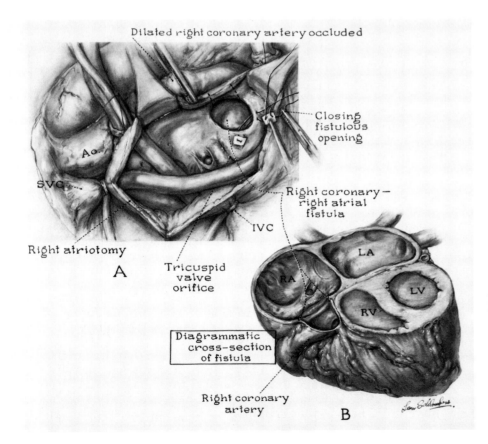

Figure 54–63. Tapes are secured around the superior and inferior venae cavae to eliminate venous return to the right atrium. The heart is then fibrillated and the right atrium is opened. The large fistulous opening is identified and closed by using interrupted nonabsorbable pledgeted sutures (*A*). The site of entry into the right coronary fistula is shown in *B*. (From Lowe, J. E., and Sabiston, D. C., Jr.: Congenital coronary malformations. *In* Cohn, L. [ed]: Modern Technics in Surgery, Cardiac-Thoracic Surgery. Mt. Kisco, NY, Futura Publishing Co., 1981.)

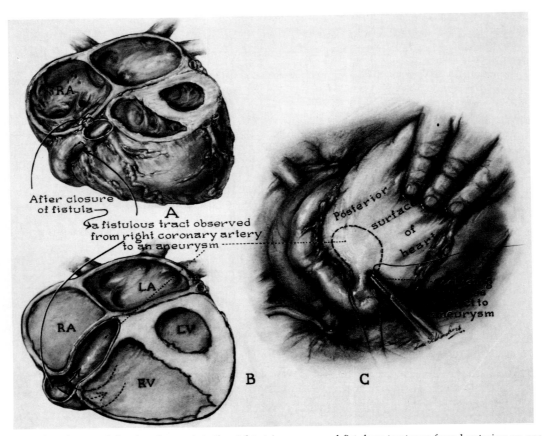

Figure 54–64. After closure of the site of entry into the right atrium, a second fistulous tract was found entering an aneurysm over the posterior surface of the heart (*A* and *B*). This fistulous tract was closed by using multiple transfixion sutures (*C*). (From Lowe, J. E., and Sabiston, D. C., Jr.: Congenital coronary malformations. *In* Cohn, L. [ed]: Modern Technics in Surgery, Cardiac-Thoracic Surgery. Mt. Kisco, NY, Futura Publishing Co., 1981.)

Thirty patients with congenital coronary artery fistulas have been evaluated at the Duke University Medical Center. These patients were between 6 weeks and 76 years of age, with a mean of 32 years and equal distribution between males and females. Half of the patients came to surgical attention because of symptoms such as congestive heart failure, angina, or failure to thrive. The remainder were asymptomatic and came to operation after evaluation of asymptomatic heart murmurs or cardiomegaly found on a routine chest film. Twenty-three of these patients have had operative repair. All procedures were done through a median sternotomy, and 14 patients had suture obliteration of the fistula without bypass (61%). Seven patients had cardiopulmonary bypass to open the recipient cardiac chamber and successfully occlude multiple draining fistulous tracts (30%). Two patients had saphenous vein bypass grafting after fistula obliteration in order to reconstitute distal coronary flow (9%). The mean time of follow-up for these 23 patients has been 10 years. There were no operative deaths, and all patients are well and do not have evidence of recurrent fistula formation, although one patient with a complex fistula of the circumflex coronary artery to the right ventricle has a small residual shunt (Lowe and Sabiston, 1982).

Urrutia-S and associates (1983) reported similar surgical results in 56 patients with an overall survival of 98.3%.

CONGENITAL ORIGIN OF THE LEFT CORONARY ARTERY FROM THE PULMONARY ARTERY

Abbott (1908) first described a left coronary artery originating from the pulmonary artery. Abrikossoff (1911) reported a 5-month-old infant who died of congestive heart failure and was found to have an aneurysm of the left ventricle at post-mortem examination. Photomicrographs of the ventricle revealed infarction, including areas of calcification. Bland and colleagues (1933) described the electrocardiographic changes in an infant with this malformation and showed for the first time that a diagnosis could be established during life.

It is generally recognized that the prognosis for most patients with origin of the left coronary artery from the pulmonary artery is poor. It has been estimated that 95% of patients with this anomaly die within the first year of life unless surgical therapy is undertaken (Keith, 1959).

The pathophysiology of this malformation was poorly understood for many years, but evidence in the past has now made this aspect relatively straight-forward. Numerous studies of post-mortem speci-mens clearly reveal the presence of many collaterals that originate from the right coronary artery and connect to the left coronary artery. If the right coro-nary artery is injected in post-mortem specimens, branches of the left coronary artery fill easily and in significant amounts (Case et al, 1958). It has also been observed at the time of operation that occlusion of the left coronary artery at its anomalous origin from the pulmonary artery causes an increase in pressure within the artery, suggesting that flow orig-inates from the right coronary artery by collaterals (Sabiston et al, 1960a, 1960b). Of additional signifi-cance is the fact that blood withdrawn from the left coronary artery at operation has been fully saturated with oxygen. Collectively, these findings are sound evidence that the direction of blood flow is from the right coronary artery by collaterals into the left cor-onary artery and then into the pulmonary artery. The resultant symptoms and clinical manifestations are secondary to left ventricular myocardial ischemia, which results either from inadequate collateral flow from the right coronary artery to the left coronary artery or from a steal of adequate collateral flow into the low-pressure pulmonary arterial system.

Clinical Manifestations

The clinical manifestations of origin of the left coronary artery from the pulmonary artery become apparent in infancy in most patients with this mal-formation. The infant usually appears to be normal at birth, because the pulmonary arterial pressure at this age is elevated and allows perfusion of the left coronary artery from the pulmonary artery. Never-theless, symptoms may be present at birth, especially if there are associated cardiac malformations. Symp-toms are most likely to occur during the first few months of life as left ventricular ischemia becomes more pronounced. When symptoms appear, the course is usually one of progressive deterioration. Unless operative therapy is undertaken, progres-sively worsening left ventricular dysfunction occurs, usually leading to death in infancy. Although most patients with this malformation develop symptoms in infancy (95%), a rare patient will survive to adult life with few, if any, symptoms (Abbott, 1927). In a collected review, Harthorne and associates (1966) reported 28 adults with this condition and Moodie and associates (1983) studied 10 adult patients with this malformation and provided long-term follow-up after surgical correction.

Symptoms. It was originally believed that symp-toms resulted from poorly oxygenated blood from the pulmonary artery flowing into the left coronary arterial system. As described earlier, however, var-ious studies have shown that blood flow is actually from the right coronary artery via collaterals into the left coronary artery and subsequently into the pul-monary artery. Symptoms result either from poor collateral flow from the right coronary artery or secondary to a steal phenomenon of blood passing through well-developed collaterals into the left cor-onary arterial system with drainage into the pulmo-nary artery. Because of the low pressures in the pulmonary artery, blood flow is selectively shunted into the pulmonary system instead of perfusing left ventricular myocardium. Two of the earliest and most characteristic symptoms are tachypnea and dyspnea. Coughing, wheezing, and cyanosis usually follow. One of the interesting findings that may be present has been described as the "angina of feeding," in which the infant shows evidence of pain during and immediately after feeding. As congestive heart failure worsens, cyanosis and pallor become apparent.

Physical Examination. The characteristic find-ings on physical examination include a rapid respi-ratory rate, tachycardia, and cardiac enlargement. A murmur is not usually present early in life, and congenital origin of the left coronary artery from the pulmonary artery is one of the few malformations that in infancy can cause congestive heart failure without a murmur. In older infants and children, mitral regurgitation develops secondarily either to left ventricular dilatation (Burchell and Brown, 1962) or to chronic ischemia or infarction, which results in papillary muscle dysfunction. The liver is character-istically enlarged, and the spleen is palpable in a smaller number of patients. Occasionally, patients first present with signs of cardiovascular collapse and shock similar to those manifested by adults with sudden coronary artery occlusion.

Evaluation

Chest Films. The chest film shows cardiomegaly, especially involving the left ventricle. Evidence of congestive heart failure may be present as well. Aneurysmal dilatation may result from marked thin-ning of the left ventricular wall. In many cases, the left border of the heart extends to the lateral rib margin. As a result of left ventricular failure, the pulmonary vascular markings are usually exagger-ated.

Electrocardiography. Considerable emphasis has been placed on the changes that occur in the electro-cardiogram leading to the establishment of a diag-nosis. Bland and associates (1933) first described myocardial ischemia on the electrocardiogram of an infant with this condition. Based on this work, con-genital origin of the left coronary artery from the pulmonary artery has also been referred to as Bland-White-Garland syndrome. Generally, it is possible to make a relatively firm diagnosis on the basis of electrocardiographic changes. Tachycardia is almost always present. The T waves are characteristically inverted in the standard limb leads, and slight ST segment elevation may be noted in lead I. The T waves in the precordial leads, especially V_5 and V_6, are usually inverted, and deep Q waves are frequently present. The body surface potential distribution has also been helpful in diagnosis and in providing evidence of improved coronary blood flow after operative therapy (Flaherty et al., 1967).

Noninvasive Techniques. Noninvasive tests to diagnose anomalous origin of the left coronary from the pulmonary artery include two-dimensional echocardiography (Fisher et al, 1981), thallium scans (Finley et al, 1978), and, most recently, pulsed-wave Doppler echocardiography (King et al, 1985). Too few patients have thus far been reported to determine whether these techniques can eliminate the need for preoperative cardiac catheterization. However, available results suggest that noninvasive studies can be used to accurately assess and monitor postoperative patients (Fyfe et al, 1987).

Angiocardiography. The right side of the heart is usually normal. The pulmonary vasculature may show slight engorgement and enlargement. The most striking feature is enlargement of the left atrium and particularly of the left ventricle. The wall of the left ventricle may be quite thin, especially the anterolateral aspect near the apex. A true ventricular aneurysm with paradoxical pulsations may be present, and mitral insufficiency is relatively common. Contrast medium passing into the aorta demonstrates a single right coronary artery, although selective coronary arteriography is more reliable for precise demonstration of this feature.

Aortography. Injection of contrast medium into a catheter passed into the proximal aorta (or when possible directly into the right coronary ostium) shows the classic findings. Contrast medium enters the right coronary artery as it originates from the aorta and passes through dilated collaterals that communicate with the left coronary artery. The contrast material can then be followed into the left circumflex and anterior descending coronary arteries, where it converges to enter the left main coronary artery, with ultimate drainage into the pulmonary artery. This finding is impressive and conclusive, and large amounts of radiopaque contrast medium can be seen flowing freely into the pulmonary artery. Thus, retrograde flow of blood in the left coronary artery can be convincingly shown in such a study, and this finding establishes an objective diagnosis (Fig. 54–65).

Cardiac Catheterization. Cardiac catheterization is also helpful in establishing the diagnosis. The right ventricular and pulmonary artery pressures may be elevated. Moreover, it is usually possible to show a left-to-right shunt at the pulmonary artery level by injection of contrast material. Although the oxygen saturation may sometimes show a significant increase from the right ventricle to the pulmonary artery, this increase is not always present, even when it can be shown that the left coronary artery arises from the pulmonary artery.

The ejection fraction in patients with anomalous origin of the left coronary artery has been determined in eight preoperative patients in whom it ranged from 0.13 to 0.72. Among those who died, the ejection fraction was less than 0.36 but in the survivors the ejection fraction was more than 0.55 (Menke et al, 1972).

Pathology. The major pathologic features of this condition are apparent at the time of operation. The left ventricle is characteristically greatly dilated, and the wall is thin. The left coronary artery is larger than normal, and numerous collateral vessels connect the right and left coronary arteries. These are usually tortuous and thin walled. The right coronary artery arises in its normal position and is also enlarged. Its branches tend to be more tortuous than usual as they emit various collateral vessels. With time, and especially in adults, the right coronary artery may become quite large and increasingly tortuous. Similarly, the left coronary artery may also become quite enlarged, up to 10 mm or more in diameter at its origin. The left coronary artery arises from the left or posterior cusp of the pulmonary artery. The branches and course of the anterior descending and circumflex branches are usually otherwise normal. On section, the left ventricle may be very thin and in areas is totally replaced by scar tissue (Fig. 54–66). Various degrees of subendocardial fibroelastosis may be present. Calcification is often present in the fibrotic portion of the left ventricle. Infarction of the ventricle may involve the papillary muscle, producing mitral insufficiency. If the left ventricle is dilated, the mitral ring may be sufficiently enlarged to prevent normal coaptation of the valve leaflets, also resulting in mitral insufficiency.

Surgical Management

It is now recognized that the prognosis for patients with origin of the left coronary artery from the pulmonary artery is generally poor when symptoms appear. Several surgical procedures were formerly advocated to improve the flow of blood in the left coronary artery, including a systemic-pulmonary anastomosis in an effort to increase both the oxygenation and pressure in the pulmonary artery; the production of a higher pressure in the left coronary artery by creating a coarctation of the pulmonary artery; and the creation of an increased blood supply to the left ventricle from the pericardium and other structures by means of irritants. Each of these operations has been attempted, but results have been disappointing.

Because it has been shown that blood flow in the left coronary artery is reversed or retrograde (blood flows from the normal right coronary artery through numerous dilated collateral vessels into the left coronary artery), an arteriovenous fistula is created, thus depriving the left ventricular myocardium of a supply of blood that is badly needed. This

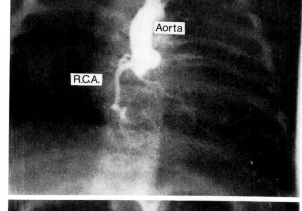

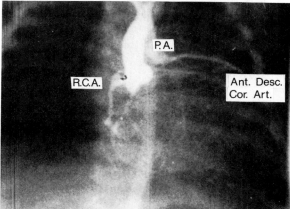

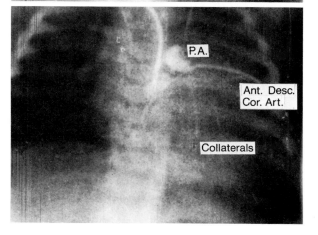

Figure 54–65. Several cine frames taken from a series illustrating coronary arterial filling during aortography. *A,* Filling of the right coronary artery as it arises normally from the aorta. Note that its size is slightly greater than normal. *B,* Filling of the branches of the left coronary artery through collaterals from the right coronary artery. *C,* Filling of the pulmonary artery by retrograde flow from the left coronary artery. (From Sabiston, D. C., Jr., and Orme, S. K.: Congenital origin of the left coronary artery from the pulmonary artery. J. Cardiovasc. Surg., *9*:543, 1968.)

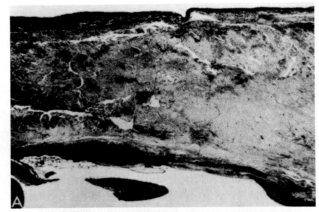

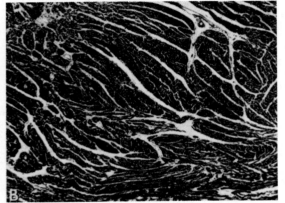

Figure 54–66. *A,.* Histologic section of full thickness of left ventricle. Note that the left ventricular wall is almost totally replaced with scar tissue. The section represents the full thickness of the ventricle and is magnified 12 times, showing the extreme thinness of the left ventricle. *B,* Histologic section of right ventricular myocardium in the same patient showing normal cardiac muscle. (From Sabiston, D. C., Jr., and Orme, S. K.: Congenital origin of the left coronary artery from the pulmonary artery. J. Cardiovasc. Surg., *9:*543, 1968.)

phenomenon has been shown by selective arteriography, in which the contrast medium can be followed from the right coronary artery into the left coronary artery with ultimate drainage into the main pulmonary artery. At the time of operation, blood aspirated from the left coronary artery and its branches is fully saturated with oxygen, indicating that it has a systemic arterial source. In addition, occlusion of the vessel at its origin causes a marked rise in the pressure within the left coronary artery. If the blood flow were actually from the pulmonary artery, a fall in the pressure would be expected. These observations led to the conclusion that ligation of the coronary artery would represent a logical procedure in the surgical treatment of this condition.

Two basic approaches are available for the surgical treatment of origin of the left coronary artery from the pulmonary artery. Simple ligation at the site of origin from the pulmonary artery is effective treatment if there are enough collaterals from the right coronary artery to adequately supply the left coronary arterial system. This approach is usually reserved for small infants, in whom the left coronary

artery is too small for a direct anastomosis. Ligation prevents the steal of right coronary collateral flow into the low-pressure pulmonary artery system. The major disadvantage of this form of therapy is that the patient has a one-coronary-artery system. The long-term fate of even large collaterals from the right coronary artery is unknown, and atherosclerotic coronary artery disease later in life involving the right coronary artery would affect flow throughout the entire coronary arterial system. Simple ligation, however, may be life-saving, and reconstruction of a two-coronary-artery system can be accomplished at a later time.

Rarely, a child may manifest severe symptoms during early life, with later remission of symptoms apparently due to the development of adequate collaterals (Ihenacho et al, 1973). An infant with a left ventricular aneurysm in congestive heart failure has been reported; treatment consisted of resection of the aneurysm and ligation of the abnormal left coronary artery at its origin (Turina et al, 1974). A combination procedure, resection of a left ventricular aneurysm and introduction of a saphenous vein graft from the aorta to the anterior descending coronary artery, has also been reported in a young child with anomalous origin of the left coronary artery from the pulmonary artery (Flemma et al., 1975).

If collateral flow from the right coronary artery is inadequate or if the patient is an older infant, a child, or an adult with large enough vessels, the initial repair can be designed to reconstruct a two-coronary-artery system. At present, this is best accomplished by either ligation and saphenous vein bypass grafting or ligation and left or right subclavian artery-left coronary artery anastomosis (Meyer et al, 1968). In younger children and infants, the latter form of therapy has technical advantages, because in this group, the subclavian artery is usually larger than autologous saphenous vein (Stephenson et al, 1981). Direct reimplantation of the left coronary artery to the aorta has also been reported (Grace et al, 1977). Finally, a two-coronary-artery system can also be created by intrapulmonary conduits from the left coronary ostia to the aorta. Segments of saphenous vein, free subclavian arterial grafts, flaps of pulmonary artery, pericardial tubes, and prosthetic conduits have all been successfully used, but their long-term patency rates are unknown.

Simple ligation is best accomplished through a left third interspace anterior thoracotomy. The pericardium is opened, and particular care is taken to avoid stretching or contusion of the phrenic nerve. Careful dissection near the posterior sinus of Valsalva of the pulmonary artery is necessary to ensure that the origin is identified. The left coronary artery is then clamped at its site of origin, and if this is tolerated, it is permanently obliterated, using multiple transfixion sutures, and divided. Left subclavian artery-left coronary artery anastomosis is also done through this incision, and the anastomosis is accomplished using interrupted sutures of 7–0 Prolene or Tycron (Fig. 54–67). If a two-coronary-artery system

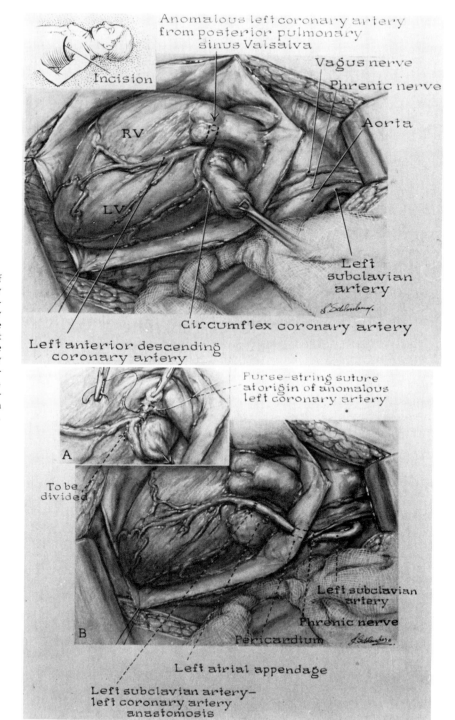

Figure 54–67. *A*, Congenital origin of the left coronary artery from the pulmonary artery. Through a left anterior third interspace thoracotomy, the left coronary artery is occluded at its site of origin with suture ligatures and is then divided. *B*, The left subclavian artery is then anastomosed to the left coronary artery in end-to-end fashion by using interrupted 7–0 nonabsorbable sutures. (From Lowe, J. E., and Sabiston, D. C., Jr.: Congenital coronary malformations. *In* Cohn, L. [ed]: Modern Technics in Surgery, Cardiac-Thoracic Surgery. Mt. Kisco, NY, Futura Publishing Co., 1981.)

is to be reconstructed by using saphenous vein, a median sternotomy is done, and the procedure is usually done with cardiopulmonary bypass.

The best form of surgical treatment for this disorder is unknown. In patients who survive beyond the age of 1 year, the proper form of treatment is controversial. These patients have been successfully treated by ligation of the left coronary artery (Baue et al, 1967; Roche, 1967; Sabiston et al, 1968), and others have been treated by anastomosis of the left coronary artery to the aorta either directly (Grace et al, 1977), by means of a venous autograft or a prosthetic graft (Cooley et al, 1966), or by intrapulmonary conduits from the aorta (passing through the pulmonary artery) to the ostia of the left coronary artery (Arciniegas et al, 1980; Takeuchi et al, 1979). Although the single best form of surgical therapy for this disorder is unknown, simple ligation in neonates with adequate right coronary artery collateral flow is generally recommended. In older infants, children, or neonates with inadequate flow, the authors' procedure of choice is ligation and immediate left or right subclavian artery-left coronary artery anastomosis. Stephenson and colleagues (1981) reported excellent results after using this procedure in six patients between the ages of 2 and 76 months. In older children and adults, a two-coronary-artery system can be reconstructed by using saphenous vein or internal mammary artery bypass grafting. It should be emphasized, however, that although the authors' initial experience as well as that of others with left subclavian artery-left coronary artery anastomosis (Pinsky et al, 1973) and saphenous vein interposition grafting has been good (Lowe and Sabiston, 1981), the long-term results in significant numbers of patients are unknown. In patients with adequate collateral flow from the right coronary artery to the left coronary system, immediate reconstruction assumes that vein graft or subclavian shunt flow is greater than intrinsic collateral flow. If this is not the case, the hemodynamics continue to favor collateral flow into the left coronary arterial system, which may result in subsequent vein graft or subclavian shunt failure (Anthony et al, 1975; Pinsky et al, 1976). Clinically, patients may continue to do well even with occluded vein grafts or subclavian shunts because of right coronary collateral flow.

The authors have evaluated 35 patients with anomalous origin of the left coronary artery from the pulmonary artery, and 25 have been treated surgically. These patients (20 females and 15 males) were between 1 month and 61 years of age. Nineteen had severe congestive heart failure, five had angina, and two infants came to attention because of failure to thrive. The remaining nine patients were evaluated for cardiac murmurs of uncertain cause, cardiomegaly, or unexplained dyspnea. All ten patients not operated on died within several hours to several months after diagnosis. Of the 25 patients who have had surgical repair, 14 had simple ligation at the origin of the left coronary from the pulmonary artery,

with five operative deaths (36%). Six patients have been treated with ligation followed by saphenous vein bypass grafting, and no operative deaths occurred. One patient was treated with ligation and left subclavian-left coronary anastomosis and has done well. Early in the authors' experience, two patients were treated with de-epicardialization and are long-term survivors. One early patient had pulmonary-aortic anastomosis and died shortly after operation, and one patient died during thoracotomy before a planned simple ligation. Among these 25 patients there were seven deaths, an overall operative mortality of 28%. Because of the 95 to 100% mortality in those treated nonoperatively, surgical therapy is definitely indicated (Lowe and Sabiston, 1982).

CONGENITAL ORIGIN OF THE RIGHT CORONARY ARTERY FROM THE PULMONARY ARTERY

Brooks (1886) originally described this rare malformation in two cadavers studied in the anatomic dissection laboratory at the University of Dublin. Both lesions occurred in adults, neither of whom had evidence of heart disease. Brooks noted dilated collaterals from the left coronary artery feeding the right coronary artery and correctly postulated, based on this observation, that flow in the right coronary artery might actually be retrograde into the pulmonary artery.

Clinical Manifestations

The clinical manifestations of this condition are usually minimal or absent. In the 17 cases collected from the literature (reviewed by Tingelstad and associates [1972]), the abnormal artery was discovered in individuals whose ages ranged from 17 to 90 years. The malformation was thought to have been associated with death in only two cases. One of these was a 17-year-old female who died suddenly and in whom autopsy showed complete occlusion of the left coronary artery by thrombus with evidence of left ventricular infarction. The only other reported death occurred in a 55-year-old woman who presented with angina and congestive heart failure. In three additional patients, the anomaly was found in association with other congenital malformations.

Even though origin of the right coronary artery from the pulmonary artery is a rare anomaly with a benign natural history in most patients, it can lead to myocardial ischemia, infarction, congestive heart failure, and myocardial fibrosis (Coe et al, 1982; Ross et al, 1987; Saenz et al, 1986). Because it can be safely corrected when diagnosed, operative correction is indicated.

Evaluation

In the rare patient with this condition who comes to medical attention, the diagnosis is established by aortography and selective coronary arteriography. The left coronary artery is found to be dilated, and large intercoronary collaterals feed the right coronary artery. As Brooks correctly suggested, flow in the right coronary artery is retrograde, emptying into the pulmonary artery. Compared with patients who have the more frequently occurring malformation of origin of the left coronary artery from the pulmonary artery, patients with origin of the right coronary artery from the pulmonary artery usually have no electrocardiographic or radiographic abnormalities. The diagnosis is therefore established only in those who have selective coronary arteriography. Two-dimensional echocardiography has been used to diagnose this malformation, which was confirmed later by coronary arteriography (Saenz et al, 1986; Worsham et al, 1985).

Surgical Management

A fascinating case has been reported of a 12-year-old boy who was asymptomatic but had a to-and-fro systolic and diastolic murmur along the left sternal border in the third intercostal space. The chest films showed slight cardiac enlargement and normal pulmonary vasculature. Mild left ventricular hypertrophy was shown on the scalar electrocardiogram. An aortogram showed a dilated left coronary artery arising normally from the left sinus of Valsalva of the aorta, and the right coronary artery was filled through tortuous intercoronary anastomoses from the left coronary artery and drained into the main pulmonary artery. At operation, a narrow rim of tissue from the pulmonary artery was removed with the origin of the right coronary artery, and this was successfully reimplanted into the ascending aorta (Tingelstad et al, 1972). This represents the ideal form of surgical management and has also been done successfully by Bregman and colleagues (1976), Coe and associates (1982), and van Meurs-van Woezik and co-workers (1984). Other alternatives include simple ligation at the site of anomalous origin (Rowe and Young, 1960), with or without saphenous vein bypass grafting.

CONGENITAL ORIGIN OF BOTH CORONARY ARTERIES FROM THE PULMONARY ARTERY

Twenty-five infants in whom both coronary arteries arose from the pulmonary artery have been reported. These patients have been reviewed in detail by Heifetz and colleagues (1986). The survival time ranged from 9 hours to 7 years. The patient who lived to the age of 7 years was able to do so because of severe pulmonary hypertension secondary to a ventricular septal defect and congenital mitral stenosis (Feldt et al, 1965). The pressure in the pulmonary artery was sufficient to force blood into the myocardial capillary bed, and under these circumstances, the child lived for an amazingly long time. This malformation has been diagnosed by cardiac catheterization, and surgical repair has been attempted (Goldblatt et al, 1984; Keeton et al, 1983; Ogasawara et al, 1985).

CONGENITAL ANEURYSMS OF THE CORONARY ARTERIES

In 1812, Bougon first reported an aneurysm of the coronary arteries. These lesions have been reported from infancy (Crocker et al, 1957) to adult life. Congenital aneurysms of the coronary arteries are rare and constituted only 15% of coronary artery aneurysms reported in 89 patients (Daoud et al, 1963). Other causes of aneurysms of the coronary arteries include atherosclerosis, mycotic aneurysms, syphilis, rheumatic heart disease, and mucocutaneous lymph node syndrome (Kawasaki's disease).

These lesions are most often asymptomatic until complications occur. Complications include thrombosis or embolization with subsequent myocardial ischemia or infarction or actual rupture of the aneurysm. Wei and Wang (1986) reported a 26-year-old woman who presented with a 3-month history of cough, shortness of breath, and vomiting. The patient was found to have a giant congenital right coronary aneurysm measuring 15 cm in diameter. The aneurysm was excised, and symptoms resolved completely. An intramural coronary aneurysm has also been reported and produced reversed flow during systole owing to bulging of the thin-walled chamber into the left ventricular cavity. The narrow neck of the aneurysm was closed successfully at operation. An example of a congenital coronary artery aneurysm involving the left circumflex vessel is shown in Figure 54–68A. In this patient, a mural thrombus occurred in the aneurysm; it embolized and produced acute myocardial infarction. The aneurysm was resected and a saphenous vein autograft was inserted (Fig. 54–68B and C) (Ebert et al, 1971). Surgical management of a coronary aneurysm is indicated if the aneurysm is symptomatic, especially if there is evidence of emboli arising from the aneurysm, producing myocardial ischemia in the distal coronary bed.

MEMBRANOUS OBSTRUCTION OF THE OSTIUM OF THE LEFT MAIN CORONARY ARTERY

Hypoplasia or atresia of the coronary arteries in infancy and childhood has been reported and usually causes severe impairment of ventricular function and sudden death. Congenital atresia of the left main

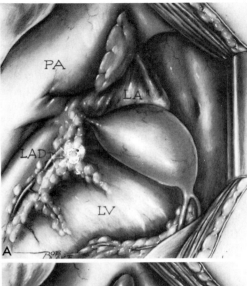

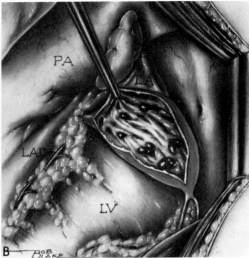

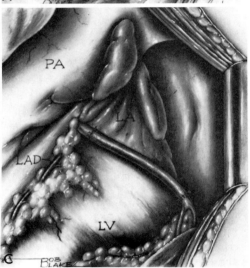

Figure 54–68. *A*, Congenital aneurysm of the left circumflex coronary artery as seen at operation in a 31-year-old woman who presented with an acute myocardial infarction with subsequent disabling angina. (PA = pulmonary artery; LAD = left anterior descending coronary artery; LV = left ventricle; LA = left atrium.) *B*, Numerous small fresh thrombi are shown adherent to the rough, irregular surface of the aneurysm. The proximal opening into the aneurysm was a discrete, mildly dilated vessel of good quality and normal-appearing intima. The distal branches of the circumflex coronary artery are of normal size. *C*, The entire aneurysm was excised, and an interposition graft of saphenous vein was placed. There was only minimal discrepancy in the size of the saphenous vein graft and the ends of the circumflex coronary artery. A continuous 7–0 nonabsorbable suture was used at each anastomosis. (From Ebert, P. A., Peter, R. H., Gunnells, J. C., and Sabiston, D. C., Jr.: Resecting and grafting of coronary artery aneurysms. Circulation, 43:593, 1971. By permission of the American Heart Association, Inc.)

coronary artery has been reported in nine patients, all of whom presented with signs and symptoms of myocardial ischemia, congestive heart failure, or both. Histopathologic studies in these patients showed that the left main coronary had been replaced by fibromuscular tissue and that the left coronary ostium was absent. These conditions are not surgically correctable. However, three patients have been reported with membranous obstruction at the ostium of the left main coronary artery, associated with a normal distal coronary artery. The first patient was a 6-month-old infant who died with myocardial infarction, and the diagnosis was established at the time of autopsy (Verney et al, 1969). Josa and associates (1981) reported two cases diagnosed at the time of operation. One patient, a 2-year-old child, was being operated on for congenital aortic stenosis and was found to have a membrane markedly obstructing the ostium of the left main coronary artery. The second patient was an 8-year-old boy with Type I truncus arteriosus; he also had membranous obstruction of the ostium of the left main coronary artery at operation. Both of these patients showed

evidence of myocardial ischemia preoperatively, and after excision of the membrane at operation, the symptoms were totally relieved. Grossly, the membranous structure appeared to be continuous with the aortic intima, and histologic studies revealed that its structure was similar to that of normal aortic root media. These two examples indicate the importance of careful evaluation of the origin and distribution of the coronary arteries in patients with congenital heart disease, especially when the signs and symptoms of ischemia and heart failure are disproportionate to the congenital lesion being evaluated (Josa et al, 1981).

Lea and associates (1986) reported a patient with congenital ostial stenosis of the right coronary artery that was repaired successfully by vein patch angioplasty.

Selected Bibliography

Abrikossoff, A.: Aneurysma des linken Herzventrikels mit abnormer Abgangsstelle der linken Koronararterie von der Pulmonalis bei einem fünfmonatlichen Kinde. Virchows Arch. (Pathol. Anat.), 203:413, 1911.

The classic description of anomalous origin of the left coronary artery from the pulmonary artery is made in this historic paper. Both the gross and microscopic illustrations are excellent. The author describes in detail the clinical manifestations and postmortem findings.

Daniel, T. M., Graham, T. P., and Sabiston, D. C., Jr.: Coronary artery-right ventricular fistula with congestive heart failure: Surgical correction in the neonatal period. Surgery, 67:985, 1970.

In this review, almost 200 patients with coronary arteriovenous fistulas are reported. The incidence of congestive heart failure was 14%. Approximately half of all patients with isolated arteriovenous fistulas were symptomatic. The age of onset of dyspnea, congestive heart failure, bacterial endocarditis, and angina pectoris is reviewed.

Ebert, P. A., Peter, R. H., Gunnells, J. C., and Sabiston, D. C., Jr.: Resecting and grafting of coronary artery aneurysm. Circulation, 43:593, 1971.

This paper describes an aneurysm of the circumflex coronary artery containing a thrombus that later embolized and produced myocardial infarction. A review of the problem, the clinical manifestations, and management are discussed.

Feldt, R. H., Ongley, P. A., and Titus, J. L.: Total coronary arterial circulation from pulmonary artery with survival to age seven: Report of a case. Mayo Clin. Proc., 40:539, 1965.

This paper presents the amazing report of a child who survived to 7 years of age with a coronary circulation arising solely from the pulmonary artery. This case report is clearly a fascinating one and is an example of the marked compensatory power of the coronary circulation.

Heifetz, S. A., Robinowitz, M., Mueller, K. H., and Virmani, R.: Total anomalous origin of the coronary arteries from the pulmonary artery. Pediatr. Cardiol., 7:11, 1986.

Four patients with total anomalous origin of the coronary arteries from the pulmonary artery are presented and compared with 21 previously reported patients. Of the 19 patients in whom a clinical history was available, 16 were symptomatic before 3 days of age. All patients died, 60% before 2 weeks of age. Longer survival was associated with additional cardiovascular malformations that resulted in pulmonary hypertension, increased oxygen saturation, or both. Cardiomegaly was present in 56% of patients, and most had myocardial fibrosis or infarction. Surgical correction has been attempted in two patients, but both attempts failed secondary to severe pre-existent myocardial injury.

Lea, J. W., IV, Page, D. L., and Hammon, J. W.: Congenital ostial stenosis of the right coronary artery repaired by vein patch angioplasty. J. Thorac. Cardiovasc. Surg., 92:796, 1986.

This is the first report of a patient with congenital ostial stenosis of the right coronary artery in which successful repair was accomplished by saphenous vein patch angioplasty. A biopsy from the region of stenosis revealed markedly thickened intima containing well-oriented fibrous tissue, whereas the media contained smooth muscle cells in mild disarray separated focally by mucoid material. There was no evidence of atheromatous involvement.

Lowe, J. E., and Sabiston, D. C., Jr.: Congenital coronary malformations. In Cohn, L. (ed): Modern Technics in Surgery, Cardiac-Thoracic Surgery. Mt. Kisco, NY, Futura Publishing Co., 1981.

This review presents the surgical techniques used to correct congenital coronary artery fistulas, anomalous origin of the left or right coronary artery from the pulmonary artery, and congenital coronary artery aneurysms. The details of the preoperative eval-

uation, anesthetic management, and postoperative care are also reviewed.

Lowe, J. E., Oldham, H. N., Jr., and Sabiston, D. C., Jr.: Surgical management of congenital coronary artery fistulas. Ann. Surg., 194:371, 1981.

This paper reports the clinical manifestations of 28 patients with congenital coronary artery fistulas seen at one institution and summarizes the results of surgical management in 22 patients. An additional 258 patients reported earlier are also reviewed. The natural history and pathophysiology of coronary fistulas are discussed, and the reason for early surgical intervention is presented.

Sabiston, D. C., Jr., and Orme, S. K.: Congenital origin of the left coronary artery from the pulmonary artery. J. Cardiovasc. Surg., 9:543, 1968.

In this report, 23 patients with origin of the left coronary artery from the pulmonary artery are described. The youngest patient was 1 day of age and the oldest patient was 31 years of age. The natural history, clinical findings, laboratory data, and ultimate course are presented.

Stephenson, L. W., Edmunds, L. H., Jr., Friedman, S., et al: Subclavian-left coronary artery anastomosis (Meyer operation) for anomalous origin of the left coronary artery from the pulmonary artery. Circulation, 64 (Suppl. II):130, 1981.

Six patients, ages 2 to 76 months, had subclavian to coronary artery anastomosis for anomalous origin of the left coronary artery from the pulmonary artery. Five of the six patients had congestive heart failure and ongoing ischemia. All six had cardiomegaly, and preoperative left ventricular ejection fractions averaged 0.46 ± 0.171. Five patients survived operation and were alive at 8 to 92 months after operation, and four of the five anastomoses were patent at postoperative cardiac catheterization. None of the surviving patients have required cardiac medications, and all of them are symptom free at follow-up. In addition to subclavian-left coronary anastomosis, multiple other surgical options including intrapulmonary shunts are discussed in detail.

Wei, J., and Wang, D.: A giant congenital aneurysm of the right coronary artery. Ann. Thorac. Surg., 41:322, 1986.

The authors report a 26-year-old patient who presented with shortness of breath and a chronic cough. A chest film showed a huge mass on the right ventricular border, and the patient was admitted with a tentative diagnosis of mediastinal tumor. Coronary arteriography showed a giant coronary aneurysm arising from the right coronary artery. At the time of operation, the aneurysm measured 15 cm in diameter. The aneurysm was resected, and histologic examination of the aneurysmal wall showed no evidence of atheromatous change. The patient recovered, and symptoms resolved completely.

Bibliography

Abbott, M. E.: Congenital cardiac disease. In Osler, W. (ed): Modern Medicine, Vol. 4. Philadelphia, Lea & Febiger, 1908.
Abbott, M. E.: Congenital cardiac disease. In Osler, W. (ed): Modern Medicine, 3rd ed. Philadelphia, Lea & Febiger, 1927.
Abrikossoff, A.: Aneurysma des linken Herzventrikels mit abnormer Abgangsstelle der linken Koronararterie von der Pulmonalis bei einem fünfmonatlichen Kinde. Virchows Arch. (Pathol. Anat.). 203:413, 1911.
Anthony, C. L., Jr., McAllister, H. A., Jr., and Cheitlin, M. D.: Spontaneous graft closure in anomalous origin of the left coronary artery. Chest, 68:586, 1975.
Arciniegas, E., Farooki, Z. Q., Haimi, M., and Green, E. W.: Management of anomalous left coronary artery from the pulmonary artery. Circulation, 62 (Suppl. I):168, 1980.

Barton, C. W., Snider, A. R., and Rosenthal, A.: Two-dimensional and Doppler echocardiographic features of left circumflex coronary artery to right ventricle fistula: Case report and literature review. Pediatr. Cardiol., 7:167, 1986.

Baue, A. E., Baum, S., Blakemore, W. S., and Zinsser, H. F.: A later stage of anomalous coronary circulation with origin of the left coronary artery from the pulmonary artery. Circulation, 36:878, 1967.

Bjork, G., and Crafoord, C.: Arteriovenous aneurysm on the pulmonary artery simulating patent ductus arteriosus botalli. Thorax, 2:65, 1947.

Bland, E. F., White, P. D., and Garland, J.: Congenital anomalies of coronary arteries: Report of an unusual case associated with cardiac hypertrophy. Am. Heart J., 8:787, 1933.

Bougon: Bibl. Med., 37:183, 1812. Cited by Packard, M., and Wechsler, H. F.: Aneurysm of the coronary arteries. Arch. Intern. Med., 43:1, 1929.

Bregman, D., Brennan, J., Singer, A., et al: Anomalous origin of the right coronary artery from the pulmonary artery. J. Thorac. Cardiovasc. Surg., 72:626, 1976.

Brooks, H. St. J.: Two cases of an abnormal coronary artery of the heart arising from the pulmonary artery. J. Anat. Physiol., 20:26, 1886.

Burchell, H. B., and Brown, A. L., Jr.: Anomalous origin of coronary artery from the pulmonary artery masquerading as mitral insufficiency. Am. Heart J., 63:388, 1962.

Case, R. B., Morrow, A. G., Stainsby, W., and Nestor, J. O.: Anomalous origin of the left coronary artery: The physiologic defect and suggested surgical treatment. Circulation, 17:1062, 1958.

Coe, J. Y., Radley-Smith, R., and Yacoub, M.: Clinical and hemodynamic significance of anomalous origin of the right coronary artery from the pulmonary artery. Thorac. Cardiovasc. Surg., 30:84, 1982.

Cooley, D. A., Hallman, G. L., and Bloodwell, R. D.: Definitive surgical treatment of anomalous origin of left coronary artery from pulmonary artery: Indications and results. J. Thorac. Cardiovasc. Surg., 52:798, 1966.

Crocker, D. W., Sobin, S., and Thomas, W. C.: Aneurysms of the coronary arteries. Report of three cases in infants and review of the literature. Am. J. Pathol., 33:819, 1957.

Daniel, T. M., Graham, T. P., and Sabiston, D. C., Jr.: Coronary artery-right ventricular fistula with congestive heart failure: Surgical correction in the neonatal period. Surgery, 67:985, 1970.

Daoud, A. S., Pankin, D., Tulgan, H., and Florentin, R. A.: Aneurysms of the coronary artery. Am. J. Cardiol., 11:228, 1963.

Ebert, P. A., Peter, R. H., Gunnells, J. C., and Sabiston, D. C., Jr.: Resecting and grafting of coronary artery aneurysm. Circulation, 43:593, 1971.

Feldt, R. H., Ongley, P. A., and Titus, J. L.: Total coronary arterial circulation from pulmonary artery with survival to age seven: Report of a case. Mayo Clin. Proc., 40:539, 1965.

Finley, J. P., Holman-Giles, R., Gilday, D. L., et al: Thallium-201 myocardial imaging in anomalous left coronary artery arising from the pulmonary artery: Applications before and after medical and surgical treatment. Am. J. Cardiol., 42:675, 1978.

Fisher, E. A., Sepehri, B., Lendrum, B., et al: Two-dimensional echocardiographic visualization of the left coronary artery in anomalous origin of the left coronary artery from the pulmonary artery. Circulation, 63:698, 1981.

Flaherty, J. T., Spach, M. S., Boineau, J. P., et al: Cardiac potentials on body surface of infants with anomalous left coronary artery (myocardial infarction). Circulation, 36:345, 1967.

Flemma, R. J., Marx, L., Litwin, S. B., and Gallen, W.: Left ventricular aneurysmectomy in infancy: Treatment of anomalous left coronary artery. Ann. Thorac. Surg., 19:457, 1975.

Fyfe, D. A., Sade, R. M., Gillette, P. C., and Kline, C. H.: Pre- and postoperative Doppler echocardiographic evaluation of anomalous left coronary artery arising from the pulmonary artery. J. Ultrasound Med., 6:101, 1987.

Goldblatt, E., Adams, A. P. S., Ross, I. K., et al: Single-trunk anomalous origin of both coronary arteries from the pulmonary artery. J. Thorac. Cardiovasc. Surg., 87:59, 1984.

Grace, R. R., Paolo, A., and Cooley, D. A.: Aortic implantation of anomalous left coronary artery arising from pulmonary artery. J. Cardiol., 39:608, 1977.

Griffiths, S. P., Ellis, K., Hordof, A. J., et al: Spontaneous complete closure of a congenital coronary artery fistula. J. Am. Coll. Cardiol., 2:1169, 1983.

Harthorne, J. W., Scannell, J. G., and Dinsmore, R. E.: Anomalous origin of the left coronary artery: Remediable cause of sudden death in adults. N. Engl. J. Med., 275:660, 1966.

Heifetz, S. A., Robinowitz, M., Mueller, K. H., and Virmani, R.: Total anomalous origin of the coronary arteries from the pulmonary artery. Pediatr. Cardiol., 7:11, 1986.

Ihenacho, H. N. C., Singh, S. P., Astley, R., and Parsons, C. G.: Case report. Anomalous left coronary artery: Report of an unusual case with spontaneous remission of symptoms. Br. Heart J., 35:562, 1973.

Josa, M., Danielson, G. K., Weidman, W. H., and Edwards, W. D.: Congenital ostial membrane of left main coronary artery. J. Thorac. Cardiovasc. Surg., 81:338, 1981.

Keeton, B. R., Keenan, D. J. M., and Monro, J. L.: Anomalous origin of both coronary arteries from the pulmonary trunk. Br. Heart J., 49:397, 1983.

Keith, J. D.: The anomalous origin of the left coronary artery from the pulmonary artery. Br. Heart J., 21:149, 1959.

King, D. H., Danford, D. A., Huhta, J. C., and Gutgesell, H. P.: Noninvasive detection of anomalous origin of the left main coronary artery from the main pulmonary trunk by pulsed Doppler echocardiography. Am. J. Cardiol., 55:608, 1985.

Krause, W.: Z. Rationelle Med., 24, 1865.

Lea, J. W., IV, Page, D. L., and Hammon, J. W., Jr.: Congenital ostial stenosis of the right coronary artery repaired by vein patch angioplasty. J. Thorac. Cardiovasc. Surg., 92:796, 1986.

Liberthson, R. R., Sagar, K., Behocoben, J. P., et al: Congenital coronary arteriovenous fistula. Circulation, 59:849, 1979.

Lowe, J. E., Oldham, H. N., Jr., and Sabiston, D. C., Jr.: Surgical management of congenital coronary artery fistulas. Ann. Surg., 194:371, 1981.

Lowe, J. E., and Sabiston, D. C., Jr.: Congenital coronary malformations. In Cohn, L. (ed): Modern Technics in Surgery, Cardiac-Thoracic Surgery. Mt. Kisco, NY, Futura Publishing Co., 1981.

Lowe, J. E., and Sabiston, D. C., Jr.: Surgical correction of congenital malformations of the coronary circulation. South. Med. J., 75:1508, 1982.

Mahoney, L. T., Schieken, R. M., and Lauer, R. M.: Spontaneous closure of a coronary artery fistula in childhood. Pediatr. Cardiol., 2:311, 1982.

Menke, J. A., Shaher, R. M., and Wolff, G. S.: Ejection fraction in anomalous origin of the left coronary artery from the pulmonary artery. Am. Heart J., 84:325, 1972.

Meyer, W., Stefanik, G., Stiles, Q. R., et al: A method of definitive surgical treatment of anomalous origin of left coronary artery. J. Thorac. Cardiovasc. Surg., 56:104, 1968.

Moodie, D. S., Fyfe, D., Gill, C. C., et al: Anomalous origin of the left coronary artery from the pulmonary artery (Bland-White-Garland syndrome) in adult patients: Long-term follow-up after surgery. Am. Heart J., 106:381, 1983.

Ogasawara, K., Aizawa, T., Fujii, J., et al: A case with fistulas from both coronary arteries and the left bronchial artery to the pulmonary artery. Jpn. Heart J., 26:597, 1985.

Ogden, J. A.: Congenital anomalies of the coronary arteries. Am. J. Cardiol., 25:474, 1970.

Pickoff, A. S., Wolff, G. S., Bennett, V. L., et al: Pulsed Doppler echocardiographic detection of coronary artery to right ventricle fistula. Pediatr. Cardiol., 2:145, 1982.

Pinsky, W. W., Fagan, L. R., Kraeger, R. R., et al: Anomalous left coronary artery. J. Thorac. Cardiovasc. Surg., 65:810, 1973.

Pinsky, W. W., Fagan, L. R., Mudd, J. F. G., and Willman, V. L.: Subclavian-coronary artery anastomosis in infancy for the Bland-White syndrome. J. Thorac. Cardiovasc. Surg., 72:15, 1976.

Reeder, G. S., Tajik, A. J., and Smith, H. C.: Visualization of coronary artery fistula by two-dimensional echocardiography. Mayo Clin. Proc., *55*:185, 1980.

Roche, A. H. G.: Anomalous origin of the left coronary artery from the pulmonary artery in the adult. Am. J. Cardiol., *20*:561, 1967.

Ross, T. C., Latham, R. D., and Craig, W. E.: Anomalous origin of the right coronary artery from the main pulmonary artery: Incidental finding in a case of dilated cardiomyopathy. South. Med. J., *80*:783, 1987.

Rowe, G. G., and Young, W. P.: Anomalous origin of the coronary arteries with special reference to surgical treatment. J. Thorac. Cardiovasc. Surg., *39*:777, 1960.

Sabiston, D. C., Jr., Floyd, W. L., and McIntosh, H. D.: Anomalous origin of the left coronary artery from the pulmonary artery in adults. Arch. Surg., *97*:963, 1968.

Sabiston, D. C., Jr., Neill, C. A., and Taussig, H. B.: The direction of blood flow in anomalous left coronary artery arising from the pulmonary artery. Circulation, 22:591, 1960a.

Sabiston, D. C., Jr., and Orme, S. K.: Congenital origin of the left coronary artery from the pulmonary artery. J. Cardiovasc. Surg., *9*:543, 1968.

Sabiston, D. C., Jr., Pelargonio, S., and Taussig, H. B.: Myocardial infarction in infancy: The surgical management of a complication of congenital origin of the left coronary artery from the pulmonary artery. J. Thorac. Cardiovasc. Surg., *40*:321, 1960b.

Sabiston, D. C., Jr., Ross, R. S., Criley, J. M., et al: Surgical management of congenital lesions of the coronary circulation. Ann Surg., *157*:908, 1963.

Saenz, C. B., Taylor, J. L., Soto, B., et al: Acute myocardial infarction in a patient with anomalous right coronary artery. Am. Heart J., *112*:1092, 1986.

Satomi, G., Endo, M., Takao, A., and Nakamura, K.: A case of right coronary artery to left ventricle fistula: Two-dimensional echocardiographic study. Pediatr. Cardiol., *4*:229, 1983.

Slater, J., Lighty, G. W., Jr., Winer, H. E., et al: Doppler echocardiography and computed tomography in diagnosis of left coronary arteriovenous fistula. J. Am. Coll. Cardiol., *4*:1290, 1984.

Sones, F. M., and Shirey, E. K.: Collateral arterial channels in living human with coronary artery disease. Circulation, *22*:815, 1960.

Stephenson, L. W., Edmunds, L. H., Friedman, S., et al: Subclavian-left coronary artery anastomosis (Meyer operation) for anomalous origin of the left coronary artery from the pulmonary artery. Circulation, *64* (Suppl. II):130, 1981.

Takeucki, S., Imamura, H., Katsumoto, K., et al: New surgical method for repair of anomalous left coronary artery from pulmonary artery. J. Thorac. Cardiovasc. Surg., *78*:7, 1979.

Tedeschi, C. G., and Helpern, M. M.: Heterotopic origin of both coronary arteries from the pulmonary artery: Review of literature and report of a case not complicated by associated defects. Pediatrics, *14*:53, 1954.

Tingelstad, J. B., Lower, R. R., and Eldredge, W. J.: Anomalous origin of the right coronary artery from the main pulmonary artery. Am. J. Cardiol., *30*:670, 1972.

Turina, M., Real, F., Meier, W., and Senning, Å.: Left ventricular aneurysmectomy in a 4-month-old infant. Alternative method of treatment of anomalous left coronary artery. J. Thorac. Cardiovasc. Surg., *67*:915, 1974.

Urrutia-S, C. O., Falaschi, G., Ott, D. A., and Cooley, D. A.: Surgical management of 56 patients with congenital coronary artery fistulas. Ann. Thorac. Surg., *35*:300, 1983.

van Meurs-van Woezik, H., Serruys, P. W., Reiber, J. H. C., et al: Coronary artery changes 3 years after reimplantation of an anomalous right coronary artery. Eur. Heart J., *5*:175, 1984.

Verney, R. N., Monnet, P., Arnaud, P., et al: Infarctus du myocarde chéz un nourrisson de cinq mois—ostium coronaire gauche punctiforme. Ann. Pédiatr. (Paris), *16*:260, 1969.

Wei, J., and Wang, D.: A giant congenital aneurysm of the right coronary artery. Ann. Thorac. Surg., *41*:322, 1986.

Wenger, N. K.: Rare causes of coronary heart disease. *In* Hurst, J. W. (ed.): The Heart. New York, McGraw-Hill, 1978.

Worsham, C., Sanders, S. P., and Burger, B. M.: Origin of the right coronary artery from the pulmonary trunk: Diagnosis by two-dimensional echocardiography. Am. J. Cardiol., *55*:232, 1985.

V SURGICAL MANAGEMENT OF CORONARY ARTERY DISEASE

1 Utilization of the Internal Mammary Arteries for Coronary Artery Bypass

J. Scott Rankin
L. Richard Smith

Two decades after the general clinical introduction of coronary artery bypass, this operation has become established as one of the most effective in history. In 1987, approximately 300,000 coronary revascularizations were done in the United States alone, and the procedure has been shown to improve the survival and well-being of most patients with coronary artery disease (Califf et al, 1989). Operative techniques are still evolving and clinical results continue to improve, despite the worsening of the average patient characteristics (Pryor et al, 1987, 1988).

A significant recent modification of this procedure is the routine use of internal mammary artery (IMA) grafting (Beggerly et al, 1987; Miller et al,

1981). This trend began in the early 1980s when it became apparent that long-term patency of IMA grafts was superior to that of venous conduits. Several studies showed improved clinical results in patients who had IMA operations, and many new methods extended the application of IMA grafting to most anatomic situations.

Most surgeons would agree that this trend has improved the clinical outlook of surgically treated patients. However, the extent to which IMA grafts should be used is still debated. It is generally acknowledged that a single left IMA is the minimal acceptable utilization in routine practice. However, some authors suggest that more frequent use of multiple IMA procedures will further improve clinical results. The purpose of this section is (1) to review the development and current understanding of the IMA as a conduit for coronary revascularization, (2) to describe in detail the standardized operative techniques, and (3) to assess recent clinical results of IMA procedures with special reference to the question of multiple IMAs.

HISTORICAL ASPECTS

Like many procedures in cardiovascular surgery, arterial bypass of the coronary circulation was first done experimentally by Carrel in 1910. A free graft of carotid artery was interposed between the descending thoracic aorta and the left coronary artery by using vascular anastomotic techniques, but the animal died of ventricular fibrillation. Although limitations in circulatory support precluded success, Carrel understood the clinical implications of this work. Murray (1940, 1953) experimented with coronary suture anastomosis and, in 1954, reported successful coronary bypass in dogs with both in-situ subclavian and free carotid arteries (Murray et al, 1954). Two papers published in 1956 described experimental IMA-to-coronary bypass (Absolon et al, 1956; Thal et al, 1956), and a succession of animal studies followed (Baker and Grindlay, 1959; Ballinger et al, 1964; Hall et al, 1961; Julian et al, 1957; Mamiya et al, 1961; Moore and Riberi, 1958).

In 1964, Spencer and associates combined microsurgical anastomotic techniques with cardiopulmonary bypass and hypothermic cardiac arrest to achieve a controlled operative field and excellent long-term patency of IMA-coronary grafts (Spencer et al, 1964a, 1964b). Kolessov from the Soviet Union reported six clinical cases of IMA bypass without coronary angiography or cardiopulmonary bypass (Kolessov, 1967). Green and associates initiated the first modern clinical series of left IMA grafts to the left anterior descending coronary artery (LAD) in 1968 and showed excellent postoperative patency (Green et al, 1968, 1970). Loop and associates (1973, 1986a) and Barner (Barner, 1973) later advocated the use of free IMA conduits, and bilateral and sequential IMA techniques were described later (Barner et al, 1985; Galbut et al, 1985; Harjola et al, 1984; Kabbani et al, 1983; Kamath et al, 1985; Kay, 1987; Lytle et al, 1983, 1986; McBride and Barner, 1983; Orszulak et al, 1986; Schimert et al, 1975; Tector et al, 1984, 1986; Tector and Schmahl, 1984).

Because of the popularity of saphenous vein grafts in the early 1970s, the more complicated and technically demanding IMA bypass did not emerge as a routine procedure, with a few exceptions (Barner et al, 1982; Green, 1972; Hutchinson et al, 1974; Jones et al, 1978; Loop et al, 1977; Tector et al, 1976). In the early 1980s, however, increased knowledge of limitations in long-term vein graft patency (Bourassa et al, 1986) and several studies showing excellent IMA performance changed the situation. By 1983 it became clear that IMA grafts should be used routinely, and this concept has been largely accepted by the medical community (Bashour et al, 1986; Gibson and Loop, 1986; Lewis and Dehmer, 1985; Olearchyk and Magovern, 1986; Speiser et al, 1983; Spencer, 1986).

GRAFT PATENCY

The long-term patency of IMA grafts in the coronary position has been shown to be superior to that of venous conduits (Barner et al, 1982; Cosgrove et al, 1985c; Geha and Baue, 1979; Grondin, 1984; Grondin et al, 1984; Jones et al, 1978, 1980; Loop et al, 1986a, 1986b; Lytle et al, 1984, 1985; Okies et al, 1984; Siegel and Loop, 1976; Singh et al, 1983; Tector et al, 1976, 1983). In most studies, early IMA patency was approximately 95%, but, more important, 10-year functional patency was almost 90%, compared with 25 to 50% for vein grafts. The propensity for saphenous veins to develop late postoperative graft atherosclerosis was largely responsible for this difference, while IMAs remained relatively free of disease. Although most long-term patency studies involved patients with recurrent symptoms or highly selected subgroups, the superiority of IMA grafts was so significant and consistent that this principle almost certainly is correct.

The biologic explanation for superior IMA graft performance is not clear. The IMA is a smaller conduit and is more closely approximate to the diameter of the coronary artery. For an equivalent flow volume, blood velocity is greater, which may reduce stasis. Vascular turbulence may be less with the IMA because transitional differences in geometry from the graft to the coronary artery are negligible and because arterial grafts have no varicosities or valves. The elastic and collagen support of the IMA wall is suited to arterial pressures, which may damage vein graft structure (Barbour and Roberts, 1984; Kalan and Roberts, 1987; Sims, 1983). The incidence of atherosclerosis in the native IMA is low (Kay et al, 1976; Singh, 1983), and the IMA is a living graft (Singh, 1985; Singh and Sosa, 1984; Singh et al, 1986). Thin-walled elastic arteries, such as the IMA, have few vasa vasorum to the arterial wall and receive most of their nutrition from luminal diffusion (Landymore and Chapman, 1987). Thus, the biologic processes of the vessel remain intact after grafting, even when the IMA is used as a free graft (Loop et al, 1986a). Potentially vital vascular mechanisms include (1) intact vasomotor activity (Dobrin, 1984; Jett et al, 1987; Lee et al, 1986; Schmidt, et al, 1980), (2) the capacity to enlarge with increased flow demands (Singh, 1985), and (3) an intact endothelium that produces prostacyclin compounds, fibrinolysins, or undefined substances (Chaikhouni et al, 1986; Mehta and Roberts, 1983; Subramanian et al, 1986). These factors, individually or in combination, may contribute to the excellent long-term patency of mammary artery bypass grafts.

INDICATIONS FOR INTERNAL MAMMARY ARTERY GRAFTING

In early series, a common indication for use of IMAs was the absence of suitable saphenous veins. IMA conduits have been thought to be better than other alternatives, such as cephalic veins (Prieto et al, 1984; Stoney et al, 1984), venous allografts (Gelbfish et al, 1986; Silver et al, 1982), or synthetic materials (Sapsford et al, 1981). As long-term patency data became available and IMA use expanded, other considerations became apparent. Young adults with coronary artery disease, almost by definition, have accelerated atherogenic diathesis and are more likely to have early vein graft failure. In the Cleveland Clinic study (Lytle et al, 1984) of patients who had coronary bypass at age 35 or younger, 4-year vein graft patency was only 56%, compared with 93% for IMAs. Persistent smoking, hyperlipemia, diabetes, and a positive family history of coronary artery disease negatively affected long-term survival. Thus, increased use of IMA grafts in young patients may be especially important.

Diabetes mellitus is a significant risk factor influencing the late results of coronary revascularization. In one series in which primarily saphenous veins were used (Salomon et al, 1983), perioperative mortality and complications such as sternal infections and strokes were significantly more frequent in diabetics. Even more significant was a direct association between diabetes and decreased long-term survival. After 8 to 10 years, the survival of diabetic patients was 15 to 20% lower than that of nondiabetics and the quality of survival was significantly worse, although the patients were similar in other baseline characteristics. This suboptimal prognosis was at least partly due to accelerated atherosclerosis in native vessels and in vein grafts. Therefore, increased use of IMAs with their better long-term patency may be advantageous for diabetics.

In patients who have a reoperation for vein graft failure, every effort should be made to use IMA conduits (Lytle et al, 1987). Because these patients have already had a negative result with venous grafts, reutilization of primarily venous material appears to be illogical. IMA grafts significantly reduce the incidence of reoperation (Cosgrove et al, 1986); thus, use of IMA conduits in reoperative cases may significantly decrease the likelihood of eventual third or fourth procedures.

In difficult anatomic situations (e.g., saphenous veins of poor quality in the elderly, small coronary vessels in women, or diffusely diseased but important coronary arteries) better patency and overall clinical success may be obtained with IMA grafts (Olearchyk and Magovern, 1986). In patients with severe ascending aortic calcification or Type I aortic dissections with associated coronary disease, proximal vein graft anastomoses are often precluded. IMA grafts increase the versatility with which these difficult problems can be managed.

In the authors' practice, unstable angina or severe left ventricular dysfunction do not contraindicate the use of IMA, although it is critical to ensure adequate graft function and myocardial protection (Rankin et al, 1984, 1985). Acute evolving myocardial infarction that requires emergency surgical revascularization does not always contraindicate IMA grafting. If a reperfusion catheter (Kereiakes et al, 1987) has been placed, the operation can be approached in a stable fashion, and IMA grafts can be constructed. A single IMA graft can be used even without a reperfusion catheter if the patient is otherwise stable, because IMA dissection adds only an extra 10 to 15 minutes to the ischemic period. With extreme hemodynamic compromise, however, more rapid revascularization with saphenous vein grafts would appear prudent. Finally, children who require coronary bypass for Kawasaki's disease (Kitamura et al, 1985) tend to have late vein graft occlusion; IMA conduits function much better (Hirose et al, 1986) in these patients and even enlarge with time in proportion to the child's growth (Kitamura et al, 1987).

In terms of patency, few clinical situations exist in which IMA conduits are not superior to vein grafts and probably also to percutaneous balloon angioplasty (Acinapura et al, 1985; Finci et al, 1987). If IMA grafts are better, one might reason that IMAs they should be used as much as possible and in most situations. This concept has led several authors to advocate more frequent use of bilateral, sequential, and free IMA grafts (Barner, 1973; Barner et al, 1985; Galbut et al, 1985; Harjola et al, 1984; Jones et al, 1986, 1987; Kabbani et al, 1983; Loop et al, 1986a; Lytle et al, 1986; McBride and Barner, 1983; Orszulak et al, 1986; Rankin et al, 1986b; Russo et al, 1986; Sauvage et al, 1986; Schimert et al, 1975; Tector, 1986; Tector et al, 1984, 1986). Other factors, however, must be considered. IMA grafting, especially with multiple IMAs, requires more operative time and *may* have a higher complication rate. An in-depth analysis of early risks versus long-term benefits is required to establish the propriety of routine multiple IMA procedures. This topic is discussed in more detail in later sections.

DRAWBACKS OF MAMMARY GRAFTING

Several potential problems of IMA grafting should be emphasized. The most important problem is operative recognition of the "inadequate mammary graft." Use of an IMA with inadequate flow for bypass of a critically jeopardized and important coronary artery may result in perioperative myocardial infarction and circulatory failure. If an inadequate IMA graft is suspected at the conclusion of cardiopulmonary bypass, the preferred approach is to rearrest the heart and to construct a distal vein graft to the coronary artery. However, routine operative testing of IMA grafts, including quantitative flow measurement, should almost eliminate this problem.

Inadequate IMA grafts are due to intimal flaps secondary to operative injury, spasm (Sarabu et al, 1987), unrecognized subclavian artery stenosis, anomalous arterial origins (Tartini et al, 1985), intrinsic atherosclerotic obstruction, and occlusion of the subclavian artery by the intra-aortic balloon pump (Rodigas and Bridges, 1986). Each of these problems can be identified by routine IMA flow testing and can thus be avoided. IMA occlusion by an intimal flap or spasm usually reflects operative trauma and can be prevented by more gentle handling of the IMA pedicle during chest wall dissection. The incidence of IMA injury decreases with the experience of the surgeon, but injury can occur rarely even with the most experienced surgeon. Routine flow testing should be an integral part of IMA procedures.

With either subclavian stenosis or intrinsic atherosclerotic disease, the IMA can still be used as a free graft if sufficiently long segments are available. Subclavian stenosis that develops late postoperatively can lead to the "coronary steal syndrome," which is managed with subclavian bypass from the carotid or contralateral subclavian artery (Bashour et al, 1984; Valentine et al, 1987). If the IMA is not properly positioned, it can be tented up and can become obstructed by expansion of the upper lobe of the lung. Strict attention to maintaining the IMA in a lateral mediastinal position, parallel to the phrenic nerve and medial to the upper lobe of the lung, prevents this complication.

OPERATIVE TECHNIQUE

Several successful techniques for IMA grafting have been described. This section describes the authors' method, which is simple, safe, and expeditious. In studies from this center (Rankin et al, 1986b), the technique has been critically evaluated with postoperative angiography and has been shown to produce 98% early postoperative IMA patency and acceptable clinical results. Although a surgeon may choose not to use multiple IMA techniques routinely, detailed familiarity with complex IMA methods is probably important, for example, when alternative conduits are required.

As the sternotomy is completed, intravenous heparin is administered so that blood shed during IMA dissection may be returned to the oxygenator. With exposure provided by the Favaloro retractor, the IMA is transected in the rectus sheath, and the distal branch is controlled with a metal clip. Early transection of the IMA helps to identify the vessel and prevents the forceful retraction and damage that can occur when the vessel is left as a sling. Narrow mammary pedicles are dissected from the chest wall, primarily by using low-energy electrocautery and working toward the apex of the chest. Excessive cauterization of the chest wall and intercostal nerves is avoided to reduce the possibility of a chronic chest wall dysesthesia syndrome. Care is taken to retract the mammary artery gently and to divide the small branches at some distance from the main IMA. In the superior aspect of the dissection, the IMA pedicle is left attached medially to the thymus to prevent phrenic nerve injury, but the graft is dissected completely from the chest wall anteriorly and laterally to the level of the subclavian vein. All proximal branches are divided to prevent competitive flow (Pelias et al, 1985). Above the level of the inferior thymus, sharp dissection and metallic clips are used rather than electrocautery to prevent electrical injury to the phrenic or recurrent laryngeal nerves (Phillips and Green, 1987), both of which can lie close to the IMA at the apex. After topical infiltration of papaverine solution by forceful spraying with a 25-gauge needle, the pedicle is wrapped with a sponge soaked in papaverine and placed in the pleural space while cardiopulmonary bypass is instituted.

As systemic cooling is begun, the locations of the distal coronary anastomoses are identified; the thymic fat pads are excised, and the pericardial edges are divided laterally with scissors to within 2 cm of the phrenic nerves. Proximal dissection of the IMA pedicles and the lateral pericardial incisions allows the grafts to lie along the lateral mediastinum, adjacent to the phrenic nerve and medial to the lung. This course provides the shortest distance to the heart, prevents stretching of the graft by lung inflation, and may decrease the likelihood of IMA injury if reoperation is required (Baillot et al, 1985). The distance to the coronary anastomotic site is measured with allowance for a gentle curve of the pedicle without tension. If extra IMA length is needed, the mammary vein and medial thymic attachments are divided, again with a sharp technique. Occasionally, the endothoracic fascia and adjacent pedicle tissue are incised transversely at multiple levels to attain extra length (Cosgrove et al, 1985b). After the necessary graft length and the anastomotic plan have been determined, the mammary artery is marked at the appropriate level with methylene blue.

The IMA pedicle is then transected a few millimeters beyond the planned anastomotic site, and free flow from the papaverine-dilated IMA is measured on cardiopulmonary bypass by allowing the artery to bleed into a 50-ml syringe for 20 to 30 seconds. IMA flow ranges from 50 to 250 ml/min at a mean arterial pressure of 50 to 60 mm Hg and can be used to estimate the "flow capacity" of the graft. A flow rate of 50 ml/min is acceptable for small coronary vessels, but flows that approach 100 ml/min or more are required for large LAD arteries or sequential grafts. Chest wall or sternal retraction during the procedure can influence radial artery pressure (Kinzer et al, 1985) and IMA flow (Graham et al, 1984). If a free IMA graft is planned, flow is still measured in situ before disconnecting the graft to ensure adequate function. If a question of free IMA adequacy remains, the proximal aortic anastomosis can be done first and flow can be measured in the eventual anatomic position.

To a certain extent, the flow rate is evaluated relative to the coronary vessel that is being grafted; a small IMA with a flow of 50 ml/min would be acceptable for a woman with a small LAD but inadequate for larger coronary arteries. If measured flow seems to be marginal, the IMA is discarded or is used to graft a secondary vessel, such as a diagonal. With satisfactory harvesting techniques and papaverine infiltration, IMA performance should be adequate for the primary vessel in approximately 95% of patients. If flows are extremely low despite a good-sized IMA, an intimal flap or an undiagnosed proximal subclavian or IMA obstruction must be suspected. The location of an intimal tear can sometimes be identified by palpating the IMA while it is flowing freely. The artery is fully distended with pressure to the point of the tear, but beyond the tear the wall is collapsed. After transection of the IMA proximal to the injury, good flow is usually established. If adequate length remains to reach the coronary artery, the IMA is left in situ; if not, it is used as a free graft. In patients with diagnosed subclavian artery obstruction, which is indicated by bruits and brachial artery pressure differentials, the IMAs can be used as free grafts. With less significant subclavian obstruction, IMA flow is measured, and the decision to convert the IMA to a free graft is based on the observed flow. Thus, measuring IMA flow capacity and matching graft flow to the coronary vessel under consideration prevent the disastrous results of inadequate graft performance. Assessment of the stream of blood alone is not as certain and often does not correlate with the measured flow.

After cardioplegic arrest, a 3- to 4-mm coronary arteriotomy is done, and the IMA pedicle is transected cleanly at the predetermined level. The interior of the IMA orifice is inspected, and if a small branch that may cause bleeding is visualized, the artery is transected again proximal to the branch. For large, thick-walled, or calcified coronary arteries such as the proximal LAD or right coronary artery (RCA), a small ellipse is removed from the arterial wall. The mammary pedicle is turned *180 degrees* so that the pleura lies away from the epicardium, and the IMA is then beveled on its undersurface for 2 to 3 mm. Care is taken not to strip the pedicle tissue from around the artery or to touch the arterial wall with instruments. The pedicle is grasped by the assistant (Fig. 54–69), and the suture line is begun on the side opposite the surgeon with 7-0 or 8-0 polypropylene and a 8- to 12-suture running technique. After the heel sutures have been placed, the anastomosis is tightened and the toe sutures are completed. The most important IMA (usually to the LAD) is constructed as the last graft. The clamp on the IMA is released, and the suture is tied as flow is established into the coronary artery. The myocardium should warm rapidly (Robicsek, 1985), become pink, and begin to contract within 30 seconds. In unusual cases in which this does not occur, an anastomotic error or other problem must be assumed and the suture line revised. Other factors that should be considered

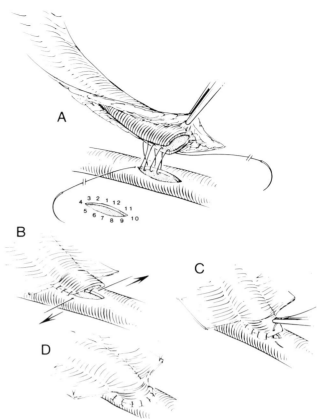

Figure 54–69. Technique of end-to-side IMA-coronary anastomosis. Stitches 1 to 6 are placed with the IMA elevated off the coronary *(A)*. The assistant grasps the pedicle with a forceps in the right hand and controls the suture loops with a forceps in the left hand. After stitch 6, the suture line is tightened *(B)*, and the remaining toe sutures are placed *(C). D,* The pedicle is sutured to the epicardium. For smaller coronary arteries, the IMA is beveled less, and (most commonly) 10 stitches (omitting 3 and 5) or 8 stitches (omitting 3, 5, 9, and 11) are used.

are unsuspected distal coronary occlusive disease and IMA performance that is inadequate for flow requirements. If either factor is suspected, the coronary artery is explored more carefully with calibrated probes, and then a different grafting site is chosen or a vein graft is inserted. Having the myocardium of the grafted region begin to beat with flow through only the most important IMA is an *absolute final requirement* that prevents the disastrous consequences of an inadequate bypass to a critical vessel such as the LAD (Rankin et al, 1986b).

Sequential IMA grafting (Fig. 54–70) is most often used with the diagonal-LAD combination but is satisfactory for multiple vessels in the circumflex or right systems as well. A good-sized IMA with a measured flow greater than 100 ml/min and ample pedicle length to reach the distal vessel without tension are required for sequential grafting. After both coronary arteries are opened and their suitability for sequential grafting is determined, the distance from the proximal to the distal IMA anastomotic site is determined as the intercoronary distance plus 1

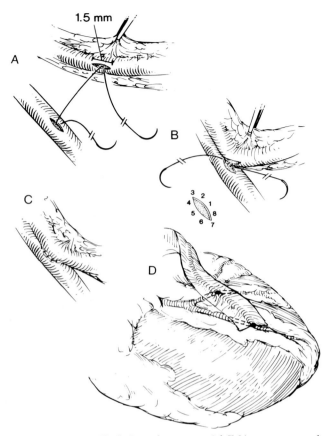

Figure 54–70. Technique for sequential IMA-coronary grafting. See text for details.

cm. To do the side-to-side anastomosis, the underside (chest wall side) of the IMA is freed of adventitia and is opened with a microsurgical knife (No. 5910 Beaver Eye Blade, Rudolph Beaver, Inc., Waltham, Mass). With microsurgical scissors, short (1.5 to 2 mm) longitudinal arteriotomies are made in both the IMA and the coronary artery; each opening tends to stretch during the anastomosis. An 8-suture running technique is used with 8-0 polypropylene; suturing begins on the side opposite the surgeon and proceeds counterclockwise. The distal anastomosis of the pedicle is then completed in an end-to-side manner, and the graft is opened. A parallel technique is used for diagonal-LAD combinations, but for circumflex sequentials both proximal and distal anastomoses are turned 90 degrees. The pedicle is sutured carefully to the epicardium proximally and distally to prevent torsion or kinking around the anastomotic sites. For anastomosis of smaller coronary arteries or for sequential grafts, microsurgical instruments are used. Before cardiopulmonary bypass is discontinued, the IMA pedicles, the anastomoses, and especially the tips of the pedicles are inspected for bleeding, and any obvious branches are clipped. When the lungs are first inflated, care is taken to position the IMA pedicles medial to the upper lobes.

Three general types of IMA grafts are used. With

the *in-situ left IMA* (LIMA) (Fig. 54–71), single or as many as three sequential anastomoses can be constructed to the LAD or circumflex systems. Most sequential grafts have two distal anastomoses; for a rare triple sequential graft, good coronary vessels and a very good IMA with high flow are required. The *in-situ right IMA* (RIMA) (Fig. 54–72) is anastomosed as a simple graft to the LAD, to the RCA, to the posterior descending (PD) coronary artery, or, less commonly, to the high circumflex marginal artery (CMA) over the top of the pulmonary artery. With adequate mobilization of the RIMA pedicle, the PD artery can be reached in most patients. Occasionally, a pledget-supported traction suture between the right atrioventricular groove and right lateral aorta is required to maintain a RIMA-PD graft without tension as the right atrium expands with filling. *Free IMA* grafts (Fig. 54–73) with simple or sequential distal anastomoses can be constructed to all three coronary systems. The proximal aortic anastomosis of free IMA grafts is done by using a method similar to that used for vein grafts (Fig. 54–74), except that 7-0 polypropylene suture is used and only a 2.5 to 3-mm circular aortotomy is made. For this delicate anastomosis, a soft, nondiseased aorta is desirable. Arteriographic appearances of the various types of IMA grafts are shown in Figure 54–75. Mammary-to-mammary circle grafts (Gold et al, 1985) or intercoronary IMA bridge grafts are not used at present, and RIMA grafts to the CMA via the transverse sinus (Puig et al, 1984) have been discontinued because of their propensity for retroaortic compression (Rankin et al, 1986b).

Three factors are considered when choosing the coronary arteries to be grafted with IMAs. First, the size and flows of the mammary grafts are matched to the coronary arteries, which was described earlier. Second, the IMAs are used to revascularize the vessels with the largest regions of normally functioning myocardium. This concept, in practice, translates into using an IMA for the LAD in most patients. If the anterior wall is infarcted, a vein graft may be selected for the LAD, and the RIMA and LIMA pedicles may be used for the viable RCA and CMA regions. Thus, IMA grafts are made not to the best vessels but to the *best myocardium*. In fact, the IMAs are often chosen for small or diffusely diseased coronary arteries, if the regional myocardium is judged to be important for the long-term maintenance of ventricular function. It is anticipated that IMA grafts will maintain better long-term patency to these vessels than will veins. An example of this problem is the diffusely diseased or segmented LAD. If a good-sized LIMA with high flow is available, up to three sequential anastomoses are made along the LAD, with the mammary artery ending at the apex. With a smaller LIMA, the mammary artery is usually used to graft to the distal LAD, and a vein is chosen for the intermediate segment. In the authors' opinion, sequential IMA grafting, with its excellent patency, is preferable to extensive endarterectomy for LAD revascularization in this setting.

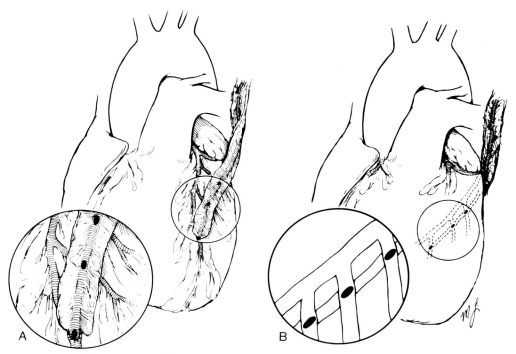

Figure 54–71. Methods of in-situ left IMA grafting. See text for details.

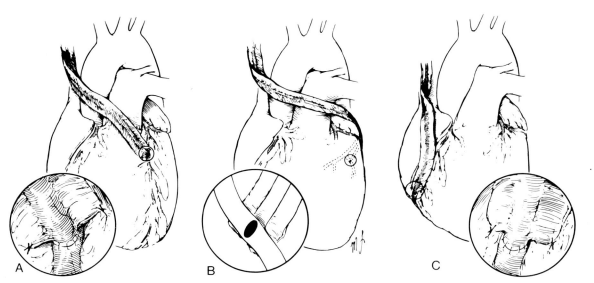

Figure 54–72. Techniques of in-situ right IMA grafting. See text for details.

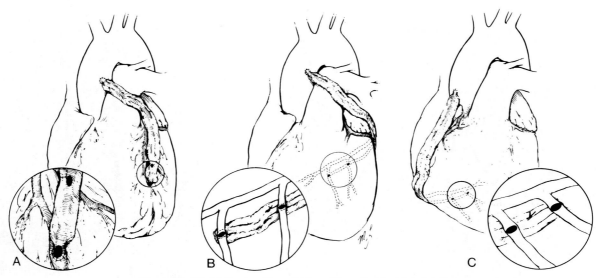

Figure 54–73. Methods of free IMA grafting. See text for details.

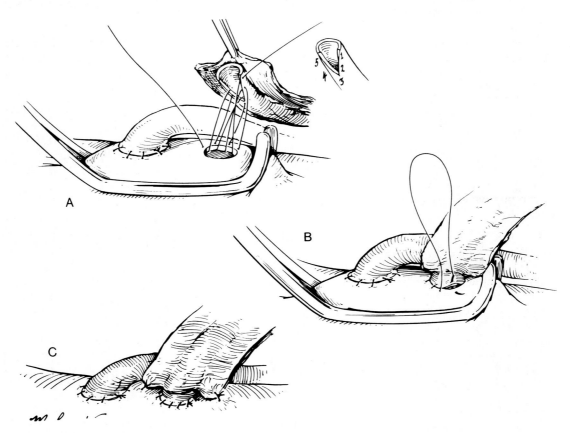

Figure 54–74. Proximal aortic anastomosis for free IMA grafting. See text for details.

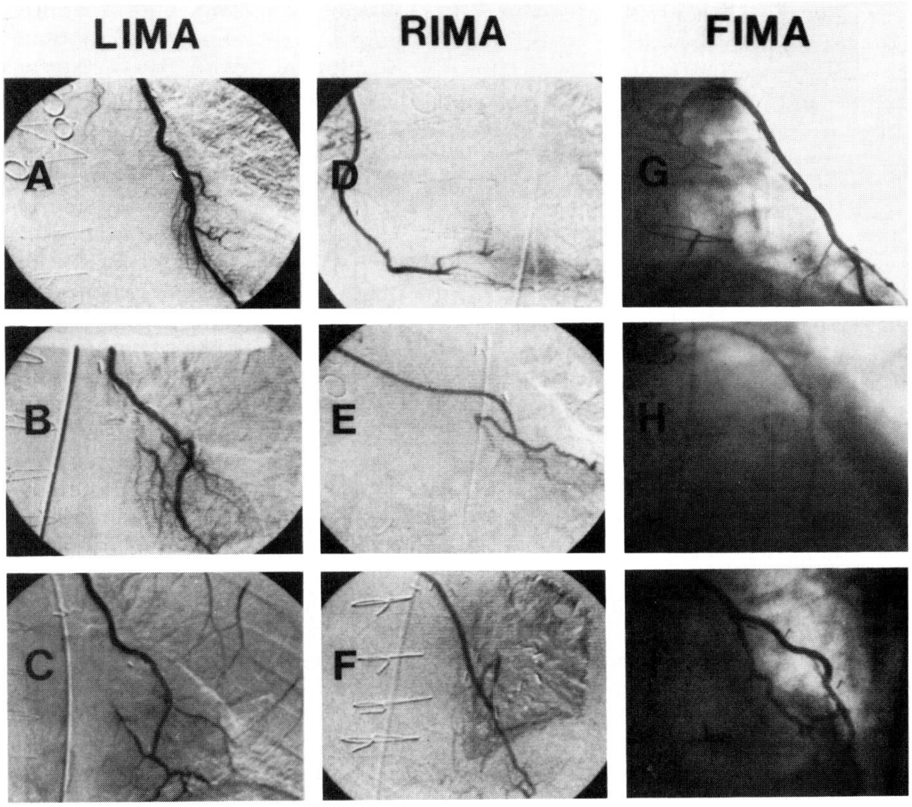

LIMA   RIMA   FIMA

Figure 54–75. Radiographic images of IMA grafts as defined in the authors' practice. *A* to *F* represent images obtained with digital subtraction angiography; *G* and *I* are frames from standard selective arteriograms; *H* is an unsubtracted digital arteriogram. *A,* Simple left IMA to LAD; *B,* Sequential left IMA to diagonal/LAD; *C,* Sequential left IMA to the first and second CMAs; *D,* Right IMA to RCA; *E,* Right IMA to CMA; *F,* Right IMA to LAD; *G,* Free IMA to LAD; *H,* Free IMA to CMA; and *I,* Sequential free IMA to the first and second CMAs.

The third factor that should be considered is technical feasibility. For example, an optional diagonal artery that courses lateral on the anterior wall is more difficult to sequence to the LAD than a more medial diagonal artery. In this situation, it may be easier and safer to construct a vein graft to the lateral optional diagonal and a simple LIMA to the LAD. Technical ease should not be the only factor considered, however. With bilateral IMA dissection and liberal use of free and sequential grafts, at least the two most important regions of the left ventricle, and often more, can be revascularized with IMA conduits in most patients.

THERAPEUTIC RESULTS

Mammary Graft Patency

IMA grafts have excellent patency in the coronary position, and the numerous reports of long-term graft patency have already been reviewed. Several studies have also shown adequate flow reserve of both simple and sequential IMA grafts (Hodgson et al, 1986; Johnson et al, 1986; Schmidt et al, 1980; Siegel and Loop, 1976). Reports on the intermediate-term patency characteristics of the newer IMA grafts have become available from a number of centers. The authors' study is representative of most and involved an 85% recatheterization rate for 207 consecutive patients who had coronary bypass (Rankin

et al, 1986b). The overall angiographic patency of 338 IMA grafts 1 to 32 weeks postoperatively was 98.6%. By comparison, vein graft patency in the same patients was 91%.

Simple LIMA grafts to the LAD had excellent patencies. The more complex types of IMA grafts also showed good performance, which was almost independent of the type of graft (Table 54–11). The patencies of sequential IMA anastomoses, RIMA grafts to the RCA or LAD, and free IMA conduits

TABLE 54–11. INDIVIDUAL GRAFT PATENCY RATES

Bypass Grafts*	Total No.	No. Patent	Percentage Patent
Simple SVG	285	262	92
Sequential SVG	218	196	90
Left IMA to LAD	110	109	99
Left IMA to CMA	14	14	100
Right IMA to RCA	20	19	95
Right IMA to LAD	10	10	100
Right IMA to CMA via TS	20	18†	90
Sequential left IMA to LAD	134	133	99
Sequential left IMA to CMA	15	15	100
Simple free IMA	9	9	100
Sequential free IMA	6	6	100

*SVG = saphenous vein graft; IMA = internal mammary artery; LAD = left anterior descending coronary artery; CMA = circumflex marginal artery; RCA = right coronary artery; TS = transverse sinus.

†Three of the 18 transverse sinus grafts showed slow flow.

were all exceptional when the selection and construction techniques described in this section were used. The difference between IMA and vein graft patency in the first postoperative year was significant, and this difference may become greater over time because of the more rapid vein graft attrition.

In this series, the one exception was the RIMA-to-CMA graft through the transverse sinus (Puig et al, 1984), which seemed to be predisposed to retroaortic graft obstruction (Rankin et al, 1986b). Because of this finding, the transverse sinus RIMA graft was abandoned in favor of other techniques, including free IMA bypass. RIMA grafts to the LAD, RCA, or CMA (lying anterior to the pulmonary artery) appeared to be satisfactory and are now used routinely.

One report (Huddleston et al, 1986) describing suboptimal RIMA patency is in direct conflict with the authors' results. As discussed by Green (1987), this disparity may reflect either a different study design that involved symptomatic patients or technical problems with use of the RIMA. One would not expect a biologic difference between the right and left mammary arteries, which suggests that technical factors may have been important. Most RIMA grafts in the reported series were used to revascularize diagonal or secondary arteries, which is not a contemporary utilization pattern. The results of most other studies, like the authors' results, indicate that complex mammary grafting yields excellent patency rates. This concept has led to increased use of bilateral, sequential, and free IMA grafts in many centers (Barner, 1973; Barner et al, 1985; Dion et al, 1988; Galbut et al, 1985; Harjola et al, 1984; Jones et al, 1987; Kabbani et al, 1983; Kamath et al, 1985; Loop et al, 1986a; Lytle et al, 1983; McBride and Barner, 1983; Orszulak et al, 1986; Rankin et al, 1986b; Russo et al, 1986; Sauvage et al, 1986; Schimert et al, 1975; Tector, 1986; Tector and Schmahl, 1984; Tector et al, 1984, 1986).

Operative Mortality and Morbidity

Complex IMA procedures are more technically demanding and usually require more operative time than saphenous vein bypasses. Therefore, operations with multiple IMAs have an inherent potential for increased complications, morbidity, and mortality. The use of new operative methods also involves a learning curve and, at least initially, may have an increased probability of complications. This problem can be minimized by introducing new methods individually (e.g., sequential or free IMA grafting) and by not combining techniques until each one has been mastered. Routine postoperative graft angiography helps to provide immediate feedback during periods of technical development.

Experienced surgeons can apply complex mammary methods without excessive operative morbidity or mortality (Barner et al, 1985; Cosgrove et al, 1985d,

1988; Galbut et al, 1985; Jones et al, 1986, 1987; Lytle et al, 1983, 1986; Rankin et al, 1986b; Russo et al, 1986; Sauvage et al, 1986; Tector et al, 1986). In many reports, including the authors' series, multiple mammary grafting in elective cases was associated with less than 1% hospital mortality. Urgent or emergency IMA procedures done in this population for unstable angina, postinfarction angina, or acute evolving myocardial infarction resulted in a hospital mortality of 3%, which compares favorably with vein graft operations (Rankin et al, 1984, 1986a). In emergency cases where immediate adequacy of revascularization is critical, careful IMA flow testing and graft selection are especially important.

Morbidity may be influenced by mammary grafting. Early reoperation rates for bleeding may be slightly higher, and postoperative blood loss may be greater because of more extensive IMA and chest wall dissection (Cosgrove et al, 1988). Blood conservation techniques, including autotransfusion (Cosgrove et al, 1985a), are useful after IMA procedures to minimize transfusion requirements. Perioperative myocardial infarction rates for IMA grafting are now approximately 2% (Rankin et al, 1985), and enhanced IMA patency may have a role in achieving low infarction rates. A higher incidence of postoperative respiratory insufficiency has occasionally been associated with bilateral IMA grafting but may have been caused by electrocautery injury to both phrenic nerves. This complication can be almost completely avoided with proper operative technique. Use of IMA grafts in patients with ascending aortic atherosclerosis may decrease morbidity by decreasing the incidence of cerebral embolization and stroke.

The relationship between bilateral IMA dissection and postoperative sternotomy infection is controversial (Breyer et al, 1984; Cosgrove et al, 1985d, 1988; Grmoljez and Barner, 1978; Grossi et al, 1985; Nkongho et al, 1984; Sarr et al, 1984; Stoney et al, 1978). Many studies of multiple mammary grafting reported no increased incidence of sternal infections. Others suggested that bilateral sternal devascularization predisposes to mediastinitis, especially in diabetics, and the results may vary from one center to another. Environmental or technical factors may contribute to these differences, and it is difficult to make definite conclusions on the basis of current data. The available evidence indicates that bilateral IMA dissection *may* predispose to sternal wound infection to some extent. In most contemporary analyses, the incidence of deep sternal infections with bilateral IMA grafting is increased minimally, if at all. With current management methods (Arnold and Pairolero, 1979; Herrera and Ginsberg, 1982; Pairolero and Arnold, 1984; Scully et al, 1985; Tobin et al, 1983) this complication should rarely cause mortality (Cheung et al, 1985; Nahai et al, 1982), and the projected long-term benefits due to enhanced graft patency could outweigh this early risk of infection. Conversely, if mediastinitis and other complications occur significantly more often with bilateral IMA grafting in a particular hospital, the early risks may exceed the benefits. The routine use of complex IMA grafts is an individual choice that depends on multiple factors: (1) the surgeon's interest and ability, (2) the risks encountered in a particular hospital environment, and (3) the observed long-term benefits. The understanding of many of these factors is evolving, and the exact role of routine multiple IMA grafting awaits the results of further clinical research.

Long-Term Survival

Several studies have examined the effect of IMA procedures on long-term patient survival (Cameron et al, 1988; Cosgrove et al, 1985c). Loop and associates (1986b) assessed 10-year survival and cardiac events in 5,931 patients who had coronary revascularization for non-left main coronary disease in the 1970s. Of the total, 60% had only vein graft operations, and 40% had an IMA graft in addition. There were significant differences between the groups that reflected operative selection biases: patients who had IMA grafts less often had left ventricular dysfunction, multivessel disease, severe angina, advanced age, and incomplete revascularization. In addition, IMA procedures were used more often in the later years of the study. After an attempt to adjust for differences in baseline risk factors by using the Cox proportional

hazards model, improved survival was observed with IMA grafting in most anatomic subsets (Fig. 54–76) and in patients with ventricular dysfunction (Fig. 54–77). IMA grafting significantly decreased the incidences of subsequent reoperation (Fig. 54–78) and nonfatal cardiac events (Cosgrove, et al, 1986).

Similar findings were reported by Green's group for 748 patients who were followed for 15 years postoperatively (Cameron et al, 1986). Survival appeared to be improved in patients who received IMA grafts, and multiple IMAs afforded an additional benefit (Fig. 54–79). Again, the incidence of reoperation was lower in the patients who had IMA grafts (Fig. 54–80), and event-free survival was enhanced (Fig. 54–81). As in Loop's study, selection biases produced significant differences in baseline characteristics; patients who had IMA grafts less often had ventricular impairment, left main disease, or incomplete revascularization. After adjustment for these baseline differences by using the Cox model, the long-term clinical benefits of IMA grafting still appeared to be significant. Operative mortality and complications were equivalent between groups, except that perioperative infarction was less common in patients with IMA grafts. Similar results have been presented from the CASS registry (Cameron et al, 1988).

It is important to analyze these studies critically. A significant concern with all retrospective analyses

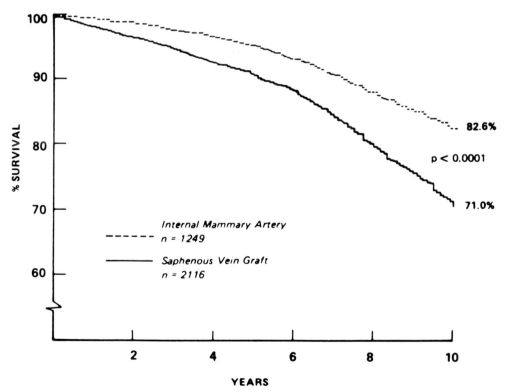

Figure 54–76. Unadjusted raw survival data for patients with three-vessel disease who were selected for coronary grafting with and without IMA use in the Cleveland Clinic series.

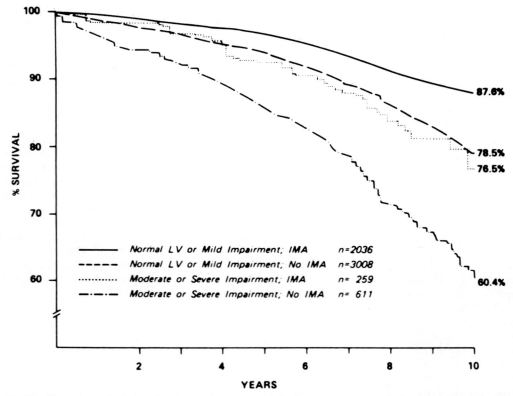

Figure 54–77. Unadjusted survival data for four subgroups who had coronary revascularization with and without IMA in the Cleveland Clinic series.

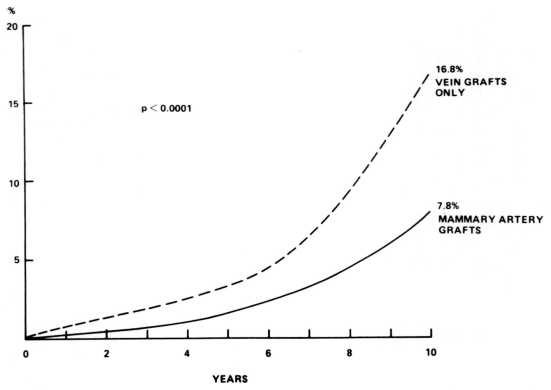

Figure 54–78. Reoperation rates versus postoperative years for patients who had vein grafts only compared with patients who had at least one IMA graft.

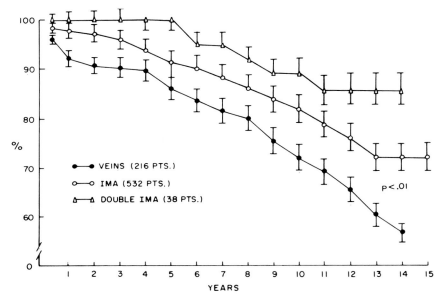

Figure 54–79. Raw survival data over time after coronary bypass for patients who received vein grafts only, one IMA, or double IMAs.

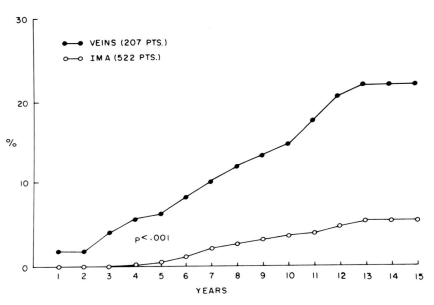

Figure 54–80. Reoperation requirement over time for the patients represented in Figure 54–79.

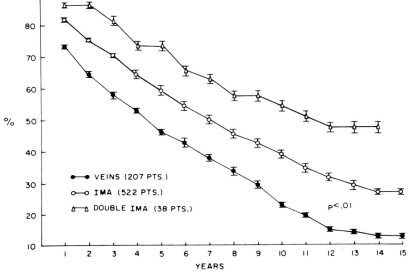

Figure 54–81. Event-free survival over time for patients who received vein grafts only, one IMA, or double IMAs.

is the influence of biases used in the selection of patients on the subsequent results (Swenson, 1986). In each study that showed improved survival with IMA grafting, two important biases existed. First, patients who received IMA grafts had *significantly* less severe risk factors and therefore a better prognosis, and it is not clear that statistical techniques can adjust for these *serious* baseline differences. Second, IMA grafts tended to be done more often in later years, so that the general improvements in surgical results with time (Pryor et al, 1987) might independently improve the prognosis for patients with IMA grafting. Thus, the results of these studies must be considered to be preliminary.

In an effort to determine differences in clinical outcome between predominant single IMA grafting and routine multiple IMA grafting, two surgeons in this center began simultaneous prospective clinical trials of routine single versus multiple IMA grafting in 1984, based on the intention to treat. The surgeons had similar previous clinical results and used a common operative technique during the study. A modified St. Thomas's cardioplegia solution and topical hypothermia were used for myocardial protection, and cardiopulmonary bypass was done with single venous cannulation, systemic hypothermia at 24° C, and aortic venting. Distal graft anastomoses were constructed first during the period of cardioplegia, sequential grafts were used commonly by both surgeons, and identical running polypropylene anastomotic techniques were used (Rankin et al, 1986a). The surgeons had similar philosophies of operative selection and previous referral profiles so that the relative distribution of patients was based hypothetically on random clinical consultation. One surgeon used predominantly single IMA grafting during the period (Group I); the other attempted to maximize distal IMA anastomoses with frequent bilateral, sequential, and free IMA grafts (Group II). A randomized prospective study would have been impossible in this center, and this design was a potentially valid method of testing the hypothesis that multiple compared with single IMA grafting provides significant clinical benefits. It should be emphasized that intention to treat (i.e., philosophy of single versus multiple IMA) was the basis of subgrouping rather than ultimate therapy.

A total of 1,063 patients had coronary revascularization during the period, 420 in Group I and 643 in Group II with similar time distributions. No differences were noted in the incidence of preoperative risk factors between groups (Table 54–12), which supports the validity of this type of clinical allocation process. Variables that reflected operative technique, including clamp time per graft, bypass time per graft, and number of grafts per patient, were similar. The distribution of single versus multiple IMA grafts between groups reflected the different operative philosophies (see Table 54–12). For example, 74% of patients in Group I with multivessel or left main disease received a single IMA and adjunctive vein

TABLE 54–12. SINGLE VERSUS MULTIPLE IMA COMPARISON

	Group I	Group II
	Preoperative Risk Factors	
No. of patients	420	643
MVD/LMD	89%	91%
Elective	53%	52%
USA/PIA	41%	43%
AEMI	6%	5%
>65 years	33%	34%
Mean EF	0.5 ± 0.10	0.49 ± 0.11
EF <0.4	26%	26%
Age	60 ± 10 years	60 ± 10 years
	Operative Variables	
ALL PATIENTS		
No IMA	16%	3%
Single IMA	73%	30%
Multiple IMA	11%	67%
Any IMA	84%	97%
SINGLE VESSEL DISEASE		
IMA used	90%	97%
MVD/LMD		
No IMA	14%	3%
Single IMA	74%	26%
Multiple IMA	12%	71%

	Postoperative Results			
SUBGROUPS	30-DAY SURVIVAL	3-YEAR SURVIVAL	30-DAY SURVIVAL	3-YEAR SURVIVAL
Overall	96	92	98	92
Elective	98	95	99	93
USA/PIA*	93	89	97	90
Age ≥65	92	87	97	91
Age <65	98	95	99	93
EF ≥0.4	96	94	99	94
EF <0.4	96	91	96	91
Nondiabetic	97	93	98	92
Diabetic	91	88	97	89

	Group I	Group II
REOP. RATE (3-YEAR)	0.2%	0.8%
STERNAL INFECTION	2.1%	1.0%

AEMI = acute evolving myocardial infarction; EF = ejection fraction; IMA = internal mammary artery; LMD = left main disease; MVD = multivessel disease; PIA = postinfarction angina*; Reop. = repeat coronary bypass; USA = unstable angina.
*As defined narrowly (Rankin et al, 1984).

grafts, whereas 71% of patients with multivessel or left main disease in Group II had multiple IMA grafts with proportionally less use of saphenous vein.

Overall 30-day and 3-year survivals, 3-year reoperation rate, and incidence of sternal infections did not differ significantly between groups (see Table 54–12). When the multivariable Cox proportional hazards model was used and all relevant variables were taken into account, overall long-term survival for 3 postoperative years was not statistically or clinically different between groups (Fig. 54–82). Similar analyses of group survival relative to operative risk factors (Rankin et al, 1988) of age, ejection fraction, acute presentation, and the presence of diabetes are shown in Figures 54–83 and 54–84. In no subset was a significant survival benefit of multiple IMA grafting observed, at least during the first

Single/Multiple IMA Comparison

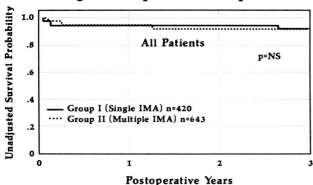

Figure 54–82. Raw unadjusted survival for 3 postoperative years for comparable groups of patients who had predominantly single IMA and adjunctive vein grafts (Group I) versus those who had predominantly multiple IMA and adjunctive vein grafts (Group II). Multivariable Cox model analysis showed no significant difference in survival between the two treatment strategies for 3 postoperative years.

3 postoperative years. It is possible that most of the clinical benefits of IMA grafting are provided by a single IMA graft and further use is associated, on average, with diminished clinical returns. Alternatively, many of the potential clinical advantages of multiple IMA grafting would be expected in later years, and 3 years of follow-up may be inadequate

Single/Multiple IMA Comparison

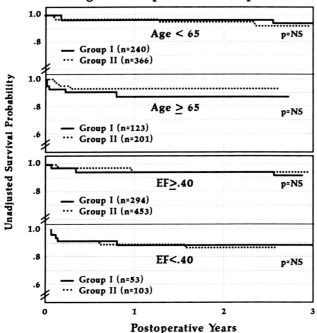

Figure 54–83. Unadjusted survival curves for patients who received single versus multiple IMA grafts with subgroups defined according to age and ejection fraction.

Single/Multiple IMA Comparison

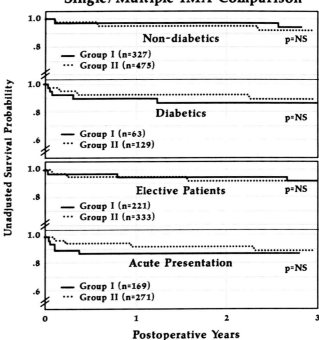

Figure 54–84. Unadjusted survival curves for patients who received single versus multiple IMA grafts subgrouped according to the presence of diabetes or acute presentation.

to test the hypothesis. However, this comparison illustrates the importance of attempting to eliminate as many clinical selection biases as possible and suggests that conclusions about single versus multiple IMA grafts are premature at present.

CONCLUSION

The development of IMA-to-coronary artery bypass and the routine application of this procedure to the general population of patients with coronary disease constitute major advances in cardiac surgery. At present, most coronary revascularizations should probably include at least one IMA graft, and multiple IMA procedures are becoming more popular. Early results suggest that the long-term survival and well-being of patients will improve with routine use of IMA grafting, but more follow-up time and analysis of prognostic variables will be necessary to understand this topic fully.

Bibliography

Absolon, K. B., Aust, J. B., Varco, R. L., and Lillehei, C. W.: Surgical treatment of occlusive coronary artery disease by endarterectomy or anastomotic replacement. Surg. Gynecol. Obstet., 103:180, 1956.

Acinapura, A. J., Cunningham, J. N., Jr., Jacobowitz, I. J., et al: Efficacy of percutaneous transluminal coronary angioplasty compared with single-vessel bypass. J. Thorac. Cardiovasc. Surg., 89:35, 1985.

Arnold, P. G., and Pairolero, P. C.: Use of *pectoris major* muscle flaps to repair defects of anterior chest wall. Plast. Reconstr. Surg., 63:205, 1979.

Baillot, R. G., Loop, F. D., Cosgrove, D. M., and Lytle, B. W.: Reoperation after previous grafting with the internal mammary artery: Technique and early results. Ann. Thorac. Surg., 40:271, 1985.

Baker, N. H., and Grindlay, J. H.: Technic of experimental systemic-to-coronary-artery anastomosis. Staff Meetings of the Mayo Clinic, 34:497, 1959.

Ballinger, W. F., Padula, R. T., Fishman, N. H., and Camishion, R. C.: Operations upon coronary arteries: Evaluation of absorbable intraluminal gelatin tubes, sutures, and tissue adhesive. J. Thorac. Cardiovasc. Surg., 48:790, 1964.

Barbour, D. J., and Roberts, W. C.: Additional evidence for relative resistance to atherosclerosis of the internal mammary artery compared to saphenous vein when used to increase myocardial blood supply. Am. J. Cardiol., 56:488, 1984.

Barner, H. B.: The internal mammary artery as a free graft. J. Thorac. Cardiovasc. Surg., 66:219, 1973.

Barner, H. B., Standeven, J. W., and Reese, J.: Twelve-year experience with internal mammary artery for coronary artery bypass. J. Thorac. Cardiovasc. Surg., 90:668, 1985.

Barner, H. B., Swartz, M. T., Mudd, J. G., and Tyras, D. H.: Late patency of the internal mammary artery as a coronary bypass conduit. Ann. Thorac. Surg., 34:408, 1982.

Bashour, T. T., Crew, J., Kabbani, S. S., et al: Symptomatic coronary and cerebral steal after internal mammary-coronary bypass. Am. Heart J., 108:177, 1984.

Bashour, T. T., Hanna, E. S., and Mason, D. T.: Myocardial revascularization with internal mammary artery bypass: An emerging treatment of choice. Am. Heart J., 111:143, 1986.

Beggerly, C. E., Austin, E. H., and Chitwood, W. R., Jr.: Current coronary artery surgery practices: A national survey. J. Am. Coll. Cardiol., 9:123A, 1987.

Bourassa, M. G., Campeau, L., Lespérance, J., and Solymoss, B. C.: Atherosclerosis after coronary artery bypass surgery: Results of recent studies and recommendations regarding prevention. Cardiology, 73:259, 1986.

Breyer, R. H., Mills, S. A., Hudspeth, A. S., et al: A prospective study of sternal wound complications. Ann. Thorac. Surg., 37:412, 1984.

Califf, R. M., Harrell, F. E., Lee, K. L., et al: The evolution of medical and surgical therapy for coronary artery disease: A 15-year perspective. J.A.M.A., 261:2077, 1989.

Cameron, A., Davis, K. B., Green, G. E., et al: Clinical implications of internal mammary artery bypass grafts: The Coronary Artery Surgery Study experience. Circulation, 77:815, 1988.

Cameron, A., Kemp, H. G., and Green, G. E.: Bypass surgery with the internal mammary artery graft: 15 year follow-up. Circulation, 74:III-30, 1986..

Carrel, A.: On the experimental surgery of the thoracic aorta and the heart. Ann. Surg., 52:83, 1910.

Chaikhouni, A., Crawford, F. A., Kochel, P. J., et al: Human internal mammary artery produces more prostacyclin than saphenous vein. J. Thorac. Cardiovasc. Surg., 92:88, 1986.

Cheung, E. H., Craver, J. M., Jones, E. L., et al: Mediastinitis after cardiac valve operations. J. Thorac. Cardiovasc. Surg., 90:517, 1985.

Cosgrove, D. M., Amiot, D. M., and Meserko, J. J.: An improved technique for autotransfusion of shed mediastinal blood. Ann. Thorac. Surg., 40:519, 1985a.

Cosgrove, D. M., and Loop, F. D.: Techniques to maximize mammary artery length. Ann. Thorac. Surg., 40:78, 1985b.

Cosgrove, D. M., Loop, F. D., Lytle, B. W., et al: Determinants of 10-year survival after primary myocardial revascularization. Ann. Surg., 202:480, 1985c.

Cosgrove, D. M., Loop, F. D., Lytle, B. W., et al: Does mammary artery grafting increase surgical risk? Circulation, 72(Suppl. II):II-170, 1985d.

Cosgrove, D. M., Loop, F. D., Lytle, B. W., et al: Predictors of reoperation after myocardial revascularization. J. Thorac. Cardiovasc. Surg., 92:811, 1986.

Cosgrove, D. M., Lytle, B. W., Loop, F. D., et al: Does bilateral internal mammary artery grafting increase surgical risk? J. Thorac. Cardiovasc. Surg., 95:850, 1988.

Dion, R., Verhelst, R., Rousseau, M., et al: Sequential mammary grafting. Clinical, functional and angiographic assessment 6 months postoperatively: in 231 consecutive patients. J. Thorac. Cardiovasc. Surg., 98:80, 1989.

Dobrin, P. B.: Mechanical behavior of vascular smooth muscle in cylindrical segments of arteries in vitro. Ann. Biomed. Eng., 12:497, 1984.

Finci, L., Segesser, L., Meier, B., et al: Comparison of multivessel coronary angioplasty with surgical revascularization with both internal mammary arteries. Circulation, 76:V-1, 1987.

Galbut, D. L., Traad, E. A., Dorman, M. J., et al: Twelve-year experience with bilateral internal mammary artery grafts. Ann. Thorac. Surg., 40:264, 1985.

Geha, A. S., and Baue, A. E.: Early and late results of coronary revascularization with saphenous vein and internal mammary artery grafts. Am. J. Surg., 137:456, 1979.

Gelbfish, J., Jacobowitz, I. J., Rose, D. M., et al: Cryopreserved homologous saphenous vein: Early and late patency in coronary artery bypass surgical procedures. Ann. Thorac. Surg., 42:70, 1986.

Gibson, C. F., and Loop, F. D.: Choice of internal mammary artery or saphenous vein graft for myocardial revascularization. Cardiology, 73:235, 1986.

Gold, J. P., Shemin, R. J., DiSesa, V. J., et al: Multiple-vessel coronary revascularization with combined in situ and free sequential internal mammary arteries. J. Thorac. Cardiovasc. Surg., 90:301, 1985.

Graham, J. E., Peter, M., and Mathai, J.: Significant improvement in flow through a potential internal mammary graft after partial approximation of the sternum. J. Thorac. Cardiovasc. Surg., 88:454, 1984.

Green, G. E.: Internal mammary artery-to-coronary artery anastomosis: Three-year experience with 165 patients. Ann. Thorac. Surg., 14:260, 1972.

Green, G. E.: Technical factors influencing IMA graft patency (Letter). Ann. Thorac. Surg., 44:104, 1987.

Green, G. E., Stertzer, S. H., Gordon, R. B., and Tice, D. A.: Anastomosis of the internal mammary artery to the distal left anterior descending coronary artery. Circulation, 41,42:II-79, 1970.

Green, G. E., Stertzer, S. H., and Reppert, E. H.: Coronary arterial bypass grafts. Ann. Thorac. Surg., 5:443, 1968.

Grmoljez, P. F., and Barner, H. B.: Bilateral internal mammary artery mobilization and sternal healing. Angiology, 29:272, 1978.

Grondin, C. M.: Late results of coronary artery grafting: Is there a flag on the field? J. Thorac. Cardiovasc. Surg., 87:161, 1984.

Grondin, C. M., Campeau, L., Lespérance, J., et al: Comparison of late changes in internal mammary artery and saphenous vein grafts in two consecutive series of patients 10 years after operation. Circulation, 70:I-208, 1984.

Grossi, E. A., Culliford, A. T., Krieger, K. H., et al: A survey of 77 major infectious complications of median sternotomy: A review of 7,949 consecutive operative procedures. Ann. Thorac. Surg., 40:214, 1985.

Hall, R. J., Khouri, E. M., and Gregg, D. E.: Coronary-internal mammary artery anastomosis in dogs. Surgery, 50:560, 1961.

Harjola, P. T., Frick, M. H., Harjula, A., et al: Sequential internal mammary artery (IMA) grafts in coronary artery bypass surgery. Thorac. Cardiovasc. Surg., 32:288, 1984.

Herrera, H. R., and Ginsberg, M. E.: The pectoralis major myocutaneous flap and omental transposition for closure of infected median sternotomy wounds. Plast. Reconstr. Surg., 70:465, 1982.

Hirose, H., Kawashima, Y., Nakano, S., et al: Long-term results in surgical treatment of children 4 years old or younger with coronary involvement due to Kawasaki disease. Circulation, 74:I-77, 1986.

Hodgson, J. M., Singh, A. K., Drew, T. M., et al: Coronary flow reserve provided by sequential internal mammary artery grafts. J. Am. Coll. Cardiol., 7:32, 1986.

Huddleston, C. B., Stoney, W. S., Alford, W. C., et al: Internal mammary artery grafts: Technical factors influencing patency. Ann. Thorac. Surg., 42:543, 1986.

Hutchinson, J. E., III, Green, G. E., Mekhjian, H. A., and Kemp, H. G.: Coronary bypass grafting in 376 consecutive patients, with three operative deaths. J. Thorac. Cardiovasc. Surg., 67:7, 1974.

Jett, G. K., Arcidi, J. M., Dorsey, L. M. A., et al: Vasoactive drug effects on blood flow in internal mammary artery and saphenous vein grafts. J. Thorac. Cardiovasc. Surg., 94:2, 1987.

Johnson, A. M., Kron, I. L., Watson, D. D., and Gibson, R. S.: Evaluation of flow reserve in internal mammary artery bypass grafts. J. Thorac. Cardiovasc. Surg., 92:822, 1986.

Jones, E. L., Lattouf, O., Lutz, J. F., and King, S. B.: Important anatomical and physiological considerations in performance of complex mammary-coronary artery operations. Ann. Thorac. Surg., 43:469, 1987.

Jones, E. L., Lutz, J. F., King, S. B., et al: Extended use of the internal mammary artery graft: Important anatomic and physiologic considerations. Circulation, 74:III-42, 1986.

Jones, J. W., Oschner, J. L., Mills, N. L., and Hughes, L.: Clinical comparison with saphenous vein and internal mammary artery as a coronary graft. J. Thorac. Cardiovasc. Surg., 80:334, 1980.

Jones, J. W., Ochsner, J. L., Mills, N. L., and Hughes, L.: The internal mammary bypass graft: A superior second coronary artery. J. Thorac. Cardiovasc. Surg., 75:625, 1978.

Julian, O. C., Lopez-Belio, M., Moorehead, D., and Lima, A.: Direct surgical procedures of the coronary arteries: Experimental studies. J. Thorac. Surg., 34:654, 1957.

Kabbani, S. S., Hanna, E. S., Bashour, T. T., et al: Sequential internal mammary-coronary artery bypass. J. Thorac. Cardiovasc. Surg., 86:697, 1983.

Kalan, J. M., and Roberts, W. C.: Comparison of morphologic changes and luminal sizes of saphenous vein and internal mammary artery after simultaneous implantation for coronary arterial bypass grafting. Am. J. Cardiol., 60:193, 1987.

Kamath, M. L., Matysik, L. S., Schmidt, D. H., and Smith, L. L.: Sequential internal mammary artery grafts. J. Thorac. Cardiovasc. Surg., 89:163, 1985.

Kay, E. B.: Internal mammary artery grafting (Letter). J. Thorac. Cardiovasc. Surg., 94:312, 1987.

Kay, H. R., Korns, M. E., Flemma, R. J., et al: Atherosclerosis of the internal mammary artery. Ann. Thorac. Surg., 21:504, 1976.

Kereiakes, D. J., Abbottsmith, C. W., Callard, G. M., and Flege, J. B.: Emergent internal mammary artery grafting following failed percutaneous transluminal coronary angioplasty: Use of transluminal catheter reperfusion. Am. Heart. J., 113:1018, 1987.

Kinzer, J. B., Lichtenthal, P. R., and Wade, L. D.: Loss of radial artery pressure trace during internal mammary artery dissection of coronary artery bypass graft surgery. Anesth. Analg., 64:1134, 1985.

Kitamura, S., Kawachi, K., Morita, R., et al: Excellent patency and growth capacity of internal mammary artery (IMA) grafts in pediatric coronary artery bypass surgery; new evidence of a "live conduit." Circulation, 76(Suppl IV):1395, 1987.

Kitamura, S., Kawachi, K., Oyama, C., et al: Severe Kawasaki heart disease treated with an internal mammary artery graft in pediatric patients. J. Thorac. Cardiovasc. Surg., 89:860, 1985.

Kolessov, V. I.: Mammary artery-coronary artery anastomosis as method of treatment for angina pectoris. J. Thorac. Cardiovasc. Surg., 54:535, 1967.

Landymore, R. W., and Chapman, D. M.: Anatomical studies to support the expanded use of the internal mammary artery graft for myocardial revascularization. Ann. Thorac. Surg., 44:4, 1987.

Lee, C. N., Orszulak, T. A., Schaff, H. V., and Kaye, M. P.: Flow capacity of the canine internal mammary artery. J. Thorac. Cardiovasc. Surg., 91:405, 1986.

Lewis, M. R., and Dehmer, G. J.: Coronary bypass using the internal mammary artery. Am. J. Cardiol., 56:480, 1985.

Loop, F. D., Irarrazaval, M. J., Bredee, J. J., et al: Internal mammary artery graft for ischemic heart disease: Effects of revascularization on clinical status and survival. Am. J. Cardiol., 39:516, 1977.

Loop, F. D., Lytle, B. W., Cosgrove, D. M., et al: Free (aortocoronary) internal mammary artery graft: Late results. J. Thorac. Cardiovasc. Surg., 92:827, 1986a.

Loop, F. D., Lytle, B. W., Cosgrove, D. M., et al: Influence of the internal mammary artery graft on 10-year survival and other cardiac events. N. Engl. J. Med., 314:1, 1986b.

Loop, F. D., Spampinato, N., Cheanvechai, C., and Effler, D. B.: The free internal mammary artery bypass graft. Ann. Thorac. Surg., 15:50, 1973.

Lytle, B. W., Cosgrove, D. M., Loop, F. D., et al: Perioperative risk of bilateral internal mammary artery grafting: Analysis of 500 cases from 1971 to 1984. Circulation, 74:III-37, 1986.

Lytle, B. W., Cosgrove, D. M., Saltus, G. L., et al: Multivessel coronary revascularization without saphenous vein: Long-term results of bilateral internal mammary artery grafting. Ann. Thorac. Surg., 36:540, 1983.

Lytle, B. W., Kramer, J. R., Golding, L. R., et al: Young adults with coronary atherosclerosis: 10 year results of surgical myocardial revascularization. J. Am. Coll. Cardiol., 4:445, 1984.

Lytle, B. W., Loop, F. D., Cosgrove, D. M., et al: Long-term (5 to 12 years) serial studies of internal mammary artery and saphenous vein coronary bypass grafts. J. Thorac. Cardiovasc. Surg., 89:248, 1985.

Lytle, B. W., Loop, F. D., Cosgrove, D. M., et al: Fifteen hundred coronary reoperations. J. Thorac. Cardiovasc. Surg., 93:847, 1987.

Mamiya, R. T., Cooper, T., Willman, V. L., et al: Distal relocation of the origin of the left coronary artery by subclavian left coronary anastomosis. Surg. Gynecol. Obstet., 113:599, 1961.

McBride, L. R., and Barner, H. B.: The left internal mammary artery as a sequential graft to the left anterior descending system. J. Thorac. Cardiovasc. Surg., 86:703, 1983.

Mehta, J., and Roberts, A.: Human vascular tissues produce thromboxane as well as prostacyclin. Am. J. Physiol., 244:R839, 1983.

Miller, D. W., Ivey, T. D., Bailey, W. W., et al: The practice of coronary artery bypass surgery in 1980. J. Thorac. Cardiovasc. Surg., 81:423, 1981.

Moore, T. C., and Riberi, A.: Maintenance of coronary circulation during systemic-to-coronary artery anastomosis. Surgery, 43:245, 1958.

Murray, G.: Heparin in surgical treatment of blood vessels. Arch. Surg., 40:307, 1940.

Murray, G.: Surgery of coronary heart disease. Angiology, 4:526, 1953.

Murray, G., Porcheron, R., Hilario, J., and Roschlau, W.: Anastomosis of a systemic artery to the coronary. Can. Med. Assoc. J., 71:594, 1954.

Nahai, F., Morales, L., Bone, D. K., and Bostwick, J.: Pectoralis major muscle turnover flaps for closure of the infected sternotomy wound with preservation of form and function. Plast. Reconstr. Surg., 70:471, 1982.

Nkongho, A., Luber, J. M., Bell-Thompson, J., and Green, G. E.: Sternotomy infection after harvesting of the internal mammary artery. J. Thorac. Cardiovasc. Surg., 88:788, 1984.

Okies, J. E., Page, U. S., Bigelow, J. C., et al: The left internal mammary artery: The graft of choice. Circulation, 70:I-213, 1984.

Olearchyk, A. S., and Magovern, G. J.: Internal mammary artery grafting. J. Thorac. Cardiovasc. Surg., 92:1082, 1986.

Orszulak, T. A., Schaff, H. V., Chesebro, J. H., and Holmes, D. R., Jr.: Initial experience with sequential internal mammary artery bypass grafts to the left anterior descending and diagonal coronary arteries. Mayo Clin. Proc., 61:3, 1986.

Pairolero, P. C., and Arnold, P. G.: Management of recalcitrant median sternotomy wounds. J. Thorac. Cardiovasc. Surg., 88:357, 1984.

Pelias, A. J., DelRossi, A. J., Tacy, L., and Wolpowitz, A.: A case of postoperative internal mammary steal. J. Thorac. Cardiovasc. Surg., 90:794, 1985.

Phillips, T. G., and Green, G. E.: Left recurrent laryngeal nerve injury following internal mammary artery bypass. Ann. Thorac. Surg., 43:440, 1987.

Prieto, I., Basile, F., and Abdulnour, E.: Upper extremity vein graft for aortocoronary bypass. Ann. Thorac. Surg., 37:218, 1984.

Pryor, D. B., Harrell, F. E., Rankin, J. S., et al: Trends in the presentation, management and survival of patients with coronary artery disease: The Duke Database for Cardiovascular Disease. In Luepker, R. V., and Higgins, M. (eds): Trends in Coronary Heart Disease Mortality: The Influence of Medical Care. New York, Oxford University Press, 1988.

Pryor, D. B., Harrell, F. E., Rankin, J. S., et al: The changing survival benefits of coronary revascularization over time. Circulation, 76:V-13, 1987.

Puig, L. B., Neto, L. F., Rati, M., et al: A technique of anastomosis of the right internal mammary artery to the circumflex artery and its branches. Ann. Thorac. Surg., 38:533, 1984.

Rankin, J. S., and Sabiston, D. C., Jr.: Physiology of the coronary circulation and intraoperative myocardial protection. In Sabiston, D. C., Jr. (ed): A Textbook of Surgery. Philadelphia, W. B. Saunders Company, 1986a.

Rankin, J. S., Newman, G. E., Bashore, T. M., et al: Clinical and angiographic assessment of complex mammary artery bypass grafting. J. Thorac. Cardiovasc. Surg., 95:832, 1986b.

Rankin, J. S., Newman, G. E., Muhlbaier, L. H., et al: The effects of coronary revascularization on left ventricular function in ischemic heart disease. J. Thorac. Cardiovasc. Surg., 90:818, 1985.

Rankin, J. S., Newton, J. R., Califf, R. M., et al: Clinical characteristics and current management of medically refractory unstable angina. Ann. Surg., 200:457, 1984.

Rankin, J. S., Smith, L. R., Muhlbaier, L. H., et al: The importance of acute clinical presentation to survival prognosis after coronary artery bypass. Circulation, 78:II-477, 1988.

Robicsek, F.: A simple test to determine the efficiency of mammary artery grafts during operation. Ann. Thorac. Surg., 39:388, 1985.

Rodigas, P. C., and Bridges, K. G.: Occlusion of left internal mammary artery with intra-aortic balloon: Clinical implications. J. Thorac. Cardiovasc. Surg., 91:142, 1986.

Russo, P., Orszulak, T. A., Schaff, H. V., and Holmes, D. R.: Use of internal mammary artery grafts for multiple coronary artery bypasses. Circulation, 74:III-48, 1986.

Salomon, N. W., Page, U. S., Okies, J. E., et al: Diabetes mellitus and coronary artery bypass. J. Thorac. Cardiovasc. Surg., 85:264, 1983.

Sapsford, R. N., Oakley, G. D., and Talbot, S.: Early and late patency of expanded polytetrafluoroethylene vascular grafts in aorta-coronary bypass. J. Thorac. Cardiovasc. Surg., 81:860, 1981.

Sarabu, M. R., McClung, J. A., Fass, A., and Reed, G. E.: Early postoperative spasm in left internal mammary artery bypass grafts. Ann. Thorac. Surg., 44:199, 1987.

Sarr, M. G., Gott, V. L., and Townsend, T. R.: Mediastinal infection after cardiac surgery. Ann. Thorac. Surg., 38:415, 1984.

Sauvage, L. R., Wu, H. D., Kowalsky, T. E., et al: Healing basis and surgical techniques for complete revascularization of the left ventricle using only the internal mammary arteries. Ann. Thorac. Surg., 42:449, 1986.

Schimert, G., Vidne, B. A., and Lee, A. B.: Free internal mammary artery graft: An improved technique. Ann. Thorac. Surg., 19:474, 1975.

Schmidt, D. H., Blau, F., Hellman, C., et al: Isoproterenol-induced flow responses in mammary and vein bypass grafts. J. Thorac. Cardiovasc. Surg., 80:319, 1980.

Scully, H. E., Leclerc, Y., Martin, R. D., et al: Comparison between antibiotic irrigation and mobilization of pectoral muscle flaps in treatment of deep sternal infections. J. Thorac. Cardiovasc. Surg., 90:523, 1985.

Siegel, W., and Loop, F. D.: Comparison of internal mammary artery and saphenous vein bypass grafts for myocardial revascularization. Circulation, 54:III-1, 1976.

Silver, G. M., Katske, G. E., Stutzman, F. L., and Wood, N. R.: Umbilical vein for aortocoronary bypass. Angiology, 33:450, 1982.

Sims, F. H.: A comparison of coronary and internal mammary arteries and implications of the results in the etiology of arteriosclerosis. Am. Heart J., 105:560, 1983.

Sims, F. H.: The internal mammary artery as a bypass graft? Ann. Thorac. Surg., 44:2, 1987.

Singh, R. N.: Atherosclerosis and the internal mammary arteries. Cardiovasc. Intervent. Radiol., 6:72, 1983.

Singh, R. N.: Physiological nature of the internal mammary artery grafts. Cathet. Cardiovasc. Diagn., 11:427, 1985.

Singh, R. N., Beg, R. A., and Kay, E. B.: Physiological adaptability: The secret of success of the internal mammary artery grafts. Ann. Thorac. Surg., 41:247, 1986.

Singh, R. N., and Sosa, J. A.: Internal mammary artery: A "live" conduit for coronary bypass. J. Thorac. Cardiovasc. Surg., 87:936, 1984.

Singh, R. N., Sosa, J. A., and Green, G. E.: Long-term fate of the internal mammary artery and saphenous vein grafts. J. Thorac. Cardiovasc. Surg., 86:359, 1983.

Speiser, K., Rothlin, M., and Turina, M.: Comparison between internal mammary artery implantation and aorto-coronary vein bypass grafting in coronary artery disease with significant left anterior descending stenosis. Thorac. Cardiovasc. Surg., 31:54, 1983.

Spencer, F. C.: The internal mammary artery: The ideal coronary bypass graft? N. Engl. J. Med., 314:50, 1986.

Spencer, F. C., Eiseman, B., Yong, N. K., and Prachuabmoh, K.: Experimental coronary arterial surgery with hypothermia and cardiopulmonary bypass. Circulation, 29(Cardiovasc. Surg. Suppl.):140, 1964a.

Spencer, F. C., Yong, N. K., and Prachuabmoh, K.: Internal mammary-coronary artery anastomoses performed during cardiopulmonary bypass. J. Cardiovasc. Surg. (Torino), 5:292, 1964b.

Stoney, W. S., Alford, W. C., Burrus, G. R., et al: Median sternotomy dehiscence. Ann. Thorac. Surg., 26:421, 1978.

Stoney, W. S., Alford, W. C., Burrus, G. R., et al: The fate of arm veins used for aorta-coronary bypass grafts. J. Thorac. Cardiovasc. Surg., 88:522, 1984.

Subramanian, V. A., Hernandez, Y., Tack-Goldman, K., et al: Prostacyclin production by internal mammary artery as a factor in coronary artery bypass grafts. Surgery, 100:376, 1986.

Swenson, L. J.: Survival after internal-mammary (thoracic)-artery grafting. N. Engl. J. Med., 314:1453, 1986.

Tartini, R., Steinbrunn, W., Kappenberger, L., et al: Anomalous origin of the left thyrocervical trunk as a cause of residual pain after myocardial revascularization with internal mammary artery. Ann. Thorac. Surg., 40:302, 1985.

Tector, A. J.: Fifteen years' experience with the internal mammary artery graft. Ann. Thorac. Surg., 42(Suppl.):S22, 1986.

Tector, A. J., Davis, L., Gabriel, R., et al: Experience with internal mammary artery grafts in 298 patients. Ann. Thorac. Surg., 22:515, 1976.

Tector, A. J., and Schmahl, T. M.: Techniques for multiple internal mammary artery bypass grafts. Ann. Thorac. Surg., 38:281, 1984.

Tector, A. J., Schmahl, T. M., and Canino, V. R.: The internal mammary artery graft: The best choice for bypass of the diseased left anterior descending coronary artery. Circulation, 68:II-214, 1983.

Tector, A. J., Schmahl, T. M., and Canino, V. R.: Expanding the use of the internal mammary artery to improve patency in coronary artery bypass grafting. J. Thorac. Cardiovasc. Surg., 91:9, 1986.

Tector, A. J., Schmahl, T. M., Canino, V. R., et al: The role of the sequential internal mammary artery graft in coronary surgery. Circulation, 70:I-222, 1984.

Thal, A., Perry, J. F., Miller, F. A., and Wangensteen, O. H.: Direct suture anastomosis of the coronary arteries in the dog. Surgery, 40:1023, 1956.

Tobin, G. R., Mavroudis, C., Howe, W. R., and Gray, L. A.: Reconstruction of complex thoracic defects with myocutaneous and muscle flaps. J. Thorac. Cardiovasc. Surg., 85:219, 1983.

Valentine, R. J., Fry, R. E., Wheelan, K. R., et al: Coronary-subclavian steal from reversed flow in an internal mammary artery used for coronary bypass. Am. J. Cardiol., 59:719, 1987.

2 Prinzmetal's Variant Angina and Other Syndromes Associated with Coronary Artery Spasm

James E. Lowe

In 1768, William Heberden described chest pain associated with effort, eating, or anxiety. He called this pain angina pectoris from the Greek word *anchein*, meaning "to choke." Subsequently, it was shown that the pain of angina pectoris is associated with myocardial ischemia, although the neurophysiology of how this pain is perceived is still unknown.

Since Heberden's original description of angina pectoris, several anginal syndromes have been described that have different clinical implications. Until relatively recently, it was thought that the pathophysiology in these syndromes was related to various degrees of subtotal or totally obstructive atherosclerotic coronary artery disease and that clinically identifiable subgroups of patients had similar degrees of obstruction at certain anatomic sites that resulted in similar degrees of myocardial ischemic dysfunction.

Although Osler (1910) postulated that coronary vasospasm was a cause of angina pectoris, most pathologists and clinicians at the time, including Herrick (1912), thought that atherosclerotic obstruction alone was responsible for both angina and myocardial infarction. In 1959, Prinzmetal and associates reported 32 patients with a different type of anginal syndrome that could not be explained solely by the degree of atherosclerotic coronary artery disease thought to be present. Prinzmetal suggested that transient coronary artery spasm was occurring in this subgroup. Subsequently, coronary artery spasm was documented in many other patients and was associated with various clinical presentations, which will be discussed.

Coronary arterial spasm is a sudden increase in coronary vascular tone with localized or diffuse vasoconstriction. The degree of vasoconstriction is an abnormal vascular phenomenon and should be distinguished from normal coronary vasomotor changes. Although spasm is most often identified in large extramural coronary arteries, there is evidence that it may also occur in small resistance arterioles. Recognition of patients with coronary artery spasm and selection of appropriate therapeutic interventions are two problems that challenge both cardiologists and cardiovascular surgeons.

CLASSIFICATION OF ANGINAL SYNDROMES

Since Heberden's original description of angina pectoris, it has been shown that there are various subgroups of patients with different types of angina, which must be identified because they have different clinical courses. *Stable angina* is the pain syndrome described by Heberden and is associated with effort, anxiety, or eating. Although the frequency of attacks can increase over time, this type of angina is usually predictable and stable over long periods. *Unstable angina* is a rapidly progressing pain syndrome that often results in myocardial infarction unless it is relieved by medical therapy or coronary artery bypass grafting. *Variant angina* is a distinctly different pain syndrome caused by coronary artery spasm, which can occur in normal coronary arteries or, more commonly, in coronary arteries with atherosclerotic lesions. Unlike stable and unstable angina, variant angina is not brought on by effort, eating, or anxiety. *Atypical angina* is a vague term that has various meanings. To some physicians, it represents chest pain secondary to coronary artery disease (with or without concomitant spasm) with a different kind of pain pattern, for example, pain that radiates into the right side of the chest or right arm; others use the term to refer to chest pain that may not even be related to coronary disease. Finally, angina occurs in patients with congenital coronary arterial malformations such as coronary artery fistulas or anomalous origin of the left coronary artery from the pulmonary artery. In these patients, angina results not from atherosclerotic disease or spasm but from a "steal" of normal coronary flow into the recipient cardiac chamber.

Each of these anginal syndromes is referred to by various names. Stable angina is referred to as typical angina, classic angina, or Heberden's angina. Stable angina is also known as effort angina because of its association with exercise, eating, or anxiety, and Maseri and associates (1978a) called it secondary angina because it appears to be secondary to fixed obstructive atherosclerotic coronary artery disease.

TABLE 54–13. ANGINAL SYNDROMES

STABLE ANGINA
  Heberden's angina
  Classic angina
  Typical angina
  Effort angina
  Secondary angina

UNSTABLE ANGINA
  Preinfarction angina
  Crescendo angina

VARIANT ANGINA
  Prinzmetal's angina
  Vasospastic angina
  Angina decubitus
  Primary angina

ATYPICAL ANGINA

ANGINA SECONDARY TO A STEAL PHENOMENON
(Congenital coronary fistulas and anomalous origin of the left
coronary artery from the pulmonary artery)

Unstable angina is also known as preinfarction or crescendo angina because of its rapid progression. Stenosis of the left main coronary artery is one anatomic cause of this type of pain, and its clinical recognition is important because survival can be improved by coronary artery bypass grafting. Variant angina is also known as Prinzmetal's angina, vasospastic angina, and angina decubitus, because it usually occurs at rest, and Maseri and associates (1978a) called it primary angina because it is caused by spasm of the coronary arteries and is not secondary to atherosclerotic disease alone. For clarification, the terminology used to describe these various anginal syndromes is summarized in Table 54–13.

PRINZMETAL'S VARIANT ANGINA

Stable angina, or classic Heberden's angina, is a distinct syndrome with two major clinical manifestations. First, the pain occurs when more work is demanded of the heart and the pain is relieved by rest or administration of nitroglycerin. Second, the electrocardiogram during an episode of pain often shows ST-segment depression in certain leads without reciprocal elevation. Prinzmetal and associates (1959) reported 32 patients, 20 of whom were personally observed, with a different anginal syndrome. They referred to this syndrome as "a variant form of angina pectoris." Prinzmetal noted that this form of angina appeared to occur at rest or during ordinary activity and was not brought on by exercise, eating, or emotional stress. The pain was in the same location as classic angina, although the duration was usually longer and the pain was more severe. Attacks often occurred at the same time each day or night, and the waxing and waning of the pain were of equal duration. Nitroglycerin promptly relieved the pain of variant angina but, unlike the situation in classic angina, the electrocardiogram often showed ST-segment elevation similar to that in patients with acute myocardial infarction (Fig. 54–85). The ST-segment elevations were usually related to the distribution of one large coronary artery. Testing of these patients showed that exercise could cause ST-segment depression but did not result in pain unless the patient also had angina secondary to fixed obstructive disease. Dysrhythmias were common during the pain of variant angina, and transient Q waves were occasionally observed. Prinzmetal observed that infarction occurred in some patients weeks or months later in areas of previous ST-segment elevation. Finally, Prinzmetal noted that the pain of variant angina was often relieved by myocardial infarction, whereas the pain of stable angina often increased after myocardial infarction. These observations are still the classic clinical criteria for establishing a diagnosis of variant angina.

Prinzmetal also noted that "it is not uncommon for both the variant and classic forms of angina pectoris to occur together in the same patient." This clinically significant observation is discussed in detail later. It has been well documented that coronary artery spasm is most common in patients with concomitant atherosclerotic coronary artery disease, but a number of patients have variant angina and coronary arteries that appear to be normal on arteriography. This subgroup of patients with "normal coronary arteries" and variant angina have been referred to as patients with a "variant of the variant" anginal syndrome of Prinzmetal (Cheng et al, 1973; Guazzi et al, 1976).

Finally, in his classic manuscript Prinzmetal postulated that "temporary increased tonus of a large coronary artery is suggested as the cause of pain in the variant form of angina." Arteriographic evidence of coronary artery spasm during an attack of Prinzmetal's variant angina was shown by Oliva and associates in 1973 (Fig. 54–86).

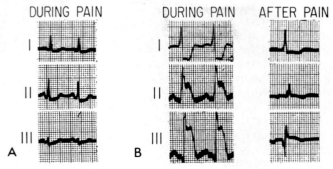

Figure 54–85. Comparison of electrocardiographic characteristics of classic angina pectoris and the variant form. *A,* Classic angina pectoris: ST segments show depression without reciprocal ST elevation. Electrocardiogram obtained after exercise. *B,* Variant form of angina pectoris: During spontaneous pain, ST segments show elevation in leads II and III with reciprocal ST depression in lead I. Immediately after pain, the electrocardiogram returns to normal or to prepain pattern. (From Prinzmetal, M., Kennamer, R., Merliss, R., et al: Angina pectoris. I: A variant form of angina pectoris. Am. J. Med., 27:375, 1959.)

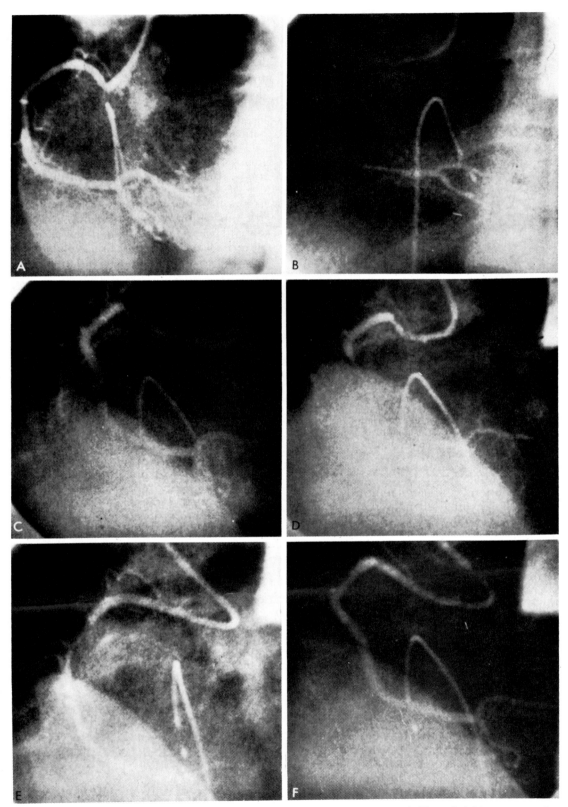

Figure 54–86. Documentation of coronary spasm during episodes of variant angina. *A,* Normal right coronary artery while the patient was pain-free, without electrocardiographic changes. *B,* During a spontaneous attack of angina, with electrocardiographic changes and spasm of a long segment of the midportion of the right coronary artery. *C,* During an injection while the patient was pain-free, showing a normal vessel (spasm could not be induced by the catheter or the contrast medium). *D,* Spasm of a long segment extending into the distal right coronary artery and posterior descending artery during the next attack of pain. *E,* During a subsequent but separate attack of angina, when a segmental area of spasm is noted. *F,* Within 2 minutes the angina subsided, and the vessel appeared normal.

Illustration continued on following page

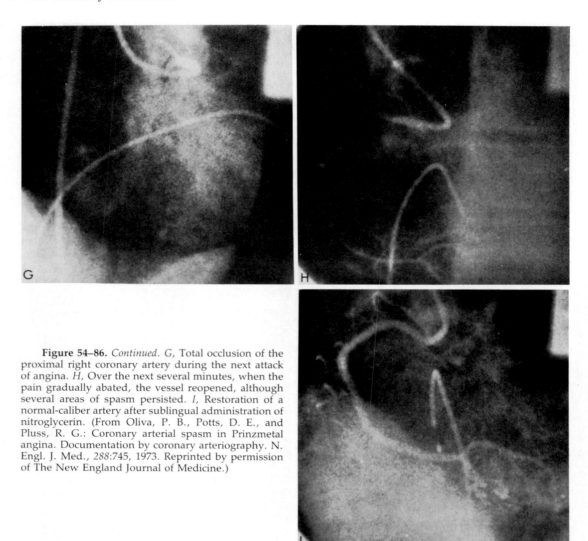

Figure 54–86. *Continued. G*, Total occlusion of the proximal right coronary artery during the next attack of angina. *H*, Over the next several minutes, when the pain gradually abated, the vessel reopened, although several areas of spasm persisted. *I*, Restoration of a normal-caliber artery after sublingual administration of nitroglycerin. (From Oliva, P. B., Potts, D. E., and Pluss, R. G.: Coronary arterial spasm in Prinzmetal angina. Documentation by coronary arteriography. N. Engl. J. Med., *288*:745, 1973. Reprinted by permission of The New England Journal of Medicine.)

Since Prinzmetal's initial observations and the demonstration of coronary artery spasm in patients with variant angina by Oliva and associates, various other syndromes have been recognized in which coronary spasm is responsible for the clinical manifestations or at least contributes to the clinical course of events. These syndromes are discussed later.

Diagnosis and Incidence

It is accepted that coronary artery spasm may occur in both normal and diseased coronary arteries, but, until recently, spasm was considered to be a rare phenomenon. The clinical significance of coronary artery spasm has been underrated by some because of its rarity during selective coronary arteriography (0.26 to 0.93%) and the frequent absence of associated symptoms when spasm is documented (Demany et al, 1968; Lavine et al, 1973; O'Reilly et al, 1970). Chahine and associates (1975) reviewed 274 consecutive coronary angiograms obtained during a

1-year period and documented eight cases of spasm (3%). This incidence, which was higher than that reported earlier, was attributed to a systematic prospective search for the phenomenon and avoidance of vasodilators and premedication before arteriography. Although many cases of arteriographically demonstrated spasm are related to catheter tip irritation, Chahine suggested that catheter-induced spasm may occur only in patients with a predisposition to spasm. Spasm is often not specifically looked for because most patients with spasm also have fixed obstructive coronary lesions, which are thought to explain their symptoms. Clinically, it is often difficult to obtain an electrocardiogram during an episode of spontaneous chest pain because attacks may be infrequent and often occur during sleep. Numerous provocation tests have been studied, but only ergonovine appears to be diagnostically useful. Ergonovine is an ergot alkaloid and smooth muscle constrictor. Conti and associates (1979), Oliva (1979), and Waters and associates (1986) observed that ergonovine produces spasm in nearly all patients with

Prinzmetal's angina and has diagnostic value if carefully administered during cardiac catheterization. However, deaths after ergonovine administration have been reported, and this test is not universally accepted (Buxton et al, 1980). Yasue and associates (1986) reported that intracoronary injection of acetylcholine is useful for provocation of coronary spasm in susceptible arteries. Further clinical investigations will be required to determine whether acetylcholine is safer than ergonovine in the test for variant angina.

When spasm is looked for, the incidence appears to increase dramatically. Maseri and associates (1978b) reported that the incidence of variant angina in their experience increased from 2% to more than 10% of patients admitted for evaluation of anginal pain when systematic measures were used for its detection. These authors proposed that variant angina is only one manifestation of coronary artery spasm and that spasm contributes to practically all phases of ischemic heart disease.

Although the true incidence of variant angina is unknown, coronary artery spasm may be more common than was previously assumed and may contribute to the clinical manifestations of various syndromes in addition to variant angina.

Natural History

Myocardial infarction and death from infarction or ventricular arrhythmias are common in patients with documented variant angina. Benivoglio and associates (1974) reviewed 90 cases reported between 1959 and 1972 for which long-term follow-up data were available. As pointed out by Raizner and Chahine (1980), this group of patients is most representative of the natural history of variant angina because, in 1972, the pathophysiology of the syndrome was not fully appreciated and appropriate therapy was not in widespread use. Of these 90 patients, 22 (24%) developed acute myocardial infarction within several months after the onset of variant angina, and 13 patients (14%) died suddenly. Catastrophic events, therefore, occurred in 38% of the group, usually soon after onset of symptoms. Stenson and associates (1975) observed that variant angina first seen after acute myocardial infarction has an even higher mortality (33%). Although the incidence of myocardial infarction and death in patients with variant angina has decreased with more aggressive medical and surgical therapy, patients with Prinzmetal's angina should be considered to be a high-risk subgroup of patients with ischemic heart disease. Infarction or death of patients with variant angina usually occurs soon after symptoms or electrocardiographic changes. In survivors, long phases of complete remission are common (Cipriano et al, 1981; Madias, 1986; Severi et al, 1980). As a rule, patients with variant angina and concomitant significant coronary artery disease are at greater risk than the less common group of patients with variant angina and normal coronary arteries (Madias, 1986; Selzer et al, 1976).

OTHER SYNDROMES ASSOCIATED WITH CORONARY ARTERY SPASM

In addition to Prinzmetal's variant angina, coronary artery spasm may contribute to the clinical manifestations observed in various ischemic heart disease syndromes (Table 54–14).

"Silent" Variant Angina. Since Prinzmetal's original description of variant angina in 1959, a number of patients have been reported who have ST-segment elevation and documented coronary artery spasm without chest pain (Bodenheimer et al, 1974; Gorfinkel et al, 1973; Guazzi et al, 1970; Lasser and de la Paz, 1973; Maseri, 1987; Prohkov et al, 1974). Clinically, these patients are difficult to identify because their symptoms are often vague and not directly referable to the heart or they present with a catastrophic event such as acute myocardial infarction or a life-threatening arrhythmia. This subgroup of patients with variant angina were said to have "silent" variant angina (Prohkov et al, 1974) because they have all of the hallmarks of Prinzmetal's angina with the important exception of no accompanying chest pain.

Partial Spasm Mimicking Stable Angina. ST-segment elevation, chest pain, and documented coronary artery spasm are the classic clinical criteria for a diagnosis of Prinzmetal's angina. Maseri and associates (1975) reported two patients and Chahine and associates (1975) reported a third patient with documented partial coronary artery spasm who had pain both at rest and with exercise. Compared with Prinzmetal's angina, the episodes of pain were associated with ST-segment depression that mimicked the usual electrocardiographic findings in classic angina secondary to fixed obstructive atherosclerotic coronary disease. Because most patients with coronary artery spasm have concomitant atherosclerotic disease, the importance of spasm in explaining a patient's clinical course is perhaps often overlooked.

Coronary Artery Spasm and Stable Angina. A number of patients with variant angina at rest have

TABLE 54–14. SYNDROMES ASSOCIATED WITH CORONARY ARTERY SPASM

Prinzmetal's angina
"Silent" variant angina
Partial coronary artery spasm mimicking stable angina
Stable angina and coronary artery spasm
Preinfarction angina
Acute myocrdial infarction
Sudden death
Nitrate withdrawal
Perioperative arrest after myocardial revascularization
Other vasospastic disorders
  Raynaud's phenomenon
  Migraine headaches
  Peripheral venous spasm

classic effort-induced angina with characteristic ST-segment depression in the same leads that demonstrated ST-segment elevation at rest (Maseri et al, 1977). Because of advances in the medical treatment of coronary artery spasm, identification of these patients is important so that appropriate treatment can be instituted to maximize control of the most important contributor to the chest pain syndrome. As discussed later, beta-blockers can exacerbate spasm in some patients and may be contraindicated in patients with both fixed obstructive disease and vasospastic disease in which spasm is the predominant feature.

Coronary Artery Spasm Resulting in Preinfarction Angina. Patients with Prinzmetal's angina can develop a worsening pain syndrome and can have subsequent myocardial infarction. Distinct from this group are patients with long-standing stable angina or with recent onset of angina who have definite severe atherosclerotic coronary disease and later develop an accelerating pain syndrome that leads to infarction unless medical or surgical therapy is given. A number of patients who have been observed to have stable, fixed obstructive disease by serial coronary angiograms progress to preinfarction angina. Linhart and associates (1972) and Bolooki and associates (1972) reported patients with atherosclerotic coronary artery disease and preinfarction angina who had ST-segment elevation with episodes of pain without evidence of subsequent myocardial infarction. These findings suggest that the addition of spasm to long-standing fixed obstructive disease resulted in preinfarction angina. The patients in both reports were successfully managed by coronary artery bypass grafting. These observations do not implicate spasm in all cases of preinfarction angina but suggest that in some patients, the addition of spasm to fixed obstructive disease can explain the transition from stable to unstable or preinfarction angina.

Coronary Artery Spasm Resulting in Acute Myocardial Infarction. It is well documented that coronary artery spasm can result in acute myocardial infarction in patients with variant angina and normal coronary arteries (Johnson and Detwiler, 1977; King et al, 1973) as well as patients without antecedent signs or symptoms of variant angina who have atherosclerotically diseased vessels (Oliva and Breckinridge, 1977). In a study reported by Oliva and Breckinridge in 1977, 15 patients who presented with acute myocardial infarction underwent coronary arteriography within 6 hours after the onset of infarction. Coronary angiograms were obtained before and after administration of nitroglycerin. Six of the patients (40%) had coronary artery spasm superimposed on a high-grade atherosclerotic lesion. The involved coronary artery remained patent after the initial relief of spasm in two patients who were maintained on sublingual nitrates and heparin. The authors concluded that their results show the occurrence of spasm in significant numbers of patients with acute myocardial infarction but do not establish the impor-

tance of spasm in the pathophysiology of acute myocardial infarction or whether relief of spasm has a beneficial or harmful effect on myocardium rendered ischemic for a prolonged period before reperfusion. This important study emphasizes the need for further investigations of the role of spasm in patients with acute myocardial infarction, because of the possible therapeutic implications.

Coronary Artery Spasm After Acute Myocardial Infarction. Stenson and associates (1975) identified an interesting group of 9 patients out of a total of 57 patients who presented with acute myocardial infarction during a 1-year period. These 9 patients (16%) had episodes of angina more than 24 hours after initial infarction, associated with transient ST-segment elevation. Seven of these patients (78%) had a second myocardial infarction within 2 weeks to 4½ months after their first infarction. Three of the 9 patients died after reinfarction, an overall mortality of 33%. All of these patients had severe atherosclerotic coronary artery disease in addition to clinical evidence for coronary artery spasm. None had symptoms of variant angina before their first infarction. Thus, spasm became manifest in these patients after infarction and appears to have greatly increased subsequent morbidity and mortality.

Coronary Artery Spasm Resulting in Sudden Death. A number of patients who die suddenly have normal coronary arteries at post-mortem examination. Presumably, they died of an arrhythmia of uncertain etiology or died secondary to vasospasm and severe ischemia or vasospasm that initiated an arrhythmia. Cheng and associates (1973) described four patients with variant angina and normal coronary arteries at the time of catheterization. Because Prinzmetal originally postulated that spasm was most likely to be associated with atherosclerotic lesions, Cheng suggested that spasm in normal coronary arteries was a variant of Prinzmetal's angina and coined the term "a variant of the variant" angina to describe the condition. When one of these patients, a 60-year-old man with angina associated with ST-segment elevation, had coronary arteriography, no atherosclerotic disease was revealed. The patient later developed ventricular fibrillation and died. Post-mortem examination confirmed that he had completely normal coronary arteries and strongly implicated coronary artery spasm as being the cause of sudden death.

In further support of coronary artery spasm as the underlying mechanism in certain cases of sudden death are numerous reports of ventricular fibrillation in patients with documented coronary artery spasm. Prohkov and associates (1974) reported a patient who presented with ventricular fibrillation. The patient was successfully resuscitated and coronary arteriography showed total spasm of the right coronary artery, which resolved after sublingual administration of nitroglycerin. Because the patient's coronary arteries were free of atherosclerotic lesions and before ventricular fibrillation the patient had no symptoms of angina, the authors referred to this as "silent" variant angina and suggested that coronary artery spasm should be considered to be a cause of sudden death syndrome. Cipriano and associates (1981) reported the clinical course of 25 patients with coronary artery spasm documented by arteriography. Ventricular tachycardia occurred in 7 patients (28%) and led to death in 1 patient. Four of the 7 patients had absent or minimal atherosclerotic coronary disease, and 3 had severe atherosclerotic disease in addition to spasm. Waters and associates (1982) reported that myocardial infarction can occur in the absence of severe fixed lesions and despite apparent clinical improvement with administration of calcium channel blockers. Collectively, these reports show that spasm in both normal and diseased coronary arteries can result in life-threatening arrhythmias and the sudden death syndrome.

Coronary Artery Spasm and the Nitrate Withdrawal Syndrome. Lange and associates (1972) described clinical, angiographic, and hemodynamic findings for 9 patients who presented with nonatheromatous ischemic heart disease induced by chronic industrial exposure to nitroglycerin and subsequent withdrawal. This group represented almost 5% of a group of 200 workers who had similar exposure. Five of these patients had coronary arteriography, which showed reversible spasm with no atherosclerotic coronary artery disease. Two patients died suddenly, most likely secondary to reflex coronary artery spasm after nitrate withdrawal. The authors suggested that long-term exposure to nitroglycerin resulted in chronic vasodilatation, which evoked a homeostatic vasoconstrictive response that resulted in severe spasm and ischemia after nitrate withdrawal.

Coronary Artery Spasm Resulting in Perioperative Arrest. Pichard and associates (1980) reported a patient who had both angina at rest and effort-induced angina. Before the angina became worse the patient had an 8-year history of stable angina. Exercise testing showed ST-segment elevation in leads AV_L and V_2 to V_4 in addition to a short run of ventricular tachycardia. Cardiac catheterization showed 70% obstruction of the right coronary artery in its proximal third, with 90% obstruction in the left anterior descending artery proximal to the first septal perforator and 50% obstruction at the origin of a posterolateral circumflex branch. The left main coronary artery was normal, and the ejection fraction was 90%. Because of his severe obstructive disease and increased angina, the patient had uncomplicated internal mammary-to-left anterior descending coronary artery grafting and saphenous vein bypass grafting to the right coronary and posterolateral circumflex coronary arteries. He was easily separated from cardiopulmonary bypass in normal sinus rhythm and showed evidence of good left ventricular contractility. However, as the chest was being closed, the patient developed rapid atrial fibrillation followed by ventricular arrhythmias and hypotension. He required multiple countershocks and reinstitution of cardiopulmonary bypass support.

The patient was eventually stabilized and again weaned from bypass uneventfully and moved to the intensive care unit. Two hours later, he again became hypotensive, with increased left atrial pressures and associated ST-segment elevation on monitor leads. These changes progressed to rapid atrial fibrillation and recurrent ventricular tachycardia, which degenerated to ventricular fibrillation refractory to external countershock and intravenous lidocaine and procainamide. The chest was reopened; there was no evidence of tamponade, and all three grafts were patent. With internal massage, the patient was stabilized again and the chest was closed, only to be reopened again 40 minutes later for resuscitation because of another episode of refractory ventricular fibrillation. The patient remained refractory to all resuscitative agents until papaverine (1 mg) was injected into each graft and nitrol paste (2%) was applied to the skin, after which he had successful cardioversion. An intra-aortic balloon pump was inserted, and the patient subsequently made an uneventful recovery. Serial postoperative electrocardiograms showed no evidence of postoperative myocardial infarction. Thirteen days postoperatively, repeat cardiac catheterization showed that all three grafts were patent. The native coronary circulation and ejection fraction were unchanged from findings before operation. When the internal mammary artery graft was injected with contrast medium, the patient developed ST-segment elevation without chest pain or arrhythmias. Repeat internal mammary artery visualization showed severe, diffuse spasm of the entire left anterior descending coronary artery, which resolved after administration of nitroglycerin. The patient was subsequently maintained on nitroglycerin and aspirin without further problems and returned to work 6 weeks after operation.

Retrospectively, it appears that this patient had fixed obstructive disease and manifested spasm when his angina increased. Spasm persisted during the perioperative period and resulted in the course of clinical events reported. Based on these observations, the authors suggest that coronary artery spasm be considered strongly in the differential diagnosis of perioperative hemodynamic deterioration in patients after coronary artery bypass graft surgery, especially in the presence of ST-segment elevation or intractable ventricular arrhythmias. Buxton and associates (1981) reported six patients who had similar problems immediately after myocardial revascularization. These reports suggest that coronary artery spasm after coronary artery bypass grafting may be more than a rare phenomenon. Lemmer and Kirsh (1988) reviewed in detail published reports of coronary spasm in the postoperative period and identified important predisposing factors, which are discussed later.

Coronary Artery Spasm Associated with Other Vasospastic Disorders. There is some evidence, although not conclusive, that coronary artery spasm is more common in patients with other vasospastic diseases such as Raynaud's phenomenon, progressive systemic sclerosis, peripheral venous spasm, and migraine headaches. Robertson and Oates (1978) described three patients with both variant angina and Raynaud's phenomenon. One patient had continuous electrocardiographic monitoring for 26 days, and 569 episodes of ST-segment elevation occurred without chest pain ("silent" variant angina). None of these patients had simultaneous chest pain with attacks of Raynaud's phenomenon, and although a cool environment could trigger signs of Raynaud's phenomenon, it was unrelated to episodes of variant angina. Spasm in normal coronary arteries that results in myocardial infarction and sudden death has been associated with progressive systemic sclerosis in patients who previously had Raynaud's phenomenon (Bulkley et al, 1978). Miller and associates (1981) studied 62 patients with variant angina and noted a statistically increased incidence of both Raynaud's phenomenon and migraine headaches compared with patients with atherosclerotic coronary disease without signs or symptoms of variant angina. This study did not show that the prevalence of Raynaud's phenomenon in women with variant angina was statistically higher than that in men with variant angina, although Raynaud's phenomenon is five times more common in women than in men (Coffman and Cohen, 1981).

Dagenais and associates (1970) described a 15-year-old female with tetralogy of Fallot with severe peripheral venous spasm observed during cardiac catheterization. In association with venous spasm, the patient developed simultaneous chest pain and ST-segment elevation, which resolved at the same time that the venous spasm resolved.

Because Raynaud's phenomenon, migraine headaches, and peripheral venous spasm sometimes appear to be triggered by emotional stress, it was suggested that investigations into the etiology of variant angina should include the possibility of a central neurogenic trigger mechanism (Coffman and Cohen, 1981).

PATHOPHYSIOLOGY OF CORONARY ARTERY SPASM

Spasm can occur in both normal and atherosclerotically diseased coronary arteries and it is an important component in various ischemic heart disease syndromes other than Prinzmetal's variant angina. Furthermore, spasm can completely or partially occlude a coronary artery, involve one or more vessels, and be diffuse or segmental in nature (Conti et al, 1979). Cannon and Epstein (1988) described patients with angiographically normal coronary arteries who had increased sensitivity to vasoconstrictor stimuli only within coronary arterioles. They called this syndrome "microvascular angina" and found that symptoms were improved by calcium antagonists. Despite the wealth of clinical information about Prinzmetal's angina and the apparently ubiquitous nature of spasm in other coronary syndromes, little

is known about the exact pathogenesis of coronary spasm.

Two general areas of investigation appear to be promising; one involves the study of neurogenic mechanisms and the other involves humoral and metabolic factors that affect vascular smooth muscle tone. A number of clinical studies and studies of animals can be cited to show that either of these possibilities is important in the pathogenesis of coronary spasm. It may eventually be shown that both mechanisms are interrelated or that either can be important in specific groups of patients with spasm.

Neurogenic Mechanisms

Considerable evidence suggests that neurogenic stimulation that originates centrally or via the autonomic nervous system is important in the etiology of coronary artery spasm.

Central Nervous System. There may be an increased incidence of variant angina in patients with generalized vasospastic disorders such as Raynaud's phenomenon, progressive systemic sclerosis, peripheral venous spasm, and migraine headaches. Because these disorders can be triggered by emotional stress, it has been suggested that variant angina may also be initiated by perceived stress (Coffman and Cohen, 1981). Melville and associates (1969) showed that severe coronary constriction can result from electrical stimulation of the central nervous system in monkeys. Also, two reports described patients with subarachnoid hemorrhage who had transient and repeated episodes of ST-segment elevation with reciprocal ST-segment depression, presumably secondary to coronary artery spasm (Goldman et al, 1975; Toyama et al, 1979). However, Cipriano and associates (1979) showed that ergonovine can cause coronary artery spasm in susceptible, totally denervated, transplanted human hearts, which suggests that the final trigger mechanism is within intramyocardial autonomic receptors or that a humoral trigger mechanism is of primary importance.

Autonomic Nervous System. SYMPATHETIC INFLUENCES. A network of autonomic nerve fibers that supply coronary arteries is demonstrated by electron microscopic and histochemical studies. Both parasympathetic and sympathetic components of the autonomic nervous system have been implicated in coronary artery spasm.

Sympathetic nerves in large numbers connect with the smooth muscle cells of coronary arteries. Beta-adrenergic stimulation results in coronary arterial dilatation by both direct and indirect mechanisms. Stimulation of smooth muscle $beta_2$-receptors directly dilates coronary arteries. Stimulation of $beta_1$-receptors results in metabolically mediated dilatation due to an increase in heart rate and contractility. Alpha-sympathetic receptor stimulation causes coronary arterial constriction. The balance between alpha and $beta_1$-$beta_2$ sympathetic discharge is thought to account for a component of normal coronary arteriolar resistance or "tone." Kelley and Feigl (1978) showed in dogs that alpha-receptor-induced coronary constriction can be produced by pretreatment with propranolol to block beta vasodilatory sympathetic responses, followed by intracoronary injection of norepinephrine and simultaneous electrical stimulation of the left stellate ganglion. The increase in large vessel resistance was approximately 60% of the total observed for the entire coronary bed, which suggests that sympathetically mediated coronary vasoconstriction affects distal small vessels and not just large epicardial vessels.

Ricci and associates (1979) showed that coronary artery spasm in eight patients was rapidly reversed by intravenous administration of the alpha-adrenergic blocker phentolamine. In four additional patients with recurrent episodes of coronary spasm, oral administration of the alpha-adrenergic blocker phenoxybenzamine prevented symptoms of spasm during a 1-year period of follow-up. Also some patients with vasospastic angina have had attacks triggered by exposure to a cold environment, and it has been suggested that the stress of cold exposure activates alpha-sympathetic discharge that results in coronary artery spasm. To test this hypothesis, Mudge and associates (1976) exposed susceptible patients to cold after intravenous administration of the alpha-adrenergic blocker phentolamine. The results showed that coronary vasoconstriction could be prevented in this group by pretreatment with phentolamine. It has not been possible to document increased alpha-sympathetic tone in patients susceptible to spasm. Robertson and associates (1979) found normal levels of urinary and plasma catecholamines and metabolite levels of catecholamines in three patients with coronary artery spasm. They obtained blood samples from two patients at the onset and termination of spontaneous episodes of ST-segment elevation and found no significant changes in catecholamine levels. There was no evidence for a generalized increase in sympathetic discharge in patients during episodes of coronary artery spasm. These data, however, do not exclude the possibility that alpha-beta$_1$, beta$_2$ sympathetic imbalance is operative in patients with coronary artery spasm.

PARASYMPATHETIC INFLUENCES. Compared with the dense network of sympathetic fibers that supply coronary arteries, parasympathetic fibers are found in much smaller numbers in the heart (Hillis and Braunwald, 1978). There is evidence that increased activity of the parasympathetic system can trigger spasm. The fact that patients with variant angina usually have attacks of coronary artery spasm at rest supports this theory, because parasympathetic activity is maximal at rest and is suppressed during exercise.

Both sympathetic and parasympathetic fibers are found in parasympathetic vagal ganglia that innervate the heart. Stimulation of the vagus (parasympathetic) nerve or intracoronary injection of its neu-

rotransmitter, acetylcholine, results in coronary vasodilatation (Berne et al, 1965; Blesa and Ross, 1970; Blumenthal et al, 1968; Feigl, 1969; Hackett et al, 1972; Levy and Zieske, 1969). However, in addition to causing direct vasodilatation, acetylcholine appears to cause release of norepinephrine from postganglionic sympathetic nerve endings in the heart (Blumenthal et al, 1968; Burn, 1967; Cabrera et al, 1966; Dempsey and Cooper, 1969; Levy, 1971). Normally, coronary blood flow is regulated primarily by metabolic requirements of the heart (an increase in myocardial oxygen consumption causes coronary vasodilatation), and neurogenic control is less important. Excess parasympathetic activity causes decreases in heart rate, blood pressure, and myocardial contractility, all of which lead to reduced myocardial oxygen consumption and thus eliminate metabolic factors that normally control coronary vascular tone.

Yasue and associates (1974) and Endo and associates (1976) postulated that increased parasympathetic activity stimulates alpha-sympathetic nerves in parasympathetic ganglia, which can cause severe coronary artery spasm under resting conditions. Yasue and associates (1974) studied 10 patients with Prinzmetal's angina and found that administration of the parasympathomimetic drug methacholine could induce spasm and the parasympathetic blocker atropine could prevent attacks of spasm. Epinephrine provoked attacks of spasm in some patients if resting parasympathetic tone appeared to be increased but had little effect if resting parasympathetic tone was normal. Administration of the beta-adrenergic blocker propranolol could not prevent attacks, but administration of the alpha-adrenergic blocker phenoxybenzamine could prevent spasm. The authors concluded that excessive parasympathetic activity may exist in patients who are prone to coronary artery spasm, that increased parasympathetic activity selectively stimulates alpha sympathetic fibers in parasympathetic ganglia, and that alpha-adrenergic stimulation is the final common pathway to coronary artery spasm. This work is supported by the observation that attacks of variant angina usually occur in patients at rest when baseline parasympathetic tone is increased. Further support for this theory was provided by the observations of Nowlin and associates (1965) and Murao and associates (1972), who reported that attacks of variant angina in susceptible individuals are associated with the rapid eye movement (REM) period of sleep. REM sleep is triggered by acetylcholine, which indicates increased parasympathetic activity, and is suppressed by atropine, which blocks acetylcholine release. Yasue and associates (1986) reported that intracoronary injection of acetylcholine resulted in coronary spasm in patients with variant angina.

In summary, the studies described suggest that parasympathetic-sympathetic imbalance in the autonomic nervous system of patients with coronary artery spasm may be an important trigger mechanism (Fig. 54–87). Whether higher-level central nervous

NEUROGENIC IMBALANCES RESULTING IN
CORONARY SPASM

CENTRAL NERVOUS SYSTEM

↓ ? Stress

HYPOTHALAMUS

↓

AUTONOMIC NERVOUS SYSTEM
Parasympathetic ⇌ Sympathetic Imbalance

Increased ACH   Beta adrenergic stimulation   Increased alpha
                                                             adrenergic stimulation

CORONARY   CORONARY
VASODILATATION   SPASM

Figure 54–87. Schematic representation of postulated para-sympathetic-sympathetic imbalances leading to increased alpha-sympathetic activity and coronary spasm. Heavy *arrows* indicate direction of the imbalance.

system input is related to this imbalance is unknown. The only evidence against neurogenic mechanisms is the fact that denervated hearts susceptible to spasm can still be provoked to show coronary artery spasm by administration of agents such as ergonovine (Clark et al, 1977). However, ergonovine appears to work by stimulation of alpha receptors in coronary arteries, thus this evidence does not disprove the theories that postulate that the final pathway in the initiation of coronary artery spasm involves alpha receptor activity in coronary arteries.

Humoral-Metabolic Mechanisms

Platelet–Prostaglandin–Vessel Wall Interactions. The role of prostaglandins in initiating and mediating various physiologic responses is under intense investigation. It has been suggested that platelet-prostaglandin and coronary vessel wall interactions are important in the pathophysiology of myocardial ischemia. It is generally accepted that platelet aggregation on atherosclerotic plaques can initiate thrombosis, and there is evidence that platelets may also be involved in the initiation of coronary artery spasm. Platelets release thromboxane A_2 as they aggregate. Thromboxane A_2 is a powerful endogenous vasoconstrictor as well as a stimulator for further platelet aggregation. Within vessel walls a prostaglandin, prostacyclin (PGI_2), is normally synthesized which has biologic actions that directly oppose those of thromboxane A_2. Specifically, PGI_2 causes vasodilatation and inhibits platelet aggregation (Bunting et al, 1976; Dusting et al, 1978). It has been suggested that the balance between PGI_2 release and thrombox-

ane release contributes to normal coronary vascular tone and the stimulation or inhibition of platelet aggregation (Boullin et al, 1979; Dusting et al, 1978; Moncada et al, 1977). This balance may be disrupted in coronary artery disease. Studies in both humans and animals showed that atherosclerotic coronary arteries have a decreased ability to synthesize prostacyclin (D'Angelo et al, 1978; Dembinska-Kiec et al, 1977). Furthermore, platelets from patients who survive acute myocardial infarction synthesize increased quantities of thromboxane A_2 (Szczeklik et al, 1978). These studies suggest that in coronary artery disease, an imbalance between prostacyclin release and thromboxane release favors vasoconstriction and platelet aggregation. Increased thromboxane release can cause vasoconstriction but has not been proved to cause coronary artery spasm. However, Lewy and associates (1979) and Tada and associates (1981) reported increased levels of thromboxane B_2, the major metabolite of thromboxane A_2, in patients with Prinzmetal's angina. Whether thromboxane release initiated spasm or was secondary to spasm and platelet aggregation is unknown.

Synthesis of both thromboxane and prostacyclin begins with arachidonic acid, a free fatty acid. The metabolism of arachidonic acid and the possible relationship between platelets, prostaglandins, and vessel walls in initiating coronary artery spasm are shown schematically in Figure 54–88.

Hydrogen Ion-Calcium Ion Imbalances. Contraction of vascular smooth muscle depends on the

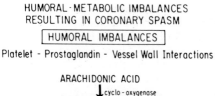

HUMORAL-METABOLIC IMBALANCES
RESULTING IN CORONARY SPASM
HUMORAL IMBALANCES
Platelet - Prostaglandin - Vessel Wall Interactions

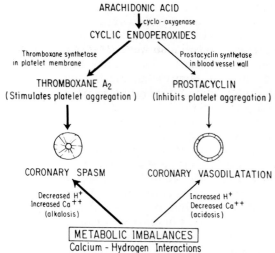

ARACHIDONIC ACID
↓ cyclo - oxygenase
CYCLIC ENDOPEROXIDES

Thromboxane synthetase   Prostacyclin synthetase
in platelet membrane   in blood vessel wall

THROMBOXANE A_2 PROSTACYCLIN
(Stimulates platelet aggregation)   (Inhibits platelet aggregation)

CORONARY SPASM   CORONARY VASODILATATION

Decreased H^+ Increased H^+
Increased Ca^{++} Decreased Ca^{++}
(alkalosis)   (acidosis)

METABOLIC IMBALANCES
Calcium - Hydrogen Interactions

Figure 54–88. Schematic representation of humoral-metabolic imbalances that have been postulated to initiate coronary spasm. Heavy *arrows* indicate direction of the imbalance. (Adapted from Conti, C. R., Pepine, C., and Curry, R. C.: Coronary artery spasm: An important mechanism in the pathophysiology of ischemic heart disease. Curr. Probl. Cardiol., 4:1, 1979. Reproduced with permission.)

presence of calcium ions, which are necessary for the activation of myofibrillar ATPase (Bohr, 1973; Fleckenstein et al, 1976). Physiologically, hydrogen ions exert a potent calcium antagonist action by competition with calcium ions for transport across cell membranes as well as for binding sites at the myofibrillar level (Fleckenstein et al, 1976). It appears that vasoconstriction can occur if calcium ion concentration increases or hydrogen ion concentration decreases. Vasodilatation is produced by decreased transmembrane calcium flux or increased hydrogen ion concentration. Yasue and associates (1978) gave nine patients with documented Prinzmetal's angina an infusion of 100 ml of TRIS buffer over a 5-minute period, followed by hyperventilation for a second 5-minute period. Arterial pH increased from normal values to 7.65 with this protocol, and eight of the nine patients developed ST-segment elevation. With the onset of alkalosis and ST-segment elevation, simultaneous coronary angiograms revealed spasm. The patients were then pretreated with the calcium blocker diltiazem and the experimental protocol was done again. After pretreatment with diltiazem, alkalosis did not induce attacks of Prinzmetal's angina. Because hydrogen ion production decreases at rest, particularly during sleep, when metabolism slows, and the respiratory rate often increases during REM sleep, alkalosis may result. Prinzmetal's angina is more likely to occur at rest and during periods of REM sleep, and the authors suggest that hydrogen ion-calcium ion imbalances may trigger coronary artery spasm (see Fig. 54–88).

MANAGEMENT OF PATIENTS WITH CORONARY ARTERY SPASM

Coronary artery spasm appears to be an important component in various syndromes other than Prinzmetal's angina, and appropriate therapy must be carefully individualized. Most patients with coronary artery spasm also have atheromatous disease, and it is important to try to identify the relative contribution of each of these processes so that successful treatment can be given. A rational approach to therapy must also take into account that over time, the clinical manifestations of ischemia may at one point be secondary to spasm and later be due to increased atherosclerotic disease with concomitant spasm. Appropriate therapy, therefore, involves both medical and surgical interventions (Table 54–15).

Medical Therapy

Nitroglycerin effectively terminates acute attacks of coronary artery spasm and should be given at the onset of symptoms. Maintenance therapy is directed toward prevention of recurrent attacks of spasm by the addition of long-acting nitrates. Patients should be warned about the possible provocation of spasm

TABLE 54–15. THERAPY FOR CORONARY ARTERY SPASM

MEDICAL THERAPY
  Calcium antagonists (nifedipine, verapamil, diltiazem, perhexiline maleate)
  Nitrates
  Nonsteroidal anti-inflammatory agents (aspirin, indomethacin, dipyridamole, sulfinpyrazone, ibuprofen)
  Alpha-adrenergic blockers (phentolamine, phenoxybenzamine)
  Beta-adrenergic blockers (selected patients with atherosclerotic disease and spasm)

SURGICAL THERAPY (selected patients only)
  Coronary artery bypass grafting
  Cardiac denervation

by drugs such as Cafergot, an ergot alkaloid used to treat migraine headaches and environmental influences such as sudden exposure to cold. Patients have been reported who developed coronary spasm after alcohol ingestion (Takizawa et al, 1984), emotional stress (Schiffer et al, 1980), extradural anesthesia (Krantz et al, 1980), biliary colic (Antonelli and Rosenfeld, 1987), hyperventilation (Hisano et al, 1984), aspirin ingestion (Miwa et al, 1983), calcium injection (Boulanger et al, 1984), phenylephrine eyedrop administration (Alder et al, 1981), and cytotoxic chemotherapy (Kleiman et al, 1987; Shachor et al, 1985). These reports show the importance of a careful history in identifying possible "trigger events" in individual patients with variant angina. Although nitroglycerin and other nitrates are often effective, breakthrough attacks are common, and most patients require more than just nitrate therapy for control.

Most patients with coronary artery spasm have concomitant atheromatous disease and beta-adrenergic blockers have been tried with various success rates. Evidence summarized by Conti and associates (1979) suggests that beta-blockers are "effective, occasionally useful, ineffective or possibly harmful" in patients with attacks of coronary artery spasm. Theoretically, beta-blockade can initiate spasm by allowing alpha-adrenergic sympathetic activity to predominate with subsequent vasoconstriction. However, in patients with ischemia due to fixed obstructive disease as well as intermittent spasm, beta-blockers, such as propranolol, may be an important adjunct to medical therapy. Therapy with beta-blockers should be initiated slowly and under careful supervision. Patients have been reported who have variant angina that does not respond to calcium channel blocking drugs but does respond to combined calcium channel and beta-blocking drugs (Bourmayan et al, 1983).

There are isolated reports that alpha-adrenergic receptor blocking agents prevented coronary artery spasm. Mudge and associates (1976) showed that administration of the alpha-adrenergic blocker phentolamine can block reflex coronary constriction caused by exposure to cold. Tzivoni and associates (1983) reported beneficial effects with the selective alpha$_1$-blocker prazosin, whereas Winniford and associates (1983) found that prazosin treatment resulted in no improvement in symptoms or decrease in episodes of spasm identified by Holter monitoring. To date, no large clinical trials have investigated the efficacy of various alpha-blockers. Because the final pathogenesis of spasm may well involve alpha-adrenergic receptors, alpha-blockers deserve further clinical investigation.

Humoral theories suggest that platelet-vessel wall interactions are important in the pathogenesis of spasm, and drugs such as aspirin, indomethacin, sulfinpyrazone, dipyridamole, and ibuprofen are being investigated. These drugs are nonsteroidal anti-inflammatory agents that appear to inhibit platelet aggregation and prevent release of the potent vasoconstrictor thromboxane A_2 from platelet membranes. However, in some patients coronary spasm has been induced by anti-inflammatory agents such as aspirin. Coronary arteries synthesize PGI_2, which causes vasodilatation, and aspirin suppresses the synthesis of prostaglandins by blocking cyclo-oxygenase. Therefore, it is postulated that, in certain patients, aspirin therapy can result in vasoconstriction and coronary spasm (Miwa et al, 1983).

At present, the most promising breakthrough in the treatment of Prinzmetal's angina and other syndromes that involve coronary artery spasm is the addition of calcium antagonists (Fig. 54–89). These agents are powerful vasodilators, and a large number of clinical studies indicate impressive results in prevention of coronary artery spasm. Nitroglycerin causes vasodilatation by blocking calcium influx into smooth muscle cells of large epicardial coronary arteries, and adenosine preferentially dilates smaller intramyocardial coronary branches, also by blockade

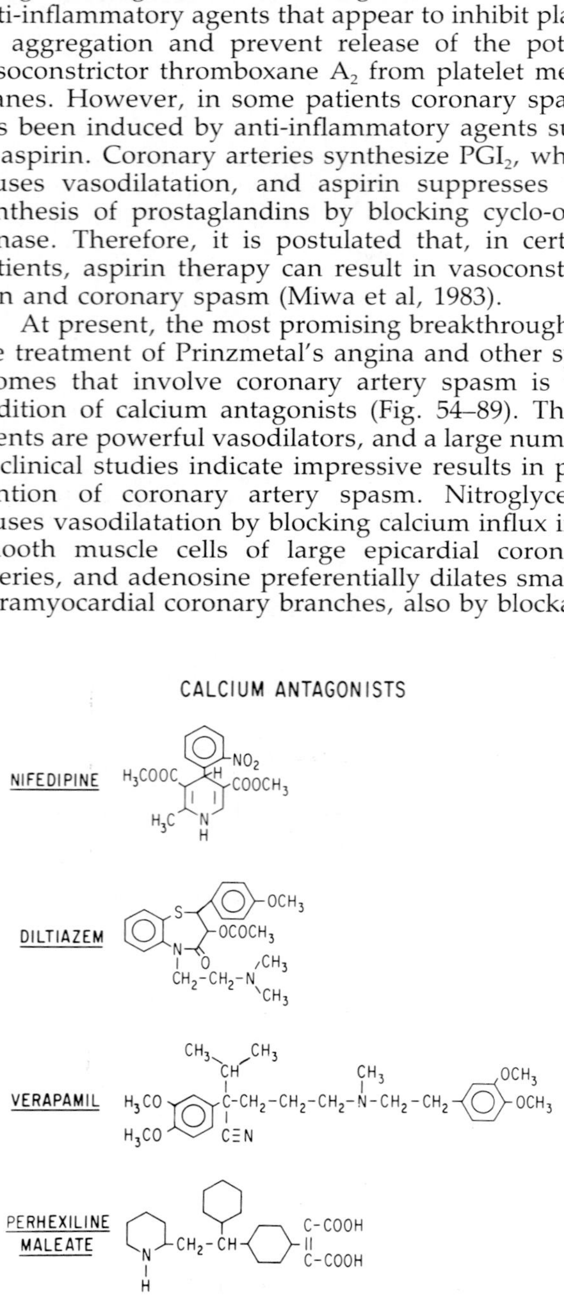

of calcium influx (Harder et al, 1979). Calcium antagonists, including nifedipine, verapamil, diltiazem, and perhexiline maleate, appear to dilate both large epicardial and small intramural coronary arteries. It is thought that the primary beneficial effect of these agents is via their vasodilatory actions, but diltiazem and verapamil are also potent inhibitors of platelet aggregation (Shinjo et al, 1978).

Increasing numbers of patients are being treated with calcium blockers, and initial reports show impressive efficacy. Endo and associates (1975) reported 35 patients with variant angina (16 with spasm and atherosclerotic disease and 19 with spasm in normal coronary arteries). Twenty-six patients were treated medically, with one death and persistence of symptoms in most patients. Addition of nifedipine to the treatment regimen of the remaining 25 patients resulted in complete relief of symptoms in each case. Antman and associates (1980) studied 127 patients with coronary spasm and found that nifedipine (40 to 160 mg/day) significantly decreased mean weekly anginal attacks from 16 to 2 ($p <0.001$). Encouraging results have been reported for verapamil (Johnson et al, 1981; Severi et al, 1979), diltiazem (Feldman et al, 1979; Pepine et al, 1981; Rosenthal et al, 1980; Schroeder et al, 1982), and perhexiline maleate (Conti et al, 1979; Raabe, 1979). Kimura and Kishida (1981) found that the efficacy rates of nifedipine, diltiazem, and verapamil were 94, 90.8, and 85.7%, respectively, in 286 patients with variant angina. Rutitzky and associates (1982) reported that amiodarone is effective in the prevention of coronary spasm. However, amiodarone has many toxic side effects and should be used only in patients refractory to calcium channel antagonists. In most of these reports, calcium antagonists have proved most efficacious when used with long-acting nitrates. Although long-term follow-up must be awaited, the addition of calcium blockers to the medical therapy of coronary artery spasm appears to be a major contribution that will decrease subsequent morbidity and mortality.

Surgical Therapy

Coronary artery bypass grafting is very effective in relieving angina in patients with obstructive coronary artery disease and prolongation of life results in specific subgroups such as those with left main coronary artery disease or severe three-vessel disease with impaired left ventricular function. Furthermore, numerous large series show that these benefits can be achieved with very low operative morbidity and mortality. Surgical intervention in the management of patients with coronary artery spasm is a more complex issue.

Since the initial report by Silverman and Flamm in 1971 of two patients with coronary disease and variant angina treated by bypass grafting, numerous small series have been reported with various results. Conti and associates (1979) and Raizner and Chahine

Figure 54–89. Structural formulas of the commonly used calcium antagonists.

TABLE 54–16. RESULTS OF MEDICAL TREATMENT OF PRINZMETAL'S ANGINA*

| No. of Patients | Atheromatous Coronary Disease | | Asymptomatic or Improved (%) | Same or Worse (%) | Myocardial Infarction (%) | Died (%) |
	None (%)	One or More Arteries Involved (%)				
275	22	78	47	47	23	6

*Adapted from Raizner, A. E., and Chahine, R. A.: The treatment of Prinzmetal's variant angina with coronary bypass surgery. *In* Hurst, J. W. (ed): Update II: The Heart—Bypass Surgery for Obstructive Coronary Disease, Chapter 9. New York, McGraw-Hill, 1980.

(1980) reviewed the results of coronary artery bypass grafting in patients with variant angina with both normal and atherosclerotically diseased coronary arteries. As shown in Tables 54–16 to 54–19, these reviews indicated that:

1. Coronary artery bypass grafting is generally contraindicated in patients with variant angina who do not have concomitant significant atherosclerotic disease.

2. Coronary artery bypass grafting may be an important adjunct to the medical treatment of patients with variant angina and concomitant atherosclerotic disease.

Addition of calcium blockers to the medical treatment of variant angina may control spasm so effectively that patients with concomitant atherosclerotic disease may have bypass grafting with morbidity and mortality that approach those achieved in patients with obstructive disease alone (Schick et al, 1982). At present, the effect of calcium antagonist therapy on the selection of patients for bypass grafting is an unsettled issue. In general, patients with variant angina and normal coronary arteries should be treated medically, and those with significant obstructive disease and variant angina should be considered for operation only if they are refractory to medical therapy or, more ideally, if medical therapy is successful in relieving spasm but the patient remains symptomatic secondary to significant obstructive disease.

In addition to coronary bypass grafting, various other procedures have been used to prevent coronary spasm. Bertrand and associates (1981b) used extensive cardiac denervation (plexectomy) followed by

coronary bypass grafting in 30 patients with two operative deaths (6.7%). Twenty-eight patients on no medical therapy were followed for an average of 23 months and only two patients had recurrent attacks of angina. Similar results were reported by Betriu and associates (1983) and DiPaolo and associates (1985). Cardiac denervation was also accomplished by autotransplantation (Bertrand et al, 1981b; Clark et al, 1977) with mixed results. Sussman and associates (1981) placed bypass grafts distal to areas of focal spasm followed by proximal ligation of the native coronary. Both patients were asymptomatic without anginal medication at 24 and 66 months. The authors recommend this approach only in patients who are completely refractory to calcium antagonists.

Management of Coronary Artery Spasm After Coronary Artery Bypass Grafting

Although the importance of spasm in patients with atherosclerotic coronary artery disease and angina is becoming more apparent, its role is often overlooked, and spasm may first be recognized in the perioperative period. A dramatic example is the case report of Pichard and associates (1980), which was cited earlier. This report and that of six additional patients described by Buxton and associates (1981) show that coronary artery spasm after coronary artery bypass grafting can result in cardiac arrest. A number of cardiovascular surgeons have had similar unreported experiences, and this phenomenon may be frequent enough to require further investigation.

TABLE 54–17. RESULTS OF CORONARY BYPASS GRAFTING IN PATIENTS WITH PRINZMETAL'S ANGINA AND ATHEROSCLEROTIC CORONARY ARTERY DISEASE*

No. of Patients	Asymptomatic or Improved (%)	Same or Worse (%)	Myocardial Infarction (%)	Died (%)
90	73	19	12	8

*Adapted from Raizner, A. E., and Chahine, R. A.: The treatment of Prinzmetal's variant angina with coronary bypass surgery. *In* Hurst, J. W. (ed): Update II: The Heart—Bypass Surgery for Obstructive Coronary Disease, Chapter 9. New York, McGraw-Hill, 1980.

TABLE 54–18. RESULTS OF MEDICAL THERAPY IN PATIENTS WITH PRINZMETAL'S ANGINA AND "NORMAL" CORONARY ARTERIES*

No. of Patients	Asymptomatic or Improved (%)	Same or Worse (%)	Myocardial Infarction (%)	Died (%)
41	66	27	7	7

*Adapted from Raizner, A. E., and Chahine, R. A.: The treatment of Prinzmetal's variant angina with coronary bypass surgery. *In* Hurst, J. W. (ed): Update II: The Heart—Bypass Surgery for Obstructive Coronary Disease, Chapter 9. New York, McGraw-Hill, 1980.

TABLE 54–19. RESULTS OF CORONARY ARTERY BYPASS GRAFTING IN PATIENTS WITH PRINZMETAL'S ANGINA AND "NORMAL" CORONARY ARTERIES*

No. of Patients	Asymptomatic or Improved (%)	Same or Worse (%)	Myocardial Infarction (%)	Died (%)
8	50	25	13	25

*Adapted from Raizner, A. E., and Chahine, R. A.: The treatment of Prinzmetal's variant angina with coronary bypass surgery. *In* Hurst, J. W. (ed): Update II: The Heart—Bypass Surgery for Obstructive Coronary Disease, Chapter 9. New York, McGraw-Hill, 1980.

As suggested by Pichard and associates (1980), coronary artery spasm should be suspected perioperatively in the patient who has myocardial revascularization and displays ventricular arrhythmias or hemodynamic instability associated with ST-segment elevation. Prompt therapy with coronary vasodilators may be lifesaving.

An excellent review of coronary spasm after coronary surgery has been published by Lemmer and Kirsh (1988). The authors found that preoperative angina at rest was an important factor in the development of postoperative native coronary spasm. Also, in 79% of patients with postoperative spasm, inferior electrocardiographic changes indicated right coronary artery involvement. The right coronary artery was angiographically free of significant obstruction and was not grafted at the time of operation. Infusion of catecholamine, especially dopamine, in-

TABLE 54–20. MANAGEMENT OF EARLY POST–CORONARY ARTERY BYPASS CORONARY ARTERY SPASM*

Situation	Management plan
Preoperative	1. Identify patients at risk 2. Maintain oral calcium channel antagonists until time of operation
Intraoperative	1. Inject intragraft nitroglycerin (0.2-mg increments) 2. Administer sublingual nifedipine (10-mg increments) or intravenous verapamil (2.5- to 5.0-mg increments) 3. Avoid vasoconstricting agents
Postoperative Patient stable	1. Perform cardiac catheterization 2. If spasm present, inject nitroglycerin (0.2-mg increments) directly into coronary artery or vein graft
Patient unstable	1. Quickly exclude other causes of deterioration 2. Administer sublingual nifedipine or intravenous verapamil 3. If patient is severely hypotensive or arrested, perform emergency sternotomy for open cardiac massage and direct injection into vein grafts

*Reprinted with permission from The Society of Thoracic Surgeons (The Annals of Thoracic Surgery, Vol. 46, 1988, p. 108)

duced postoperative spasm. The authors emphasize that reluctance to use vasodilating agents must be overcome, even if hypotension is present, when evidence of postoperative coronary spasm is apparent. The management of perioperative coronary spasm is shown in Table 54–20.

RESULTS OF THERAPY FOR VARIANT ANGINA

Conti and associates (1979) and Raizner and Chahine (1980) reviewed in detail the results of medical and surgical therapy for variant angina. As shown in Tables 54–16 and 54–17, there is only a slight difference in mortality between patients with variant angina and coronary artery disease treated medically and patients treated by coronary artery bypass grafting. These groups are not directly comparable, however; as shown in Table 54–16, 22% of medically treated patients had no significant atherosclerotic coronary disease. However, there appears to be a decrease in symptoms in patients with variant angina and coronary disease who had successful coronary artery bypass grafting (73% asymptomatic or improved compared with 47% asymptomatic or improved with medical therapy).

Tables 54–18 and 54–19 compare medical and surgical results in the treatment of variant angina in patients without significant coronary artery disease. These data indicate that coronary artery bypass grafting is contraindicated in this subgroup of patients and that medical therapy, although not ideal, is superior. If spasm can be controlled effectively by calcium antagonists, selection of patients who would benefit from coronary artery bypass grafting or possible cardiac denervation procedures may become more objective. It is hoped that these agents will also decrease the incidence of perioperative myocardial infarction as well as operative mortality secondary to the persistence of spasm.

Selected Bibliography

Cannon, R. O., and Epstein, S. E.: "Microvascular angina" as a cause of chest pain with angiographically normal coronary arteries. Am. J. Cardiol., 61:1338, 1988.

It has long been recognized that coronary vasospasm can occur in large epicardial coronary arteries. This clinical investigation is the first to show that some patients can develop angina secondary to an increased sensitivity to vasoconstrictor stimuli of small coronary arterioles. The authors called this vasospastic disorder "microvascular angina" and suggested that it is caused by a basic derangement of cellular calcium regulation, because this group of patients responded favorably to calcium antagonist agents.

Kimura, E., and Kishida, H.: Treatment of variant angina with drugs: A survey of 11 cardiology institutes in Japan. Circulation, 63:844, 1981.

This clinical study summarizes data from 11 cardiology institutes in Japan to determine the effectiveness of various calcium antagonists in variant angina. There were 286 patients available for comparison. The efficacy rates of nifedipine, diltiazem, and verapamil were 94, 90.8, and 85.7%, respectively. Regardless of the presence or absence of organic coronary lesions, the agents were effective in 92.3% of patients with normal or almost normal coronary arteries and 82.6% of patients with stenosis of more than 50% of the luminal diameter.

Lemmer, J. H., and Kirsh, M. M.: Coronary artery spasm following coronary artery surgery. Ann. Thorac. Surg., 46:108, 1988.

This is an excellent review of perioperative coronary artery spasm after myocardial revascularization procedures. The literature on perioperative coronary spasm is reviewed and methods of prevention, diagnosis, and treatment are discussed in detail. Preoperative angina at rest appears to be an important factor in patients who have postoperative coronary spasm. Anatomically, the presence of a relatively normal, dominant right coronary artery may also indicate risk for early postoperative spasm. Acute hypotension is often the first sign of coronary artery spasm, and conventional treatment methods may increase the vasospastic reaction. Peripheral intravenous nitroglycerin effusion has often been unsuccessful. Intragraft or intracoronary nitroglycerin injection or administration of calcium channel-blocking drugs, or both, has been effective in reversing the coronary artery spasm and ventricular dysfunction. The authors emphasize that reluctance to use vasodilating agents must be overcome, even if confronted with hypotension, when evidence for postoperative spasm is present.

Maseri, A.: Role of coronary artery spasm in symptomatic and silent myocardial ischemia. J. Am. Coll. Cardiol., 9:249, 1987.

A detailed discussion of the diagnosis, treatment, and pathophysiology of vasospastic angina is presented. Maseri and associates have contributed greatly to our understanding of the clinical manifestations of coronary artery spasm and have accumulated convincing evidence that spasm may contribute to practically all aspects of ischemic heart disease.

Oliva, P. B., Potts, D. E., and Pluss, R. G.: Coronary arterial spasm in Prinzmetal angina. Documentation by coronary arteriography. N. Engl. J. Med., 288:745, 1973.

This manuscript is among the first to show convincingly that the clinical and electrocardiographic manifestations of variant angina are secondary to transient episodes of coronary artery spasm. Evidence is presented that the severity of coronary artery spasm can vary from one attack to another and that spasm can be diffuse or segmental.

Prinzmetal, M., Kennamer, R., Merliss, R., et al: Angina pectoris. I: A variant form of angina pectoris. Am. J. Med., 27:375, 1959.

This classic article describes the clinical manifestations of 32 patients with a different kind of anginal syndrome referred to as variant angina. Unlike typical angina, variant angina is not associated with effort, eating, or anxiety. Prinzmetal correctly postulated that "temporary increased tonus of a large coronary artery" occurred in these patients during episodes of chest pain. The clinical manifestations of variant angina, initially described by Prinzmetal, are still the criteria for establishing a diagnosis of vasospastic angina. Variant angina is commonly referred to as Prinzmetal's angina in recognition of this major contribution.

Raizner, A. E., and Chahine, R. A.: The treatment of Prinzmetal's variant angina with coronary bypass surgery. In Hurst, J. W. (ed): Update II: The Heart—Bypass Surgery for Obstructive Coronary Disease, Chapter 9. New York, McGraw-Hill, 1980.

This review summarizes the results of medical and surgical therapy for Prinzmetal's angina. The evidence presented indicates that patients with spasm and insignificant coronary artery disease are best treated medically and that some patients with spasm and significant atherosclerotic coronary disease are candidates for myocardial revascularization.

Walling, A., Waters, D. D., Miller, D. D., et al: Long-term prognosis of patients with variant angina. Circulation, 76:990, 1987.

The long-term prognosis of variant angina and the factors that influence it were determined in 217 consecutive patients. Cardiac death occurred in 30 patients and an additional 54 experienced a nonfatal myocardial infarction. Survival at 1 and 5 years was 95 and 89%, respectively. Survival without infarction was 83 and 69%. Coronary disease and the degree of disease activity were strong predictors of survival. Survival at 1 year was 99%, and survival at 5 years was 95 and 94%, respectively, for patients with one-vessel disease and patients without stenosis of 70% or greater. Survival at 1 and 5 years was only 87 and 77% for patients with multivessel disease. Treatment with nifedipine, diltiazem, or verapamil significantly improved survival without infarction compared with other medical treatment. Myocardial infarction occurred most commonly soon after diagnosis in patients with a short history of angina at rest. Late coronary events were almost never preceded by resting angina.

Bibliography

Alder, A. G., McElwain, G. E., and Martin, J. H.: Coronary artery spasm induced by phenylephrine eyedrops. Arch. Intern. Med., 141:1384, 1981.

Ambrosio, G.: Calcium-channel blockers in vasospastic angina—a review. Postgrad. Med. J. (Suppl. 3), 59:26, 1983.

Antman, E., Muller, J., Goldberg, S., et al: Nifedipine therapy for coronary artery spasm. N. Engl. J. Med., 302:1269, 1980.

Antonelli, D., and Rosenfeld, T.: Variant angina induced by biliary colic. Br. Heart J., 58:417, 1987.

Ascher, E. K., Stauffer, J. E., and Gaasch, W. H.: Coronary artery spasm, cardiac arrest, transient electrocardiographic Q waves and stunned myocardium in cocaine-associated acute myocardial infarction. Am. J. Cardiol., 61:939, 1988.

Bentivoglio, L. G., Ablaza, S. G. G., and Greenberg, L. F.: Bypass surgery for Prinzmetal angina. Arch. Intern. Med., 134:313, 1974.

Berne, R. M., Degust, H., and Levy, M. N.: Influence of the cardiac nerves on coronary resistance. Am. J. Physiol., 208:763, 1965.

Bertrand, M. E., Lablanche, J. M., and Tilmant, P. Y.: Treatment of Prinzmetal's variant angina. Am. J. Cardiol., 47:174, 1981a.

Bertrand, M. E., Lablanche, J. M., Tilmant, P. Y., et al: Complete denervation of the heart (autotransplantation) for treatment of severe, refractory coronary spasm. Am. J. Cardiol., 47:1375, 1981b.

Betriu, A., Pomar, J. L., Bourassa, M. G., and Grondin, C. M.: Influence of partial sympathetic denervation on the results of myocardial revascularization in variant angina. Am. J. Cardiol., 51:661, 1983.

Blesa, M. I., and Ross, G.: Cholinergic mechanism on the heart and coronary circulation. Br. J. Pharmacol., 38:93, 1970.

Blumenthal, M. R., Wang, H. H., Markee, S., and Wang, S. G.: Effects of acetylcholine on the heart. Am. J. Physiol., 214:1280, 1968.

Bodenheimer, M., Lipski, J., Donoso, E., and Dack, S.: Prinzmetal's variant angina: A clinical and electrocardiographic study. Am. Heart J., 87:304, 1974.

Bohr, D. F.: Vascular smooth muscle updated. Circ. Res., 32:665, 1973.

Bolooki, H., Vargas, A., Gharamani, A., et al: Aortocoronary bypass graft for preinfarction angina. Chest, 61:312, 1972.

Boulanger, M., Maille, J., Pelletier, G. B., and Michalk, S.: Vasospastic angina after calcium injection. Anesth. Analg., 63:1124, 1984.

Boullin, D., Bunting, S., Blasp, W., et al: Responses of human and baboon arteries to prostaglandin endoperoxides and biologically generated and synthetic prostacyclin: Their relevance to cerebral arterial spasm in man. Br. J. Clin. Pharmacol., 7:139, 1979.

Bourmayan, C., Artigou, J. Y., Barrillon, A. G., et al: Prinzmetal's variant angina unresponsive to calcium channel-blocking drugs but responsive to combined calcium channel- and beta-blocking drugs. Am. J. Cardiol., 51:1792, 1983.

Bulkley, B., Klacsmann, P., and Hutchins, G.: Angina pectoris, myocardial infarction, and sudden death with normal coronary arteries: A clinicopathologic study of 9 patients with progressive systemic sclerosis. Am. Heart J., 95:563, 1978.

Bunting, S., Gryglewski, R., Moncada, S., and Vane, J.: Arterial walls generate from prostaglandin endoperoxides a substance (prostaglandin X) which relaxes strips of mesenteric and coeliac arteries and inhibits platelet aggregation. Prostaglandins, 12:897, 1976.

Burn, J. H.: Release of noradrenaline from the sympathetic postganglionic fiber. Br. Med. J., 2:197, 1967.

Buxton, A. E., Goldberg, S., and Hirschfield, J. W.: Refractory ergonovine-induced coronary vasospasm: Importance of intracoronary nitroglycerin. Am. J. Cardiol., 46:329, 1980.

Buxton, A. E., Goldberg, S., Harken, A., et al: Coronary artery spasm immediately after myocardial revascularization: Recognition and management. N. Engl. J. Med., 304:1249, 1981.

Cabrera, R., Cohen, A., Middleton, S., et al: The immediate source of noradrenaline released in the heart by acetylcholine. Br. J. Pharmacol., 27:46, 1966.

Cannon, R. O., and Epstein, S. E.: "Microvascular angina" as a cause of chest pain with angiographically normal coronary arteries. Am. J. Cardiol., 61:1338, 1988.

Chahine, R., Raizner, A., Ishimori, T., et al: The incidence and clinical implications of coronary artery spasm. Circulation, 52:972, 1975.

Cheng, T. O., Bashour, T., Kelser, G. A., et al: Variant angina of Prinzmetal with normal coronary arteriograms. A variant of the variant. Circulation, 47:476, 1973.

Cipriano, P., Guthaner, D., Orlick, A., et al: The effects of ergonovine maleate on coronary arterial size. Circulation, 59:82, 1979.

Cipriano, P., Koch, F., Rosenthal, S. J., and Schroeder, J. S.: Clinical course of patients following the demonstration of coronary artery spasm by angiography. Am. Heart J., 101:127, 1981.

Clark, D. A., Quint, R. A., Mitchell, R. L., and Angell, W. W.: Coronary artery spasm. Medical management, surgical denervation, and autotransplantation. J. Thorac. Cardiovasc. Surg., 73:332, 1977.

Coffman, J. D., and Cohen, R. A.: Vasospasm—ubiquitous? N. Engl. J. Med., 304:780, 1981.

Conti, C. R., Pepine, C. J., and Curry, R. C.: Coronary artery spasm: An important mechanism in the pathophysiology of ischemic heart disease. Curr. Probl. Cardiol., 4:1, 1979.

Dagenais, G., Gundel, W., and Conti, C.: Peripheral venospasm associated with signs of transient myocardial ischemia. Am. Heart J., 80:544, 1970.

D'Angelo, V., Ville, S., Mysliwiec, M., et al: Defective fibrinolytic and prostacyclin-like activity in human atheromatous plaques. Thromb. Haemost., 39:535, 1978.

Demany, M., Tambe, A., and Zimmerman, H.: Coronary arterial spasm. Dis. Chest., 53:714, 1968.

Dembinska-Kiec, A., Gryglewski, T., Zmuda, A., and Gryglewski, R. J.: The generation of prostacyclin by arteries and by the coronary vascular bed is reduced in experimental atherosclerosis in rabbits. Prostaglandins, 14:1025, 1977.

Dempsey, P. J., and Cooper, T.: Ventricular cholinergic receptor systems: Interaction with adrenergic systems. J. Pharmacol. Exp. Ther., 167:282, 1969.

DiPaolo, C., Kerin, N. Z., Rubenfire, M., and Levine, F.: Surgical treatment of medically refractory variant angina pectoris: Segmental coronary resection with aortocoronary bypass and plexectomy. Am. J. Cardiol., 56:792, 1985.

Dusting, G., Chapple, D., Hughes, R., et al: Prostacyclin (PG₂) induced coronary vasodilatation in anaesthetized dogs. Cardiovasc. Res., 12:720, 1978.

Endo, M., Hirosawa, K., Kaneko, N., et al: Prinzmetal's variant angina: Coronary arteriogram and left ventriculogram during angina attack induced by methacholine. N. Engl. J. Med., 294:252, 1976.

Endo, M., Kanda, I., Hosoda, S., et al: Prinzmetal's variant form of angina pectoris. Circulation, 52:33, 1975.

Feigl, E. O.: Parasympathetic control of coronary blood flow in dogs. Circ. Res., 25:509, 1969.

Feldman, R. L., Pepine, C. J., Whittle, J., and Conti, C. R.: Short- and long-term responses to diltiazem in patients with variant angina. Am. J. Cardiol., 49:554, 1982.

Fleckenstein, A., Nakayama, K., Fleckenstein-Grün, G., and Byon, Y. K.: Interactions of hydrogen ions, calcium antagonistic drugs and cardiac glycosides with excitation-contraction coupling of vascular smooth muscle. In Betz, E. (ed): Ionic Actions on Vascular Smooth Muscle. Berlin, Springer-Verlag, 1976, p. 117.

Goldman, M., Rogers, E., and Rogers, M.: Subarachnoid hemorrhage: Association with unusual electrocardiographic changes. J.A.M.A., 234:957, 1975.

Gorfinkel, H. J., Inglesby, T. V., Lansing, A. M., and Goodin, R. R.: ST-segment elevation, transient left-posterior hemiblock, and recurrent ventricular arrhythmias unassociated with pain: A variant of Prinzmetal's anginal syndrome. Ann. Intern. Med., 79:795, 1973.

Guazzi, M., Fiorentini, C., Polese, A., and Magrini, F.: Continuous electrocardiographic recording in Prinzmetal's variant angina pectoris: A report of four cases. Br. Heart J., 32:611, 1970.

Guazzi, M., Olivari, M., Polese, A., et al: Repetitive myocardial ischemia of Prinzmetal type without angina pectoris. Am. J. Cardiol., 37:923, 1976.

Hackett, J. G., Abboud, F. M., Mark, A. L., et al: Coronary vascular responses to stimulation of chemoreceptors and baroreceptors: Evidence for reflex activation of vagal cholinergic innervation. Circ. Res., 31:8, 1972.

Harder, D., Belardinelli, L., Sperelakis, N., et al: Differential effects of adenosine and nitroglycerin on the action potentials of large and small coronary arteries. Circ. Res., 44:176, 1979.

Heberden, W.: Some account of a disorder of the breast. Medical Transactions of the Royal College of Physicians of London, 2:59, 1772.

Herrick, J. B.: Clinical features of sudden obstruction of the coronary arteries. J.A.M.A., 59:2015, 1912.

Hillis, L., and Braunwald, E.: Coronary artery spasm. N. Engl. J. Med., 299:695, 1978.

Hisano, K., Matsuguchi, T., Oatsubo, H., et al: Hyperventilation-induced variant angina. Am. Heart J., 108:423, 1984.

Johnson, A. D., and Detwiler, J. H.: Coronary spasm, variant angina, and recurrent myocardial infarctions. Circulation, 55:947, 1977.

Johnson, S. M., Mauritson, D. R., Willerson, J. T., and Hillis, L. D.: Comparison of verapamil and nifedipine in the treatment of variant angina pectoris: Preliminary observations in 10 patients. Am. J. Cardiol., 47:1295, 1981.

Kelley, K., and Feigl, E.: Segmental alpha-receptor mediated vasoconstriction in the canine coronary circulation. Circ. Res., 43:908, 1978.

Kimura, E., and Kishida, H.: Treatment of variant angina with drugs: A survey of 11 cardiology institutes in Japan. Circulation, 63:844, 1981.

King, S., Mansour, K., Hatcher, C., et al: Coronary artery spasm producing Prinzmetal's angina in myocardial infarction in the absence of coronary atherosclerosis. Ann. Thorac. Surg., 16:337, 1973.

Kleiman, N. S., Lehane, D. E., Geyer, C. E., Jr., et al: Prinzmetal's angina during 5-fluorouracil chemotherapy. Am. J. Med., 82:566, 1987.

Krantz, E. M., Viljoen, J. F., and Gilbert, M. S.: Prinzmetal's variant angina during extradural anaesthesia. Br. J. Anaesth., 52:945, 1980.

Lange, R., Reid, M., Tresch, D., et al: Nonatheromatous ischemic heart disease following withdrawal from chronic industrial nitroglycerin exposure. Circulation, 46:666, 1972.

Lasser, R. T., and de la Paz, N. D.: Repetitive transient myocardial ischemia, Prinzmetal type, without angina pectoris, presenting with Stokes-Adams attacks. Chest, 64:350, 1973.

Lavine, P., Kimbiris, D., and Linhart, J.: Coronary artery spasm during selective coronary arteriography: A review of 8 years experience (Abstract). Circulation, 48(Suppl. 4):89, 1973.

Lemmer, J. H., Jr., and Kirsh, M. M.: Coronary artery spasm following coronary artery surgery. Ann. Thorac. Surg., 46:108, 1988.

Levy, M. N.: Sympathetic-parasympathetic interactions in the heart. Circ. Res., 29:437, 1971.

Levy, M. N., and Zieske, H.: Comparison of the cardiac effects of vagus nerve stimulation and of acetylcholine infusions. Am. J. Physiol., 216:890, 1969.

Lewy, R., Smith, J., Silver, M., et al: Detection of thromboxane B_2 in the peripheral blood of patients with Prinzmetal's angina. Prostaglandins Med., 2:243, 1979.

Linhart, J. W., Beller, B. M., and Talley, R. C.: Preinfarction angina: Clinical, hemodynamic and angiographic evaluation. Chest, 61:312, 1972.

Madias, J. E.: The long-term outcome of patients who suffered and survived an acute myocardial infarction in the midst of recurrent attacks of variant angina. Clin. Cardiol., 9:277, 1986.

Maseri, A.: Role of coronary artery spasm in symptomatic and silent myocardial ischemia. J. Am. Coll. Cardiol., 9:249, 1987.

Maseri, A., Klassen, G. A., and Lesch, M. (eds): Primary and Secondary Angina Pectoris. New York, Grune & Stratton, 1978a.

Maseri, A., L'Abbate, A., Pesola, A., et al: Coronary vasospasm in angina pectoris. Lancet, 1:713, 1977.

Maseri, A., Mimmo, R., Chierchia, S., et al: Coronary spasm as a cause of acute myocardial ischemia in man. Chest, 68:625, 1975.

Maseri, A., Severi, S., Nes, M. D., et al: "Variant" angina: One aspect of a continuous spectrum of vasospastic myocardial ischemia. Am. J. Cardiol., 42:1019, 1978b.

Melville, K., Garvey, H., Shister, E., et al: Central nervous system stimulation and cardiac ischemic changes in monkeys. Ann. N.Y. Acad. Sci., 156:241, 1969.

Miller, D., Waters, D. D., Warnica, W., et al: Is variant angina the coronary manifestation of a generalized vasospastic disorder? N. Engl. J. Med., 304:763, 1981.

Miwa, K., Kambara, H., and Kawai, C.: Effect of aspirin in large doses on attacks of variant angina. Am. Heart J., 105:351, 1983.

Moncada, S., Higgs, E., and Vane, J.: Human arterial and venous tissues generate prostacyclin (prostaglandin X), a potent inhibitor of platelet aggregation. Lancet, 1:18, 1977.

Mudge, G., Grossman, W., Miles, R., et al: Reflex increase in coronary vascular resistance in patients with ischemic heart disease. N. Engl. J. Med., 295:1333, 1976.

Murao, S., Harumi, K., Katayama, S., et al: All-night polygraphic studies of nocturnal angina pectoris. Jpn. Heart J., 13:295, 1972.

Nowlin, J. B., Troyer, W. G., Collens, W. S., et al: The association of nocturnal angina pectoris with dreaming. Ann. Intern. Med., 63:1040, 1965.

Oliva, P. B.: Coronary artery spasm: An important mechanism in the pathophysiology of ischemic heart disease (Editorial Comment). Curr. Probl. Cardiol., 4:1, 1979.

Oliva, P. B., and Breckinridge, J.: Arteriographic evidence of coronary arterial spasm in acute myocardial infarction. Circulation, 56:366, 1977.

Oliva, P. B., Potts, D. E., and Pluss, R. G.: Coronary peripheral spasm in Prinzmetal angina. Documentation by coronary arteriography. N. Engl. J. Med., 288:745, 1973.

O'Reilly, R., Spellberg, R., and King, T.: Recognition of proximal right coronary artery spasm during coronary arteriography. Radiology, 95:305, 1970.

Osler, W.: The Lumleian lectures on angina pectoris. Lancet, 1:699, 1910.

Pepine, C. J., Feldman, R. L., Whittle, J., et al: Effect of diltiazem in patients with variant angina: A randomized double-blind trial. Am. Heart J., 101:719, 1981.

Pichard, A. D., Ambrose, J., Mindrich, B., et al: Coronary artery spasm and perioperative cardiac arrest. J. Thorac. Cardiovasc. Surg., 80:249, 1980.

Prinzmetal, M., Kennamer, R., Merliss, R., et al: Angina pectoris.

I: A variant form of angina pectoris. Am. J. Med., 27:375, 1959.

Prohkov, V. K., Mookherjee, S., Schiess, W., and Obeid, A. L.: Variant anginal syndrome, coronary artery spasm and ventricular fibrillation in absence of chest pain. Ann. Intern. Med., 81:858, 1974.

Raabe, D.: Treatment of variant angina pectoris with perhexiline maleate. Chest, 75:152, 1979.

Raizner, A. E., and Chahine, R. A.: The treatment of Prinzmetal's variant angina with coronary bypass surgery. In Hurst, J. W. (ed): Update II: The Heart—Bypass Surgery for Obstructive Coronary Disease, Chapter 9. New York, McGraw-Hill, 1980.

Ricci, D., Orlick, A., Cipriano, P., et al: Altered adrenergic activity in coronary arterial spasm. Insight into mechanism based on study of coronary hemodynamics and the electrocardiogram. Am. J. Cardiol., 43:1073, 1979.

Robertson, D., and Oates, J.: Variant angina and Raynaud's phenomenon (Letter). Lancet, 1:452, 1978.

Robertson, D., Robertson, R., Nies, A., et al: Variant angina pectoris: Investigation of indexes of sympathetic nervous system functioning. Am. J. Cardiol., 43:1080, 1979.

Rosenthal, S. J., Ginsburg, R., Lamb, I. H., et al: Efficacy of diltiazem for control of symptoms of coronary arterial spasm. Am. J. Cardiol., 46:1027, 1980.

Rutitzky, B., Girotti, A. L., and Rosenbaum, M. B.: Efficacy of chronic amiodarone therapy in patients with variant angina pectoris and inhibition of ergonovine coronary constriction. Am. Heart J., 103:38, 1982.

Schick, E. C., Davis, Z., Lavery, R. M., et al: Surgical therapy for Prinzmetal's variant angina. Ann. Thorac. Surg., 33:359, 1982.

Schiffer, F., Hartley, H., Schulman, C. L., and Abelmann, W. H.: Evidence for emotionally induced coronary arterial spasm in patients with angina pectoris. Br. Heart J., 44:62, 1980.

Schroeder, J. S., Feldman, R. L., Giles, T. D., et al: Multiclinic controlled trial of diltiazem for Prinzmetal's angina. Am. J. Med., 72:227, 1982.

Selzer, A., Langston, M., Ruggeroli, C., and Cohn, K.: Clinical syndrome of variant angina with normal coronary arteriogram. N. Engl. J. Med., 295:1343, 1976.

Severi, S., Davies, T., L'Abbate, L., and Maseri, A.: Long-term prognosis of variant angina with medical management. Circulation, 60(Suppl. 2):250, 1979.

Severi, S., Davies, G., Maseri, A., et al: Long-term prognosis of "variant" angina with medical treatment. Am. J. Cardiol., 46:226, 1980.

Shachor, J., Beker, B., Geffen, Y., and Bruderman, I.: Acute ECG changes during cyclophosphamide infusion in a patient with bronchogenic carcinoma. Cancer, 69:734, 1985.

Shinjo, A., Sasaki, Y., Inamasu, M., and Morita, T.: In vivo effects of the coronary vasodilator diltiazem on human and rabbit platelets. Thromb. Res., 13:941, 1978.

Silverman, M., and Flamm, M.: Angina pectoris. Anatomic findings and prognostic implications. Ann. Intern. Med., 75:339, 1971.

Stenson, R. E., Flamm, M. D., Zaret, B. L., and McGowan, R. L.: Transient ST-segment elevation with postmyocardial infarction angina: Prognostic significance. Am. Heart J., 89:449, 1975.

Sussman, E. J., Goldberg, S., Poll, D. S., et al: Surgical therapy of variant angina associated with nonobstructive coronary disease. Ann. Intern. Med., 94:771, 1981.

Szczeklik, A., Gryglewski, R. J., Musial, J., et al: Thromboxane generation and platelet aggregation in survivors of myocardial infarction. Thromb. Haemost., 40:66, 1978.

Tada, M., Kuzuya, T., Inoue, M., et al: Elevation of thromboxane B_2 levels in patients with classic and variant angina pectoris. Circulation, 64:1107, 1981.

Takizawa, A., Yasue, H., Omote, S., et al: Variant angina induced by alcohol ingestion. Am. Heart J., 107:25, 1984.

Toyama, Y., Tanaka, H., Nuruki, K., and Shirao, T.: Prinzmetal's variant angina associated with subarachnoid hemorrhage: A case report. Angiology, 30:211, 1979.

Tzivoni, D., Keren, A., Benhorin, J., et al: Prazosin therapy for refractory variant angina. Am. Heart J., 105:262, 1983.

Waters, D. D., Crean, P. A., Roy, D., and Theroux, P.: Problems related to the detection of myocardial ischemia. Can. J. Cardiol., (Suppl. A):173A, 1986.

Waters, D. D., Szlachcic, J., Miller, D., and Theroux, P.: Clinical characteristics of patients with variant angina complicated by myocardial infarction or death within 1 month. Am. J. Cardiol., 49:658, 1982.

Winniford, M. D., Filipchuk, N., and Hillis, L. D.: Alpha-adrenergic blockade for variant angina: A long-term, double-blind, randomized trial. Circulation, 67:1185, 1983.

Yasue, H., Nagao, M., Omote, S., et al: Coronary arterial spasm and Prinzmetal's variant form of angina induced by hyper-ventilation and TRIS-buffer infusion. Circulation, 58:56, 1978.

Yasue, H., Omote, S., Takizawa, A., et al: Exertional angina pectoris caused by coronary arterial spasm: Effects of various drugs. Am. J. Cardiol., 43:647, 1979.

Yasue, H., Touyama, M., Shimamoto, M., et al: Role of autonomic nervous system in the pathogenesis of Prinzmetal's variant form of angina. Circulation, 50:534, 1974.

Yasue, J., Horio, Y., Nakamura, N., et al: Induction of coronary spasm by acetylcholine in patients with variant angina: Possible role of the parasympathetic nervous system in the pathogenesis of coronary spasm. Circulation, 74:955, 1986.

3 Repeat Coronary Artery Bypass Grafting for Myocardial Ischemia

Floyd D. Loop

The evolution of coronary bypass surgery is marked by changes in the clinical spectrum of patients and in the practice of surgery, including reoperations. The mean age of surgical candidates is increasing; 40% or more of patients operated on for the first time are in the Medicare age group, 65 years or older. Among all patients having coronary bypass, cigarette smoking and hypertension are found less frequently than in earlier years, but diabetes and peripheral vascular disease are encountered significantly more often today than 10 years ago, and more patients are women. As discussed elsewhere in this text, these latter patient characteristics affect operative risk. Advanced age contributes to a greater prevalence of extensive coronary atherosclerosis. Almost all patients operated on today have more than one severely obstructed major coronary artery, and most have three-vessel involvement. Coronary artery balloon angioplasty has almost eliminated patients with one-vessel disease from immediate surgical consideration, a fact that further increases the percentage of multivessel cases. Abnormal findings on the initial arteriogram, elevated serum lipid levels, hypertension, diabetes, obesity, and cigarette smoking all are acknowledged risk factors for progressive disease; unfortunately, they are unreliable in predicting the rate of progression (Bruschke et al, 1981; Kramer et al, 1981).

The indications for primary and reoperative coronary artery surgery have been refined in the last 15 years mainly as a result of randomized trials and observational studies. Angina is still the principal reason for initial and subsequent coronary artery operations. However, this angina is no longer the intractable type that is resistant to all forms of medical therapy; instead, earlier surgical consideration is given to patients with persistent pain or discomfort that, despite a good medical program, interferes with the patient's life-style. Symptoms should correlate with objective evidence of ischemia, and with few exceptions, most surgical candidates and almost all patients having reoperation have multivessel coronary atherosclerosis. Particular attention should be given to lesions in the anterior descending artery. Subtotal obstruction in the proximal anterior descending coronary artery, above the first diagonal, and especially at or above the first septal perforator, is recognized as prognostically dangerous and more likely to cause fatal myocardial infarction than any other vessel closure (Klein et al, 1986; Schuster et al, 1981). Patients with severe proximal stenoses in all major coronary vessels combined with exercise test or scintigraphic proof of ischemia should be considered for bypass grafting. Among these patients with multivessel disease, left ventricular dysfunction (defined as an ejection fraction of less than 0.5) is best treated surgically (Passamani et al, 1985). Patients referred for bypass grafting should fit these criteria clinically and angiographically.

Selection criteria have evolved toward including more difficult cases; however, just as the patients have changed, so too has the operation. In the late 1970s, myocardial protection advanced with the use of cold potassium cardioplegia. This addition reduced mortality and morbidity and allowed the performance of more grafts per patient. The luxuries of time and a dry, motionless field have accelerated the trend toward arterial bypass grafting and have provided greater safety when coronary artery surgery is combined with other cardiac reconstructive procedures.

Traditionally, assessment of outcome after coronary artery surgery reveals relief of symptoms and improved long-term survival. However, coronary bypass is done for a degenerative disease and, like many other operations, does not provide a cure. The clinical result depends on the anatomic result, which tends to deteriorate over time. After the first postoperative year, a 5% or greater rate of angina recurrence may accrue annually and is almost always related to bypass graft closure, progressive atherosclerosis in ungrafted vessels, or, less frequently, development of lesions beyond the distal graft sites.

Later on, mainly after the fifth to seventh postoperative year, vein graft atherosclerosis becomes the dominant reason for graft closure. These events weigh heavily on the incidence of reoperation, which increases with time.

INCIDENCE OF REOPERATION

Incidence estimates for coronary artery reoperation are based on experience in coronary bypass surgery during the 1970s (Loop et al, 1983). Five years after the initial operation, only 3% of patients had been reoperated on (Cosgrove et al, 1986; Foster et al, 1984), and early reoperations were attributed to technical problems that resulted in graft stenosis or closure (Culliford et al, 1979). The cumulative rate of reoperation escalated to 11 and 17% at 10 and 12 years, respectively (Fig. 54–90). A 4% annual risk of reoperation was found at 12 years. This incidence may be altered by demographics, conduits used in the first operation, and new therapies, notably coronary artery balloon angioplasty, which affects the surgical case-mix initially and thus may influence reoperations. Prototypic variations in catheter interventions (e.g., atherectomy devices, stents, and laser ablation) may further delay operation and reduce reoperation rates, but their impact now is only speculative.

One factor that definitely modifies the probability of reoperation is the choice of conduits used during the first operation. Late patency of the internal thoracic (mammary) arterial graft is significantly greater than that of a vein graft done to the anterior descending coronary artery. Internal thoracic artery graft patency up to 12 years is consistently greater than 90% in all years surveyed (Loop et al, 1986), whereas vein graft patency declines to approximately 60% at 10 years (Campeau et al, 1984; Lytle et al, 1985). Of patent grafts, approximately half show evidence of luminal irregularity connoting vein graft atherosclerosis. The number of diseased or occluded vein grafts at 10 years is double that recorded during the first 5 years.

Fibrinolysis is greater; lipolysis is slower; and prostacyclin production is diminished in vein grafts compared with internal thoracic artery grafts (Grondin, 1986b). The internal thoracic artery may differ from the radial and gastroepiploic arteries in that it may have a more impermeable internal elastic membrane, which may limit smooth muscle cell migration (Sims, 1987). As in many small arteries, it is nourished principally from the lumen and not by the vasa vasorum. These observations may explain why veins tend to deteriorate and this particular arterial graft is relatively immune to late atherosclerosis.

This sustained patency of the internal thoracic artery graft has decreased the incidence of coronary artery reoperation (Cameron et al, 1986; Loop et al, 1986). A single thoracic arterial graft anastomosed to the anterior descending coronary artery solely or combined with aortocoronary vein grafts to other

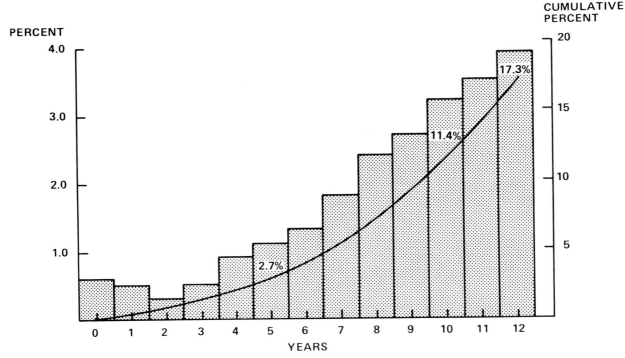

Figure 54–90. The annual incidence of reoperation *(bars)* is compared with the cumulative incidence of reoperation *(curve)* up to 12 years after the first coronary bypass operation. Although the risk for reoperation is low at 5 years (3%), it reaches 17% at 12 years, a linearized rate of 4% per year. This experience is compiled from patients who had coronary bypass surgery at the Cleveland Clinic during the 1970s.

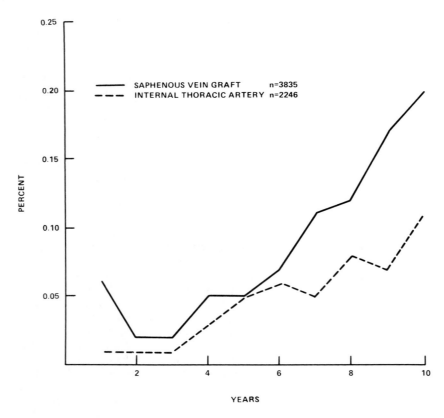

Figure 54–91. The conditional reoperation rate is shown for patients who had vein grafts only, compared with patients who had one internal thoracic artery graft to the anterior descending artery, either alone or combined with vein grafts to other arteries. Patients who had only vein grafts had twice the incidence of reoperation during the first 10 years. (Based on data from Loop, F. D., Lytle, B. W., Cosgrove, D. M., et al: Influence of the internal-mammary-artery graft on 10-year survival and other cardiac events. N. Engl. J. Med., *314*:1, 1986.)

major coronary vessels reduced the rate of reoperation by half during the first decade after primary operation (Fig. 54–91).

Graft thrombosis usually develops within 3 to 6 months after bypass surgery and is usually attributed to technical error, poor distal runoff, and vein graft damage (Shark and Kass, 1981). Serial angiograms showed that of vein grafts found to be stenotic 1 year postoperatively, 60% progressed to complete occlusion by the time of the second postoperative angiogram, a mean of 7 years later (Lytle et al, 1985). Atherosclerotic narrowing along the graft course, which is usually encountered after the fifth postoperative year, frequently progresses rapidly to complete occlusion, suggesting that even early vein graft atherosclerosis has an unstable history and a poor prognosis for continuing graft patency. Vein grafts that were patent at the first postoperative arteriogram but stenotic or occluded at the second postoperative arteriogram were associated with lengthening interval between arteriograms, diabetes, and hyperlipidemia, and these patients had significantly more cardiac events than patients without progressive graft disease. Thrombosis superimposed on a ruptured atheromatous plaque may cause acute late thrombotic graft occlusion (Walts et al, 1982). Hyperlipoproteinemia has been identified as being the major risk factor in progressive atherosclerosis and is implicated in vein graft failure (Barboriak et al, 1978). Preliminary reports indicate that aspirin and dipyridamole or even aspirin alone significantly increases early vein graft patency up to 1 year postoperatively

(Brown et al, 1985; Chesebro et al, 1982; Goldman et al, 1988; Lorenz et al, 1984). No correlation has been found between administration of antiplatelet agents postoperatively and reduction in vein graft atherosclerosis.

What variables present at the first operation influence the probability of reoperation? Multivariate regression analysis indicates that performance of vein grafts only, incomplete revascularization, and young age at first operation are important predictors of reoperation (Cosgrove et al, 1986; Fox et al, 1987; Lytle et al, 1987). Patients who received no arterial grafts were twice as likely to have subsequent reoperation as were those who had one internal thoracic artery graft solely or in combination with vein grafts. At present, the durability of the arterial graft is the most important variable responsible for lowering the reoperation rate. Because most patients with one-vessel disease and some with two-vessel disease are treated initially by nonsurgical therapy and many patients with multivessel disease now receive more than one arterial graft initially, the escalating rate of reoperation may be slowed, perhaps indefinitely. The most effective method of countering vein graft failure is to use the internal thoracic artery during the first coronary bypass operation.

INDICATIONS FOR REOPERATION

Clinical indications for coronary artery reoperation follow the same guidelines as those applied to primary operation. The differences are that the selection process is more conservative for reoperation and that functional disability seems to carry more weight in decision-making than pathoanatomy. Based on the higher risk involved, this practice of recommending reoperation for only very symptomatic patients is cautious and probably justified. However, arteriographic findings and the perception of myocardial jeopardy frequently underlie recommendations for primary operation (Alderman et al, 1982).

Angiographic indications for reoperation are more complex than those for primary operation and have been categorized into three groups: (1) graft closure (or dysfunction), (2) progressive atherosclerosis, and (3) a combination of both graft closure (or dysfunction) and progressive disease. Early graft failure caused by technical errors from conduit twisting, kinks, short grafts producing "tenting" of the distal anastomosis, or vein grafts traumatized by high distention pressures during preparation or long storage in saline is encountered less frequently today. Grafts constructed to small vessels with poor arterial runoff are also found less often. Graft closure mainly applies to aortocoronary saphenous vein grafts; arterial grafts close less frequently. As reoperation experience has accumulated, late vein graft obstruction has become the predominant angiographic reason for reoperation (Loop et al, 1983). Age at first operation, gender, and artery bypassed did not predict graft closure, but as mentioned earlier, elevated plasma lipid levels have been implicated in vein graft narrowing. Risk factors associated with atherosclerosis in native vessels, notably hypercholesterolemia, may affect atherosclerosis in aortocoronary vein bypass grafts (Neitzel et al, 1986). Graft failure more than 5 years postoperatively is most often attributed to vein graft atherosclerosis (Loop et al, 1983; Lytle et al, 1985). In the author's experience, late graft failure accounted for 82% of reoperative angiographic indications (1982 to 1984). Progressive atherosclerosis applies mainly to progressive arterial lesions in previously ungrafted coronary arteries. New or progressive lesions beyond distal graft anastomoses that require revision appear less frequently (Bourassa et al, 1978). Progressive atherosclerosis per se is encountered significantly less often than graft failure as an angiographic indication for reoperation. Both graft obstruction or narrowing and progressive atherosclerosis account for approximately a third of the angiographic indications, and their incidence together has not changed appreciably over time.

These angiographic groupings, however, do not take the whole patient into account. Few patients face reoperation in the first 5 postoperative years. The interval between operations is increasing; most occur between the fifth and tenth year (now closer to the tenth year), and reoperations beyond the tenth year are increasing in frequency. Thus, candidates for reoperation are often considerably older than they were before the first operation and show an increased prevalence of diabetes, more diffuse atherosclerosis

(often in more than one arterial system), and significantly more left main coronary artery stenosis. During this sometimes lengthy interval between operations, most patients have had additional cardiac events that may further increase operative risk. A third of the author's patients having reoperation had a perceptible deterioration in left ventricular performance in the interim. Despite this incidence, patients who have had previous bypass surgery tend to have smaller myocardial infarctions than their counterparts who have not been operated on but who have a myocardial infarction (Crean et al, 1985). Coronary artery surgery may offer protection by bypassing the major vessels so that more minor vessels are involved in the myocardial infarction.

In the author's most recent reoperation series (1982 to 1984), the clinical spectrum has shifted significantly to greater operative risk factors. Age 70 years or older, female gender, three-vessel disease, left main coronary artery stenosis 50% or greater, abnormal left ventricular function, and graft failure as the principal angiographic indication occurred with significantly greater frequency in this latest cohort than in earlier groups of patients dating back to 1968. Also, the author has more recently seen more patients with a patent internal thoracic artery graft, usually to the anterior descending artery, who face reoperation because of closed or diseased vein grafts to other major coronary arteries (Fig. 54–92). Patency of an internal thoracic artery graft is not a contraindication for reoperation, but it does require experience in reoperations to avoid injuring it.

Advanced age is not a contraindication to first or subsequent coronary artery surgery, but chronologic age cannot be dismissed as a risk factor. An accurate assessment of physiologic age is important and includes prior activity, attitude toward operation, which encompasses an understanding of the potential risks and benefits, and finally, comorbidity (Loop et al, 1988). Associated diseases include hypertension, diabetes, pulmonary disease, peripheral vascular atherosclerosis, and cancer, none of which contraindicates operation but must be evaluated in the appraisal of the whole patient. Some patients reach a point in their aging process where additional higher-risk, expensive surgical therapy is not warranted based on a meager potential for effective rehabilitation.

The reoperation candidate may be referred for percutaneous transluminal coronary angioplasty (PTCA). This conservative approach may be recommended for early or late graft stenosis or dilatation of previously ungrafted vessels. Early results are generally good. Stenoses of distal anastomoses are recognized and treated at an early stage; however, the success rate of less than 50% for dilatation of aortic anastomoses and lesions in the graft body is significantly less than the success rate for native vessels (Douglas et al, 1984). PTCA for intimal hyperplasia frequently results in restenosis from fibrocellular proliferation. Dilatation after the first post-

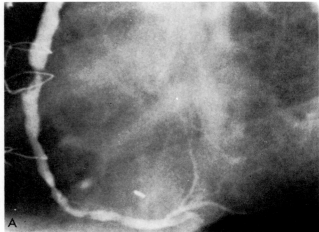

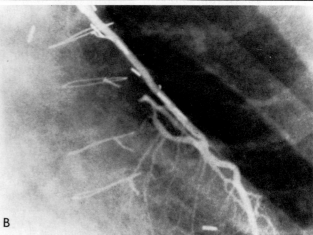

Figure 54–92. Diffuse atherosclerosis of vein grafts occurs with increased frequency after the fifth postoperative year. *A,* Diffuse atherosclerosis in a 7-year-old vein bypass graft to the right coronary artery. *B,* A normal-appearing internal thoracic artery graft to the left anterior descending coronary artery in the same patient.

bypass year carries a risk of atheroembolism because these vein graft plaques are vulnerable to disruption and embolism of relatively large fragments (Saber et al, 1988). PTCA applied to the stenotic internal thoracic artery may result in a high primary success rate, few complications, and sustained clinical improvement (Shimshak et al, 1988). Overall, PTCA in patients who have had coronary artery surgery is moderately successful for relief of angina, but improvement is less than that achieved in patients undergoing PTCA without bypass surgery and similar to that of PTCA for multivessel disease (Reed et al, 1989).

Emergency reoperation for failed angioplasty has a higher risk of mortality than emergency primary operation. These patients should be informed that reoperation under emergency circumstances is not the same as a planned elective reoperation. No reports have addressed urgent or emergency reoperation after failed angioplasty, but something is known

about emergency primary operation in that setting. Not only is risk elevated, but the probability of perioperative myocardial infarction is high (Golding et al, 1986) and the patient is likely to receive only vein grafts. Although results of emergency operation are improving (Ferguson et al, 1988), the patient having reoperation represents one of the most demanding technical challenges. In time, better methods of support will stabilize the hemodynamic state before emergency re-entry.

PREOPERATIVE ASSESSMENT

Patients and their families should be apprised of reoperative risk. Because the profile of the candidate for reoperation is changing, the surgeon must pay particular attention to risk among the increased numbers of patients having reoperation who are 70 years or older, women, patients with left main stenosis 50% or greater, those with patent but atherosclerotic vein grafts, and patients with abnormal left ventricular function. Statistical analysis of the author's experience through 1984 indicates that elderly patients with progressive or unstable anginal disability and those with severe left main coronary artery stenosis face a significantly higher operative risk during reoperation (Loop and Cosgrove, 1986). Operative risk factors may change with time and depend on the accuracy of clinical, angiographic, and operative variables entered into the univariate and multivariate regression analyses. The reoperation experience of the institution and its surgeons' results provide objective evidence that certain variables may increase risk and serve as a background for preoperative discussion. Patients should understand that although risk assessment is only an educated estimate, the risk of coronary artery reoperation is probably two to three times that of the first operation.

Major morbidity is generally higher with reoperation, specifically perioperative myocardial infarction, respiratory complications, and bleeding requiring exploration. However, stroke, wound, renal, and gastrointestinal complications occur with about the same frequency as in the first operation. Obviously, morbidity differs among institutions, but it behooves surgeons to be aware of their experience regarding mortality and morbidity in these more complicated coronary artery bypass operations.

The risk assessments are aided by a thorough review of the patient's history. What were the indications for the first operation, and are they different for the second operation? What procedure was done initially? It may make a difference technically if the patient had Beck's talc poudrage, Vineberg's implant, or coronary endarterectomy. Wherever possible, previous hospital records and the original operative note should be surveyed for co-morbid illnesses, technical problems, or perioperative complications. The surgeon should ask the patients if they have copies of missing or inaccessible records (Bahn and Annest, 1986).

The patient's physical appearance is important, not only as part of a standard physical examination but also for information that could affect surgical technique. Persons with small body surface area (<1.7 m²) are likely to require more blood and blood products. Women with previous mastectomy may have had chest wall irradiation, which could affect wound healing and precludes internal thoracic artery use, and consequently may have atherosclerosis of the ascending aorta. In the author's experience, previous mediastinitis may not affect re-entry or adhesion formation; however, when the sternum has been destroyed by osteomyelitis and removed and replaced with a muscle flap, re-entry presents a problem that must be solved on an individual basis or may not be amenable to midline re-entry. The responsible surgeon should be cognizant of peripheral vascular disease and previous arterial reconstruction, both of which could affect femoral cannulation and intra-aortic balloon insertion.

A carotid bruit requires further investigation to confirm or disprove significant internal carotid disease. When present in a neurologically asymptomatic patient, these lesions, unless subtotal, are often ignored and the coronary artery reoperation takes precedence; however, the patient should be informed of the findings and plan for follow-up. A history of neurologic problems in a patient with documented carotid disease may require a strategy that takes into account the severity and bilaterality of the lesion, current cardiac symptoms, coronary pathoanatomy, and magnitude of the planned cardiac reoperation. When the condition is stable, carotid endarterectomy sometimes may be staged first. In patients with dangerous coexisting carotid and coronary disease, simultaneous operation may be required, but the additional potential for stroke should be conveyed to the patient.

Of the laboratory tests reviewed, the preoperative lateral chest film may reveal proximity of the cardiac structures and the overlying sternum (Fig. 54–93), and a posteroanterior view may show the location of a viable internal thoracic artery graft that could modify the plan of re-entry. Routine coagulation tests have not been found to be helpful in predicting postoperative bleeding. Discontinuation of aspirin and other antiplatelet drugs 10 or more days (Ferraris et al, 1988) and anticoagulants 2 to 3 days preoperatively is indicated. Predeposit of blood for possible autologous use should be encouraged for patients who are in stable condition, are having elective operation, and do not have serious comorbid diseases or anemia that contraindicates blood donation.

A thorough review of the most recent cine coronary arteriogram may reveal vein graft atherosclerosis, especially when the vein graft was placed more than 5 years previously. The course of mild vein graft atherosclerosis is not known, but severe atherosclerotic vein graft narrowing may progress rapidly to closure. It is not unusual to see complete occlusion of a vein graft that was perceptibly atherosclerotic

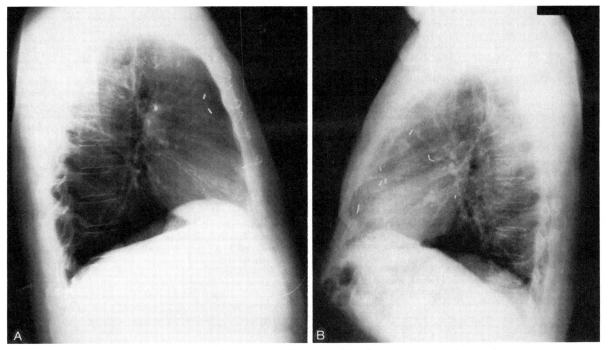

Figure 54–93. Lateral chest films showing differences in adherence of cardiac structures to the overlying sternum. *A,* A typical reoperation patient, who may show some adherence of the right ventricle to the sternum, mainly in the lower third of the sternum. *B,* Dense adherence of an enlarged heart to the sternum. This finding alerts the surgeon that re-entry could be hazardous. Femoral artery exposure or femoral-femoral cannulation should be considered before operation.

but open on the prereoperative film that was obtained only a few weeks earlier. The observation that an atherosclerotic vein graft is still patent should be communicated to the patient because it constitutes a potential source of morbidity, even mortality, in the reoperation. Even when the reoperation is expertly done, atherosclerotic emboli may lodge in the microcirculatory system and cause myocardial infarction. The question is whether a graft that looks normal 5 or more years after the first operation should be replaced, and this is easier to answer if another vein graft is atherosclerotic in the same patient. The decision is also made easier if the old but normal-appearing vein graft perfuses the anterior descending artery and could be replaced with an internal thoracic artery graft. This is more of a dilemma 5 years or so after the first operation but is less of an issue 7 to 10 years after the operation, when most vein grafts show atherosclerosis. In discussing whether functioning grafts will be replaced, the surgeon should point out that another factor is the quality of the new vein available or the viability of the internal thoracic artery graft. Patients with minimal atherosclerosis in vein grafts as shown by arteriography generally have more diffuse atherosclerosis in the vein graft when it is removed. Angiographic studies tend to underestimate the severity of atherosclerotic degeneration, and because of the propensity of atherosclerotic disease in grafts to progress unpredictably, some surgeons have recommended routine replacement of all saphenous vein grafts at the time of reoperation if done 5 or more years after the initial procedure (Marshall et al, 1986).

As experience with reoperation grows, problems with heparin and protamine have been recognized. Protamine sensitivity is discussed in the section on technical aspects of reoperation. A syndrome termed heparin-induced platelet activation has already been described (Kappa et al, 1987). Although the condition is still rare, these patients have previously been exposed to heparin, usually continuous heparin therapy over days, and have had severe thrombocytopenia or thrombosis. A low platelet count preoperatively ($<50,000/mm^3$) or history of thromboembolism during previous heparin administration should alert the surgeon. Heparin-dependent platelet aggregation is analyzed by platelet aggregation and ^{14}C-serotonin release. When re-exposed to heparin, the patient could experience thrombocytopenia, intravascular thrombosis, arterial emboli, and hemorrhage. Surveillance of the platelet count does not prevent thrombosis (King and Kelton, 1984). Aspirin may prevent platelet aggregation in vitro, but it has not been consistently efficacious in vivo. A stable analog of prostacyclin appears to stimulate adenylcyclase and to elevate intracellular levels of cyclic adenosine monophosphate. Starting prostacyclin analog as an infusion preoperatively and continuing it throughout the operation until the administration of protamine has led to a successful outcome (Addonizio et al, 1987; Schrör et al, 1981.)

Finally, the pre-reoperative arteriogram should be reviewed again immediately before the reoperation. A clear strategy for re-entry, cannulation, and grafting should be formulated at the outset. Reoperation that is based on a plan for prevention is the best method to avoid complications.

REOPERATION TECHNIQUES

As experience in coronary artery reoperation is gained, a trend toward more complete revascularization has developed—that is, grafts done to all major coronary vessels narrowed 50% or more in diameter (nondominant right coronary arteries excluded). Consequently, more grafts per patient having reoperation have been done in recent years, but still fewer than on the first operation because of diffuse coronary atherosclerosis, new transmural scar, and the fact that some grafts are open and functioning well. In reoperations, the mean number of grafts per patient is slightly more than two (Loop et al, 1983; Schaff et al, 1983) compared with three or more bypass grafts in primary operations. There is a trend toward more use of the internal thoracic artery among patients having reoperation.

In the immediate preoperative period, premedication protocols are essentially the same as in patients having primary operation and depend on age and clinical stability. Transdermal nitroglycerin ointment is advocated by many anesthesia groups. Packed red blood cells should be available when the patient arrives in the operating room. Most anesthesiologists insert two large-bore peripheral intravenous catheters, one of which may be a pulmonary artery catheter. Although thermodilution pulmonary artery catheters are used inconsistently in primary coronary operations, most anesthesiologists and surgeons believe that the greater risk of hemodynamic instability with repeat operation requires serial recording of filling pressures and cardiac output (Camann et al, 1987). Placement of a pulmonary artery thermistor and a left atrial line postoperatively is an alternative method.

A radial arterial monitoring line almost always suffices, but a brachial line may be preferred because of greater accuracy. Some anesthesiologists prefer to insert a catheter in the arm opposite the side of internal thoracic artery dissection to avoid subclavian artery or arm compression by the sternal retractor. Five-lead electrocardiographic monitoring is standard. Continuous monitoring of V_5 and lead II is preferred to cover the range of potential ischemia. Narcotic anesthesia may be preferred to inhalation agents, especially in patients with left ventricular dysfunction and to facilitate ventilation during the period of intubation.

It may be prudent to expose the femoral vessels in patients with dense adherence of cardiac structures to the sternum, in patients having their second or later reoperation, in patients with evidence of a patent right internal thoracic artery crossing the midline or vein graft adhering to the sternotomy, in patients who have received mediastinal irradiation, in patients with aneurysms of the ascending aorta or aortic arch, and in some elderly patients, especially cachectic women who have long-standing mitral or tricuspid valve dysfunction and have fragile osteoporotic sternums. In selected cases, the surgeon should cannulate the femoral artery and vein before reopening the sternum. Cardiopulmonary bypass could be initiated through the femoral artery, which would provide some support if catastrophic bleeding occurred. In cannulating the femoral vein, a long cannula may be advanced into the vena cava or right atrium. A second venous cannula may be placed through the right atrium after the sternotomy.

A number of safeguards may prevent bleeding associated with re-entry (Loop, 1984). (1) Appreciate that a high-risk situation exists. (2) In the most hazardous circumstance, cannulate the femoral vessels before opening the sternum. (3) Use a nitrogen-powered oscillating saw at low power and first divide the outer sternal table only. (4) Simultaneously retract the sternum outward with rakes (Fig. 54–94) and request that the anesthesiologist deflate the lungs. (5) Avoid probing retrosternally, which may result in penetration of a thin right ventricle. (6) When the sternum is divided, mobilize each side 2 to 4 cm before inserting a retractor. (7) Also mobilize the innominate vein. (8) If hemorrhage occurs, gently compress the site until good exposure is obtained and sound repair is possible. Large rents may require a patch to alleviate tension on the suture line.

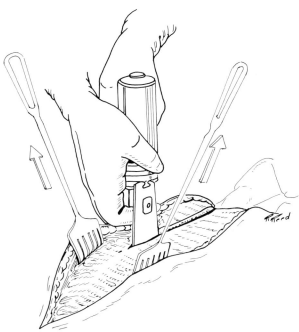

Figure 54–94. Sternotomy is done with a nitrogen-powered oscillating saw. The anesthesiologist deflates the lungs while an assistant simultaneously pulls outward with rakes fastened to subcutaneous tissue. The objective of these maneuvers is to move the sternum away from the underlying structures.

If only the circumflex or posteroventricular right coronary arterial branches require grafting, some surgeons (Burlingame et al, 1988; Faro et al, 1982; Ungerleider et al, 1985) advocate a left thoracotomy for reoperative coronary bypass. The technique limits versatility in grafting and should be considered only in unusual situations. It requires femoral artery and left atrial or pulmonary artery cannulation. Proximal anastomoses are done on the descending aorta or subclavian artery, and the site should be marked for future catheterization. In the rare case of reoperation in the presence of a tracheostoma, a bilateral thoracotomy approach separates the stoma from the operative field (Marshall et al, 1988).

Various synthetic and bioprosthetic membranes have been used to reduce pericardial and mediastinal adhesions. None have worked consistently, and they may be detrimental in the midst of infection. Even pericardial closure is no guarantee that adhesion formation will be reduced. Preliminary experience in congenital heart patients with a polytetrafluoroethylene membrane 0.1 mm thick is encouraging in that patients reoperated on within 2 years showed only filmy adhesions (Amato et al, 1989). The behavior of this plastic membrane during infection is not known. A case may be made for a pericardial substitute in congenital heart surgical therapy (Harada et al, 1988) and perhaps in selected young patients who are likely to have reoperation, but routine use is not required (Heydorn et al, 1988). At this time, surgeons are unlikely to encounter pericardial substitutes in patients having reoperation.

After conventional sternotomy, the objective is to confine dissection to exposure of the right atrium and aorta. A plane around the right atrium is entered by dividing adhesions between the right ventricular margin and the diaphragm. The guiding principles for entering and developing planes include sharp rather than blunt dissection, which may tear cardiac structures. The surgeon advances superiorly to expose the aorta. At this junction, heparin is administered. Some surgeons will already have procured lower-extremity vein for the reoperation bypass; others prefer to wait until heparin is given. Removal of the lower-extremity vein during cannulation shortens the storage time. Gentle technique in procurement, avoidance of distention, and storing the specimen filled with dilute papaverine reduces endothelial sloughing. Agreement has not been reached about the optimal storage medium. If the internal thoracic arteries and greater saphenous veins do not supply adequate conduits, the next choice is the lesser saphenous veins. Arm veins and synthetic conduits offer significantly lower patency rates. The gastroepiploic artery holds promise, but its versatility as an in-situ conduit is limited, and the patency of in-situ and free gastroepiploic arteries as coronary artery bypass grafts is too preliminary to recommend them for routine use.

Heparin dosage cannot always be predicted, and activated clotting time should be maintained at greater than 400 seconds. A consistently reliable and practical method for anticipating the extremes of heparin responsiveness has not been identified (Gravlee et al, 1987). In most cases, the aorta can be recannulated for insertion of the arterial perfusion line and a two-stage right atrial-inferior vena caval cannula is inserted for venous drainage. In patients who have poor left ventricular function or who require reoperative coronary bypass combined with other cardiac operations, the surgeon may use two caval cannulas, caval tourniquets, and a left atrial or left atrioventricular vent. This full cannulation results in lower septal temperature and consistent decompression.

The preferred cardioplegic solution may be delivered antegrade into the aortic root and retrograde through a coronary sinus balloon catheter. The double-lumen retrograde catheter may be inserted through a right atrial purse-string and advanced into the coronary sinus without opening the right atrium. Cardioplegia administered retrograde through the cardiac venous system provides excellent myocardial protection (Weisel et al, 1983) and is efficacious in patients who have (1) diffuse coronary atherosclerosis, (2) poor left ventricular function, (3) open internal thoracic artery grafts, and (4) patent atherosclerotic vein grafts.

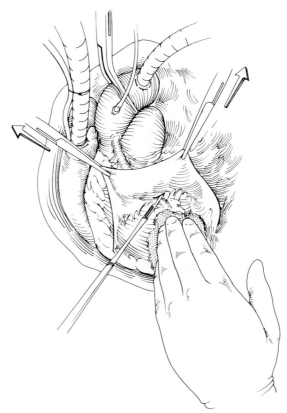

Figure 54–96. The most anterior leaf of pericardium is grasped, and with gentle countertraction, a flap of pericardium is raised by sharp dissection to expose the anterior descending coronary artery.

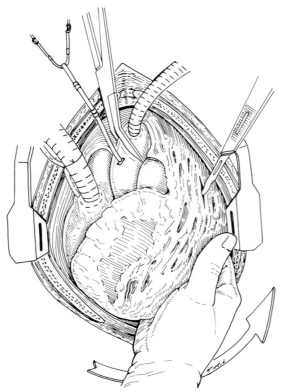

Figure 54–95. After cannulation and institution of cardiopulmonary bypass and cardioplegia, dissection begins inferiorly to mobilize the cold, flaccid heart. When the surgeon frees the posterolateral surface of the left ventricle, the pericardium may be opened anteriorly to gain access to the pericardial space.

Based on the author's experience with reoperation core cooling is recommended, followed by aortic cross-clamping and cardioplegia delivery *before* mobilizing the left ventricle. Trying to dissect out the beating heart is more traumatic than freeing the cold, flaccid heart. Dissection begins inferiorly and is extended down along the diaphragmatic surface of the left ventricular wall between the heart and the diaphragm (Fig. 54–95). The dissection proceeds first inferiorly and then posterolaterally. The surgeon may gently sweep the right hand around the posterolateral surface, up anteriorly under the pericardium, which may then be opened toward the left ventricular apex. The pericardium may be dissected back sharply to expose the anterior descending coronary artery (Fig. 54–96).

The regrafting sequence is important, and priorities should be established. Reoperation in patients with occluded atherosclerotic vein grafts should not produce embolism, but atheroembolism from still patent atherosclerotic vein grafts is a real hazard. Even mild atherosclerosis in vein grafts constitutes a hazard for embolization (Fig. 54–97). Rather than use angiographic studies, which underestimate the extent of atherosclerotic involvement of these grafts, some surgeons have recommended replacing all vein grafts more than 5 years old because almost all vein

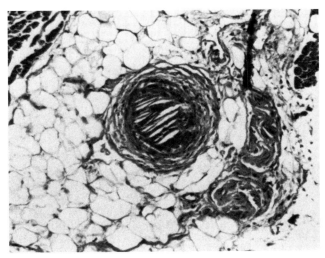

Figure 54–97. Atherosclerotic debris has occluded the coronary arterial branch vessel. This event may cause infarction in the distribution perfused by the patent atherosclerotic vein graft. Death has resulted from massive atheroembolism.

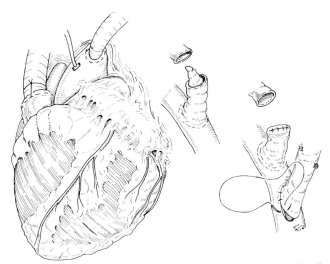

Figure 54–98. An atherosclerotic vein graft is divided distally near the old anastomosis. A new distal anastomosis is done, and the stump of the old graft is oversewn.

grafts explanted before that time show evidence of atherosclerosis. Reoperation mortality and incidence of myocardial infarction have been reduced by minimal graft handling, prompt ligation of grafts before cardioplegic infusion, and performance of all anastomoses (distal and proximal) under one period of cross-clamping (Grondin et al, 1984; Keon et al, 1982). To avoid atheroembolism from these atherosclerotic grafts that are still open (occluded vein grafts generally pose no threat), the surgeon must avoid touching the graft. This is another important reason for mobilizing the cold, flaccid left ventricle rather than the beating heart, which requires more manipulation.

In the author's experience, the first dose of cardioplegic solution may be given via the aortic root and down the old vein graft if it is patent. Subsequent doses are administered at 15- to 20-minute intervals throughout the reoperation. After the left ventricle is mobilized, the atherosclerotic graft should be divided distally (Fig. 54–98) and oversewn after the distal anastomosis is completed. The cardioplegic solution may be administered into the graft through a side-arm cannula, or the graft may be connected to the aorta and the root can be reperfused. Proximal anastomoses may frequently be done at the site of an old graft aortic anastomosis (Fig. 54–99). The entire grafting procedure may be done under one period of aortic cross-clamping (Salerno, 1982). In patients having reoperation, it is easier to construct aortic anastomoses with the aorta fully clamped. After regrafting arteries perfused by open atherosclerotic vein grafts, attention is turned to other vessels. Priorities in the grafting process should be established from the start of the operation.

In patients who are having reoperation and who have a patent internal thoracic artery graft to the anterior descending artery, the procedure is essen-

tially the same except that during mobilization of the left side of the heart, the arterial conduit must be identified so that a small bulldog clamp may be temporarily applied to it (Fig. 54–100) (Baillot et al, 1985). This maneuver is necessary so that continued blood flow through the thoracic artery does not rewarm the myocardium or wash out the effect of cardioplegia. After this maneuver, additional cardioplegia is done to cool the area supplied by the patent thoracic artery. If thoracic artery perfusion of the coronary bed is allowed during the operation,

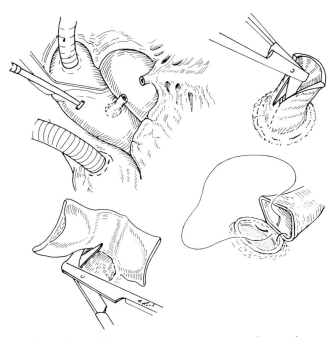

Figure 54–99. The new proximal anastomosis frequently may be centered at the site of the previous vein graft aortic anastomosis. This maneuver conserves space on the aorta in cases of multiple grafting.

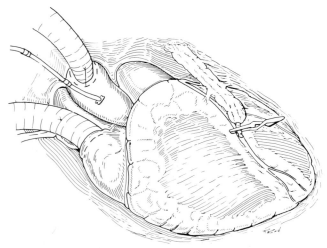

Figure 54–100. The patent internal thoracic artery graft has been located and is clamped temporarily to stop blood flow to the anterior descending distribution. Failure to temporarily occlude the internal thoracic artery graft usually results in continued myocardial metabolic activity and less than optimal myocardial protection in that region.

myocardial protection may be less than optimal because of continued electrical activity in that region.

Approximately 20% of all transfusions result in some adverse effect (Walker, 1987). Eighty to 90% of hepatitis that occurs as a result of operation is the non-A, non-B type; half of these patients have chronic hepatitis, and approximately 10% have late cirrhosis. Blood conservation should be practiced throughout the operation (Cosgrove et al, 1979; Thurer and Hauer, 1982; Utley et al, 1981). Patients having reoperation have greater transfusion requirements than first-operation patients because of bleeding adhesions and the generally longer period of cardiopulmonary bypass. Nevertheless, blood conservation has resulted in a reduction of bank blood or blood products from eight units in the earliest reoperation experience to two units today. During the last 5 years, the author's patients having coronary reoperation have received an average of 2.1 units of packed cells per patient versus 0.7 units for primary revascularization. The following methods may be used to reduce transfusion requirements in all cardiac operations: (1) Secure hemostasis throughout the procedure; persistent oozing requires greater use of cardiotomy suction with attendant hemolysis. (2) Restrict total crystalloid infusion, preferably to less than 1 liter to minimize dilutional anemia. (3) Use a regionally heparinized blood processing system to collect intraoperative blood shed before heparinization and after protamine; these cells are washed, concentrated, and transfused at the end of the procedure. (4) Allow normovolemic anemia (25 to 30% hematocrit), depending on preoperative left ventricular function. (5) Transfuse all oxygenator contents at the conclusion of the procedure. (6) Transfuse shed mediastinal and pleural cavity blood postoper-

atively. This blood may be collected in the cardiotomy reservoir and transfused without washing or concentration (Cosgrove et al, 1985).

When the aorta is unclamped, cardiopulmonary bypass perfusion is continued until the patient is normothermic and cardiac activity has fully recovered. During this interval of support, hemostasis is obtained and, when indicated, temporary pacemaker wires and additional monitor lines are applied. Anastomoses should be inspected, posterolateral and other bleeding sites should be electrocoagulated or oversewn, and management should be discussed with the anesthesiologist while the patient is on pump support. At this time, all major bleeding points should be controlled. Anastomotic or other bleeding that requires control by lifting or retraction of the heart after decannulation may have devastating consequences.

Protamine administration requires careful monitoring. The cardiovascular effects of protamine are those of vasodilatation and negative inotropism. Three types of adverse response have been identified: (1) hypotensive, (2) anaphylactoid, and (3) catastrophic pulmonary vasoconstriction (Gupta et al, 1988; Horrow, 1988). Patients who have neutral protamine Hagedorn (NPH) insulin-dependent diabetes and those with allergies to fish (commercial protamine is prepared from the sperm of salmon) should be administered protamine cautiously (Stewart et al, 1984). These patients are susceptible to protamine reactions that simulate anaphylaxis. Anyone who has previously received protamine is suspect, although major adverse reactions among nondiabetic patients are rare. The NPH insulin-dependent diabetic patient may have had a long exposure to protamine and thus may have an allergic reaction when rechallenged with a large dose. The use of alternate routes for protamine delivery is conjectural. The safest approach is to administer a test dose, and if no signs of allergy are noted, protamine is given slowly to neutralize heparin.

After protamine is delivered and clot formation is established, hemostatic agents may be useful. Raw sites, especially over the anterior right ventricle, may be managed effectively by a cellulose gauze. Anastomotic oozing may be controlled by fibrin glue applied as a topical hemostatic agent (Borst et al, 1982). This sealant is best used after heparin has been reversed by protamine. Fibrin sealant is useful particularly to control oozing in small-vessel anastomoses, and no adverse reactions or transmission of viral infection has been documented when used topically (Rousou et al, 1989).

An organized, methodical cleanup phase can be accomplished expeditiously; random cauterization and purposeless movement should be minimized. Pleural chest tubes are best inserted at the time of pleural entry. If the pleura has been entered earlier, extensive lysis of adhesions should be avoided because many are vascular. Dense pleural adhesions may bar entry, and in those cases, drainage by mediastinal tubes only is indicated. A heavy No. 6 stainless-steel wire ensures tight sternal approximation and prevents dehiscence even if respiratory complications ensue. Interrupted sutures are recommended for fascial and subcutaneous closure, and interrupted monofilament or braided plastic is preferable for skin closure for diabetic patients, obese patients, those with bilateral internal thoracic artery grafting, and patients with previous mastectomy. In the early phase of postoperative management, attention to afterload reduction, judicious volume replacement, and maintenance of normal hemodynamic parameters help to ensure a favorable outcome. Antiplatelet drugs are indicated whenever possible to enhance vein graft patency (Chesebro et al, 1982). Of all the management techniques, none is more effective than the performance of a complete revascularization operation without untoward intraoperative events.

CLINICAL RESULTS

Despite evidence of a worsening clinical profile of patients having reoperation, early results are improving. After coronary bypass surgery began in 1967, several years elapsed before publication of the first reports of reoperation. Adam and colleagues (1972) and Johnson and associates (1972) reported an operative mortality rate of approximately 10% and higher morbidity in patients requiring second procedures. Higher risk in coronary artery reoperation was attributed to greater extent of coronary atherosclerosis, interim left ventricular damage, accidents during re-entry, technical difficulty caused by adhesions, and longer pump oxygenator time. In the mid-1970s, other reports confirmed that reoperation was more hazardous, but early relief of angina approached that achieved after the first operation (Benedict et al, 1974; Londe and Sugg, 1974; Macmanus et al, 1975; Skow et al, 1973; Stiles et al, 1976; Thomas et al, 1976; Winkle et al, 1975).

This initial experience in coronary artery reoperations has been steadily improved on, particularly in the 1980s. Operative mortality has been at least halved (Foster et al, 1984), and morbidity, which is still higher than for primary operation, has been significantly reduced (Loop et al, 1983; Lytle et al, 1987; Schaff et al, 1983). In 1,500 consecutive coronary artery reoperations through 1984, the overall operative (hospital) mortality was 3%, and in recent reports, it has ranged from 3 to 5% (Foster et al, 1984; Schaff et al, 1983). Logistic regression analysis of a number of clinical, angiographic, and operative variables indicated that advanced age, left main arterial narrowing 50% or greater, severe angina, and incomplete revascularization at reoperation were risk factors implicated in hospital death. In addition to left main coronary artery disease, open but stenotic grafts are believed by some investigators (Schaff et al, 1983) to pose a higher surgical risk because graft injury or

manipulation leading to embolism of atherosclerotic material could compromise myocardial blood supply. Atheroemboli originate in aortocoronary vein bypass grafts and also occur during angioplasty and cause myocardial infarction or death. This observation emphasizes the point that any manipulation, external or internal, may disrupt the fragile debris and cause an embolic myocardial infarction (Case Records of Massachusetts General Hospital, 1987). In the hospital the deaths of most patients after coronary artery reoperation are related to myocardial dysfunction; even in the most recent series, 82% of early deaths were from cardiac causes (Lytle et al, 1987). Major morbidity in reoperation series (Foster et al, 1984; Loop et al, 1983) has been due to perioperative myocardial infarction (6 to 8%), stroke (1 to 2%), reoperation for bleeding (4 to 5%), respiratory distress (2 to 3%), wound complication (1%), and renal failure (<1%).

After reoperation, relief of angina is less than after the first operation (Cameron et al, 1988; Loop et al, 1983; Schaff et al, 1983), mainly because of high recurrence of angina in the first year postoperatively. Rather than studying freedom from angina per se, which is approximately 50% at 10 years after reoperation (Lytle et al, 1987), angina should be included in an assessment of cardiac events. Cardiac events are analyzed in terms of event-free survival, and the end-points depend on which cardiac events are included in the follow-up. In 1982, Schaff and colleagues (1983) calculated that angina-free survival was 40% at 3 years, 28% at 5 years, and 26% at 7 years. Freedom from New York Heart Association Class III or IV angina was 73% at 3 years and 63% at 5 to 7 years. Thus, a relatively high proportion of patients having reoperation had mild angina 5 years postoperatively, but severe angina was uncommon. In one report, a low serum cholesterol level was the best correlate of an improved symptomatic response after the *first* operation (Lamas et al, 1986). However, after a reoperation, the principal correlate of a better symptomatic response was normal or almost normal left ventricular *ejection fraction*. Lytle and colleagues (1987) determined that event-free survival (freedom from severe recurring angina, myocardial infarction, or another reoperation) was 48% at 10 years (Fig. 54–101). These results indicate that palliation after coronary artery reoperation is satisfactory but not as good as generally achieved after the first procedure.

Information about reoperation graft patency is scant because not many patients who have one or more coronary reoperations will be restudied by postoperative angiography unless they have recurrent symptoms of angina that substantially affect lifestyle. Nevertheless, records of 256 patients were compiled from a reoperation series of 1,500 patients who had angiography after reoperation (Lytle et al, 1987). Recurrent symptoms or cardiac events led to repeat angiography in 73%. Patency of both vein and internal thoracic artery grafts was almost the same as that reported after the first operation—70% for

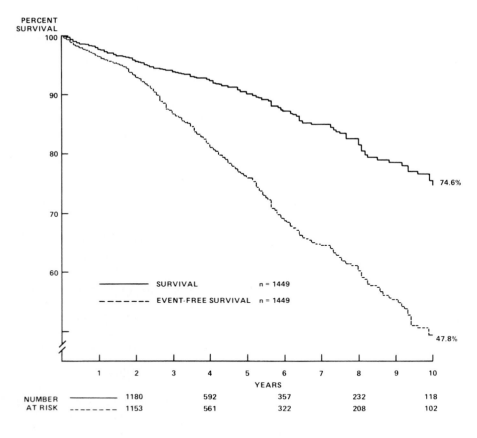

Figure 54–101. Ten-year actuarial survival after coronary artery reoperation. The 10-year actuarial survival is 75% *(top curve)*, and the 10-year event-free survival is 48%. (Adapted from Lytle, B. W., Loop, F. D., Cosgrove, D. M., et al: Fifteen hundred coronary reoperations: Results and determinants of early and late survival. J. Thorac. Cardiovasc. Surg., *93*:851, 1987.)

SURVIVAL

Longevity after coronary reoperation must be considered to be a continuum of survival that begins with the first coronary operation. These patients were operated on initially for angina in most cases, but they tended to be a decade or more younger than the average surgical candidate today. Furthermore, these patients, who were operated on originally in the 1970s, tended to have less extensive coronary atherosclerosis, had normal left ventricular function, or had incomplete revascularization (i.e., not all significantly narrowed major coronary arteries received bypass grafts). This profile is different today. In the 1980s, the average age of surgical patients has increased, 75% or more have three-vessel disease, and left ventricular performance is impaired in more than half. Complete revascularization is achieved in 90% or more, and one or both internal thoracic artery grafts are more liberally used. The point made here is that both the patient and the operation have changed in the last 10 years, and these changes affect the incidence and outcome of reoperations.

In this continuum, the patient has survived the first operation and later on, at various intervals but mainly after the fifth postoperative year, has a cardiac event that initiates re-evaluation and a reoperation. These patients have shown 5-year and 10-year actuarial survival rates of 90 and 75%, respectively (see Fig. 54–101). However, their survival rate is more impressive if one takes into account their longevity beginning with the first operation. From an analysis of 1,500 consecutive reoperation patients, advanced age, hypertension, and abnormal left ventricular function are found to adversely affect late survival (Lytle et al, 1987) (Fig. 54–102). The angiographic indication for reoperation (i.e., graft closure, progressive atherosclerosis, or a combination of these two indications) did not affect survival. Data on subsets indicate a 3-year survival of 85% for patients 70 years or older and a 5-year survival of 82% for patients with severely impaired left ventricular function. Preliminary data indicate that a new internal thoracic artery graft to the anterior descending coronary artery favorably influences 5-year survival after reoperation; however, this improvement is not as striking as after the first operation, probably because of more diffuse arterial disease and intervening worse left ventricular function.

Results of two or more coronary artery reoperations indicate even higher mortality and morbidity than that cited earlier. For hospital survivors, however, the outlook was reasonably good, with 87% alive 5 years later (Brenowitz et al, 1988).

vein grafts and 91% for internal thoracic artery grafts at an average of 4 years postoperatively.

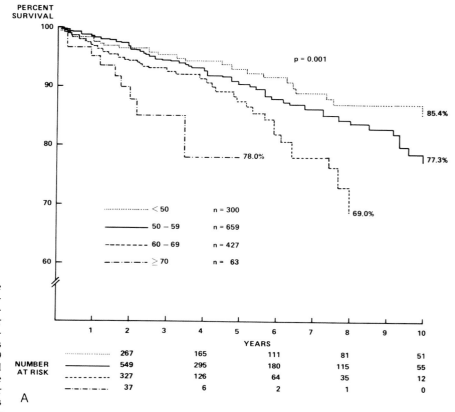

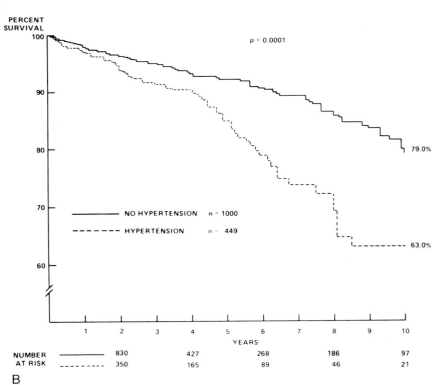

Figure 54–102. Late survival of the 1,449 in-hospital survivors of coronary reoperation according to (A) age at reoperation expressed in decades; (B) presence or absence of hypertension; and (C) left ventricular function. A, Five-year survival rates of patients less than 50 years, 50 to 59 years, and 60 to 69 years were 93, 91, and 87%, respectively. The 3-year survival rate of patients 70 years or older was 85%. For hypertensive patients (B), survival rates were 85 and 63% at 5 and 10 postoperative years compared with 92 and 79% for normotensive patients.

Illustration continued on following page

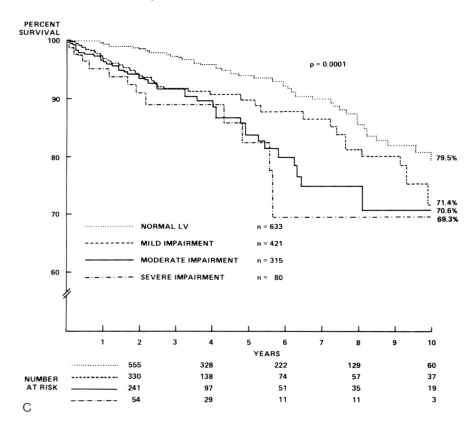

Figure 54–102 *Continued (C)* Reoperation patients were grouped according to left ventricular (LV) function graded subjectively according to the preoperative left ventricular angiogram. Survival rates at 5 years were 94, 90, 84, and 82%, respectively, for patients with normal left ventricular function and mild, moderate, and severe impairment. Ten-year survival rates for patients with normal LV function, mild, or moderate impairment were 80, 71, and 71%, respectively. (From Lytle, B. W., Loop, F. D., Cosgrove, D. M., et al: Fifteen hundred coronary reoperations: Results and determinants of early and late survival. J. Thorac. Cardiovasc. Surg., 93:853, 1987.)

REHABILITATION

The surgeon should advise the patient to eat a prudent, low-fat diet, monitor serum lipid levels, keep diabetes and hypertension under good control, stop smoking completely (Hermanson et al, 1988), maintain ideal weight, exercise as monitored through a cardiovascular rehabilitation program, and modify Type A behavior. Reduction of serum lipids is an attainable goal for most patients. Although bypass surgery has no effect on the underlying cause of the disease, secondary prevention that modifies risk factors may reduce recurrent coronary heart disease and death (Siegel et al, 1988). Dietary recommendations should be individualized to the specific lipoprotein abnormality and ideal body weight (Lavie et al, 1988). The patient may begin with the American Heart Association's Step-One Diet, which lowers the total fat and saturated fat in the diet to 30 and 10% of total calories, respectively, by restricting the cholesterol intake to 300 mg/day or less. If this diet is unsuccessful after 3 months, a Step-Two Diet in which saturated fats are restricted to 7% of total calories and cholesterol is held to 200 mg/day may be appropriate. A registered dietitian with a particular interest in heart disease can help to provide the patient with advice and encouragement. Patients who do not respond to dietary efforts and who have lipoprotein abnormalities are candidates for drug therapy. All of the lipid-lowering drugs are expensive and potentially have major side effects. The 3-hy-

droxy-3-methylglutaryl coenzyme A reductase inhibitor (e.g., lovastatin) is the most promising of these agents, but the long-term efficacy and safety of this drug is not yet known.

Although regression of the complicated plaque has been considered to be a rare event, the advent of new lipid-lowering agents may slow down the progression of disease and may even make regression of coronary atherosclerosis a reality (Sheperd and Packard, 1988). The Cholesterol-Lowering Atherosclerosis Study showed that aggressive lowering of low-density lipoprotein cholesterol with an increase in the high-density fraction produced beneficial changes, which was documented by serial arteriography, both in native coronary arteries and in venous bypass grafts (Blankenhorn et al, 1987). These and other clinical trials were done in middle-aged men, and the extrapolation to women and elderly persons must be kept in perspective. An optimal weight and exercise in keeping with norms for age and previous activity are part of any rehabilitation plan. At least 3 months of supervised exercise training is recommended for patients who desire strenuous exercise such as jogging, tennis, and handball (Thompson, 1988). This advice applies particularly to patients who have reoperation, who must be at higher risk because of more diffuse coronary atherosclerosis and abnormal left ventricular function.

Because platelet function inhibition appears to improve vein graft patency up to 1 year after coronary bypass surgery (Chesebro et al, 1982), aspirin/dipyridamole or aspirin alone is prescribed indefinitely for patients who tolerate salicylates and have not had peptic ulcer disease or blood dyscrasia and are not receiving anticoagulants. As mentioned earlier, no information exists about the effect of antiplatelet agents on the development of vein graft atherosclerosis. There is no reason to believe that the new vein grafts are any more immune to atherosclerosis than the first ones. Ten years after the first or subsequent coronary bypass operation, even if no cardiac events have occurred, another coronary arteriogram is advisable.

Selected Bibliography

Camann, W. R., Wojtowicz, S. R., and Mark, J. B.: Reoperation for coronary artery bypass grafting: Anesthetic challenge. J. Card. Anes., 1:458, 1987.

This comprehensive review article addresses anesthesia management during coronary artery reoperation. The discussion includes intravascular access monitoring, preoperative preparation, and anesthetic techniques.

Cosgrove, D. M., Loop, F. D., Lytle, B. W., et al: Predictors of reoperation after myocardial revascularization. J. Thorac. Cardiovasc. Surg., 92:811, 1986.

The incidence of reoperation, which rose to 17% at 12 years, is reported along with an analysis of patient descriptors to predict reoperation. The most important predictor of reoperation-free survival after the first operation was the presence or absence of an internal thoracic artery graft.

Grondin, C. M.: Graft disease in patients with coronary bypass grafting: Why does it start? Where do we stop? J. Thorac. Cardiovasc. Surg., 92:323, 1986.

A superb review of coronary artery and vein graft atherosclerosis. Theories regarding vein graft atherosclerosis are timely, as is the author's technique of intraoperative avoidance of atheroembolism.

Lytle, B. W., Loop, F. D., Cosgrove, D. M., et al: Fifteen hundred coronary reoperations: Results and determinants of early and late survival. J. Thorac. Cardiovasc. Surg., 93:847, 1987.

The Cleveland Clinic Foundation's consecutive experience with 1,500 coronary artery reoperations is grouped into eras that show changes in patient characteristics and results. Multivariate analyses identify operative risk and predictors of survival up to 10 years.

Marshall, W. G., Jr., Saffitz, J., and Kouchoukos, N. T.: Management during reoperation of aortocoronary saphenous vein grafts with minimal atherosclerosis by angiography. Ann. Thorac. Surg., 42:163, 1986.

This article emphasizes the fact that angiography underestimates the severity of vein graft atherosclerosis. During reoperation, explanted grafts showed diffuse atherosclerosis. Because of the propensity of atherosclerotic vein grafts to progress to occlusion unpredictably, these investigators recommend routine replacement of aortocoronary saphenous vein grafts 5 years or more after the initial procedure, irrespective of angiographic findings.

Schaff, H. V., Orszulak, T. A., Gersh, B. J., et al: The morbidity and mortality of reoperation for coronary artery disease and analysis of late results with use of actuarial estimate of event-free interval. J. Thorac. Cardiovasc. Surg., 85:508, 1983.

This Mayo Clinic report surveys survival and cardiac events after repeat myocardial revascularization. They noted a 60% freedom from major cardiac events and relief of severe symptoms 5 years after reoperation. Actuarial estimates of event-free intervals are the best method of analysis.

Bibliography

Adam, M., Geisler, G. F., Lambert, C. J., and Mitchel, B. F., Jr.: Reoperation following clinical failure of aorta-to-coronary artery bypass vein grafts. Ann. Thorac. Surg., 14:272, 1972.

Addonizio, V. P., Jr., Fisher, C. A., Kappa, J. R., and Ellison, N.: Prevention of heparin-induced thrombocytopenia during open heart surgery with Iloprost (ZK 36374). Surgery, 102:796, 1987.

Alderman, E. L., Fisher, L., Maynard, C., et al: Determinants of coronary surgery in a consecutive patient series from geographically dispersed medical centers: The Coronary Artery Surgery Study. Circulation, 66(Suppl. I):6, 1982.

Amato, J. J., Cotroneo, J. V., Galdieri, R. J., et al: Experience with the polytetrafluoroethylene surgical membrane for pericardial closure in operations for congenital cardiac defects. J. Thorac. Cardiovasc. Surg., 97:929, 1989.

Bahn, C. H., and Annest, L. S.: Reoperation without medical records: Avoidable? J. Thorac. Cardiovasc. Surg., 91:139, 1986.

Baillot, R. G., Loop, F. D., Cosgrove, D. M., and Lytle, B. W.: Reoperation after previous grafting with the internal mammary artery: Technique and early results. Ann. Thorac. Surg., 40:271, 1985.

Barboriak, J. J., Barboriak, D. P., Anderson, A. J., et al: Risk factors in patients undergoing a second aorta-coronary bypass procedure. J. Thorac. Cardiovasc. Surg., 76:111, 1978.

Benedict, J. S., Buhl, T. L., and Henney, R. P.: Re-revascularization of the ischemic myocardium. Arch. Surg., 108:40, 1974.

Blankenhorn, D. H., Nessim, S. A., Johnson, R. L., et al: Beneficial effects of combined colestipol-niacin therapy on coronary atherosclerosis and coronary venous bypass grafts. J.A.M.A., 257:3233, 1987.

Borst, H. G., Haverich, A., Walterbusch, G., and Maatz, W.: Fibrin adhesive: An important hemostatic adjunct in cardiovascular operations. J. Thorac. Cardiovasc. Surg., 84:548, 1982.

Bourassa, M. G., Lespérance, J., Corbara, F., et al: Progression of obstructive coronary artery disease 5 to 7 years after aortocoronary bypass surgery. Circulation, 58(Suppl. I):100, 1978.

Brenowitz, J. B., Johnson, W. D., Kayser, K. L., et al: Coronary artery bypass grafting for the third time or more: Results of 150 consecutive cases. Circulation, 78(Suppl. I):166, 1988.

Brown, B. G., Cukingnan, R. A., DeRouen, T., et al: Improved graft patency in patients treated with platelet-inhibiting therapy after coronary bypass surgery. Circulation, 72:138, 1985.

Bruschke, A. V. G., Wijers, T. S., Kolsters, W., and Landmann, J.: The anatomic evolution of coronary artery disease demonstrated by coronary arteriography in 256 nonoperated patients. Circulation, 63:527, 1981.

Burlingame, M. W., Bonchek, L. I., and Vazales, B. E.: Left thoracotomy for reoperative coronary bypass. J. Thorac. Cardiovasc. Surg., 95:508, 1988.

Camann, W. R., Wojtowicz, S. R., and Mark, J. B.: Reoperation for coronary artery bypass grafting: Anesthetic challenge. J. Card. Anes., 1:458, 1987.

Cameron, A., Kemp, H. G., Jr., and Green, G. E.: Bypass surgery with the internal mammary artery graft: 15 year follow-up. Circulation, 74(Suppl. III):30, 1986.

Cameron, A., Kemp, H. G., Jr., and Green, G. E.: Reoperation for coronary artery disease: 10 years of clinical follow-up. Circulation, 78(Suppl. I):158, 1988.

Campeau, L., Enjalbert, M., Lespérance, J., et al: The relation of risk factors to the development of atherosclerosis in saphenous-vein bypass grafts and the progression of disease in the native circulation: A study 10 years after aorto-coronary bypass surgery. N. Engl. J. Med., 311:1329, 1984.

Case Records of the Massachusetts General Hospital: Case 6–1987. N. Engl. J. Med., *316*:321, 1987.

Chesebro, J. H., Clements, I. P., Fuster, V., et al: A platelet-inhibitor-drug trial in coronary-artery bypass operations: Benefit of perioperative dipyridamole and aspirin therapy on early postoperative vein-graft patency. N. Engl. J. Med., *307*:73, 1982.

Cosgrove, D. M., Amiot, D. M., and Meserko, J. J.: An improved technique of autotransfusion of shed mediastinal blood. Ann. Thorac. Surg., *40*:519, 1985.

Cosgrove, D. M., Loop, F. D., Lytle, B. W., et al: Predictors of reoperation after myocardial revascularization. J. Thorac. Cardiovasc. Surg., *92*:811, 1986.

Cosgrove, D. M., Thurer, R. L., Lytle, B. W., et al: Blood conservation during myocardial revascularization. Ann. Thorac. Surg., *28*:184, 1979.

Crean, P. A., Waters, D. D., Bosch, X., et al: Angiographic findings after myocardial infarction in patients with previous bypass surgery: Explanations for smaller infarcts in this group compared with control patients. Circulation, *71*:693, 1985.

Culliford, A. T., Girdwood, R. W., Isom, O. W., et al: Angina following myocardial revascularization: Does time of recurrence predict etiology and influence results of operation? J. Thorac. Cardiovasc. Surg., *77*:889, 1979.

Douglas, J. S., Gruentzig, A. R., King, S. B., III, et al: Percutaneous transluminal coronary angioplasty in patients with prior coronary bypass surgery. J. Am. Coll. Cardiol., *2*:745, 1983.

European Coronary Surgery Study Group: Long-term results of prospective randomised study of coronary artery bypass surgery in stable angina pectoris. Lancet, *2*:1173, 1982.

Faro, R. S., Javid, H., Najafi, H., and Serry, C.: Left thoracotomy for reoperation for coronary revascularization. J. Thorac. Cardiovasc. Surg., *84*:453, 1982.

Ferguson, T. B., Jr., Muhlbaier, L. H., Salai, D. L., and Wechsler, A. S.: Coronary bypass grafting after failed elective and failed emergent percutaneous angioplasty. J. Thorac. Cardiovasc. Surg., *95*:761, 1988.

Ferraris, V. A., Ferraris, S. P., Lough, F. C., and Berry, W. R.: Preoperative aspirin ingestion increases operative blood loss after coronary artery bypass grafting. Ann. Thorac. Surg., *45*:71, 1988.

Foster, E. D., Fisher, L. D., Kaiser, G. C., et al: Comparison of operative mortality and morbidity for initial and repeat coronary artery bypass grafting: The Coronary Artery Surgery Study (CASS) Registry experience. Ann. Thorac. Surg., *38*:563, 1984.

Fox, M. H., Gruchow, H. W., Barboriak, J. J., et al: Risk factors among patients undergoing repeat aorta-coronary bypass procedures. J. Thorac. Cardiovasc. Surg., *93*:56, 1987.

Golding, L. A. R., Loop, F. D., Hollman, J. L., et al: Early results of emergency surgery following coronary angioplasty. Circulation, *74*(Suppl. III):26, 1986.

Goldman, S. G., Copeland, J., Moritz, T., et al: Improvement in early saphenous vein graft patency after coronary artery bypass surgery with antiplatelet therapy: Results of a Veterans Administration Cooperative Study. Circulation, *77*:1324, 1988.

Gravlee, G. P., Brauer, S. D., Roy, R. C., et al: Predicting the pharmacodynamics of heparin: A clinical evaluation of the Hepcon System 4. J. Card. Anes., *1*:379, 1987.

Grondin, C. M.: Graft disease in patients with coronary bypass grafting (Editorial). J. Thorac. Cardiovasc. Surg., *92*:323, 1986a.

Grondin, C. M.: The removal of still functioning albeit old grafts: Not in our genes? Ann. Thorac. Surg., *42*:122, 1986b.

Grondin, C. M., Pomar, J. L., Hébert, Y., et al: Reoperation in patients with patent atherosclerotic coronary vein grafts: A different approach to a different disease. J. Thorac. Cardiovasc. Surg., *87*:379, 1984.

Gupta, K. G., Veith, F. J., Ascer, E., et al: Anaphylactoid reactions to protamine: An often lethal complication in insulin-dependent diabetic patients undergoing vascular surgery. J. Vasc. Surg., *9*:342, 1988.

Harada, Y., Imai, Y., Kurosawa, H., et al: Long-term results of the clinical use of an expanded polytetrafluoroethylene surgical membrane as a pericardial substitute. J. Thorac. Cardiovasc. Surg., *96*:811, 1988.

Hermanson, B., Omenn, G. S., Kronmal, R. A., et al: Beneficial six-year outcome of smoking cessation in older men and women with coronary artery disease: Results from the CASS Registry. N. Engl. J. Med., *319*:1365, 1988.

Heydorn, W. H., Ferraris, V. A., and Berry, W. R.: Pericardial substitutes: A survey. Ann. Thorac. Surg., *46*:567, 1988.

Horrow, J. C.: Protamine allergy. J. Card. Anes., *2*:225, 1988.

Johnson, W. D., Hoffman, J. F., Jr., Flemma, R. J., and Tector, A. J.: Secondary surgical procedure for myocardial revascularization. J. Thorac. Cardiovasc. Surg., *64*:523, 1972.

Kappa, J. R., Horn, M. K., III, Fisher, C. A., et al: Efficacy of Iloprost (ZK36374) versus aspirin in preventing heparin-induced platelet activation during cardiac operations. J. Thorac. Cardiovasc. Surg., *94*:405, 1987.

Keon, W. J., Heggtveit, H. A., and Leduc, J.: Perioperative myocardial infarction caused by atheroembolism. J. Thorac. Cardiovasc. Surg., *84*:849, 1982.

King, D. J., and Kelton, J. G.: Heparin-associated thrombocytopenia. Ann. Intern. Med., *100*:535, 1984.

Klein, L. W., Weintraub, W. S., Agarwal, J. B., et al: Prognostic significance of severe narrowing of the proximal portion of the left anterior descending coronary artery. Am. J. Cardiol., *58*:42, 1986.

Kramer, J. R., Matsuda, Y., Mulligan, J. C., et al: Progression of coronary atherosclerosis. Circulation, *63*:519, 1981.

Lamas, G. A., Mudge, G. H., Jr., Collins, J. J., Jr., et al: Clinical response to coronary artery reoperations. J. Am. Coll. Cardiol., *8*:274, 1986.

Lavie, C. J., Gau, G. T., Squires, R. W., and Kottke, B. A.: Management of lipids in primary and secondary prevention of cardiovascular diseases. Mayo Clin. Proc., *63*:605, 1988.

Londe, S., and Sugg, W. L.: The challenge of reoperation in cardiac surgery. Ann. Thorac. Surg., *17*:157, 1974.

Loop, F. D.: Catastrophic hemorrhage during sternal reentry. Ann. Thorac. Surg., *37*:271, 1984.

Loop, F. D., and Cosgrove, D. M.: Repeat coronary bypass surgery: Selection of cases, surgical risks, and long-term outlook. Mod. Concepts Cardiovasc. Dis., *55*:31, 1986.

Loop, F. D., Lytle, B. W., Cosgrove, D. M., et al: Coronary artery bypass graft surgery in the elderly: Indications and outcome. Cleve. Clin. J. Med., *55*:23, 1988.

Loop, F. D., Lytle, B. W., Cosgrove, D. M., et al: Influence of the internal-mammary-artery graft on 10-year survival and other cardiac events. N. Engl. J. Med., *314*:1, 1986.

Loop, F. D., Lytle, B. W., Gill, C. C., et al: Trends in selection and results of coronary artery reoperations. Ann. Thorac. Surg., *36*:380, 1983.

Lorenz, R. L., Schacky, C. V., Weber, M., et al: Improved aortocoronary bypass patency by low-dose aspirin (100 mg daily). Lancet, *1*:1261, 1984.

Lytle, B. W., Cosgrove, D. M., Easley, K., et al: Clinical implications of late stenoses in saphenous vein to coronary bypass grafts. J. Am. Coll. Cardiol., *7*:34A, 1986.

Lytle, B. W., Loop, F. D., Cosgrove, D. M., et al: Fifteen hundred coronary reoperations: Results and determinants of early and late survival. J. Thorac. Cardiovasc. Surg., *93*:847, 1987.

Lytle, B. W., Loop, F. D., Cosgrove, D. M., et al: Long-term (5 to 12 years) serial studies of internal mammary artery and saphenous vein coronary bypass grafts. J. Thorac. Cardiovasc. Surg., *89*:248, 1985.

Macmanus, Q., Okies, J. E., Phillips, S. J., and Starr, A.: Surgical considerations in patients undergoing repeat median sternotomy. J. Thorac. Cardiovasc. Surg., *69*:138, 1975.

Marshall, W. G., Meng, R. L., and Ehrenhaft, J. L.: Coronary artery bypass grafting in patients with a tracheostoma: Use of a bilateral thoracotomy incision. Ann. Thorac. Surg., *46*:465, 1988.

Marshall, W. G., Saffitz, J., and Kouchoukos, N. T.: Management during reoperation of aortocoronary saphenous vein grafts with minimal atherosclerosis by angiography. Ann. Thorac. Surg., *42*:163, 1986.

Neitzel, G. F., Barboriak, J. J., Pintar, K., and Qureshi, I.: Atherosclerosis in aortocoronary bypass grafts: Morphologic study and risk factor analysis 6 to 12 years after surgery. Arteriosclerosis, *6*:594, 1986.

Passamani, E., Davis, K. B., Gillespie, M. J., et al: A randomized trial of coronary artery bypass surgery: Survival of patients with a low ejection fraction. N. Engl. J. Med., 312:1665, 1985.

Reed, D. C., Beller, G. A., Nygaard, T. W., et al: The clinical efficacy and scintigraphic evaluation of post-coronary bypass patients undergoing percutaneous transluminal coronary angioplasty for recurrent angina pectoris. Am. Heart J., 117:60, 1989.

Rousou, J., Levitsky, S., Gonzalez-Lavin, L., et al: Randomized clinical trial of fibrin sealant in patients undergoing resternotomy or reoperation after cardiac operations: a multicenter study. J. Thorac. Cardiovasc. Surg., 97:194, 1989.

Saber, R. S., Edwards, W. D., Holmes, D. R., Jr., et al: Balloon angioplasty of aortocoronary saphenous vein bypass grafts: A histopathologic study of six grafts from five patients, with emphasis on restenosis and embolic complications. J. Am. Coll. Cardiol., 12:1501, 1988.

Salerno, T. A.: Single aortic cross-clamping for distal and proximal anastomoses in coronary surgery: An alternative to conventional techniques. Ann. Thorac. Surg., 33:518, 1982.

Schaff, H. V., Orszulak, T. A., Gersh, B. J., et al: The morbidity and mortality of reoperation for coronary artery disease and analysis of late results with use of actuarial estimate of event-free interval. J. Thorac. Cardiovasc. Surg., 85:508, 1983.

Schrör, K., Darius, H., Matzky, R., and Ohlendorf, R.: The antiplatelet and cardiovascular actions of a new carbacyclin derivative (ZK36374) equipotent to PGI_2 in vitro. Naunyn Schmiedebergs Arch. Pharmacol., 316:252, 1981.

Schuster, E. H., Griffith, L. S., and Bulkley, B. H.: Preponderance of acute proximal left anterior descending coronary arterial lesions in fatal myocardial infarction: A clinicopathologic study. Am. J. Cardiol., 47:1189, 1981.

Shark, W. M., and Kass, R. M.: Repeat myocardial revascularization in coronary disease therapy: Consideration of primary bypass failures and success of second graft surgery. Am. Heart J., 102:303, 1981.

Sheperd, J., and Packard, C. J.: Regression of coronary atherosclerosis: Is it possible? Br. Heart J., 59:149, 1988.

Shimshak, T. M., Giorgi, L. V., Johnson, W. L., et al: Application of percutaneous transluminal coronary angioplasty to the internal mammary artery graft. J. Am. Coll. Cardiol., 12:1205, 1988.

Siegel, D., Grady, D., Browner, W. S., and Hulley, S. B.: Risk factor modification after myocardial infarction. Ann. Intern. Med., 109:213, 1988.

Sims, F. H.: The internal mammary artery as a bypass graft? Ann. Thorac. Surg., 44:2, 1987.

Skow, J. R., Carey, J. S., Plested, W. G., and Mulder, D. G.: Saphenous vein bypass as a secondary cardiac procedure. Arch. Surg., 107:34, 1973.

Stewart, W. J., McSweeney, S. M., Kellett, M. A., et al: Increased risk of severe protamine reactions in NPH insulin-dependent diabetics undergoing cardiac catheterization. Circulation, 70:788, 1984.

Stiles, Q. R., Lindesmith, G. G., Tucker, B. L., et al: Experience with fifty repeat procedures for myocardial revascularization. J. Thorac. Cardiovasc. Surg., 72:849, 1976.

Thomas, C. S., Jr., Alford, W. C., Jr., Burrus, G. R., et al: Results of reoperation for failed aortocoronary bypass grafts. Arch. Surg., 111:1210, 1976.

Thompson, P. D.: The benefits and risks of exercise training in patients with chronic coronary artery disease. J.A.M.A., 259:1537, 1988.

Thurer, R. L., and Hauer, J. L.: Autotransfusion and blood conservation. Curr. Probl. Surg., 19:97, 1982.

Ungerleider, R. M., Mills, N. L., and Wechsler, A. S.: Left thoracotomy for reoperative coronary artery bypass procedures. Ann. Thorac. Surg., 40:11, 1985.

Utley, J. R., Moores, W. Y., and Stephens, D. B.: Blood conservation techniques. Ann. Thorac. Surg., 31:482, 1981.

Walker, R. H.: Special report: Transfusion risks. Am. J. Clin. Pathol., 1987.

Walts, A. E., Fishbein, M. C., Sustaita, H., and Matloff, J. M.: Ruptured atheromatous plaques in saphenous vein coronary artery bypass grafts: A mechanism of acute, thrombotic, late graft occlusion. Circulation, 65:197, 1982.

Weisel, R. D., Hoy, F. B. Y., Baird, R. J., et al: Improved myocardial protection during a prolonged cross-clamp period. Ann. Thorac. Surg., 36:664, 1983.

Winkle, R. A., Alderman, E. L., Shumway, N. E., and Harrison, D. C.: Results of reoperation for unsuccessful coronary artery bypass surgery. Circulation, 51, 52(Suppl. 1):61, 1975.

4 Kawasaki's Disease

Thomas A. D'Amico
David C. Sabiston, Jr.

Kawasaki's disease is a multisystemic disorder of undetermined etiology that is an important cause of cardiovascular disease in children. Described in Japan by Kawasaki in 1967, the disorder was first presented in English in 1974 (Kawasaki et al, 1974). This acute illness presents with fever, sterile conjunctivitis, cervical lymphadenopathy, and vasculitic mucocutaneous changes. Although usually indolent and self-limiting, in its advanced stage the syndrome is characterized by coronary and peripheral artery aneurysms, coronary stenoses, mitral valve insufficiency, and left ventricular dysfunction (Kitamura et al, 1977). In Kawasaki's original description, the syndrome was thought to be limited to Japanese children. The syndrome was recognized in the United States in 1973 (Melish et al, 1976) and has been described since then throughout North America (Fetterman and Hashida, 1974; Landing and Larson, 1977; Russell et al, 1975), Europe (Becker, 1976; Corbeel et al, 1977; Della Porta and Alberti, 1977; Scopes and Hulse, 1977; Stephenson, 1977; Valaes, 1975), Australia (Carter et al, 1976), and the Pacific, in addition to approximately 70,000 cases in Japan alone (Hicks and Melish, 1986).

Kawasaki's disease exclusively affects prepubertal children; most of the patients are under 5 years of age and half are under 2 years. The reported male:female ratio is 3:2. Various causative agents have been proposed, but the etiology of Kawasaki's syndrome is still unclear. The pathophysiology has been well described, but the infrequent progression to severe cardiovascular manifestations is not well understood. Current therapy consists of antiplatelet and anti-inflammatory agents, as well as surgical intervention in patients with advanced disease. An ideal treatment that ameliorates the early inflammatory symptoms, arrests the vasculitic progression, and prevents the formation of coronary aneurysms has not yet been discovered.

CLINICAL MANIFESTATIONS

Symptoms

Kawasaki's original description of the clinical features of the syndrome has been consistently supported by others. The diagnostic criteria, including the principal symptoms and associated findings, are shown in Table 54–21 (Hicks and Melish, 1986; Kawasaki et al, 1974). The diagnosis of Kawasaki's disease is secured by the presence of five of the six major criteria. The presentation of this syndrome is acute, and the symptoms evolve during a period of a few days. Although there are atypical presentations (Canter et al, 1981), Kawasaki's disease is usually seen in a stereotypical clinical pattern that leads to a particular diagnosis.

The principal presenting symptom is fever, which usually has an abrupt onset, may be prolonged or intermittent, and does not respond to antibiotics (Fukushige et al, 1980). The fever lasts from 7 to 14 days but may persist in more severe cases. The appearance of fever is often accompanied by the presence of congested ocular conjunctivae, bilateral and sterile, a condition that does not respond to ocular preparations. After the appearance of conjunctivitis, several changes in the lips and oral cavity occur. Commonly, there is a reddening of the lips,

---

TABLE 54–21. PRINCIPAL SYMPTOMS AND ASSOCIATED FINDINGS IN KAWASAKI'S DISEASE

Principal Symptoms (5 of 6 needed for diagnosis)
1. Fever
2. Conjunctivitis
3. Changes in the mouth and oral cavity—at least one of the following:
   Dry, chapped, fissured, or reddened lips
   Prominent, reddened tongue
   Diffuse reddening of oral mucosa
4. Changes of the extremities—at least one of the following:
   Reddening of the palms and soles
   Indurative edema of the hands or feet
   Desquamation of fingertips or toes
5. Polymorphous truncal rash
6. Nonpurulent cervical adenopathy

Associated Findings
Arthralgia
Arthritis
Aseptic meningitis
Diarrhea
Hydrops of the gallbladder
Jaundice
Myocarditis
Pericarditis
Proteinuria
Urethritis

---

which may then become dry and fissured. The tongue may appear prominently, with protuberant papillae ("strawberry tongue"), or there may only be diffuse reddening of the oropharyngeal mucosa.

By the third day of the illness, a polymorphous macular erythematous rash appears. The rash begins with reddening of the palms and soles; individual lesions may coalesce as the rash progresses proximally to spread over the trunk, usually over 48 hours. As the rash resolves, secondary changes in fingers and toes appear. A unique desquamation begins at the junction of the nails and the skin on the tips of the digits. In less than 50% of patients, nonpurulent cervical lymphadenopathy develops.

Physical Examination

The principal physical findings are easily recognized. Elicitation of the more subtle physical findings early in the course of Kawasaki's disease may facilitate the prompt diagnosis of its numerous complications.

Examination of the heart may reveal tachycardia, distant heart sounds, or a gallop, suggestive of myocarditis or congestive failure. A holosystolic apical murmur signifies mitral valve insufficiency, which may be secondary to cardiomegaly, endocarditis, or papillary muscle dysfunction. Palpation of the peripheral arteries, especially in the axillary and inguinal regions, may reveal an aneurysm (Fig. 54–103). Palpation of the abdomen may show hepatomegaly, secondary to congestive heart failure, or right upper quadrant tenderness, secondary to hydrops of the gallbladder. Auscultation of the abdomen may reveal the bruit of an aneurysm of the renal, celiac, mesenteric, or iliac arteries. Neurologic examination may show meningeal signs, as well as emotional lability, irritability, stupor, or coma, secondary to aseptic meningitis.

Laboratory Studies

Leukocytosis is invariably present and is often accompanied by a shift to the left. Anemia and thrombocytosis may be present. Other findings include an increase in the red blood cell sedimentation rate, C-reactive protein, alpha$_2$-globulin, and alpha$_1$-antitrypsin and a negative antistreptolysin O (ASO) antibody assay.

The electrocardiogram is abnormal in 70% of patients. The most common findings are sinus tachycardia, prolonged PQ and QR intervals, second-degree atrioventricular block, decreased voltage, ST segment changes, and T wave changes (Onouchi et al, 1975).

Etiology

Kawasaki's disease is the main cause of acquired heart disease in children in the United States and

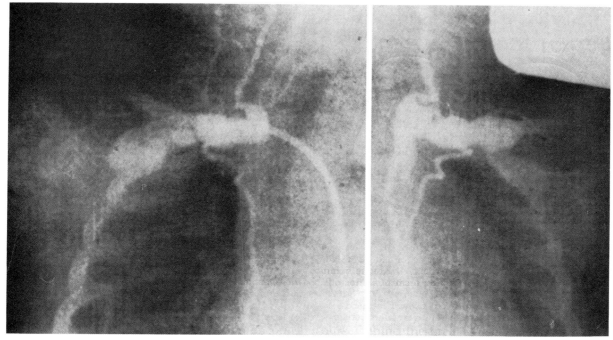

Figure 54–103. Arteriogram of a 3-month-old infant with Kawasaki's disease. Right and left subclavian arterial injections show large tortuous fusiform aneurysms of the right and left distal subclavian arteries that extend into both axillary arteries with complete distal obstruction of the right and decreased flow to the left brachial artery. (From Fukushige, J., Nihill, M. R., and McNamara, D. G.: Spectrum of cardiovascular lesions in mucocutaneous lymph node syndrome: Analysis of eight cases. Am. J. Cardiol., *45*:98, 1980.)

Japan (Rowley and Shulman, 1987). Despite the prevalence of the disorder, investigations of the etiology have been unsuccessful; the pathogenesis of Kawasaki's syndrome has not yet been discovered. Many clinical aspects of the syndrome imply a communicable causative factor. The acute presentation of fever, rash, conjunctivitis, and lymphadenopathy in children suggests an infectious illness. That the disease exclusively affects children and spares adults suggests a mechanism of acquired immunity. Epidemiologic evidence supports the theory of an infectious etiology. In addition to geographic areas where it appears to be endemic, such as Japan, seasonal epidemic outbreaks are common.

The search for a single causative agent has been unsuccessful. Possibilities include mercury poisoning (Orlowski and Mercer, 1980), mite-associated antigens (Fujimoto et al, 1982; Furosho et al, 1981), rickettsiae (Carter et al, 1976; Hamashima et al, 1973), spirochetes (Marchette et al, 1987), *Propionibacterium* (Kato et al, 1983), lactobacilli (Lehman et al, 1985), *Borrelia* (Marchette et al, 1987), *Pseudomonas* (Kerin et al, 1983), and Epstein-Barr virus (Osato, 1987), all without confirmation. The lack of evidence for person-to-person transmissibility has made it difficult to isolate a single etiologic factor. Variable immunity or low communicability could explain this phenomenon.

Investigation of peripheral blood lymphocytes isolated from the acute stage of Kawasaki's disease showed increased helper T lymphocyte activity and decreased suppressor T lymphocyte activity, which suggests a retroviral component in the etiology of Kawasaki's disease (Shulman and Rowley, 1986). Reverse transcriptase, which synthesizes DNA from a template of RNA, is the hallmark of retroviral activity. Analysis of supernatants from cultures of lymphocytes from patients with Kawasaki's syndrome showed significantly increased reverse transcriptase activity compared with controls. Although this finding has been confirmed by multiple laboratories (Burns et al, 1986; Melish, 1987), there has been no conclusive evidence of a specific viral agent.

Pathology

The pathologic basis of Kawasaki's disease is the progression of a nonspecific vasculitis that involves the microvasculature of the aorta and its major branches and is manifested by endarteritis of the vasa vasorum of the coronary, brachiocephalic, celiac, renal, and iliofemoral systems. As the inflammatory process of the intima and adventitia progresses, aneurysms form in these vessels and lead to stenosis, thromboembolism, ischemia, rupture, or asymptomatic healing. Pathologic analysis of hearts affected by Kawasaki's disease has helped to elucidate the pathophysiology of the vasculitis (Fujiwara et al, 1978, 1988). Kawasaki's disease can be described in four stages: acute, subacute, convalescent, and chronic (Table 54–22) (Fujiwara and Hamashima, 1978).

TABLE 54–22. THE FOUR STAGES OF KAWASAKI'S DISEASE

Stage	Duration	Symptoms	Pathology
I	0–9 days	Fever Conjunctivitis Mucocutaneous changes	Myocarditis Perivasculitis of arterioles, capillaries, and venules Intimal inflammation of medium and large arterioles
II	10–20 days	Fever Palpable aneurysms	Panvasculitis Coronary and peripheral aneurysms, with early thrombosis
III	21–31 days	Arthritis (most symptoms resolved)	Coronary aneurysms Thrombosis and stenosis
IV	>40 days	Angina	Scarring Fibrosis Intimal thickening

The acute phase, characterized by perivasculitis, corresponds to the febrile period and usually involves the first 10 days of the illness. During this period the oral changes, skin changes, and conjunctivitis also develop. On presentation, the patient may also have arthritis, myocarditis, pericarditis, mitral insufficiency, and meningitis. At this stage the perivasculitis affects the small vessels—arterioles, capillaries, and venules. There may be inflammation in the intima of medium and large arteries, as well as in the atrioventricular conduction system, but aneurysmal dilatation and stenoses are not observed at this stage. Death in the acute phase is usually secondary to advanced myocarditis but is rare (Fujiwara et al, 1987).

During the subacute phase, typically the second 10 days of the illness, most of the clinical findings may resolve, although fever and irritability often persist. Examination of arteries during this phase shows perivasculitis of the major coronary arteries, aneurysmal development, and early platelet thrombus formation (Fig. 54–104). Thrombotic occlusion may develop and cause myocardial ischemia, and thromboembolism may ensue with subsequent myocardial infarction (Fig. 54–105). Myocarditis persists in the subacute stage, and coagulation necrosis may be found in the myocardium (especially in papillary muscles) and in the conduction system. Pericarditis may also persist, and endocarditis and valvulitis may develop. Death in the subacute stage is often caused by a ruptured coronary artery aneurysm.

The convalescent stage, which extends into the second month, is characterized by decreased arterial inflammation. Granulation changes are seen in this stage, as internal proliferation within the aneurysm may ameliorate luminal defects. Aneurysmal dilatation may persist and produce progressive stenosis and further risk of thromboembolism. Death in this stage is usually secondary to diffuse myocardial ischemia. The disease rarely enters a chronic phase during which scarring continues, as does myocardial ischemia secondary to coronary stenoses. Resolution of the myocarditis may cause fibrous myocardial changes and endocardial fibroelastosis.

Natural History

A spectrum of cardiovascular manifestations may occur in Kawasaki's disease, although they are usually self-limited and benign (Table 54–23) (Kato et al, 1987). Myocarditis, diagnosed clinically and by electrocardiographic criteria, is present in as many

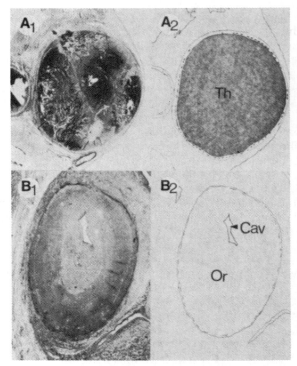

Figure 54–104. *A,* Coronary aneurysm with fresh occlusive thrombi, stained with elastic van Gieson's stain (*A₁,* original magnification ×6; *A₂,* magnified 10 times by enlarger and sketched). *B,* Coronary aneurysms with organization or intimal thickening, stained with elastic van Gieson's stain (*B₁,* original magnification ×10; *B₂,* magnified 10 times by enlarger and sketched). *Perforated line* indicates remnant elastic interna. (Cav = cavity; Or = organization; Th = thrombi.) (From Fujiwara, T., Fujiwara, H., and Hamashima, Y.: Frequency and size of coronary arterial aneurysm at necropsy in Kawasaki disease. Am. J. Cardiol., *59*:808, 1987.)

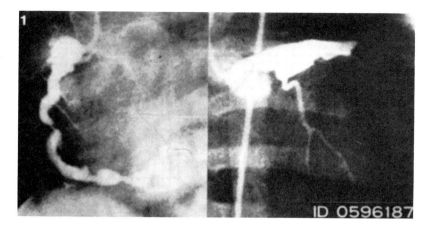

Figure 54–105. Cross-section of the heart shows areas of acute myocardial infarction in the posterior part of the ventricular septum and posterior walls of both ventricles, including the left ventricular papillary muscle. Old myocardial infarction is found in the posterior part of the ventricular septum. (From Suzuki, A., Kamiya, T., Ono, Y., et al: Indication of aortocoronary bypass for coronary arterial obstruction due to Kawasaki disease. Heart Vessels, *1*:94, 1985.)

as 30% of patients. One study, in which endomyocardial biopsies were taken during cardiac catheterization for coronary arteriography, showed inflammatory changes in each of 201 cases (Kato et al, 1979). In the acute phase, myocarditis may cause exercise intolerance, congestive heart failure, or death, secondary to ischemia or diffuse hypokinesia (Kitamura et al, 1977).

The most serious complication of Kawasaki's disease is the formation of coronary artery aneurysms, which has an incidence of 20 to 40% in the subacute phase (Kato et al, 1975; Kegel et al, 1977). The aneurysms may be asymptomatic or may not present symptoms until years later. Serial angiographic studies have shown "resolution" of aneurysms that are discovered as early as the second week; pathologic analysis has shown that angiographic resolution may be caused by intimal proliferation rather than by healing, which leaves these arteries at further risk for stenosis and thromboembolism (Bierman and Gersony, 1987; Nakano et al, 1986).

Coronary artery aneurysms result from inflammatory changes in the intima and adventitia, caused by perivasculitis of the major coronary arteries. As in atherosclerotic coronary artery disease, the most common locations for lesions are at the bifurcation of the left anterior descending (LAD) and circumflex vessels (found in 74% of patients with coronary aneurysms) and at the origin of the right coronary artery (RCA) (48%) (Nakanishi et al, 1985; Suma et al, 1981). Within the aneurysm, turbulence and stagnation produce platelet aggregation and thrombosis.

Advanced thrombosis causes critical stenoses in the coronary arteries, the most common indication for surgical intervention. Thromboembolic phenomena are also common and sometimes produce acute myocardial infarction.

The diagnosis of Kawasaki's disease should be accompanied routinely by selective coronary angiography for detection of aneurysms (Fig. 54–106). Echocardiography has been used to detect coronary aneurysms with 85% success (Bierman and Gersony, 1987). Analysis of these results has shown groups of patients who are most likely to develop aneurysms and who require serial echocardiograms, selective angiography, and possibly surgical intervention (Table 54–24) (Koren et al, 1986; Nakano et al, 1986).

Mitral insufficiency is a complication in approximately 10% of patients with Kawasaki's disease. Mitral regurgitation may be secondary to valvulitis, endocarditis, or cardiomegaly but is most often as-

TABLE 54–23. CARDIAC MANIFESTATIONS OF KAWASAKI'S DISEASE

Coronary aneurysms (20–40%)
Myocarditis (20–30%)
Mitral regurgitation (10%)
Aortic insufficiency (5%)
Valvulitis (1%)
Myocardial infarction (3%)
Sudden death (<1%)

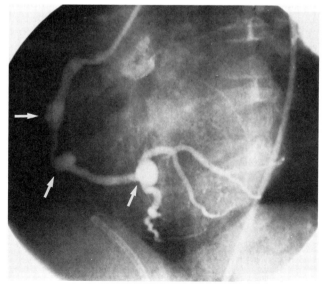

Figure 54–106. Coronary arteriogram shows three aneurysms of the right coronary artery in a 10-year-old boy with Kawasaki's disease.

TABLE 54–24. RISK FACTORS FOR THE DEVELOPMENT OF CORONARY ANEURYSMS IN KAWASAKI'S DISEASE

Male
Age under 1 year
Duration of fever greater than 16 days
White blood cell count greater than 30
Red blood cell sedimentation rate greater than 100
Elevated C-reactive protein
Thrombocytosis

sociated with papillary muscle dysfunction secondary to coronary stenosis and myocardial ischemia. In patients with documented coronary stenoses, papillary dysfunction occurs in 50%, compared with approximately 8% in patients without coronary involvement.

Myocardial infarction, a rare complication of Kawasaki's disease, may occur after diffuse ischemia or a thromboembolic event. Myocardial ischemia is due to profound fibrotic changes or is secondary to multiple stenotic lesions. The presence of collateral circulation usually preserves ventricular function, despite multiple stenotic lesions; however, left ventricular hypertrophy associated with diffuse hypokinesia sometimes develops.

Treatment

The mortality of Kawasaki's disease before 1976 was 1 to 2%. Since 1976 the mortality has decreased to approximately 0.5% (Suma et al, 1982), because of earlier diagnosis and the evolution of effective treatment modalities, including surgical intervention. Optimal therapy depends ultimately on the discovery of the etiology of Kawasaki's disease. Early diagnosis and recognition of the appearance of the cardiovascular complications are critical in the successful management of patients with Kawasaki's disease, because death from congestive failure may occur in the first week. When the disease is diagnosed, children are given a regimen of aspirin, 100 mg/kg/day, which is continued until defervescence. Thereafter, they are maintained on aspirin, 10 mg/kg/day, for 8 weeks or until the red blood cell sedimentation rate is normal. In children who develop aneurysms, low-dose aspirin therapy may be continued indefinitely; the risk of associated salicylate complications, including Reye's syndrome, is low.

Treatment with intravenous gamma globulin has been initiated (Newburger et al, 1986; Stiehm et al, 1987). A cooperative study compared aspirin therapy alone for 14 days with the combination of intravenous gamma globulin for 4 days and aspirin for 14 days. A decreased incidence of cardiovascular complications at 14 days (8 versus 23.1%) and at 49 days (3.8 versus 17.7%) was reported in the group treated with both aspirin and gamma globulin. The dosage schedule of gamma globulin was based on experience with thrombocytopenic purpura. Further studies are required to determine the optimal dose.

Advanced cardiovascular complications require surgical intervention. Surgical treatment has included Vineberg's procedure (Kitamura et al, 1983), coronary artery bypass grafting (CABG) with autologous saphenous vein grafts (SVG) (Kitamura et al, 1976; Sandiford et al, 1980), CABG with homologous SVG (Konishi et al, 1979), CABG with a right subclavian artery graft (Mains et al, 1983), CABG with internal mammary artery grafts (IMAG) (Hirose et al, 1986; Ino et al, 1987; Kitamura et al, 1985), CABG with coronary artery aneurysmectomy (Suma et al, 1982), mitral valve repair (Konishi et al, 1978), and mitral valve replacement (Kitamura et al, 1980).

The first use of bypass grafting for obstructive coronary aneurysms in Kawasaki's disease was reported in 1976 by Kitamura. The procedure involved a 4-year-old boy with coronary aneurysms that obstructed the LAD and the RCA, which were diagnosed 10 months after presentation with Kawasaki's disease. Early follow-up showed the patient doing well. General problems with CABG became apparent with experience, however. Further use of homologous and autologous SVG showed frequent early occlusion of the grafts. In many cases, the distal coronary arteries appeared to be too small to accept vein grafts. In many children, autogenous SVG are not available. The potential for SVG to grow as the heart grows and the thoracic cavity expands is unknown.

Alternative graft choices were sought. Mains and associates (1983) reported the successful use of a right subclavian artery bypass to the LAD. Kitamura and associates (1985) described the first successful use of an IMAG to treat coronary aneurysms in Kawasaki's disease. Before the use of arterial bypass grafts, venous graft closure at 1 year was greater than 50%. With the use of IMAG, patency is now 85% at 1 year, and late patency is nearly 60%. In a study by Hirose and associates (1986) of children over 5 years, the early patency rate with IMAG was 100% and overall early patency with both IMAG and SVG was 83%. In that study, late patency of the IMAG was 50%, compared with 38% for the SVG. A more recent study by Kitamura (personal communication, 1988) showed 100% early and late patency (more than 1 year) of the IMAG, compared with 90% early patency and 50% late patency of the SVG. In children younger than 8 years of age, patency of the SVG was 65%, compared with 87% in children older than 8 years of age (Kitamura et al, 1988).

TABLE 54–25. INDICATIONS FOR CARDIAC CATHETERIZATION IN KAWASAKI'S DISEASE

1. Severe symptoms at onset
2. Symptoms of ischemic heart disease
3. Symptoms of congestive heart failure
4. Coronary calcifications evident on chest films
5. Persistent coronary aneurysms by repeat echocardiograms

TABLE 54–26. OPERATIVE CRITERIA FOR CORONARY ARTERY BYPASS GRAFTING IN KAWASAKI'S DISEASE

1. Progressive coronary lesions, shown by selective arteriography
2. No distal coronary aneurysms with stenosis
3. Localized aneurysm with significant stenosis in the left main coronary artery
4. Significant stenosis in two coronary arteries
5. Presence of collateral vessels arising from coronary artery with an aneurysm
6. Progressive stenosis in the left anterior descending coronary artery
7. Presence of left ventricular aneurysm

The use of IMAG provides greater patency and the potential for growth, both elongation and dilatation. The indications for cardiac catheterization are shown in Table 54–25 (Takeuchi et al, 1981). The operative indications are shown in Table 54–26 (Suzuki et al, 1985).

Mitral valve insufficiency in Kawasaki's disease is most often due to papillary muscle dysfunction, secondary to myocarditis and ischemia. Mitral regurgitation as a complication of this disorder is associated with high mortality when accompanied by poor left ventricular function. Survival is increased with the correction of valvular dysfunction, and both mitral valve repair and mitral valve replacement have been done. Surgical correction, in the presence of myocarditis and compromised left ventricular function, presents a more difficult problem than is usually encountered with valve replacement for rheumatic disease. Experience with ineffective valve repair has shown that mitral valve replacement is the most certain means of ensuring the management of severe mitral insufficiency, despite the absence of valvulitis.

CONCLUSION

Kawasaki's disease is a fascinating disorder with many cardiovascular manifestations. Aspects of this disease yet to be explained include its etiology, selectivity for children, and ability to progress to severe stages in view of its usually benign and self-limited nature.

Bibliography

Becker, A. E.: Kawasaki disease (Letter). Lancet, 1:864, 1976.
Bierman, F. Z., and Gersony, W. M.: Kawasaki disease: Clinical perspective. J. Pediatr., 111:789, 1987.
Burns, J. C., Geha, R. S., Schneeburger, E. E., et al: Polymerase activity in lymphocyte culture supernatants from patients with Kawasaki disease. Nature, 323:814, 1986.
Canter, C. E., Bower, R. J., and Strauss, A. W.: Atypical Kawasaki disease with aneurysm. Pediatrics, 68:885, 1981.
Carter, R. F., Haynes, M. E., and Morton, J.: Rickettsia-like bodies and splenitis in Kawasaki disease (Letter). Lancet, 2:1254, 1976.
Corbeel, L., Delmotte, B., Standaert, L., et al: Kawasaki disease in Europe (Letter). Lancet, 1:797, 1977.
Della Porta, G., and Alberti, A.: Kawasaki disease in Europe. Lancet, 2:797, 1977.
Fetterman, G. H., and Hashida, Y.: Mucocutaneous lymph node syndrome: A disease widespread in Japan which demands our attention. Pediatrics, 54:268, 1974.
Fujimoto, T., Kato, H., Ichoise, E., et al: Immune complex and mite antigen in Kawasaki disease. Lancet, 2:980, 1982.
Fujiwara, H., and Hamashima, Y.: Pathology of the heart in Kawasaki disease. Pediatrics, 61:100, 1978.
Fujiwara, H., Kawai, C., and Hamashima, Y.: Clinicopathologic study of the conduction systems in 10 patients with Kawasaki's disease (mucocutaneous lymph node syndrome). Am. Heart J., 96:744, 1978.
Fujiwara, T., Fujiwara, H., and Hamashima, Y.: Frequency and size of coronary arterial aneurysm at necropsy in Kawasaki disease. Am. J. Cardiol., 59:808, 1987.
Fujiwara, T., Fujiwara, H., and Nakano, H.: Pathologic features of coronary arteries in children with Kawasaki disease in which coronary arterial aneurysm was absent at autopsy. Circulation, 78:345, 1988.
Fukushige, J., Nihill, M. R., and McNamara, D. G.: Spectrum of cardiovascular lesions in mucocutaneous lymph node syndrome: Analysis of eight cases. Am. J. Cardiol., 45:98, 1980.
Furosho, K., Ohba, T., Soeda, T., et al: Possible role for mite antigen in Kawasaki disease. Lancet, 2:194, 1981.
Hamashima, Y., Kishi, K., and Tasaka, K.: Rickettsia-like bodies in infantile acute febrile mucocutaneous lymph-node syndrome. Lancet, 2:42, 1973.
Hicks, R. V., and Melish, M. E.: Kawasaki syndrome. Pediatr. Rheum., 33:1151, 1986.
Hirose, H., Kawashima, Y., Nakano, S., et al: Long-term results in surgical treatment of children 4 years old or younger with coronary involvement due to Kawasaki disease. Circulation, 74:I-77, 1986.
Ino, T., Iwahara, M., Boku, H., et al: Aortocoronary bypass surgery for Kawasaki disease. Pediatr. Cardiol., 8:195, 1987.
Kato, H., Kitamura, S., and Kawasaki, T.: Guidelines for the treatment and management of cardiovascular sequelae in Kawasaki disease. Heart Vessels, 3:50, 1987.
Kato, H., Koike, S., Yamamoto, M., et al: Coronary aneurysms in infants and young children with acute febrile mucocutaneous lymph node syndrome. J. Pediatr., 86:892, 1975.
Kato, H., Koike, S., Tanaka, C., et al: Coronary heart disease in children with Kawasaki syndrome. Jpn. Circ. J., 43:469, 1979.
Kato, H., Fujimoto, T., Inoue, O., et al: Variant strain of P. acnes: A clue to the etiology of Kawasaki syndrome. Lancet, 2:1383, 1983.
Kawasaki, T.: M.C.L.S.—Clinical observation of 50 cases. Jpn. J. Allerg., 16:178, 1967.
Kawasaki, T., Kosaki, F., Okawa, S., et al: A new infantile acute febrile mucocutaneous lymph node syndrome (MLNS) prevailing in Japan. Pediatrics, 54:271, 1974.
Kegel, S. M., Dorsey, T. J., Rowen, M., and Taylor, W. F.: Cardiac death in mucocutaneous lymph node syndrome. Am. J. Cardiol., 40:282, 1977.
Kerin, G., Barzilay, Z., Alpert, G., et al: Mucocutaneous lymph node syndrome (Kawasaki disease) in Israel. Acta Pediatr. Scand., 72:455, 1983.
Kitamura, S., Kawachi, K., Harima, R., et al: Surgery for coronary heart disease due to mucocutaneous lymph node syndrome (Kawasaki disease). Am. J. Cardiol., 51:444, 1983.
Kitamura, S., Kawashima, Y., Fujita, T., et al: Aortocoronary bypass grafting in a child with coronary artery obstruction due to mucocutaneous lymph node syndrome. Circulation, 53:1035, 1976.
Kitamura, S., Seki, T., Kawachi, K., et al: Excellent patency and growth potential of internal mammary artery graft in pediatric coronary artery bypass surgery. Circulation, 78:I-129, 1988.
Kitamura, S., Kawashima, Y., Kawachi, K., et al: Left ventricular function in patients with coronary arteritis due to acute febrile mucocutaneous lymph node syndrome or related diseases. Am. J. Cardiol., 40:156, 1977.
Kitamura, S., Kawachi, K., Oyama, C., et al: Severe Kawasaki heart disease treated with an internal mammary artery graft

in pediatric patients. J. Thorac. Cardiovasc. Surg., 89:860, 1985.

Kitamura, S., Kawashima, Y., Kawachi, K., et al: Severe mitral regurgitation due to coronary arteritis of mucocutaneous lymph node syndrome. J. Thorac. Cardiovasc. Surg., 80:629, 1980.

Konishi, Y., Tatsuta, N., Miki, S., et al: Mitral insufficiency secondary to mucocutaneous lymph node syndrome. Jpn. Circ. J., 42:901, 1978.

Konishi, Y., Tatsuta, N., Miki, S., et al: Simultaneous surgical treatment of tetralogy of Fallot and coronary artery aneurysm due to mucocutaneous lymph node syndrome in a 4 year old child. Jpn. Circ. J., 43:749, 1979.

Koren, G., Sasson, L., Rose, V., and Rowe, R.: Kawasaki disease: Review of risk factors for coronary aneurysms. J. Pediatr., 108:388, 1986.

Landing, B. H., and Larson, E. J.: Are infantile periarteritis nodosa with coronary involvement and fatal mucocutaneous lymph node syndrome the same? Comparison of 20 patients from North America with patients from Hawaii and Japan. Pediatrics, 59:651, 1977.

Lehman, T. J. A., Walker, S. M., Mahnovski, V., et al: Coronary arteritis in mice following the systemic infection of Group B *Lactobacillus casei* cell walls in aqueous suspension. Arthr. Rheum., 28:652, 1985.

Mains, C., Wiggins, J., Groves, B., and Clarke, D.: Surgical therapy for a complication of Kawasaki's disease. Ann. Thorac. Surg., 35:197, 1983.

Marchette, N. J., Melish, M. E., James, J. F., et al: Spirochaetal studies in Kawasaki syndrome. In Shulman, S. T. (ed): Kawasaki Disease: Proceedings of the Second International Kawasaki Disease Symposium. New York, Alan R. Liss, 1987.

Melish, M.: Retroviruses and Kawasaki disease. In Shulman, S. T. (ed): Kawasaki's disease: Proceedings of the Second International Kawasaki Disease Symposium. New York, Alan R. Liss, 1987.

Melish, M. E., Hicks, R. V., and Larson, E.: Kawasaki syndrome in the United States. Am. J. Dis. Child., 130:599, 1976.

Nakanishi, T., Takao, A., Nakazawa, M., et al: Mucocutaneous lymph node syndrome: Clinical, hemodynamic and angiographic features of coronary obstructive disease. Am. J. Cardiol., 55:662, 1985.

Nakano, H., Ueda, K., Saito, A., et al: Scoring method for identifying patients with Kawasaki disease at high risk of coronary artery aneurysms. Am. J. Cardiol., 58:739, 1986.

Newburger, J. W., Takahashi, M., Burns, J. C., et al: The treatment of Kawasaki syndrome with intravenous gamma globulin. N. Engl. J. Med., 315:341, 1986.

Onouchi, Z., Tomizawa, N., Goto, M., et al: Cardiac involvement and prognosis in acute mucocutaneous lymph node syndrome. Chest, 68:297, 1975.

Orlowski, J. P., and Mercer, R. D.: Urine mercury levels in Kawasaki disease. Pediatrics, 66:633, 1980.

Osato, T.: Kawasaki disease and Epstein-Barr virus. In Shulman, S. T. (ed): Kawasaki Disease: Proceedings of the Second International Kawasaki Disease Symposium. New York, Alan R. Liss, 1987.

Rowley, A. H., and Shulman, S. T.: The search for the etiology of Kawasaki disease. Pediatr. Infect. Dis. J., 6:506, 1987.

Russell, A. S., Zargoza, A. S., and Shea, R.: Mucocutaneous lymph node syndrome in Canada. Can. Med. Assoc. J., 112:1210, 1975.

Sandiford, F. M., Vargo, T. A., Sheh, J. Y., et al: Successful triple coronary bypass in a child with multiple coronary aneurysms due to Kawasaki's disease. J. Thorac. Cardiovasc. Surg., 79:283, 1980.

Scopes, J. W., and Hulse, H. A.: Mucocutaneous lymph node syndrome (Letter). Br. Med. J., 1:511, 1977.

Shulman, S. T., and Rowley, A. H.: Does Kawasaki disease have a retroviral etiology? Lancet, 2:545, 1986.

Stephenson, S. R.: Kawasaki disease in Europe. Lancet, 1:373, 1977.

Stiehm, E. R., Ashida, E., Kim, K. S., et al: Intravenous immunoglobulins as therapeutic agents. Ann. Intern. Med., 107:367, 1987.

Suma, K., Takeuchi, Y., Shiroma, K., et al: Cardiac surgery of eight children with Kawasaki disease (mucocutaneous lymph node syndrome). Jpn. Heart J., 22:605, 1981.

Suma, K., Takeuchi, Y., Shiroma, K., et al: Early and late postoperative studies in coronary arterial lesions resulting from Kawasaki's disease in children. J. Thorac. Cardiovasc. Surg., 84:224, 1982.

Suzuki, A., Kamiya, T., and Ono, Y.: Indication of aortocoronary by-pass for coronary arterial obstruction due to Kawasaki disease. Heart Vessels, 1:94, 1985.

Takeuchi, Y., Suma, K., Shiroma, K., et al: Surgical experience with coronary arterial sequelae of Kawasaki disease in children. J. Cardiovasc. Surg., 22:231, 1981.

Valaes, T.: Mucocutaneous lymph node syndrome in Athens, Greece (Letter). Pediatrics, 55:295, 1975.

5 Left Ventricular Aneurysm

Alden H. Harken

HISTORICAL ASPECTS

Sauerbruch was apparently the first to operate on a patient with a cardiac aneurysm (Sauerbruch and O'Shaughnessy, 1937). He diagnosed a mediastinal tumor, but at the time of operation he found that the mass contained blood. The sac was opened and was found to communicate with the right ventricle. Sauerbruch placed two fingers into this communication to control the bleeding and ligated the neck of the sac as he withdrew the fingers. Beck (1944) analyzed this procedure and concluded that Sauerbruch operated on a false aneurysm of the right ventricle. In 1944 Beck buttressed a ventricular aneurysm with strips of fascia lata.

Early reports of cardiac aneurysms were complicated by failure to distinguish generalized cardiomegaly from aneurysm formation. Sternberg (1914) catalogued descriptions of cardiac enlargement by Baillow in 1538 and Lancisius in 1740. Schlichter and associates (1954) attributed the first reports of ventricular aneurysm to Dominicus Gusmanus Galeati (1751) and John Hunter (1757). Hunter's description identified aneurysmal thinning of the left ventricular apex "lined with a thrombus just the shape of the pouch in which it lay." In 1827, Cruveilhier recognized that a ventricular aneurysm was myocardial fibrosis, but the pathogenesis of the fibrosis was unclear (Rokitansky, 1844). Several cases of left ventricular aneurysm were suspected ante mortem

(Voelcker, 1902), and Cohnheim and Shulthess-Rechberg (1881) traced the etiology of ventricular aneurysm to myocardial infarction. By 1914, Sternberg recognized the sequence of angina, myocardial infarction, and ventricular aneurysm. Sternberg correctly diagnosed ventricular aneurysm based on the concept of coronary artery occlusion and even predicted the feasibility of radiologic confirmation.

In the early 20th century, radiographs greatly facilitated diagnosis, and Sezary and Alibert first visualized an aneurysm in 1922. Ten years later, mural calcification was shown radiologically. Paradoxical systolic ventricular motion was observed fluoroscopically (Schwedel et al, 1950), and Dolly and associates demonstrated a ventricular aneurysm by angiography in 1951.

With a diagnosis established, Bailey initiated the surgical approach to left ventricular aneurysms (Likoff and Bailey, 1955); through a left thoracotomy, a large clamp was applied to the bulging, beating aneurysm and the adjacent ventricle was plicated below the instrument. Cooley and associates (1958) used cardiopulmonary bypass to establish the current open heart technique of aneurysmectomy. By 1973, Loop and associates had established indications and provided surgical rehabilitation for a large group of patients with left ventricular aneurysms.

PATHOPHYSIOLOGY

Ventricular aneurysm is almost always secondary to transmural myocardial infarction. Tennant and Wiggers (1935) showed the effect of coronary occlusion on regional myocardial contraction. Infarction and aneurysm are more common in the left ventricle than in the right ventricle. Congenital, traumatic, or ischemic aneurysms of the right ventricle exist but are uncommon.

Functional aneurysm formation, regional left ventricular dyskinesia, and dilatation often follow acute myocardial infarction (Eaton et al, 1979). Acute regional left ventricular dilatation is functionally similar to a chronic ventricular aneurysm (Cabin and Roberts, 1980). At this stage, structure does not parallel function (Hutchins and Bulkley, 1978). Meizlish and associates (1984) obtained radionuclide angiocardiograms of 51 patients immediately after acute anterior myocardial infarction. Functional aneurysms developed in 18 of the patients within 48 hours.

The pathologic process of acute myocardial infarction leads directly to the three clinical signs of left ventricular aneurysm: (1) left ventricular dysfunction, (2) mural thrombosis, and (3) ventricular arrhythmias.

Left Ventricular Dysfunction. As a thin layer of necrotic muscle and fibrous tissue replaces the contracting myocardium, paradoxical systolic motion "steals" left ventricular stroke volume and thus decreases cardiac output (Alpert and Braunwald, 1980; Swan et al, 1972). In accordance with Laplace's law, wall tension increases as the ventricle dilates, and factors that further increase global or regional ventricular dilatation increase rapidly.

Mural Thrombosis. Transmural or subendocardial infarction transforms the smooth endocardium into a microscopically rough surface susceptible to thrombus formation (Weiss, 1975). Endothelial injury promotes release of thromboxanes, which induce platelet release and aggregation (Didisheim and Foster, 1978). Platelet involvement is indicated by increased levels of circulating platelet factor four (PF-4), a marker of platelet activation (Handin et al, 1978). Conformational changes in the left ventricle may produce relative stasis that contributes to thrombus formation (Rosenthal and Braunwald, 1980), but aneurysm formation is not essential to the development of an endocardial clot (Cabin and Roberts, 1980).

Ventricular Arrhythmias. The thin wall of a left ventricular aneurysm and the jeopardized adjacent border consist of a mixture of fibrous tissue, necrotic muscle, and viable myocardium (Schlichter et al, 1954). The electrophysiologic properties of conduction and refractoriness in these tissues are different (Spear et al, 1979). The conditions for re-entrant ventricular arrhythmias are satisfied when two or more electrically heterogeneous pathways (with respect to conduction and refractoriness) are connected proximally and distally (Wellens, 1975). An impulse must travel in only one direction along one of these pathways (unidirectional block). When the impulse reaches the distal connection, it may return along the originally blocked pathway. If conduction of the impulse is sufficiently slow to permit repolarization of the origin, the impulse may re-enter the circuit. Normal hearts contain a network of interarterial anastomotic channels 50 to 100 μ in diameter. In patients with coronary occlusive disease, these coronary collaterals become quite extensive (Gorlin, 1976). Subsequent myocardial infarction with multiple zones of pericollateral salvage produces a heterogeneously injured zone that predisposes to re-entrant arrhythmias.

Esoteric Aneurysms

In 1676, Borrich described the first aneurysmal dilatation of a cardiac chamber, a right atrial aneurysm. Left atrial aneurysms, which are less common, have been described as "giant dog ears" (Galeati, 1757) and as aneurysms that follow mitral valvuloplasty (Fojo-Echevarria et al, 1955). Right ventricular aneurysms occur and tend to be ischemic in origin (Stansel et al, 1963) and may also be congenital. Iatrogenic "patch" or pseudoaneurysms are a complication of right ventricular closure after surgical repair of a congenital defect. Cardiac diverticular (Arnold, 1894) and congenital aneurysms (Klein, 1889) have been associated with hypoplasia of the aorta. Left ventricular aneurysm secondary to an aberrant coronary artery arising from the pulmonary artery was diagnosed in a 2-month-old child (Schlichter et al, 1954). Syphilitic ventricular aneurysms due to gummatous myocarditis or syphilitic coronary ostial stenosis are mentioned in the older literature (Basset-Smith, 1908; Bricout, 1912). Small mycotic aneurysms secondary to bacterial endocarditis were identified (Schlichter et al, 1954). Rare pseudoaneurysms of the right ventricle (Stansel et al, 1963) and the left ventricle (Lyons and Perkins, 1958) were due to traumatic disruption and containment. False left ventricular aneurysm secondary to ischemia, cardiac rupture, and containment is more common (Vlodaver et al, 1975) and shares the hemodynamic and thromboembolic complications of a true aneurysm.

NATURAL HISTORY

Left ventricular function is an important cardiac prognostic indicator (Gay, 1986; Peyton and Sabiston, 1987). An association between congestive heart failure, angiographic evidence of regional left ventricular dysfunction, and poor prognosis (regardless of medical or surgical therapy) has been reported (Cohn and Braunwald, 1980). Of the many risk factors related to prognosis in ischemic heart disease, left ventricular function is the dominant variable. Pathologic studies show a poor prognosis for patients with left ventricular aneurysms. Of 102 patients with pathologically proven aneurysms, only 27% survived for 3 years and 12% survived for 5 years (Schlichter et al, 1954). Schattenberg and associates (1970) reported 76% mortality in 39 months in a similar group of patients. Proudfit (1979) reported that 74 patients with angiographically proven left ventricular aneurysms had a 5-year survival of 47% and a 10-year survival of 18%. Results of aneurysmectomy are almost entirely dependent on the quantity and quality of residual contracting ventricle (Cooperman et al, 1975; Lee et al, 1977).

In a classic study by Bruschke and associates (1973), 490 patients were studied angiographically and treated medically, with a follow-up of 5 to 9 years. Survival depended primarily on the extent of coronary disease and left ventricular function. In the 15 years since publication of that series, medical therapy has improved greatly, and the older data do not represent current medical standards. For ethical, moral, perhaps legal, and certainly practical reasons, however, it will not be possible to improve on this study. Patients are necessarily selected for operation after angiographic documentation of left main coronary artery disease (Murphy et al, 1977) or triple-vessel disease (European Coronary Surgery Study Group, 1979), even with regional ventricular dysfunction.

Grondin and associates (1979) confirmed poor 10-year survival of symptomatic patients with left ventricular aneurysm but reported an actuarial survival of 90% at 10 years for a small group of asymptomatic patients. One wonders why the latter group was catheterized. Prolongation of life as an isolated indication for operation in patients with left ventricular aneurysm is controversial. In symptomatic patients with medically intractable ventricular failure, angina, thromboemboli, and ventricular arrhythmias, the role of surgical therapy is clearer.

Meizlish and associates (1984) isolated left ventricular aneurysm as a risk factor and separated this parameter from ventricular dysfunction as a prognostic variable. This group studied 51 patients with acute anterior myocardial infarction and identified 18 patients with left ventricular aneurysms (Group I) and 33 patients with no aneurysm (Group II). Left ventricular ejection fraction was comparable in both groups (27 versus 31%). The 1-year mortality in Group I was 11 deaths (61%) and in Group II was 3 deaths (9%). Six of the deaths in the group with aneurysms were sudden and were presumably due to arrhythmias.

DIAGNOSIS

Physical Examination. A ventricular aneurysm may be suspected from the history and physical signs but is never confirmed by physical examination. Multiple physical signs, such as enlargement of transverse cardiac fullness and forceful cardiac impulse concurrent with a weak peripheral pulse, are indicators of left ventricular aneurysm (Schlichter et al, 1954). Libman (1932) emphasized that a distinct pulsation independent of the apical impulse and associated with a gallop rhythm and a dull first heart sound was pathognomonic of an aneurysm.

Contrast Ventriculography. Regional contractility can be localized by superimposing the angiographic outlines of end diastole (Herman et al, 1967). There is a spectrum of ventricular function from normal to grossly paradoxical. Akinesia exists when parts of the diastolic and systolic ventriculographic silhouettes share a common line. Dyskinesia is present when the end-systolic silhouette protrudes outside the end-diastolic outline. The nonischemic ventricle should have synchronous and symmetric shortening of all segments (Sniderman et al, 1973). Coronary artery disease typically produces regional rather than global damage, thus it is mandatory to use biplane (at least two views) ventriculography (Cohn et al, 1974).

With current surgical techniques, almost any patient can survive operation, but that does not mean that the patient will be functionally better. Interventional angiography with inotropic stimulation (Horn et al, 1974), afterload reduction (Helfant et al, 1974), or postextrasystolic potentiation (Dyke et al, 1974) has been developed to assess regional "contractile reserve." These tests permit the surgeon to obtain information concerning functional response to aneurysmectomy and myocardial revascularization.

Echocardiography. Echocardiography provides a

precise, noninvasive, and almost universally available assessment of intracardiac structures. In M-mode echocardiography a beam of ultrasound is emitted from a transducer placed on the patient's chest. Echoes arise from an interface in tissue density, such as blood to muscle. The spatial resolution (± 1 to 2 mm) and temporal resolution ($\pm$ milliseconds) of the M mode are high, but the "tunnel vision" of the echo beam gives a narrow image of intracardiac structures (Parisi et al, 1980). Two-dimensional echocardiograms display a planar beam of echoes in a slice-like tomographic fashion. Regional left ventricular dysfunction (Fortuin and Pawsey, 1977) may distinguish true aneurysms and pseudo-aneurysms (Gatewood and Nanda, 1980) with or without intraventricular thrombus (see Fig. 54–112). An echocardiographic method of quantifying three-dimensional endocardial surface area has been developed (Guyer et al, 1986a, 1986b). Cross-sectional echocardiography gives tomographic views of the heart in multiple planes that are readily standardized to internal cardiac landmarks (Triulzi et al, 1984). These techniques delineate the entire left ventricle.

Gated Blood-Pool Scintigraphy. This high-resolution method assesses regional and global left ventricular function noninvasively. The technique is 96% accurate in detecting left ventricular aneurysm compared with contrast left ventriculography (Winzelberg et al, 1980). Real-time radionuclide cineangiography is useful for the evaluation of patients with coronary artery disease and its sequels (Borer et al, 1977). Advocates of this technique note that it is safe, simple, noninvasive and therefore comfortable for the patient, inexpensive compared with cardiac catheterization, and accurate (Borer et al, 1980). The correlation between radionuclide cineangiography and contrast ventriculography is good. In a study by Friedman and Cantor (1979), the radionuclide scintigram correctly identified all of 54 apical and antero-apical aneurysms and one inferior aneurysm. Scintigraphy did not detect one of six anterior aneurysms and two of three posterobasal aneurysms. Conversely, in 74 patients with angiograms negative for aneurysm, there were two false-positive radionuclide results. The overall accuracy of gated heart scintigraphy was therefore 96%. The relative "blind" zone appears to be the posterobasal region. Radionuclide cineangiography has a role as a screening procedure for patients with suspected left ventricular aneurysm.

Magnetic Resonance Imaging. The clinical use of magnetic resonance imaging (MRI) is restricted to the delineation of pathologic anatomy (Higgins, 1986). Technologic challenges are associated with spectroscopic evaluations of ventricular function. Proton, ^{31}P and ^{13}C nuclear magnetic resonance (NMR) techniques have been used with surface coils (Bottomly et al, 1984) and with catheter NMR probes (Kantor et al, 1984) to examine cardiac structure and bioenergetic profile. Flowing blood in the cardiovascular system generates a negligible NMR signal, thus there is substantial natural contrast between blood and cardiac chambers (Higgins, 1986). Gated NMR images show left ventricular wall thinning, bulging, and thrombus. The spin echo technique has provided useful left ventricular images based on T_1 and T_2 relaxation times and proton density (Zeitler et al, 1986).

SURGICAL INDICATIONS

Hospital deaths of patients who have left ventricular aneurysmectomy have been related to New York Heart Association class, age, preoperative angina, preoperative dyspnea, preoperative diuretic dose, ejection fraction, left ventricular end-diastolic pressure, end-diastolic volume, and extent of occlusive coronary artery disease (Barratt-Boyes et al, 1984). The accepted indications for surgical intervention are (1) congestive heart failure with or without angina, (2) systemic arterial emboli, and (3) medically refractory ventricular tachyarrhythmias (Peyton and Sabiston, 1987).

Congestive Heart Failure and Angina. The decrease in left ventricular function associated with myocardial infarction is related to the volume of muscle damage (Pfeffer et al, 1979). Because of the virtual absence of oxygen reserve, contractility decreases significantly 4 to 6 seconds after the cessation of blood flow (Harden et al, 1979). In a normothermic working heart, some cells are irreversibly damaged after 20 minutes of ischemia (Jennings and Ganote, 1974). With continued ischemia, four sequential contraction abnormalities result (Forrester et al, 1976): (1) *dyssynchrony*, dissociation of electrical and mechanical events in the same muscle region; (2) *hypokinesia*, decreased muscle shortening; (3) *akinesia*, absence of muscle shortening; and (4) *paradoxical motion*, systolic muscle bulging. By 6 to 8 hours, edema and cellular infiltration increase left ventricular wall stiffness (decrease compliance), which improves function by decreasing paradoxical systolic wall motion (Vokonas et al, 1976). As pump function deteriorates, cardiac output, stroke volume, blood pressure, and contractility (dp/dt) are decreased (Pfeffer et al, 1979). Rackley and associates (1977) correlated clinical measurements of left ventricular dysfunction with left ventricular angiography in humans. A decrease in ejection fraction could be detected when 10% of the ventricle contracted abnormally, and an increase in left ventricular end-diastolic pressure and volume occurred when 15% of the ventricle was involved. When 25% of the ventricle contracted abnormally, patients had congestive failure; 40% involvement was associated with shock.

There is evidence that ischemic injury and reperfusion injury may be distinguishable (Brown et al, 1988b) and that the latter is mediated by circulating oxidants (Brown et al, 1988a). Ultimately, myocardial ischemia occurs when oxygen demand exceeds supply, and wall motion abnormalities are seen in all patients after clinical infarction (Wynne et al,

1977). The peri-ischemic "border zone" may contract weakly, and a compensatory increase in the force of contraction was described in surrounding nonischemic muscle (Katz, 1973). Braunwald and Sobel (1980) identified the increase in wall tension associated with left ventricular dilatation as a primary determinant of myocardial oxygen consumption, and Harken and associates (1981) used a high-precision fluorophotographic technique to show the sensitivity of the peri-ischemic border zone (thus infarct volume) to alterations in oxygen demand. According to Laplace's law, wall tension (force/cm) is the product of intraventricular pressure and radius. An increase in global or regional left ventricular dimensions results in increases in wall tension and muscle oxygen demand. Clinically, the largest cross-sectional wall tension at the equator of the ventricle is presented as circumferential wall stress (Mirsky, 1979) (dyne/cm² × 10³).

Laplace's law:
$$\text{Tension} = \text{pressure} \times \text{radius}$$

Mirsky's modification:
$$CWS = (PY)(1 - Y^2/2X^2 - H/2Y + H^2/8X^2/H)$$

where H is wall thickness, P is left ventricular pressure (dyne/cm²), and X and Y are the horizontal and vertical axes (cm) of the ventricle. Circumferential wall stress, and thus myocardial oxygen consumption, is a function of left ventricular dimensions. The reason for surgical aneurysmectomy in congestive heart failure is based on the principle that a smaller ventricular chamber will pump more efficiently while consuming less oxygen.

Systemic Arterial Emboli. Endocardial thrombosis often accompanies myocardial infarction (Handin et al, 1978). Mural thrombus is identified (Fig. 54–107) at autopsy (Schlichter et al, 1954) or operation (Rao et al, 1974) in approximately half of the patients with a left ventricular aneurysm. In approximately half of these patients, systemic emboli occur (Schlichter et al, 1954). Many emboli may be "silent" or not evident clinically. In a study of 500 patients, Davies and associates (1976) found that half of the emboli identified at autopsy were cerebral. Not all intraventricular clotting is obvious. Thrombus that is apparent is a relative indication for operation.

Ventricular Tachyarrhythmias. The common denominator of left ventricular aneurysm and ventricular irritability is myocardial ischemia, and they often coexist. When a rhythm originates in the ventricle, the pattern of ventricular activation is aberrant (wide QRS complex). The mechanism of premature ventricular contractions or ventricular tachycardia is enhancement of automatic rhythms, re-entry, or both (Harken, 1988). Automatic ventricular rhythms due to local myocardial irritability are common in the perioperative and peri-infarction periods. These rhythms are exacerbated by hypokalemia, catecholamines, or digitalis (Kastor et al, 1981). A re-entrant rhythm may occur when two or more electrically heterogeneous (with respect to conduction and refractoriness) pathways are connected proximally and distally (Figs. 54–108 and 54–109). An impulse must travel in only one direction along one of these pathways (unidirectional block). When the impulse arrives at the distal connection, it may return by the initially blocked pathway. If conduction of the impulse is sufficiently slow to allow the originally blocked site to recover excitability, the impulse may re-enter the circuit. A re-entrant arrhythmia may be induced by an electrophysiologic technique of specially timed paced beats called programmed stimulation. This technique permits pharmacologic testing and eventual mapping of re-entrant rhythms such as ventricular tachycardia. Automatic arrhythmias cannot be induced and therefore cannot be tested or mapped. Operation is a therapeutic option for re-entrant ventricular tachycardia. Currently, there is no evidence to support a surgical approach for au-

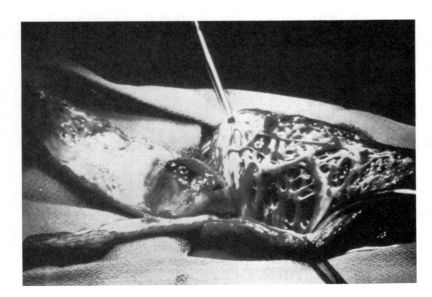

Figure 54–107. Intraoperative photograph of a left ventricular aneurysm opened to show a mural thrombus. Note also the junction between the thin-walled fibrous aneurysmal wall and the muscular trabeculations of viable ventricular endocardium.

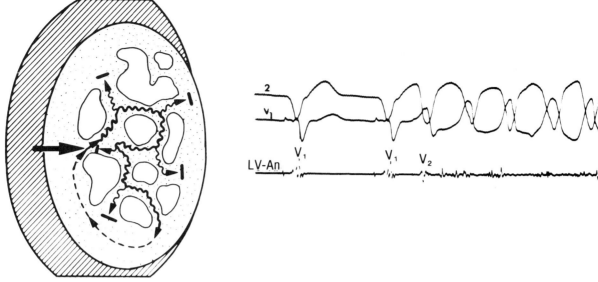

Figure 54–108. Boineau and Cox (1973) introduced this concept of re-entrant arrhythmias. Heterogeneous myocardial ischemia and damage serve as a potential re-entrant circuit. The wave front enters the heterogeneous zone and is slowed, which produces a fragmented afterpotential. Further heterogeneity and slower conduction produce a longer afterpotential. The ischemic zone is sufficiently complex to fragment and slow the wave front so that it may re-enter and sustain a re-entrant arrhythmia.

tomatic ventricular tachycardia and no reason to operate for isolated premature ventricular contractions.

Each year, one-third of a million Americans die suddenly. Education of civilians in cardiopulmonary resuscitation and the implementation of emergency medical systems have increased the salvage in cata-

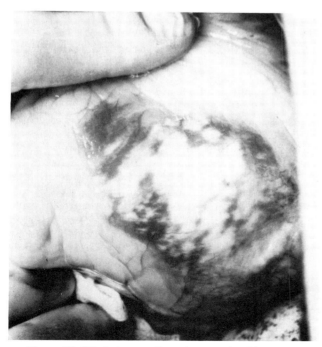

Figure 54–109. Intraoperative photograph of heterogeneous postinfarction myocardial scar that predisposes to re-entrant arrhythmias (see Fig. 54–108).

strophic situations. Patients who survive episodes of recurrent ventricular tachycardia are given pharmacologic testing during programmed induction of arrhythmia (Kastor et al, 1981). If the rhythm cannot be suppressed with high doses of antiarrhythmic agents, these patients are candidates for excision of the re-entrant circuit.

Ventricular Rupture. Although ventricular rupture occurs in 10% of patients with fatal acute myocardial infarction (Bjorck et al, 1960), late rupture of a mature aneurysm almost never occurs (Vlodaver et al, 1975). The incidence of cardiac rupture is high only during the acute phase of infarct evolution. During this phase, the pathophysiologic and technical risks of surgical intervention are prohibitively high. Avoidance of possible ventricular rupture for acute and certainly for chronic left ventricular aneurysms therefore is not routinely an indication for operation.

ANEURYSMECTOMY TECHNIQUE

All preoperative medications are continued until operation (Fullerton and Harken, 1988). A left ventricular aneurysm is repaired through a standard median sternotomy. The aorta is cannulated, and a single venous cannula is sufficient unless an associated ventricular septal defect is suspected. A postinfarction left ventricular aneurysm often presents with dense pericardial adhesions. Cardiopulmonary bypass decompresses the heart and facilitates "takedown" of the adhesions. The patient is cooled. The heart is allowed to cool until it fibrillates. The aorta is then cross-clamped to prevent left ventricular distention. With proper decompression, the aneurysmal zone should collapse, while viable left ventricle remains firm. A linear incision is made in the collapsed aneurysm while cold, blood-potassium cardioplegic solution is infused into the aortic root. Cold saline solution is then poured directly into the left ventricle and over the epicardial surface. If coronary bypass or valve replacement is to be done concurrently, the ventricular aneurysm is always opened first, which provides optimal ventricular decompression and permits thorough epicardial and endocardial cooling.

The entire ventricle is then inspected for mural thrombus (see Fig. 54–107). Thrombus should be removed and the underlying endocardium should be cleaned with a sponge. The ventricular cavity is irrigated again with iced saline solution to recool the myocardium and to remove any residual thrombus. Coronary bypass grafting or valvular procedure is done at this time in a cold, flaccid, decompressed heart. The aneurysmal edge is trimmed and a 1-cm fibrous rim is left. The aneurysm is closed with 0 monofilament sutures in a horizontal mattress manner over long felt buttresses (Fig. 54–110). Felt strips that are at least 1 cm wide facilitate closure. Separate

sutures are begun at either end, brought to the middle, and tied. Before tying this row, the ventricle is filled with blood by inflating the lungs. The atrial appendage should be inverted. A second row of 0 monofilament sutures is placed in an over-and-over technique at both ends and tied over a felt buttress in the middle (see Fig. 54–110). Closed in this manner, the ventriculotomy does not bleed (Fig. 54–111). Seemingly minor traction on the felt buttresses, however, can tear the heart at the lateral junction between the ventricle and the suture line. This tearing typically occurs on the right ventricular side in older patients. Repair of this complication requires recooling and decompression of the heart. Sutures placed (even with pledgets) into a firm, beating ventricle are prone to tear. It is thought that myocardial reperfusion injury is real and is mediated by toxic oxygen metabolites and calcium (Brown, 1988b). Red blood cells contain antioxidants that can minimize reperfusion injury (Brown, 1988a). Before removing the cross-clamp, the author reperfuses the aortic root with hypocalcemic, (0.25 mg/dl) hyperkalemic (9 mEq/l), normothermic blood cardioplegic solution for 10 minutes (Brown, 1989).

Jatene (1985) considered that closing a left ventricular aneurysmectomy incision in a linear manner (see Fig. 54–110) not only distorted the ventricle but also significantly impaired left ventricular function. This group has attempted to *reconstruct* the ventricular geometry with a Dacron patch. The orifice of the aneurysm is concentrically anchored externally with sutures over Teflon bolsters. The patch shape should duplicate that of the original infarcted area.

Variations

Antunes (1987) described a transatrial approach for the correction of submitral left ventricular aneurysms. Akins (1986) reported excellent results of left ventricular aneurysmectomy during hypothermic fibrillatory arrest without aortic occlusion. Inferior aneurysms are more difficult to expose but should be repaired in an identical manner. Some landmarks are worthy of attention. The aneurysm may be adjacent to the mitral valve posteriorly. The mitral annulus is a firm anchor for one end of the closure, and inclusion of the mitral annulus typically does not distort the mitral valve or lead to mitral regurgitation. The posterior descending coronary artery is characteristically occluded in the presence of an inferior aneurysm. This artery and its adjacent vein may therefore be included in the aneurysm repair with impunity. Occasionally, the posterior papillary muscle has been infarcted and replaced by firm scar, which does not necessarily mean that it is no longer an adequate support for the mitral valve. The blood supply to the papillary muscle is derived from its center and from the lateral wall (Estes et al, 1966).

If the indication for operation is recurrent sustained ventricular tachycardia, the left ventricular endocardium should be mapped when the aneurysm

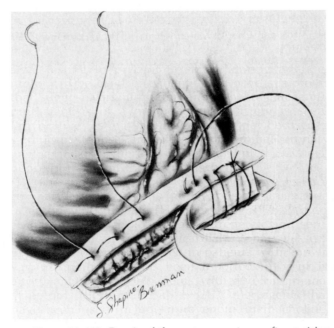

Figure 54–110. Repair of the aneurysmectomy after excision involves reapproximation of the fibrous rims of the aneurysm. In closing an anteroapical or posterior aneurysm, the left anterior descending or posterior descending coronary artery is typically occluded and may be included in the repair with impunity. The aneurysm is closed with 0 monofilament suture in a horizontal mattress fashion over long felt strips. Separate sutures are placed at either end, brought to the middle, and tied. A secondary row of 0 monofilament suture is placed in an over-and-over fashion at both ends and tied over a felt buttress in the middle. When closed in this manner, the ventriculotomy is less likely to bleed. Seemingly minor traction on the felt buttresses, however, can tear the heart at the lateral junction between the ventricle and the suture line, which typically occurs on the right ventricular side in older patients.

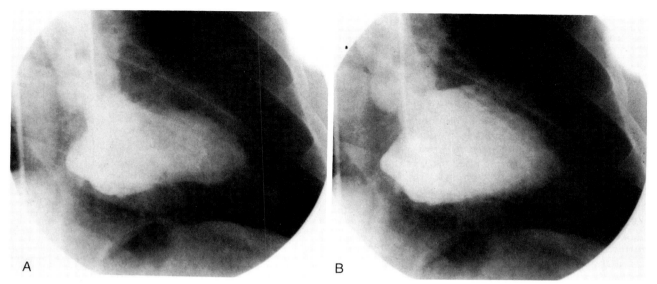

Figure 54–111. Contrast ventriculogram of a patient with an anteroapical left ventricular aneurysm. Note that during systole *(A)* and diastole *(B)* no intraventricular thrombus is evident. Forty-eight hours later, this patient had left ventricular aneurysmectomy and a 4 × 4 cm intraventricular thrombus was found at the time of operation. Contrast ventriculography, radionuclide ventriculography, echocardiography, and tagged platelet studies have been disappointing in identifying intraventricular clot.

is opened (Harken et al, 1980). After the area of earliest activation is located, this endocardial zone is peeled back beyond the aneurysmal edge into grossly viable myocardium (Horowitz et al, 1980b).

SURGICAL RESULTS

A surgical procedure is indicated when the result would be better than the natural history of the disease. Global left ventricular dysfunction is an ominous prognostic risk factor. Left ventricular aneurysm has been dissociated from global ventricular dysfunction as an independent and grave prognostic indicator (Meizlish et al, 1984). The 1-year mortality of patients with a left ventricular aneurysm after an anterior myocardial infarction was 61%. Patients who developed a detectable aneurysm within 48 hours of a myocardial infarction had 80% mortality. Surgical results are superior to available medical therapy.

As with most surgical procedures, results of left ventricular aneurysmectomy depend on coexistent disease. Barratt-Boyes and associates (1984) examined a 13-year surgical experience and reported 15% hospital and 30% 1-year mortality. Harken and associates (1980a) reported 6.7% hospital mortality, and Akins (1986) reported 2% hospital mortality with ventricular irritability predictive of both early and late deaths.

The rapid evolution of medical and surgical therapy for patients with ischemic cardiac disease has confounded attempts to characterize and compare results. It is impractical and perhaps unethical to randomize patients prospectively after catheterization that shows left ventricular aneurysm and differing ventricular dysfunction, noncomparable coronary artery disease, variable associated valvular

lesions, and myriad concurrent risk factors. Formerly, medical management of patients with post-infarction aneurysms was associated with a very poor prognosis. In the autopsy series of Schlichter and associates (1954), three-quarters of patients with documented ventricular aneurysms died in 3 years; only 12% were alive 5 years after the precipitating myocardial infarction. Medical therapy is now better. Only the prospective study by Meizlish and associates (1984) of angiographically proven candidates for operation who were treated medically would provide the answers. Comparative information is available, but examination of the results of aneurysmectomy is simplified by categorizing the patients with respect to the indication for operation.

Enthusiasm for aneurysm resection in patients with angina with congestive failure (Cooperman et al, 1975) or without congestive failure (Lefemine et al, 1977) is based on subjective clinical improvement and a decrease in expected late mortality compared with studies of the natural history (Borer et al, 1980). The presence of left ventricular aneurysm burdens nonaneurysmal myocardial fibers and increases systolic shortening and thus myocardial oxygen uptake. When an aneurysm involves more than 25% of the ventricular surface, myocardial fiber shortening limits are exceeded. The ventricle dilates and stiffens, stroke volume decreases, end-diastolic pressure increases, and congestive heart failure with or without ischemia ensues (Klein et al, 1967). Aneurysmectomy reverses this process at least partially.

Some groups (Bjorck et al, 1960; Spencer et al, 1971) have reported disappointing symptomatic relief and marginal influence on expected long-term survival. Conversely, Froehlich and associates (1980) examined 18 patients, of whom 13 had concurrent angina and congestive failure and 11 had aneurysm resection. Only 50% of the noncontractile area visualized on contrast ventriculography was resected. There was a marked discrepancy between substantial symptomatic relief and marginal objective functional improvement. Patients improved from New York Heart Association Functional Class 3.6 before operation to Class 2.3 ($p < 0.005$) after aneurysmectomy. Only 4 patients in this series had either an increase in ejection fraction or a decrease of more than 10% in end-diastolic volume, and there were no operative deaths. Others (Cullhed et al, 1975) have documented a decrease in both end-diastolic and end-systolic heart volume postoperatively, with an increase in left ventricular ejection fraction. In the authors' series (Martin et al, 1982) of 62 patients examined with preoperative and postoperative cardiac catheterization, symptomatic relief was associated with an increase in ejection fraction from 28 to 39% ($p < 0.001$) and a decrease in left ventricular end-diastolic pressure from 17 to 14 mm Hg ($p < 0.005$).

With rapidly evolving medical therapy it is difficult to compare aneurysmectomy and endocardial excision for ventricular tachycardia. However, in patients with left ventricular dysfunction and ventricular tachycardia not controllable with drugs, 80% mortality is anticipated during the first year (Kastor et al, 1981). When ventricular tachycardia is suppressible with drugs, one-third to one-half of patients are expected to survive for the first year. With surgical aneurysmectomy and endocardial resection, 80% of patients are expected to survive for the first year (Harken et al, 1980b; Kastor et al, 1981).

Selected Bibliography

Barratt-Boyes, B. G., White, H. D., Agnew, T. M., et al: The results of surgical treatment of left ventricular aneurysms. J. Thorac. Cardiovasc. Surg., *87*:87, 1984.

This is an excellent and critically evaluated series in which hospital mortality in patients who have surgical therapy for left ventricular aneurysm is related to New York Heart Association class, age, preoperative angina, preoperative dyspnea, preoperative diuretic dose, ejection fraction, left ventricular end-diastolic pressure, end-diastolic volume, and extent of occlusive coronary artery disease.

Boineau, J. P., and Cox, J. L.: Slow ventricular activation in acute myocardial infarction: A source of re-entrant premature ventricular contractions. Circulation, *48*:702, 1973.

This study was the first to suggest that a heterogeneous pattern of myocardial ischemia (see Fig. 54–109) led to zones of slow conduction that predisposed to re-entrant ventricular arrhythmias (see Fig. 54–108). Automatic and re-entrant arrhythmias are explained and related to fragmentation of intramyocardial potentials.

Brown, J. M., Grosso, M. A., Terada, L. S., et al: Erythrocytes decrease myocardial hydrogen peroxide levels and reperfusion injury. Am. J. Physiol., *256*:H588, 1989.

The authors distinguish ischemic from reperfusion injury and show that the latter is at least partially mediated by an "oxidant burst" during early myocardial reperfusion. This injury leads to mechanical dysfunction and electrical instability and should be prevented. Warm blood-cardioplegic reperfusion decreases both hydrogen peroxide levels and reperfusion injuries.

Harken, A. H., Horowitz, L. N., and Josephson, M. E.: Comparison of standard aneurysmectomy and aneurysmectomy with directed endocardial resection for the treatment of recurrent sustained ventricular tachycardia. J. Thorac. Cardiovasc. Surg., *80*:527, 1980.

This is the only comparative study that relates standard aneurysmectomy to electrophysiologically directed endocardial excision plus aneurysmectomy in the treatment of ventricular tachycardia. It is a retrospective, nonrandomized comparison of 19 patients treated with standard aneurysmectomy and 30 patients treated with aneurysmectomy plus directed endocardial excision. The operative mortality in the group who had standard aneurysmectomy was 42%, and 79% of patients (15 of 19) still had spontaneous ventricular tachycardia postoperatively. The operative mortality in the electrophysiologically directed group was 6.7% (2 of 30), and 10% (3 of 30) had ventricular tachycardia inducible with postoperative programmed stimulation.

Higgins, C. B.: Overview of MR of the heart—1986. Am. J. Roentgenol., *146*:907, 1986.

An overview of anatomy, global ventricular function, left ventricular regional function, blood flow, myocardial tissue characterization, and spectroscopy available with magnetic resonance techniques in 1986.

Martin, J. L., Untereker, W. J., Harken, A. H., et al: Aneurysmectomy and endocardial resection for ventricular tachycardia: Favorable hemodynamic and antiarrhythmic results in patients with global left ventricular dysfunction. Am. Heart J., *103*:960, 1982.

Results are presented for a large series of patients who had left ventricular aneurysmectomy with both preoperative and postoperative contrast ventriculography. Sixty-two patients were catheterized before and after aneurysmectomy. Ejection fraction increased from 28 ± 8% to 39 ± 10% ($p < 0.001$), and left ventricular end-diastolic pressure decreased from 17 ± 8 to 14 ± 5 mm Hg ($p < 0.005$). Objectively, aneurysmectomy improves left ventricular function.

Meizlish, J. L., Berger, H. J., Plankey, M., et al: Functional left ventricular aneurysm formation after acute anterior transmural myocardial infarction. N. Engl. J. Med., *311*:1001, 1984.

The incidence, natural history, and prognostic implications of an anterior transmural myocardial infarction are critically examined. The authors obtained serial radionuclide angiocardiograms of patients after an anterior myocardial infarction. Patients with and without aneurysms had comparable depression of left ventricular function (31 versus 27% ejection fraction). The 1-year mortality was very different (61 versus 9%).

Schlichter, J., Hellerstein, H. K., and Katz, L. N.: Aneurysm of the heart: A correlative study of 102 proved cases. Medicine, *33*:43, 1954.

A classic clinicopathologic correlation of 102 confirmed cases of left ventricular aneurysm treated nonoperatively. The history, diagnosis, pathology, and prognosis are reviewed in detail. The authors indicate that three-quarters of patients are dead in 3 years and that there is a 12% 5-year survival. This study is still the classic example of the natural history of medically treated left ventricular aneurysm. It will never be repeated.

Bibliography

Akins, C. W.: Resection of left ventricular aneurysm during hypothermic fibrillatory arrest without aortic occlusion. J. Thorac. Cardiovasc. Surg., *91*:610, 1986.
Alpert, J. S., and Braunwald, E.: Pathological and clinical manifestations of acute myocardial infarction. In Braunwald, E. (ed): Heart Disease: A Textbook of Cardiovascular Medicine. Philadelphia, W. B. Saunders Company, 1980, p. 1309.
Antunes, M. J.: Submitral left ventricular aneurysms. J. Thorac. Cardiovasc. Surg., *94*:241, 1987.

Arnold, J.: Ueber angeborene Divertikel des Herzens. Virchows Arch. (Pathol. Anat.), 137:318, 1894.

Barratt-Boyes, B. G., White, H. D., Agnew, T. M., et al: The results of surgical treatment of left ventricular aneurysms. J. Thorac. Cardiovasc. Surg., 87:87, 1984.

Basset-Smith, P. W.: Aneurysm of the heart due to syphilitic gummata. Br. Med. J., 2:1060, 1908.

Beck, C. S.: Operation for aneurysm of the heart. Ann. Surg., 120:34, 1944.

Bjorck, G., Morgensen, L., Nyquist, O., et al: Studies of myocardial rupture with cardiac tamponade in acute myocardial infarction. Concours Med., 82:2637, 1960.

Boineau, J. P., and Cox, J. L.: Slow ventricular activation in acute myocardial infarction: A source of re-entrant premature ventricular contractions. Circulation, 48:702, 1973.

Borer, J. S., Bacharach, S. L., Green, M. V., et al: Real time radionuclide cineangiography in the noninvasive evaluation of global and regional left ventricular function at rest and during exercise in patients with coronary artery disease. N. Engl. J. Med., 296:839, 1977.

Borer, J. S., Jacobstein, J. G., Bacharach, S. L., and Green, M. V.: Detection of left ventricular aneurysm and evaluation of effects of surgical repair: The role of radionuclide cineangiography. Am. J. Cardiol., 45:1103, 1980.

Bottomly, B. A., Foster, P. B., and Darrow, R. D.: Depth resolved surface coil spectroscopy (dress) for in vivo proton, phosphorus-31 and carbon-13 NMR. J. Magnet. Reson., 59:338, 1984.

Braunwald, E., and Sobel, B. E.: Coronary blood flow and myocardial ischemia. In Braunwald, E. (ed): Heart Disease: A Textbook of Cardiovascular Medicine. Philadelphia, W. B. Saunders Company, 1980, p. 1279.

Bricout, C.: Syphilis du coeur. These, Paris, 1912, p. 45.

Brown, J. M., Grosso, M. A., Whitman, G. J., et al: Cardiac oxidase systems mediate oxygen metabolite reperfusion injury. Surgery, 104:266, 1988a.

Brown, J. M., Terada, L. S., Grosso, M. A., et al: Xanthine oxidase produces hydrogen peroxide which contributes to reperfusion injury of ischemic isolated rat hearts. J. Clin. Invest., 81:1556, 1988b.

Bruschke, A. V. G., Proudfit, W. F., and Sones, F. M.: Progress study of 490 consecutive non-surgical cases of coronary disease followed 5 to 9 years. II: Ventriculographic and other correlation. Circulation, 47:1154, 1973.

Cabin, H. S., and Roberts, W. C.: True left ventricular aneurysm and healed myocardial infarction: Clinical and necropsy observations including quantification of degrees of coronary artery narrowing. Am. J. Cardiol., 46:754, 1980.

Cohn, P. F., and Braunwald, E.: Chronic coronary artery disease. In Braunwald, E. (ed): Heart Disease: A Textbook of Cardiovascular Medicine. Philadelphia, W. B. Saunders Company, 1980, p. 1387.

Cohn, P. F., Gorlin, R., Adams, D. F., et al: Comparison of biplane and single-plane left ventriculography in patients with coronary artery disease. Am. J. Cardiol., 33:1, 1974.

Cooley, D. A., Collins, H. A., Morris, G. C., and Chapman, D. W.: Ventricular aneurysm after myocardial infarction. Surgical excision with use of temporary cardiopulmonary bypass. J.A.M.A., 167:557, 1958.

Cooperman, M., Stinson, E. B., Griepp, R. B., and Shumway, N. E.: Survival and function after left ventricular aneurysmectomy. J. Thorac. Cardiovasc. Surg., 69:321, 1975.

Cruveilhier, J.: Essai sur l'anatomie pathologique en général, et sur les transformations et productions organiques en particulier. Nouvelle Bibliotheque Med., 2:72, 1827.

Cullhed, I., Delius, W., Bjork, L., et al: Resection of left ventricular aneurysm—late results. Acta Med. Scand., 197:241, 1975.

Davies, M. J., Woolf, N., and Robertson, W. B.: Pathology of acute myocardial infarction with particular reference to occlusive coronary thrombi. Br. Heart J., 38:659, 1976.

Didisheim, P., and Foster, V.: Actions and clinical status of platelet suppressive agents. Semin. Hematol., 15:55, 1978.

Dolly, C. H., Dotter, C. T., and Steinberg, H.: Ventricular aneurysm in a 29-year-old man studied angiocardiographically. Am. Heart J., 42:894, 1951.

Dyke, S. H., Cohn, P. F., Gorlin, E., and Sonnenblick, E. H.: Detection of residual myocardial function in coronary artery disease using postextrasystolic potentiation. Circulation, 50:694, 1974.

Eaton, L. W., Weiss, J. L., Bulkley, B. H., et al: Regional cardiac dilatation after acute myocardial infarction: Recognition by two dimensional echocardiography. N. Engl. J. Med., 300:57, 1979.

Estes, E. H., Dalton, F. M., Entman, M. L., et al: The anatomy and blood supply of the papillary muscles of the left ventricle. Am. Heart J., 71:356, 1966.

European Coronary Surgery Study Group: Coronary artery bypass surgery in stable angina pectoris: Survival at two years. Lancet, 1:889, 1979.

Fojo-Echevarria, P., Muniz-Sotolongo, J. C., and Aixala, R.: Aneurysma de la auticula izquierda como sequela de comisurotomia. Revista Cubana de Cardiologia, 16:377, 1955.

Forrester, J. S., Wyatt, H. L., DaLuz, P. L., et al: Functional significance of regional ischemic contraction abnormalities. Circulation, 54:64, 1976.

Fortuin, N. J., and Pawsey, C. G. K.: The evaluation of left ventricular function by echocardiography. Am. J. Med., 63:1, 1977.

Friedman, M. L., and Cantor, R. E.: Reliability of gated heart scintigrams for detection of left ventricular aneurysm: Concise communication. J. Nucl. Med., 20:720, 1979.

Froehlich, R. T., Falsetti, H. L., Doty, D. B., and Marcus, M. L.: Prospective study of surgery for left ventricular aneurysm. Am. J. Cardiol., 45:923, 1980.

Fullerton, D., and Harken, A. H.: Preoperative cardiac assessment. In Wilmore, D., Brennan, M., Harken, A., et al (eds): Care of the Surgical Patient. New York, Scientific American, 1989.

Galeati, D. G.: DeBononiensi scientiarum et atrium instituto atque academia commentarii. De Morbis Duobus, 4:25, 1757.

Gatewood, R., and Nanda, N.: Differentiation of left ventricular pseudoaneurysm from true aneurysm with two dimensional echocardiography. Am. J. Cardiol., 46:869, 1980.

Gay, W. A.: Ventricular aneurysm. In Sabiston, D. C., Jr. (ed): Textbook of Surgery: The Biologic Basis of Modern Surgical Practice. Philadelphia, W. B. Saunders Company, 1986, p. 2310.

Gorlin, R.: Coronary collaterals. In Coronary Artery Disease. Philadelphia, W. B. Saunders Company, 1976, p. 59.

Grondin, P., Kretz, J. G., Bical, O., et al: Natural history of saccular aneurysms of the left ventricle. J. Thorac. Cardiovasc. Surg., 77:57, 1979.

Guyer, D. E., Foale, R. A., Gillam, L. D., et al: An echocardiographic technique for quantifying and displaying the extent of left ventricular dyssynergy. J. Am. Coll. Cardiol., 8:830, 1986b.

Guyer, D. E., Gibson, T. C., Gillam, L. D., et al: A new echocardiographic model for quantifying three dimensional endocardial surface area. J. Am. Coll. Cardiol., 8:819, 1986a.

Handin, R. I., McDonough, M., and Lesch, M.: Elevation of platelet factor four in acute myocardial infarction: Measurement of radioimmunoassay. J. Lab. Clin. Med., 91:340, 1978.

Harden, W. R., Barlow, C. H., Simson, M. J., and Harken, A. H.: Temporal relation between the onset of cell anoxia and ischemic contractile failure. Am. J. Cardiol., 44:741, 1979.

Harken, A. H.: Cardiac arrhythmias. In Wilmore, D., Brennan, M., Harken, A., et al (eds): Care of the Surgical Patient. New York, Scientific American, 1988.

Harken, A. H., Horowitz, L. N., and Josephson, M. E.: Comparison of standard aneurysmectomy and aneurysmectomy with directed endocardial resection for the treatment of recurrent sustained ventricular tachycardiac. J. Thorac. Cardiovasc. Surg., 80:527, 1980a.

Harken, A. H., Horowitz, L. N., and Josephson, M. E.: The surgical treatment of ventricular tachycardia. Ann. Thorac. Surg., 30:499, 1980b.

Harken, A. H., Simson, M. B., Weststein, L. W., et al: Early ischemia following complete coronary ligation in the rabbit, dog, pig and monkey. Am. J. Physiol., 241:202, 1981.

Helfant, R. H., Pine, R., Meister, S. G., et al: Nitroglycerine to unmask reversible asynergy: Correlation with post-coronary bypass ventriculography. Circulation, 50:108, 1974.

Herman, M. V., Heinle, R. A., Klein, M. D., and Gorlin, R.: Localized disorders in myocardial contraction: Asynergy and its role in congestive heart failure. N. Engl. J. Med., 277:222, 1967.

Higgins, C. B.: Overview of magnetic resonance of the heart. Am. J. Roentgenol., 146:907, 1986.

Horn, H. R., Teichholz, L. E., Cohn, P. F., et al: Augmentation of left ventricular contraction pattern in coronary artery disease by inotropic catecholamine: The epinephrine ventriculogram. Circulation, 49:1063, 1974.

Horowitz, L. N., Harken, A. H., Kastor, J. A., and Josephson, M. E.: Ventricular resection guided by epicardial and endocardial mapping for the treatment of recurrent ventricular tachycardia. N. Engl. J. Med., 302:589, 1980.

Hunter, J.: An account of the dissection of morbid bodys. A manuscript copy in the Library of the Royal College of Surgeons, No. 32, 1757, pp. 30–32.

Jatene, A. D.: Left ventricular aneurysmectomy: Resection or reconstruction. J. Thorac. Cardiovasc. Surg., 89:321, 1985.

Jennings, R. B., and Ganote, C. E.: Structural change in myocardium during acute ischemia. Circ. Res., 35(Suppl. 3):156, 1974.

Kantor, H. L., Briggs, R. W., and Balaban, R. S.: In vivo 31-P nuclear magnetic resonance measurements in canine heart using a catheter coil. Circ. Res., 55:261, 1984.

Kastor, J. A., Horowitz, L. N., Harken, A. H., and Josephson, M. E.: Clinical electrophysiology of ventricular tachycardia. N. Engl. J. Med., 304:1004, 1981.

Katz, A. M.: Effects of ischemia on the contractile processes of heart muscle. Am. J. Cardiol., 32:456, 1973.

Klein, G. I.: Zur Aetiologie der aneurysmen der pars membranacea septi ventriculorum cordis und deren ruptur. Virchows Arch. (Pathol. Anat.), 118:57, 1889.

Klein, M. D., Herman, M. V., and Gorlin, R.: A hemodynamic study of left ventricular aneurysm. Circulation, 35:614, 1967.

Lee, D. C., Johnson, R. A., Boucher, C. A., et al: Angiographic predictors of survival following left ventricular aneurysmectomy. Circulation, 56(Suppl. 2):12, 1977.

Lefemine, A. R., Govindarajan, R., Ramaswamy, K., et al: Left ventricular wall resection for aneurysm and akinesia due to coronary artery disease: Fifty consecutive patients. Ann. Thorac. Surg., 23:461, 1977.

Libman, E.: Affections of the coronary arteries. Interst. Postgrad. Med. Assoc. North Am., 2:405, 1932.

Likoff, W., and Bailey, C. P.: Ventriculoplasty: Excision of myocardial aneurysm. J.A.M.A., 158:915, 1955.

Loop, F. D., Effler, D. B., Navia, J. A., et al: Aneurysms of the left ventricle: Survival and results of a ten year experience. Ann. Surg., 178:399, 1973.

Lyons, C., and Perkins, R.: Resection of a left ventricular aneurysm secondary to a cardiac stab wound. Ann. Surg., 147:256, 1958.

Martin, J., Untereker, W. J., Harken, A. H., et al: Aneurysmectomy and endocardial resection for ventricular tachycardia: Favorable hemodynamic and antiarrhythmic results in patients with global left ventricular dysfunction. Am. Heart J., 103:960, 1982.

Meizlish, J. L., Berger, H. J., Plankey, M., et al: Functional left ventricular aneurysm formation after acute anterior transmural myocardial infarction. N. Engl. J. Med., 311:1001, 1984.

Mirsky, I.: Elastic properties of the myocardium: A quantitative approach with physiological and clinical applications. In Berne, L. M. (ed): Handbook of Physiology. Vol. I: The Heart. Bethesda, MD, American Physiological Society, 1979, p. 501.

Murphy, M. L., Hultgren, H. N., Detre, K., et al: Treatment of chronic stable angina. N. Engl. J. Med., 297:621, 1977.

Parisi, A. F., Moynihan, P. F., Ray, B. J., and Pietro, D. A.: Two dimensional echocardiography. J. Cardiovasc. Med., 5:39, 1980.

Peyton, R. B., and Sabiston, D. C., Jr.: Ventricular aneurysm. In Sabiston, D. C., Jr. (ed): Essentials of Surgery. Philadelphia, W. B. Saunders Company, 1987, p. 1124.

Pfeffer, M. A., Pfeffer, J. M., Fishbein, M. C., et al: Myocardial infarct size and ventricular function in rats. Circ. Res., 44:503, 1979.

Proudfit, W. L.: Personal communication. Cited in Grondin, P., Kretz, J. G., Bical, O., et al: Natural history of saccular aneurysms of the left ventricle. J. Thorac. Cardiovasc. Surg., 77:57, 1979.

Rackley, C. E., Russell, R. O., Jr., Mantle, J. A., and Rogers, W. J.: Modern approach to the patient with acute myocardial infarction. Curr. Probl. Cardiol., 1:49, 1977.

Rao, G., Zikria, E. A., Miller, W. H., et al: Experience with sixty consecutive ventricular aneurysm resections. Circulation, 49(Suppl. 2):149, 1974.

Rokitansky, C.: Handbuch der Pathologischen Anatomie, Vol. II. Vienna, Braumuller and Seidel, 1844, p. 449.

Rosenthal, D. S., and Braunwald, E.: Hematologic oncologic disorders and heart disease. In Braunwald, E. (ed): Heart Disease: A Textbook of Cardiovascular Medicine. Philadelphia, W. B. Saunders Company, 1980, p. 1771.

Sauerbruch, F., and O'Shaughnessy, L.: Thoracic Surgery. Baltimore, William Wood & Co., 1937, p. 245.

Schattenberg, T. T., Giuliana, E. R., Campion, B. C., and Danielson, G. K., Jr.: Post-infarction ventricular aneurysm. Mayo Clin. Proc., 45:13, 1970.

Schlichter, J., Hellerstein, H. K., and Katz, L. N.: Aneurysm of the heart: A correlative study of 102 proved cases. Medicine, 33:43, 1954.

Schwedel, J. B., Samet, P., and Mednick, H.: Electrokymographic studies of abnormal left ventricular pulsations. Am. Heart J., 40:410, 1950.

Sezary, A., and Alibert, T.: Aneurysm in wall of heart. Bull. Mem. Soc. Med. Hosp. Paris, 46:172, 1922.

Sniderman, A. D., Marpole, D., and Fallen, E. L.: Regional contraction patterns in the normal and ischemic left ventricle in man. Am. J. Cardiol., 31:484, 1973.

Spear, J. F., Horowitz, L. N., Hodess, A. B., et al: Cellular electrophysiology of human myocardial infarction. I: Abnormalities of cellular activation. Circulation, 59:247, 1979.

Spencer, F. C., Green, G. E., Tice, D. A., et al: Coronary artery bypass grafts for congestive heart failure: A report of experience with 40 patients. J. Thorac. Cardiovasc. Surg., 62:529, 1971.

Stansel, J. C., Jr., Julian, O. C., and Dye, W. S.: Right ventricular aneurysm. J. Thorac. Cardiovasc. Surg., 46:66, 1963.

Sternberg, M.: Das chronische partielle herzaneurysma. Vienna and Leipzig, Franz Deuticke, 1914.

Swan, H. J. C., Forrester, J. S., Diamond, G., et al: Hemodynamic spectrum of myocardial infarction and cardiogenic shock. Circulation, 45:1097, 1972.

Tennant, R., and Wiggers, C. J.: Effect of coronary occlusion on myocardial contraction. Am. J. Physiol., 112:351, 1935.

Triulzi, M. O., Gillam, L. D., Gentile, F., et al: Normal adult cross-sectional echocardiographic valves: Linear dimensions and chamber areas. Echocardiography, 1:403, 1984.

Vlodaver, Z., Coe, J. I., and Edwards, J. E.: True and false left ventricular aneurysms: Propensity for the latter to rupture. Circulation, 51:567, 1975.

Voelcker, A. F.: Aneurysm of the heart. Trans. Pathol. Soc. (Lond.), 53:409, 1902.

Vokonas, P. S., Pirzada, F. A., and Hood, W. B., Jr.: Experimental myocardial infarction. XII: Dynamic changes in segmental mechanical behavior of infarcted and non-infarcted myocardium. Am. J. Cardiol., 37:853, 1976.

Weiss, H. J.: Platelet physiology and abnormalities of platelet function. N. Engl. J. Med., 293:531, 1975.

Wellens, H. J. J.: Observations of the pathophysiology of ventricular tachycardia in man. Arch. Intern. Med., 135:473, 1975.

Winzelberg, G. G., Strauss, H. W., Bingham, J. B., and McKusick, K. A.: Scintigraphic evaluation of left ventricular aneurysm. Am. J. Cardiol., 46:1138, 1980.

Wynne, J., Birnholz, J., Fineberg, H., and Alpert, J. S.: Assessment of regional left ventricular wall motion in acute myocardial infarction by two-dimensional echocardiography. Circulation, 56(Suppl. 2):152, 1977.

Zeitler, E., Kaiser, W., and Schuierer, G.: Magnetic resonance imaging of aneurysms and thrombi. Cardiovasc. Intervent. Radiol., 8:321, 1986.

6 Assisted Circulation

Eldred D. Mundth

HISTORICAL ASPECTS

The development of a relatively safe and effective method of circulatory assistance, including ventricular assist devices and the total artificial mechanical heart, represents an extraordinary example of the success of careful research and a multidisciplinary approach of physiology, bioengineering, clinical medicine, and operative procedures. The concept of prolonged assisted circulation for support of the failing heart evolved simultaneously with the development of cardiopulmonary bypass (CPB) devices for use in open heart operations (Gibbon, 1954). Early investigators envisioned prolonged CPB for support of the failing heart, thus enabling sufficient myocardial functional recovery to allow gradual weaning from circulatory assistance and survival of the patient. Stuckey and associates (1957) used brief periods of CPB in three patients in cardiogenic shock; one patient survived. Connolly and associates (1958) proposed venoarterial bypass without an oxygenator for treatment of cardiogenic shock, hoping to effectively benefit the failing heart without severely depressing peripheral arterial oxygen saturation and also eliminating problems associated with blood-gas interface reactions (Lee et al, 1961). Although venoarterial partial bypass relieved right ventricular failure and reduced left ventricular volume work, it did not relieve left ventricular work significantly until almost total bypass was achieved.

Clauss and associates (1961), working as an effective surgical-medical and bioengineering team, first developed the concept of arterial counterpulsation. Withdrawal of arterial blood from a cannula during ventricular systole and pulsatile return of blood to the arterial system during diastole were achieved with phasing of counterpulsation controlled by electrocardiographic (ECG) gating (Fig. 54–112). Arterial counterpulsation, when properly phased, reduced left ventricular pressure work by 20 to 40%, as reported by Soroff and associates (1963) and Rosensweig and Chatterjee (1968). However, clinical use of this device was not particularly effective in patients with cardiogenic shock and was not associated with improved survival (Sugg et al, 1970). It was noted in the laboratory and clinically that when arterial counterpulsation was attempted in the presence of severe hypotension, rapid withdrawal of blood was difficult to achieve during systole, thus resulting in collapse of the artery, preventing adequate volume withdrawal, and causing severe mechanical trauma to the blood.

Another approach to assisted circulation was developed during this time by Senning and associates (1962). A left atrial-arterial bypass system using a percutaneously introduced cannula was placed in the left atrium by transatrial septal puncture. By using this approach, myocardial oxygen consumption could be moderately reduced with significant reduction of left ventricular preload, causing decreased left ventricular wall tension, although little change was noted in left ventricular tension-time index or myocardial contractility (Chiu et al, 1969). Litwak and associates (1976) effectively used a similar left atrial-arterial left-sided heart assist system for postcardiotomy cardiogenic shock to allow satisfactory weaning from CPB.

Perhaps the most simple yet ingenious device to achieve arterial diastolic counterpulsation is the intra-aortic balloon pump (IABP), introduced by Moulopoulos and co-workers (1962). The intra-aortic balloon is introduced in most cases via the common femoral artery, and effective diastolic counterpulsation is achieved with compressed gas-driven volume

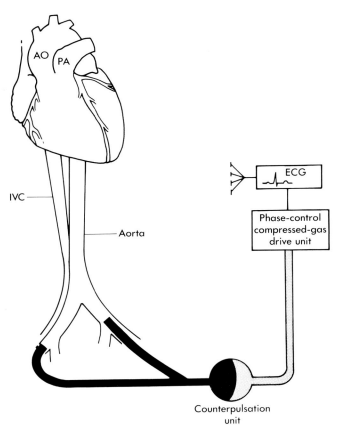

Figure 54–112. Arterioarterial diastolic counterpulsation circulatory assistance device. During systole, arterial blood is withdrawn from cannulas in the iliac arteries (inserted via bilateral common femoral arterial cannulation) and reinfused under pressure during early diastole by a compressed-gas drive unit phased with the patient's ECG. (AO = aorta; PA = pulmonary artery; IVC = inferior vena cava.)

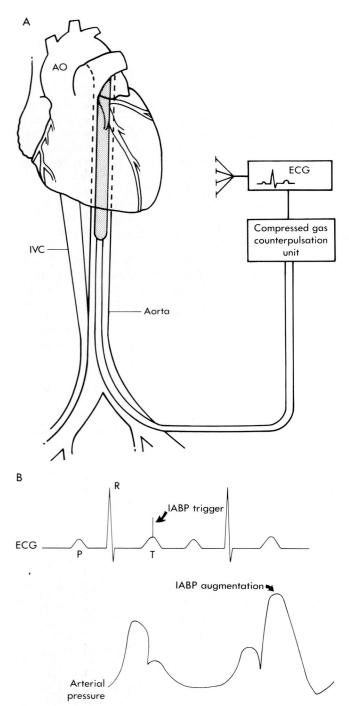

Figure 54–113. IABC assist device. An elongated balloon mounted on a catheter is introduced via the common femoral artery into the descending thoracic aorta, and diastolic counterpulsation is phased with the patient's ECG and inflation-deflation of the balloon using compressed gas. Optimal efficiency in IABC assistance is achieved with inflation timed with the dicrotic notch of the arterial pressure and deflation occurring just before isometric left ventricular contraction, thus optimizing left ventricular afterload reduction.

displacement of an elongated catheter-mounted balloon electronically gated to the ECG (Fig. 54–113). Refinement of a clinically applicable and effective IABP was described by Buckley and associates (1970) and by Bregman and co-workers (1970). IABP counterpulsation has continued to be the primary mode of circulatory assistance in most clinical situations because of its physiologic effectiveness, minimal invasiveness, relative ease and safety of use, and scope of clinical applicability.

Continued technologic advances in biocompati-

ble surfaces, efficient and compact pumping chambers, and successful cardiac transplantation have stimulated development of extracorporeal ventricular assist devices as well as the total artificial heart (Deutsch, 1979; DeVries et al, 1984; Golding et al, 1982; Norman et al, 1981; Pennington et al, 1985a; Pierce et al, 1981). Although hemodynamically more effective in supporting left ventricular function than are the counterpulsation devices, the ventricular assist devices are inherently more invasive and currently are relatively limited in use to investigative

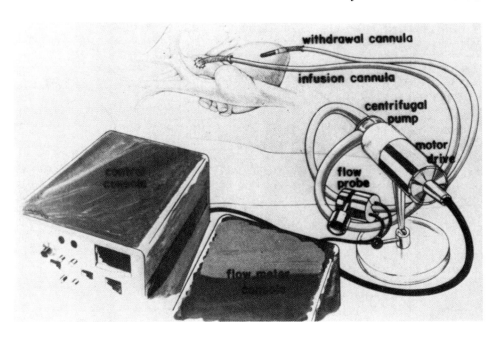

Figure 54–114. Medtronic centrifugal pump ventricular assist device shown with withdrawal cannula in the left ventricular apex and infusion cannula in the ascending aorta. Currently, the preferred cannulation is left atrial to aorta. (From Pennington, D. G., Bernhard, W. F., Golding, L. R., et al: Long-term follow-up of postcardiotomy patients with profound cardiogenic shock treated with ventricular assist devices. Circulation, 72[Suppl. 2]:216, 1985. By permission of the American Heart Association, Inc.)

clinical trials. In current clinical practice, the ventricular assist devices (left ventricular assist device [LVAD] and right ventricular assist device [RVAD]) (Figs. 54–114 and 54–115) are generally reserved for patients who have failed to wean from CPB after cardiac surgical procedures and in those patients in whom IABP counterpulsation (IABC) has not been sufficiently effective to maintain circulation. The extracorporeal artificial heart as typified by the Jarvik-7 device has been clinically used primarily as a variable-duration temporizing support measure for patients awaiting cardiac transplantation (Griffith et al, 1987; Jarvik et al, 1978).

Continued research on autologous, conditioned, fatigue-resistant skeletal muscle as a potential biologic ventricular assist device shows that a skeletal muscle surrounding a ventricle can effectively pump blood at physiologic arterial pressures at 15 to 20% of the experimental animal's cardiac output for as long as 8 hours (Mannion et al, 1987). Other studies using a totally implantable mock circulation with the conditioned fatigue-resistant skeletal muscle ventricular preparation have indicated that the ventricle can continuously pump at physiologic pressures of 104 mm Hg and continuous flow of 206 ml/min 2 weeks after implantation and continuous function (Acker et

Figure 54–115. The Pierce-Donarchy ventricular assist device shown with the polyurethane blood sac. Atrial cannulation for withdrawal is now preferred. (From Pennington, D. G., Bernhard, W. F., Golding, L. R., et al: Long-term follow-up of postcardiotomy patients with profound cardiogenic shock treated with ventricular assist devices. Circulation, 72[Suppl. 2]:216, 1985. By permission of the American Heart Association, Inc.)

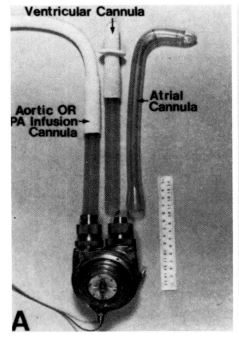

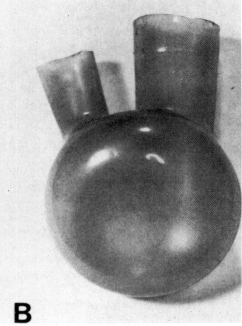

al, 1986). Whether an autologous, conditioned, fatigue-resistant skeletal muscle ventricle could be effective for clinical use requires further investigation.

PHYSIOLOGIC CONSIDERATIONS

Circulatory failure to any variable degree is caused by cardiac pump failure or peripheral vascular collapse. In most cases, circulatory failure necessitating the use of circulatory assistance occurs as a result of cardiac pump failure. In rare cases, circulatory failure occurs as a result of primary vasomotor peripheral arterial collapse, such as with toxic septicemia or profound metabolic disorders. In almost all clinical applications, the use of circulatory assist devices is temporary, and major emphasis is directed to correction of the underlying cause of circulatory failure.

To understand properly the mechanism of the beneficial effect of assisted circulation, when it is clinically indicated, and how to successfully manage patients in need of circulatory assistance, it is imperative to have a thorough understanding of normal and pathologic cardiac physiology. The principal roles of assisted circulation are essentially twofold: (1) assist circulation by augmenting cardiac output and maintaining the arterial blood pressure in a physiologically acceptable range (assist the mechanically failing heart) and (2) reduce myocardial ischemia and prevent progression of ischemia-related pathophysiologic changes while maintaining acceptable circulatory hemodynamics. The most common causes of the mechanically failing heart clinically are critical valvular heart disease and complications of severe myocardial ischemia and infarction.

Mechanically, the biophysics of cardiac function and circulation indicate that the right side of the heart and the left side of the heart are two pumps in series. The outputs of each pump (i.e., the left and right sides of the heart) must be equal, because an imbalance of output or failure of one places an untenable strain on the other and leads to progressive biventricular and circulatory failure (Burton, 1972). Balance to a significant degree can be achieved by compensatory physiologic mechanisms such as the Starling mechanism, but with progressive disease states or postcardiotomy cardiogenic shock, the pathophysiologic changes can overcome the compensatory mechanisms. This important physiologic concept has particularly appeared in recent experience with the clinical use of ventricular assist devices (Pennington et al, 1985b; Pierce, 1979).

Starling's law states that the work performance of the heart is directly proportional to the ventricular preload in terms of a pressure-volume relationship within a certain physiologic range (Fig. 54–116). By increasing ventricular volume loading and, by definition, simultaneously increasing ventricular end-diastolic filling pressure, the ventricular stroke volume and developed pressure increase. This relationship

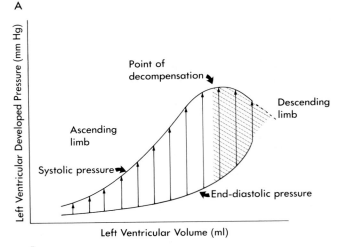

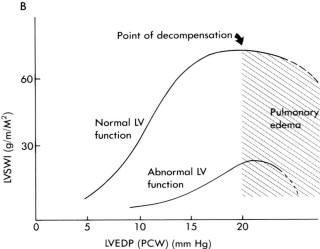

Figure 54–116. The Frank-Starling relationship (Starling's law). *A*, Increased ventricular end-diastolic volume results in increased ventricular developed pressure *(vertical arrows)* until overdistention and decompensation occur when further volume increases result in progressively declining developed pressure. *B*, The Starling mechanism, as it is evaluated in humans when blood pressure and stroke volume vary, is shown here. Clinically measurable physiologic parameters such as cardiac output, heart rate, mean arterial blood pressure, and pulmonary capillary wedge pressure (PCW) (closely equivalent to left ventricular end-diastolic pressure [LVEDP]) allow plotting left ventricular stroke work index (LVSWI, $g/m/M^2$) versus PCW. Normal left ventricular (LV) function with decompensation occurring at high filling (PCW) pressures (e.g., high output cardiac failure) is shown in the upper curve. A shift in the LV function curve down and to the right showing an abnormal LV function curve, which occurs in severe ischemic or valvular heart disease, is shown in *B*. The shaded area representing left-sided filling pressures (PCW) over 20 mm Hg is often associated clinically with pulmonary edema.

indicates that a pathologic state causing an increase in ventricular end-diastolic volume and pressure can be compensated by an increased cardiac output and developed pressure until the compensatory mechanism fails (the ventricle dilates to the point where it enters onto the descending limb of the Starling curve) (see Fig. 54–116). This compensatory mechanism is based primarily on the changes in force of contraction of the myocardial fibrils related to the diastolic resting length. With increased myocardial fibrillar diastolic resting length and tension, maximal fibrillar tension increases until resting length approaches twice its initial resting length. Stretch beyond this point causes decompensation with progressive loss of maximal active tension and concomitant increase in resting tension. When pathophysiologic changes progress to the point where either the left or the right ventricle pressure-volume relationships enter onto the descending limb of the Starling curve, progressive ventricular failure occurs, with clinical evidence of congestive failure and diminished cardiac output. These progressive pathologic changes can occur in disease states such as critical aortic stenosis, which causes a sharp increase in the required left ventricular developed pressure to achieve ejection, or severe ischemic heart disease, which results in decreased myocardial contractility and a shift of the Starling curve down and to the right (Fig. 54–117). Chronic pathologic processes such as left ventricular hypertrophy and left ventricular chamber dilatation also affect resting diastolic ventricular pressure-volume relationships. The normal end-diastolic ventricular pressure-volume curve shifts upward and to the left, reflecting significant loss of ventricular compliance (Fig. 54–118), based on the law of Laplace:

$$T = \frac{P \times R}{h}$$

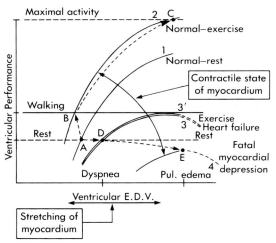

Figure 54–117. Starling's left ventricular function curves representing normal left ventricular function at rest and exercise (*upper curves* representing significant rise in ventricular performance with relatively small incremental increases in ventricular end-diastolic volume). Depressed left ventricular function that may occur with profound myocardial ischemia or myocardial infarction (*lower curves* showing marked deterioration in ventricular function with progressive loss of myocardial contractility even with relatively small increases in ventricular end-diastolic volume). Uninterrupted, a progressive deterioration in myocardial contractility leads to increased heart failure, low cardiac output, and eventually, fatal myocardial depression. (From Braunwald, E., Ross, J., Jr., and Sonnenblick, E. H.: Control of cardiac performance and cardiac output: A synthesis. *In* Braunwald, E., Ross, J., and Sonnenblick, E. H.: Mechanisms of Contraction of the Normal and Failing Heart. Boston, Little, Brown and Co., 1968.)

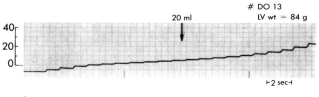

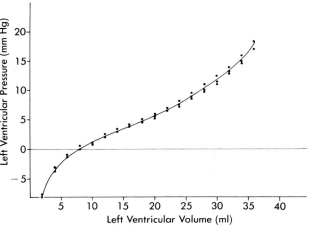

Figure 54–118. Pressure-volume relations in the potassium-arrested normal canine left ventricle showing normal compliance within a physiologic range of left ventricular diastolic (resting) volumes (flatter midportion of the lower curve) with progressive loss of ventricular compliance with increased ventricular distention at excessively high volumes (progressively increased pressures for smaller incremental volume increases). (From Ross, J., Jr., Covell, J. W., Sonnenblick, E. H., and Braunwald, E.: Contractile state of heart characterized by force-velocity relations in variably after-loaded and isovolumic beats. Circ. Res., *18*:149, 1966. By permission of the American Heart Association, Inc.)

where T = ventricular wall tension (dyne/cm), P = intraventricular pressure (dyne/cm), R = intracavitary radius (cm), and h = ventricular wall thickness (cm).

Although inotropic and afterload–preload-reducing pharmacologic agents can effectively change the Starling left ventricular function curve upward and to the left in clinical pathologic cardiac disease states by enhancing myocardial contractility and reducing elevated ventricular diastolic pressure and volume, the degree of functional improvement in patients with profound ventricular failure may be insufficient to affect recovery. It is in this clinical situation that circulatory assistance may be beneficial in achieving recovery, if the underlying pathologic process can be resolved or significantly mitigated during the time of circulatory assistance.

In most clinicopathologic disease states in which progressive ventricular failure threatens recovery, whether occurring secondary to progressive myocardial ischemia due to coronary artery occlusive disease or as a consequence of valvular heart disease, a pathophysiologic vicious cycle of events leads to progressive ventricular power failure (Fig. 54–119). The complex inter-relationship and interdependence of physiologic parameters result in a common pathway of progressive ventricular dysfunction characterized by increases in ventricular volume, resting

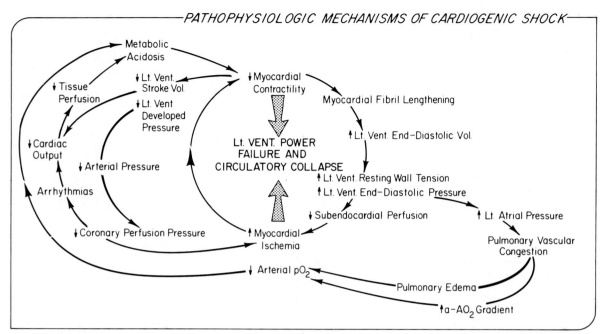

Figure 54–119. Schematic representation of the vicious cycle of pathophysiologic mechanisms of progressive left ventricular power failure. Progressive myocardial ischemia resulting in decreased myocardial contractility not only leads to a decrease in left ventricular stroke volume, cardiac output, and arterial pressure but also to myocardial fibril lengthening, increased left ventricular end-diastolic volume and pressure eventually leading to congestive failure, hypoxemia, and progressive subendocardial ischemia (see also Fig. 54–117).

pressure, and wall tension advancing to myocardial ischemia, reduced contractility, and falling cardiac output and arterial pressure. Progressive myocardial ischemia results when an increasing imbalance occurs between myocardial oxygen demand and supply (Fig. 54–120). The resultant decrease in myocardial contractility associated with the metabolic consequence of reduced myocardial high-energy phosphate stores (creatine phosphate and adenosine triphosphate) leads to a decrease in the velocity and extent of myofibrillar shortening and subsequent lengthening in the resting state to achieve the same active fiber-length tension (Frank-Starling mecha-

nism). The consequent increase in ventricular wall tension (law of Laplace) results in increased oxygen demand and consumption if oxygen delivery can meet the demand. Particularly when significant coronary artery occlusive disease or abnormalities of myocardial blood flow distribution to the subendocardium are present, such as after prolonged CPB and in aortic cross-clamp-induced global myocardial ischemia, oxygen delivery may be inadequate to meet the demand and progressive ventricular power failure ensues (see Fig. 54–119).

The principal determinant of myocardial oxygen consumption has been shown to be left ventricular

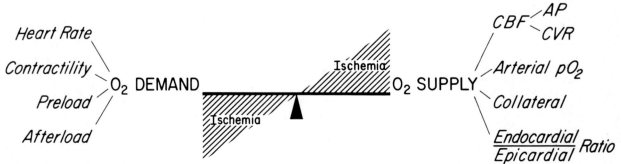

Figure 54–120. Schematic illustration of factors that influence myocardial oxygen demand (consumption) and myocardial oxygen supply. Any pathologic state that results in negatively altering determinants of myocardial oxygen supply contributes to myocardial ischemia as well as to excessive myocardial oxygen demand. A continuing imbalance between myocardial oxygen supply and demand results in progressive ischemia and, if profound for a sufficiently long period, will result in myocardial infarction. (AP = mean aortic pressure; CBF = coronary blood flow; CVR = coronary vascular resistance.)

pressure work (Sarnoff et al, 1958) (Fig. 54–121). Volume work (left ventricular stroke work) and heart rate, although significant, have a lesser contribution to myocardial oxygen demand. The findings of Graham and associates (1968) indicated that myocardial oxygen demand primarily depends on two physiologic variables: (1) left ventricular peak wall stress and (2) the intrinsic contractile state of the muscle, neither of which is directly correlated with ventricular stroke work or performance. Because myocardial contractility is depressed with progressive myocardial ischemia, a therapeutic attempt to reduce myocardial contractility to decrease myocardial oxygen demand, such as with beta-adrenergic blockade by using propranolol, could have an adverse effect on ventricular performance. Thus, therapeutically, reduction of myocardial oxygen demand is better accomplished by reduction of peak left ventricular wall stress or left ventricular afterload while attempting to maintain or improve contractility.

Optimal therapeutic management of severe left ventricular power failure associated with myocardial ischemia involves (1) reduction of myocardial oxygen consumption, (2) augmentation of coronary blood flow, and (3) improvement of ventricular performance. Although inotropic agents such as dobutamine, dopamine, isoproterenol, epinephrine, and norepinephrine increase myocardial contractility, cardiac output, heart rate, and arterial pressure, they cause an increase in myocardial oxygen demand, frequently under conditions in which myocardial oxygen delivery cannot be enhanced. Any attempted therapeutic

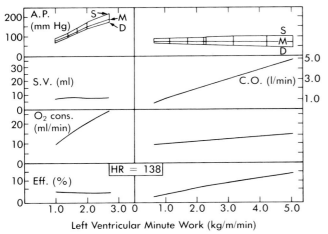

Figure 54–121. Relationship of myocardial oxygen consumption (demand) relative to increases in mean aortic pressure (afterload pressure work) with constant cardiac output compared with increases in cardiac output (volume work) with constant mean aortic pressure (afterload). Pressure work clearly is much more costly in terms of myocardial oxygen demand than volume work. Therapeutic interventions to relieve progressive myocardial ischemia thus should preferentially attempt to achieve reduction and stabilization of left ventricular afterload. (From Sarnoff, S. J., Braunwald, E., Welch, G. H., et al: Hemodynamic determinants of oxygen consumption of the heart with special reference to the tension-time index. Am. J. Physiol., 192:148, 1958.)

intervention that increases myocardial oxygen consumption may cause further myocardial ischemia and eventual deterioration despite temporary hemodynamic improvement. An effective therapeutic approach must be directed toward (1) reduction of left ventricular afterload and left ventricular wall tension, (2) augmentation of myocardial perfusion with normal distribution of flow, and (3) maintenance of physiologically adequate cardiac output.

Circulatory assistance by partial CPB, ventricular assistance, or IABC has been relatively effective in achieving all three physiologically therapeutic objectives. Left ventricular bypass and IABC reduce myocardial oxygen consumption in a direct linear relationship to reduction of peak left ventricular pressure (afterload) and ventricular tension-time index (Laks et al, 1977; Pennock et al, 1979; Powell et al, 1970). Clinical application of IABC in the treatment of progressive ventricular failure has been shown to significantly reduce left ventricular afterload and preload associated with increased cardiac output and hemodynamic improvement (Buckley et al, 1970). In the experimental study by Powell and associates (1970), IABC significantly increased coronary blood flow in the failing ischemic ventricle and also decreased left ventricular afterload, causing reduced left ventricular end-diastolic pressure and volume with resultant decreased wall tension (law of Laplace). This study further showed that IABC in the normal heart caused no significant change in coronary blood flow or left ventricular performance (cardiac output and developed pressure) but did cause reduction of left ventricular peak systolic pressure and left ventricular end-diastolic pressure independent of changes in coronary blood flow.

There is little evidence that circulatory assist devices directly augment coronary blood flow (Jett et al, 1981; Port et al, 1984; Williams et al, 1982). Although circulatory assistance, including IABC, may increase coronary blood flow in cardiogenic shock as a result of increased mean arterial pressure as well as diastolic arterial pressure, total coronary blood flow tends to be autoregulatory even in disease states, and the changes noted in total flow with circulatory assistance are related primarily to changes in myocardial oxygen demand. There is, however, good evidence that IABC may improve zonal myocardial perfusion, particularly of the subendocardial zone, by improving the endocardial viability ratio (EVR) (Fig. 54–122), defined as

$$EVR = \frac{DPTI}{TTI} = \frac{\text{diastolic pressure-time index}}{\text{time-tension index}} = \frac{\text{supply}}{\text{demand}}$$

It is questionable whether IABC can increase regional coronary blood flow to an ischemic region or improve subendocardial perfusion in the ischemic zone more than transiently. Cox and associates (1975) found initial improvement in ischemic zone perfusion with IABC but noted that the effect was transient. Similarly, Willerson and colleagues (1976) showed an

EFFECTS OF IABP ON MYOCARDIAL OXYGEN SUPPLY (DPTI) AND DEMAND (TTI)

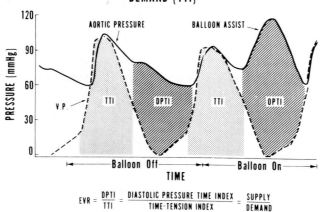

$$EVR = \frac{DPTI}{TTI} = \frac{DIASTOLIC\ PRESSURE\ TIME\ INDEX}{TIME\text{-}TENSION\ INDEX} = \frac{SUPPLY}{DEMAND}$$

Figure 54–122. Relationship of left ventricular time-tension index (TTI) and diastolic pressure-time index (DPTI) and the effect of diastolic counterpulsation achieved by IABP. The area beneath the ventricular pressure *(broken line)* represents the myocardial oxygen demand or TTI, whereas the area under the aortic pressure curve during diastole represents the driving force for myocardial oxygen supply (coronary blood flow) and the ratio of supply to demand (supply/demand) reflects an indication of endocardial viability (EVR = DPTI/TTI) because the subendocardial zone is the most sensitive myocardial zone in terms of developing ischemia. (From Bolooki, H.: Clinical Application of Intra-aortic Balloon Pump, 2nd ed. Mt. Kisco, NY, Futura Publishing Co., 1984.)

acute 20% increase in regional coronary blood flow to an ischemic myocardial zone. Subsequently, Jett and co-workers (1981) found no persistent increase in collateral blood flow to a region of myocardial ischemia 15 minutes after instituting IABC or pharmacologic interventions alone. However, by combining IABC with pharmacologic agents (mannitol, isosorbide dinitrate, or propranolol), collateral blood flow to the ischemic region was persistently improved during the period of treatment. These studies as well as the clinical experience of Sterling and associates (1984) and Fuchs and colleagues (1983) suggest that combined mechanical circulatory support and pharmacologic management in the treatment of myocardial ischemia are superior to either method alone. The studies of Weiss and co-workers (1984), using radionuclide ventriculograms, showed improved contractility and regional ejection fraction in ischemic areas in patients with acute myocardial infarction shock treated by IABC. The mechanism proposed improved perfusion to ischemic but not completely infarcted myocardium in the peri-infarction zone.

Attempts to reduce the extent of myocardial injury and to improve prognosis in acute myocardial infarction by instituting circulatory assistance by using IABC early in the course of evolving myocardial infarction were a logical extension of the potential indications for circulatory assistance. Experimental studies by Maroko and associates (1972) and Roberts and colleagues (1978) suggested that IABC started within 3 hours after acute coronary artery occlusion

could significantly reduce expected infarct size. Other studies (Haston and McNamara, 1979; Laas et al, 1980) using IABC in the experimental model have not substantiated a significant effect on infarct size. The clinical studies of a relatively small group of patients (Leinbach et al, 1978) suggested that IABC begun within 6 hours of onset of infarction could reduce the expected infarct size in patients with acute evolving anterior myocardial infarction, particularly in patients without total occlusion of the coronary artery in the distribution of the infarct. However, a recent randomized controlled trial of IABC in early myocardial infarction complicated by left ventricular failure indicated no significant modification of infarct size, mortality, or morbidity (O'Rourke et al, 1981). Similarly, a randomized prospective clinical trial comparing combined IABC and intravenous nitroglycerin for 4 to 5 days with routine treatment in patients with estimated extensive myocardium at risk for infarction as evidenced by a thallium defect score of 7 units or greater showed no significant differences in mortality or clinical outcome (Flaherty et al, 1985). In both of the latter studies the mean time that elapsed from the onset of infarction pain to the start of IABC was more than 6 hours. With established infarction (more than 6 hours after onset of persistent pain), circulatory assistance probably cannot modify the extent of infarction, but it may be effective in preventing extension of infarction to jeopardized ischemic myocardium by reducing left ventricular afterload and by possibly augmenting coronary blood flow to adjacent areas. Currently, clinical efforts to modify potential myocardial infarct size in acute evolving myocardial infarction (less than 6 hours from onset) are primarily limited to urgent therapeutic intervention using thrombolytic agents (streptokinase and tissue plasminogen activator), emergency percutaneous transluminal coronary angioplasty (PTCA), or surgical revascularization.

Refractory and potentially life-threatening ventricular arrhythmias associated with acute myocardial ischemia or infarction may be partially controlled by circulatory assistance (IABC) if that is the only intervention that is effective in controlling ischemia. Clinical experience with IABC in the management of refractory ventricular tachyarrhythmias associated with acute myocardial ischemia has been relatively small but encouraging (Hanson et al, 1980; Mundth et al, 1973). Reduction in left ventricular workload and myocardial oxygen consumption with consequent resolution of active myocardial ischemia appears to be the mechanism for effective circulatory assistance in the management of ventricular irritability.

CLINICAL INDICATIONS FOR AND RESULTS OF ASSISTED CIRCULATION

Clinical indications for the use of assisted circulation have continued to evolve during the past several years, particularly as related to (1) selection of patients, (2) changing methods of insertion of the intra-aortic balloon, and (3) type of circulatory assist device to be used (IABP versus ventricular assist device). Although the incidence of use and indications for assisted circulation vary considerably between institutions; overall, the trend nationally has been a gradual increase in use but a modest decrease in incidence per institution per patient admitted. In a composite experience of 440 patients treated with IABC during a 12-year period, Bolooki (1984) reported that the indications for IABC were 43% for postcardiotomy cardiogenic shock, 23% for myocardial infarction cardiogenic shock, 20% for elective prophylactic preoperative use, and 14% for miscellaneous indications. Pennington and associates (1983) reported that the overall incidence for instituting assisted circulation in 5,546 patients having cardiac surgical procedures during a period of 9 years (1973 to 1982) was 6.8%. With the development of more effective intraoperative myocardial preservation techniques, the incidence of intraoperative use of assisted circulation for postcardiotomy cardiogenic shock has decreased significantly. Similarly, the incidence of cardiogenic shock complicating acute myocardial infarction has decreased significantly as a result of improved medical therapy during the evolution of acute infarction. The general consensus is that early intracoronary or intravenous thrombolytic therapy in the course of evolving acute myocardial infarction has frequently prevented massive infarction and the potential complication of cardiogenic shock. Earlier and more effective medical management of patients with unstable angina using a combined therapeutic approach including intravenous nitrates, beta-adrenergic blocking agents, and calcium channel blockers frequently interrupts and resolves unstable myocardial ischemia (Mundth, 1976a). In medically refractory patients, IABC is indicated early in the clinical course with consideration of emergency cardiac catheterization and, in some cases, urgent coronary artery bypass revascularization or PTCA. Results with these approaches have been excellent (Alcan et al, 1983; Mundth et al, 1975; Pennington et al, 1983; Weintraub et al, 1979).

An analysis of the pooled data of five recent clinical series including 1,764 patients revealed that the most common indication for assisted circulation using IABC was intraoperative postcardiotomy cardiogenic shock (49%). Other indications for IABC were postmyocardial infarction cardiogenic shock (22%), medically refractory unstable angina (both preinfarction and postinfarction (15%), postoperative cardiogenic shock (7%), and preoperative elective IABC for severe left ventricular dysfunction or critical left main coronary artery disease (7%). Excluding more specialized modes of assisted circulation such as ventricular assist or total artificial heart devices, the current indications for assisted circulation using IABC are shown in Table 54–27.

TABLE 54–27. CURRENT INDICATIONS FOR ASSISTED CIRCULATION USING INTRA-AORTIC BALLOON COUNTERPULSATION

Postcardiotomy cardiogenic shock (inability to wean from CPB after cardiac procedures)
Complications of acute myocardial infarction:
  1. Cardiogenic shock secondary to left ventricular power failure
  2. Acute postinfarct ventricular septal defect with progressive left ventricular failure and cardiogenic shock
  3. Acute postinfarct papillary muscle rupture, mitral regurgitation, induced left ventricular failure, and cardiogenic shock
Myocardial ischemia refractory to medical therapy:
  1. Unstable preinfarction angina
  2. Unstable postinfarction angina
  3. Refractory ventricular tachyarrhythmias
Postoperative cardiogenic shock
Preoperative prophylaxis:
  1. Severe left ventricular dysfunction
  2. Critically severe left main coronary artery stenosis with unstable angina syndrome or associated with dominant right coronary artery proximal occlusion
  3. Combined severe valvular and coronary artery disease with severe left ventricular dysfunction or unstable angina syndrome
Failed coronary angioplasty with unstable myocardial ischemia (preoperative)

POSTCARDIOTOMY CARDIOGENIC SHOCK

Although more effective intraoperative myocardial preservation techniques have resulted in a significant decrease in the incidence of postcardiotomy cardiogenic shock and failure to wean from CPB, the increased numbers of high-risk patients with increasingly complex operative procedures have maintained this complication as the major indication for assisted circulation.

Postoperative left or right ventricular power failure occurs usually as a result of multiple factors, including (1) the preoperative hemodynamic status of the left ventricle, (2) the presence or absence of unstable myocardial ischemia preoperatively, (3) the incidence of complications during induction of anesthesia, (4) the duration of aortic cross-clamping (global myocardial ischemia period), (5) the effectiveness of hypothermic cardioplegia and myocardial preservation, (6) the degree of completeness and technical success of the surgical procedure, (7) the physiologic adequacy of CPB and metabolic management, and, undoubtedly, other unknown factors.

The reversibility of postcardiotomy ventricular power failure appears to depend primarily on whether a potentially reversible acute ischemic injury has occurred and on prompt, effective intervention by using pharmacologic and circulatory assist support (Buckley et al, 1973; Park et al, 1986; Pennington et al, 1985a; Phillips and Bregman, 1977). The best clinical results also appear to be associated with reducing the time delay before instituting assisted circulation when a patient has shown difficulty in being weaned from CPB and with the use of biventricular assistance when there is evidence of significant right ventricular dysfunction. Although survival may be diminished when postcardiotomy cardiogenic shock develops in patients with preoperatively known severe left or right ventricular dysfunction, overall results indicate little correlation between successful CPB weaning or survival and preoperative ventricular function (Pennington et al, 1985b). Postoperative right ventricular failure was not necessarily related to preoperative right ventricular dysfunction, and perioperative myocardial injury appeared to be the major factor in the development of postoperative ventricular failure (Pennington et al, 1985a). Other researchers (McEnany et al, 1978; Scanlon et al, 1976) reported that the greatest likelihood of success by using only IABC for postcardiotomy cardiogenic shock occurred in patients with left ventricular hypertrophy and an identifiable intraoperative ischemic event. Sturm and associates (1981) reported improved survival for IABP treatment of postoperative low-output syndrome in patients with only coronary artery disease compared with patients with valvular disease or combined valvular and coronary artery disease. Similarly, Downing and associates (1986) reported relatively poor early (50%) and late 1-year survival (38%) in patients with valvular disease requiring IABC for postcardiotomy cardiogenic shock and difficult weaning from CPB. In most series, the prompt use of IABC for postcardiotomy cardiogenic shock resulted in successful weaning from CPB in 75 to 85% of patients, with a hospital survival of approximately 55% (Bolooki, 1984; Buckley et al, 1973; Golding et al, 1980; Kaiser et al, 1976; Macoviak et al, 1979; Scanlon et al, 1976). The overall survival rate of 55% is reasonably impressive, considering the expected almost 100% mortality of patients who fail to wean readily from CPB despite inotropic support. The late follow-up of hospital survivors in this group of patients showed a 2-year actuarial survival of 96%, with excellent symptomatic relief and functional status (Golding et al, 1980). This clinical experience clearly emphasizes the potential reversibility of postcardiotomy cardiogenic shock when circulatory support is instituted promptly, providing maintenance of physiologically adequate circulation with simultaneous reduction of left and right ventricular workload.

As clinical experience has been gained, it has been shown that if a patient cannot be weaned satisfactorily from CPB by using inotropic drug support and vasodilatory afterload-reducing agents, circulatory assistance should be started promptly to achieve the optimal potential for survival (Phillips and Bregman, 1977). The degree of hemodynamic deterioration at the time of institution of assisted circulation was predictive of survival by Norman and associates (1977). They found that hemodynamically defined Class A patients (cardiac index CI >2.1 l/min/m² and systemic vascular resistance [SVR]* <2,100 dyn-sec/cm⁵) on IABC assistance had an 80% survival, whereas Class C patients (CI <2.1 l/min/m² with SVR >2,100 dyn-sec/cm⁵ or CI <1.2 l/min/m² regardless of SVR) all expired despite continued IABC if they remained in hemodynamically defined Class C for 12 hours. Sturm and associates (1981) achieved a significant improvement in survival from postcardiotomy cardiogenic shock by combining pharmacologic management with IABC and careful volume (preload) adjustment. Inotropic support with intravenous dopamine or dobutamine plus afterload reduction with intravenous sodium nitroprusside in ten patients during IABC support resulted in a significant increase in CI from a mean of 1.6 to 2.5 l/min/m² (p <0.01) and a decrease in SVR from 2,774 to 1,439 dyn-sec/cm⁵ (p <0.02). Hemodynamic Class C patients were successfully reassigned to Class A, and all were later weaned from IABC and pharmacologic support.

Predominant right ventricular power failure has increasingly been recognized as being a significant cause of postcardiotomy cardiogenic shock. Perioperative right ventricular power failure may occur from ischemic injury in the distribution of the right coronary artery circulation as a result of profound interventricular septal dysfunction or inadequate right ventricular myocardial preservation during intraoperative global ischemia. With profound cardiogenic shock due to severe right ventricular power failure, left ventricular failure usually soon ensues if it is not already present. Conventional IABC may significantly benefit right ventricular failure but, not infrequently, is insufficient to allow successful weaning of the patient from CPB, particularly if a large component of left ventricular failure is not present.

Pulmonary arterial balloon counterpulsation (PABC) has been shown experimentally and clinically to improve right ventricular output in the presence of right ventricular failure (Flege et al, 1984; Jett et al, 1983; Opravil et al, 1984; failure (Flege et al, 1984; Jett et al, 1983; Miller et al, 1980; Moran et al, 1984; Spence et al, 1985). In experimental studies with profound right ventricular failure, PABC has resulted in a significant increase in cardiac output, reduction in peak right ventricular systolic pressure, decrease in right ventricular end-diastolic pressure and mean right atrial pressure, decrease in right ventricular systolic pressure-time index, associated with increased right ventricular stroke work index and aortic systolic pressure (Jett et al, 1983; Opravil et al, 1984; Spence et al, 1985). Clinical applications have shown similar hemodynamic benefit, by allowing weaning from CPB, but overall salvage and long-term recovery

---

*SVR = $\dfrac{(BP - CVP \times 80)}{CO}$

Normal range = 1,100 to 1,500 dyn-sec/cm⁵
where BP = mean arterial blood pressure (mm Hg), CVP = mean central venous pressure (mm Hg), and CO = cardiac output (l/min).

are still relatively low in the small series reported (two of seven; Flege et al, 1984; Miller et al, 1980; Moran et al, 1984; Symbas et al, 1985) (Fig. 54–123). Recent experimental studies have shown that although PABC improves hemodynamics significantly compared with passive flow through the pulmonary artery, because of a right atrial to left atrial pressure gradient, the CI achieved with PABC in studies of profound right ventricular failure was marginally adequate (Gaines et al, 1984; Jett et al, 1987; Spence et al, 1985). Use of a RVAD significantly improved hemodynamic indices in these experimental studies and in many cases improved cardiac indices to a level for potential recovery (Gaines et al, 1984; Jett et al, 1987). Currently, in most institutions using ventricular assist devices for postcardiotomy cardiogenic shock for refractory shock despite IABC, right ventricular or biventricular assist is initiated in patients with any significant degree of right ventricular failure.

Despite the potential effectiveness of IABC and pharmacologic support for management of postcar-

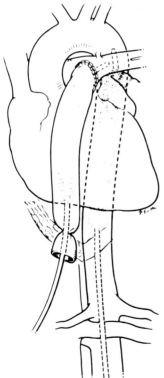

Figure 54–123. PABC along with IABC for severe right ventricular power failure in patients with severe biventricular failure and postcardiotomy shock. The intra-aortic balloon is inserted by a standard common femoral artery approach. The pulmonary artery balloon catheter is inserted via a 20-mm woven Dacron graft sewn to the main pulmonary artery after making a pulmonary arteriotomy. Balloon counterpulsation within the distally occluded pulmonary artery graft reservoir results in effective counterpulsation in the relatively short main pulmonary artery. (Reprinted with permission from The Society of Thoracic Surgeons [The Annals of Thoracic Surgery, Vol. 39, 1985, p. 437.])

diotomy cardiogenic shock, approximately 15% of patients cannot be effectively weaned from CPB. In a retrospective study of 14,168 patients having cardiac procedures during a 4-year period at the Texas Heart Institute, McGee and associates (1980) reported that 326 patients (2.3%) had difficulty in weaning from CPB and were managed by IABC and pharmacologic support; 94 patients (29%) failed to respond. In this series, 21 patients had implantation of an abdominal left ventricular apical-aortic assist device (LVAD), and three survived. Subsequent clinical investigations have been accomplished primarily with two types of ventricular assist devices: the vortex centrifugal pump, which was typified by the Biomedicus vortex centrifugal pump,* or the Medtronic centrifugal pump† and the Pierce-Donarchy ventricular assist device.‡ Pierce and co-workers (1981) reported the clinical use of Pierce-Donarchy ventricular assist devices in 14 patients because of inability to be weaned from CPB despite IABC support. LVAD was used in ten patients, biventricular assist in three patients, and isolated RVAD plus IABC in one patient. Ventricular assistance was continued 1 hour to 8 days, with two surviving patients of four weaned from the ventricular assist device. Failures were associated with progressive right ventricular failure, excessive bleeding, or critical inflow obstruction at the apical ventricular cannulation site. Golding and associates (1982) reported six patients treated with a Medtronic centrifugal pump LVAD after failing to be weaned from CPB despite IABC and pharmacologic support. LVAD support was continued for 72 to 168 hours, and five of the six patients could be weaned from the LVAD device. Two patients survived after approximately 72 hours of LVAD support. Subsequently, Pennington and associates (1985a), Park and colleagues (1986), and Zumbro and co-workers (1987) have reported improved results, particularly related to earlier application and increased early use of biventricular assistance in patients showing right ventricular failure as well as left ventricular power failure (Table 54–28). Significant complications of bleeding, neurologic complications, respiratory insufficiency, renal failure, and sepsis were frequent.

These data suggest that approximately one-third of patients with severe postcardiotomy cardiogenic shock refractory to IABC and failure to wean from CPB can be salvaged with left ventricular assistance, right ventricular assistance, or biventricular assistance. Improved results achieving almost 50% long-term survival have been associated with earlier institution of ventricular assistance and more frequent use of biventricular assistance (Park et al, 1986; Pennington et al, 1985a). Prediction of survival appears to be more related to the type and extent of perioperative myocardial injury than to the patient's pre-

*Biomedicus, Inc., Eden Prairie, MN.
†Medtronic Corp., Minneapolis, MN.
‡Thoratex Corp., Berkeley, CA.

TABLE 54–28. CLINICAL RESULTS IN MECHANICAL VENTRICULAR ASSIST FOR POSTCARDIOTOMY CARDIOGENIC SHOCK*

Type of Device	No. of Patients	No. Weaned	No. Discharged From Hospital
LVAD	80	42 (52%)	25 (31%)
RVAD	11	7 (64%)	6 (54%)
Biventricular	20	10 (50%)	4 (20%)
Total	111	59 (54%)	35 (32%)

*Pooled data from Golding and associates (1982), Pennington and associates (1985a), Park and associates (1986), and Zumbro and associates (1987).

operative ventricular functional status. Recent experimental studies have suggested that IABC plus inotropic support and left ventricular assistance provides adequate support of the circulation, but after 3 hours of assisted circulation significant differences were seen. Significantly greater decreases in left ventricular compliance and systolic function were noted in association with histologic evidence of greater myocardial necrosis in the IABC group compared with the group with early institution of an LVAD (Mickleborough et al, 1987). Further improvement in patient salvage and long-term survival may also be expected with reduction of the high incidence of the serious complications that have been associated with ventricular assistance. In most clinical series reported, multiorgan failure occurred in approximately 80% of patients with postcardiotomy shock who were treated with ventricular assistance. Use of heparin-bonded tubing and low-dose heparin may help to reduce the prevalent excess bleeding problems and thus the severe pulmonary complications of multiple transfusions.

COMPLICATIONS OF ACUTE MYOCARDIAL INFARCTION

Despite the decrease in the incidence of cardiogenic shock complicating acute myocardial infarction with current techniques of medical management including early invasive therapy with thrombolytic agents, PTCA, or urgent surgical revascularization, the occurrence of postinfarction cardiogenic shock is usually an indication for circulatory assistance (Bolooki, 1984; McEnany et al, 1978).

Current concepts for management of patients who have developed postinfarction cardiogenic shock recommend use of assisted circulation, predominantly IABC, for supportive therapy in preparation for more definitive management including urgent coronary artery bypass revascularization or PTCA (Goldberger et al, 1986; Mundth, 1977; Sanfelippo, 1986). In recent years, IABC combined with pharmacologic support and operative intervention has produced significant improvement, particularly when the combined treatment is begun early in the

course of postinfarction shock (DeWood et al, 1980; Mundth and Austen, 1978; Pierri et al, 1980; Sanfelippo, 1986). The mortality for severe postinfarction (hemodynamic Class C) cardiogenic shock treated medically is still high, greater than 90% (Bolooki, 1984; Leinbach et al, 1973; Norman et al, 1977). Similarly, mortality with medical therapy plus IABC for patients with profound postinfarction cardiogenic shock (Class IV) with hemodynamic balloon dependence has remained essentially 100% (Bolooki, 1984). Bolooki reported that of 30 balloon-dependent patients with cardiogenic shock treated by IABC plus pharmacologic support, all died within 40 days of onset of shock; 26 patients died in less than 1 week. Even in Class II and III patients with cardiogenic shock successfully weaned from IABC, less than 45% were alive after 6 months. Results for combined IABC and revascularization for profound cardiogenic shock, however, have shown significant improvement in long-term survival, which is now almost 50 to 60% (Bolooki, 1984; Mundth and Austen, 1978).

Postinfarction cardiogenic shock may result from extensive left ventricular infarction with primary ventricular power failure, from acute ventricular septal rupture, or from papillary muscle rupture. In all patients, the development of cardiogenic shock is characterized by (1) CI less than 2 l/min/m², (2) hypotension with mean arterial pressure less than 60 mm Hg, and (3) elevated pulmonary capillary wedge pressure greater than 20 mm Hg. Cardiogenic shock usually occurs as a progressive vicious cycle of pathophysiologic events (see Fig. 54–119). Successful therapeutic intervention depends on interruption of these events by preventing further ischemic myocardial damage and by improving myocardial perfusion, thus facilitating improved myocardial function of ischemic but viable myocardium (Mundth, 1976a,b). IABC has been shown to achieve these therapeutic goals, with reversal of cardiogenic shock temporarily in at least 75% of patients (Bolooki, 1984; DeWood et al, 1980; Dunkman et al, 1972; Weiss et al, 1984). The most important hemodynamic parameters determining prognosis in cardiogenic shock have been CI, left ventricular preload (pulmonary capillary wedge pressure), and SVR. Combined IABC and pharmacologic support (inotropic drugs plus afterload-reducing agents) have been very effective in the treatment of severe left ventricular power failure but rarely can achieve long-term recovery in patients with profound Class IV (Class C) cardiogenic shock. In this category of patients, urgent surgical intervention with coronary artery revascularization or repair of mechanical defects such as ventricular septal defect, mitral regurgitation secondary to papillary muscle rupture, or acute left ventricular aneurysm is essential to achieve success (Mundth, 1977). Although the results of IABC and early surgical intervention for cardiogenic shock resulting from mechanical complications of myocardial infarction appear to be slightly better than for cardiogenic shock secondary to left ventricular power failure alone, the difference does not appear to be significant (Goldberger et al, 1986; Mundth and Austen, 1978).

Long-term follow-up of patients with postinfarction cardiogenic shock treated by prompt institution of assisted circulation and surgical intervention has indicated overall acceptable results in terms of survival and functional status (Pierri et al, 1980; Radford et al, 1981). Pierri and associates (1980) reported 47% survival of 34 patients 2 years after IABC and urgent coronary bypass. Exercise testing in 13 of the 16 surviving patients revealed substantial exercise capacity with minimal residual symptoms, and six patients returned to their former occupations. The acceptable early and late survival and functional status in these patients support the reason for early institution of assisted circulation and surgical management in carefully selected patients with cardiogenic shock complicating acute myocardial infarction. Improvement in ventricular assist devices and in the effective use of percutaneously introduced assist devices may produce even better results, particularly with prompt intervention using ventricular assistance in patients with profound cardiogenic shock.

MYOCARDIAL ISCHEMIA REFRACTORY TO MEDICAL THERAPY

Unstable angina is a common diagnostic term with various definitions including crescendo angina and angina that do not respond readily to conventional outpatient medication. Although *preinfarction angina* is a term that can be applied only retrospectively, numerous clinical studies have indicated that an identifiable clinical syndrome of unstable angina is associated with an increased incidence of subsequent acute myocardial infarction and death (Cox et al, 1973; Gazes et al, 1973; Swan, 1974). The current accepted definition of unstable angina includes three parameters: (1) one or more prolonged episodes (> 30 minutes) of chest pain at rest, (2) documentation of ST-T wave ECG changes of ischemia during pain, and (3) exclusion of acute myocardial infarction on the basis of serial ECG tracings and serum creatine phosphokinase-MB enzymes (Russell et al, 1978).

The sine qua non of effective treatment of unstable angina is to achieve prompt relief of myocardial ischemia. Medical therapy in many cases is effective by using intravenous nitroglycerin, afterload reducing agents, adrenergic blocking agents, and calcium channel blockers. When myocardial ischemia remains refractory to the various modes of medical therapy, the use of assisted circulation, particularly in the form of IABC, has proved to be very successful (Aroesty et al, 1979; Fuchs et al, 1983; Gold et al, 1973; Maroko et al, 1972; Williams et al, 1982). Gold and associates (1973) indicated that recurrent episodes of myocardial ischemia were completely resolved by IABC in more than 75% of patients. Nichols and associates (1973) showed significant improve-

ment in abnormal left ventricular contractility during IABC by using multigated nuclear cardiac scanning techniques. To achieve permanent resolution, relatively urgent coronary artery bypass revascularization or PTCA is required (Mundth et al, 1975; Weintraub and Aroesty, 1976). The overall clinical results of combined IABC and urgent revascularization have been excellent for this higher-risk group, with an operative mortality of 1.7 to 5% and a low perioperative infarction incidence of 2.2 to 6.6% (Langou et al, 1978; Levine et al, 1978; Weintraub et al, 1979). Long-term follow-up of patients has indicated excellent functional results and relatively low late mortality. Weintraub and associates (1979) reported more than 90% of patients classified in New York Heart Association functional Class I or II at a mean follow-up time of 31 months. Levine and co-workers (1978) reported a 4.5% late mortality over a mean 38-month follow-up period, with 93% of the surviving patients having no significant angina.

Currently, the accepted approach to patients with medically refractory unstable angina is prompt intervention to interrupt myocardial ischemia with IABC followed by prompt invasive intervention to improve myocardial perfusion. In selected patients, PTCA may be the preferred technique, particularly in patients with one- or two-vessel coronary artery disease. In patients with multivessel coronary artery disease, significant left main disease, or anatomic lesions unsuitable for PTCA, urgent coronary bypass revascularization is indicated. Although difficult to prove, this approach has undoubtedly decreased the incidence of myocardial infarction in patients with unstable or "preinfarction" angina.

Unstable angina that is refractory to medical treatment after myocardial infarction is managed similarly. Although one would expect the risk, and thus mortality, of revascularization to be higher in this group of patients, clinical experience has shown that the risk is little different from that in patients with unstable angina without infarction when IABC and reperfusion are instituted promptly (Bardet et al, 1977; Levine et al, 1978; Mundth, 1976a,b). Brundage and associates (1980) reported similarly low operative mortality for urgent revascularization without IABC but did note a higher perioperative myocardial infarction rate of 13.6%. When not contraindicated because of a high potential for balloon-related complications, IABC is preferable for the preoperative and perioperative management of patients with postinfarction refractory and unstable angina, in terms of reducing both perioperative myocardial injury and operative mortality.

Medically refractory ventricular ectopy with malignant ventricular tachyarrhythmia associated with intermittent severe myocardial ischemia may be benefited by assisted circulation by virtue of resolution of the severe ischemia. Assisted circulation in this situation has generally been accomplished with IABC (Hanson et al, 1980; Mundth et al, 1973). Because of the recurrent nature of myocardial ischemia, prompt revascularization achieved by coronary artery bypass grafts or PTCA is indicated (Hanson et al, 1980). Current surgical approaches use preoperative electrophysiologic mapping, particularly in postinfarction patients, to attempt to localize irritable ectopy trigger foci and facilitate operative obliteration by combined coronary artery revascularization and subendocardial myocardial resection (Guiraudon et al, 1978; Harken et al, 1979). In the experience of Hanson and associates (1980), refractory ventricular irritability after infarction was improved by IABC in 86% of patients and totally resolved in 55%. Sixty-eight per cent of the patients with ventricular irritability treated by IABC required surgical intervention because of recurrent refractory ventricular irritability or hemodynamic deterioration when IABC weaning was attempted. Operative survival was 47%, with no late deaths in the combined IABC surgically treated patients at an average follow-up of 46 months. Clearly, assisted circulation may be of considerable benefit in the management of patients with ischemia-related refractory ventricular arrhythmias.

CARDIOGENIC SHOCK POSTOPERATIVELY OR AFTER FAILED CORONARY ANGIOPLASTY (PTCA)

Similar indications apply to postoperative cardiogenic shock after failed PTCA as with postcardiotomy cardiogenic shock. Postoperative cardiogenic shock usually occurs in the intensive care unit, and if excessive bleeding with hypotension or cardiac tamponade is excluded, the usual cause is related to or is a result of severe myocardial ischemia (Bolooki, 1984; Buckley et al, 1973). Delayed occurrence of cardiogenic shock in a patient successfully weaned from CPB may be secondary to an acute ischemic event, such as acute coronary artery bypass occlusion or coronary/graft spasm, but may also occur gradually as a result of intraoperative myocardial ischemic injury or inadequate myocardial preservation. Determining the exact cause of postoperative cardiogenic shock may be difficult, and the essential task is to attempt to reverse the hemodynamic deterioration. Prompt institution of circulatory assistance when pharmacologic inotropic support and correction of metabolic disorders have been accomplished is essential to improve cardiac output and correct hypotension before further deterioration and potential cardiac arrest occur. Stabilization can usually be achieved with IABC. When hemodynamic deterioration continues despite IABC, surgical exploration is generally indicated to assess coronary bypass graft function of the previous coronary artery revascularization or allow use of ventricular assist devices. In some cases, thrombectomy of an acutely thrombosed coronary bypass graft with the adjunct of IABC support facilitates recovery. On occasion, revision of the graft may be required with full CPB support. In

any case, early intervention with assisted circulation allows the best potential for a staged, controlled approach and for eventual recovery. In some cases when coronary artery spasm is suspected as being a cause of profound postoperative cardiogenic shock, assisted circulation with IABC has allowed transport of the patient to the cardiac catheterization laboratory for acute diagnostic study and intracoronary administration of nitroglycerin to counteract severe coronary artery spasm.

Assisted circulation with IABC has been a helpful adjunct for management of patients with failed PTCA who have developed acute ischemia or evolving myocardial infarction, usually caused by acute coronary artery dissection or occlusion. Prompt institution of IABC is beneficial in stabilizing hemodynamic deterioration or resolving ischemia and reducing the extent of myocardial injury in these patients in the interval from the onset of ischemic injury in the catheterization laboratory to the time of emergent surgical coronary revascularization (Alcan et al, 1983). The author recommends that IABC be promptly instituted in the absence of specific contraindications in all patients in whom PTCA has failed and severe myocardial ischemia or hemodynamic deterioration develops.

ELECTIVE PREOPERATIVE ASSISTED CIRCULATION

Elective preoperative insertion of the IABP as a prophylactic measure is still controversial (Cooper et al, 1977b; Craver et al, 1979; Mundth, 1976; Rajai et al, 1978). The primary indication for consideration of elective prophylactic preoperative IABC is severe left ventricular dysfunction associated with low cardiac output or critical left main coronary artery disease. Poor left ventricular function preoperatively (left ventricular ejection fraction <30%), particularly when associated with a CI of less than 2 l/min/m^2, has been associated with increased operative mortality in many reported series, with improved results using elective preoperative IABC (Bolooki, 1984; Feola et al, 1977; Hochberg et al, 1983; Manly et al, 1976; Zubiate et al, 1977). Bolooki (1984) indicated a reduction of mortality in this category of patients, from 14% to less than 7%, when elective preoperative IABC was used.

Elective use of IABC in patients with critical left main coronary artery disease or with unstable angina that does not respond to medical therapy is more controversial (Cooper et al, 1977b; Craver et al, 1979; Rajai et al, 1978). The tendency in recent years has been toward decreased use for these indications in most institutions and has been related to improved results of coronary bypass in these patients as a result of advances in anesthesia management, improved myocardial preservation technique, and improved surgical techniques.

The significant incidence of major complications of IABC in large series has mandated careful selection of indications for its use despite significant improvement in techniques of insertion including percutaneous insertion, guidewire insertion with central lumen balloon catheter, and small-diameter balloon catheters (Goldberger et al, 1986; Harvey et al, 1981; Hauser et al, 1982; McEnany et al, 1978; Pennington et al, 1983).

In the author's opinion, the principal indications for elective preoperative IABC are limited to the following:

1. Severe left ventricular dysfunction with left ventricular ejection fraction less than 30% *associated* with low CI, less than 2.

2. Critical (> 80%) left main coronary artery stenosis *associated* with occlusion of a dominant right coronary artery and demonstrated unstable angina.

3. Absence of contraindication such as severe arterial occlusive disease of the lower extremities, abdominal aortic aneurysm, or inability to use heparin anticoagulation safely.

TECHNICAL ASPECTS OF ASSISTED CIRCULATION

Undoubtedly, the most significant technical developments in the field of assisted circulation are the improvements in the design and the biocompatible materials used in ventricular assist devices during the last several years. Surgeons now have the opportunity to use effective and increasingly safe devices for ventricular and biventricular support. Another important development in circulatory assistance was the refinement of a relatively safe and effective percutaneous method for intra-aortic balloon catheter insertion with or without a guidewire-directed central lumen catheter (Bregman and Casarella, 1980; Lundell et al, 1981; Subramanian et al, 1980). The development of the percutaneous technique of IABP catheter insertion greatly expanded the clinical use of IABC that previously required a surgical team to insert the balloon catheter by exposure of the common femoral artery. Since this development, most balloon catheters have been inserted by cardiologists or, in some cases by surgeons, in a cardiac catheterization laboratory, in critical care units, or in operating rooms with fluoroscopic control when available. Although the percutaneous balloon catheter was designed to improve the ease of insertion and also to decrease the complications associated with surgical insertion, its clinical use in greater numbers and diverse types of patients has failed to reduce the rate of complications and has paradoxically increased the incidence of major complications (Grayzel, 1982; Hauser et al, 1982; McCabe et al, 1978). Numerous technical pitfalls have resulted in the persistent considerable complication rate of 15 to 20% and include (1) inadvertent puncture and catheter insertion through the superficial femoral artery, causing an increased incidence of vascular ischemia; (2) elevation of atheromatous plaque, arterial wall injury, or distal ischemia caused by the more rigid percutaneous catheter; and (3) potential aortic dissection or puncture with possibly disastrous results, also because of the rigid catheter.

In approximately 5 to 10% of patients, the balloon catheter cannot be successfully inserted by the femoral artery approach (Harvey et al, 1981; McEnany et al, 1978). When postcardiotomy cardiogenic shock occurs with consequent difficulty in weaning from CPB, transthoracic IABP insertion has been accomplished successfully in those patients in whom IABP insertion via the femoral artery route has been impossible (Bonchek and Olinger, 1981; Gueldner and Lawrence, 1975; McGeehan et al, 1987). By using a vascular partially occlusive clamp, a 10-mm polytetrafluoroethylene (PTFE) prosthetic graft is sutured to the ascending aorta after an aortotomy is made. The balloon is then inserted through the PTFE graft, and the distal end of the graft is ligated tightly around the balloon catheter. The balloon catheter can be brought out through the lower portion of the incision. In the intensive care unit, removal is accomplished with a relatively minor procedure done through the lower portion of the incision below the sternum (McGeehan et al, 1987). McGeehan and colleagues reported 39 patients who required transthoracic IABC when percutaneous attempts failed. Overall survival was 44%; 81% survived after successful weaning from IABC support. Complications occurred in 13%, including cerebrovascular accident, balloon rupture, and mediastinitis, in descending order of occurrence.

Another, perhaps simpler, approach to transthoracic IABP insertion uses simple purse-string sutures, which may be tied tightly or like a tourniquet and placed in the proximal portion of the aortic arch (Balderman et al, 1980; Bonchek and Olinger, 1981; Melvin and Goldman, 1982). Although they facilitate insertion, particularly in a patient with multiple bypass grafts and aortic cannulation for CPB, these techniques mandate a second sternotomy for removal.

COMPLICATIONS OF ASSISTED CIRCULATION

Although the complications of assisted circulation are similar regardless of the device or system used, some complications are specific to the type of assist device used (e.g., IABP versus ventricular assist devices). The overall complication rate in patients who require circulatory assistance tends to be high because many of these patients are critically ill. In general, this discussion is directed toward complications related to assist devices and not overall complications such as multiorgan failure from prolonged low cardiac output.

COMPLICATIONS OF INTRA-AORTIC BALLOON COUNTERPULSATION

The incidence of major complications related to IABP insertion and IABC varies in different clinical series, from 8 to 30% (Bolooki, 1984; Goldberger et al, 1986; Goldman et al, 1982; Grayzel, 1982; Harvey et al, 1981; Hauser et al, 1982; Leinbach et al, 1982; Martin et al, 1983; McEnany et al, 1978; Pennington et al, 1983; Vignola et al, 1981). Major complications in order of frequency are shown in Table 54–29.

Ischemic complications of the limbs paradoxically have not been decreased by use of the percutaneous IABP catheter technique, but rather have increased (Goldberger et al, 1986; Harvey et al, 1981; Martin et al, 1983). IABP-related complications occurred in 31% of patients with the percutaneous route versus 10% with the surgical route (Goldberger et al, 1986). It has become clear that with the increased ease and success of percutaneous insertion that more patients with significant peripheral vascular disease have had successful percutaneous IABP placement, but a substantial number of these patients developed vascular complications of IABC (Goldberger et al, 1986; Hauser et al, 1982; Martin et al, 1983). Although transient limb ischemia may resolve on removal of the IABP catheter, approximately 60% of patients with significant limb ischemia during IABC will require surgical intervention and vascular repair (Todd et al, 1983).

The use of heparin anticoagulation during IABC is controversial. Some authors have recommended low-molecular-weight dextran without heparinization (Harvey et al, 1981; Pennington et al, 1983; Perler et al, 1983; Todd et al, 1983), particularly in postoperative patients. Other physicians (Bemis et al, 1981; Vignola et al, 1981) have recommended heparinization in all patients, maintaining the activated clotting time approximately 1 1/2 to 2 times normal. Although the incidence of major vascular complications varies in the reported series, it is 7 to 15% when heparin anticoagulation is not used postoperatively (Pennington et al, 1983; Perler et al, 1983; Todd et al, 1983), whereas the incidence is approximately 5% when heparinization is used exclusively (Grayzel et al, 1981; Hauser et al, 1982). Vignola and associates (1981)

reported femoral arterial thrombosis in 5 of 54 patients (10.2%), but on analyzing the data found that in two patients with this complication no heparin was used and anticoagulation was inadequate in three patients. Femoral arterial thrombosis did not occur in 49 patients who were adequately anticoagulated. In the author's opinion, heparin anticoagulation should be used at therapeutic levels in all patients with IABC, including postoperative patients. In the postoperative period, an intravenous heparin drip is initiated as soon as cumulative chest tube drainage is less than 100 ml/hr, when the patient's partial thromboplastin time is less than 30 seconds, and preferably within 2 to 4 hours postoperatively.

A useful technique for facilitating subsequent IABP insertion for patients having cardiac catheterization and coronary angiographic study is to obtain a limited abdominal aortogram outlining the aortoiliofemoral arterial anatomy before withdrawing the angiographic catheter. This technique facilitates selection of the preferred side for IABP insertion if required and is useful particularly in patients with critical disease when it is quite likely that IABC will be used (Bahn et al, 1979, Bemis et al, 1981, Vignola et al, 1981). The use of a longer (16-inch) introducer sheath for IABP has also resulted in a significant decrease in the number of arterial injuries precipitating subsequent limb ischemia, arterial dissection, or perforation (Bemis et al, 1981; Grayzel, 1982; Vignola et al, 1981). Similarly, the use of a central lumen, wire-guided IABP catheter has reduced the incidence of arterial injury and dissection as reported by Leinbach and associates (1982), but does not eliminate the potential for limb ischemia secondary to iliofemoral arterial thrombosis (5% in this series of patients).

When the use of IABC seems to be essential for successful management of a critically ill patient with known severe peripheral vascular disease, it is this author's opinion that the IABP should be inserted some hours before a contemplated surgical procedure so that the limb can be carefully observed. If progressive ischemia occurs, it may be necessary to construct a crossover femoral-femoral bypass graft before operation to prevent progressive ischemia to the point of loss of viability of the limb during the cardiac procedure. Progressive loss of viability of an extremity during cardiac operations can have an extremely deleterious effect associated with progressively severe metabolic acidosis and release of negatively inotropic anaerobic metabolites.

In a necropsy study of 45 patients who died after institution of IABC, Isner and associates (1980) found that 36% had significant complications of IABP insertion at necropsy, including aortic dissection, arterial perforation, thrombi, and emboli. Of the significant complications found, only 4 of 20 (20%) were clinically diagnosed before death. These authors concluded that the incidence of complications from the use of IABC noted clinically most likely underestimates the actual frequency. Gottlieb and associates (1984), in examining a multivariate risk factor analysis

TABLE 54–29. MAJOR COMPLICATIONS OF IABC

Complication	Frequency (%)
Limb ischemia	5–18
Insertion site hemorrhage	2–4
Infection	1–2
Aortic or iliac artery perforation	1–2
Aortic dissection	1
Renal artery embolism or thrombosis	1
Mesenteric infarction	1
Spinal cord ischemic injury (embolism or aortic dissection)	0.5–1
Gas embolization from balloon rupture	0.5
Cerebrovascular accident	0.5

of patients having IABC, concluded that the major risk factor for complications were (1) evidence of pre-existing peripheral vascular disease (claudication, femoral bruit, absent pedal pulses), (2) use of the percutaneous approach for IABP insertion, and (3) female gender.

Other major complications related to vascular problems include mesenteric infarction, renal failure secondary to renal artery occlusion (Baciewicz et al, 1982), spinal cord infarction and paraplegia (Gottlieb et al, 1984; Harris et al, 1986; Harvey et al, 1981; Rose et al, 1984; Tyros and Willman, 1978) and cerebrovascular accident (Gottlieb et al, 1984). The incidence of complications relative to the technique of IABP catheter insertion in a series of 206 patients, such as that reported by Gottlieb and associates (1984), is shown in Table 54–30.

The incidence of major complications in the range of 10 to 30% in the reported series of patients treated with IABP clearly indicates the need for extreme care in selecting patients for IABC. This form of assisted circulation is not without potentially serious and even life-threatening complications. The decision to use IABC must be based on selection of individual patients and not on a stereotyped response to the type of cardiac disease, pathologic anatomy, or hemodynamic indices.

COMPLICATIONS OF VENTRICULAR ASSIST DEVICES

Because of the predominant clinical use of ventricular assist devices for postcardiotomy cardiogenic shock with failure to wean from CPB, a major complication is excessive bleeding (Pennington et al, 1985a; Zumbro et al, 1987). Heparinization is generally continued during use of ventricular assistance, with maintenance of the activated clotting time approximately two times control to prevent potential

TABLE 54–30. INCIDENCE OF MAJOR COMPLICATIONS OF IABC IN 206 PATIENTS: COMPARISON OF THE PERCUTANEOUS AND SURGICAL ROUTES OF IABP CATHETER INSERTION*

Complication	Total (206 Patients)	Percutaneous Route (105 Patients)	Surgical Route (101 Patients)
All major complications	56 (27%)	32 (30%)	24 (24%)
All vascular complications	42 (20%)	28 (27%)	14 (14%)
requiring operation	21 (11%)	14 (13%)	7 (7%)
Infection	13 (6%)	3 (3%)	10 (10%)
Renal failure	9 (4%)	7 (7%)	2 (2%)
Cerebrovascular accident	4 (2%)	2 (2%)	2 (2%)
Mesenteric infarction	2 (1%)	1 (1%)	1 (1%)
Death due to IABP	1 (0.5%)	1 (1%)	0

*From Gottlieb, S. O., Brinker, J. A., Borkon, A. M., et al: Identification of patients at high risk for complications of intraaortic balloon counterpulsation: A multivariate risk factor analysis. Am. J. Cardiol., 53:1135, 1984.

thromboembolic complications (Park et al, 1986; Pierce et al, 1981; Zumbro et al, 1987). Re-exploration for excessive bleeding was required in 30 to 45% of patients on ventricular assistance. No definite pattern of coagulopathy was found, but thrombocytopenia and fibrinolysis did occur.

Multiple transfusions were thought to contribute to the significant incidence of respiratory failure with increased intrapulmonary shunting. Prolonged ventilatory support also contributed to a higher incidence of pulmonary infection and sepsis, although this condition was not specifically related to ventricular assistance. Renal failure, primarily related to these critical patients' multiorgan system involvement, occurred in 32 to 61% of patients treated with ventricular assistance. Dialysis was required in almost 50% of these cases. Central nervous system depression, including cerebrovascular assistance, occurred in 6 to 18% in reported series and in most all cases was thought to be the result of prolonged cardiogenic shock and multiorgan system disease.

Device-related complications were reported by Pennington and associates (1985a) in 45% of patients with ventricular assistance. Thrombus in the pump occurred in 16%, cyanosis related to pumping in 10%, systemic emboli in 65%, mechanical device failure in 6.5%, hemolysis in 3%, and inflow cannula obstruction of the device in 3%. It is evident that the surgeon has to expect potential multiple major complications in patients who have ventricular assistance. However, if survival without ventricular assistance is projected to be essentially zero because of inability to wean from CPB, the reported salvage rates of 25 to 45% seem to justify the continued selective application of ventricular assisted circulation.

FUTURE CONSIDERATIONS

Although improved techniques for insertion of the IABP catheter, including the percutaneous approach, use of a central lumen catheter with a guidewire, and the longer introducer sheath, have facilitated the ease, timeliness, and rate of successful IABP insertion, these have not reduced the incidence of IABP-related complications, particularly complications related to limb ischemia. Despite the significant reduction in arterial injuries by using these newer techniques, the relatively significant size of the IABP catheter and its potential for obstruction of arterial flow, particularly in diseased vessels, can easily cause progressive limb ischemia. Consequently, smaller-diameter (< No. 9.5 French) catheters and introducer sheaths have the potential for reducing limb ischemia complications.

The percutaneous insertion technique poses the hazard of inadvertently introducing the IABP catheter through the smaller superficial femoral artery rather than through the larger common femoral artery. Accidental insertion of the IABP catheter and introducer sheath into a small-diameter and diseased superficial femoral artery greatly increases the risk of distal limb ischemia. The reduced incidence of major limb ischemia in a series of patients with surgically rather than percutaneously introduced IABP catheters may well reflect this potential technical problem, because exposure of the common femoral artery essentially ensures correct placement. Vascular surgeons have frequently noted during vascular reparative or reconstructive procedures that the thrombotic occlusion is related to a dislodged atherosclerotic plaque in the proximal superficial femoral artery at the point of the inadvertent distal IABP catheter insertion. Increased awareness of the potential for incorrect placement of the IABP catheter by the percutaneous technique will probably have a significant potential for reducing complications of limb ischemia.

Many ischemic limb complications occur soon after the balloon catheter is removed even when palpable or Doppler-identified pedal pulses are noted just before removal. Thrombotic occlusion of the femoral artery in this clinical setting is thought to occur when a semiadherent clot on the catheter just below the catheter-mounted balloon is stripped off and lodges in the smaller distal common femoral, superficial, and profunda femoral arteries when the balloon is removed. This author strongly believes that therapeutic anticoagulation with heparin should prevent this potential complication in most cases.

New developments in biocompatible materials with very low thrombogenicity or effective heparin bonding to the surfaces may facilitate a significant decrease in thromboembolic complications in both ventricular assist devices and the intra-aortic balloon. At present, the safest approach appears to be effective systemic heparinization.

The most recent studies of patients requiring assisted circulation have clearly shown that earlier institution of a circulatory assist device is associated with both a reduced incidence of multiorgan system failure and improved salvage. In addition, accurate physiologic monitoring of both left *and* right ventricular function is essential for making an early and correct decision with regard to whether single ventricular assistance or biventricular assistance is required. Increased awareness of the importance of adequate right ventricular performance has allowed an increased salvage of patients by using right or biventricular assistance.

It is exciting to consider the potential of autologous, conditioned, fatigue-resistant skeletal muscle that might serve as a dynamic muscle patch to replace akinetic, acutely infarcted, or scarred ventricular wall which would function via electrical pacing electronically gated to the patient's ECG. Considerably more investigation is required.

Selected Bibliography

Acker, M. A., Hammond, R. L., Mannion, J. D., et al: An autologous biologic motor pump. J. Thorac. Cardiovasc. Surg., 92:733, 1986.

Latissimus dorsi skeletal muscle ventricles were studied after electrical preconditioning for 6 weeks by connecting the ventricles to an implanted mock circulation allowing chronic pressure-flow measurements. The skeletal muscle ventricles were activated by motor nerve stimulation by using an implanted generator. The ventricles pumped continuously against a mean afterload of 80 mm Hg with a 40 to 50 mm Hg preload and maintained a systolic pressure of 104 ± 1 mm Hg and continuous flow of 206 ± 16 ml/min for more than 2 weeks. Two of the ventricles were allowed to pump continuously for 5 and 9 weeks. One ventricle generated pressure up to 205 mm Hg, and the other ventricle generated to 160 mm Hg after this period. These studies suggest the feasibility of a conditioned skeletal muscle ventricle for use as an auxiliary pump for chronic end-stage cardiac failure.

Gottlieb, S. O., Brinker, J. A., Borkon, A. M., et al: Identification of patients at high risk for complications of intraaortic balloon counterpulsation: A multivariate risk factor analysis. Am. J. Cardiol., 53:1135, 1984.

In a group of 206 patients having IABC, risk factors for vascular complications (most common major complication of IABP) were analyzed. The percutaneous insertion of the balloon catheter was used in 105 patients, and surgical cutdown was used in 101 patients. Vascular complications occurred in 20.4% (42 patients), and vascular surgical intervention was required in 10.2%. Multivariate analysis showed that the major risk factors for vascular complications were (1) pre-existing peripheral vascular disease with a history of claudication, (2) absent pedal pulses or femoral bruit, (3) the use of the percutaneous approach for IABP insertion, and (4) female gender. Patients with peripheral vascular disease (PVD) had a threefold greater incidence of major vascular complications, irrespective of the method of IABP insertion. The combination of PVD and the percutaneous insertion approach resulted in a 31% incidence of major vascular complications. In all patients without evidence of PVD, women had an almost fourfold greater incidence of major vascular complications than men, and this complication was attributed to their smaller iliofemoral vessels.

Grayzel, J.: Clinical evaluation of the Percor percutaneous intra-aortic balloon: Cooperative study of 722 cases. Circulation, 66(Suppl. I):223, 1982.

The results of clinical experience with use of IABC by using the percutaneous route of insertion was studied in 722 patients from a national cooperative study. Eighty-eight per cent of the participating clinicians reported that percutaneous insertion was easier than surgical insertion, but 12.6% were unable to insert the IABP catheter successfully. Peripheral ischemia occurred in 5.3% of patients; bleeding complications occurred in 1.9% with 2% requiring surgical repair, emboli in 3.6%, arterial dissection in 1.9%, perforation in 1.1%, local femoral artery thrombosis in 1%, and dislodged arterial plaque in 1.1%. The surgeon can conclude that although the percutaneous method of insertion of the IABP catheter allows easier and more timely use of IABC in a potentially greater number of patients considered for circulatory assistance, the incidence of major complications is still substantial. Careful selection of patients for IABC on an individual basis is essential to achieve good clinical results.

McEnany, M. T., Kay, H. R., Buckley, M. J., et al: Clinical experience with intra-aortic balloon pump support in 728 patients. Circulation, 58(Suppl. I):124, 1978.

Short-term and longer-term results in all patients treated by IABC at the Massachusetts General Hospital for 8 years were analyzed. Of the 747 patients analyzed, the overall in-hospital survival was 57% (including patients treated medically only and surgically treated patients in addition to IABC). The overall improvement in survival between 1974 and 1976, from 57 to 65%, was attributed to (1) broader indications for and earlier insertion of IABP and (2) earlier definitive surgical treatment of the underlying cardiac disease. The predominant indication for IABC was postcardiotomy cardiogenic shock (30%), and next in frequency were unstable angina (23%), postinfarction cardiogenic shock (20%), and other categories including preoperative elective insertion, ventricular septal defect, acute mitral regurgitation, left ventricular aneurysm, and ventricular tachyarrhythmia (28%). The rate of major complications remained fairly constant at 8.5% throughout the study (surgical insertion of IABP), and IABP-related mortality was 0.8%. The most frequent major complication encountered was vascular (9.4%).

Mundth, E. D., and Austen, W. G.: Surgical treatment of acute cardiac ischemia. *In* Hayase, S., and Murao, S. (eds): Proceedings of the VIII World Congress of Cardiology, Tokyo. Amsterdam, Excerpta Medica, 1978.

This study reviews an 8-year experience with the use of IABC with definitive cardiac surgical treatment in the management of patients with (1) postinfarction cardiogenic shock as a result of "pure" left ventricular power failure, (2) unstable angina preinfarction and postinfarction, and (3) cardiogenic shock secondary to postinfarction ventricular septal rupture and papillary muscle rupture with acute mitral regurgitation. IABC was found to relieve medically refractory, unstable myocardial ischemia in 80% of patients and had an acceptably low operative mortality of 5% and a perioperative myocardial infarction incidence of 2%. The combination of assisted circulation using IABC and urgent revascularization with or without infarctectomy for postinfarction cardiogenic shock secondary to left ventricular power failure resulted in 50% hospital survival of 60 patients in this category with only four late deaths in the survivors during a 5-year postoperative follow-up period. All 60 patients in this group were in Stage IV cardiogenic shock, when the mortality with conventional therapy was almost 100%.

The hospital survival of patients with cardiogenic shock secondary to ventricular septal rupture treated by IABC plus surgical correction (closure of the ventricular septal defect plus coronary artery revascularization) was 55% in 20 patients. The hospital survival of 30 patients with cardiogenic shock secondary to acute mitral regurgitation associated with papillary muscle rupture having IABC and operation (mitral valve replacement plus coronary artery revascularization) was 57%. This study indicates that this approach to life-threatening complications of myocardial ischemia results in a significant improvement in hospital survival and is associated with good long-term results.

Park, S. B., Liebler, G. A., Burkholder, J. A., et al: Mechanical support of the failing heart. Ann. Thorac. Surg., 42:627, 1986.

Results of mechanical ventricular assist in 41 patients with postcardiotomy ventricular failure were analyzed. Left, right, and biventricular assists were used during this study from 1980 to 1985. The incidence of postcardiotomy ventricular failure necessitating mechanical ventricular assistance was 0.7%. The duration of assistance ranged from 20 to 69 hours, with a mean of 41 hours in long-term survivors, a mean of 68 hours in short-term survivors, and 35 hours in nonsurvivors. Thirteen of 41 were long-term survivors (32%); 20% of these were weaned successfully from assist but were not hospital survivors, and 48% could not be weaned from ventricular assistance and died. During the last year of the study (1985), survival increased to 57% (4 of 7 patients) and was attributed to (1) earlier institution of assist, (2) maintenance of better assist blood flow rates near physiologic levels, and (3) use of biventricular assistance when there was a significant element of combined biventricular power failure. The cause of death in nonsurvivors was progressive deterioration of cardiac function associated with multiorgan failure in all cases.

Pennington, D. G., Merjavy, J. P., Swartz, M. T., et al: The importance of biventricular failure in patients with postoperative cardiogenic shock. Ann. Thorac. Surg., 39:16, 1985.

Thirty patients having mechanical ventricular assistance for postcardiotomy ventricular failure were analyzed from 1978 to 1984. The status of preoperative ventricular function was not predictable in terms of which patients were likely to require ventricular assist devices. The most common cause of postcardiotomy cardiogenic shock requiring ventricular assistance was perioperative myocar-

dial ischemic injury. Twenty patients received a LVAD, and of four with isolated left ventricular failure, three were weaned from the LVAD and two survived. None of the 16 patients who had biventricular failure and who were treated with LVAD alone were weaned. Ten patients with biventricular failure were treated with biventricular assist devices; five patients were successfully weaned and three survived. This study clearly showed that biventricular failure is common in postcardiotomy cardiogenic shock and is usually a result of perioperative ischemic biventricular injury. In this group of patients, the best chance for success in survival is the early institution of biventricular assistance.

Sanfelippo, P. M., Baker, N. H., Ewy, H. G., et al: Experience with intra-aortic balloon counterpulsation. Ann. Thorac. Surg., 41:36, 1986.

Six hundred thirty-seven patients undergoing IABC were studied for 11 years, and the early and late results were analyzed. Overall hospital survival was 48%, with 32% survival of 228 patients with left ventricular power failure, 66% of 134 patients with unstable ischemia, and 52% of 275 patients in whom IABP was used in conjunction with cardiac surgical procedures. Complications of limb ischemia occurred in 10.4%; unsuccessful insertion occurred in 1.3%; and wound infection occurred in 0.2%. No IABP-related deaths occurred. Follow-up of survivors was 93%, with 69% surviving for 3 years or more. Sixty-three per cent were free of angina; 52% were free of significant cardiac failure; and 56% considered themselves to have a normal activity level. Thirty-eight per cent of the patients continued their previous occupations; 36% retired; and 24% were disabled with respect to their previous occupation. This study clearly indicates the efficacy of assisted circulation by using IABC in the management of difficult clinical problems in patients with life-threatening myocardial ischemia syndromes with expected high mortality. It indicates not only improved early survival but also excellent long-term survival and functional status.

Spence, P. A., Weisel, R. D., and Salerno, T. A.: Right ventricular failure: Pathophysiology and treatment. Surg. Clin. North Am., 65:689, 1985.

This report reviews the pathophysiology of right ventricular failure and modes of treatment. Right ventricular failure can occur with normal pulmonary artery pressures, particularly when an ischemic injury to the right ventricle is associated with left ventricular and septal dysfunction. However, right ventricular failure most commonly develops in the presence of increased pulmonary vascular resistance and is often associated with concomitant left ventricular failure. Right ventricular function is critically dependent on left ventricular septal motion. When septal motion is normal, right ventricular output has been shown to remain adequate despite fairly extensive right ventricular free-wall damage. The most common cause of postoperative right ventricular failure is an acute increase in pulmonary vascular resistance with limited right ventricular functional reserve associated with left ventricular and septal wall dysfunction. The cause of acute right ventricular functional depression is most likely to be right ventricular ischemic injury or inadequate right ventricular myocardial protection during global ischemia intraoperatively.

Treatment consists of pharmacologic management and mechanical assistance. The use of inotropic agents such as isoproterenol or amiodarone with pulmonary vasodilator effects as well as positive inotropic effects is beneficial in most cases. However, if right ventricular dysfunction is profound, with persistent low cardiac output despite pharmacologic treatment, mechanical circulatory assistance using IABC plus PABC or a right ventricular assist device is indicated. When the right ventricle is profoundly depressed, mechanical right ventricular assistance rather than PABC is required to achieve any degree of success.

Williams, D. O., Korr, K. S., Gewirtz, H., and Most, A. S.: The effect of intra-aortic balloon counterpulsation on regional myocardial blood flow and oxygen consumption in the presence of coronary artery stenosis in patients with unstable angina. Circulation, 66:593, 1982.

This study was undertaken in six patients with unstable angina who required IABC in addition to medical therapy to relieve myocardial ischemia. IABC results in a significant reduction in peak systolic aortic (left ventricular) pressure, rate-pressure product, and end-diastolic aortic pressure and increase in peak and mean diastolic pressure. Myocardial oxygen consumption significantly declined, indicating a significant reduction in myocardial oxygen demand associated with a reduction in regional coronary artery blood flow correlated with the reduction in peak left ventricular (aortic) systolic pressure. This study, as well as others alluded to in the literature, suggests that IABC results in alleviation of myocardial ischemia primarily by reduction of myocardial oxygen demand as a consequence of reducing cardiac work and myocardial oxygen demand.

Bibliography

Acker, M. A., Hammond, R. L., Mannion, J. D., et al: An autologous biologic pump motor. J. Thorac. Surg., 92:733, 1986.

Alcan, K. E., Stertzer, S. H., Wallsh, E., et al: The role of intra-aortic balloon counterpulsation in patients undergoing percutaneous transluminal coronary angioplasty. Am. Heart J., 105:527, 1983.

Aroesty, J. M., Weintraub, R. M., Paulin, S., and O'Grady, G. P.: Medically refractory unstable angina pectoris. II: Hemodynamic and angiographic effects of intra-aortic balloon counterpulsation. Am. J. Cardiol., 43:833, 1979.

Baciewicz, F. A., Jr., Kaplan, B. M., Murphy, T. E., and Neiman, H. L.: Bilateral renal artery thrombotic occlusion: A unique complication following removal of a transthoracic intraaortic balloon. Ann. Thorac. Surg., 33:631, 1982.

Bahn, C. H., Vitikaineu, K. J., Anderson, C. L., and Whitney, R. B.: Vascular evaluation for balloon pumping. Ann. Thorac. Surg., 27:474, 1979.

Balderman, S. C., Bhayana, J. N., and Pifarre, R.: Technique for insertion of the intraaortic balloon through the aortic arch. J. Cardiovasc. Surg., 21:614, 1980.

Bardet, J., Rigand, M., Kahn, J. C., et al: Treatment of post-myocardial infarction angina by intra-aortic balloon pumping and emergency revascularization. J. Thorac. Cardiovasc. Surg., 74:299, 1977.

Bemis, C. E., Mundth, E. D., Mintz, G. S., et al: Comparison of technique for intraaortic balloon insertion (Abstract). Am. J. Cardiol., 47:417, 1981.

Bolooki, H.: Clinical Application of Intra-aortic Balloon Pump, 2nd ed. Mt. Kisco, NY, Futura Publishing Co., 1984.

Bonchek, L. I., and Olinger, G. N.: Direct ascending aortic insertion of the "percutaneous" intra-aortic balloon catheter in the open chest: Advantages and precautions. Ann. Thorac. Surg., 32:512, 1981.

Bregman, D., and Casarella, W. J.: Percutaneous intra-aortic balloon pumping: Initial clinical experiences. Ann. Thorac. Surg., 29:153, 1980.

Bregman, D., Kripke, D. C., and Goetz, R. H.: The effect of synchronous unidirectional intra-aortic balloon pumping on hemodynamics and coronary blood flow in cardiogenic shock. Trans. Am. Soc. Artif. Intern. Organs, 16:439, 1970.

Brundage, B. H., Ullyst, D. J., Winokur, S., et al: The role of aortic balloon pumping in postinfarction angina: A different perspective. Circulation, 62(Suppl. I):119, 1980.

Buckley, M. J., Craver, J. M., Gold, H. K., et al: Intra-aortic balloon pump assist for cardiogenic shock after cardiopulmonary bypass. Circulation, 48(Suppl. 3):90, 1973.

Buckley, M. J., Leinbach, R. C., Kastor, J. A., et al: Hemodynamic evaluation of intra-aortic balloon pumping in man. Circulation, 46(Suppl. 2):130, 1970.

Burton, A. C.: The law of the heart. In Burton, A. C. (ed): Physiology and Biophysics of the Circulation, 2nd ed. Chicago, Year Book Medical Publishers, 1972.

Chiu, C. J., Dennis, C., and Harris, B.: Response of myocardial fiber length to left heart bypass. J. Surg. Res., 9:241, 1969.

Clauss, R. H., Birtwell, W. C., Albertal, G., et al: Assisted circulation. I: The arterial counterpulsator. J. Thorac. Cardiovasc. Surg., 41:447, 1961.

Connolly, J. E., Bacaner, M. B., Bruns, E. L., et al: Mechanical support of the circulation in acute heart failure. Surgery, 44:225, 1958.

Cooper, G. N., Singh, A. K., Christian, F. C., et al: Preoperative intra-aortic balloon support in surgery for left main coronary stenosis. Ann. Surg., 185:242, 1977a.

Cooper, G. N., Singh, A. K., Vargas, L. L., and Karlson, K. E.: Preoperative intra-aortic balloon assist in high-risk revascularization patients. Am. J. Surg., 133:463, 1977b.

Cox, J. L., Daniel, T. M., and Boineau, J. P.: The electrophysiologic time course of acute myocardial ischemia and the effects of early coronary artery reperfusion. Circulation, 48:971, 1973.

Cox, J. L., Pass, H. I., Anderson, R. N., et al: Augmentation of coronary collateral blood flow in acute myocardial infarction. Surg. Forum, 26:238, 1975.

Craver, J. M., Kaplan, J. A., Jones, E. L., et al: What role should the intra-aortic balloon have in cardiac surgery? Ann. Surg., 189:769, 1979.

Deutsch, M.: The ellipsoid left ventricular assist device: Experimental and clinical results. In Unger, E. (ed): Assisted Circulation. Berlin, Springer-Verlag, 1979, p. 127.

DeVries, W. C., Anderson, J. L., Joyce, L. D., et al: Clinical use of the total artificial heart. N. Engl. J. Med., 310:273, 1984.

DeWood, A. M., Notske, R. N., Hensley, G. R., et al: Intraaortic balloon counterpulsation with or without reperfusion for myocardial infarction shock. Circulation, 61:1105, 1980.

Downing, T. P., Miller, D. C., Stofer, R., and Shumway, N. E.: Use of the intraaortic balloon pump after valve replacement: Predictive indices, correlative parameters, and patient survival. J. Thorac. Cardiovasc. Surg., 92:210, 1986.

Dunkman, W. B., Leinbach, R. C., Buckley, M. J., et al: Clinical and hemodynamic results of intra-aortic balloon pumping and surgery for cardiogenic shock. Circulation, 46:465, 1972.

Feola, M., Wiener, L., Walinsky, P., et al: Improved survival after coronary bypass surgery in patients with poor left ventricular function: Role of intra-aortic balloon counterpulsation. Am. J. Cardiol., 39:1021, 1977.

Flaherty, J. T., Becker, L. C., Weiss, J. L., et al: Results of a randomized prospective trial of intraaortic balloon counterpulsation and intravenous nitroglycerin in patients with acute myocardial infarction. J. Am. Coll. Cardiol., 6:434, 1985.

Flege, J. B., Wright, C. B., and Reisinger, T. J.: Successful balloon counterpulsation for right ventricular failure. Ann. Thorac. Surg., 37:167, 1984.

Fuchs, R. M., Brin, K. P., Brinker, J. A., et al: Augmentation of regional coronary blood flow by intra-aortic balloon counterpulsation in patients with unstable angina. Circulation, 68:117, 1983.

Gaines, W. E., Pierce, W. S., Prophet, G. A., and Holtzman, K.: Pulmonary circulatory support: A quantitative comparison of four methods. J. Thorac. Cardiovasc. Surg., 88:958, 1984.

Gazes, P. C., Mobley, E. M., Faris, H. M., et al: Preinfarctional (unstable) angina—a prospective study: Ten year follow-up. Circulation, 48:331, 1973.

Gibbon, J. H., Jr.: Application of a mechanical heart and lung apparatus to cardiac surgery. Minn. Med., 37:171, 1954.

Gold, H. K., Leinbach, R. C., Sanders, C. A., et al: Intraaortic balloon pumping for control of recurrent myocardial ischemia. Circulation, 47:1197, 1973.

Goldberger, M., Tabak, S. W., and Shah, P. K.: Clinical experience with intra-aortic balloon counterpulsation in 112 consecutive patients. Am. Heart J., 111:497, 1986.

Golding, L. R., Jacobs, G., Groves, L. K., et al: Clinical results of mechanical support of the failing left ventricle. J. Thorac. Cardiovasc. Surg., 83:597, 1982.

Golding, L. R., Loop, F. D., Mohan, P., et al: Late survival following use of intraaortic balloon pump in revascularization operations. Ann. Thorac. Surg., 30:48, 1980.

Goldman, B. S., Hill, T. J., Rosenthal, G. A., et al: Complications associated with use of the intra-aortic balloon pump. Canad. J. Surg., 25:153, 1982.

Gottlieb, S. O., Brinker, J. A., Borkon, A. M., et al: Identification of patients at high risk for complications of intraaortic balloon counterpulsation: A multivariate risk factor analysis. Am. J. Cardiol., 53:1135, 1984.

Grayzel, J.: Clinical evaluation of the Percor percutaneous intraaortic balloon: Cooperative study of 722 cases. Circulation, 66(Suppl. I):223, 1982.

Griffith, B. P., Hardesty, R. L., Kormos, R. L., et al: Temporary use of the Jarvik-7 total artificial heart before transplantation. N. Engl. J. Med., 316:130, 1987.

Gueldner, T. L., and Lawrence, G. H.: Intraaortic balloon assist through cannulation of ascending aorta. Ann. Thorac. Surg., 19:88, 1975.

Guiraudon, G., Fontaine, G., and Frank, R.: Encircling endocardial ventriculotomy: A new surgical treatment for life-threatening ventricular arrhythmias resistant to medical treatment following myocardial infarction. Ann. Thorac. Surg., 26:438, 1978.

Hanson, E. C., Levine, F. H., Kay, H. R., et al: Control of postinfarction ventricular irritability with the intraaortic balloon pump. Circulation, 62(Suppl. I):130, 1980.

Harken, A. H., Josephson, M. E., and Horowitz, L. N.: Surgical endocardial resection for the treatment of malignant ventricular tachycardia. Ann. Surg., 190:456, 1979.

Harris, R. E., Reimer, K. A., Barbara, J. C., et al: Spinal cord infarction following intraaortic balloon support. Ann. Thorac. Surg., 42:206, 1986.

Harvey, J. C., Goldstein, J. E., McCabe, J. C., et al: Complications of percutaneous intraaortic balloon pumping. Circulation, 64(Suppl. II):114, 1981.

Haston, H. H., and McNamara, J. J.: The effects of intraaortic balloon counterpulsation on myocardial infarct size. Ann. Thorac. Surg., 28:335, 1979.

Hauser, A. M., Gordon, S., Gangadharon, V., et al: Percutaneous intraaortic balloon counterpulsation. Clinical effectiveness and hazards. Chest, 82:422, 1982.

Hochberg, M. S., Parsonnet, V., Gielchinsky, I., and Hussain, S. M.: Coronary bypass grafting in patients with ejection fractions below forty percent: Early and late results in 466 patients. J. Thorac. Cardiovasc. Surg., 86:519, 1983.

Isner, J. M., Cohen, S. R., Virmani, R., et al: Complications of the intraaortic balloon counterpulsation device: Clinical and morphologic observations in 45 necropsy patients. Am. J. Cardiol., 45:260, 1980.

Jarvik, R. K., Olsen, D. B., Lawson, J., et al: Recent advances with the total artificial heart. N. Engl. J. Med., 298:404, 1978.

Jenning, A., Dennis, C., Moreno, J. R., and Hall, D. P.: Atrial septal puncture without thoracotomy for total left heart bypass. Acta Chir. Scand., 132:267, 1962.

Jett, G. K., Dengle, S. K., Barnett, P. A., et al: Intraaortic balloon counterpulsation: Its influence alone and combined with various pharmacologic agents on regional myocardial blood flow during experimental acute coronary occlusion. Ann. Thorac. Surg., 31:144, 1981.

Jett, G. K., Picone, A. L., and Clark, R. E.: Circulatory support for right ventricular dysfunction. J. Thorac. Cardiovasc. Surg., 94:95, 1987.

Jett, G. K., Siwek, L. G., Picone, A. L., et al: Pulmonary artery balloon counterpulsation for right ventricular failure. J. Thorac. Cardiovasc. Surg., 86:364, 1983.

Kaiser, G. C., Marco, J. D., Barnes, H. B., et al: Intraaortic balloon assistance. Ann. Thorac. Surg., 21:487, 1976.

Laas, J., Campbell, C. D., Takanashi, Y., et al: Failure of intraaortic balloon pumping to reduce experimental myocardial infarct size in swine. J. Thorac. Cardiovasc. Surg., 80:85, 1980.

Laks, H., Ott, R. A., Standeven, J. W., et al: The effect of left atrium-to-aortic assistance on infarct size. Circulation, 56(Suppl. 2):38, 1977.

Langou, R. A., Geha, A. S., Hammond, G. L., and Cohen, L. S.: Surgical approach for patients with unstable angina pectoris: Role of the response to initial medical therapy and intraaortic balloon pumping in perioperative complications after aortocoronary bypass grafting. Am. J. Cardiol., 42:629, 1978.

Lee, W. H., Jr., Krumhaar, E., Fonkalsrud, E. W., et al: Denaturation of plasma proteins as a cause of morbidity and death after intracardiac operations. Surgery, 50:29, 1961.

Leinbach, R. C., Gold, H. K., Buckley, M. J., et al: Reduction of myocardial injury during acute infarction by early application of intraaortic balloon pumping and propranolol. Circulation, 48(Suppl. 4):100, 1973.

Leinbach, R. C., Gold, H. K., Harper, R. W., et al: Early intraaortic balloon pumping for anterior myocardial infarction without shock. Circulation, 58:204, 1978.

Leinbach, R. C., Goldstein, J., Gold, H. K., et al: Percutaneous wire-guided balloon pumping. Am. J. Cardiol., 49:1707, 1982.

Levine, F. H., Gold, H. K., Leinbach, R. C., et al: Management of acute myocardial ischemia with intraaortic balloon pumping and coronary bypass surgery. Circulation, 58(Suppl. 1):69, 1978.

Litwak, D. S., Koffsky, R. M., Jurado, R. A., et al: Use of left heart assist device after intracardiac surgery: Technique and clinical experience. Ann. Thorac. Surg., 21:191, 1976.

Lundell, D. C., Hammond, G. L., Geha, A. S., et al: Randomized comparison of the modified wire-guided and standard intraaortic balloon catheters. J. Thorac. Cardiovasc. Surg., 81:297, 1981.

Macoviak, J., Stephenson, L. W., Edmunds, L. H., Jr., et al: The intraaortic balloon pump: An analysis of five years experience. Ann. Thorac. Surg., 29:451, 1979.

Manly, J. C., King, J. F., Zeft, H. J., and Johnson, W. D.: The "bad" left ventricle: Results of coronary surgery and effect on late survival. J. Thorac. Cardiovasc. Surg., 72:841, 1976.

Mannion, J. D., Acker, M. A., Hammond, R. L., et al: Power output of skeletal muscle ventricles in circulation: Short-term studies. Circulation, 76:155, 1987.

Maroko, P. R., Bernstein, E. F., Libby, P., et al: Effects of intraaortic balloon counterpulsation on the severity of myocardial ischemic injury following acute coronary artery occlusion. Circulation, 45:1150, 1972.

Martin, R. S., Mancure, A. C., Buckley, M. J., et al: Complications of percutaneous intra-aortic balloon insertion. J. Thorac. Cardiovasc. Surg., 85:186, 1983.

McCabe, J. C., Abel, R. M., Subramanian, V. A., and Gay, W. A., Jr.: Complications of intra-aortic balloon insertion and counterpulsation. Circulation, 57:769, 1978.

McEnany, M. T., Kay, H. R., Buckley, M. J., et al: Clinical experience with intraaortic balloon pump support in 728 patients. Circulation, 58(Suppl. 1):124, 1978.

McGee, M. G., Zillgit, S. L., Trono, R., et al: Retrospective analysis of the need for mechanical circulatory support (intraaortic balloon pump/abdominal left ventricular assist device or partial artificial heart) after cardiopulmonary bypass: A 44 month study of 14,168 patients. Am. J. Cardiol., 46:135, 1980.

McGeehan, W., Sheikh, F., Donahoo, J. S., et al: Transthoracic intraaortic balloon pump support: Experience in 39 patients. Ann. Thorac. Surg., 44:26, 1987.

Melvin, K. N., and Goldman, B. S.: Intraoperative placement of the percutaneous intraaortic balloon pump through the ascending aorta. Ann. Thorac. Surg., 33:636, 1982.

Mickleborough, L. L., Rebeyka, I., Wilson, G. J., et al: Comparison of left ventricular assist and intra-aortic balloon counterpulsation during early reperfusion after ischemic areas of the heart. J. Thorac. Cardiovasc. Surg., 93:597, 1987.

Miller, D. C., Moreno-Cabral, R. J., Stinson, E. B., et al: Pulmonary artery balloon counterpulsation for acute right ventricular failure. J. Thorac. Cardiovasc. Surg., 80:760, 1980.

Moran, J. M., Opravil, M., Gorman, A. J., et al: Pulmonary artery balloon counterpulsation for right ventricular failure. II: Clinical experience. Ann. Thorac. Surg., 38:254, 1984.

Moulopoulos, S. D., Topaz, S., and Kolff, W. J.: Diastolic balloon pumping (with carbon dioxide) in the aorta: Mechanical assistance to the failing circulation. Am. Heart J., 63:669, 1962.

Mundth, E. D.: Mechanical and surgical interventions for the reduction of myocardial ischemia. Circulation, 53(Suppl. 1):1, 176, 1976a.

Mundth, E. D.: Preoperative intraaortic balloon pump assistance. Ann. Thorac. Surg., 22:603, 1976b.

Mundth, E. D.: Surgical treatment of cardiogenic shock and of acute mechanical complications following myocardial infarction. In Rahmitoola, S. H. (ed): Coronary Bypass Surgery. Philadelphia, F. A. Davis Co., 1977, pp. 241–264.

Mundth, E. D., and Austen, W. G.: Surgical treatment of acute cardiac ischemia. In Hayase, D., and Murao, S. (eds): Proceedings of VIII World Congress of Cardiology. Amsterdam, Excerpta Medica, 1978, p. 359.

Mundth, E. D., Buckley, M. J., Daggett, W. M., et al: Surgical intervention for pre-infarction angina. Adv. Cardiol., 15:59, 1975.

Mundth, E. D., Buckley, M. J., DeSanctis, R. W., et al: Surgical treatment of ventricular irritability. J. Thorac. Cardiovasc. Surg., 66:943, 1973.

Nichols, A. B., Pohost, G. M., Gold, H. K., et al: Left ventricular function during intra-aortic balloon pumping assessed by multigate cardiac blood pool imaging. Circulation, 58(Suppl. 1):176, 1973.

Norman, J. C., Cooley, D. A., Igo, S. R., et al: Prognostic indices for survival during post-cardiotomy intraaortic balloon pumping: Methods of scoring and classification with implications for left ventricular assist device utilization. J. Thorac. Cardiovasc. Surg., 74:709, 1977.

Norman, J. C., Duncan, J. M., Frazier, O. H., et al: Intracorporeal (abdominal) left ventricular assist devices or partial artificial hearts: A five year clinical experience. Arch. Surg., 116:1441, 1981.

Opravil, M. O., Gorman, A. J., Krejcie, T. C., et al: Pulmonary artery balloon counterpulsation for right ventricular failure. I: Experimental results. Ann. Thorac. Surg., 38:242, 1984.

O'Rourke, M. F., Norris, R. N., Campbell, T. J., et al: Randomized controlled trial of intraaortic balloon counterpulsation in early myocardial infarction with acute heart failure. Am. J. Cardiol., 47:815, 1981.

Park, S. B., Liebler, G. A., Burkholder, J. A., et al: Mechanical support of the failing heart. Ann. Thorac. Surg., 42:627, 1986.

Pennington, D. G., Bernhard, W. F., Golding, L. R., et al: Long-term follow-up of postcardiotomy patients with profound cardiogenic shock treated with ventricular assist devices. Circulation, 72(Suppl. 2):216, 1985a.

Pennington, D. G., Merjavy, J. P., Swartz, M. T., et al: The importance of biventricular failure in patients with postoperative cardiogenic shock. Ann. Thorac. Surg., 39:16, 1985b.

Pennington, D. G., Swartz, M., Codd, J. E., et al: Intraaortic balloon pumping in cardiac surgical patients: A nine year experience. Ann. Thorac. Surg., 36:125, 1983.

Pennock, J. L., Pae, W. E., Jr., Pierce, W. S., and Waldhausen, J. A.: Reduction of myocardial infarct size: Comparison between left atrial and left ventricular bypass. Circulation, 59:275, 1979.

Perler, B. A., McCabe, C. J., Abbott, W. M., and Buckley, M. J.: Vascular complications of intra-aortic balloon counterpulsation. Arch. Surg., 118:957, 1983.

Phillips, P. A., and Bregman, D.: Intraoperative application of intraaortic balloon counterpulsation determined by clinical monitoring of the endocardial viability ratio. Ann. Thorac. Surg., 23:45, 1977.

Pierce, W. S.: Clinical left ventricular bypass: Problems of pump inflow obstruction and right ventricular failure. Trans. Am. Soc. Artif. Intern. Organs, 2:1, 1979.

Pierce, W. S., Parr, G. V. S., Myers, J. L., et al: Ventricular assist pumping in patients with cardiogenic shock after cardiac operations. N. Engl. J. Med., 305:1606, 1981.

Pierri, M. K., Zema, M., Kligfield, P., et al: Exercise tolerance in late survivors of balloon pumping and surgery for cardiogenic shock. Circulation, 62(Suppl. I):138, 1980.

Port, S. C., Patel, S., and Schmidt, D. H.: Effects of intraaortic balloon counterpulsation on myocardial blood flow in patients with severe coronary artery disease. J. Am. Coll. Cardiol., 3:1367, 1984.

Powell, W. J., Jr., Daggett, W. M., Magro, A. E., et al: Effects of intra-aortic balloon counterpulsation on cardiac performance, oxygen consumption, and coronary blood flow in dogs. Circ. Res., 26:753, 1970.

Radford, N. J., Johnson, R. A., Daggett, W. M., et al: Ventricular septal rupture: A review of clinical and physiologic features and analysis of survival. Circulation, 64:545, 1981.

Rajai, H. R., Hartman, C. W., Innes, B. J., et al: Prophylactic use of intra-aortic balloon pump in aortocoronary bypass for patients with left-main coronary artery disease. Ann. Surg., 187:118, 1978.

Roberts, A. J., Alonso, D. R., Combes, J. R., et al: Role of delayed intraaortic balloon pumping in treatment of experimental myocardial infarction. Am. J. Cardiol., 141:1202, 1978.

Rose, D. M., Jacobowitz, I. J., Acinapura, A. J., and Cunningham, J. N., Jr.: Paraplegia following percutaneous insertion of an intraaortic balloon. J. Thorac. Cardiovasc. Surg., 87:788, 1984.

Rosensweig, J., and Chatterjee, S.: Restoration of normal cardiac metabolism and hemodynamics after coronary occlusion. Ann. Thorac. Surg., 6:146, 1968.

Russell, R. O., Jr., Resnekou, L., Woek, M., et al: Unstable angina pectoris: National cooperative study group to compare surgical and medical therapy. Am. J. Cardiol., 42:839, 1978.

Sanfelippo, P. M., Baker, N. H., Ewy, H. G., et al: Experience with intraaortic balloon counterpulsation. Ann. Thorac. Surg., 41:36, 1986.

Sarnoff, S. J., Braunwald, E., Welch, G. H., et al: Hemodynamic determinants of oxygen consumption of the heart with special reference to the tension-time index. Am. J. Physiol., 192:148, 1958.

Scanlon, P. J., O'Connell, J., Johnson, S. A., et al: Balloon counterpulsation following surgery for ischemic heart disease. Circulation, 54(Suppl. 3):90, 1976.

Senning, A., Dennis, C., Moreno, J. R., and Hall, D. P.: Atrial septal puncture without thoracotomy for total left heart bypass. Acta Chir. Scand., 132:267, 1962.

Soroff, H. S., Levine, H. J., Sacks, B. F., et al: Assisted circulation. II: Effects of counterpulsation on left ventricular oxygen consumption and hemodynamics. Circulation, 27:722, 1963.

Spence, P. A., Weisel, R. O., Easdown, J., et al: The hemodynamic effects and mechanism of action of pulmonary artery balloon counterpulsation in the treatment of right ventricular failure during left heart bypass. Ann. Thorac. Surg., 39:329, 1985.

Spence, P. A., Weisel, R. D., and Salerno, T. A.: Right ventricular failure: Pathophysiology and treatment. Surg. Clin. North Am., 65:689, 1985.

Sterling, R. P., Taegtmeyer, H., Turner, S. A., et al: Comparison of dopamine and dobutamine therapy during intraaortic balloon pumping for the treatment of post-cardiotomy low-output syndrome. Ann. Thorac. Surg., 38:37, 1984.

Stuckey, J. H., Newman, M. M., Dennis, C., et al: The use of the heart-lung machine in selected cases of acute myocardial infarction. Surg. Forum, 8:342, 1957.

Sturm, J. T., Fuhrman, T. N., Sterling, R., et al: Combined use of dopamine and nitroprusside therapy in conjunction with intra-aortic balloon pumping for the treatment of post-cardiotomy low-output syndrome. J. Thorac. Cardiovasc. Surg., 82:13, 1981.

Subramanian, V. A., Goldstein, J. E., Sos, T. A., et al: Preliminary clinical experience with percutaneous intraaortic balloon pumping. Circulation, 62(Suppl. I):123, 1980.

Sugg, W. L., Rea, M. J., Webb, W. R., and Ecker, R. R.: Cardiac assistance (counterpulsation in 10 patients): Clinical and hemodynamic observations. Ann. Thorac. Surg., 9:1, 1970.

Swan, H. J. C.: Functional basis of the hemodynamic spectrum associated with myocardial infarction. In Gunnar, R. M., Loeb, H. S., and Rahimtoola, S. H. (eds): Shock in Myocardial Infarction. New York, Grune & Stratton, 1974.

Symbas, P. N., McKeown, P. P., Santora, A. H., and Vlasis, S. E.: Pulmonary artery balloon counterpulsation for treatment of intraoperative right ventricular failure. Ann. Thorac. Surg., 39:437, 1985.

Todd, G. J., Bregman, D., Voorhees, A. B., and Reemtsma, K.: Vascular complications associated with percutaneous intraaortic balloon pumping. Arch. Surg., 118:963, 1983.

Tyros, D. H., and Willman, V. L.: Paraplegia following intraaortic balloon assistance. Ann. Thorac. Surg., 25:164, 1978.

Vignola, P. A., Swaye, P. S., and Gosselin, A. J.: Guidelines for effective and safe percutaneous intraaortic balloon pump insertion and removal. Am. J. Cardiol., 48:660, 1981.

Weintraub, R. M., and Aroesty, J. M.: The role of intraaortic balloon pumping and surgery in the treatment of preinfarction angina. Chest, 69:707, 1976.

Weintraub, R. M., Aroesty, J. M., Paulin, S., et al: Medically refractory unstable angina pectoris. I: Long-term follow-up of patients undergoing intraaortic balloon counterpulsation and operation. Am. J. Cardiol., 43:877, 1979.

Weintraub, R. M., Voukydis, P. C., Aroesty, J. M., et al: Treatment of preinfarction angina with intraaortic balloon counterpulsation and surgery. Am. J. Cardiol., 34:809, 1974.

Weiss, A. T., Engel, S., Gotsman, C. J., et al: Regional and global left ventricular function during intra-aortic balloon counterpulsation in patients with acute myocardial infarction shock. Am. Heart J., 108:249, 1984.

Willerson, J. T., Watson, J. T., and Platt, M. R.: Effect of hypertonic mannitol and intraaortic counterpulsation on regional myo-cardial blood flow and ventricular performance in dogs during myocardial ischemia. Am. J. Cardiol., 37:514, 1976.

Williams, D. O., Korr, K. S., Gewirtz, H., and Most, A. S.: The effect of intraaortic balloon counterpulsation on regional myo-cardial blood flow and oxygen consumption in the presence of coronary artery stenosis with unstable angina. Circulation, 66:593, 1982.

Zubiate, P., Kay, J. H., and Mendez, A. M.: Myocardial revascu-larization for the patient with drastic impairment of function of the left ventricle. J. Thorac. Cardiovasc. Surg., 73:84, 1977.

Zumbro, G. L., Kitchens, W. R., Shearer, G., et al: Mechanical assistance for cardiogenic shock following cardiac surgery, myocardial infarction, and cardiac transplantation. Ann. Thorac. Surg., 44:11, 1987.

7 Partial Ileal Bypass for Control of Hyperlipidemia and Atherosclerosis

Henry Buchwald
Christian T. Campos

The efforts of the cardiovascular surgeon have been directed primarily to management of the complications of atherosclerosis. Coronary artery bypass, certain valve repairs or replacements, and cardiac transplantation benefit individuals with severe, or end-stage, cardiac atherosclerosis. Peripheral arterial bypass procedures using venous or prosthetic conduits, aneurysm resection with graft replacement, endarterectomy, and balloon or laser angioplasty are all aimed toward amelioration of atherosclerotic cardiovascular disease. These procedures are, at best, palliative. Until recently, limited concern has been directed to the underlying disease process, and strategies to alter the course of atherosclerosis have rarely been contemplated.

Atherosclerosis is not synonymous with aging but is a true disease process. It occurs rarely in certain undeveloped areas of the world but is endemic in the United States and Western Europe. In industrialized nations, it is uncommon for humans to be free of atherosclerosis (Keys, 1970). Atherosclerotic cardiovascular disease (coronary, cerebral, or peripheral vascular disease) is the leading cause of morbidity and mortality in the United States. In 1987, the mortality from ischemic heart disease (210.9 deaths per 100,000 people) exceeded the rate in any other disease category, including malignancy, and accounted for almost one-fourth of all deaths in the United States in 1987 (Table 54–31) (National Center for Health Statistics, 1988). Although a decline in mortality from cardiovascular disease has occurred since the 1970s (Stern, 1979), a slowing of this downward trend may be occurring. The 1987 mortality from ischemic heart disease is nearly identical to the 217.4 per 100,000 mortality observed in 1986 (National Center for Health Statistics, 1987a).

The morbidity due to atherosclerotic cardiovas-cular disease is also overwhelming. More than 10 million Americans have a history of myocardial infarction or angina pectoris. Diseases of the circulatory system were the principal discharge diagnoses in 5,563,000 of the 34,256,000 hospital discharges re-corded in the United States in 1986, far exceeding the observed frequency of any other disease category (National Center for Health Statistics, 1987b). The American Heart Association estimated that cardio-vascular disease cost Americans almost 46.2 billion dollars in 1981 (American Heart Association, 1981). Clearly, the pain, incapacitation, emotional impact, economic hardship, and career deprivation resulting from cardiovascular disease create problems of substantial magnitude for those concerned with the management of atherosclerosis.

It is evident that atherosclerosis has its onset in infancy and perhaps even in utero (Adlersberg, 1951). Hemodynamically significant lesions are present in American men in their early twenties. In autopsies conducted on American casualties during the Korean conflict, 77.3% of men with a mean age of 22.1 years had some degree of coronary athero-sclerosis, and 15.3% had a luminal narrowing of greater than 50% in one or more coronary arteries (Enos et al, 1953). During the Vietnamese conflict, coronary atherosclerosis, determined by postmortem angiography and gross pathologic examination, was present in 45% of cases, and severe disease, defined by the presence of single plaques more than 1 cm in greatest diameter or confluent, multiple, smaller plaques, was seen in 5% (McNamara et al, 1971). Although these figures vary greatly, the high prevalence of significant coronary artery disease in asymptomatic, otherwise healthy, young men is an alarming finding.

Atherosclerosis has been present since antiquity.

TABLE 54–31. DEATH RATES AND PERCENTAGE OF TOTAL DEATHS FOR THE 15 LEADING CAUSES OF DEATH IN THE UNITED STATES IN 1986*

Rank	Cause of Death	Death Rate	Percentage of Total Deaths
	All causes	870.8	100.0
1	Diseases of the heart	318.7	36.6
2	Malignant neoplasms	193.3	22.2
3	Cerebrovascular diseases	61.3	7.0
4	Accidents and adverse effects	39.7	4.6
	Motor vehicle accidents	20.1	2.3
	Other accidents and adverse effects	19.5	2.2
5	Chronic obstructive pulmonary disease and allied conditions	31.3	3.6
6	Pneumonia and influenza	29.2	3.4
7	Diabetes mellitus	15.1	1.7
8	Suicide	13.1	1.5
9	Chronic liver disease and cirrhosis	10.9	1.2
10	Atherosclerosis	9.2	1.1
11	Nephritis, nephrotic syndrome, and nephrosis	9.0	1.0
12	Homicide and legal intervention	8.9	1.0
13	Septicemia	7.7	0.9
14	Conditions originating in the perinatal period	7.5	0.9
15	Congenital anomalies	5.1	0.6
	All other causes	110.8	12.7

*From the National Center for Health Statistics: Annual summary of births, marriages, divorces, and deaths, United States, 1986. Monthly Vital Statistics Report. Vol. 35, No. 13. DHHS Pub. No. (PHS) 87-1120. Hyattsville, MD, Public Health Service, Aug. 24, 1987.

Death rates per 100,000 population based on a 10% sample of deaths. Causes of death according to the Ninth Revision, International Classification of Diseases, 1975.

An autopsy done by Smith (1933) on the mummy of the pharaoh Memephtah, the nemesis of Moses in the Bible, disclosed a fragment of aorta that remained after the preparative evisceration. Microscopic examination by Shattock (1908) showed typical advanced atherosclerotic lesions with extensive deposits of calcium phosphate. Ruffer (1911) published an extensive account of the presence of classic atherosclerotic lesions in mummies embalmed between 1580 B.C. and 525 A.D. (Fig. 54–124). Leonardo da Vinci initially described and accurately depicted atherosclerotic lesions (Heydenreich, 1954) and suggested that sudden death might be due to thickening and narrowing of "the blood vessels which supply the musculature of the heart, with resultant failure of blood flow to the heart."

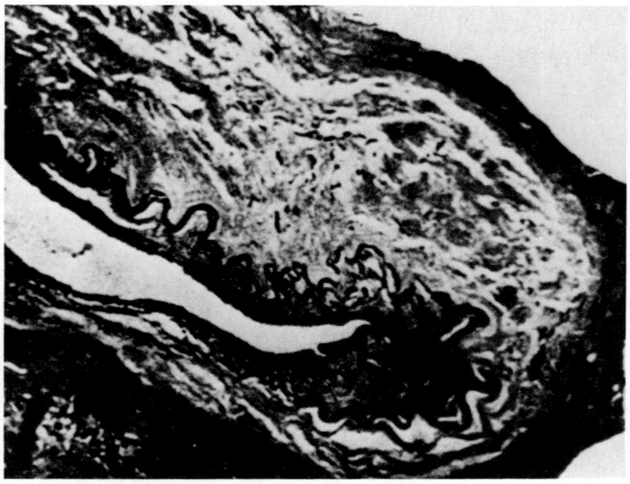

CLASSIFICATION OF THE HYPERLIPOPROTEINEMIAS

In the past, the designations familial hypercholesterolemia, familial hypertriglyceridemia, and familial xanthomatosis were used to describe severe, hereditary forms of hyperlipidemia. Acquired hypercholesterolemia and hypertriglyceridemia indicated less florid manifestations of this spectrum of conditions. Fredrickson and Lees (1965) more effectively categorized lipid elevations as functions of lipoprotein abnormalities. Their classification, which was later revised by them and also by others (Beaumont et al, 1970), provides a standard nomenclature that continues to be relevant to discussions of the hyperlipoproteinemias. In this schema, the hyperlipoproteinemias are divided into five phenotypes (Fig. 54–125):

Type I. Type I hyperchylomicronemia is due to a deficiency of lipoprotein lipase with the resultant inability to clear circulating chylomicrons derived from intestinally absorbed fatty acids and cholesterol.

Type II. Type II hyperbetalipoproteinemia is further subdived into Type II-A (without concomitant hyperprebetalipoproteinemia) and Type II-B (with associated hyperprebetalipoproteinemia). Type II hy-

Figure 54–124. Far-advanced, arterial atherosclerotic lesion from an ancient Egyptian mummy (Heidenhain's iron—hematoxylin stain; ×260). Photograph from a slide, University of Minnesota Rare References Library.

perlipoproteinemia is characterized by an increased concentration of low-density lipoproteins (LDLs) (density 1.006 to 1.063 g/ml, Sf 0 to 20, beta mobility on electrophoresis). These LDLs are rich in cholesterol. In Type II-A hyperlipoproteinemia, the ratio of total plasma cholesterol to triglycerides is greater than 1.5. Individuals with Type II-A are most synonymous with patients previously classified as having primary hypercholesterolemia. In Type II-B hyperlipoproteinemia, in addition to elevations in the LDL and total plasma cholesterol levels, increased triglyceride levels in association with an increased concentration of the triglyceride-rich, very low density lipoproteins (VLDLs) (density 0.94 to 1.006 g/ml, Sf 20 to 400, prebeta mobility on electrophoresis) are present. Both Type II phenotypes arise from an inherited, dominant gene with incomplete penetrance. In heterozygous Type II-A patients, the total plasma cholesterol level is between 300 and 400 mg/dl. These patients often manifest overt atherosclerotic coronary artery disease in early adulthood. Homozygous Type II-A patients, with total plasma cholesterol levels in excess of 300 mg/dl and often greater than 1,000 mg/dl, are severely limited by atherosclerosis as children and rarely survive beyond the third decade of life.

Type III. Type III is an uncommon hyperlipoproteinemia resulting from a block in the metabolic conversion of VLDL to LDL. An abnormal intermediate lipoprotein, characterized as a "floating beta lipoprotein" and identified on electrophoresis as a broad beta band extending from the beta position into the prebeta position, is present in the plasma. Both the total plasma cholesterol and triglyceride concentrations are elevated, with the ratio of cholesterol to triglycerides generally around 1.0 (range of 0.3 to > 2).

Type IV. Type IV hyperprebetalipoproteinemia is due to either excessive production or inadequate clearance of VLDLs. This lipoprotein phenotype is characterized by elevated VLDL and triglyceride levels, normal total plasma cholesterol and LDL concentrations, and increased prebeta band staining on electrophoresis. The Type II and Type IV hyperlipoproteinemias account for most lipoprotein abnormalities in the general population. Although patients with Type IV hyperlipoproteinemia are at increased risk for pancreatitis, it is not clear whether their risk of atherosclerosis is elevated. When atherosclerosis occurs in patients with Type IV hyperlipoproteinemia, it is generally late in onset and presents with a more diffuse and peripheral distribution of lesions than in Type II patients, whose disease is generally early in onset and predominantly coronary in distribution.

Type V. Type V is a rare hyperlipoproteinemia

Type	Cholesterol	Triglycerides	Chylomicrons	LDL	VLDL	Other
I	Normal	Increased	Increased	Decreased	Normal or Slightly Increased	HDL Decreased
II$_a$	Increased	Normal	Normal	Increased	Normal	
II$_b$	Usually Increased	Increased	Normal	Increased	Increased	
III	Increased	Increased	Normal	Sf 0-12 Decreased Sf 12-20 Increased	Sf 100-400 Increased	"Floating" Beta Present
IV	Normal or Increased	Increased	Normal	Normal or Decreased	Increased	HDL may be Decreased
V	Increased	Increased	Increased	Usually Decreased	Increased	HDL may be Decreased

Figure 54–125. Classification of the hyperlipoproteinemias (Adapted from Fredrickson, D. S., and Lees, R. S.: System for phenotyping hyperlipoproteinemia. Circulation, *31*:321, 1965.)

characterized by the presence of hyperchylomicronemia, increased VLDL levels, normal LDL concentrations, increased total plasma cholesterol and triglyceride levels, and increased staining of the prebeta band and the presence of chylomicrons on electrophoresis. The ratio of cholesterol to triglycerides is generally between 0.15 and 0.6 in individuals with Type V hyperlipoproteinemia.

An alternative classification system, based on lipid analysis in patients and in their relatives, has been developed by Goldstein and associates (1973). The presence of elevated total plasma cholesterol or triglyceride levels suggesting a genetic pattern of inheritance serves as the basis for classification of individuals into one of five categories (Table 54–32). Sporadic hypertriglyceridemia reflects exogenous factors and is considered to be nongenetic. Polygenic hypercholesterolemia is manifested by an elevated total plasma cholesterol level but may also include an elevated plasma triglyceride level reflecting a combination of genetic and environmental influences. The monogenetic hyperlipidemias with a clear familial inheritance pattern include (1) familial hypercholesterolemia with isolated elevation of the total plasma cholesterol, (2) familial hypertriglyceridemia characterized by isolated elevation of the triglyceride concentration, and (3) familial combined hyperlipidemia with elevations of both the total plasma cholesterol and triglyceride levels. This classification system is most helpful for genetic counseling of hyperlipidemic individuals and is useful in selecting appropriate therapy for individual patients.

LIPID-ATHEROSCLEROSIS THEORY

Risk factors for the development of atherosclerotic cardiovascular disease have been well established by large-scale epidemiologic analyses. Studies such as the Framingham Study (Kannel and Gordon, 1974) have clearly focused attention on cigarette smoking, hypertension, diabetes, and hypercholesterolemia as the primary risk factors for atherosclerosis. The cholesterol-atherosclerosis relationship has been further defined with LDL cholesterol elevations associated with increased risk (The Pooling Project Research Group, 1978) and high-density lipoprotein (HDL) cholesterol elevation thought to be protective against atherosclerosis development (Gordon et al,

1977). Other secondary cardiovascular risk factors include sex, race, family history, level of physical activity, obesity, plasma triglyceride concentration, and personality type (Gotto and Farmer, 1988).

The role of hypercholesterolemia in the development of atherosclerosis has been extensively evaluated in experimental models and in humans. Since Anitschkow and Chalatow (1913) first induced atherosclerosis in rabbits fed a cholesterol-enriched diet and concluded that cholesterol was an essential ingredient for atherosclerosis, experimental analyses in various species have confirmed the causal relationship between cholesterol and experimental atherosclerosis.

The Seven Countries Study (Keys, 1970), data from the World Health Organization (Simons, 1986), and recent analysis of the screening results from the Multiple Risk Factor Intervention Trial (Martin et al, 1986) have clearly shown that, in humans, coronary artery disease mortality increases with the total plasma cholesterol level (Fig. 54–126). These experimental and epidemiologic observations have led to the proposal of the lipid (cholesterol)-atherosclerosis theory, which states that atherosclerosis is a disease of multiple causes in which altered lipid metabolism, primarily manifested as hypercholesterolemia, has a crucial and operant role (Davignon, 1978; Frantz and Moore, 1969; Glueck and Kwiterovich, 1978).

If elevated total plasma cholesterol is causally related to the development of atherosclerosis, does a reduction in total plasma cholesterol result in a decreased incidence of atherosclerosis and its clinical manifestations? Tests of this corollary of the lipid-atherosclerosis theory abound. Many of these studies have been inconclusive or negative. Although evidence is accumulating that total plasma cholesterol reduction is associated with slower progression of existing atherosclerosis and a lower incidence of de-novo lesions assessed angiographically (Blankenhorn et al, 1987) and although it appears that decreasing total plasma cholesterol can decrease the incidence of multiple, clinical, coronary artery disease endpoints when they are combined (Frick et al, 1987; Lipid Research Clinics Program, 1984a), no study has yet shown that lowering of total plasma cholesterol is associated with increased longevity in treated versus untreated patients. The results of several of the major primary (studies in patients without clinical evidence of atherosclerosis) and secondary (studies

TABLE 54–32. CLASSIFICATION OF THE HYPERLIPOPROTEINEMIAS ACCORDING TO INHERITANCE PATTERN*

Disorder	Cholesterol	Triglyceride	Mode of Inheritance
Sporadic hypertriglyceridemia	Normal	Elevated	Nongenetic
Polygenic hypercholesterolemia	Elevated	Normal to elevated	Polygenic
Familial hypercholesterolemia	Elevated	Normal	Autosomal dominant
Familial hypertriglyceridemia	Normal	Elevated	Autosomal dominant
Familial combined hyperlipidemia	Elevated	Elevated	Autosomal dominant

*Adapted from Goldstein, J. L., Schrott, H. G., Hazzard, W. R., et al: Genetic analysis of lipid levels in 176 families and a delineation of a new inherited disorder: Combined hyperlipidemia. J. Clin. Invest., 52:1544, 1973.

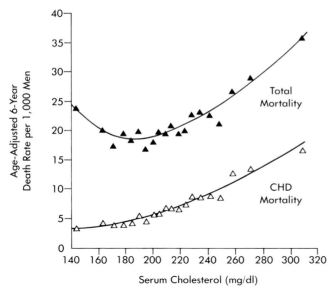

Figure 54–126. Age-adjusted 6-year total and coronary heart disease (CHD) mortality per 1,000 men screened for the Multiple Risk Factor Intervention Trial according to serum cholesterol. (From Martin, M. J., Hulley, S. B., Browner, W. S., et al: Serum cholesterol, blood pressure, and mortality: Implications from a cohort of 361,622 men. Lancet, 2:933, 1986.)

in patients with manifest atherosclerosis, i.e., post-myocardial infarction) intervention trials are reviewed here.

CLINICAL TRIALS OF THE LIPID-ATHEROSCLEROSIS THEORY

Numerous well-designed trials have used dietary restriction of fat and cholesterol or pharmacologic

intervention to examine the potential effects of total plasma cholesterol reduction on overall mortality and cardiovascular disease end-points (Table 54–33). The Los Angeles Veterans Administration Study (Dayton et al, 1969) compared a conventional American diet containing 40% of calories as fat and 650 mg of cholesterol per day with an experimental diet substituting vegetable oils for almost two-thirds of the animal fat (polyunsaturated/saturated fat ratio = 1.7) and 365 mg of cholesterol per day in 846 men living in a Veterans Administration domicile. The experimental group had a 20% reduction of total plasma cholesterol; the group on the conventional diet had a 7% total plasma cholesterol reduction. Sudden death or death from a definite myocardial infarction occurred in 65 members of the control group (15.4%) and in 52 men in the experimental group (12.3%). This difference, although favorable, was not statistically significant.

The Minnesota Coronary Survey (Brewer et al, 1975; Frantz et al, 1975), another hospital-based, primary intervention trial, compared a standard diet with an experimental diet containing 38% fat, with a polyunsaturated/saturated fat ratio of 1.6, and 166 mg of cholesterol per day in 9,449 institutionalized patients. A 13% lower total plasma cholesterol level was achieved with the experimental diet; however, no statistically significant differences in overall mortality, cause-specific mortality, or the incidence of myocardial infarction were observed between the two groups.

The Multiple Risk Factor Intervention Trial was a randomized, primary intervention trial evaluating stepwise treatment of hypertension, counseling for smoking cessation, and dietary modification. The diet in the intervention group limited saturated fat to 8% of the daily caloric consumption. Daily cholesterol

TABLE 54–33. TOTAL CHOLESTEROL RESULTS OF THE MAJOR CLINICAL TRIALS OF THE LIPID-ATHEROSCLEROSIS THEORY

	Number of Subjects	Sex	Age	Follow-up (Years)	Total Cholesterol Effect (%)
Dietary Intervention					
Los Angeles Veterans Administration Study	846	M	55–89	8	−13
Minnesota Coronary Survey	9,449	M & F	21–100	1–5	−13
Multiple Risk Factor Intervention Trial (MRFIT)*	12,866	M	35–57	7	−2
Leiden Intervention Trial	39	M & F	33–59	2	−10
Pharmacologic Intervention					
Coronary Drug Project	8,341	M	30–64	6.2	−6.5 (clofibrate) −9.9 (niacin)
WHO Cooperative Clofibrate Trial	15,745	M	30–55	5.3	−9 (clofibrate)
Lipid Research Clinics–Coronary Primary Prevention Trial (LRC-CPPT)	3,806	M	35–59	7.4	−8.5 (cholestyramine)
Helsinki Heart Study	4,081	M	40–55	5	−11 (gemfibrozil)
NHLBI Type II Coronary Intervention Trial	116	M & F	21–55	5	−17 (cholestyramine)
Cholesterol-Lowering Atherosclerosis Study	162	M	40–59	2	−26 (cholestipol + niacin)
Surgical Intervention					
The Program on the Surgical Control of the Hyperlipidemias (POSCH)	838	M	30–64	7	−23.9 (partial ileal bypass)

*Smoking cessation and antihypertensive therapy were also used in MRFIT.

intake was reduced to less than 250 mg. Dietary intervention in this large, noninstitutionalized population led to a meager 2% reduction of total plasma cholesterol. Overall mortality and mortality due to coronary heart disease were not statistically different between the intervention and the usual care groups (Multiple Risk Factor Intervention Trial Research Group, 1982).

The Coronary Drug Project was a secondary intervention trial that assessed the effects of nicotinic acid (niacin), clofibrate, dextrothyroxine, and two dosage levels of estrogen on overall mortality in 30- to 64-year-old men who survived a documented myocardial infarction. The estrogen and dextrothyroxine treatment arms were prematurely discontinued because of adverse and occasionally lethal effects of these agents (The Coronary Drug Project Research Group, 1970, 1972, 1973). In comparison with placebo-treated controls, 1.8 g/day of clofibrate lowered the total plasma cholesterol level 6.5%, and 3 g/day of niacin reduced the total plasma cholesterol level 9.9% (The Coronary Drug Project Research Group, 1975). No significant differences in overall or cause-specific mortality versus placebo were noted with either agent. A follow-up report 9 years after the conclusion of the Coronary Drug Project showed an 11% lower overall mortality in the niacin-treated group than in the placebo group (Canner et al, 1986). It is not clear whether this overall mortality benefit, many years after discontinuing niacin therapy, is due to an early favorable effect of niacin in decreasing nonfatal reinfarction or is a result of the early cholesterol-lowering effect of this drug, or both.

In the World Health Organization Cooperative Clofibrate Trial, men with mild to moderate hypercholesterolemia were treated with placebo or 1.6 g/day of clofibrate. A 9% lower total plasma cholesterol was achieved with clofibrate; however, no significant reduction in coronary heart disease mortality was observed. A significantly increased noncardiovascular disease mortality was seen in the clofibrate group, leading to the recommendation that clofibrate not be routinely used in the treatment of hypercholesterolemia (Committee of Principal Investigators: WHO Clofibrate Trial, 1980, 1984).

The Lipid Research Clinics Coronary Primary Prevention Trial (LRC-CPPT) compared the effects of placebo and 24 g/day of cholestyramine in 3,806 men with Type II hyperlipoproteinemia (Lipid Research Clinics Program, 1984a, 1984b). At 7-year follow-up, total plasma cholesterol was reduced 8.5% and LDL cholesterol was lowered 12.6% in the cholestyramine group compared with the controls. These reductions were significantly smaller than anticipated, primarily because of the high noncompliance rate in the intervention group. Twenty-seven per cent of the patients assigned to cholestyramine treatment were taking less than 2 g/day of the resin after 7 years of treatment. Overall mortality was not significantly reduced by cholestyramine treatment. A 19% lower incidence of the combined primary end-points—death due to

coronary heart disease and definite, nonfatal myocardial infarction—was observed in the cholestyramine group (p < 0.05, one-sided t-test). This favorable result provides evidence in support, but does not provide definitive proof, of the lipid-atherosclerosis theory. Unfortunately, the high noncompliance rate associated with cholestyramine treatment limited the cholesterol reduction observed in this trial. No significant differences in overall or cause-specific mortality were observed, and statistically significant results could be obtained only by combining the incidences of primary end-points and by using a one-sided test of statistical significance.

The Helsinki Heart Study (Frick et al, 1987) was a primary intervention trial involving 4,081 men with non-HDL cholesterol levels greater than 200 mg/dl comparing treatment with gemfibrozil (600 mg twice daily) to placebo. Total plasma cholesterol was 11% lower, LDL cholesterol was 10% lower, and HDL cholesterol was 10% higher in the gemfibrozil group. No significant reductions in 5-year overall or cause-specific mortality were observed with gemfibrozil therapy. The combined number of cardiac end-points (nonfatal myocardial infarctions, fatal myocardial infarctions, sudden cardiac deaths, and unwitnessed deaths) was significantly lower (p < 0.02) in the gemfibrozil group ($n = 56$) than in the placebo group ($n = 84$). Like the LRC-CPPT, the Helsinki Heart Study was unable to show significant decreases in overall mortality, in cause-specific mortality, or in individual coronary heart disease end-points after lipid modification. Only by combining numerous coronary heart disease end-points could a statistically significant result be obtained. This trial also provides evidence for, but does not prove, the lipid-atherosclerosis theory.

Several studies have examined the effects of lipid modification on arteriographically documented coronary artery disease (see Table 54–33). The National Heart, Lung, and Blood Institute Type II Coronary Intervention Study compared the effects of cholestyramine treatment (24 g/day) with placebo therapy on the angiographic progression of coronary artery disease 5 years after initiating treatment (Brensike et al, 1984; Levy et al, 1984). Total plasma cholesterol was reduced 17%, LDL cholesterol was lowered 26%, and HDL cholesterol was increased 8% compared with the controls in this secondary intervention trial. Definite progression (at least one lesion with definite progression and no lesion with regression) occurred in 25.4% of the cholestyramine group and in 35.1% of the placebo group. This difference, although favorable, was not statistically significant. By combining definite and probable progression (at least one lesion with probable progression and no lesion with regression or definite progression) and by using a one-sided test of significance, a statistically significant difference between the cholestyramine group (32.2%) and the placebo group (49.1%) was found (p = 0.03). From these results, it was concluded that lipid modification may retard the rate of progression of coronary artery disease in patients with Type II hyperlipoproteinemia.

In a small, nonrandomized study in Leiden in the Netherlands, the effects of a 2-year, vegetarian diet, with a polyunsaturated/saturated fat ratio of at least 2 and containing less than 100 mg/day of cholesterol, were assessed with respect to the angiographic progression of coronary artery disease (Arntzenius et al, 1985). Total serum cholesterol and the ratio of total to HDL cholesterol were reduced significantly by 10 and 8.5%, respectively. Disease progression at 2 years was present in patients whose ratio of total to HDL cholesterol was higher than the median throughout the trial. No coronary lesion progression was observed in patients with a ratio of total to HDL cholesterol below the median or in patients with initially higher values that were significantly lowered with diet.

The strongest evidence that total plasma cholesterol reduction may be associated with improvement in the course of coronary heart disease assessed angiographically has come from the Cholesterol-Lowering Atherosclerosis Study (CLAS). In this study (Blankenhorn et al, 1987), 162 men, who had previously had coronary artery bypass surgery and had total plasma cholesterol levels between 185 mg/dl and 350 mg/dl, were randomly assigned to dietary intervention (polyunsaturated/saturated fat ratio = 2 and less than 250 mg/day of cholesterol) or to dietary intervention plus 29.5 g/day of colestipol hydrochloride and 4.3 g/day of niacin. High drug dosages were used, and patients with total plasma cholesterol reductions of 30 to 40% in the drug group and 7 to 8% in the diet group were selected for this 2-year study. Compared with the control group, total plasma cholesterol was 22% lower, LDL cholesterol was 38% lower, and HDL cholesterol was 35% higher in the colestipol-niacin group at 2 years. Significant reductions in the average number of lesions per subject that progressed and in the percentage of patients with the development of new lesions in their native coronary arteries were observed after lipid modification. The percentages of patients with new lesions or any adverse changes in their coronary artery bypass grafts were also significantly reduced by combined colestipol-niacin therapy. Atherosclerosis regression, indicated by improvement in a global coronary artery disease score, was noted in 16.2% of the colestipol–niacin-treated patients versus 2.4% of the placebo-treated group (one-sided p = 0.002). These results strongly support the conclusion that lipid modification is correlated with improvement in the angiographic course of coronary artery disease and suggest that regression of atherosclerosis may even be possible. The CLAS trial was not designed to examine the effects of lipid modification on clinical end-points or to correlate angiographic changes with subsequent coronary artery disease events. No significant differences in overall mortality, cause-specific mortality, or individual coronary artery disease end-points were noted between the placebo and the intervention groups in this trial.

The Program on the Surgical Control of the Hyperlipidemias (POSCH) is the one ongoing intervention trial that can potentially provide definitive proof of the lipid-atherosclerosis theory (Buchwald et al, 1982, 1985). Between 1975 and 1983, 838 survivors of a single, documented myocardial infarction with total plasma cholesterol levels of 220 mg/dl or greater, or LDL cholesterol levels of 140 mg/dl or greater if the total plasma cholesterol was between 200 mg/dl and 219 mg/dl, were enrolled in this multicenter, secondary intervention study. Patients in the control group received instruction in the American Heart Association prudent diet therapy for hypercholesterolemia. Intervention group participants received dietary counseling and, in addition, had a partial ileal bypass operation. POSCH is scheduled to conclude in 1990, when all patients will have been monitored for at least 7 years (mean follow-up = 9.6 years). Overall mortality is the primary trial end-point. Deaths are categorized as being atherosclerotic or nonatherosclerotic. Secondary end-points include fatal and nonfatal myocardial infarctions, other clinical events, new electrocardiographic abnormalities or changes in treadmill exercise test performance, alterations in Doppler assessment of peripheral pulses, and changes in serial coronary and peripheral arteriograms. All participants in POSCH are scheduled to have coronary and peripheral arteriography at baseline and 3, 5, and 7 or 10 years after entrance into the trial. Thus, in this definitive test of the lipid-atherosclerosis theory, POSCH will assess the relationship of lipid modification achieved by partial ileal bypass to overall and cause-specific morbidity and mortality. Furthermore, the progression of coronary and peripheral vascular disease, assessed angiographically, will be correlated with specific clinical cardiovascular disease end-points.

THERAPY FOR THE HYPERLIPOPROTEINEMIAS

Although definitive evidence to support the necessity for lipid reduction in the management and prevention of atherosclerotic cardiovascular disease is lacking, animal experimental data and the results of the previously reviewed clinical trials of the lipid-atherosclerosis theory support the prudence of attempting atherosclerosis risk modification by plasma lipid reduction. Plasma lipid modification has become the focus of a national public health initiative in the United States. Through previous efforts, primarily the educational activities of the American Heart Association, eating habits in the United States have already changed significantly. The current American diet contains fewer eggs; less butter, cream, and whole milk; less animal fat, beef, and other red meat,

TABLE 54–34. RECOMMENDATIONS OF THE NATIONAL CHOLESTEROL EDUCATION PROGRAM FOR THE EVALUATION AND TREATMENT OF HYPERCHOLESTEROLEMIA IN ADULTS*

Cholesterol Level	CHD† Risk	Recommendation
< 200 mg/dl	Low	Repeat lipid screening every 5 years
200–239 mg/dl without CHD or other CHD risk factors‡	Moderate	Restrict dietary fat, cholesterol, and calories (if overweight) Repeat lipid determination annually
200–239 mg/dl with CHD or at least two other CHD risk factors‡	High	Restrict dietary fat, cholesterol, and calories (if overweight) If LDL remains > 190 mg/dl after diet or if LDL was > 160 mg/dl and CHD was already present, pharmacologic therapy is advocated Repeat lipid determinations at least annually
> 240 mg/dl	High	Same as above

*Adapted from The Expert Panel: Report of the National Cholesterol Education Program Expert Panel on detection, evaluation, and treatment of high blood cholesterol in adults. Arch. Intern. Med., *148*:36, 1988.
†CHD = coronary heart disease.
‡For a complete list of CHD risk factors, see the text.

and more vegetable and polyunsaturated fats, fish, and poultry than were consumed earlier.

The recent report of the Expert Panel on Detection, Evaluation, and Treatment of High Blood Cholesterol in Adults has been widely circulated by the National Cholesterol Education Program (Cleeman and Lenfant, 1987; The Expert Panel, 1988). The recommendations in this report serve as guidelines for the evaluation and treatment of hypercholesterolemia in adults (Table 54–34). Determination of total plasma cholesterol at 5-year intervals is advocated for all adults at least 20 years of age. Based on the result of this test, individuals are placed into risk strata. Individuals with total plasma cholesterol levels less than 200 mg/dl are at low risk, and repeat cholesterol testing at 5-year intervals is recommended. Individuals who have total plasma cholesterol levels between 200 and 239 mg/dl and who do not have overt coronary heart disease or other risk factors (male sex, history of coronary heart disease before 55 years of age in a parent or sibling, smoking more than 10 cigarettes per day, hypertension, diabetes mellitus, ≥ 30% overweight, HDL cholesterol < 35 mg/dl, or a history of definite cerebrovascular or occlusive peripheral vascular disease) are considered to be at moderate risk. For this group, dietary restriction of saturated fat, cholesterol, and calories (if overweight) is recommended along with annual plasma lipid analysis. Individuals who have total plasma cholesterol levels between 200 and 239 mg/dl and have overt coronary heart disease or at least two coronary heart disease risk factors and individuals with total cholesterol levels of 240 mg/dl or greater plasma are considered to be at high risk. For them, a complete lipoprotein profile is advocated, along with dietary restriction of saturated fat, cholesterol, and calories (if obese). If the LDL cholesterol level remains greater than 190 mg/dl after dietary intervention or if the LDL cholesterol was initially greater than 160 mg/dl and coronary heart disease was al-

ready present, more aggressive intervention with pharmacologic agents is recommended. The authors believe that partial ileal bypass should also be considered in these high-risk individuals in place of, or in addition to, pharmacologic therapy.

Dietary and Pharmacologic Therapy

Nonpharmacologic measures, including dietary restriction of saturated fats and cholesterol, exercise, and weight loss, still constitute the principal therapy for hypercholesterolemia. The following general dietary guidelines are well established. Total fats should contribute less than 30% of total daily caloric intake. The ratio of polyunsaturated to saturated fat should be at least 1.5. Finally, the daily intake of cholesterol should be less than 300 mg. The American Heart Association has advocated a progressive dietary approach for hypercholesterolemia that is universally accepted (Ad Hoc Committee to Design a Dietary Treatment of Hyperlipoproteinemia, 1984). The Phase I diet is recommended for the general population and contains less than 300 mg/day of cholesterol, with less than 30% of the daily caloric intake supplied by fats, and with a polyunsaturated/saturated fat ratio of 1. The Phase II and Phase III diets are recommended for persistently high total plasma cholesterol levels. The Phase III diet contains between 100 and 150 mg/day of cholesterol, with less than 20% of the daily caloric intake supplied by fats, and with a polyunsaturated/saturated fat ratio between 1 and 2 (Table 54–35).

Cholestyramine, colestipol, nicotinic acid, gemfibrozil, probucol, and lovastatin are currently accepted pharmacologic agents for the treatment of hypercholesterolemia refractory to dietary intervention. Cholestyramine and colestipol are quaternary ammonium salts that bind bile salts in the intestine, leading to increased bile salt loss in the stool (Levy,

TABLE 54–35. COMPOSITION OF THE AMERICAN HEART ASSOCIATION PHASE I, II, AND III DIETS*

	Phase I	Phase II	Phase III
Fat (% of total calories)	30	25	20
Carbohydrate (% of total calories)	55	60	65
Protein (% of total calories)	15	15	15
Cholesterol (mg)	300	200–250	100–150
P/S ratio†	1	1	1–2

*Adapted from Ad Hoc Committee to Design a Dietary Treatment of Hyperlipoproteinemia: AHA Special Report: Recommendation for treatment of hyperlipidemia in adults. Circulation, 69:1065, 1984. By permission of the American Heart Association, Inc.

†P/S ratio = ratio of polyunsaturated to saturated fat.

1980). Hepatic synthesis of bile acids from cholesterol is increased. Depletion of the hepatic cholesterol pool results in increased LDL receptor activity with increased removal of LDL cholesterol from the plasma. The bile acid sequestrants are difficult to administer because of frequent side effects and numerous drug interactions. The major side effects are gastrointestinal and include constipation, bloating, nausea, and flatulence. These resins bind concomitantly administered drugs such as digitalis, phenobarbital, thiazide diuretics, warfarin, thyroxine, tetracycline, and beta-blockers and lead to variable absorption of these agents. Decreased absorption of fat-soluble vitamins and folic acid has also been noted. Cholestyramine and colestipol have been reported to produce a 15 to 30% lowering of LDL cholesterol; however, primarily because of poor long-term compliance with daily resin administration, only an 8.5% reduction in total plasma cholesterol was achieved after 7 years of treatment with cholestyramine in the LRC-CPPT. Despite close medical supervision including compliance counseling, 27% of patients assigned to the cholestyramine regimen in this trial were taking less than one-half a packet of drug each day (one-twelfth of the recommended daily dose).

Nicotinic acid (niacin) decreases hepatic production of VLDL cholesterol and results in decreased LDL cholesterol formation (Grundy et al, 1981). This agent also inhibits the release of fatty acids by inhibiting lipolysis in adipose tissue and leads to decreased hepatic triglyceride synthesis. Total and LDL cholesterol reductions of 25% and HDL cholesterol increases of 20 to 40% have been observed (Shepherd et al, 1979). However, in the Coronary Drug Project, nicotinic acid treatment led to only a 9.9% lower total plasma cholesterol. The use of nicotinic acid is limited primarily by cutaneous flushing and gastrointestinal symptoms. Flushing and pruritus occur within an hour of drug administration as a result of prostaglandin-mediated capillary dilation. This side effect is persistent in 10 to 15% of patients (Eder, 1965). Elevations of liver function test results and gastritis can occur, requiring monitoring of liver function and contraindicating use of this agent in patients with a history of peptic ulcer disease. Other side effects

include hyperpigmentation, impaired glucose tolerance, and hyperuricemia.

Gemfibrozil, a fibric acid derivative, appears to reduce incorporation of free fatty acids into triglycerides (Samuel, 1983). Cholesterol excretion into bile also appears to increase with this agent. Gemfibrozil is highly effective in lowering triglycerides, reducing these levels by as much as 50%. HDL cholesterol has been increased by as much as 20% with this agent (Lewis, 1982). In the Helsinki Heart Study, gemfibrozil led to an 11% decrease in total plasma cholesterol, a 10% decrease in LDL cholesterol, and a 10% increase in HDL cholesterol. The most common side effects of this drug are nausea, gastrointestinal discomfort, myositis, and impaired glucose tolerance. Gemfibrozil can also potentiate the anticoagulant effects of warfarin and increase biliary lithogenicity.

Probucol, a lipophilic *bis*-phenol, lowers both LDL and HDL cholesterol levels (Mellies et al, 1980). LDL cholesterol can be reduced up to 15%. However, the 20 to 25% reductions in HDL cholesterol with this agent are of concern, because HDL cholesterol appears to be protective against atherosclerosis. The mechanisms of action of probucol are unclear, with cholesterol synthesis reportedly lower in combination with decreased cholesterol absorption and increased cholesterol excretion (Nestel and Billington, 1981). In LDL receptor-deficient rabbits, probucol enhanced plasma LDL cholesterol clearance by the macrophage or scavenger pathway. The side effects of this agent are primarily gastrointestinal and include diarrhea, flatulence, abdominal pain, and nausea. These are generally mild and occur in less than 5% of patients. Probucol may prolong the Q-T interval and should not be used in patients with electrocardiographic evidence of ventricular irritability, patients with an initially prolonged Q-T interval, or patients who are taking other drugs that might prolong the Q-T interval.

Lovastatin is a member of a new class of cholesterol-lowering agents that includes compactin, simvastatin, pravastatin, and SRI-62320. These drugs act as competitive inhibitors of 3-hydroxy-3-methylglutaryl-coenzyme A (HMG-CoA) reductase, the enzyme controlling the rate-limiting step in cholesterol biosynthesis (Grundy, 1988). Lovastatin received Food and Drug Administration approval in 1987. The clinical experience with these agents is limited, and their long-term safety and efficacy have not yet been established. The HMG-CoA reductase inhibitors decrease cholesterol biosynthesis (Grundy and Bilheimer, 1984). Lower cholesterol levels lead to increased synthesis of LDL cholesterol receptors, increased uptake of plasma LDL cholesterol by these receptors, and further reduction of plasma LDL cholesterol levels. Lovastatin, at a dose of 20 mg twice daily, reduced LDL cholesterol by 25 to 30%. At a dose of 40 mg twice daily, LDL cholesterol reductions of 35 to 40% are possible (Havel et al, 1987; Illingworth and Sexton, 1984). Lovastatin is not effective in patients with receptor-negative, homozygous, familial hypercholesterolemia (Uauy et al, 1988). This fact provides evidence that the principal action of these drugs is to increase the number of LDL receptors, augmenting LDL receptor-mediated plasma LDL cholesterol clearance. In the limited clinical experience with lovastatin, side effects have included changes in bowel function, headaches, nausea, fatigue, insomnia, and skin rashes. Approximately 2% of patients have developed increased hepatic transaminase levels requiring discontinuation of lovastatin therapy (Tobert, 1987). Careful monitoring of liver function is recommended. Myositis of uncertain cause with greatly elevated creatine phosphokinase and potassium levels has been encountered (East et al, 1988; Edelman and Witztum, 1989). Rhabdomyolysis leading to acute renal failure has occurred in patients treated with lovastatin in combination with immunosuppressive therapy after cardiac transplantation (Norman et al, 1988). Finally, the potential for cataract induction is of concern. In the Lovastatin Study Group II trial, 13 of 101 patients receiving lovastatin for 18 weeks developed lens opacities that were not present at baseline (Hunninghake et al, 1988; The Lovastatin Study Group II, 1986). Until the lens opacity issue is clearly resolved, baseline and frequent lens examinations are advocated. The HMG-CoA reductase inhibitors are an exciting and potentially major addition to the pharmacologic armamentarium for the treatment of hypercholesterolemia. Until the long-term safety and efficacy of these agents are established, however, careful use of the HMG-CoA reductase inhibitors appears to be prudent.

New drugs are continually being introduced for the treatment of hyperlipoproteinemia. Clinicians must be wary of using these agents before their efficacy and side effects are clearly determined. Estrogen therapy was once advocated but subsequently abandoned when its use caused feminization in men, intravascular coagulation, and increased mortality. Clofibrate appeared to be promising but was rejected when toxic side effects became apparent. Dextrothyroxine was once used but is no longer recommended because of an increased incidence of adverse cardiovascular effects including angina pectoris and arrhythmias. Finally, neomycin has been found to have cholesterol-lowering effects; however, the potential for serious ototoxicity and nephrotoxicity has severely limited the use of neomycin in the treatment of hypercholesterolemia.

Surgical Therapy: Partial Ileal Bypass

Historical Aspects

On May 29, 1963, the authors did the first partial ileal bypass operation specifically for cholesterol reduction in humans. More than 600 partial ileal bypass procedures have now been done. Other institutions in the United States and abroad currently have programs evaluating this method of lowering cholesterol

(Balfour and Kim, 1974; Chalstrey et al, 1982; Clot et al, 1971; Kelly et al, 1982; Macarone-Palmiere et al, 1978; Russell et al, 1979; Schouten and Beynen, 1986; Schouten et al, 1985; Sodal et al, 1970; Strisower et al, 1968a, 1968b; Vaislic et al, 1984; Van Niekerk et al, 1984). Because this method of lowering lipids is surgical, it has encountered resistance from the non-surgical medical community. Nevertheless, this reluctance is slowly fading and an increasing number of patients has been evaluated for partial ileal bypass, particularly individuals who have had inadequate cholesterol reduction after dietary or pharmacologic intervention.

Metabolic Rationale

From 1962 to 1964, the first experiments designed to develop the metabolic rationale for partial ileal bypass were done at the University of Minnesota (Buchwald and Gebhard, 1964, 1968; Buchwald et al, 1974b; Gebhard and Buchwald, 1970). Studies using New Zealand White rabbits and pigs, and retrospective analyses of patients who had had ileal resections for causes other than carcinoma (e.g., incarcerated hernia or Crohn's ileitis), showed that both cholesterol absorption from the intestinal tract and whole blood cholesterol concentration were significantly reduced, without concomitant weight loss, after diversion or resection of substantial lengths of distal small bowel. Additional studies showed that although the entire small intestine is capable of cholesterol absorption, preferential cholesterol uptake occurs in the distal half of the small bowel with normal bowel continuity. Transit time in the small intestine also strongly influences quantitative cholesterol absorption.

The data with respect to absorption sites for bile acids are less clear than the experimental findings for cholesterol absorption. They have often been contradictory. The authors have shown that bypass of the distal third of the small bowel interferes with the enterohepatic bile acid cycle and results in a loss of bile acids in the feces at a rate at least three times normal (Buchwald and Gebhard, 1968). Thus, partial ileal bypass alters body cholesterol homeostasis by causing (1) a direct drain on the body cholesterol pool from increased fecal loss of normally absorbed exogenous (dietary) and endogenous (biliary and intestinally secreted) cholesterol and (2) an indirect drain on the cholesterol pool resulting from increased hepatic conversion of body cholesterol to its metabolic end-product, bile acids, in order to maintain the normal bile acid reservoir (Fig. 54–127).

In 1965, the authors developed a reproducible rabbit model of myocardial infarction by feeding rabbits a diet high in cholesterol for prolonged periods (Buchwald, 1965b). By using this model, it was shown in adult rabbits (Buchwald, 1965a) and in infant rabbits (Buchwald et al, 1972) that partial ileal bypass prevents hypercholesterolemia and atherosclerosis despite consumption of a severely athero-

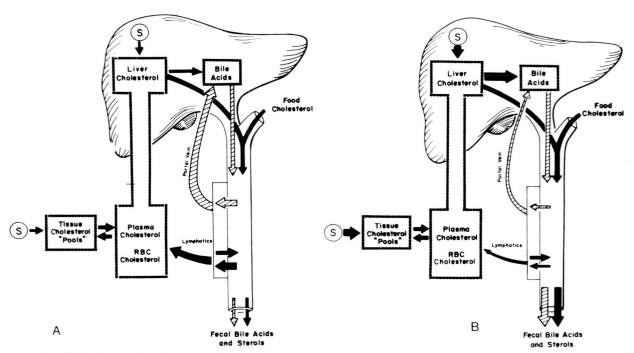

Figure 54–127. Before partial ileal bypass *(A)*, most exogenous cholesterol and bile and mucosally secreted cholesterol are absorbed from the distal small intestine. Similarly, most secreted bile acids are reabsorbed by the ileum. After partial ileal bypass *(B)*, there is a sharp decrease in intestinal absorption and an increase in fecal cholesterol and bile acid excretion. Cholesterol synthesis greatly increases to replenish the bile acid reservoir. The overall effect is reduction in the plasma cholesterol concentration and in the miscible body cholesterol pool.

genic (2% added cholesterol) diet for 4 months. In rabbits with established hypercholesterolemia and atherosclerosis, the operation lowers the total plasma cholesterol below normal and reduces cholesterol accumulation in xanthomata despite maintenance on the 2% cholesterol diet. In addition, partial ileal bypass arrests and even reverses the atherosclerotic process—the plaque lesions evolve from a proliferative phase to a scarring or healing phase with quantitatively less cholesterol content. In infant rabbits, loss of absorption from the bypassed segment does not interfere with structural growth or normal body weight gain. Finally, adaptive mechanisms do not lead to increased cholesterol or bile salt absorption over time.

Other investigators have confirmed these findings in dogs (Scott et al, 1966) and in rhesus monkeys (Shepard et al, 1968). Scott and associates have shown that partial ileal bypass achieved twice the circulating cholesterol reduction as a daily 1.5 mg/kg dose of cholestyramine in rhesus monkeys (Younger et al, 1969). With all animals on the same atherogenic diet, the average serum cholesterol concentration was 803 mg/dl in the untreated control animals, 418 mg/dl in the monkeys treated with cholestyramine, and 175 mg/dl in the animals that had a partial ileal bypass. In addition, significantly less aortic atherosclerosis was noted in monkeys treated by partial ileal bypass than in monkeys treated with cholestyramine and in

the untreated controls. In studies using white Carneau pigeons (Gomes et al, 1971), birds with naturally occurring atherosclerosis, partial ileal bypass reduced the severity of aortic atherosclerosis without interfering with normal growth and weight gain. Regression of atherosclerotic plaques after partial ileal bypass was also noted in this experimental preparation.

These laboratory experiments have been complemented by the evaluation of human cholesterol dynamics after partial ileal bypass using radioisotope techniques (Moore et al, 1969, 1970). Cholesterol absorption from the intestine is reduced by 60% after partial ileal bypass. This reduced cholesterol absorption has been maintained for 10 years after the operation. A 3.8-fold increase in total fecal steroid excretion, with a greater increase in bile acid excretion (4.9-fold) than in neutral steroid excretion (2.7-fold), has been observed. This increased steroid excretion has also been maintained for as long as 10 years. Compensatory cholesterol and bile acid absorptive adaptation by the nonbypassed small intestine apparently does not occur. Thus, the effects of partial ileal bypass on the cholesterol and the bile acid enterohepatic cycles appear to remain unchanged over time.

Other homeostatic mechanisms in humans do change in response to the increased loss of cholesterol and bile acids. A 5.7-fold increase in the syn-

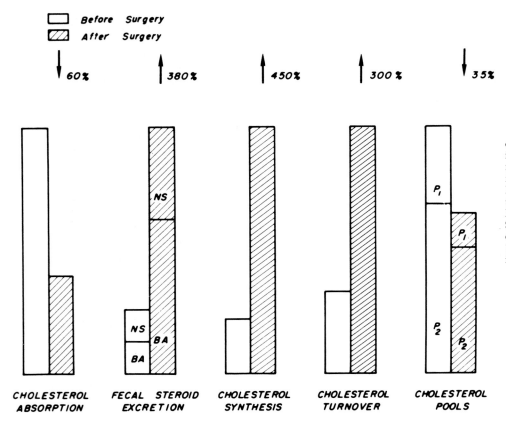

Figure 54–128. Changes in cholesterol dynamics after partial ileal bypass. (NS = neutral steroids; BA = bile acids; P_1 = freely miscible cholesterol pool; P_2 = less freely miscible cholesterol pool.) (From Buchwald, H., Moore, R. B., and Varco, R. L.: Surgical treatment of hyperlipidemia. Circulation, 49(Suppl. 1):1, 1974. By permission of the American Heart Association, Inc.)

thesis rate of cholesterol occurs after partial ileal bypass. This effect is also maintained for as long as 10 years. The cholesterol turnover rate increases greatly. One year after partial ileal bypass, the total exchangeable cholesterol pool is reduced by about one-third. This lowering is reflected in both the freely miscible cholesterol pool (plasma, red blood cells, liver, intestinal mucosa) and the less freely miscible pool (fat stores, muscle, organs). The less freely miscible cholesterol pool includes cholesterol deposited in arterial walls. Loss of cholesterol from the less freely miscible cholesterol pool reflects a loss of cholesterol from atherosclerotic plaques. The effects of partial ileal bypass on cholesterol dynamics are summarized in Figure 54–128.

Operative Technique

The abdomen is generally entered through a transverse, right lower quadrant incision approximately 2 cm below the umbilicus (Fig. 54–129). When an additional procedure (e.g., cholecystectomy) is planned, an upper transverse or a midline abdominal incision is preferred. After routine abdominal exploration, the length of the entire small bowel is determined along the mesenteric border with a calibrated umbilical tape. This intestinal length, measured from the ileocecal valve to the ligament of Treitz under general anesthesia, varies between 400 and 700 cm. The bowel is transected 200 cm proximal to the

ileocecal valve or at a point one-third the length of the small bowel if the total length is greater than 600 cm, allowing 25 cm for the duodenal length. The distal end of the divided ileum is closed. The proximal end is anastomosed, end-to-side, into the anterior taenia of the cecum approximately 6 cm above the inverted appendiceal stump. The appendix, if present, is routinely removed. The cecum is retained to maximize the colonic, water-absorptive surface. The anastomosis is made distal to the ileocecal valve to minimize ileal absorption of cholesterol and bile acids. The closed end of the bypassed distal bowel is sutured to the anterior taenia of the cecum, between the anastomosis and the appendiceal stump, to prevent intussusception of this segment. The small divisional and the large rotational mesenteric defects are carefully closed to prevent internal herniation. The abdomen is thoroughly irrigated and closed in layers, by using nonabsorbable, fascial sutures. No drains are used. Postoperative convalescence has averaged approximately 6 days.

Plasma Lipid and Lipoprotein Results

The authors' clinical experience with partial ileal bypass can be divided into two categories: results achieved in patients having the operation as part of the Program on the Surgical Control of the Hyperlipidemias (POSCH) and results obtained in patients outside of the POSCH trial. The intervention group in POSCH (421 patients) was counseled in the prudent diet therapy for hypercholesterolemia of the American Heart Association and had a partial ileal bypass. The control group (417 patients) was treated with restriction of dietary fat and cholesterol alone. Analysis of the lipid and lipoprotein results after partial ileal bypass in the POSCH trial provides the only controlled assessment of the lipid modification achieved by partial ileal bypass in hypercholesterolemic patients.

In the experience outside of the POSCH trial, total plasma cholesterol was reduced by an average of 41% from the preoperative, post-diet intervention baseline after partial ileal bypass (Buchwald et al, 1974c, 1974d). In combination with phenotype-specific dietary fat and cholesterol restriction, a 53% lowering of the total plasma cholesterol level has been achieved in Type II-A patients (Buchwald et al, 1968) (Fig. 54–130). In addition to its effectiveness in Type II-A individuals, partial ileal bypass significantly reduces the total plasma cholesterol level in all other lipoprotein phenotypes. These results develop rapidly, usually within 3 months of operation, and appear to be permanent. No significant rebound changes occur after the initial lipoprotein modifica-

tions achieved by partial ileal bypass. Follow-up extends beyond 20 years in several patients. Similar lipid results after partial ileal bypass have been reported by other investigators (Balfour and Kim, 1974; Chalstrey et al, 1982; Clot et al, 1971; Grundy et al, 1971; Kelly et al, 1982; Koivisto and Miettinen, 1984; Koivisto et al, 1987; Macarone-Palmieri et al, 1978; Miettinen and Lempinen, 1977; Russell et al, 1979; Schouten and Beynen, 1986; Schouten et al, 1985; Sodel et al, 1970; Spengel et al, 1981; Strisower et al, 1968a, 1968b; Van Niekerk et al, 1984; Vaislic et al, 1984).

The lipid and lipoprotein results after partial ileal bypass in the initial 396 (196 control and 200 operative) patients in the POSCH trial with complete 5-year results have recently been reviewed (Campos et al, 1987). In comparison with the diet-treated control group, total plasma cholesterol levels were significantly lower in patients who had a partial ileal bypass: 32.7 ± 1.0% (mean ± SEM) at 3 months, 27.9 ± 1.1% at 1 year, 26.1 ± 1.1% at 2 years, 25.2 ± 1.1% at 3 years, 25.6 ± 1.1% at 4 years, and 23.9 ± 1.2% at 5 years (Fig. 54–131). LDL levels were significantly lower in the surgical patients than in the controls: 46.3 ± 1.4% at 3 months, 42.0 ± 1.5%

Figure 54–129. Operative technique: (1) measurement of the bowel along the mesenteric border; (2) division of the bowel; (3) closure of the distal end leaving the middle and corner sutures uncut; (4) end-to-side anastomosis of the proximal bowel into the anterior taenia of the cecum; (5) completed anastomosis; (6) suturing of the closed end of the bypassed bowel to the anterior taenia of the cecum by using the uncut sutures with closure of the mesenteric defects.

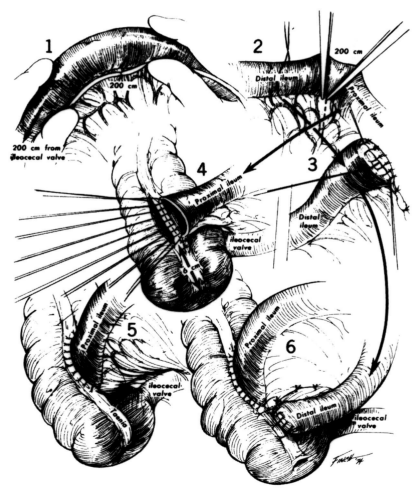

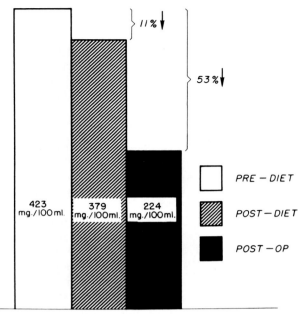

Figure 54–130. Reduction of the total plasma cholesterol level after dietary intervention and partial ileal bypass in 24 Type II-A patients. (From Buchwald, H., Moore, R. B., and Varco, R. L.: Surgical treatment of hyperlipidemia. Circulation, *49*(Suppl. 1):1, 1974. By permission of the American Heart Association, Inc.)

at 1 year, 41.6 ± 1.4% at 2 years, 39.8 ± 1.4% at 3 years, 40.4 ± 1.5% at 4 years, and 38.2 ± 1.5% at 5 years (Fig. 54–132). HDL levels were not significantly changed from the preoperative baseline in patients having a partial ileal bypass. However, in the diet-treated controls, a slow decline in HDL occurred over time; therefore, the HDL levels were significantly higher in the patients having a partial ileal bypass than in the nonoperated controls: 7.7 ± 2.3% at 1

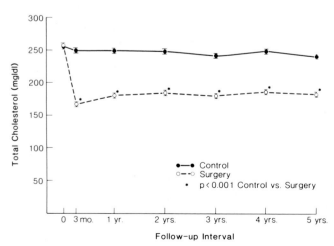

Figure 54–131. Total plasma cholesterol levels in 200 patients after partial ileal bypass and in 196 diet-treated controls in POSCH. (From Campos, C. T., Matts, J. P., Fitch, L. L., et al: Lipoprotein modification achieved by partial ileal bypass: Five-year results of the Program of the Surgical Control of the Hyperlipidemias. Surgery, *102*:424, 1987.)

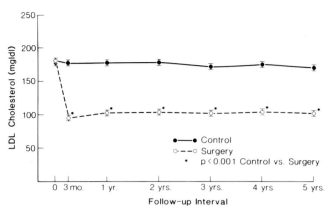

Figure 54–132. LDL cholesterol reduction in 200 patients after partial ileal bypass and in 196 diet-treated controls in POSCH. (From Campos, C. T., Matts, J. P., Fitch, L. L., et al: Lipoprotein modification achieved by partial ileal bypass: Five-year results of the Program on the Surgical Control of the Hyperlipidemias. Surgery, *102*:424, 1987.)

year, 7.4 ± 2.2% at 2 years, 7.7 ± 2.2% at 3 years, 6.7 ± 2.3% at 4 years, and 4.9 ± 2.3% at 5 years (Fig. 54–133). VLDL and triglyceride levels slowly increased after partial ileal bypass. Five years postoperatively, VLDL levels were 24 ± 7.6% higher and triglyceride levels were 21 ± 5.4% higher in the operative group than in the control group (Fig. 54–134).

The ratios of HDL to total plasma cholesterol and HDL to LDL are inversely correlated with the severity of atherosclerosis. Increases in these ratios are associated with decreased atherosclerosis risk. Five years after partial ileal bypass, the ratio of HDL to total plasma cholesterol was 44 ± 3.5% greater and the ratio of HDL to LDL was 85 ± 5.3% higher than in the nonoperated controls in POSCH (Campos et al, 1987).

Determinations of the concentrations of apolipoprotein A-I, the major carrier protein for HDL,

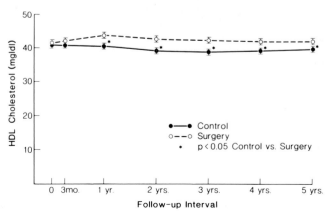

Figure 54–133. HDL cholesterol levels in 200 patients after partial ileal bypass and in 196 diet-treated controls in POSCH. (From Campos, C. T., Matts, J. P., Fitch, L. L., et al: Five-year results of the Program on the Surgical Control of the Hyperlipidemias. Surgery, *102*:424, 1987.)

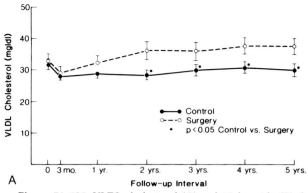
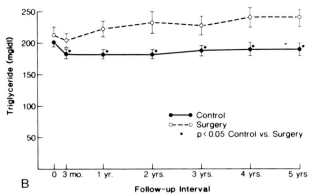

A   Follow-up Interval   **B**   Follow-up Interval

Figure 54–134. VLDL cholesterol *(A)* and triglyceride *(B)* changes in 200 patients after partial ileal bypass compared with 196 diet-treated controls in POSCH. (From Campos, C. T., Matts, J. P., Fitch, L. L., et al: Five-year results of the Program on the Surgical Control of the Hyperlipidemias. Surgery, *102*:424, 1987.)

and apolipoprotein B-100, the major carrier protein for LDL, are thought to be more predictive of the severity of atherosclerosis than measurements of HDL or LDL levels alone. Similarly, determination of the HDL-2 subfraction level is thought to provide additional predictive information, with an increase in HDL-2 correlated with decreased severity of atherosclerosis. Since 1985, measurements of apolipoprotein and HDL subfraction levels have been done in POSCH. In the subset of patients with these levels available (Table 54–36), a significantly lower apolipoprotein B-100 level and significantly higher apolipoprotein A-I and HDL-2 levels were found in patients who had a partial ileal bypass than in the diet-treated controls.

When the lipid and lipoprotein results after partial ileal bypass were examined in each of the common lipoprotein phenotypes present in the POSCH trial, total plasma cholesterol was 26.5 ± 1.2% lower in normal phenotype patients, 24.7 ± 2.2% lower in Type II-A patients, 27.8 ± 9.6% lower in Type II-B patients, and 18.3 ± 2.9% lower in Type IV patients than in diet-treated controls 5 years after operation (Fig. 54–135). Patients with a normal phenotype have hypercholesterolemia (total plasma cholesterol ≥ 220 mg/dl or LDL ≥ 140 mg/dl if the total plasma cholesterol is between 200 mg/dl and 219 mg/dl). However, the magnitude of their lipoprotein abnormality is not greater than the 90th or 95th

percentile required for assignment to a specific lipoprotein phenotype.

LDL cholesterol was reduced 39.4 ± 1.5% in normal phenotype patients, 35.4 ± 2.8% in Type II-A patients, 28.4 ± 9.1% in Type II-B patients, and 41.8 ± 3.8% in Type IV patients compared with nonoperated controls 5 years after operation (see Fig. 54–135). HDL cholesterol was 6.8 ± 2.4% higher in normal phenotype patients, 2.6 ± 5.2% lower in Type II-A patients, 20.7 ± 11.3% higher in Type II-B patients, and 1.9 ± 5.9% higher in Type IV patients 5 years after partial ileal bypass (Campos et al, 1988b).

Partial ileal bypass is equally effective in men and women with hypercholesterolemia. Compared with diet-treated controls, partial ileal bypass reduced the total plasma cholesterol 28 ± 1%, 26 ± 1%, and 24 ± 1% at 1, 3, and 5 years after operation in men and lowered the total plasma cholesterol 30 ± 3%, 27 ± 2%, and 27 ± 3% at 1, 3, and 5-year follow-up in women. LDL cholesterol was 43 ± 1%, 42 ± 1%, and 39 ± 1% lower at 1, 3, and 5 years after partial ileal bypass in men and was 42 ± 4%, 42 ± 3%, and 38 ± 4% lower 1, 3, and 5 years postoperatively in women. HDL cholesterol levels were 10 ± 2%, 8 ± 2%, and 7 ± 2% higher at 1, 3, and 5 years after partial ileal bypass in men and were 10 ± 5%, 8 ± 6%, and 9 ± 7% higher 1, 3, and 5 years postoperatively in women (Campos et al, 1988a).

TABLE 54–36. APOLIPOPROTEIN AND HDL SUBFRACTION RESULTS IN PATIENTS 4 AND 5 YEARS AFTER PARTIAL ILEAL BYPASS COMPARED WITH RESULTS IN DIET-TREATED CONTROLS IN POSCH*

Interval	Group	Apolipoprotein B-100	Apolipoprotein A-I	HDL-2	HDL-3
4 years	C(*n*=31)	137.1 ± 4.6	104.7 ± 3.8	8.1 ± 1.0	31.0 ± 0.8
	S(*n*=22)	88.7 ± 3.9†	129.0 ± 5.2†	13.0 ± 1.1†	30.5 ± 1.2
5 years	C(*n*=71)	129.6 ± 2.4	104.0 ± 2.1	7.7 ± 0.6	31.7 ± 0.6
	S(*n*=74)	94.7 ± 2.1†	125.0 ± 2.3†	11.9 ± 0.7†	31.4 ± 0.8

*From Campos, C. T., Matts, J. P., Fitch, L. L., et al: Lipoprotein modification achieved by partial ileal bypass: Five-year results of the Program on the Surgical Control of the Hyperlipidemias. Surgery, *102*:424, 1987.
†p < 0.005, control versus surgery.
Values as mean ± SEM in mg/dl. C = control; S = surgery.

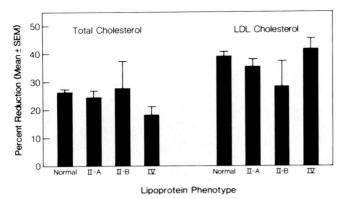

Figure 54–135. Percent reductions in total plasma cholesterol and in LDL cholesterol 5 years after partial ileal bypass in the common WHO lipoprotein phenotypes. (From Campos, C. T., Matts, J. P., Fitch, L. L., et al: Normalization of lipoproteins following ileal bypass in individual WHO lipoprotein phenotypes. Curr. Surg., 45:380, 1988.)

It is not possible to predict precisely the reductions in total plasma cholesterol or LDL cholesterol expected after partial ileal bypass in individual patients. By using stepwise linear regression analysis of numerous preoperative patient characteristics (Campos et al, 1988c), the preoperative total plasma cholesterol level was the only significant, independent, preoperative predictor of the 5-year total plasma cholesterol level (5-year total plasma cholesterol = 0.54 × baseline total plasma cholesterol + 42.3; r = 0.547; p < 0.001). The preoperative LDL level was the only significant, independent, preoperative predictor of the 5-year LDL level (5-year LDL = 0.455 × baseline LDL + 19.2; r = 0.599; p < 0.001).

Operative Morbidity and Mortality

In the authors' experience, partial ileal bypass can be done with an operative mortality of less than 1%, even though most patients have overt manifestations of atherosclerotic cardiovascular disease. Wound infections, pneumonia, pulmonary emboli, or other serious postoperative complications requiring hospitalization for more than 1 week have occurred in 2% of patients (Buchwald et al, 1974c, 1974d). Intussusception of the bypassed segment and bowel obstruction resulting from internal herniation due to inadequate closure of the divisional or rotational mesenteric defects have not occurred in this series and appear to be avoidable complications. The incidences of late bowel obstruction secondary to adhesions (2%) and late development of incisional hernia (5%) are identical to those observed after any abdominal surgical procedure.

Side Effects of Partial Ileal Bypass

Diarrhea is the most frequent side effect after partial ileal bypass. Generally, it is not persistent.

One year after operation, 86% of patients have fewer than five bowel movements per day without bowel-controlling medications (Buchwald et al, 1974d). Further intestinal adaptation occurs, and most patients have an additional increase in the firmness and consistency of their stools over time. Less than 2% of patients in this series have had operative restoration of intestinal continuity because of intractable diarrhea.

After partial ileal bypass, vitamin B_{12} absorption is either severely impaired or totally lost (Buchwald, 1964). After several years, absorptive adaptation for vitamin B_{12} occurs in approximately 50% of patients (Coyle et al, 1977; Nygaard et al, 1970). Nevertheless, it is believed prudent to provide 1,000 μg of vitamin B_{12} intramuscularly every 4 to 6 weeks after partial ileal bypass for the lifetime of the patient.

An increased incidence of calcium oxalate renal calculi has been observed after partial ileal bypass. Oral calcium was once prescribed to reduce intestinal oxalate absorption, without appreciable benefit. Patients currently are advised to avoid dietary oxalate, to maintain adequate daily fluid intake, and to take oral potassium citrate (20 mEq three times daily) to alkalize their urine. It is not clear whether this latter treatment decreases renal stone formation. The use of potassium citrate after partial ileal bypass is currently being evaluated in a randomized, placebo-controlled clinical trial. No cases of nephrocalcinosis leading to renal function impairment or loss have been noted after partial ileal bypass.

Excessive, foul-smelling flatus and the gas-bloat syndrome are occasionally encountered after partial ileal bypass. These patients generally respond to a 2-week course of oral metronidazole (250 mg three times daily). If these symptoms recur, patients are placed on oral metronidazole indefinitely (250 mg/day).

Although variable in occurrence, gastric hypersecretion after massive intestinal resection or the jejunoileal bypass for morbid obesity has been documented (Frederick et al, 1965; Osborne et al, 1966). However, laboratory and clinical studies of gastric volume and acid output in a randomly selected group of patients before and after partial ileal bypass has demonstrated no similar hypersecretory effect (Buchwald and Varco, 1971; Buchwald et al, 1974a).

Contrary to the experience frequently encountered after jejunoileal bypass for morbid obesity, no significant changes in serum electrolytes follow partial ileal bypass. Specifically, the potassium, calcium, and magnesium values remain within normal limits (Buchwald et al, 1969). A need for electrolyte supplements after partial ileal bypass has not been reported. Nutrient malabsorption has not been described after partial ileal bypass, and no long-term weight loss has occurred in these patients (Buchwald et al, 1974c).

Finally, and of considerable importance in clearly distinguishing partial ileal bypass from the jejunoileal bypass formerly used for the management of morbid

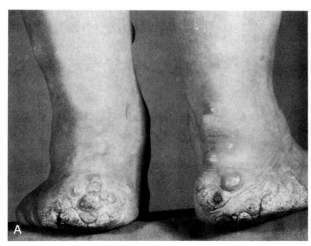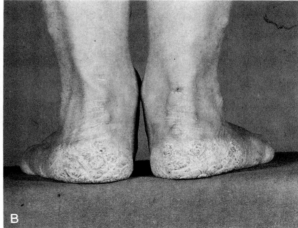

Figure 54-136. Marked regression of tendon xanthomata after partial ileal bypass (*A,* Preoperative appearance; *B,* Appearance 1 year after operation).

obesity, hepatic fatty infiltration or fibrosis leading to hepatic insufficiency in occasional patients has not occurred after partial ileal bypass (Schwartz et al, 1971).

Clinical Results

Xanthomata. Various investigators have reported a postoperative decrease in the size or even disappearance of periorbital xanthelasma, subcutaneous xanthomata (Fig. 54-136), and tendon xanthomata, particularly xanthomata of the plantar extensor tendons (Buchwald, 1970; Buchwald et al, 1974c, 1974d; Helsinger and Rootwelt, 1969). A reduction in the size of xanthomatous lesions appears to indicate that tissue lipid stores have been mobilized and are being excreted from the body. Theoretically, this lipid mobilization should also occur from arterial walls.

Angina Pectoris. Many individuals with angina pectoris have reported a reduction in the frequency of the attacks or the complete disappearance of these symptoms during comparable effort after partial ileal bypass (Buchwald et al, 1974c; Fritz and Walker, 1966; Sodal et al, 1970; Swan and McGowan, 1968). A survey of 101 patients (Buchwald et al, 1974d) showed that of the 41 individuals who were free of angina pectoris before partial ileal bypass, none developed these symptoms subsequently. Of the 60 patients with angina pectoris preoperatively, 7% stated that their condition was worse; 27% had no change; 23% reported moderate improvement, which was determined by a reduction in their use of nitroglycerin; 18% stated that they had marked improvement, which was determined by reduced use of nitroglycerin and an increase in exercise capacity; and 25% stated that they had complete remission of angina pectoris. Thus, 66% of the patients with angina pectoris before operation had subjective improvement postoperatively (Fig. 54-137). In several

of these patients, although not in all, a concomitant objective improvement in exercise tolerance without the development of ischemic ST-T wave changes was observed during treadmill exercise testing. Although difficult to quantitate, these findings may indicate improvement in circulatory hemodynamics or tissue oxygen delivery. In-vitro experiments using rabbit blood show that oxygen extraction from blood with

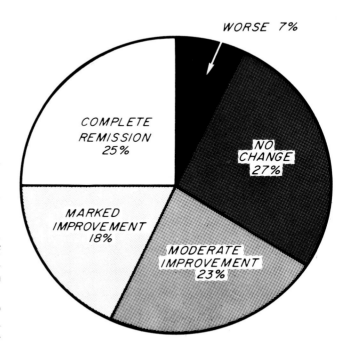

Total Improvement : 66%

Figure 54-137. Changes in patients' subjective assessment of angina pectoris after partial ileal bypass in 60 patients with angina pectoris at the time of operation. (From Buchwald, H., Moore, R. B., and Varco, R. L.: Ten years' clinical experience with partial ileal bypass in management of the hyperlipidemias. Ann. Surg., *180:*384, 1974.)

a high cholesterol content is significantly less than from blood with a low cholesterol content (Steinbach et al, 1974). A barrier to oxygen diffusion resides within the red blood cell membrane when the cholesterol content is increased. The effect of this diffusion block is to shift the oxygen-hemoglobin dissociation curve to the left. Serial treadmill exercise testing and symptom assessment are done on all POSCH patients. Final analysis of these data at the conclusion of POSCH in 1990 will definitively show whether cholesterol lowering is associated with subjective improvement in angina pectoris and objective improvement in treadmill exercise tolerance.

Serial Arteriography. Analyses of sequential arteriograms in patients with partial ileal bypass having the operation outside the POSCH trial indicate that retardation of the progression of atherosclerosis may occur as a result of the significant, sustained lipid modification accomplished by this procedure. Apparent coronary arteriographic evidence of plaque regression has been noted in several patients with partial ileal bypass 1 to 2 years (Baltaxe et al, 1969; Knight et al, 1972) and 10 years (Buchwald et al, 1983) postoperatively (Fig. 54–138). Serial coronary

and peripheral arteriograms are being obtained in all POSCH participants. Analysis of these results in 1990 will assess the effects of marked lipid modification on the angiographic course of atherosclerosis. Most important, POSCH will assess whether these angiographic results are correlated with changes in the rates of fatal and nonfatal events in aggressively treated, hypercholesterolemic patients.

Other Surgical Approaches

In 1973, Starzl and associates first described end-to-side portacaval anastomosis for management of a homozygous Type II-A hyperlipidemic patient (Starzl et al, 1973, 1983). In this patient, total plasma cholesterol was lowered from 769 to 343 mg/dl, a reduction of 55%. Total plasma cholesterol reductions of 10 to 70% have subsequently been reported after portacaval shunting (Cywes et al, 1976; Stein et al, 1975). The mechanism of cholesterol lowering after portacaval shunting is unclear. Shunting of portal venous blood, rich in nutrients, hormones, and hepatotrophic factors, away from the liver may result

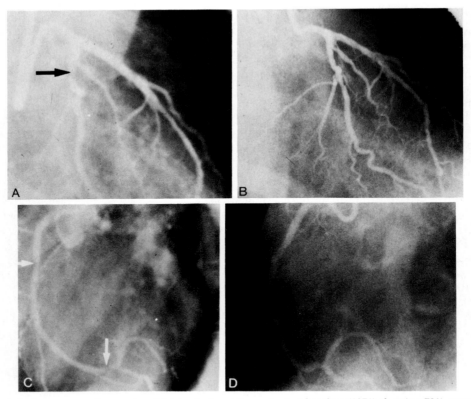

Figure 54–138. *A,* Left coronary artery system (right anterior oblique view) at baseline (1971) showing 70% stenosis of the proximal left circumflex artery *(arrow),* 30% stenosis of the first diagonal branch of the left anterior descending artery, and 30% stenosis of the second obtuse marginal branch. *B,* Left coronary artery system (right anterior oblique view) 10 years after partial ileal bypass (1981) showing 20% stenosis of the proximal left circumflex artery and no changes in the stenoses in the other segments noted at baseline. *C,* Right coronary artery (RCA) system (left anterior oblique view) at baseline (1971) showing 90% spasm (with underlying stenosis of unknown extent) of the proximal RCA, 45% stenosis of the middle segment of the RCA *(upper arrow),* and 80% stenosis of the distal RCA *(lower arrow). D,* RCA system (left anterior oblique view) 10 years after partial ileal bypass (1981) showing 20% stenosis of the proximal RCA, 20% stenosis of the middle segment of the RCA, and 50% stenosis of the distal RCA.

in decreased lipoprotein synthesis. Portacaval shunting is currently used only in selected patients who have severe homozygous Type II hyperlipidemia and who have had an inadequate response to intensive dietary and pharmacologic therapy.

De Gennes and colleagues (1967) reported lowering of total plasma cholesterol by plasmapheresis. By using 800-ml exchanges every other day for 2 months, a 39% reduction in total plasma cholesterol was achieved. Smaller decreases result from less frequent plasmaphereses. Cholesterol levels return to baseline when therapy is terminated. Plasmapheresis with selective LDL absorption columns is currently being investigated (Mabuchi et al, 1987).

Starzl and colleagues (1984) did combined cardiac and hepatic transplantation in a young girl with severe homozygous Type II hyperlipidemia. Individuals with this disorder produce few or no LDL receptors and accumulate great quantities of LDL in the plasma. Because the liver is responsible for almost three-fourths of the total number of LDL receptors, successful hepatic transplantation should dramatically lower total and LDL cholesterol levels. Hepatic transplantation has now been done in combination with cardiac transplantation in several homozygous Type II patients with end-stage coronary artery disease (Shaw et al, 1985). In the initial case, total plasma cholesterol decreased 72%, from 1,079 to 302 mg/dl, within weeks of the procedure. At present, hepatic transplantation for hypercholesterolemia is limited to highly selected patients who require concomitant cardiac replacement.

CONCLUSION

Experimental and epidemiologic evidence is accumulating to support efforts to reduce elevated total plasma cholesterol and LDL cholesterol levels to diminish the risk of atherosclerotic cardiovascular disease. Partial ileal bypass is not proposed as the first-choice therapy for hyperlipidemia; however, this procedure may be the ideal treatment for certain hypercholesterolemic patients at high risk for atherosclerosis, particularly those who have failed to respond to previous dietary or pharmacologic therapy. The available data clearly show that only modest cholesterol lowering can be achieved by restriction of dietary fat and cholesterol. With the exception of high-dose HMG-CoA reductase inhibitor therapy, the long-term effects of which are unknown, no available pharmacologic agent can achieve the lipid modification accomplished by partial ileal bypass. The cholesterol reduction observed after partial ileal bypass is substantial and sustained, and follow-up extends to 25 years in several patients. Patients may or may not adhere to a diet; they may or may not take medications. However, when a partial ileal bypass has been performed, its therapeutic effects are obligatory and lasting.

Selected Bibliography

Blankenhorn, D. H., Nessim, S. A., Johnson, R. L., et al: Beneficial effects of combined colestipol-niacin therapy on coronary atherosclerosis and coronary venous bypass grafts. J.A.M.A., *257*:3233, 1987.

This final report of the Cholesterol-Lowering Atherosclerosis Study provides the most convincing evidence available that lowering of total plasma cholesterol and LDL cholesterol is beneficial. By using angiographic end-points, it was found that patients who had cholesterol reduction had less progression of existing disease and a lower incidence of de-novo lesion formation. A beneficial effect of cholesterol reduction on coronary venous bypass grafts was also shown. No beneficial effect on clinical end-points (cause-specific morbidity or mortality) was observed; however, this study was designed to assess angiographic rather than clinical end-points.

Buchwald, H., Moore, R. B., and Varco, R. L.: Surgical treatment of hyperlipidemia. Circulation, *49*(Suppl. 1):1, 1974.

This three-part monograph summarizes the authors' initial laboratory and clinical experience with partial ileal bypass. It may be useful to those interested in the initial experiments examining cholesterol and bile acid metabolism that led to the development of the partial ileal bypass procedure.

Campos, C. T., Matts, J. P., Fitch, L. L., et al: Lipoprotein modification achieved by partial ileal bypass: Five-year results of the Program on the Surgical Control of the Hyperlipidemias. Surgery, *102*:424, 1987.

This article presents the 5-year lipoprotein results of the Program on the Surgical Control of the Hyperlipidemias. The lipid responses after partial ileal bypass are compared with those achieved by dietary fat and cholesterol restriction. These data represent the only controlled assessment of the efficacy of the partial ileal bypass procedure.

Campos, C. T., Matts, J. P., Santilli, S. M., et al: Predictors of total and low-density lipoprotein cholesterol change after partial ileal bypass. Am. J. Surg., *155*:138, 1988.

This article examines the preoperative predictors of lipoprotein response 5 years after partial ileal bypass. Predictive equations that allow calculation of estimated postoperative total plasma cholesterol and LDL cholesterol levels are developed.

The Expert Panel: Report of the National Cholesterol Education Program Expert Panel on detection, evaluation, and treatment of high blood cholesterol in adults. Arch. Intern. Med., *148*:36, 1988.

This report gives detailed guidelines for the evaluation and treatment of hypercholesterolemia in adults. Dietary and pharmacologic therapies are emphasized; however, the authors believe that partial ileal bypass should have a role in the management of hypercholesterolemia in high-risk patients.

Bibliography

Ad Hoc Committee to Design a Dietary Treatment of Hyperlipoproteinemia: AHA Special Report: Recommendations for treatment of hyperlipidemia in adults. Circulation, *69*:1065A, 1984.
Adlersberg, D.: Hypercholesterolemia with predisposition to atherosclerosis: Inborn error of lipid metabolism. Am. J. Med., *11*:600, 1951.
American Heart Association: Heart Facts 1981. Dallas, American Heart Association Communications Division, 1981.

Anitschkow, N., and Chalatow, S.: Uber experimentelle Cholesterinsteatose. Zentralbl. Allg. Pathol., 24:1, 1913.

Arntzenius, A. C., Kromhout, D., Barth, J. D., et al: Diet, lipoproteins, and the progression of coronary atherosclerosis: The Leiden Intervention Trial. N. Engl. J. Med., 312:805, 1985.

Balfour, J. F., and Kim, R.: Homozygous type II hyperlipoproteinemia treatment, partial ileal bypass in two children. J.A.M.A., 227:1145, 1974.

Baltaxe, H., Amplatz, K., Varco, R. L., and Buchwald, H.: Coronary arteriography in hypercholesterolemic patients. Am. J. Roentgenol., 105:784, 1969.

Beaumont, J. L., Carlson, L. A., Cooper, G. R., et al: Classification of the hyperlipidemias and hyperlipoproteinemias. Bull. W.H.O., 43:891, 1970.

Blankenhorn, D. H., Nessim, S. A., Johnson, R. L., et al: Beneficial effects of combined colestipol-niacin therapy on coronary atherosclerosis and coronary venous bypass grafts. J.A.M.A., 257:3233, 1987.

Brensike, J. F., Levy, R. I., Kelsey, S. F., et al: Effects of therapy with cholestyramine on progression of coronary atherosclerosis: Results of the NHLBI Type II Coronary Intervention Study. Circulation, 69:313, 1984.

Brewer, E. R., Ashman, P. L., and Kuba, K.: The Minnesota Coronary Survey: Composition of the diets, adherence, and serum lipid response. Circulation, 52(Suppl. 2):269, 1975.

Buchwald, H.: Alterations in the cutaneous lesions of the hyperlipidemias following partial ileal bypass. Dermatol. Dig., 9:65, 1970.

Buchwald, H.: The effect of ileal bypass on atherosclerosis and hypercholesterolemia in the rabbit. Surgery, 58:22, 1965a.

Buchwald, H.: Myocardial infarction in rabbits induced solely by a hypercholesterolemic diet. J. Atheroscler. Res., 5:407, 1965b.

Buchwald, H.: Vitamin B12 absorption deficiency following bypass of the ileum. Am. J. Dig. Dis., 9:755, 1964.

Buchwald, H., Coyle, J. J., and Varco, R. L.: Effect of small bowel bypass on gastric secretory function: Postintestinal exclusion hypersecretion, a phenomenon in search of a syndrome. Surgery, 75:821, 1974a.

Buchwald, H., Fitch, L. L., and Varco, R. L.: Surgical intervention in atherosclerosis: Partial ileal bypass and the Program on the Surgical Control of the Hyperlipidemias (POSCH). Pharmacol. Ther., 29:93, 1985.

Buchwald, H., and Gebhard, R. L.: Effect of intestinal bypass on cholesterol absorption and blood levels in the rabbit. Am. J. Physiol., 20:567, 1964.

Buchwald, H., and Gebhard, R. L.: Localization of bile salt absorption in vivo in the rabbit. Ann. Surg., 167:191, 1968.

Buchwald, H., Gebhard, R. L., and Varco, R. L.: Relative secretion of cholesterol-4-14C in the bile and upper and lower small intestinal washings of the bile fistula rabbit. Surgery, 75:266, 1974b.

Buchwald, H., Moore, R. B., Bertish, J., and Varco, R. L.: Effect of ileal bypass on cholesterol levels, atherosclerosis and growth in the infant rabbit. Ann. Surg., 175:311, 1972.

Buchwald, H., Moore, R. B., and Frantz, I. D., Jr.: Serum uric acid, carotene and vitamin A, proteins, sugar, and electrolyte balance before and after partial ileal bypass for hyperlipidemia. Circulation, 40(Suppl. 3):4, 1969.

Buchwald, H., Moore, R. B., Lee, G. B., et al: Combined dietary, surgical, and bile salt binding resin therapy in the treatment of hypercholesterolemia. Arch. Surg., 97:275, 1968.

Buchwald, H., Moore, R. B., Matts, J. P., et al: The Program on the Surgical Control of the Hyperlipidemias: A status report. Surgery, 92:654, 1982.

Buchwald, H., Moore, R. B., Rucker, R. D., Jr., et al: Clinical angiographic regression of atherosclerosis after partial ileal bypass. Atherosclerosis, 46:117, 1983.

Buchwald, H., Moore, R. B., and Varco, R. L.: Surgical treatment of hyperlipidemia. Circulation, 49(Suppl. 1):1, 1974c.

Buchwald, H., Moore, R. B., and Varco, R. L.: Ten years clinical experience with partial ileal bypass in management of the hyperlipidemias. Ann. Surg., 180:384, 1974d.

Buchwald, H., and Varco, R. L.: Human gastric secretory studies

following distal small bowel bypass. Curr. Top. Surg. Res., 3:409, 1971.

Campos, C. T., Matts, J. P., Fitch, L. L., et al: Comparison of male and female lipoprotein results following partial ileal bypass for hypercholesterolemia. Surg. Forum, 39:193, 1988a.

Campos, C. T., Matts, J. P., Fitch, L. L., et al: Lipoprotein modification achieved by partial ileal bypass: Five-year results of the Program on the Surgical Control of the Hyperlipidemias. Surgery, 102:424, 1987.

Campos, C. T., Matts, J. P., Fitch, L. L., et al: Normalization of lipoproteins following partial ileal bypass in individual WHO lipoprotein phenotypes. Curr. Surg., 45:380, 1988b.

Campos, C. T., Matts, J. P., Santilli, S. M., et al: Predictors of total and low-density lipoprotein cholesterol change after partial ileal bypass. Am. J. Surg., 155:138, 1988c.

Canner, P. L., Berge, K. G., Wenger, N. K., et al: Fifteen year mortality in Coronary Drug Project patients: Long-term benefit with niacin. J. Am. Coll. Cardiol., 8:1245, 1986.

Chalstrey, L. J., Winder, A. F., and Galton, D. J.: Partial ileal bypass in treatment of familial hypercholesterolemia. J. R. Soc. Med., 75:851, 1982.

Cleeman, J. I., and Lenfant, C.: New guidelines for the treatment of high blood cholesterol in adults from the National Cholesterol Education Program. Circulation, 76:960, 1987.

Clot, J. P., Roufly, J., Loeper, J., and Mercadier, M.: Dérivation iléal, thérapeutique, chirurgicale des hypercholesterolémies pures majeures (à propos de deux observations). Chirurgie, 97:57, 1971.

Committee of Principal Investigators: WHO Clofibrate Trial: WHO cooperative trial on primary prevention of ischaemic heart disease using clofibrate to lower serum cholesterol: Mortality follow-up. Lancet, 2:379, 1980.

Committee of Principal Investigators: WHO Clofibrate Trial: WHO cooperative trial on primary prevention of ischaemic heart disease with clofibrate to lower serum cholesterol: Final mortality follow-up. Lancet, 2:600, 1984.

Coyle, J. J., Varco, R. L., and Buchwald, H.: Vitamin B12 absorption following human intestinal bypass surgery. Am. J. Dig. Dis., 22:1069, 1977.

Cywes, S., Davies, M. R. Q., Louw, J. H., et al: Portacaval shunt in two patients with homozygous type II hyperlipoproteinaemia. S. Afr. Med. J., 50:239, 1976.

Davignon, J.: The lipid hypothesis: Pathophysiological basis. Arch. Surg., 113:28, 1978.

Dayton, S., Pearce, M. L., Hashimoto, S., et al: A controlled clinical trial of a diet high in unsaturated fat. Circulation, 40(Suppl. 2):1, 1969.

De Gennes, J. L., Touraine, R., Maunard, B., et al: Formes homozygotes cutaneotendineuses de xanthomatose hypercholesterolémique dans une observation familiale exemplaire. Essai de plasmaphérèse à titre de traitement heroïque. Bull. Mem. Soc. Med. Paris, 118:1377, 1967.

East, C., Alivizatos, P. A., Grundy, S. M., et al: Rhabdomyolysis in patients receiving lovastatin after cardiac transplantation. N. Engl. J. Med., 318:47, 1988.

Edelman, S., and Witztum, J. L.: Hyperkalemia during treatment with HMG-CoA reductase inhibitor. N. Engl. J. Med., 320:1219, 1989.

Eder, H. A.: Drugs used in the prevention and treatment of atherosclerosis. In Goodman, L. S., and Gilman, A. (eds): The Pharmacologic Basis of Therapeutics, 3rd ed. New York, Macmillan, 1965.

Enos, W. F., Holmes, R. H., and Beyer, J.: Coronary disease among United States soldiers killed in action in Korea: Preliminary report. J.A.M.A., 152:1090, 1953.

Frantz, I. D., Jr., Dawson, E. A., Kuba, K., et al: The Minnesota Coronary Survey: Effect of diet on cardiovascular events and deaths. Circulation, 52(Suppl. 2):4, 1975.

Frantz, I. D., Jr., and Moore, R. B.: The sterol hypothesis in atherogenesis. Am. J. Med., 46:684, 1969.

Frederick, P. L., Sizer, J. S., and Osborne, M. P.: Relation of massive bowel resection to gastric secretion. N. Engl. J. Med., 272:509, 1965.

Fredrickson, D. S., and Lees, R. S.: System for phenotyping hyperlipoproteinemia. Circulation, 31:321, 1965.

Frick, M. H., Elo, O., Haapa, K., et al: Helsinki Heart Study: Primary-prevention trial with gemfibrozil in middle-aged men with dyslipidemia. N. Engl. J. Med., 317:1237, 1987.

Fritz, S. H., and Walker, W. J.: Ileal bypass in the control of intractable hypercholesterolemia. Am. Surg., 32:691, 1966.

Gebhard, R. L., and Buchwald, H.: Cholesterol absorption after reversal of the upper and lower halves of the small intestine. Surgery, 67:474, 1970.

Glueck, C. J., and Kwiterovich, P. O., Jr.: The lipid hypothesis: Genetic basis. Arch. Surg., 113:35, 1978.

Goldstein, J. L., Schrott, H. G., Hazzard, W. R., et al: Genetic analysis of lipid levels in 176 families and delineation of a new inherited disorder: Combined hyperlipidemia. J. Clin. Invest., 52:1544, 1973.

Gomes, M. M., Kottke, B. A., Bernatz, P., and Titus, J. L.: Effect of ileal bypass on aortic atherosclerosis in white Carneau pigeons. Surgery, 70:353, 1971.

Gordon, T., Castelli, W. P., Hjortland, M. C., et al: High density lipoprotein as a protective factor against coronary heart disease: The Framingham study. Am. J. Med., 62:707, 1977.

Gotto, A. M., Jr., and Farmer, J. A.: Risk factors for coronary artery disease. In Braunwald, E. (ed): Heart Disease: A Textbook of Cardiovascular Medicine, 3rd ed. Philadelphia, W. B. Saunders Company, 1988, pp. 1153–1190.

Grundy, S. M.: HMG-CoA reductase inhibitors for treatment of hypercholesterolemia. N. Engl. J. Med., 319:24, 1988.

Grundy, S. M., Ahrens, E. H., Jr., and Salen, G.: Interruption of the enterohepatic circulation of bile acids in man: Comparative effects of cholestyramine and ileal exclusion on cholesterol metabolism. J. Lab. Clin. Med., 78:94, 1971.

Grundy, S. M., and Bilheimer, D. W.: Inhibition of 3-hydroxy-3-methylglutaryl CoA reductase by mevinolin in familial hypercholesterolemia heterozygotes: Effects on cholesterol balance. Proc. Natl. Acad. Sci. USA, 81:2538, 1984.

Grundy, S. M., Mok, H. Y. I., Zech, L., and Berman, M.: Influence of nicotinic acid on metabolism of cholesterol and triglycerides in man. J. Lipid Res., 22:24, 1981.

Havel, R. J., Hunninghake, D. B., Illingworth, D. R., et al: Lovastatin (mevinolin) in the treatment of heterozygous familial hypercholesterolemia: A multicenter study. Ann. Intern. Med., 107:609, 1987.

Helsinger, N., Jr., and Rootwelt, K.: Partial ileal bypass for surgical treatment of hypercholesterolemia. Nord. Med., 82:1409, 1969.

Heydenreich, L. H.: Leonardo da Vinci, Vols. I and II. New York, Macmillan-Holbein, 1954.

Hunninghake, D. B., Miller, V. T., Goldberg, I., et al: Lovastatin: Follow-up ophthalmologic data. J.A.M.A., 259:354, 1988.

Illingworth, D. R., and Sexton, G. J.: Hypocholesterolemic effects of mevinolin in patients with heterozygous familial hypercholesterolemia. J. Clin. Invest., 74:1972, 1984.

Kannel, W. B., and Gordon, T.: The Framingham Study: An epidemiologic investigation of cardiovascular disease, Section 30. Some characteristics related to the incidence of cardiovascular disease and death: The Framingham Study. 18-year follow-up. Washington, D.C., Dept. of Health, Education, and Welfare, Pub. No. (NIH) 74-599, 1974.

Kelly, D., Lane, D., Gearly, G., et al: Partial ileal bypass in the treatment of familial hypercholesterolemia. Ir. J. Med. Sci., 151:343, 1982.

Keys, A.: Coronary heart disease in seven countries. Circulation, 41(Suppl. 1):1, 1970.

Knight, L., Scheibel, R., Amplatz, K., et al: Radiographic appraisal of the Minnesota partial ileal bypass study. Surg. Forum, 23:141, 1972.

Koivisto, P., Kuusi, T., and Miettinen, T. A.: High density lipoprotein, apoproteins A-I and A-II and postheparin plasma lipolytic enzymes after ileal bypass. Atherosclerosis, 63:181, 1987.

Koivisto, P., and Miettinen, T. A.: Long-term effects of ileal bypass on lipoproteins in patients with familial hypercholesterolemia. Circulation, 70:290, 1984.

Levy, R. I.: Drugs used in the treatment of hyperlipoproteinemia. In Goodman, A. S., Gilman, L. S., and Gilman, A. (eds): The Pharmacologic Basis of Therapeutics. New York, Macmillan, 1980, pp. 834–877.

Levy, R. I., Brensike, J. F., Epstein, S. E., et al: The influence of changes in lipid values induced by cholestyramine and diet on progression of coronary artery disease: Results of the NHLBI Type II Coronary Intervention Study. Circulation, 69:325, 1984.

Lewis, J. E.: Long-term use of gemfibrozil in the treatment of dyslipidemia. Angiology, 33:603, 1982.

Lipid Research Clinics Program: The Lipid Research Clinics Coronary Primary Prevention Trial results. I: Reduction in incidence of coronary heart disease. J.A.M.A., 251:351, 1984a.

Lipid Research Clinics Program: The Lipid Research Clinics Coronary Primary Prevention Trial results. II: The relationship of reduction in incidence of coronary heart disease to cholesterol lowering. J.A.M.A., 251:365, 1984b.

Mabuchi, H., Michishita, I., Takeda, M., et al: A new low density lipoprotein apheresis system using two dextran sulfate cellulose columns in an automated column regenerating unit (LDL continuous apheresis). Atherosclerosis, 68:19, 1987.

Macarone-Palmieri, R., Chapuis, G., and Saegesser, F.: Experience clinique à moyen terme avec le court-circuit ileal partiel pour hyperlipidémie. Schweiz. Rundsch. Med. Prax., 67:550, 1978.

Martin, M. J., Hulley, S. B., Browner, W. S., et al: Serum cholesterol, blood pressure, and mortality: Implications from a cohort of 361,662 men. Lancet, 2:933, 1986.

McNamara, J. J., Molot, M. A., Stremple, J. F., and Cutting, R. T.: Coronary artery disease in combat casualties in Vietnam. J.A.M.A., 216:185, 1971.

Mellies, M. J., Gartside, P. S., Glatfelter, L., et al: Effects of probucol on plasma cholesterol, high- and low-density lipoprotein cholesterol and apolipoprotein A-I and A-II in adults with primary familial hypercholesterolemia. Metabolism, 29:956, 1980.

Miettinen, T. A., and Lempinen, M.: Cholestyramine and ileal bypass in the treatment of familial hypercholesterolemia. Eur. J. Clin. Invest., 7:509, 1977.

Moore, R. B., Frantz, I. D., Jr., and Buchwald, H.: Changes in cholesterol pool size, turnover rate, and fecal bile acid and sterol excretion after partial ileal bypass in hypercholesterolemic patients. Surgery, 65:98, 1969.

Moore, R. B., Frantz, I. D., Jr., Varco, R. L., and Buchwald, H.: Cholesterol dynamics after partial ileal bypass. In Jones, R. J. (ed): Proceedings of the Second International Symposium on Atherosclerosis. New York, Springer-Verlag, 1970, pp. 295–300.

Multiple Risk Factor Intervention Trial Research Group: Multiple Risk Factor Intervention Trial: Risk factor changes and mortality results. J.A.M.A., 248:1465, 1982.

National Center for Health Statistics: Annual summary of births, marriages, divorces, and deaths, United States, 1986. Monthly Vital Statistics Report. Vol. 35, No. 13. DHHS Pub. No. (PHS) 87–1120. Hyattsville, MD, Public Health Service, Aug. 24, 1987a.

National Center for Health Statistics: 1986 Summary: National Hospital Discharge Survey. Advance Data from Vital and Health Statistics. No. 145. DHHS Pub. No. (PHS) 87–1250. Hyattsville, MD, Public Health Service, Sept. 30, 1987b.

National Center for Health Statistics: Births, marriages, divorces, and deaths for 1987. Monthly Vital Statistics Report. Vol. 36, No. 12. DHHS Pub. No. (PHS) 88–1120. Hyattsville, MD, Public Health Service, March 21, 1988.

Nestel, P. J., and Billington, T.: Effects of probucol on low-density lipoprotein removal and high-density lipoprotein synthesis. Atherosclerosis, 38:203, 1981.

Norman, D. J., Illingworth, D. R., Munson, J., and Hosenpud, J.: Myolysis and acute renal failure in a heart-transplant recipient receiving lovastatin. N. Engl. J. Med., 318:46, 1988.

Nygaard, K., Helsinger, N., and Rootwelt, K.: Adaptation of vitamin B$_{12}$ absorption after ileal bypass. Scand. J. Gastroenterol., 5:349, 1970.

Osborne, M. P., Frederick, P. L., Sizer, J. S., et al: Mechanism of gastric hypersecretion following massive intestinal resection: Clinical and experimental observations. Ann. Surg., *164*:622, 1966.

Ruffer, M. A.: On arterial lesions found in Egyptian mummies. J. Pathol. Bacteriol., *15*:453, 1911.

Russell, D., Fritz, V., Mieny, C., et al: Treatment of familial hypercholesterolemia by partial ileal bypass. S. Afr. Med. J., *55*:237, 1979.

Samuel, P.: Effects of gemfibrozil on serum lipids. Am. J. Med., *74*:23, 1983.

Schouten, J. A., and Beynen, A. C.: Partial ileal bypass in the treatment of familial hypercholesterolemia: A review. Artery, *13*:240, 1986.

Schouten, J. A., Beynen, A. C., Hoitsma, H. F., et al: Partial ileal bypass surgery in the treatment of familial hypercholesterolemia: Report of two cases. Neth. J. Med., *28*:356, 1985.

Schwartz, M. Z., Varco, R. L., and Buchwald, H.: Liver function and morphology following distal ileal excision in the rabbit. Surg. Forum, *22*:355, 1971.

Scott, H. W., Jr., Stephenson, S. E., Jr., Younger, R., et al: Prevention of experimental atherosclerosis by ileal bypass: Twenty-percent cholesterol diet and ¹³¹I-induced hypothyroidism in dogs. Ann. Surg., *163*:795, 1966.

Shattock, S. G.: A report on the pathological condition of the aorta of King Memephtah, traditionally regarded as the pharaoh of the Exodus. Proc. R. Soc. Med. Lond., *2*:122, 1908.

Shaw, B. W., Jr., Bahnson, H. T., Hardesty, R. L., et al: Combined transplantation of the heart and liver. Ann. Surg., *202*:667, 1985.

Shepard, G. H., Wimberly, J. E., Younger, R. K., et al: Effects of bypass of the distal third of the small intestine on experimental hypercholesterolemia and atherosclerosis in rhesus monkeys. Surg. Forum, *19*:302, 1968.

Shepherd, J., Packard, C. J., Patsch, J. R., et al: Effects of nicotinic acid therapy on plasma high density lipoprotein subfraction distribution and composition on apolipoprotein A metabolism. J. Clin. Invest., *63*:858, 1979.

Simons, L. A.: Interrelations of lipids and lipoproteins with coronary artery disease mortality in 19 countries. Am. J. Cardiol., *57*:56, 1986.

Smith, G. E.: Cited by Long, E. R.: The development of our knowledge of arteriosclerosis. *In* Cowdry, E. V. (ed): Arteriosclerosis. New York, Macmillan, 1933.

Sodal, G., Gjertsen, K. T., and Schrumpf, A.: Surgical treatment of hypercholesterolemia. Acta Chir. Scand., *136*:671, 1970.

Spengel, F. A., Jadhav, A., Duffield, R. G., et al: Superiority of partial ileal bypass over cholestyramine reducing cholesterol in familial hypercholesterolemia. Lancet, *2*:768, 1981.

Starzl, T. E., Bilheimer, D. W., Bahnson, H. T., et al: Heart-liver transplantation in a patient with familial hypercholesterolemia. Lancet, *1*:1382, 1984.

Starzl, T. E., Chase, H. P., Ahrens, E. H., Jr., et al: Portacaval shunt in patients with familial hypercholesterolemia. Ann. Surg., *198*:273, 1983.

Starzl, T. E., Chase, H. P., Putnam, C. W., and Porter, K. A.: Portacaval shunt in hyperlipoproteinemia. Lancet, *2*:940, 1973.

Stein, E. A., Mieny, C., Spitz, L., et al: Portacaval shunt in four

patients with homozygous hypercholesterolemia. Lancet, *1*:832, 1975.

Steinbach, J. H., Blackshear, P. L., Jr., Varco, R. L., and Buchwald, H.: High blood cholesterol reduces in vitro blood oxygen delivery. J. Surg. Res., *16*:134, 1974.

Stern, M. P.: The recent decline in ischemic heart disease mortality. Ann. Intern. Med., *91*:630, 1979.

Strisower, E. H., Adamson, G., and Strisower, B.: Treatment of hyperlipidemias. Am. J. Med., *45*:488, 1968a.

Strisower, E. H., Kradjian, R., Nichols, A. V., et al: Effect of bypass on serum lipoproteins in essential hypercholesterolemia. J. Atheroscler. Res., *8*:525, 1968b.

Swan, D. M., and McGowan, J. M.: Ileal bypass in hypercholesterolemia associated with heart disease. Am. J. Surg., *116*:81, 1968.

The Coronary Drug Project Research Group: The Coronary Drug Project: Initial findings leading to modifications of its research protocol. J.A.M.A., *214*:1303, 1970.

The Coronary Drug Project Research Group: The Coronary Drug Project: Findings leading to further modification of its protocol with respect to dextrothyroxine. J.A.M.A., *220*:996, 1972.

The Coronary Drug Project Research Group: The Coronary Drug Project: Findings leading to discontinuation of the 2.5 mg/day estrogen group. J.A.M.A., *226*:652, 1973.

The Coronary Drug Project Research Group: Clofibrate and niacin in coronary heart disease. J.A.M.A., *231*:360, 1975.

The Expert Panel: Report of the National Cholesterol Education Program Expert Panel on detection, evaluation, and treatment of high blood cholesterol in adults. Arch. Intern. Med., *148*:36, 1988.

The Lovastatin Study Group II: Therapeutic response to lovastatin (mevinolin) in nonfamilial hypercholesterolemia: A multicenter study. J.A.M.A., *256*:2829, 1986.

The Pooling Project Research Group: Relationship of blood pressure, serum cholesterol, smoking habit, relative weight, and ECG abnormalities to incidence of major coronary events: Final report of the Pooling Project. J. Chronic Dis., *31*:201, 1978.

Tobert, J. A.: New developments in lipid-lowering therapy: The role of inhibitors of hydroxymethylglutaryl-coenzyme A reductase. Circulation, *76*:534, 1987.

Uauy, R., Vega, G. L., Grundy, S. M., and Bilheimer, D. W.: Lovastatin therapy in receptor-negative homozygous familial hypercholesterolemia: Lack of effect on low density lipoprotein concentrations or turnover. J. Pediatr., *113*:387, 1988.

Vaislic, C. D., Grondin, P. R., Bourassa, M. G., and Campeau, L.: Partial ileal bypass in type II familial hypercholesterolemia: Eleven-year experience at the Montreal Heart Institute. Am. Surg., *50*:165, 1984.

Van Niekerk, J. L., Hendriks, T., and De Boer, H. H.: The treatment of familial hypercholesterolemia by partial ileal bypass surgery: A review of the literature. Neth. J. Med., *27*:18, 1984.

Younger, R. K., Shepard, G. H., Butts, W. H., and Scott, H. W., Jr.: Comparison of the protective effects of cholestyramine and ileal bypass in rhesus monkeys on an atherogenic regimen. Surg. Forum, *20*:101, 1969.

8 Bypass Grafting for Coronary Artery Disease

Frank C. Spencer

HISTORICAL ASPECTS

Coronary bypass grafting surgery was developed between 1967 and 1968 at three major centers in the United States: the Cleveland Clinic in Cleveland, Ohio; the University of Wisconsin in Milwaukee; and New York University in New York City. Before this time, there had been a few isolated case reports of bypass grafting, but these had had little clinical impact.

The principal credit belongs to the pioneering efforts of Favaloro, Effler, and associates at the Cleveland Clinic, where, with the development of coronary angiography by F. Mason Sones, investigation of surgical treatment of coronary disease had been their primary objective for several years. Their observation of the usefulness of the saphenous vein for bypass grafting was the first clear indication of its widespread applicability. Johnson, in Milwaukee, quickly perceived the significance of this fact and made the quantum step of extending the procedure to the left coronary artery. The magnitude of this achievement is illustrated by the fact that before 1967 operative procedures on the left coronary artery had a mortality exceeding 50% and had been almost abandoned. By 1969, Johnson reported to the American Surgical Association successful operations on the left coronary artery in 301 patients, with a mortality of 12%. This report soundly launched the modern era of coronary bypass grafting, which has grown exponentially since that time. Over 200,000 bypass operations were done in 1985.

At New York University the concept of anastomosis of the internal mammary artery to the left anterior descending coronary artery by using microsurgical technique was developed by Green and associates (1968) after earlier demonstration of the feasibility of this procedure in the laboratory (Spencer et al, 1964).

In 1967 in Russia Kolessov did an end-to-end anastomosis between the mammary artery and the coronary artery on a beating heart; the next year he did a similar end-to-side anastomosis on another patient. Kolessov was Chairman of the Department of Surgery at the first Leningrad Medical Institute between 1953 and 1976, during which time he did bypass procedures on 132 patients, performing most of these on a beating heart. His work was previously almost unknown in the United States, but his contributions are well summarized by Olearchyk (1988). This paper has also a concise summary of different historical events during the development of coronary bypass.

In the 3 decades before 1967, numerous indirect procedures were evaluated. Almost all were designed to enhance the growth of collateral circulation to the myocardium. Some were ingenious, others were bizarre; all have now been discarded. The only procedure that offered some encouragement for several years was the Vineberg procedure of implantation of the internal mammary artery into the myocardium. The artery is still patent in most cases, but the magnitude of flow through the implanted artery was disappointingly small in most patients. Thus, it is rarely done today.

In the 1970s bypass grafting was widely adopted because the operation became simpler and safer. The introduction of potassium cardioplegia greatly facilitated the performance and safety of the operation. Large randomized studies were done and were discussed in detail by Frye (1987). The three major studies were the Veterans Administration Study, the European Cooperative Study reported in 1983, and

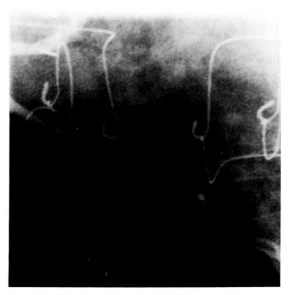

Figure 54–139. An angiogram done 10 years after insertion of a saphenous vein bypass graft to the anterior descending coronary artery. The patient was studied again because of angina found to be due to atherosclerosis developing in the circumflex coronary artery. The graft appears to be normal, with adequate flow into the anterior descending coronary artery, both antegrade and retrograde.

the Coronary Artery Surgery Study (CASS) of almost 25,000 patients between 1974 and 1979.

Several major changes occurred in the 1980s. The 1983 report of Campeau from the Montreal Heart Institute of angiographic findings in 82 patients 10 years after bypass was a sobering milestone. Previously, 5-year postoperative studies had been encouraging. However, between 5 and 10 years, significant atherosclerosis developed in a high percentage of vein grafts so that 10 years after operation, 40% of grafts were closed, 30% had significant atherosclerosis, and only 30% remained satisfactory (Fig. 54–139).

However, internal mammary grafts remained patent without adverse changes in more than 90% of patients, often showing significant enlargement, apparently dilating in response to increased "demand" in the distal coronary tree. This important report prompted world-wide surgical interest in the use of the mammary artery. Earlier, as late as 1981, the internal mammary was used in less than 15% of bypass operations. The use of bilateral mammary grafts and sequential mammary grafts soon followed (Lytle et al, 1986; Rankin et al, 1986).

Loop and associates reported in 1986, 10 years after operation, that longevity was much better in patients in whom the internal mammary was used compared with those in whom only saphenous veins had been used. These different considerations with the mammary artery were summarized by Loop in an editorial in 1986. Additional details are given by Rankin in Chapter 54V1.

Another major development was the evolution of angioplasty, first done by Gruentzig in Switzerland in 1977 and later applied worldwide with increased frequency. More than 80,000 of these procedures were done in 1985. A separate major development was the introduction of effective thrombolytic therapy, initially streptokinase and urokinase but more recently tissue plasminogen activator (TPA). This therapy first became available for clinical use in late 1987. Topol and associates summarized events with this remarkable therapy in December, 1988, and described results in 708 patients from the first three Thrombosis and Angioplasty in Myocardial Infarction (TAMI) studies.

Administration of TPA in the first few hours after onset of coronary thrombosis results in reopening of the diseased artery in approximately 75% of patients. Angioplasty can then reopen approximately 70% of the 25% group of patients who do not reopen with thrombolytic therapy. The entire field is rapidly changing at this time, and the relative role of bypass grafting, angioplasty, and thrombolysis is being investigated.

Despite these major advances, however, the basic disease, coronary atherosclerosis, has been little influenced by therapy. Almost all angiographic studies have shown some progression of atherosclerosis in the coronary circulation in the year after operation. Fortunately, effective medication is now available that drastically lowers cholesterol levels in the blood, but the long-term benefits are yet unknown.

FREQUENCY AND EPIDEMIOLOGY

Coronary atherosclerosis is the most common serious disease in the white male throughout the world. It causes more than 600,000 deaths annually in the United States. In worldwide epidemiologic studies done several years ago, the United States had the second highest frequency of coronary disease in the world, exceeded only by Finland. Japan had the lowest frequency of coronary disease (Stamler, 1978). The disease is seldom found in populations in which the average cholesterol concentration is below 200 mg/100 ml. In Japan the average cholesterol level is approximately 160 mg/100 ml. The disease is more common in men in the first five decades of life and has a ratio of almost 4:1; 1976 death statistics from the Bureau of Vital Statistics reported 644,000 deaths (360,000 men and 284,000 women). However, only 34,000 deaths occurred in women under 65 years of age compared with approximately 110,000 in men.

The frequency of deaths from coronary disease increases two to four times with each decade of life. For example, in 1976 the death rate for men between 45 and 55 years of age was 281 per 100,000 compared with 66 per 100,000 for men between 35 and 44 years of age. Between 55 and 65 years of age the number of deaths rose to 756. This striking increase with age probably indicates both the slowly progressive growth of coronary atherosclerosis combined with the inability of collateral circulation to compensate for the progressive obstruction.

Fortunately, there was a 21% decrease in mortality from major cardiovascular disease in the United States between 1958 and 1976. This reduction is still unexplained. It was discussed in detail at a 2-day conference at the National Institutes of Health in 1978. This reduction did not occur in most countries in the world. Possible explanations were considered during the 2-day conference but no definite conclusions were made. This improvement in death rate occurred before many current methods of treatment were available (e.g., beta-blockade, bypass surgery, intensive dietary therapy, and emphasis on avoidance of smoking).

ETIOLOGY AND PATHOLOGY

Etiology

Coronary atherosclerosis is apparently a disorder of lipid metabolism of unknown origin. The main risk factors associated with coronary disease are cigarette smoking, lipid disorders, diabetes, and hypertension. Obesity, lack of physical exercise, and stress are "plausible," factors but lack scientific proof. Tobacco smoking has a clear adverse effect because the death rate in smokers is approximately three times greater than that in nonsmokers. There is a strong association between cholesterol concentration in the blood and atherosclerosis, especially with cholesterol levels above 250 to 300 mg/dl. Epidemiologic studies indicate that any cholesterol level above 200 mg/dl is associated with some increase in frequency of death from coronary disease. The increased frequency with either diabetes or hypertension is well known.

Pathology

Coronary atherosclerosis is a segmental disease that usually occurs in the proximal portion of the three major coronary arteries within 5 cm of their origin from the aorta. Fortunately, the distal segments are almost always patent. The disease is principally in epicardial vessels because small endomyocardial branches are rarely involved.

The popular terminology is "single, double, or triple" vessel disease, depending on the number of vessels involved. Triple-vessel disease is seen in most patients with severe disease. A common pattern is stenosis or occlusion of the proximal right coronary artery, the anterior descending artery, and the circumflex artery. The distal right coronary artery is usually patent where it bifurcates into the posterior descending branch and the atrioventricular groove branch. The anterior descending branch is usually patent in its middle or distal thirds; one or more marginal branches of the circumflex usually remain patent. This fortunate segmental localization is the basis for bypass grafting. Numerous variations of this basic pattern exist. In the 1978 monograph by Ochsner and Mills, six different pathologic variations encountered during their experience with more than 1,000 patients are described.

Severe myocardial ischemia may produce localized myocardial necrosis, which is clinically recognized as an acute infarction; however, more subtle forms of "silent ischemia" produce progressive myocardial fibrosis, slightly analogous to the gradual trophic changes that evolve in the feet from progressive atherosclerosis in the femoral and popliteal arteries. The two dominant factors that determine the severity of disease and prognosis are the number of vessels involved (single-, double-, or triple-vessel disease) and the function of the left ventricle. Left ventricular function is customarily expressed as ejection fraction, which is measured either by cineangiography or radionuclide scanning. In general, an ejection fraction between 0.5 and 0.7 is considered to be normal. Ejection fractions between 0.4 and 0.5 represent mild depression; those between 0.3 and 0.4 represent moderate depression; and those lower than 0.3 represent severe depression of ventricular function. These different ejection fractions represent the number of grams of nonfunctioning left ventricular muscle, either from necrosis or ischemia.

Congestive heart failure appears with increased severity with an ejection fraction between 0.2 and 0.3 and is common with an ejection fraction below 0.2.

The normal left ventricular end-diastolic pressure is 12 mm Hg or less. With moderate left ventricular injury, end-diastolic pressure rises to the range of 12 to 20 mm Hg and to levels of 20 to 30 mm Hg with severe disease.

The decrease in ejection fraction, either from myocardial infarctions or from progressive fibrosis, represents the inability of the heart to compensate for the atherosclerotic occlusive process by the development of collateral circulation. Thus, bypass surgery to improve coronary flow is primarily for patients with a significant decrease in myocardial function.

The influence of ventricular function on prognosis is striking. In patients with triple-vessel disease and normal ventricular function, 5-year survival is well above 90%. With different degrees of impaired ventricular function, however, 5-year survival decreases from almost 70% with a moderate decrease to almost 40% with severely decreased function.

Clinical Considerations

Progressive myocardial ischemia usually results in one of three serious events: angina pectoris, myocardial infarction, or sudden death. Angina is the most frequent symptom, but unfortunately myocardial infarction or sudden death may appear without any preceding symptoms.

Angina results from anaerobic myocardial metabolism, typically appearing when myocardial oxygen consumption is increased from exercise, eating, or emotional stress, and subsides with rest or treatment by vasodilatation with sublingual nitroglycerin. Angina is analogous to claudication that develops in the calf muscles of the lower extremities from femoral atherosclerosis, appearing with exercise and subsiding with rest.

Unfortunately, a significant number of patients, probably at least 20%, do not have angina despite the presence of significant myocardial ischemia. The prevalence of "silent ischemia" has been recognized with increased frequency and is more common than previously realized.

"Unstable angina" is an important clinical syndrome that is intermediate between classical angina and myocardial infarction. It probably results from an acute decrease in regional myocardial blood flow, probably from thrombosis of a collateral vessel. If the regional myocardial ischemia improves, the patient may recover without permanent injury. However, if it does not, myocardial infarction or death may ensue. Thus, the condition is analogous to the patient with femoral atherosclerosis who has had intermittent claudication but who suddenly develops acute rest pain with cyanotic toes.

Myocardial infarction is the most common serious complication. More than 1 million infarcts occur in the United States annually. With current therapy, mortality is almost 10%.

Myocardial infarction usually results from acute thrombosis of a diseased coronary artery, which usually arises from a disruption of the intimal surface. The precise sequence of events that precipitate acute thrombosis is unknown, but a disruption of the intimal surface with resultant accumulation of platelets and fibrin appears to be the most plausible. The significance of the resultant infarction depends on the number of grams of myocardium injured, but at present this cannot be quantitated precisely.

Sudden death, which is defined as occurring within 1 hour after the onset of symptoms (Holmes and Davis, 1986), is the most common form of death from coronary disease. The risk of sudden death varies with the extent of the disease and the degree of impairment of ventricular function, ranging from 2% to as high as 10%. More than 400,000 deaths occur each year in the United States. Death may result from acute myocardial infarction or an arrhythmia, usually ventricular fibrillation, without infarction. The relative frequency of these two causes of death is unknown, but clearly ventricular fibrillation without massive infarction is common. This is the basis of the importance of widespread familiarity with techniques of cardiopulmonary resuscitation, which was dramatically emphasized in the 1980 report by Cobb, who described experiences from Seattle with 10 years of cardiac resuscitation outside the hospital. In that report, experiences with resuscitation in approximately 300 patients each year by trained laymen outside the hospital were described. Although most patients had coronary disease, more than one-half of the patients resuscitated did not have any signs of myocardial necrosis.

In a small percentage of patients, *congestive heart failure* develops and is the result of multiple infarctions that have destroyed more than 40% of the left ventricular muscle mass. In some patients, the clinical history includes angina and recurrent infarctions, but in others the clinical history is puzzling because of the lack of significant events. Apparently, extensive destruction of myocardium "silently" evolved from progressive ischemia. Chronic congestive failure, manifested by a right atrial pressure above 10 to 15 mm Hg, has an ominous outlook. Patients often die within 1 to 2 years. Bypass grafting has little value in these patients unless there are significant areas of ischemic but viable myocardium. Cardiac transplantation has been used with increased frequency for these patients.

LABORATORY EVALUATION

There are usually no abnormalities on physical examination. Thus, the diagnosis of coronary disease depends on a history of angina. Without angina, the disease can be detected only by routine laboratory studies, emphasizing the importance of liberal indications for these studies.

The chest film shows normal-sized heart unless previous infarctions have resulted in cardiac dilatation. The electrocardiogram is normal at rest in approximately 70% of patients. The simplest and most widely used study is the exercise electrocardiogram, the "stress test," which observes electrocardiographic signs of ischemia during graded amounts of exercise. More complex studies include radionuclide angiography to measure myocardial contractility (gated pool scan), expressed as "ejection fraction" or myocardial perfusion with radioactive thallium. Ejection fraction normally increases with exercise. With significant coronary disease, however, the ejection fraction falls with exercise, which is an important finding.

Coronary Arteriography

Cineangiography, including coronary arteriography and ventriculography, is the important laboratory study. Arteriography outlines the location and severity of disease whereas ventriculography measures ventricular function and permits calculation of ejection fraction. An angiographically severe stenosis is considered to be present when the diameter is reduced more than 70%, corresponding to a reduction in cross-sectional area near 90%. Moderate stenosis is present with a diameter reduction of 50%,

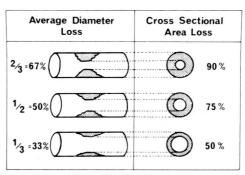

Figure 54–140. Diagrammatic presentation of the relationship between the two methods of estimating the severity of coronary artery stenosis. Reports from UAB use diameter loss, whereas those from GLH use cross-sectional area loss. (From Brandt, P. W. T., Partridge, J. B., and Wattle, W. J.: Coronary arteriography: A method of presentation of the arteriogram report and a scoring system. Clin. Radiol., 28:361, 1977.)

equivalent to a 75% reduction in cross-sectional area (Fig. 54–140) (Kirklin and Barratt-Boyes, 1986).

Regional ventricular contraction is usually evaluated from the right anterior oblique view in the cineangiogram. The left ventricular outline is divided into five segments: anterobasal, anterolateral, apical, diaphragmatic, and posterobasal. The motion of each segment may be recorded as normal, hypokinetic, akinetic, or dyskinetic. A myocardial numerical score is commonly used, ranging from No. 1 (normal function) to No. 6 (dyskinesia or paradoxical contraction). Thus, with the five segments a normal myocardial score is 5; the worst score is 30. Impaired myocardial contractility is often expressed as "left ventricular scores" above 10.

Although cineangiography is the most precise method for evaluating coronary disease, unwarranted erroneous conclusions are often reached. The two most common errors are concluding that vessels are "too small" for bypass or that regional myocardial contractility is irreversibly injured (dyskinetic or akinetic); thus bypass to this area of myocardium is futile.

Coronary arteries distal to an obstruction may appear to be small on angiography for various reasons, usually from inadequate amounts of dye entering through collateral vessels or from lack of distention of the vessel wall from normal perfusion pressure. It has been established clinically for many years that in most patients, more than 95%, a coronary artery over 1 mm internal diameter can be found distal to the area of obstruction and bypass grafting can be effectively performed. Thus, the coronary angiogram should not be used to conclude that the distal vessels "cannot be bypassed." Similarly, dyskinetic or akinetic segments may improve in function after a bypass to that area of myocardium has restored normal flow. Almost always at operation these areas of operation contain large areas of viable myocardial cells, rather than avascular scar. These considerations are discussed in detail by Kirklin and Barratt-Boyes (1986).

TREATMENT: MEDICAL, ANGIOPLASTY, OR BYPASS?

Medical Therapy

Details of medical therapy are beyond the scope of this textbook; thus, only basic essentials are described here. The most important three measures are complete cessation of cigarette smoking, control of hypertension, and modification of diet to sharply decrease the intake of lipids. Precise guidelines for daily dietary lipid intake have been well described in publications by the American Heart Association. If possible, the blood cholesterol should be lowered below 200 mg/dl, either with diet or appropriate medication.

Weight reduction and physical exercise are plausible goals, although their effectiveness has not been proven. Drug therapy includes nitrates, beta-blockade, and calcium blockers. The goal with medication is relief of angina, combined with an appropriate lipid intake and cholesterol level in the blood. At present, the effectiveness of medical therapy is difficult to measure. As stated earlier, angiography has shown a gradual but relentless progression of the coronary atherosclerotic process in most patients.

Angioplasty

This procedure was initiated in 1977 and is now widely used, although indications and contraindications are still evolving. The current status is well described in the 1988 report by Detre from the National Heart Institute Angioplasty Registry. In general, stenotic lesions judged suitable for dilatation can be treated successfully in 80 to 90% of patients. "Successful dilatation" is defined as reducing the degree of stenosis by at least 20%. Mortality ranges from less than 1% with single-vessel disease to almost 3% with triple-vessel disease; myocardial infarction occurs in 3 to 4% of patients. The stenosis recurs within 6 to 12 months in at least 20% of patients but may be successfully redilated. Five-year follow-up data are available mainly for patients in whom single angioplasty has been done but, to date, are reasonable, only a small percentage of patients requiring either bypass or repeat angioplasty. Thus, the procedure is clearly a valuable method for selected patients although the mortality and morbidity are similar to elective bypass in good-risk patients. The ultimate fate of stenotic lesions treated by angioplasty will not be known for some time.

Angioplasty is best done in a facility with immediate access to an operating room, which may be either available on short notice or on a "stand-by" basis. For unknown reasons, prompt operation and bypass, however, are still associated with a significantly higher mortality and perioperative infarction rate than elective bypass. The 1988 report by Connor

described experiences with 146 patients at the Mayo Clinic in whom bypass was started within 1 hour of failed angioplasty. Nonetheless, the operative mortality was 2.7%, and the perioperative infarction rate was 39%.

Bypass: Stable Angina of Varying Severity

There is uniform agreement that significant disease in the left main coronary, narrowing the diameter more than 50%, should be operated on promptly, even though the patient is completely asymptomatic.

There is also widespread agreement that surgical therapy is indicated in the patient with severe angina that does not respond to drug therapy. Therapeutic choices usually arise with patients with extensive disease but minimal or no angina. As discussed earlier, three large cooperative studies, the Veterans Administration Study, the European Cooperative Study, and CASS, all evaluated these questions in the 1970s. CASS includes almost 25,000 patients studied by angiography and followed for at least 5 years up to 1983. Significant coronary disease was considered to be present if the diameter was narrowed more than 70% in the three major arteries and more than 50% in the left main coronary artery. Left ventricular function was evaluated by the "left ventricular score" described earlier, based on segmental contraction of the five different ventricular segments with a normal ventricle having a score of 5. The worst ventricle had a score of 30. In the patients studied, the 4-year survival was 97% for patients without coronary disease; 92% with single-vessel disease; 84% for double-vessel disease; and 68% for triple-vessel disease.

These studies indicated that patients with few symptoms with single-vessel or double-vessel disease did not do better with operation than with medical therapy. The one exception to this generalization is patients with disease in the left anterior descending proximal to the first septal perforator, which is well known to have a worse prognosis than those with more distal disease. Also, longevity in patients with triple-vessel disease, little angina, and normal ventricular function was no better with operation than with medical therapy. A most important fact, however, is that almost 40% of patients with triple-vessel disease developed symptoms during the 5-year period of observation and "crossed-over" for surgical therapy, emphasizing that a choice of medical therapy is valid only as long as the patient has few symptoms; but this occurs in less than two of three patients treated.

With impaired ventricular function, a bypass (ejection fraction below 0.5) should be done regularly. Seven years after operation survival in the surgical group was almost 88% and was only 65% in the medical group (Passamani et al, 1985). Even with an ejection fraction less than 0.25, significant benefit occurs with bypass; 5-year survival is approximately

60% in the surgical group compared with 40% in the medical group (Kirklin and Barratt-Boyes, 1986).

Unstable Angina

As described earlier, this condition is an acute physiologic state in which the blood flow to a segment of myocardium is seriously jeopardized but necrosis has not yet occurred. It probably arises from a sudden decrease in regional blood flow. Treatment is essentially the same as for an acute infarction with immediate hospitalization in a coronary care unit. Most patients respond to acute medical therapy within a short time, but those who do not should be operated on promptly; otherwise, there is a significant hazard of myocardial infarction or death. After recovery with medical therapy, patients should be evaluated, usually with coronary arteriography, to determine if elective bypass should be done.

Acute Infarction

The availability of effective thrombolytic agents, most recently TPA, has drastically changed the treatment of acute infarctions. With favorable logistic circumstances, bypass may be done within a few hours after the onset of acute infarction, but thrombolytic therapy is simpler and safer.

A certain degree of irreversible necrosis develops in the myocardium between 30 and 60 minutes after occlusion of a coronary artery. The infarction, however, continues to evolve for several hours, probably in the marginal zones surrounding the initially complete infarction. This is probably the basis for improvement with revascularization, which is similar to removal of an acute arterial occlusion in other arteries in the body. If thrombolytic therapy is not available, immediate bypass may be considered if circumstances are such that it can be completed within a few hours after the onset of infarction.

When a massive infarction produces cardiogenic shock, mortality is well above 50%. Most of these patients have triple-vessel disease with pre-existing impaired ventricular function. The best treatment is probably immediate bypass or angioplasty, which is perhaps preceded by intra-aortic balloon support (Fig. 54–141). Significant data, however, are not yet available.

Post-Infarction Angina

A patient recovering from myocardial infarction can be safely operated on promptly. When operation is done in the first month after infarction, operative mortality is little influenced by the time lapsing since infarction (Fig. 54–142). Mortality is similar for operations done in the first few days after infarction to those done 2 to 3 weeks later. Mortality is influenced, however, by both the severity of myocardial ischemia and hemodynamic instability. In 1988, a report by Naunheim described 336 of these patients operated on within 1 month after infarction. Mortality was 2% in patients with minimal angina and 6% with angina at rest; it rose sharply to almost 10% in patients requiring a balloon pump and to almost 50% in 23 patients with cardiogenic shock (see Fig. 54–141).

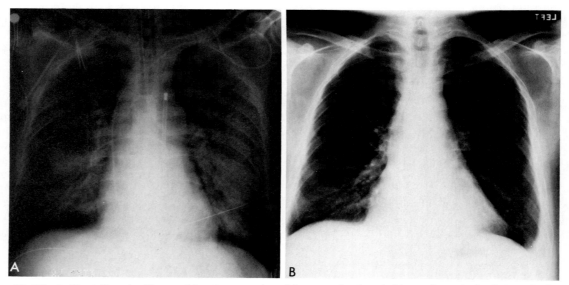

Figure 54–141. *A,* Chest film of a 65-year-old patient transferred from another hospital in cardiogenic shock 1 week after a massive myocardial infarction, receiving infusions of dopamine and norepinephrine bitartrate (Levophed). He was comatose, intubated, and in renal failure. A balloon pump was inserted promptly. *B,* Chest film before discharge from the hospital. At operation, a ruptured papillary muscle was found, and it was causing massive mitral insufficiency. The mitral valve was replaced, and the right coronary artery, which was totally obstructed, was bypassed. Blood cardioplegia was used. At catheterization 1 year later, the cardiac findings were normal, with a patent graft and a normal left atrial pressure.

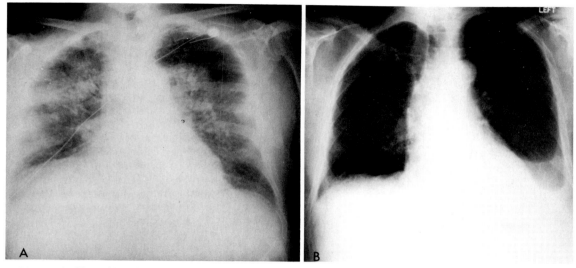

Figure 54–142. *A,* Chest film of a patient 2 weeks after myocardial infarction and 5 days after rupture of the ventricular septum. The severe pulmonary congestion is obvious. This patient was also in oliguric renal failure, with a blood urea nitrogen of 60, despite inotropic therapy with dobutamine and dopamine. *B,* Chest film before discharge from the hospital. At operation, using blood cardioplegia, an infarctectomy and a patch repair of the ruptured ventricular septum were done, which resulted in a complete recovery.

CONTRAINDICATIONS TO OPERATION

The only strong contraindication at the author's institution is chronic congestive failure with pulmonary hypertension, which is manifested by a right atrial pressure above 15 mm and hepatomegaly. These unfortunate patients have necrosis of a large amount of left ventricular muscle; thus, cardiac transplantation is the only therapy that is likely to be helpful. A similar viewpoint is expressed by Kirklin and Barratt-Boyes (1986).

Intermittent congestive failure, often manifested by intermittent pulmonary edema, is a strong indication for prompt operation. These episodes indicate a serious degree of myocardial ischemia that can easily be fatal, especially if another infarction occurs. The intermittent episodes probably evolve from acute ischemic episodes that elevate end-diastolic pressure sufficiently to produce pulmonary edema.

A severe depression of ejection fraction to the range of 0.2 or lower is still erroneously considered to be a contraindication to bypass by some surgeons although contrary experiences have been published by several groups. This erroneous concept probably evolved from surgical experiences in previous years with ineffective myocardial preservation that produced some degree of infarction during operation. At present, several reports show that some benefit occurs in most patients, no matter how low the ejection fraction, as long as chronic congestive failure is not present.

Advanced age is not a contraindication. Several reports cite excellent results in patients in their seventh or eighth decade of life, although mortality and morbidity are slightly increased.

OPERATIVE TECHNIQUE

The three major considerations with coronary bypass are: (1) prevention of myocardial infarction; (2) the method of procurement of the vascular grafts used, usually the saphenous veins and the internal mammary arteries; (3) a meticulous operative technique that constructs anastomoses with smooth intimal surfaces without stenoses.

Preoperative Therapy

A modification of the platelet inhibitor therapy reported by Chesebro in 1982 is routinely used. Dipyridamole is started 48 hours before operation, giving 100 mg four times a day, and continued until a few hours before operation. Eight to 10 hours after operation, aspirin, 325 mg, is initially given. The aspirin is then continued with a single daily dose of 325 mg for 1 year. Dipyridamole is no longer given after operation, as randomized studies have shown no additional benefit beyond that provided by aspirin alone.

Prevention of Myocardial Infarction

Careful management with cardiac drugs, especially propranolol and nitrates, is essential. Propranolol is continued until the time of operation, although the dosage may be decreased to less than 160 mg/day. If larger amounts are required, inotropic agents are usually needed for 1 to 2 days after operation. With unstable angina, intravenous nitroglycerin is invaluable, sometimes requiring unusually large amounts, even 100 to 200 μg/min. In hypertensive patients, afterload can be reduced with nitroprusside infusion to decrease peripheral vascular resistance. Monitoring of these patients is best done with a Swan-Ganz catheter to measure pulmonary artery wedge pressure, diastolic pressure, and cardiac output. With serious hemodynamic instability that cannot be stabilized with drug therapy, an intra-aortic balloon pump should be inserted that will decrease cardiac work and augment coronary blood flow by raising diastolic blood pressure. Although not often necessary, the balloon pump is a valuable form of therapy that should be used promptly if drug therapy is ineffective.

At New York University the Swan-Ganz catheter is inserted routinely after the induction of anesthesia. An occasional patient will have an alarming rise in pulmonary artery diastolic pressure from 10 to 20 mm Hg, or even 30 mm Hg, which is not detected by arterial pressure or electrocardiographic changes. This can be reversed quickly by appropriate infusion of nitroglycerin; otherwise, a subendocardial infarction will almost certainly evolve.

The importance of a precise anesthetic technique can scarcely be overemphasized. Significant myocardial ischemia from either hypertension or hypotension can usually be avoided with such a technique. In the early 1970s, the authors were astonished to find in a cooperative study among several institutions that more than 25% of patients had enzymatic changes of myocardial necrosis *before* bypass was started, a subtle myocardial injury that was later avoided with appropriate changes in anesthetic technique.

Myocardial Preservation and General Perfusion Technique

Hypothermic potassium cardioplegia with cold blood is routinely used. This technique evolved jointly from investigations in the author's laboratory with those of Buckberg at UCLA.

At operation arterial cannulation is done with a standard technique except in patients over 70 years of age or in those with atherosclerosis in the aortic arch in whom a special long aortic arch cannula is inserted to permit perfusion beyond the ostium of the left subclavian artery. Although unproven, this technique has been associated with a sharp decrease in the frequency of perioperative stroke in the last 2 to 3 years. Venous cannulation is done with two caval cannulas (preferred by the author) or by a single large cannula in the inferior vena cava and right atrium (preferred by other members of the New York University faculty). The oxygenator is usually a membrane oxygenator. A hemodilution prime is used, and a hematocrit above 20% is maintained. Perfusion rates are between 2 and 2.5 l/m² at a temperature of 30° C. The left ventricle is usually vented with a catheter inserted through the right pulmonary vein. Perfusion pressure is kept near 60 mm.

Once bypass has been established, the aortic root is clamped, and the heart is arrested by infusing cold blood (temperature near 6° C) with potassium (concentration of 25 to 30 mEq/l) into the aortic root at a rate sufficient to develop an aortic root pressure of 70 to 80 mm. This is usually an infusion rate between 200 to 350 ml/min, striving to arrest the heart as quickly as possible. A higher perfusion pressure, near 100 mm, is used with left main disease. Once the heart is arrested, perfusion pressure is maintained near 70 mm, striving to maintain a pressure sufficient to perfuse the myocardium beyond the obstructed arteries but avoiding production of myocardial edema from excessive pressure.

No fixed amount is infused but regional myocardial temperatures are measured with a thermister, infusing sufficient cold blood to lower all areas below 15° C. Usually this requires between 1,000 and 1,500 ml of blood.

Topical hypothermia is routinely used, both by intermittently flooding the operative field with cold electrolyte solution and also by a constant pericardial infusion of cold electrolyte removed by continuous sump suction, a modification of Shumway's original technique. Care is taken to keep the right side of the heart empty and wrinkled, ensuring that reflux of blood from the vena cava is not occurring.

Cold blood is reinfused for 2 to 3 minutes after each anastomosis or every 20 to 30 minutes. When blood is perfused through a vein graft after it has been anastomosed to a coronary artery, care is taken to maintain perfusion pressure near 50 mm to avoid distal myocardial edema. Potassium concentration in the infusate is usually decreased to near 15 mEq after the first or second injection, especially if blood potassium rises above 5 mEq/l.

The New York University method of myocardial preservation is extremely effective. Periods of aortic occlusion for as long as 2 hours or more are readily tolerated, even though these long periods are seldom necessary. In patients with the combination of coronary disease and multivalvular disease, periods of occlusion may be longer than 3 hours without significant myocardial injury.

The coronary sinus method of cardioplegia has been used with increasing frequency by some members of the faculty, especially with complex problems. This technique is useful particularly for patients with repeated operations in whom an internal mammary artery was used at the previous operation. Although objective data are not yet available, the technique has been satisfactory and care is taken to keep the coronary sinus pressure below 40 mm Hg while blood is infused.

Technique of Graft Procurement

The left internal mammary is used in most bypass operations, mobilizing the artery from the chest wall with a narrow strip of soft tissue and gently dilating it with an intraluminal injection of papaverine. Bilateral mammary grafts are used with increased frequency in patients with favorable anatomy under 60 years of age, although these grafts have a higher frequency of significant ischemia in the sternum. Mammary grafting is discussed in detail by Rankin in Chapter 54 V 1.

Appropriate segments of saphenous vein are removed from the lower extremity, preferring vein segments from the lower leg as long as these are larger than about 3.5 mm. Larger veins, over 6 mm, are avoided if possible, although there is no precise correlation between the size of the vein used and subsequent results. The veins, however, are carefully distended with electrolyte solution (plasmalyte), monitoring distention pressure to keep it less than 100 mm Hg. Particular care is taken to avoid veins with significant disease, manifested by scarring and thickening.

If the greater saphenous veins are not satisfactory, the lesser saphenous veins are used. The third choice is the use of cephalic veins from the arm, which have been used regularly at New York University for several years if no other veins are available, although data published by others indicate a higher frequency of late degeneration than with saphenous veins, probably because of the thinner wall. After procurement, the veins are distended and then stored in a cool plasmalyte solution containing a small amount of papaverine and heparin.

The incisions in the lower extremity are closed with figure-of-eight sutures of Dexon. The continuous suture technique was used for years but has been abandoned because of an occasional patient with significant morbidity from fat necrosis. Closure is usually deferred until after bypass and neutralization of heparin with protamine.

Grafting Technique

As stated earlier, the operative technique must be a precise one, constructing a smooth anastomosis with no disruption of the intimal surface. Ocular magnification to four times normal is used regularly with binocular loupes (Fig. 54–143). These were developed at New York University (Spencer, 1971) and quickly adopted throughout the world. A short arteriotomy (6 to 8 mm) is made beyond the site of obstruction after which the lumen is gently probed with a calibrated metal dilator, usually 1.5 to 2 mm (Fig. 54–144). This confirms patency of the distal artery. The venous anastomosis is constructed end-to-side with a continuous suture of 7-0 prolene, usually with suture "bites" about 1 mm deep and 1 mm apart (Figs. 54–145 and 54–146). Before the suture line is tied, blood is injected down the vein graft to displace any air. Subsequently, additional blood is injected for 2 to 3 minutes to perfuse the region of myocardium grafted.

The aortic anastomosis is a standard one in which grafts are placed either to the left or the right

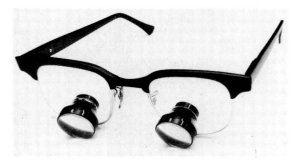

Figure 54–143. Binocular loupes that magnify to 4 power, with a focal length of 16 inches and a depth of field of 4 inches.

of the midline. Initially, a small tangential clamp is applied to the anterior surface of the aorta after which a small button of aorta is removed with a 4 to 5-mm aortic punch. The anastomosis is constructed with a continuous 6-0 prolene suture.

This author's preference is for performance of distal anastomoses usually with the heart arrested, subsequently unclamping and defibrillating the aorta and attaching the proximal grafts while the heart is rewarmed and decompressed. An alternate approach

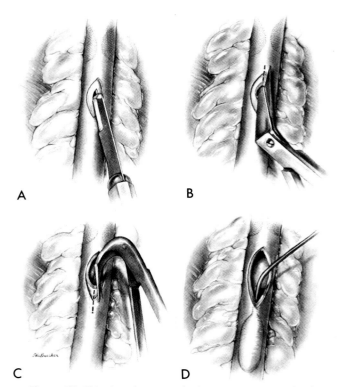

Figure 54–144. Arteriotomy. *A,* An incision is made first through the epicardium overlying the coronary artery and is then made through the entire thickness of the anterior wall with a miniblade. *B,* The arteriotomy is extended proximally with obtuse-angled Pott's scissors. *C,* The arteriotomy is extended distally with reverse acute-angle scissors. *D,* After completion of the arteriotomy, the lumen of the coronary artery is sized with calibrated obturators. (From Ochsner, J. L., and Mills, N. L.: Coronary Artery Surgery. Philadelphia, Lea & Febiger, 1978.)

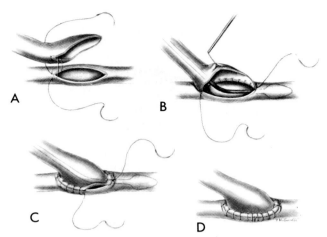

Figure 54–145. Continuous suture anastomosis. *A,* The anastomosis is begun with a double-ended mattress suture at the heel. *B,* One end of the suture is continued as an over-and-over stitch to the toe. A ball-point angle-tipped probe is used to place traction on the adventitia, thus exposing the free edge of the saphenous vein graft. *C,* The other end of the original stitch is continued on the contralateral side to the midpoint of the arteriotomy. *D,* The second suture is continued as an over-and-over stitch from the toe to meet with the original stitch at the midpoint of the arteriotomy. (From Ochsner, J. L., and Mills, N. L.: Coronary Artery Surgery. Philadelphia, Lea & Febiger, 1978.)

popularly used among the New York University faculty is to attach the proximal grafts before bypass is started. Either technique gives satisfactory results, depending primarily on the preference of the surgeon.

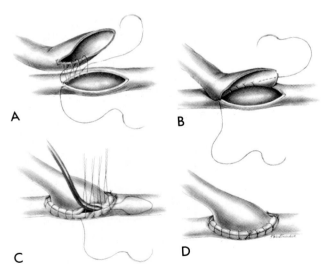

Figure 54–146. Combination continuous and interrupted suture anastomosis. *A,* The heel or proximal aspect of the anastomosis is begun as a horizontal mattress stitch, and four or five passes of the suture are done before making the suture taut. *B,* The continuous suture has been made taut for one half of a side of the anastomosis. *C,* The proximal half of the anastomosis has been completed as a continuous over-and-over stitch. The distal half is completed with multiple interrupted sutures. A calibrated dilator is passed through the anastomosis before completion to ensure patency. *D,* Completed anastomosis. (From Ochsner, J. L., and Mills, N. L.: Coronary Artery Surgery. Philadelphia, Lea & Febiger, 1978.)

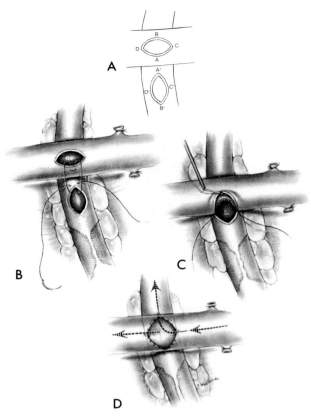

Figure 54–147. Diamond anastomosis. *A,* Diagram showing the method of alignment of the incisions in the bypass graft and coronary artery. *B,* The anastomosis is begun with a double-ended horizontal mattress suture placed at the midpoint of the venotomy and the apex of the arteriotomy. *C,* The anastomosis is continued halfway and is then interrupted by tying to another suture. The second suture is a continuous anastomosis. *D,* Completed anastomosis and continuing through the graft to the primary anastomosis. (From Ochsner, J. L., and Mills, N. L.: Coronary Artery Surgery. Philadelphia, Lea & Febiger, 1978.)

Sequential anastomoses are commonly used, although not nearly as frequently as those described by Kirklin and Barratt-Boyes (1986). The most common sequential anastomosis is to the left anterior descending, grafting the distal vessel as well as the diagonal branch. It is unusual to do more than four or five distal anastomoses. A more radical approach, with impressive data, is described by Kirklin, grafting all vessels near 1.5 mm in diameter that are narrowed more than 50% (Fig. 54–147). By using multiple sequential anastomoses, as many as eight to 10 anastomoses have been done in a few patients.

Endarterectomy is seldom done, this author preferring to graft beyond the distal obstruction. The experiences of Johnson and Brenowitz in Milwaukee, Mills in New Orleans, and several surgeons in England, are observed with interest but serious doubt exists about long-term patency (Fig. 54–148) (after 1 to 3 years) in endarterectomized vessels because of progressive cicatricial contraction of fibrous tissue. This phenomenon long ago led to abandonment of endarterectomy in the femoral popliteal system in arteries that are much larger than coronary arteries.

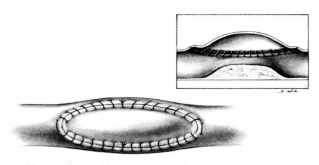

Figure 54-148. The arteriotomy is made through the stenotic lesion and into a sufficiently large lumen proximally and distally. A venous bypass graft is sutured end to side to the arteriotomy so that unobstructed flow is possible in both directions. (From Ochsner, J. L., and Mills, N. L.: Coronary Artery Surgery. Philadelphia, Lea & Febiger, 1978.)

After bypass, flow rates are measured routinely with a flowmeter, usually finding peak flows greater than 80 to 100 ml/min. Flow rates, of course, vary with the size of the vessel grafted and arterial pressure.

Subsequently, before the operative incision is closed, soft tissues are closed in the superior mediastinum to cover the grafts, leaving the pericardium open inferiorly. Pacemaker wires are routinely left in the right ventricle and right atrium for control of postoperative arrhythmias. A small plastic catheter for monitoring blood pressure is usually left in the left atrium as well as a Swan-Ganz catheter in the pulmonary artery.

POSTOPERATIVE CARE

The principal considerations in the first 12 to 24 hours after operation are cardiac output, adequacy of ventilation, postoperative bleeding, and arrhythmias. Ventilation is usually done through an indwelling endotracheal tube for a few hours, by which time the patient is usually awake sufficiently to permit extubation. Blood gas tensions are periodically monitored. Significant ventilatory problems are uncommon.

The left atrial pressure, arterial pressure, and electrocardiogram are usually displayed continuously on a monitoring screen for visual observation. The basic goal is to maintain a cardiac index between 2.5 and 3 liters, with a systolic blood pressure of 100 to 120 mm Hg. Some degree of hypertension is common and responds to appropriate infusions of nitroprusside or nitroglycerin. Blood volume is adjusted by infusion of appropriate fluids, depending on both blood loss and the degree of vasoconstriction or vasodilatation present. Left atrial pressure is usually maintained between 8 and 12 to 15 mm Hg.

If an adequate cardiac output is not present with a satisfactory left atrial pressure and a peripheral vascular resistance near 1,000 units, inotropic agents, usually dobutamine (5 to 10 μg/kg/min) and epinephrine (2 to 6 μg/min) are used. With the myocardial

preservation technique described, a low cardiac output after an uncomplicated bypass is uncommon and is usually due to some cause other than diffuse myocardial injury.

Significant postoperative bleeding is uncommon, the usual blood loss ranging from 300 to 700 ml in the first 24 hours. If significant bleeding continues despite a normal activated clotting time, transfusions of platelets or fresh frozen plasma are given. The unusual patient with a blood loss of more than 1 liter is usually returned to the operating room for exploration regardless of the hemodynamic status. This approach not only excludes a discrete site of bleeding but also removes intrapericardial clots that could cause tamponade.

A patient with a low cardiac output not responding to infusion of fluid or inotropic agents is usually promptly returned to the operating room. One of four causes can then be readily excluded. These causes include thrombosis of a bypass graft, tamponade, swollen myocardium compressed within the pericardium, or diffuse myocardial injury. The first three of these four causes can be corrected by appropriate surgical maneuvers. The fourth cause, myocardial depression, is uncommon and is usually diagnosed in the operating room by exclusion of the other three factors; it is then treated by insertion of an intra-aortic balloon pump. A balloon pump is almost never inserted empirically in the recovery room because of the difficulty of excluding pericardial tamponade or myocardial compression from edema. Minor arrhythmias are common and are usually treated by infusion of lidocaine (1 to 2 mg/min) or procainamide. Supplemental potassium therapy may be needed for hypokalemia. Electrical pacing is used for transient bradycardia. Significant tachycardia is usually treated with small amounts of propranolol.

A small perioperative infarction occurs in less than 5% of patients, usually diagnosed from the appearance of Q waves on the electrocardiogram. Myocardial enzymes are measured regularly (the CPK-MB enzyme), although the precise significance of these measurements is uncertain. If a significant possibility of an infarction exists, the ejection fraction is usually measured with a radionuclide gated pool scan before the patient is discharged from the hospital.

Fortunately, with modern techniques most patients recover uneventfully and are discharged from the hospital within 7 to 9 days after operation.

Early Results

Operative Mortality and Morbidity. Operative mortality in good-risk patients is almost 1%, similar to that reported in many centers throughout the United States. Significant risk factors have been defined in several publications. A 1988 report identified 21 statistically significant risk factors found in a combined study from 15 surgical centers of more than 7,000 patients having operation. The more significant of these were advanced age, severity of angina, number of vessels diseased, left ventricular function (ejection fraction), signs of heart failure or hemodynamic instability, and priority of operation (elective, urgent, or emergent).

At New York University patients are often referred from other centers because of significant risk factors, often considering the patient "inoperable," usually because of depressed ventricular function or diffuse vascular disease. Even in these high-risk patients, however, with the techniques described, operative mortality is seldom greater than 4 to 5%.

Significant Operative Complications. The four most serious operative complications are myocardial infarction, stroke, renal failure, and wound infection. Myocardial infarction was discussed in the preceding paragraphs. A stroke is the most disabling complication, fortunately decreasing in frequency at New York University in recent years to a range of 1 to 2%. This may possibly be related to the special cannula and technique used with patients with known atherosclerotic disease in the aortic arch and carotid arteries. Preliminary experiences with this technique were reported by Culliford in 1986. Concomitant procedures for coexisting carotid and coronary disease are rarely done, and the combined procedure is reserved only for the unusual patient with acutely symptomatic coronary and carotid disease. The authors no longer believe that asymptomatic carotid disease, even though hemodynamically significant, is a significant cause of perioperative stroke. Preferably, the most symptomatic disease is treated first, followed within a few days by treatment of the other disease. This conservative policy, a reversal of procedures in earlier years, has been associated with a decreased frequency of stroke and lends credence to the theory that most strokes may arise from atheroma in the transverse aortic arch, not from the carotid arteries.

Wound infection is fortunately rare, less than 1% of elective operations. It occurs more frequently in older patients, especially those with diabetes. Bilateral mammary grafts are avoided in these patients because of the higher frequency of sternal complications from the resultant ischemia.

Renal failure of significant degree is fortunately rare. Hemodialysis via catheters in the subclavian vein is used in the uncommon patient whose blood urea nitrogen rises above 90 mg/dl.

Relief of Angina. Immediate relief of angina is the most dramatic feature of coronary bypass, prompt and complete relief occurring in most patients with complete revascularization. This familiar dramatic result is responsible for the rapid rise in frequency of bypass grafting after its introduction in 1967 to 1968.

Long-Term Results

Patency of Vein Grafts. With appropriate technique, combined with preoperative antiplatelet ther-

apy, a patency rate greater than 90% can be anticipated in the first month after operation, decreasing slightly in subsequent months but remaining at or above 90% a year after operation (Fig. 54–149) (Bourassa et al, 1986). Limited data are now available because angiograms are seldom done after operation unless complications occur.

A degree of intimal thickening characteristically occurs in the first several months after operation, which is apparently a normal histologic response of the vein to arterial pressure. This process, called a "remodeling" by Barrett-Boyes, continues to where within a few months the diameter of the vein decreases to more closely resemble that of the distal coronary artery. More severe degrees of fibromuscular hyperplasia, perhaps resulting in thrombosis, may be a result of excessive accumulation of platelets with their stimulus for proliferation of smooth muscle.

Between 1 and 5 years after operation, vein grafts occlude at a rate between 2 and 3% per year to where patency 5 years after operation is in the range of 70 to 80%. The frequency of occlusion appears to be related partly to the technique of vein procurement and loss of intimal surface. In a 1984 report by Chesebro and associates, 1 year of antiplatelet therapy decreased the frequency of late occlusion from 25% to 11% in the group of 343 patients studied with angiography 11 to 18 months after operation.

As mentioned earlier, atherosclerosis appears with increased frequency in vein grafts between 5 and 10 years after operation so that 10 years after operation approximately 40% of grafts are closed, 30% show severe atherosclerosis, and only about 30% remain in satisfactory condition. The ultimate fate of this 30% is yet unknown, but the trend is clearly not favorable. As stated earlier, recognition of this fact in the last few years has led to widespread use of different combinations of mammary grafts as well as a continued search for other satisfactory autogenous arteries.

Long-term patency of internal mammary grafts, more than 90% 10 years after operation, is discussed in a separate section by Rankin.

Recurrent Angina. Angina returns in 10 to 15% of patients within 5 years after operation, and in approximately 50% of patients within 10 years. This recurrence of angina almost always indicates occlusion of a previously functioning graft or the development of significant disease in the native coronary circulation. Fortunately, these patients can be treated by reoperation when necessary. This procedure is done now with increased frequency, fortunately with an operative risk and morbidity little greater than that with elective bypass. Repeat operations are discussed in a separate section by Loop.

Exercise Tolerance and Changes in Ventricular Function. With effective revascularization of all significantly diseased coronary arteries, patients have almost normal exercise capacity within 2 to 3 months after operation, depending on the degree of ventricular function that existed before operation. This is

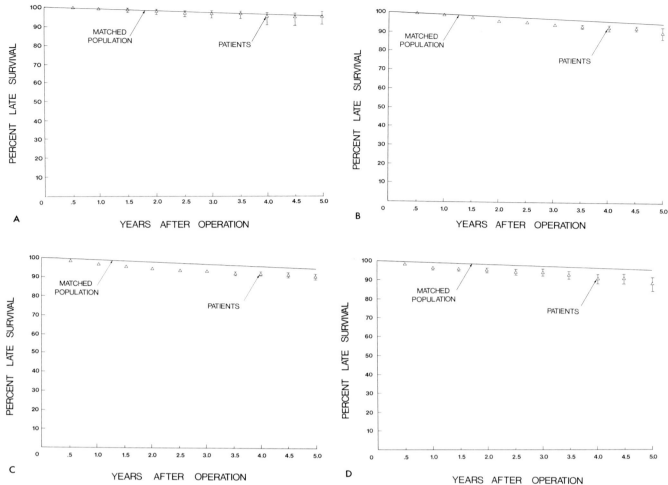

Figure 54–149. *A,* The actuarial survival of 182 patients surviving coronary bypass grafting for single-vessel disease. The vertical bar represents one standard error. Thus, the life expectancy of a patient with single-vessel disease after leaving the hospital is the same as that of the matched general population at 5 years. *B,* The five-year actuarial survival of 508 patients who survived coronary bypass grafting for double-vessel disease. The life expectancy at 5 years is about 5% less than that of the matched general population. *C,* The 5-year actuarial survival of 863 patients surviving bypass grafting for triple-vessel disease. The life expectancy 5 years after operation is about 6% less than that of the matched general population. *D,* The 5-year survival of 247 patients surviving operation for left main coronary artery disease. The 5-year life expectancy is approximately 7% less than that of the matched general population.

best confirmed by a stress test before strenuous physical exercise is done. This ability to return to a normal life-style is one of the great attractions of bypass operations.

Ventricular function improves promptly after effective bypass, with a normal response of a rise in ejection fraction with exercise. Barratt-Boyes stated that improvements in hypokinetic and dyskinetic segments have continued for several months after operation.

Progression of Atherosclerosis. As stated earlier, serial angiographic studies after operation show a continued progression of atherosclerosis that varies in rate and severity. Cessation of the atherosclerotic process, however, is almost unknown, and represents a continuing challenge to medical therapy.

Progression of disease occurs at different rates in the native coronary arteries and in grafted coronary arteries, both proximal and distal to the site of anastomosis. Progression is most rapid in the grafted coronary artery proximal to the site of anastomosis, apparently from changes in blood flow. Progression distal to the anastomosis is uncommon. Kroncke in 1988 reported findings in angiograms done 5 years after initial study in the more than 200 patients originally evaluated in the randomized Veterans Administration Study of Bypass Surgery. In 1986, Bourassa also analyzed their findings of the frequency of atherosclerotic changes after bypass and found that antilipid therapy had not yet been shown to have significant benefit.

Capacity to Return to Work. As stated earlier, with effective bypass, ventricular function improves to the point at which work capacity is actually better than that existing before operation. Thus, there is rarely a cardiac reason for not returning to work unless revascularization was ineffective, either from operative injury or thrombosis of a graft. Failure to return to work is usually for socioeconomic reasons, not cardiac reasons. This, of course, varies with the

LIFE-TABLE SURVIVAL CURVES

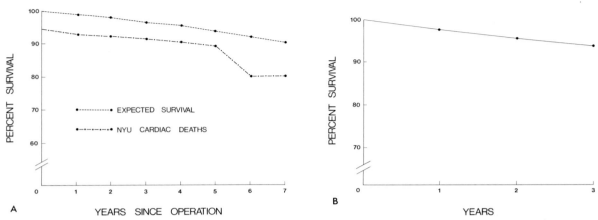

Figure 54–150. *A,* The 7-year actuarial survival of the first 1174 patients having bypass at New York University Medical Center (1968 to 1975) compared with that of the matched general population. The average operative mortality rate was 5%, declining to between 1 and 2% during the later part of the study. The significant points are that the mortality rate between 1 and 4 years after operation was only 1.4% per year, the same as that for the general population, and the mortality rate between 3 and 5 years after operation was identical to that between 1 and 3 years after operation. *B,* The 3-year survival for 249 patients having three or more bypass grafts at New York University Medical Center between 1972 and 1974.

working status of patients who have had surgical therapy. At New York University, operation is often done for patients limited in their capacity to work because of angina. Most of these patients return to work within 2 to 3 months after operation.

Arrhythmias. Compared with the effectiveness of bypass for relief of angina, arrhythmias are often unchanged after operation and carry with them the unpredictable hazard of sudden death. Surgical therapy for arrhythmias is discussed later and thus the topic is only briefly mentioned here.

The ability of bypass surgery to protect from sudden death depends on whether the arrhythmias are arising from reversible myocardial ischemia; an irritable focus, such as a scar from a previous infarction, or a combination of the two. The report by Tresch and associates in 1985 described a long-term follow-up of 49 survivors of prehospital cardiac arrest who had bypass surgery. Three- and 5-year survivals subsequently were 82 and 72%, respectively.

This subject was also analyzed in the CASS data (1986) by Holmes, who found a marked protection from sudden death with operation in the high-risk patient with three-vessel disease and significant impairment of ventricular function. With current techniques, a proper evaluation and treatment of the patient for both myocardial ischemia and arrhythmic foci has the potential for yielding much better results in the future.

Increase in Longevity with Coronary Bypass. In the first 1,100 patients operated on at New York University between 1968 and 1975, the 5-year survival rate, including operative deaths, was 88%, and only 49 cardiac deaths occurred after the patients were discharged from the hospital. After discharge from the hospital, the average mortality was 1.5% per year

for the next 5 years, a rate almost identical to that of a matched group of a similar age and sex. The similarity of survival (Fig. 54–150) between the two groups strongly indicated the significant influence of bypass on longevity.

The beneficial influence of effective bypass grafting on mortality can also be inferred by noting that the surgical results 5 years after bypass are similar for patients with single-, double-, or triple-vessel disease compared with the significant difference in mortality for patients treated medically with single-, double-, or triple-vessel disease. This effect is discussed in detail by Kirklin and Barratt-Boyes (1986).

The different major randomized trials in coronary artery bypass surgery, which are well summarized by Frye in 1987, have shown that prognosis in coronary disease depends on more than 10 subsets of disease, depending on the number of vessels involved. These subsets include single-, double-, triple-vessel and left main disease combined with the degree of impairment of ventricular function. These studies have clearly delineated certain major groups with a striking improvement in longevity 5 years after operation. The more familiar groups include those with left main disease and triple-vessel disease with different degrees of impaired left ventricular function. A separate group consists of those with severe or even unstable angina. A less familiar group, documented more precisely in recent years, consists of patients with triple-vessel disease and significant "silent" ischemia, or patients with double-vessel disease, including disease in the proximal anterior descending coronary artery.

The ultimate influence on longevity depends on continued patency of the bypass grafts. Thus, a more widespread use of multiple mammary anastomoses may result in even greater influence on longevity than that shown in previous years when most bypasses were done with saphenous veins. A few reports exist of small groups of patients studied for more than 10 years after bilateral mammary grafting, all of which show a low frequency of late cardiac death. (Geha et al, 1987; Green et al, 1971; Galbut et al, 1985).

Selected Bibliography

Baumann, F. G., Catinella, F. P., Cunningham, J. N., Jr., and Spencer, F. C.: Vein contraction and smooth muscle cell extensions as causes of endothelial damage during graft preparation. Ann. Surg., 194:199, 1981.

A striking phenomenon with removal of a saphenous vein is the development of spasm. This concentric contraction of the vessel, with contraction of the internal elastic membrane, may rupture the endothelial lining with exposure of the underlying vessel wall to elements in the blood. Thus, the graft is no longer a tube completely lined with endothelium and is more susceptible to thrombosis. This paper demonstrates with electron microscopy the mechanism of this phenomenon. It can be minimized by the use of papaverine at the time of removal of the saphenous vein.

An additional 7% of the patients died, and the 5-year survival rate was 88%. This actuarial survival curve parallels that of a matched population of similar age and sex, and thus, this is one of the first papers that shows the strong likelihood that bypass grafting greatly increases longevity.

Bounos, E. P., Mark, D. B., Pollock, B. G., et al: Surgical survival benefits for coronary disease patients with left ventricular dysfunction. Circulation, 78 (Suppl. I):I-151, 1988.

In a group of 710 patients with an ejection fraction of less than 40%, 301 patients were treated surgically. Three-year surgical survival was 86% compared with a medical survival of only 68%. The greatest surgical benefits occurred in the patients with the most severe left ventricular dysfunction, contradicting the common opinion that patients with severe impairment of ventricular function benefit little from bypass.

CASS Principal Investigators and Their Associates: Coronary Artery Surgery Study (CASS): A randomized trial of coronary artery bypass surgery: Survival data. Circulation, 68:939, 1983.

This important report was one of the first from the extensive CASS of patients between 1975 and 1979, including almost 25,000 patients. This report discussed 780 patients with stable coronary disease with good ventricular function. During a period of 5 years, the longevity was very good in both medical and surgical groups (almost 93%). Thus, there was no benefit from performance of elective bypass.

An important point, however, is that these conclusions were valid only for patients whose angina did not increase in severity. In patients with triple-vessel disease, more than 7% of the patients each year developed symptoms and were treated with a bypass operation; thus within 5 years, 38% had had a bypass, emphasizing the importance of continued periodic evaluation.

Catinella, F. P., Cunningham, J. N., Jr., Srungaram, R. K., et al: Cold blood should not be used for vein preparation prior to coronary bypass grafting. J. Thorac. Cardiovasc. Surg., 82:904, 1981.

There is an increasing amount of data that indicate that the method of handling the saphenous vein at the time of coronary bypass grafting is crucial and determines both early and long-term patency and possibly also the susceptibility of the vein to atherosclerosis.

This paper indicates that cold blood is actually harmful. The cold causes a contraction of the vein with disruption of the endothelium, and the platelets in the blood then accumulate and initiate a thrombotic reaction. Moderately cold plasmanate is superior.

Chesebro, J. H., Clements, I. P., Fuster, V., et al: A platelet-inhibitor-drug trial in coronary-artery bypass operations: Benefit of perioperative dipyridamole and aspirin therapy on early postoperative vein graft patency. N. Engl. J. Med., 307:73, 1982.

This important report was the first to show the significant influence of preoperative antiplatelet therapy on patency rate of vein grafts following operation. With some modifications, this therapeutic regimen has now been widely adopted throughout the United States.

Cobb, L. A., Werner, J. A., and Trobaugh, G. B.: Sudden cardiac death. I: A decade's experience with out-of-hospital resuscitation. Mod. Concepts Cardiovasc. Dis., 49:31, 1980.

This remarkable paper from Seattle summarizing several years' experience with resuscitation of patients who develop cardiac arrest outside the hospital should be studied in detail. The data are especially significant because of the 600,000 deaths that occur annually in the United States, approximately two-thirds occur outside the hospital. The data are remarkable in that only one-fifth of the patients resuscitated had a transmural infarction, and more than half had no signs of myocardial necrosis whatsoever. About 75% of the patients had triple-vessel disease, indicating that the event causing ventricular fibrillation was an arrhythmia, not an infarction. The implications for prompt cardiopulmonary resuscitation, as well as for the long-term monitoring for malignant arrhythmias, are clear.

European Coronary Surgery Study Group: Prospective randomised study of coronary artery bypass surgery in stable angina pectoris: Second interim report. Lancet, 2:491, 1980.

The most important question with coronary bypass grafting is its influence on longevity. This randomized study is probably the best of its kind in the world. It was the first to conclusively show a significant difference in 5-year survival in patients with triple-vessel disease and good ventricular function. Patients with triple-vessel disease had a 5-year survival rate of 95% after operation and one of 85% after medical therapy.

Froelicher, V., Jensen, D., Sullivan, M.: A randomized trial of the effects of exercise training after coronary artery bypass surgery. Arch. Intern. Med., 145:689, 1985.

This carefully designed study randomized 53 patients after bypass surgery to determine the influence of a specific exercise program in the year after bypass. Although about one-third of the patients had signs or symptoms of residual ischemia after revascularization, little benefit from the exercise program could be shown.

Isom, O. W., Spencer, F. C., Glassman, E., et al: Does coronary bypass increase longevity? J. Thorac. Cardiovasc. Surg., 75:28, 1978.

This paper reports experiences at New York University with the first 1174 patients operated on between 1968 and 1975. The overall operative mortality rate was 5%. In the subsequent 5 years, an additional 7% of the patients died, an 88% 5-year survival rate. This actuarial survival curve parallels that of a matched population of similar age and sex, and thus, this was one of the first papers to show the strong likelihood that bypass grafting greatly increased longevity.

Loop, F. D., Cosgrove, D. M., Lytle, B. W., et al: An eleven year evolution of coronary arterial surgery (1967–1978). Ann. Surg., 190:444, 1979.

This paper summarizes much of the extensive experience at the Cleveland Clinic for a period of several years. Graft patency rates for four different groups, each studied around 20 months after operation, ranged from 77 to 87%. The 5-year survival rate for these four groups ranged from 89 to 92%.

Loop, F. D., Lytle, B. W., Cosgrove, D. M., et al: Influence of internal mammary artery grafts on 10 year survival and other cardiac events. N. Engl. J. Med., *314*:1, 1986.

This important paper was one of the first to show the significant influence of internal mammary artery grafting on longevity 10 years after operation. This influence is not apparent 5 years after operation but appears later on as significant disease develops in vein grafts. Another reason for the difference may be that the internal mammary artery often enlarges. The studies presented in the paper included more than 2,300 patients with an internal mammary graft, 855 of whom had postoperative catheterization. Patency of the internal mammary 10 years after operation was 96%. Catheterization studies also found that patency rate was similar both 1 year and 10 years after operation, which indicates the absence of a significant frequency of late occlusion.

Lytle, D. W., Cosgrove, D. M. K., et al: Perioperative risk of bilateral internal mammary artery grafting: Analysis of 500 cases 1971 to 1984. Circulation, *71* (Suppl. 3):37, 1986.

This significant report clearly showed that bilateral internal mammary artery grafting could be done with little increase in mortality or morbidity. During the year preceding this report, 25% of all patients having bypass had bilateral mammary grafts.

Mock, M. B., Fisner, L. D., Holmes, D. R., Jr., et al: Comparison of effects of medical and surgical therapy on survival in severe angina pectoris and two-vessel coronary artery disease with and without left ventricular dysfunction: A coronary artery surgery study registry study. Am. J. Cardiol., *61*:1198, 1988.

In a group of about 2,000 patients in the CASS with double-vessel disease, 1,317 were treated with bypass grafting. A definite benefit from surgical intervention was shown in the patients who either had severe left-ventricular dysfunction or severe angina, with one or two proximal stenoses. Six-year survival was 78% in the surgical group and 49% in the medical group.

Passamani, E., Davis, K. B., Gillespie, M. J., et al: A randomized trial of coronary artery bypass surgery: Survival of patients with a low ejection fraction. N. Engl. J. Med., *312*:1665, 1985.

This study evaluated by randomization the influence of operation on 780 patients with an ejection fraction between 0.34 and 0.5. Seven years later, there was a significant benefit from operation in those with triple-vessel disease. Of the surgical group 88% were alive compared with 65% of the medical group.

Spencer, F. C.: The internal mammary artery: The ideal coronary bypass graft? (Editorial). N. Engl. J. Med., *314*:50, 1986.

This editorial by the author summarized the sequence of events that led to the performance of the first successful internal mammary artery bypass graft in people in the United States by Green and Tice at New York University in 1986. More than a decade later, after 1980, internal mammary grafts were used in less than 15% of bypass operations done in the United States, but after the demonstration of the serious deterioration of vein grafts between 5 and 10 years after operation, internal mammary artery grafting was widely accepted as indicated in almost all patients having bypass.

Topol, E. J., Califf, R. M., George, B. S., et al: Insights derived from the thrombolysis and angioplasty in myocardial infarction (TAMI) trials. J. Am. Coll. Cardiol., *12*:24-A, 1988.

This report describes experiences with the first three TAMI studies in 708 patients. In general, thrombolysis therapy reopened the thrombosed vessel in almost 80% of patients. With patent vessels, immediate angioplasty had no advantage over deferred angioplasty. If vessels remained occluded, however, angioplasty was successful in more than 50%. Morbidity was significant, however, because 14 patients developed a stroke, five of which were from intracranial hemorrhage. Bleeding was significant; approximately 30% of the patients required transfusion of at least two units of blood.

Weiner, D. A., Ryan, T. A., McCabe, C. H., et al: Comparison of coronary artery bypass surgery and medical therapy in patients with exercise-induced silent myocardial ischemia: A report from the coronary artery surgery study (CASS) registry. J. Am. Coll. Cardiol., *12*:595, 1988.

Six hundred ninety-two patients were studied, 268 of whom underwent surgical therapy. Definite benefit from operation was found in the group with triple-vessel disease and impaired ventricular function, because the 7-year survival was 90% in the surgical group and only 37% in the medical group.

Bibliography

Baumann, F. G., Catinella, F. P., Cunningham, J. N., Jr., and Spencer, F. C.: Vein contraction and smooth muscle cell extensions as causes of endothelial damage during graft preparation. Ann. Surg., *194*:199, 1981.

Berg, R. J., Selinger, S. L., Leonard, J. J., et al: Surgical management of acute myocardial infarction. Cardiovasc. Clin., *12*:61, 1982.

Bonow, R. O., and Epstein, S. E.: Indications for coronary artery bypass surgery in patients with chronic angina pectoris: Implications of the multicenter randomized trials. Circulation, *72* (Suppl. V):V-23, 1985.

Bounos, E. P., Mark, D. B., Pollock, B. G., et al: Surgical survival benefits for coronary disease patients with left ventricular dysfunction. Circulation, *78* (Suppl. I):8-151, 1988.

Bourassa, M. G., Campeau, L., Lespérance, J., et al: Atherosclerosis after coronary artery bypass surgery: Results of recent studies and recommendations regarding prevention. Cardiology, *73*:259, 1986.

Boyd, A. D., Tremblay, R. E., Spencer, F. C., and Bahnson, H. T.: Estimation of cardiac output soon after intracardiac surgery with cardiopulmonary bypass. Ann. Surg., *150*:613, 1959.

Brenowitz, J. B., Kayser, K. L., and Johnson, W. D.: Results of coronary artery endarterectomy and reconstruction. J. Thorac. Cardiovasc. Surg., *95*:1, 1988.

Cameron, A., Davis, K. A., Green, G. E., et al: Clinical implications of internal mammary artery bypass grafts: The coronary artery surgery study experience. Circulation, *77*:815, 1988.

Cameron, A., Kemp, H. G., et al: Bypass surgery with the internal mammary artery graft: 15-year follow-up. Circulation, *74* (Suppl. 3):30, 1986.

CASS Principal Investigators and Their Associates: Coronary artery surgery study (CASS): A randomized trial of coronary artery bypass surgery: Survival data. Circulation, *68*:939, 1983.

Catinella, F. P., Cunningham, J. N., Jr., Srungaram, R. K., et al: Cold blood should not be used for vein preparation prior to coronary bypass grafting. J. Thorac. Cardiovasc. Surg., *82*:904, 1981.

Chatterjee, K.: Is there any long-term benefit from coronary artery bypass surgery? J. Am. Coll. Cardiol., *12*:881, 1988.

Chesebro, J. H., Clements, I. P., Fuster, V., et al: A platelet-inhibitor-drug trial in coronary-artery bypass operations: Benefit of perioperative dipyridamole and aspirin therapy on early postoperative vein graft patency. N. Engl. J. Med., *307*:73, 1982.

Chesebro, J. H., Fuster, V., Elveback, L. R., et al: Effect of dipyridamole and aspirin on late vein graft patency after coronary bypass operations. N. Engl. J. Med., *310*:209, 1984.

Cobb, L. A., Werner, J. A., and Trobaugh, G. B.: Sudden cardiac death. I: A decade's experience with out-of-hospital resuscitation. Mod. Concepts Cardiovasc. Dis., *49*:31, 1980a.

Cobb, L. A., Werner, J. A., and Trobaugh, G. B.: Sudden cardiac death. II: Outcome of resuscitation; management; and future directions. Mod. Concepts Cardiovasc. Dis., 49:37, 1980b.

Connor, A. R., Vlietstra, R. E., Schaff, H. V., et al: Early and late results of coronary artery bypass after failed angioplasty. J. Thorac. Cardiovasc. Surg., 96:191, 1986.

Culliford, A. T., Colvin, S. B., Rohrer, K., et al: The atherosclerotic ascending aorta and transverse arch: A new technique to prevent cerebral injury during bypass: Experiences with 13 patients. Ann. Thorac. Surg., 41:27, 1986.

Cunningham, J. N., Jr., Adams, P. X., Knopp, E. A., et al: Preservation of ATP, ultrastructure, and ventricular function after aortic cross-clamping and reperfusion: Clinical use of blood potassium cardioplegia. J. Thorac. Cardiovasc. Surg., 78:708, 1979.

Cunningham, J. N., Jr., Catinella, F. P., and Spencer, F. C.: Blood cardioplegia—Experience with prolonged cross-clamping. In Engleman, R. E., and Levitzky, S. (eds): A Textbook of Clinical Cardioplegia. Mt. Kisco, New York, Futura Publishing Co., 1982.

Daggett, W. M., Guyton, R. A., Mundth, E. D., et al: Surgery for post-myocardial infarct ventricular septal defect. Ann. Surg., 186:260, 1977.

Detre, K., Holubkov, R., Kelsley, S., et al: Percutaneous transluminal coronary angioplasty in 1985–1986 and 1977–1981. N. Engl. J. Med., 318:265, 1988.

Ernst, S. M. P. G., Van der Feltz, T. A., Bal, E. T., et al: Long term angiographic follow up, cardiac events, and survival in patients undergoing percutaneous transluminal coronary angioplasty. Br. Heart J., 57:220, 1987.

European Coronary Surgery Study Group: Prospective randomised study of coronary artery bypass surgery in stable angina pectoris. Second interim report. Lancet, 2:491, 1980.

European Coronary Surgery Study Group: Long-term results of prospective randomised study of coronary artery bypass surgery in stable angina pectoris. Lancet, 2:1173, 1982.

Froelicher, V., Jensen, D., and Sullivan, M.: A randomized trial of the effects of exercise training after coronary artery bypass surgery. Arch. Intern. Med., 145:689, 1985.

Frye, R. L., Fisher, L., Schaff, H. V., et al: Randomized trial in coronary artery bypass surgery. Prog. Cardiovasc. Dis., 30:1, 1987.

Galbut, D. L., Traad, E. A., Dorman, M. J., et al: Twelve-year experience with bilateral internal mammary artery grafts. Ann. Thorac. Surg., 40:264, 1985.

Gay, W. A., Jr., and Ebert, P. A.: Functional, metabolic, and morphologic effects of potassium-induced cardioplegia. Surgery, 74:284, 1973.

Geha, A. S., Hammond, G. L., Stephan, R. N., et al: Long-term outcome of revascularization of the anterior coronary arteries with crossed double internal mammary versus saphenous vein grafts. Surg., 102:667, 1987.

Gersh, B. J., Kronmal, R. A., Schaff, H. V., et al: Comparison of coronary artery bypass surgery and medical therapy in patients 65 years of age or older. N. Engl. J. Med., 313:217, 1985.

Green, G. E., Spencer, F. C., Tice, D. A., and Stertzer, S. H.: Arterial and venous microsurgical bypass grafts for coronary artery disease. J. Thorac. Cardiovasc. Surg., 60:491, 1970.

Green, M. V., Ostrow, H. G., Douglas, M. A., et al: High temporal resolution ECG-gauged scintigraphic angiocardiography. J. Nucl. Med., 16:95, 1975.

Guyton, R. A., Arcidi, R. M., Jr., Langford, D. A., et al: Emergency coronary bypass for cardiogenic shock. Circulation, 76 (Suppl. V):V-22, 1987.

Hamby, R. I., Aintablian, A., Handler, M., et al: Aortocoronary saphenous vein bypass grafts: Long-term patency, morphology, and blood flow in patients with patent grafts early after surgery. Circulation, 60:901, 1979.

Harken, A. H., Josephson, M. E., and Horowitz, L. N.: Surgical endocardial resection for the treatment of malignant ventricular tachycardia. Ann. Surg., 190:456, 1979.

Hellman, C. K., Kamath, M. L., Schmidt, D. H., et al: Improvement in left ventricular function after myocardial revascularization: Assessment by first-pass rest and exercise nuclear angiography. J. Thorac. Cardiovasc. Surg., 79:645, 1980.

Holmes, D. R., and Davis, K. B.: The effect of medical and surgical treatment on subsequent sudden cardiac death in patients with coronary artery disease: A report from the coronary artery surgery study. Circulation, 73:1254, 1986.

Huddleston, C. B., Stoney, W. S., Alford, W. C., Jr., et al: Internal mammary artery grafts: Technical factors influencing patency. Ann. Thorac. Surg., 42:543, 1986.

Hurst, J. W., King, S. B., III, Logue, R. B., et al: Value of coronary bypass surgery. Controversies in cardiology, Part I. Am. J. Cardiol., 42:308, 1978.

Isom, O. W., Spencer, F. C., Glassman, E., et al: Does coronary bypass increase longevity? J. Thorac. Cardiovasc. Surg., 75:28, 1978.

Isom, O. W., Spencer, F. C., Glassman, E., et al: Long-term survival following coronary bypass surgery in patients with significant impairment of left ventricular function. Circulation, 51 (Suppl. 1):141, 1975.

Johnson, W. D., Flemma, R. J., Lepley, D., Jr., and Ellison, E. H.: Extended treatment of severe coronary artery disease: A total surgical approach. Ann. Surg., 170:460, 1969.

Jones, E. L., Craver, J. M., Kaplan, J. A., et al: Criteria for operability and reduction of surgical mortality in patients with severe left ventricular ischemia and dysfunction. Ann. Thorac. Surg., 25:413, 1978.

Jones, E. L., Craver, J. M., King, S. B., et al: Clinical, anatomic and functional descriptors influencing morbidity, survival and adequacy of revascularization following coronary bypass. Ann. Surg., 192:390, 1980.

Kaiser, G. C.: CABG 1984: Technical aspects of bypass surgery. Circulation, 72:V-46, 1985.

Kay, P. H., Brooks, N., Magee, P., et al: Bypass grafting to the right coronary with and without endarterectomy: Patency at one year. Br. Heart J., 54:489, 1985.

Kent, J. M., Borer, J. S., Green, M. V., et al: Effects of coronary-artery bypass on global and regional left ventricular function during exercise. N. Engl. J. Med., 298:1434, 1978.

Kirklin, J. W., and Barratt-Boyes, B. G.: Cardiac Surgery. New York, John Wiley & Sons, 1986.

Kirklin, J. W., Kouchoukos, N. T., Blackstone, E. H., and Oberman, A.: Research related to surgical treatment of coronary artery disease. Circulation, 60:1613, 1979.

Kolessov, V. I.: Mammary artery-coronary artery anastomosis as a method of treatment for angina pectoris. J. Thorac. Cardiovasc. Surg., 54:535, 1967.

Kroncke, G. M., Kosolcharoen, P., Clayman, J. A., et al: Five-year changes in coronary arteries of medical and surgical patients of the Veterans Administration randomized study of bypass surgery. Circulation, 78 (Suppl. I):I-144, 1988.

Landymore, R. W., Tice, D., Trehan, N., and Spencer, F. C.: Does topical hypothermia prevent sublethal intraoperative injury during coronary artery bypass surgery? Presented at American Association for Thoracic Surgery Meeting, Washington, D. C., May 1981.

Lawrie, G. M., Morris, G. C., Jr., Chapman, D. W., et al: Patterns of patency of 596 vein grafts up to seven years after aorta-coronary bypass. J. Thorac. Cardiovasc. Surg., 73:443, 1977.

Loop, F. D., Cosgrove, D. M., Lytle, B. W., et al: An eleven year evolution of coronary arterial surgery (1967–1978). Ann. Surg., 190:444, 1979.

Loop, F. D., Lytle, B. W., Cosgrove, D. M., et al: Coronary artery bypass graft surgery in the elderly: Indications and outcome. Cleve. Clin. J. Med., 55:23, 1988.

Loop, F. D., Lytle, B., Cosgrove, D. M., et al: Influence of internal mammary artery grafts on 10 year survival and other cardiac events. N. Engl. J. Med., 314:1, 1986.

Lytle, B. W., Cosgrove, D. M., Loop, F. D., et al: Perioperative risk of bilateral internal mammary artery grafting: Analysis of 500 cases 1971 to 1984. Circulation, 74 (Suppl. 3):37, 1986.

Miller, D. W., Jr., Ivey, T. D., Bailey, W. W., et al: The practice of coronary artery bypass surgery in 1980. J. Thorac. Cardiovasc. Surg., 81:423, 1981.

Mock, M. B., Fisher, L. D., Holmes, D. R., Jr., et al: Comparison of effects of medical and surgical therapy on survival in severe angina pectoris and two-vessel coronary artery disease with and without left ventricular dysfunction: A coronary artery surgery study registry study. Am. J. Cardiol., 61:1198, 1988.

Mock, M. B., Ringqvist, I., Fisher, L. D., et al: Survival of medically treated patients in the Coronary Artery Surgery Study (CASS) Registry. Circulation, 66:562, 1982.

Naunheim, K. S., Kern, M. J., McBride, L. R., et al: Coronary artery bypass surgery in patients aged 80 years or older. Am. J. Cardiol., 59:804, 1987.

Naunheim, K. S., Kesler, K. A., Kanper, K. R., et al: Coronary artery bypass for recent infarction: Predictors of mortality. Circulation, 78 (Suppl. 1):I-122, 1988.

Nelson, G. R., Cohn, P. F., and Gorlin, R.: Prognosis in medically treated coronary artery disease: Influence of ejection fraction compared to other parameters. Circulation, 52:408, 1975.

Newman, D. C., and Hicks, R. G.: Combines carotid and coronary artery surgery: A review of the literature. Ann. Thorac. Surg., 45:574, 1988.

Ochsner, J. L., and Mills, N. L.: Coronary Artery Surgery. Philadelphia, Lea & Febiger, 1978.

Ochsner, J. L., Mills, N. L., and Bethea, M. C.: Operative technique of myocardial revascularization. World J. Surg., 2:767, 1978.

Olearchyk, A. S.: Coronary revascularization: Past, present and future. JUMANA (J. Ukr. Med. Assoc. North Am.), 35:3, 1988.

Passamani, E., Davis, K. B., Gillespie, M. J., et al: A randomized trial of coronary artery bypass surgery: Survival of patients with a low ejection fraction. N. Engl. J. Med., 312:1665, 1985.

Perler, B. A., Burdick, J. F., and Williams, G. M.: The safety of carotid endarterectomy at the time of coronary artery bypass surgery: Analysis of results in a high risk patient population. J. Vasc. Surg., 2:558, 1985.

Principal Investigators of CASS and Associates: The National Heart, Lung, and Blood Institute Coronary Artery Surgery Study (CASS). Circulation, 63(Part II):I-1, 1981.

Rahimtoola, S. H., Grunkemeier, G. L., and Starr, A.: Ten year survival after coronary artery bypass surgery for angina in patients aged 65 years and older. Circulation, 74:509, 1986.

Rankin, J. S., Newman, G. E., Bashore, T. M., et al: Clinical angiographic assessment of complex mammary artery bypass grafting. J. Thorac. Cardiovasc. Surg., 92:832, 1986.

Read, R. C., Murphy, M. L., Hultgren, H. N., and Takaro, T.: Survival of men treated for chronic stable angina pectoris: A cooperative randomized study. J. Thorac. Cardiovasc. Surg., 75:1, 1978.

Report of ad hoc committee on risk factors for coronary artery bypass surgery. Ann. Thorac. Surg., 45:348, 1988.

Rerych, S. K., Scholz, P. M., Sabiston, D. C., Jr., et al: Effects of exercise training on left ventricular function in normal subjects: A longitudinal study by radionuclide angiography. Am. J. Cardiol., 45:244, 1980.

Rifkind, B. M., and Levy, R. I.: Testing the lipid hypothesis. Clinical trials. Arch. Surg., 113:80, 1978.

Rossi, N. P., Koepke, J. A., and Spencer, F. C.: Histologic changes in long-term autologous arterial patch grafts in coronary arteries. Surgery, 57:335, 1965.

Sauvage, L. R., Wu, H. D., Kowalsky, T. E., et al: Healing basic and surgical techniques for complete revascularization of the left ventricle using only the internal mammary arteries. Ann. Thorac. Surg., 42:449, 1985.

Schulman, S. P., Achuff, S. C., Griffith, L. S. C., et al: Prognostic cardiac catheterization variables in survivors of acute myocardial infarction: A five year prospective study. J. Am. Coll. Cardiol., 11:1164, 1988.

Sheldon, W. C., and Loop, F. D.: Coronary artery bypass surgery: The Cleveland Clinic experience, 1967–1982. Postgrad. Med., 75:108, 1984.

Spencer, F. C.: Binocular loupes (microtelescopes) for coronary artery surgery. J. Thorac. Cardiovasc. Surg., 62:163, 1971.

Spencer, F. C.: The influence of coronary bypass on ventricular function. Consensus Meeting on Coronary Artery Bypass Surgery, Medical and Scientific Aspects, N.I.H., Bethesda, MD, December 1980.

Spencer, F. C.: The internal mammary artery: The ideal coronary bypass graft? (Editorial). N. Engl. J. Med., Vol. 314, 1986.

Spencer, F. C., Green, G. E., Tice, D. A., et al: Coronary artery bypass grafts for congestive heart failure: A report of experiences with 40 patients. J. Thorac. Cardiovasc. Surg., 62:529, 1971.

Spencer, F. C., Isom, O. W., Glassman, E., et al: The long-term influence of coronary bypass grafts on myocardial infarction and survival. Ann. Surg., 180:439, 1974.

Spencer, F. C., Yong, N. K., and Prachuabmoh, K.: Internal mammary-coronary artery anastomoses performed during cardiopulmonary bypass. Cardiovasc. Surg., 5:292, 1964.

Stamler, J.: Dietary and serum lipids in the multifactorial etiology of atherosclerosis. Arch. Surg., 113:21, 1978.

Stiles, Q. R.: Use of a punch to obtain a consistently uniform venotomy for rapid coronary anastomoses. J. Thorac. Cardiovasc. Surg., 82:154, 1981.

Topol, E. J., Califf, R. M., George, B. S., et al: Insights derived from the thrombolysis and angioplasty in myocardial infarction (TAMI) trials. J. Am. Coll. Cardiol., 12:24A, 1988.

Tresch, D. D., Wetherbee, J. N., Siegel, R., et al: Long-term follow-up of survival of prehospital sudden cardiac death treated with coronary bypass surgery. Am. Heart J., 110:1139, 1985.

U. S. Department of Health, Education and Welfare: Proceedings of the Conference on the Decline in Coronary Heart Disease Mortality. NIH Publication 79-1610. Washington, D.C., U. S. Government Printing Office, May 1979.

Weiner, D. A., Ryan, T. A., McCabe, C. H., et al: Comparison of coronary artery bypass surgery and medical therapy in patients with exercise-induced silent myocardial ischemia: A report from the coronary artery surgery study (CASS) registry. J. Am. Coll. Cardiol., 12:595, 1988.

VI DIETARY AND PHARMACOLOGIC MANAGEMENT OF ATHEROSCLEROSIS

Fredrick L. Dunn
Pamela B. Morris

Although coronary heart disease continues to be one of the leading causes of morbidity and mortality in the United States, convincing evidence now indicates that the development and progression of atherosclerosis can be retarded. Since the mid-1960s, there has been a dramatic reduction in the age-adjusted mortality from ischemic heart disease (Fig. 54–151) (Levy, 1981; Stern, 1979). From 1963 to 1982, the overall death rate from cardiovascular disease declined 36% nationwide (Kannel and Thom, 1984). The decline in mortality has coincided with aggressive approaches to management of cardiovascular risk factors and healthier life-styles (Goldman and Cook, 1984; Pyorala et al, 1985; Stamler, 1985), as

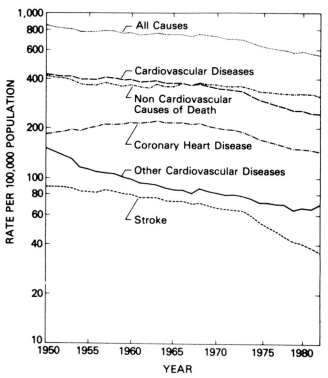

Figure 54–151. Decline in mortality due to cardiovascular diseases. (From Kannel, W. B., and Thom, T. J.: Declining cardiovascular mortality. Circulation, *70*:331, 1984. By permission of the American Heart Association, Inc.)

well as improved techniques of medical and surgical management of patients with cardiovascular disease (Beaglehole, 1986; Gillum et al, 1983). The approach to treatment of patients with coronary heart disease must therefore include not only the most recent medical and surgical interventions, but also vigorous attempts to modify those cardiac risk factors known to have an important part in the development and progression of atherosclerosis.

The use of coronary artery bypass as an effective technique for restoration of blood flow beyond an area of coronary artery obstruction is an important intervention for many patients with coronary atherosclerosis. Cardiac surgery has been estimated to account for a significant portion of the decline in mortality from coronary heart disease (Beaglehole, 1986; Goldman and Cook, 1984; Neutze and White, 1987). In addition, refinements in operative techniques have led to improved survival in surgically treated patients (Pryor et al, 1987). However, coronary artery bypass alone neither cures the underlying disease nor significantly affects the progression of atherosclerosis. Long-term follow-up of patients who have coronary revascularization procedures indicates that atherosclerosis can recur in the grafts as well as progress in nongrafted vessels and is related to persistence of cardiac risk factors (Atkinson et al, 1985; Campeau et al, 1984; Fitzgibbon et al, 1987; Neitzel et al, 1986). Substantial evidence now indi-

cates that progression of the atherosclerotic disease process can be retarded and that regression of pathologic lesions can sometimes be effected (Blankenhorn, 1981; Blankenhorn and Brooks, 1981; Glueck, 1986). Recent data in humans indicate that dietary restrictions of saturated fat and cholesterol combined with aggressive lipid-lowering treatment after coronary bypass can significantly retard progression of atherosclerosis in native arteries and bypass grafts and can cause some regression of lesions in native vessels (Blankenhorn et al, 1987). The performance of coronary revascularization identifies a patient at high risk for progression of atherosclerosis and emphasizes the importance of diagnosing and treating cardiovascular risk factors to prevent both graft occlusion and accelerated atherosclerosis in the nongrafted native vessels.

ATHEROSCLEROSIS

Pathology

The distribution of atherosclerotic plaques in the human arterial tree follows certain distinctive patterns (Strong et al, 1972). Involvement is usually more extensive in the abdominal aorta, the proximal coronary arteries, the thoracic aorta including the femoral and popliteal arteries, and the carotid arteries, with relative sparing of the renal, mesenteric, and pulmonary arteries (Glagov and Ozoa, 1968). These variations in plaque distribution may be due to hemodynamic forces or localized conditions of the architecture of the arterial wall.

The lesions of artherosclerosis involve primarily the intima, the innermost layer of the arterial wall. Three different types of pathologic lesions have been described: the fatty streak, the fibrous plaque, and the complicated lesion (Ross, 1986). Although more advanced atherosclerotic lesions are most commonly recognized in the aging population, pathology examinations have shown clear evidence of early lesions in young, asymptomatic individuals (Newman et al, 1986).

The process of atherosclerosis begins in childhood with the appearance of fatty streaks, usually by the age of 10. These yellow, sessile lesions are characterized by lipid-laden macrophages and smooth muscle cells. They result in no clinical manifestations and do not inevitably lead to more advanced lesions of atherosclerosis.

The fibrous plaque is characteristic of more advanced atherosclerosis, generally appearing in the third decade of life in populations at risk. Clinical manifestations are common, because smooth muscle cell proliferation within the intima causes elevation of the lesion and protrusion into the vascular lumen (Ross, 1981). In addition, extracellular and intracellular accumulation of lipids is accompanied by deposition of a new connective tissue matrix. The relationship between the fibrous plaque and fatty streaks

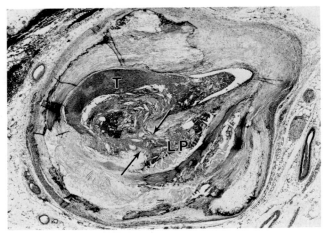

Figure 54–152. Coronary atherosclerosis complicated by plaque rupture and thrombosis (T). The fibrous cap of the plaque has ruptured *(arrows)*, allowing acellular debris from the lipid pool (LP) to extrude into the lumen. The lumen had already been narrowed by 85 to 90% by the concentric plaque and is now completely occluded by plaque debris and superimposed thrombus. (From Reimer, K. A., and Jennings, R. B.: Myocardial ischemia, hypoxia, and infarction. *In* Fozzart, H. A. (ed): The Heart and Cardiovascular System. New York, Raven Press, 1986, p. 1133.)

is unclear, because the common anatomic sites of the fibrous plaque are different from those in which fatty streaks appear.

In the advanced complicated lesion of atherosclerosis, tissue reaction in areas adjacent to the fibrous plaque results in hemorrhage, calcification, cell necrosis, and mural thrombosis. The complicated lesion occurs with increased frequency with age and is commonly associated with occlusive vascular disease and its clinical sequelae. Thus, the focal lesions of atherosclerosis are characterized by tissue proliferation, accumulation of intracellular and extracellular lipids, deposition of connective tissue matrix components, and tissue reaction causing thrombosis, ulceration, and calcification (Fig. 54–152).

Pathogenesis

Several theories of atherogenesis have been proposed to explain the characteristic accumulation of cells and extracellular material within the intima of arteries. Three of these hypotheses are (1) the response-to-injury hypothesis, (2) the lipogenic hypothesis, and (3) the monoclonal hypothesis. These theories of atherogenesis share many elements and help to explain our current understanding of the origin of atherosclerotic lesions.

Response-to-Injury Hypothesis. The response-to-injury hypothesis (Ross, 1986; Ross and Glomset, 1973; Ross and Glomset, 1976) incorporates the role of (1) the endothelium in maintaining the nonthrombogenic character of the artery and as a protective barrier for the artery wall, (2) platelets in mediating

intimal proliferation and vascular thrombotic occlusive complications, and (3) smooth muscle cells as the principal component of the lesions of atherosclerosis. This hypothesis states that the lesions of atherosclerosis occur as a response to some form of injury to arterial endothelial cells, possibly as a result of hypertensive arterial pressure, hemodynamic shear stress, hyperlipidemia, hypoxia, thrombosis, or some other form of chemical, humoral, or immunologic irritation. This focal endothelial injury leads to alterations in the relationship between endothelial cells and the underlying connective tissue substrate, causing detachment of cells and exposure of underlying collagen.

Disruption of endothelial integrity leads to platelet adherence at sites of injury and results in release of platelet constituents into the arterial wall. One of these platelet constituents, platelet-derived growth factor (PDGF), has been identified as one of a group of polypeptide hormones or growth factors known to have a critical part in cell proliferation (Ross, 1987; Ross et al, 1986). The release of PDGF at sites of endothelial injury is thought to lead to migration and proliferation of smooth muscle cells from the intima and media of the arterial wall, leading to formation of the mature atherosclerotic lesion. Protection of the endothelium or restoration of the endothelial barrier may allow the lesions to regress if the injury to the endothelium and the response to it are limited. However, chronic cycles of injury over many years result in progressive smooth muscle cell proliferation and progression to the mature lesions of occlusive arterial disease (Fig. 54–153). Traditional coronary risk factors, such as hypercholesterolemia and hypertension, are thought to have a critical role in progression of atherosclerotic lesions in the response-to-injury hypothesis by causing chronic injury or by interfering with the normal tissue healing in response to injury (Ross and Harker, 1976).

The importance of PDGF in smooth muscle cell proliferation and atherosclerosis is currently the focus of investigation. In experimental animal models of arterial injury and atherosclerosis, production of PDGF-like molecules has been shown to accompany cellular proliferation typical of atherosclerotic lesions (Walker et al, 1986). Recent data indicate that survivors of acute myocardial infarction with angiographically documented coronary atherosclerosis have increased platelet-derived mitogenic activity (Nilsson et al, 1986). This finding suggests that individual variations in growth factor activity for smooth muscle cells are one of the factors associated with development of atherosclerosis. Increased levels of PDGF gene transcript have been found in human atherosclerotic plaques isolated from carotid artery lesions (Barrett and Benditt, 1987). Smooth muscle proliferation and intimal hyperplasia also have an important part in aortocoronary vein graft disease after revascularization procedures (McCann et al, 1979). Thus, accumulating evidence indicates that factors such as PDGF controlling the migration and proliferation of

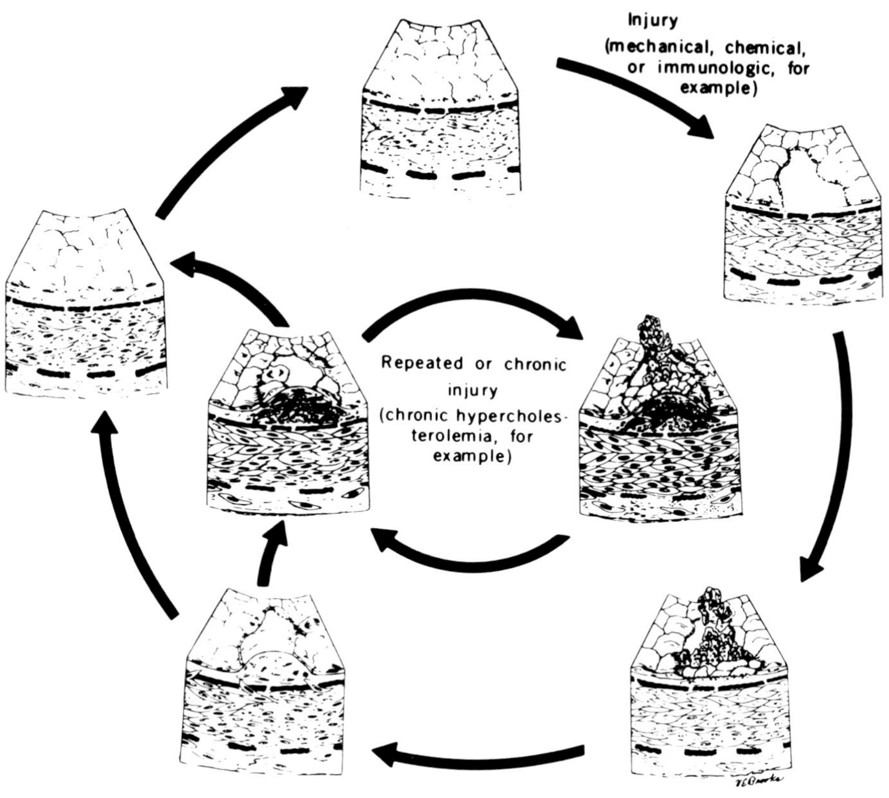

Figure 54–153. In the response-to-injury hypothesis of atherogenesis, platelet aggregation and smooth muscle cell proliferation after endothelial injury are limited (outer cycle). In the setting of chronic injury (inner cycle), smooth muscle cell proliferation and lipid deposition may continue, leading to advanced atherosclerotic lesions and subsequent clinical sequelae. (From Ross, R., and Glomset, J. A.: The pathogenesis of atherosclerosis. Reprinted by permission of the New England Journal of Medicine, 295:369, 1976.)

smooth muscle cells are important elements in the initation and progression of atherosclerosis.

In the mature atherosclerotic plaque, the cellular proliferation and accumulation of lipids and connective tissue matrix components result in thickening and scarring of the arterial wall. This damage is thought to result in localized hypoxia and alterations in cellular metabolism that may lead to the necrosis and inflammation characteristic of advanced complicated lesions.

Lipogenic Hypothesis. The lipogenic hypothesis is based on the recognition that cholesterol is a major constituent of the atherosclerotic plaque (Geer et al, 1961) and the evidence that sustained hypercholesterolemia, specifically elevation of plasma low-density lipoproteins (LDL), causes typical progressive atherosclerotic lesions in both experimental animals and humans (Frantz and Moore, 1969). Studies have shown that in the presence of elevated levels of LDL, changes in arterial wall metabolism promote a sequence of events leading to the development of advanced atherosclerotic lesions. These alterations in metabolism may cause smooth muscle cell proliferation and the production of connective tissue elements typical of atherosclerotic plaques. In the presence of elevated LDL, internalization and esterification of cholesterol are promoted, causing the proliferated smooth muscle cells to become filled with cholesterol esters (Dayton and Hashimoto, 1970; Smith, 1977). In addition, products of altered cellular metabolism may cause fibrosis, inflammation, and necrosis lead-ing to mature fibrous plaques. Because the lipogenic hypothesis shares many common elements in the response-to-injury hypothesis of atherogenesis, it is possible that the multiple lesions of progressive atherosclerosis may occur by a combination of these mechanisms.

Monoclonal Hypothesis. The monoclonal hypothesis of atherogenesis was proposed by Benditt and Benditt and suggests that each atherosclerotic lesion is a benign neoplasm derived from a single smooth muscle cell (Benditt, 1977; Benditt and Benditt, 1973). They examined the glucose-6-phosphate dehydrogenase isoenzyme content of isolated atherosclerotic plaques at autopsy. The lesions were found to be monotypic, expressing a single isoenzyme form rather than the bimorphic forms observed in undiseased, nonatherosclerotic arterial wall (Person et al, 1977). The lesion is thought to occur from cell transformation caused by mutagens, such as viruses or chemicals. This cellular transformation may make the lesion unresponsive to normal growth regulation, causing stimulation of cell replication. The progression to a mature atherosclerotic plaque occurs as proposed in the other hypotheses of atherogenesis.

LIPOPROTEIN METABOLISM

Most of the cholesterol in atherosclerotic plaques arises from the plasma (Steinberg, 1987). Cholesterol is transported in the blood as complex particles called

TABLE 54–37. PLASMA LIPOPROTEINS

Lipoprotein	Major Core Lipids	Major Apoproteins
Chylomicrons	Dietary triglyceride	B-48, C, E
VLDL	Endogenous triglyceride	B-100, C, E
Remnants	Triglyceride, cholesterol	B-100, E
LDL	Cholesterol	B-100
HDL	Cholesterol	A-I, A-II

lipoproteins. The major function of lipoproteins is to transport the two predominant lipids in the blood, cholesterol and triglyceride, from one organ or tissue to another (Goldstein et al, 1983; Havel, 1987; Schaefer and Levy, 1985). Several types of lipoproteins are present in plasma (Table 54–37), and each has a different origin and function (Fig. 54–154). These lipoproteins are classified as chylomicrons, very low-density lipoprotein (VLDL), LDL, and high-density lipoprotein (HDL). Each of these particles consists of a nonpolar lipid core (cholesterol ester and triglyceride) surrounded by a solubilizing surface layer of phospholipid, unesterified cholesterol, and apoproteins.

Chylomicrons are formed from dietary fat and cholesterol absorbed in the intestine. They are secreted into the lymph, pass through the thoracic duct, and eventually enter the systemic circulation. As chylomicrons enter capillaries, they encounter an enzyme, lipoprotein lipase, located on the surface of endothelial cells particularly in adipose tissue and muscle. The interaction of chylomicrons and lipoprotein lipase results in hydrolysis of triglyceride to fatty acids and glycerol. After lipolysis is complete, a chylomicron remnant is released into the circulation and is cleared rapidly by the liver.

VLDL is endogenously synthesized by the liver.

The core lipid in VLDL is primarily triglyceride, although approximately 20% is cholesterol. Normally, after an overnight fast, chylomicrons are cleared from the plasma and triglyceride circulates as VLDL. The metabolism of VLDL is similar to that of chylomicrons; VLDL transports triglyceride to tissues to be used as fuel or to fat for storage. After interaction with lipoprotein lipase, a VLDL remnant is produced, which can be removed by the liver or converted to LDL.

Most cholesterol in plasma is found in *LDL* (about two-thirds to three-fourths of the total cholesterol). LDL delivers cholesterol to tissues via a specific, high-affinity *LDL receptor,* which controls the uptake of cholesterol by cells (Brown and Goldstein, 1986). Cholesterol is important for the maintenance of cell membranes and as a precursor of steroid hormones and bile acids. When the cholesterol requirements of cells are met by the uptake of plasma cholesterol through the LDL receptor, there is competitive inhibition of the rate-limiting enzymes of cholesterol biosynthesis. Conversely, when plasma LDL cholesterol levels are low, synthesis of cholesterol within the cell is increased. In this manner, the LDL receptor controls intracellular cholesterol synthesis. Most LDL is cleared from the plasma by LDL receptors on the liver and to a lesser extent by extrahepatic tissues.

HDL is important for the return of cholesterol from peripheral tissues to the liver and for the normal metabolism of VLDL and chylomicrons. The origins and fates of HDL are complex. The liver and intestines secrete nascent HDL particles. These particles acquire cholesterol from VLDL and chylomicrons to become HDL_3. After esterification of plasma HDL cholesterol by the enzyme lecithin-cholesterol acyltransferase, further uptake of cholesterol from peripheral tissues transforms HDL_3 to HDL_2. HDL_2 can

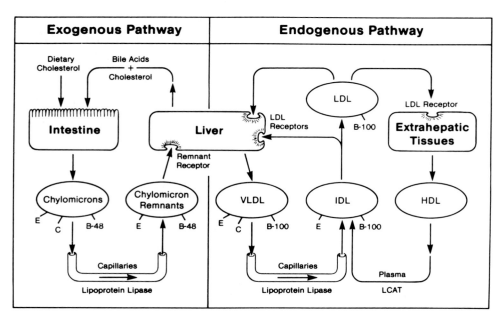

Figure 54–154. A model of our current understanding of lipoprotein metabolism, proposed by Goldstein and associates (1983). Metabolism of the lipoproteins is discussed in the text. (IDL = intermediate-density lipoprotein; LCAT = lecithin cholesterol acyltransferase.) (From Goldstein, J. L., Kita, T., and Brown, M. S.: Defective lipoprotein receptors and atherosclerosis. Lessons from an animal counterpart of familial hypercholesterolemia. Reprinted by permission of the New England Journal of Medicine, 295:288, 1983.)

transfer cholesterol to VLDL to be taken up by the liver or can deliver cholesterol directly to the liver by being reconverted to HDL_3 by hepatic triglyceride lipase.

The apolipoproteins are attracting increased interest. Apolipoproteins have several important functions, including solubilizing lipids, activating enzymes, and initiating receptor-mediated clearance of lipoproteins (Mahley et al, 1984).

Apoproteins A-I and A-II are the major apoproteins of HDL. They are found almost exclusively with HDL and may have a major part in removing excess cholesterol from the surface of cells. Measurement of apoprotein A-I levels may more accurately predict patients with coronary artery disease than HDL-C levels (Maciejko et al, 1983).

Two major proteins are found in the apoprotein B family. The smaller type, B-48, is the major structural apoprotein of chylomicrons. The larger form, B-100, is the major structural protein of VLDL and LDL. It has a critical role in the interaction of LDL with the LDL receptor. Several reports suggest that measurement of apoprotein B-100 may be useful clinically. It may be elevated in some patients with coronary heart disease and "normal" LDL levels (Sniderman et al, 1980). In addition, patients with hypertriglyceridemia who are at increased risk of developing coronary heart disease may be distinguished from those who are not at increased risk by elevated apoprotein B levels (Sniderman et al, 1982; Vega and Grundy, 1984).

Apoprotein C is found in VLDL and chylomicrons. These apoproteins regulate the activity of lipoprotein lipase. Apoprotein C-II activates lipoprotein lipase. Its absence prevents normal lipolysis and causes hypertriglyceridemia. Apoprotein C-III retards catabolism of VLDL and chylomicrons.

Apolipoprotein E is also present in VLDL and chylomicrons, which are required for normal catabolism of remnants by a specific receptor on the liver that recognizes apoprotein E. There are several isoforms of apoprotein E by electrophoresis. Studies indicate that three genes (E_2, E_3, and E_4) code for the different isoforms (Utermann et al, 1980). One of these types, E_2E_2, is associated with defective catabolism of remnants. Patients with this genotype accumulate VLDL and chylomicron remnants.

Classification of Lipid Disorders

The development of the lipoprotein phenotyping system, originally proposed by Fredrickson and colleagues (1965), emphasized the importance of relating plasma lipid disorders to altered plasma lipoprotein levels. Their classification system was based on the pattern of lipoprotein elevation found in fasting plasma using paper electrophoresis. Lipoprotein electrophoresis separates the various lipoproteins according to their migration in an electric field. By using this technique, HDL migrates the farthest and has alpha mobility. The next type is LDL, which has beta mobility, followed by VLDL, which has prebeta mobility. Chylomicrons do not migrate and remain at the origin. However, classification of patients according to their lipoprotein electrophoretic pattern is no longer considered to be useful because individual lipoprotein phenotypes are not distinct diseases. For example, increased LDL levels (Type IIa hyperlipidemia) may be due to one of several different genetic disorders (e.g., familial hypercholesterolemia, familial combined hyperlipidemia, or polygenic hypercholesterolemia) or secondary to hypothyroidism or nephrotic syndrome.

A genetic classification of hyperlipidemia in patients with coronary heart disease was first proposed by Goldstein and colleagues (1973). They tested 500 consecutive survivors of a myocardial infarction less than 60 years of age for hyperlipidemia; 31% of the survivors were hyperlipidemic. Genetic analysis of the families of the hyperlipidemic survivors indicated that 54% had a monogenic form of familial hyperlipidemia, 31% had either polygenic or sporadic hyperlipidemia, and 15% were unclassified (the families were either too small or unavailable for study). The three monogenic disorders were labeled familial hypercholesterolemia, familial hypertriglyceridemia, and familial combined hyperlipidemia.

Familial hypercholesterolemia is an autosomal dominant disorder characterized by a deficiency of the cell surface LDL receptors (Brown and Goldstein, 1986; Goldstein and Brown, 1983). Heterozygotes for this disorder (1 in 500 persons in the population) have only half of the normal number of LDL receptors, whereas homozygotes (1 in 1 million) have almost no normal LDL receptors. The LDL receptor binds plasma LDL, and this complex forms a critical step in regulating intracellular cholesterol synthesis. Normally, when this complex is internalized, it delivers cholesterol to the cell and inhibits endogenous cholesterol synthesis. When LDL receptors are totally deficient (in the homozygote), intracellular cholesterol production continues unchecked, resulting in plasma cholesterol levels of 800 to 1,000 mg/dl. In afflicted individuals, atherosclerosis usually develops before the age of 20. Heterozygotes have about one-half of the normal number of LDL receptors and usually have plasma cholesterol levels in the 350 to 450 mg/dl range. Clinically, these patients develop tendinous xanthoma, xanthelasma, and arcus cornea and typically have myocardial infarctions in their 30s and 40s.

Familial hypertriglyceridemia, another common autosomal dominant disease, is characterized by elevations of plasma VLDL levels. Fasting plasma triglyceride levels tend to be moderately elevated (250 to 500 mg/dl), and plasma cholesterol levels are often normal. This disorder appears to be genetically heterogeneous, and the underlying defect may be related to either overproduction or an inability to catabolize VLDL triglyceride (Chait et al, 1980; Dunn et al, 1985). The incidence of atherosclerosis is slightly increased in patients with familial hypertriglyceridemia (Goldstein et al, 1973), but this disorder may not be associated with premature atherosclerosis in all families (Brunzell et al, 1976).

Familial combined hyperlipidemia (also called multiple lipoprotein-type hyperlipidemia) is a third common autosomal dominant disorder. It is characterized by alterations in both VLDL and LDL metabolism and may be associated with hypercholesterolemia or hypertriglyceridemia or both (Goldstein et al, 1973). The characteristic feature of this disease is the variation of lipoprotein patterns among affected individuals in the same family and in the same individual at different times. The primary defect appears to be an overproduction of apoprotein B (Brunzell et al, 1983; Chait et al, 1980; Kissebah et al, 1984). Patients usually have a strong family history of premature coronary artery disease, affecting women as well as men.

Familial dysbetalipoproteinemia (formerly Type III hyperlipidemia) is a relatively uncommon but important disorder characterized by increases in plasma VLDL and chylomicron remnants. Clinically, it is associated with tuberous xanthoma and xanthoma of the palmar creases and is characterized by premature atherosclerosis of the coronary arteries, the internal carotids, and the abdominal aorta and its branches (Morganroth et al, 1975). An abnormal apoprotein E (E_2E_2) interferes with the normal metabolism of VLDL and chylomicrons, leading to increased plasma cholesterol and triglyceride levels (Mahley and Angelin, 1984). This diagnosis is suggested by the finding of a broad beta pattern on lipoprotein electrophoresis, indicating the presence of remnants. Confirmation requires specialized laboratory procedures (Brown et al, 1983). This diagnosis should be considered in any patient with peripheral vascular disease and elevations of both plasma cholesterol and triglycerides.

A number of different disorders can cause marked hypertriglyceridemia associated with elevated plasma chylomicrons (Brunzell and Bierman, 1982), which have been termed the *chylomicronemia syndrome* (formerly Type V hyperlipidemia). The hyperchylomicronemia often reflects a combination of a monogenic and secondary cause of hypertriglyceridemia. Patients with familial hypertriglyceridemia or familial combined hyperlipidemia may develop plasma triglyceride levels in excess of 1,000 mg/dl in response to excess alcohol consumption, poorly controlled diabetes mellitus, ingestion of birth control pills or estrogen, or the development of hypothyroidism. However, some individuals in certain families develop severe hypertriglyceridemia in the absence of known exacerbating factors (Greenberg et al, 1977). When plasma chylomicron levels are very high, these patients may develop eruptive xanthoma and pancreatitis.

Most patients with increases in plasma cholesterol or triglyceride levels do not have a monogenic disorder, but rather have a polygenic sporadic or secondary form of hyperlipidemia. Most cases of

hyperlipidemia are due to a combination of various dietary and environmental factors in a genetically predisposed individual. In addition, various *secondary hyperlipidemias* can be identified. The most common form is associated with diabetes mellitus. The increases in VLDL and sometimes chylomicrons are secondary to poorly controlled diabetes and can be corrected with improved diabetic control (Dunn, 1988). Hypothyroidism may cause increased LDL levels. Because the clinical signs and symptoms of hypothyroidism can be subtle, it is often prudent to screen for low plasma thyroxine levels in hypercholesterolemic individuals. Alcohol and estrogens are common secondary causes of hypertriglyceridemia (VLDL and chylomicrons). Glucocorticoids and progestins can result in hypercholesterolemia due to elevated LDL. The nephrotic syndrome may cause elevated LDL levels, whereas uremia is a cause of increased VLDL. Liver disease may cause various alterations, including increased VLDL with hepatitis and hypercholesterolemia with primary biliary cirrhosis and biliary obstruction.

EPIDEMIOLOGY OF ATHEROSCLEROSIS

Hyperlipidemia

During the last 30 years, several large epidemiologic studies have identified the nature of coronary heart disease risk factors and their relative importance (Bottinger and Carlson, 1980; Kannel et al, 1976; Kornitzer et al, 1980; Multiple Risk Factor Intervention Trial [MRFIT] Research Group, 1982; Pooling Project Research Group, 1978; Thelle et al, 1976). Risk factors that can be classified as unmodifiable include increased age, male sex, and family history of coronary heart disease. Modifiable risk factors are appropriate targets for intervention efforts and include hypercholesterolemia, hypertension, cigarette smoking, diabetes mellitus, low HDL-C levels, and severe obesity (Superko et al, 1985).

Hypercholesterolemia. Although the association between hypercholesterolemia and coronary heart disease has been known for more than 20 years, it has only recently been shown that lowering elevated plasma cholesterol levels with diet or drugs can reduce the risk of coronary atherosclerosis. Because almost half of the American population is at increased risk of developing coronary heart disease as a result of elevated cholesterol levels, the detection and treatment of hypercholesterolemia has become a major public health concern.

Various different types of evidence have contributed to the concept of the cholesterol-coronary heart disease connection. Studies of laboratory animals have shown the relationship between high cholesterol levels and the development of atherosclerosis (St. Clair, 1983). Several animal species developed

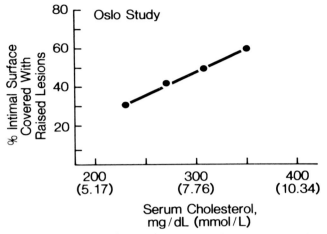

Figure 54–155. Relation of premortem plasma cholesterol level to severity of atherosclerosis at autopsy in Oslo Study (Solberg and Strong, 1983). Atherosclerosis is expressed as percentage of surface of coronary arteries covered with raised atherosclerotic lesion. (From Grundy, S. M.: Cholesterol and coronary heart disease: A new era. J.A.M.A., 256:2849. Copyright 1986, American Medical Association.)

atherosclerosis when fed diets that raise cholesterol levels, and the atherosclerosis can regress when cholesterol is lowered with diet or drugs. In humans, premature atherosclerosis can result from very high cholesterol levels even in the absence of other cardiovascular risk factors (i.e., homozygous familial hypercholesterolemia).

Several large surveys reveal a positive correlation between the level of plasma cholesterol and the risk of coronary artery disease. In a prospective autopsy study (Solberg and Strong, 1983), a positive correlation was found between the premortem plasma cho-

lesterol level and the severity of atherosclerosis (expressed as percentage of surface of coronary arteries covered with raised atherosclerotic lesions) (Fig. 54–155). Prospective studies of individuals within populations, (Goldbourt et al, 1985; Kannel et al, 1971; Pooling Project Research Group, 1978), as well as comparisons between populations (Keys, 1970), have uniformly shown that the plasma cholesterol level is predictive of coronary artery disease. In the Framingham study, for individuals younger than 50 years, cholesterol levels were related directly to overall as well as to cardiovascular mortality (Anderson, 1987).

In one of the largest prospective studies, the MRFIT (Stamler et al, 1986), more than 350,000 men between the ages of 35 and 57 years were monitored for 6 years (Fig. 54–156). A curvilinear relationship between plasma cholesterol and coronary death rate was observed. If a risk ratio of 1 is assigned for a cholesterol level of 200 mg/dl, then at 250 mg/dl the risk is doubled, and at 300 mg/dl it is doubled again. Because most cholesterol in plasma is transported in LDL, it is generally believed that this lipoprotein is primarily responsible for the correlation between the plasma cholesterol level and coronary heart disease (Grundy, 1986a).

HDL Cholesterol. Another important predictor of cardiovascular risk is the HDL level (Castelli et al, 1977; Gordon et al, 1977; Miller and Miller, 1975; Rhoads et al, 1976). The HDL fraction of cholesterol is a relatively small portion of the total plasma cholesterol level, usually about 20 to 25%. This fraction, unlike total cholesterol levels, however, is inversely related to cardiovascular risk. As HDL-C levels decrease, the risk of coronary heart disease increases and as HDL-C levels increase, the risk decreases. In the Framingham study, the average

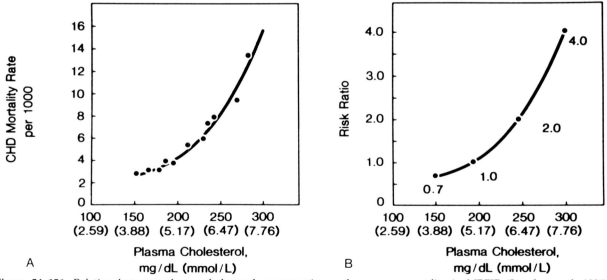

Figure 54–156. Relation between plasma cholesterol concentration and coronary mortality in MRFIT (Stamler et al, 1986). *A*, Coronary mortality for all individuals who were normotensive at screening expressed as yearly rates per 1,000. *B*, Coronary mortality expressed by risk ratios. (From Grundy, S. M.: Cholesterol and coronary heart disease: A new era. J.A.M.A., 256:2849. Copyright 1986, American Medical Association.)

HDL-C level was 45 mg/dl in middle-aged men and 55 mg/dl in middle-aged women. In both sexes, small increases or decreases of HDL-C (±5 to 10 mg/dl) significantly decreased or increased, respectively, the cardiovascular risk. Some epidemiologists have recommended using the ratio of total cholesterol to HDL-C levels to determine relative cardiac risk (Kannel et al, 1979), even though total cholesterol and HDL-C are independent risk factors.

Triglycerides. The relationship between high plasma triglyceride levels and coronary heart disease remains controversial (Carlson and Bottiger, 1981; Hulley et al, 1980). Some patients with hypertriglyceridemia are at increased cardiovascular risk; others are not. Although increases in plasma triglyceride levels often identify high-risk patients, epidemiologic studies have suggested that the increased risk is not necessarily due to the hypertriglyceridemia, but correlates best with other cardiovascular risk factors, such as obesity, low HDL-C levels, associated hypercholesterolemia, or diabetes mellitus. Hypertriglyceridemia may also be a marker of an individual with a genetic form of hyperlipidemia, such as familial combined hyperlipidemia or dysbetalipoproteinemia, which is associated with premature atherosclerosis.

Hypertension

Hypertension is one of the most common cardiovascular disorders in the United States. Epidemiologic studies have shown consistently that it is strongly associated with a greater incidence of cardiovascular and cerebrovascular disease and complications (Keys, 1980; Pooling Project Research Group, 1978). Elevations in both systolic and diastolic blood pressure are powerful predictors of mortality from all causes, from coronary heart disease, and from stroke. Hypertension has also been associated with the development of fibrointimal hyperplasia in saphenous vein grafts after coronary artery bypass (Atkinson et al, 1985). Although antihypertensive drug treatment is clearly effective in preventing cardiovascular complications in moderate and severe hypertension (Veterans Administration Cooperative Study Group on Antihypertensive Agents, 1967), the appropriate management of mild hypertension (diastolic blood pressure of 90 to 94 mm Hg) in otherwise healthy individuals is still controversial (Fries, 1986; Kaplan, 1983). Results of therapeutic trials in patients with mild hypertension are conflicting, and side effects of drug therapy outweigh potentially benefical effects on mortality and cardiovascular complications in some studies (MRFIT Trial, 1982).

Cigarette Smoking

All of the major longitudinal studies that have analyzed the relationship between cigarette smoking and coronary heart disease have found a substantial risk that is dose dependent and independent of the effects of other coronary risk factors (Pooling Project Research Group, 1978). Men who are between the ages of 45 and 60 and who smoke more than one pack of cigarettes daily have three to four times the risk of a major coronary event compared with nonsmokers. The relationship between cigarette smoking and ischemic heart disease is complex; it can be detected within individual populations but is not always apparent in international comparisons (Keys, 1970). It has been proposed that the risk of coronary artery disease in smokers is inter-related with the level of serum cholesterol, which varies widely across populations (Stamler, 1967). The influence of cigarette smoking on the development of coronary artery disease is most prominent in countries in which the mean serum cholesterol level is highest. In women, the risks of myocardial infarction in smokers versus nonsmokers are particulary high and have a consistent dose-response relationship (Rosenberg et al, 1980). The risk is significantly increased when cigarette smoking is combined with oral contraceptive use (Shapiro et al, 1979). Cigarette smoking has also been associated with angiographic progression of atherosclerosis in saphenous vein grafts after coronary artery bypass procedures (Fitzgibbon et al, 1987). Cessation of tobacco use is clearly beneficial in a program for prevention of ischemic heart disease. Persons younger than 65 who continue to smoke have more than twice the risk of coronary events than those who cease smoking (Friedman et al, 1981).

Diabetes Mellitus

Accelerated coronary and peripheral arterial atherosclerosis is one of the most common and serious chronic complications of long-term diabetes (Kannel and McGee, 1984; Krolewski et al, 1987). Although diabetic patients have a high incidence of other cardiovascular risk factors such as hyperlipidemia, hypertension, and obesity, even when these associated risk factors are taken into consideration, diabetic patients still have a two- to three-fold increase in cardiovascular disease compared with nondiabetic persons. The increased risk of atherosclerosis is particularly striking in women. Many factors appear to contribute to the increased risk, including alterations in platelet function, clotting factors, arterial smooth muscle cell metabolism, and possibly blood pressure regulation (Colwell et al, 1981). In addition, changes in plasma lipoprotein metabolism in diabetes are still important in terms of explaining the accelerated atherosclerosis (Dunn, 1988). The risk of coronary artery disease in diabetes appears to be most closely correlated with increases in plasma triglyceride and glucose levels (Donahue et al, 1987; West et al, 1983). Even mild abnormalities of glucose metabolism, such as in impaired glucose tolerance, increase the risk of coronary heart disease (Fuller et al, 1980).

Other Coronary Risk Factors

Other risk factors associated with coronary artery disease include male sex, positive family history of premature coronary artery disease, Type A behavior pattern, and severe obesity. Lack of physical activity has also received attention as a risk factor for ischemic heart disease. Several recent prospective epidemiologic studies suggest that physical fitness and regular physical activity are associated with a reduced risk of heart disease (Brand et al, 1979; Ekelund et al, 1986; Morris et al, 1980; Paffenbarger et al, 1986). Four randomized prospective trials have examined the effects of exercise in patients with heart disease for secondary prevention of cardiac events (Kallio et al, 1979; Rechnitzer et al, 1983; Shaw, 1981; Wilhelmsen et al, 1975). Three of these studies showed trends toward a reduction in coronary deaths, although the results did not achieve statistical significance. However one interprets the evidence, regular exercise has clear beneficial effects in the management of other coronary risk factors, such as hyperlipidemia, hypertension, obesity, and diabetes, and remains an important component of comprehensive strategies for risk factor modification.

The relationship between alcohol consumption and ischemic heart disease continues to be controversial (Fraser, 1986). At moderate to high levels of alcohol consumption, an increase in cardiovascular mortality and sudden death is noted. In addition, these levels of consumption are associated with a definite elevation in blood pressure that may prove detrimental (Klatsky et al, 1977). Evidence that alcohol consumption might be protective against cardiovascular disease is usually found in subjects with low alcohol consumption levels. Although alcohol has been shown to increase HDL levels, the clinical relevance of this observation is not known (Castelli et al, 1977b). At this time, there is little evidence to support advising patients to drink alcohol for prevention of cardiovascular disease.

PROGRESSION OF ATHEROSCLEROSIS

Primary Prevention Studies

Since 1980, a number of studies have clearly showed that it is possible to prevent coronary artery disease by reducing cardiovascular risk factors, particularly elevated plasma cholesterol levels. One of the first, the Oslo Heart Trial, involved both smoking cessation and treatment with a low-cholesterol diet in 1,200 hypercholesterolemic, normotensive middle-aged men. At the end of 5 years, the intervention group reduced their cigarette consumption by 45% and their cholesterol levels by 13%. The incidence of myocardial infarction and sudden death in the intervention group decreased 47%, compared with the control group. Unfortunately, a similarly designed

study in the United States, the MRFIT, was not successful in showing a beneficial effect of cardiac risk factor reduction (MRFIT Research Group, 1982). The MRFIT studied the effect of smoking cessation, low-cholesterol diet modification, and antihypertensive therapy in 12,000 otherwise healthy high-risk men (high cholesterol, hypertensive or cigarette smokers). Part of the reason for the negative result in the MRFIT study was that there was only a 2% difference in mean cholesterol levels between the intervention and the control groups, and antihypertensive drug treatment may have had adverse effects in this study (Oslo Study Research Group, 1983).

Probably the most significant study in terms of showing the benefit of treatment for hypercholesterolemia was the Lipid Research Clinics-Coronary Primary Prevention Study (Lipid Research Clinics Program, 1984). This was a multicenter, randomized, placebo-controlled, double-blind trial testing the efficacy of cholesterol lowering with the bile acid resin cholestyramine in reducing the risk of coronary artery disease in 3,800 otherwise healthy middle-aged men with hypercholesterolemia. The treatment group had an 8.5% greater reduction in total cholesterol and a 12.6% reduction in LDL than the placebo group. After an average of 7.4 years, this difference resulted in a 19% decrease in coronary artery disease death and nonfatal myocardial infarction. Moreover, those participants with a 25% reduction in total cholesterol had a 49% decrease in the incidence of coronary artery disease compared with the control subjects.

In a similarly designed primary prevention study, the Helsinki Heart Study (Frick et al, 1987) used another lipid lowering agent, gemfibrozil. Four thousand middle-aged hypercholesterolemic men entered a randomized, double-blind, placebo-controlled protocol. After 5 years, a 34% reduction in the incidence of fatal and nonfatal myocardial infarction and cardiac death was noted in the gemfibrozil group compared with the placebo group. This improvement was believed to be related to the 8% reduction in total cholesterol and LDL, 35% decrease in triglycerides, and 10% increase in HDL observed in the treatment group compared with the controls.

Secondary Prevention Studies

Another major area of study has been the effect of treatment of hyperlipidemia in patients with pre-existing coronary artery disease. The Coronary Drug Project examined the long-term effects of various lipid-lowering agents in men with previous myocardial infarctions. Three of the five treatment regimens (two estrogen regimens and dextrothyroxine) were discontinued early because of adverse effects, and no benefits were found with clofibrate treatment. Initial reports showed a modest benefit with niacin treatment in decreasing recurrent myocardial infarction but did not decrease total mortality (Coronary Drug Project Research Group, 1975). However, after

15 years of follow-up (9 years after termination of the trial), all-cause mortality in the niacin group was 11% lower than in the placebo group (Canner et al, 1986). This late benefit of niacin was thought to be due to the earlier cholesterol-lowering effect of niacin on nonfatal reinfarction translating into a mortality benefit over subsequent years.

Four investigations have used coronary angiograms to monitor the effect of lipid lowering on progression of coronary atherosclerosis. Nikkila and colleagues (1984) studied the effect of treatment with clofibrate or nicotinic acid in 24 hyperlipidemic subjects with coronary artery disease who had coronary angiography. Repeated coronary angiograms after 7 years of hyperlipidemic treatment showed a correlation between the progression of arterial obstruction and decreased response to lipid lowering. A second study, the Leiden Intervention Trial (Arntzenius et al, 1985), examined the effect of 2 years of a low-cholesterol diet on progression of coronary artery lesions in patients with stable angina pectoris. Also using coronary angiograms, they reported that decreasing total cholesterol/HDL ratios were correlated with less progression of coronary lesion growth.

The third study, the National Heart, Lung, and Blood Institutes Type II Coronary Intervention Study (Brensike et al, 1984; Levy et al, 1984), was a randomized double-blind, placebo-controlled trial in 143 patients with existing coronary artery disease and hypercholesterolemia. The extent of coronary artery disease during 5 years was angiographically compared in patients treated with a low-cholesterol diet and cholestyramine to patients treated with diet and placebo. A significant decrease in progression of coronary artery disease was found in the cholestyramine-treated group compared with the placebo group, and this finding was related to the decrease in LDL and increase in HDL levels.

The most impressive and significant results were reported by the Cholesterol-Lowering Atherosclerosis Study (CLAS) (Blankenhorn et al, 1987). The researchers tested the effect of hyperlipidemic treatment with combined colestipol and niacin in middle-aged men who had had successful coronary bypass procedure. One hundred sixty-two nonsmoking, normotensive men, aged 40 to 59 years, with cholesterol levels between 185 and 350 mg/dl were randomized into drug versus placebo groups and had coronary angiography at baseline and after 2 years. In the drug treatment group, there was a 26% reduction in total cholesterol, a 43% reduction in LDL, and 37% increase in HDL. A significant reduction was noted in the average number of lesions that progressed per subject and the percentage of subjects with new lesions in the native vessels. In the bypass grafts, there was also a reduction in the number of new lesions as well as any adverse change in the bypass grafts in the drug treatment group. Furthermore, 16.2% of the colestipol-niacin treated group showed improvement in their coronary angiograms after 2 years, compared with only 2.4% of the placebo-treated group.

Thus, these studies clearly show the benefit of cardiac risk factor reduction, particularly the benefit of lowering elevated cholesterol levels in high-risk patients. Not only can lowering elevated cholesterol levels help to prevent the development of coronary artery disease, but aggressive treatment of even moderate elevations of plasma cholesterol levels may slow the progression and recurrence of coronary atherosclerosis and in some cases might cause mild regression of pre-existing disease. Because hyperlipidemia is one of the most important predictors of recurrence of atherosclerosis in coronary bypass grafts (Campeau et al, 1984; Lie et al, 1977; Neitzel et al, 1986), these findings of the potential benefit of lipid-lowering treatment are particularly important to thoracic surgeons in designing a postcoronary bypass rehabilitation program.

TREATMENT OF HYPERLIPIDEMIA

Who Should Be Treated

In 1984, the National Institutes of Health (NIH) convened a Consensus Development Conference on Lowering Blood Cholesterol. After reviewing the evidence relating cholesterol levels to coronary heart disease, the panel unanimously concluded that elevated blood cholesterol levels represent a major cause of coronary artery disease and that lowering blood cholesterol levels reduces the risk of coronary atherosclerosis. The panel recommended that moderate-risk adults (cholesterol greater than the 75th percentile for age) be treated with a low-cholesterol diet and that high-risk adults (cholesterol greater than the 90th percentile) be considered for drug treatment if not responsive to a low-cholesterol diet.

In 1985, the National Cholesterol Education Program (NCEP) was initiated by the National Heart, Lung, and Blood Institute to reduce the prevalence of elevated blood cholesterol in patients in the United States. As part of the overall cholesterol education program, in October of 1987, a panel of experts (Adult Treatment Panel) issued a set of guidelines for clinicians to use for treating high blood cholesterol (National Cholesterol Education Program, 1988). The panel developed recommendations for total and LDL cholesterol cutoff points that slightly modified the NIH Consensus Development Conference recommendations.

The NCEP recommended that all adults older than 20 years and children of families with premature atherosclerosis should be tested for their serum cholesterol. This initial blood sample for serum cholesterol screening can be obtained at any time of the day and does not require fasting. Acute illness, myocardial infarction, or operative intervention can lower cholesterol levels, thus these patients should have their serum lipids remeasured 8 to 12 weeks later. The actual levels considered to be elevated is no longer age and sex adjusted. Current recommendations by the NCEP for total serum cholesterol levels are as follows:

Desirable: <200 mg/dl
Borderline high: 200 to 239 mg/dl
High: >240 mg/dl

If serum cholesterol is less than 200 mg/dl, no further evaluation is needed and the patient should be advised to have a repeat serum cholesterol test in 5 years. Patients with a cholesterol greater than 200 mg/dl and coronary heart disease or other cardiovascular risk factors or with cholesterol greater than 240 mg/dl should have a complete assessment of their lipid status (Table 54–38). This assessment requires a fasting sample of blood and measurement of total cholesterol, triglycerides, HDL, and calculated LDL. The NCEP further recommends that decisions about treatment of patients with hypercholesterolemia be based primarily on the LDL levels according to the following categories:

Desirable: <130 mg/dl
Borderline high: 130–159 mg/dl
High: >160 mg/dl

High-risk patients should begin a program of dietary therapy. High-risk patients are defined by the NCEP as those who have an average LDL level greater than 160 mg/dl or who have a level of 130 to 159 mg/dl and high-risk status (Table 54–39). Patients are considered to have a high-risk status if they have definite coronary artery disease or two or more other cardiovascular risk factors: male sex, family history of premature coronary heart disease, cigarette smoking, hypertension, low HDL-C levels (<35 mg/dl), diabetes mellitus, or severe obesity (>30% overweight). Drug therapy should be reserved for patients who, after an adequate trial of dietary therapy, have (1) an LDL level greater than 190 mg/dl or (2) who have coronary artery disease or two or more other cardiovascular risk factors (high-risk status) and a LDL level greater than 160 mg/dl. The goal of therapy is to reduce the LDL level to less than 160 mg/dl, except in patients with high-risk status, when the goal should be less than 130 mg/dl.

These recommendations by the NCEP (Table 54–40) will probably become the standard of care for treatment of hypercholesterolemia in patients with and without coronary artery disease. However, it is important to realize that there is still considerable disagreement about the exact level of plasma total and cholesterol LDL to begin treatment and the goal

TABLE 54–38. LIPOPROTEIN ANALYSIS

12-hour fast
Measure total cholesterol (TC), triglycerides (TG), and HDL-C
Estimate LDL-C = TC − TG/5 − HDL-C
Average of two to three measurements

TABLE 54–39. CRITERIA FOR HIGH-RISK STATUS (NATIONAL CHOLESTEROL EDUCATION PROGRAM)

Definite coronary heart disease
Two or more other cardiovascular risk factors:
  Male sex
  Family history of premature coronary heart disease
  Cigarette smoking
  Hypertension
  HDL-C < 35 mg/dl
  Diabetes mellitus
  Cerebrovascular or peripheral vascular disease
  Severe obesity (≥30% overweight)

of therapy. For instance, the results of the CLAS study suggest that patients with coronary bypass grafts might benefit from more aggressive treatment than that recommended by the NCEP.

Treatment of hypertriglyceridemia and isolated low HDL levels remains controversial. The NIH Consensus Conference on Treatment of Hypertriglyceridemia (1984) recommended that fasting triglyceride levels should not be considered to be elevated unless greater than 250 mg/dl and that these levels should be treated only in patients with associated high cholesterol levels, family history of premature atherosclerosis, or other significant cardiovascular risk factors. However, other physicians have recommended treatment of triglyceride levels if greater than 200 mg/dl, particularly in patients with coronary artery disease (European Atherosclerosis Society Study Group, 1987; Gotto and Farmer, 1988). Although the level of HDL is inversely related to risk of coronary artery disease, there is no direct evidence that raising low HDL levels in patients with otherwise normal plasma lipid levels reduces cardiovascular risk. A strong statistical association has been found between elevated triglyceride and low HDL levels, and treatment of hypertriglyceridemia often increases HDL.

Diet Therapy

Diet modification is the first step in the management of hyperlipidemia. Even when drugs are re-

TABLE 54–40. CLASSIFICATION OF HYPERLIPIDEMIA (NATIONAL CHOLESTEROL EDUCATION PROGRAM)

Total cholesterol	
<200 mg/dl	Desirable
200–239 mg/dl	Borderline high
≥240 mg/dl	High
LDL cholesterol	
<130 mg/dl	Desirable
130–159 mg/dl	Borderline high-risk
≥160 mg/dl	High-risk
Triglycerides	
<250 mg/dl	Normal
250–500 mg/dl	Borderline hypertriglyceridemia
≥500 mg/dl	Definite hypertriglyceridemia

quired, dietary therapy is important to achieve the maximal benefit from drug treatment. In addition, some patients are unusually responsive to dietary changes and may be able to achieve a therapeutic goal with diet alone. The diet currently recommended by the American Heart Association limits cholesterol intake to less than 300 mg/day, total fat calories to less than 30% of daily intake, and saturated fat to less than 10%. This diet is called a Step I AHA Diet. If after 3 months the desired response is not obtained, the diet should be advanced to a Step II diet (cholesterol less than 200 mg/day and saturated fat less than 7% of calories). In obese patients who are also hypertriglyceridemic, it is particularly important to emphasize weight loss and alcohol restriction. It is also useful to refer patients to a registered dietitian for help in adhering to the dietary therapy. Dietary therapy should be used for 6 months before considering the use of drugs.

Three dietary habits typically contribute to elevated lipid levels in the American population: (1) high intake of cholesterol, which suppresses the synthesis of hepatic LDL receptors; (2) high intake of saturated fats, which reduces the activity of LDL receptors; and (3) obesity and excess caloric intake, which cause an overproduction of VLDL by the liver and increased conversion of VLDL to LDL (Grundy, 1986a). Recent studies suggest that except in patients with very severe hyperlipidemia, very low-fat diets are not necessary for an adequate cholesterol-lowering response (Grundy et al, 1986). There is a tendency to allow increased amounts of monounsaturated fats (olive and canola) in cholesterol-lowering diets. This appears to be as effective for lowering LDL-C levels as very low-fat diets but does not raise triglyceride levels or decrease HDL-C levels, which sometimes occurs with the very low-fat diets (Grundy, 1986b). Fish oils have also received considerable attention. They inhibit the synthesis of VLDL triglycerides but do not lower LDL-C levels any more than other unsaturated fats (Nestel et al, 1984; Phillipson et al, 1985). They should not be recommended for the general public until further studies of their long-term effects and toxicity are conducted.

Pharmacologic Treatment

Patients who do not adequately respond to dietary therapy are candidates for drug therapy. Several effective and safe drugs are available for the treatment of hyperlipidemia. However, correct selection of a hypolipidemic agent requires knowledge of the elevated lipoprotein responsible for the hyperlipidemia (Table 54–41). If the major problem is elevated total cholesterol levels, an agent that affects LDL metabolism is used. If triglyceride levels are raised, drugs that affect VLDL metabolism are appropriate.

The drugs of first choice for the treatment of hypercholesterolemia are the two bile acid resins, cholestyramine and colestipol. These agents have

TABLE 54–41. EFFECT OF HYPOLIPIDEMIC DRUGS ON LIPOPROTEINS

Drug	Effect LDL	VLDL	HDL
Bile acid resins Cholestyramine Colestipol	↓	↑	±
Nicotinic acid	↓	↓	↑
Lovastatin	⇓	±	↑
Probucol	↓	±	↓
Fibric acids Clofibrate	±	↓	±
Gemfibrozil	±	↓	↑

been used in long-term clinical trials and have been shown to reduce the risk of coronary heart disease (Lipid Research Clinics Program, 1984). In addition, they appear to be free of serious long-term adverse effects. These anion-exchange resins bind bile acids in the intestine, preventing reabsorption in the terminal ileum. The normal enterohepatic circulation of bile acids is interrupted, thus decreasing the return of bile acids to the liver. As a result, the liver increases conversion of cholesterol into bile acids. Depletion of the hepatic pool of cholesterol results in an increase in LDL receptor activity in the liver, thus stimulating removal of LDL from the plasma and lowering plasma LDL levels (Brown and Goldstein, 1986). These agents may increase hepatic VLDL production and cause hypertriglyceridemia in some patients (Kane et al, 1981). The usual daily dose of cholestyramine is 16 to 24 g, and that of colestipol is 20 to 30 g, given in two divided doses with meals. Some patients may respond to lower doses. The most common side effects are bloating, nausea, and constipation. These agents can also bind and impair absorption of certain medications given concurrently, particularly digitalis, thyroxine, phenobarbital, and warfarin.

Nicotinic acid (niacin) effectively lowers elevated VLDL and LDL levels (Knopp et al, 1985). It inhibits the secretion of VLDL from the liver and thus secondarily lowers LDL levels. It also suppresses the mobilization of free fatty acids from adipose tissue. In some patients with low HDL, it can substantially increase HDL levels. Side effects include cutaneous flushing, worsening of glucose tolerance in diabetes, hyperuricemia, abnormal liver function studies, pruritus, skin rashes, and reactivation of peptic ulcer. The dose required for effective lipid lowering is often 2 to 3 g/day, but the drug should initially be started at a low dosage (100 mg three times a day with meals) and increased gradually as tolerated. The flushing can be mitigated by low doses of aspirin.

A new class of drugs for lowering LDL competitively inhibits the rate-limiting enzyme for cholesterol biosynthesis, HMG-CoA reductase. These drugs increase LDL receptor activity in the liver and the rate of receptor-mediated removal of LDL and VLDL remnants from plasma (Brown and Goldstein, 1986). Lovastatin (formerly mevinolin) has been most extensively studied and was released by the Food and Drug Administration in September of 1987. These agents are very effective and have minimal side effects. Mean reduction in total LDL and cholesterol of 20 to 35% has been reported (Lovastatin Study Group II, 1986), and when it is combined with a bile acid resin, a 50 to 60% reduction in LDL-C has been observed (Grundy et al, 1985; Illingworth, 1984; Vega and Grundy, 1987). The usual dose is 20 mg once a day with the evening meal to 40 mg twice a day. Adverse effects include elevation of hepatic transaminase enzymes, possible increased risk of lens opacitis, and myositis. The long-term safety of these agents is unknown.

Probucol is moderately effective in reducing LDL-C, but it also decreases HDL-C (Atmeh et al, 1983). The mechanism of action of probucol appears to be an increase in LDL catabolism by non-receptor-mediated pathways (Kesaniemi and Grundy, 1984a). Probucol may also inhibit the oxidation and tissue deposition of LDL (Carew et al, 1987; Parthasarathy et al, 1986). The recommended dose is 500 mg twice a day. It is generally well tolerated, although patients occasionally develop nausea or diarrhea. It also causes a mild prolongation of the Q-T interval in some patients and should not be used in patients with ventricular arrhythmias or with an initially prolonged Q-T interval. It is particularly effective when used in combination with other agents, such as bile acid resins (Dujovne et al, 1984).

The two fibric acid derivatives currently available in the United States are clofibrate and gemfibrozil. These agents are most effective in lowering elevated triglyceride (VLDL) levels. Their effect on cholesterol levels varies: In patients with elevated LDL-C, they cause a moderate reduction; but in some patients with low or "normal" LDL-C levels, they may cause an increase in LDL-C levels (Vega and Grundy, 1985). Gemfibrozil also increases HDL-C levels (Saku et al, 1985). Both agents increase lipoprotein lipase activity and promote VLDL clearance. Gemfibrozil also decreases VLDL production (Kesaniemi and Grundy, 1984b). The use of clofibrate has been curtailed because of the finding of adverse long-term effects in a large clinical trial (World Health Organization, 1980). Side effects include abdominal discomfort, myalgias, and increased incidence of gallstones. These agents are very effective in the treatment of patients with accumulation of VLDL remnants. In patients with familial combined hyperlipidemia, the combination of gemfibrozil and a bile acid resin can be very effective.

Surgical treatment of hyperlipidemia is usually reserved for patients with familial hypercholesterolemia who do not respond to medical management. Partial ileal bypass has been used to lower elevated LDL levels in patients with heterozygous familial hypercholesterolemia, but complications include diarrhea, steatorrhea, and decreased intestinal calcium absorption (Foergeman et al, 1982; Thompson and Gotto, 1973). This procedure can be considered in patients in whom drug therapy is not tolerated. In patients with homozygous familial hypercholesterolemia, ileal bypass is ineffective. Portacaval shunt has been successful in some children but is considered experimental (Starzl et al, 1983). One 6-year-old girl was treated with combined heart and liver transplantation (Bilheimer et al, 1984). The heart transplantation was necessary because she had had several previous myocardial infarctions and congestive heart failure. The new liver provided efficient LDL receptors and was able to lower plasma LDL levels to almost normal levels.

PLATELETS AND THROMBOSIS

Complex interactions between the arterial wall and blood platelets, often leading to the formation of thrombi, are now known to be important in the development and progression of ischemic heart disease. The vascular endothelium has an important part in the prevention of thrombosis. The luminal surface of the arterial endothelium forms a protective barrier, providing a nonreactive interface between blood elements such as platelets and the artery wall (Fig. 54–157) (Ross, 1981). Vascular endothelium is thromboresistant through several mechanisms, including production of a heparin-like glycosaminoglycan, synthesis of prostacyclin (Moncada, et al, 1977; Moncada and Vane, 1979), secretion of plasminogen activator, and uptake and clearance of thrombi and vasoactive amines (Gimbrone, 1976). The dynamic interplay between the endothelial barrier, vascular injury, and platelet activation and thrombus formation is an important regulatory mechanism involved in normal vascular function and repair (Schwartz et al, 1981).

In the normal vessel wall, platelet activation is essential to hemostasis, the normal response of the blood to vascular injury (Frishman and Miller, 1986). When a vessel is injured, activated platelets adhere to the exposed endothelial surface (see Fig. 54–157) and release active constituents, including platelet Factor IV, beta-thromboglobulin, and PDGF. There is subsequent platelet aggregation, thrombus formation, and stabilization of the thrombus by the action of thrombin on fibrinogen. In the presence of minor vascular injury, platelet thrombi are transported peripherally as microemboli. Severe vascular injury may result in larger thrombus formation and a significant risk of arterial thromboembolism.

Platelets are involved in atherogenesis by means of platelet aggregation and thrombus formation and by release of growth factors stimulating intimal smooth muscle cell proliferation (Fuster and Chesebro, 1982). Several lines of evidence have confirmed the role of platelets in the initiation and progression of atherosclerotic lesions. In an experimental animal model of atherosclerosis, induction of thrombocytopenia after vascular injury significantly inhibited development of atherosclerotic lesions (Friedman et al,

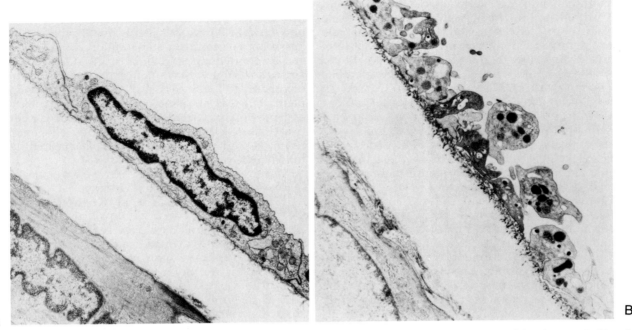

A

B

Figure 54–157. *A,* Normal vascular endothelium provides thromboresistance and a protective permeability barrier. *B,* Vascular injury and endothelial denudation results in platelet adhesion and degranulation. (From Harker, L. A., and Ross, R.: Seminars in Thrombosis and Hemostasis, Vol. 5, No. 3. New York, Thieme Medical Publishers, Inc., 1979. Reprinted by permission.)

1977). Platelet survival time is reduced in patients with atherosclerosis, presumably because of increased platelet aggregation and consumption during atherogenesis (Fuster et al, 1981). Traditional coronary risk factors including diabetes (Sagel et al, 1975), hypertension (Mehta and Mehta, 1981), hypercholesterolemia (Carvalho et al, 1974), and tobacco use (Davis and Davis, 1981) all have been shown to cause increased platelet aggregation.

Coronary artery bypass procedures have been considered to represent an accelerated model of atherogenesis. Platelets have etiologic importance in this pathologic process as well as in progression of disease in native arteries postoperatively. Thrombosis, fibrointimal hyperplasia, and typical advanced atherosclerotic lesions cause saphenous vein graft stenosis and occlusion in a significant number of patients (Grondin, 1986). Mechanical or technical factors that are related to operative technique and that provoke platelet activation and thrombosis are the major causes of graft closure in the early postoperative period (Fuster and Chesebro, 1986). In the late postoperative period, fibrointimal hyperplasia with smooth muscle cell proliferation is thought to be a platelet-dependent process due to release of PDGF (Fig. 54–158) (Atkinson et al, 1985; Neitzel et al, 1986). Platelets probably also have a decisive role in the subsequent development of atherosclerotic lesions within vein grafts as well as in the progression of disease in native coronary arteries. Increased circulating levels of active platelet constituents, such as platelet Factor IV and beta-thromboglobulin, have been found in patients having coronary artery bypass compared with controls who do not have symptomatic ischemic heart disease (Al-Mondhiry et al, 1985). Antiplatelet therapy reduces lipid intake in experimental vein grafts in normolipemic and hyperlipemic monkeys, suggesting an important role for these agents in the prevention of atherosclerosis in human vein bypass grafts (Bonchek et al, 1982). Recent long-term comparative studies of internal mammary artery conduits with saphenous vein grafts have clearly shown higher patency rates for the internal mammary artery graft. Increased production of prostacyclin by the internal mammary artery is thought to contribute to its patency (Subramanian et al, 1986).

PATHOGENESIS OF VEIN GRAFT OCCLUSION

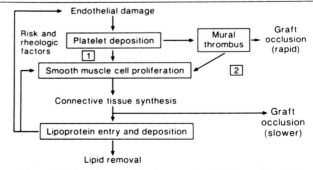

Figure 54–158. Proposed pathogenesis of vein graft occlusion and the role of platelets and platelet constituents. (From Chesebro, J. H., Lam, J. Y. T., and Fuster, V.: The pathogenesis and prevention of aortocoronary vein bypass graft occlusion and restenosis after arterial angioplasty: Role of vascular injury and platelet thrombosis deposition. Reprinted with permission from the American College of Cardiology [Journal of the American College of Cardiology Vol. 8, No. 6, 1986, pp. 57B–66B.])

ANTIPLATELET THERAPY

The role of platelets in thrombosis and atherogenesis has promoted much interest in the identification of drugs that suppress platelet function and that may prove useful in prevention of the complications of atherosclerosis. Drugs that modify platelet behavior may do so through several mechanisms (Fig. 54–159). One of the most important categories of drugs is those that inhibit enzymes of the arachidonate pathway, including aspirin, ibuprofen, indomethacin, naproxen, and sulfinpyrazone. These agents inhibit steps in platelet aggregation that depend on thromboxane A_2 synthesis. Aspirin irreversibly inactivates platelet cyclo-oxygenase by acetylating this enzyme at its active site (Fuster and Chesebro, 1981). Platelets from patients taking aspirin fail to synthesize thromboxane A_2 and show reduced platelet aggregability. One dose of aspirin inhibits cyclo-oxygenase for the lifetime of the platelet, and platelet function is fully restored only after new platelets are released into the circulation. Aspirin also affects the synthesis of prostacyclin by the vessel wall, and this effect is partly responsible for the thromboresistance of vascular endothelium. This inhibition is less prolonged than in platelets, because the endothelial cells are capable of resynthesizing cyclo-oxygenase despite irreversible inactivation of this enzyme (Jaffe and Weksler, 1979). The dose of aspirin required for its antiplatelet effects is quite small, usually 325 mg/day or less (Preston et al, 1981). The amount of aspirin that affects vascular production of prostacyclin is under investigation. It was originally thought that endothelial cells were inhibited only by higher doses of aspirin, but recent studies have suggested that the effects of low-dose aspirin on prostacyclin production in the vascular wall may be more prolonged (Preston et al, 1981). The dose of aspirin recommended for prevention of thromboembolic complications of atherosclerosis varies depending on the clinical manifestation of disease, ranging from 325 mg every other day for primary prevention of acute myocardial infarction to as much as 1.3 to 1.5 g/day for prevention of transient ischemic attacks and stroke.

Sulfinpyrazone is a competitive inhibitor of cyclo-oxygenase with reversible effects on platelet function (Ali and McDonald, 1978). It has been shown to prolong platelet survival time but does not affect platelet aggregation nor prolong bleeding time. The usual daily dose is 800 mg/day given at frequent intervals.

Dipyridamole is an inhibitor of platelet phosphodiesterase, causing decreased breakdown of cyclic adenosine monophosphate (cAMP). The resultant elevation of cyclic cAMP in platelets decreases adherence to sites of vascular injury, inhibits platelet aggregation, and reduces release of granule contents into the vessel wall (Fitzgerald, 1987). It has been proposed that dipyridamole has potentially synergistic antithrombotic properties when given with aspirin because it interferes with different aspects of platelet function. However, in many clinical situations it is unclear that the addition of dipyridamole to aspirin therapy provides any additional benefit in prevention of thromboembolic events. Usually, 200 to 300 mg/day of dipyridamole is given in three to four divided doses.

Several clinical studies have assessed the value of antiplatelet therapy in the prevention of cardiovascular disease and the prevention of thromboembolic complications (Fuster et al, 1987). Although most clinical studies examining the role of aspirin therapy for the primary prevention of ischemic heart disease have been inconclusive, the preliminary results of the Physicians' Health Study were published when the board monitoring the data determined that there was a definite beneficial effect in the treatment group (Physicians' Health Study Research Group, 1988). This double-blind controlled trial of aspirin for the primary prevention of cardiovascular disease showed a significant 23% reduction in nonfatal myocardial infarctions, nonfatal strokes, and all-cause vascular deaths when aspirin (325 mg/day) was given every other day with an average follow-up of 4.8 years. A more critical review of the design, conduct,

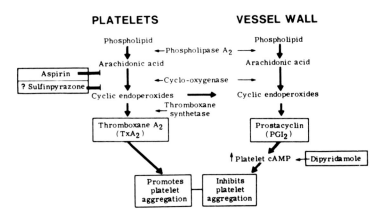

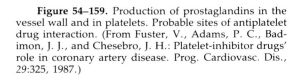

Figure 54–159. Production of prostaglandins in the vessel wall and in platelets. Probable sites of antiplatelet drug interaction. (From Fuster, V., Adams, P. C., Badimon, J. J., and Chesebro, J. H.: Platelet-inhibitor drugs' role in coronary artery disease. Prog. Cardiovasc. Dis., 29:325, 1987.)

and analysis of this study is in progress, but the findings suggest that aspirin therapy may be useful in carefully selected patients for the prophylaxis of cardiovascular events.

At least ten drug trials have been conducted to assess the value of antiplatelet agents for secondary prevention of myocardial infarction and coronary mortality. Six large prospective, randomized, double-blind, placebo-controlled clinical trials have evaluated the role of aspirin therapy in secondary prevention after myocardial infarction (Aspirin Myocardial Infarction Study Research Group, 1980; Breddin et al, 1979; Coronary Drug Project Research Group, 1976; Elwood et al, 1974; Elwood and Sweetnam, 1979; Persantine-Aspirin Reinfarction Study Group, 1980). Each trial demonstrated a trend toward reduced all-cause mortality in the treated patients, although these differences were not statistically significant. The trials differed in the dose of aspirin used, the number of patients enrolled, the enrollment of female patients, duration of patient follow-up, and time from myocardial infarction before initiation of therapy. Statistical methods for pooling of data suggest an approximate 16% reduction in cardiovascular mortality with aspirin therapy and a 21% reduction in recurrent infarction (Peto, 1980). However, the practice of pooling data from clinical trials in this fashion has been the subject of criticism (Goldman and Feinstein, 1979). In October of 1985, the Food and Drug Administration approved the use of one aspirin tablet (325 mg) daily for prevention of reinfarction or death in survivors of acute myocardial infarction, based on its detailed review of the evidence.

The significant incidence of early postoperative thrombotic occlusion of saphenous vein grafts and the subsequent platelet-mediated intimal smooth muscle cell proliferation provide clear rationale for antiplatelet therapy in improving graft patency after coronary artery bypass. After initial contradictory results, more recent studies have shown the effectiveness of antiplatelet therapy in the prevention of bypass graft occlusion. In the evaluation of data available, certain technical and clinical variables known to affect graft patency must be taken into account. Technical factors such as endothelial damage during harvesting of the vein graft, low flow in the vein graft, small lumen size of the grafted coronary artery, and associated endarterectomy have been shown to result in reduced graft patency rates (Chesebro et al, 1982). Clinical variables such as tobacco use, hyperlipidemia, hypertension, and diabetes have an important role in long-term occlusion of saphenous vein grafts (Campeau et al, 1984; Fuster and Chesbro, 1986). No fewer than ten trials of antiplatelet therapy after coronary artery bypass procedures have been conducted. All of the clinical trials showing a benefit of antiplatelet therapy in reduction of graft occlusion started drug administration before or on the second postoperative day (Baur et al, 1982; Chesebro et al, 1982; Chesebro et al, 1984; Chevigne et al, 1984; Limet et al, 1987; Lorenz et al, 1984;

Mayer et al, 1981; Pirk et al, 1986). None of the trials initiating therapy more than 3 days postoperatively showed any beneficial effects (McEnany et al, 1982; Pantely et al, 1979; Sharma et al, 1983). The positive effect on graft patency appears to persist for at least 1 year (Chesebro et al, 1986). The evaluation of long-term effects of therapy after 1 year must include the presence of risk factors predisposing to progression of atherosclerosis. Therapy with dipyridamole started 2 days before operation (100 mg four times a day) and given on the morning of operation and 1 hour after the procedure (100 mg), then continued at a lower dose (75 mg three times a day), plus aspirin (325 mg three times a day) added 7 hours postoperatively has been found to be extremely effective in improving both early vein graft patency and patency rates at 1 year. It is currently recommended that antithrombotic therapy be started before or as soon as possible postoperatively, because platelet aggregation and the genesis of thrombi within grafts can begin during or within hours of operation. The relative importance of the combination of both aspirin and dipyridamole compared with either drug alone remains to be determined by larger clinical trials (Fitzgerald, 1987).

REHABILITATION OF THE CORONARY PATIENT

The accumulating evidence that the progression of atherosclerosis can be retarded makes a comprehensive strategy for risk factor modification essential in the care of patients with coronary artery disease. An ideal setting for such a comprehensive approach to high-risk patients is the cardiac rehabilitation program (Wenger, 1986). Important components of a comprehensive rehabilitation program include nutritional and dietary consultation for control of obesity, hyperlipidemia, and diabetes; psychological consultation for behavior modification, stress management, evaluation of depression, and other emotional consequences of cardiovascular disease; consultation for smoking cessation; medical management as indicated for control of hypertension, diabetes, hyperlipidemia, and other potential risk factors such as ventricular dysfunction and cardiac arrhythmias; and educational and vocational counseling for patients and their families.

Individually prescribed physical activity is also an important component of the rehabilitative approach. Medically supervised exercise is ideally recommended for most patients, because long-term compliance, motivation, and patient reassurance are often improved in such a setting. However, in appropriate patients similar benefits can be achieved in home-based exercise programs (DeBusk et al, 1985; Hands et al, 1987; Stevens and Hanson, 1984). The exercise prescription for each patient includes the frequency, intensity, duration, and type of exercise to be done (American College of Sports Medicine,

1986). The frequency of aerobic exercise recommended to achieve the desired training effect is generally three to five sessions a week, each lasting 30 to 60 minutes with appropriate warm-up and cool-down periods. The intensity of prescribed exercise is based on standard exercise treadmill testing for the safest and most effective results. The aerobic phase of exercise should approximate 60 to 80% of the highest safely achieved heart rate during testing. Lower levels of exercise have also been shown to result in a training effect, particularly in debilitated, physically unfit, or elderly individuals.

Increases in functional capacity (Ehsani et al, 1981; Froelicher et al, 1984; Hands et al, 1987; Stevens and Hanson, 1984), improvement in symptoms due to an increase in the threshold for angina (Redwood et al, 1972), and a subjective improvement in quality of life (Goff and Dimsdale, 1985; Tomporowski and Ellis, 1986) are the major beneficial effects of a regular exercise program in patients with coronary artery disease. Beneficial effects on plasma lipids include reduction in triglycerides and elevation of HDL (Hartung et al, 1981; Haskell et al, 1980; Heath et al, 1983). Regular aerobic exercise has also been shown to lower blood pressure and may be a potentially nonpharmacologic method for control of blood pressure in carefully selected patients (Jennings et al, 1986). Most studies have found no significant changes in left ventricular function or myocardial perfusion as a result of training programs (Cobb et al, 1982; Hands et al, 1987). Rehabilitative physical activity has been safe and feasible for most cardiac patients with angina pectoris (Thompson, 1985), after myocardial infarction (DeBusk et al, 1985; Sennet et al, 1984), and after percutaneous transluminal angioplasty and coronary revascularization (Sennett et al, 1984; Stevens and Hanson, 1984), as well as in patients with left ventricular dysfunction (Conn et al, 1982).

Changes in the care of patients with coronary artery disease in recent years reflect the substantial evidence that the development and progression of atherosclerotic cardiovascular disease can be modified by intensive dietary, pharmacologic, and lifestyle interventions. The incorporation of prevention and rehabilitation into standard medical care will potentially restrict the morbidity and mortality associated with atherosclerotic cardiovascular disease and reduce the economic consequences of long-term care of cardiac patients.

Selected Bibliography

Blankenhorn, D. H., Nessim, S. A., Johnson, R. L., et al: Beneficial effects of combined colestipol-niacin therapy on coronary atherosclerosis and coronary venous bypass graft. J.A.M.A., 257:3233, 1987.

This study shows the effect of aggressive lowering of cholesterol with diet and drugs on coronary bypass grafts. After only 2 years of treatment, there was a significant improvement in the coronary angiograms of the bypass grafts and native vessels in the group treated with cholesterol-lowering drugs compared with the group treated with only a cholesterol-lowering diet.

Brown, M. S., and Goldstein, J. L.: A receptor-mediated pathway for cholesterol homeostasis. Science, 231:34, 1986.

This article is adapted from the lecture delivered by Drs. Brown and Goldstein when they received the Nobel Prize in Physiology and Medicine. It describes their attempts to understand the disease familial hypercholesterolemia and how it eventually led them to a better understanding of cellular cholesterol regulation and to the discovery of LDL receptor. The authors also explain how pharmacologic manipulation of the LDL receptor can reduce the risk of atherosclerosis.

Fraser, G. E.: Preventive Cardiology. New York, Oxford University Press, 1986.

This text provides a comprehensive review of cardiovascular epidemiology and a detailed survey of risk factors for coronary heart disease. Intervention strategies for prevention of cardiovascular disease and rehabilitative programs for long-term management are evaluated. This book contains a thorough review of the medical literature in the field of preventive cardiology.

Fuster, V., Adams, P. C., Badimon, J. J., and Chesebro, J. H.: Platelet-inhibitor drugs' role in coronary artery disease. Prog. Cardiovasc. Dis., 24:325, 1987.

The role of platelets and antiplatelet therapy in three coronary artery disease processes is described: coronary artery disease, aortocoronary vein graft disease, and restenosis after coronary angioplasty. The current understanding of the pharmacology of platelet inhibitor drugs and their mechanisms of action in the prevention of atherogenesis and thrombosis formation is reviewed.

Grundy, S. M.: Cholesterol and coronary heart disease: A new era. J.A.M.A., 256:2849, 1986.

This article is an excellent review of the relationship between cholesterol and coronary heart disease. It has a particularly informative section on the reasons for current dietary recommendations. Much of the material reviewed in this article was the basis for the recommendation by the National Cholesterol Education Program.

Report of the National Cholesterol Education Program Expert Panel on detection, evaluation and treatment of high blood cholesterol in adults. Arch. Intern. Med., 148:36, 1988.

This is the report of the Adult Treatment Panel of the National Cholesterol Education Program. It provides the new guidelines for the treatment of hypercholesterolemia in adults. The reason for their recommendations is presented and also a detailed discussion of their new classification system. In addition, specific recommendations are made with regard to the use of diet and drugs for the treatment of hypercholesterolemia.

Ross, R.: The pathogenesis of atherosclerosis—an update. N. Engl. J. Med., 314:488, 1986.

This review of our current understanding of the pathogenesis of atherosclerosis is presented by one of the major investigators in the field. It has a particularly informative section on the role of platelets and PDGF in atherosclerosis. The author also discusses his revised response-to-injury hypothesis.

Schaefer, E. J., and Levy, R. I.: Pathogenesis and management of lipoprotein disorders. N. Engl. J. Med., 312:1300, 1985.

This article is a comprehensive review of our current understanding of normal and abnormal lipoprotein metabolism. The authors present an approach to patients with lipid disorders based on our understanding of abnormal lipoprotein metabolism.

Stamler, J.: The marked decline in coronary heart disease mortality rates in the United States, 1968–1981: Summary of findings and possible explanations. Cardiology, 72:11, 1985.

The decline in coronary heart disease mortality and the relation to risk factor modification and developments in medical and surgical care are discussed. Data are presented to support an aggressive approach to coronary risk reduction both in community-based efforts as well as in the care of individuals at risk for atherosclerosis.

Superko, H. R., Wood, P. F., and Haskell, W. L.: Coronary heart disease and risk factor modification: Is there a threshold? Am. J. Med., 78:826, 1985.

This article is an excellent review of our current understanding of coronary heart disease risk factors and how modification may have an important part in the control and alteration of the atherosclerotic process. A comprehensive review of epidemiologic and arteriographic studies is presented and also a discussion of the issue of threshold levels of modification that may be required before some benefit is obtained.

Bibliography

Ali, M., and McDonald, J. W. D.: Reversible and irreversible inhibition of platelet cyclooxygenase and serotonin release by nonsteroidal anti-inflammatory drugs. Thromb. Res., 13:1057, 1978.

Al-Mondhiry, H., Pierce, W. S., and Pennack, J. L.: Platelet release in coronary heart disease: Effect of antiplatelet drugs and coronary artery bypass graft. J. Lab. Clin. Med., 105:397, 1985.

American College of Sports Medicine: Principles of exercise prescription. In Blair, S. N., Gibbons, L. W., Painter, P., et al: Guidelines for Exercise Testing and Prescription. Philadelphia, Lea & Febiger, 1986.

Anderson, K. M., Castelli, W. P., and Levy, D.: Cholesterol and mortality: 30 years of follow-up from the Framingham study. J.A.M.A., 257:2176, 1987.

Arntzenius, A. C., Kromhout, D., Barth, J. D., et al: Diet, lipoprotein, and the progression of coronary atherosclerosis. The Leiden Intervention Trial. N. Engl. J. Med., 312:805, 1985.

Aspirin Myocardial Infarction Study Research Group: A randomized controlled trial of aspirin in persons recovered from myocardial infarction. J.A.M.A., 243:661, 1980.

Atkinson, J. B., Forman, M. B., Vaughn, W. K., et al: Morphologic changes in long-term saphenous vein bypass grafts. Chest, 88:341, 1985.

Atmeh, R. H., Stewart, J. M., Boag, D., et al: Hypolipidemic action probucol: A study of its effects on high and low density lipoproteins. J. Lipid Res., 24:588, 1983.

Barrett, T. B., and Benditt, E. P.: Sis (platelet-derived growth factor B-chain) gene transcript levels are elevated in human atherosclerotic lesions compared to normal artery. Proc. Natl. Acad. Sci. U.S.A., 84:1099, 1987.

Baur, H. R., Van Tassel, R. A., Pierach, C. A., and Gobel, F. L.: Effects of sulfinpyrazone on early graft closure after myocardial revascularization. Am. J. Cardiol., 49:420, 1982.

Beaglehole, R.: Medical management and the decline in mortality from coronary heart disease. Br. Med. J., 292:33, 1986.

Benditt, E. P.: Implications of the monoclonal character of human atherosclerotic plaques. Am. J. Pathol., 86:693, 1977.

Benditt, E. P., and Benditt, J. M.: Evidence for a monoclonal origin of human atherosclerotic plaques. Proc. Natl. Acad. Sci. U.S.A., 70:1753, 1973.

Bilheimer, D. W., Goldstein, J. L., Grundy, S. C., et al: Liver transplantation provides low density lipoprotein receptors and lowers plasma cholesterol in a child with homozygous familial hypercholesterolemia. N. Engl. J. Med., 311:1658, 1984.

Blankenhorn, D. H.: Will atheroma regress with diet and exercise? Am. J. Surg., 141:644, 1981.

Blankenhorn, D. H., and Brooks, S. H.: Angiographic trials of lipid-lowering therapy. Arteriosclerosis, 1:242, 1981.

Blankenhorn, D. H., Nessim, S. A., Johnson, R. L., et al: Beneficial effects of combined colestipol-niacin therapy on coronary atherosclerosis and coronary venous bypass grafts. J.A.M.A., 257:3233, 1987.

Bonchek, L. I., Boerboom, L. E., Olinger, G. N., et al: Prevention of lipid accumulation in experimental vein bypass grafts by antiplatelet therapy. Circulation, 66:338, 1982.

Bottinger, L. E., and Carlson, L. A.: Risk factors for ischaemic vascular death in men in the Stockholm Prospective Study. Atherosclerosis, 36:389, 1980.

Brand, R. T., Paffenbarger, R. S., Sholtz, R. I., et al: Work activity and fatal heart attack studied by multiple logistic risk analysis. Am. J. Epidemiol., 110:52, 1979.

Breddin, K., Loew, D., Lechner, K., et al: Secondary prevention of myocardial infarction: Comparison of acetylsalicylic acid, phenprocoumon and placebo. A multicenter two-year prospective study. Thromb. Haemost., 40:225, 1979.

Brensike, J. F., Levy, R. I., Kelse, S. F., et al: Effects of therapy with cholestyramine on progression of coronary arteriosclerosis: Results of the NHLBI Type II Coronary Intervention Study. Circulation, 69:313, 1984.

Brown, M. S., and Goldstein, J. L.: A receptor-mediated pathway for cholesterol homeostasis. Science, 232:34, 1986.

Brown, M. S., Goldstein, J. L., and Fredrickson, D. S.: Familial type 3 hyperlipoproteinemia (dysbetalipoproteinemia). In Stanbury, J. B., Wyngaarden, J. B., Fredrickson, D. S., et al (eds): The Metabolic Basis of Inherited Disease, 5th ed. New York, McGraw-Hill Book Co., 1983.

Brunzell, J. D., Albers, J. J., Chait, A., et al: Plasma lipoproteins in familial combined hyperlipidemia and monogenic familial hypertriglyceridemia. J. Lipid Res., 24:147, 1983.

Brunzell, J. D., and Bierman, E. L.: Chylomicronemia syndrome: Interaction of genetic and acquired hypertriglyceridemia. Med. Clin. North Am., 66:455, 1982.

Brunzell, J. D., Schrott, H. H., Motulsky, A. G., and Bierman, E. L.: Myocardial infarction in the familial forms of hypertriglyceridemia. Metabolism, 25:313, 1976.

Campeau, L., Enjalbert, M., Lesperance, J., et al: The relation of risk factors to the development of atherosclerosis in saphenous-vein bypass grafts and the progression of disease in the native circulation. N. Engl. J. Med., 311:1329, 1984.

Canner, P. L., Berge, K. G., Wenger, N. K., et al: Fifteen year mortality in Coronary Drug Project patients: Long-term benefit with niacin. J. Am. Coll. Cardiol., 8:1245, 1986.

Carew, T. E., Schwenke, D. C., and Steinberg, D.: Antiatherogenic effect of probucol unrelated to its hypocholesterolemic effect: Evidence that antioxidants in vivo can selectively inhibit low density lipoprotein degradation in macrophage-rich fatty streaks and slow the progression of atherosclerosis in the Watanabe heritable hyperlipidemic rabbit. Proc. Natl. Acad. Sci. U.S.A., 84:7725, 1987.

Carlson, L. A., and Bottiger, L. E.: Serum triglycerides, to be or not to be a risk factor for ischaemic heart disease? Atherosclerosis, 39:287, 1981.

Carvalho, A. C. A., Coleman, R. W., and Lees, R. L.: Clofibrate reversal of platelet hypersensitivity in hyperbetalipoproteinemia. Circulation, 50:570, 1974.

Castelli, W. P., Doyle, J. T., Gordon, T., et al: HDL cholesterol and other lipids in coronary heart disease: The Cooperative Lipoprotein Phenotyping Study. Circulation, 55:767, 1977a.

Castelli, W. P., Gordon, T., Hjorsland, M. C., et al: Alcohol and blood lipids. Lancet, 2:153, 1977b.

Chait, A., Albers, J. J., and Brunzell, J. D.: Very low density lipoprotein overproduction in genetic forms of hypertriglyceridemia. Eur. J. Clin. Invest., 10:17, 1980.

Chesebro, J. H., Clements, I. P., Fuster, V., et al: A platelet-inhibitor-drug trial in coronary-artery bypass operations: Benefits of perioperative dipyridamole and aspirin therapy on early post-operative vein-graft patency. N. Engl. J. Med., 307:73, 1982.

Chesebro, J. H., Fuster, V., Elveback, L. R., et al: Effect of dipyridamole and aspirin on late vein-graft patency after coronary bypass operations. N. Engl. J. Med., 310:209, 1984.

Chesebro, J. H., Lam, J. Y. T., and Fuster, V.: The pathogensis and prevention of aortocoronary vein bypass graft occlusion and restenosis after arterial angioplasty: Role of vascular injury and platelet thrombus deposition. J. Am. Coll. Cardiol., 8:57B, 1986.

Chevigne, M., David, J. L., Rigo, P., and Limet, R.: Effect of ticlopidine on saphenous vein bypass patency rates: A double blind study. Ann. Thorac. Surg., 37:371, 1984.

Cobb, F. R., Williams, R. S., McEwan, P., et al: Effects of exercise training on ventricular function in patients with recent myocardial function. Circulation, 66:100, 1982.

Colwell, J. A., Lopes-Virella, M., and Halushka, P. V.: Pathogenesis of atherosclerosis in diabetes mellitus. Diabetes Care, 4:121, 1981.

Conn, E. H., Williams, R. S., and Wallace, A. G.: Exercise responses before and after physical conditioning in patients with severely depressed left ventricular function. Am. J. Cardiol., 49:296, 1982.

Coronary Drug Project Research Group: Aspirin in coronary heart disease. J. Chron. Dis., 29:625, 1976.

Coronary Drug Project Research Group: Clofibrate and niacin in coronary heart disease. J.A.M.A., 231:360, 1975.

Davis, J. W., and Davis, R. F.: Prevention of cigarette smoking-induced platelet aggregate formation by aspirin. Arch. Intern. Med., 73:227, 1981.

Dayton, S., and Hashimoto, S.: Origin of cholesteryl oleate and other esterified lipids of rabbit atheroma. Atherosclerosis, 12:371, 1970.

DeBusk, R. F., Haskell, W. L., Miller, N. H., et al: Medically directed at-home rehabilitation soon after clinically uncomplicated acute myocardial infarction: A new model for patient care. Am. J. Cardiol., 55:251, 1985.

Dujovne, C. A., Krehbiel, P., Decoursey, S., et al: Probucol with colestipol in the treatment of hypercholesterolemia. Ann. Intern. Med., 100:477, 1984.

Donahue, R. P., Abbott, R. D., Reed, D. M., and Yano, K.: Postchallenge glucose concentration and coronary heart disease in men of Japanese ancestry: Honolulu Heart Program. Diabetes, 36:689, 1987.

Dunn, F. L.: Treatment of lipid disorders in diabetes mellitus. Med. Clin. North Am., 72:1379, 1988.

Dunn, F. L., Grundy, S. M., Bilheimer, D. W., et al: Impaired catabolism of very low-density lipoprotein-triglyceride in a family with primary hypertriglyceridemia. Metabolism, 34:316, 1985.

Ehsani, A. A., Heath, G. W., Hagberg, J. M., et al: Effects of 12 months of intense exercise training on ischemic ST-segment depression in patients with coronary artery disease. Circulation, 64:1116, 1981.

Ekelund, L. G., Haskell, W. H., Johnson, J. L., et al: Physical fitness as predictor of cardiovascular mortality in asymptomatic men: The Lipid Research Clinic Prevalence Follow-Up Study (Abstract). Circulation, 74(Suppl. II):397, 1986.

Elwood, P. C., Cochrane, A. L., Burr, M. L., et al: A randomized controlled trial of acetylsalicylic acid in the secondary prevention of mortality from myocardial infarction. Br. Med. J., 1:436, 1974.

Elwood, P. C., and Sweetnam, P. M.: Aspirin and secondary mortality after myocardial infarction. Lancet, 2:1313, 1979.

European Atherosclerosis Society Study Group: Strategies for the prevention of coronary heart disease: A policy statement of the European Atherosclerosis Society. Eur. Heart. J., 8:77, 1987.

Fiell, M. L., and Spaet, T. H.: The effect of thrombocytopenia on experimental atherosclerotic lesion formation in rabbits. J. Clin. Invest., 60:1191, 1977.

Fitzgerald, G. A.: Dipyridamole. N. Engl. J. Med., 316:1247, 1987.

Fitzgibbon, G. M., Hamilton, M. G., Leach, A. J., et al: Coronary artery disease and coronary bypass grafting in young men: Experience with 138 subjects 39 years of age and younger. J. Am. Coll. Cardiol., 9:977, 1987.

Foergeman, O., Meinertz, H., Hylander, E., et al: Effects and side-effects of partial ileal bypass surgery for familial hyper-cholesterolemia. Gut, 23:558, 1982.

Frantz, I. D., Jr., and Moore, R. B.: The sterol hypothesis in atherogenesis. Am. J. Med., 46:684, 1969.

Fraser, G. E.: Preventive Cardiology. New York, Oxford University Press, 1986.

Fredrickson, D. S., Levy, R. I., and Lees, R. S.: Fat transport in lipoproteins—an integrated approach to mechanisms and disorders. N. Engl. J. Med., 276:32, 94, 148, 215, 273, 1967.

Frick, M. H., Elo, O., Haapa, K., et al: Helsinki Heart Study: Primary-prevention trial with gemfibrozil in middle-aged men with dyslipidemia. N. Engl. J. Med., 317:1237, 1987.

Friedman, G. D., Petitti, D. B., Bawol, R. D., and Siegelaub, A. B.: Mortality in cigarette smokers and quitters. N. Engl. J. Med., 304:1407, 1981.

Friedman, R. J., Stemerman, M. B., Wenz, B. I., et al: The effect of thrombocytopenia on experimental atherosclerotic lesion formation on rabbits. J. Clin. Invest., 60:1191, 1977.

Fries, E. D.: Borderline mild systemic hypertension: Should it be treated? Am. J. Cardiol., 58:642, 1986.

Frishman, W. H., and Miller, K. P.: Platelets and antiplatelet therapy in ischemic heart disease. In O'Rourke, R. A. (ed): Current Problems in Cardiology. Chicago, Year Book Medical Publishers, 1986.

Froelicher, V., Jensen, D., Genter, F., et al: A randomized trial of exercise training in patients with coronary heart disease. J.A.M.A., 252:1291, 1984.

Frosser, C., Pollock, M. L., Anholon, J. D., et al: Work capacity and left ventricular function during rehabilitation after myocardial revascularization surgery. Circulation, 69:748, 1984.

Fuller, J. H., Shipley, M. J., Rose, G., Jarrett, R. J., and Keen, H.: Coronary-heart-disease risk and impaired glucose tolerance: The Whitehall Study. Lancet, 1:1373, 1980.

Fuster, V., Adams, P. C., Badimon, J. J., and Chesebro, J. H.: Platelet-inhibitor drugs role in coronary artery disease. Prog. Cardiovasc. Dis., 29:325, 1987.

Fuster, V., and Chesebro, J. H.: Antithrombotics therapy: Role of platelet inhibitor drugs. II: Pharmacologic effects of platelet inhibitor drugs. Mayo Clin. Proc., 56:185, 1981.

Fuster, V., and Chesebro, J. H.: Pathogenesis of atherosclerosis: The role of platelets and thrombosis. In Kowan, H. C., and Bowie, E. J. W. (eds): Thrombosis. Philadelphia, W. B. Saunders Company, 1982.

Fuster, V., and Chesebro, J. H.: Role of platelets and platelet inhibitors in aortocoronary artery vein-graft disease. Circulation, 73:227, 1986.

Fuster, V., Chesebro, J. H., Frye, R. L., and Elveback, L. R.: Platelet survival and the development of coronary artery disease in the young: The effects of a cigarette smoking, strong family history, and medical history. Circulation, 63:546, 1981.

Geer, J. C., McGill, H. C., Jr., and Strong, J. P.: The fine structure of human atherosclerotic lesions. Am. J. Pathol., 38:263, 1961.

Gillum, R. F., Folson, A., Luepker, R. V., et al: Sudden death and acute myocardial infarction in a metropolitan area, 1970–1980: The Minnesota Heart Survey. N. Engl. J. Med., 309:1353, 1983.

Gimbrone, M. A., Jr.: Culture of vascular endothelium. In Spaet, T. H. (ed): Progress in Hemostasis and Thrombosis. New York, Grune & Stratton, 1976.

Glagov, S., and Ozoa, A.: Significance of the relatively low incidence of atherosclerosis in the pulmonary, renal and mesenteric arteries. Ann. N.Y. Acad. Sci., 149:940, 1968.

Glueck, C. J.: Role of risk factor management in progression and regression of coronary and femoral artery atherosclerosis. Am. J. Cardiol., 57:356, 1986.

Goff, D., and Dimsdale, J. E.: The psychological effects of exercise. J. Cardiopulmonary Rehabil., 5:234, 1985.

Goldbourt, V., Holtzman, E., and Neufeld, H. N.: Total and high density lipoprotein cholesterol in the serum and risk of mortality: Evidence of a threshold effect. Br. Med. J., 290:1239, 1985.

Goldman, L., and Cook, F. C.: The decline in ischemic heart disease mortality rates: An analysis of the comparative effects of medical interventions and changes in lifestyle. Ann. Intern. Med., 101:825, 1984.

Goldman, L., and Feinstein, A. R.: Anticoagulants and myocardial infarction: The problems of pooling, drowning and floating. Ann. Intern. Med., 90:92, 1979.

Goldstein, J. L., and Brown, M. S.: Familial hypercholesterolemia. *In* Stanbury, J. B., Wyngarden, J. B., Fredrickson, D. S., et al (eds): The Metabolic Basis of Inherited Disease, 5th ed. New York, McGraw-Hill Book Co., 1983, p. 672.

Goldstein, J. L., Hazzard, W. R., Schrott, H. G., et al: Hyperlipidemia in coronary heart disease. J. Clin. Invest., 52:1533, 1973.

Goldstein, J. L., Kita, T., and Brown, M. S.: Defective lipoprotein receptors and atherosclerosis: Lessons from an animal counterpart of familial hypercholesterolemia. N. Engl. J. Med., 309:288, 1983.

Gordon, T., Castelli, W. P., Hjortlan, M. C., et al: High density lipoprotein as a protective factor against coronary heart disease: The Framingham Study. Am. J. Med., 62:707, 1977.

Gotto, A. M., and Farmer, J. A.: Risk factors for coronary artery disease. *In* Braunwald, E. (ed): Heart Disease: A Textbook of Cardiovascular Medicine, 3rd ed. Philadelphia, W. B. Saunders Company, 1988, p. 1155.

Greenberg, B. H., Blackwelder, W. C., and Levy, R. I.: Primary type V hyperlipoproteinemia: A descriptive study in 32 families. Ann. Intern. Med., 87:526, 1977.

Grondin, C. M.: Graft disease in patients with coronary bypass grafting. J. Thorac. Cardiovasc. Surg., 92:323, 1986.

Grundy, S. M.: Cholesterol and coronary heart disease: A new era. J.A.M.A., 256:2849, 1986a.

Grundy, S. M.: Comparison of monounsaturated fatty acids and carbohydrates for lowering plasma cholesterol. N. Engl. J. Med., 314:745, 1986b.

Grundy, S. M., Nis, D., Whelan, M. F., and Franklin, L.: Comparison of three cholesterol-lowering diets in normolipidemic men. J.A.M.A., 256:2351, 1986.

Grundy, S. M., Vega, G. L., and Bilheimer, D. W.: Influence of combined therapy with mevinolin and interruption of bile-acid reabsorption on low density lipoproteins in heterozygous familial hypercholesterolemia. Ann. Intern. Med., 103:339, 1985.

Hands, M. E., Briffa, T., Henderson, K., et al: Functional capacity and left ventricular function: The effect of supervised and unsupervised exercise rehabilitation soon after coronary artery bypass graft surgery. J. Cardiopulmonary Rehabil., 7:578, 1987.

Hartung, G. H., Squires, W. G., and Gotto, A. M., Jr.: Effect of exercise training on plasma high-density lipoprotein cholesterol in coronary disease patients. Am. Heart J., 101:181, 1981.

Haskell, W. L., Taylor, H. L., Wood, P. D., et al: Strenuous physical activity, treadmill exercise test performance, and plasma high-density lipoprotein cholesterol. Circulation, 62(Suppl. IV):53, 1980.

Havel, R. J.: Origin, metabolic rate, and metabolic function of plasma lipoproteins. *In* Steinberg, D., and Olefsky, J. M. (eds): Hypercholesterolemia and Atherosclerosis: Pathogenesis and Prevention. New York, Churchill-Livingstone, 1987, p. 117.

Heath, G. W., Ehsani, A. A., Hagberg, J. M., et al: Exercise training improves lipoprotein lipid profiles in patients with coronary artery disease. Am. Heart J., 105:889, 1983.

Hjermann, I., Holme, I., Velve, B. K., and Leren, P.: Effect of diet and smoking intervention on the incidence of coronary heart disease. Lancet, 2:1303, 1981.

Hulley, S. B., Rosenman, R. H., Bawol, R. D., and Brand, R. J.: Epidemiology as a guide to clinical decision: The association between triglyceride and coronary heart disease. N. Engl. J. Med., 302:1383, 1980.

Illingworth, D. R.: Mevinolin plus colestipol in therapy for severe heterozygous familial hypercholesterolemia. Ann. Intern. Med., 101:598, 1984.

Jaffe, E., and Weksler, B. B.: Recovery of endothelial cell prostacyclin production after inhibition by low doses of aspirin. J. Clin. Invest., 63:532, 1979.

Jennings, G., Nelson, L., Nestel, P., et al: The effects of changes in physical activity on major cardiovascular risk factors, hemodynamics, sympathetic function, and glucose utilization in man: A controlled study of four levels of activity. Circulation, 73:30, 1986.

Kallio, V., Hamalainen, H., Hakkila, J., et al: Reduction in sudden deaths by a multifactorial intervention program after acute myocardial infarction. Lancet, 2:1091, 1979.

Kane, J. P., Malloy, M. J., Tun, P., et al: Normalization of low-density-lipoprotein levels in heterozygous familial hypercholesterolemia with a combined drug regimen. N. Engl. J. Med., 304:251, 1981.

Kannel, W. B., Castelli, W. P., and Gordon, T.: Cholesterol in the prediction of atherosclerotic disease: New prespective based on the Framingham study. Ann. Intern. Med., 90:85, 1979.

Kannel, W. B., Castelli, W. P., Gordon, T., and McNamar, P. M.: Serum cholesterol, lipoproteins, and the risk of coronary heart disease. Ann. Intern. Med., 74:1, 1971.

Kannel, W. B., and McGee, D. L.: Diabetes and cardiovascular disease: The Framingham study. J.A.M.A., 241:780, 1984.

Kannel, W. B., McGee, D., and Gordon, T.: A general cardiovascular risk profile: The Framingham study. Am. J. Cardiol, 38:46, 1976.

Kannel, W. B., and Thom, T. J.: Declining cardiovascular mortality. Circulation, 70:331, 1984.

Kaplan, N. M.: Hypertension: Prevalence, risks and effect of therapy. Ann. Intern. Med., 98:705, 1983.

Kesaniemi, Y. A., and Grundy, S. M.: Influence of probucol on cholesterol and lipoprotein metabolism in man. J. Lipid Res., 25:780, 1984a.

Kesaniemi, Y. A., and Grundy, S. M.: Influence of gemfibrozil and clofibrate on metabolism of cholesterol and plasma triglycerides in man. J.A.M.A., 251:2241, 1984b.

Keys, A. (ed): Coronary heart disease in seven countries. Circulation, 41(Suppl. 1):1, 1970.

Keys, A.: Seven Countries: A Multivariate Analysis of Death and Coronary Heart Disease. Cambridge, MA, Harvard University Press, 1980.

Kissebah, A. H., Alfarsi, S., and Evans, D. J.: Low density lipoprotein metabolism in familial combined hyperlipidemia: Mechanism of the multiple phenotypic expression. Arteriosclerosis, 4:614, 1984.

Klatsky, A. L., Friedman, G. D., Siegelaub, A. B., et al: Alcohol consumption and blood pressure. N. Engl. J. Med., 296:1194, 1977.

Knopp, R. H., Ginsberg, J., Albers, J. J., et al: Contrasting effects of unmodified and time-release forms of niacin on lipoproteins in hyperlipidemic subjects: Clues to mechanism of action of niacin. Metabolism, 34:642, 1985.

Kornitzer, M., De Backer, G., Dramaix, M., and Thilly, C.: The Belgian heart disease prevention project. Circulation, 61:18, 1980.

Krolewski, A. S., Kosinski, E. J., Warram, J. H., et al: Magnitude and determinants of coronary artery disease in juvenile-onset, insulin-dependent diabetes mellitus. Am. J. Cardiol., 59:750, 1987.

Levy, R. I.: Declining mortality in coronary heart disease. Arteriosclerosis, 1:312, 1981.

Levy, R. I., Brensike, J. F., Epstein, S. E., et al: The influence of changes in lipid values induced by cholestyramine and diet on progression of coronary artery disease: Results of the NHLBI Type II Coronary Intervention Study. Circulation, 69:325, 1984.

Lie, J. T., Laurie, G. M., and Morris, G. C.: Aortocoronary bypass saphenous vein graft atherosclerosis: Anatomic study of 99 vein grafts from normal and hyperlipoproteinemic patients up to 75 months postoperatively. Am. J. Cardiol., 40:906, 1977.

Limet, R., David, J. L., Magotteaux, P., et al: Prevention of aortocoronary bypass graft occlusion: Beneficial effect of ticlopidine on early and late patency rates of venous coronary bypass grafts: A double-blind study. J. Thorac. Cardiovasc. Surg., 94:773, 1987.

Lipid Research Clinics Program: The Lipid Research Clinics Coronary Primary Prevention Trial results. I: Reduction of incidence of coronary heart disease. II: The relationship of reduction in incidence of coronary heart disease to cholesterol lowering. J.A.M.A., 251:351, 1984.

Lorenz, R. L., Weber, M., Kotyur, J., et al: Improved aortocoronary bypass patency by low dose aspirin (100 mg daily): Effects on platelet aggregation and thromboxane formation. Lancet, 1:1261, 1984.

Lovastatin Study Group II: Therapeutic response to lovastatin (Mevinolin) in nonfamilial hypercholesterolemia. A multicenter study. J.A.M.A., 251:351, 1984.

Maciejko, J. J., Holmes, D. R., Kottke, B. A., et al: Apolipoprotein A-I as a marker of angiographically assessed coronary-artery disease. N. Engl. J. Med., 309:385, 1983.

Mahley, R. W., and Angelin, B.: Type III hyperlipoproteinemia: Recent insights into the genetic defect of familial dysbetalipoproteinemia. Adv. Intern. Med., 29:385, 1984.

Mahley, R. W., Innerarity, T. L., Rall, S. C., Jr., and Weisgraber, K. H.: Plasma lipoproteins: Apolipoprotein structure and function. J. Lipid Res., 25:1277, 1984.

Matson, F. H., and Grundy, S. M.: Comparison of effects of dietary saturated, monounsaturated and polyunsaturated fatty acids on plasma lipids and lipoproteins in man. J. Lipid Res., 26:194, 1985.

May, G. S., Eberlein, K. A., Furberg, C. D., et al: Secondary prevention after myocardial infarction: A review of long-term trials. Prog. Cardiovasc. Dis., 24:331, 1982.

Mayer, J. E., Maj, M. C., Lindsay, W. G., et al: Influence of aspirin and dipyridamole therapy on patency of coronary artery bypass grafts. Ann. Thorac. Surg., 31:204, 1981.

McCann, R. L., Larson, R. M., Mitchener, J. S., III, et al: Intimal thickening and hyperlipidemia in experimental primate vascular autografts. Ann. Surg., 189:62, 1979.

McEnany, M. T., Salzman, E. W., Mundth, E. D., et al: The effect of antithrombotic therapy on patency rates of saphenous vein coronary artery bypass grafts. J. Thorac. Cardiovasc. Surg., 83:81, 1982.

McGill, H. C.: Morphologic development of the atherosclerotic plaque. In Lauer, R. M., and Shekell, R. B. (eds): Childhood Prevention of Atherosclerosis and Hypertension. New York, Raven Press, 1980.

Mehta, J., and Mehta, P.: Platelet function in hypertension and effect of therapy. Am. J. Cardiol., 47:331, 1981.

Miller, G. J., and Miller, N. E.: Plasma high density lipoprotein concentration and development of ischaemic heart disease. Lancet, 1:16, 1975.

Moncada, S., Higgs, E. A., and Vane, J. R.: Human arterial and venous tissue generate prostacyclin, a potent inhibitor of platelet aggregation. Lancet, 2:18, 1977.

Moncada, S., and Vane, J. R.: Arachiodonic and acid metabolites and the interactions between platelets and blood vessel walls. N. Engl. J. Med., 300:1142, 1979.

Morganroth, J., Levy, R. I., and Fredrickson, D. S.: The biochemical, clinical and genetic features of type III hyperlipoproteinemia. Ann. Intern. Med., 82:158, 1975.

Morris, J. N., Pollard, R., Everitt, M. G., et al: Vigorous exercise in leisure-time: Protection against coronary heart disease. Lancet, 2:1207, 1980.

Multiple Risk Factor Intervention Trial (MRFIT) Research Group: Multiple Risk Factor Intervention Trial: Risk factor changes and mortality results. J.A.M.A., 248:1465, 1982.

National Cholesterol Education Program: Report of the National Cholesterol Education Program Expert Panel on detection, evaluation and treatment of high blood cholesterol in adults. Arch. Intern. Med., 148:36, 1988.

National Institutes of Health Consensus Conference: Lowering blood cholesterol to prevent heart disease. J.A.M.A., 253:2080, 1985.

National Institutes of Health Consensus Conference: Treatment of hypertriglyceridemia. J.A.M.A., 251:1196, 1984.

Neitzel, G. F., Barboriak, J. J., Pintar, K., and Qureshi, I.: Atherosclerosis in aortocoronary bypass grafts—morphologic study and risk factor analysis 6 to 12 years after surgery. Arteriosclerosis, 6:594, 1986.

Nestel, P. J., Connor, W. E., Reardon, M. F., et al: Suppression by diets rich in fish oil of very low density lipoprotein production in man. J. Clin. Invest., 74:82, 1984.

Neutze, J. M., and White, H. D.: What contribution has cardiac surgery made to the decline in mortality from coronary heart disease? Br. Med. J., 294:405, 1987.

Newman, W. P., Freedman, D. S., Voors, A. W., et al: Relation of serum lipoprotein levels and systolic blood pressure to early atherosclerosis: The Bogalusa Heart Study. N. Engl. J. Med., 314:138, 1986.

Nikkila, E. A., Viikinkoski, P., Valle, M., and Frick, M. H.: Prevention of progression of coronary atherosis by treatment of hyperlipidemia: A seven year prospective angiographic study. Br. Med. J., 289:220, 1984.

Nilsson, J., Svensson, J., Hamstern, A., and deFaire, V.: Increased platelet-derived mitogenic activity in plasma of young patients with coronary atherosclerosis. Atherosclerosis, 61:237, 1986.

Oslo Study Research Group: MRFIT and the Oslo Study. J.A.M.A., 249:893, 1983.

Paffenbarger, R. S., Jr., Hyde, R. T., Wing, A. L., and Hsieh, C. C.: Physical activity, all-cause mortality, and longevity of college alumni. N. Engl. J. Med., 314:605, 1986.

Pantely, G. S., Goodnight, S. H., Jr., Rahimtoola, S. H., et al: Failure of antiplatelet and anticoagulant therapy to improve patency of grafts after coronary bypass: A controlled, randomized study. N. Engl. J. Med., 301:962, 1979.

Parthasarathy, S., Young, S. G., Witztum, J., et al: Probucol inhibits oxidative modification of low density lipoprotein. J. Clin. Invest., 77:641, 1986.

Persantine-Aspirin Reinfarction Study Research Group: Persantine and aspirin in coronary heart disease. Circulation, 62:449, 1980.

Person, T. A., Kramer, E. C., Soley, K., and Hepinstall, R. H.: The human atherosclerotic plaque. Am. J. Pathol., 86:657, 1977.

Peto, R.: Aspirin after myocardial infarction (Editorial). Lancet, 1:1172, 1980.

Phillipson, B. E., Rothrock, D. W., Connor, W. E., et al: Reduction of plasma lipids, lipoproteins, and apoproteins by dietary fish oils in patients with hypertriglyceridemia. N. Engl. J. Med., 312:1210, 1985.

Physicians' Health Study Research Group: Preliminary report: Findings from the aspirin component of the ongoing Physicians' Health Study. N. Engl. J. Med., 318:262, 1988.

Pirk, J., Vojacek, J., Kovac, J., et al: Improved patency of aortocoronary bypass by antithrombotic drugs. Ann. Thorac. Surg., 42:312, 1986.

Pooling Project Research Group: Relationship of blood pressure, serum cholesterol, smoking habit, relative weight and ECG abnormalities to incidence of major coronary events: Final report of the Pooling Project Research Group. J. Chronic Dis., 31:201, 1978.

Preston, F. E., Whipps, W., Jackson, C. A., et al: Inhibition of prostacyclin platelet thromboxane A_2 after low dose aspirin. N. Engl. J. Med., 304:76, 1981.

Pryor, D. B., Harrell, F. E., Rankin, J. S., et al: The changing survival benefits of coronary revascularization over time. Circulation, 76(Suppl. 5):13, 1987.

Pyorala, K., Epstein, F. H., and Kornitzer, M.: Changing trends in coronary heart disease mortality: Possible explanations. Cardiology, 72:5, 1985.

Rechnitzer, P. A., Cunningham, P. A., Andrew, G. M., et al: Relation of exercise to the recurrent rate of myocardial infarction in men. Cardiology, 51:65, 1983.

Redwood, D. R., Rosing, D. R., and Epstein, S. E.: Circulatory and symptomatic effects of physical training in patients with coronary artery disease and angina pectoris. N. Engl. J. Med., 286:959, 1972.

Reimer, K. A., and Jennings, R. B.: Myocardial ischemia, hypoxia, and infarction. In Fozzard, H. A. (ed): The Heart and Cardiovascular System. New York, Raven Press, 1986, p. 1133.

Rhoads, G. C., Culbrandsen, C. L., and Kagen, A.: Serum lipoprotein and coronary heart disease in a population study of Hawaii on Japanese men. N. Engl. J. Med., 294:293, 1976.

Rosenberg, L., Shapiro, S., Kaufman, D. W., et al: Cigarette smoking in relation to the risk of myocardial infarction in young women. Int. J. Epidemiol., 9:57, 1980.

Ross, R.: Atherosclerosis: A problem of the biology of arterial wall cells and their interactions with blood components. Arteriosclerosis, 1:293, 1981.

Ross, R.: The pathogenesis of atherosclerosis—an update. N. Engl. J. Med., 314:488, 1986.

Ross, R.: Platelet-derived growth factor. Ann. Rev. Med., 38:71, 1987.

Ross, R., and Glomset, J. A.: Atherosclerosis and the arterial smooth muscle cell. Science, 180:1332, 1973.

Ross, R., and Glomset, J. A.: The pathogenesis of atherosclerosis. N. Engl. J. Med., 295:369, 1976.

Ross, R., and Harker, L.: Hyperlipidemia and atherosclerosis. Science, 193:1094, 1976.

Ross, R., Raines, E. W., and Bowen-Pope, D. F.: The biology of platelet-derived growth factor. Cell, 46:155, 1986.

Sagel, J., Colwell, J. A., Crook, L., and Laimins, M.: Increased platelet aggregation in early diabetes mellitus. Ann. Intern. Med., 82:733, 1975.

Saku, K., Gartside, P. S., Hynd, B. A., and Kashyap, M. L.: Mechanism of action of gemfibrozil on lipoprotein metabolism. J. Clin. Invest., 75:1702, 1985.

St. Clair, R. N.: Atherosclerosis regression in animal models: Current concepts of cellular and biochemical mechanisms. Prog. Cardiovasc. Dis., 26:109, 1983.

Schaefer, E. J., and Levy, R. I.: Pathogenesis and management of lipoprotein disorders. N. Engl. J. Med., 312:1300, 1985.

Schwartz, S. M., Gajduske, C. M., and Selden, S. C.: Vascular wall growth control: The role of the endothelium. Arteriosclerosis, 1:107, 1981.

Sennett, S. M., Pollock, M. L., Pels, A. E., et al: Medical problems of cardiac patients in an outpatient cardiac rehabilitation program. Med. Sci. Sports Exerc., 16:149A, 1984.

Shapiro, S., Rosenberg, L., Seone, P., et al: Oral contraceptive use in relation to myocardial infarction. Lancet, 1:743, 1979.

Sharma, G. V. R. K., Khuri, S. F., Josa, M., et al: The effect of antiplatelet therapy on saphenous vein coronary artery bypass graft patency. Circulation, 68(Suppl. II):218, 1983.

Shaw, L.: Effects of a prescribed supervised exercise program on mortality and cardiovascular morbidity in patients after myocardial infarction. Am. J. Cardiol., 48:39, 1981.

Shepherd, J., Packard, C. J., Bicker, S., et al: Cholestyramine promotes receptor mediated low density lipoprotein catabolism. N. Engl. J. Med., 302:1219, 1980.

Smith, E. B.: Molecular interactions in human atherosclerotic plaques. Am. J. Pathol., 86:665, 1977.

Sniderman, A., Shapiro, S., Marpole, D., et al: Association of coronary atherosclerosis with hyperapobetalipoproteinemia (increased protein but normal cholesterol levels in human plasma low density lipoproteins). Proc. Natl. Acad. Sci. U.S.A., 77:604, 1980.

Sniderman, A. D., Wolfson, C., Ten, B., et al: Association of hyperapobetalipoproteinemia with endogenous hypertriglyceridemia and atherosclerosis. Ann. Intern. Med., 97:833, 1982.

Solberg, L. A., and Strong, J. P.: Risk factors and atherosclerotic lesions: A review of autopsy studies. Arteriosclerosis, 3:187, 1983.

Stamler, J.: Lectures on Preventive Cardiology. New York, Grune & Stratton, 1967.

Stamler, J.: The marked decline in coronary heart disease mortality rates in the United States, 1968–1981: Summary of findings and possible explanations. Cardiology, 72:11, 1985.

Stamler, J., Wentworth, D., and Neaton, J.: Is the relationship between serum cholesterol and risk of death from coronary heart disease continuous and graded? J.A.M.A., 256:2823, 1986.

Starzl, T. E., Chase, H. P., Ahrens, E. H., Jr., et al: Portacaval shunt in patients with familial hypercholesterolemia. Ann. Surg., 198:273, 1983.

Steinberg, D.: Lipoproteins and the pathogenesis of atherosclerosis. Circulation, 76:508, 1987.

Stern, M. P.: The recent decline in ischemic heart disease mortality. Ann. Intern. Med., 91:630, 1979.

Stevens, R., and Hanson, P.: Comparison of supervised and unsupervised exercise training after coronary bypass surgery. Am. J. Cardiol., 53:1524, 1984.

Strong, J. P., Eggen, D. A., and Oalmann, M. C.: The natural history, geographic pathology, and epidemiology of atherosclerosis. In Wissler, R. W., and Geer, J. C. (eds): The Pathogenesis of Atherosclerosis. Baltimore, Williams & Wilkins, 1972.

Subramanian, V. A., Hernandez, Y., Tack-Goldman, K., et al: Prostacyclin production by internal mammary artery as a factor in coronary artery bypass grafts. Surgery, 100:376, 1986.

Superko, H. R., Wood, R. F., and Haskell, W. L.: Coronary heart disease and risk factor modification: Is there a threshold? Am. J. Med., 78:826, 1985.

Thelle, D. S., Forde, O. H., Try, K., and Lehmann, E. H.: The Tromso Heart Study: Methods and main results of the cross-sectional study. Acta Med. Scand., 200:107, 1976.

Thompson, G. R., and Gotto, A. M.: Ileal bypass in the treatment of hyperlipoproteinemia. Lancet, 2:35, 1973.

Thompson, P. D.: The cardiovascular risks of cardiac rehabilitation. J. Cardiopulmonary Rehabil., 5:321, 1985.

Tomporowski, P. O., and Ellis, N. R.: Effects of exercise on cognitive processes: A review. Psychol. Bull., 99:338, 1986.

Utermann, G., Langenbeck, U., Beisiegel, U., and Weber, W.: Genetics of the apolipoprotein E system in man. Am. J. Hum. Genet., 32:399, 1980.

Vega, G. L., and Grundy, S. M.: Comparison of apolipoprotein B to cholesterol in low density lipoproteins of patients with coronary heart disease. J. Lipid Res., 25:580, 1984.

Vega, G. L., and Grundy, S. M.: Gemfibrozil therapy in primary hypertriglyceridemia associated with coronary heart disease. J.A.M.A., 253:2398, 1985.

Vega, G. L., and Grundy, S. M.: Treatment of primary moderate hypercholesterolemia with lovastatin (mevinolin) and colestipol. J.A.M.A., 257:33, 1987.

Veterans Administration Cooperative Study Group on Anti-hypertensive Agents: Effects of treatment on morbidity in hypertension. I: Results in patients with diastolic blood pressure averaging 115 through 129 mm Hg. J.A.M.A., 202:1028, 1967.

Walker, L. N., Bowen-Pope, D. F., Ross, R., and Reidy, M. A.: Production of platelet-derived growth factor-like molecules by cultured arterial smooth muscle cells accompanies proliferation after arterial injury. Proc. Natl. Acad. Sci. U.S.A., 83:7311, 1986.

Wenger, N. K.: Rehabilitation of the coronary patient: Status 1986. Prog. Cardiovasc. Dis., 29:181, 1986.

West, K. M., Ahuja, M. M. S., Bennett, P. H., et al: The role of circulating glucose and triglyceride concentrations and their interactions with other "risk factors" as determinants of arterial disease in nine diabetic population samples from the WHO multinational study. Diabetes Care, 6:361, 1983.

Wilhelmsen, L., Sanne, H., Elmfeldt, D., et al: A controlled trial of physical training after myocardial infarction. Prev. Med., 4:491, 1975.

World Health Organization (WHO): Cooperative trial on primary prevention of ischemic heart disease using clofibrate to lower serum cholesterol. Lancet, 2:379, 1980.

CHAPTER 55

THE SURGICAL MANAGEMENT OF CARDIAC ARRHYTHMIAS

James L. Cox

Surgical intervention is now recognized as being an integral part of the armamentarium to treat almost all types of cardiac arrhythmias. The development of specific surgical techniques has paralleled the evolution of understanding of the anatomic basis of arrhythmias and the availability of progressively more sophisticated methods for their electrophysiologic evaluation.

There are certain fundamental differences between the anatomic-electrophysiologic substrates responsible for supraventricular tachycardias and those associated with ventricular tachycardias; therefore, the surgical approaches to these two categories of arrhythmias differ. Although the electrophysiology of most supraventricular tachycardias is well understood, the anatomic substrate of the tachycardia is not visible to the surgeon (e.g., accessory pathways, dual atrioventricular [AV] node pathways, Mahaim's fibers, and atrial cell rests). This inability to visualize the abnormal anatomy responsible for supraventricular tachycardias dictates a dependence on accurate electrophysiologic mapping for successful surgical results. Although the electrophysiologic basis of ventricular tachycardia is not as well understood, the anatomic substrate (endocardial fibrosis) is usually apparent to the surgeon. This fact has led many teams to abandon the intraoperative mapping of ventricular tachycardia, a practice that has had a detrimental effect on the development of more effective surgical therapy for these relatively common disorders. In contradistinction, it is believed that every patient who requires operation for a cardiac arrhythmia should have that arrhythmia studied preoperatively, intraoperatively, and postoperatively as thoroughly as possible. Only by this approach can recent surgical progress be continued.

In addition to the development of surgical techniques to treat cardiac arrhythmias, during the last decade, antitachycardia devices, especially the automatic internal cardioverter-defibrillator (AICD), have evolved. The availability and effectiveness of the AICD have narrowed the indications for ventricular tachycardia procedures, but the indications for su-

praventricular tachycardia operations have continued to broaden. Because arrhythmia procedures are rapidly becoming an important part of the specialty, cardiac surgeons will be expected to become more familiar with the anatomy and electrophysiology relating to these common disorders of the heart.

BASIC ELECTROPHYSIOLOGIC CONCEPTS

The introduction of the microelectrode by Draper and Weidmann (1957) led to general acceptance of the theory that normal cardiac cells generate upstrokes by a rapid, voltage-dependent, transient inflow of sodium ions (*rapid channel*). The resultant transmembrane action potential recorded by a microelectrode from normal myocardial cells has five distinct phases (Fig. 55–1). Phase 0 represents the sharp upstroke recorded during depolarization of the cell, when sodium ions pass rapidly into the cell. Phases 1 and 2 occur immediately after completion of cellular depolarization, during which time the cell is absolutely refractory to further depolarization. During phase 3, the cell begins to repolarize as sodium ions transfer out of the cell and potassium ions flow inward to re-establish the resting transmembrane potential (phase 4). Reuter (1967) showed a slow inward current of calcium ions during the plateau (phase 2) of the transmembrane action potential. Because the kinetics of activation, inactivation, and reactivation of sinoatrial (SA) node and AV node cells and of certain abnormal cells with low resting transmembrane potentials are considerably slower than those for the inward sodium current, the *slow channel* of calcium ion influx is considered to be a major factor in the activation of these cells. SA node cells probably operate with a mixed dependence on rapid and slow currents (Strauss et al, 1977). Although spontaneous phase 4 depolarization (characteristic of pacemaker cells) is due in part to deactivation of a fast potassium current (McAllister et al, 1975), the sensitivity of SA node cells to slow-channel

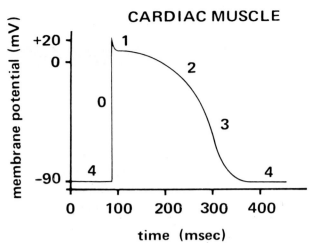

CARDIAC MUSCLE

Figure 55–1. The cardiac action potential (shown here for Purkinje fiber) lasts for more than 300 msec and consists of five phases. Phase 0 (upstroke) corresponds to depolarization in skeletal muscle, and phase 3 (repolarization) corresponds to repolarization in that tissue. Phases 1 (early repolarization) and 2 (plateau) have no clear counterpart in skeletal muscle, whereas phase 4 (diastole) corresponds to the resting potential. (From Katz, A. M.: Cardiac action potential. *In* Katz, A. M. [ed]: Physiology of the Heart. New York, Raven Press, 1977.)

blocking agents (Zipes and Fisher, 1974) suggests that the background inward current may be the slow calcium current rather than a sodium current. Although these ionic currents form the basis for normal cardiac impulse generation and conduction, pathologic changes in myocardial cells may lead to a detrimental interplay between the rapid and slow currents and thus to the two basic types of cardiac rhythm disturbances, automatic arrhythmias and reentrant arrhythmias.

The appearance of automaticity in pathologic myocardial cells is believed to develop on the same electrochemical basis that evokes spontaneous activity in normal pacemaker cells. Injured cells show *spontaneous phase 4 depolarization*, which may result in atrial or ventricular premature systoles or, if repetitive, in atrial or ventricular tachycardia.

The physiologic basis for re-entrant arrhythmias is slightly more complex because several different types of re-entry may occur, depending on the type of anatomic-electrophysiologic abnormality present. The simplest type of re-entry is that of a *circus movement*, first described by Mines (1914) (Fig. 55–2). In this type of re-entrant arrhythmia, it is essential that a unidirectional block develop at some point in a contiguous conducting circuit. If the course of the circuit is sufficiently long (or the refractory period sufficiently short) to allow previously depolarized tissue to repolarize before the electrical wave front traverses the circuit, the wave front will always be preceded by excitable tissue, and the arrhythmia may continue indefinitely. This type of re-entrant mechanism (usually called macro-re-entry) is responsible for the reciprocating tachycardia of Wolff-Parkinson-White (WPW) syndrome, certain types of atrial flutter, and certain unusual types of ventricular tachycardia in which the re-entrant circuit involves various branches of the His-Purkinje system.

Re-entrant arrhythmias associated with ischemic heart disease may occur on the basis of macro-re-entry or micro-re-entry, the latter requiring two conditions for the development of sustained re-entry: unidirectional block and slow conduction. Unidirectional block has the same role in micro-re-entry as it does in macro-re-entry—that is, it dictates that the wave front of depolarization be propagated in only one direction around the circuit. Although some asymmetry of conduction exists in normal myocardial

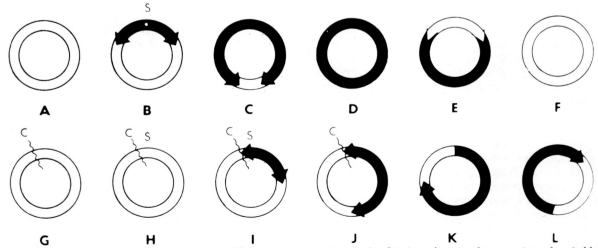

Figure 55–2. Role of unidirectional block in establishing circus movement. Application of a stimulus to a ring of excitable tissue (*unshaded area*) in the absence of block (*B*) initiates an impulse (*shaded area*) that depolarizes the entire ring (*D*). Mutual cancellation of the impulses moving in opposite directions (*C*) allows the tissue to repolarize completely (*E,F*). However, if unidirectional block is established by temporary clamping of the tissue (*C* in *G–J*), the impulse propagated in the clockwise direction can continue to travel around the ring (*K,L*), thus establishing a circus movement. (From Katz, A.M.: The arrhythmias. III: Tachycardia, flutter and fibrillation, concealed conduction. *In* Katz, A. M. [ed]: Physiology of the Heart. New York, Raven Press, 1977.)

tissue owing to differences in the passive or active properties of cells, local unidirectional block is an extreme form. This asymmetry is exaggerated by conditions that depress excitability, such as high local extracellular potassium concentrations existing in ischemic myocardium. In addition, myocardial fibrosis, which reduces the ability of an electrical impulse to be propagated by increasing the resistance, can cause unidirectional block when the fibrosis is distributed asymmetrically.

Because of the comparatively long distances traversed by an electrical impulse in macro-re-entrant circuits (e.g., in WPW syndrome), slow conduction in a portion of these circuits is not an absolute requisite for the development of sustained re-entry. However, in micro-re-entrant circuits, the actual distance traversed by the electrical impulse may be so short (e.g., perhaps involving only a few cells) that sustained re-entry cannot occur unless conduction velocity is decreased in some portion of the circuit. Four physiologically interdependent factors influence conduction velocity in myocardial tissue: (1) action potential amplitude, (2) rate of depolarization of the action potential, (3) threshold, and (4) electrical resistance. In regions of ischemia, myocardial cells become partially depolarized because some of the intracellular potassium is replaced with sodium. This results in partial inactivation of the rapid sodium channels and, therefore, decreases both action potential amplitude and the rate of depolarization. These partially depolarized tissues can conduct a propagated action potential, although extremely slowly and usually with decrement. These conductive properties, which elicit slowly propagated waves of depolarization, have the features of the slow inward current transported mainly by calcium ions. Thus, calcium-mediated slow responses are regarded as having an important, if not exclusive, role in the genesis of micro-re-entrant arrhythmias (Katz, 1977). The conditions necessary for the development of sustained micro-re-entrant arrhythmias may occur in an ischemic limb of distal Purkinje fibers or in an ischemic strand of myocardial muscle (Fig. 55–3).

Clinical differentiation between automatic and re-entrant arrhythmias is important in patients who require surgical intervention because automatic arrhythmias are frequently suppressed by general anesthesia. However, the ability to discriminate between these two types of arrhythmias is limited clinically. Current practice involves the use of rapid burst pacing or programmed electrical stimulation. With the latter technique, regular pacing stimuli (S_1) are introduced at a given cycle length, and a premature stimulus (S_2) is delivered in late diastole. The premature stimulus is introduced progressively until it no longer elicits a depolarization, thus delineating the refractory period of the tissue being stimulated. If the arrhythmia is not induced by this single premature impulse delivered at different intervals throughout electrical diastole, double premature stimuli (S_2, S_3) are introduced, with S_3 being delivered

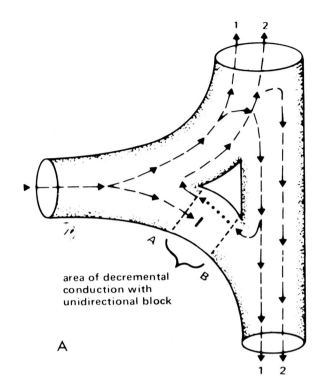

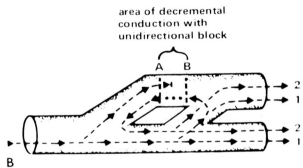

Figure 55–3. Re-entry at the point of impingement of a Purkinje fiber on the ventricular myocardium (*A*) and within a strand of cardiac muscle (*B*). In both situations, a region of decremental conduction with unidirectional block (A–B) blocks antegrade conduction of the normal impulse (1) but allows this impulse to traverse the depressed region in the retrograde direction (*broken line*) after a delay. This retrograde impulse re-enters the myocardium proximal to the region of decremental conduction after the proximal tissue has recovered from the normal impulse, thus allowing the retrograde impulse to initiate a premature systole (2). (From Katz, A. M.: The arrhythmias. II: Abnormal impulse formation and reentry, premature systoles, pre-excitation. *In* Katz, A. M. [ed]: Physiology of the Heart. New York, Raven Press, 1977.)

at progressive intervals beginning 50 to 100 msec longer than the effective refractory period of the tissue. This sequence is repeated until the arrhythmia is initiated. The same programmed single, double, and triple stimuli may be delivered to terminate the arrhythmia. Clincally, arrhythmias that respond to programmed electrical stimulation are considered to be re-entrant arrhythmias, and those that do not respond are classified as being automatic arrhythmias. Although this clinical classification is strictly empiric, it is useful because it provides (1) a method of assessing medical management, (2) a reason for using pacemaker devices, and (3) some assurance that the arrhythmia can be invoked for investigative purposes at the time of operation.

ANATOMY OF THE CARDIAC CONDUCTION SYSTEM AND RELATED STRUCTURES

The SA node is a small subepicardial group of highly specialized cells located in the sulcus terminalis just lateral to the junction of the superior vena cava and the right atrium (Anderson and Becker, 1978). The cells are arranged around a central SA node artery arising from either the right or left coronary system and passing either anterior or posterior to the superior vena cava. Studies suggest that the SA node consists of three distinct regions, each responsive to a separate group of neural and circulatory stimuli (Boineau et al, 1977). The inter-relationship of these three regions determines the ultimate output of the SA node. Under normal conditions, only these cells in the heart are capable of spontaneous phase 4 depolarization, thus establishing the SA node as the site of origin of the normal cardiac impulse.

The existence of specialized conduction pathways between the SA node and the AV node has been a subject of controversy for many years. Most experts now agree, however, that although an electrical impulse emanating from the SA node travels to the AV node preferentially through the crista terminalis and the limbus of the fossa ovalis, these muscle bundles do not represent specialized, insulated conduction tracts comparable with the ventricular bundle branches. Although electrical impulses travel more rapidly through these thick atrial muscle bundles, surgical transection will not block internodal conduction.

The AV junctional area is the most complex anatomic portion of the cardiac conduction system. From a functional standpoint, the AV node should be considered to be the area in which there occurs a normal delay in AV conduction. This area corresponds anatomically with a group of AV junctional cells that are histologically distinct from the working myocardium (Anderson and Becker, 1976). As an atrial impulse approaches the AV nodal area, it traverses a transitional zone of specialized cells located anteriorly in the base of the atrial septum slightly to the right of and cephalad to the central fibrous body. This transition zone surrounds the atrial aspect of the compact AV node, where the major conduction delay occurs. The lower, longitudinal portion of the compact AV node penetrates the central fibrous body immediately posterior to the membranous portion of the intra-atrial septum and becomes the bundle of His. The AV node, transitional zone, and penetrating bundle are contained within the triangle of Koch, an anatomically discrete region bounded by the tendon of Todaro, the tricuspid valve annulus, and the thebesian valve of the coronary sinus (Fig. 55–4). There is little danger of surgical damage to AV conduction if this triangle is avoided in all procedures.

When the penetrating portion of the AV node traverses the central fibrous body, it becomes the bundle of His. The anatomy in this area is complicated by the fact that the junction of the right-sided heart chambers occupies a different spatial plane from the junction of the left-sided heart chambers, the annulus of the tricuspid valve being situated more toward the ventricular apex than that of the mitral valve (Anderson and Becker, 1979). The bundle of His travels along the posteroinferior rim of the membranous portion of the interventricular septum.

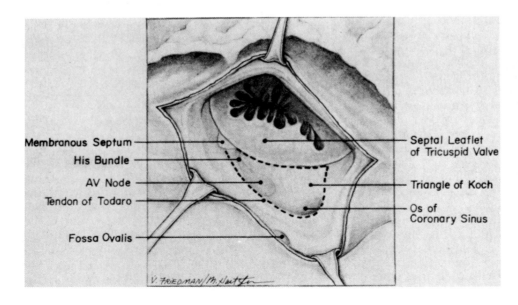

Membranous Septum
His Bundle
AV Node
Tendon of Todaro
Fossa Ovalis

Septal Leaflet of Tricuspid Valve
Triangle of Koch
Os of Coronary Sinus

V. FRIEDMAN/M.

Figure 55–4. The right atrial septum viewed through a longitudinal right atriotomy. The patient's head is to the left and the feet are to the right. The boundaries of the triangle of Koch are the tendon of Todaro, the tricuspid valve annulus, and a line connecting the two at the level of the os of the coronary sinus. Within the triangle of Koch resides the AV node and proximal portion of the bundle of His, which enters the ventricular septum immediately posterior to the membranous portion of the interatrial septum. (From Cox, J. L., Holman, W. L., and Cain, M. E.: Cryosurgical treatment of atrioventricular node reentry tachycardia. Circulation, 76:1329, 1987. By permission of the American Heart Association, Inc.)

The right bundle branch proceeds subendocardially toward the base of the medial papillary muscle and descends toward the ventricular apex, partly crossing the cavity of the ventricle in the moderator band. At the lower level of the membranous interventricular septum, the bundle of His emits a broad band of fasciculi, forming the left bundle branch that extends down the left side of the septum 1 to 2 cm, where it divides into a smaller anterior and a larger posterior radiation. The medial aspects of these radiations usually become intermeshed distally to form three anastomosing nets of fibers—anterior, middle, and posterior. When the left side of the ventricular septum is seen through the aortic valve, the danger area from the standpoint of the conduction tissue is immediately subjacent to the right coronary-noncoronary commissure.

The distal branches of the conduction system terminate in an intermediate zone between the Purkinje cells and the myocardium, where the cells gradually lose Purkinje characteristics and assume the characteristics of working ventricular myocardia.

Of particular importance to cardiac surgeons involved with conduction abnormalities are the relationships of the various structures and potential spaces comprising the junction of the atrial septum, the ventricular septum, the AV groove, and the fibrous skeleton of the heart. The cardiac skeleton is strongest at the central fibrous body where the annuli of the mitral, tricuspid, and aortic valves meet (Fig. 55–5). Because the tricuspid annulus is more apical in position than the mitral annulus, the anterior part of the central fibrous body extends into the ventricles beneath the attachment of the tricuspid valve and forms the interventricular component of the membranous septum between the aortic outflow tract and the right atrium. Likewise, immediately posterior to the membranous septum, the right atrial wall is in potential communication with the inlet portion of the left ventricle.

The mitral and aortic valve annuli contribute significantly to the structural integrity of the fibrous skeleton and are further strengthened at their left junction to form the left fibrous trigone. The left anterior portion of the central fibrous body is designated as the right fibrous trigone. The AV groove between these two trigones represents the site of continuity between the anterior leaflet of the mitral valve and the aortic valve annulus and is the only area in the AV groove where atrial muscle is not in juxtaposition to ventricular muscle. Thus, accessory AV pathways are not found between the left and right fibrous trigones.

SUPRAVENTRICULAR TACHYARRHYTHMIAS

Wolff-Parkinson-White Syndrome

Anatomic-Electrophysiologic Basis

The WPW syndrome is characterized by an abnormal muscular connection between the atrium and ventricle (accessory AV connection or accessory pathway). It is believed that these accessory muscle bundles result from incomplete separation of the fetal atria and ventricles during the "pinching-off" process that occurs when the fibrous annulus of the heart develops. Normally, the only remaining connection between the atria and ventricles after formation of the annulus fibrosus is the bundle of His. Thus, if the separation is incomplete, an abnormal connection persists between the atria and ventricles, and the anatomic substrate for the WPW syndrome remains. The region of the annulus fibrosus where the atria and ventricles are not continuous during fetal development is between the right and left fibrous trigones—that is, where the anterior leaflet of the mitral valve is in continuity with the annulus of the aortic valve (Figs. 55–5 and 55–16). This anatomic development is believed to explain why accessory pathways do not occur between the right and left fibrous trigones. The persistent accessory pathways in patients with the WPW syndrome are capable of conducting electrical activity. However, these patients also have a normal bundle of His connecting the atria to the ventricles electrically and, thus, have two routes by which an electrical impulse may travel between the atria and ventricles. When patients with the WPW syndrome are in normal sinus rhythm, the SA node impulse activates the atria normally. After activating the atria, the electrical wave front propagates to the ventricles across both the bundle of His and the accessory pathway (Fig. 55–6). However, this antegrade (atrial-to-ventricular) conduction is delayed before entering the bundle of His because of the normal conduction delay that occurs in the AV node. Because there is no AV node proximal to the accessory pathway to delay conduction, the electrical activity reaches the ventricle first at the site of insertion of the accessory pathway onto the ventricle (see

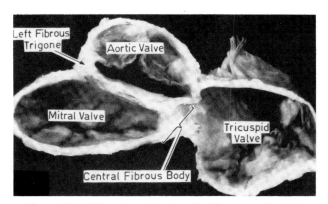

Figure 55–5. Dissection showing the fibrous cardiac skeleton after it has been removed from the ventricles. (From Anderson, R. H., and Becker, A. E.: Cardiac anatomy for the surgeon. *In* Davidson, G. K. [ed]: Cardiovascular Surgery. Hagerstown, MD, Harper & Row, 1979.)

Fig. 55–6B). The initial activation of the ventricle at a site remote from the bundle of His causes an early deflection off the baseline of the standard electrocardiogram (ECG), resulting in a delta wave. As the electrical wave front propagates down the ventricle from the site of ventricular insertion of the accessory pathway, the electrical activity passing through the normal AV node-bundle of His complex eventually emerges and passes rapidly down the bundle branches (see Fig. 55–6C). The fusion of the wave front from the bundle of His and the wave front from the accessory pathway (Fig. 55–6D) causes the QRS complex to be wide. Thus, during normal sinus rhythm, the standard ECG in patients with the WPW syndrome shows (1) a short P-R interval because of the lack of a delay in conduction from the atrium to the ventricle across the accessory pathway, (2) a delta wave due to eccentric activation of the ventricle across the accessory pathway, and (3) a wide QRS complex due to fusion of the electrical activity propagating from the bundle of His and that propagating from the accessory pathway (Fig. 55–7). These are the three ECG findings described by Wolff, Parkinson, and White, who noted that patients with this type of ECG had a high incidence of supraventricular tachycardia (Wolff et al, 1930).

Although antegrade conduction across an accessory pathway causes an abnormal ECG, it does not result in tachycardia. For tachycardia to occur, antegrade conduction across the accessory pathway must be blocked (Fig. 55–8A). Antegrade block in an accessory pathway may result from various causes, including premature atrial or ventricular beats and

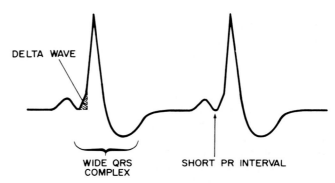

Figure 55–7. Typical ECG during normal sinus rhythm in a patient with the WPW syndrome.

sudden changes in the autonomic input to the heart. When antegrade block occurs in the accessory pathway with the patient in normal sinus rhythm, the sinus impulse activates the atria normally. The electrical activity propagates through the AV node-bundle of His complex normally and activates the ventricles normally. However, when the electrical activity reaches the AV groove at the base of the heart, it encounters a bundle of muscle, the accessory pathway, that has not yet been depolarized. As a result, the electrical activity simply propagates across the accessory pathway retrogradely (from the ventricle to the atrium) and quickly reactivates the atria. The atrial activation wave front then passes normally through the AV node-bundle of His complex again and reactivates the ventricle. In this manner, a macro-re-entrant circuit is established around which electrical activity can propagate as fast as four times per second or 240 times per minute (see Fig. 55–8B). Thus, the patient progresses from a normal sinus rhythm, for example 80 beats per minute (with an abnormal ECG), to a single premature beat, to a supraventricular tachyardia (reciprocating tachycardia) of 240 beats per minute.

Historical Aspects

Gaskell (1833) first showed that electrical activity propagated from the atrium to the ventricle by way of myocardial tissue rather than nerves in his studies

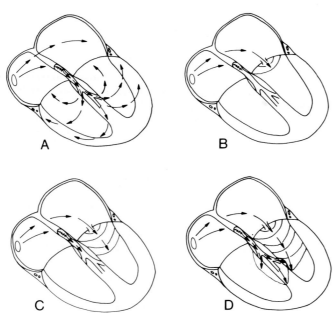

Figure 55–6. A, Normal spread of electrical activation in the heart during sinus rhythm. The electrical impulse is delayed approximately 100 msec in the AV node. B–D, Spread of electrical activation during sinus rhythm in the WPW syndrome with an accessory pathway in the left free-wall position.

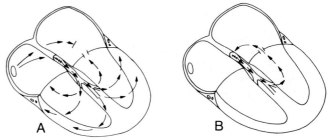

Figure 55–8. A, Antegrade conduction block across the accessory pathway in a patient with the WPW syndrome. B, Reciprocating tachycardia in a patient with the WPW syndrome.

on the turtle heart. Kent (1893) identified muscular connections between the atria and ventricles of mammals but erroneously concluded that these connections were multiple and that they represented the normal pathways of AV conduction. Despite this misconception, his name serves as the eponym for the accessory AV connections responsible for the WPW syndrome (Kent bundles).

Perhaps the most important work delineating the specialized conduction system of the heart was reported when Tawara, working in Aschoff's laboratory in Germany, identified and characterized the AV node, bundle of His, bundle branches, and Purkinje system (Aschoff, 1906). Keith and Flack (1906) identified the SA node as the heart's normal pacemaker.

During the 1920s, Paul Dudley White, one of the great teachers and clinical cardiologists of this century, noted that a small group of young, apparently normal patients with ventricular pre-excitation on standard ECG had frequent episodes of paroxysmal tachycardia. During a visit to London, he discovered that Parkinson, an English physician, had identified a similar series of patients. White suggested that Wolff, one of White's fellows, combine their series and report these observations, which they did (Wolff et al, 1930). Neither the ventricular pre-excitation nor the bouts of tachycardia were explained, however, until Wolferth and Wood (1933) reported a patient with the same clinical syndrome and suggested that the ECG abnormalities were due to accessory pathways between the atrium and ventricle similar to those previously described by Kent. Although they accepted Kent's erroneous hypothesis that these accessory pathways were normal and occurred on the right free wall, Wolferth and Wood directed attention to the region in a patient with the syndrome. This patient died, and they fortuitously were able to document an accessory pathway histologically at autopsy, which they reported in 1943.

Although the basis for the WPW syndrome was suspected, the issue remained controversial for many years. The explanation became slightly clearer in 1967, however, when Durrer, of Amsterdam, the generally acknowledged father of modern clinical electrophysiology, did intraoperative mapping in a patient with the WPW syndrome and showed electrical conduction across the AV groove in the region of ventricular pre-excitation (Durrer and Roos, 1967). Burchell, of the Mayo Clinic, did intraoperative mapping in a patient who had the WPW syndrome and who was having closure of an atrial septal defect. After identifying the suspected site of the accessory pathway on the right free wall, he was able to abolish ventricular pre-excitation by injecting procainamide into the AV groove at that site (Burchell et al, 1967). Although the pre-excitation returned postoperatively, this procedure showed for the first time that a surgical technique might be capable of permanently interrupting conduction across an accessory pathway, thus curing the WPW syndrome. The first

surgical attempt at permanent ablation followed several months later, when Sealy, of Duke University, successfully divided a right free-wall accessory pathway in a 31-year-old fisherman (Cobb et al, 1968). Sixteen years later, Sealy published the following comment, which gives some insight into the role frequently occurring by serendipity in the advance of medical science:

Had Kent not published what are now considered to be incorrect observations, Wood and colleagues might never have found the right free-wall pathway. Had the fisherman's anomalous pathway been anyplace other than the right free-wall, I would not likely have found it at operation.

SEALY, 1984.

Indications for Operation

The major indication for surgical intervention in the WPW syndrome is medical refractoriness. Other common indications include patient intolerance to drug therapy, detrimental side effects of antiarrhythmic agents, and poor patient compliance. Major additions to these surgical indications include (1) recurrent supraventricular tachycardia in young, otherwise healthy patients and (2) spontaneous atrial fibrillation that conducts rapidly enough antegrade across the accessory pathway to allow the induction of ventricular fibrillation from the atrium. The inclusion of young patients whose arrhythmias might be controlled with antiarrhythmic agents clearly represents a liberalization of previous surgical indications. However, operation for the WPW syndrome is no longer an experimental procedure, and because of safety and curative nature, it should be considered to be the conservative alternative to a lifetime of dependence on antiarrhythmic drugs.

Preoperative Electrophysiologic Evaluation

All patients who are to be subjected to operation for the WPW syndrome should first have an endocardial catheter electrophysiologic study. The purposes of the preoperative study are (1) to document that the arrhythmia is supraventricular in origin, (2) to evaluate the response of the supraventricular tachycardia to programmed electrical stimulation to determine if it is re-entrant or automatic, (3) to establish the conduction properties of the normal specialized conduction tissue, (4) to document that the etiology of the arrhythmia is on the basis of the WPW syndrome rather than some other type of supraventricular tachycardia, and (5) to define the location of the accessory pathway responsible for the WPW syndrome.

Intraoperative Electrophysiologic Mapping

The computerized intraoperative mapping system currently used at Barnes Hospital was developed in 1984 (Witkowski and Corr, 1984). The system is presently capable of recording 160 bipolar electrograms simultaneously, analyzing the data, and displaying it in various forms within 2 minutes after data acquisition. Analog data recorded from the heart enter the front-end system located in the operating theater, where each electrogram is individually filtered and digitized. The digitized data are then transferred across a fiberoptic cable to a remote computer facility located approximately 1,500 meters away. The personnel in the operating theater and those in the computer facility are connected by both an audio system (headphones) and a video camera and display system for constant communication during the mapping procedure. Only 16 channels of the mapping system are used for patients having operation for WPW syndrome, but all 160 channels are used to map atrial flutter, atrial fibrillation, ectopic atrial tachycardias, and ventricular tachyarrhythmias.

The computerized mapping system has precluded the need to use cardiopulmonary bypass for the intraoperative mapping of patients with WPW syndrome. Epicardial pacing and sensing electrodes are sutured onto the atrium and ventricle near the suspected site of the accessory pathway. The band

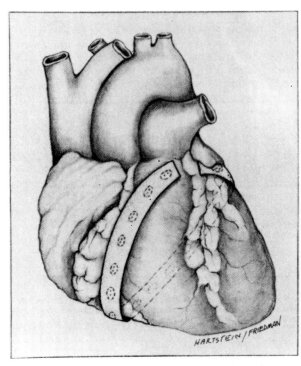

Figure 55–10. Diagrammatic sketch showing the placement of the band electrode around the ventricular side of the AV groove in a patient with the WPW syndrome during stable antegrade pre-excitation. (From Cox, J. L.: Intraoperative computerized mapping techniques. *In* Brugada, P., and Wellens, H. J. J. [eds]: Cardiac Arrhythmias: Where to Go From Here? Mount Kisco, NY, Futura Publishing Co., 1987.)

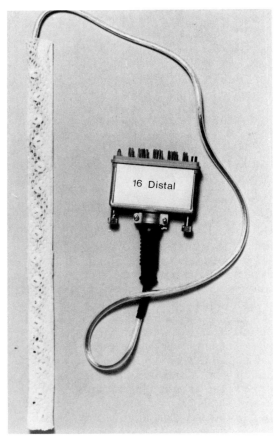

Figure 55–9. Epicardial band containing 16 bipolar button electrodes. (From Kramer, J. B., Corr, P. B., Cox, J. L., et al: Arrhythmia and conduction disturbances: Simultaneous computer mapping to facilitate intraoperative localization of accessory pathways in patients with Wolff-Parkinson-White syndrome. Am. J. Cardiol., 56:571, 1985.)

electrode (Fig. 55–9) (Kramer et al, 1985) is placed around the ventricular side of the AV groove (Fig. 55–10), and electrograms are recorded simultaneously from the 16 bipolar electrodes during normal sinus rhythm and during atrial pacing (see Fig. 55–6B). Two minutes later, three digitized tracings from the standard ECG are displayed simultaneously on the color graphics terminals in the operating theater and in the computer facility. The adjustable window is positioned over the pre-excited QRS complex (Fig. 55–11), and the computer is commanded to display the activation sequence of the 16 electrodes during the time interval encompassed by the window. The 16 digitized electrograms are then displayed automatically on the graphics terminals, and the point of rapid deflection (local activation time) is marked automatically by a vertical cursor on each electrogram (Fig. 55–12). The electrogram recorded from the electrode located nearest the site of the ventricular insertion of the accessory pathway shows the earliest activation. This method of graphics display is helpful particularly in detecting the presence of multiple accessory pathways that are capable of conducting in the antegrade direction.

The band electrode is then moved to the atrial side of the AV groove (Fig. 55–13), and reciprocating tachycardia is induced with programmed electrical stimulation (see Fig. 55–8B). Only a few cycles of

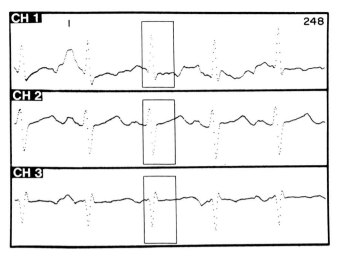

Figure 55–11. Hard copy of the color graphics terminal display of three digitized standard ECG leads used to select the desired pre-excited QRS complex (*inside window*). The window can be narrowed or enlarged and can be moved to any portion of the QRS complex. (From Cox, J. L.: Intraoperative computerized mapping techniques. *In* Brugada, P., and Wellens, H. J. J. [eds]: Cardiac Arrhythmias: Where to Go From Here? Mount Kisco, NY, Futura Publishing Co., 1987.)

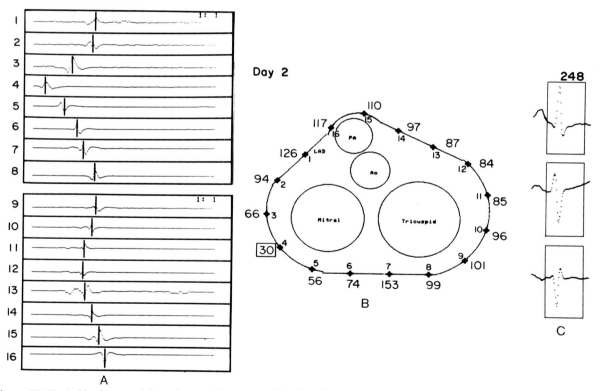

Figure 55–12. *A,* Hard copy of the color graphics terminal display showing the activation sequence of the 16 electrodes contained in the band. Because this is an antegrade ventricular pre-excitation map and the band has been placed on the ventricular side of the AV groove, the electrode showing the earliest activation (electrode number 4) is located at the site of the ventricular insertion of the accessory pathway. *B* and *C,* Hard copy of the color graphics terminal display showing the activation sequence of the base of the ventricles during stable antegrade pre-excitation. The designated window is displayed on the right side of the screen. The activation sequence is related to a sketch of the base of the heart, and the earliest site of ventricular activity during stable antegrade pre-excitement is enclosed in a box. (Modified from Cox, J. L.: Intraoperative computerized techniques. *In* Brugada, P., and Wellens, H. J. J. [eds]: Cardiac Arrhythmias: Where to Go From Here? Mount Kisco, NY, Futura Publishing Co., 1987.)

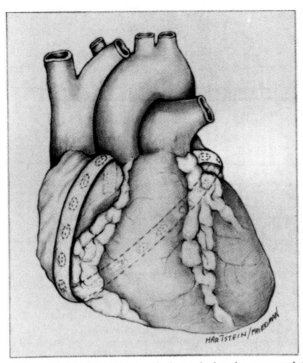

Figure 55–13. Once the band electrode has been moved to the atrial side of the AV groove as demonstrated in this diagram, reciprocating tachycardia is induced and a retrograde atrial map is performed. (From Cox, J. L.: Intraoperative computerized mapping techniques. *In* Brugada, P., and Wellens, H. J. J. [eds]: Cardiac Arrhythmias: Where to Go From Here? Mount Kisco, NY, Futura Publishing Co., 1987.)

is detected during the computerized mapping procedure, the patient is placed on cardiopulmonary bypass, a right atriotomy is performed, and endocardial mapping of the right atrium and atrial septum is completed by using the hand-held single-point mapping system before proceeding with surgical dissection.

Surgical Technique

Accessory AV connections may be located anywhere around the annulus fibrosus of the heart except between the right and left fibrous trigones (Fig. 55–16). However, from a surgical standpoint, their locations are classified as (1) left free wall, (2) right free wall, (3) anterior septal, and (4) posterior septal. In decreasing order of frequency, accessory pathways are located in the left free wall, posterior septal, right free wall, and anterior septal positions (Cox et al, 1985b). Twenty per cent of the patients in the author's series have had multiple (two, three, or four) accessory pathways.

The objective of operative procedures for the WPW syndrome is to divide the accessory pathways responsible for the syndrome. By definition, these strands of conducting tissue must connect to the atrium on one end and to the ventricle on the other end. In addition, both the atrial and ventricular connections must be located between the annulus of one of the AV valves and the epicardial reflection that covers the AV groove fat pad (Fig. 55–17A). This arrangement dictates that all accessory pathways must course through the AV groove fat pad unless they are located immediately adjacent to the valve annulus or immediately beneath the epicardium. Physiologically, an accessory pathway is analogous

tachycardia are allowed to occur, because hemodynamic compromise is common and the patients are not on cardiopulmonary bypass. Atrial electrograms are recorded from the bipolar electrodes on the band, and again the digitized ECG tracings are displayed. Because only the retrograde atrial data are of interest, the window is positioned over that portion of the ECG tracing that contains the retrograde P wave (Fig. 55–14). The computer then displays the activation sequence of the atrial electrograms recorded during reciprocating tachycardia (Fig. 55–15). Because the band electrode is usually too long for the atrial aspect of the AV groove, the distal three to five electrodes on the band are usually not in contact with the atria and are therefore ignored. This display of the atrial data is especially important because it shows unsuspected concealed accessory pathways that would have remained undetected until this point in the mapping procedure. When reciprocating tachycardia cannot be induced, the retrograde atrial map is recorded during ventricular pacing.

The antegrade and retrograde mapping techniques described are capable of detecting not only free-wall pathways but also anterior septal and posterior septal accessory pathways. However, if either

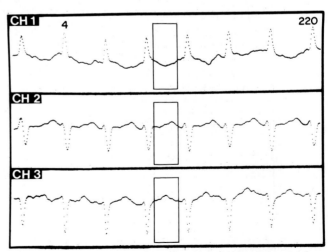

Figure 55–14. Hard copy of the color graphics terminal display showing the window centered over the suspected site of the retrograde P wave (following QRS complex) during reciprocating tachycardia. (From Cox, J. L.: Intraoperative computerized mapping techniques. *In* Brugada, P., and Wellens, H. J. J. [eds]: Cardiac Arrhythmias: Where to Go From Here? Mount Kisco, NY, Futura Publishing Co., 1987.)

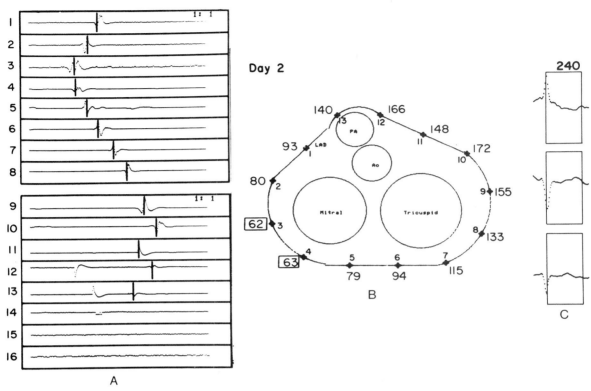

Figure 55–15. *A,* Hard copy of the color graphics terminal display showing the activation sequence of the base of the atrium during reciprocating tachycardia as determined by the band electrode array. The distal three electrograms were not in contact with the heart and are therefore to be ignored. *B* and *C,* Hard copy of the color graphics terminal display showing the retrograde atrial activation sequence of the base of the atrium during reciprocating tachycardia superimposed on a diagrammatic sketch of the base of the heart. Electrodes 3 and 4 activate almost simultaneously, indicating that the insertion of the atrial end of the accessory pathway is located midway between these two electrodes. (Modified from Cox, J. L.: Intraoperative computerized mapping techniques. *In* Brugada, P., and Wellens, H. J. J. [eds]: Cardiac Arrhythmias: Where to Go From Here? Mount Kisco, NY, Futura Publishing Co., 1987.)

Figure 55–16. Diagram of the superior view of the heart with the atria cut away, showing the boundaries of each of the four anatomic areas where accessory pathways can occur in the Wolff-Parkinson-White syndrome. The boundaries of the *left free-wall* space are the mitral valve annulus and the ventricular epicardial reflection and extend from the left fibrous trigone to the posterior septum. The boundaries of the *posterior septal* space are the tricuspid valve annulus, the mitral valve annulus, the posterior superior process of the left ventricle, and the ventricular epicardial reflection. The boundaries of the *right free-wall* space are the tricuspid valve annulus and the epicardial reflection extending from the posterior septum to the anterior septum. The boundaries of the *anterior septal* space are the tricuspid valve annulus, the membranous portion of the interatrial septum, and the ventricular epicardial reflection. All accessory AV connections must insert into the ventricle *somewhere* within these anatomic boundaries. (From Cox, J. L., Gallagher, J. J., and Cain, M. E.: Experience with 118 consecutive patients undergoing surgery for Wolff-Parkinson-White syndrome. J. Thorac. Cardiovasc. Surg., *90:*490, 1985.)

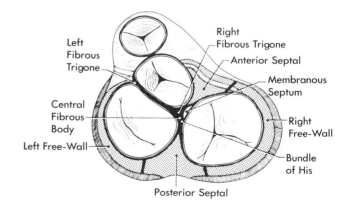

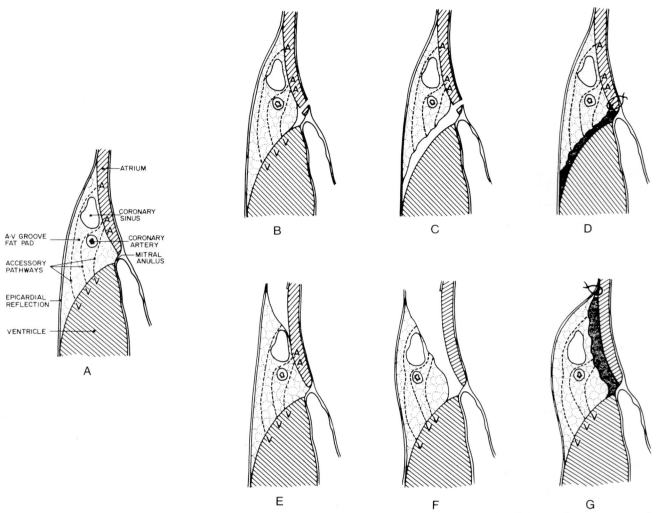

Figure 55–17. A cross-section of the posterior left heart showing the different depths at which left free-wall pathways can be located in relation to the mitral annulus and epicardial reflection (*A*). The endocardial surgical technique is shown in *B* to *D* and the epicardial technique in *E* to *G*.

to a wire that conducts electrical activity, and as such, it is unimportant which end of the wire is divided because division at either end will permanently interrupt conduction.

Two approaches are commonly used to divide accessory AV connections (see Fig. 55–17). The endocardial technique is designed to divide the ventricular end of the accessory pathway, and the epicardial technique is directed toward division of the atrial end of the pathway. Although some controversy has arisen regarding which approach is preferable (Cox, 1986; Guiraudon et al, 1986a), excellent results can be obtained with both techniques (Cox et al, 1985b; Guiraudon et al, 1986b; Klein et al, 1984).

LEFT FREE-WALL ACCESSORY PATHWAYS

Endocardial Technique. Accessory pathways on the left free wall are approached through a left atriotomy after the heart has been arrested with cold potassium cardioplegia. A supra-annular incision is placed 2 mm above the mitral valve annulus (see Fig. 55–17B) extending from the left fibrous trigone to the posterior septum (Fig. 55–18A and B). The entire space is dissected completely in every patient regardless of the precise location of the accessory pathway within the space because early operative experience proved that more localized dissections were followed by an unacceptable recurrence rate (Gallagher et al, 1984b). Recurrences are believed to occur because the anatomic connections between the atrium and ventricle within a given space frequently are broad bands and electrical conduction occurs predominantly over only one specific and precise portion of that broad band in some patients. If only that portion of the connection that is predominantly conducting electrical activity is divided, another part of the broad connection, either dormant or blocked preoperatively, may begin to conduct postoperatively. Three observations lend credibility to this hypothesis: (1) The plane of dissection between the AV groove fat pad and the ventricle is always abnormal at the site of an accessory pathway in that the fat is tightly adherent to the muscle; this region of abnormal adherence varies from 0.5 cm in width to as much as two-thirds of the entire anatomic space. (2) When early reoperations for failed procedures were common, as many as four separate operations were required before the accessory pathway was finally divided; the last operation invariably included dissection of the entire anatomic space. (3) Since initiating dissection of the entire anatomic space in every patient in 1981, not a single reoperation has been required and no patient has had an early or late recurrence. The principle of dissecting the entire anatomic space in every patient regardless of the precise location of the accessory pathway within that particular space is applied not only to left free-wall accessory pathways but also to those occurring in the posterior septal, right free-wall, and anterior septal spaces.

After the supra-annular incision is placed, a plane of dissection is established between the underlying AV groove fat pad and the top of the left ventricle throughout the length of the supra-annular incision (see Fig. 55–18C). It is important to extend this plane of dissection all the way to the epicardial reflection off the posterior left ventricle to be certain

to divide any accessory pathway that might be located in the subepicardial position in the AV groove (see Figs. 55–17C and 55–18D). After this dissection, it is still theoretically possible for a small accessory pathway located immediately adjacent to the valve annulus to be intact unless the annulus has been cleaned meticulously with a sharp nerve hook or knife. To preclude this possibility, the two ends of the supra-annular incision are then squared off (Fig. 55–19C) so that even if such a juxta-annular pathway survives the dissection the small rim of atrial tissue to which it would be attached will be isolated from the remainder of the heart and therefore the potential conduction circuit will be interrupted. This dissection exposes the entire left free-wall space and each of its boundaries; therefore, there is no other site in this space where an accessory pathway could insert onto the ventricle.

Epicardial Technique. The epicardial approach to left free-wall accessory pathways incorporates dissection from the atrial side of the AV groove. The epicardial reflection off the atrium is opened, and a plane of dissection is established between the AV groove fat pad and the atrial wall (see Fig. 55–17E). The plane of dissection is extended to the level of the posterior mitral valve annulus and carried slightly onto the top of the posterior left ventricle (see Fig. 55–17F). This dissection necessarily divides the atrial end of all accessory pathways in this region except those that are located immediately adjacent to the

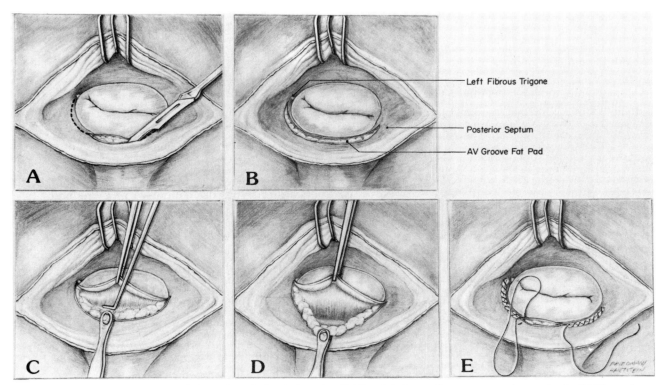

Figure 55–18. Surgeon's view of the endocardial technique for dividing left free-wall accessory pathways in the WPW syndrome. (Modified from Cox, J. L., Gallagher, J. J., and Cain, M. E.: Experience with 118 consecutive patients undergoing surgery for Wolff-Parkinson-White syndrome. J. Thorac. Cardiovasc. Surg., *90*:490, 1985.)

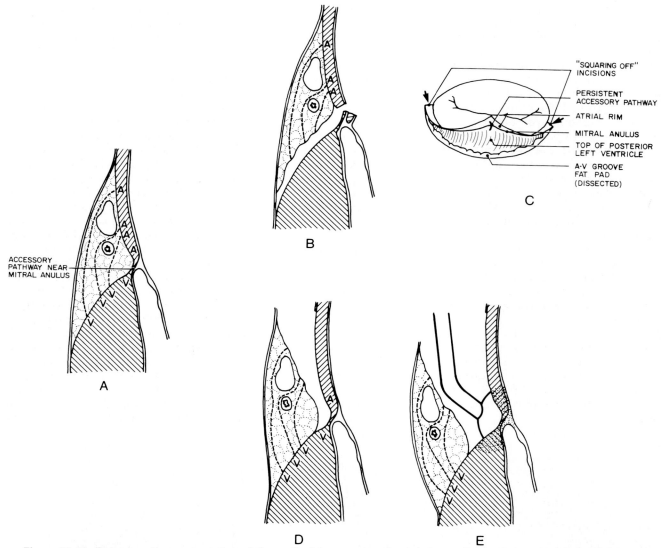

ACCESSORY
PATHWAY NEAR
MITRAL ANULUS

A

B

"SQUARING OFF"
INCISIONS

PERSISTENT
ACCESSORY PATHWAY

ATRIAL RIM

MITRAL ANULUS

TOP OF POSTERIOR
LEFT VENTRICLE

A-V GROOVE
FAT PAD
(DISSECTED)

C

D

E

Figure 55–19. Diagrammatic representation of the method for ensuring that left free-wall accessory pathways located near the mitral annulus (*A*) are deactivated using the endocardial technique (*B, C*) and the epicardial technique (*D, E*).

mitral valve annulus. Advocates of this technique state that the ventricular pre-excitation caused by antegrade conduction across the accessory pathway disappears in almost every case during this dissection (Guiraudon et al, 1986b), indicating that the pathway has been divided. Despite this observation, they recommend placement of one or more cryolesions at the level of the mitral valve annulus to destroy any accessory pathways located immediately adjacent to the valve annulus that might have survived the dissection (see Fig. 55–19*E*). Although cryosurgery is unnecessary if the pathway has already been divided by the dissection (i.e., ventricular pre-excitation has disappeared), this technique has nevertheless been labeled a "cryosurgical technique" by its advocates (Klein et al, 1984). Moreover, to expose the atrial side of the AV groove on the left side of the heart (the

most common site of accessory pathways), it is necessary to elevate the apex of the heart out of the pericardium. In most patients, this maneuver causes hypotension to such an extent that cardiopulmonary bypass must be instituted to maintain stable hemodynamics. Despite the fact that almost all of these patients require total cardiopulmonary bypass, this technique has also been called a "closed heart procedure" (Guiraudon et al, 1986a, 1986b). Moreover, one should remember that to obtain a true perspective of the atrial dissection with this technique, Figure 55–17*E, F, G* and Figure 55–19*D* and *E* should be turned upside down.

POSTERIOR SEPTAL ACCESSORY PATHWAYS

In the past, posterior septal accessory pathways were considered to be the most difficult to divide successfully, and because the bundle of His is located in this space, the dissection was frequently complicated by inadvertent heart block (Gallagher et al, 1984b). However, since 1981, posterior septal pathways have proved to be perhaps the easiest to treat surgically, and the problem of postoperative heart block is now of historical interest only (Cox et al, 1985b).

Normothermic cardiopulmonary bypass is instituted and a right atriotomy is done to expose the triangle of Koch (see Fig. 55–4). The position of the bundle of His is identified with a hand-held electrode (Fig. 55–20A), and the right atrial endocardium is mapped during induced reciprocating tachycardia to confirm the findings of the computerized epicardial mapping. A supra-annular incision is placed 2 mm above the posterior medial tricuspid valve annulus beginning well posterior to the bundle of His (see Fig. 55–20B). The supra-annular incision is extended in a counterclockwise direction well onto the free wall of the posterior right atrium (see Fig. 55–20C). This latter extension is important for two reasons: (1) It provides a larger incision for better exposure in the depths of the posterior septal space near the posterior-superior process of the left ventricle and (2) it simplifies identification of the epicardial reflection off the posterior right ventricle, a landmark that is to be followed across the crux of the heart to the posterior left ventricle during dissection of the posterior septal space.

When the fat pad occupying the posterior septal space has been identified through the supra-annular incision (see Fig. 55–20D), a plane of dissection is established between the fat pad and the top of the posterior ventricular septum (Fig. 55–20E). Before cardioplegic arrest is begun, this plane is developed in the *anterior* portion of the posterior septal space closest to the bundle of His, approaching the central body from the posterior direction. The junction of the posterior medial mitral and triscupid valve annuli forms a V at the posterior edge of the central fibrous body, and the fat pad comes to a point at the apex of that V (see Fig. 55–16). The apex of the V is always posterior to the bundle of His, although the distance between the apex of the V and the bundle of His may vary. However, as long as the dissection in this region remains posterior to the central fibrous body, the bundle of His will not be damaged. When the anterior point of the fat pad is gently dissected away from the apex of the V (i.e., away from the posterior edge of the central fibrous body), the mitral valve annulus comes into view at the point where it joins the tricuspid valve to form the central fibrous body. The heart is usually arrested with cold potassium cardioplegia at this time, but it is not absolutely necessary to do so. If the plane of dissection is relatively bloodless and easily identified, the entire posterior septal space can be dissected with the heart beating. However, if the plane is extremely vascular from the beginning, it is acceptable to perform the entire dissection under cardioplegic arrest. In the past, surgeons were reluctant to do the latter for fear of injuring the bundle of His during the dissection, but with a more complete understanding of the

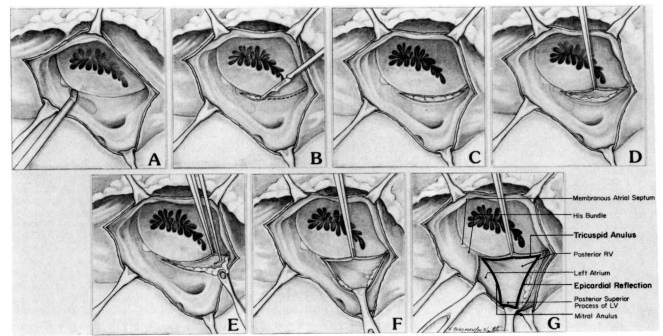

Figure 55–20. Endocardial technique for surgical division of posterior septal accessory pathways in the WPW syndrome. (Modified from Cox, J. L., Gallagher, J. J., and Cain, M. E.: Experience with 118 consecutive patients undergoing surgery for Wolff-Parkinson-White syndrome. J. Thorac. Cardiovasc. Surg., *90*:490, 1985.)

anatomic relationships between the posterior edge of the central fibrous body (the apex of the V) and the bundle of His, this is no longer a concern.

Because the epicardial reflection off the posterior right ventricle has already been identified (see Fig. 55–20F), visualization of the mitral valve annulus in the anterior portion of the posterior septal space (see Fig. 55–20G) completes the identification of the boundaries of dissection of the space. The plane of dissection between the fat pad and the top of the posterior ventricular septum is developed completely by following the mitral annulus over to the posterior-superior process of the left ventricle and by following the epicardial reflection from the posterior right ventricle, across the posterior crux, onto the posterior left ventricle. It is essential to divide all structures penetrating the posterior ventricular septum in the posterior septal space, including, if necessary, the AV node artery. It has been found that the AV node artery does leave the fat pad to enter the posterior ventricular septum within the posterior septal space in approximately 50% of patients with posterior septal accessory pathways. In every case, it has been ligated and no AV node dysfunction has resulted. On the contrary, the author has on several occasions been contacted by surgeons who have done perfect dissections of the posterior septal space, except that a penetrating AV node artery has been spared, and the accessory pathway has reappeared postoperatively. On each of these occasions, an immediate reoperation to divide the AV node artery (with the accompanying accessory pathway) cured the patient.

RIGHT FREE-WALL PATHWAYS

Right free-wall accessory pathways are the one condition in which the epicardial technique without cardioplegic arrest is probably as easy to perform as the endocardial technique with cardioplegic arrest. The epicardial technique can usually be applied in these patients without cardiopulmonary bypass, making it a true closed heart procedure in this case. However, the author prefers to open the right atrium to do endocardial mapping because there is frequently a larger amount of fat in the AV groove on the right side, making the epicardial mapping less than optimal. After the accessory pathway is localized, the heart is cardioplegically arrested and a supra-annular incision is placed 2 mm above the tricuspid valve annulus around the entire free right wall (see Fig. 55–16). A plane of dissection is established between the underlying AV groove fat pad and the top of the right ventricle throughout the length of the supra-annular incision. This dissection plane is developed all the way to the epicardial reflection off the ventricle so that the entire right ventricular free wall that is in contact with the AV groove fat pad is free of any penetrating fibers from the fat pad.

Two additional potential problems with right free-wall dissections do not exist on the left side: (1)

The plane of dissection between the AV groove fat pad and the heart (atrium or ventricle) is not as well defined on the right, and (2) the atrium and ventricle tend to "fold over" on each other at the tricuspid annulus (Fig. 55–21). The latter condition results in right-sided pathways that appear to be located in a more endocardial position than those on the left side, but in fact they are not. Because of the folding over of the right atrial and ventricular walls at the annular level, the AV groove fat pad does not actually touch the true tricuspid valve annulus as it does the mitral annulus on the left. Therefore, when the fat pad is dissected away from the tricuspid annulus using the epicardial technique, the ventricular pre-excitation usually remains. This observation has been reported on several occasions by the advocates of the epicardial technique, who have erroneously attributed it to a more endocardial location of right free-wall pathways (Guiraudon et al, 1986b). Just as is the case on the left, right-sided accessory pathways must connect to the atrium somewhere between the valve annulus and the atrial epicardial reflection and to the ventricle somewhere between the valve annulus and the ventricular epicardial reflection. Unlike the left side, however, the folded over anatomy of the tricuspid annulus simply precludes the division of accessory pathways located adjacent to the annulus by dissection of the fat pad away from the heart. To interrupt these right free-wall accessory pathways that reside too close to the valve annulus to be divided by routine dissection, one of three adjunctive measures must be added to the dissection: (1) mechanical

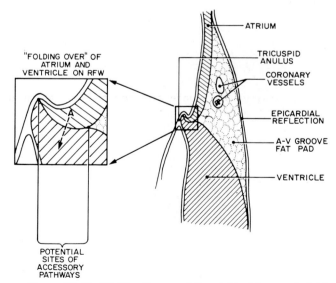

Figure 55–21. "Folding" over of the right atrium and right ventricle near the tricuspid annulus on the right free wall. Note that simple dissection of the AV groove fat pad away from the ventricle (endocardial technique) or atrium (epicardial technique) will not divide accessory pathways connecting the atrium and ventricle if they are near the tricuspid annulus. This is a common location for right free-wall accessory pathways, accounting for the erroneous concept that they are endocardial pathways.

"unfolding" of the atrium and ventricle so that the true valve annulus can be seen and freed of any adjacent fibers connecting the atrium and ventricle (applicable to both the epicardial and endocardial techniques), (2) application of a cryolesion to the tissues near the valve annulus to destroy the juxta-annular accesssory pathway (applicable to both techniques), or (3) squaring off of the supra-annular incision at both ends to isolate the atrial rim of tissue to which a juxta-annular accessory pathway would connect (applicable to the endocardial technique).

Finally, it is noteworthy that the folding over of the atrium and ventricle at the level of the tricuspid annulus is much more pronounced in patients with Ebstein's anomaly, a condition present in 14% of the patients in the author's series. This is true whether the patient has the classic Ebstein's anomaly or only the forme fruste of the disease.

ANTERIOR SEPTAL ACCESSORY PATHWAYS

Epicardial mapping is excellent for documenting existence of an anterior septal pathway, but it does not localize these pathways precisely because of the large fat pad covering both the atrium and ventricle in the anterior septal space. Therefore, endocardial mapping is especially important in these patients, particularly because in the author's experience these pathways are more frequently located adjacent to the bundle of His (anteriorly) than are posterior septal pathways (posteriorly) (see Fig. 55–16). After retrograde endocardial mapping is completed, a supra-annular incision is placed just anterior to the bundle of His 2 mm above the tricuspid annulus and extended to a clockwise direction well onto the right anterior free wall. The initial incision frequently abolishes ventricular pre-excitation, but whether or not pre-excitation persists, the entire anterior septal space is dissected (see Fig. 55–16). After the initial supra-annular incision is completed, a plane of dissection is established between the fat pad occupying the anterior septal space and the top of the right ventricle. This plane of dissection is developed completely to the aorta medially and to the epicardial reflection off the ventricle anteriorly. During this dissection, the fat pad must be retracted very gently to avoid injury to the proximal right coronary artery, which courses through the fat pad before entering the AV groove of the anterior right free wall. In addition, when the anteromedial portion of the anterior septal space is being dissected, extreme care should be taken to avoid injury to the aorta. This is actually the external surface of the right coronary sinus of Valsalva beneath the orifice of the right coronary artery, and it therefore is quite thin.

Surgical Results

The incidence of successful surgical correction of the WPW syndrome now approaches 100%, with an operative mortality for elective, uncomplicated cases that ranges from 0 to .5% (Cox et al, 1985b; Guiraudon et al, 1986b). No early or late recurrences have followed use of the endocardial technique in the author's series (Cox et al, 1985b), and the recurrence rate after the epicardial technique is small (Guiraudon et al, 1986b). Moreover, the inadvertent creation of heart block is no longer a problem. Whether the surgeon uses the endocardial or the epicardial approach, these surgical results require liberalization of the previous limited surgical indications for this curable congenital cardiac abnormality.

Paroxysmal Supraventricular Tachycardia

Concealed Accessory Atrioventricular Connection

Accessory AV connections may be "manifest" or "concealed." If an accessory pathway is capable of conducting in the antegrade (atrial-to-ventricular) direction thus causing a delta wave on the standard ECG, it is said to be manifest—that is, its presence is apparent electrocardiographically (see Figs. 55–6 and 55–7). The retrograde (ventricular-to-atrial) conduction characteristics of such a pathway determine the heart rate and frequency of occurrence of the associated reciprocating tachycardia. Some patients harbor accessory AV connections that are capable of conducting in the *retrograde direction only*. Because antegrade conduction across the accessory pathway does not occur, the ventricles are activated only through the normal AV node bundle of His complex and the standard ECG is normal. Therefore, these accessory pathways are said to be concealed. Because these accessory pathways are capable of conducting in the retrograde direction, however, reciprocating tachycardia can occur just as it does in the classic WPW syndrome (see Fig. 55–8B). Thus, from a clinical standpoint, the only difference between patients with manifest accessory pathways and those with concealed accessory pathways is the appearance of the standard ECG during normal sinus rhythm. The former have an ECG characteristic of the WPW syndrome, and the latter have a normal ECG.

Paroxysmal supraventricular tachycardia (PSVT) is a contemporary term for what was earlier called paroxysmal atrial tachycardia. PSVT is a clinical condition in which supraventricular tachycardia occurs suddenly in a patient who otherwise has a *normal* ECG. Two abnormalities account for essentially all PSVT: a concealed accessory AV connection and AV node re-entry. In patients with a concealed accessory pathway, the absence of antegrade conduction across the pathway precludes the necessity of performing antegrade ventricular mapping intraoperatively. Thus, only retrograde atrial mapping is performed, and these maps are recorded during ventricular pacing or during induced reciprocating tachycardia (see Figs. 55–13 to 55–15). The surgical technique used to divide concealed accessory pathways is the same as for patients with the classic WPW syndrome.

Atrioventricular Node Re-entry

AV node re-entry tachycardia is caused by a re-entrant circuit that is confined to the AV node or to the perinodal tissues of the lower atrial septum. The anatomic-electrophysiologic basis for this re-entrant circuit is the presence of two conduction routes, one slow and one fast, through the AV node, the so-called dual AV node conduction pathways (Fig. 55–22).

Before 1982, the only surgical therapy available for patients with medically refractory AV node re-entry tachycardia was elective cryoablation of the bundle of His (Sealy et al, 1981). This operation did not ablate AV node re-entry, but it did confine the tachycardia to the atria, thus relieving the patient's symptoms of tachycardia. Obviously, a ventricular pacemaker was necessary after cryoablation of the bundle of His. In 1982, a closed chest technique was developed for permanent ablation of the bundle of

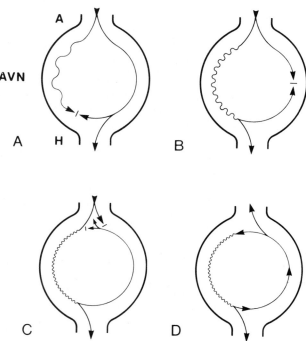

Figure 55–22. Schematic presentation of impulse propagation along the fast and slow conducting pathways in AV node re-entry. The sinus or paced atrial impulse preferentially negotiates the bundle of His via the fast pathway (A). Owing to longer refractoriness of the fast pathway, an atrial premature beat may block it (B) while engaging the bundle of His via the slow pathway and then retrogradely penetrate the fast pathway (B). Depending on the recovery of tissue ahead, the returning impulse may produce a single echo (Ae) beat (C) or sustained arrhythmia (D). D, The situation during sustained intranodal reciprocation is shown, with activation of the atrium and bundle of His shown to be incidental. (A = atrium; AVN = AV node; H = bundle of His.) (From Akhtar, M.: Supraventricular tachycardias: Electrophysiologic mechanisms, diagnosis, and pharmacologic therapy. In Josephson, M. E., and Wellens, H. J. J. [eds]: Tachycardias: Mechanisms, Diagnosis, Treatment. Philadelphia, Lea & Febiger, 1984.)

His in which 200 to 500 joules were delivered through a bundle of His catheter (Scheinman et al, 1982). This procedure effectively replaced surgical cryoablation of the bundle of His for the treatment of medically refractory AV node re-entry tachycardia because it did not require an open heart operation. However, because cryoablation or catheter ablation of the bundle of His replaces one problem (tachycardia) with another (heart block), a surgical technique capable of interrupting the actual re-entrant circuit responsible for AV node re-entry tachycardia without blocking normal AV conduction was developed. This was accomplished by placing multiple discrete (3 mm) cryolesions around the triangle of Koch (see Fig. 55–4) to alter the input pathways of the AV node, resulting in permanent prolongation of AV conduction in experimental animals (Holman et al, 1982). Subsequent studies documented that in the presence of dual AV node conduction pathways, this discrete cryosurgical procedure was capable of selectively ablating only one of the pathways of conduction, thus leaving normal AV conduction intact while interrupting the anatomic-electrophysiologic substrate responsible for AV node re-entry tachycardia (Holman et al, 1984, and 1986). After the salutory effects of this approach in experimental animals were developed and characterized, this procedure was applied to patients with AV node re-entry tachycardia (Cox, 1983b; Cox et al, 1987).

The heart is exposed through either a median sternotomy or a right anterior thoracotomy in the fourth intercostal space. The aorta and both venae cavae are cannulated for cardiopulmonary bypass, and epicardial plaque electrodes are sutured to the right atrium and right ventricle. After incremental atrial pacing and induction and termination of AV node re-entry tachycardia, normothermic cardiopulmonary bypass is instituted and a right atriotomy is done. A hand-held probe is used to confirm that the bundle of His is in its normal position at the apex of the triangle of Koch (see Fig. 55–20A). Atrial pacing is then instituted, and the AV interval is monitored on a beat-to-beat basis. A nitrous oxide cryoprobe with a 3-mm-diameter tip is then placed over the tendon of Tadaro at the upper edge of the os of the coronary sinus (Fig. 55–23A). Cryothermia is applied at a temperature of −60° C for 2 minutes. Three more cryolesions are placed along the tendon of Todaro, moving sequentially toward the apex of the triangle of Koch near the bundle of His (sites 2, 3, and 4 in Fig. 55–23B). Cryothermia is applied at each site for 2 minutes or until transient heart block occurs. In the author's experience, the placement of the first four cryolesions does not result in significant prolongation of the AV interval.

Cryolesions are then placed along the annulus of the tricupsid valve, beginning just beneath the os of the coronary sinus (sites 5, 6, 7, and 8 in Fig. 55–23B). Prolongation of the AV interval usually occurs first during application of cryothermia at sites 7 or 8. It is important to apply cryothermia to each of these

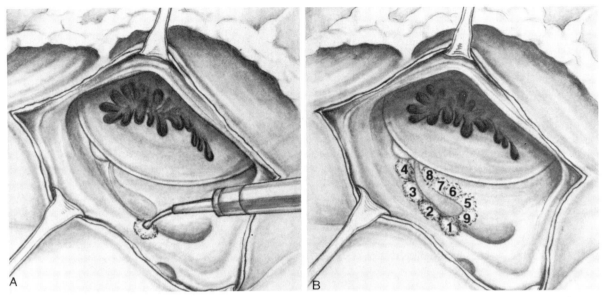

Figure 55–23. Discrete cryosurgical procedure for the treatment of AV node re-entry tachycardia. A 3-mm cryoprobe is used to place nine cryolesions around the periphery of the AV node (*B*), beginning at the upper edge of the os of the coronary sinus (*A*). (Modified from Cox, J. L., Holman, W. L., and Cain, M. E.: Cryosurgical treatment of atrioventricular node reentry tachycardia. Circulation, 76:1329, 1987. By permission of the American Heart Association, Inc.)

sites for the full 2 minutes, if possible, because permanent tissue injury cannot be ensured otherwise (Mazur, 1968). Fortunately, the AV interval prolongs in a linear fashion during cryothermia application, allowing the electrophysiologist to notify the surgeon of the degree of AV interval prolongation with each succeeding beat. As the AV interval prolongs to approximately 200 to 300 msec, one can expect complete AV block to occur within the next few beats. Cryothermia is terminated instantly on the development of complete AV block, and the tip of the cryoprobe is irrigated immediately with copious amounts of warm saline. AV conduction invariably resumes within two to three beats, and the AV interval returns to its control value during the ensuing 10 to 15 beats. The cryoprobe is then moved slightly more peripherally until cryothermia can be applied for the full 2 minutes to a given site without causing heart block. In this manner, the cryoprobe serves as a "reversible knife" and permanent AV block is precluded, because the cryothermia would have to be applied for a more protracted interval to result in permanent conduction block.

After cryolesions are placed at sites 1 through 9 (see Fig. 55–23*B*), thus encircling the AV node, cryolesions are also placed at as many sites within the triangle of Koch as possible without creating permanent AV block, using the same end-point of temporary block as described previously. However, having placed the first nine cryolesions, it is usually impossible to apply cryothermia to additional sites within the triangle of Koch for 2 minutes without causing temporary block. In essence, the objective of this operation is to cryoablate as much of the peri-

nodal tissue as possible without causing permanent AV conduction block. This approach is feasible only because of the unique nature of cryosurgery, which allows a definitive end-point (complete heart block) to be reached but only on a temporary, reversible basis.

In patients with AV node re-entry tachycardia and concomitant WPW syndrome, the latter problem must be surgically corrected first before any attempt is made to treat the AV node re-entry. Correction of the WPW syndrome initially is essential because the discrete cryosurgical procedure for AV node re-entry depends on the ability to monitor exclusive conduction through the AV node-bundle of His complex on a beat-to-beat basis. If the patient has a functioning accessory pathway that conducts in the antegrade direction, it is impossible to monitor the effects of cryosurgical modification of normal AV conduction during atrial pacing because the atrial impulse travels preferentially across the accessory pathway to the ventricles.

Application of the discrete cryosurgical procedure has resulted in the selective ablation of only one of the two AV node conduction pathways present and has effected a permanent cure of the AV node re-entry tachycardia in all 23 patients in the author's series. No operative deaths have occurred. Results of the immediate and late postoperative electrophysiologic studies have shown smooth AV node conduction curves through the remaining single conduction pathway and no inducible AV node re-entry tachycardia. Moreover, all patients have maintained normal conduction through the AV node-bundle of His complex, with no recurrent tachycardia during a

7-year follow-up. Ross and colleagues (1985) have also reported excellent results with surgical dissection in the region of the AV node in several patients with AV node re-entry tachycardia.

Automatic Atrial Tachycardia

Automatic atrial tachycardias are frequently suppressed by general anesthesia, and as a result, intraoperative mapping to localize the site of origin may not be possible. However, if the arrhythmia persists intraoperatively so that it can be localized precisely, simple surgical excision or isolation of that part of the atrium or local cryoablation cures the problem

(Gallagher et al, 1984a). If the arrhythmogenic myocardium cannot be localized intraoperatively, elective cryoablation of the bundle of His has previously been the only alternative. Because of a desire to avoid having to resort to ablation of the bundle of His, alternative surgical techniques that leave normal AV conduction intact while isolating the arrhythmogenic atrial myocardium from the remainder of the heart have been developed.

Automatic *left atrial tachycardias* usually originate in the body of the left atrium. Because the SA node, internodal conduction routes, and AV node-bundle of His complex reside either in the right atrium or atrial septum, a technique has been developed to isolate the entire left atrium from the remainder of

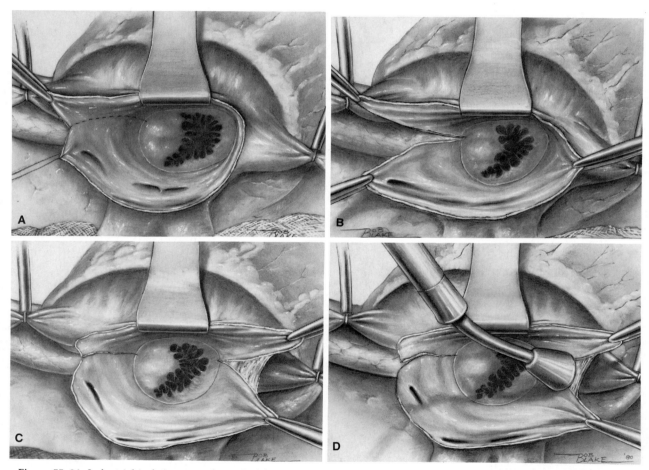

Figure 55–24. Left atrial isolation procedure. *A,* After a standard left atriotomy incision, the interatrial septum is retracted gently, and the atriotomy is extended anteriorly (dashed line) across Bachmann's bundle to the level of the mitral valve annulus just to the left of the right fibrous trigone. *B,* The anterior extension of the standard left atriotomy has been completed. The base of the aorta and its juxtaposition with the anterior leaflet of the mitral valve are demonstrated. Note that the anterior atriotomy extends across the mitral valve annulus. The main body of the left atrium has been separated anteriorly from the remainder of the heart. *C,* The transmural left atriotomy is extended posteriorly to the level of the coronary sinus. The remaining portion of the incision is made through the endocardium and extends across the mitral valve annulus posteriorly just to the left of the interatrial septum. At this point, electrical activity continues to be propagated in a 1:1 fashion between the right and left atria because of the presence of interatrial muscular connections accompanying the coronary sinus. *D,* A cryoprobe is positioned over the endocardial aspect of the posterior atriotomy, and its temperature is decreased to −60° C for 2 minutes. This cryolesion ablates the endocardial interatrial fibers accompanying the coronary sinus. A similar cryolesion is created on the epicardial aspect of the AV groove on the opposite side of the coronary sinus to ablate all remaining interatrial epicardial connections. The left atriotomy is closed with a continuous 4-0 nonabsorbable suture. (From Williams, J. M., Ungerleider, R. M., Lofland, G. K., and Cox, J. L.: Left atrial isolation: New technique for the treatment of supraventricular arrhythmias. J. Thorac. Cardiovasc. Surg., *80*:373, 1980.)

the heart, which then persists in normal sinus rhythm regardless of the presence or absence of tachycardia in the left atrium (Fig. 55–24) (Williams et al, 1980). After the left atrial isolation procedure, patients remain in normal sinus rhythm despite the presence of an incessant tachycardia confined to the left atrium (Fig. 55–25). A 7-year follow-up has shown no adverse sequelae from this procedure.

Right atrial tachycardias may occur on the basis of either automaticity or re-entry and are usually confined to the body of the right atrium. In the author's experience, the suppression of these arrhythmias by general anesthesia is slightly less of a problem intraoperatively than it is with left atrial automatic tachycardias. As mentioned earlier, if the automatic atrial tachycardias spontaneously occur intraoperatively or if the re-entrant atrial tachycardias can be induced intraoperatively, they can be mapped by electrophysiologic means and cryoablated. However, if the tachycardia cannot be induced intraoperatively, the surgeon has previously had to resort to ablation of the bundle of His with insertion of a permanent pacemaking system. A procedure has been developed to isolate the body of the right atrium while leaving the atrial pacemaker complex in continuity with the atrial septum and the ventricles (Fig. 55–26) (Harada et al, 1988). This technique was considerably more difficult to develop than was the left atrial

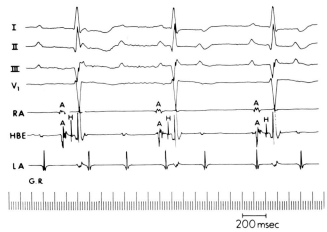

Figure 55–25. Postoperative recordings after surgical exclusion of the left atrium. Recordings from the top down are surface ECG leads I to III, V₁, bipolar catheter recordings of the right atrium (RA) and the bundle of His (HBE), and a bipolar recording obtained by permanent electrodes sutured to the left atrial (LA) appendage. The right and left atria are dissociated. Right atrial activity proceeds from the catheter positioned in the high right atrium to the atrial septum as recorded on the bundle of His catheter, followed by conduction to the ventricle. An irregular left atrial tachycardia is present, which fails to propagate to either the right atrium or to the ventricles. Note that the surface P wave correlates with left atrial activity, although the ventricles are responding to activity initiated in the right atrium. (From Gallagher, J. J., Cox, J. L., German, L. D., and Kasell, J. H.: Nonpharmacologic treatment of supraventricular tachycardia. *In* Josephson, M. E., and Wellens, H. J. J. [eds]: Tachycardias: Mechanisms, Diagnosis, Treatment. Philadelphia, Lea & Febiger, 1984.)

isolation procedure because of the complexities of the atrial pacemaker tissue and the anatomic variation of its blood supply. Nevertheless, the author has now isolated the right atrium in three patients, with cure of the tachycardia and no adverse sequelae during an 18-month follow-up (Fig. 55–27).

Atrial Flutter and Atrial Fibrillation

Studies by Boineau and associates (1980, 1984) of atrial flutter and by Allessie and colleagues (1984) of atrial fibrillation have documented that both of these supraventricular tachyarrhythmias are most likely to occur on the basis of macro-re-entrant circuits. This new information provides for the first time a "target" for the surgeon and will undoubtedly lead to the development of specific procedures to ablate these two arrhythmias. The detrimental hemodynamic effects of atrial flutter and atrial fibrillation, as well as the thromboembolic complications associated with both arrhythmias, appear to require the development of these surgical procedures. Surgical ablation of these arrhythmias appears particularly appropriate in patients having isolated mitral valve replacement, 60% of whom suffer from chronic atrial flutter/fibrillation (Salomon et al, 1977).

The earlier approach to this problem was to evaluate the potential beneficial effects of either a complete or partial left atrial isolation procedure. Experimentally, the complete left atrial isolation procedure has been shown to ablate chronic atrial flutter/fibrillation, but it results in a loss of synchrony of contraction of the left atrium. Incomplete isolation of the left atrium has proved to be unsatisfactory for the control of atrial flutter/fibrillation. However, the new knowledge and insights gained from the studies by Boineau and Allessie and their co-workers have encouraged the development of intraoperative computerized mapping techniques to identify the re-entrant circuits responsible for atrial flutter and atrial fibrillation (Canavan et al, 1988a, 1988b). The ability to map these complex arrhythmias will almost certainly lead to the development of specific surgical techniques for their ablation.

VENTRICULAR TACHYARRHYTHMIAS

Nonischemic Ventricular Tachycardia

The most common tachyarrhythmias arising in the ventricles are those associated with ischemic heart disease, but many types of ventricular tachycardia occur in the absence of coronary artery disease. Nonischemic ventricular tachycardias usually arise in the right ventricle, and although they are extremely resistant to medical therapy, newly developed surgical isolation techniques are proving to be most effective in their management. These arrhythmias have been classified into five categories based on their pathologic or clinical characteristics.

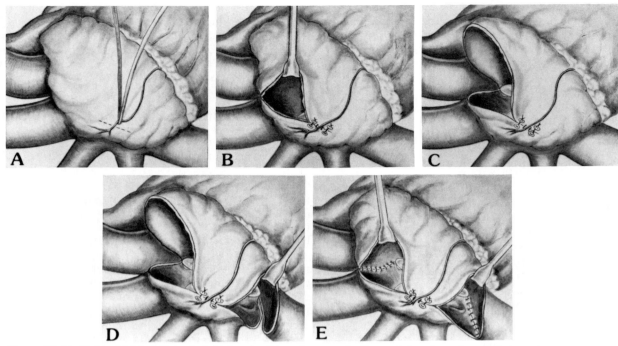

Figure 55–26. Right atrial isolation: *A,* Initially, the SA node artery is dissected free from the atrial tissue 5 mm anterior to the crista terminalis. A 2-cm incision parallel to the crista terminalis is placed beneath the artery. *B,* The incision beneath the SA node artery is closed with a continuous nonabsorbable 5-0 suture, and care is taken not to damage the artery. The small pledgets are used above and below the artery to reinforce the incision. The right atriotomy is then extended to a point anterior to the junction of the superior vena cava and the base of the right atrial appendage. *C,* The atriotomy is extended along the anterior limbus of the fossa ovalis to the anteromedial tricuspid valve annulus, just anterior to the membranous interatrial septum. *D,* Caudad extension of the right atriotomy around the posterior right atrial-inferior vena cava junction to the posterior-lateral tricuspid valve annulus. A cryolesion (−60° C for 2 minutes) is placed at the end of the incision to ensure complete interruption of connecting atrial muscle fibers between the body of the right atrium and the remainder of the heart. *E,* The atriotomy is closed with a continuous 4-0 nonabsorbable suture. (From Harada, A., D'Agostino, H. J., Jr., Schuessler, R. B., et al: Right atrial isolation: A new surgical treatment for supraventricular tachycardia. I.: Surgical technique and electrophysiologic effects. J. Thorac. Cardiovasc. Surg., *95*:643, 1988.)

Idiopathic ventricular tachycardia refers to an arrhythmia in patients in whom the only clinical manifestation of cardiac disease is the arrhythmia. Both the macroscopic appearance of the heart at operation and the pathologic data acquired at the time of autopsy in these patients fail to show any evidence of primary cardiac disease. The only abnormality noted is global dilatation of the heart secondary to functional post-tachycardia heart failure. If these patients require operation, they first have intraoperative electrophysiologic mapping during ventricular tachycardia in an effort to localize the apparent site of origin of the arrhythmia. Initial surgical approaches included simple ventriculotomy, exclusion procedures, and cryoablation, but the results were poor, primarily because many of these arrhythmias arise within the ventricular septum (Guiraudon et al, 1981). More recent approaches have included local isolation procedures if the site of origin is in the right ventricular free wall (Cox, 1983b; Cox et al, 1985a) and multipoint map-guided cryoablation if in the septum.

A small group of patients have ventricular tachycardia due to *nonischemic cardiomyopathy.* This group comprises patients with angiographic and catheter data indicating some type of abnormal myocardial contractility associated with recurrent ventricular tachycardia. These patients usually show a diffuse dilatation of both ventricles with widespread patchy myocardial fibrosis. These tachyarrhythmias frequently arise in the right ventricle, and the author's approach to these patients has been to use a combination of surgical isolation and cryoablation of the apparent site of origin of the arrhythmia. One patient, a 16-year-old female with coxsackievirus myocarditis, was documented to have intermittent ventricular tachycardia for 7 years after initial viral infection. Preoperative electrophysiologic studies indicated that the ventricular tachycardia arose from the pulmonary infundibulum near the level of the pulmonic valve annulus. However, the intraoperative electrophysiologic studies showed that the tachycardia arose in the high right ventricular septum between the crista supraventricularis and the pulmonic valve annulus. A combination of surgical isolation and cryoablation of the apparent site of origin of the ventricular tachycardia (Fig. 55–28) resulted in cessation of the arrhythmia. The patient has remained free of ventricular tachycardia for 10 years and has required no antiarrhythmic medication.

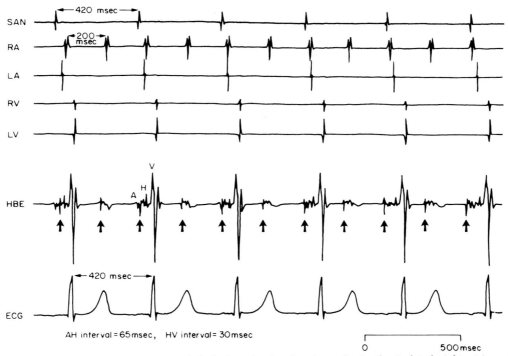

Figure 55–27. Postoperative electrograms recorded during simulated tachycardia in the isolated right atrium. Tachycardia is simulated by rapid right atrial pacing at a cycle length of 200 msec and is confined to the isolated right atrium. The simulated right atrial tachycardia does not affect sinus rhythm or the normal conduction sequence in the remainder of the heart. *Arrows* mark right atrial pacing spikes reflected in the bundle of His electrogram. (SAN = SA node; RA = right atrium; LA = left atrium; RV = right ventricle; LV = left ventricle; HBE = bundle of His electrogram; A = atrial depolarization; H = bundle of His depolarization; V = ventricular depolarization.) (From Harada, A., D'Agostino, H. J., Jr., Schuessler, R. B., et al: Right atrial isolation: A new surgical treatment for supraventricular tachycardia. I: Surgical technique and electrophysiologic effects. J. Thorac. Cardiovasc. Surg., *95*:643, 1988.)

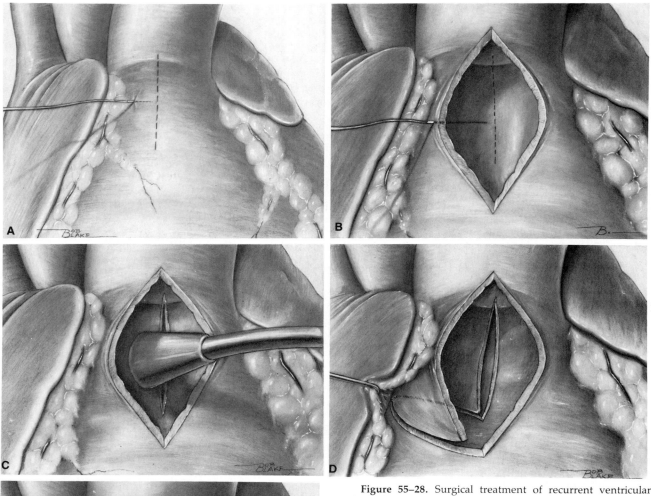

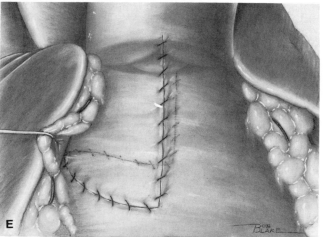

Figure 55–28. Surgical treatment of recurrent ventricular tachycardia in a 16-year-old female with nonischemic cardiomyopathy secondary to coxsackievirus myocarditis. Initial intraoperative electrophysiologic mapping indicated that the ventricular tachycardia arose from the free wall of the pulmonary outflow tract near the AV groove and just proximal to the level of the pulmonic valve annulus. An intramural needle electrode was inserted at that epicardial site and was passed transmurally so that its tip was positioned in the interventricular septum between the crista supraventricularis and the pulmonic valve annulus. Intramural electrograms were recorded from electrode contacts located every millimeter along the needle shaft. Earliest ventricular activation during ventricular tachycardia occurred at the electrode contact point at the tip of the needle shaft, indicating that the ventricular tachycardia was originating in the supracristal portion of the interventricular septum. *A*, A longitudinal incision was made on the free wall of the pulmonary outflow tract, beginning just distal to the level of the pulmonic valve annulus and extending proximally, as shown by the broken line. This free-wall incision did not alter the ventricular tachycardia.

B, The pulmonary outflow tract has been opened, and the needle electrode is seen intramurally in the supracristal portion of the interventricular septum. A counterincision was made on the posterior wall of the pulmonary outflow tract beginning just distal to the pulmonic valve annulus and extending proximally to the level of the crista supraventricularis (*broken line*). This incision was transmural, and the aortic root could be visualized through this posterior incision. This counterincision did not alter the ventricular tachycardia. *C*, A cryoprobe was positioned over the site of earliest activation during ventricular tachycardia, and the myocardium was frozen at −60° C for 2 minutes. This cryolesion resulted in cessation of the ventricular tachycardia. *D*, The proximal ends of the anterior and posterior ventriculotomies were then connected by a transmural semicircular incision around the left side of the pulmonary outflow tract, as shown. This resulted in total isolation of the segment of the pulmonary outflow tract that contained the arrhythmogenic myocardium. *E*, The incisions were closed with a continuous 3-0 nonabsorbable suture, as shown. The patient has remained free of ventricular tachycardia for 4 years after this surgical procedure. (From Cox, J. L., Bardy, G. H., Damiano, R. J., et al: Right ventricular isolation procedures for nonischemic ventricular tachycardia. J. Thorac. Cardiovasc. Surg., *90*:212, 1985.)

Fontaine and associates (1979) described a previously unrecognized form of cardiomyopathy localized to the right ventricle, which they called *arrhythmogenic right ventricular dysplasia*. This syndrome is a congenital cardiomyopathy characterized by transmural infiltration of adipose tissue resulting in weakness and aneurysmal bulging of the infundibulum, apex, or posterior basilar region of the right ventricle. The syndrome is characterized clinically by intractable ventricular tachycardia originating from one or all of the three pathologic areas of the right ventricle (Fig. 55–29). Because the origin of the tachycardia is in the right ventricle, the standard ECG shows a pattern consistent with left bundle branch block during the tachycardia. Right ventricular angiography should be done in all patients who have ventricular tachycardia with a left bundle branch block pattern. In patients with arrhythmogenic right ventricular dysplasia, the right ventricle appears enlarged; ventricular bulges or frank aneurysms are seen in the infundibulum, the apex, or the basal portion of the inferior wall; and right ventricular contractility is usually greatly decreased. Hypertrophic muscular bands in the infundibulum and anterior right ventricular wall result in apparent pseudodiverticula, the so-called feathering appearance of the right ventricular outflow tract.

The author's current approach to these patients uses a transmural encircling ventriculotomy that effectively isolates the arrhythmogenic myocardium from the remainder of the heart (Cox et al, 1985a). The operation shown in Figure 55–30 was done on a 69-year-old man who was in continuous ventricular tachycardia for 28 days before operation. Preoperative electrophysiologic studies showed that the tachycardia originated from the posterior basilar region of the right ventricle. Preoperative right ventricular angiography showed feathering of the right ventricular outflow tract and aneurysmal bulging of the infun-

dibulum, apex, and posterior basilar region of the right ventricle. Intraoperative electrophysiologic studies showed that the tachycardia arose in the posterior basilar region of the right ventricle adjacent to an electrically silent area on the anterior right ventricle measuring 2 × 3 cm. In these cases, the surgeon must recognize the possibility that the actual site of origin of the ventricular tachycardia may be in the electrically silent region and that it appears to arise from the border of the silent region only because a certain critical mass of synchronously depolarized myocardium is essential to produce an electrogram large enough to be detected by the exploring electrode. Because the three pathologically abnormal regions of the right ventricle in arrhythmogenic right ventricular dysplasia may show electrical silence on epicardial mapping, every attempt should be made to isolate the entire pathologic area giving rise to the tachycardia from the remainder of the heart. The surgically isolated pedicle shown in Figure 55–30*B* is based on a vascular supply originating from the right coronary artery. The incision is begun in the AV groove at the level of the tricuspid annulus and is extended around the arrhythmogenic region of the myocardium and returned to the level of the tricuspid annulus inferiorly. At both ends of the incision, a cryolesion is placed to ensure complete separation of all ventricular myocardial fibers on either side of the incision. In the operation shown in Figure 55–30, a separate incision was extended to the right ventricular apex because of a discrete aneurysm in that location. In making such an incision in the right ventricle, care is taken to avoid the base of the papillary muscles, but should it be necessary, the incision can be extended around the base of a papillary muscle. The incision is closed in two layers with a continuous suture. The patient whose operation is shown in Figure 55–30 has remained free of ventricular arrhythmias for 9 years after operation and has received no antiarrhythmic medication.

Although Fontaine's original description of arrhythmogenic right ventricular dysplasia suggested that the cardiomyopathy was confined to three discrete areas of the right ventricle, intraoperative mapping of these patients has suggested that the entire right ventricular free wall may be arrhythmogenic in certain cases. In the author's experience, as many as seven different sites of origin of tachycardia may be found in these patients, each site giving rise to a different morphologic type of ventricular tachycardia. Computerized intraoperative mapping systems are able to localize these tachycardias only if each of them can be induced at the time of operation—an unrealistic expectation. As a result of these problems, the author has resorted occasionally to surgical isolation of the entire right ventricular free wall to relieve the life-threatening sequelae of arrhythmogenic dysplasia (Cox, 1983b). Isolation of the entire right ventricular free wall (Fig. 55–31) represents a logical extension of the two localized right ventricular isolation procedures described earlier (see Figs. 55–

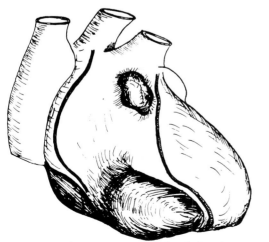

Figure 55–29. Diagrammatic sketch of the three areas of pathologic involvement in arrhythmogenic right ventricular dysplasia. (Courtesy of Dr. G. Fontaine.)

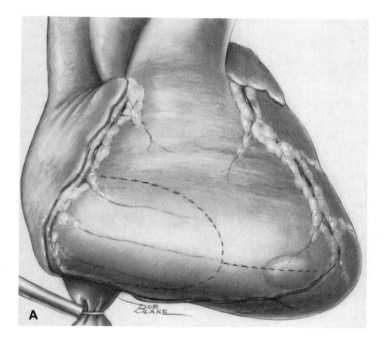

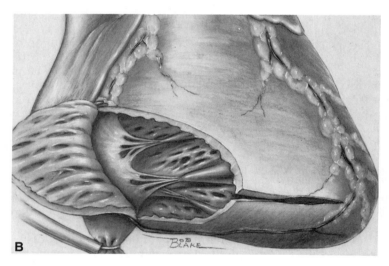

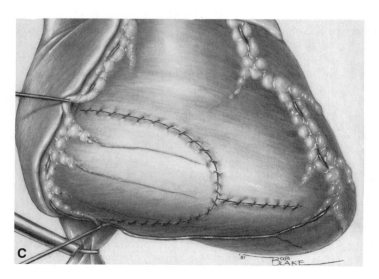

Figure 55–30. *A,* Appearance of the right ventricle in a patient with arrhythmogenic right ventricular dysplasia. Note the three coronary arteries coursing from the AV groove across the surface of the right ventricle. The acute margin of the right ventricle corresponded to the location of the middle coronary artery shown in this drawing. An area approximately 2 × 3 cm near the upper coronary artery was electrically silent. Epicardial mapping during ventricular tachycardia showed the earliest site of activation to be located near the lower edge of this electrically silent region just below the midsegment of the middle coronary region on the posterior basilar region of the right ventricle. A transmural ventriculotomy was placed around the electrically silent area and included the apparent site of origin of the ventricular tachycardia on the posterior basilar region of the heart (*broken line*). The two ends of this incision were based at the AV groove, where cryolesions were applied to ensure isolation of the arrhythmogenic region of myocardium from the remainder of the heart. In addition, a second transmural incision was made from the apex of the semicircular incision to the apex of the right ventricle to include the small saccular aneurysm in that region. *B,* The isolated pedicle of right ventricular myocardium containing the electrically silent area and the apparent site of origin of the ventricular tachycardia has been reflected to show the internal anatomy of the right ventricle. Note the extension of the incision to the right ventricular apex to open the small aneurysm located in that region. *C,* The transmural encircling ventriculotomy around the arrhythmogenic region of the right ventricle and the simple ventriculotomy through the right ventricular apical aneurysm have been closed with a continuous 3-0 nonabsorbable suture. After completion of this procedure for arrhythmogenic right ventricular dysplasia, the isolated pedicle was paced at a rapid rate, but the paced impulses were not conducted to the remainder of the heart. In addition, the remainder of the right ventricle was then paced rapidly, but those paced impulses were not conducted into the isolated pedicle, confirming total isolation of the arrhythmogenic right ventricular myocardium from the remainder of the heart. (From Cox, J. L.: Surgery for cardiac arrhythmias. *In* Harvey, W. P. [ed]: Current Problems in Cardiology, Vol. 8, No. 4. Chicago, Year Book Medical Publishers. Copyright © 1983. Reproduced with permission.)

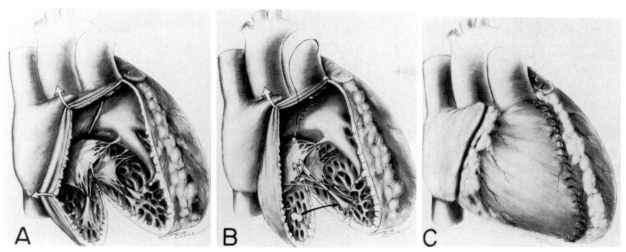

Figure 55-31. Right ventricular disconnection procedure. *A*, A transmural right ventriculotomy is placed parallel to and 5 mm from the interventricular septum, extending from just across the pulmonic valve annulus anteriorly to the tricuspid valve posteriorly. It is necessary to divide several large infundibular muscular bundles and to divide the moderator band of the right ventricle. Although the entire incision is transmural, special care must be taken to avoid injury to the right coronary artery lying in the AV groove at the posterior extent of this incision. After identification of the location of the bundle of His and right bundle branch, a second transmural incision is placed from the posterior pulmonic valve annulus to the anterior medial tricuspid valve annulus, exposing the underlying aortic root. If the tricuspid portion of this incision is placed too far anteriorly, the bundle of His may be inadvertently divided. *B*, After completion of the two transmural incisions, the papillary muscle attached to the anterior leaflet of the tricuspid valve is divided at its base and reimplanted on the lower ventricular septum using interrupted 3-0 pledgeted Prolene suture. Cryolesions are placed at each end of the anterior-posterior ventriculotomy and at each end of the ventriculotomy between the posterior pulmonic valve annulus and the anterior medial suture, followed by closure of the long free-wall ventriculotomy with continuous 3-0 nonabsorbable suture (*C*). (*A* and *B*, Modified from Cox, J. L.: Surgery for cardiac arrhythmias. *In* Harvey, W. P. [ed]: Current Problems in Cardiology, Vol. VIII, No. 4. Chicago, Year Book Medical Publishers, Inc. Copyright © 1983. Reproduced with permission.)

28 and 55-30), but it should be reserved for only the most dire circumstances. For example, the procedure shown in Figure 55-31 was done in 1982 on a 16-year-old male who had received full cardiopulmonary resuscitation (CPR) more than 250 times. In addition, an automatic internal defibrillator had been earlier implanted at another institution, one of the first such devices implanted clinically. He had continued to require frequent CPR and, as a result, had a right ventricular isolation procedure and removal of the automatic defibrillator. Although the follow-up of these patients documents excellent control of tachycardia (Fig. 55-32), the right ventricle may have progressive dilatation postoperatively, and for this reason, cardiac transplantation would likely be done today.

Uhl's syndrome is a rare congenital cardiomyopathy that, from the anatomic point of view, may be considered to be a more complete form of arrhythmogenic right ventricular dysplasia. The right ventricle is extremely dilated, but the tricuspid valve remains in a normal position, thus differentiating it from Ebstein's anomaly. The main characteristic of Uhl's syndrome is the complete absence of myocardium in the right ventricular free wall, resulting in the endocardial and epicardial layers being in direct contact without interposition of myocardial fibers. Since Uhl's description of this cardiomyopathy in 1952, the descriptive term *parchment heart* has been applied to the abnormality. Although Uhl's syndrome usually leads to rapid cardiac failure in the first months or years of life, an adult form of this condition occurs in which associated ventricular tachycardia is the dominant feature.

Jervell and Lange-Nielsen (1957) described a clinical entity consisting of a *long Q-T interval*, congenital deafness, and syncopal attacks due to ventricular fibrillation after emotional or physical stresses. The absence of congenital deafness characterizes the otherwise identical Romano-Ward syndrome (Romano et al, 1963; Ward, 1964). The prolongation of the Q-T interval in both of these syndromes has been considered to be congenital in origin, and both syndromes are recognized to contribute to sudden death in children (Fraser and Froggatt, 1966; Schwartz et al, 1975). However, in 1978, Schwartz and Wolf showed that certain patients who sustained acute myocardial infarction subsequently developed Q-T interval prolongation and after that had a significantly higher rate of sudden death. Although the pathogenesis of the long Q-T syndrome is poorly understood, James and associates (1978) demonstrated the presence of focal neuritis and neural degeneration within the specialized conduction system and the ventricular myocardium. They suggested the possibility that a chronic viral infection or some noninfectious degenerative process of the cardiac nerves might be responsible for the prolongation of the Q-T interval and the associated fatal ventricular arrhythmias.

Ventricular tachycardia that occurs in association with the long Q-T syndrome is frequently of a distinct type called *torsades de pointes*. This term is derived

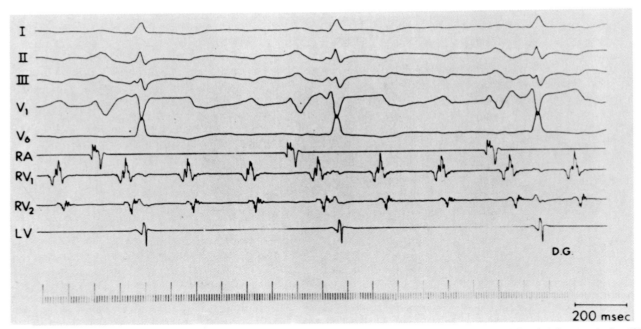

Figure 55–32. Surface recordings and intracardiac electrograms in a 16-year-old male during an episode of right ventricular (RV) tachycardia after the right ventricular isolation procedure. The limb lead (I-III) and precordial lead (V_1 and V_6) electrograms showed normal sinus rhythm in the remainder of the heart documented by right atrial (RA) activity preceding each left ventricular (LV) complex. (From Cox, J. L., Bardy, G. H., Damiano, R. J., et al: Right ventricular isolation procedures for non-ischemic ventricular tachycardia. J. Thorac. Cardiovasc. Surg., *90*:212, 1985.)

from the appearance of the ventricular tachycardia on a standard ECG, on which the polarity of the tachycardia is inconstant (Fig. 55–33). The ECG features of torsades de pointes are unique and may be described as follows (Dessertenne, 1966; Krikler and Curry, 1976; Kulbertus, 1978): (1) The episodes are generally initiated by a ventricular ectopic beat late after the preceding sinus complex; (2) the successive QRS complexes during tachycardia show an "undulating series of rotations" (Wellens et al, 1975) of the electrical axis; and (3) the episodes most frequently cease spontaneously. In addition, the arrhythmia is usually preceded by variations in the T wave during the last several beats before development of the tachycardia. One of the most frequent causes of torsades de pointes is the administration of medications that prolong ventricular repolarization, particularly quinidine (Kulbertus, 1980).

These observations support the concept that torsades de pointes represents an abnormality in myocardial *repolarization*, compared with most other types of ventricular tachycardia, which are thought to be abnormalities in myocardial *depolarization*. As a result, the surgical treatment of recurrent ventricular tachycardia associated with the long Q-T syndrome has centered around efforts to modify cardiac innervation. The classic studies of Yanowitz and co-workers (1966) showed that unilateral alterations in sympathetic tone altered not only the shape of the T wave but also its duration (Q-T interval). Their study of animals showed that resection of the right stellate ganglion or stimulation of the left stellate ganglion resulted in prolonged Q-T intervals and increased T wave amplitude. Conversely, resection of the left stellate ganglion or stimulation of the right stellate ganglion produced increased T wave negativity without measurable changes in the Q-T interval. These observations have led to the hypothesis that the ECG changes after unilateral alterations of sympathetic tone provide a functional explanation for the ECG

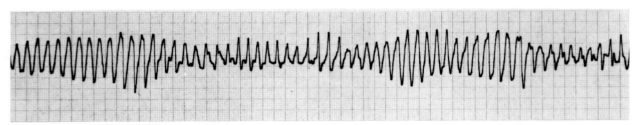

Figure 55–33. Torsades de pointes. This type of ventricular tachycardia, which is usually associated with the long Q-T syndrome, is characterized by rhythmic changes in the polarity of successive QRS complexes.

abnormalities in patients with lesions of the central nervous system as well as in patients with the long Q-T syndrome. Left stellate ganglion resection has been reported to abolish symptoms in many patients with the long Q-T syndrome (Malliani et al, 1980; Moss and McDonald, 1971; Schwartz et al, 1975; Smith and Gallagher, 1979). However, the author's experience (Benson and Cox, 1982) and that of others (Bhandari et al, 1984) have been characterized by early success and late failure.

Ischemic Ventricular Tachycardia

Acute myocardial infarction results in the non-uniform juxtaposition of normal and abnormal myocardium, a favorable anatomic substrate for the development of either automatic or re-entrant arrhythmias. Although ventricular irritability, tachycardia, and fibrillation frequently occur during the initial and early phases of acute myocardial infarction, these manifestations of acute ischemic injury are usually transient and tend to respond to medical management. With the subsequent progression of acute ischemic injury to cell death, the substrate for automaticity (primarily cellular membrane instability due to ischemia) disappears and leaves a scar in the place of injured myocardium. The interlacing pattern of the remaining scar and normal myocardium, especially at the periphery of the myocardial infarcts or aneurysms, may harbor local areas of slow conduction, unidirectional block, uneven refractoriness, and nonuniform repolarization, the electrophysiologic substrates for the development of re-entrant circuits (Boineau and Cox, 1973, 1982; Cox, 1983a). The ventricular tachyarrhythmias that develop as a result of these chronic changes in ischemically injured myocardium are frequently intractable and may not respond to pharmacologic agents. Thus, a surgical solution to these recalcitrant arrhythmias has been sought for almost 3 decades.

Historical Aspects

Lewis (1909) was apparently the first to recognize the relationship between ventricular aneurysm and ventricular tachycardia when he suggested the need for a controlled method of inducing tachycardia so that it could be studied in a systematic manner. In the absence of such a technique even 50 years later, Couch (1959) did a simple aneurysmectomy specifically for the treatment of intractable ventricular tachycardia. Durrer and colleagues (1967) of Amsterdam, and Coumel and associates (1967) of Paris, described the technique of programmed electrical stimulation, precisely the procedure desired by Lewis to induce and terminate tachycardia in a reproducible manner for purposes of diagnosis and evaluation of interventional therapy.

Experimental studies in the mid- and late 1960s documented the heterogeneity of tissue injury in

acute myocardial infarction (Cox et al, 1968), and the re-entrant basis of ischemic ventricular tachyarrhythmias was confirmed (Boineau and Cox, 1973; Cox et al, 1969; Durrer et al, 1971; El-Sherif et al, 1977; Han et al, 1970; Scherlag et al, 1974; Waldo and Kaiser, 1973). Thus, with the advent of coronary bypass procedures in the late 1960s, it appeared that ischemic ventricular tachycardia would be corrected easily by this new procedure because the basis for the arrhythmia (myocardial ischemia) could be alleviated by myocardial revascularization. During the 1970s, however, it became apparent that neither revascularization nor resection of the injured myocardium resulted in acceptable cure rates, and in addition, the operative mortality reported when these procedures were done primarily for control of ventricular tachycardia was prohibitively high (Boineau and Cox, 1982). Although the demonstration that ischemic ventricular tachyarrhythmias occurred on a re-entrant basis improved our concept of the arrhythmia, there remained a profound ignorance of the uncharted interplay between the autonomic nervous system, endogenous humoral stimulants, intracellular electrophysiology, extracellular electrophysiology, the specialized conduction system, coronary artery disease, myocardial ischemia and infarction, and normal myocardial conduction, all of which undoubtedly have a role in the genesis and perpetuation of ischemic ventricular tachyarrhythmias.

Because myocardial revascularization and resection are ineffective for controlling inschemic ventricular tachycardia, several groups began to approach the problem more directly. Daniel and colleagues (1969) and Kaiser and associates (1969) independently reported intraoperative mapping in patients with ischemic heart disease to localize the area of ischemic injury. Fontaine and associates (1974) did intraoperative mapping before doing a standard aneurysmectomy, but Wittig and Boineau (1975) and Gallagher and colleagues (1975) first reported the use of intraoperative mapping specifically to guide the attempted surgical ablation of ischemic ventricular tachycardia. Guiraudon and colleagues (1978) described the encircling endocardial ventriculotomy (EEV), a procedure successfully used to ablate ventricular tachycardia in five patients. Shortly thereafter, Harken and associates (Josephson et al, 1979) described the endocardial resection procedure, modifications of which remain the mainstay for the treatment of ischemic ventricular tachycardia.

Preoperative Electrophysiologic Evaluation

All patients who are to undergo surgical therapy for ventricular tachyarrhythmias should first have an endocardial catheter electrophysiologic study. The objectives of the preoperative study are (1) confirmation that the arrhythmia is ventricular rather than supraventricular in origin; (2) demonstration that the ventricular arrhythmia can be induced and terminated by programmed electrical stimulation techniques (i.e., that it is a re-entrant arrhythmia); and (3) localization of the region of origin of the ventricular tachycardia by "catheter mapping" when possible. In addition to having the preoperative electrophysiologic study, patients with ventricular tachyarrhythmias routinely have cardiac catheterization and coronary angiography before surgical intervention.

The preoperative electrophysiologic study may show that the arrhythmia is ventricular tachycardia of a single morphologic type, indicating that it is originating from a single region in the left or right ventricle. After induction, these *monomorphic ventricular tachycardias* are usually sustained for a sufficient length of time to allow endocardial catheter mapping to determine the site of origin. However, monomorphic ventricular tachycardia may be nonsustained, thus precluding adequate mapping during the preoperative electrophysiologic study. The preoperative study may also document the arrhythmia to be *polymorphic ventricular tachycardia*. This term is applied not only to ventricular tachycardia that originates from several different regions of the left ventricle giving rise to different morphologic types of tachycardia, but it is also applied to tachycardia that originates from one general region of the left ventricle but is characterized electrophysiologically by excessive fragmentation such that individual depolarization complexes may be difficult to identify. Polymorphic ventricular tachycardia may also be either sustained or nonsustained, and it commonly deteriorates rather quickly into ventricular fibrillation. Electrophysiologic deterioration to ventricular fibrillation may be the result of primary electrical instability or may occur because of hemodynamic compromise associated with the onset of polymorphic ventricular tachycardia. The third type of ventricular tachyarrhythmia that may be identified by the preoperative electrophysiologic study is *primary ventricular fibrillation*. This arrhythmia is characterized by the absence of any type of induced ventricular tachycardia before the onset of ventricular fibrillation after programmed electrical stimulation.

Surgical Indications and Contraindications

Decisions regarding surgical intervention for ischemic ventricular tachycardia are based on various clinical factors and must be individualized for each patient. Because no surgical technique exists for the ablation of primary ventricular fibrillation, the author implants the AICD in all patients with this unusual problem. It is important to realize, however, that even though ventricular fibrillation may be the primary diagnosis in a patient who has been resuscitated from an episode of sudden death, an electrophysiologic study usually confirms that the episode of fibrillation is preceded by at least a short course of ventricular tachycardia, most commonly of the polymorphic type described earlier. These patients are considered to have primary ventricular tachycar-

dia, not ventricular fibrillation, which is believed to be a secondary problem that will be alleviated if the ventricular tachycardia can be controlled.

Polymorphic ventricular tachycardia was considered earlier to be a contraindication to operation because of its complex nature and the attendant difficulty in mapping it at operation. However, the availability of computerized intraoperative mapping systems has provided a method of identifying the area or areas of arrhythmogenic myocardium, even with this fleeting, changing type of ventricular tachyarrhythmia.

Perhaps the major contraindication to operation is left ventricular dysfunction so severe that it precludes any reasonable possibility of surviving an operative procedure. Before the advent of the AICD, there was no viable alternative to operation in these patients if their arrhythmia could not be controlled pharmacologically. However, it is now preferable to implant the AICD in these patients because of the lower operative mortality associated with this relatively simple procedure. One extra benefit of this selection of patients who will not have operative intervention for ventricular tachycardia should be an improvement in the operative mortality of the remaining patients who do have operation.

Finally, the question of whether or not the antiarrhythmic agent amiodarone is associated with a higher operative mortality or postoperative complication rate is controversial. This question depends partly on the conduction of the operation for ventricular tachycardia. For example, in the author's experience, amiodarone has caused the low-output syndrome postoperatively only in patients who require cardioplegic arrest for performance of some portion of the operative procedure. Because all ventricular tachycardia procedures are done in the normothermic beating heart, amiodarone is not a problem unless it is also necessary to do a coronary artery bypass procedure, in which case cardioplegic arrest would be used after completion of the specific tachycardia procedure. In the latter case, it is preferable to discontinue amiodarone for a minimum of 4 weeks before operation. If that is not feasible, the coronary bypass procedure is done during ventricular fibrillation. Only under the most unusual of circumstances, however, will cardioplegic arrest be used in patients who take amiodarone.

Intraoperative Electrophysiologic Mapping

In patients having operation for ventricular tachyarrhythmias, the first step intraoperatively is to do detailed electrophysiologic mapping procedures to guide the specific surgical technique that is to be used. As mentioned earlier, all 160 channels of the computerized system are used to map the heart in patients with ventricular tachycardia. The sock electrode array (Fig. 55–34) is first used to determine the epicardial activation sequence during sinus rhythm and during induced ventricular tachycardia. The sock

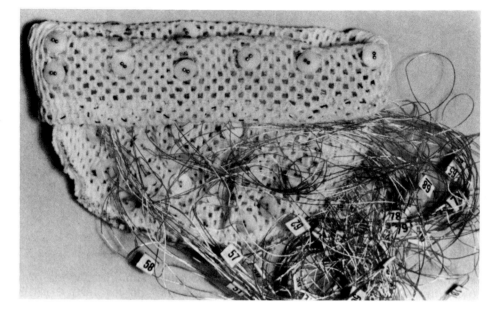

Figure 55–34. The sock electrode array. The 96 bipolar electrodes are maintained in contact with the epicardial surface of the ventricles by a nylon mesh stocking. (From Cox, J. L.: Surgical management of cardiac arrhythmias. *In* Samet, P., and El-Sherif, N. (eds): Cardiac Pacing and Electrophysiology, 3rd ed. Orlando, Grune & Stratton, 1988.)

electrode array presently used contains 96 electrodes. The earliest site of epicardial breakthrough is automatically cursored in red by the computer for rapid detection of the region of most interest (Fig. 55–35). The epicardial data are not used to identify the site to be ablated but rather are used to guide the subsequent placement of plunge needle electrodes to further delineate the specific site of arrhythmogenesis. The epicardial map is helpful not only as an initial screening device that can be obtained in 2 to 3

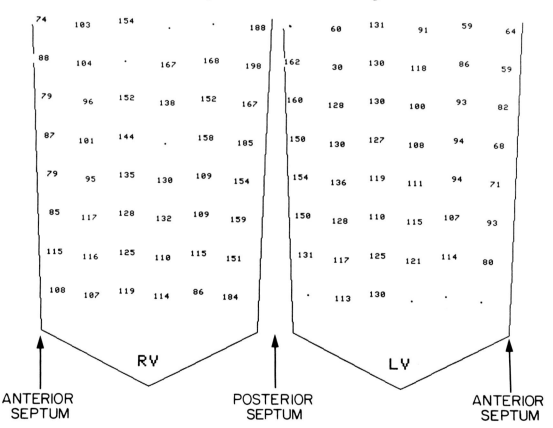

Figure 55–35. Hard copy of the color graphics terminal display of data recorded from the 96 epicardial electrodes in the sock electrode array during induced ventricular tachycardia. The epicardial data show that the earliest area of epicardial breakthrough is over the upper anterior ventricular septum. (From Cox, J. L.: Intraoperative computerized mapping techniques. *In* Brugada, P., and Wellens, H. J. J. [eds]: Cardiac Arrhythmias: Where to Go From Here? Mount Kisco, NY, Futura Publishing Co., 1987.)

minutes, but it is most useful in characterizing non-clinical arrhythmias that may be induced during programmed electrical stimulation.

When the epicardial activation sequence during ventricular tachycardia has been established, multiple plunge needle electrodes containing four bipolar pairs of contacts along the needle shaft are inserted into the ventricle in the region of earliest epicardial activation (Fig. 55–36). If the epicardial map has suggested that the tachycardia is arising from the ventricular septum, a right atriotomy is done and as many as 15 right-angle needle electrodes are inserted into the ventricular septum from the right side. Access is gained across the tricuspid valve. As many as 60 transmural data points are thus provided from the ventricular septum without the necessity for doing a ventriculotomy. As many as 25 other needle electrodes can be placed in or near the arrhythmogenic region, yielding a total of 160 endocardial, intramural, and epicardial data points simultaneously from the septum and free wall without doing a ventriculotomy. It has been shown on many occasions by various researchers that a ventriculotomy frequently alters the electrophysiologic milieu sufficiently to prevent further inducibility of the ventricular tachycardia, thus precluding further mapping and necessitating a nonguided ("blind") operation to be performed.

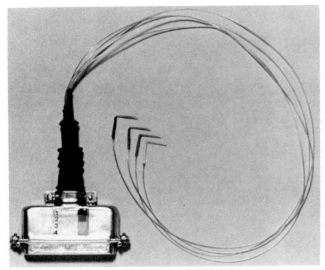

Figure 55–36. One bay of four needle electrodes. Each needle shaft contains four bipolar electrodes to record data from four different layers of the ventricular free wall or septum; thus, this one bay carries signals recorded from 16 individual sites in the heart. By inserting multiple needle electrodes, endocardial maps of the left or right ventricles (in addition to intramural and epicardial maps) can be constructed without a ventriculotomy.

Direct Surgical Procedures for the Treatment of Ischemic Ventricular Tachycardia

The EEV was the first technique introduced specifically for the control of refractory ischemic ventricular tachycardia (Guiraudon et al, 1978). Guiraudon considered that because the re-entrant circuits responsible for the tachycardia were suspected to reside at or near the junction of the endocardial fibrosis associated with the infarct or aneurysm and normal myocardium (Fig. 55–37A), and because a standard aneurysmectomy did not remove this area (see Fig. 55–37B), the surgeon should not expect the latter to be effective in ablating the arrhythmia. He therefore advocated placing an endocardial incision around the entire circumference of the infarct or aneurysm just outside the junction of the fibrosis and normal myocardium (see Fig. 55–37C). This incision was a deep one extending to very near the epicardium on the free wall and 1 cm deep on the septum. The objective of the encircling endocardial incision was to interrupt the re-entrant circuit or to encompass it entirely in hope of isolating it from the remainder of the ventricle. Although the EEV was extremely effective in controlling ventricular tachycardia, its effectiveness stemmed from the fact that the encompassed myocardium was made more ischemic, thus suppressing the re-entrant circuit causing the tachycardia (Ungerleider et al, 1982a, 1982b). In addition, because increased ischemia caused by

the EEV resulted in poorer left ventricular function (Ungerleider et al, 1982c), the EEV was associated with an unacceptable incidence of postoperative low-output syndrome and operative mortality (Cox et al, 1982). The EEV as originally described, therefore, is no longer used for the treatment of ventricular tachycardia.

Josephson and colleagues (1979) introduced the concept of first localizing the site of origin of ventricular tachycardia by endocardial mapping and then resecting the endocardial fibrosis in the arrhythmogenic region in hope of either interrupting or removing the re-entrant circuit causing the ventricular tachycardia (see Fig. 55–37D). This technique, called by various names, including the *local endocardial resection procedure* (ERP) and *subendocardial resection* (SER), involved removing approximately 10 cm^2 of fibrosis from one quadrant of the infarct or aneurysm. Moran and associates (1982) later modified the local ERP so that all of the endocardial fibrosis was removed regardless of the location of the arrhythmogenic tissue (the *extended endocardial resection procedure*, or EERP). Endocardial cryosurgery to ablate arrhythmogenic tissue that was located near the aortic or mitral valve annuli or on the base of the papillary muscles that was not amenable to treatment by the EEV, ERP, or EERP techniques was advocated (see Fig. 55–37E) (Cox et al, 1982).

Ostermeyer and associates (1984, 1987) have used a partial EEV technique in which an endocardial incision is placed only in the region of arrhythmogenesis with excellent results. In addition, superior results have been reported with a technique that combines wide endocardial resection with endocar-

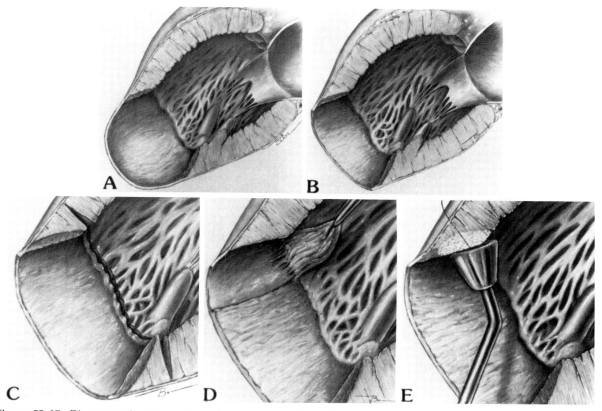

Figure 55–37. Diagrammatic cross-section of an anterior left ventricular aneurysm showing more proximal extension of the associated fibrosis at the endocardial level than at the epicardial level (*A*). Because the re-entrant circuits responsible for ischemic ventricular tachycardia occur most commonly at the junction of this endocardial fibrosis and normal myocardium, a standard left ventricular aneurysm resection (*B*) does not ablate or remove them. The encircling endocardial ventriculotomy (*C*), localized endocardial (or "subendocardial") resection (*D*), and endocardial cryoablation (*E*) all were introduced specifically to ablate ventricular tachycardia associated with left ventricular aneurysms or infarcts. (Modified from Cox, J. L.: Anatomic-electrophysiologic basis for the surgical treatment of refractory ischemic ventricular tachycardia. Ann. Surg., *198*:119, 1983.)

dial cryosurgery (Krafchek et al, 1986a, 1986b), the approach that most closely resembles the one currently employed by the author. The site of origin of the ventricular tachycardia is localized as described earlier. Then, with the heart in the normothermic beating state, preferably during ventricular tachycardia, the ventricle is opened through the infarct or aneurysm and all of the associated endocardial fibrosis is resected except that which extends onto the base of the papillary muscles (Fig. 55–38). After resecting all visible endocardial fibrosis, endocardial cryolesions are applied to the sites of origin of the tachycardia. The cryothermia is applied only after removal of the endocardial scar because, in the author's experience, approximately 10% of patients still have inducible ventricular tachycardia intraoperatively after removal of all visible endocardial fibrosis. This indicates that the actual site of origin of the tachycardia in these patients is deeper in the myocardium than the visible border of the endocardial fibrosis and that therefore the myocardium beneath the fibrosis must be destroyed to ablate the tachycardia. In those cases in which one site of origin is a scarred papillary muscle, one or more cryolesions are

placed directly on the base of the involved papillary muscle without removing the scar (Figs. 55–39 and 55–40). More than 75 papillary muscles have been cryoablated without a single case of mitral valve regurgitation, an experience that is consistent with experimental studies showing that cryoablation of papillary muscles does not cause subsequent papillary muscle dysfunction. This experience argues strongly against the practice of resecting papillary muscles for ventricular tachycardia that has been reported earlier (Moran et al, 1983).

When EERP and subsequent endocardial cryoablation have been completed, programmed electrical stimulation is applied in an attempt to reinduce the arrhythmia. If ventricular tachycardia is still inducible, it is again mapped and cryoablation of the remaining arrhythmogenic myocardium is done. If the arrhythmia is no longer inducible, the surgeon considers that it has been permanently ablated. If other procedures are to be done, such as coronary bypass grafting, they are then done under cardioplegic arrest. It is important to note, however, that cardioplegia is absolutely not administered until the ventricular tachycardia has been satisfactorily ablated.

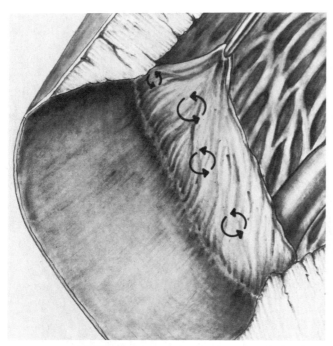

Figure 55–38. Diagrammatic sketch of an extended endocardial resection procedure (EERP) in an anterior left ventricular aneurysm. The principle involved in this procedure is the same as that for a localized ERP (see Fig. 51–37D), but in this procedure *all* of the endocardial fibrosis associated with the aneurysm is resected except that involving the papillary muscles. (From Cox, J. L.: Surgical treatment of ischemic and nonischemic ventricular tachyarrhythmias. *In* Cohn, L. H. [ed]: Modern Technics in Surgery. Mount Kisco, NY, Futura Publishing Co., 1985.)

The reason for this strict approach is that the cardioplegia itself may temporarily alter the delicate reentry circuits causing the tachycardia; therefore, if the antitachycardia procedure is done under cardioplegic arrest, it is impossible to determine intraoperatively whether the surgical procedure has ablated the arrhythmia. This point is often ignored when considering the factors that predispose to postoperative recurrences, and it emphasizes the importance of the manner in which the operative procedure is conducted. The author believes that the practice of doing ventricular tachycardia procedures under cardioplegic arrest is the major reason for the high reinducibility rates at the time of the postoperative electrophysiologic study reported in most series.

Selle and colleagues (1986) and Svenson and associates (1987) have reported promising results by using the Nd-YAG laser to ablate arrhythmogenic myocardium after endocardial mapping. Major advantages of this technique are that it is easy and quick to do and can also be applied in the normothermic beating heart. As described earlier, this allows immediate reapplication of programmed stimulation to determine the efficacy of the procedure without the introduction of any intervening variables; therefore, it is not surprising that the patients have had no spontaneous or reinducible ventricular tachycardia postoperatively.

Role of the Automatic Internal Cardioverter-Defibrillator and Intraoperative Mapping in the Surgical Management of Ventricular Tachycardia

Although various operative techniques have proved to be reasonably effective for the control of ischemic ventricular tachycardia, the cumulative experience of the previous decade indicates that high operative mortality and postoperative reinducibility rates have persisted (Miller et al, 1984a, 1984b, 1985).

Because the postoperative reinducibility rate of ventricular tachycardia is excessive, some authors have recommended the routine placement of AICD patches at the time of operation so that if the arrhythmia can be reinduced at the time of the postoperative electrophysiologic study, an AICD unit can be implanted without the need for another thoracotomy (Platia et al, 1986). Others have suggested that because the operative mortality for ventricular tachycardia procedures is so high, perhaps the map-guided (and nonguided) direct surgical procedures should be abandoned altogether in favor of simple coronary artery bypass grafting and routine implantation of an AICD (Fonger et al, 1987).

Although both of these suggestions may have some merit, they are based on the assumption that neither the operative mortality associated with direct surgical procedures nor the postoperative reinduci-

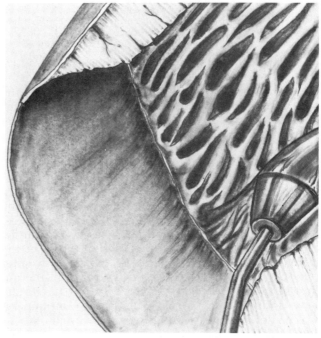

Figure 55–39. After all of the endocardial scar is resected as a preliminary measure, endocardial cryolesions are placed at the site or sites of origin of the ventricular tachycardia as determined by intraoperative mapping. In addition, any remaining scar on the papillary muscle is cryoablated as shown. (From Cox, J. L.: Surgical treatment of ischemic and nonischemic ventricular tachyarrhythmias. *In* Cohn, L. H. [ed]: Modern Technics in Surgery. Mount Kisco, NY, Futura Publishing Co., 1985.)

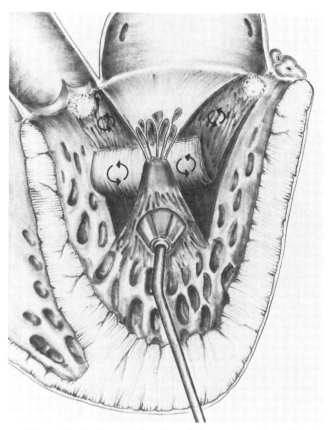

Figure 55–40. Extended endocardial resection of the fibrosis associated with a posterior myocardial infarction or aneurysm and cryoablation of the lower two-thirds of the posterior papillary muscle. The endocardial fibrosis is resected to within 5 mm of the aortic and mitral valve annuli. Because the site of origin of ventricular tachycardia is frequently adjacent to the junction of the aortic and mitral valve annuli, endocardial cryolesions (*white circles*) are applied at the base of the aortic and mitral valve annuli to ablate any re-entrant circuits that might reside in the remaining endocardial fibrosis immediately beneath the valve annuli. In addition, endocardial cryolesions are applied to the site or sites of origin of ventricular tachycardia as determined by intraoperative mapping, but only *after* removal of all endocardial scar. (From Cox, J. L.: Surgical treatment of ischemic and nonischemic ventricular tachyarrhythmias. *In* Cohn, L. H. [ed]: Modern Technics in Surgery. Mount Kisco, NY, Futura Publishing Co., 1985.)

bility rate can be decreased to acceptable levels. Paradoxically, this assumption overlooks the potential importance of the AICD in decreasing the operative mortality associated with the direct surgical procedures now done. One of the major reasons for the high operative mortality in the past was the lack of a viable therapeutic option in patients who had medically refractory ventricular tachycardia and such severe left ventricular dysfunction that there was little hope of their surviving an operation. Despite the obvious risk in such patients, if antiarrhythmic agents were ineffective, there was little choice but to proceed with operation. The results in these patients were considerably different from those attained in patients with more reasonable left ventricular function. The AICD now provides the previously unavailable therapeutic option for patients who have medically refractory ventricular tachycardia and who

are not surgical candidates. Because these patients who are prohibitively high operative risks will no longer be subjected to operation, the mortality for operative procedures should decrease in the future.

The postoperative reinducibility rate should also be decreased in the future by the increasing availability of multipoint intraoperative mapping systems and by the avoidance of cardioplegic arrest or other variables that prevent the accurate intraoperative assessment of the efficacy of the specific surgical procedure in curing ventricular tachycardia. Doing an endocardial resection for ventricular tachycardia without mapping is analogous to doing a coronary artery bypass procedure for angina pectoris without angiography. Approximately 50% of patients with ventricular tachycardia can be cured by these blind resections (Swerdlow et al, 1986), and it is reasonable to expect that a similar cure rate for angina pectoris could be accomplished by bypassing all coronary arteries in every patient. However, if the surgeon expects to accomplish optimal cure rates for either condition, the abnormality must be defined more precisely. The cure rates for map-guided ventricular tachycardia procedures in some series now exceed 90% (Ostermeyer et al, 1987; Svenson et al, 1987), an indication that blind surgical procedures for this life-threatening arrhythmia should be abandoned except in unusual or emergency situations.

Because multipoint mapping systems are not yet available in all institutions and because patients with refractory ventricular tachycardia are frequently incapable of being transferred to centers that are thus equipped, surgeons must still deal with the questions of how patients are to be selected for ventricular tachycardia procedures, which surgical technique should be used, and how the surgical procedure should be conducted. In the absence of other indications for operation, the decision regarding surgical intervention for ventricular tachycardia should be made only after the patient has failed all medical therapy except amiodarone (Fig. 55–41). Before initiating amiodarone therapy, an assessment is made of the operative risks and of the likelihood of success. In practical terms, this assessment is based primarily on the status of the patient's left ventricular function, but the morphologic type of tachycardia must also be considered.

If the patient's left ventricular function is considered to be compatible with reasonable operative risk, a surgical course should be pursued at this point, but if the ventricular dysfunction poses a prohibitive operative risk, amiodarone therapy should be initiated. The subsequent treatment plan for the latter patients is discussed later.

When the decision has been made to pursue surgical therapy, the choices outlined in Figure 55–41 are made at various steps in the procedure. The importance of doing intraoperative mapping and of avoiding cardioplegic arrest is apparent, because this is the only combination that allows the surgeon to do programmed electrical stimulation to assess the efficacy of the surgical technique intraoperatively. If

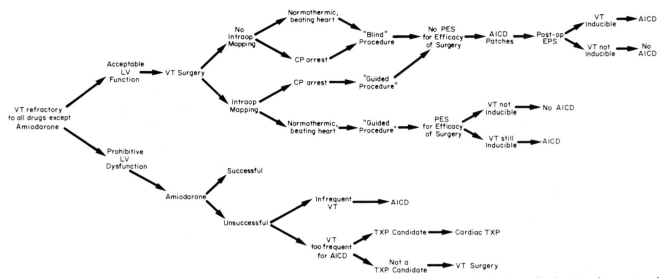

Figure 55–41. Algorithm for the selection and treatment of patients with ischemic ventricular tachycardia that is refractory to all antitachycardia drugs except amiodarone. The decision regarding operation or amiodarone is made at this point because of the increased risk of operation in patients who are taking amiodarone. (Modified from Cox, J. L.: Patient selection and results of surgery for refractory ischemic ventricular tachycardia. Circulation, 79:I-163, 1989. By permission of the American Heart Association, Inc.)

such a map-guided procedure is done in the normothermic beating heart and, on completion, ventricular tachycardia cannot be induced, the likelihood of inducing the arrhythmia 7 to 10 days later during the postoperative electrophysiologic study is less than 2% in the author's experience. The lack of inducibility at the time of the postoperative study portends a much better prognosis on long-term follow-up, because patients in whom ventricular tachycardia is not inducible are less likely to develop spontaneous recurrence of ventricular tachycardia (Kienzle et al, 1983; Swerdlow et al, 1986). In addition, if the tachycardia is noninducible postoperatively, further medical therapy is unnecessary.

If nonguided operation is done, AICD patches should be placed when the procedure has been completed because of the likelihood that ventricular tachycardia will still be inducible at the time of the postoperative electrophysiologic study. If the arrhythmia is inducible, an AICD can then be connected to the patches without the need for another thoracotomy. If no tachycardia is inducible, it is not necessary to insert an AICD unless the patient has a spontaneous recurrence later. Likewise, if map-guided operation is done under cardioplegic arrest, programmed electrical stimulation (PES) after completion of the procedure is ineffective in determining whether the operation has ablated the ventricular tachycardia, which is evidenced by the 25% reinducibility rate postoperatively. The lack of inducibility intraoperatively after completion of the procedure in patients who have inducible tachycardia 7 to 10 days later indicates that although the surgical procedure was guided by intraoperative mapping, the site of arrhythmogenesis was not ablated. It is reasonable

to conclude that the reason that the arrhythmia could not be reinduced by PES intraoperatively after the surgical procedure is that the cardioplegia temporarily suppressed the offending re-entrant circuit and that it had "recovered" by the time of the postoperative study. Thus, if a ventricular tachycardia procedure is done under cardioplegic arrest, even though it is map guided, AICD patches should be placed at the end of the procedure so that an AICD can be implanted in the 25% of patients who will still have inducible tachycardia at the time of the postoperative electrophysiologic study.

As mentioned earlier, the initial decision to treat ventricular tachycardia with amiodarone should be based primarily on the fact that the patient's left ventricular dysfunction represents a prohibitive operative risk. If amiodarone is unsuccessful in controlling the tachycardia, which is frequently the case (Fogoros et al, 1983; Rasmussen et al, 1982), the next logical step would be to implant an AICD. However, if the patient has frequent episodes of tachycardia despite amiodarone therapy, the AICD may not be a viable option because the present units are capable of delivering only 150 total discharges before requiring replacement. In addition, the experience of receiving electrical cardioversions on a frequent basis is not a pleasant one. If these patients are candidates, they should be considered for cardiac transplantation. However, if they are not transplant candidates, there is no alternative but to subject them to a ventricular tachycardia procedure. This group of patients (1) have already been deemed inoperable, (2) have failed amiodarone therapy, (3) have tachycardia episodes so frequently that AICDs have little value, and (4) are not cardiac transplant candidates. These considerations explain the inordinately high operative mortality that has been associated with ventricular tachycardia operative procedures. Thus, if this group can be kept to a minimum in the future, the current operative mortality reported for ventricular tachycardia surgery should decrease dramatically.

Selected Bibliography

Anderson, R. H., Becker, A. E.: Cardiac anatomy for the surgeon. *In* Danielson, G. K. (ed): Lewis' Practice of Surgery, Chapter 16. New York, Harper & Row, 1979.

This chapter is an excellent, concise description of the anatomy of the heart pertinent to the cardiac surgeon. Most of the diagrams are drawn in the view in which they appear during cardiac procedures. The anatomy of the AV junctional area and of the normal cardiac conduction system is described particularly well.

Cobb, F. R., Blumenschein, S. D., Sealy, W. C., et al: Successful surgical interruption of the bundle of Kent in a patient with Wolff-Parkinson-White syndrome. Circulation, *38*:1018, 1968.

This is the first description of the successful surgical treatment of the WPW syndrome. Although current surgical techniques differ significantly from those described in this original article, this report represents a milestone in the surgical treatment of cardiac arrhythmias.

Cox, J. L.: Anatomic-electrophysiologic basis for the surgical treatment of refractory ischemic ventricular tachycardia. Ann. Surg., *198*:119, 1983.

This article describes the anatomic abnormalities underlying the electrophysiologic derangements that are believed to be responsible for refractory ischemic ventricular tachycardia. The article also describes the basis for each of the direct surgical procedures currently used to treat ischemic ventricular tachycardia.

Cox, J. L., Gallagher, J. J., and Cain, M. E.: Experience with 118 consecutive patients undergoing surgery for the Wolff-Parkinson-White syndrome. J. Thorac. Cardiovasc. Surg., *90*:490, 1985.

This article describes the current method for performing the endocardial technique for surgical division of accessory pathways in patients with the WPW syndrome. In addition, the authors' surgical results using the endocardial approach are reported.

Guiraudon, G. M., Klein, G. J., Sharma, A. D., et al: Closed-heart technique for Wolff-Parkinson-White syndrome: Further experience and potential limitations. Ann. Thorac. Surg., *42*:651, 1986.

In this article, the authors describe the surgical results and potential limitations of the epicardial approach to accessory pathways in patients with the WPW syndrome. Cryosurgery is usually added to surgical dissection in the AV groove to interrupt electrical conduction across accessory pathways.

Bibliography

Akhtar, M.: Supraventricular tachycardias: Electrophysiologic mechanisms, diagnosis, and pharmacologic therapy. *In* Josephson, M. E., Wellens, H. J. J. (eds): Tachycardias: Mechanisms, Diagnosis, Treatment. Philadelphia, Lea & Febiger, 1984.

Allessie, M. A., Lammers, W. J. E. P., Bonke, I. M., and Hollen, J.: Intra-atrial reentry as a mechanism for atrial flutter induced by acetylcholine and rapid pacing in the dog. Circulation, 70:123, 1984.

Anderson, R. H., and Becker, A. E.: Anatomy of conducting tissue revisited. Br. Heart J., *40*(Suppl):2, 1978.

Anderson, R. H., and Becker, A. E.: Cardiac anatomy for the surgeon. *In* Danielson, G. K. (ed): Lewis' Practice of Surgery, Chapter 16. New York, Harper & Row, 1979.

Anderson, R. H., and Becker, A. E.: Morphology of the human atrioventricular junction area. *In* Wellens, H. J. J., Lie, K. I., Janse, M. J., et al (eds): The Conduction System of the Heart: Structure, Function and Clinical Implications. Philadelphia, Lea & Febiger, 1976, p. 264.

Aschoff, K. A. L.: A discussion on some aspects of heart-block. Br. Med. J., 2:1103, 1906.

Benson, D. W., Jr., and Cox, J. L.: Surgical treatment of cardiac arrhythmias. *In* Roberts, N. K., and Gelband, H. (eds): Cardiac Arrhythmias in the Neonate, Infant and Child, 2nd ed. East Norwalk, Appleton & Lange, 1982, pp. 341–366.

Bhandari, A. K., Scheinman, M. M., Morady, F., et al: Efficacy of left cardiac sympathectomy in the treatment of patients with the long QT syndrome. Circulation, 70:1018, 1984.

Boineau, J. P., and Cox, J. L.: Rationale for a direct surgical approach to control ventricular arrhythmias. Am. J. Cardiol., 49:381, 1982.

Boineau, J. P., and Cox, J. L.: Slow ventricular activation in acute myocardial infarction: A source of re-entrant premature ventricular contractions. Circulation, *48*:702, 1973.

Boineau, J. P., Mooney, C., Hudson, R., et al: Observations on re-entrant excitation pathways and refractory period distribution in spontaneous and experimental atrial flutter in the dog. *In* Kulbertus, H. E. (ed): Re-Entrant Arrhythmias. Baltimore, MD, University Park Press, 1977, pp. 79–98.

Boineau, J. P., Schuessler, R. B., Mooney, C. R., et al: Natural and evoked atrial flutter due to circus movement in dogs. Am. J. Cardiol., 45:1167, 1980.

Boineau, J. P., Wylds, A. C., Autry, L. J., et al: Mechanisms of atrial flutter as determined from spontaneous and experimental models. *In* Josephson, M. E., and Wellens, H. J. J. (eds): Tachycardias: Mechanisms, Diagnosis and Treatment. Philadelphia, Lea & Febiger, 1984, pp. 91–111.

Burchell, H. B., Frye, R. L., Anderson, M. W., et al: Atrial-ventricular and ventricular-atrial excitation in Wolff-Parkinson-White syndrome (type B): Temporary ablation at surgery. Circulation, 36:663, 1967.

Canavan, T. E., Schuessler, R. B., Boineau, J. P., et al: Computerized global eletrophysiologic mapping of the atrium in patients with the Wolff-Parkinson-White syndrome. Ann. Thorac. Surg., 46:223, 1988a.

Canavan, T. E., Schuessler, R. B., Cain, M. E., et al: Computerized global electrophysiologic mapping of the atrium in a patient with multiple supraventricular tachyarrhythmias. Ann. Thorac. Surg., 46:232, 1988b.

Cobb, F. R., Blumenschein, S. D., Sealy, W. C., et al: Successful surgical interruption of the bundle of Kent in a patient with Wolff-Parkinson-White syndrome. Circulation, 38:1018, 1968.

Couch, O. A., Jr.: Cardiac aneurysm with ventricular tachycardia and subsequent excision of aneurysm. Circulation, 20:251, 1959.

Coumel, P., Cabarol, C., Fabiato, A., et al: Tachycardia permanente par rythme réciproque. Arch. Mal. Coeur, 60:1830, 1967.

Cox, J. L.: Anatomic-electrophysiologic basis for the surgical treatment of refractory ischemic ventricular tachycardia. Ann. Surg., *198*:119, 1983a.

Cox, J. L.: Intraoperative computerized mapping techniques. *In* Brugada, P., Wellens, H. J. J. (eds): Cardiac Arrhythmias: Where to Go From Here? Mount Kisco, NY, Futura Publishing Co., 1987.

Cox, J. L.: Manuscript reviewer's comment. J. Thorac. Cardiovasc. Surg., 92:411, 1986.

Cox, J. L.: Patient selection criteria and results of surgery for refractory ischemic ventricular tachycardia. Circulation, 79:I-163, 1989.

Cox, J. L.: Surgery for cardiac arrhythmias. Chicago, Year Book Medical Publishers, Vol. 8, No. 4, July 1983.

Cox, J. L.: Surgical management of cardiac arrhythmias. *In* Samet, P., and El-Sherif, N. (eds): Cardiac Pacing and Electrophysiology, 3rd ed. Orlando, Grune & Stratton, 1988b.

Cox, J. L.: Surgical treatment of ischemic and non-ischemic ventricular tachyarrhythmias. *In* Cohn, L.H. (ed): Modern Technics in Surgery. Mount Kisco, NY, Futura Publishing Co., 1985.

Cox, J. L., Bardy, G. H., Damiano, R. J., et al: Right ventricular isolation procedures for non-ischemic ventricular tachycardia. J. Thorac. Cardiovasc. Surg., *90*:212, 1985a.

Cox, J. L., Daniel, T. M., Sabiston, D. C., Jr., and Boineau, J. P.: Desynchronized activation in myocardial infarction—a reentry basis for ventricular arrhythmias (Abstract). Circulation, *39*(Suppl. 3):63, 1969.

Cox, J. L., Gallagher, J. J., and Cain, M. E.: Experience with 118 consecutive patients undergoing surgery for the Wolff-Parkinson-White syndrome. J. Thorac. Cardiovasc. Surg., *90*:490, 1985b.

Cox, J. L., Gallagher, J. J., and Ungerleider, R. M.: Encircling endocardial ventriculotomy (EEV) for refractory ischemic ventricular tachycardia. IV: Clinical indications, surgical technique, mechanism of action, and results. J. Thorac. Cardiovasc. Surg., *83*:865, 1982.

Cox, J. L., Holman, W. L., and Cain, M. E.: Cryosurgical treatment of atrioventricular node reentry tachycardia. Circulation, *76*:1329, 1987.

Cox, J. L., McLaughlin, V. W., Flowers, N. C., and Horan, L. G.: The ischemic zone surrounding acute myocardial infarction: Its morphology as detected by dehydrogenase staining. Am. Heart J., *76*:650, 1968.

Daniel, T. M., Cox, J. L., Sabiston, D. C., Jr., and Boineau, J. P: Epicardial and intramural mapping activation of the human heart: A technique for localizing infarction and ischemia of the myocardium (Abstract). Circulation, *49*(Suppl. III):66, 1969.

Dessertenne, F.: La tachycardie ventriculaire à deux foyers opposés variables. Arch. Mal. Coeur, *59*:263, 1966.

Draper, M. H., and Weidmann, S.: Cardiac resting and action potentials recorded with an intracellular electrode. J. Physiol., *115*:74, 1957.

Durrer, D., and Roos, J. P.: Epicardial excitation of the ventricles in a patient with Wolff-Parkinson-White syndrome (type B): Temporary ablation at surgery. Circulation, *35*:15, 1967.

Durrer, D., Schoo, L., Schuilenburg, R. M., and Wellens, H. J. J.: The role of premature beats in the initiation and the termination of supraventricular tachycardia in the Wolff-Parkinson-White syndrome. Circulation, *36*:644, 1967.

Durrer, D., van Dam, R. T., Freud, G. E., and Janse, M. J.: Reentry and ventricular arrhythmias in local ischemia and infarction of the intact dog heart. Proc. K. Ned. Akad. Wet. Ser. Biol. Med. Sci., *74*:321, 1971.

El-Sherif, N., Scherlag, B. J., Lazzara, R., and Hopen, R. R.: Reentrant ventricular arrhythmias in the late myocardial infarction period. I: Conduction characteristics of the infarction zone. Circulation, *55*:686, 1977.

Fogoros, R. N., Anderson, K. P., Winkle, R. A., et al: Amiodarone: Clinical efficacy and toxicity in 96 patients with recurrent, drug-refractory arrhythmias. Circulation, *68*:88, 1983.

Fonger, J. D., Guarnieri, T., Griffith, L. S. C., et al: Impending sudden cardiac death: Treatment with myocardial revascularization and automatic implantable cardioverter defibrillator. Presented at the Twenty-third Annual Meeting of The Society of Thoracic Surgeons, Toronto, Ontario, Canada, September 22, 1987.

Fontaine, G., Frank, R., and Guiraudon, G.: Surgical treatment of resistant re-entrant ventricular tachycardia by ventriculotomy: A new application of epicardial mapping (Abstract). Circulation, *50*(Suppl. III):82, 1974.

Fontaine, G., Guiraudon, G., and Frank, R.: Management of chronic ventricular tachycardia. *In* Narula, O. S. (ed): Inno-

vations in Diagnosis and Management of Cardiac Arrhythmias. Baltimore, Williams & Wilkins, 1979.

Fraser, G. R., and Froggatt, P.: Unexpected cot deaths. Lancet, *2*:56, 1966.

Gallagher, J. J., Cox, J. L., German, L. D., and Kasell, J. H.: Nonpharmacologic treatment of supraventricular tachycardia. *In* Josephson, M. E., and Wellens, H. J. J. (eds): Tachycardias: Mechanisms, Diagnosis, and Treatment. Philadelphia, Lea & Febiger, 1984a, pp. 271–285.

Gallagher, J. J., Oldham, H. N., Jr., Wallace, A. G., et al: Ventricular aneurysm with ventricular tachycardia: Report of a case with epicardial mapping and successful resection. Am. J. Cardiol., *35*:696, 1975.

Gallagher, J. J., Sealy, W. C., Cox, J. L., et al: Results of surgery for pre-excitation caused by accessory atrioventricular pathways in 267 consecutive cases. *In* Josephson, M.E., and Wellens, H. J. J. (eds): Tachycardias: Mechanisms, Diagnosis, and Treatment. Philadelphia, Lea & Febiger, 1984b, pp. 259–269.

Gaskell, W. H.: On the innervation of the heart, with especial reference to the heart of the tortoise. J. Physiol., *4*:43, 1883.

Guiraudon, G., Fontaine, G., Frank, R., et al: Encircling endocardial ventriculotomy: A new surgical treatment of life-threatening ventricular tachycardias resistant to medical treatment following myocardial infarction. Ann. Thorac. Surg., *26*:438, 1978.

Guiraudon, G., Fontaine, G., Frank, R., et al: Surgical treatment of ventricular tachycardia guided by ventricular mapping in 23 patients without coronary artery disease. Presented at the 17th Annual Meeting of the Society of Thoracic Surgery, January, 1981.

Guiraudon, G. M., Klein, G. J., Sharma, A. D., et al: Surgical ablation of posterior septal accessory pathways in the Wolff-Parkinson-White syndrome by a closed heart technique. J. Thorac. Cardiovasc. Surg., *92*:406, 1986a.

Guiraudon, G. M., Klein, G. J., Sharma, A. D., et al: Closed-heart technique for Wolff-Parkinson-White syndrome: Further experience and potential limitations. Ann. Thorac. Surg., *42*:651, 1986b.

Han, J., Gael, B. G., and Hansen, C. S.: Re-entrant beats induced in the ventricle during coronary occlusion. Am. Heart J., *80*:778, 1970.

Harada, A., D'Agostino, H. J., Jr., Schuessler, R. B., et al: Right atrial isolation: A new surgical treatment for supraventricular tachycardia. I: Surgical technique and electrophysiologic effects. J. Thorac. Cardiovasc. Surg., *95*:643, 1988.

Holman, W. L., Ikeshita, M., Lease, J. G., et al: Alteration of antegrade atrioventricular conduction by cryoablation of periatrioventricular nodal tissue. J. Thorac. Cardiovasc. Surg., *88*:67, 1984.

Holman, W. L., Ikeshita, M., Lease, J. G., et al: Cryosurgical modification of retrograde atrioventricular conduction: Implications for the surgical treatment of atrioventricular node reentry tachycardia. J. Thorac. Cardiovasc. Surg., *91*:826, 1986.

Holman, W., Ikeshita, M., Lease, J. G., et al: Elective prolongation of atrioventricular conduction by multiple discrete cryolesions: A new technique for the treatment of paroxysmal supraventricular tachycardia. J. Thorac. Cardiovasc. Surg., *84*:554, 1982.

James, T. N., Froggatt, P., Atkinson, W. J., Jr., et al: De subitaneis mortibus XXX: Observations on the pathophysiology of the long Q-T syndromes with special reference to the neuropathology of the heart. Circulation, *57*:1221, 1978.

Jervell, A., and Lange-Nielsen, F.: Congenital deaf-mutism, functional heart disease with prolongation of the Q-T interval, and sudden death. Am. Heart J., *54*:59, 1957.

Josephson, M. E., Harken, A. H., and Horowitz, L. N.: Endocardial excision—a new surgical technique for the treatment of recurrent ventricular tachycardia. Circulation, *60*:1430, 1979.

Kaiser, G. A., Waldo, A. L., Harris, P. D., et al: New method to delineate myocardial damage at surgery. Circulation, *39*(Suppl. 1):83, 1969.

Katz, A. M.: The arrhythmias. II: Abnormal impulse formation and re-entry, premature systoles, pre-excitation. *In* Katz, A. M. (ed): Physiology of the Heart. New York, Raven Press, 1977, p. 331.

Kent, A. F. S.: Researches on structure and function of mammalian heart. J. Physiol., *14*:233, 1893.

Kienzle, M. G., Doherty, J. U., Roy, D., et al: Subendocardial resection for refractory ventricular tachycardia: Effects on ambulatory electrocardiogram, programmed stimulation and ejection fraction, and relation to outcome. J. Am. Coll. Cardiol., *2*:853, 1983.

Klein, G. J., Guiraudon, G. M., Perkins, D. G., et al: Surgical correction of the Wolff-Parkinson-White syndrome in the closed heart using cryosurgery: A simplified approach. J. Am. Coll. Cardiol., *3*:405, 1984.

Krafchek, J., Lawrie, G. M., Roberts, R., et al: Surgical ablation of ventricular tachycardia: Improved results with a map-directed regional approach. Circulation, *73*:1239, 1986a.

Krafchek, J., Lawrie, G. M., and Wyndham, C. R.: Cryoablation of arrhythmias from the interventricular septum: Initial experience with a new bioventricular approach. J. Thorac. Cardiovasc. Surg., *91*:419, 1986b.

Kramer, J. B., Corr, P. B., Cox, J. L., et al: Arrhythmia and conduction disturbances: Simultaneous computer mapping to facilitate intraoperative localization of accessory pathways in patients with Wolff-Parkinson-White syndrome. Am. J. Cardiol., *56*:571, 1985.

Krikler, D. M., and Curry, P. V. L.: Torsades de pointes: An atypical ventricular tachycardia. Br. Heart J., *38*:117, 1976.

Kulbertus, H. E.: La torsades de pointes. Rev. Med. Liege, *33*:63, 1978.

Kulbertus, H. E.: The arrhythmogenic effects of anti-arrhythmic agents. *In* Befeler, B. (ed): Selected Topics in Cardiac Arrhythmias. Mount Kisco, NY, Futura Publishing Co., 1980, p. 113.

Lewis, T.: The experimental production of paroxysmal tachycardia and the effects of ligation of the coronary arteries. Heart, *1*:98, 1909.

Malliani, A., Schwartz, P. J., and Zanchetti, A.: Neural mechanisms and life-threatening arrhythmias. Am. Heart J., *100*:705, 1980.

Mazur, P.: Physical-chemical factors underlying cell injury in cryosurgical freezing. *In* Rand, R.W., Rinfret, P.R., and Von Leden, H. (eds): Cryosurgery. Springfield, IL, Charles C Thomas, 1968, p. 32.

McAllister, R. E., Noble, D., and Tsien, R. W.: Reconstruction of the electrical activity of cardiac Purkinje fibers. J. Physiol., *251*:1, 1975.

Miller, J. M., Kienzle, M. G., Harken, A. H., and Josephson, M. E.: Morphologically distinct sustained ventricular tachycardias in coronary artery disease: Significant and surgical results. J. Am. Coll. Cardiol., *4*:1073, 1984a.

Miller, J. M., Kienzle, M. G., Harken, A. H., and Josephson, M. E.: Subendocardial resection for ventricular tachycardia: Predictors of surgical success. Circulation, *70*:624, 1984b.

Miller, J. M., Marchlinski, F. E., Harken, A. H., et al: Subendocardial resection for sustained ventricular tachycardia in the early period after acute myocardial infarction. Am. J. Cardiol., *55*:980, 1985.

Mines, G. R.: On circulating excitations in heart muscle and their possible relation to tachycardia and fibrillation. Trans. R. Soc. Can., *8*:43, 1914.

Moran, J. M., Kehoe, R. F., Loeb, J. M., et al: Extended endocardial resection for the treatment of ventricular tachycardia and ventricular fibrillation. Ann. Thorac. Surg., *34*:538, 1982.

Moran, J. M., Kehoe, R. F., Loeb, J. M., et al: The role of papillary muscle resection and mitral valve replacement in the control of refractory ventricular arrhythmia. Circulation, *68*(Suppl. II):154, 1983.

Moss, A. J., and McDonald, J.: Unilateral cervicothoracic sympathetic ganglionectomy for the treatment of long Q-T interval syndrome. N. Engl. J. Med., *285*:903, 1971.

Ostermeyer, J., Borggrefe, M., Breithardt, G., et al: Direct operations for the management of life-threatening ischemic ventricular tachycardia. J. Thorac. Cardiovasc. Surg., *94*:848, 1987.

Ostermeyer, J., Breithardt, G., Borggrefe, M., et al: Surgical treatment of ventricular tachycardias: Complete versus partial encircling endocardial ventriculotomy. J. Thorac. Cardiovasc. Surg., *87*:517, 1984.

Platia, E. V., Griffith, L. S., Watkins, L., Jr., et al: Treatment of malignant ventricular arrhythmias with endocardial resection and implantation of the automatic cardioverter-defibrillator. N. Engl. J. Med., *314*:213, 1986.

Rasmussen, K., Winkle, R., Ross, D., et al: Antiarrhythmic efficacy of amiodarone in recurrent ventricular tachycardia evaluated by multiple electrophysiological and ambulatory ECG recordings. Acta Med. Scand., *212*:367, 1982.

Reuter, H.: The dependence of slow inward current in Purkinje fibers on the extracellular calcium concentration. J. Physiol., *192*:479, 1967.

Romano, C., Gemme, G., and Pongiglione, R.: Aritmie cardiache rare dell'eta pediatrica. Clin. Pediatr., *45*:656, 1963.

Ross, D. L., Johnson, D. C., Denniss, A. R., et al: Curative surgery for atrioventricular junctional ("A-V nodal") reentrant tachycardia. J. Am. Coll. Cardiol., *6*:1383, 1985.

Salomon, N., Stinson, E., Randall, B., and Shumway, N.: Patient related risk factors as predictors of results following isolated mitral valve replacement. Ann. Thorac. Surg., *24*:519, 1977.

Scheinman, M. M., Morady, F., Hess, D. S., and Gonzalez, R.: Catheter-induced ablation of the atrioventricular junction to control refractory supraventricular arrhythmias. J.A.M.A., *248*:851, 1982.

Scherlag, B. J., El-Sherif, N., Hopen, R. R., and Lazzara, R.: Characterization and localization of ventricular arrhythmias resulting from myocardial ischemia and infarction. Circ. Res., *35*:372, 1974.

Schwartz, P. J., Periti, M., and Malliani, A.: The long Q-T syndrome. Am. Heart J., *89*:378, 1975.

Sealy, W.C.: The Wolff-Parkinson-White syndrome and the beginnings of direct arrhythmia surgery. Ann. Thorac. Surg., *38*:176, 1984.

Sealy, W. C., Gallagher, J. J., and Kasell, J. H.: His bundle interruption for control of inappropriate ventricular responses to atrial arrhythmias. Ann. Thorac. Surg., *32*:429, 1981.

Selle, J. G., Svenson, R. H., Sealy, W. C., et al: Successful clinical laser ablation of ventricular tachycardia: A promising new therapeutic method. Ann. Thorac. Surg., *42*:380, 1986.

Smith, W., and Gallagher, J. J.: Q-T prolongation syndromes. Pract. Cardiol., *5*:118, 1979.

Strauss, H. C., Prystowsky, E. N., and Scheinman, N. M.: Sinoatrial and atrial electrogenesis. Prog. Cardiovasc. Dis., *19*:385, 1977.

Svenson, R. H., Gallagher, J. J., Selle, J. G., et al: YAG laser photocoagulation: A successful new map-guided technique for the intraoperative ablation of ventricular tachycardia. Circulation, *76*:1319, 1987.

Swerdlow, C. D., Mason, J. W., Stinson, E. B., et al: Results of operations for ventricular tachycardia in 105 patients. J. Thorac. Cardiovasc. Surg., *92*:105, 1986.

Uhl, H. S.: A previously undescribed malformation of the heart: Almost total absence of the myocardium of the right ventricle. Bull. Johns Hopkins Hosp., *91*:197, 1952.

Ungerleider, R. M., Holman, W. L., Stanley, T. E., III, et al: Encircling endocardial ventriculotomy (EEV) for refractory ischemic ventricular tachycardia. I: Electrophysiologic effects. J. Thorac. Cardiovasc. Surg., *83*:840, 1982a.

Ungerleider, R. M., Holman, W. L., Stanley, T. E., III, et al: Encircling endocardial ventriculotomy (EEV) for refractory ischemic ventricular tachycardia. II: Effects on regional myocardial blood flow. J. Thorac. Cardiovasc. Surg., *83*:850, 1982b.

Ungerleider, R. M., Holman, W. L., Calcagno, D., et al: Encircling endocardial ventriculotomy (EEV) for refractory ischemic ventricular tachycardia. III: Effects on regional left ventricular function. J. Thorac. Cardiovasc. Surg., *83*:857, 1982c.

Waldo, A. L., and Kaiser, G. A.: A study of ventricular arrhythmias associated with acute myocardial infarction in the canine heart. Circulation, *47*:1222, 1973.

Ward, O. C.: New familial cardiac syndrome in children. J. Ir. Med. Assoc., *54*:103, 1964.

Wellens, H. J. J., Duren, D. R., Liem, K., and Lie, K. I.: Effects of digitalis in patients with paroxysmal atrioventricular nodal tachycardia. Circulation, 52:779, 1975.

Williams, J. M., Ungerleider, R. M., Lofland, G. K., and Cox, J. L.: Left atrial isolation: New technique for the treatment of supraventricular arrhythmias. J. Thorac. Cardiovasc. Surg., 80:373, 1980.

Witkowski, F. X., and Corr, P. B.: An automated simultaneous transmural cardiac mapping system. Am. J. Physiol., 247:H661, 1984.

Wittig, J. H., and Boineau, J. P.: Surgical treatment of ventricular arrhythmias using epicardial transmural and endocardial mapping. Ann. Thorac. Surg., 20:117, 1975.

Wolferth, C. C., and Wood, F. C.: The mechanism of production of short P-R intervals and prolonged QRS complexes in patients with presumably undamaged hearts: Hypothesis of an accessory pathway of auriculo-ventricular conduction (bundle of Kent). Am. Heart J., 8:297, 1933.

Wolff, L., Parkinson, J., and White, P. D.: Bundle branch block with short PR interval in healthy young people prone to paroxysmal tachycardia. Am. Heart J., 5:685, 1930.

Wood, F. C., Wolferth, C. C., and Geckler, G. D.: Histologic demonstration of accessory muscular connections between auricle and ventricle in a case of short P-R interval and prolonged QRS complex. Am. Heart J., 25:454, 1943.

Yanowitz, F., Preston, J. B., and Abildskov, J. A.: Functional distribution of right and left stellate innervation to the ventricles. Circ. Res., 18:416, 1966.

Zipes, D. P., and Fisher, J. C.: Effects of agents which inhibit the slow channel on sinus node automaticity and atrioventricular induction in the dog. Circ. Res., 34:184, 1974.

CHAPTER 56

TUMORS OF THE HEART

Peter Van Trigt
David C. Sabiston, Jr.

Primary neoplasms of the heart are rare forms of cardiac disease. These tumors range in clinical presentation from the more common myxoma, which can usually be cured, to the rare cardiac sarcoma, which is associated with a uniformly poor outcome. These tumors are of great interest because of their low incidence and protean clinical manifestations and because the benign form represents a potentially curable form of serious cardiac disease that can be diagnosed accurately by echocardiography.

Cardiac tumors have been recognized since the report by Columbus from Padua in 1562. In 1934 Barnes and associates made the first antemortem clinical diagnosis of a primary sarcoma of the heart by using electrocardiography and biopsy of a metastatic nodule. In 1936 Beck successfully removed an intrapericardial teratoma (Beck, 1942). In 1945 Mahaim published a classic monograph that described 413 tumors of the heart and pericardium. Angiography was first used clinically to show an intracardiac myxoma in 1951 (Goldberg et al, 1952), and Bahnson and Newman (1953) removed a large right atrial myxoma in 1952, but the patient died 24 days later. The first successful resection of a left atrial myxoma was done in 1954 by Crafoord with use of cardiopulmonary bypass (Crafoord, 1955). The introduction of echocardiography in 1968 provided a noninvasive technique that allowed accurate diagnosis of cardiac neoplasms (Schattenberg, 1968). Before that time, 90% of tumors were diagnosed at autopsy or as an unexpected finding at cardiac operation.

INCIDENCE

Primary cardiac tumors are rare; the incidence at autopsy is variously reported between 0.002 and 0.3% (Silverman, 1980). These neoplasms are often difficult to diagnose because of their varied clinical presentation. Approximately 75% of primary tumors of the heart are benign, and half of those are myxomas (Table 56–1). The approximately 25% of primary cardiac neoplasms that are malignant are almost always a form of sarcoma (Table 56–2). Malignant neoplasms are more common in adults and constitute less than 10% of primary cardiac tumors in children.

Patients with myxomas have the most favorable prognosis and have a 90% or greater survival after resection. The survival for other benign tumors is approximately 50%, and survival is less than 10% for primary cardiac malignancies. Reports of several large series reviewed the incidence and clinical characteristics of cardiac neoplasms (Bloor and O'Rourke, 1984; Goldman et al, 1986; Poole et al, 1984; Silverman, 1980); the largest collection was reported from the Armed Forces Institute of Pathology (AFIP), which has more than 500 specimens (McAllister and Fenoglio, 1978).

MYXOMA

Myxoma is the most frequent primary tumor of the heart and constitutes 27% of all tumors and cysts of the heart in the AFIP series. In adults, half of all benign cardiac tumors are myxomas. Myxomas occur less often in children and represent 10% of all pediatric benign tumors (Table 56–3). These lesions are

TABLE 56–1. BENIGN CARDIAC NEOPLASMS IN ADULTS*

Tumor	No.	Percent
Myxoma	118	49
Lipoma	45	19
Papillary fibroelastoma	42	17
Hemangioma	11	5
AV node mesothelioma	9	4
Fibroma	5	2
Teratoma	3	1
Granular cell tumor	3	1
Neurofibroma	2	<1
Lymphangioma	2	<1
Rhabdomyoma	1	<1
Total	241	100

*From McAllister, H. A., Jr., and Fenoglio, J. J., Jr.: Tumors of the cardiovascular system. *In* Hartman, W. H., and Cowan, W. R. (eds): Atlas of Tumor Pathology. Washington, DC, Armed Forces Institute of Pathology, 1978.

TABLE 56–2. PRIMARY MALIGNANT CARDIAC NEOPLASMS IN ADULTS*

Tumor	No.	Percent
Angiosarcoma	39	33
Rhabdomyosarcoma	24	21
Mesothelioma	19	16
Fibrosarcoma	13	11
Lymphoma	7	6
Osteosarcoma	5	4
Thymoma	4	3
Neurogenic sarcoma	3	2
Leiomyosarcoma	1	<1
Liposarcoma	1	<1
Synovial sarcoma	1	<1
Total	117	100

*From McAllister, H. A., Jr., and Fenoglio, J. J., Jr.: Tumors of the cardiovascular system. *In* Hartman, W. H., and Cowan, W. R. (eds): Atlas of Tumor Pathology. Washington, DC, Armed Forces Institute of Pathology, 1978.

the most significant cardiac tumors, not only because of their relative frequency but also because the potential for total cure after surgical removal is high (Bulkley and Hutchins, 1979). Myxoma arises from the endocardium as a polypoid, often pedunculated, tumor that extends into a cardiac chamber. Cardiac myxomas are derived from multipotential mesenchymal cells of the subendocardial layer and imitate primitive mesenchyme. Most experts consider that atrial myxomas are true neoplasms on the basis of histologic, ultrastructural, electron microscopic, and tissue culture studies, although in the past some physicians thought that cardiac myxomas developed from organized thrombi and underwent myxomatous degeneration (Salyer et al, 1975). Myxomas occur in patients at all ages, but the incidence is greatest in patients in the third to sixth decades, and there is a slight predominance in women. A familial tendency for cardiac myxoma has been found and rarely is associated with a constellation of findings that include multiple pigmented skin lesions, myxoid fibroadenoma of the breasts, and pigmented nodular adrenocortical disease.

Most myxomas arise singly in the atria and approximately 75% occur in the left atrium (Sabiston

and Hattler, 1983). The remainder usually occur in the right atrium (20%) or in the ventricles (less than 10%). Multiple or multicentric myxoma occurs in 5% of patients. Atrial myxomas are commonly attached to the septum in the region of the fossa ovalis; the next most common site is the posterior atrial wall. Most ventricular myxomas do not arise from the interventricular septum. Rarely they arise from the mitral or aortic valve leaflet tissue (Gosse et al, 1986; Hajar et al, 1986; Sandrasgra et al, 1979). Bilateral atrial tumors usually arise from corresponding sites on opposite sides of the interatrial septum and represent growth in both directions from a single focus within the atrial septum (Imperio et al, 1980).

Pathology

Although myxomas differ in clinical presentation, most myxomas have a similar macroscopic and microscopic character (Wold and Lie, 1980). These tumors are soft, gelatinous, and polypoid clusters often with a pedunculated attachment to the endocardium (Fig. 56–1). The average diameter is 5 to 6 cm, but they can range in size from 0.5 to 15 cm. Areas of hemorrhage are often apparent in gross surgical specimens. True sessile myxomas with a wide-based attachment are less common.

Microscopically, these neoplasms consist of a myxoid matrix comprised of a basophilic ground substance rich in mucopolysaccharides (Fig. 56–2). Within the myxoid matrix are polygonal cells, which are often stellate and sometimes multinuclear (Ferrans and Roberts, 1973). The cells may be single or occur in clusters and form vascular-like channels that simulate primitive capillaries. Ultrastructurally, these polygonal cells resemble multipotential mesenchymal cells. Other cellular elements include plasma cells, lymphocytes, and mast cells. Foci of calcification are seen in 10% of myxomas (Fig. 56–3).

Malignant Potential

Although myxomas are considered to be benign neoplasms, their recurrence and metastatic potential

TABLE 56–3. BENIGN CARDIAC NEOPLASMS IN CHILDREN*

Tumor	0 to 1 Year		1 to 15 Years	
	No.	Percent	No.	Percent
Rhabdomyoma	28	62	35	45.0
Teratoma	9	21	11	14.0
Fibroma	6	13	12	15.5
Hemangioma	1	2	4	5.0
AV node mesothelioma	1	2	3	4.0
Myxoma	—	—	12	15.5
Neurofibroma	—	—	1	1.0
Total	45	100	78	100

*From McAllister, H. A., Jr., and Fenoglio, J. J., Jr.: Tumors of the cardiovascular system. *In* Hartman, W. H., and Cowan, W. R. (eds): Atlas of Tumor Pathology. Washington, DC, Armed Forces Institute of Pathology, 1978.

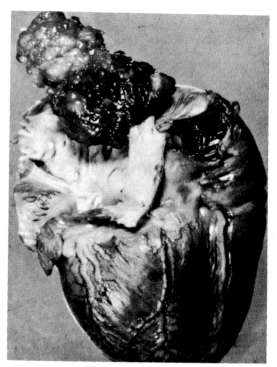

Figure 56–1. Large, friable, gelatinous myxoma located in the left atrium, attached to the atrial septum. Extreme care must be taken during surgical removal to avoid operative embolization. (From McAllister, H. A., and Fenoglio, J. J.: Tumors of the cardiovascular system. In Hartman, W. H., and Cowan, W. R. (eds): Atlas of Tumor Pathology. Washington D.C., Armed Forces Institute of Pathology, 1978.)

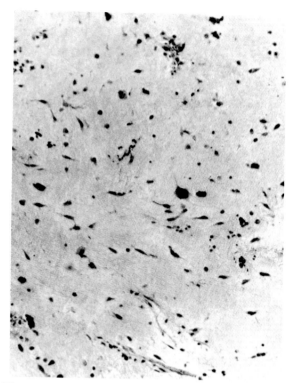

Figure 56–2. Histologic section of atrial myxoma showing polygonal cells dispersed throughout a lightly staining acid mucopolysaccharide matrix.

have been noted (Gerbode et al, 1967; Hannah et al, 1982; Markel et al, 1986; McAllister, 1979; Read et al, 1974). McAllister and Fenoglio (1978) thought that cardiac myxomas initially considered to be malignant were actually examples of sarcomas with extensive areas of myxoid degeneration (liposarcoma, rhabdomyosarcoma) or multicentric benign myxomas. Attum and associates (1987) reviewed 57 cases of malignant myxomas or "myxoid imitators" documented in the literature between 1933 and 1985. Recurrence of the tumor or metastases occurred in approximately 50% of the patients reviewed. The mortality in this group of patients was 47% and surgical excision was attempted in all except five patients. Eight patients had myxoma associated with multiple mycotic cerebral aneurysms that were thought to occur by invasive transgression of arterial walls with replacement of the muscularis by embolic myxomatous tissue. In a separate review of 16 series with a total of 194 patients with atrial myxoma who survived operation, the recurrence rate for "benign" myxoma was 7% (Gray and Williams, 1985). The authors emphasize the importance of follow-up of all patients after resection of cardiac myxoma with serial two-dimensional echocardiography because of the possibility of recurrent tumor. Myxomas that arose from extraseptal locations were thought to be more likely to recur, and the microscopic appearance of the primary tumor

is not predictive of the tendency to recur or metastasize (Martin et al, 1987).

Syndrome of "Complex" Cardiac Myxoma

A group of patients from the Mayo Clinic had unusual biologic behavior of cardiac myxomas, including development at an early age, atypical location

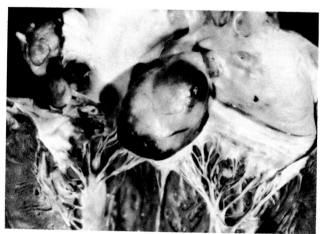

Figure 56–3. Although most myxomas are polypoid and friable, a significant number are round and smooth and may be confused with ball-thrombi.

of the myxomas, and a high risk for recurrence of myxomas (Powers et al, 1979). Of 85 patients evaluated at the Mayo Clinic for cardiac myxoma, 5 had unusual associated findings that included multiple pigmented skin lesions, myxoid fibroadenomas of the breast, skin myxomas, and primary pigmented nodular adrenocortical disease (a cause of Cushing's syndrome) (Carney et al, 1985). Four of these five patients had multiple cardiac myxomas and three of the four patients who had surgical excision had recurrent myxomas. The occurrence of multiple and recurrent myxomas in patients with the complex was significantly higher than in the 80 patients with sporadic myxomas (Jones et al, 1986). The authors commented that the myxomas that occur with this complex of findings can be familial, and because of the high risk of recurrence screening of patients after resection and screening of asymptomatic family members are indicated (Carney et al, 1985; McCarthy et al, 1986; Powers et al, 1979).

Clinical Presentation

Atrial myxoma produces various clinical presentations that can be categorized into three main types: (1) obstructive manifestations, which are due to tumor occlusion or interference with flow through the atrioventricular valves and simulate mitral and tricuspid valve disease; (2) embolic manifestations; and (3) constitutional manifestations, which simulate a systemic disease.

Before an accurate noninvasive diagnostic modality (two-dimensional echocardiography) was available, most myxomas were diagnosed postmortem. Echocardiography combined with a higher clinical index of suspicion has allowed earlier diagnosis and successful surgical removal in most patients (O'Neil et al, 1979; Sutton et al, 1980).

In the AFIP series of 130 cases, 44% of patients with myxomas were seen with signs and symptoms of obstructive valvular disease (McAllister, 1979). In this group, 30% had an initial history of systemic embolization and 12% had no previous symptoms. The clinical features of cardiac myxoma are summarized in Table 56–4 and are relevant particularly to left atrial myxoma. Patients with myxoma may have none, some, or all of the classic manifestations, but the various features are seldom associated and the clinical diagnosis can be difficult to make.

As a result of obstruction of flow by the tumor, left atrial myxomas often mimic mitral stenosis and the most common symptom is dyspnea or left-sided heart failure (Panidis et al, 1986). If the pedicle of the myxoma is large, the tumor may intermittently obstruct the mitral orifice and cause syncope or sudden death. Careful examination may show positional hemodynamic alterations that include the classic early diastolic sound or "tumor plop." This sound is best heard at the apex and may be confused with the opening snap of a pliable mitral stenosis, but the

TABLE 56–4. CLINICAL PRESENTATION OF CARDIAC MYXOMA IN 131 PATIENTS*

Signs and symptoms of mitral valve disease	57
Embolic phenomena	36
No cardiac symptoms—incidental findings	16
Signs and symptoms of tricuspid valve disease	6
Sudden unexpected death	5
Pericarditis	4
Myocardial infarction	3
Signs and symptoms of pulmonary valve disease	2
Fever of undetermined origin	2

*From McAllister, H. A., Jr., and Fenoglio, J. J., Jr.: Tumors of the cardiovascular system. *In* Hartman, W. H., and Cowan, W. R. (eds): Atlas of Tumor Pathology. Washington, DC, Armed Forces Institute of Pathology, 1978.

tumor plop generally occurs later and has a much lower intensity.

In addition to heart failure and dyspnea, other complaints involve ill-defined chest pain. Hemoptysis is often found in mitral stenosis but is unusual in patients with left atrial myxoma despite the increase in pulmonary vascular resistance that often occurs with left atrial myxomas (Selzer et al, 1972).

Right atrial myxomas are often larger than left atrial myxomas and may produce obstruction of the tricuspid orifice that results in the clinical presentation of tricuspid stenosis. Alternatively, the tumor may damage the leaflets and cause tricuspid insufficiency. This lesion may also be confused clinically with constrictive pericarditis, pulmonary hypertension, and Ebstein's anomaly (Currey et al, 1967).

Systemic emboli occur in approximately one-third of patients with cardiac myxoma. Embolization is common because of the friability of the tumor and the intracavitary location. In many patients the embolus is the initial clinical presentation and in most cases involves the cerebrovascular circulation (DeSousa et al, 1978). Emboli to lower extremity arteries occur next in frequency, and other sites include the renal arteries, abdominal aorta, and coronary arteries. After embolization of friable myxomatous material, a diagnosis of cardiac myxoma can be made by histologic examination of the surgical specimen removed at thrombectomy. The first antemortem diagnosis of a left atrial myxoma was made by examining peripheral arterial tumor emboli (Goldberg et al, 1952). Embolic episodes in young patients with normal sinus rhythm should arouse suspicion of cardiac myxoma in the absence of active endocarditis. Pulmonary emboli from right atrial myxomas occur similar to emboli in the systemic circulation. Whereas typical pulmonary thromboembolic disease usually resolves after anticoagulation or through the natural fibrinolytic mechanism, tumor defects can remain occlusive for a long time and may give rise to pulmonary hypertension from vascular obstruction. Paradoxical embolism from a right atrial myxoma in association with atrial septal defect has been reported (Powers et al, 1979).

Myxomas can present with unusual constitutional symptoms, most commonly increased red blood cell sedimentation rate, fever, anemia, weight loss, and protein abnormalities (usually increased serum immunoglobulin levels). The association of fever, anemia, and increased sedimentation rate with myxoma was described by MacGregor and Cullen in 1959. Constitutional manifestations noted since then include leukocytosis, arthralgias, thrombocytopenia, and Raynaud's phenomenon. Most patients have one or more of these symptoms at some stage during the illness and the constitutional symptoms may occur long before obstructive or embolic symptoms. Generally, the constitutional symptoms and serum protein abnormalities vanish after tumor resection (Hattler et al, 1970).

Mechanisms proposed for the constitutional manifestations include hemorrhage and degeneration within the tumor, microembolism, and an immunologic response to the release of tumor fragments that leads to an increase in immunoglobulins (Currey et al, 1967). The probable cause of the increase in sedimentation rate is the hypergammaglobulinemia, but no qualitative abnormalities in globulins have been documented.

Because of the protean clinical manifestations of cardiac myxoma, a high index of suspicion is needed in the clinical approach to diagnosis (Silverman and Sabiston, 1981). The differential diagnosis for a left atrial myxoma includes mitral stenosis, mitral regurgitation, infective endocarditis, acute rheumatic fever, collagen vascular disorders (polyarteritis no-

dosa), and Wegener's granulomatosis (Leonhardt and Kullenberg, 1977). Right atrial myxoma may be difficult to distinguish clinically from isolated rheumatic tricuspid stenosis or regurgitation, constrictive pericarditis, Ebstein's anomaly, carcinoid syndrome, chronic pulmonary emboli, or pulmonary hypertension.

DIAGNOSTIC TESTS

The impact of noninvasive screening tests, specifically two-dimensional echocardiography, on the diagnosis and management of cardiac neoplasms is shown in the Mayo Clinic review of 40 patients with atrial myxoma evaluated from 1957 to 1977. Before the introduction of echocardiography in 1968, the diagnosis was made preoperatively or antemortem in only 37% of patients, compared with 90% of patients treated after 1968 (Sutton et al, 1980). Other major diagnostic techniques that help in evaluating cardiac neoplasms before surgical intervention are computed tomography, magnetic resonance imaging, and cineangiography.

Echocardiography

Since use of two-dimensional echocardiography has become routine, almost 100% of atrial myxomas have been diagnosed noninvasively (Goldman et al,

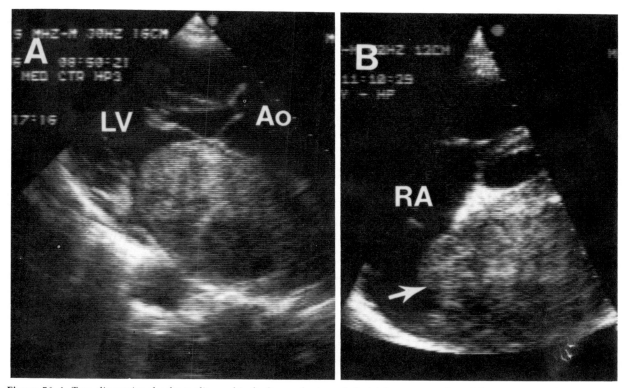

Figure 56–4. Two-dimensional echocardiographic findings of a large left atrial myxoma, viewed by a parasternal long axis image (*A*) and a parasternal short axis image (*B*). *A,* The myxoma is seen to occlude the mitral valve orifice. Almost the entire left atrium is filled. *B,* A portion of the myxoma bulges (*arrow*) through the fossa ovalis. (Courtesy of Joseph A. Kisslo, M.D., Duke University Medical Center.)

1986). In efficacy and accuracy, preoperative diagnosis by echocardiography is superior to diagnosis by cardiac catheterization and angiography. In the Mayo Clinic review (Sutton et al, 1980), the diagnosis was not made in one-third of the patients who had catheterization. Also, patients with myxomas are at risk of catheter-induced embolization. Most authors agree that the preoperative diagnosis of a myxoma can be based solely on echocardiography and that catheterization is not indicated (Dein et al, 1987; Silverman, 1980).

The M-mode of echocardiography was developed first and rapidly became helpful in diagnosis of atrial myxoma. The characteristic finding from M-mode echocardiography is the presence of a mass of echoes behind the anterior mitral leaflet a few milliseconds after maximal opening. The layered mass of echoes fills the space between the anterior and posterior mitral leaflets throughout the rest of diastole and then returns to the left atrial cavity during systole.

Two-dimensional echocardiography provides real-time imaging of the entire heart and specifically allows visualization of the entire left atrium, right atrium, interatrial septum, atrioventricular (AV) valve, orifices, both ventricles, and the venae cavae (Fig. 56–4). This method is superior to M-mode

echocardiography because it provides quantitative information about tumor size, position in the heart, mobility, and effect on valvular and ventricular function (Figs. 56–5 and 56–6). With the resolution and spatial orientation of two-dimensional echocardiography, the attachment site of the tumor and the stalk can be well visualized (DePace et al, 1981). Even very small valvular papillary fibroelastomas (0.5 cm) have been localized accurately (McFadden et al, 1987). Myxoma can be detected in all cardiac chambers, and biatrial and multiple tumors have been detected with this technique (Tway et al, 1981). Two-dimensional echocardiography also provides an excellent means of follow-up to detect late tumor recurrence (Fig. 56–7).

Generally, two-dimensional echo imaging provides a safe and accurate diagnosis and obviates the need for cardiac catheterization for most patients (Dunningham et al, 1981). Other atrial masses that can usually be discriminated from myxoma include thrombi, vegetations, and metastatic tumor (Panidis et al, 1984). Echo imaging is also useful in the detection of other intramural ventricular lesions but cannot be used alone to determine the malignant nature or histologic characteristics of these lesions. Intraoperative transesophageal echocardiography (Fig. 56–8) combined with color-flow Doppler imaging has been used to plan the surgical approach, including selection of the right atrial site for cannulation (Mora et al, 1987).

Computed Tomography and Magnetic Resonance Imaging

Myxomas and other cardiac tumors have been visualized with high resolution by computed tomography (CT) and magnetic resonance imaging (MRI). Although CT scanning times are too long to detect motion of the heart, there is excellent tissue discrimination (based on density or specific gravity of the tissue) and primary or secondary cardiac tumors (such as liposarcomas) can be distinguished from normal cardiac tissue (Chaloupka et al, 1986). CT imaging is not useful for the diagnosis of myxoma, which is similar in tissue density to normal cardiac tissue, but it gives the best evaluation of the extra-cardiac mediastinal structures, which are usually not imaged by echocardiography (Shin et al, 1987).

MRI is a newer technique that enables high-resolution tomography in three dimensions. It is nonionizing and provides intravascular and soft-tissue contrast without the need for contrast medium. Electrocardiographic gating allows high-resolution imaging of cardiac morphology (Figs. 56–9 and 56–10) and has made MRI a promising technique for the evaluation of cardiac neoplasms (Camesas et al, 1986). In a review of 14 patients with intracavitary cardiac tumors diagnosed initially by echocardiography who subsequently had MRI, the MRI contributed important additional information about the tumor's

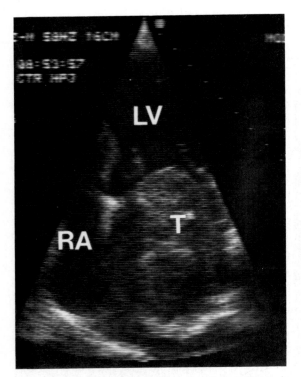

Figure 56–5. Apical four-chamber view of the patient shown in Figure 56–4. The myxoma (T) is seen to prolapse through and occlude the mitral valve orifice in diastole. The point of attachment was diffusely over the atrial septum, which required almost complete atrial septectomy and repair with a pericardial patch. (Courtesy of Joseph A. Kisslo, M.D., Duke University Medical Center.)

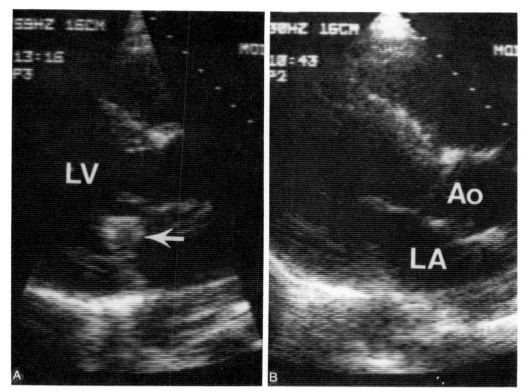

Figure 56–6. *A,* Parasternal long axis view from a patient with a left atrial myxoma attached to the posterior left atrial wall (*arrow*). *B,* The same patient is shown 1 day later after the onset of right lower extremity pain. The tumor was found in the right iliac artery. (Courtesy of Joseph A. Kisslo, M.D., Duke University Medical Center.)

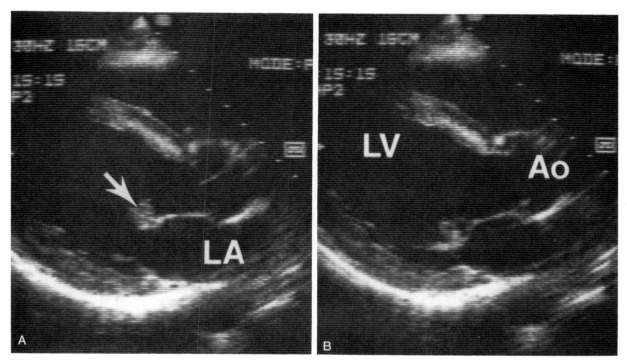

Figure 56–7. *A,* Paired parasternal long axis images in diastole and systole. *B,* The arrow indicates a small myxoma on the tip of the anterior mitral valve leaflet. The myxoma was removed with primary excision and repair of the anterior mitral leaflet. (Courtesy of Joseph A. Kisslo, M.D., Duke University Medical Center.)

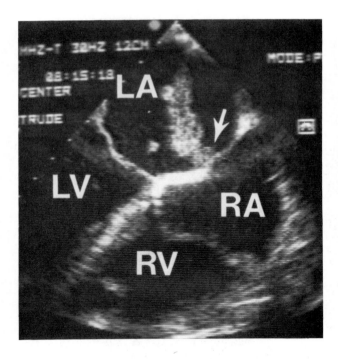

Figure 56–8. Transesophageal two-dimensional echocardiogram showing a left atrial myxoma attached at the fossa ovalis (*arrow*).

relationship to normal intracardiac structures or extension to adjacent vascular and mediastinal structures (Freedberg et al, 1988). The information was especially helpful for tumors other than myxomas (e.g., angiosarcoma, metastatic melanoma, malignant thymoma, and hypernephroma) (Gindea et al, 1987). In a separate review by Go, MRI was found to provide better definition of tumor prolapse, secondary valvular obstruction, and cardiac chamber size than two-dimensional echo imaging. Although two-dimensional echocardiography is still the technique of choice in the initial evaluation of intracardiac tumors, MRI can be an important adjunct in the

diagnostic evaluation of cardiac tumors (Gomes et al, 1987).

Cineangiography

Before echocardiography, angiocardiography was the standard preoperative test used to confirm the diagnosis of myxoma and other cardiac tumors. Injection of contrast material allows visualization of intracavitary filling defects, and mobile myxomas may be seen to traverse right and left AV valves during the cardiac cycle (Fig. 56–11). Small atrial ball-

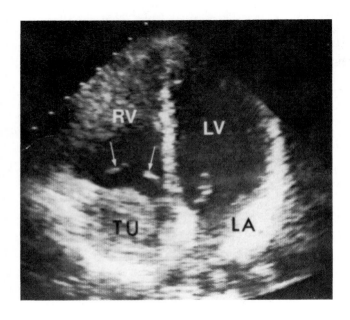

Figure 56–9. Apical four-chamber echocardiogram showing a large sessile tumor (angiosarcoma) in the right atrium of a 29-year-old woman who presented with superior vena caval syndrome.

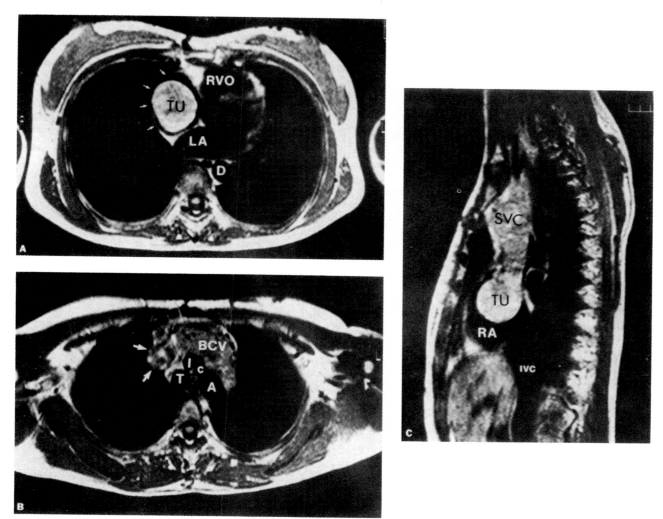

Figure 56–10. Magnetic resonance tomograms from the patient in Figure 56–9 show the intravenous extension of the tumor (Tu). *A,* Axial image through the atria shows a high-signal tumor mass with right atrium (*arrows*). (D = descending aorta, LA = left atrium, RVO = right ventricular outflow tract.) *B,* Axial image at the level of the aortic arch (A) and great vessels shows tumor mass within superior vena cava (*arrows*) and brachiocephalic vein (BCV). *C,* Sagittal image shows tumor within the right atrium extending into the superior vena cava (SVC). (From Freedberg, R. S., Kronzon, I., Rumancik, W. M., and Liebeskind, D.: Contribution of magnetic resonance imaging to the evaluation of intracardiac tumors diagnosed by echocardiography. Circulation, *77:*96, 1988. By permission of the American Heart Association, Inc.)

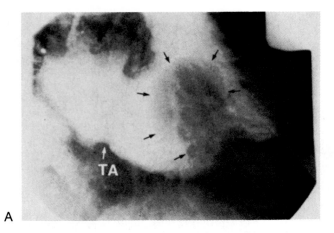

A

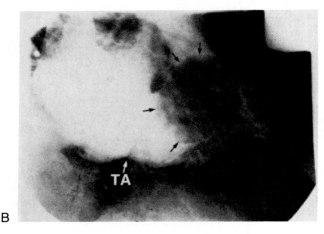

B

Figure 56–11. Cineangiographic appearance of a large liposarcoma within the right ventricle (*arrows*) after contrast injection in the right atrium. *A,* The large smooth pedunculated tumor is attached to the right ventricular apex. *B,* Systole. The pedunculated tumor almost fills the right ventricular outflow tract. (TA = tricuspid annulus.) (From Godwin, J.D., Axel, L., Adams, J. R., et al: Computed tomography: A method for diagnosing tumors of the heart. Circulation, *63*:448, 1981. By permission of the American Heart Association, Inc.)

thrombi may be mistaken for myxomas and small intramural tumors may not be visualized. Selective coronary angiography may also show neovascularization of a tumor, but this is not commonly found. With angiography, morbidity and mortality are associated with catheter-induced embolization of the tumor (Seifert et al, 1986). Trans-septal injection techniques are not recommended for left atrial myxomas, which most often arise from the fossa ovalis and are best visualized during the levo phase of a pulmonary artery injection. At present, the role of angiography is small; it should be used if the echocardiogram is normal but the clinical presentation is highly suggestive or if there is some doubt about the echocardiographic findings.

Other Diagnostic Tests

Phonocardiography, gated radionucleotide cardiac imaging, and plain chest films are sometimes helpful, but the contribution of these screening tests is outweighed heavily by the advantages and accuracy of two-dimensional echocardiography (Come et al, 1981).

SURGICAL MANAGEMENT OF MYXOMAS

After the diagnosis of cardiac myxoma, operation should proceed on an urgent basis; up to 8% of patients with myxoma die while they await operation (Chitwood, 1988). Intracardiac neoplasms are best managed by complete excision under direct vision with use of cardiopulmonary bypass and hypothermic cardioplegic arrest (Castenada and Varco, 1968; Okada et al, 1986) (Figs. 56–12 and 56–13). Recurrence of myxoma has been documented (Gerbode et al, 1967; Read et al, 1974) and should be prevented by complete resection with removal of an adequate margin of normal endocardium, atrial septum, or atrial wall. Tumor manipulation should be minimal during cannulation and before aortic cross-clamping and cardioplegic arrest to prevent intraoperative tumor dislodgment and embolization. Most patients do well after resection, and operative mortality is less than 3% (Dein et al, 1987; Hanson et al, 1985). Probably the greatest risk for perioperative mortality and morbidity is tumor embolization to the cerebral or coronary circulation.

The surgical approach for resection of cardiac

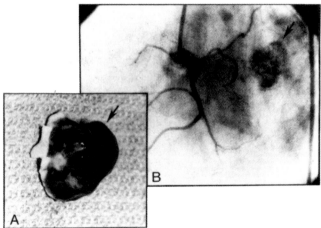

Figure 56–12. *A,* A small left atrial myxoma shown after resection. *B,* Right coronary injection shows filling of tumor vessels. The myxoma *(arrow)* was an incidental finding at cardiac catheterization. (From Chitwood, W. R.: Cardiac neoplasms—current diagnosis, pathology and therapy. J. Cardiac Surg., 3:119, 1988.)

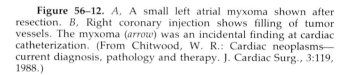

myxoma is usually a median sternotomy; a right anterolateral thoracotomy through the fourth intercostal space is selected for a better cosmetic result in younger women (Fig. 56–14). The patient is placed on cardiopulmonary bypass with perfusion temperature maintained at 28 to 30° C. Minimal tumor manipulation during cannulation and institution of full cardiopulmonary bypass is required to minimize risk of embolization. The myxoma is then removed through the appropriate atriotomy; right atrial myxomas are usually more easily exposed and more expeditiously resected. For surgical removal of myxomas attached to the atrial septum, part of the atrial septal wall to which the pedicle of the tumor is attached must be removed en bloc with the pedicle of the tumor. The defect is closed either primarily or with a native pericardial or prosthetic patch.

Exposure and resection of left atrial myxomas are usually more difficult. Most surgeons approach these tumors through a left atriotomy made posterior to the interatrial groove in a manner similar to mitral valve exposure (Guiloff et al, 1986). The interatrial septum is positioned anteriorly and exposure is fa-

cilitated by use of special atrial retractors. For large myxomas with a broad-based attachment to the atrial septum, the neoplasm is better exposed with a right atriotomy and a trans-septal approach. With this method, access is provided to the atrial septum, mitral valve, and free atrial wall, and left atrial myxomas can be readily resected with an adequate button of normal tissue. Removal of a large tumor base usually requires patch closure. Biatrial incisions are recommended by some surgeons to allow adequate examination of all cardiac chambers. Biatrial myxomas usually arise from a common site in the interatrial septum that extends on each side. Both myxomas may be removed through separate atrial incisions or through a single atrial incision with a second septal incision.

Prognosis after surgical excision is usually excellent (Hattler et al, 1970; Silverman, 1980). Regression of all preoperative symptoms including the constitutional symptoms of the myxoma syndrome has been documented for periods of more than 15 years.

Right ventricular myxomas are best excised through a right ventriculotomy because they usually

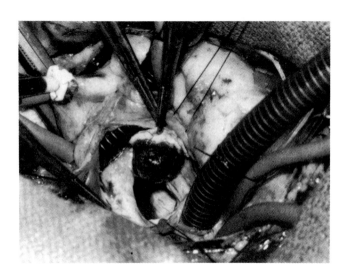

Figure 56–13. The left atrial myxoma shown in Figure 56–12 is being removed by a trans-septal right atrial approach, with excellent exposure allowed under cardioplegic arrest.

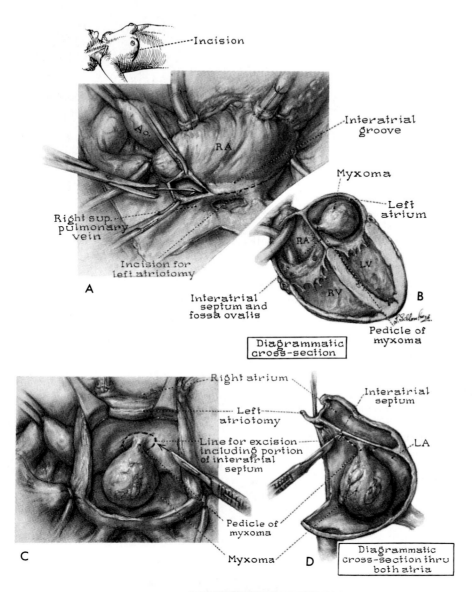

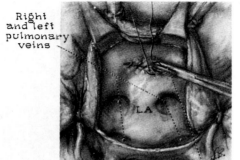

Figure 56–14. Surgical technique for removal of a left atrial myxoma. *A,* The aorta is clamped and cardioplegic arrest is achieved. The left atrial myxoma is approached through a left atriotomy. *B,* The myxoma arises from the interatrial septum near the fossa ovalis. *C,* The myxoma is exposed and a portion of the atrial septum is excised around the attachment of the pedicle. *D,* If the tumor has a large, broad-based attachment to the atrial septum, the neoplasm is better exposed by a right atrial approach. The fossa ovalis is more easily exposed through a right atriotomy, and the base of the tumor can be readily excised. *E,* The atrial septal defect created by excision of the tumor is closed primarily. With large defects, a patch closure may be required. (From Silverman, N. A., and Sabiston, D. C., Jr.: Cardiac neoplasms. *In* Sabiston, D. C., Jr. [ed]: Textbook of Surgery, 13th ed. Philadelphia, W. B. Saunders Company, 1986.)

arise from the infundibular wall. Removal of left ventricular myxomas is usually attempted through an aortotomy with retraction of the aortic valve (Palazzuoli et al, 1986). An apical ventriculotomy is sometimes necessary to remove larger tumors. Valvular reconstruction or replacement is sometimes necessary for adequate resection of large tumors.

RHABDOMYOMA

Rhabdomyomas are the most common cardiac tumors in childhood and the second most common benign cardiac tumors at all ages (after myxomas). Ninety per cent occur in children less than 15 years of age and 30 to 50% are associated with tuberous sclerosis (mental retardation, convulsions, speech defects). Up to 90% of these tumors are multiple and occur mainly in the left and right ventricles; 30% involve the atria (Fig. 56–15). These tumors are usually deep within the myocardium and present with recurrent tachyarrhythmias. The tumors also can extend within a cavity and obstruct the cardiac chamber or respective valve orifice (Fig. 56–16). The gross appearance of these tumors is pale yellow to white with a range in size from 5 mm to 2.5 cm. The lesions are well circumscribed from the surrounding myocardium but are not encapsulated. Microscopically, rhabdomyomas consist of large ovoid, vacuolated cells with abundant glycogen (Kidder, 1950). Classic spider cells are found characteristically and consist of centrally placed cytoplasmic bodies that contain the nucleus, from which myofibrils project radially to the periphery of the cells (Landing and Farger, 1956). Because of the multicentric pattern and the

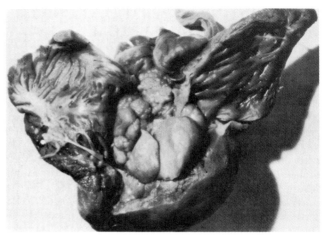

Figure 56–16. Rhabdomyoma that fills the right ventricle of a newborn infant. The multicentric origin of the tumor is shown. (From Fenoglio, J. J. et al: Cardiac rhabdomyoma: A clinicopathologic and electron microscopic study. Am. J. Cardiol., 38:241, 1976.)

high incidence in children, rhabdomyomas are thought to be hamartomas rather than true neoplasms and are probably derived from fetal cardiac myoblasts. Because of the multiple locations, poor encapsulation, and deep myocardial location, surgical resection can be difficult (Corono et al, 1984). However, because tuberous sclerosis is rare in the symptomatic intracavitary rhabdomyoma and there is evidence that rhabdomyomas do not undergo mitosis after birth, these patients should be considered to be surgical candidates, and reports of small series show acceptable results of surgical treatment in selective cases (Corono et al, 1984; Reece et al, 1984). The goal of resection is to alleviate the obstructive symptoms, preserve ventricular and valvular function, and prevent injury to the conduction system.

FIBROMA

Cardiac fibromas almost always occur in a solitary location, usually in the ventricular septum or ventricular myocardium. These tumors are more common in children but have been reported in all age groups (17 patients were reported in the AFIP series). Fibromas are the second most common primary cardiac tumors in the pediatric age group. Grossly, they appear as firm, nonencapsulated masses 3 to 7 cm in diameter. The central part of the tumor consists of hyalinized fibrous tissue with multiple foci of cystic degeneration and calcification. Most fibromas invade the conduction system and patients often die suddenly of arrhythmia. Successful resection of a septal fibroma has been reported (Reece et al, 1983). A 17-year-old patient with an unresectable fibroma was treated successfully with cardiac transplantation (Jamieson et al, 1981).

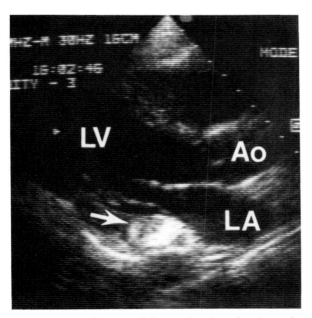

Figure 56–15. Parasternal long axis view showing a large rhabdomyoma in the posterior wall of the left ventricle (arrow).

LIPOMATOUS HYPERTROPHY OF THE ATRIAL SEPTUM

This lesion, also called *interatrial lipoma*, is a nonencapsulated mass of adipose tissue in the atrial septum that develops in continuity with the epicardial fat. The condition is thought to be due to hypertrophy of primordial fat rather than a true neoplasm. It is most common in patients over 60 years of age and usually in obese individuals. The fatty tissue bulges subendocardially into the right atrium and ranges from 1 to 8 cm in diameter. Microscopically, the lesion consists of fat cells that surround separate myocardial cells. The condition is manifested clinically with supraventricular arrhythmias and is associated occasionally with sudden death (Isner et al, 1982). Lipomas other than lipomatous hypertrophy of the atrial septum occur throughout the heart but are much less common and are usually asymptomatic (McAllister and Fenoglio 1978).

MESOTHELIOMA

Primary mesotheliomas occur most commonly in the region of the AV node. These neoplasms occur usually in adult women and, because of their location, can cause partial or complete heart block. The neoplasm consists of nests of mesothelial cells arranged in a multicystic pattern, and the central portion of the cyst is composed of amorphous colloid material. Grossly, the neoplasms appear as elevated nodules in the atrial septum close to the AV node. The preferred treatment is with an AV pacemaker; surgical excision would uniformly result in heart block. Ventricular fibrillation has been reported to develop after cardiac pacing, and a combination of cardiac pacing and antiarrhythmic therapy is indicated for the treatment of this lesion (McAllister and Fenoglio, 1978).

PAPILLARY FIBROELASTOMA

Papillary fibroelastomas are derived from the endocardium, most commonly valvular endocardium. The neoplasm is most common in adults, is usually asymptomatic clinically, and is an incidental finding at post-mortem examination. Occasionally, this tumor embolizes to obstruct a coronary artery or produce a transient ischemic attack (McFadden, 1986).

Other benign tumors reported to arise from the heart are hemangioma, teratoma, chemodectoma, neurilemoma, granular cell myoblastoma, and bronchogenic cysts (Hui et al, 1987; Leithiser et al, 1986; Stowers et al, 1987; Villafane et al, 1987). These neoplasms are rare or have only minor clinical significance.

MALIGNANT PRIMARY CARDIAC TUMORS

Of all primary cardiac tumors, approximately 25% are malignant. Almost all primary cardiac malignancies are sarcomas; the most common are angiosarcomas (33%) followed by rhabdomyosarcomas (20%), and the remainder are mesotheliomas or malignant fibrous histiocytomas (Laya et al, 1987). Malignant tumors occur usually after the fourth decade of life and, in contrast to myxomas, occur with approximately the same incidence in men and women. The right atrium is involved most commonly, and patients usually show symptoms of congestive heart failure, arrhythmias, myocardial ischemia, or hemopericardium (Kilma et al, 1987). Rapidly progressive congestive heart failure of recent onset refractory to medical therapy is characteristic of a malignant cardiac tumor. By the time the tumor is diagnosed, regional extension or distant metastases have usually occurred and preclude resection (Movahed and Wait, 1986). Most patients die within the first year after the diagnosis. The role of surgery is usually to establish the diagnosis and to guide adjunctive therapy. The differentiating features of benign and malignant primary cardiac tumors are shown in Table 56–5.

Clinical and pathologic findings for the largest series of malignant primary cardiac tumors from a single institution was reported from the Cleveland Clinic (Bear and Moodie, 1987). Malignant primary cardiac tumors were found between 1956 and 1986 in 11 patients with a mean age of 44 years and were approximately equally distributed in men and women. No patient was asymptomatic on initial presentation and most patients had respiratory symptoms and chest pain. Angiosarcoma was the most frequent type of tumor (four patients), followed by malignant fibrous histiocytoma (three patients), rhabdomyosarcoma (two patients), mesothelioma (one patient), and primary lymphoma (one patient). Of the patients, 70% had surgical biopsy and in 30% surgical excision was attempted. Ten of the patients died within the year after diagnosis; the single long-term survivor had primary lymphoma of the heart, which was treated with radiation. Associated findings in this series were a normochromic, normocytic anemia in ten patients and cardiac enlargement seen on the chest film in eight patients. Postsurgical chemotherapy or radiation therapy had little effect on survival except for the patient with a non-Hodgkin's lymphoma, who was well 6 years after treatment.

Angiosarcoma is the most common malignant primary cardiac tumor and occurs two to three times more often in men than in women, almost always in the adult age group. The tumor arises from the right atrium in 80% of reported cases and is usually associated with a rapid clinical onset and progressive deterioration (Janigan et al, 1986). In approximately 75% of patients, either right ventricular failure or

TABLE 56–5. CHARACTERISTICS OF BENIGN AND MALIGNANT PRIMARY CARDIAC TUMORS

Characteristics	Benign	Malignant
Incidence	80%	20%
Pathologic type	Mainly myxoma	All are sarcomas
Location	Usually left atrial, multiple sites uncommon	Usually right atrial, multiple sites common
Age	30 to 60 years	30 to 70 years, rare under 30 years
Sex (female:male ratio)	3:1	1:1
Arrhythmias	Uncommon	Common due to intramyocardial invasion
Pericardial effusion	Unusual	Common—usually bloody
Diagnosis	Echocardiography	Echocardiography, CT scan, some require open biopsy
Prognosis	Excellent after resection	Fatal within 6 months to 2 years
Management	Surgical excision	Combined approach (excision, chemotherapy, radiation therapy) Cardiac transplantation

pericardial disease is found (Chitwood, 1988). Other common symptoms are fever, chest pain, hemoptysis, and malaise. Surgical resection is rarely possible because of distant metastases and frequent pericardial involvement (Percy et al, 1987). Despite adjunctive chemotherapy or radiation therapy, 90% of patients die within 9 to 12 months of diagnosis of the tumor (Dein et al, 1987; Wiske et al, 1986).

Rhabdomyosarcoma, the next most common malignant tumor of the heart, occurs equally in both sexes. There is no predilection for any cardiac chamber and the neoplasm is multicentric in 60% of patients (Becker et al, 1985). These lesions are rare in children and follow malignant teratomas in frequency. Rhabdomyosarcoma is usually seen with intracavitary extension, and most patients have partial or almost complete obstruction of one of the heart valves, most commonly the mitral or pulmonic valves. Unlike benign tumors, these malignant tumors invade the cardiac valves and often destroy them. Pericardial involvement due to direct tumor extension is common. The histologic diagnosis is based on the presence of rhabdomyoblasts, which may be difficult to locate, and electron microscopy is usually required to identify the muscular origin of the tumor. Most patients die within 1 year after diagnosis of the tumor, but excision of the main tumor mass followed by combined radiation therapy and chemotherapy may be indicated in selected patients.

Fibrosarcoma and malignant fibrous histiocytoma are malignant mesenchymal tumors that are primarily fibroblastic in differentiation. These tumors constitute only 10% of primary cardiac malignancies, although malignant fibrous histiocytoma is one of the more common soft-tissue sarcomas. Cardiac involvement is commonly in the left atrium (Lee et al, 1987) and the incidence is higher in young women in whom it may be confused with left atrial myxoma (Smith, 1986). Although radiation and chemotherapy have had minimal success, no therapy has been effective for treating malignant fibroblastic tumors of the heart and the prognosis is uniformly poor. Primary lymphoma of the heart has been reported (Chou et al, 1983; Gelman et al, 1986) and associated with acquired immunodeficiency syndrome (Constantino et al, 1987) and is best treated by radiation therapy.

In summary, malignant primary cardiac tumors are associated with poor long-term survival, because of the advanced local involvement of the tumor at presentation and the fact that most patients already have distal metastases. With two-dimensional echocardiography, noninvasive imaging of these tumors early in their course may allow earlier diagnosis, earlier institution of aggressive surgical resection and advanced chemotherapy, and a potential for better survival. For patients with localized disease but with extensive cardiac involvement, cardiac transplantation may have a role in the future.

METASTATIC TUMORS OF THE HEART

The most common neoplastic process that involves the heart is metastatic deposits from primary tumors elsewhere in the body. Metastatic tumors of the heart are up to 40 times more frequent than primary tumors of the heart (Fine, 1968; Hallahan et al, 1986; Hanfling, 1960). The incidence of metastatic cardiac disease in patients with known malignancies is approximately 10% (Hanfling, 1960). An increase in cardiac metastases noted in later series may be related to prolonged survival after surgical and adjunctive therapy. Almost every type of malignant tumor from all organs has been reported to spread to the heart and pericardium (Pillai et al, 1986). Up to 50% of patients with leukemia have cardiac involvement (Fine, 1968), and other malignancies that commonly metastasize to the heart include melanoma, carcinoma of the lung, and carcinoma of the breast. In 418 cases of lung carcinoma reported by Strauss and associates (1977), the incidence of cardiac metastases was 25%. The parts of the heart affected by metastatic tumors in decreasing order of frequency are pericardium, myocardium, and endocardium. When the heart is affected, metastatic disease is usually found to be widespread throughout the body. The clinical diagnosis of metastatic heart disease is usually not made because only 10% of the patients have symptoms attributable to metastases to the heart. Symptoms that do arise are overshadowed by the primary disease. Symptoms of congestive heart failure without an apparent cause of development of an arrhythmia in a patient with known malignant disease may indicate cardiac involvement of the tumor (Cates et al, 1986). The most frequent clinical expression of secondary cardiac malignancy is pericardial effusion and cardiac tamponade. Also, solid tumor growth may impinge on structures of the heart and cause various symptoms and signs (Cohen et al, 1986).

Metastatic disease usually involves the ventricular chambers more often than the atria and is reported by some authors to be slightly more common on the right side of the heart (Smith, 1986). Malignant involvement of the heart may occur by retrograde invasion from lymphatic channels, by hematogenous routes, or by direct invasion from adjacent mediastinal structures. Most patients with carcinoma of the breast and lung have cardiac involvement by lymphatic spread rather than by direct extension (McAllister and Fenoglio, 1978). Metastases from sarcomas, leukemias, and melanomas (Fig. 56–17) are most commonly by hematogenous routes (Ali, 1987). Intrathoracic primary tumors such as esophageal, breast, and lung carcinomas may extend directly into the pericardial and cardiac tissue, and up to 50% of lymphomas involve the heart by direct extension (Armstrong et al, 1986; Balasubramanyam et al, 1986).

Surgical treatment for metastatic cardiac malignancies is indicated for relief of ventricular obstruction caused by isolated lesions or for relief of cardiac tamponade caused by malignant pericardial effusion. Before surgical resection of metastatic disease is considered, primary tumors should be well controlled and the metastatic focus is potentially resectable. Renal cell carcinoma with tumor extension into the right atrium has been treated efficaciously with surgical removal (Novick and Cosgrove, 1980). Patients with moderate to large symptomatic malignant pericardial effusions can be treated effectively with a subxyphoid pericardial window. The procedure can be done easily under local anesthesia, has minimal morbidity in these debilitated patients with metastatic disease, and significantly alleviates symptoms of cardiac tamponade. In a review of four series with a total of 100 patients with malignant cardiac tamponade treated by subxyphoid pericardiotomy, Press and Livingston (1987) found that all the patients had relief of tamponade and there were only three recurrences and no fatalities. The survival of patients varied from 1 week to more than 8 years and depended on the progression of malignancy elsewhere in the body, although generally, of patients with malignant effusions treated with subxyphoid pericardiotomy, approximately 50% die within 3 months from progression of the primary disease. Left anterior thoracotomy with creation of a pleuropericardial window provides effective decompression of malignant pericardial effusions, but this procedure requires general anesthesia and may be poorly tolerated by debilitated hemodynamically unstable patients with advanced cancer. Mortality and significant morbidity of 10 to 15% can be expected from this procedure (Gregory et al, 1985).

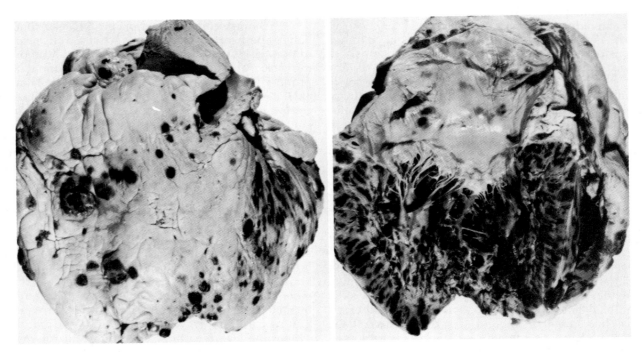

Figure 56–17. Metastatic melanoma. Dark tumor nodules are clearly seen distributed throughout the myocardium. The mode of metastasis is usually hematogenous spread. (From McAllister, H. A., and Fenoglio, J. J., Jr.: Tumors of the cardiovascular system. *In* Hartman, W. H., and Cowan, W. R. (eds): Atlas of Tumor Pathology. Washington, D.C., Armed Forces Institute of Pathology, 1978.)

Radiation therapy is beneficial in 60% of patients with malignant pericardial effusion (Cham et al, 1975). In this series, 38 patients with neoplastic effusions were treated with 2500 to 3000 rads of external-beam radiation for 3 to 4 weeks. The median duration of improvement was approximately 4 months. In an alternative approach to delivering radiotherapy, Martini and associates (1977) instilled radioactive chromic phosphate intrapericardially in a series of 28 patients. With this technique of pericardiocentesis followed by pericardial infusion of the radioactive agent, effusions were controlled successfully in 70% of the patients, and the efficacy of this approach has been documented by others (Maher and Buckman, 1986).

Selected Bibliography

Chitwood, W. R., Jr.: Cardiac neoplasms: Current diagnosis, pathology and therapy. J. Cardiac Surg., 3:119, 1988.

A well-illustrated review that examines almost all diagnostic, pathologic, and therapeutic aspects of benign and malignant cardiac tumors. The various surgical approaches for removal of resectable neoplasms are detailed.

Dein, J. R., Frist, W. N., Stinson, E. B., et al: Primary cardiac neoplasms. J. Thorac. Cardiovasc. Surg., 93:502, 1987.

A contemporary surgical series of 42 patients who had resection of cardiac neoplasms between 1961 and 1986. All 34 patients with benign lesions had resection with excellent results. All gross tumor was removed in four of eight patients with malignant tumors.

DePace, N. L., Soulen, R. L., Kotler, M. N., and Mintz, G. S.: Two-dimensional echocardiographic detection of intra-atrial masses. Am. J. Cardiol., 48:957, 1981.

This paper reviews the role of two-dimensional echocardiographic detection of masses in the left atrium and the distinguishing features of atrial thrombus, myxoma, and malignant tumors as studied by two-dimensional echocardiography.

Harvey, W. P.: Clinical aspects of cardiac tumors. Am. J. Cardiol., 21:328, 1968.

A classic description of the signs and symptoms that should alert the clinician to the presence of a cardiac neoplasm. Detailed descriptions of representative cases are especially informative.

McCallister, H. A., Jr.: Primary tumors and cysts of the heart and pericardium. Curr. Prob. Cardiol., 4:1, 1979.

A comprehensive review of the vast experience of the Armed Forces Institute of Pathology with more than 500 primary cardiac tumors. The review is well illustrated and supported by pertinent tables and provides excellent clinical correlations.

Bibliography

Ali, M. K.: Right ventricular metastatic sarcoma. Am. J. Clin. Oncol. (CCT), 10:270, 1987.

Armstrong, W. F., Buck, J. D., Hoffman, R., and Waller, B. F.: Cardiac involvement by lymphoma: Detection and follow-up by two-dimensional echocardiography. Am. Heart J., 112:627, 1986.

Attum, A. A., Johnson, G. S., Masri, Z., et al: Malignant clinical behavior of cardiac myxomas and "myxoid imitators." Ann. Thorac. Surg., 44:217, 1987.

Bahnson, H. T., and Newman, E. V.: Diagnosis and surgical removal of intracavitary myxoma of the right atrium. Bull. Johns Hopkins Hosp., 93:150, 1953.

Balasubramanyam, A., Waxman, M., Kazal, H. L., and Lee, M. H.: Malignant lymphoma of the heart in acquired immune deficiency syndrome. Chest, 90:243, 1986.

Barnes, A. R., Beaver, D. C., and Snell, A. M.: Primary sarcoma of the heart: Report of a case with electrocardiographic and pathological studies. Am. Heart J., 9:480, 1934.

Bear, P. A., and Moodie, D. S.: Malignant primary cardiac tumors: The Cleveland Clinic Experience, 1956 to 1986. Chest, 92:860, 1987.

Beck, C. S.: An intrapericardial teratoma and a tumor of the heart: Both removed operatively. Ann. Surg., 116:161, 1942.

Becker, R. C., Hobbs, R. E., and Ratliff, N. B.: Cardiac rhabdomyosarcoma: Case report with review of clinical and pathologic features. Cleve. Clin. Q., 51:83, 1985.

Bloor, C. M., and O'Rourke, R. A.: Cardiac tumors: Clinical presentation and pathologic correlations. In Current Problems in Cardiology, Chicago, Year Book Medical Publishers, 1984.

Bulkley, B. H., and Hutchins, M.: Atrial myxomas: A fifty year review. Am. Heart J., 97:639, 1979.

Camesas, A. M., Lichtstein, E., Kramer, J., et al: Complementary use of two-dimensional echocardiography and magnetic resonance imaging in the diagnosis of ventricular myxoma. Am. Heart J., 114:440, 1986.

Carney, J. A., Gordon, H., Carpenter, P. C., et al: The complex of myxomas, spotty pigmentation, and endocrine overactivity. Medicine, 64:270, 1985.

Carney, J. A.: Differences between nonfamilial and familial cardiac myxoma. Am. J. Surg. Pathol., 9:53, 1985.

Castenada, A. R., and Varco, R. L.: Tumors of the heart: Surgical considerations. Am. J. Cardiol., 21:357, 1968.

Cates, C. U., Virmani, R., Vaughn, W. K., and Robertson, R. M.: Electrocardiographic markers of cardiac metastasis. Am. Heart J., 112:1297, 1986.

Chaloupka, J. C., Fishman, E. K., and Siegelman, S. S.: Use of CT in the evaluation of primary cardiac tumors. Cardiovasc. Intervent. Radiol., 9:132, 1986.

Cham, W. C., Freiman, A. H., Carstens, P. H. B., et al: Radiation therapy of cardiac and pericardial metastases. Radiology, 114:701, 1975.

Chitwood, W. R., Jr.: Cardiac neoplasms: Current diagnosis, pathology, and therapy. J. Cardiac Surg., 3:119, 1988.

Chou, S.-T., Arkles, L. B., Gill, G. D., et al: Primary lymphoma of the heart: A case report. Cancer, 52:744, 1983.

Cohen, D. E., Mora, C., and Keefe, D. L.: Echocardiographic findings of metastatic chondrosarcoma involving the left atrium. Am. Heart J., 111:993, 1986.

Columbus, MR: De Re Anatomica, Libri XV. Paris, 1562.

Come, P. C., Riley, M. F., Markis, J. E., and Malagold, M.: Limitations of echocardiographic techniques in evaluation of left atrial masses. Am. J. Cardiol., 48:947, 1981.

Constantino, A., West, T. E., Gupta, M., and Loghmanee, F.: Primary cardiac lymphoma in a patient with acquired immune deficiency syndrome. Cancer, 60:2801, 1987.

Corono, A., Catena, G., and Marcelletti, C.: Cardiac rhabdomyoma: Surgical treatment in the neonate. J. Thorac. Cardiovasc. Surg., 87:725, 1984.

Crafoord, C.: Mitral stenosis and mitral insufficiency. In Lam, C. R. (ed): International Symposium on Cardiovascular Surgery, Henry Ford Hospital, Detroit. Philadelphia, W. B. Saunders Company, 1955, p. 203.

Currey, H. L. F., Matthew, J. A., and Robinson, J.: Right atrial myxoma mimicking a rheumatic disorder. Br. Med. J., 1:547, 1967.

Dein, J. R., Frist, W. H., Stinson, E. B., et al: Primary cardiac neoplasms: Early and late results of surgical treatment in 42 patients. J. Thorac. Cardiovasc. Surg., 93:502, 1987.

DePace, N. L., Soulen, R. L., Kotler, M. N., and Mintz, G. S.: Two dimensional echocardiographic detection of intraatrial masses. Am. J. Cardiol., 48:954, 1981.

DeSousa, A. L., Muller, J., Campbell, R. L., et al: Atrial myxoma: A review of neurological complications, metastases, and recurrences. J. Neurol. Neurosurg. Psychiatry, 41:1119, 1978.

Dunninghan, A., Oldham, H. N., Serwer, G. A., et al: Left atrial myxoma: Is cardiac catheterization essential? Am. J. Dis. Child., 135:420, 1981.

Ferrans, V. J., and Roberts, W. C.: Structural features of cardiac myxomas. Hum. Pathol., 4:111, 1973.

Fine, G.: Neoplasms of the pericardium and heart. In Gould, S. E. (ed): Pathology of the Heart and Blood Vessels. Springfield, IL, Charles C Thomas, 1968.

Freedberg, R. S., Kronzon, I., Rumancik, W. M., and Liebeskind, D.: The contribution of magnetic resonance imaging to the evaluation of intracardiac tumors diagnosed by echocardiography. Circulation, 77:96, 1988.

Gelman, K. M., Ben-Ezra, J. M., Steinschneider, M., et al: Lymphoma with primary cardiac manifestations. Am. Heart J., 111:808, 1986.

Gerbode, F., Kerth, W. J., and Hill, J. D.: Surgical management of tumors of the heart. Surgery, 61:94, 1967.

Gindea, A. J., Steele, P., Rumancik, W. M., et al: Biventricular cavity obliteration by metastatic malignant melanoma: Role of magnetic resonance imaging in the diagnosis. Am. Heart J., 114:1249, 1987.

Go, R. T., O'Donnell, J. K., Underwood, D. A., et al: Comparison of gated MRI and 2D echocardiography of intracardiac neoplasms. Am. J. Radiol., 145:21, 1985.

Goldberg, H. P., Glenn, F., Dotter, C. T., and Steinberg, I.: Myxoma of the left atrium. Diagnosis made during life with operative and postmortem findings. Circulation, VI:762, 1952.

Goldman, A. P., Kotler, M. N., and Parry, R. A.: Atrial tumors. In Kapoor, A. (ed): Cancer and the Heart. New York, Springer-Verlag, 1986.

Gomes, A. S., Lois, J. F., Child, J. S., et al: Cardiac tumors and thrombus: Evaluation with MR imaging. Am. J. Roentgenol. 149:895, 1987.

Gosse, P., Herpin, D., Roudaut, R., et al: Myxoma of the mitral valve diagnosed by echocardiography. Am. Heart J., 111:803, 1986.

Gray, I. R., and Williams, W. G.: Recurring cardiac myxoma. Br. Heart J., 53:645, 1985.

Gregory, J. R., McMurtrey, M. H., and Mountain, C. F.: A surgical approach to the treatment of pericardial effusion in cancer patients. Am. J. Clin. Oncol., 8:317, 1985.

Guiloff, A. K., Flege, J. B., Callard, G. M., et al: Surgery of left atrial myxomas: Report of eleven cases and review of the literature. J. Cardiovasc. Surg., 27:194, 1986.

Hajar, R., Roberts, W. C., and Folger, G. M., Jr.: Embryonal botryoid rhabdomyosarcoma of the mitral valve. Am. J. Cardiol., 57:376, 1986.

Hallahan, D. E., Vogelzang, N. J., Borow, K. M., et al: Cardiac metastases from soft-tissue sarcomas. J. Clin. Oncol., 4:1662, 1986.

Hanfling, S. M.: Metastatic cancer to the heart: Review of the literature and report of 127 cases. Circulation, 22:474, 1960.

Hannah, H., III, Eisemann, G., Hiszchnskyj, R., et al: Invasive atrial myxoma: Documentation of malignant potential of cardiac myxomas. Am. Heart J., 104:881, 1982.

Hanson, E. C., Gill, C. C., Razavi, M., et al: The surgical treatment of atrial myxomas. J. Thorac. Cardiovasc. Surg., 89:298, 1985.

Hattler, B. G., Fuchs, J. C. A., Cosson, R., et al: Atrial myxomas: An evaluation of clinical and laboratory manifestations. Ann. Thorac. Surg., 10:65, 1970.

Hui, G., McAllister, H. A., and Angelini, P.: Left atrial paraganglioma: Report of a case and review of the literature. Am. Heart J., 113:1230, 1987.

Imperio, J., Summels, D., Krasnow, N., and Piccone, V. A.: The distribution patterns of biatrial myxomas. Ann. Thorac. Surg., 29:469, 1980.

Isner, J., Swan, C. S., II, Mikus, J. P., and Carter, B. L.: Lipomatous hypertrophy of the interatrial septum: In vivo diagnosis. Circulation, 66:470, 1982.

Jamieson, S. W., Gaudiani, V. A., Reitz, B. A., et al: Operative treatment of an unresectable tumor on the left ventricle. J. Thorac. Cardiovasc. Surg., 81:797, 1981.

Janigan, D. T., Husain, A., and Robinson, N. A.: Cardiac angiosarcomas: A review and a case report. Cancer, 57:852, 1986.

Jones, K. L., Wolf, P. L., Jensen, P., et al: The Gorlin syndrome: A genetically determined disorder associated with cardiac tumor. Am. Heart J., 111:1013, 1986.

Kidder, L. A.: Congenital glycogenic tumors of the heart. Arch. Pathol., 49:55, 1950.

Kilma, T., Milam, J. D., Bossart, M. I., and Cooley, D. A.: Rare primary sarcomas of the heart. Arch. Pathol. Lab. Med., 110:1155, 1986.

Landing, B. H., and Farger, S.: Tumors of the cardiovascular system. In Atlas of Tumour Pathology, Sec. III, Fasc. VII. Washington, D.C., U.S. War Department, 1956.

Laya, M. B., Mailliard, J. A., Bewtra, C., and Levin, H. S.: Malignant fibrous histiocytoma of the heart: A case report and review of the literature. Cancer, 59:1026, 1987.

Lee, J., Cheung, K. L., Wang, R., et al: Malignant fibrous histiocytoma of left atrium. J. Thorac. Cardiovasc. Surg., 3:450, 1987.

Leithiser, R. E., Jr., Fyfe, D., Weatherby, E., III, et al: Prenatal sonographic diagnosis of atrial hemangioma. Am. J. Roentgenol., 147:1207, 1986.

Leonhardt, E. T. G., and Kullenberg, K. P. G.: Bilateral atrial myxomas with multiple arterial aneurysms: A syndrome mimicking polyarteritis nodosa. Am. J. Med., 62:792, 1977.

MacGregor, G. A., and Cullen, R. A.: Syndrome of fever, anemia, and high sedimentation rate with atrial myxoma. Br. Med. J., 2:991, 1959.

McAllister, H. A., Jr.: Primary tumors and cysts of the heart and pericardium. In Current Problems in Cardiology. Chicago, Year Book Medical Publishers, 1979.

McAllister, H. A., Jr., and Fenoglio, J. J., Jr.: Tumors of the cardiovascular system. In Hartman, W. H., and Cowan, W. R. (eds): Atlas of Tumor Pathology, Sec. Series, Fasc. 15. Washington, DC, Armed Forces Institute of Pathology, 1978.

McCarthy, P. M., Piehler, J. M., Schaff, H. V., et al: The significance of multiple, recurrent, and "complex" cardiac myxomas. J. Thorac. Cardiovasc. Surg., 91:389, 1986.

McFadden, P. M., and Lacy, J. R.: Intracardiac papillary fibroelastoma: An occult cause of embolic neurologic deficit. Ann. Thorac. Surg., 43:667, 1987.

Mahaim, I.: Les tumeurs et les polyps du coeur: Étude anatomoclinique. Paris, Masson et Cie, 1945.

Maher, E. R., and Buckman, R.: Intrapericardial instillation of bleomycin in malignant pericardial effusion. Am. Heart J., 111:613, 1986.

Markel, M. L., Armstrong, W. F., Waller, B. F., and Mahomet, Y.: Left atrial myxoma with multicentric recurrence and evidence of metastases. Am. Heart J., 111:409, 1986.

Martini, N., Freiman, A. H., Watson, R. C., et al: Intrapericardial instillation of radioactive chromic phosphate in malignant pericardial effusion. Am. J. Roentgenol., 128:639, 1977.

Martin, L. W.: Wasserman, A. G., Goldstein, H., et al: Multiple cardiac myxomas with multiple recurrences: Unusual presentation of a "benign" tumor. Ann. Thorac. Surg., 44:77, 1987.

Mora, F., Mindich, B. P., Guarino, T., and Goldman, M. E.: Improved surgical approach to cardiac tumors with intraoperative two-dimensional echocardiography. Chest, 91:142, 1987.

Movahed, A., and Wait, J.: Carcinoma of the heart presenting as myocardial infarction. Am. Heart J., 112:1329, 1986.

Novick, A., and Cosgrove, D.: Surgical approach for removal of renal cell carcinoma extending into the vena cava and right atrium. J. Urol., 123:977, 1980.

O'Neil, M. B., Grehl, T. M., and Hurley, E. J.: Cardiac myxomas: A clinical diagnostic challenge. Am. J. Surg., 138:68, 1979.

Okada, M., Ohta, T., Yasuoka, S., et al: Surgical management of intracavitary cardiac tumors: A review of fifteen patients and current status in Japan. J. Cardiovasc. Surg., 27:641, 1986.

Palazzuoli, V., Mondillo, S. Angelini, G. D., et al: Myxoma of the left ventricle. Thorac. Cardiovasc. Surg., 34:271, 1986.

Panidis, I. P., Kotler, M. N., Mintz, G. S., and Ross, J.: Clinical and echocardiographic features of right atrial masses. Am. Heart J., 107:745, 1984.

Panidis, I. P., Mintz, G. S., and McAllister, M.: Hemodynamic consequences of left atrial myxomas as assessed by Doppler ultrasound. Am. Heart. J., *111*:927, 1986.

Percy, R. F., Perryman, R. A., Amornmarn, R., et al: Prolonged survival in a patient with primary angiosarcoma of the heart. Am. Heart J., *113*:1228, 1987.

Pillai, R., Blauth, C., Peckham, M., et al: Intracardiac metastases from malignant teratoma of the testis. J. Thorac. Cardiovasc. Surg., *92*:118, 1986.

Poole, G. V., Breyer, R. H., Holliday, R. H., et al: Tumors of the heart: Surgical considerations. J. Cardiovasc. Surg., *25*:5, 1984.

Powers, J. C., Falkoff, M., Heinle, R. A., et al: Familial cardiac myxoma: Emphasis on unusual clinical manifestations. J. Thorac. Cardiovasc. Surg., *77*:782, 1979.

Press, O. W., and Livingston, R.: Management of malignant pericardial effusion and tamponade. J.A.M.A., *257*:1088, 1987.

Read, R. C., White, J. H., Murphy, M. L., et al: The malignant potentiality of left atrial myxoma. J. Thorac. Cardiovasc. Surg., *6*:857, 1974.

Reece, I. H., Cooley, D. A., Frazier, O. H., et al: Cardiac tumors: Clinical spectrum and prognosis of lesions other than classical benign myxoma in 20 patients. J. Thorac. Cardiovasc. Surg., *88*:439, 1984.

Reece, I. H., Houston, A. B., and Pollick, J. C.: Inter-ventricular fibroma: Echocardiograph diagnosis and successful surgical removal in infancy. Br. Heart J. *50*:590, 1983.

Sabiston, D. C., Jr., and Hattler, B. G., Jr.: Tumors of the heart. *In* Sabiston, D. C., Jr., and Spencer, F. C. (eds): Gibbon's Surgery of the Chest. Philadelphia, W. B. Saunders Company, 1983.

Salyer, W. R., Page, D. L., and Hutchins, G. M.: The development of the cardiac myxoma and the papillary endocardial lesions from mural thrombus. Am. Heart J., *89*:4, 1975.

Sandrasagra, F. A., Oliver, W. A., and English, T. A. H.: Myxoma of the mitral valve. Br. Heart J., *42*:221, 1979.

Schattenberg, T. T.: Echocardiographic diagnosis of left atrial myxoma. Mayo Clin. Proc., *43*:620, 1968.

Seifert, P., Chomka, E. V., Stagl, R., et al: Application of the cine computed tomographic scan for precise localization of the origin of an atrial myxoma: Surgical implications. Ann. Thorac. Surg., *42*:469, 1986.

Selzer, A., Sakai, E. J., and Popper, R. W.: Protean clinical manifestations of primary tumors of the heart. Am. J. Cardiol., *52*:9, 1972.

Shin, M. S., Kirklin, J. K., Cain, J. B., and Ho, K. J.: Primary angiosarcoma of the heart: CT characteristics. Am. J. Roentgenol., *148*:267, 1987.

Silverman, N. A.: Primary cardiac tumors. Ann. Surg., *191*:127, 1980.

Silverman, N. A., and Sabiston, D. C., Jr.: Cardiac neoplasms. *In* Sabiston, D. C., Jr. (ed): Textbook of Surgery. Philadelphia, W. B. Saunders Company, 1981.

Smith, C.: Tumors of the heart. Arch. Pathol. Lab. Med., *110*:371, 1986.

Stowers, S. A., Gilmore, P., Stirling, M., et al: Cardiac pheochromocytoma involving the left main coronary artery presenting with exertional angina. Am. Heart J., *114*:423, 1987.

Strauss, B. L., Matthews, M. J., Cohen, M. N., et al: Cardiac metastases in lung cancer. Chest, *71*:607, 1977.

Sutton, M. G. St. J., Mercier, L.-A., Giuliana, E. R., and Lie, J. T.: Atrial myxomas: A review of clinical experience in 40 patients. Mayo Clin Proc., *55*:371, 1980.

Tway, K. P., Shah, A. A., and Rahimtoola, S. H.: Multiple biatrial myxomas demonstrated by two-dimensional echocardiography. Am. J. Med., *71*:896, 1981.

Villafane, J., Saltz, M., Kaiser, G., et al: A rare right atrial tumor presenting with cyanosis in a newborn. Am. Heart J., *113*:1036, 1987.

Wiske, P. S., Gillam, L. D., Blyden, G., and Weyman, A. E.: Intracardiac tumor regression documented by two-dimensional echocardiography. Am. J. Cardiol., *58*:186, 1986.

Wold, L. E., and Lie, J. T.: Cardiac myxomas: A clinicopathological profile. Am. J. Pathol., *101*:219, 1980.

CHAPTER 57

TRANSPLANTATION
I HEART AND LUNG TRANSPLANTATION*

Bruce A. Reitz

The conceptual simplicity of replacing the cardiopulmonary axis has been recognized since the early 1900s. Carrel and later Demikhov and Marcus mentioned the possibility of heart-lung transplantation to replace diseased organs (Carrel, 1907; Demikhov, 1962; Marcus et al, 1951). The operation requires only a right atrial (inflow) anastomosis and aortic (outflow) anastomoses, with a connection at the trachea (airway). The surgical procedure is easier in some ways than isolated heart replacement, which explains why heart and lung transplantation was technically feasible before orthotopic heart replacement. However, technical simplicity was offset by the reality of severe difficulties with transplantation of lung tissue.

HISTORICAL ASPECTS

Almost all the later developments in cardiovascular surgery were anticipated by the experiments of Alexis Carrel. This French-born American surgeon developed many techniques for vascular surgery, and his life and work provide fascinating reading. Among his studies was the transplantation of both heart and lung, as described in the following manner:

We attempted also to make the transplantation of the lungs together with the heart. Both lungs, the heart, the aorta, and vena cava of a cat one week old were extirpated and put into the neck of a large adult cat. The aorta was anastomosed to the peripheral end of the carotid, and the vena cava to the peripheral end of the jugular vein. The coronary circulation was immediately re-established and the auricles began to beat. The lungs became red and after a few minutes, effective pulsations of the ventricles appeared. But the lungs soon became edematous, and distention of the right part of the heart occurred. This accident seems difficult of prevention. A phlegmon of the neck terminated this observation two days later.

CARREL, 1907

Although this experiment had little success, it and other observations by Carrel predicted the eventual use of transplantation of organs. For these outstanding accomplishments, Carrel received the Nobel Prize in 1912, the first such award to a scientist working in an American laboratory. Many people have speculated why his work was not applied by other surgeons at the time, but no good answers have been found (Comroe, 1979).

In the mid-1940s in Russia, Demikhov and Sinitsyn began their ingenious experiments that showed the technical feasibility of intrathoracic heterotopic heart transplants. Demikhov was also able to devise a method for transplanting the heart-lung bloc before the advent of cardiopulmonary bypass and hypothermia techniques.

Demikhov's work was first reported in the West in 1962 with the publication of his book *Experimental Transplantation of Vital Organs*, which documents the work of an extremely innovative surgeon. However, Demikhov thought that the failure of all transplanted organs was secondary to technical factors and that immunology did not have a role. He failed to realize that, because of variations in donor and recipient matching, favorable long-term function can occasionally occur despite immunologic rejection.

Demikhov achieved some remarkable firsts, including the first successful heart-lung transplant. By removing the heart-lung bloc at normothermia and maintaining a heartbeat, he was able to transfer the heart and both lungs, or the heart and one lung, into a recipient dog. One variation of this experiment is shown in Figure 57–1. Demikhov accomplished the

*This chapter (including Figures and Tables) has been reprinted in part from Baumgartner, W.A., Reitz, B.A., and Achuff, S.C. (eds): Heart and Heart-Lung Transplantation. Philadelphia, W. B. Saunders Company, 1990.

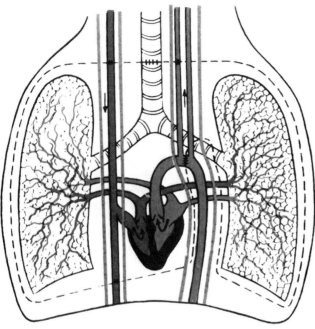

Figure 57–1. The points of transection and reanastomosis of the heart-lung bloc, as performed by Demikhov in dogs during the late 1940s.

transfer by alternating one of two venous inflow anastomoses (the superior or inferior vena cava) with one of two outflow anastomoses (the brachiocephalic artery or the transverse aortic arch just distal to the brachiocephalic artery) and then the trachea. Thus, he replaced the heart and lungs of the recipient animal while both the donor and recipient hearts and lungs continued to function with a circulation. As his surgical technique improved, animal survival increased. In his 15th experiment, the animal was removed alive from the operating table. The notes from this experiment relate that after the chest was closed "spontaneous respiration was resumed, but respirations were infrequent and deep, 7 per minute. Later, respirations ceased, and the animal died shortly thereafter." Other experiments confirmed that the respiratory pattern was very deep and the animals used the muscles of the abdominal wall and neck, with their mouths open. These changes in respiratory pattern were associated later with complete cardiopulmonary denervation in the dog.

In all, Demikhov subjected 67 dogs to replacement of the heart together with the lungs. Although many dogs died on the operating table or within 24 hours after operation, 8 survived more than 48 hours and 2 survived 5 and 6 days, respectively. His experiments proved that the operation was feasible from the point of view of surgical technique. The animal that survived longest is shown in Figure 57–2. In a prophetic statement, Demikhov noted:

In the surgery of the future, when the causes of the complications and failures attending these operations have *been studied and overcome, transplantation of the heart, together with the lungs, will find its application in irreversible forms of cardiopulmonary insufficiency.*

In 1953, Neptune and associates from Hahnemann Medical College in Philadelphia and Marcus and associates from the Chicago Medical School presented papers on experimental heart-lung transplantation in the same volume of the Archives of Surgery. Neptune and associates (1953) reported what they thought was the first successful replacement of the heart and both lungs by using hypothermia and circulatory arrest. In their three experiments, one animal survived as long as 6 hours and had satisfactory blood pressure, spontaneous respiration, and return of reflexes. They concluded that this preparation was an "ideal way of obtaining a completely denervated heart, as well as lungs, for physiologic study."

Marcus and associates (1953) described heterotopic heart-lung transplantation to the intra-abdominal aorta and vena cava of a recipient animal. In eight animals, they sutured the superior and inferior venae cavae of the donor heart and lung to the distal inferior vena cava of the recipient, the brachiocephalic artery of the donor to the proximal abdominal aorta, and the transverse aortic arch to the distal abdominal aorta. The trachea was then exteriorized and mechanically ventilated. Nitrogen was given to the recipient's own trachea, and circulation was maintained by administering oxygen to the trachea of the donor. The experimental preparation is shown in Figure 57–3. They were able to maintain the recipient for approximately 75 minutes after the heart of the host animal had died.

Marcus and associates described a second experiment. While the heart and lung preparation was functioning in the abdominal position, the chest of the host was entered and the main pulmonary artery was occluded temporarily to empty the left side of the heart. The heart was then opened with an incision in the left atrial appendage, and the mitral valve was manipulated under direct vision. After 7 minutes of intracardiac exposure, the atrium was closed and

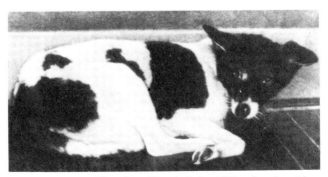

Figure 57–2. The dog "Damka" in 1951, after heart-lung transplantation by Demikhov. The dog survived for 6 days and died of pulmonary failure, probably as a result of allograft rejection, although this was not appreciated by Demikhov.

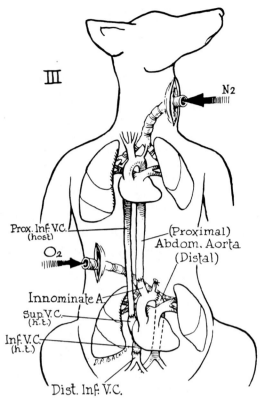

Figure 57–3. The use of a heterotopic heart-lung transplant to support the host as reported by Marcus and associates. (From Marcus, E., Wong, S. N. T., and Luisada, A. A.: Homologous heart grafts. A.M.A. Arch. Surg., 66:179, 1953. Copyright 1953, American Medical Association.)

the heart was allowed to beat again. Thus, the authors had devised a method for open intracardiac surgery with a donor heart and lungs used as the pump oxygenator.

In 1957, Webb and Howard reported the use of a pump oxygenator to do heart-lung transplantation in dogs. They could restore the heart to relatively normal function, and the animals lived from 75 minutes to 22 hours. They anticipated later technical difficulties, as they noted continued bleeding from the extensive raw surfaces that developed during the dissection and none of the animals returned to spontaneous normal respiration. They also reported four attempts at autotransplantation of the heart and lung, but although cardiac function was sufficient, the animals were unable to breathe spontaneously. In other experiments in which heart transplantation alone was done, there was an immediate return to spontaneous respiration, which again suggested that cardiopulmonary denervation was not well tolerated by dogs. Webb and Howard concluded that transplantation of the heart and both lungs was not practical, because of respiratory paralysis. They suggested that transplantation of the heart with one lung would prevent respiratory paralysis by retaining one innervated lung.

The next encouraging report was from Lower and associates (1961), who had previously reported the first significant survival after orthotopic heart transplantation in the dog and now turned to complete heart-lung replacement. They emphasized the need for preservation of the recipient's phrenic and vagus nerves and careful ligation of bronchial vessels. The donor organs were immersed in cold saline solution at 4° C for topical hypothermia, and anastomoses were done at the aorta, trachea, and both venae cavae. Six animals resumed spontaneous respiration, although the respiratory pattern showed increased tidal volume and low respiratory rate. This now familiar pattern is typical of a dog with cardiopulmonary denervation. Two of the animals survived for as long as 4 days postoperatively. The authors concluded that the lung could survive without a bronchial arterial supply, but the question of prolonged survival after pulmonary denervation remained unanswered.

In a study of heart-lung transplantation in dogs, Longmore and associates (1969) introduced the concept of a single inflow anastomosis at the right atrium. One dog survived for 25 hours. A coauthor, Cooper (1969), wrote a historical review as part of the study. Clearly, although surgical technique was capable of heart-lung transplantation, cardiopulmonary denervation had to be overcome.

Insight into the breathing difficulties after denervation came from the experiments of Nakae and associates (1967), who did different types of cardiopulmonary autotransplantation in several species of animals. First, they divided the great vessels, vena cava and trachea, and divided all other tissue that connected the heart and lungs with the surrounding structures. In dogs who had this type of denervation, the breathing pattern was extremely slow and abnormal, as in dogs who had heart-lung transplantation. When mediastinal denervation was complete but without transection of the great vessels, the breathing pattern was also abnormal. In a third group, complete mediastinal denervation without tracheal transection also resulted in an abnormal breathing pattern, and the animals died of respiratory failure. In a final group, the major vessels were divided without pulmonary denervation, and these dogs resumed spontaneous respiration with a normal respiratory pattern. The procedure was repeated in cats with the same results. Finally, when the experiments were done in monkeys, a relatively normal respiratory pattern was resumed despite pulmonary denervation; deaths were due to technical factors such as bleeding or air leakage and not to respiratory insufficiency.

Proof of these physiological experiments came in 1972 with reports by Castaneda and associates at the University of Minnesota. They operated on primates to avoid respiratory difficulties and performed autotransplants to avoid allograft rejection. In a series of 40 baboons, 6 survived for more than a month and several survived for more than 1 year after operation. In addition, they examined the pulmonary ventilation and perfusion and circulatory hemodynamics in baboons and found that in all respects they were normal (Castaneda et al, 1972a, 1972b). The authors predicted that heart-lung transplantation would be successful in patients.

Primate studies were begun in 1978 by Reitz and associates at Stanford University (Reitz et al, 1980). The initial experiments in small cynomolgus monkeys were with autotransplants. Hypothermia and circulatory arrest was the technique used first; later, cardiopulmonary bypass was found to give better results (Reitz et al, 1981). Animals given autotransplants had normal cardiopulmonary function and long-term survival.

In the late 1970s, cyclosporine was studied in several laboratories, and it was suggested that this immunosuppressive drug could prevent allograft rejection. A small amount of the material was available in the Stanford laboratory and it was used for the treatment of monkeys after heart-lung allotransplantation; these were the first animals to receive lung transplants with cyclosporine for immunosuppression. The drug prevented allograft rejection without obvious toxicity, and several animals survived for more than 1 year after heart-lung allotransplantation (Reitz et al, 1980). Several of these animals lived for more than 5 years after allotransplantation (Harjula et al, 1987). The early results suggested that the degree of rejection was similar in the heart and lung and that the clinically useful endomyocardial biopsy might be sufficient after the rejection. Later clinical experience proved that pulmonary rejection could occur without cardiac rejection, but the survival of these animals gave encouragement for a new clinical trial.

CLINICAL HEART-LUNG TRANSPLANTATION

Three early attempts at heart-lung transplantation were made in the late 1960s. The first attempt was by Cooley and associates in September 1968. The recipient was a 2½-month-old child with atrioventricular canal defect and pulmonary hypertension. The child died of pulmonary insufficiency 14 hours after operation and there was evidence of pulmonary consolidation (Cooley et al, 1969). In December 1969 Lillehei and associates transplanted the heart and lungs of a 50-year-old woman into a 43-year-old man with terminal emphysema. The patient was extubated on the first postoperative day and was ambulatory for several days before he developed severe bronchopneumonia. He died 8 days after the transplantation (Lillehei, 1970). A third human heart-lung transplantation was done by Barnard in 1971 but was not reported until 1982 (Losman et al, 1982). This patient developed a tracheobronchial fistula and intractable pneumonia but survived for 23 days. These results were similar to those of

isolated lung transplantations at that time, and the ability of Lillehei and Barnard's patients to breathe spontaneously was evidence that heart-lung denervation would not preclude the patients' survival, as it had in dogs.

A new clinical trial of heart-lung transplantation began at Stanford in 1981. The first patient was Mary Gohlke, who was 45 years old and who had end-stage primary pulmonary hypertension. The donor for the procedure was brought to the transplant center to minimize the ischemic time, and the heart-lung transplantation was done by the method developed earlier in the laboratory. The patient's thorax with heart and lungs removed is shown in Figure 57–4. She was treated with a combination of cyclosporine and azathioprine for 14 days, and then azathioprine was discontinued and prednisone was added. An acute rejection episode 10 days after the transplantation required intubation and ventilatory assistance, but ultimately she was discharged from the hospital in good condition and was very well for more than 5 years after transplantation (Reitz et al, 1982).

Since March 1981 there has been a significant increase in the number of heart-lung transplantations. Five transplantations were done in 1981 (all at Stanford University) and more than 130 worldwide in 1987. Altogether, more than 400 heart-lung transplantations were done by mid-1988. A review of 239 patients during the period 1981 to 1986 showed that 17 centers reported performance of the procedure— 11 in the United States and 2 each in Canada, England, and Europe (Griffith, 1987). The number of patients reported to the International Society for Heart Transplantation (ISHT) Registry in 1988 is shown in Figure 57–5 and indicates the growth in the number of procedures (Fragomeni and Kaye,

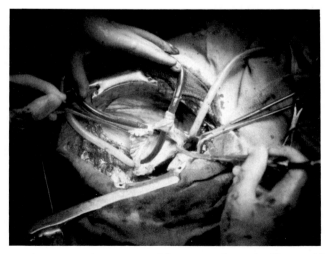

Figure 57–4. Appearance of the empty chest of a 45-year-old patient with primary pulmonary hypertension who received a heart-lung transplant in March 1981. The aortic clamp is to the right; the cuff of right atrium is easily seen with the cannulas inserted into the venae cavae.

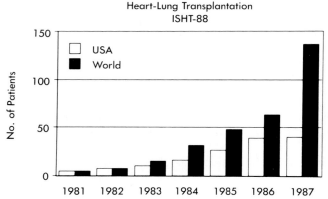

Heart-Lung Transplantation
ISHT-88

Figure 57–5. The number of heart-lung transplantations done in the United States and worldwide from 1980 to 1987 and reported to the International Society for Heart Transplantation Registry. (From Fragomeni, L. S., and Kaye, M. P.: The Registry of the International Society for Heart Transplantation: 5th Official Report, 1988. J. Heart Transplant., 7:249, 1988.)

1988). The level of heart-lung transplantation activity in the United States was relatively constant between 1986 and 1987 (40 and 41, respectively) and reflected the scarcity of heart-lung donors.

The increased clinical experience with this procedure and with transplantation in general has improved results and has shown the areas of major problems. Heart-lung transplantation is restricted by the small number of available donors, lack of methods for adequate preservation of pulmonary tissue, technical problems with bleeding at the time of the operative procedure, an increased incidence of pulmonary infections, and late complications of chronic rejection manifested as bronchiolitis obliterans. These specific problem areas are addressed in relation to further topics in this chapter.

RECIPIENT DIAGNOSIS

Many patients with end-stage disease of both the heart and lungs can potentially be treated by heart and lung replacement. These include patients with congenital abnormalities of the heart and lung, such as univentricular heart with pulmonary atresia or end-stage Eisenmenger's syndrome due to a ventricular septal defect. Patients with other primary lung diseases that result in severe secondary right-sided heart failure are ideally treated by heart-lung replacement. Patients with primary parenchymal lung disease or pulmonary vascular disease and only mild or absent right ventricular dysfunction could be treated by single or double lung replacement or by heart and lung transplantation. Further experience with all of these procedures will determine which patients should receive combined heart-lung replacement. Optimal use can be made of donor resources, as the feasibility of heart donation from a heart-lung recipient (Baumgartner et al, submitted) and the use of both the heart and a double or single lung from a

single donor (Brodman et al, 1985) have been shown. In either case, two recipients benefit from a single donor of thoracic organs.

The most common indication for heart-lung transplantation is primary pulmonary hypertension, which was the diagnosis for 49% of patients reported to the ISHT Registry in 1988. The second most frequent diagnosis is congenital heart disease or Eisenmenger's syndrome, which is responsible for 38% of procedures. Various primary lung diseases, severe cardiomyopathy with resultant pulmonary vascular disease, and retransplantation for bronchiolitis obliterans account for the remainder of the procedures. Among the pulmonary diseases treated successfully by transplantation are cystic fibrosis, emphysema, eosinophilic granuloma, fibrosing alveolitis, primary pulmonary fibrosis, pulmonary lymphangioleiomyomatosis, and pulmonary sarcoidosis.

CONSIDERATIONS FOR SELECTION OF RECIPIENTS

The illnesses that lead to the need for heart-lung transplantation are generally chronic and debilitating, although patients can be maintained at a very low level of functional activity for longer periods than is generally possible with primary cardiac disease. For example, patients with cystic fibrosis are often treated successfully for multiple episodes of infection, receive chronic oxygen therapy, and greatly limit activities to prolong survival. It is often difficult to schedule intervention, because transplant procedures are generally restricted to patients with a life expectancy of 6 months to 1 year. Helpful criteria are the presence of a marked functional disability and an unacceptable quality of life, the occurrence of repeated syncopal episodes, and other life-threatening complications such as massive hemoptysis. When symptoms of severe right-sided heart failure lead to hepatic or renal decompensation, transplantation should be considered.

These patients tend to be younger than those considered for heart transplantation. The average age of patients reported to the ISHT Registry was 32.7 years, compared with 42.5 years for heart recipients. Whereas most heart recipients are male (83%), most heart-lung recipients are female (58%). The requirements for heart-lung recipients are similar to those for patients requiring heart transplant. Patients should be psychologically stable, have a good family support structure, and be reliable in following a complex medical program. The way in which they have adapted to their end-stage heart and pulmonary disease is often a good indication of their ability to handle post-transplant complications and problems.

In a few centers, heart-lung transplantation has been extended to pediatric patients with congenital heart disease or cystic fibrosis. These recipients should have extremely strong family support to be able to adapt to the frequent medical follow-up procedures and possibly invasive procedures such as endomyocardial biopsy or bronchoscopy.

Heart-lung transplantation should be done before complete multiorgan system failure and severe malnutrition occur. Many chronically ill patients are found in this category in their end stage. This problem can arise when patients have been on a waiting list for a potential donor. Every effort should be made to maximize nutrition, including consideration of a feeding gastrostomy for continuous adminstration of nutritional supplements. Because of the magnitude of the operative procedure and potential problems with postoperative bleeding, severe hepatic failure must be avoided.

Most centers consider extensive previous cardiac or thoracic surgery to be a contraindication to heart-lung transplantation. The presence of previous thoracotomies has increased the morbidity and mortality after transplantation, although many patients of this type have had successful transplants. However, if a center wishes to achieve the best 1-year survival results and to maximize the benefit from available donors, previous cardiac or thoracic surgery should be a relative contraindication.

In patients selected for transplantation, routine pretransplant screening is done for ABO blood group, the presence of preformed antibodies (by screening against 50 random donors), HLA and DR tissue types, titers of antibodies against cytomegalovirus (CMV), herpes simplex virus, and toxoplasmosis. A portable anteroposterior chest film is used to obtain measurements of the transverse and vertical dimensions of the thoracic cavity for comparison with similar measurements of potential donors.

SELECTION AND MANAGEMENT OF DONORS

There are fewer suitable donors for lung transplantation than for kidney or heart transplantation. Brain death may be associated with neurogenic pulmonary edema. Similarly, aspiration is frequent during severe trauma and resuscitation, prolonged ventilatory support may predispose to nosocomial infection, and direct thoracic trauma may result in pulmonary contusion. Probably less than 20% of potential cadaver donors have lungs that are suitable for transplantation. In 1987 there were 1,436 heart transplant procedures at 109 centers in the United States and only 41 heart-lung transplant procedures. These numbers reflect the difficulty in obtaining suitable lungs for transplantation and the pressure from multiple transplant centers for the use of hearts for urgent heart recipients even if the donor's lungs are suitable for heart-lung transplantation. The scarcity of heart-lung donors will continue to be a major limiting factor in meeting the clinical need.

The ideal heart-lung donor must meet the criteria for cardiac donation and must also have a clear chest film, an arterial oxygen tension of more than 300 mm

Hg, and an inspired oxygen concentration of 100%. The sputum should be free of gross purulence, and occasionally bronchoscopy is indicated for evaluation.

The lung volumes of the donor can be estimated from the anteroposterior portable chest film as shown in Figure 57–6. Generally, the measurements should not be more than 4 cm greater than similar measurements of the recipient and preferably should be smaller than the measurements of the recipient.

HEART-LUNG PRESERVATION

Routinely successful extended preservation of the lung is difficult to achieve. Although much work has been done on preservation of single lungs for transplantation, the need for immediate, adequate pulmonary function leaves little margin for any inadequacy in preservation. Transportation of the donor to the transplant center and on-site procurement were considered to be essential between 1981 and 1984 (Hardesty and Griffith, 1985; Reitz, 1982). Many laboratories tried to perfect methods to allow preservation for more than 4 hours to make distant procurement successful. As with heart transplantation, adequate preservation techniques would expand the pool of potential donors and would make donation simpler for the referring hospital and the donor's family. Several different techniques have been used at different centers to achieve satisfactory distant procurement.

There is evidence that oxygen free radicals released by tissue damage, perhaps from white blood

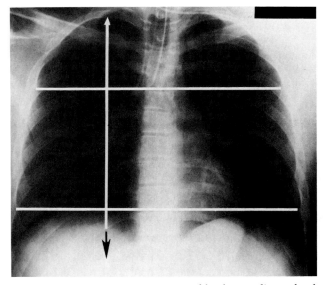

Figure 57–6. Anteroposterior portable chest radiograph of a potential heart-lung transplant donor. The transverse diameter of the chest is measured at the aortic knob, and at the widest portion of the chest is measured at the top of the diaphragm. The vertical dimension from the apex to a line drawn between both costophrenic angles is also measured, and all of these measurements are compared with similar measurements of the potential recipient.

cells, are responsible for the injury to the lung (McCord, 1983). The oxygen free radicals, when released in the extracellular space, directly injure cells of the endothelial or epithelial layer of the lung. Trapped neutrophils are apparently an important source of oxygen free radicals and of lysozymes. The role of recruited white cells in injury to the lung after preservation was shown by Hall and associates (1987). In their experiments with an isolated, perfused, rabbit heart-lung preparation, reperfusion injury after up to 24 hours of cold storage was prevented by removing white blood cells from the blood reperfusion medium. After a 5-hour period of ischemia, reperfusion of blood containing white blood cells caused significant lung injury.

The common result of inadequate pulmonary preservation is an abnormal increase in extravascular pulmonary water. As the alveolocapillary barrier membrane between the intravascular compartment and the pulmonary interstitium is damaged, the water content of the interstitial compartment increases. Compared with pulmonary edema due to cardiac causes, this fluid has a higher protein concentration and is an exudate as opposed to a transudate. Extravascular lung water accumulates at lower critical hydrostatic pressures than those in pulmonary edema of cardiac origin because of increased membrane permeability. The amount of extravascular pulmonary water correlates with other measures of

lung function including airway compliance (which decreases), gas exchange (which deteriorates), and pulmonary vascular resistance (which increases).

As in preservation of other organs, most methods of preservation of the lung rely on deep hypothermia. Hypothermia is generally induced by pulmonary arterial flush, but simple topical hypothermia has been used for preservation of the lung (Todd et al, 1988). The perfusion medium can be crystalloid solution, usually an intracellular-type solution (Baldwin et al, 1987a), or more blood-like in composition (Wheeldon et al, 1988). With any type of flush solution, the concomitant administration of a potent pulmonary vasodilator allows more uniform distribution and more rapid cooling of the perfusion medium. The perfusion solutions and methods of administration used in several active transplant programs are summarized in Table 57–1.

An interesting step toward clinical heart-lung preservation was the initial use of the autoperfusing, normothermic, heart-lung preparation. The concept was first described by Martin in 1883 (Sewall, 1911) and was used by Starling in his classic experiments (Knowlton and Starling, 1912–1913). Demikhov (1962) used this type of preparation as a method of heart-lung preservation during the operation. Robicsek and associates (1963) showed the utility of the heart-lung autoperfusing preparation as a means of extracorporeal preservation of the heart. Hardesty

TABLE 57–1. PRESERVATION METHODS FOR HEART-LUNG AND LUNG TRANSPLANTATION

Centers	References	Pretreatment	Perfusion Solution	Inflation During Storage	Storage
Toronto Lung Transplant Group, Canada	(Todd et al, 1988)	None	None	Collapsed	Collins' solution, 4° C, ice chest
Papworth Hospital, Cambridge, England	(Wheeldon et al, 1988)	Prostacyclin, 10 to 20 ng/kg/min, infused into pulmonary artery 10 to 20 minutes before removal	Ringer's, 700 ml 20% SPA,* 200 ml 20% mannitol, 100 ml Prostacyclin, 20 μg Donor blood, 400 ml CPD,† 63 ml	50% with room air	Saline solution, 4° C, maintained by eutectoid techniques
Harefield Hospital, London, England	(Yacoub et al, 1988)	None	Cold blood by means of CPB	50% with room air	Cold blood from oxygenator, 4° C, ice chest
Johns Hopkins Hospital, Baltimore, MD	(Baumgartner et al, 1988)	Isoproterenol, 0.02 μg/kg/min, 10 to 20 minutes before bypass	Cold blood by means of CPB	50% with room air	Collins' solution, 4° C, ice chest
University of Pittsburgh, Pittsburgh, Pennsylvania, (1984–1986)	(Hardesty and Griffith, 1987)	None	Autoperfusion with donor blood	Continuous ventilation with room air	37° C in sterile container
Stanford University, Stanford, CA and University of Pittsburgh (1987–present)	(Baldwin et al, 1987a)	Prostaglandin E₁, 10 to 80 ng/kg/min, 15 minutes before removal	60 ml/kg Collins' solution with added 50% dextrose (65 ml/l) Magnesium sulfate, 12 mEq/l	50% with room air	Physiol Solution (Abbott Laboratories), 4° C, ice chest

*SPA = salt-poor albumin.
†CPD = citrate phosphate dextrose.

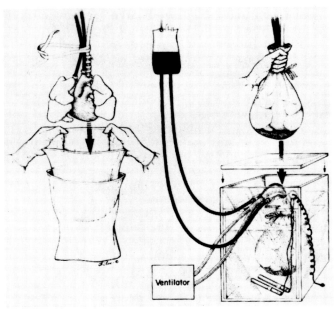

Figure 57–7. The autoperfusion method of Hardesty and Griffith from the University of Pittsburgh. This technique was used for 20 heart-lung procurements between 1984 and 1986.

liver. The chest is entered through a midline sternotomy incision that is extended into the abdomen. Both pleural spaces are entered anteriorly, and the pericardium is removed back to both phrenic nerves. The femoral artery is cannulated for arterial return and a single venous cannula is placed in the right atrial appendage for systemic venous return as shown in Figure 57–8. After cardiopulmonary bypass is begun, profound cooling is continued, to lower body temperature to approximately 12 to 15° C. During bypass, ventilation is stopped to facilitate the dissection. The ascending aorta and pulmonary artery are separated, and the innominate artery is ligated and divided. Similarly, the innominate vein is ligated and divided to give good exposure of the upper mediastinum and help in dissection of the trachea. Both venae cavae are dissected free. When the patient has been cooled to approximately 12° C, the aorta is cross-clamped and 500 ml of standard cold cardioplegia solution is instilled into the aortic root. The lung is not separately perfused at this time. Cardiopulmonary bypass is discontinued and the

and Griffith (1987) at the University of Pittsburgh adapted this technique to clinical heart-lung transplant procedures and reported successful heart-lung preservation with distant procurement for 20 patients during a 20-month period. They considered that the technique provided adequate preservation in most cases and allowed them to increase the number of potential donors for transplant procedures. The apparatus for autoperfusion preservation is shown in Figure 57–7.

The autoperfusing preparation is complicated and cumbersome. Simpler methods that rely primarily on static hypothermic preservation are easier to maintain and less susceptible to bacterial contamination. Almost all centers that use distant procurement rely on hypothermic static preservation.

The technique favored by the author is the use of cardiopulmonary bypass for total body hypothermia in the donor. Simple perfusion of cold blood is used to induce both heart and lung hypothermia, and then the heart is stopped with cold cardioplegia solution by standard techniques. The graft is explanted and transported with cold storage (Baumgartner et al, in press). When this technique was compared with the other commonly used methods, it was more reliable (Fraser et al, 1988).

OPERATIVE TECHNIQUE FOR DONOR HEART-LUNG REMOVAL

The donor is prepared for operation similarly to other cadaver heart donors. Multiple-organ harvesting is feasible and includes removal of kidneys and

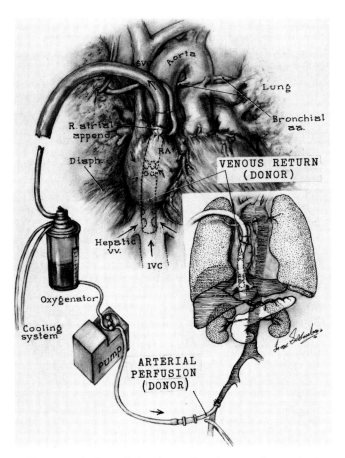

Figure 57–8. Cannulation for cardiopulmonary bypass in the heart-lung transplant donor. The donor is cooled to approximately 12° C before the organs are harvested for transplantation. (From Baumgartner, W. A., Williams, G. M., Fraser, C. D., et al: Cardiopulmonary bypass with profound hypothermia: An optimal preservation method for multi-organ procurement. Transplantation. © by Williams & Wilkins (in press).)

patient's blood volume is drained into the bypass circuit. The ascending aorta and the superior vena cava are transected. The trachea is then divided high in the mediastinum, with approximately 6 to 8 cm of trachea left above the carina. Dissection continues down the posterior aspect of the trachea, and a good amount of adventitial tissue is left attached to the posterior aspect of the heart-lung bloc. The heart-lung bloc is dissected free from the esophagus. Both pulmonary ligaments are divided inferiorly. Posterior hilar attachments are divided. The heart-lung bloc is then removed, the trachea is clamped, and the entire graft can be immersed in cold Euro-Collins' solution. The graft is wrapped in gauze pads, placed in several plastic bags within a sterile plastic container, and then placed in an ice chest. The graft is then ready for transportation to the transplant center.

Both on-site heart-lung procurement with this technique and distant procurement with ischemic times of more than 4½ hours have resulted in satisfactory early pulmonary function. In the author's experience, reimplantation response has been minimal and less than that seen when the lung graft was perfused with Euro-Collins' solution with short ischemic times. The same technique has been used extensively by Yacoub and the group at Harefield Hospital in many distant heart-lung transplant procedures (Yacoub et al, 1988).

OPERATIVE PROCEDURE

The operative procedure to replace the heart and lungs is one of the most fascinating and challenging procedures for cardiothoracic surgeons. The anatomy that is visualized and the areas of the thorax that are dissected are not commonly seen in other procedures. Careful attention to details can simplify the procedure in even the most challenging patient.

Patients with primary pulmonary hypertension are usually the ideal candidates for transplantation. These patients generally have not had previous cardiac or thoracic surgery or large mediastinal collaterals due to cyanosis. Patients with congenital heart disease and pulmonary atresia or severe cyanosis due to Eisenmenger's syndrome may have large mediastinal bronchial collaterals, which require careful ligation. The most challenging aspect of the procedure is the removal of the heart and lungs so that injury to the phrenic, recurrent laryngeal, and vagus nerves is avoided. Attention to hemostasis is also necessary, because after implantation of the graft, exposure of many of the areas of dissection is difficult.

The patient is prepared for operation with the usual monitoring lines. After the induction of anesthesia, the chest and both groins are prepared and draped in a sterile manner. A standard median sternotomy incision is made, and both pleural spaces are opened anteriorly. A portion of the pericardium

is removed anteriorly, but a large segment of pericardium is left laterally to support the heart later and to protect the phrenic nerves. The ascending aorta and both venae cavae are dissected free and encircled with tapes. If the patient can tolerate further manipulation, the phrenic nerve on the right is then dissected free by incising the pericardium just posterior to the phrenic nerve and anterior to the right pulmonary veins. Alternatively, the right phrenic nerve is left in situ, and the opening for the right lung is made by opening the left atrium through the orifices of the right superior and inferior pulmonary veins, after cardiopulmonary bypass is started and the heart and right lung are removed.

Cannulation is done routinely in the high ascending aorta, and the superior and inferior venae cavae are cannulated separately. When cardiopulmonary bypass is instituted, the patient is cooled to approximately 30° C. The aorta is cross-clamped, and a small amount of cardioplegia is given to induce cardiac arrest. When the operation was first done on patients, an effort was made to remove the heart and lungs en bloc. When monkeys were operated on, it was relatively easy to dissect and remove the heart and lungs together. Experience showed that this was relatively difficult and unnecessary in the human thorax, and soon a technique of sequential removal of the heart and lungs was used.

The heart is excised at the ascending aorta just above the aortic valve, through the main pulmonary artery and the atrioventricular groove along the right atrium, and across into the left atrium (Fig. 57–9). This procedure is similar to the standard cardiectomy for cardiac transplantation.

At this point, the left phrenic nerve can easily be dissected free by incising the pericardium anterior to the left pulmonary veins. Both the right and left phrenic nerves are now freed, and there is good access to both pleural spaces. The pulmonary ligaments are divided inferiorly and the pulmonary artery and vein are divided in each hilum by using electrocautery, which is shown in Figure 57–10. The right and left bronchi are skeletonized, and a stapling device (TIA surgical stapler, 4.8 mm) is used to occlude them. Cutting the bronchus distally allows the lung to be removed easily and avoids contamination from the open bronchus.

The final step in preparing the recipient is to open the pericardium at the superior part of the pericardial space just anterior to the right and left bronchi, which allows dissection back to the carina. In this area it is important to stay right on the bronchus, use electrocautery if possible, and avoid injury to the vagus nerve as it passes posterior to the bronchus and anterior to the esophagus, which is shown in Figure 57–11. The vascular lymph nodes in this area may be very large, particularly in patients with cystic fibrosis.

A portion of the pulmonary artery is left intact adjacent to the underside of the aorta in the region of the ligamentum arteriosus, which minimizes dam-

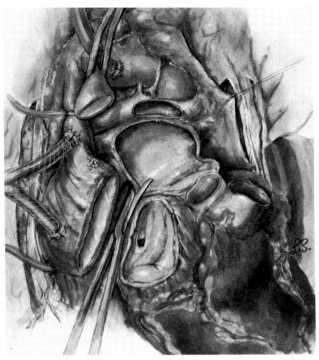

Figure 57–9. Cannulation for cardiopulmonary bypass is done in the usual manner: a cannula in the high ascending aorta and a separate vena caval cannula through the right atrium. Cardiectomy is similar to that for standard cardiac transplantation, with an adequate cuff of right atrium left in the recipient for later anastomosis.

age to the recurrent laryngeal nerve. The portion of right pulmonary artery that is left in place can be opened anteriorly and used to wrap the anterior tracheal suture line to separate it from the aorta. The trachea is not opened until just before implantation of the graft to minimize bronchial spillage into the mediastinum.

The donor heart and lung graft is then prepared for implantation. The graft is removed from its sterile container and brought to the operative field in a basin with cold saline. The trachea is excised several rings above the carina, and the superior tracheal segment with the clamp attached is then removed from the field. The tracheobronchial tree is aspirated with a sucker that is later discarded. At the same time, a culture is taken directly from the trachea. The trachea is then trimmed back so that only one complete cartilaginous ring is left just above the carina. The author often uses a syringe full of normal saline to irrigate the bronchi and visualize them for retained secretions or any foreign body that might have been aspirated by the donor.

The graft is then lowered into the chest, with the right lung placed below the right atrial cuff and the right phrenic nerve (Fig. 57–12). Cold saline and gauze pads soaked in cold saline are placed over the lung and heart to maintain hypothermia during implantation. The recipient trachea is opened just above the carina, with all the adventitial peritracheal tissue

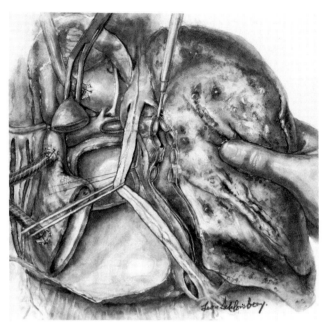

Figure 57–10. The left phrenic nerve is freed from the hilum of the left lung. The inferior ligament is divided, together with the pulmonary artery and veins, by using the electrocautery. The left bronchus is transected after closure of the proximal segment with a stapling device. A similar maneuver is then done on the right lung.

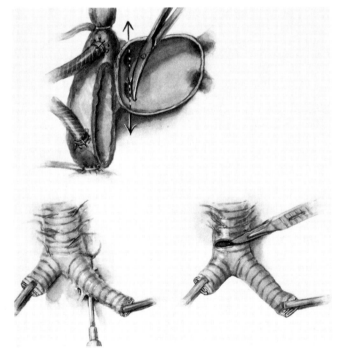

Figure 57–11. An alternative method of providing access to the right pleural space. The right superior and inferior pulmonary veins can be opened together and the opening is extended by incising the atrial wall superiorly and inferiorly, which creates a space for passing the right lung of the donor into the right thorax. The right and left bronchi are freed by grasping the closed ends of the bronchi and dissecting with an electrocautery. Care must be taken to protect the vagus nerve, which passes just anterior to the esophagus in this area. The recipient's trachea is divided one cartilaginous ring above the tracheal bifurcation.

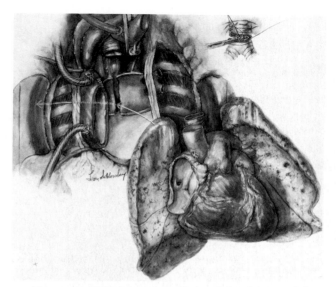

Figure 57–12. Implantation of the donor heart and lungs begins with placement of the right lung below the right atrial cuff. The tracheas are joined with a running 3-0 polypropylene suture that begins with the posterior wall.

that is adjacent to the superior tracheal segment left in place. Small bronchial vessels may require a Liga clip or suture; use of electrocautery at the cut edge of the trachea is avoided. The tracheal anastomosis with a running suture of 3-0 polypropylene is started on the left side of the trachea and the posterior row is sewn from inside. The same suture is continued anteriorly from outside the trachea. There should be a fairly close size match between donor and recipient, but any disparity can usually be accommodated by the flexibility of the membranous part of the trachea. These bites usually go around at least one cartilaginous ring, and the donor trachea slightly invaginates into the recipient trachea in most cases. When the tracheal anastomosis is complete, the chest is irrigated with several liters of ice-cold saline for topical cooling of the graft and to help remove any contamination from the trachea. Omental wrapping of the tracheal anastomosis is advocated by the group at the University of Pittsburgh.

The donor right atrium is then opened as in a standard cardiac transplant. The inferior vena cava is opened laterally and then brought up toward the right atrial appendage to make a right atrial cuff that is similar in size to the recipient right atrial opening. The right atria of the donor and recipient should be inspected for the presence of a patent foramen ovale, or an atrial septal defect, which is repaired if found. A very long (54-inch) 3-0 polypropylene suture is then used for a continuous anastomosis of the right atrium (Fig. 57–13). The superior vena cava was ligated earlier, and the ligation is reinforced with a mattress suture. The patient is then rewarmed to 37° C.

In the case of heart donation from a heart-lung recipient (domino donor), the author modifies the

procedure by cannulating the vena cava directly and dividing the vena cava at removal of the heart. The donor heart-lung is then implanted with separate superior and inferior caval anastomoses as shown in Figure 57–14.

The donor aorta is trimmed to the appropriate length, and a 4-0 polypropylene suture is used for aortic anastomosis. After the anastomosis the patient is placed in a slightly head-down position, the ascending aorta and pulmonary artery are aspirated for air, and the caval tapes and aortic clamp are removed. The author usually begins a slow infusion of isoproterenol (0.02 µg/kg/min) with initial reperfusion, which increases the heart rate slightly and decreases pulmonary vascular resistance. The tracheal tube is aspirated with sterile technique, and ventilation is resumed with an inspired oxygen concentration of 50%. When the patient's body temperature is almost normal and heart and lung function is satisfactory, cardiopulmonary bypass is discontinued and decannulation is done routinely. Temporary pacing wires are applied to the donor right atrium and ventricle and brought out through the skin below the incision. Right-angled chest tubes are left in the right and left pleural spaces, and protamine and any required clotting factors are administered. The appearance of the chest just before closure is shown in Figure 57–15.

By decreasing the tidal volume and using hand ventilation, it is possible to rotate the right or left

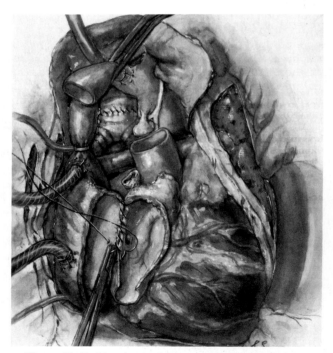

Figure 57–13. The donor right atrium is joined to the right atrial cuff of the recipient with a long, running suture of 3-0 polypropylene. The right atrium of the graft has been opened in a manner similar to that for standard cardiac transplantation, with ligation of the superior vena cava and protection of the region of the sinoatrial node (*stippled area*).

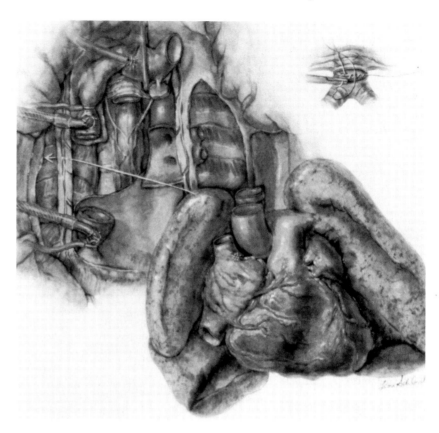

Figure 57–14. Modification of the heart-lung transplant procedure when the recipient has donated the heart for another heart transplant operation. The venae cavae are cannulated separately, with right-angled cannulas, and separate superior and inferior vena caval anastomoses are required. Otherwise, the implantation is the same as the one described earlier.

lung out into the midportion of the incision to observe the posterior mediastinum on that side and assess any bleeding from adhesions in either pleural space. The author uses large amounts of saline at 37° C to irrigate both pleural spaces and the medias-

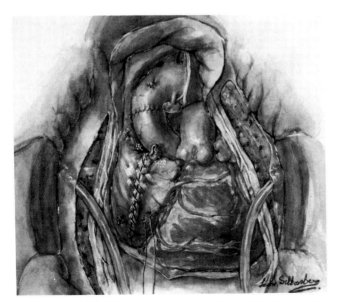

Figure 57–15. The completed operation with all cannulas removed. Chest tubes are inserted into both the right and left pleural space, and temporary pacing wires are applied to the donor right atrium. The sternotomy wound is closed in the usual manner with wire suture.

tinum. When hemostasis is satisfactory, the wound is closed routinely with multiple stainless-steel sternal wires.

In most cases the operation proceeds normally, but unexpected adhesions and scarring, together with coagulopathy due to preoperative hepatic congestion, can result in substantial bleeding. In the author's experience, this is most frequent in patients who had previous cardiac surgery and in older patients with cystic fibrosis who had severe pleural scarring. Blood and coagulation factors are required more frequently than for heart transplantation. Cell saving and re-infusion of shed blood can be very useful.

POSTOPERATIVE MANAGEMENT

Intensive Care Unit

The immediate postoperative care of the heart-lung transplant recipient is similar to that of other patients who have cardiac surgery. Patients are allowed to awaken from anesthesia and are monitored closely for hemodynamic stability and chest tube drainage. Endotracheal suctioning is done routinely when appropriate, and the patient is weaned from the ventilator by standard protocols. When blood gases and ventilatory mechanics are satisfactory, the patient is extubated. Attention is given to fluid balance to avoid overhydration and encourage diuresis of the usual accumulation of fluid.

As soon as possible, the patient is allowed to sit in a chair and begin ambulation. A physical therapist works with the patient to encourage mobilization and rehabilitation.

Immunosuppression

All patients with normal renal function receive cyclosporine before transplantation as an oral dose of 10 mg/kg. On release of the aortic cross-clamp, 500 mg of methylprednisolone is administered. No other steroids are given for the next 2 to 3 postoperative weeks unless acute rejection occurs. The patient is started on cyclosporine at 10 mg/kg/day in two divided doses or 2 to 4 mg/kg intravenously with a constant infusion for 24 hours if oral intake is not possible. The serum levels of cyclosporine are regulated by high-performance liquid chromatographic assay of whole blood, with trough levels between 100 and 200 ng/ml in the first 3 months and 50 to 150 ng/ml more than 3 months after transplantation. In addition, azathioprine is begun immediately after operation at 2 mg/kg and is continued on a daily basis if the white blood cell count is greater than 4,000/mm^3.

The author has also used rabbit antithymocyte globulin (10 mg/kg/day) for the first 3 to 4 postoperative days, and this additional drug is preferred by other centers as well. Recently, OKT3 (monoclonal antibody preparation) has been advocated as an alternative for the first 14 days.

Between 2 and 3 weeks after transplantation, low-dose prednisone is started at 0.2 mg/kg/day and the triple-drug regimen of cyclosporine, azathioprine, and prednisone is continued for the long term. Triple-drug protocols are associated with improved late survival and a lower incidence of renal dysfunction.

DIAGNOSIS OF REJECTION

Detection of acute rejection is rare in the first postoperative week. Although rejection can be manifested in the heart and lungs simultaneously, most rejection episodes are heralded by pulmonary changes. The number of rejection episodes in heart-lung transplant patients is considerably less than the number in patients who receive only a heart transplant. In a comparison of heart-lung transplant and heart transplant patients over similar periods, Baldwin and associates (1987b) showed a highly significant difference in the time to the first rejection episode and in the incidence of rejection in the first month after transplantation. This finding was confirmed by most other centers that do heart-lung transplantation. Cardiac rejection after the first 2

months is almost never seen, which is determined by serial endomyocardial biopsies in a large number of patients (Glanville et al, 1987). Therefore, clinical symptoms, the chest film, pulmonary function, and bronchoscopy are commonly used to prove heart-lung allograft rejection.

The clinical onset of rejection in the heart-lung transplant patient is often heralded by a slight increase in temperature and a diffuse interstitial infiltrate on the chest film, which may be accompanied in the early post-transplant course by serous pleural effusions. There is usually no increase in cough or sputum associated with infiltrate, and a bronchoscopy at this time shows a slight erythema of the donor trachea and absence of purulent secretions and is frequently associated with Leu-7 positive lymphocytes on bronchial biopsy (Hruban et al, 1988). The Papworth Hospital group first described the use of histology in the bronchial biopsy to make the diagnosis of rejection (Stewart et al, 1988). If infection is excluded, a therapeutic trial of intravenous methylprednisolone helps to establish the diagnosis of pulmonary rejection. The author recommends a 3-day protocol of 1 g intravenously in adults and lower doses in smaller patients. Generally, this therapy reverses the infiltrate and improves compliance and oxygenation. The chest film of a 7-year-old patient 10 days after heart-lung transplantation with the diagnosis of rejection is shown in Figure 57–16. The second film shows the patient 3 days later after treatment with methylprednisolone. Additional or more resistant episodes of rejection can be treated with rabbit antithymocyte globulin or monoclonal (OKT3) antibody, as with resistant heart transplant rejection.

In a study of right ventricular endomyocardial biopsies after heart-lung transplantation. Glanville and associates (1987) at Stanford showed a striking reduction in the frequency of acute rejection after the third postoperative month. A total of 159 biopsies from 35 patients showed an incidence of acute rejection after 4 months of only 1.9%. Fully 40% of the transplant recipients had no evidence of acute rejection in any biopsy postoperatively. These results are in sharp contrast to those for patients who have heart transplant alone, and Glanville and associates recommended that right ventricular endomyocardial biopsy for surveillance be omitted after the first 6 weeks and done only for specific indications. Findings in the author's patients are similar, and this policy has been adopted.

REIMPLANTATION RESPONSE

A diffuse interstitial infiltrate on the chest film in the early postoperative period was often called a "reimplantation response" (Veith, 1978). Experience has shown that this finding can usually be attributed to a specific cause, such as inadequate preservation and reperfusion injury or onset of pulmonary rejec-

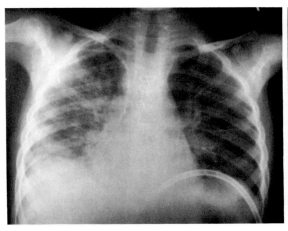 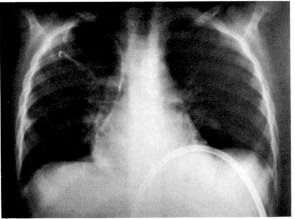

Figure 57–16. Posteroanterior chest films of a 7-year-old patient after heart-lung transplantation for cystic fibrosis. On the left is the film 10 days after transplantation when the diagnosis of rejection was made. The film on the right shows the patient 3 days later after treatment with intravenous methylprednisolone.

tion. Most patients now do not have any abnormality that cannot be explained on this basis, although some interstitial edema due to lack of adequate pulmonary lymphatics in the first few weeks after transplantation is still a possibility.

INFECTIOUS COMPLICATIONS

The major causes of morbidity and mortality after heart-lung transplantation are infectious complications. The incidence of infectious complications early and late after transplantation in both heart and heart-lung transplant recipients at Johns Hopkins Hospital is shown in Table 57–2. There are more than three times as many infections after heart-lung transplantation, and this incidence is associated with a higher late mortality. CMV infection, particularly in patients who had negative exposure to CMV before transplantation and received a heart-lung graft from a patient who had been exposed to CMV, results in high morbidity and mortality (Burke et al, 1986). The Papworth group now requires negative CMV serology in the donor if the recipient has negative CMV serology. The author favors prophylactic treatment of the recipient with acyclovir and human immune globulin in this case.

Patients who have heart-lung transplantation for cystic fibrosis do not appear to have an increased incidence of infectious complications, although the

total number of patients is still small and further experience is required (Scott et al, 1988).

BRONCHIOLITIS OBLITERANS

The major long-term complication for heart-lung transplant patients is the development of a chronic lung disease characterized as bronchiolitis obliterans. The disease is histologically similar to other types of bronchiolitis obliterans, which is often considered to have an immune mechanism. This complication develops in approximately one-third of patients who survive more than 6 months. Clinical manifestations of bronchiolitis obliterans include a cough and progressive dyspnea. Interstitial pulmonary infiltrates are seen on the chest film and an obstructive pattern is seen in pulmonary function tests. Serial measurements of FEV_1 in patients with bronchiolitis obliterans are shown in Figure 57–17. Histologically, the airway disease begins as tough subgranulation tissue that protrudes into distal airway lumina and is slowly replaced by dense fibrous connective tissue.

The evidence suggests that bronchiolitis obliterans is a manifestation of chronic pulmonary allograft rejection. The disease is found in patients with the greatest degree of HLA mismatch (Harjula et al, 1987) and in the earliest stages responds to an increase in immunosuppression (Allen et al, 1986). Direct epithelial injury by infectious agents such as CMV may

TABLE 57–2. INFECTIOUS COMPLICATIONS FOLLOWING HEART AND HEART-LUNG TRANSPLANTATION (JULY 1983 TO JULY 1988)

Operation	No. of Patients	Mean Follow-up (months)	No. of Infections	Percentage of Pulmonary Infections	Infection Episodes per Patient-Month
Heart transplants	91	23	126	25	0.06
Heart-lung transplants	10	18	33	55*	0.20*

*Difference is significant at $p \ll 0.05$.

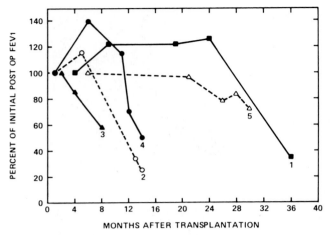

Figure 57–17. Forced expiratory volume in 1 second (FEV₁) of 5 patients who developed bronchiolitis obliterans after heart-lung transplantation. The decrease in flow rates occurred between 4 and 36 months after transplantation. The rapid decline in pulmonary function was correlated with symptoms of dyspnea. (From Burke, C. M., Theodore, J., Dawkins, K. D., et al: Post-transplant obliterative bronchiolitis and other late lung sequelae in human heart-lung transplantation. Chest, *86*:824, 1984.)

also result in bronchiolitis (Dummer et al, 1985). Other infections have also been implicated, but it is difficult to ascertain whether the infection is primary or secondary. Bronchiolitis is also associated with the development of coronary artery disease in the transplanted heart, which is thought to be due to chronic cardiac allograft rejection. No patient has been reported with severe coronary artery disease in the heart with a heart-lung transplant and absence of bronchiolitis.

The best surveillance technique at present is to provide the patient with a portable spirometer, so that expiratory flow can be checked frequently between clinic visits. Any deterioration or change in clinical condition is quickly correlated with a chest film and fiberoptic bronchoscopy with bronchial biopsy to assess the presence of infection or changes characteristic of bronchiolitis obliterans or rejection. Rejection is treated aggressively and the existing chronic immunosuppressive protocol is optimized. Early aggressive immunosuppressive augmentation has been the only successful treatment of this relentlessly progressive disease. Despite this approach, patients often go on to severe symptomatic deterioration. The author performed a retransplantation in one patient and had a second patient who died before retransplantation because of this complication. At present, bronchiolitis is the major obstacle to the long-term therapeutic benefit of heart-lung transplantation.

Late airway disease in patients who have heart-lung transplant may also be manifested as chronic bronchiectasis. Several patients have had chronic bronchial infection that required frequent hospitalizations and treatment with antibiotics, including suppressive prophylactic treatment.

LATE RESULTS

The overall survival of patients who have heart-lung transplants is less than that of heart transplant recipients, primarily because of higher operative mortality. In the patients reported to the ISHT, actuarial survival 1 year after transplantation was 51.6% between 1981 and 1985 and 62.5% between 1986 and 1987. The actuarial curve is shown in Figure 57–18. Overall survival is improving with experience.

Individual centers with more experience generally have better survival results. For example, a Stanford University report indicates 70% 1-year survival (Starnes et al, 1987), and the Papworth Hospital group reports 78% 1-year survival (English and Wallwork, 1987). Patient selection is important, and survival of patients with primary pulmonary hypertension is better than that of patients with congenital heart disease and much better than that of patients with diffuse pulmonary disease from various causes. The status of the recipient before transplantation and the quality of the donor organs, particularly in relation to donor-transmitted infections, are major determinants of long-term results.

A review of 239 patients from 17 centers showed 104 deaths both early and late after transplantation (Griffith, 1987). Of these, 39% were due to infection, 24% to operative bleeding, 11.6% to cardiopulmonary failure (primarily poor pulmonary preservation), and 10.6% to the late development of bronchiolitis obliterans. Only 3.8% were due to tracheal dehiscence, and the rest were due to various other causes. Other late complications after transplantation are similar to those described for heart transplant patients. Hypertension and decreased renal function are typical of patients who take cyclosporine. Other problems such as pancreatitis or problems that require surgical care

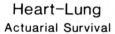
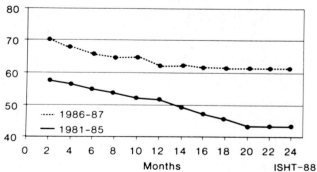

Figure 57–18. Actuarial survival of heart-lung transplant recipients reported to the International Society for Heart Transplantation. The upper curve represents patients who received transplants in 1986 and 1987, and the lower curve represents patients who received transplants between 1981 and 1985. (From Fragomeni, L. S., and Kaye, M. P.: The Registry of the International Society for Heart Transplantation: 5th Official Report, 1988. J. Heart Transplant., *7*:249, 1988.)

are similar to those of patients with heart transplants (Aziz et al, 1985; Steed et al, 1985).

Patient survival will increase as the selection of donors and recipients is improved and the incidence of early donor-transmitted pneumonia is decreased. Further improvement requires a better understanding of bronchiolitis obliterans and methods of prevention. Experimental and clinical studies of the immunologic changes that occur in the lung are necessary.

LATE PULMONARY FUNCTION

Within several months after successful heart-lung transplantation, the physical activity of recipients is usually unrestricted. Most patients have a significantly improved clinical status compared with their long debilitating illnesses before transplantation. Serial study of pulmonary function early after transplantation shows a decrease in most pulmonary volumes that results in a moderately severe restrictive ventilatory defect but shows a great improvement in the arterial oxygen tension and gas exchange (Theodore et al, 1984). Pulmonary function improves over time, and studies at 1 and 2 years show that gas exchange and ventilation are essentially normal (Theodore et al, 1987). These results show that denervation of the heart and lungs, disruption of the bronchial circulation and pulmonary lymphatics, and graft ischemia at the time of transplantation do not seriously limit the long-term result. The overall functional capacity of the heart and lungs is more than adequate to meet the activities of normal life, which is documented by Theodore and associates.

FUTURE DEVELOPMENTS

Further improvements in immunosuppression and perhaps the development of selective immune tolerance will be necessary before heart-lung transplantation can achieve the goal of restoring heart and lung function without significant late morbidity or mortality. It is remarkable that the present results can be obtained by using broad-spectrum immunosuppression with multiple agents. As the management problems are resolved, the major problem of donor availability will remain. Xenotransplantation may be the alternative that ultimately overcomes this limitation. Heart and lung transplantation will continue to be the only therapy for patients with end-stage heart and lung disease, because of the inherent complexities of mechanical replacement of this organ system.

Selected Bibliography

Fragomeni, L. S., and Kaye, M. P.: The Registry of the International Society for Heart Transplantation: 5th Official Report, 1988. J. Heart Transplant., 7:249, 1988.

The accumulated experience up to the end of 1987 is reported from the members of the International Society for Heart Transplantation. The annual report is presented at the spring meeting of the society, and the 1988 report includes 41 patients who received transplants in the United States and 136 patients who received transplants at centers outside the United States in 1987. The most significant finding of the 1988 report is an improvement in the actuarial survival. Patients operated on from 1981 to 1985 had 51.6% survival at 1 year, and patients operated on from 1986 to 1987 had 62.3% survival at 1 year. This improvement is undoubtedly due to increased experience with the procedure.

Fraser, C. D., Tamura, F., Kontos, G. J., et al: Evaluation of current organ preservation methods for heart-lung transplantation. Transplant. Proc., 20:987, 1988.

Many laboratories have studied variables of lung preservation for heart-lung transplantation. This study compares the methods reported to be successful for clinical heart-lung procurement and preservation—the working autoperfused heart-lung preparation, flush perfusion with modified Euro-Collins' solution and pretreatment with prostaglandin E_1 infusion, and core cooling with cardiopulmonary bypass for simple hypothermic preservation. These techniques were examined in calves who had orthotopic heart-lung transplantation and then had analysis of heart and lung function as well as histology. Adequate acute organ function was provided by all preservation methods, but core cooling appeared to be slightly better in terms of low extravascular pulmonary water and histology of the pulmonary grafts.

Glanville, A. R., Imoto, E., Baldwin, J. C., et al: The role of right ventricular endomyocardial biopsy in the long-term management of heart-lung transplant recipients. J. Heart Transplant., 6:357, 1987.

This report details the experience with right ventricular endomyocardial biopsy in patients who received heart-lung transplants at Stanford. During 670 patient-care months, 35 patients had a total of 447 biopsies. After the fourth postoperative month, only 3 of 159 biopsies showed any evidence of acute cardiac rejection. Moreover, 14 of the patients (40%) had no biopsy that showed cardiac rejection. Late after heart-lung transplantation, the cardiac biopsy is no longer helpful in detecting allograft rejection. Obliterative bronchiolitis developed in the absence of findings on cardiac biopsy, which indicates that chronic lung rejection cannot be detected by this method.

Griffith, B. P.: Cardiopulmonary transplantation—growing pains. Int. J. Cardiol., 17:119, 1987.

This review of cardiopulmonary transplantation summarizes the results from 17 centers worldwide and includes 239 procedures. Griffith reviews the accumulated experience with emphasis on the practice at the University of Pittsburgh. At the time of the publication, 135 of 239 patients had survived between more than 1 and less than 5 years.

Reitz, B. A., Wallwork, J. L., Hunt, S. A., et al: Heart-lung transplantation: Successful therapy for patients with pulmonary vascular disease. N. Engl. J. Med., 306:557, 1982.

This is the first report of the Stanford series of heart-lung transplantations, which began in March 1981. After laboratory demonstration of the feasibility of heart-lung transplantation with cyclosporine for immunosuppression, a 45-year-old woman with primary pulmonary hypertension had successful heart-lung transplantation. Subsequently, a patient with Eisenmenger's syndrome due to a ventricular septal defect had heart-lung transplantation that resulted in a dramatic improvement in his clinical condition. These patients were the first to have therapeutic transplantation of pulmonary tissue and contributed to enthusiasm about the immunosuppressive agent cyclosporine.

Scott, J., Hutter, J., Stewart, S., et al: Heart-lung transplantation for cystic fibrosis. Lancet, 2:192, 1988.

The Papworth Hospital experience with heart-lung transplantation in six patients with cystic fibrosis is reported. Five of the recipients were alive from 3 to 29 months after the operation. There was no evidence of recurrence of pulmonary disease typical of cystic fibrosis and no increase in infectious complications over those normally seen with heart-lung transplantation.

Stewart, S., Higenbottam, T. W., Hutter, J. A., and Wallwork, J.: Histopathology of transbronchial biopsies in heart-lung transplantation. Transplant. Proc., 20:764, 1988.

This report from Papworth Hospital near Cambridge, England, details the use of frequent transbronchial biopsy for the histologic study of rejection of the lung. This technique helped to detect clinically significant rejection after the results of immunosuppressive treatment and has been adopted by most centers that do heart-lung transplantation.

Theodore, J., Morris, A. J., Burke, C. M., et al: Cardiopulmonary function at maximum tolerable constant work rate exercise following human heart-lung transplantation. Chest, 92:433, 1987.

Parameters of heart and lung function were measured at rest and during maximum tolerable exercise in 16 patients who had had successful heart-lung transplantation. Ten patients were studied 1 year after transplantation and six patients were studied 2 years after transplantation. Exercise capacity was significantly greater than the preoperative value. Cardiorespiratory function at maximal exercise was well maintained, and the authors concluded that overall functional capacities of the transplanted heart and lungs are more than adequate for the activities of normal life.

Bibliography

Allen, M. D., Burke, C. M., McGregor, C. G. A., et al: Steroid-responsive bronchiolitis after human heart-lung transplantation. J. Thorac. Cardiovasc. Surg., 92:449, 1986.

Aziz, S., Bergdahl, L., Baldwin, J. C., et al.: Pancreatitis after cardiac and cardiopulmonary transplantation. Surgery, 97:653, 1985.

Baldwin, J. C., Frist, W. H., Starkey, T. D., et al.: Distant graft procurement for combined heart and lung transplantation using pulmonary artery flush and simple topical hypothermia for graft preservation. Ann. Thorac. Surg., 43:670, 1987a.

Baldwin, J. C., Oyer, P. E., Stinson, E. B., et al: Comparison of cardiac rejection in heart and heart-lung transplantation. J. Heart Transplant., 6:352, 1987b.

Baumgartner, W. A., Traill, T. A., Cameron, D. E., et al.: Unique aspects of heart and lung transplantation exhibited in the "domino-donor" operation. J.A.M.A., submitted.

Baumgartner, W. A., Williams, G. M., Fraser, C. D., et al: Cardiopulmonary bypass with profound hypothermia: An optimal preservation method for multi-organ procurement. Transplantation, in press.

Brodman, R. F., Veith, F. J., Goldsmith, J., et al: Multiple organ procurement from one donor. J. Heart Transplant., 4:254, 1985.

Burke, C. M., McCormick, S., O'Connell, B. M., et al: Cytomegalovirus infection in heart-lung transplant recipients. J. Heart Transplant., 5:267, 1986.

Carrel, A.: The surgery of blood vessels. Johns Hopkins Hosp. Bull., 18:18, 1907.

Castaneda, A. R., Arnar, O., Schmidt-Habelmann, P., et al: Cardiopulmonary autotransplantation in primates (baboons): Late functional results. J. Cardiovasc. Surg., 37:523, 1972a.

Castaneda, A. R., Zamora, R., Schmidt-Habelmann, P., et al: Cardiopulmonary autotransplantation in primates (baboons): Late functional results. Surgery, 72:1064, 1972b.

Comroe, J. H.: Who was Alexis WHO? Cardiovascular diseases. Bull. Texas Heart Inst., 6:251, 1979.

Cooley, D. A., Bloodwell, R. D., Hallman, G. L., et al: Organ transplantation for advanced cardiopulmonary disease. Ann. Thorac. Surg., 8:300, 1969.

Cooper, D. K. C.: Transplantation of the heart and both lungs. I: Historical review. Thorax, 24:383, 1969.

Demikhov, V. P.: Experimental Transplantation of Vital Organs. New York. Consultant Bureau, 1962.

Dummer, J. S., White, L. T., Ho, M., et al: Morbidity of cytomegalovirus infection in recipients of heart or heart-lung transplants who received cyclosporine. J. Infect. Dis., 152:1182, 1985.

English, T. A. H., and Wallwork, J.: Heart and heart-lung transplantation: Papworth Hospital 1979–1987. In Terasaki, P. I. (ed): Clinical Transplantation 1987. Los Angeles, UCLA Tissue Typing Laboratory, 1987.

Fragomeni, L. S., and Kaye, M. P.: The Registry of the International Society for Heart Transplantation.: 5th Official Report, 1988. J. Heart Transplant., 7:249, 1988.

Fraser, C. D., Tamura, F., Kontos, G. J., et al: Evaluation of current organ preservation methods for heart-lung transplantation. Transplant. Proc., 20:987, 1988.

Glanville, A. R., Imoto, E., Baldwin, J. C., et al: The role of right ventricular endomyocardial biopsy in the long-term management of heart-lung transplant recipients. J. Heart Transplant., 6:357, 1987.

Griffith, B. P.: Cardiopulmonary transplantation—growing pains. Int. J. Cardiol., 17:119, 1987.

Griffith, B. P., Hardesty, R. L., Trento, A., et al: Heart-lung transplantation: Lessons learned and future hopes. Ann. Thorac. Surg., 43:6, 1987.

Hall, T. S., Breda, M. A., Baumgartner, W. A., et al: The role of leukocyte depletion in reducing injury to the lung after hypothermic ischemia. Curr. Surg., 44:137, 1987.

Hardesty, R. L., and Griffith, B. P.: Autoperfusion of the heart and lungs for preservation during distant procurement. J. Thorac. Cardiovasc. Surg., 93:11, 1987.

Hardesty, R. L., and Griffith, B. P.: Procurement for combined heart-lung transplantation: Bilateral thoracotomy with sternal transection, and profound hypothermia. J. Thorac. Cardiovasc. Surg., 89:795, 1985.

Harjula, A., Baldwin, J., Henry, D., et al: Minimal lung pathology on long-term primate survivors of heart-lung transplantation. Transplantation, 44:852, 1987.

Hruban, R. H., Beschorner, W. E., Baumgartner, W. A., et al: Diagnosis of lung allograft rejection by bronchial intra-epithelial Leu-7 positive lymphocytes. J. Thorac. Cardiovasc. Surg., 96:939, 1988.

Knowlton, F. P., and Starling, E. H.: The influence of variations in temperature and blood-pressure on the performance of the isolated mammalian heart. J. Physiol. 44:206, 1912–1913.

Lillehei, C. W.: Discussion of Wildevuur, C. R. H., Benfield, J. R. A review of 23 human lung transplantations by 20 surgeons. Ann. Thorac. Surg., 9:489, 1970.

Longmore, D. B., Cooper, D. K. C., Hall, R. W., et al: Transplantation of the heart and both lungs. II: Experimental cardiopulmonary transplantation. Thorax, 241:391, 1969.

Losman, J. G., Campbell, C. D., Replogle, R. L., et al: Joint transplantation of the heart and lungs. Past experience and present potentials. J. Cardiovasc. Surg., 23:440, 1982.

Lower, R. R., Stofer, R. C., Hurley, E. J., et al: Complete homograft replacement of the heart and both lungs. Surgery, 50:842, 1961.

Marcus, E., Wong, S. N. T., and Luisada, A. A.: Homologous heart grafts. AMA Arch. Surg., 66:179, 1953.

Marcus, E., Wong, S. N. T., and Luisada, A. A.: Homologous heart grafts: Transplantation of the heart in dogs. Surg. Forum, 2:212, 1951.

McCord, J. M.: The biochemistry and pathophysiology of superoxide. Physiologist, 26:156, 1983.

Nakae, S., Webb, W. R., Theodorides, T., et al: Respiratory function following cardiopulmonary denervation in dog, cat and monkey. Surg. Gynecol. Obstet., 125:1285, 1967.

Neptune, W. B., Cookson, B. A., Bailey, C. P., et al: Complete homologous heart transplantation. Arch. Surg., 66:174, 1953.

Reitz, B. A.: Heart-lung transplantation: A review. J. Heart Transplant., 1:291, 1982.

Reitz, B. A., Burton, N. A., Jamieson, S. W., et al: Heart and lung transplantation, autotransplantation and allotransplantation in primates with extended survival. J. Thorac. Cardiovasc. Surg., 80:360, 1980.

Reitz, B. A., Pennock, J. L., and Shumway, N. E.: Simplified operative method for heart and lung transplantation. J. Surg. Res., 31:1, 1981.

Reitz, B. A., Wallwork, J. L., Hunt, S. A., et al: Heart-lung transplantation: Successful therapy for patients with pulmonary vascular disease. N. Engl. J. Med., 306:557, 1982.

Robicsek, F., Sawyer, P. W., and Taylor, F. H.: Simple method of keeping the heart "alive" and functioning outside the body for prolonged periods. Surgery, 53:525, 1963.

Scott, J., Hutter, J., Stewart, S., et al: Heart-lung transplantation for cystic fibrosis. Lancet, 2:192, 1988.

Sewall, H.: Henry Newell Martin: Professor of biology in Johns Hopkins University, 1876–1893. Johns Hopkins Hosp. Bull., 22:327, 1911.

Starnes, V. A., Baldwin, J. C., and Harjula, A.: Combined heart and lung transplantation: The Stanford experience. J. Appl. Cardiol., 2:71, 1987.

Steed, D. L., Brown, B., Reilly, J. J., et al: General surgical complications in heart and heart-lung transplantation. Surgery, 98:739, 1985.

Stewart, S., Higgenbottam, T. W., Hutter, J. A., et al: Histopathology of transbronchial biopsies in heart-lung transplantation. Transplant. Proc., 20:764, 1988.

Theodore, J., Jamieson, S. W., Burke, C. M., et al: Physiologic aspects of human-lung transplantation: Pulmonary function status of the post-transplanted lung. Chest, 86:349, 1984.

Theodore, J., Morris, A. J., Burke, C. M., et al: Cardiopulmonary function at maximum tolerable constant work rate exercise following human heart-lung transplantation. Chest, 92:433, 1987.

Todd, T. R., Goldberg, M., Koshal, A., et al: Separate extraction of cardiac and pulmonary grafts from a single organ donor. Ann. Thorac. Surg., 46:356, 1988.

Veith, F. J.: Lung transplantation. Surg. Clin. North Am., 58:357, 1978.

Webb, W. R., and Howard, H. S.: Cardiopulmonary transplantation. Surg. Forum, 8:313, 1957.

Wheeldon, D. R., Wallwork, J., Bethune, D. W., et al: Storage and transport of heart and heart-lung donor organs with inflatable cushions and eutectoid cooling. J. Heart Transplant., 7:265, 1988.

Yacoub, M. H., Khaghani, A., Banner, N., et al: Distant organ procurement for heart-lung transplantation. (Presented) XII International Congress of the Transplantation Society, Sydney, 1988.

II CARDIAC TRANSPLANTATION

William A. Gay, Jr.
John B. O'Connell

Cardiac transplantation is "a medically reasonable and necessary service" for appropriately selected patients with end-stage heart disease (Health Care Finance Administration, 1987). Several centers have reported 2-year survival of more than 80% after cardiac transplantation in patients with a predicted 1-year survival of less than 50% (Bolman et al, 1988; Frazier et al, 1988; Renlund et al, 1987a). The number of transplantations and the number of centers offering this service have increased dramatically in the last 5 years. Approximately 120 heart transplantations were done in the United States in 1982, compared with more than 1,400 in 1987 (M. P. Kaye, personal communication, 1988). A study concluded that approximately 15,000 persons annually could benefit from cardiac transplantation in the United States and that the limiting factor is the number of available donor organs (Evans et al, 1986).

In this chapter, the important events in the development of cardiac transplantation and the present status of the procedure are discussed. Emphasis is placed on the selection and management of recipients, donor evaluation, management, and organ recovery; operative techniques; and postoperative management.

HISTORICAL ASPECTS

Pien Ch'iao, a Chinese physician who lived during the latter years of the Chou dynasty (1121 to 249 B.C.), is said to have exchanged the hearts of two men, Kung Hu and Ch'i Ying, to establish equilibrium between strong and weak forces (yang and yin). The two were later maintained on "supernatural drugs" and, except for initial confusion about whose wife and children belonged to whom, they remained well (Wong and Wu Lien-Teh, 1936). In 1905 Carrel and Guthrie described a technique for heterotopic transplantation of hearts in experimental animals. Demikov in the Soviet Union (Demikov, 1962) and Reemtsma in the United States (Reemtsma, 1964) used the heterotopic model to study organ function and to observe the rejection process. Lower and Shumway (1960) reported a method for the orthotopic transplantation of canine hearts. In 1967, Barnard performed the first successful orthotopic human heart transplantation. In the next few years, about 150 human cardiac transplant procedures were done in centers around the world, but most of the recipients died within the first year after transplantation of rejection or opportunistic infection. Although the technical aspects of cardiac transplantation appeared to have been satisfactorily addressed, the procedure was abandoned in the early 1970s in all but a few centers.

Between 1970 and 1980 the centers that remained active in the heart transplant area studied the basic principles of organ transplantation in general and cardiac transplantation in particular. The technique of percutaneous endomyocardial biopsy, which allowed surveillance of myocardial histology and facilitated early diagnosis of rejection before deterioration of cardiac function, was developed (Caves et al, 1973). An organized system of grading the histologic manifestations of rejection was described (Billingham, 1979).

In 1959 it was reported that animals given the antimetabolite 6-mercaptopurine were unable to synthesize humoral antibody after an appropriate antigen challenge (Schwartz et al, 1959). Azathioprine, an imidazole derivative of 6-mercaptopurine with a more predictable gastrointestinal absorption pattern, blocks the conversion of inosine monophosphate to adenosine and guanidine monophosphates and thus inhibits the synthesis of purines. Early immune suppression regimens included azathioprine in addition to corticosteroids (Lower et al, 1965; Reemtsma et al, 1962). In 1976 the polyclonal lymphocytolytic agent antithymocyte globulin (ATG) was introduced (Bieber et al, 1976), and ATG is still a mainstay in early prophylaxis and in the treatment of acute rejection. In some centers, antilymphoblast globulin (ALG) has been used. Cyclosporine A, an endecapeptide fungal metabolite, was shown to have immunosuppressive properties (Borel et al, 1976); was studied in the laboratory (Calne et al, 1978; Jamieson et al, 1979; Kostakis et al, 1977); and was then used clinically, first in renal, hepatic, and pancreatic transplantation (Calne et al, 1981). Use of cyclosporine as part of the immune suppression regime in cardiac transplantation (Bolman et al, 1985; Borel, 1983; Oyer et al, 1982) led to greatly improved survival, an increase in the number of transplant operations, and an increase in the number of centers doing such operations.

SELECTION AND MANAGEMENT OF RECIPIENTS

Etiology

Although criteria for selection of recipients have traditionally been restrictive because of the unpredictable results and limited accessibility, improvements in survival and increases in the number of cardiac transplant programs have resulted in liberalization of these criteria (Copeland et al, 1987). Generally, cardiac transplantation should be limited to patients with terminal cardiac disease who are unable to do the minimal activity of an acceptable life-style and who cannot achieve palliation or prolongation of life with conventional medical or surgical therapy (Table 57–3). Most recipients have cardiomyopathy or end-stage coronary artery disease, but cardiac transplantation is also being offered to selected patients with complex forms of congenital heart disease for whom repair or palliation is not possible (Table 57–4) (Addonizio and Rose, 1987; Bailey et al, 1986; Fricker et al, 1987).

Patients with cardiomyopathy and cardiac dilatation were originally considered to be ideal candidates for cardiac transplantation because of the young age of onset of illness and the poor prognosis of the condition (O'Connell and Gunnar, 1982). Improved management of congestive heart failure in these patients, however, may prolong survival by decreasing the incidence of death from progressive cardiac failure without altering the incidence of sudden unexpected death. The prognosis is variable, but 2-year survival of approximately 50% from onset of symptoms is the accepted standard. Poor prognostic indicators include age of onset above 55 years, New York Heart Association Class IV symptoms, marked cardiomegaly detected radiographically and echocardiographically, ejection fraction less than 20%, cardiac index less than 3 l/min/m², and left ventricular end-diastolic pressure greater than 20 mm Hg. Symptomatic ventricular tachycardia is considered a poor prognostic indicator by most investigators. Even when these poor prognostic indicators are taken into account in consideration of risks and benefits, patients deemed too well for transplantation may still have unacceptably high mortality (Stevenson et al, 1987). It has been recommended that patients with an ejection fraction less than or equal to 25% be considered candidates for transplantation, even if their symptoms are relatively mild. Patients with cardiomyopathy and severe ventricular arrhythmia refractory to all modes of antiarrhythmic therapy and not altered by an automatic implantable cardioverter/defibrillator may be considered for cardiac transplantation.

TABLE 57–3. CRITERIA FOR HEART TRANSPLANT RECIPIENTS

1. Severe, progressive heart disease unable to be improved or significantly palliated by medical or surgical therapy
2. Age less than 65 years
3. Pulmonary vascular resistance less than 4 Wood units (with or without therapy)
4. Absence of other organ dysfunction (e.g., liver, kidneys) not reversible and related to cardiac disease
5. Absence of other life-threatening conditions not related to cardiac disease (i.e., active malignancy, active systemic infection, diabetes with end-organ dysfunction)
6. Strong support system
7. Absence of substance abuse
8. Ability to adhere to complex medical regimen

TABLE 57–4. ETIOLOGY OF END-STAGE HEART DISEASE IN 150 CARDIAC TRANSPLANT RECIPIENTS

Disease	Percent
Ischemic heart disease	49.7
Cardiomyopathy	40.8
Valvular heart disease	3.4
Congenital heart disease	1.4
Rejection of previous transplant	2.7
Other	2.0
Total	100.0

Patients with selected etiologic subtypes of cardiomyopathy have had cardiac transplantation, but little is known about the results. For example, patients with myocarditis proved by biopsy may be considered to be candidates for cardiac transplantation, but it may be advantageous to wait until active myocardial inflammation regresses spontaneously or is modified by immunosuppressive therapy because the myocyte damage is immunologic in origin (O'Connell, 1987). If cardiac transplantation is done in the presence of active immune-mediated heart disease, early and severe cardiac allograft rejection is possible. Also, because biopsy-proven myocarditis sometimes regresses spontaneously, extended hemodynamic support to ascertain the degree of reversibility of the myocardial dysfunction may be warranted before transplantation is considered. In severe fulminant cases, cardiac transplantation may be required urgently.

Patients with amyloid heart disease, another etiologic subtype, have recently had cardiac transplantation (Conner et al, 1986). In the past, the systemic nature of this condition and the possibility of recurrence in the recipient heart were considered to be contraindications for cardiac transplantation. However, patients without evidence of renal, gastrointestinal, hepatic, or peripheral nerve involvement may have successful cardiac transplantation, although long-term results have not been reported.

The other common condition that requires cardiac transplantation is refractory left ventricular dysfunction secondary to end-stage ischemic heart disease. Patients with refractory arrhythmia or angina pectoris with lesser degrees of left ventricular dysfunction may also be candidates for cardiac transplantation. Patients with angina should be considered only when use of antianginal agents has been maximized and coronary arteriography shows that revascularization is not possible. For patients with symptomatic congestive heart failure and coronary artery disease, diagnostic evaluation should include documentation that left ventricular dysfunction is irreversible. Generally, thallium exercise testing should be used to show irreversible perfusion abnormalities or reversible lesions that cannot be revascularized. With these criteria, most patients with coronary artery disease who are considered for transplantation will have had previous coronary artery bypass. Although there are more transplant patients with dilated cardiomyopathy than with coronary artery disease (Kaye, 1987), there is a trend for an increased number of patients with coronary artery disease to have this procedure as the acceptable age is extended to the seventh decade.

Patients with valvular heart disease who have acceptable pulmonary vascular resistance are candidates for transplantation when left ventricular dysfunction becomes refractory. Generally, patients with end-stage valvular heart disese may be more debilitated and have a greater degree of cardiac cachexia because of the chronic nature of their condition.

Nutritional factors must be considered before such patients are accepted and attention to nutrition must be included in perioperative care.

As children with complex forms of congenital heart disease who have successful palliative procedures become older, left ventricular dysfunction may become greater and cardiac transplantation may be considered if they have a protected pulmonary vasculature. The operation often must be tailored to the individual anatomy and vascular access for biopsy must be considered. Several centers reported encouraging results in transplantation of neonates with severe forms of congenital heart disease, such as hypoplastic left heart syndrome (Bailey et al, 1986; Mavroudis et al, in press).

With greater long-term survival, more individuals will require retransplantation for allograft arteriosclerosis. Although cyclosporine and other selective immunosuppressive drugs have increased early survival, there is no evidence that the rate of development of graft arteriosclerosis has decreased (Renlund et al, 1989). Coronary artery lesions can be detected by routine coronary angiography in most patients within the first 3 years after cardiac transplantation (Gao et al, 1988). Until the immunology of chronic vascular rejection is better understood, allograft arteriosclerosis will require cardiac retransplantation in a greater percentage of patients. Retransplantation should be done only when the graft arteriosclerosis results in ischemia or left ventricular dysfunction in candidates who are otherwise acceptable.

Analysis of the mortality in cardiac transplantation according to the etiology of heart disease by the Registry of the International Society for Heart Transplantation (Kaye, 1987) showed no difference between patients with cardiomyopathy and coronary artery disease. The mortality was higher for patients with congenital heart disease, valvular heart disease, or allograft rejection, but this result may be an artifact because relatively few procedures are performed in patients with these etiologies.

Age

In the past, patients over 50 to 55 years old were excluded from cardiac transplantation, because of the lack of donor availability and the nonspecific potency of immunosuppression. As potent immunosuppressive agents with corticosteroid-sparing effects were developed and the supply of donor organs increased, patients in the early pediatric population and adults over 55 years of age were considered to be candidates for cardiac transplantation. The survival of patients between 55 and 65 years of age who have cardiac transplantation is similar to if not better than that of younger patients (Carrier et al, 1986; Renlund et al, 1987b), which may be explained by a decreased incidence of acute allograft rejection due to T-lymphocyte senescence and decreased immunoreactivity to allograft antigens. From a medical perspective, a candidate between 55 and 65 years old who is physiologically youthful should not be excluded from transplantation on the basis of age. However, with age there is an increased frequency of noncardiac complications such as transient ischemic attacks due to cerebrovascular disease, diverticular disease, and prostatic complications.

Cardiac transplantation is also being offered to younger children and neonates with greater frequency. The experience is not as extensive as in the adult population, and definitive statements about survival are not possible. When cardiac transplantation is considered for infants and children, the morbidity associated with immunosuppressive therapy and the difficulties of vascular access for biopsy should be considered.

Pulmonary Hypertension

As part of the routine evaluation, right-sided heart catheterization must be done for all potential recipients and pulmonary vascular resistance must be calculated (Gay, 1988). Although resting pulmonary vascular resistance may be above the traditional threshold of 6 to 8 Wood units, the peak pulmonary artery pressure and pulmonary vascular resistance may be decreased with intensive medical management of congestive heart failure and incremental doses of nitroprusside. If the pulmonary artery pressure falls below 60 mm Hg or the pulmonary vascular resistance falls below 3 Wood units, orthotopic cardiac transplantation can be done. When pulmonary vascular resistance and pulmonary artery pressure are at the upper limits, a donor whose body size is at least equal to that of the recipient should be selected. In some centers, heterotopic cardiac or heart-lung transplantation is considered for recipients with high pulmonary vascular resistance.

Other Criteria

If the recipient has had a recent pulmonary embolism or infarction, cardiac transplantation should be delayed until healing occurs. If delay is not possible, the operation is feasible but pulmonary infection often occurs (Young et al, 1986). The pulmonary infarct can sometimes be resected at the time of transplantation to minimize this complication. Diabetes is a relative contraindication. In some centers, selected insulin-dependent diabetics without evidence of renal, neuropathic, gastrointestinal, or microangiopathic disease are successfully transplanted by using immune suppression protocols with minimal corticosteroid therapy (Badellino et al, 1988). The long-term prognosis of these patients has yet to be determined, and selection criteria must be stringent to ensure the greatest possibility of long-term allograft survival. Intrinsic diseases of the liver, kidneys, or central nervous system are relative contrain-

dications. Generally, patients with end-stage congestive heart failure have abnormalities in glomerular filtration because of decreased renal blood flow. Efforts should be made to ensure that these abnormalities are not due to intrinsic renal disease, because of the additive nephrotoxicity of cyclosporine. Similarly, liver disease should be evaluated and irreversible changes are considered a contraindication for cardiac transplantation. When possible, biopsy of these organs may help resolve these issues. Active peptic ulcer disease is a relative contraindication and efforts must be made to allow healing of ulcers. If transplantation is necessary in an otherwise ideal candidate, intensive antacid and H_2 blocker therapy may allow healing to continue after the procedure. Active systemic infection is a contraindication because of the possibility of dissemination after immunosuppression. Patients with malignancy should not be considered for cardiac transplantation because the immunosuppression may inhibit the natural immune responses that prevent proliferation of such lesions. A history of a malignancy cured by medical or surgical management is not an absolute contraindication for cardiac transplantation. The type of tumor, severity, and residual effects must be considered before a decision is made.

Psychosocial Criteria

Candidates for cardiac transplantation should have strong psychologic support systems and be able to tolerate the stress of living away from their family for long periods, prolonged hospitalizations, and toxicity from immunosuppressive agents (Christopherson, 1987). Candidates should have shown the ability to comply with complex medical regimens. All patients should be screened for psychosocial acceptability, but standardized criteria are not available and acceptability is determined on a case-by-case basis. Patients who suffer from alcohol or substance abuse should be evaluated by drug rehabilitation experts and should have a compulsive treatment protocol with which they are compliant. Ideally, compliance should be tested for several weeks to months before the transplant, but when this is not feasible a frank discussion with the patient is necessary before acceptance. In patients with previous psychiatric histories, psychiatric evaluation is mandatory. Generally, any endogenous psychotic state that could be exacerbated by environmental stress or corticosteroid administration is a contraindication for cardiac transplantation.

Immunologic Assessment

Immunologic assessment of all patients who have cardiac transplantation should include screening for the presence of lymphocytotoxic antibodies to allograft antigens. In most centers, this is done by mixing serum from the recipient with lymphocytes from a random panel of donors and calculating the per cent of reactive antibody. A cardiac transplant recipient is thought to be sensitized if there is more than 5 to 10% reactive antibody. Some centers require a specific cross-match with the donor if the recipient is sensitized, but this may be unnecessary because the likelihood of a positive cross-match is low (O'Connell et al, 1988). In the presence of a positive cross-match, alterations of immunosuppression to focus on humoral immune responses have been successful.

The National Heart Transplant Study found that of more than 1,000 patients referred for cardiac transplantation, 350 were accepted; however, 280 never had the procedure. Of this 280, 59% died waiting and 31% refused the procedure (Evans and Maier, 1986). Although there is a trend toward less rigid criteria for cardiac transplantation, the disparity between donor organ availability and recipient need suggests that medically sound guidelines should be developed and followed.

Recipient Management

When a candidate is accepted for transplantation, the major challenge for the medical team is to sustain adequate perfusion until a compatible donor is identified (Renlund et al, 1989b). In general, less use of instrumentation and shorter hospitalization reduce the risk of infection. Hospitalization with intravenous lines should be minimized. In most patients, however, intravenous therapy is needed because of the lack of predictably effective oral agents for inotropic support. Clinical study of a class of orally active phosphodiesterase inhibitors has shown promising early results. One of these agents, enoximone, was effective in providing inotropic support to patients who depended earlier on intravenous inotropes (Weber et al, 1986).

If oral therapy does not sustain adequate perfusion, intravenous drugs are required. The drug of choice is dobutamine, which has beta-agonist inotropic properties without significant peripheral vascular effects. This drug is most effective when infused at doses up to 10 μg/kg/min and there is no benefit from further increments. If it is difficult to maintain systemic blood pressure, dopamine up to a maximal dose of 5 μg/kg/min may be added to dobutamine. At higher doses of dopamine, the arrhythmogenic and renal vasoconstrictive effects may predominate and have deleterious effects on organ perfusion. If blood flow is still inadequate with intravenous dobutamine and dopamine, mechanical assistance should be considered.

The use of mechanical assistance devices increases the risk of infectious complications, and these circulatory aids should be used for the shortest time possible. Intra-aortic balloon counterpulsation uses volume displacement to effect afterload reduction and diastolic augmentation. Inotropic agents and

other vasoactive drugs are often used with intra-aortic balloon pumping to improve hemodynamics. If left ventricular ejection is severely compromised, because of inadequate ventricular contractility or a rapid or irregular heart rate, intra-aortic balloon pumping will not be effective and some other form of support is needed.

A left or right ventricular assist device (LVAD or RVAD) diverts blood around the ventricle by removing the blood from the atrium or from the ventricle itself and returning it to the appropriate great vessel. There are two basic types of ventricular assist devices: those that move blood into a sac or diaphragm and then pump it back into the circulation by means of a volume displacement system, usually air or gas, and those that move blood by passing it through a centrifugal pump with electrically driven rotator cones and impellers (Magovern et al, 1987). The pumping mechanism of most ventricular assist devices is external, but prosthetic ventricles have also been placed in the heterotopic internal position and used for circulatory support in patients who await transplantation (Farrar et al, 1988). Neither short-term nor long-term survival after transplantation has been affected by the use of circulatory assist devices (Bolman et al, 1987; Farrar et al, 1988; O'Connell et al, 1988). Pneumatically powered orthotopically placed total artificial hearts have also been used successfully for circulatory support in patients who await suitable donor organs. The present survival of these patients is approximately 50% and probably reflects the severity of the existing cardiac disease and some extracardiac organ dysfunction (D. Olsen, personal communication, 1988).

EVALUATION OF CARDIAC DONORS

Acceptable cardiac donors are young individuals who die of a traumatic or medical cerebral insult and are pronounced brain dead by neurologic specialists according to acceptable criteria (Table 57-5) (Emery et al, 1986). A detailed history and physical examination should be obtained, and any history of drug use, cardiac arrhythmia, or previous cardiac symptoms must be considered before acceptance of the donor. Physical examination by a cardiologist should be obtained if possible. Because of the effects of increased intracranial pressure on catecholamine re-

TABLE 57-5. DONOR CRITERIA

1. Meets requirements for brain death
2. Consent from next of kin
3. ABO compatible with recipient
4. Approximately same size as recipient
5. Absence of history of cardiac disease
6. Normal echocardiogram
7. Age under 35 or
   men between 35 and 45 with normal coronary angiogram;
   women between 40 and 45 with normal coronary angiogram
8. Normal heart by visual inspection at recovery

lease and subsequent distribution of myocardial blood flow, the ST segments and T waves on the electrocardiogram are often abnormal in donors with normal cardiac function. Tachycardia and arrhythmias do not necessarily indicate intrinsic cardiac abnormalities. Cardiac donors are acceptable to age 45, but in men over 35 years and women over 40 years, coronary angiography should be considered routinely before acceptance. Younger donors may require coronary angiography if their history suggests coronary artery disease. There is a reluctance to accept donors over age 45 because of the reported increased incidence of allograft arteriosclerosis with older donor hearts (Billingham, 1987), but the medical necessity and the age of the intended recipient should be considered before an older donor is excluded.

Generally, hemodynamic monitoring is done with a radial arterial line and a central venous pressure or a pulmonary artery catheter, and hydration is required in most donors. Because the neurologic injury typically results in depletion of volume from diabetes insipidus and there is a tendency to attempt reduction of cerebral edema when these patients are treated before brain death, early hemodynamic support is achieved primarily with vasopressors, particularly dopamine. After the declaration of brain death, management of donors should focus on volume replacement and weaning from catecholamines. Prolonged infusion of dopamine at doses of 10 μg/kg/min or more has been considered a contraindication to acceptance of the heart for cardiac transplantation. When echocardiography is available, allograft function can be assessed noninvasively, and as many as 29% of donors who would have been excluded by conventional criteria are acceptable when normal left ventricular function is evident (Gilbert et al, 1988). If a donor organ is questionable on the basis of noninvasive evaluation, direct visualization of the heart by the harvesting surgical team is essential before acceptance. In that case, the recipient should be prepared but not under anesthesia until the cardiac surgeon in the donor hospital has inspected the donor heart.

When the heart is acceptable for transplantation, other systemic conditions must be considered. Systemic infection that has been treated with broad-spectrum antibiotics is not a contraindication for cardiac transplantation, as these infections rarely affect the myocardium. Hepatitis surface antigen positivity and the presence of human immunodeficiency virus (HIV) in the donor are contraindications to acceptance of the organ for transplantation.

Donor/Recipient Matching

In most cases, a donor within 20% of the recipient's body weight is acceptable. If the recipient's pulmonary vascular resistance is at the high end of acceptable limits, a larger donor may be chosen.

ABO compatibility is required, but ABO identical organs are preferred because they may be less likely to induce rejection than organs that are merely ABO compatible. Blood from the donor should be tested for viral titers, particularly for cytomegalovirus (CMV), because the incidence of clinically significant CMV infection approaches 100% when an organ from a CMV-positive donor is procured for a CMV-negative recipient. This information is available only retrospectively and therefore cannot be used to control organ allocation. Donor lymphocytes should be harvested for a donor-specific cross-match, which should be done for all patients. Recipients with preformed reactive antibody titers (PRA) greater than 5% may have a positive cross-match and require alteration of immunosuppressive therapy, but this occurs uncommonly.

Donor Organ Recovery

There are far more potential recipients for cardiac allografts than donors, and hearts recovered for transplantation must be handled in a way that maximizes their usefulness (Gilbert et al, in press). The logistics of organ retrieval must be carefully coordinated and the technical aspects of the procedure accomplished with dispatch and attention to detail. When the donor and recipient are in the same hospital the excision of the donor heart and its implantation can take place almost simultaneously, which minimizes organ ischemia time. Most often, a suitable organ becomes available at a distant institution and close coordination of activities that take place simultaneously at two different locations is necessary. Because the heart is usually only one of several transplantable organs that are being recovered, donor cardiectomy must be coordinated with the excision of kidneys, liver, and pancreas, which sometimes involves several transplant surgical teams from distant locations (Brodman et al, 1985; Starzl et al, 1984). Because the final decision about the suitability of the organ for transplantation is made at the time of recovery, many institutions have an experienced senior surgeon lead the organ recovery team, usually accompanied by a surgical resident and a transplant coordinator.

Organ ischemic time begins when the aortic cross-clamp is placed in the donor and ends when the aortic clamp is released in the recipient. The upper limit of tolerable ischemia in the transplant setting is not known (Copeland et al, 1973), but most cardiac transplant teams attempt to limit organ ischemic time to 4 hours or less. In the authors' experience with approximately 230 transplants, ischemic time has ranged from 55 to 380 minutes and no acute organ dysfunction was related to this interval. However, it should be the primary goal of the organ recovery teams to excise the transplantable organs in the best possible condition and deliver them to the sites of implantation expeditiously.

Multiple organs are recovered by using a midline incision from the sternal notch to the pubis, sometimes with bilateral transverse extensions at or slightly above the level of the umbilicus. The sternum is incised longitudinally, the pericardium opened widely, and the heart inspected for the presence of any unsuspected anomalies or injuries, such as contusions. The condition of the heart and its acceptability for transplantation are then reported to the implanting team, with an estimate of the timing of the rest of the harvesting procedure to coordinate activities and minimize organ ischemia time. The intrapericardial portions of the superior and inferior venae cavae are dissected free and encircling transfixion sutures of 2-0 Dacron are placed about the superior vena cava well cephalad to the area of the sinoatrial node. These sutures are not tied until later. Any catheters that enter the heart, such as flow-guided pulmonary artery lines, are removed at this time. The aorta and pulmonary artery are separated, and the pulmonary artery is dissected free to a point distal to its bifurcation. A purse-string suture of 3-0 Dacron is placed in the adventitia of the aorta as far distal as practical, but not so far as to prevent placement of the aortic cross-clamp beyond it.

When all the organ recovery teams have completed preliminary dissection, the donor is given 20,000 to 50,000 units of heparin and the inferior vena cava is divided slightly above the level of the diaphragm and allowed to bleed into the pericardium. As the arterial pressure of the donor falls with the acute blood loss, the aorta is clamped as far cephalad as possible, and 1,000 ml of cold crystalloid potassium cardioplegic solution (Table 57–6) is infused into the aortic root through a 14-gauge catheter inserted through the purse-string suture. The superior vena cava is then doubly ligated by tying the previously placed transfixion sutures, and the cava is divided between the ligatures. The donor heart is then excised by first dividing the right then the left pulmonary veins at their entrance into the pericardium and then dividing the left and right pulmonary arteries just distal to the bifurcation of the main pulmonary artery. Finally, the aorta is transected distal to the cardioplegic needle but proximal to the aortic cross-clamp. The excised heart is rinsed thoroughly with iced saline, placed into two concentric sterile plastic bags, and packed beneath crushed ice in a portable ice chest for transport to the implant team.

ORGAN IMPLANT

The timing of operation in the cardiac recipient is carefully coordinated with that of the donor. The heart is exposed by a midline sternotomy in most cases. Exposure can be difficult in patients who have had previous cardiac surgery, and the common femoral artery is often used for arterial cannulation in these patients. When the heart is exposed, preparations are made for arterial and bicaval cannulation,

TABLE 57–6. CARDIOPLEGIA SOLUTION

1,000 ml of 5% dextrose in ¼ normal saline containing
   20 mEq of KCl
   5 mEq of NaHCO₃
Kept iced at 4° C

heparin is administered, cannulation is done, and cardiopulmonary bypass is started. Ideally, bypass is started just before the arrival of the donor heart. Because the heart is to be excised and bypass time is usually short, there is no need for cardioplegia or more than moderate hypothermia; the body temperature is maintained at 30 to 32° C. Cardiectomy is done by first incising the left and then the right atrium inferiorly and laterally just on the atrial aspect of the atrioventricular groove. The atrial septum is then incised from its most inferior aspect, with a generous remnant left posteriorly. Finally, the great vessels are divided immediately above the commissures of the semilunar valves. The atrial, aortic, and pulmonary arterial cuffs are then appropriately trimmed. The visceral pericardium binding the aortic and pulmonary arterial cuffs is opened for greater mobility.

The donor heart is then prepared by first opening into the left atrium by connecting the orifices of the pulmonary veins and then trimming residual left atrial tissue to facilitate a good fit with the left atrial cuff in the recipient. The anastomoses are shown in Figure 57–19. The left atria are connected with a continuous suture of 3-0 polypropylene and, after the right atrium of the donor heart is opened along its lateral wall, the right atria are joined with a similar suture. The aortic and pulmonary arterial cuffs are trimmed and sized and then joined with continuous sutures of 4-0 polypropylene for each. All air is evacuated from the heart and from the aortic root, the cross-clamp is released, and perfusion of the transplanted heart is resumed. The heart usually develops an effective rhythm spontaneously, but defibrillation is sometimes required. Temporary pacing wires are attached to the right atrium and the right ventricle, to be used for synchronized atrioventricular pacing or as electrocardiographic leads to obtain epicardial electrograms.

Orthotopic placement of the heart is sometimes not possible or practical and heterotopic placement is used. The presence of severely increased pulmonary vascular resistance is considered by some to be an indication for heterotopic placement (Barnard et al, 1981), because attempts at orthotopic transplantation may result in the development of acute right ventricular failure. The technique for heterotopic transplantation differs significantly from the orthotopic procedure (Fig. 57–20). The inferior vena cava and the right pulmonary veins of the donor heart must be ligated or oversewn at the time of organ recovery. Also, the recovery team should obtain as much length of aorta and superior vena cava as possible. The left atrial anastomosis is done first; an

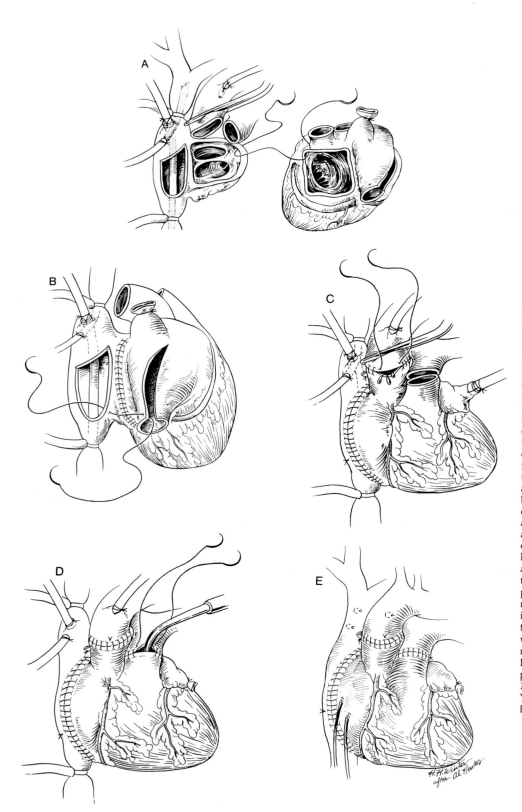

Figure 57–19. Operative technique for human cardiac transplantation. *A,* Cannulation technique is similar to routine cardiac procedures with central cannulation. Tapes have been placed around the superior and inferior venae cavae, and the aorta has been cross-clamped to exclude the heart from the circulation. The recipient's heart has been excised at the atrioventricular groove. The superior vena cava of the donor's heart has been ligated. The left atrial anastomosis has been started. *B,* The left atrial anastomosis has been completed. The incision in the right atrium of the donor heart is curved away from the superior vena cava and the adjacent sinoatrial node. The right atrial anastomosis is begun at the inferior border of the atrial septum. *C,* The right atrial anastomosis is completed. A perfusion catheter has been inserted into the left atrium through which cold (4° C) normal saline is infused to further cool the left ventricular cavity as well as displace air. The aortic anastomosis is being completed. *D,* The aortic cross-clamp has been released after completion of the aortic anastomosis. The perfusion catheter has been removed from the left atrium, and the pulmonary anastomosis is completed with the heart fibrillating. *E,* The bypass cannulas have been removed. Pacing wires have been inserted on the right atrium of the donor heart. (Reproduced with permission from Baumgartner, W. A., Reitz, B. A., Oyer, P. E., et al: Cardiac homotransplantation. Curr. Probl. Surg., *16*:1, 1979. Copyright © 1979 by Year Book Medical Publishers, Inc., Chicago.)

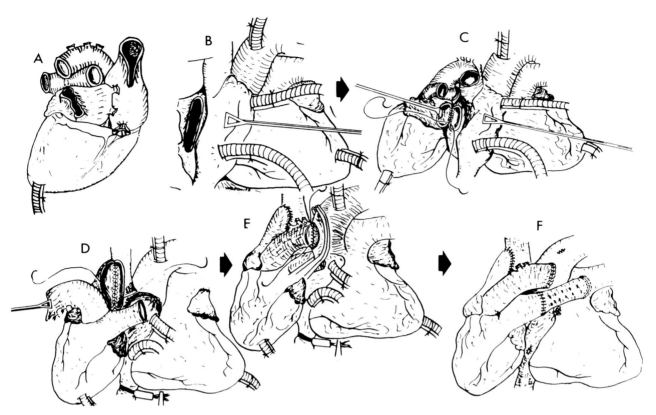

Figure 57–20. The heterotopic cardiac transplant. *A,* Posterior view of the donor after preparation for anastomosis. *B,* Left atriotomy. *C,* Left atrial anastomosis. *D,* Right atrial anastomosis. *E,* Aortic anastomosis. *F,* Completed anastomosis with a pulmonary-to-pulmonary arterial graft. (Reproduced with permission from Barnard, C. N., and Wolpowitz, A.: Heterotopic versus orthotopic heart transplantation. Transplant. Proc., *11:*309, 1979.)

opening is made in the donor left atrium by connecting the orifices of the two left pulmonary veins and then incising the left atrium of the recipient near the interatrial groove just anterior to the entrance of the right pulmonary veins. The left atria are connected with continuous 3-0 polypropylene. Next, the superior vena cava of the donor heart is anastomosed from end to side to that of the recipient with 5-0 polypropylene. An end-to-side anastomosis is then created between the aortae and a short length of prosthetic graft or aortic homograft is used to connect the two pulmonary arteries.

PERIOPERATIVE MONITORING

Because of the risk of infection in the immunosuppressed patient, invasive monitoring techniques are used minimally in cardiac transplantation. Immediately before anesthesia, a radial arterial line is placed. As soon as the patient is asleep, a Foley catheter is placed in the bladder and a large-bore catheter (a triple-lumen device) is inserted in the left internal jugular vein (the right jugular is saved for later percutaneous endomyocardial biopsies). No flow-guided catheter is placed in the pulmonary artery; if one is already in place, it is removed. If indicated on clinical grounds, a pulmonary arterial

catheter can be inserted after the donor heart has been implanted.

Most cardiac transplant recipients are anticoagulated with warfarin at the time of transplantation, because of dilated cardiomyopathy, the existence of mural thrombi from prior myocardial infarctions, the presence of atrial fibrillation, or a combination of the above. An effort is made to restore a normal coagulation profile preoperatively with vitamin K and fresh frozen plasma, but most patients remain therapeutically anticoagulated at the time of operation. Additional fresh frozen plasma and sometimes platelet transfusions may be required in the early postoperative period. Chest drains that allow reinfusion of mediastinal and pleural drainage after it has been filtered are also useful, because drainage may be considerable for the first few hours. If excessive chest tube drainage continues after the coagulation indices have returned to normal, surgical exploration for hemostasis is indicated.

POSTOPERATIVE MANAGEMENT

Hemodynamic Support

The transplanted heart is a denervated organ and, when appropriately volume loaded, increases its output largely by increases in heart rate (Cannon et al, 1973). Before cardiopulmonary bypass is discontinued, an intravenous drip of isoproterenol is started at 0.1 µg/min and the dosage is increased incrementally until the heart rate reaches 100 to 110 beats per minute. This rate gives satisfactory cardiac output without excessive ventricular irritability. Isoproterenol may also be beneficial because of its bronchodilatory action. The drug can usually be discontinued after several days.

In recipients who have pulmonary vascular resistances above 3.0 Wood units despite aggressive preoperative treatment, there is an increased risk of acute right ventricular failure in the transplanted heart. The reason is that the donor right ventricle is unaccustomed to pumping blood against high pulmonary resistance. Every effort is made to obtain a heart from a donor of equal or larger body size and to minimize organ ischemic time when it is known that the recipient has increased pulmonary vascular resistance. Right ventricular failure is seen with elevated venous pressure, dilatation of the right ventricle, and low or normal pulmonary wedge pressure. In this setting, the combination of nitroprusside at 5 to 10 µg/kg/min and the synthetic catecholamine dobutamine at 3 to 10 µg/kg/min has been effective. Prostaglandin E_1, a vasoactive product of the enzymatic conversion of cyclooxygenase, has been effective as a selective pulmonary vasodilator (Armitage et al, 1987). It is recommended that a bolus of 25 to 75 µg be administered into a central vein or directly into the pulmonary artery and followed by an intravenous infusion of 0.1 µg/kg/min. Effectiveness of the drug is shown by a decrease in the pulmonary artery pressure with improved cardiac output and systemic oxygenation.

Other agents that are useful immediately after transplantation are dopamine, an l-norepinephrine precursor; the phosphodiesterase inhibitor enoximone; and, rarely, the combination of epinephrine and calcium chloride (1 mg epinephrine and 1 g $CaCl_2$ in 500 ml of 5% dextrose and water [D/W]). When enoximone is used intravenously, care should be taken to ensure that the patient has adequate intravascular volume as determined by a left ventricular filling pressure of 15 mm Hg or greater. A loading infusion of enoximone is begun at 90 µg/kg/min for a maximum of 20 minutes, and the infusion is decreased or terminated if the heart rate increases by 15% or more or the systolic blood pressure decreases by 20% or more. The maintenance dose is 7 to 10 µg/kg/min but should not exceed 250 mg in 24 hours.

Except when hyperacute rejection occurs, which is very rare immediately after the operation, mechanical circulatory support is seldom necessary. If the recipient required support by intra-aortic balloon counterpulsation preoperatively, it is probably prudent to continue this support for 12 to 24 hours after transplantation and to remove the balloon electively when coagulation indices are normalized. Rarely, a right or left ventricular assist device is required after transplantation and may be connected in the standard manner with atrial uptake and return to the appropriate great artery. However, external instrumentation should be minimal in these patients, who are soon to be immunocompromised.

Immunosuppression

The major nonoperative complications are rejection and the predisposition to infection from potent immunosuppression. Although the approach to immunosuppression varies from center to center, the goal of immunosuppression in the early postoperative period is to allow successful wound healing and induce tolerance to the allograft. Cyclosporine is the cornerstone of all immunosuppressive regimens (Cohen et al, 1984; Kahan, 1987). This drug, first approved by the Food and Drug Administration in 1983 for use in transplantation of solid organs, acts primarily by inhibiting the production of interleukin-2 and thus attenuating the recruitment of cytotoxic T lymphocytes. Early use of this agent resulted in a high incidence of acute renal failure because large preoperative loading doses were used. Cyclosporine is now given in lower doses (2 to 8 mg/kg/day), and in many protocols therapy is started only when postoperative hemodynamic stability has been achieved. This approach avoids high peak and trough levels at a time when liver and renal function may not be optimal because of compromised organ perfusion. Early immunoprophylaxis also includes corticosteroids in various doses, and most immunosuppressive regimens prescribe a high early corticosteroid dose that decreases to a maintenance prednisone level of 0.15 to 0.20 mg/kg/day. Cyclosporine and prednisone alone result in 80% survival at 1 year, and addition of azathioprine to this regimen (triple therapy) increases survival to 85 to 90% at 1 year (Kaye, 1987). Azathioprine is typically given at 2 mg/kg to maintain the white blood cell count between 4,000 and 6,000 per cubic millimeter.

Cytolytic therapy is commonly incorporated in the first 1 to 2 weeks to intensify T-cell immunosuppression. The most common agent for this purpose is equine antithymocyte globulin, but antilymphoblast globulins and rabbit antithymocyte globulin are also used for immunoprophylaxis. These agents are given perioperatively and continued for 1 to 2 weeks. The murine monoclonal antibody against the human CD3 T-cell antigen (OKT3) was shown to decrease the incidence of rejection when compared with a protocol based on equine ATG (Bristow et al, 1988). In addition, significantly more patients were maintained on steroid-free protocols after they received the OKT3-based immunoprophylaxis. The patients who had OKT3 had fewer side effects and infectious complications as well as a decrease in the hypercholesterolemia that accompanies high-dose corticosteroids.

In the patient who has a positive donor-specific cross-match, early immunosuppression is directed toward decreasing humoral antibody load and B-lymphocyte proliferation. Cyclophosphamide may be substituted for azathioprine and plasmapheresis may be done to decrease antibody load. Because there is little experience with highly sensitized cardiac transplant recipients, no firm recommendations can be given for managing patients with a positive retrospective cross-match.

Diagnosis of Rejection

Cytoimmunological monitoring with quantitation of lymphocyte subpopulations and interleukin-2 receptors and echocardiographic detection of abnormalities of systolic and diastolic function have been proposed as noninvasive techniques that aid in the diagnosis of rejection, but the endomyocardial biopsy remains the standard (Billingham, 1982). Although pathologic criteria vary, the histologic definition of rejection includes the intensity and characteristics of the inflammatory infiltrate, evidence of myocyte damage, and changes in microvascular integrity. The histologic abnormalities precede left ventricular dysfunction, and surveillance endomyocardial biopsy allows rejection to be diagnosed before end-organ dysfunction occurs. Hence, immunosuppression may be intensified to a lesser degree than is required in other solid-organ allografts, where rejection is diagnosed only after allograft dysfunction is identified. A typical protocol for endomyocardial biopsy recommends weekly procedures for 6 to 8 weeks with a gradual increase in the interval between biopsies to 3 to 4 months (Table 57–7).

Treatment of Rejection

When the histologic diagnosis of rejection is established, the degree of intensification of immunosuppression depends on the severity of histologic change and the presence of hemodynamic compromise. Most episodes of rejection can be managed by increasing the dose of oral corticosteroids or giving

TABLE 57–7. SCHEDULE FOR ENDOMYOCARDIAL BIOPSIES

Biopsy Number	Time
1	5 to 7 days after transplantation
2–6	Weekly
7–11	Every 2 weeks
12–14	Every 4 weeks
15–18	Every 6 weeks
19–21	Every 8 weeks
22, 23	Every 12 weeks

Thereafter, every 6 months
Rejection, 5 to 7 days after treatment begins
Coronary arteriography done annually

a short course of high-dose (pulse) intravenous corticosteroid. With more severe rejection, cytolytic therapy with antithymocyte or antilymphoblast globulin or OKT3 may be required. The incidence of rejection is highest in the first 4 to 6 months and then tapers off to a state of relative immune tolerance. At that time, the quantity of immunosuppressive agents may be reduced to decrease the risk of infection. Maintenance immunosuppression usually includes corticosteroid, cyclosporine, and azathioprine in low doses and in various combinations. Aggressive early immunosuppression may make it possible to minimize or eliminate the long-term use of corticosteroids and thus to decrease their side effects (Renlund et al, 1987c; Yacoub et al, 1985).

Complications of Immunosuppression

The complications of immunosuppressive agents must be assessed to individualize immunosuppression. Corticosteroids may lead to a cushingoid appearance, osteoporosis, cataracts, thinning of the skin and capillary fragility, peptic ulcer disease, and the development of overt diabetes mellitus in previously borderline diabetics. Azathioprine is rarely hepatotoxic but is usually well tolerated. When cyclosporine was introduced in high doses and combined with multiple intensive immunosuppressive agents, a high incidence of lymphoma was identified (Penn, 1987). This unusual lymphoma begins as a polyclonal lymphocyte proliferation stimulated by Epstein-Barr virus and presents atypically with primary gastrointestinal or cerebral involvement. As the dose of cyclosporine has decreased, the incidence of lymphoma and all malignancies in patients who have cardiac transplants is not different from that in patients with renal and liver transplant; lymphoma occurs in 6% of transplant patients at any time after operation. Hypertension is so common in patients who receive cyclosporine that it is unusual for a patient who takes the agent not to be hypertensive (Thompson et al, 1986). The hypertension tends to have a reversed diurnal variation with the highest pressures recorded early in the morning and is unresponsive to many conventional antihypertensive drugs although usually responsive to beta-adrenergic and calcium channel blockade. Cyclosporine nephrotoxicity occurs most often when the drug is administered in high loading doses. Most patients who have chronic maintenance cyclosporine have a decrease in glomerular filtration to approximately 50% of normal. Less common side effects are seizures, hirsutism, and gingival hyperplasia.

The most frequent complications of immunosuppressive agents are infections (Andreone et al, 1986). The use of cyclosporine has decreased the incidence of life-threatening bacterial and fungal infections, but viral infections, particularly CMV, are still a major source of morbidity (Hofflin et al, 1987). Pneumocystis may be a common cause of interstitial pneumonia after cardiac transplantation. The treatment for pneumocystis pneumonia is trimethoprim-sulfamethoxazole, and the antiviral agent ganciclovir is effective in gastrointestinal ulceration and interstitial pneumonia due to CMV infection. An aggressive approach to the treatment of interstitial pneumonia is mandatory for successful recovery of the cardiac transplant recipient.

Coronary Arteriosclerosis

The major complication that prevents long-term survival after cardiac transplantation is the development of coronary artery disease (Billingham, 1987; Renlund et al, 1989c). This form of coronary artery disease is distinct from atherosclerosis in patients who do not have transplants. Allograft coronary artery disease appears to begin in the distal vessels and progress proximally. It is rarely found at bifurcations of major epicardial vessels and, therefore, is not amenable to percutaneous transluminal coronary angioplasty or coronary artery bypass grafting. This form of coronary arteriosclerosis is clinically silent because of the denervated state of the heart and presents as left ventricular dysfunction or arrhythmia in the absence of chest pain. Annual coronary angiography is done routinely to screen for this complication. Histologically, these vessels have concentric fibrous narrowing without the classic eccentric atherosclerotic plaque. Most recipients have evidence of coronary artery disease by 3 years. Although the etiology of this state is unclear, it probably represents chronic vascular rejection in an atherogenic milieu (e.g., hypertension, hypercholesterolemia). Treatment has not prevented the development of this complication and it is the major cause for consideration of retransplantation after the first 6 postoperative months.

RESULTS AND FUTURE CONSIDERATIONS

Improved immunosuppression and use of surveillance endomyocardial biopsy have resulted in a 1-year survival of more than 85% and comparable 2- and 3-year survivals (Fig. 57–21). The causes of death are essentially unchanged; infection and rejection predominate. Patients who have successful cardiac transplantation are usually functionally rehabilitated without cardiac symptoms. Less than 50% return to full-time employment, either because they are unable to re-enter the workforce for economic reasons or because society and employers refuse to accept their normal activity level.

Clinical research should be directed toward the development of more specific immunosuppressive protocols to further decrease the incidence of infection and rejection. Monoclonal antibody therapy with OKT3 has led to improvement in the management

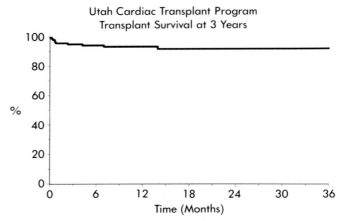

Utah Cardiac Transplant Program
Transplant Survival at 3 Years

Figure 57–21. Actuarial survival in one cardiac transplant program: 92% at 1 year and 90% at 2 and 3 years ($n = 143$ transplants).

of rejection with excellent survival in patients who receive this therapy prophylactically. At one center where 147 such operations were done and an OKT3-based prophylactic protocol was used, in the first 36 months the actuarial survival was 92% at 1 year and 90% at 3 years. As new monoclonal antibodies directed toward lymphocyte receptors (anti-TAC directed toward the interleukin-2 receptor) or blocking antibodies directed toward allograft antigens are developed, the specificity of immunosuppression will increase and the requirement for nonspecific immunosuppression and thus the risk of infection will decrease. Despite the possibility of improved management of early postoperative complications, little is known about the pathogenesis of allograft coronary artery disease. When research directed toward the resolution of this problem is fruitful, the long-term prognosis of these patients will be enhanced.

The disparity between the number of organs needed for transplantation and the number available for this purpose requires attention. Progress continues to be made in the specificity of immunosuppressive agents and in tissue typing and cross-matching, but long-term survival in grafts between disparate species has not been reliably achieved (Bailey et al, 1985; Sadeghi et al, 1987). Similarly, experience with the orthotopically placed total artificial heart has been disappointing (DeVries, 1988; D. Olsen, personal communication, 1988). With approximately 15,000 patients in need of cardiac replacement in the United States and at most about 2,500 transplantable hearts available, the areas of cardiac xenografting and permanent mechanical replacement deserve further investigation.

Selected Bibliography

Bolman, R. M., Elick, B., Olivari, M. T., et al: Improved immunosuppression for heart transplantation. J. Heart Transplant., 4:315, 1985.

Because of concern about the reported nephrotoxicity of the immune suppressant cyclosporine A, the authors embarked on a trial of triple-drug therapy. The regimen consisted of cyclosporine A, in lower doses than reported earlier, with azathioprine and prednisone. The article describes the initial results of this trial, which were quite good. This regimen has become standard for immunosuppression in many centers.

Gilbert, E. M., Krueger, S. K., Murray, J. L., et al: Echocardiographic evaluation of potential cardiac transplant donors. J. Thorac. Cardiovasc. Surg. 95:1003, 1988.

By use of echocardiography to evaluate ventricular function in potential heart donors, almost one-third of hearts that were unacceptable by conventional criteria were successfully recovered and transplanted. The authors describe methods for donor evaluation that have proved to be successful. At this time, when the number of donor organs available for transplantation is the critical factor that controls the number of transplants done, every method possible must be used to recover suitable organs.

Starzl, T. E., Hakala, T. R., Shaw, B. W., Jr., et al: A flexible procedure for multiple cadaveric organ procurement. Surg. Gynecol. Obstet., 158:223, 1984.

In this beautifully illustrated article the authors describe in detail a method commonly used for multiple-organ recovery. At present, recovery of multiple transplantable organs from one donor is the best way to provide as many organs as possible to the recipient pool, which is much larger than the donor pool.

Yacoub, M., Alivizatos, P., Hadley-Smith, R., et al: Cardiac transplantation. Are steroids really necessary? J. Am. Coll. Cardiol., 5:533, 1985.

In this incisive and provocative article, the authors challenge the conventional view that long-term maintenance corticosteroid therapy is necessary for survival after cardiac transplantation. Deletion of maintenance steroids from the immunosuppressive regimen would not only decrease the incidence of infectious complications but also make cardiac transplantation a more realistic option for a wider spectrum of patients (e.g., diabetics and children).

Bibliography

Addonizio, L. J., and Rose, E. A.: Cardiac transplantation in children and adolescents. J. Pediatr., 111:1034, 1987.
Andreone, P. A., Olivari, M. T., Elick, B., et al: Reduction of infectious complications following heart transplantation with triple-drug immunotherapy. J. Heart Transplant., 5:13, 1986.
Armitage, J., Hardesty, R., and Griffith, B.: Prostaglandin E₁: An effective treatment of right heart failure after orthotopic heart transplantation. J. Heart Transplant., 6:348, 1987.
Badellino, M., Nairns, B., Fucci, P., et al: Influence of diabetes mellitus on the course of cardiac transplantation (Abstract). J. Am. Coll. Cardiol., 11:103A, 1988.
Bailey, L., Concepcion, W., Shattuck, H., and Huang, L.: Method of heart transplantation for treatment of hypoplastic left heart syndrome. J. Thorac. Cardiovasc. Surg., 92:1, 1986.
Bailey, L. L., Jang, J., Johnson, W., and Jolley, W. B.: Orthotopic cardiac xenografting in the newborn goat. J. Thorac. Cardiovasc. Surg., 89:242, 1985.
Barnard, C. N.: The operation. S. Afr. Med. J., 41:1271, 1967.
Barnard, C. N., Barnard, M. S., Cooper, D. K. L., et al: The present status of heterotopic cardiac transplantation. J. Thorac. Cardiovasc. Surg., 81:433, 1981.
Bieber, C. P., Griepp, R. B., Oyer, P. E., et al: Use of rabbit antithymocyte globulin in cardiac transplantation: Relationship of serum clearance rates to clinical outcome. Transplant, 22:478, 1976.
Billingham, M. E.: Some recent advances in cardiac pathology. Hum. Pathol., 10:367, 1979.
Billingham, M. E.: Diagnosis of cardiac rejection by endomyocardial biopsy. J. Heart Transplant., 1:25, 1982.
Billingham, M. E.: Cardiac transplant atherosclerosis. Transplant. Proc., 19(Suppl. 5):19, 1987.
Bolman, R. M., Cance, C., Spray, T., et al: The changing face of cardiac transplantation: The Washington University Program, 1985–1987. Ann. Thorac. Surg., 45:192, 1988.
Bolman, R. M., Elick, B., Olivari, M. T., et al: Improved immunosuppression for heart transplantation. J. Heart Transplant., 4:315, 1985.
Bolman, R. M., III, Spray, T. L., Cox, J. L., et al: Heart transplantation in patients requiring preoperative mechanical support. J. Heart Transplant., 6:273, 1987.
Borel, J., Feurer, C., Gubler, H. U., and Stahelin, H.: Biological effects of cyclosporine A: A new lymphocytic agent. Agents Actions, 6:468, 1976.
Borel, J. F.: Cyclosporine: Historical perspectives. Transplant. Proc., 15(Suppl. 1):3, 1983.
Bristow, M. R., Gilbert, E. M., Renlund, D. G., et al: Use of OKT3 monoclonal antibody in cardiac transplantation: Review of the initial experience. J. Heart Transplant., 7:1, 1988.
Brodman, R. F., Veith, F. J., Goldsmith, J., et al: Multiple organ procurement from one donor. J. Heart Transplant., 4:254, 1985.
Calne, R. Y., Rolles, K., White, D. J. G., et al: Cyclosporine A in clinical organ grafting. Transplant. Proc., 13:349, 1981.
Calne, R. Y., White, D. J. G., Rolles, K., et al: Prolonged survival of pig orthotopic heart grafts treated with cyclosporine A. Lancet, 1:1183, 1978.
Cannon, D. S., Graham, A. F., and Harrison, D. C.: Electrophysiologic studies in the denervated transplanted human heart. Response to atrial pacing and atropine. Circ. Res., 32:268, 1973.
Carrel, A., and Guthrie, C. C.: The transplantation of veins and organs. Am. J. Med., 11:1101, 1905.
Carrier, M., Emery, R. W., Riley, J. E., et al: Cardiac transplantation in patients over 50 years of age. J. Am. Coll. Cardiol., 8:285, 1986.
Caves, P. K., Stinson, E. B., Billingham, M. E., and Shumway, N. E.: Percutaneous transvenous endomyocardial biopsy in human heart recipients. Ann. Thorac. Surg., 16:325, 1973.
Christopherson, L. K.: Cardiac transplantation: A psychological perspective. Circulation, 75:57, 1987.
Cohen, D. J., Loertscher, R., Rubin, M. F., et al: Cyclosporine: A new immunosuppressive agent for organ transplantation. Ann. Intern. Med., 101:667, 1984.
Conner, R., Hosenpud, J., Norman, D., et al: Recurrence of amyloidosis in a cardiac allograft (Abstract). J. Heart Transplant., 5:385, 1986.
Copeland, J. G., Emery, R. W., Levinson, M., et al: Selection of patients for cardiac transplantation. Circulation, 75:2, 1987.
Copeland, J. G., Jones, M., Spragg, R., and Stinson, E. B.: In vitro preservation of canine hearts for 24 to 48 hours followed by successful orthotopic transplantation. Ann. Surg., 178:687, 1973.
Demikov, V. P.: Experimental Transplantation of Vital Organs. New York, Consultants Bureau, 1962.
DeVries, W. C.: The permanent artificial heart. Four case reports. J.A.M.A., 259:847, 1988.
Emery, R. W., Cork, R. C., Levinson, M. M., et al: The cardiac donor. A six-year experience. Ann. Thorac. Surg., 41:356, 1986.
Evans, R. W., and Maier, A. M.: Outcome of patients referred for cardiac transplantation. J. Am. Coll. Cardiol., 8:1312, 1986.
Evans, R. W., Mannien, R. L., Garrison, L. P., and Maier, A. M.: Donor availability as the primary determinant of the future of heart transplantation. J.A.M.A., 255:1892, 1986.
Farrar, D. J., Hill, J. D., Gray, L. A., et al: Heterotopic prosthetic ventricles as a bridge to cardiac transplantation. N. Engl. J. Med., 318:333, 1988.
Frazier, O. H., Macris, M. P., Duncan, J. M., et al: Cardiac transplantation in patients over 60 years of age. Ann. Thorac. Surg., 45:129, 1988.
Fricker, F. J., Griffith, B. P., Hardesty, R. L., et al: Experience with heart transplantation in children. Pediatrics, 79:138, 1987.

Gao, S. Z., Johnson, D., Schroeder, J. S., et al: Transplant coronary artery disease: Histopathologic correlations with angiographic morphology (Abstract). J. Am. Coll. Cardiol, 11:153A, 1988.

Gay, W. A.: Cardiac transplantation—a surgical perspective. J. Cardiothorac. Anesth., 2:513, 1988.

Gilbert, E. M., Krueger, S. K., Murray, J. L., et al: Echocardiographic evaluation of potential cardiac transplant donors. J. Thorac. Cardiovasc. Surg., 95:1003, 1988.

Health Care Finance Administration (HCFA), Department of Health and Human Services Medicare Program: Criteria for Medicare coverage of heart transplants. Federal Register, 52:10935, 1987.

Hofflin, J. M., Potasman, I., Baldwin, J. C., et al: Infectious complications in heart transplant recipients receiving cyclosporine and corticosteroids. Ann. Intern. Med., 106:209, 1987.

Jamieson, S. W., Burton, N. A., Bieber, C. P., et al: Cardiac allograft survival in primates treated with cyclosporine A. Lancet, 1:545, 1979.

Kahan, B. D.: Immunosuppressive therapy with cyclosporine for cardiac transplantation. Circulation, 75:40, 1987.

Kaye, M. P.: The Registry of the International Society for Heart Transplantation. Fourth Official Report—1987. J. Heart Transplant., 6:63, 1987.

Kostakis, A. J., White, D. J. G., and Calne, R. Y.: Prolongation of rat heart allograft survival by cyclosporine A. I.R.C.S. Med. Sci., 5:280, 1977.

Lower, R. R., and Shumway, N. E.: Studies on orthotopic transplantation of the canine heart. Surg. Forum, 11:18, 1960.

Lower, R. R., Dong, E. J., and Shumway, N. E.: Long-term survival of cardiac homografts. Surgery, 58:110, 1965.

Magovern, G. J., Park, S. B., Magovern, G. J., Jr., et al: Mechanical circulatory assist devices. Texas Heart Inst. J., 14:276, 1987.

Mavroudis, C., Kline, J. B., Harrison, H. L., et al: Infant orthotopic heart transplantation. J. Thorac. Cardiovasc. Surg., 96:912, 1988.

O'Connell, J. B.: The role of myocarditis in end-stage dilated cardiomyopathy. Texas Heart Inst. J., 14:268, 1987.

O'Connell, J. B., and Gunnar, R. M.: Dilated-congestive cardiomyopathy: Prognostic features and therapy. J. Heart Transplant., 2:7, 1982.

O'Connell, J. B., Renlund, D. G., DeWitt, C. W., and Bristow, M. R.: Cardiac transplantation in sensitized recipients without a prospective crossmatch (Abstract). J. Heart Transplant., 7:74, 1988.

O'Connell, J. B., Renlund, D. G., Lee, H. R., et al: Newer techniques of immunosuppression in cardiac transplantation. In Emery, R. W., and Prizker, M. (eds): Cardiac Surgery: State of the Art Reviews. Philadelphia, Hanley and Belfus, 2:607, 1988.

O'Connell, J. B., Renlund, D. G., Robinson, J. A., et al: Effect of preoperative hemodynamic support on survival following cardiac transplantation. Circulation, 76(II):257, 1987.

Oyer, P. E., Stinson, E. B., Jamieson, S. W., et al: One year experience with cyclosporine A in clinical heart transplantation. Heart Transplant., 1:285, 1982.

Penn, I.: Cancers following cyclosporine therapy. Transplantation, 43:32, 1987.

Reemtsma, K.: The heart as a test organ in transplantation studies. Ann. N.Y. Acad. Sci., 120:778, 1964.

Reemtsma, K., Williamson, W. E., Jr., Iglesias, F., et al: Studies in homologous canine heart transplantation: Prolongation of survival with a folic acid antagonist. Surgery, 52:127, 1962.

Renlund, D. G., Bristow, M. R., Burton, N. A., et al: Survival following cardiac transplantation: What are acceptable standards? Western J. Med., 146:627, 1987a.

Renlund, D. G., Bristow, M. R., Crandall, B. G., et al: Hypercholesterolemia after cardiac transplantation: Amelioration by corticosteroid-free maintenance immunosuppression. J. Heart Transplant., 8:214, 1989.

Renlund, D. G., Bristow, M. R., Lee, H. R., and O'Connell, J. B.: Medical aspects of cardiac transplantation. J. Cardiothorac. Anesthesia, 2:500, 1988.

Renlund, D. G., Gilbert, E. M., O'Connell, J. B., et al: Age-associated decline in cardiac allograft rejection. Am. J. Med., 83:391, 1987.

Renlund, D. G., O'Connell, J. B., Gilbert, E. M., et al: Feasibility of discontinuation of corticosteroid maintenance therapy in heart transplantation. J. Heart Transplant., 6:71, 1987c.

Sadeghi, A. M., Robbins, R. C., Smith, C. R., et al: Cardiac xenotransplantation in primates. J. Thorac. Cardiovasc. Surg., 93:809, 1987.

Schwartz, R., Dameshek, N.: Drug-induced immunological tolerance. Nature, 183:1682, 1959.

Starzl, T. E., Hakala, T. R., Shaw, B. W., Jr., et al: A flexible procedure for multiple cadaveric organ procurement. Surg. Gynecol. Obstst., 158:223, 1984.

Stevenson, L. W., Fowler, M. B., Schroeder, J. S., et al: Poor survival of patients in idiopathic cardiomyopathy considered too well for transplantation. Am. J. Med., 83:871, 1987.

Thompson, M. E., Shapiro, A. P., Johnsen, S.-M., et al: The contrasting effects of cyclosporine A and azathioprine on arterial blood pressure and renal function following cardiac transplantation. Int. J. Cardiol., 11:219, 1986.

Weber, K. T., Janicki, J. S., and Jain, M. C.: Enoximone (MDL17,043), a phosphodiesterase inhibitor, in the treatment of advanced, unstable chronic heart failure. J. Heart Transplant., 6:105, 1986.

Wong, K. C., and Wu Lien-Teh: History of Chinese Medicine, 2nd ed. Shanghai, National Quarantine Service, 1936.

Yacoub, M., Alivizatos, P., Radley-Smith, R., et al: Cardiac transplantation: Are steroids really necessary? J. Am. Coll. Cardiol., 5:533, 1985.

Young, J. N., Yazbeck, J., Esposito, G., et al: The influence of acute preoperative pulmonary infarction on the results of heart transplantation. J. Heart Transplant., 5:20, 1986.

III LUNG TRANSPLANTATION

Joel D. Cooper

HISTORICAL ASPECTS

In the last two decades, transplantation of the kidney, liver, and heart has become clinically well established and has provided a therapeutic option for individuals with irreversible failure of these organs. Lung transplantation has been less progressive, notwithstanding considerable interest and research activity in this field for several decades. Several problems, unique to the lung, have impeded progress both experimentally and clinically. The lung is a very fragile organ with intimate approximation of the air spaces and the capillaries so that even a relatively minor insult can lead to significant malfunction. This malfunction can jeopardize the survival of the lung transplant recipient who depends on the immediate function of the organ. The systemic arterial supply to the lung, the fine network of bronchial vessels, is interrupted and is not restored at the time of transplantation, thus the bronchial anastomosis is rendered ischemic. The lung is exposed to the atmosphere, which increases the risk of infection, and this liability is all the greater with the immunosuppression necessary to prevent rejection.

Metras in France (1950) and Hardin and Kittle in the United States (1954) showed the technical feasibility of lung transplantation in canines and used a technique that has not changed substantially. Most experimental work has been conducted in dogs by using either a reimplantation model in which the lung is severed and reattached or allotransplantation, which is the implantation of a lung from another dog. Reimplantation eliminates factors that relate to rejection and provides an observatory period of those factors associated with the technical aspects of the procedure as well as the effects of lymphatic, neural, and bronchial artery interruption. Early experiments suggested that there was a significant increase in pulmonary vascular resistance in the transplanted organ. Subsequently, it was shown that with meticulous anastomotic technique for the pulmonary arterial and venous attachments, the vascular resistance of the transplanted organ was almost normal (Alican et al, 1971; Benfield and Coon, 1971; Daicoff et al, 1970; Vieth and Richards, 1969; Waldhausen et al, 1967). Similarly, it has become apparent that interruption of the lymphatic connections, the vagal nerves, and the bronchial arteries does not cause significant physiologic derangement. Progress in lung transplantation has been impeded partly by the lack of a suitable experimental model analogous to the clinical situation. With unilateral lung transplantation in the dog, the function of the remaining native lung is sufficient to sustain the animal, and physiologic malfunction of the transplanted lung may not be apparent. However, unilateral transplantation with immediate ligation of the contralateral pulmonary artery, or contralateral pneumonectomy, requires that the transplanted lung immediately accept the entire cardiac output that is not analogous to the clinical situation. This may lead to pulmonary edema in the immediate post-transplant period, especially if lung preservation is not optimal.

Early malfunction of a transplanted lung has often been attributed to the "reimplantation response." This response is attributed variably to the effects of lymphatic, neural, or bronchial artery interruption along with possible effects due to ischemia and reperfusion. With increased clinical experience, it has become evident that this response is not inevitable and likely occurs primarily from ischemic or reperfusion injury.

Accurate diagnosis of lung rejection is still elusive, and, in the absence of reliable diagnostic criteria, excessive immunosuppression may be used resulting in an increased risk of infectious complications. The combination of exposure to bacterial contamination from the atmosphere and ischemia of the donor airway due to interruption of the bronchial circulation, together with the use of immunosuppression, has not surprisingly, led to significant problems with pulmonary sepsis and poor healing of the airway anastomosis.

Finally, the effects of organ ischemia on posttransplant function have been difficult to identify because of numerous other factors that lead to posttransplant malfunction. Thus, the period of safe ischemic time, between extraction of the lung and restoration of circulation, has been difficult to ascertain.

In summary, early malfunction of the transplanted lung may be attributed to numerous ill-defined factors and this, together with the lack of a clinically relevant animal model, has contributed to the slow progress made with lung transplantation compared with other organ transplants.

HUMAN LUNG TRANSPLANTATION

In 1963, Hardy and co-workers reported the first human lung transplant. The recipient survived for 18 days and died of renal failure. This experience showed the technical feasibility of lung transplantation and stimulated worldwide interest in the field. During the next 20 years, approximately 40 lung or lobe transplants were done worldwide with little clinical success. Only one recipient survived long enough to be discharged from the hospital. This recipient was a 23-year-old man who had a right lung transplant for an advanced form of silicosis (Derom et al, 1971). The patient was discharged from the hospital 8 months after transplantation and died 2 months later from chronic rejection and pulmonary sepsis.

The report of a successful combined heart-lung transplant by the Stanford group in 1981 provided an important stimulus for further efforts in lung transplantation (Reitz et al, 1982). This report confirmed that an individual can function satisfactorily solely on transplanted lung tissue, which was suggested earlier by the 10-month survival of Derom's patient (1971). The combined heart-lung transplant was attempted initially by Cooley and associates (1969) and later by Lillehei (1970) and Barnard (Barnard and Cooper, 1981), all without success. By using the new immunosuppressant drug, cyclosporine, the Stanford group was able to achieve repeated clinical success with the heart-lung transplant procedure in patients with right-sided heart failure and pulmonary hypertension. The author's initial experience with unilateral lung transplantation was in 1978 when a right lung transplant was done in a ventilator-dependent patient who had inhalation burns (Nelems et al, 1980). The recipient died in the third week of disruption of the bronchial anastomosis. A review of world experience to that date showed that only nine patients had survived for more than 2 weeks after unilateral lung transplantation and that six of these nine patients, including the author's patient, died within the first month of bronchial anastomotic disruption. After this experience, a laboratory program to evaluate factors affecting bronchial anastomotic healing after lung transplantation was undertaken. The initial experiments involved canine lung autotransplantation with severing and immediate reattachment of the lung. Half of the animals received no postoperative immunosuppressants, whereas the other half received standard immunosuppression with azathioprine and prednisone. The animals that were treated showed significant bronchial anastomotic complications, including ischemia, necrosis, and disruption of the anastomosis, similar to complications reported earlier after human lung transplantation (Lima et al, 1981). The untreated animals showed primary healing of the bronchial anastomosis although narrowing of the bronchus distal to the anastomosis was a frequent occurrence, which was attributed to ischemia.

Later experiments showed that the adverse effect on bronchial healing in the immunosuppressed animals related entirely to the prednisone and that the use of azathioprine did not prejudice bronchial healing. Further experiments using cyclosporine rather than prednisone indicated that bronchial healing in these animals did not differ from untreated animals.

In an attempt to rapidly restore bronchial arterial blood supply after transplantation, a pedicle of omentum brought into the chest with its blood supply intact was used by the author and was wrapped around the bronchial anastomosis after its completion. These studies showed rapid restoration of bronchial blood supply by means of omental collaterals and resulted in improved anastomotic healing after transplantation (Dubois et al, 1984; Morgan et al, 1983).

ORGANIZATION OF A TRANSPLANT PROGRAM FOR END-STAGE LUNG DISEASE

Development of a program of transplantation for end-stage lung disease requires individuals with expertise in pulmonary medicine, pulmonary anesthesia, rehabilitation, physiotherapy, hematology, immunology, infectious disease, nutrition, intensive care, psychiatry, and nursing. The surgical team requires expertise in all aspects of pulmonary and airway operative procedures, respiratory care, and intensive care.

SELECTION OF RECIPIENTS FOR SINGLE LUNG TRANSPLANTATION

The author believes that patients with end-stage pulmonary fibrosis are the most ideal candidates for unilateral lung transplantation. The poor compliance and increased vascular resistance of the native lung ensures that both ventilation and perfusion are preferentially diverted to the transplanted lung. Patients with bilateral pulmonary sepsis, either acute or chronic, appear to be poorly suited for unilateral lung transplantation because the remaining infected lung would not only contaminate the transplanted lung but would also serve as a focus for systemic infection, especially after institution of immunosuppression. There has also been concern that unilateral transplantation for emphysema might not be ideal. The contralateral native lung may show hyperexpansion and air trapping resulting in a shift of the mediastinum and restriction of ventilation to the transplant. However, the author and others have recently had success with lung transplantation for emphysema, but long-term follow-up is lacking.

Because of the severe shortage of suitable donor lungs, it has been necessary to adopt slightly arbitrary guidelines for the selection of recipients. These guidelines are based on risk factors that may adversely affect success. Thus, the author has excluded individuals over 60 years of age, patients who depend on a ventilator, and individuals with hepatic or renal disease, insulin-dependent diabetes, or a history of previous malignancy.

Patients with end-stage pulmonary fibrosis are frequently treated with high-dose prednisone in an attempt to reduce the progression of the disease. Because of the experimental evidence indicating the adverse effects of routine prednisone administration in the early postoperative period, all transplant recipients are weaned entirely from steroids for at least 1 month before transplantation. Most patients with end-stage pulmonary fibrosis who need a transplant have inactive disease, and thus these patients can generally be weaned from steroids without adverse effect.

Attempts to identify recipients who are likely to die within 12 to 18 months have been made. These individuals usually depend on oxygen, show progressive deterioration of pulmonary function, and have increasing oxygen requirements. Noninvasive monitoring of oxygen saturation during a standardized exercise protocol has proved useful in documenting the progression of the disease.

Patients with end-stage pulmonary fibrosis generally have excellent respiratory muscle strength due to the chronic workload of ventilating the fibrotic lungs. These patients usually have a moderate degree of pulmonary hypertension, and cor pulmonale is not present. Right ventricular function is evaluated noninvasively by using echocardiography and nuclear angiography.

Prospective transplant recipients have psychological testing, and any recipients who have significant psychosocial problems are excluded because of the considerable stress that the preoperative assessment, long waiting period, and postoperative recovery impose. In addition, the need for strict patient compliance and cooperation is essential to ensure a satisfactory long-term result.

SELECTION OF DONORS

The lack of suitable lungs from donors is a major obstacle to more widespread application of lung transplantation and impedes progress that depends on a concentrated experience. Lungs are more difficult to obtain than other organs, due to the susceptibility of the lungs to infection and edema, especially in the presence of brain death. The author's requirements are that the donor chest film should be entirely clear; the arterial oxygen tension should exceed 300 mm Hg with 100% oxygen and 5 cm of positive end-expiratory pressure; and that bronchoscopy reveals no purulent secretions or suggestion of aspiration of gastric contents.

To minimize ischemic injury to the lung, initially only donors available in the author's hospital were used. With increased experience, this policy has been abandoned, and most lungs from donors are now removed from other centers and transported for implantation.

Vertical and transverse radiologic dimensions of the chest are used for appropriate size matching. Because lateral films are generally unavailable for the donor, the dimensions from the portable anterior-posterior film must be used. Accurate comparison with the intended recipient is thus not possible. Together with the radiologic dimensions, the body weight, height, and chest circumference of the donor and the recipient are compared in an attempt to assess the suitability of the match. Initially, the author sought a donor lung of approximately the same size as the recipient's chest but later realized it would be more appropriate to select a lung based on the predicted normal size for the height and weight of the recipient. The recipient's chest is contracted because of the fibrotic "shrunken" lungs and soon expands to a more normal configuration when a larger lung is inserted. The accommodation of the recipient's chest to a larger donor lung is facilitated if the left side is used for the transplantation. The left diaphragm readily distends and the mediastinum easily shifts toward the right (Fig. 57–22).

Lung transplantation can be done readily on either side, but for technical reasons the left side is preferred when possible. The right pulmonary veins enter the left atrium near the interatrial groove, which makes it slightly more difficult to place an atrial clamp proximal to the veins on this side. This maneuver is accomplished more easily on the left side. For the same anatomic reason, separate extraction of the donor's heart is easier when the left lung is used. A satisfactory cuff of left atrium can easily be left surrounding the pulmonary veins without jeopardizing the amount of atrial cuff remaining on the heart for cardiac transplantation. This can be accomplished with use of the right lung but is more difficult. If the recipient has had a major thoracotomy or pleurodesis on the left side, a right lung transplant is preferred.

Suitable donors are selected on the basis of ABO blood compatibility. Histocompatibility matching is

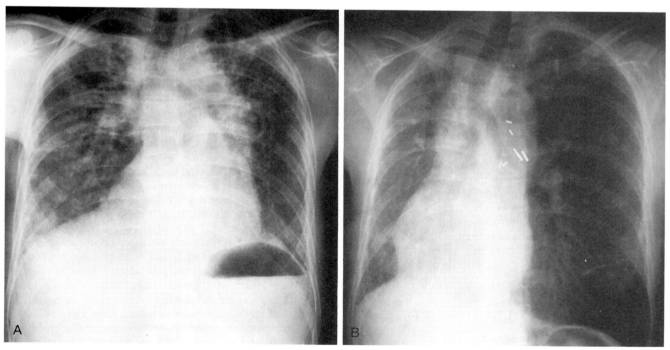

Figure 57–22. Preoperative (*A*) and postoperative (*B*) chest film from a patient who has had left lung transplant for end-stage pulmonary fibrosis. An oversized donor lung was used. The postoperative film, taken 2 months after the procedure, shows the diaphragmatic descent and mediastinal shift that allowed accommodation of the transplanted lung.

done only in retrospect because the effect of this matching is still uncertain and the delay in obtaining prospective cross-matching jeopardizes the use of lungs from many unstable donors.

PREPARATION OF THE DONOR

Currently, most lungs from donors are removed in conjunction with multiple organ removal for transplantation. A method for removing the heart for cardiac transplantation without jeopardizing the use of the lungs has been developed (Todd et al, 1988). The heart is removed before the lungs, leaving a small cuff of left atrium attached to the donor lung. The superior and inferior venae cavae, the ascending aorta, the common pulmonary artery, and the contralateral pulmonary veins are divided immediately after inflow occlusion and cardioplegic arrest. This leaves the heart attached only to the pulmonary veins of the donor lung. Careful division of the left atrium is then accomplished leaving an adequate cuff on the heart as well as surrounding the two pulmonary veins. This separate excision of the heart requires only a few minutes more than is ordinarily required for cardiac excision without the use of the lungs. After the heart is removed, the trachea is clamped or stapled at its mid-point and is divided. The lungs and most of the pericardium are extracted en bloc and are immersed in a bag containing 4°C Collins' solution. The bag is placed on ice for transportation. By using this simple technique, satisfactory results with ischemic periods of up to 5 hours have been obtained by the author. Other centers have used the technique of flushing the pulmonary circulation with a cold electrolyte solution or cooling the entire donor with the use of cardiopulmonary bypass. The author anticipates that flush techniques will be developed which are superior to simple immersion and which will extend the period of safe ischemia to up to 12 hours or longer. Limited success with these techniques in animals has been reported earlier from several centers (Haverich et al, 1985; Pinsker et al, 1981; Veith et al, 1976).

Just before implantation, the donor lung is trimmed from the specimen dividing the donor bronchus two rings proximal to the upper lobe takeoff and the pulmonary artery at its origin from the common pulmonary artery. The atrial cuff made at the time of cardiac extraction usually requires no revision. A large flap of pericardium is left attached to the hilum of the donor lung, which provides an alternate route for the development of collateral circulation to the lung.

RECIPIENT PROCEDURE

The lung transplant is done with the aid of one-lung anesthesia. Cardiopulmonary bypass is always available on a standby basis and has been required in approximately 25% of the author's patients. For left lung transplantation, a bronchus-blocking balloon (Fogerty No. 14 venous occlusion catheter) is positioned in the left main bronchus, and a standard endotracheal tube is inserted into the trachea. Subsequent inflation of the balloon permits ventilation of the right lung only. For right lung transplantation, a left-sided Robertshaw double-lumen tube is used.

The recipient procedure is initiated with the patient in the supine position. Through a small upper midline abdominal incision, the omentum is mobilized sufficiently to permit easy accessibility to the hilum of the lung, which generally requires only mobilization of the omentum from the transverse colon. A retrosternal tunnel is then created, and the apex of the omental pedicle is placed there for later withdrawal into the chest when thoracotomy is done. The abdomen is then closed. If a trial of one-lung anesthesia during this procedure indicates the need for cardiopulmonary bypass, the femoral vessels on the side of the transplant can be prepared at the same time as the omental dissection.

The patient is then placed in position for lateral thoracotomy, and the chest, abdomen, and ipsilateral groin area are prepared and draped. Alternatively, the patient can be placed in the position for thoracotomy with preparation of the omentum initially, followed by thoracotomy without the need to reposition and redrape. On entering the chest, the adhesions are divided and cautery is used as much as possible. The pulmonary artery is encircled intrapericardially. On the left side, the ligamentum arteriosum is divided to facilitate subsequent proximal clamping of the pulmonary artery. On the right side, exposure of the proximal pulmonary artery is facilitated by division of the azygous vein and forward retraction of the superior vena cava. The pulmonary artery is clamped temporarily to determine if the transplant procedure can be done without the need for bypass. This is possible if the blood pressure is stable, contralateral pulmonary pressure does not rise significantly, and arterial blood gases are satisfactory during the period of temporary pulmonary occlusion. The pulmonary clamp is removed after this trial. The pulmonary veins are isolated lateral to the pericardium, and the bronchus is mobilized just proximal to the upper lobe bronchus. Care is taken to avoid unnecessary dissection around the recipient main bronchus. After complete hilar mobilization, cardiopulmonary bypass is started if necessary; otherwise, the pulmonary clamp is replaced and the lungs are extracted. The first branch of the pulmonary artery is divided between ligatures and division of the pulmonary artery occurs just distal to this point providing additional length, as well as a slightly reduced caliber, especially if the recipient pulmonary artery is large. In addition, the divided first branch of the pulmonary artery helps to orient the pulmonary artery at the time of anastomosis to the donor pulmonary artery.

The two pulmonary veins are ligated extrapericardially and are divided between ligatures. The bronchus is divided just proximal to the upper lobe bronchus (Fig. 57–23).

After the recipient lung is removed, the pericardium is opened circumferentially around the stumps of the pulmonary veins and a Satinsky clamp is placed as centrally as possible on the left atrium without impinging on the contralateral pulmonary veins. On the right side, it may be necessary to dissect into the interatrial groove for a short distance to mobilize sufficient left atrium for satisfactory placement of a Satinsky clamp.

The previously placed ligatures on the pulmonary venous stumps are removed, and an incision is made between the two veins to create a suitable atrial cuff. This cuff is then made to match the size of the donor atrial cuff (Fig. 57–24).

The previously prepared donor lung is then positioned posteriorly in the chest. The atrial anastomosis is done first. The back wall is done from in front by using a continuous 3-0 polypropylene suture. The front wall of the atrial anastomosis is done similarly without the need to reposition or to handle the lung (Fig. 57–25*A*). The donor and recipient pulmonary arteries are then trimmed, if necessary, and the proper orientation is determined. This is facilitated by aligning the first branch of the recipient pulmonary artery and the first branch of the donor pulmonary artery to ensure that no rotation of the donor artery occurs. The back wall of the pulmonary anastomosis is done with a continuous 5-0 polypropylene suture. The anterior wall is then completed

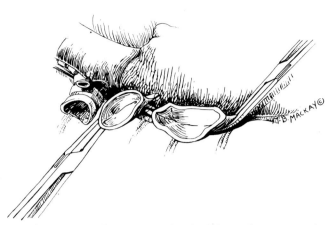

Figure 57–24. Preparation of right hilum of recipient. The stumps of the divided pulmonary veins are connected to make an atrial cuff.

in a similar manner, but the running suture is left untied at this point to permit subsequent flushing and back bleeding through the anastomosis (Fig. 57–25*B*).

Before removing the vascular clamps, the bronchial anastomosis is done with interrupted 4-0 absorbable sutures with the knots placed exteriorly as much as possible. On completion of the bronchial anastomosis, the left atrial clamp is gradually released. Back bleeding through the untied pulmonary artery suture line should occur within several minutes and may be helped by gentle inflation of the lung. When back bleeding has occurred, or after 3 to 5 minutes if no back bleeding has occurred, the pulmonary artery clamp is loosened momentarily to flush the pulmonary artery. The pulmonary artery suture line is then ligated; the pulmonary artery clamp is removed; and circulation is restored to the transplanted lung.

The omentum is retrieved from its retrosternal position, brought inferior to the hilum of the lung, and wrapped completely around the bronchus. The omentum is sutured to itself to avoid subsequent displacement (Fig. 57–26).

A free edge of the donor pericardium, which is left attached to the hilum of the lung, is sutured to the omentum. In animals, this procedure is associated with development of collateral circulation from the omentum through pericardial vessels to the bronchial circulation at the hilum of the lung.

Two chest tubes are placed, and the chest is closed in standard manner. The average blood loss for this procedure has been one unit of blood. Even when cardiopulmonary bypass is required, bleeding has not been a problem because complete dissection of the recipient lung can be done usually before the administration of heparin. The bronchial anastomosis is assessed endoscopically before termination of the procedure.

If temporary occlusion of the pulmonary artery, before excision of the recipient's lung, shows the

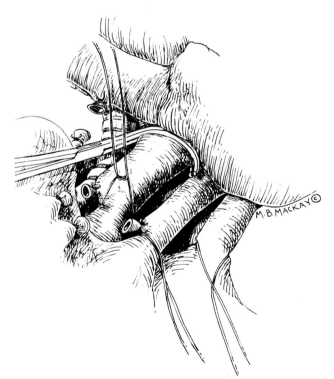

Figure 57–23. Preparation of recipient hilum for right lung transplant. The pulmonary artery is clamped as proximal as possible. The pulmonary veins are divided peripherally.

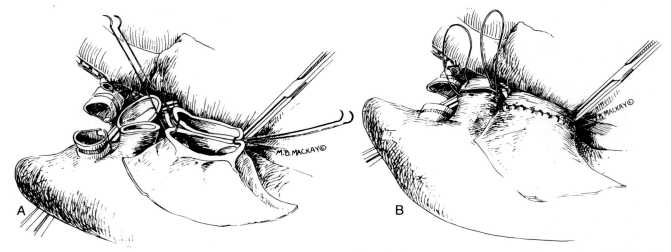

Figure 57–25. *A*, The posterior portion of the atrial anastomosis is done first by using a running monofilament suture. The anterior portion of the anstomosis is then completed. *B*, The pulmonary artery anastomosis is done with a running monofilament suture that is interrupted at the corners. The suture line is not tied until after the bronchial anastomosis has been completed, and the atrial clamp has been removed to permit backbleeding.

need for extracorporeal support, partial venoarterial bypass is begun through the femoral vessels. This procedure is initiated after the lung has been completely mobilized and continues until circulation is restored to the transplanted lung.

IMMUNOSUPPRESSION

As a result of laboratory studies showing the adverse effect of daily prednisone on bronchial healing, the author's initial immunosuppressive strategy is designed to avoid routine use of prednisone if possible. Cyclosporine and azathioprine are administered from the time of transplant, and antilymphocyte globulin is used for the first 7 to 14 days. During this time, suspected rejection episodes are treated with intravenous bolus doses of methylprednisone

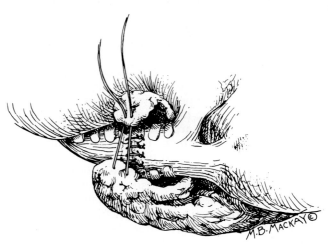

Figure 57–26. After completion of the bronchial anastomosis, the omentum is brought inferiorly and posteriorly to the hilum of the lung and is used to completely encircle the bronchus.

sodium succinate, 500 mg to 1 g intravenously for 3 successive days. At 2 to 3 weeks, if the thoracotomy wound is healing well and if bronchoscopy reveals a satisfactory bronchial anastomosis, oral prednisone is begun in a dose of 0.5 mg/kg/day. After that time, maintenance immunosuppression is done with cyclosporine, azathioprine, and prednisone. At 3 months after transplant, the dose of prednisone is gradually tapered to a dose of 15 mg on alternate days.

DIAGNOSIS OF REJECTION

The diagnosis of rejection remains imprecise and is based on a combination of suggestive signs and symptoms including deterioration in arterial oxygenation, pyrexia, decreased exercise tolerance, or decreased oxygen saturation with exercise, increased fatigue, development of a radiologic infiltrate or hilar flare, together with the absence of any alternative cause of deterioration, such as fluid overload or infection. Sequential quantitative lung perfusion scans have helped with the diagnosis of rejection. A relative decrease in perfusion to the transplanted lung has frequently been observed in association with rejection episodes and reverses within hours after a bolus of steroid.

The single most useful diagnostic measure in diagnosing rejection is the response to a pulse dose of intravenous methylprednisolone. Improvement in oxygenation, reduction in temperature, improvement in exercise tolerance, and sense of well-being occur within hours. Radiologic alterations, if present, generally improve during a 12- to 24-hour period. Similarly, improvement in the quantitative perfusion scan is usually apparent within 24 hours.

Most recipients have had two or three significant rejection episodes in the first 3 weeks. The first episode commonly occurs at 5 days, but may occur as early as 48 hours after transplant. Almost all episodes of acute rejection occur within the first 6 weeks. Chronic rejection, however, has developed in some patients within the first year. The author has not recognized the development of obliterative bronchiolitis to date after single lung transplant.

The function of the transplanted lung improves gradually during the initial 3 weeks, and this improvement is paralleled by the increase in perfusion to the transplanted lung. At 7 days, perfusion of the transplanted lung has ranged from 47 to 87% of the total pulmonary flow and likely depends on the status of the transplanted lung and on the pulmonary vascular resistance in the native lung. In some recipients, flow to the transplanted lung has been over 80% of the total when first measured 3 days after transplantation, which indicates the ability of the transplanted lung to accept most of the cardiac output without adverse effect. At 3 weeks, perfusion to the transplanted lung has ranged between 64 and 90% with a mean of 72%. A further increase in the relative perfusion of the transplanted lung occurs during the ensuing weeks.

Long-term function of the transplanted lung has generally been excellent with little or no deterioration for follow-up periods exceeding 4 years (Cooper et al, 1989).

PHYSICAL REHABILITATION

Patients with end-stage fibrotic lung disease and oxygen dependency have very limited physical reserve and tend to desaturate quickly with exercise. This leads to a sedentary existence that results in further progressive deterioration of muscular strength. A program of graded exercise and muscular training should begin before operation and includes treadmill walking, cycling, and weight training, all with careful monitoring of pulse and oxygen saturation. This monitoring ensures that the patients are exercising within safe limits and that adequate oxygen flows are being administered. The author has observed a significant improvement in exercise performance preoperatively in patients who have this rehabilitation, and this is reflected in an accelerated postoperative recovery. An active exercise program is started generally 3 to 4 weeks after transplantation and is maintained for a minimum of 3 months. Improvement in overall performance continues for 6 to 12 months, and most recipients are able to return to their regular employment 4 to 6 months after transplantation.

The 6-minute walk test is a convenient index of overall performance both preoperatively and postoperatively. For this test, the patients are instructed to walk as quickly and comfortably as possible on a level course for 6 minutes. The patients are allowed to rest if necessary, and oxygen administration, preoperatively, is administered with a light-weight portable tank. The frequency of rests, the total distance

covered, and the pre-effort and post-effort pulse and respiratory rate are recorded. In the author's experience, the mean distance covered in the 6-minute walk test has increased from 346 m preoperatively (with oxygen administration) to 462 m at 1 month (room air) and 649 m at 3 months (room air) post-transplant.

BRONCHIAL HEALING

No patient has died as a result of complications of bronchial anastomotic healing. Primary healing has occurred in most cases; two patients have developed partial necrosis of the donor bronchus, possibly related to numerous pulse doses of steroids for rejection episodes. In both cases, a late bronchostenosis developed and required treatment with dilatation after implantation of a silicone stent.

DOUBLE LUNG TRANSPLANTATION

Initially the single lung program has been restricted to patients with fibrotic lung disease. For patients with bilateral sepsis, such as cystic fibrosis, single lung transplantation would lead to contamination of the transplant lung from the remaining native lung. For chronic obstructive lung disease, unilateral lung transplantation might be followed by further expansion of the opposite emphysematous lung with crowding and restricted ventilation of the transplanted lung. Theoretically, unilateral lung transplantation and excision of the contralateral lung would address these problems, but would be associated with a high operative and perioperative risk. The author has chosen instead to develop a procedure for simultaneous en-bloc bilateral pulmonary transplantation, a procedure analogous to the combined heart-lung transplant, without the need to transplant the heart. The concept of simultaneous en-bloc bilateral pulmonary transplant was shown in dogs by Vanderhoeft and co-workers (1972). That procedure, however, done through a right thoracotomy, is not suitable for clinical use. The technique that the author has employed utilizes a median sternotomy, bilateral pneumonectomy, and implantation of the double-lung bloc with three anastomoses, namely the trachea, the common pulmonary artery, and a cuff of donor left atrium containing the pulmonary veins (Dark et al, 1986; Patterson et al, 1988; Toronto Lung Transplant Group, 1988).

TECHNIQUE OF OPERATION

The extraction technique for double-lung transplant, like that for single lung transplant, generally includes initial removal of the heart for separate transplantation followed by removal of the double-lung bloc (Todd et al, 1988). Before the heart is extracted, dissection of the interatrial groove is useful to provide extra margin between the right pulmonary veins and the attachment of the right and left atria. After in-flow occlusion and cardioplegia, the superior and inferior venae cavae are divided and the superior vena cava is completely dissected free from the right pulmonary artery, down to the point where the vena cava joins the right atrium. The aorta is divided in the usual manner, and the common pulmonary artery is divided midway between the pulmonic valve and the pulmonary artery bifurcation. Beginning at a point between the left pulmonary veins and the coronary sinus, a left atriotomy is made and extended carefully so as to leave a cuff of left atrium surrounding the four pulmonary veins while maintaining an adequate margin of left atrium on the heart for cardiac transplantation. After the heart has been extracted, the trachea is stapled at its mid-point and the two lungs are removed from the chest en bloc and immersed in cold Collins' solution for preservation (Fig. 57–27).

The recipient procedure is done through a median sternotomy with the incision extended into the upper abdomen. The omentum is mobilized for subsequent use, and a small diaphragmatic window is created several centimeters anterior to the esophageal hiatus through which the omentum is later passed into the posterior mediastinum (Fig. 57–28).

Before institution of cardiopulmonary bypass, the aorta and pulmonary artery are encircled, the venae cavae are isolated, the right pulmonary artery is isolated between the vena cava and the aorta, and pleural adhesions are dissected free as much as possible with the use of cautery.

Cardiopulmonary bypass is started by using double caval cannulation through the right atrium. From this point on, the procedure is conducted with the use of cardiopulmonary bypass, but the aorta is

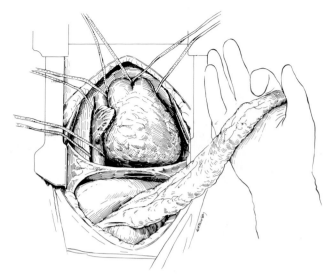

Figure 57–28. For a double lung transplant, the sternotomy incision is extended into the upper abdomen for mobilization of the omentum. An opening is made in the midportion of the diaphragm for subsequent passage of the omentum into the posterior mediastinum.

not cross-clamped and the heart remains beating. The left pulmonary veins are stapled inside the pericardium, (Fig. 57–29), the left pulmonary artery is similarly stapled, and the left lung is excised within the left pleura, dividing the left main bronchus between staple lines (Fig. 57–30). The right pulmonary veins and pulmonary artery are then stapled within the mediastinum (Fig. 57–31) after which a right pneumonectomy is done through the pleural space. The right main bronchus is divided between staple lines (Fig. 57–32). The distal trachea and both bronchial stumps are then dissected free. This procedure can be done either through the right pleural space or through the mediastinum (Fig. 57–33).

The posterior pericardial attachments around the transverse sinus are divided so that a hand can be passed freely from below, behind the heart up to the superior mediastinum, anterior to the esophagus. Pleural pericardial windows are created by enlarging the openings through which the pulmonary veins entered the pericardium (Fig. 57–34). The omentum is passed through the previous fenestration in the diaphragm and behind the heart to the superior mediastinum (Fig. 57–35). The donor trachea, which is left as long as a handle, is similarly passed behind the heart and is withdrawn into the superior mediastinum between the aorta and the superior vena cava. An umbilical tape, sutured to the trachea, facilitates this maneuver (Fig. 57–36). Each lung is directed through the appropriate pleural pericardial window into the pleural spaces. The recipient trachea is divided two rings above the carina, and the carina and main bronchial stumps are excised. The donor trachea is divided again two rings above the carina, and an end-to-end tracheal anastomosis is constructed between the donor and recipient by using

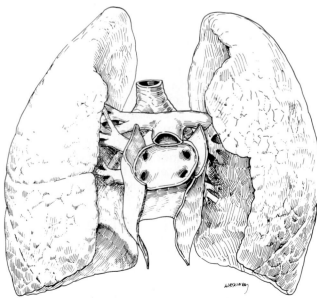

Figure 57–27. Double lung graft showing the two lungs together with the trachea, common pulmonary artery, and back wall of the left atrium containing the four pulmonary veins.

Text continued on page 1963

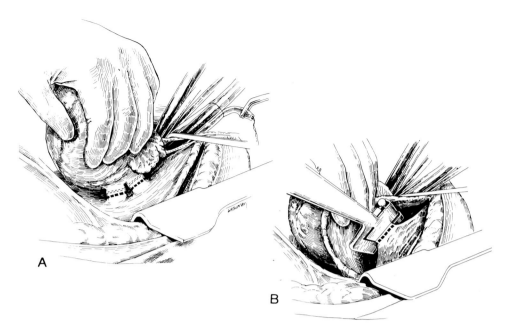

Figure 57–29. After institution of cardiopulmonary bypass, the left lung is removed. The pulmonary veins are stapled intrapericardially (*A*) and the pulmonary artery is stapled either extrapericardially (*B*) or intrapericardially.

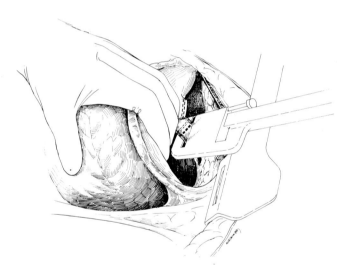

Figure 57–30. The left main bronchus is divided between staple lines to avoid contamination. The left lung is then removed from the chest.

Figure 57–31. The right pulmonary artery is stapled in the mediastinum between the superior vena cava and the aorta. It is later divided lateral to the pericardium. The pulmonary veins are stapled within the pericardium and divided lateral to the staple lines.

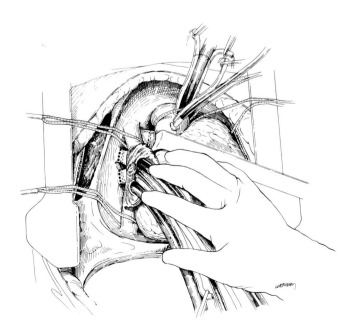

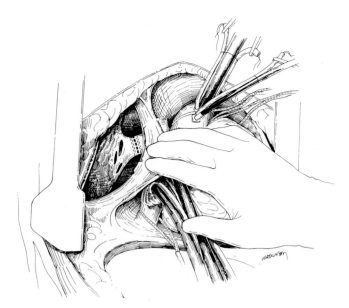

Figure 57–32. The right main bronchus is divided between staple lines after which the right lung is removed.

Figure 57–33. The right bronchial stump is grasped with a clamp and pulled into the right pleural space. The right and left bronchi and carina are dissected free, taking great care to ensure that the bronchial vessels are adequately secured. After the dissection the airway retracts back into the mediastinum where it is subsequently divided just above the carina for the tracheal anastomosis.

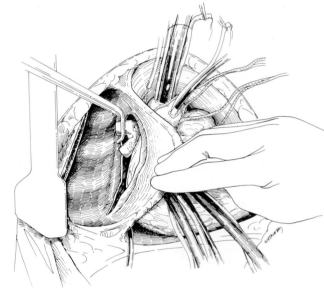

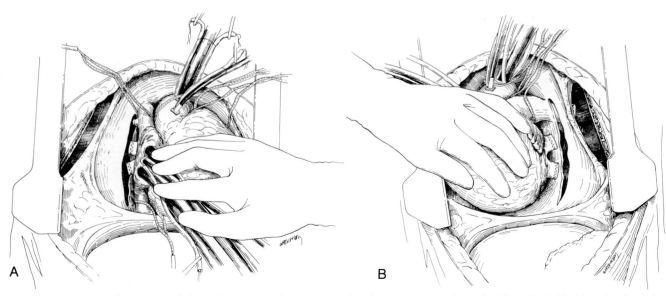

A

B

Figure 57–34. A pleuropericardial window is created posterior to the phrenic nerve on the right (*A*) and left (*B*) sides. On the right the azygous vein can be divided to allow maximal enlargement of the window.

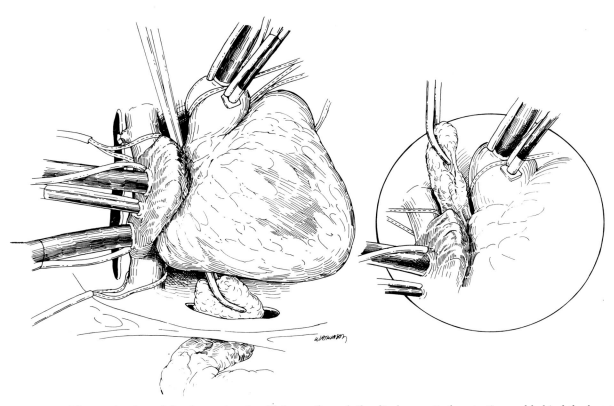

Figure 57–35. The previously mobilized omentum is withdrawn through the diaphragmatic fenestration and behind the heart into the superior mediastinum before insertion of the double lung bloc.

Figure 57–36. With the apex of the heart elevated, the double lung bloc is inserted into the posterior mediastinum and each lung is directed through its respective pleuropericardial windows into the pleural space. An umbilical tape (not shown here) attached to the trachea facilitates withdrawal of the trachea into the superior mediastinum after the lungs have been properly positioned.

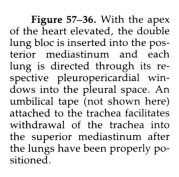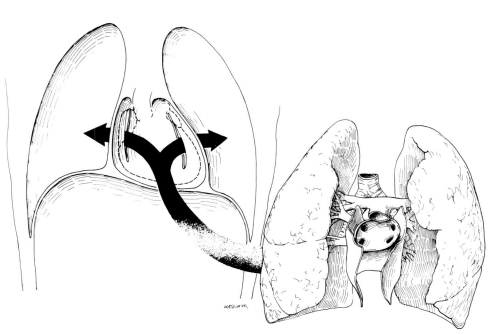

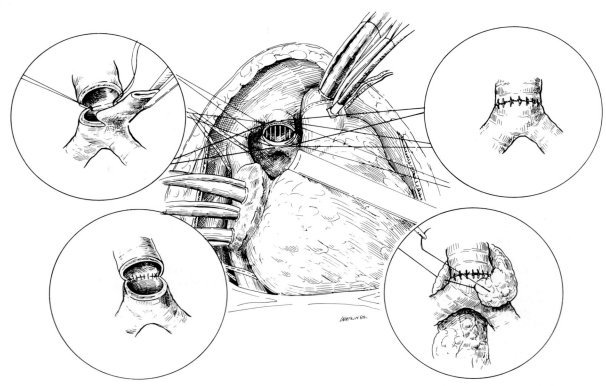

Figure 57–37. The recipient trachea is divided just above the carina with removal of the carina and proximal bronchial stumps. The donor trachea is divided just above the carina (*upper left*) and the posterior portion of the tracheal anastomosis is done with a running monofilament suture (*lower left*). The cartilaginous portion of the tracheal anastomosis is done with interrupted absorbable sutures (*upper right*), after which the omentum is securely wrapped completely around the tracheal anastomosis (*lower right*).

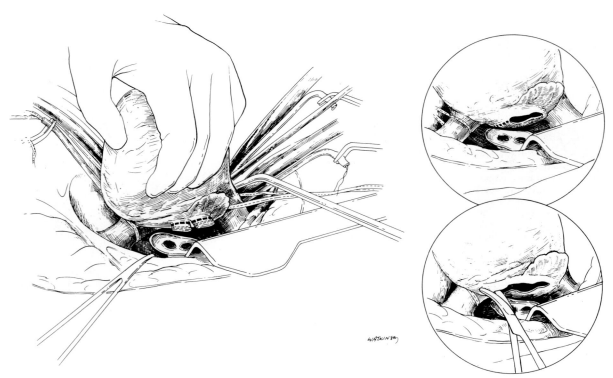

Figure 57–38. With the apex of the heart elevated, an opening is created in the back of the left atrium. Initially the stumps of the left pulmonary veins are excised (*upper right*) and the opening in the atrium is extended by incision of the back wall of the atrium transversely (*lower right*). Further enlargement can be obtained by incision in the atrial appendage, if necessary.

running monofilament for the membranous trachea and interrupted absorbable sutures for the cartilaginous portion (Fig. 57–37).

At this point, the aorta is cross-clamped and cardioplegia solution is delivered through the aortic root to arrest the heart. Up to this point, coronary sinus blood has been drained through the caval cannulas, with the tourniquets around the cavae left loose. In addition, a right ventricular drain, placed through the right atrium can be used. After cardioplegic arrest, the right ventricular drain is no longer required, and the caval tourniquets can be secured. The apex of the heart is elevated and rotated toward the right, exposing the back of the recipient left atrium. The stumps of the left pulmonary veins are excised creating a left atriotomy (Fig. 57–38), which is extended by division of the back wall of the left atrium toward the right pulmonary veins and creates a left atrial cuff that is anastomosed to the donor cuff with running monofilament suture (Fig. 57–39). The heart is returned to its normal position. The recipient pulmonary artery is transected proximal to the bifurcation, and an end-to-end pulmonary artery anastomosis is constructed between the donor and recipient pulmonary arteries (Fig. 57–40). Thus, the transplant procedure is completed.

This operation has been used in nine patients—seven patients with obstructive lung disease; one patient with primary pulmonary hypertension; and

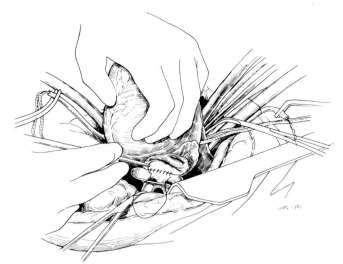

Figure 57–39. The donor atrial cuff is anastomosed to the back of the left atrium by using a running monofilament suture.

one patient with cystic fibrosis. Eight of these patients, including the patient with cystic fibrosis, did well for periods of up to 18 months (Cooper et al, 1989). The patient with primary pulmonary hypertension showed immediate improvement of right ventricular function but died as a result of ischemic necrosis of the airway. Two other patients developed

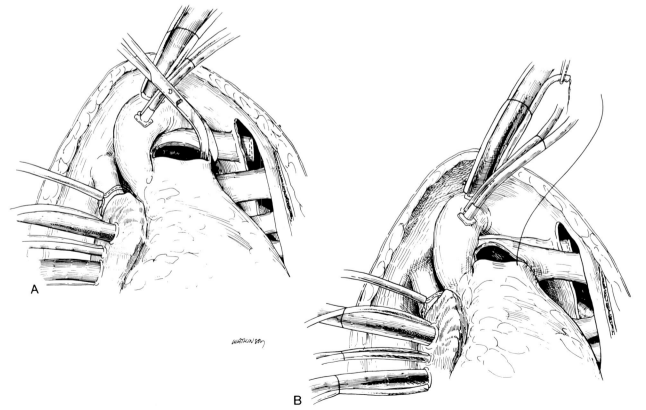

Figure 57–40. The common pulmonary artery of the recipient is transected several centimeters above the pulmonic valve (A). It is not necessary to excise the distal portion of the common pulmonary artery or the right and left pulmonary artery stumps. An end-to-end anastomosis is created between the donor and the recipient pulmonary arteries (B).

late airway complications, presumably as a result of ischemia, but are clinically well after dilatation and insertion of a silicone rubber stent. Retrograde collateral flow in the bronchial arteries from the pulmonary circulation is more tenuous at the tracheal level than at the bronchial level used for single lung transplant, and thus ischemic airway problems were anticipated. The omental wrap has been used for all double-lung transplants and has prevented gross disruption, or the formation of an abscess or fistula, when primary airway healing has not occurred. A technique for directly restoring bronchial artery flow to the trachea is currently being developed. Bilateral bronchial anastomoses rather than tracheal anastomosis has also been used by the author and others with success.

SUMMARY

Transplantation for end-stage lung disease is still at an early stage, but recent success suggests that transplantation for end-stage interstitial lung disease can achieve the same degree of success shown with other organ transplantation. Many problems must still be solved and include improved methods of immunosuppression, the ability to accurately diagnose rejection, and the need to secure more transplantable lungs from the available donors. This will require improved means for donor maintenance, to avoid deterioration of the lung both before and after declaration of brain death, and the ability to preserve lungs for 12 hours or more to allow transportation of suitable lungs from greater distances.

The author prefers the use of single lung transplantation for pulmonary fibrosis; double lung transplantation for patients with emphysema or cystic fibrosis when right ventricular function is preserved; and combined heart-lung transplantation for individuals who have a combination of pulmonary hypertension and irreversible right-sided heart failure. It is anticipated that single-lung or double-lung transplantation may also be appropriate for individuals with primary pulmonary hypertension before the occurrence of irreversible right-sided heart failure and tricuspid regurgitation. Methods for successfully applying unilateral transplant for emphysema have been developed recently.

Success with lung transplantation has been achieved because of the experimental and clinical contributions of numerous investigators during a 40-year period. The demonstration of clinical success with the various types of lung transplantation should provide additional stimulus for rapid advances in the future.

Bibliography

Alican, F., Cayirli, M., Isin, E., and Hardy, J. D.: Left lung replantation with immediate pulmonary artery ligation. Ann. Surg., 174:34, 1971.

Barnard, C. N., and Cooper, D. K. C.: Clinical transplantation of the heart: A review of 13 years' personal experience. J.R. Soc. Med., 74:670, 1981.

Benfield, J. R., and Coon, R.: The role of the left atrial anastomosis in pulmonary replantation. J. Thorac. Cardiovasc. Surg., 61:847, 1971.

Cooley, D. A., Bloodwell, R. D., Hallman, G. L., et al: Organ transplantation for advanced cardiopulmonary disease. Ann. Thorac. Surg., 8:30, 1969.

Cooper, J. D., Patterson, G. A., Grosman, R., and the Toronto Transplant Group: Double lung transplant for advanced chronic lung disease. Am. Rev. Resp. Dis., 139:303, 1989.

Daicoff, G. R., Allen, P. D., and Streck, C. J.: Pulmonary vascular resistance following lung reimplantation and transplantation. Ann. Thorac. Surg., 9:569, 1970.

Dark, J. H., Patterson, G. A., Al-Jilaihawi, A. N., et al: Experimental en bloc double-lung transplantation. Ann. Thorac. Surg., 42:394, 1986.

Derom, F., Barbier, F., Ringoir, S., et al: Ten month survival after lung homotransplantation in man. J. Thorac. Cardiovasc. Surg., 61:835, 1971.

Dubois, P., Choiniere, L., and Cooper, J. D.: Bronchial omentopexy in canine lung allotransplantation. Ann. Thorac. Surg., 38:211, 1984.

Goldberg, M., Lima, O., Morgan, E., et al: A comparison between cyclosporin A and methylprednisolone plus azathioprine on bronchial healing following canine lung allotransplantation. J. Thorac. Cardiovasc. Surg., 85:821, 1983.

Hardin, C. A., and Kittle, C. F.: Experiences with transplantation of the lung. Science, 119:97, 1954.

Hardy, J. D., Webb, W. R., Dalton, M. L., and Walker, G. R.: Lung homotransplantation in man. J.A.M.A., 186:1065, 1963.

Haverich, A., Scott, W. C., and Jamieson, S. W.: Twenty years of lung preservation—a review. Heart Trans., 4:234, 1985.

Lillehei, C. W.: Discussion of Wildevuur, C. R. H., and Benfield, J. R.: A review of 23 human lung transplantations by 20 surgeons. Ann. Thorac. Surg., 9:489, 1970.

Lima, O., Cooper, J. D., Peters, W. J., et al: Effects of methylprednisolone and azathioprine on bronchial healing following lung autotransplantation. J. Thorac. Cardiovasc. Surg., 82:211, 1981.

Metras, H.: Note preliminaire sur la graffe totale du poumon chéz le chien. Fr. Acad. Sci., Oct. 30, 1950, p. 1176.

Morgan, W. E., Lima, O., Goldberg, M., et al: Improved bronchial healing in canine left lung reimplantation using omental pedicle wrap. J. Thorac. Cardiovasc. Surg., 85:139, 1983.

Nelems, J. M., Rebuck, A. S., Cooper, J. D., et al: Human lung transplantation. Chest, 78:569, 1980.

Patterson, G. A., Cooper, J. D., Goldman, B., et al: Technique of successful clinical double lung transplantation. Ann. Thorac. Surg., 45:626, 1988.

Pinsker, K. L., Kamholz, S. L., Montefusco, C., et al: Long-term functional adequacy of canine lung autografts after 24 hour preservation. Transplant. Proc., 13:715, 1981.

Reitz, B. A., Wallwork, J. L., Hunt, S. A., et al: Heart-lung transplantation: Successful therapy for patients with pulmonary vascular disease. N. Engl. J. Med., 3067:557, 1982.

Todd, T. R., Goldberg, M., Koshal, A., et al: Separate extraction of cardiac and pulmonary grafts from a single organ donor. Ann. Thorac. Surg., 46:356, 1988.

Vanderhoeft, P., Dubois, A., Lauvan, N., et al: Block allotransplantation of both lungs with pulmonary trunk and left atrium in dogs. Thorax, 278:415, 1972.

Veith, F. J., Crane, R., Torres, M., et al: Effective preservation and transportation of lung transplants. J. Thorac. Cardiovasc. Surg., 72:97, 1976.

Veith, F. J., and Richards, K.: Lung transplantation with simultaneous contralateral pulmonary artery ligation. Surg. Gynecol. Obstet., 129:768, 1969.

Waldhausen, J. A., Daly, W. J., Baez, M., and Giammona, S. T.: Physiologic changes associated with autotransplantation of the lung. Ann. Surg., 165:580, 1967.

CHAPTER 58

THE ARTIFICIAL HEART

William S. Pierce

HISTORICAL ASPECTS

Having developed the first successful artificial kidney in the early 1940s, Kolff, Professor of Research Surgery at the Cleveland Clinic, directed attention to the development of an artificial heart. In 1958, 5 years after the successful clinical use of the heart-lung machine for open heart operations, Akutsu and Kolff (1958) reported that two compact vinyl pumps, powered by an external air compressor, had been used to replace the function of the canine heart for a short period. Various ingenious pump designs were later evaluated (Akutsu et al, 1960; Pierce et al, 1965), but problems related to abnormal physiology, thrombus formation, and device failure precluded animal survival for more than a few hours. With additional experience, investigators found that the air-powered pumps appeared to be the easiest to control and the calf, with its large chest size and docile nature, was the optimal animal model (Nosé et al, 1965). One decade after the initial studies from Kolff's laboratory, the calf's survival for 3 to 5 days was reported (Klain et al, 1971). This feat, which earlier had seemed impossible, served as a source of further encouragement to investigators. Attention was focused on improved pump designs, use of biocompatible materials for device fabrication, and the construction of more reliable power consoles. Annual progress was made and, by 1975, calves that appeared normal with implanted, pneumatically powered artificial hearts were maintained. The calves were able to stand, eat, and do limited treadmill exercise (Honda et al, 1975; Lawson et al, 1975). The longest reported survival time was 100 days and since then it has gradually increased to 357 days (Pierce, 1986).

In 1969 (Cooley et al, 1969), and again in 1981 (Cooley, 1982), pneumatic artificial hearts were used to support the circulation of patients whose hearts had been removed for 39 and 64 hours, respectively, while suitable donor hearts were identified. In both cases, heart transplantation was done, but neither patient survived. Clearly, both the artificial hearts and the transplant techniques needed improvement. However, an important concept was proved: That a pneumatic artificial heart could provide adequate circulatory support to a critically ill patient awaiting a compatible donor (Pennock et al, 1982a). The use of the artificial heart in these cases is referred to as a "bridge" to transplant. Important refinements have been made in artificial hearts and in cardiac transplantation techniques since then (Pennock et al, 1982b), and reasonable clinical results have been achieved by using the artificial heart as a "bridge" in critically ill patients.

In 1983, DeVries and associates, working in Kolff's laboratory at the University of Utah, believed that the pneumatic artificial heart had been developed to a level that could benefit patients with end-stage heart disease when all other conventional methods of treatment had been exhausted. In a historic operation done on December 2, 1982, in a 61-year-old dentist with end-stage cardiac disease (DeVries et al, 1984), Dr. Clark received a pneumatic artificial heart that was designed at the University of Utah and was referred to as a Jarvik 7, named for Robert Jarvik, a co-investigator in Kolff's laboratory. Although the patient's postoperative course was characterized by multiple complications, his condition gradually improved so that he could eat, talk with his family, and walk a few steps with the attached bulky pneumatic power unit. After 112 days he died of multiple-systems failure. DeVries (1988) later implanted three Jarvik 7 hearts as permanent replacement at the Humana Heart Institute International with the survival of patients for almost 2 years. Problems of stroke and infection in addition to the cumbersome percutaneous pneumatic tubes and the external power unit, however, have detracted from the advisability of continuing to replace hearts with the currently available pneumatic prostheses.

PNEUMATIC ARTIFICIAL HEART

System Components

The pneumatic artificial hearts being evaluated now use a pneumatic pressure console, positioned external to the patient, to generate pulses of air or

1965

carbon dioxide that are transmitted by flexible tubing across the chest wall to energize the implanted blood pumps (Atsumi et al, 1981; Bücherl et al, 1985; Hughes et al, 1985; Jarvik et al, 1978; Pierce et al, 1981) (Fig. 58–1). These pumps are modified diaphragm pumps that have rigid outer housings and a flexible inner, or blood contacting, bladder (Fig. 58–2). Internal tilting disk valves similar to those used for heart valve replacement ensure unidirectional blood flow. The internal design of the blood pump is crucial to minimizing hemolysis and preventing thromboemboli. In most blood pumps that are being developed, the blood pump bladder is made of flawlessly smooth surfaced, seam-free segmented polyurethane (Boretos and Pierce, 1967). This elastomeric material provides an excellent flexion life and reasonably good thrombus resistance, if attention has been paid to bladder design. Bladder discontinuities must be minimized and adequate surface shear rates must be obtained to minimize the evacuation of blood from the ventricles. The left and right pumps are separate entities and have detachable atrial and arterial suture cuffs to facilitate implantation.

A pneumatic power console activates the artificial heart by providing timed pulses of gas that compress the bladder and alternately apply gentle

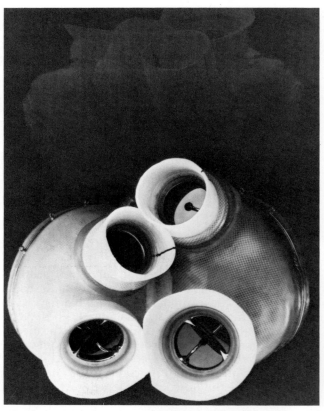

Figure 58–2. The Jarvik 7 artificial heart. The prosthetic left ventricle (*left side of photograph*) has a mitral valve (*lower*) and aortic valve (*upper*). The prosthetic right ventricle (*right side of photograph*) has a tricuspid inlet valve (*lower*) and a pulmonary valve (*upper*). The valves are of the tilting disk Hall-Medtronic type. The air ports are not seen in this view. (Photograph courtesy of Symbion, Inc.)

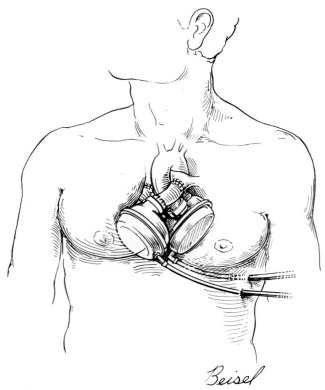

Figure 58–1. The pneumatic artificial heart as it is used in clinical application. The ventricles are implanted within the pericardial sac. A separate power line transmits the pressure and vacuum pulses to actuate each ventricle. (From Gaines, W. E., Donachy, J. H., Rosenberg, G., et al: Studies leading to an artificial heart for clinical application. Contemp. Surg., 24:41, 1984.)

suction to aid in filling the pump (Ross et al, 1972) (Fig. 58–3). The output of the power console is attached to each ventricle of the artificial heart through 2-m to 3-m flexible tubes that traverse the skin. The power unit provides a controlled systolic pressure of 120 to 250 mm Hg for a preset time, and a diastolic vacuum of 0 to −50 mm Hg for a preset time. In some designs, the pumping frequency and ratio between systolic and diastolic times can be preset. As investigators (Coleman et al, 1972; Rosenberg et al, 1978) have gained experience with this system, they have recognized the importance of monitoring left drive unit pressure or gas flow (Fig. 58–4). Complete pump emptying and filling can be detected by the contour of tracings from the air lines. Moreover, abnormal conditions, such as inlet restriction, outlet obstruction, and valve malfunction can be detected (Fig. 58–5). The Utah group (Nielson et al, 1983) developed a microcomputerized cardiac output monitor and diagnostic unit (COMDU) to help to assess pump function based on left air-line flow.

High reliability of the pneumatic power console has been a primary consideration in design. Consoles incorporate a number of safety systems that include

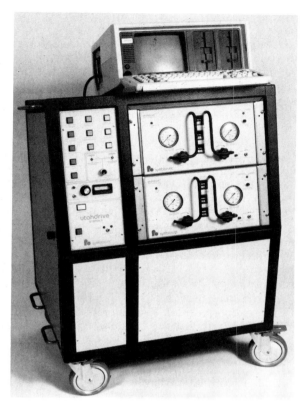

Figure 58–3. The power unit designed for the Jarvik 7 artificial heart provides a separate air pulse for the right and left ventricle. The right side of the console has controls for systolic pressure, diastolic vacuum, and time for each phase that can be set independently for each ventricle. The left side of the console has a monitoring function. The unit contains an emergency power supply and an alarm system. (Photograph courtesy of Symbion, Inc.)

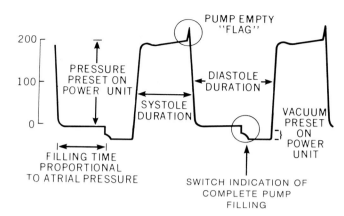

Figure 58–4. An idealized pressure tracing from a transducer implanted in the left power line. Visual inspection can detect complete pump filling and emptying and other parameters. The filling time can be related to the atrial pressure. Vertical scale is in mm Hg. (From Pierce, W. S., Myers, J. L., Donachy, J. H., et al: Approaches to the artificial heart. Surgery, *90*:137, 1981.)

a spare power unit, an emergency AC power source, and a series of visible and audible alarms to indicate failure of the console to generate an adequate drive pressure and loss of electrical power. Because of the need for reliability, redundancy, and safety measures, the power consoles are bulky and heavy and, accordingly, severely limit the mobility of experimental animals or patients. To alleviate this problem, Heimes and Klasen (1982) designed a small, portable battery powered unit capable of providing sufficient pneumatic power to maintain an artificial heart for several hours (Fig. 58–6). The unit was small enough that it could be carried by the patient. Unfortunately, the safety systems of the larger console were, of necessity, minimized.

Control of the output of the blood pumps is required to ensure an adequate left ventricular output, atrial pressures of below 15 mm Hg, and a similar, but not identical, output of both prosthetic ventricles. In the most commonly used control system, each ventricle is set at a rate that prevents complete pump filling (Kwan Gett et al, 1969). The systolic console pressure is set sufficiently high to ensure complete ventricle emptying under all conditions. Any factor, such as exercise, that increases

venous return causes more complete pump filling. In this system, pump output is related to filling pressure and has some of the aspects of output control of the natural heart, often referred to as the Frank-Starling principle (Hennig et al, 1978). Although this system works well, the change in output achieved is small and is in the range of 10 to 20%. Larger increments of output require manual increases in pump rates (Takatani et al, 1982).

Automatic electronic control of cardiac output has been achieved with a system in which each pump is controlled by using a feedback control system (Landis et al, 1977). The pumps always fill and empty completely with this method of control. The left pump rate changes automatically to maintain the arterial blood pressure within a preset normal range. The right pump rate changes automatically to maintain the left atrial pressure within a normal range.

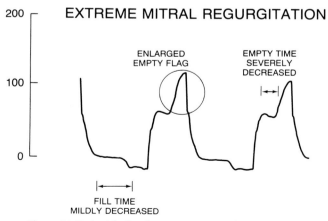

Figure 58–5. An idealized pressure tracing from the left power line of an artificial heart with a malfunctioning (regurgitant) mitral valve. Note particularly the large "empty" flag and the short empty time. Urgent reoperation would be required to restore valve function and to improve forward flow. Vertical scale is in mm Hg.

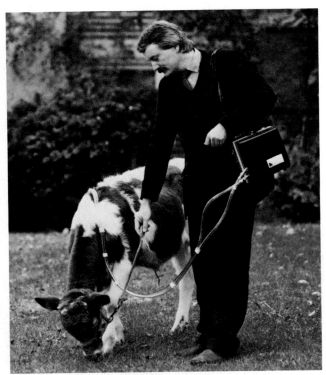

Figure 58–6. The Heimes' drive unit is much smaller and lighter in weight than the conventional consoles. The unit is shown attached to the calf with an artificial heart through two 3-m vinyl tubes. (Photograph courtesy of Symbion, Inc.)

This control system provides an automatic increase in output in response to exercise. Some technique is required to measure aortic pressure and left atrial pressure either directly or indirectly. These measurements are best derived indirectly from the pneumatic power line (Rosenberg et al, 1978) rather than by the use of direct implanted transducers or by indwelling catheters, thus obviating problems associated with the electrical instability of transducers and the risks of sepsis associated with vascular access catheters.

Animal Studies

A few surgical research laboratories both in the United States and abroad have programs to study pneumatic artificial hearts in experimental animals. Most implants are done in 60-kg to 100-kg calves through a right thoracotomy (Olsen et al, 1977). The animals are supported on cardiopulmonary bypass for the 2 hours required for cardiectomy and the implantation of the blood pumps. At the completion of the operation, they are put into a restraining cage and usually stand within 2 or 3 hours after operation. The calves eat and have a return of normal body function within 12 hours. The animals must be constantly observed to ensure that the pneumatic drive lines are not injured or distracted. Treadmill exercise begins several weeks after operation. The animals

remain alert, well, and active and gain weight rapidly.

Detailed hemodynamic and clinical chemistry observations have been made in these animals for many months after heart replacement and they show no evidence of organ dysfunction. The animals do, however, have a mild anemia with a hematocrit in the range of 28 to 30% (Hughes et al, 1985; Razzeca et al, 1978; Shaffer et al, 1979), which is most likely to be a result of the four mechanical valves used in the device. Despite satisfactory maintenance of the circulation, animal survival is generally limited to 6 or 7 months, although one calf survived for almost 1 year (Aufiero et al, 1987).

Survival of animals with artificial hearts implanted in the 1960s was limited by mechanical failures and thromboemboli (Klain et al, 1971). Improved design, the use of smooth surfaced polyurethane pumping bladders, and better understanding of the interactions between the prosthetic device and the host animal increased survival time during the 1970s by several months. Better inlet port design and the use of smooth surfaced inlet connectors largely eliminated the earlier problems of inlet port pannus growth (Jarvik et al, 1981; Pae et al, 1985). As a result, animals now commonly live for 6 to 7 months after artificial heart implantation (Fig. 58–7). Problems that lead to the termination of animal studies include (1) infection, (2) elastomer bladder calcification, and (3) relatively inadequate cardiac output as a result of rapid growth.

Bloodstream infection is a serious and, sometimes, lethal complication in animals with mechanical hearts (Fields et al, 1983; Murray et al, 1983). Infection occurring soon after implantation is due to improper operative technique. The presence of intravascular catheters and percutaneous drive lines poses a constant threat of infection, which can be minimized but not eliminated. Moreover, studies have shown decreased host resistance in animals with implanted pneumatic hearts (Paping et al, 1978). Accordingly, minimal use of vascular access catheters with removal of those used when no longer required is recommended. To reduce the risk of sepsis associated with the percutaneous tubes, considerable research effort has been directed toward developing a bacterial seal between the external environment and the patient. The two best techniques currently available to inhibit bacterial invasion are wrapping the implanted segment of tube with Dacron velour fabric (Hall et al, 1975) and using the Utah skin button (Hastings et al, 1981). The latter device consists of two concentric tubes; the drive line passes through the inner one and the adjacent surfaces are sealed with adhesive. The outer tube is covered with velour and is passed through the opening in the skin. Drive line entrance sites must be kept clean, and tension and movement at the skin site must be minimized. Systemic antibiotics are used similar to their use in clinical medicine.

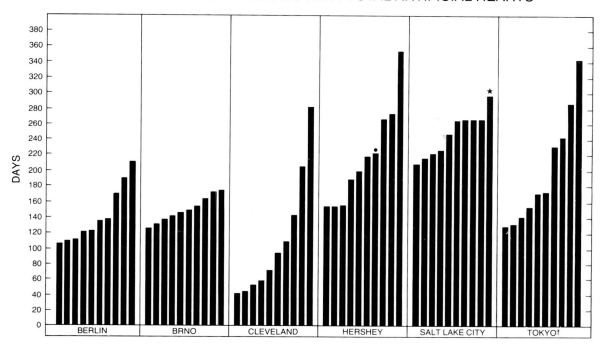

Figure 58–7. This bar graph shows the maximal survival times achieved by the major groups doing artificial heart research in experimental animals. No animal has lived for 1 year after artificial heart implantation. (Modified from Pierce, W. S.: The artificial heart, 1986: Partial fulfillment of a promise. Trans. Am. Soc. Artif. Intern. Organs, 32:5, 1986.)

Elastomer bladder calcification was not an anticipated problem but began to be observed as animal survival lengthened beyond 3 months (Coleman et al, 1981). Dystrophic calcification has been observed on pump bladders made of various materials including segmented polyurethane, segmented polyurethane-polydimethyl siloxane copolymer, Dacron flock-lined polyurethane, and gluteraldehyde-treated, gelatin-coated polyolefin. Areas of the pump bladder subject to high mechanical stress tended particularly to have calcification (Whalen et al, 1980). The calcific deposits densely adhered to the polymer and caused stiffening, flexion failure, and perforation of the bladder. This dystrophic calcification may have an etiology similar to that which occurs in biologic prosthetic valves and occurs most often in young patients (Ferrans et al, 1980). Clinical experience with blood pumps in adults suggests that calcification does not present a major problem, at least during use of the device for several years. Both warfarin sodium, which blocks the formation of gamma-carboxyglutamic acid containing protein, and diphosphonates, which inhibit crystal formation, have been used in studies on calves and appear to improve, but not eliminate, calcification of the bladder (Hughes et al, 1984; Levy et al, 1983; Pierce et al, 1980).

The first successful uses of implanted artificial hearts were in calves weighing 60 to 100 kg, which continue to serve as the most widely used animal model. Their chest size is ample and both the cardiac output and the size of their vessels are similar to that of an adult human. The animals are uniform in size, tolerate anesthesia well, and are docile and easy to care for. They grow rapidly, however, gaining 0.4 to 1 kg/day, and quickly outgrow the artificial heart so that no calf with an implant has yet to survive for 1 year. Moreover, the use of an immature animal appears to increase the likelihood and severity of pump bladder calcification. There is considerable interest among investigators in using an adult animal model whose weight is close to that of an adult human. A subhuman primate might appear to be ideal, but the only species large enough for clinical-sized devices is the baboon, which is dangerous to handle, costly, and an endangered species. The best alternatives to the calf appear to be the mature goat (Atsumi et al, 1981; Gaines et al, 1985) and sheep (Murray et al, 1985). Successful heart replacement in these species is a formidable undertaking with results that do not approach those in the calf. Alternatives are an important challenge to research scientists in this field.

INDICATIONS FOR CLINICAL USE OF THE ARTIFICIAL HEART

Temporary or Bridge Use

Cardiac transplantation has evolved into an effective, lifesaving procedure for a selected group of patients with end-stage cardiomyopathy. However, a suitable donor heart must be made available to the transplant candidate as soon as possible. In 1988, the scarcity of donor hearts resulted in an average waiting period of approximately 3 weeks, and some patients had to wait even longer. As many as 20% of the candidates die before a compatible heart becomes available. A number of treatment modalities help to maintain the circulation in a transplant candidate who has an inadequate cardiac output, including hospitalization with bed rest, optimized drug programs, intravenous infusions of inotropic agents, and the use of the intra-aortic balloon. Even with these regimens, however, a patient may have inadequate hemodynamic indices to support life and may be a candidate for a left ventricular assist pump, biventricular assist pumps, or the artificial heart (Pennock et al, 1986). During the last 4 years, an artificial heart has been used successfully as a bridge to transplantation in a number of patients and has supported their circulation until a suitable donor heart could be identified. Hemodynamic criteria for the use of the bridge technique include a cardiac output index of below 1.8 l/min/m², a mean arterial pressure of less than 60 mm Hg, a mean left atrial pressure of more than 25 mm Hg, and a urine output of less than 10 ml/min (Griffith et al, 1987; Levinson et al, 1986). Certain transplant candidates develop intractable arrhythmias with less severe deterioration of hemodynamic indices and may also be helped with the artificial heart bridge.

Permanent Heart Replacement

A large population of patients exist with end-stage heart disease and are not transplant candidates because they have diabetes mellitus that requires insulin, mild to moderate elevation in pulmonary vascular resistance, or are beyond the age that is acceptable for transplantation. The life expectancy of New York Heart Association Class IV patients with impaired hemodynamic indices is measured in months (Franciosa et al, 1983). Other than drug programs, the physician has little to offer these patients; however, understandably, the availability of an artificial heart has raised their hopes. Although most surgeons do not believe that the pneumatic artificial heart in its present state of development is suitable for the permanent support of the circulation, the area is controversial and five patients, who are not transplant candidates, have been accepted for permanent heart replacement (DeVries et al, 1984;

DeVries, 1988). The hemodynamic criteria for the use of the artificial heart in these patients are similar to those generally accepted as a bridge device.

CLINICAL IMPLANTATION OF THE ARTIFICIAL HEART

Technique

Before implantation of a pneumatic artificial heart in the human chest, the surgeon must be certain that the intrathoracic space is large enough. The Jarvik 7 100-ml stroke and the Penn State clinical heart are suitable for patients who weigh 70 kg or more and who have enough space between the sternum and spine to accommodate the device (Jarvik et al, 1986). For slightly smaller males and for females, the Jarvik 7 70-ml stroke pump may fit within the available space and certainly would provide an adequate cardiac output index.

An implantation procedure is frequently followed by complications of sepsis (Griffith et al, 1988). Before operation, active infection must be eradicated, and extraordinary care must be taken during every step of the procedure to ensure strict asepsis.

The operation is begun with a standard median sternotomy (DeVries and Joyce, 1983; Richenbacker et al, 1986). Ascending aortic and bicaval cannulation is done, and cardiopulmonary bypass is started. The patient's temperature is lowered to 22° C. The ventricles are excised by dividing both great arteries above the valves and dividing the heart at the atrioventricular junction, leaving full atrial remnants. The operation is almost identical to that done for heart transplantation (Fig. 58–8). The left atrial cuff is trimmed and double sewn (Fig. 58–9). The prosthetic left ventricle is brought onto the operative field, and the length of the aortic graft is determined. The graft is cut to fit and is sutured to the aorta. Both anastomoses are inspected to ensure that no leaks are present; this step is important because suture lines are difficult to visualize after the ventricles are in place (see Fig. 58–9). Any leaks observed at this early stage are readily controlled by using pledgeted polypropylene mattress sutures.

The left pump is brought onto the operative field. A stab wound is then made in the skin to the left of the umbilicus and a tunnel is created, similar to that used for the placement of a chest tube, from the apex of the pericardium, through the diaphragm, and out through the stab wound. The left drive line is passed through this tunnel and the left pump is positioned within the pericardial sac. The union nuts on the left atrial cuff and on the aortic cuff are aligned and tightened (Fig. 58–10). De-airing of the prosthetic left ventricle is done by passing a Swan-Ganz catheter through the atrial anastomosis and across the prosthetic mitral valve; the tip is positioned in the highest portion of the pump bladder. Place-

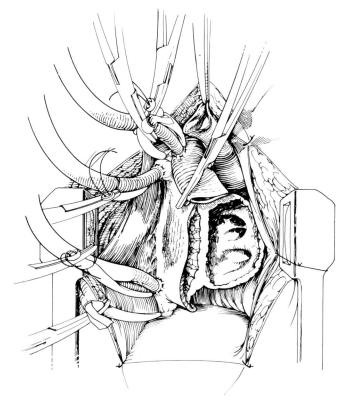

Figure 58–8. The chest has been opened through a median sternotomy; cardiopulmonary bypass has been started, and the heart (ventricles) has been excised. Both venae cavae have been cannulated, and occlusive snares have been placed. The arterial perfusion cannula is positioned in the ascending aorta, distal to an occlusive clamp. (From Richenbacher, W. E., Pennock, J. L., Pae, W. E., Jr., et al: Artificial heart implantation for end-stage heart disease. J. Cardiac Surg. *1*:1, 1986.)

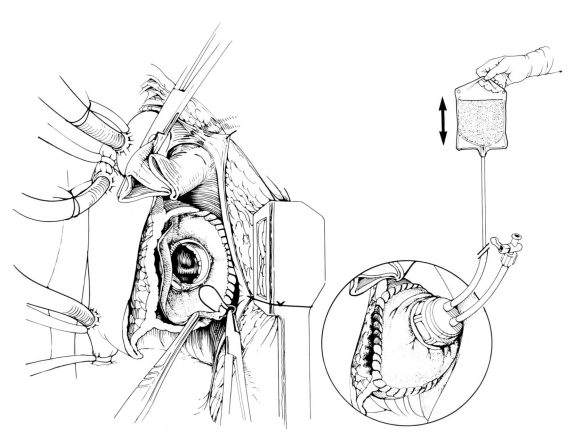

Figure 58–9. The left atrial connector is trimmed and doubly sutured to the left atrial remnant with 4-0 polypropylene suture. This anastomosis is difficult to visualize after both ventricles have been implanted. The *insert* indicates a technique to distend the completed suture line and identify any leaks, which are readily repaired at this stage of the operation. (From Richenbacher, W. E., Pennock, J. L., Pae, W. E., Jr., et al: Artificial heart implantation for end-stage heart disease. J. Cardiac Surg., *1*:1, 1986.)

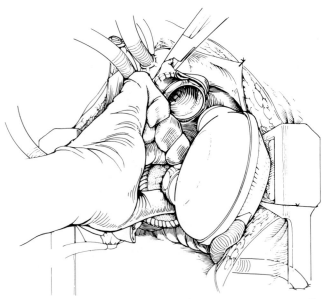

Figure 58–10. After suturing the left atrial and aortic cuffs, the surgeon passes the left drive line through a skin tunnel. The union nuts on the cuffs facilitate a tight seal to the pump. De-airing is done and slow pumping of the left ventricle is begun. (From Richenbacher, W. E., Pennock, J. L., Pae, W. E., Jr., et al: Artificial heart implantation for end-stage heart disease. J. Cardiac Surg., *1*:1, 1986.)

ment of the catheter is facilitated by passing it through the valve before seating the threaded atrial connector. When the de-airing catheter is positioned within the blood sac and both connectors are firmly seated, air is withdrawn as the sac fills with blood. After all air has been removed from the blood pump, the catheter is withdrawn and the entry site is repaired with a pledgeted polypropylene suture. The aortic cross-clamp is then removed, and the left pump is pulsed slowly. The suture lines are inspected again for bleeding.

The right pump is then brought onto the operative field to determine the proper length for the pulmonary arterial graft. This conduit is cut to length and anastomosed to the pulmonary artery with a running suture of 4-0 polypropylene. The right atrial skirt is trimmed and anastomosed to the right atrial remnant by using a double row of 4-0 polypropylene sutures. The right atrial anastomosis is then observed for leaks. At this point the patient is warmed to 37° C. A second stab wound is created to the left of the umbilicus and a tunnel is formed that leaves the pericardium midway between the left drive line and the inferior vena cava. The drive line is passed through the tunnel, and the right pump is connected (Fig. 58–11). The central venous pressure is raised to 10 mm Hg, the caval snares are loosened, and air is removed from the right blood sac as it was from the left one.

Ventilation of the patient is resumed. Right ventricular pumping is initiated, and cardiopulmonary bypass is gradually discontinued. Again, all anasto-

moses are inspected carefully for evidence of leaks. When an index of 2.4 l/min/m^2 has been reached, the atrial cannulas are removed and the insertion sites are oversewn with pledgeted polypropylene mattress sutures (Fig. 58–12). The patient is transfused to a central venous pressure of 10 to 15 mm Hg and the arterial cannula is removed. The previously placed aortic purse-string sutures are tightened. Mediastinal chest tubes are positioned, and the sternotomy is closed in the usual manner.

The postoperative care of a patient with an implanted artificial heart is similar to the care given to patients who have had open heart surgery. Atrial, pulmonary, arterial, and aortic pressures are readily maintained within narrow limits, which are determined by drive unit pumping parameters. A cardiac output index of between 2.2 and 2.6 l/min/m^2 is fairly easily maintained. An alpha agent such as neosynephrine is sometimes required to maintain an adequate arterial blood pressure. A low dose infusion of dopamine (3 mg/kg/min) to promote adequate renal perfusion and urine output has been given.

There is no uniform agreement with regard to the optimal drug program needed to minimize the risk of thromboembolic complications. For a patient with a permanent artificial heart who will not have

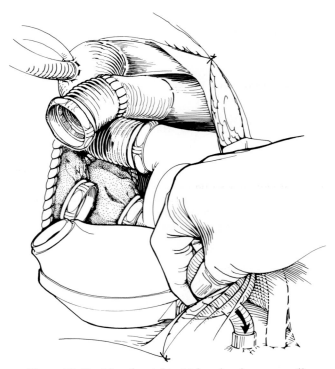

Figure 58–11. After the right atrial and pulmonary cuffs are sutured to the respective sites, the surgeon passes the right drive line through the preformed skin tunnel. The union nuts on the right cuffs are threaded to the right pump. De-airing is accomplished and right ventricle pumping is begun. (From Richenbacher, W. E., Pennock, J. L., Pae, W. E., Jr., et al: Artificial heart implantation for end-stage heart disease. J. Cardiac Surg., *1*:1, 1986.)

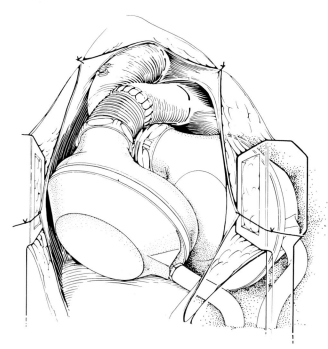

Figure 58–12. This drawing shows the proper placement of the two pumps within the pericardial sac after removal of the arterial and venous cannulas. (From Richenbacher, W. E., Pennock, J. L., Pae, W. E., Jr., et al: Artificial heart implantation for end-stage heart disease. J. Cardiac Surg., 1:1, 1986.)

subsequent cardiac transplantation, an acceptable drug program includes the use of low molecular weight dextran (5%) at 20 ml/hr begun when drainage from the chest tube has decreased to less than 50 ml/hr (Bygdeman and Eliasson, 1967). On the third or fourth postoperative day, warfarin sodium is administered, much in the same way as it is for patients with a prosthetic heart valve (Harker and Schlicter, 1970). When the prothrombin time is between 20 and 25 seconds, the dextran can be discontinued. The best use of drugs is less clear in the patient in whom the artificial heart has been implanted as a bridge to transplantation. In these patients, adequate coagulation parameters must be restored within a few hours of identifying a suitable donor organ. For this

group of patients, a continuous intravenous heparin drip to maintain the activated clotting time between 150 and 250 seconds combined with dipyridamole 75 mg by mouth every 6 hours, may be a reasonable therapy.

Patients with an artificial heart have a high likelihood of developing septic complications due to the presence of the large foreign body, percutaneous drive lines, and long operative times. Accordingly, meticulous attention must be directed toward preserving complete asepsis. After operation, these patients are kept in reverse isolation and are given intravenous antibiotics (cefamandole nafate, 1 g every 6 hours). Pulmonary toilet is vigorous and extubation is done when clinically indicated. Strict aseptic technique is observed when handling vascular catheters. Central and peripheral lines are changed every 2 to 3 days, and the urinary catheter is removed as soon as an adequate urine output is maintained. The percutaneous drive lines used are covered with Dacron velour and sutured to the skin at their exit sites; every effort is made to minimize motion at these sites so that fibrous tissue growth into the velour is encouraged. These areas are cleansed with hydrogen peroxide and covered with povidone-iodine ointment daily. Surveillance cultures are obtained and any positive cultures are promptly investigated. Avoiding sepsis in the bridge patients is the key to subsequent successful cardiac transplantation later (Griffith et al, 1988).

Results

From 1981 to 1987, 93 pneumatic artificial hearts have been implanted in patients. In 88 patients, the implanted devices were intended to be temporary (Table 58–1). Of these implants, 40 were done in 1987. The average age of the patients was 40 years, and they were categorized according to their diagnosis: cardiomyopathy (57 patients), patients who had a failed graft after a heart transplant (16 patients), patients who had open heart operations and could not be weaned from the pump oxygenator (9 patients), and a miscellaneous or status unknown group

TABLE 58–1. ARTIFICIAL HEART AS A BRIDGE FOR TRANSPLANTATION: CLINICAL EXPERIENCE 1981 to 1987*

Cardiac Diagnosis	No. of Patients	Days On Device†	Patients Dead Before Transplant	Transplants Performed	No. of Patients Who Died	No. of Patients Still Alive
Cardiomyopathy						
Idiopathic	14	2 weeks	2	12	1	11
Ischemic	26	2 weeks	6	20	11	9
Miscellaneous or unknown	17	2 weeks	2	15	9	6
Transplant rejection	16	9 weeks	7	9	5	4
Nonweanable CPB‡	9	4 days	1	8	5	3
Miscellaneous	6	1 week	2	4	4	0
Total	88		20	68	35	33

*Data provided by Don B. Olsen, DVM, University of Utah Artificial Heart Research Laboratory.
†Approximations.
‡CPB = cardiopulmonary bypass.

(six patients) (see Table 58–1). Most prostheses used (76) were of the Jarvik 7 design and were implanted at approximately 20 centers in the United States and abroad. The remainder were custom-made devices that were developed by physician-engineer teams and were usually used at the same institution in which they were made. The preimplant condition of the patients varied from stable but severe end-stage heart failure, where a semielective artificial heart implant was done, to a patient in extremis who had the circulation supported by external cardiac massage. Accordingly, the results might be expected to differ greatly in such a wide spectrum of patients. A number of patients have had relatively uncomplicated implantations and have been weaned from the respirator. These patients have been able to eat, converse, and walk around their rooms. If the patient's condition was satisfactory and a suitable donor heart was identified, the prosthesis was removed and transplantation was done. The length of stay in the hospital has been increased by the use of the bridge device, but the outcome has been excellent. Unfortunately, some patients have had various problems after implantation including the sequelae of inadequate circulation before implantation generally manifested as multisystem failure. Other problems included bleeding, infection, and thromboembolism and were caused by the interaction between the host and the device. While the timing of transplantation in such a patient is based on the status of organ function and on the availability of a donor organ, experience indicates that the best results are obtained when the artificial heart is kept in place for less than 1 week.

The most representative results of the artificial heart as a bridge are in the cardiomyopathy group (see Table 58–1). Fifty-seven of these implants were done, and ten patients died before transplantation (18%). Of the 47 patients who received transplants, 21 died. Thus, the survival rate after transplantation was 26 of 47 (55%) patients, whereas the overall survival rate was 26 of 57 (46%) patients. When one considers the novelty of the artificial heart and the magnitude of the staged procedure, these results are certainly acceptable. With additional experience in the selection of patients and improvements in the artificial heart, the results will also improve.

Five patients with end-stage heart disease, who were not considered to be transplant candidates, have had a Jarvik 7 artificial heart permanently implanted. One death occurred 10 days after implantation as a result of cardiac tamponade. Several patients have done reasonably well and are able to eat, sit in a chair, and take walks with the help of someone to move the power unit. The compact Heimes' power unit has been used for as long as several hours with the artificial heart functioning well. One patient was able to ride outdoors in a specially equipped van. However, the occurrence of strokes, poor nutrition, or infection led ultimately to their gradual "down hill" course and death. Two

patients lived for more than 1 year while the longest survivor lived for 622 days. Most observers believe that pneumatic hearts have not been developed to their fullest potential. Although improvements in their design will reduce the incidence of thromboembolic complications, the problem of infection appears intimately related to the percutaneous power lines, which are intrinsic components of the pneumatic artificial heart. The electric motor driven artificial heart will overcome most of the problems associated with the pneumatically driven ones.

ELECTRICALLY POWERED ARTIFICIAL HEART FOR PERMANENT HEART REPLACEMENT

Experience with the pneumatically powered heart, both in the laboratory and in the clinical setting, has confirmed the disadvantage of percutaneous passage of the power lines. A major breakthrough in the transmission of energy in the form of pressurized fluid across the skin does not appear to be imminent. However, investigators (Schuder et al, 1961) have recognized for decades that electrical energy can be transmitted across the intact skin by inductive coupling, a principle widely used in transformers and other commonly used electrical devices. Such a system was used clinically by Glenn and associates (1959) to energize pacemakers. However, the low power requirement of a pacemaker and reliable implantable batteries quickly made the inductively coupled pacemaker obsolete. A power requirement of more than a million times that of a pacemaker eliminates from consideration an artificial heart solely dependent on an implantable battery. Accordingly, the permanent artificial heart now under development in several laboratories consists of two implantable blood pumps activated by a miniature electric motor. Energy for the system is supplied continuously to a primary coil on the surface of the skin by either house current or a wearable external battery. The secondary coil, positioned under the skin and energized by the primary coil, actuates the electric motor. An element of safety and comfort is provided by a sophisticated implantable rechargeable battery. This implanted battery powers the heart for only about 30 minutes, which is sufficient time for the external coil to be changed and for minor power interruptions to be rectified. Although the principle of operation and design plans for the electrically powered hearts are well formulated, these plans have only recently resulted in the fabrication of hardware and institution of animal studies.

The electric heart under development at the University of Utah (Jarvik et al, 1978, 1981) is based on a modification of the Jarvik 7 pneumatically powered ventricles (Fig. 58–13). In this design, a high-speed, reversing, brushless DC motor is coupled to an axial flow pump, located between the two ventri-

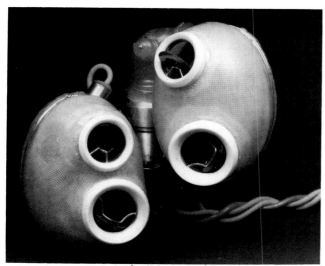

Figure 58-13. The electrohydraulic artificial heart being developed at the University of Utah. The axial flow pump, positioned between the two blood pumps, pressurizes the hydraulic fluid and alternately actuates the right and left ventricles. (Photograph provided by Donald B. Olsen, DVM, University of Utah.)

cles. This motor-pump unit is positioned within a short conduit that joins what were the pneumatic ports of the two ventricles. The system is filled with silicone hydraulic fluid. Axial flow pumping in one direction activates the left blood pump while axial rotation in reverse activates the right pump. The volume of hydraulic fluid pumped closely approximates the stroke volume of the pump. The system uses a clever design module that is a small size and has few moving parts. The requirement of rapidly reversing the high-speed motor, however, places extreme loads on the miniature bearings, which may limit the functional life of the energy converter.

The Penn State University electric heart (Rosenberg et al, 1984, 1985) uses two pusher plate actuated ventricles (Fig. 58–14). A low-speed, reversing, brushless DC motor with a motion translator is positioned between the two ventricles. The most efficient long-life motion translator available is a roller screw, which functions in a manner similar to a nut rotating on a threaded shaft. In this application, the nut rotates and the shaft moves to and fro for a distance of 25 mm. Again, as in the University of Utah design, the two ventricles pump alternately. This design requires a larger, heavier motor than the hydraulic system design. The 2-year functional life design criterion appears to be well within the design specifications for the roller screw and associated bearings.

The output of the electric artificial heart can be varied by changing the stroke or the pumping rate. As with the pneumatic heart, the change in output can occur secondary to change in filling pressure or in response to an electronic control based on atrial or arterial pressures, or their analogs.

One reason why electrically powered hearts have

lagged far behind their pneumatic counterparts is related to their complexity of control. In any design of an artificial heart, provision must be made to prevent atrial collapse in the event that there is inadequate blood to fill the ventricle. In the pneumatic design, a preset low diastolic (filling) vacuum ensures against atrial collapse; the hydraulic or mechanical types of electric heart must rely on other techniques. In the hydraulic design, a pressure sensor is used in the hydraulic fluid behind each ventricle which, through appropriate electronic circuity, promptly slows or stops and reverses axial pump movement when a significant negative pressure is registered. In the pusher plate design (Landis et al, 1980), the bladder is not attached to the pusher plate; this enables the pusher plate to travel a full distance without obligatory bladder filling. Incomplete or slow bladder filling, in turn, provides a signal to the control system that automatically decreases the pump rate to a level at which a full to empty cycle will result. A system of this type that is closed to the atmosphere requires a volume displacement device to allow minor variations in the output of each ventricle and compensation for normal variation in atmospheric pressure (Lee et al, 1984). The compliance chamber consists of a flexible, gas-containing sac that is connected to the gas space of the motor heart (Fig. 58–15). The compliance chamber is covered with Dacron velour.

The transcutaneous energy transmission system (TETS) consists of a primary coil of Litz wire energized at 150 kHz. The secondary coil is implanted under the skin and provides energy to power the motor and associated electronics and to recharge the implanted batteries. The energy required for the

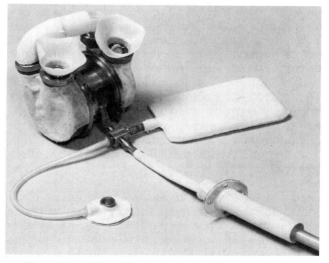

Figure 58–14. The roller screw motor driven artificial heart is being developed at The Penn State University. The brushless DC motor and the roller screw unit are positioned between the two ventricles. The transcutaneous electrical line, compliance chamber, and percutaneous access port are also shown. (From Pierce, W. S.: The artificial heart, 1986: Partial fulfillment of a promise. Trans. Am. Soc. Artif. Intern. Organs, 32:1, 1986).

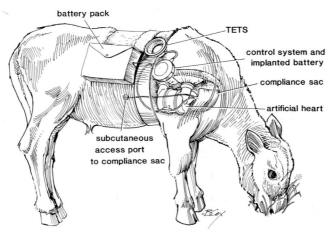

Figure 58–15. The Penn State electric heart is being evaluated in the calf. The placement of the pump is shown within the thorax. The compliance sac and its subcutaneous access port, the location of the transcutaneous energy transmission system (TETS), the control system with the implanted battery, and the external battery pack are also shown. (From Rosenberg, G., Snyder, A. J., Weiss, W. J., et al: Power requirements for an electric motor-driven total artificial heart. IEEE/Ninth Annual Conference of the Engineering in Medicine and Biology Society, Vol. 1, p. 188. © 1987 IEEE.)

electric heart can be transmitted, with the coils 5 to 10 mm apart (simulated skin thickness), with a 70% efficiency and no noticeable rise in skin temperature or nutritional effect on the interpositioned skin. Important information can be transmitted to and from the implanted electronics by modulation of the 150-kHz power signal, which allows the assessment of device function and battery condition and adjustment of operating modes.

The power input required for the electric heart is between 10 and 20 watts and is provided easily by conventional house current. For portable function, the heart must be powered by an external, rechargeable battery pack. In addition to the batteries, such a pack must include the electronics required for recharging them and a system to indicate the power available and the "health" of the battery. At present, NiCd batteries represent the best type of batteries available. Approximately one pound of battery is required for each hour of heart function. Development of higher energy density batteries is a current focus of industrial research; advances in this area will result in a lighter power pack for the patients to carry.

Extensive bench studies are now being done with the electric hearts and are confirming adequate maintenance of pressure and flow during various mock circulatory loop conditions. In-vitro fatigue testing is an important part of the evaluation of these hearts. Results generally indicate that failures before the anticipated design life of 2 years frequently occur because of mechanical malfunction or the effect of moisture effects on electronic circuitry. Minor, but important, design changes continue to be made to remedy these problems.

Animal implant studies are being done with iterations of the electric hearts to develop and evaluate appropriate implantation techniques and to evaluate the in-vivo function of the devices (see Fig. 58–15). Both systems, exclusive of the TETS, have been used successfully for heart replacement, resulting in animals that have normal hemodynamic parameters, eat well, and appear to be comfortable. The longest period of survival after heart replacement with the Utah device was limited to approximately 1 month with cessation of pumping due to loss of hydraulic oil. Improved sealing techniques and overall design modifications are now being made to extend the duration of animal studies with this device.

Experience with the Penn State device has also been marred by early failures. However, several animals have lived for more than 2 months and one animal has lived for more than 7 months (Fig. 58–16) (Rosenberg et al, 1984). This latter animal, a benchmark, has been important in advancing research in this field. The animal grew normally and was able to exercise on a treadmill. Its death was due to the failure of an external electrical circuit component. Necropsy examination showed good organ preservation and no evidence of thromboemboli. Furthermore, no significant wear was observed in the mechanical pump components.

Both research groups now plan additional animal implant studies with improved hearts. Energy transmission via the TETS system is also included in these future studies.

Progress in the development of the electric heart is not limited by lack of basic knowledge or by the unavailability of any particular component. Research-

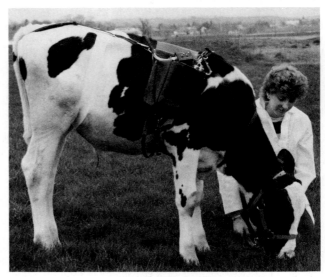

Figure 58–16. A calf with a motor driven artificial heart is shown here. The implanted components are similar to those shown in Figure 58–15, although the controller is not implanted and electrical energy is supplied through a percutaneous wire. This animal lived for 222 days with the electric heart.

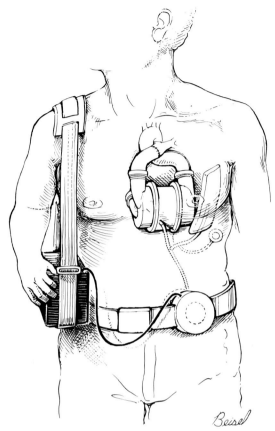

Figure 58–17. The implantable electric heart is shown as it is proposed for human use. The artificial heart and associated compliance sac are positioned within the thorax. The compliance sac is accessed through a subcutaneous port. The external battery is carried in a shoulder case. Electrical energy is transferred by using inductive coupling techniques via a belt-located primary and secondary coil. (From Rosenberg, G., Snyder, A., Landis, D. L., et al: An electric motor-driven total artificial heart: Seven months' survival in the calf. Trans. Am. Soc. Artif. Intern. Organs, *30*:69, 1984.)

ers are attuned particularly to adopting any advances in electronics, batteries, super conductors, ultra-high-strength magnets, and elastomers and to adapting them to the electric heart. Based on current progress, the best estimates suggest that the electric heart will be available for clinical application almost at the end of the 20th century (Fig. 58–17).

Selected Bibliography

DeVries, W. C.: The permanent artificial heart: Four case reports. J.A.M.A., *259*:849, 1988.

This article provides a detailed summary of four patients who had permanent artificial hearts implanted. The blood pumps were able to maintain an adequate circulation for prolonged periods. Most of the problems that have occurred in animal studies with the Jarvik 7 heart have been seen when the device was used in the clinical setting.

Griffith, B. P., Hardesty, R. L., Kormos, R. L., et al: Temporary use of the Jarvik-7 total artificial heart before transplantation. N. Engl. J. Med. *316*:130, 1987.

A number of transplant centers have used the artificial heart as an interim circulatory support device while a patient is awaiting transplantation. The University of Pittsburgh group has described their experience with the Jarvik 7 heart in this important article. The use of this artificial heart poses a risk of thromboembolus and infarction. Accordingly, the best results occurred in the patients when the artificial heart was used for the shortest period.

Pierce, W. S.: The artificial heart—1986: Partial fulfillment of a promise. Trans. Am. Soc. Artif. Intern. Organs, *32*:5, 1986.

This review article describes the different artificial hearts being developed and the progression that has occurred as these devices have moved from the research laboratory to being applied clinically.

Bibliography

Akutsu, T., Houston, C. S., and Kolff, W. J.: Artificial hearts inside the chest, using small electro-motors. Trans. Am. Soc. Artif. Intern. Organs, *6*:299, 1960.

Akutsu, T., and Kolff, W. J.: Permanent substitutes for valves and hearts. Trans. Am. Soc. Artif. Intern. Organs, *4*:230, 1958.

Atsumi, K., Fujimasa, I., Imachi, K., et al: Three goats survived for 288 days, 243 days, and 232 days with hybrid total artificial heart (HTAH). Trans. Am. Soc. Intern. Organs, *27*:77, 1981.

Aufiero, T. X., Magovern, J. A., Rosenberg, G., et al: Long-term survival with a pneumatic total artificial heart (pTAH). Trans. Am. Soc. Artif. Intern. Organs, *33*:157, 1987.

Boretos, J. W., and Pierce, W. S.: Segmented polyurethane: A new elastomer for biomedical application. Science, *158*:1481, 1967.

Bücherl, E. S., Hennig, E., Frank, B. J., et al: Status of the artificial heart programs in Berlin. World J. Surg., *9*:103, 1985.

Bygdeman, S., and Eliasson, R.: Effect of dextrans on platelet adhesiveness and aggregation. Scand. J. Clin. Lab. Invest., *20*:17, 1967.

Coleman, D. L., Lim, D., Kessler, T., and Andrade, J. D.: Calcification of nontextured implantable blood pumps. Trans. Am. Soc. Artif. Intern. Organs, *27*:97, 1981.

Coleman, S. J., Bornhorst, W. J., LaFarge, C. G., and Carr, J. G.: Pneumatic waveform diagnostics of implanted ventricular assist pumps. Trans. Am. Soc. Artif. Intern. Organs, *18*:176, 1972.

Cooley, D. A.: Staged cardiac transplantation: Report of three cases. Heart Trans., *1*:145, 1982.

Cooley, D. A., Liotta, D., Hallman, G. L., et al: Orthotopic cardiac prosthesis for two-staged cardiac replacement. Am. J. Cardiol. *24*:723, 1969.

DeVries, W. C.: The permanent artificial heart: Four case reports. J.A.M.A., *259*:849, 1988.

DeVries, W. C., and Joyce, L. D.: The artificial heart. CIBA Clinical Symposia, *35*:4, 1983.

DeVries, W. C., Anderson, J. L., Joyce, L. D., et al: Clinical use of the total artificial heart. N. Engl. J. Med., *310*:273, 1984.

Ferrans, V. J., Boyce, S. W., Billingham, M. D., et al: Calcific deposits in porcine bioprostheses—structure and pathogenesis. Am. J. Cardiol., *46*:721, 1980.

Fields, A., Harasaki, H., Sands, D., and Nose, Y.: Infection in artificial blood pump implantation. Trans. Am. Soc. Artif. Intern. Organs, *29*:532, 1983.

Franciosa, J. A., Wilen, M., Ziesche, S., and Cohn, J. N.: Survival in men with severe chronic left ventricular failure due to either coronary heart disease or idiopathic dilated cardiomyopathy. Am. J. Cardiol., *51*:831, 1983.

Gaines, W. E., Pierce, W. S., Prophet, G. A., and Holtzman, K. L.: The goat: An animal model for implantable blood pumps. ASAIO J., *8*:135, 1985.

Glenn, W. W. L., Mauro, A., Longo, E., et al: Remote stimulation of the heart by radio frequency transmission. N. Engl. J. Med., 261:948, 1959.

Griffith, B. P., Hardesty, R. L., Kormos, R. L., et al: Temporary use of the Jarvik-7 total artificial heart before transplantation. N. Engl. J. Med., 316:130, 1987.

Griffith, B. P., Kormos, R. L., Dummer, J. S., and Hardesty, R. L.: The artificial heart: Infection-related morbidity and its effect on transplantation. Ann. Thorac. Surg., 45:409, 1988.

Hall, C. W., Adams, L. M., and Ghidoni, J. J.: Development of skin interfacing cannula. Trans. Am. Soc. Artif. Int. Organs, 21:281, 1975.

Harker, L. A., and Schlicter, S. J.: Studies of platelet and fibrinogen kinetics in patient with prosthetic heart valves. N. Engl. J. Med., 283:1302, 1970.

Hastings, W. L., Aaron, J. L., Deneris, J., et al: A retrospective study of nine calves surviving five months on the pneumatic total artificial heart. Trans. Am. Soc. Artif. Intern. Organs, 27:71, 1981.

Heimes, H. P., and Klasen, F.: Completely integrated wearable TAH-drive unit. Int. J. Artif. Organs, 5:157, 1982.

Hennig, E., Grosse-Siestrup, C., Krautzberger, W., et al: The relationship of cardiac output and venous pressure in long surviving calves with total artificial hearts. Trans. Am. Soc. Artif. Intern. Organs, 24:616, 1978.

Honda, T., Nagai, I., Nitta, S., et al: Evaluation of cardiac function and venous return curves in awake, unanesthetized calves with an implanted total artificial heart. Trans. Am. Soc. Artif. Intern. Organs, 21:362, 1975.

Hughes, S. D., Butler, M. D., Holmberg, D. L., et al: Comparative hematological data from animals implanted with a total artificial heart containing different valves. Trans. Am. Soc. Artif. Intern. Organs, 31:224, 1985.

Hughes, S. D., Coleman, D. L., Dew, P. A., et al: Effects of coumadin on thrombus and mineralization in total artificial hearts. Trans. Am. Soc. Artif. Intern. Organs, 30:75, 1984.

Jarvik, R. K.: The total artificial heart. Sci. Am., 244:74, 1981.

Jarvik, R. K., DeVries, W. C., Semb, B. K. H., et al: Surgical positioning of the Jarvik-7 artificial heart. J. Heart Transplant., 5:185, 1986.

Jarvik, R. K., Kessler, T. R., McGill, L. D., et al: Determinants of pannus formation in long-surviving artificial heart calves, and its prevention. Trans. Am. Soc. Artif. Intern. Organs, 27:90, 1981.

Jarvik, R. K., Smith, L. M., Lawson, J. H., et al: Comparison of pneumatic and electrically powered total artificial hearts in vivo. Trans. Am. Soc. Artif. Intern. Organs, 24:593, 1978.

Klain, M., Mrava, G. L., Tajima, K., et al: Can we achieve over 100 hours' survival with a total mechanical heart? Trans. Am. Soc. Artif. Intern. Organs, 17:437, 1971.

Kwan-Gett, C. S., Wu, Y., Collan, R., et al: Total replacement artificial heart and driving system with inherent regulation of cardiac output. Trans. Am. Soc. Artif. Intern. Organs, 15:245, 1969.

Landis, D. L., Pierce, W. S., Rosenberg, G., et al: Long-term in vivo automatic electronic control of the artificial heart. Trans. Am. Soc. Artif. Intern. Organs, 23:519, 1977.

Landis, D. L., Rosenberg, G., Donachy, J. H., and Pierce, W. S.: Automatic control for the artificial heart. IEEE 1980 Frontiers of Engineering in Health Care, 1:305, 1980.

Lawson, J. H., Olsen, D. B., Hershgold, E., et al: A comparison of polyurethane and silastic artificial hearts in 10 long survival experiments in calves. Trans. Am. Soc. Artif. Intern. Organs, 21:368, 1975.

Lee, S., Rosenberg, G., Donachy, J. H., et al: The compliance problem: A major obstacle in the development of implantable blood pumps. Artif. Organs, 8:82, 1984.

Levinson, M. M., Smith, R. G., Cork, R., et al: Three recent cases of the total artificial heart before transplantation. J. Heart Transplant, 5:215, 1986.

Levy, R. J., Schoen, F. J., Levy, J. T., et al: Biologic determinants of dystrophic calcification and osteocalcin deposition in glutaraldehyde-preserved porcine aortic valve leaflets implanted subcutaneously in rats. Am. J. Pathol., 113:143, 1983.

Murray, K. D., Hughes, S., Bearnson, D., and Olsen, D. B.: Infection in total artificial heart recipients. Trans. Am. Soc. Artif. Intern. Organs, 29:539, 1983.

Murray, K. D., and Olsen, D. B.: The use of calves and sheep as total heart recipients. ASAIS J., 8:128, 1985.

Nielsen, S. D., Willshaw, P., Nanas, J., and Olsen, D. B.: Non-invasive cardiac monitoring and diagnostics for pneumatic pumping ventricles. Trans. Am. Soc. Artif. Intern. Organs, 29:589, 1983.

Nosé, Y., Topaz, S., SenGupta, A., et al: Artificial hearts inside the pericardial sac in calves. Trans. Am. Soc. Artif. Intern. Organs, 11:255, 1965.

Olsen, D. B., Fukumasu, H., Kolff, J., et al: Implantation of the total artificial heart by lateral thoracotomy. Artif. Organs. 1:1, 1977.

Pae, W. E., Rosenberg, G., Donachy, J. H., et al: A solution to inlet pannus formation in the pneumatic artificial heart. Trans. Am. Soc. Artif. Intern. Organs, 31:12, 1985.

Paping, R., Webster, L. R., Stanley, T. H., et al: White blood cell phagocytosis after artificial heart implantation. Trans. Am. Soc. Artif. Intern. Organs, 24:578, 1978.

Pennock, J. L., Oyer, P. E., Reitz, B. A., et al: Cardiac transplantation in perspective for the future. J. Thorac. Cardiovasc. Surg., 83:168, 1982b.

Pennock, J. L., Pierce, W. S., Campbell, D. B., et al: Mechanical support of the circulation followed by cardiac transplantation. J. Thorac. Cardiovasc. Surg., 92:994, 1986.

Pennock, J. L., Wisman, C. B., and Pierce, W. S.: Mechanical support of the circulation prior to cardiac transplantation. Heart Transplantation, 1:299, 1982a.

Pierce, W. S.: The artificial heart—1986: Partial fulfillment of a promise. Trans. Am. Soc. Artif. Intern. Organs, 32:5, 1986.

Pierce, W. S., Donachy, J. H., Rosenberg, G., and Baier, R. E.: Calcification inside artificial hearts: Inhibition by warfarin-sodium. Science, 208:601, 1980.

Pierce, W. S., Gardner, B. N., Morris, L., et al: Total heart replacement by a single intrathoracic blood pump. J. Surg. Res., 5:387, 1965.

Pierce, W. S., Myers, J. L., Donachy, J. H., et al: Approaches to the artificial heart. Surgery, 90:137, 1981.

Razzeca, K. J., Hodges, M. R., Peters, J. L., et al: Insignificant blood damage in calves with a total artificial heart up to six months. Trans. Am. Soc. Artif. Intern. Organs, 24:581, 1978.

Richenbacher, W. E., Pennock, J. L., Pae, W. E., Jr., and Pierce, W. S.: Artificial heart implantation for end-stage cardiac disease. J. Cardiac Surg., 1:3, 1986.

Rosenberg, G., Cleary, T. J., Snyder, A. L., et al: A totally implantable artificial heart design. Trans. Am. Soc. Mech. Eng., 85-WA/DE-11, 1985.

Rosenberg, G., Landis, D. L., Phillips, W. M., et al: Determining arterial pressure, left atrial pressure, and cardiac output from the left pneumatic drive line of the total artificial heart. Trans. Am. Soc. Artif. Intern. Organs, 24:341, 1978.

Rosenberg, G., Snyder, A., Landis, D. L., et al: An electric motor-driven total artificial heart: Seven months survival in the calf. Trans. Am. Soc. Artif. Intern. Organs, 30:69, 1984.

Ross, J. N., Jr., Akers, W. W., O'Bannon, W., et al: Problems encountered during the development and implantation of the Baylor-Rice orthotopic cardiac prosthesis. Trans. Am. Soc. Artif. Organs, 18:168, 1972.

Schuder, J. C., Stephenson, H. E., Jr., and Townsend, J. F.: Energy transfer into a closed chest by means of stationary coupling coils and a portable high-power oscillator. Trans. Am. Soc. Artif. Intern. Organs, 7:327, 1961.

Shaffer, L. J., Donachy, J. H., Rosenberg, G., et al: Total artificial heart implantation in calves with pump of an angled port design. Trans. Am. Soc. Artif. Intern. Organs, 25:254, 1979.

Takatani, S., Harasaki, H., Koike, S., et al: Optimum control mode for a total artificial heart. Trans. Am. Soc. Artif. Intern. Organs, 28:148, 1982.

Whalen, R. L., Snow, J. L., Harasaki, H., and Nosé, Y.: Mechanical strain and calcification in blood pumps. Trans. Am. Soc. Artif. Intern. Organs, 26:487, 1980.

INDEX

Dopamine, action of, 141, *141*
 as inotrope, 142t
 in cardiac surgery, 213–214, 213t–214t
 in cardiogenic shock, 168–169, 171
 in heart donor management, 1942
 in heart transplantation, 1941, 1946
 in pediatric patients, 374, 375t
 in pericardiectomy, 1245
 in renal failure prevention, 232
 in septic shock, 180
Dopamine agonists/antagonists, after cardiac surgery, 212t
Doppler echocardiography, 1089–1090, *1090–1092,* 1092
 color-flow, 1092
  applications of, 1098–1099; Color Plates: Figs. 31–104 to 31–110
 continuous-wave, 1090, *1092*
  applications of, 1097–1098, *1097–1098*
 in patent ductus arteriosus, 1130
 in tricuspid atresia, 1465
 pulsed-wave, 1090–1091, *1092*
  applications of, 1097–1098, *1097*
Doppler flowmeter, in coronary blood flow determination, 1673
Dorsal sympathectomy, in thoracic outlet syndrome, 551–552
Down's syndrome, atrioventricular canal in, 1257
Doxorubicin, in lung carcinoma, 569–570
 in pleural mesothelioma, 491
Doxycycline, esophageal injury from, 866
Draping, surgical, 189
Dressler's syndrome, 465
Drug(s). See also specific drug.
 abuse of, heart transplantation and, 1940
 esophageal injury from, 866
 information on, in database, 326
 interactions of, 238, 239t
 reactions to, in cardiac care, 237–239, 239t
Ductus arteriosus, anatomy of, 1129
 aneurysm of, 1131
 anomalies of, 1129
 aortic coarctation and, 1135
 closure of, 1129
 patent. See *Patent ductus arteriosus.*
 prolonged patency of, 1129
 rupture of, 1131
Ductus arteriosus sling, 1158
"Ductus bump," 1131
Duke centerline method of cardiac wall motion analysis, 1013, *1014*
Duke University Medical Center TMR (The Medical Record) database, 319
Dumbbell tumor, mediastinal, 512
Dumon-Gilliard prosthesis, in esophageal carcinoma, 92, *93*
Duplication (enteric) cyst, mediastinal, 531–532, *532*
Duromedic prosthetic valve, assessment of, 1018
Dust inhalation, diffuse infiltrative lung disease in, 649–650, *649–650*
DVI pacing, 1617–1618, *1618*
Dysbetalipoproteinemia, familial, 1844
Dysphagia, in achalasia, 859
 in esophageal spasm, 878
 in esophageal stricture, 898
 in hiatal hernia, 898
 in lung carcinoma, 559
 in tracheal reconstruction, 358
 postvagotomy, 883, 952–955, *953–954*
 sideropenic, 881
Dysphagia lusoria, 825, 883, 1151, 1153
Dyspnea, in coronary artery fistula, 1690, *1691*
 in emphysema, 806
 in lung carcinoma, 559, 559t

Dyspnea *(Continued)*
 in mitral stenosis, 1514
 in pleural disease, 483
 in pleural effusion, 458
 in pneumothorax, 447–448, *447–448*

Eaton-Lambert syndrome, 976
Ebstein's anomaly, 1485–1492
 anatomy of, 1485, *1485*
 angiography in, 1487
 cardiac arrhythmia in, 1487
 cardiac catheterization in, 1486–1487
 clinical features of, 1486
 definition of, 1485, *1485*
 diagnosis of, 1486–1487
 echocardiography in, 1487
 electrocardiography in, 1486
 hemodynamics of, 1485–1486
 in tricuspid atresia, 1462
 incidence of, 1486
 left-sided, 1485
 mitral regurgitation in, 1392, 1396
 natural history of, 1486–1487
 pathophysiology of, 1485–1486
 roentgenography in, 1486
 surgical treatment of, historical aspects of, 1487–1489
  results of, 1489t, *1488,* 1490, 1491
  techniques for, *1488,* 1489, *1490,* 1491
 tricuspid valvular prolapse in, 1017
Echinococcosis, of lung, 642, *643*
 of pericardium, 1235
Echocardiography, 1087–1106
 A-mode, 1087, *1087,* 1089, *1089*
 applications of, 1092–1093
 as cardiac catheterization replacement, 1102, Color Plate: Fig. 31–117
 back scatter in, in myocardial ischemia study, 1101
 B-mode, 1089, *1089*
 bubbles in, 1094–1096, 1101
 color-flow Doppler, 1092, 1098–1099, Color Plates: Figs. 31–104 to 31–110
  with transesophageal method, 1100
 continuous-wave Doppler, 1090, *1092,* 1097–1098, *1097–1098*
 contrast agents in, 1101–1102, *1102*
 Doppler. See *Doppler echocardiography.*
 historical aspects of, 1087, *1087–1088*
 in aortic regurgitation, 1574, *1575*
 in aortic root abscess, 1099
 in aortic stenosis, 1369, 1571, *1571*
 in atrioventricular canal, 1304
 in cardiac function assessment, 1093–1094
 in cardiac neoplasms, 1905–1906, *1905–1908*
 in cardiac structure studies, 1094–1097, *1094–1096*
 in cardiac trauma, 1102, Color Plate: Fig. 31–117
 in congenital disease, 1095, 1097
 in cor triatriatum, 1291
 in coronary artery bypass, 1101–1102, *1102*
 in coronary artery disease, 1093–1094
 in coronary artery-pulmonary artery connection, 1698
 in coronary artery visualization, 1096
 in Ebstein's anomaly, 1487
 in ejection fraction determination, 1093
 in end-diastolic area determination, 1093
 in end-systolic area determination, 1093
 in endocarditis, 1095, *1096*
 in endomyocardial biopsy, 1097
 in foreign body location, 1094, *1094–1095*
 in great artery transposition, 1404

Embolism *(Continued)*
in cardiac myxoma, 1904
paradoxical, 713–714
pulmonary. See *Pulmonary embolism.*
tumor, 714–715
Embolization technique, in pulmonary arteriovenous malformation, 801, *801,* 842–843, *844,* 845
Embryonal cell carcinoma, mediastinal, 521–522
Emepronium bromide, esophageal injury from, 866
Emerson ventilators, for infant use, 296t
modes on, 282t
Emesis. See *Vomiting.*
Emphysema (mediastinal). See *Pneumomediastinum.*
Emphysema (pulmonary), 801–809
alpha₁-antitrypsin and, 802, *808,* 809
"blue bloater" (Type B), 803–804, 804t
bronchiectasis in, 616
bullous, 804–809
clinical manifestations of, 805, *806*
definition of, 804
in periacinar form, 805–806, *807*
large, 804, *805*
pneumothorax in, 805, *806*
surgical treatment of, 805–809, *806–808*
objectives of, 806–807
patient selection in, 806
results of, 807, 809
technique for, 806–807
versus bleb, 804
versus pneumothorax, 447–448, *448–449*
centrilobular, 802
classification of, by acinus involvement, 802–803
clinical, 803
clinical manifestations of, 777–778, *778,* 778t, 803, *803–804,* 804t
compensatory, 803
congenital interstitial, 785, *786*
definition of, 801
diffuse obstructive, 803–804, *803–804,* 804t
bulla formation in, *807*
distal acinar, 803
dry (Type A), 803–804, 804t
familial, 802
forced expiratory volume in, 5, *5*
in chronic obstructive pulmonary disease, 803–804, *803–804,* 804t
in mechanical ventilation, 300
of infants, 297
incidence of, 801–802
infantile lobar, 777–780, *778–780,* 778t
interstitial, 785, *786*
irregular, 803
lung elasticity in, 6, *7*
lung transplantation in, 1952
lung volume in, 4
obstructive, mechanism of, *69*
panacinar, 802–803
panlobular, 802–803
paraseptal, 803
pathogenesis of, 802
pathology of, 803–804
"pink puffer" (Type A), 803–804, 804t
prognosis of, 803–804
proximal acinar, 802
smoking and, 802
treatment of, 804
wet (Type B), 803–804, 804t
Emphysema (subcutaneous), in mechanical ventilation, 283
in pneumothorax, 390
Empyema, 467–480
acute, 467, 469–470, *470–471*
amebic, 642
antibiotics in, 468–469, 474–475

Empyema *(Continued)*
bronchopleural fistula in, 468–469, 476–479, *478–479*
calcification in, 486
chronic, 467, 472–474, *473–474*
clinical presentation of, 468–469, *468*
definition of, 467
diagnosis of, 469, *469*
drainage of, 472, *473–474,* 474–475, 477–478
rib resection in, 190–191, *190*
spontaneous, 468
etiology of, 467, 467t
extrapleural pneumonectomy in, 705–706, *705*
fibrothorax in, 480
historical aspects of, 444
in coccidioidomycosis, 629, *631*
in hemothorax, 391, *394–395*
in lung resection, in tuberculosis, 706
in tuberculosis, 469, 485–486, 695
incidence of, 467, 467t
irrigation of, 474–475, *474–475*
management of, 469–476
acute, 469–470, *470–471*
chronic, 472–474, *473–474*
postpneumonectomy, 474–476, *474–476*
posttraumatic, 476
transitional, 469–470, *470–471*
metastatic abscess from, 469
organisms causing, 467, 467t, 474
pathogenesis of, 467–468, 467t
phases of, 467
pleural effusion in, 462
pleural fluid pH in, 463
pneumothorax with, 451
postpneumonectomy, 474–476, *474–476*
postpneumonic, 467–469, 467t, *468*
posttraumatic, 476
shape of, 469, *469*
sterilization of, 474–475, *474–475*
thoracentesis in, 470
thoracoplasty in, 475–476, *476*
thoracotomy in, 476
transitional, 467, 469–470, *470–471*
tube thoracostomy in, 470, *471,* 472
tuberculous, 484
versus lung abscess, 469, *469*
Empyema necessitatis, 468
Empyemectomy, 472–474, *473–474*
Encainide, in ventricular arrhythmias, 220t
Encircling endocardial ventriculotomy, in ventricular tachycardia, 1892
Endarterectomy. See also *Carotid endarterectomy.*
in coronary artery bypass, 1830, *1831*
in occlusive disease, of aortic arch branches, 1223, 1224t, 1225, *1225–1226,* 1227
End-diastolic area, determination of, echocardiography in, 1093
Endocardial viability ratio, cardiac assist device effects on, 1783–1784, *1784*
Endocarditis, aortic aneurysm with, 1179
aortic regurgitation in, 1573, *1573*
echocardiography in, 1095, *1096*
in aortic coarctation, 1137
in coronary artery fistula, 1690, *1691*
in mitral valve replacement, 1527–1528
in patent ductus arteriosus, 1131
in ventricular septal defect, 1318
of aortic valve, valve replacement during, 1584–1585
of tricuspid valve, 1509–1510
prosthetic valve. See under *Prosthetic valve.*
Endocardium, resection of, in ventricular tachycardia, 1892–1894, *1893–1895*
Endocrinopathy, after cardiac surgery, 234–236, *236*

Heparin (*Continued*)
  in pulmonary embolism, 711, 721, 723
  in valve replacement, 1550
  in vascular grafting, 1560
  in vascular shunt coating. See *Shunt (tube), heparinized vascular.*
  in ventricular assist device use, 1793
  platelet activation induced by, 1748
  side effects of, 1561
  thrombolytic therapy with, 1053
  uses of, 1561
Heparin effect, after cardiac surgery, 224, *224*
Hepaticobronchial fistula, in amebic abscess, 642
Hepatitis, after blood transfusion, 225
Hepatojugular reflex, in constrictive pericarditis, 1238
Hepatorenal syndrome, 159
Hereditary hemorrhagic telangiectasia, pulmonary arteriovenous malformation in, 799–801, *799–801*, 840–841
Hernia, Bochdalek's, 958–959
  hiatal. See *Hiatal hernia.*
  Larrey's (Morgagni's), 959–960, *960*
  Morgagni's, 959–960, *960*
  of colon, 398
  of diaphragm. See under *Diaphragm.*
  of lung, congenital, 768
  of stomach, 398, *398*
  paraesophageal. See under *Hiatal hernia.*
  retrosternal (Morgagni's), 959–960, *960*
  sliding. See under *Hiatal hernia.*
  subcostosternal (Morgagni's), 959–960, *960*
Herpes virus infection, esophageal, in AIDS, 680
Hexylcaine, in bronchoscopy, 72
Hiatal hernia, 890–956
  acid perfusion test in, 901
  acid-load test in, 899, 901
  Allison repair of, 902–903
  anatomic considerations in, esophagus, 890–891
    gastroesophageal junction, 891–892
  axial (sliding, Type I), 892–893, *892*
    symptoms of, 897
    versus paraesophageal hernia, 923–924, *924*
  barium swallow in, 898–899
  cardia function and, 895–896
  clinical presentation of, 897–898
  combined (Type III), 893, 923
  diagnosis of, 898–901, *900*
  dysphagia in, 897–898
  esophageal anatomy and, 890–891
  esophageal function and, 893–896
  esophagitis and, 896–897
  esophagoscopy in, 88
  gastroesophageal reflux and, 827–828, *827*, 890, 896–897
  Hill repair in, 915–922, *916*, *919–921*, 920t–921t
  incidence of, postvagotomy, 950–951
  manometry in, 899, *900*
  Mark IV antireflux repair of, 902–909, *903*, *906–908*
  multiorgan (Type IV), 893
  Nissen fundoplication in, 910–914, *911–912*
  paraesophageal, 923–930
    anatomy of, 924–925, *924*
    clinical manifestations of, 925–927, *925–927*
    complications of, 926
    diagnosis of, 927–928, *928*
    iatrogenic, in peptic stricture repair, *946*, 947
    incarceration in, 925, 928–930
    incidence of, 923
    pathophysiology of, 923–925, *924–925*
    treatment of, 928–930, *928–929*, 929t
    versus parahiatal hernia, 923
    versus sliding hernia, 923–924, *924*
  pathophysiology of, postvagotomy, 951–952

Hiatal hernia (*Continued*)
  peptic stricture and. See *Peptic stricture.*
  pH monitoring in, 901
  postvagotomy, 950–952, *951*
  prevention of, postvagotomy, 952
  regurgitation in, 898
  rolling (Type II), *892*, 893, *894*
    symptoms of, 897–898
  sliding (axial, Type I), *892*, 893
    symptoms of, 897
    versus paraesophageal hernia, 923–924, *924*
  treatment of, postvagotomy, 952
  types of, 892–893, *892*
High-density lipoproteins. See *Lipoproteins, HDL.*
High-frequency mechanical ventilation, 57, 280–281
  in infants, 297
Hill repair, 915–922
  complications of, 921–922
  indications for, 916–917
  preoperative evaluation in, 917–918
  principles of, 915–916, *916*, 921
  results of, 920–921, 921t
  technique of, 918–920, *919–921*, 920t
His bundle, ablation of, in paroxysmal supraventricular tachycardia, 1878
  anatomy of, 1864–1865, *1864*
Histiocytoma, of heart, 1915
  of lung, 595
Histoplasma capsulatum, 626–628, *626–627*
Histoplasmosis, 626–628
  chronic cavitary, 628
  clinical manifestations of, 627–628
  diagnosis of, 628
  disseminated, 628
  epidemiology of, 624–625
  etiology of, 626–627
  geographic distribution of, 626, *626*
  in AIDS, 678–679
  incidence of, 626
  of mediastinum, 501, 503, 628, *628*
  of trachea, 343
  solitary nodule in, 627, *627*
  treatment of, 628
HIV. See *Acquired immunodeficiency syndrome; Human immunodeficiency virus.*
Hoarseness, in lung carcinoma, 559
  in thoracic aortic aneurysm, 1184
Hodgkin's lymphoma, mediastinal, 523, *524*
Homograft valve, in aortic valve disease, 1590
Homoiothermy, 375
Hopkins rod-lens optical system, in bronchoscopy, 69, *70*
Hormone abnormalities, in cardiac surgery, 234–236, *236*
Hospital information systems, 317–318, *318*
HpD phototherapy, bronchoscopy in, 82
HTLV-III. See *Human immunodeficiency virus.*
Human chorionic gonadotropin, in germ-cell tumors, 520–521
  in mediastinal neoplasms, 510
Human immunodeficiency virus, action of, 672–673
  antigen shedding by, 672–673
  culture of, 673, 673t
  in body fluids, 672
  life cycle of, 672
  structure of, 671–672
  T-cell destruction by, 672–673
Human immunodeficiency virus infection, acute, 671, 673
  asymptomatic period of, 671, 673–674
    hilar adenopathy in, 679
  classification of, 674, 674t
  cytomegaloviral infection in, 677
  diagnosis of, 672, 673, 673t
  epidemiology of, 674–675

Lung(s) *(Continued)*
  mobilization of, in fibrothorax, 480–482
  monosporiosis of, 640
  mucormycosis of, 637–638, *637*
  neoplasms of. See also *Lung carcinoma.*
    benign, bronchoplasty in. See *Bronchoplasty.*
      classification of, 588, 588t
      clinical features of, 588–589
      diagnosis of, 589
      incidence of, 588
      inflammatory, 595–596
      neurogenic, 593, *593*
      of developmental origin, 593–595, *594*
      of epithelial origin, 589–590
      of mesodermal origin, 590–593, *591–592*
    pneumothorax in, 451
    with tuberculosis, lung resection in, 702
  neurilemmoma of, 593, *593*
  neurofibromatosis of, 593
  nitrogen distribution in, 26–27, *27*
  nocardiosis of, 623–624, *625*
  of infant, 288–289, 288t, 291, 291t
  of pediatric patients, 372–373, *373*
  osteochondroma of, 591
  papilloma of, 589
  paracoccidioidomycosis of, 639, *639*
  parasitic infections of, 640–644, *640–641, 643*
  perfusion of. See *Ventilation-perfusion relationships.*
  plasma cell granuloma of, 595
  pleural covering of. See *Pleura.*
  pleural effusion under, 461–462
  Pneumocystis carinii infection of. See *Pneumocystis carinii* infection.
  polyps of, 589
  pressure-volume curve and, 7
  pseudolymphoma of, 595
  "pump," after blood transfusion, 183–184
  reexpansion of, after pneumonectomy, 482
  reimplantation response of, in heart-lung transplantation, 1932–1933
  right isomerism of (asplenia syndrome), 769, *770*
  sequestration anomalies in. See *Pulmonary sequestration.*
  shock. See *Adult respiratory distress syndrome.*
  solitary nodule in, in histoplasmosis, 627, *627*
  static elastic recoil pressure of, 6–7, *7*
  stiff, in adult respiratory distress syndrome, 182
  sugar tumor of, 595
  teratogenic effects on, 765
  teratoma of, 595
  thymoma of, 595
  translucent, 772, *772*
  transplantation of. See under *Transplantation.*
  trilobed, 768
  tuberculosis of. See under *Tuberculosis.*
  tumorlets of, 589–590
  unilobar, 775, *776*
  vascular abnormalities of, 795–801
    arteriovenous connections, 799–801, *799–801*
    venous drainage, 797, *798*, 799
  vasoconstriction in, in diaphragmatic hernia, 959
  venous anomalies of, 797, *798*, 799
  ventilation of. See *Ventilation.*
  ventilation of single. See *Anesthesia, one-lung.*
  volume of. See *Pulmonary volume.*
  "wet." See *Adult respiratory distress syndrome.*
  xanthoma of, 595
Lung abscess, 618–624
  air-fluid level in, 619, *620*
  anesthesia in, 622
  chronic, 619, *621*
  clinical presentation of, 619
  diagnosis of, 619–620, *620*
  drainage of, 622
  historical aspects of, 618–619

Lung abscess *(Continued)*
  mortality in, 622
  pathogenesis of, 619
  treatment of, 620–622, *621*, 621t
  versus empyema, 469, *469*
Lung carcinoma, adeno-, pathology of, 556
  after pneumonectomy, 557–558
  alveolar cell, 556–557, *564–565*
  anaplastic, pathology of, 555
  asbestos and, 554–555
  asymptomatic, 558–560, 559t
  bacille Calmette-Guérin in, 571–572
  bilateral, 557, 565
  biopsy in, 561
  bone marrow examination in, 562
  bronchiolar (alveolar cell), pathology of, 556
  bronchoplasty in. See *Bronchoplasty.*
  bronchoscopy in, 76–79, *77–78*
  chemotherapy in, 569–570
    from testicular metastasis, 610
    with immunotherapy, 572
  chest films in, 560–561, *560–565*
  chest pain in, 559
  chest wall invasion of, 568
  classification of, 555–556
  clinical manifestations of, 558–560, 559t
  clubbing of fingers in, 559
  "coin lesion" in, 556
  computed tomography in, 561
  cough in, 559
  cytology in, 556
  "dense core granules" in, 570, *571*
  diagnosis of, 76–78, *77–78*, 556, 560–563, *560–565*, 570, *571*
  differential diagnosis of, 562–563
  dual primary, 557
  dysphagia in, 559
  dyspnea in, 559
  electron microscopy in, 570, *571*
  endobronchial, 76, *77*
  eosinophilia in, 560
  giant-cell, 557
  growth of, *562*
  hemoptysis in, 559
  historical aspects of, 554–555, *555*
  hoarseness in, 559
  hormonal aspects of, 559–560
  hypertrophic pulmonary osteoarthropathy in, 559
  immunology of, 570–572, *572*, 600–603, 602t
  immunotherapy in, 571–572, *572*, 601–602, 602t
  incidence of, 554
  inoperability of, 563, 567–568, 568t
  laser therapy in, 572–573
  lung scan in, 561
  mediastinoscopy in, 561–562
  metastasis from, 555–558, *557–558*, 558t
    operability and, 563, 565, 567–568, 568t
    physical findings in, 560
  natural history of, 573–574, *573*
  neuromyopathy in, 560
  oat-cell, chemotherapy in, 569–570
    pathology of, 556
    resection in, 570
  occult, 77–78, 561
  occupational causes of, 554–555
  palliation of, 568–569, 571–572
  paraneoplastic syndrome in, 602–603
  pathology of, 555–558, *557–558*, 558t
  peribronchial, 77
  pericardial effusion in, 567
  peripheral, 77, *560*
  peritoneovenous shunt in, 558
  photodynamic detection of, 78
  physical findings in, 560
  pleural effusion in, 559